Pathology of the Lung

Pathology of the Lung

Edited by

William M. Thurlbeck, M.B., F.R.C.P.C., F.R.C.Path.
Professor of Pathology
University of British Columbia
Pathologist
British Columbia's Children's Hospital
Consultant Pathologist
U.B.C. Health Sciences Center Hospital
  and Shaughenessy Hospital
Vancouver, British Columbia
Canada

1988
Thieme Medical Publishers, Inc.,
Georg Thieme Verlag, Stuttgart • New York

Thieme Medical Publishers, Inc.
381 Park Avenue South
New York, New York 10016

Cover design by Wendy Ann Fredericks

PATHOLOGY OF THE LUNG
William M. Thurlbeck

Library of Congress Cataloging-in-Publication Data
Pathology of the lung.
  Includes index.
  1. Lungs—Diseases. 2. Lungs—Diseases—Diagnosis.
3. Diagnosis, Laboratory. I. Thurlbeck, William M.
[DNLM: 1. Lung—pathology. 2. Lung Diseases—
pathology. WF 600 P9275]
RC711.P38 1987   616.2'407   87-16158

Copyright © 1988 by Thieme Medical Publishers, Inc. This book, including all parts thereof, is legally protected by copyright. Any use, exploitation or commercialization outside the narrow limits set by copyright legislation, without the publisher's consent, is illegal and liable to prosecution. This applies in particular to photostat reproduction, copying, mimeographing or duplication of any kind, translating, preparation of microfilms, and electronic data processing and storage.

Important note: Medicine is an ever-changing science. Research and clinical experience are continually broadening our knowledge, in particular our knowledge of proper treatment and drug therapy. Insofar as this book mentions any dosage or application, readers may rest assured that the authors, editors, and publishers have made every effort to ensure that such references are strictly in accordance with the state of knowledge at the time of production of the book. Nevertheless, every user is requested to carefully examine the manufacturers' leaflets accompanying each drug to check on his own responsibility whether the dosage schedules recommended therein or the contraindications stated by the manufacturers differ from the statements made in the present book. Such examination is particularly important with drugs that are either rarely used or have been newly released on the market.

Some of the product names, patents, and registered designs referred to in this book are in fact registered trademarks or proprietary names even though specific reference to this fact is not always made in the text. Therefore, the appearance of a name without designation as proprietary is not to be construed as a representation by the publisher that it is in the public domain.

Printed in the United States of America.

5 4 3 2 1

TMP ISBN 0-86577-134-0
GTV ISBN 3-13-665401-3

To the memory of Dr. Charles B. Carrington

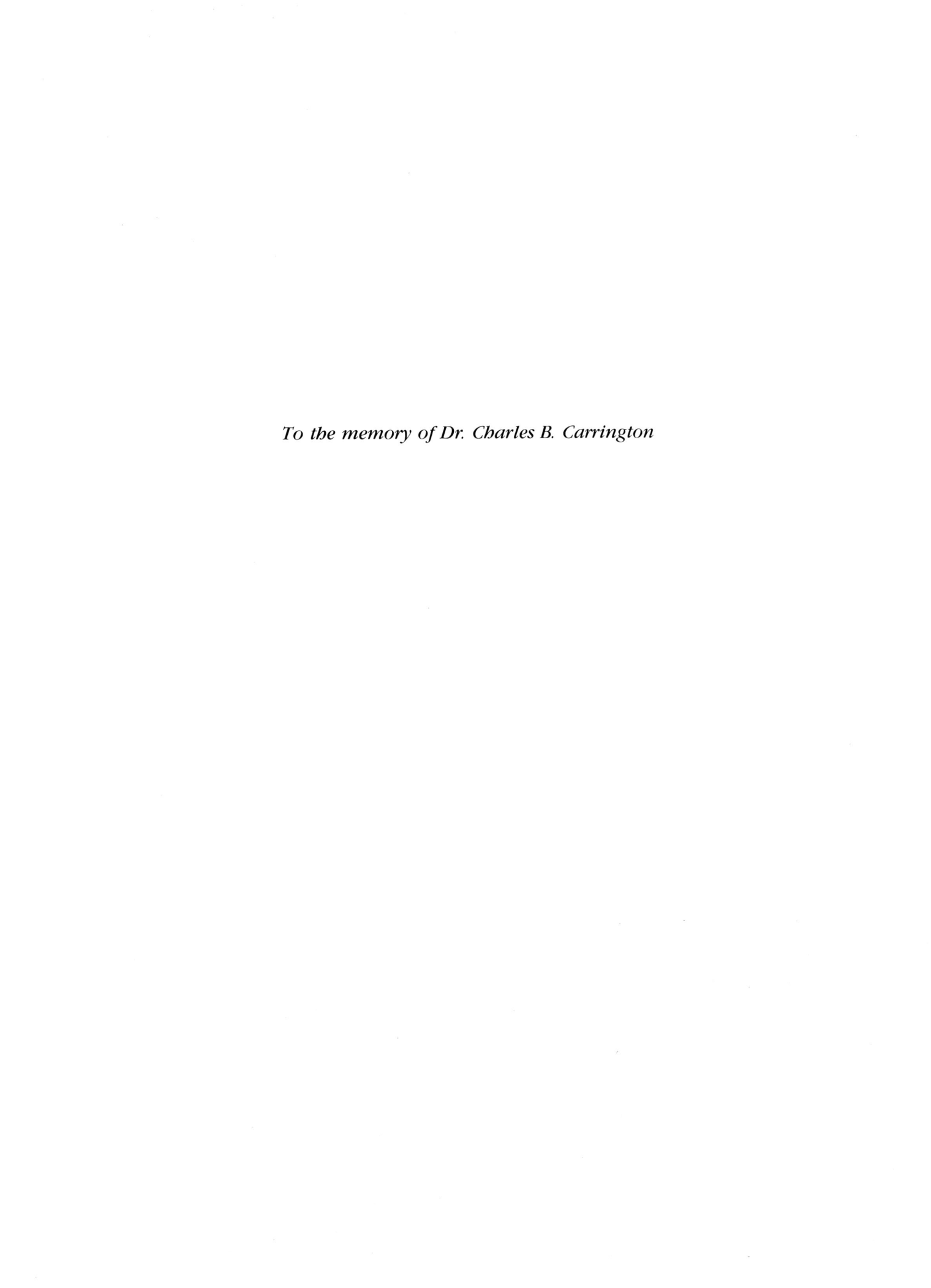

Preface

This book originates from a postgraduate course in lung pathology sponsored by the American College of Chest Physicians. Dr. Thomas Petty, Chairman of the Education Committee and President of the College, recognized the need for such a course since it appeared that trainees in chest medicine were deficient in their knowledge of pulmonary pathology. The success of this course since 1979 is a tribute to his insight. Many course attendees have suggested that it should be developed into a textbook and this is the result.

The objective of this book is to provide a comprehensive review of the pathologic basis of lung disease. The authors were requested to stress clinical features and clinical-pathologic correlations so that the book would be useful to both pathologists and chest physicians. Emphasis has also been placed on the diagnostic criteria and techniques so that the book would have a useful place in hospital pathology laboratories.

This book is meant to be practical, clinically oriented, authoritative, and up-to-date. Many of the faculty of the course are contributors, but some could not participate. An international flavor has been added by including experts from Britain who have not taught in the course. Additionally, local experts from Vancouver have also contributed. The book is very much a group effort, rather than being the work of one person. Inevitably, there will be errors of omission and overlaps between chapters. I have attempted to keep them to a minimum.

It is also inevitable that a multi-author textbook reflect the styles and attitudes of the individuals concerned. Every attempt has been made to ensure a uniform quality of presentation; the various authors put up with requests for revisions with a view to this end. If the objective was not reached, the fault is mine.

This book is dedicated to the memory of Dr. Charles B. Carrington who died late in 1985. He was a close friend of many of the authors and a direct teacher to several. He is remembered by us as being an outstanding diagnostician and lecturer and a significant contributor to the literature of human pulmonary pathology. The field of pulmonary pathology is diminished by his absence.

William M. Thurlbeck

Foreword

To chest physicians of a generation ago, active in their profession in the years immediately following the second world war, it was axiomatic that the foundation of knowledge of all disease lay in understanding its pathology. They were aware that it was the methodical study of this science that had advanced the understanding of disease in a systematic way since the turn of the century. Many went to Europe, and particularly to Germany, to master the details of pathology and bacteriology. Chest physicians of my generation embraced pulmonary physiology, and during the 1950's and 1960's saw an incredible advance in the understanding of how the lung works. In addition, clinical interest shifted from tuberculosis to chronic airflow obstruction, restrictive lung disease, and the adult respiratory distress syndrome. Now chest physicians use immunology, biochemistry, cell biology, and (somewhat paradoxically) experimental pathology as their main experimental tools.

It is common for us to observe (though I suspect that it always come as a surprise) that when we have been away from somewhere for some period, things have not stood still in our absence. It seems to be a general instinct to feel that, because we were not there, there was no right for there to be change.

This book will reveal to many physicians interested in chest disease, that while they were fascinated by physiology, or attempting to master the latest insights of immunology, or conceding that they were too old to learn the emerging jargon of biochemistry, the traditonal study of lung pathology had been steadily advancing, if rarely commanding the headlines.

Beginning with a relatively brief description of contemporary understanding of the relevant aspects of the normal human lung, *Pathology of the Lung* describes in some detail modern methods of study relevant to diagnosis made by the anatomical pathologist; such as lung biopsy and lung resection, techniques of post mortem lung inflation, microbial diagnosis, and sputum examination. One can hear Virchow repeating "Die Method is Alles."

In the chapters that follow, experts on every aspect of lung pathology, many of whom have spent years studying special groups of conditions within the totality of lung disease, describe the details of their understanding of the several conditions. It is as if we are privileged to sit in on teaching sessions designed to pass on this knowledge.

Those who do so, as I mentioned earlier, are in for several surprises. They will discover that this field of knowledge has been advancing steadily. The traditional concept that "the lung has only very limited ways of responding to injury" might still be true of a few specific conditions; for example, in the Adult Respiratory Distress Syndrome, there is a "final common path" as a consequence of different insults. But the variation in lung responses is extraordinary, and makes the subject of great interest. One has only to mention the differences between responses to silica, coal dust, asbestos, and tobacco smoke to make the point. There are still some relatively common diseases of unknown genesis like sarcoidosis; we seem to have been creeping up on the key to this condition for years. The pathology of allergic alveolitis offers puzzling clues, but the exact sequence of events has still to be described; not least of all the arbitrary way in which uniformly exposed groups respond.

In some of the sections, a historical perspective has been provided. This could not have been attempted for more than a small part of the book without it running to several volumes. However, if the reader compares the comprehensive descriptions of many of the conditions in this book with the cursory understanding that existed forty years ago, he or she will come to realize that major advances have been steadily occurring across the whole field; advances attributable to a large volume of painstaking work, and a few unpredictable but decisive steps forward.

Not only does this remarkable volume provide, as it claims, a practical working book for anatomical pathologists; but it is also an indispensible requirement for anyone wishing to develop a scholarly understanding of contemporary knowledge of lung disease. Such a foundation is in no sense eclipsed by more spectacular discoveries in other fields of study; in the end these will only be fully comprehensible in the light of the information contained in these pages. The authors and the editor are to be congratulated on giving us such a splendid volume.

It is a pleasure and a privilege to be the first to wish it well.

David V. Bates, M.D., F.R.C.P., F.R.C.P.C.
F.A.C.P., F.R.S.C.
Professor of Medicine
Department of Medicine
U.B.C. Health Sciences Center
Vancouver, British Columbia

Contributors

Frederic B. Askin, M.D.
Professor of Pathology
University of North Carolina, Chapel Hill
Director, Surgical Pathology
North Carolina Memorial Hospital
Chapel Hill, North Carolina

Charles B. Carrington, M.D. (deceased)
Professor of Pathology
Stanford University Medical Center
Stanford, California

Andrew Churg, M.D., Ph.D., F.R.C.P.C.
Professor of Pathology
University of British Columbia
Head, Anatomic Pathology
U.B.C. Health Sciences Center Hospital
Vancouver, British Columbia
Canada

Thomas V. Colby, M.D.
Associate Professor of Pathology
Mayo Medical School
Division of Surgical Pathology
Mayo Clinic
Rochester, Minnesota

Linda Ferrel, M.D.
Assistant Professor of Pathology
Co-director of Cytology
University of San Francisco
San Francisco, California

Donald Heath, M.D., D.Sc., Ph.D., F.R.C.P., F.R.C.Path.
George Holt Profesor of Pathology
University of Liverpool
Liverpool, United Kingdom

A.G. Heppleston, D.Sc., M.D., F.R.C.P., F.R.C.Path.
Emeritus Professor of Pathology
University of Newcastle upon Tyne
Institute of Occupational Medicine
Edinburgh, United Kingdom

James C. Hogg, M.D., Ph.D., F.R.C.P.C.
Professor of Pathology
University of British Columbia
U.B.C. Pulmonary Research Laboratory
St. Paul's Hospital
Pulmonary Research Laboratory
Vancouver, British Columbia
Canada

Anna-Luise A. Katzenstein, M.D.
Professor of Pathology
Division of Surgical Pathology
University of Alabama at Birmingham
Birmingham, Alabama

Charles Kuhn III, M.D.
Profesor of Pathology
Washington University
Pathologist
Barnes Hospital
St. Louis, Missouri

Roberta R. Miller, M.D., F.R.C.P.C.
Associate Pathologist
Vancouver General Hospital
Associate Member
Department of Medicine—Respiratory Division
Clinical Assistant Professor
Department of Pathology
University of British Columbia
Vancouver, British Columbia
Canada

Bill Nelems, M.D., F.R.C.S.C.
Director, Division of Thoracic Surgery
Vancouver General Hospital
Associate Professor of Surgery
University of British Columbia
Vancouver, British Columbia
Canada

Geno Saccommono, M.D., Ph.D.
Pathologist
St. Mary's Hospital and Medical Center
Chief Pathologist
Veteran Administration Medical Center
Grand Junction, Colorado

Paul Smith, B.Sc., Ph.D.
Senior Lecturer in Pathology
Department of Pathology
University of Liverpool
Liverpool, United Kingdom

Joanne L. Wright, M.D., F.R.C.P.C.
Associate Professor of Pathology
University of British Columbia
U.B.C. Pulmonary Research Laboratory
St. Paul's Hospital
Vancouver, British Columbia
Canada

Contents

1. Lung Growth 1
   William M. Thurlbeck

2. Norml Anatomy and Histology 11
   Charles Kuhn III

3. Quantitative Anatomy of the Lung 51
   William M. Thurlbeck

4. Pulmonary Defense Mechanisms 57
   James C. Hogg

5. Lung Biopsy: Handling and Diagnostic Limitations 67
   Andrew Churg

6. Gross Examination of Lung Resection Specimens 79
   Roberta R. Miller and Bill Nelems

7. Examination of the Lung: Autopsy 95
   William M. Thurlbeck

8. Microbiologic Diagnosis 101
   Anna-Luise A. Katzenstein

9. Diagnostic Cytology Techniques Including Fine Needle Aspirations:
   Practical Considerations 105
   Linda Ferrell and Geno Saccommono

10. Pulmonary Disorders in the Neonate Infant and Child 115
    Frederic B. Askin

11. Viral Infections of the Respiratory Tract 147
    Roberta R. Miller

12. Mycoplasma, Chlamydia, and Coxiella Infections of the Respiratory Tract 181
    Roberta R. Miller

13. Bacterial Infections 185
    Charles Kuhn III

14. Mycobacterial Infections and Fungal and Protozoal Disease 221
    Anna-Luise A. Katzenstein

Contents

15. Pulmonary Disease in the Immunocompromised Host ... 247
    Andrew Churg

16. Pulmonary Edema and Diffuse Alveolar Injury ... 263
    James C. Hogg and Anna-Luise A. Katzenstein

17. Pulmonary Angiitis and Granulomatosis ... 283
    Anna-Luise A. Katzenstein

18. Diffuse Pulmonary Hemorrhage ... 303
    Roberta R. Miller

19. Tumors of the Lung ... 311
    Andrew Churg

20. Infiltrative Lung Disease ... 425
    Thomas V. Colby and Charles B. Carrington

21. Chronic Airflow Obstruction ... 519
    William M. Thurlbeck

22. Extrinsic Immunologic Lung Disease ... 577
    James C. Hogg

23. Environmental Lung Disease ... 591
    A.G. Heppleston

24. Disorders of the Vascular System ... 687
    Donald Heath and Paul Smith

25. Consequences of Aspiration and Bronchial Obstruction ... 751
    Joanne L. Wright

26. Diseases of the Pleura ... 769
    Andrew Churg

27. Diagnostic Cytology ... 803
    Geno Saccomanno and Linda Ferrell

Index ... 823

Pathology of the Lung

1 Lung Growth

William M. Thurlbeck

Since this book deals with human disease, this chapter will deal primarily with human lung growth. Intrauterine lung growth and factors that affect it will first be discussed. The importance of separating various aspects of lung growth will be emphasized and then postnatal lung growth will be covered briefly.

Intrauterine Lung Development of Airways

The lung begins to develop at 26 days of fetal age when a ventral groove (the largyngotracheal groove) appears in the endodermal tube. This evaginates to form the lung bud which branches at about 26 to 28 days of age. Intrauterine lung development can be divided into five stages[1] all of which overlap to some degree (Table 1–1):

1. The first six weeks after ovulation constitute the *embryonal phase* during which the bronchial tree to just beyond segmental bronchi develops.

2. The *pseudoglandular* phase continues to the 16th week of gestation. During this phase the bronchial buds continue to bud by asymmetric dichotomy. Sixty-five to 75 percent of bronchial branching occurs between the 10th and 14th week of fetal life and by 16 weeks bronchial and bronchiolar branching is complete as far as the terminal bronchiole. Thus the conducting airways are completed by this age. The branching airways on histologic section have a very glandular appearance and the distal epithelium is lined by cuboidal or columnar epithelium containing glycogen. The intervening matrix is cellular, forming a primitive mesenchyme.

3. The *canalicular* phase starts at about 17 weeks and is characterized by the development of the vascular system, together with further division of the airways, thinning of the epithelium, and a decrease in the proportion of mesenchyme (Fig. 1–1). As the epithelium thins irregularly, a rich capillary network appears which approaches the airway epithelium. Protrusion by capillaries into the thinned epithelium produces focal areas where gas exchange is now possible (Fig. 1–2). Progressive flattening of the epithelium occurs and this becomes most complete in the airspaces just distal to the terminal bronchiole and appears to extend peripherally. Very characteristically only the terminal portions are cuboidal at a late stage. A capillary network develops and surrounds the airspaces. As the interstitium thins, the airspaces and the capillary networks that surround the air spaces approach each other. The structures distal to the terminal bronchioles, most properly termed saccules, thus have a double capillary layer between them, derived from each of the saccules. The precise sequence of events in the lung periphery is not known. At this stage, the framework of the acinus (the unit gas-exchanging part of the lung distal to the terminal bronchiole, see Chapter 2) is presumably being laid down. At about 20 weeks the number of subdivisions beyond the terminal bronchioles is small and it is easy to trace from the terminal bronchiole to the periphery of the lung through two or three saccules. The saccules develop a very characteristic appearance at about 23 weeks gestation, at which time the airspaces have a distinct sawtooth appearance (Fig. 1–3). The nature of this appearance is not clear but it is likely that it represents division of saccules to form more saccules, and hence the framework of the acinus. At the end of the canalicular phase, at about 28 weeks gestation, the structure distal to the terminal bronchiole is moderately complex, vascularization is extensive, the epithelium is thin and both type I and type II cells are present. Osmiophilic bodies may be seen and gas exchange can occur at this stage.

4. The *saccular* phase now begins (at about 28 weeks gestation) and is characterized by a dramatic increase in gas-exchanging surface area (Fig. 1–4) and lung volume, an increase in proportion of gas-exchanging lumen, and

Table 1–1. Classification of Phases of Human Intrauterine Lung Growth

Phase	Time of Occurrence	Significance
Embryonic	Day 26–day 52	Development of trachea and major bronchi
Pseudoglandular	Day 52–16 week	Development of remaining conducting airways
Canalicular	17 week–28 week	Development of vascular bed, framework of acinus, flattening of epithelium
Saccular	29 week–36 week	Increased complexity of saccules
Alveolar	36 week–term	Presence and development of alveoli

diminution of mesenchyme between the saccules. (Rats and mice are born at the beginning of this stage and the events that occur subsequently in gestation in the human occur postnatally in them.) Small crests begin to appear in the walls of the saccules at the beginning of the phase and correspond to the much better recognized and described secondary crests in rats and mice.[2,3] The crests elongate and form relatively shallow structures (Fig. 1–5) with a double capillary layer; these structures have been referred to as "subsaccules." The crests elongate further and the subsaccules become further subdivided until the smallest structures are now multifaceted structures which may or may not have a double capillary layer. Characteristically the margins of the secondary crests and the rim of the mouths of alveoli have an elastic fiber at their margin.[4] It is not clear when one can first term the smallest structures alveoli, but structures resembling alveoli can be seen at 32 weeks and alveoli are clearly present at 36 weeks in all fetuses.

5. The final stage of lung growth in the human is the *alveolar* phase continuing from 36 weeks to term (Figs. 1–6, 1–7). The number of alveoli at birth is quite variable and a range of 10 to 149 million (mean 55 million) has been described in infants, following apparently normal gestation.[1]

Development of Epithelium and Submucosal Glands

Although this has been well studied in animals, data for humans are relatively scanty. During the glandular phase, the epithelium is stratified with cylindrical cells vertically oriented and more basally situated polygonal cells.[5] Cilia first appear in the trachea and then progressively extend to the more distal airways. Ciliated cells and mucus-secreting cells are apparent by 13 weeks gestation.[5] Kultschitsky cells have been seen at 15 weeks gestation.[6] The epithelium is corregated and the secretory cells are present in the crypts. Submucosal glands appear in the trachea at 10 weeks gestation[7] and are present in bronchi at 14 weeks of age. They form from a sharply defined cluster of cells with dark nuclei along the basal lamina. These cells multiply to form a cylinder which protrudes into the submucosa, enclosed in a basement membrane continuous with the surface basement membrane.[5] A lumen develops and the duct then divides into two lateral ducts. Subsequent division forms the secretory tubules.

Development of Blood Vessels

Pulmonary Arteries

An excellent and complete review of the development of the pulmonary vascular system is available.[8] The pulmonary artery is derived from the sixth (pulmonary) branchial arch that appears at about 32 days of gestation. Two branches arise from each sixth branchial arch artery to supply the mesenchyme of lung buds. In an 11-mm embryo, approximately 40 days' gestation, the first and second branchial arches have disappeared. The third arch will form the carotid arteries and the left fourth dorsal arch will form the aorta. The left sixth arch increases in size and its distal part is destined to become the ductus arteriosus and the proximal portion part of the left pulmonary artery. The distal part of the right sixth arch and the distal part of the right dorsal aorta degenerate. The truncus arteriosus splits and rotates so that the pulmonary artery comes to lie in front of the aorta.

There are two types of pulmonary arteries: conventional arteries, that accompany airways and branch with them; and supernumerary arteries, that branch off the conventional ones at right angles and supply alveoli immediately adjacent to the bronchovascular tree. By angiography it is apparent that there is a well-defined branching pattern by 14 weeks' gestation and all preacinar branches are present at 16 weeks' gestation. At 19 to 20 weeks' gestation the branching of the conventional arteries is similar to the adult pattern, as is the distribution of elastic and partially elastic arteries. Surprisingly, supernumerary branches are present as early as 12 weeks' gestation. Elastic tissue begins to appear in the major pulmonary artery at about 12 weeks' gestation and gradually becomes more apparent with advancing gestational age but even at birth elastic fibers are thinner than in the adult. Immature muscle cells become apparent early in development and the arterial tree gradually takes on the configuration of the adult tree with elastic arteries extending to the seventh generation of an axial pathway. Muscular pulmonary arteries extend to the terminal bronchiole by 28 weeks but generally do not extend further until after birth.

Pulmonary Veins

The mesenchyme around the lung buds is vascular (even before being connected formally to branches of the

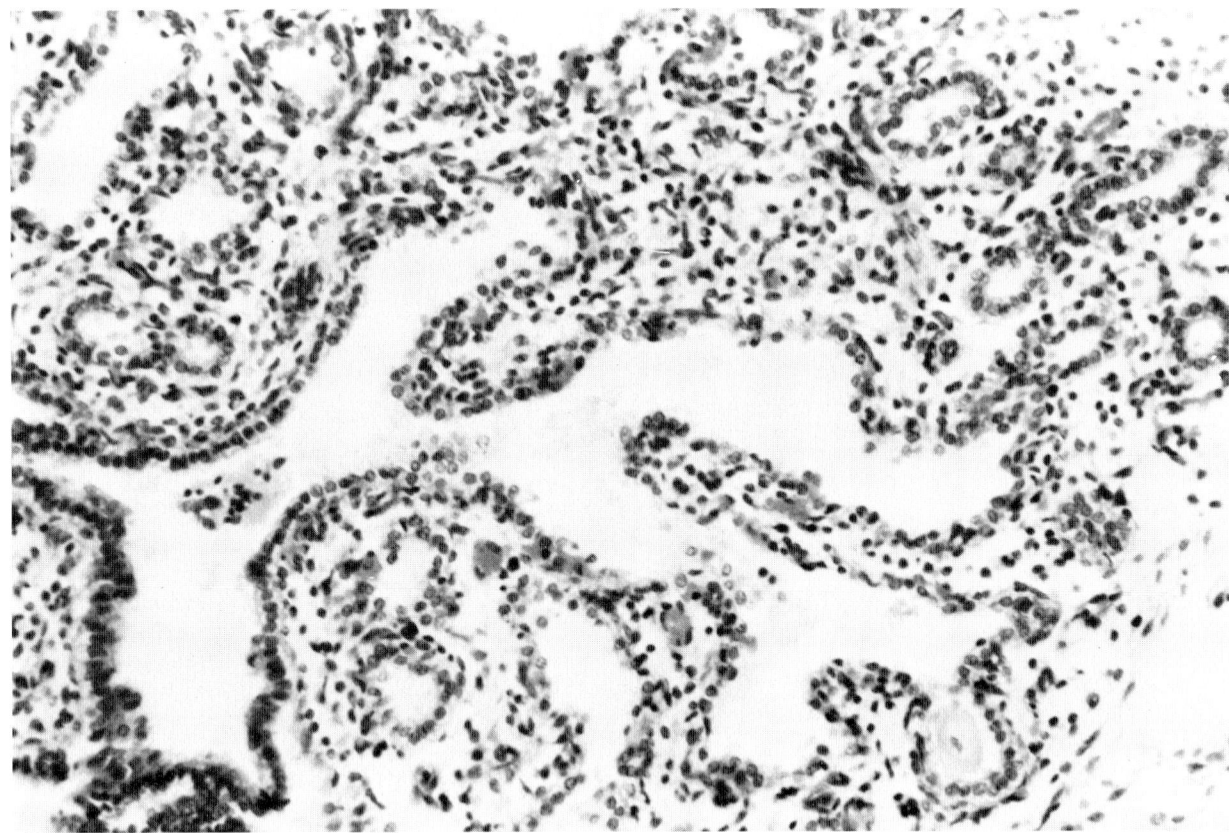

Figure 1–1. Twenty-two weeks gestation. Simple smooth-walled respiratory channels are characteristic of the canalicular phase. There is much interstitial tissue, at this stage sparsely vascular [hematoxylin and eosin (H&E, ×200). From Langston et al.[1]

pulmonary arteries and veins) and initially drains into systemic vessels. The primitive pulmonary vein develops as an evagination from the dorsal wall of the atrium in the sinoatrial region and grows to approach the lung buds. It divides several times but then, by a complex process of fusion, the two proximal branches fuse to form the left atrium and the other branches join so that there are four entrances to the left atrium, corresponding to the main pulmonary veins. The veins branch within the lung mesenchyme and join up with preexisting vascular channels that then run in the interlobular septa at some distance from the bronchoarterial tree.

Bronchial Arteries

The bronchial arteries have been little studied. Initially the lung is supplied by paired vessels from the dorsal aorta. Bronchial arteries have been described in an 8-week-old fetus and in a more complete form in a 12-week-old fetus.[9] The bronchial arteries grow along the airways and parallel the development of cartilage.

Development of Gas-Exchanging Epithelium

Gas-exchanging epithelium (saccules and alveoli) initially consists of cuboidal cells containing much glycogen. As these disappears there is concurrent appearance of lamellar bodies, and the cells then develop the characteristic morphologic features of type II cells.

Development of Connective Tissue

Early in gestation there is a complex interaction between mesoderm and endodermal branching. The airway branching pattern may be altered by applying mesoderm of a different species or site and the branching pattern that results is that of the original mesoderm. The primitive mesenchyme is also responsible for the development of mesodermal structures. Endothelial channels arise, forming a plexus of angioblastic structures which appear before the major vessels reach them. Fibroblasts differ-

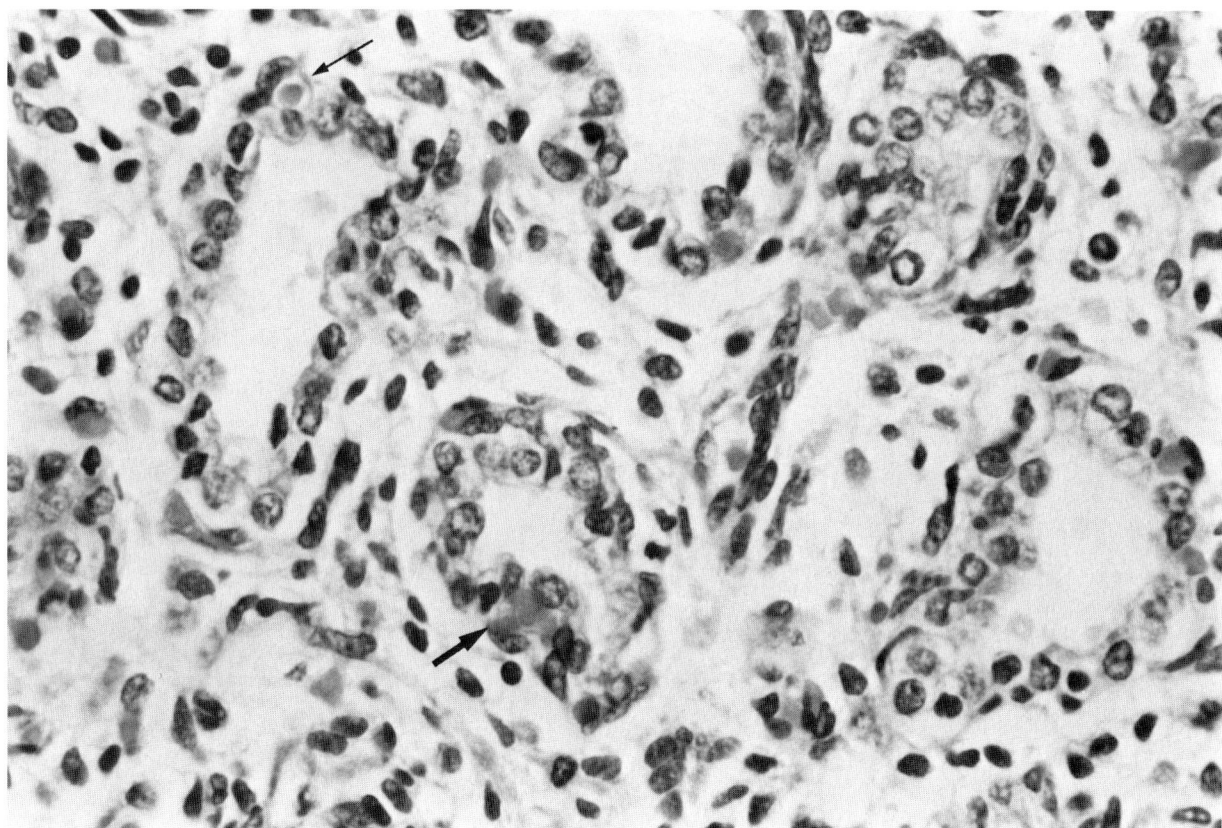

Figure 1–2. Twenty-two weeks gestation. Canalicular phase. The distal airspaces are lined by cuboidal epithelium. At one point (arrow) a capillary has reached the epithelium (H&E, ×500). From Langston et al.[1]

entiate and secrete the major connective tissue components. Collagen appears early in fetal life and is involved in the branching of the bronchial tree. It is the dominant connective tissue element in airways, blood vessels, pleura, and lobular septa throughout fetal life. Although elastin may be seen in pulmonary arteries at ten to 12 weeks of gestation, airway elastin does not appear until about the 20th to 25th week of fetal life. Elastin also appears in the pleura but the most important role of elastin is probably in the lung parenchyma where elastin appears and increases rapidly between 26 and 32 weeks' gestation. The elastin lies mainly as fibers along the free margins of the secondary crests (the saccular phase, above). It is thought that this elastin network, with associated collagen and proteoglycan matrix, is responsible for the formation of alveoli. The network forms a semirigid structure resembling a fishnet which surrounds the mouths of alveoli, and the lung parenchyma protrudes through the net to form alveoli.

Even in late gestation there may be epithelial-mesenchymal connections. There are gaps in the basement membrane in the distal airways in rats at day 18 of gestation.[10] This phenomenon has been well studied by Adamson and colleagues.[11–13] They have found that the extent of basal lamina discontinuities under cuboidal cells, the number of foot processes, and the percentage of these that penetrated the basal lamina all increased parallel with the rate of growth, differentiation, and disaturated phosphatidylcholine content in day 17 to 22 gestation in rats. Female rats develop earlier than male rats but at birth the males had caught up. Cell-to-cell contacts differed in the sexes and paralleled these changes.[11–13]

Control of Intrauterine Lung Growth

The exact definition of the term pulmonary hypoplasia is not clear. It can mean too few constituent parts such as cells or alveoli, but these have seldom been measured and the precise range of normality is imprecisely known; thus they are difficult to use as criteria in human subjects. Lung weight has been used more usually as a criterion since it is readily available at autopsy, but it seems likely that weight will underestimate the frequency of hypoplasia because of confounding weight increases due to

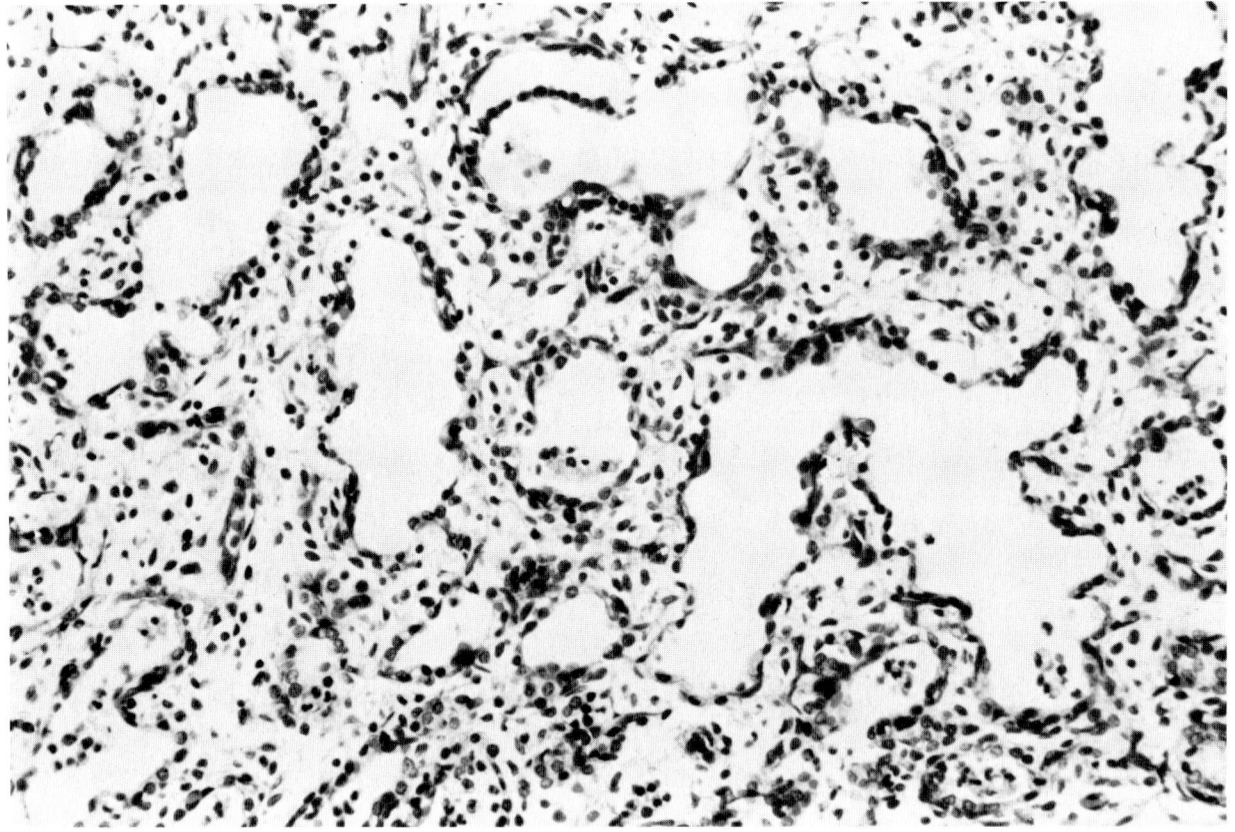

Figure 1–3. Twenty-three weeks gestation. Canalicular phase. The internal lining of the airspace has taken on a wavy configuration. Epithelium is slightly flatter than in Figure 1–1 (H&E, ×200). From Langston et al.[1]

edema and other concurrent disease. Volume is a more sensitive measure[14] but once again it is not usually available. Even with these constraints, a number of factors controlling intrauterine lung growth have become apparent.[15] The major ones are:

1. Chest wall compression or distortion due to any cause, the classical ones being diaphragmatic hernia and chest wall deformities. These, particularly diaphragmatic hernia, result in the most severe degrees of hypoplasia.
2. The amount of amniotic fluid. Oligohydramnios is a major cause of hypoplasia and hypoplasia with renal agenesis with Potter's syndrome (see Chapter 10.) is mediated through oligohydramnios. It has been suggested that polyhydramnios can produce hyperplastic hyperalveolated lungs.[16] How amniotic fluid plays its role is less clear. Experimentally tracheal ligation produces hyperplasia and tracheal drainage hypoplasia[17] so that it is tempting to think that intrapulmonary distension by lung fluid is the mechanism. There is, however, no definite evidence of the association of polyhydramnios with increased transpulmonary pres-

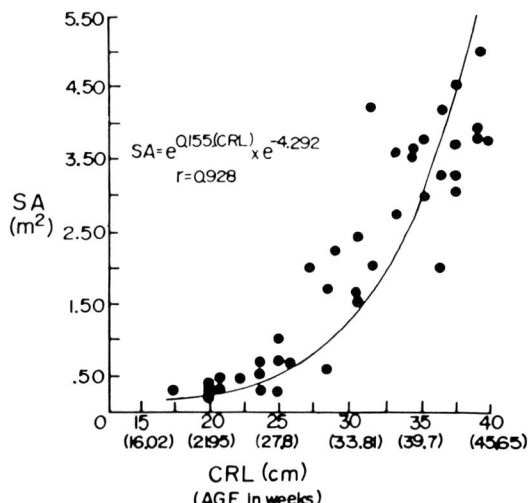

Figure 1–4. Note the rapid increase in gas-exchanging surface area (SA) with age, starting at about 28 weeks' gestation and coinciding with the commencement of the saccular phase. From Langston et al.[1]

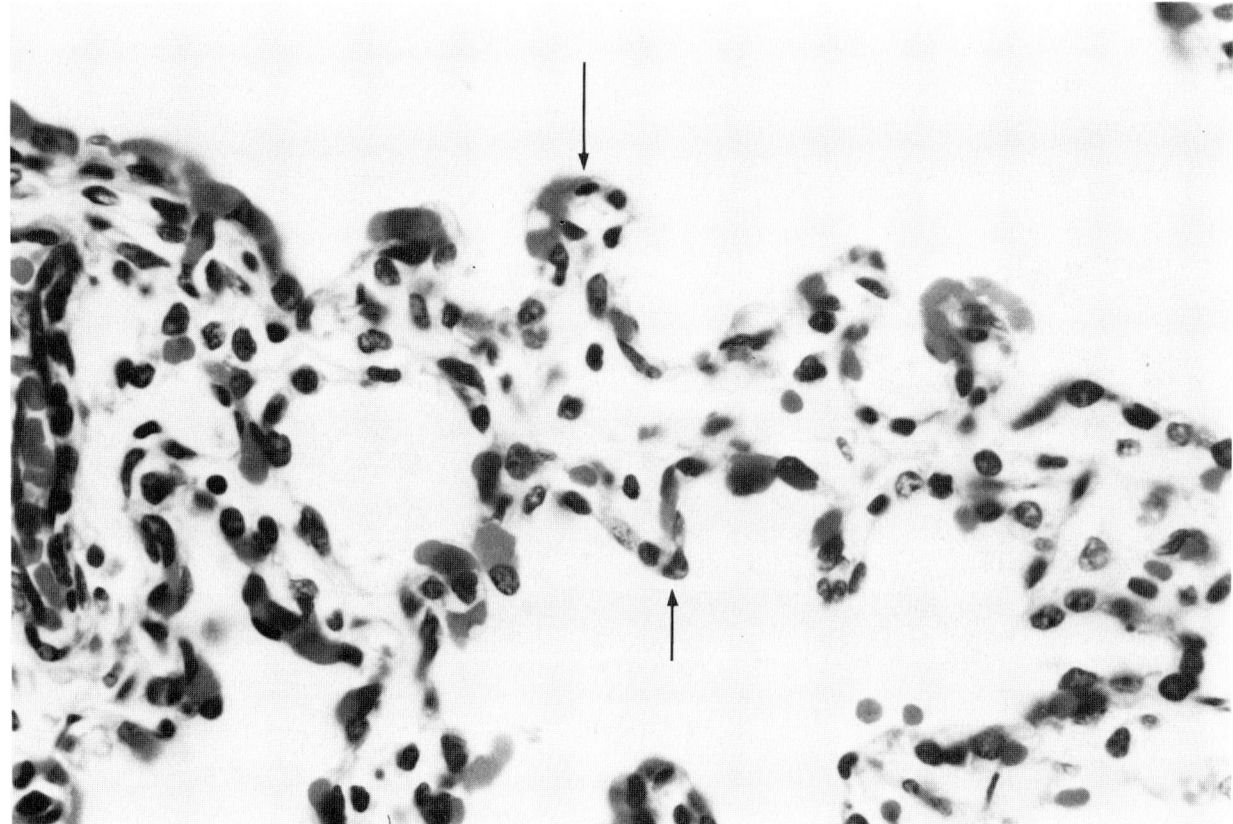

Figure 1–5. Twenty-nine weeks gestation. Saccular phase. Airspaces, top and bottom, are being subdivided by secondary crests, indicated by arrows (H&E, ×50). From Langston et al.[1]

sure (the difference between amniotic fluid pressure and intraalveolar pressure) and that of oligohydramnios with decreased pressure.

3. There is excellent evidence from experimental studies that diminished fetal respiration is associated with pulmonary hypoplasia.[15] The reverse has not been investigated, that is, whether increased fetal respiration results in pulmonary hyperplasia.

It seems likely that both the amount of amniotic fluid and fetal respiration may be sensitive to environmental perturbations such as smoking or medications. Indeed, perhaps the wide structural variation of the lung at birth[1] may be due to subtle environmental disturbances.

Maturation, Hypoplasia, and Tissue Complexity

It is all too easy to equate hypoplasia, tissue immaturity, and cellular immaturity and it is important to recognize that both normal and abnormal growth are complex, and that the various facets may proceed separately. Maturity of the cells in the lung, notably the type II cells and their ability to secret surfactant, is manipulated by a number of hormones, particularly glucocorticoids. However, with certain doses of steroids, the lung may have too few cells but type II cell maturity may be enhanced, that is, the lung cells may be hypermature but the lung hypoplastic.[18] Two other aspects of lung growth should be considered—tissue maturity and tissue complexity. By studying the light microscopic appearance of the lung, with a little experience one may guess at the duration of gestation with considerable precision. The extent of "tissue maturity" is a subjective assessment and may not take into account hypoplasia or cell maturity; indeed, perhaps these can all proceed at different rates. For example, it has never been established whether the hypoplastic lungs in diaphragmatic hernia are accompanied by a corresponding lack of tissue maturity. Tissue complexity can be assessed by the radial count of Emery and Mithal.[19] This measures the number of alveoli between the most distal respiratory bronchiole or terminal bronchiole and the periphery of the acinus. It is thus a measure of the complexity of the acinus (or more correctly the subacinus when the measurement is made from a respiratory bronchiole). It is an easy measurement to make and shows a relatively small range of normal

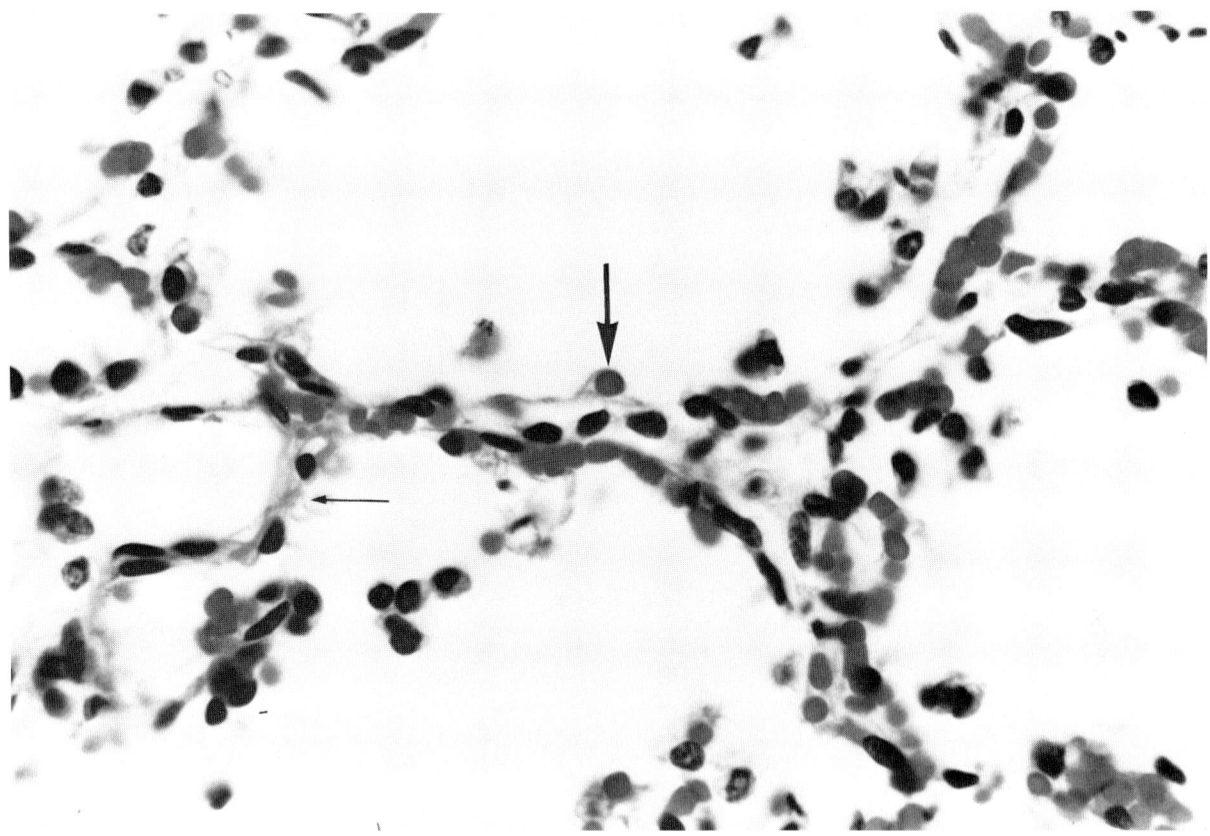

Figure 1–6. Thirty-six weeks gestation. Alveolar phase. An airspace wall is shown with a double capillary (thick arrow) and an alveolus with a thin wall and single capillary is also visible (thin arrow) (H&E, ×500). From Langston et al.[1]

both in utero and postnatally (Figs. 1–8, 1–9) as opposed to total alveolar number.[20–22]

In erythroblastosis fetalis, for example, it is possible for the lung to have normal complexity as assessed by the radial count[23] but yet be grossly hypoplastic because portions of the major airways may be missing. A rough estimate of the relative contribution of diminished alveolar complexity and absence of airway units can be made from the radial count. If the radial count is reduced by half, it would account for an eightfold (2^3) reduction in lung volume. (Since it is a linear measurement, the reduction must be cubed.) If the reduction in lung volume is greater than this then absence of units can be postulated. A direct measurement of airway development can be made by dissecting and reconstructing, from serial sections, a standard airway. The posterior segment of the upper lobe has been used successfully.[24] However, this technique is expensive and difficult (new programs are available for reconstructing serial sections that make it much easier) and the exact range of normal generations of bronchi and bronchioles has never been properly established. It is important to analyze any given case by the degree of hypoplasia or hyperplasia (whether assessed by cell number, lung weight, or volume), tissue maturity (apparent duration of gestation by appearance), tissue complexity (radial count), and cellular maturity (largely by ultrastructural appearance, surfactant activity, or disaturated phosphatidylcholine content).

Human Postnatal Lung Growth

While, as has been pointed out, there are approximately 50×10^6 alveoli at birth, the major postnatal event is alveolar multiplication and about 85 percent of alveoli are added after birth. Alveolar multiplication is extremely rapid in the first few years of life and then slows down. The time of cessation of alveolar multiplication is still not settled. The older view was that alveolar multiplication continued to 8 years of age[25]; newer data (Fig. 1–10) put this at an earlier date, perhaps 2 years of age.[22] It is not clear whether there is any clinical relevance to these observations. It might be thought that the age at which lung resection was done may affect the degree of compensatory response and that the younger the age, the better would be the response. A report suggests that this is not the case and there was no difference in response to lobectomy in children varying from 12 hours to 11 years

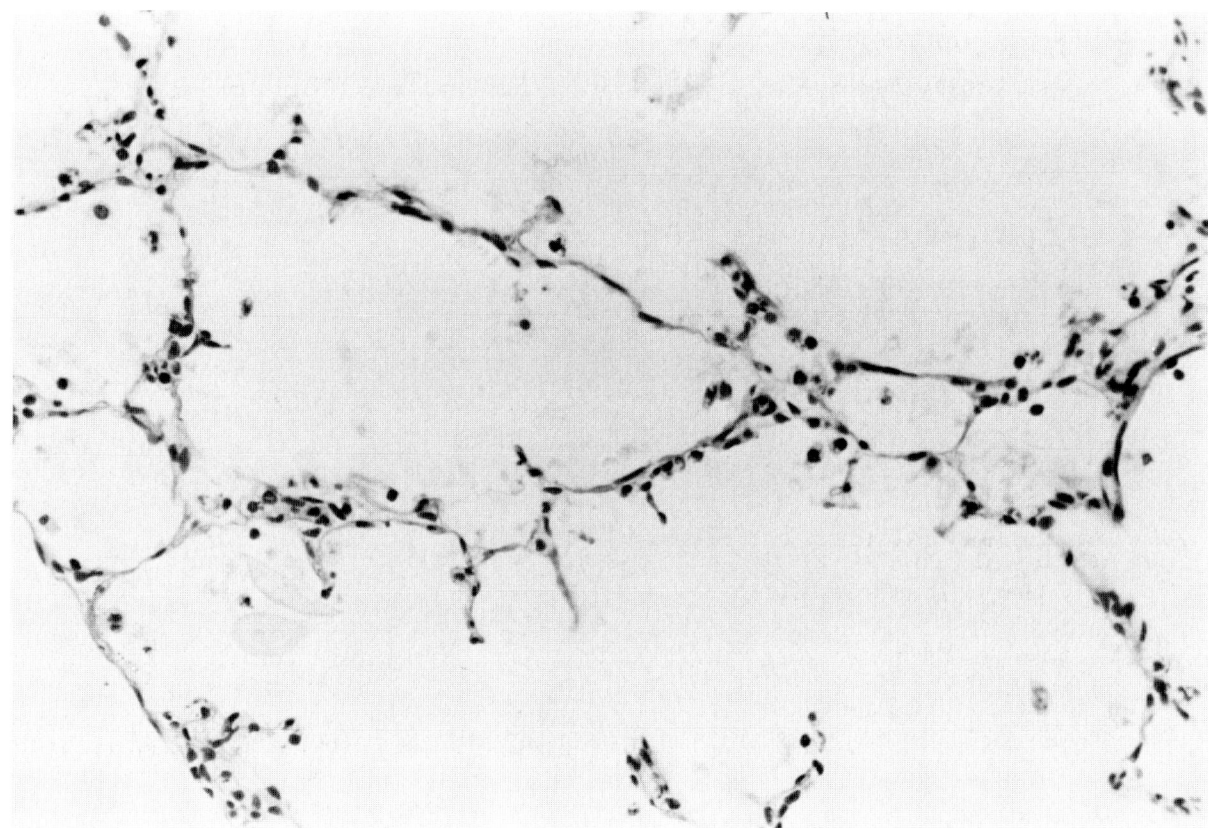

Figure 1–7. Thirty-six weeks' gestation. Alveolar phase. Thin-walled alveoli are readily visible (H&E, ×200). From Langston et al.[1]

of age.[26] As a result of alveolar multiplication, alveolar surface area increases rapidly. The precise way in which alveolar multiplication occurs is not certain. It is likely that the bulk of alveoli are added in the same way as intrauterine alveoli in the human, or postnatally in rats and mice,[2,3] that is, by subdivisions of saccules by crests. It also seems likely that there is centripetal extension of alveoli along airways since respiratory bronchioles are scarce at birth yet readily apparent in children two to three years old. The radial count increases from age 2 to 10 years.[20] Since the measurement extends from the most distal respiratory bronchiole to the edge of the acinus, the increase could come about as the most distal respiratory bronchiole moves proximally. This cannot be a major method of alveolar multiplication since, as mentioned previously in this section, direct alveolar counts show little change during this period.[22]

Not much is known about the control of human postnatal lung growth. Diminished alveolar number has been described in kyphoscoliosis of infantile onset, but not when the onset is later in childhood or early adolescence.[27–29] A diminished number of alveoli has been described in the tetralogy of Fallot.[30]

Experimental studies have given strong support to the hypothesis that the lungs can respond to increased oxygen requirement—such as increased physical activity, hypoxia, and cold—by increasing the morphologically determined diffusing capacity.[31] This in turn is primarily determined by alveolar (both epithelial and endothelial) surface area. The most effective way of doing this is by increased alveolar multiplication although the evidence for this way of increasing alveolar surface area is not particularly convincing. Perhaps the best known way of manipulating lung growth is pneumonectomy. Depending on the age and the species, the contralateral lung may develop the same weight, volume, cell, and alveolar number as control animals. The change in alveolar number is controversial.[32] Conventional wisdom is that the response is more complete in young than in old animals. The response is blunted or ablated by plombage on the pneumonectomized side, suggesting that stretch of the lung may be a major determining factor in lung growth.

Arteries

A complex set of changes occurs in the pulmonary arteries following birth. There is a rapid change in thickness of the smallest arteries as the arteries change from thick-walled fetal vessels to thin-walled infantile vessels. This change is complete by about 3 days of age.

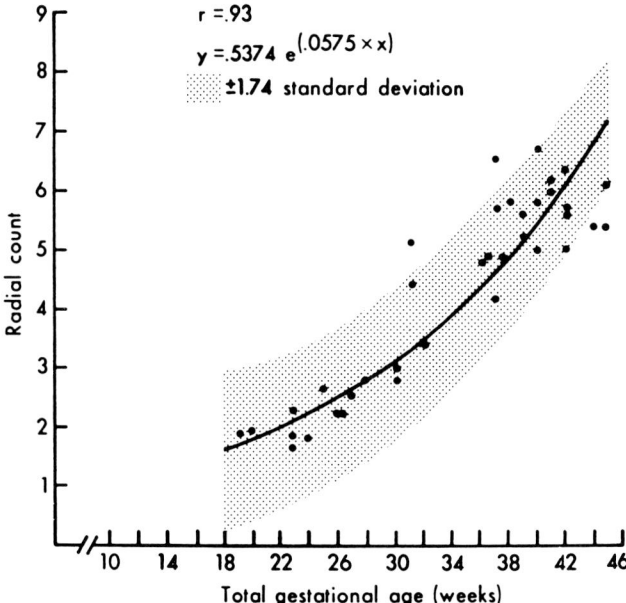

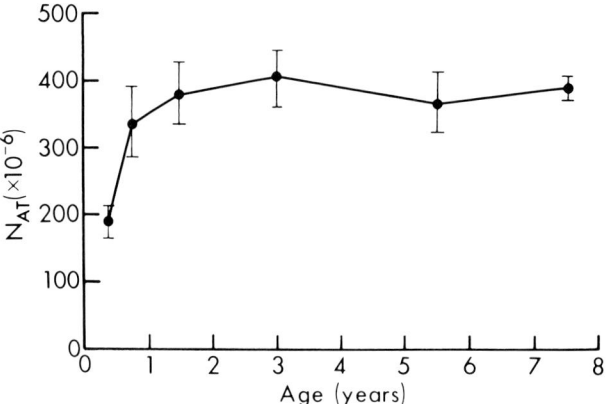

Figure 1–8. The radial count is shown during gestation and the early postnatal period. There is rapid increase in radial count from 2.7 at 28 weeks' gestation to 5.4 at 40 weeks' gestation. From Cooney and Thurlbeck.[21]

Figure 1–10. There is a rapid increase in total alveolar number postnatally with the adult complement being apparently reached by 2 years of age. The wide range is not shown—the bars indicate 1 SEM. From Thurlbeck.[22]

The distribution of elastic arteries and transitional arteries does not change; indeed, this is achieved by 19 weeks' gestation. The change in arteries is mainly one of increased dimension. There is a gradual extension of muscle into the acinus with age. At about 1 year of age muscle has extended to the respiratory bronchioles, and by three years of age to alveolar ducts, however, even at 11 years of age muscle is not found in the alveoli as it is in adults.[8] The other change is the development of numerous new branches of the pulmonary artery in the acinus. This is related to the development of alveoli, and more supernumerary arteries develop than conventional vessels. There is also increase of supernumery arteries in the preacinar region.

Connective Tissue

Little is known about postnatal collagen synthesis in humans, but in rabbits collagen synthesis is rapid in early postnatal life and then slows although collagen continues to increase as a percentage of lung weight throughout the first three months of life. In rats, elastin synthesis is most rapid in the first few weeks of life and this is accompanied by increased elastic recoil at mid- and low lung volumes.[33] Collagen synthesis continues to be rapid for another two weeks and is associated with a lesser tendency for the lung to rupture at high lung volumes.[33] There is a rapid increase in lung elastin content in the postnatal period in humans, and the adult level of 12% of lung dry weight is reached by six months of age.[34]

Laws of Lung Development

The clearest exposition of the salient features of lung development has been given by Reid.[35] These are (with some modification):

1. The bronchial and bronchiolar trees (conducting airways) are developed by the 16th week of gestation.
2. Alveoli develop mainly after birth, particularly in the first 2 years of life.
3. Preacinar arteries follow the development of the airways; intra-acinar vessels that of alveoli.

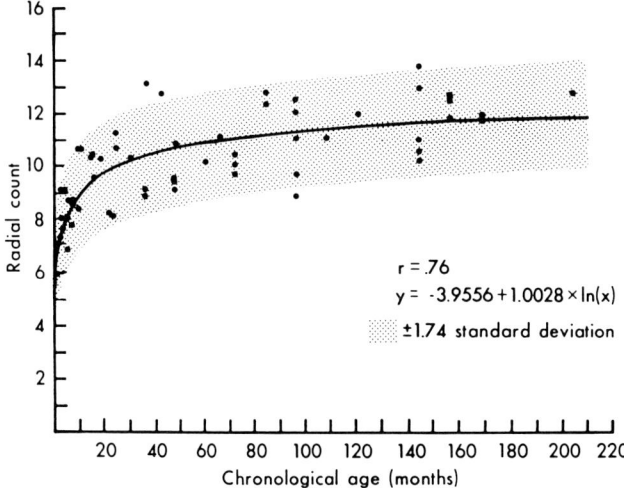

Figure 1–9. The radial count is shown from 1 month to 17 years of age. The radial count increases rapidly in the first 2 years of life and only slowly thereafter. From Cooney and Thurlbeck.[20]

References

1. Langston C, Kida K, Reed M, Thurlbeck WM: Human lung growth in late gestation and in the neonate. Am Rev Respir Dis 129:607–613, 1984.
2. Burri P: The post-natal growth of the rat lung. III. Morphology. Anat Rec 180:77–98, 1974.
3. Amy R, Bowes D, Burri PH, Thurlbeck WM: Post-natal growth of the mouse lung. J Anat 124:131–151, 1977.
4. Loosli CG, Potter EL: Pre and postnatal development of the respiratory portion of the human lung. Am Rev Respir Dis 80:5–23, 1959.
5. Bucher U, Reid L: Development of the mucus-secreting elements in the human lung. Thorax 16:219–225, 1961.
6. Rosan RC, Lauweryns JM: Mucosal cells of the small bronchioles of prematurely born human infants (1600–1700 g). Beitr Pathol 147:145–75, 1972.
7. Thurlbeck WM, Benjamin B, Reid L: Development and distribution of mucus glands in the fetal human trachea. Br J Dis Chest 55:54–64, 1961.
8. Hislop A, Reid L: Growth and development of the respiratory system—anatomical development. In Davis JA, Dobbing J (eds): *Scientific Foundations of Pediatrics*, 2nd ed. London: William Heinemann Medical Books, 1981, pp 390–432.
9. Boyden EA: The developing bronchial arteries in a fetus of the twelfth week. Am J Anat 129:357–368, 1970.
10. Grant MM, Roth N, Brody JS: Basement membrane development in fetal rats. Fed Proc 40:468, 1981.
11. Adamson IYR, King GM: Sex differences in development of fetal rat lung. I. Autoradiographic and biochemical studies. Lab Invest 50:546–560, 1984.
12. Adamson IYR, King GM: Sex differences in development of fetal rat lung. II. Quantitative morphology of epithelial-mesenchymal interactions. Lab Invest 50:461–468, 1974.
13. Adamson IYR, King GM: Sex-related differences in cellular composition and surfactant synthesis of developing fetal rat lungs. Am Rev Respir Dis 129:130–134, 1984.
14. Cooney TP, Thurlbeck WM: Lung growth and development in anencephaly and hydranencephaly. Am Rev Respir Dis, 132:596–601, 1985.
15. Wigglesworth JS, Desai R: Is fetal respiratory function a major determinant of perinatal survival? Lancet 1:264–267, 1982.
16. Cooney TP, Dimmick JE, Thurlbeck WM: Increased ascinar complexity with polyhydramnios. Pediatr Pathol, 5:183–197, 1986.
17. Alcorn D, Adamson TM, Lambert TE, et al. Morphological effects of chronic tracheal ligation and drainage in the fetal lamb lung. J Anat 123:649–660, 1977.
18. Kotas RV, Mims L, Hart L: Reversible inhibition of lung cell numbers after glucocorticoid injection. Pediatrics 53:358–361, 1974.
19. Emery JL, Mithal A: The number of alveoli in the terminal respiratory unit of man during late intrauterine life and childhood. Arch Dis Child 35:544–547, 1960.
20. Cooney TP, Thurlbeck WM: The radial alveolar count of Emery and Mithal—a re-appraisal. I. Post-natal lung growth. Thorax 37:572–579, 1982.
21. Cooney TP, Thurlbeck WM: The radial count method of Emery and Mithal: A reappraisal. II. Intrauterine and early postnatal lung growth. Thorax 37:580–583, 1982.
22. Thurlbeck WM: Postnatal human lung growth. Thorax 37:564–571, 1982.
23. Chamberlain D, Hislop A, Hey E, Reid L: Pulmonary hypoplasia in babies with severe rhesus iso-immunization: A quantitative study. J Pathol 122:43–52, 1977.
24. Hislop A, Reid L: New pathologic findings in emphysema of childhood: 1. Polyalveolar lobe. Thorax 25:682–690, 1970.
25. Dunnill MS: Postnatal growth of the lung. Growth in children. Thorax 17:329–333, 1962.
26. Frenckner B, Freyschuss U: Pulmonary function after lobectomy for congenital lobar emphysema and congenital cystic adenomatoid malformation. Scand J Thorac Cardiovasc Surg 16:293, 1982.
27. Dunnill MS: Quantitative observations on the anatomy of chronic non-specific lung disease. Med Thorac 22:261–274, 1965.
28. Davies G, Reid L: Effect of scoliosis on growth of alveoli and pulmonary arteries and on right ventricle. Arch Dis Child 46:623–632, 1971.
29. Berend N, Marlin GE: Arrest of alveolar multiplication in kyphoscoliosis. Pathology 11:485–491, 1979.
30. Rabinovitch M, Herrera-deLeon V, Castenada AR, Reid L: Growth and development of the pulmonary vascular bed in patients with tetralogy of Fallot with and without pulmonary atresia. Circulation 64:1234–1249, 1981.
31. Weibel ER: Fleischner Lecture. Looking at the lung: What can it tell us. AJR 133:1021–1031, 1979.
32. Thurlbeck WM: Postpneumonectomy compensatory lung growth. Am Rev Respir Dis 128:96–97, 1983.
33. Nardell EA, Brody JS: Determinants of the mechanical properties of the rat lung during postnatal development. J Appl Physiol 53:140–148, 1982.
34. Keeley FW, Fagan DG, Webster SI: Quantity and character of elastin in developing human lung. Parenchymal tissues of normal infants and infants with respiratory distress syndrome. J Lab Clin Med 90:981, 1977.
35. Reid L: The embryology of the lung. In de Reuck AVS, Porter R (eds): *Ciba Foundation: Symposium on Development of the Lung*. London: Churchill, 1967, pp 109–430.

2 Normal Anatomy and Histology

Charles Kuhn III

Functionally the lung consists of the acini, units specialized for gas exchange between air and blood, and conducting tissues, the airways and blood vessels that distribute the air and blood to the gas-exchanging units. Disease processes may involve acini, airways, or vessels selectively or in combination. Differing as they do in structure, function, and cellular composition, these tissues react differently in disease. Thus an understanding of lung disease requires a knowledge of the structure and function of the tissues that comprise the normal lung.[1]

Gross Anatomy

General Features

The lungs are paired, asymmetric organs roughly conical in shape. Their normal combined weight averages 850 g in men and 750 g in women.[2] The space that they occupy in the thoracic cavity is enclosed by the rib cage dorsally, laterally, and ventrally, the mediastinum medially, and the diaphragm inferiorly. The shape of the expanded lung, after removal from the body, corresponds with the cavities thus defined. The lung has three surfaces: a convex surface abutting the rib cage, more sharply curved posteriorly than anteriorly; a concave mediastinal surface; and a concave diaphragmatic surface conforming to the convexity of the diaphragm as it covers the domes of the liver and spleen. Toward the posterior portion of the mediastinal surface lies the hilum of the lung, the region in which the bronchi blood vessels, lymphatics, and nerves enter the lung (Fig. 2–1). Distinct sharp margins are formed anteriorly by the junction of the mediastinal and costal surfaces and inferiorly by the junction of the costal and diaphragmatic surfaces; the posterior transition from the costal to mediastinal surface and the junction of the mediastinal and diaphragmatic surfaces are rounded. The right lung is slightly larger than the left owing to the space required to accommodate the heart on the left side of the mediastinum, but the vertical (cephalocaudal) dimension of the right lung is less than that of the left lung due to the higher position of the right hemidiaphragm where it covers the right lobe of the liver.

The lungs can move freely within the thoracic cavity, being attached only at the two hila. The free surfaces of the lung are covered by a serous membrane, the visceral pleura, which is reflected over the hilum to cover the mediastinum, chest wall, and diaphragm as the parietal pleura. The pleural reflection at the hilum continues inferiorly as the pulmonary ligament. In vivo, the parietal and visceral pleura are normally closely apposed, lubricated by a thin film of pleural fluid, composition of which is similar to other interstitial fluids. The exact volume of pleural fluid in normal subjects is not known, but it is not more than a few milliliters.

The lungs are divided into their major subdivisions, the lobes, by clefts or fissures lined by visceral pleura (see Fig. 2–1). The right lung has three lobes. The major fissure follows an oblique course from a level above the hilum dorsally to the base of the lung anteriorly, dividing the inferior lobe from the remainder of the lung; a second (minor) fissure, nearly horizontal, separates the remainder into a superior and middle lobe. The left lung is divided into superior and inferior lobes by a single oblique fissure; it has no middle lobe. The homologous region, the anterior and inferior portion of the superior lobe, is known as the lingula owing to its tongue-like extension anteriorly into costophrenic sulcus. It is frequently partially set off from the remainder of the lobe by an incomplete fissure.

The conducting airways, which distribute air to the gas exchanging units, begin with the trachea, which originates at the larynx in the neck and descends into the mediastinum where it branches at the level of T 4–5

12 Normal Anatomy and Histology

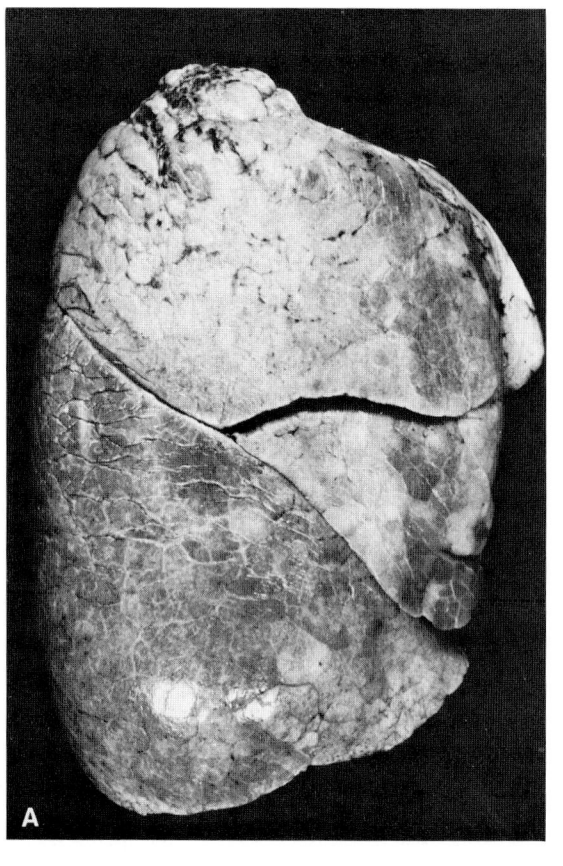

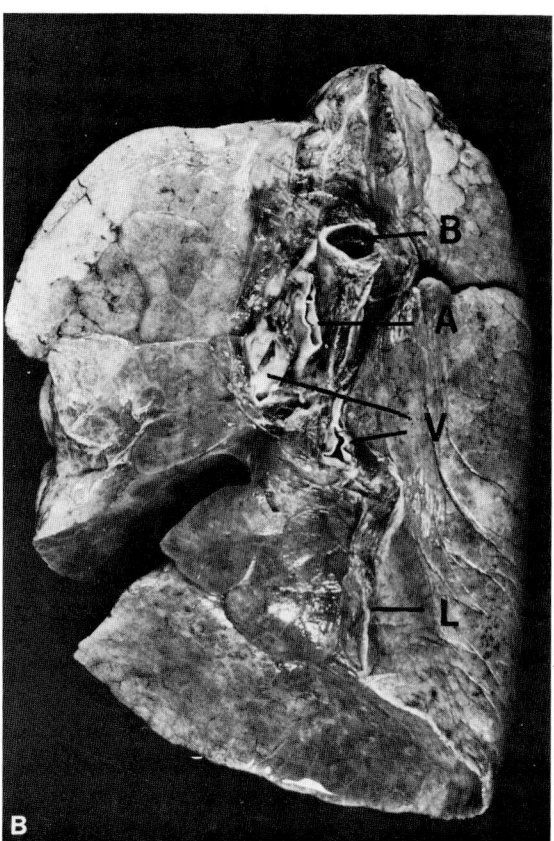

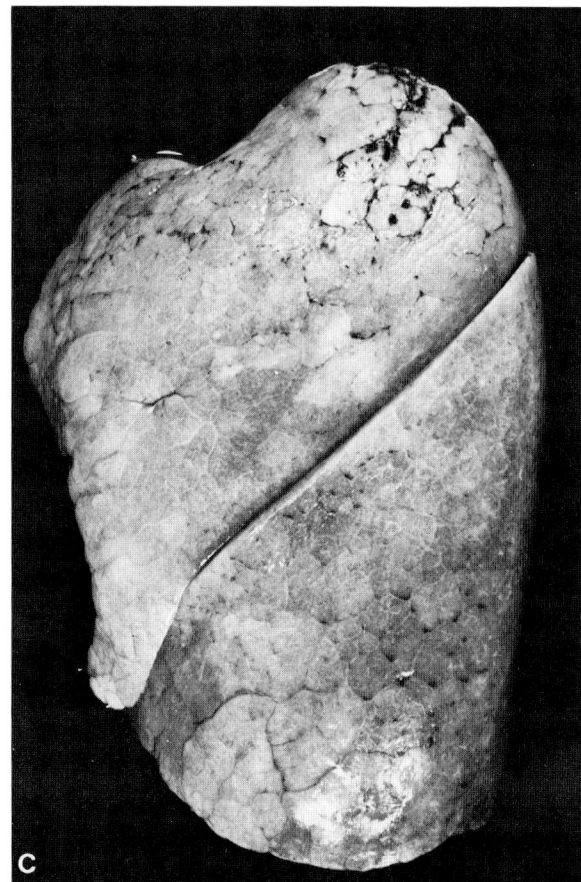

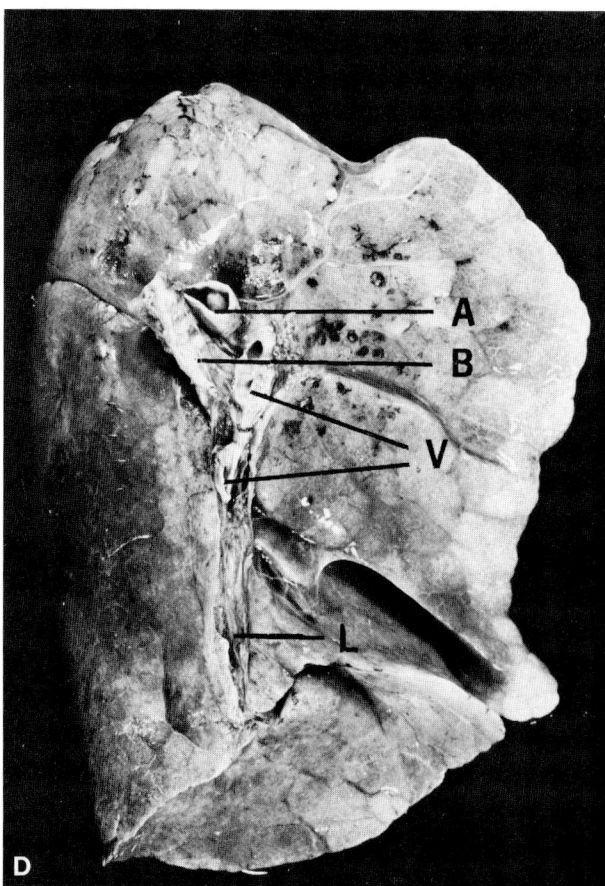

Table 2–1. Bronchopulmonary Segments

Right Lung	Left Lung
Upper lobe	Upper lobe
1. Apical	1,2. Apical-posterior
2. Posterior	3. Anterior
3. Anterior	Lingula
Middle lobe	4. Superior
4. Lateral	5. Inferior
5. Medial	Lower lobe
Lower lobe	6. Superior
6. Superior	7. Anterior-medial basal
7. Medial basal (cardiac)	8. Lateral basal
8. Anterior basal	9. Posterior basal
9. Lateral basal	
10. Posterior basal	

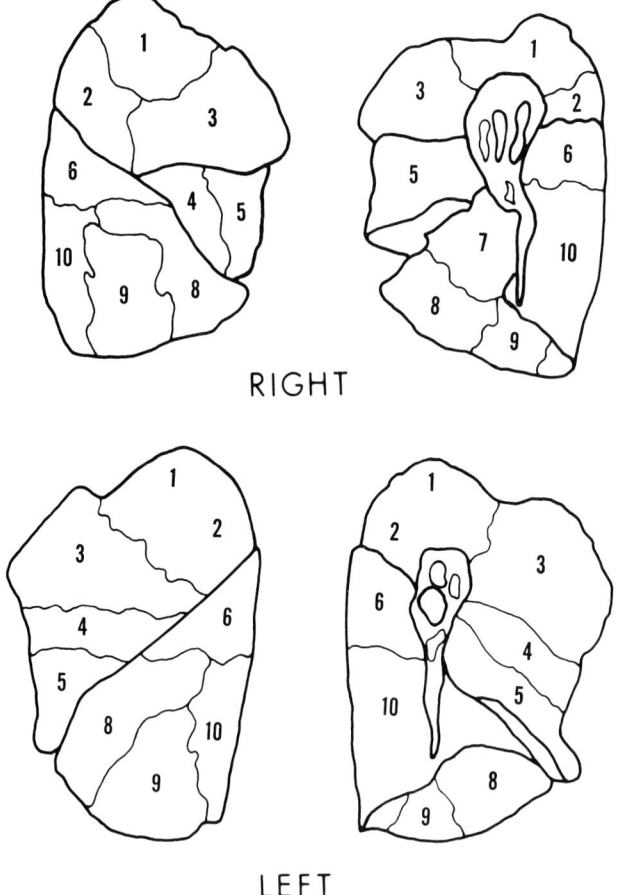

Figure 2–2. Pleural projections of the bronchopulmonary segments. Numbering is explained in Table 2–1. There is no segment number 7 in the left lung.

giving rise to the left and right main bronchi. The branching is asymmetric. The left main bronchus is narrower, longer, and given off at a greater angle than the right. The bronchus to the right upper lobe branches off the main bronchus just before they enter the lung at the hilum. Within the lung, the bronchi branch dichotomously, giving rise to progressively smaller airways. Branching is asymmetric: the two daughters of a given branching may differ both in diameter, length, and angle. The number of generations from the main bronchus to the acini varies from as few as 8 to as many as 25 depending on the region of the lung supplied.

Mixed venous blood is brought to the lung by the pulmonary artery which leaves the right ventricle of the heart anterior and to the left of the ascending aorta and branches below the aortic arch. The right main pulmonary artery passes beneath the arch of the aorta to enter the lung anterior to the right main bronchus with which it is closely associated. The left pulmonary artery passes above the main stem bronchus and lies above it in the hilus where it passes over the superior lobar bronchus coming to lie posterior to the bronchus. Within the lung, the pulmonary arteries accompany the bronchi, branching with them until they reach the acini. The pulmonary veins drain independently from the bronchi with two trunks leaving each lung at the hilus to enter the left atrium separately.

The nutrient blood supply to the bronchi, major pulmonary vessels, and part of the pleura comes from the systemic circulation via bronchial arteries which vary in number and origin. They arise either directly from the aorta or from the intercostal, internal mammary, or subclavian arteries passing along the esophagus and posterior wall of the main bronchi to enter the lung. Within the lung, they remain within the connective tissue sheath of the bronchi where they extend peripherally to the level of the bronchioles. Bronchial vessels are not found within the acini. Apparently the venous blood provided by the pulmonary artery supplies all the metabolic substrates required by the lung parenchyma, and oxygen is supplied by diffusion from the air spaces.

The venous drainage from the walls of the more peripheral bronchi enters the pulmonary veins. Bronchial veins drain only the central bronchi and nearby pleura and empty into the azygos and hemiazygos veins.

Figure 2–1. External appearance of fully inflated adult human lungs showing the normal lobe pattern. A. Lateral surface, right lung. B. Medial surface, right lung. C. Lateral surface, left lung. D. Medial surface, left lung. The hilar structures seen on the medial surfaces are the bronchi (B), pulmonary arteries (A), and pulmonary veins (V). The pleural reflection at the hilus extends inferiorly as the pulmonary ligament (L). Note that the right pulmonary artery enters the lung anterior to the bronchus, whereas the left pulmonary artery crosses over the bronchus.

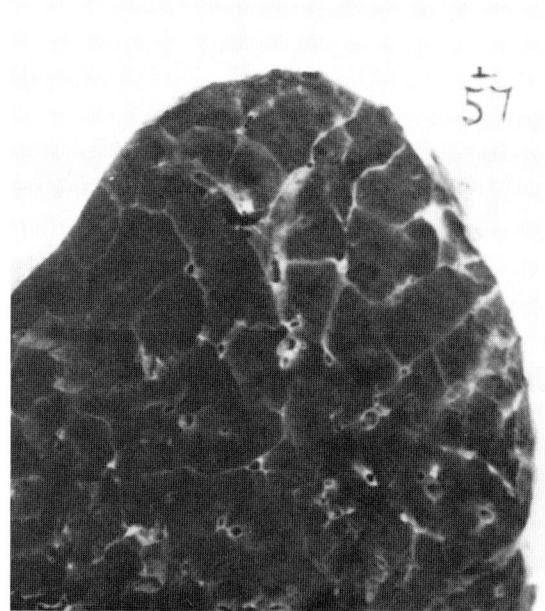

Figure 2–3. Sectioned surface of a lung showing lobules partially enclosed by connective tissue septa. The extent of development of the septa varies from lung to lung and from one region to another in the same lung.

Subunits of Lung Structure

In addition to the lobes of the lung, various subunits of lung structure are recognized. The bronchopulmonary segments are important to thoracic surgery since they are subunits of a lobe which can be resected relatively conveniently with little hemorrhage or air leakage from the raw surfaces. Generally they are the unit of lung supplied by the first generation of bronchi below the lobar bronchi, are roughly pyramidal in shape, and are pleural-based. The nomenclature of the segments is given in Table 2–1, and their pleural projections outlined in Figure 2–2. A detailed discussion of the many variations in segmental anatomy can be found in Boyden's monograph.[3]

When the pleural surface of the lung is viewed, connective septa which outline polygonal units approximately 1 cm in diameter can be seen. On the cut surface of the sliced lung, these septa extend a variable distance into the lung, incompletely enclosing units known as pulmonary lobules or secondary lobules of Miller[4] (Fig. 2–3).

The acinus is the basic unit of lung funtion, the largest structural unit of lung, all of whose elements participate in gas exchange. Thus it is the unit supplied by a single terminal bronchiole; it consists of respiratory bronchioles, alveolar ducts, alveolar sacs, and alveoli. Individual acini cannot be recognized grossly. A lobule consists of three to five acini; although it is a less meaningful structure than an acinus in terms of lung function, the lobule provides a convenient reference for gross pathology. The terminal bronchioles branch near the center of the lobules, and their acini terminate in alveolar sacs abutting the connective tissue septa. Consequently, lesions affecting the proximal portions of acini will predominate near the center of the lobules, and the lesions of the distal portions of the acini adjoin the lobular septa.

Airways

Classification

Although the conducting airways share a common plan—all are muscular tubes lined by a ciliated epithelium—they differ in detail depending on size.[5,6] The walls of airways approximately 1 mm or more in diameter are reinforced by cartilage and are called bronchi. Conducting airways without cartilage are called bronchioles. In many species, rodents for example, there is an abrupt change from the bronchioles to gas-exchanging tissue formed of alveoli. In humans and other primates, there are transitional airways called respiratory bronchioles that have a bronchiolar structure over a portion of their circumference but also have alveoli over a portion. The term terminal bronchiole is used to identify the most distal generation of bronchioles completely free of alveoli, that is, the parent generation to the respiratory bronchioles.

Bronchi

The bronchi are lined by a pseudostratified ciliated columnar epithelium which rests on a homogeneous eosinophilic membrane 1 to 3μm thick, often regarded as the basement membrane by light microscopists (Fig. 2–4). As seen by electron microscopy, the bronchial epithelium rests on a typical slender basal lamina, but a layer of closely packed collagen fibers lies just beneath it; it is the combined structure that is recognized by light microscopists as basement membrane.[7,8] Beneath the basement membrane is the lamina propria which contains loose connective tissue composed predominantly of longitudinally arranged elastic fibers.[4]

The Bronchial Wall

The smooth muscle of the bronchial wall lies just beneath the zone of elastic fibers, still close to the epithelium, and is arranged in discrete bundles, which wind down the airway wall in a spiral pattern with a rather shallow pitch. Consequently the predominant effect of contraction of the smooth muscle is airway narrowing. Loose connective tissue and bronchial glands occupy the space between the muscle and the outermost layer of the bronchi, which consists of heavy circumferential bundles of collagen fibers and hyaline cartilage. The form taken by the cartilage varies between the extrapulmonary bronchi and the intrapulmonary bronchi. In the trachea and extrapulmonary bronchi, the cartilages take the form of U-shaped

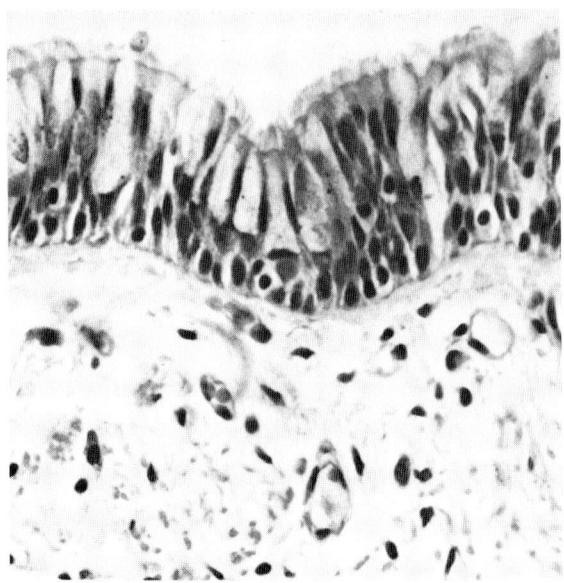

Figure 2–4. Mucosa of a major bronchus. Basal cells, goblet cells, and ciliated cells rest on a thin basement membrane (×400).

The Bronchial Mucosa

The epithelium lining the bronchi functions mainly in the production and propulsion of mucus.[9] If particulate material, such as dust or organisms, suspended in the inspired air should impact on the bronchial wall, it deposits on a thin coating of mucus, a product of specialized secretory epithelial cells found in the bronchial surface epithelium and in glands located in the connective tissue of the bronchial wall.[9] The mucus streams in a generally cephalad direction to the oropharynx, propelled by the beating of cilia in the respiratory mucosa. The rate of movement of the mucus varies with the level of the bronchial tree, being slower in peripheral bronchi and fastest in the central bronchi and trachea where particles are transported at a rate of 1 to 2 cm/min.[10] The mucous blanket is considered to have two layers: a superficial gel layer rich in macromolecules providing a viscoelastic barrier and a watery serous layer beneath it in which the cilia beat. In experimental animals in which the airways have been fixed for morphologic study using vascular perfusion to avoid disturbing secretions in the airways, the mucous blanket appears as a nearly continuous sheet 5 μm thick resting on the tips of the cilia.[11,12] In addition to mucous glycoproteins, the bronchial secretions contain antibacterial proteins such as lysozyme and lactoferrin,[13] immunoglobulins (principally IgA),[13] and locally produced proteinase inhibitors.[14] The serous layer appears empty in morphologic preparations, implying paucity of macromolecules.

In standard histologic sections, the bronchial surface epithelium consists of three principal cell types: basal, ciliated, and secretory cells (see Fig. 2–4). Round nuclei just above the basement membrane belong to the basal cells, which are small triangular cells that rest on the basal lamina and are excluded from the bronchial lumen by the neighboring columnar cells.[15] They have few organelles and are joined to the neighboring columnar cells by desmosomes associated with tonofilament bundles. Basal cells label heavily with tritiated thymidine and function as reserve cells for the other epithelial cell types, the ciliated and secretory cells.[16] Above the nuclei of the basal cells are elongated nuclei of columnar cells, ciliated and secretory. Ciliated cells are normally approximately three to five times more numerous than secretory cells.[15]

Ciliated Cells

The ciliated cells are columnar cells attached to the basal lamina and reach the bronchial lumen. They have a centrally placed oval nucleus, a surprisingly large Golgi apparatus for a nonsecretory cell, and usually several large lysosomal residual bodies lying near the Golgi apparatus just above the nucleus.[15] Mitochondria are found in all parts of the cell, but they are particularly concentrated in a zone near the apex of the cell close to the cilia which they supply with adenosine triphosphate (ATP). Ciliated cells do not take up tritiated thymidine, and their replacement probably takes place mainly from basal cells, but also from differentiation of mucus-secreting cells.

rings which are open dorsally. The intrapulmonary bronchi have irregularly shaped islands of cartilage in their walls (Fig. 2–5) that diminish in size and number progressively with the decreasing caliber of the bronchi. Their distribution was investigated in detail by Hayward and Reid,[5] who found that, in the axial bronchial pathways, there was a high density of cartilage which effectively provided circumferential support for the first four to six generations. The axial bronchi had only scattered plates for another four to six generations. Laterally branching bronchi had circumferential cartilaginous support only at their orifices and occasional cartilage plates for another five to six generations.

Horsefield[6] has pointed out that the pattern of cartilage organization is well adapted for an efficient cough mechanism. During coughing a marked positive intrathoracic pressure is first generated by forced expiration against a closed glottis; simultaneously the airways markedly narrow. When the glottis abruptly opens, the high pressure produces very rapid flows through the narrowed tubes to dislodge obstructing material. The extrapulmonary airways have no external support, and the cartilage rings enable the airways to remain open even in the presence of positive intrathoracic pressure. The intrapulmonary bronchi are resistant to collapse being tethered by the surrounding lung tissue, and the incomplete cartilaginous plates provide additional buttressing while still permitting the bronchi to narrow.

The intrapulmonary bronchi are enclosed in a sheath of loose connective tissue containing bundles of collagen fibers and adipose tissue, together with the bronchial arteries, venous trunks, lymphatics, and nerves.

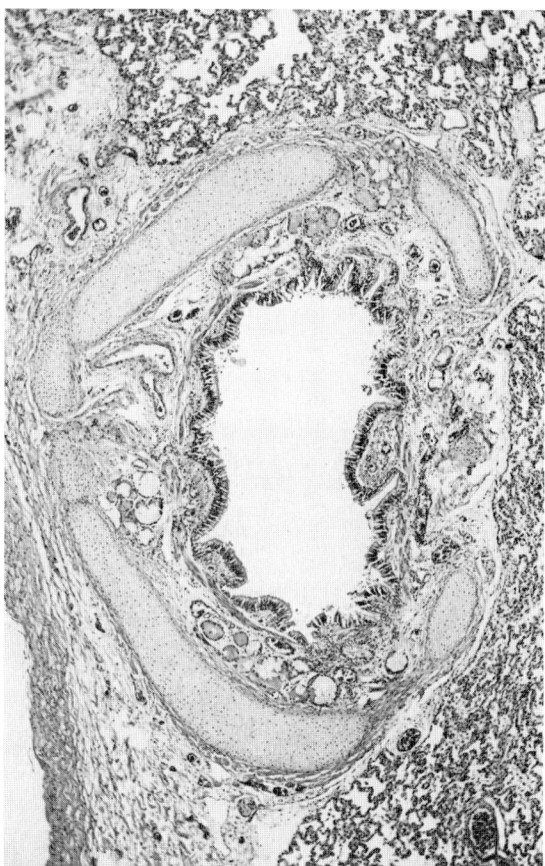

Figure 2–5. Large intrapulmonary bronchus in a child's lung. Multiple plates of cartilage completely enclose the bronchus, yet potentially permit it to vary in caliber. The pulmonary artery at the lower left occupies the same connective tissue sheath as the bronchus (×150).

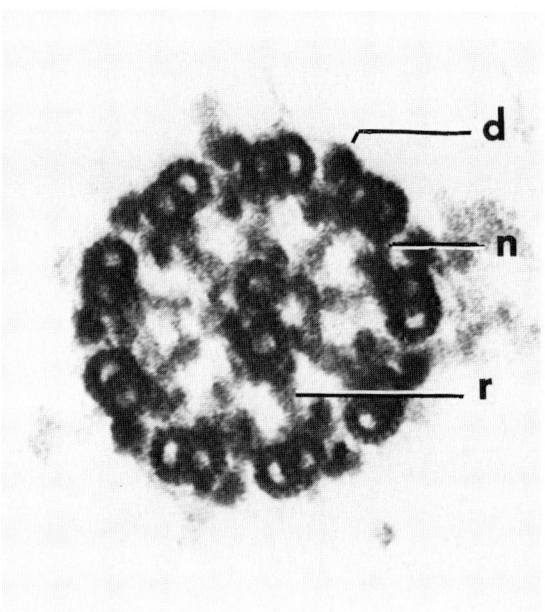

Figure 2–6. Cross-section of an axoneme of a detergent-extracted nasal cilium viewed from the tip toward the cell. The plasma membrane was removed by the extraction. The axoneme consists of nine doublet microtubules in a ring surrounding two single microtubules. d—dynein arm, n—nexin link, r—radial spoke (×250,000).

The structure and cell biology of cilia have recently been reviewed by Gibbons.[17] The cilia are membrane-covered extensions of the apex of the cell, 5 to 8 μm in length and 0.3 μm in diameter. With a few exceptions, the basic structure of cilia is similar in most eukaryotic organisms. The basic machinery of the cilium resides in the axoneme, a complicated structure which arises as an outgrowth of basal bodies, centriole-like structures anchored in the apical cytoplasm. The axoneme consists of nine peripheral microtubule pairs arranged in a circle around two central single microtubules (Fig. 2–6). Each of the peripheral doublet fibers consists of a complete 240-A microtubule composed of 13 protofilaments (the A subfiber) fused to an incomplete tubule (B subfiber) composed of 10 protofilaments.[18] In conventional electron micrographs, there are paired asymmetric arms at regular intervals of 240 A along the A subfiber which project toward the B subfiber of the neighboring doublet (see Fig. 2–6). These arms contain the majority of the adenosine triphosphatase (ATPase) activity of the cilium.[19] Ciliary ATPase is known as dynein, hence the arms are called dynein arms. Using replicas of frozen and deeply etched detergent-treated cilia, Goodenough and Heuser[20] visualized the substructure of the outer dynein arms. The main component is a globular unit (the head) that interacts with two smaller globular units, the proximal and distal feet which couple the head to the A subfiber of the doublet (Fig. 2–7). A delicate stalk, invisible in conventional micrographs, connects the head to the B subfiber of the neighboring doublet.

Each of the A subfibers is also joined on its inner aspect to the B subfiber of the neighboring doublet by a series of fine, highly extensible filaments known as nexin links. At regular intervals of 150 A along both central singlet tubules, there are paired curved projections 180 A in length, nearly perpendicular to the plane of the singlet tubules. These projections were known collectively as the central sheath before their structure was known in detail. Radially oriented spokes attached to the A subfibers of the peripheral doublet project inward to the central sheath, ending in a slight enlargement, the spoke head. The spokes are arranged in clusters of three, with an overall spacing of 900 A, so that the spacing of each group of three radial spokes exactly matches six central sheath projections.[21]

The B subfibers, dynein arms, and radial spokes terminate 10 to 20 nm from the tip of the cilium, whereas the A subfibers continue into the tip to end in an electron-dense plaque that fills the 200-A gap between the axoneme and the membrane over the tip. A cluster of five to eight bristles 250 to 300 A in length anchored to the plaque penetrates the plasma membrane forming the ciliary crown, a special glycocalyx on the tip of each

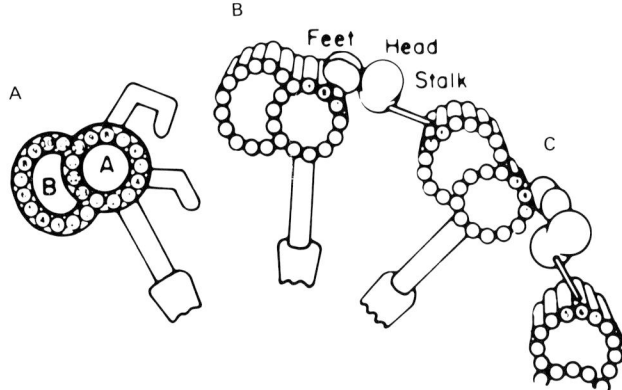

Figure 2–7. Diagram of the structure of the dynein arms based on conventional images and three-dimensional replicas of rapidly frozen cilia. A. Conventional image as seen in thin sections. The A and B subfibers of the microtubular doublet are labeled. Two angulated dynein arms and a radial spoke with spoke head are shown attached to the A subfiber. B and C show the components of the outer arm as seen in the replicas. The inner dynein arms are not illustrated, as they have not been described by this technique. B. The configuration in the absence of adenosine triphosphate (ATP). C. With ATP From Goodenough and Heuser: J Cell Biol 95:798–815, 1982. Used with permission of the Rockefeller University Press.

cilium.[22,23] The ciliary crown is strongly anionic, indicated by its ability to bind cationized ferritin and ruthenium red.[23,24] It is postulated to play a role in coupling the motile cilia to the overlying mucous blanket.

At the junction of the cilium and the apex of the ciliated cell, there is a specialized region known as the ciliary neck where there are changes in the structure of both the membrane and the axoneme.[25] In this region, the central singlet fibers terminate, radial spokes and dynein arms disappear. The doublet fibers are joined to one another and are connected to the plasma membrane by delicate Y-shaped linkers. Where the Y-shaped linkers join the membrane, freeze-fracture preparations show there are distinct circumferential rows of intramembranous particles, the ciliary necklace,[25] and cationic ferritin binding shows a concentration of anionic groups on the extracellular surface of the membrane.[24] At least one function of this complex structure must be to bind down the plasma membrane to the axoneme, thereby maintaining the separation of the individual cilia.

The basal bodies, of which the cilia are an outgrowth, are cylindrical structures approximately 0.4 μm in length located in the apex of the cell. They are composed of nine triplet microtubules, two tubules continuous with the A and B subfibers of the axonemal doublet tubules, fused to a third (C) subfiber. The triplets are twisted to an angle of 30 to 40 degrees in a "pinwheel" arrangement. Among the accessory structures attached to the basal bodies are striated rootlets, which extend a few tenths of a micron into the cytoplasm, and a lateral triangular projection 0.1 μm in length, the basal foot, which is a nucleating site for cytoplasmic microtubules.[26]

The beating of the cilia is a complex movement in which there is a rapid planar effective stroke in the direction of fluid movement in which the cilia engage the bottom of the mucous gel, followed by a slower recovery stroke in which the cilia recoil while swinging in a clockwise direction beneath the gel.[27] The plane of the effective stroke is perpendicular to the plane of the central singlet fibers, and the basal foot protrudes in the direction of the effective stroke.

Only a few aspects of the mechanisms producing ciliary movement are currently understood. The energy for ciliary beating is provided by ATP. Although dynein is activated by Ca^{++} in a calmodulin-dependent manner,[28] Mg^{++} is required for optimal dynein ATPase activity. The power for ciliary activity is produced by the sliding of the peripheral doublet tubules relative to their neighbors,[29,30] and is unaccompanied by changes in the length of the tubules.[21,31] In the presence of bound ATP, the dynein arms rest in the relaxed configuration shown schematically in Figure 2–8. Following hydrolysis of the ATP, the adenosine diphosphate and phosphate dissociate, and the dynein arms shift to the rigor configuration in Figure 2–8. The shift exerts traction on adjacent doublet through the stalk producing a small amount (~8 nm) of sliding displacement between the doublets.[20] The cycle is then repeated as another ATP molecule is hydrolyzed. At some point during the transition from rigor back to the relaxed configuration, there must be detachment of the dynein arms from the neighboring doublet, followed by reattachment at a new binding site, but it is not known how this occurs and which components of the arm detach.

The sliding is restrained by trypsin-sensitive structures, probably the nexin links and radial spokes.[32] Morphologic studies of cilia fixed during beating have shown that the radial spokes are attached to the central sheath projections in straight portions of the cilium but are free at sites of bending.[21] The spoke heads have cytochemically demonstrable ATPase activity, suggesting that the attachment or detachment is an energy-requiring process and is actively involved in converting the interdoublet sliding into the complex waveforms taken by motile cilia.

Fields of beating cilia are coordinated in metachronal waves which pass along the mucosa. The waves are thought to be brought about by mechanical interaction of cilia.[27]

Mucus-Secreting Cells

The source of the serous periciliary fluid has not been established. To date no specific cell has been associated with its secretion. The tracheobronchial epithelium actively transports ions, specifically sodium, away from the bronchial lumen and chloride toward it, while water will follow down the resultant osmotic gradient.[33] This process offers a potential mechanism for the regulation of the proper depth of periciliary sol layer, which is so critical to effective ciliary function.

The mucous gel is secreted by specific secretory cells in the tracheobronchial surface epithelium and in the glands of the submucosa. The glands are considered the

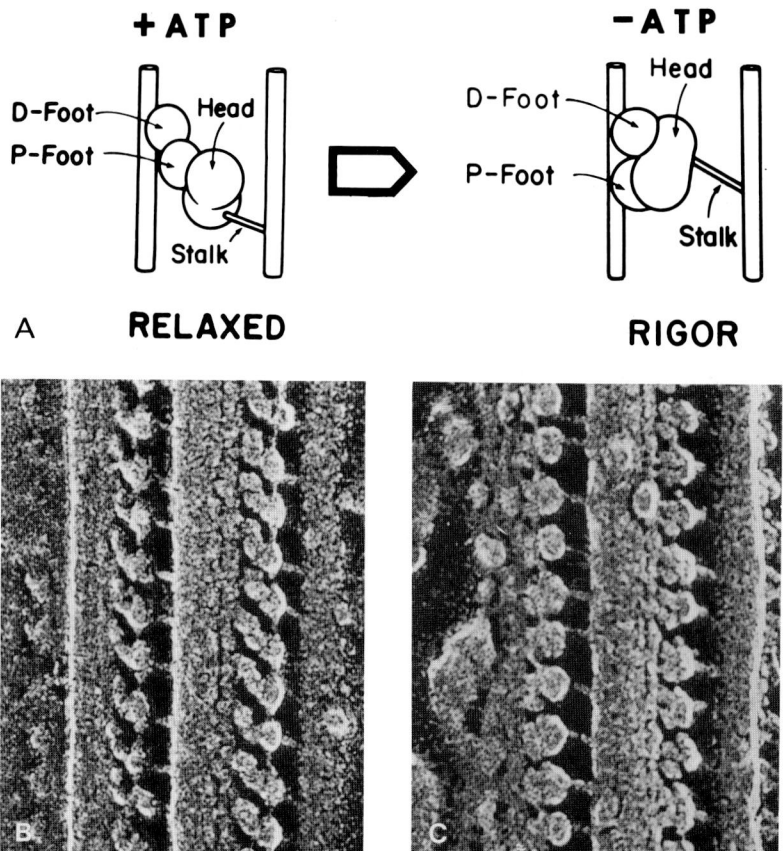

Figure 2–8. A. Schematic drawing of two configurations of the outer dynein arms. The shift from relaxed to rigor exerts traction through the stalk, producing sliding displacement of the neighboring microtubules. B and C are actual replicas illustrating the two configurations. Three microtubule doublets are seen in lateral view with two rows of outer dynein arms in the spaces between them. B. Cilium frozen in the presence of ATP and vanadate, an inhibitor that prevents release of hydrolyzed ATP (adenosine diphosphate and phosphate) from the dynein. C. Cilium frozen in the absence of ATP (both ×270,000). From Goodenough and Heuser: J Cell Biol 95:798–815, 1982. Used with permission of the Rockefeller University Press.

major source, since their volume is much greater than that of the secretory cells of the surface epithelium. Two types of secretory cells have been identified in the surface epithelium in the rat: serous cells and mucous cells.[22] In the limited number of ultrastructural studies reported in humans, serous cells have not been described in the surface epithelium. Typical goblet cells are characterized by a bulging apex distended with coalescing secretory vacuoles.[15,34] In the electron microscope, these vacuoles contain fibrillar electron-lucent material (Fig. 2–9). The apex of the goblet cells is covered by microvilli, and the cytoplasm is electron-dense and contains a considerable amount of lamellar endoplasmic reticulum compressed into the basal and lateral portions of cytoplasm. Other mucus-secreting cells share the electron-dense cytoplasm and other cytoplasmic features of the goblet cells, but have only a few small mucous-filled secretory vesicles. McDowell and collaborators[34] have called these small mucus granule cells (SMGC).

They recognized that these cells are probably not a separate type of cell but may well be mucous cells in a different phase of the secretory cycle from the goblet cells. A few bronchial columnar cells have neither cilia nor mucous granules. Such "indifferent" cells are infrequent and may represent a way station between basal cells and one or both of the differentiated columnar cell types.[34]

Mucous Glands

The mucous glands are compound tubular glands (Fig. 2–10) which lie deep to the muscle, in submucosa of the bronchi between the cartilage and surface epithelium, often extending through the gaps between cartilages to occupy the connective tissue of the adventitia. Their three-dimensional organization has been described in detail by Meyrick and colleagues.[35] The secretory tubules drain into collecting ducts which discharge into the

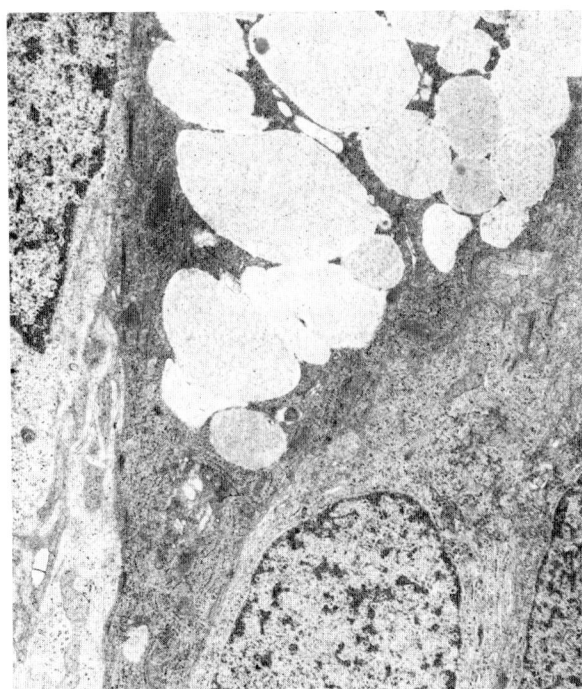

Figure 2–9. Goblet cell in the surface epithelium of a bronchus. The cytoplasm is relatively electron-dense. The apical cytoplasm is filled with coalescent vacuoles containing electron-lucent mucus (×10,000).

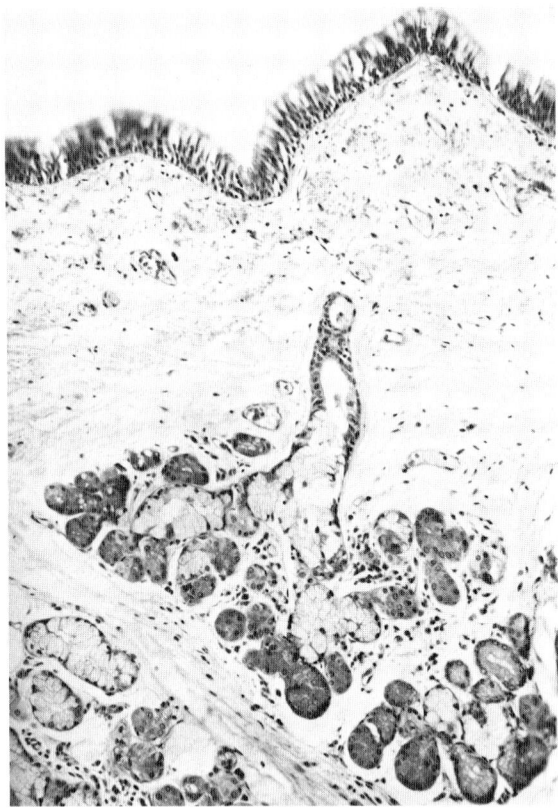

Figure 2–10. Bronchial mucous gland. The lumen of the bronchus is at the top. A duct branches, giving rise to secretory tubules lined by mucous cells in their proximal portions and serous cells in their terminal portions. The small dark cells in the interstitium between the tubules are mainly plasma cells (×100).

bronchial lumen at an estimated frequency of approximately one per square millimeter of bronchial surface in the central bronchi. The glands decrease in frequency distally, ultimately disappearing at the same level as the cartilage, at the tenth generation on the average.

Three types of cells are recognized in the secretory tubules: mucous, serous, and myoepithelial cells (Fig. 2–11). Serous cells are most numerous at the ends of the secretory tubules. Their outline is roughly triangular with a basally placed nucleus and a polarized cytoplasm. The apical portion of the cell contains large eosinophilic granules, whereas the basal portion is strongly basophilic owing to its high content of lamellar endoplasmic reticulum. The secretory granules contain acidic glycoproteins[36,37] but also contain at least two specific proteins found in bronchial secretions, lysozyme (Fig. 2–12) and antileukoprotease.[38–41] Lysozyme is an enzyme that hydrolyzes the β 1, 4 glucosidic bonds between N-acetyl muramic acid and N-acetyl glucosamine found in the cell wall of certain Gram-positive bacteria. Antileukoprotease is a low-molecular-weight protease inhibitor found in a variety of mucoid secretions. It effectively inhibits the two major proteases in polymorphonuclear neutrophil granules, elastase and cathepsin G,[14] and presumably protects the bronchi from proteolytic damage when the sputum becomes purulent. Lactoferrin is probably also a product of serous cells.[42]

Mucous cells have basally located, rather pyknotic nuclei. The entire cell is filled with secretory vesicles with pale electron-lucent fibrillar content, which compress the mitochondria and endoplasmic reticulum into a small intervening volume of electron-dense cytoplasm. The Golgi apparatus is well developed and is found near the nucleus. The apical surface of the secretory cells is covered with short microvilli. The exposed surface is increased by the presence of intercellular canaliculi.[43]

The myoepithelial cells have the cytoplasmic features of smooth muscle, notably their cytoplasm is filled with contractile microfilaments including focal, dense attachment bodies. However, like epithelium, they are enclosed within the basal lamina of the glands and are joined to the secretory cells by desmosomal junctions. Their appearance and location suggest that their function is to contract, milking the secretions toward the lumen. Cholinergic nerve endings have been identified among the various types of epithelial cells of the glands.[43]

Initially both myoepithelial and mucus-secreting cells continue to line the secretory tubules as they coalesce to form the collecting duct. At variable distances along the duct, the lining epithelium changes to cuboidal or columnar cells which are rather nondescript in the light-microscope and are characterized ultrastructurally by the possession of a microvillous apical border, a large

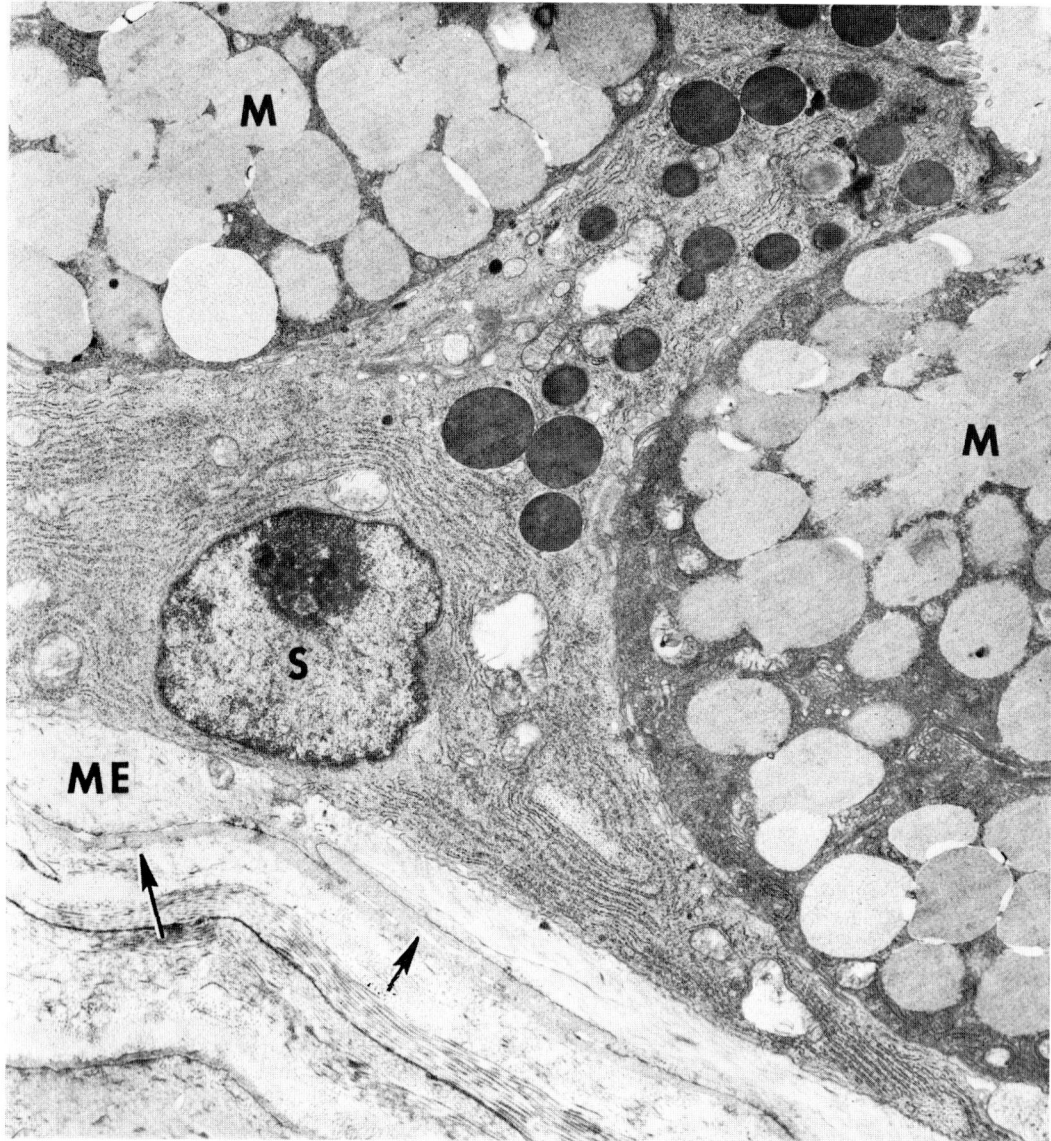

Figure 2–11. Mucous gland. The serous cell (S) has extensive endoplasmic reticulum in its basal portion and discrete apical granules. The cytoplasm of the mucous cell (M) is more dense, but the secretions are more lucent. A projection of the cytoplasm of a myoepithelial cell (ME) lies inside the basal lamina (arrows) (×6700).

perinuclear Golgi apparatus, but no apparent secretory granules (Fig. 2–13). Near the termination of the duct at the bronchial lumen, the epithelium again changes, becoming ciliated. Meyrick and Reid[43] have described columnar cells with numerous mitochondria in the ducts of the glands in several lungs resected for carcinoma; they suggest that these cells may play a role in regulating the ionic composition of the mucus, but oncocytes occur in mucous glands, apparently as an acquired abnormality,[44] and may account for the mitochondria-rich duct cells.

Plasma cells are often found in considerable numbers in the interstitial tissue around and between secretory tubules. There are nearly equal numbers of IgA- and IgG-containing plasma cells, but only few cells containing IgM.[42,45] The immunoglobulin in mucus is principally 11S secretory IgA, consisting of two IgA molecules joined by J-protein and complexed to "secretory piece." The IgA and J-piece have been identified in plasma cells, but the secretory piece, absent from plasma cells, has been localized to the endoplasmic reticulum and lateral plasma membranes of serous and mucous secretory cells.[42,46] This localization supports the hypothesis that the IgA is produced by plasma cells but complexed to secretory piece at the membrane of the epithelial cells of the secretory tubules and transported across the epithelium to the tubular lumen.

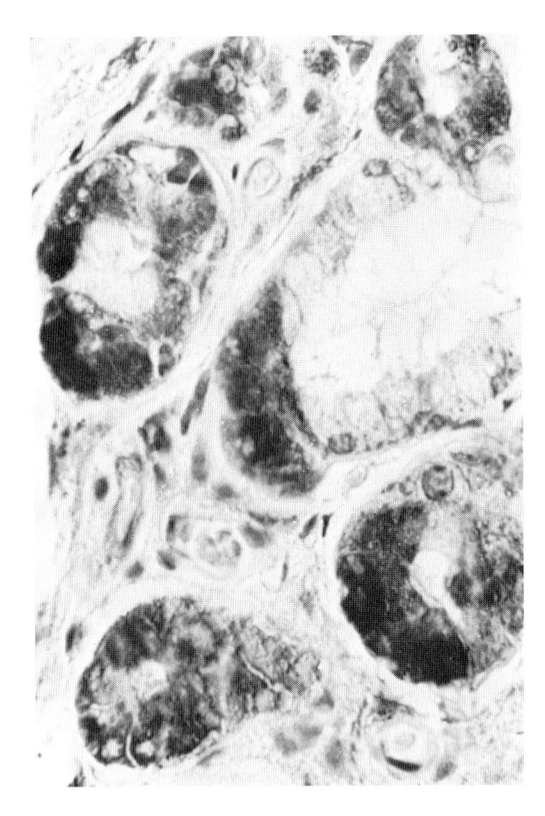

Figure 2–12. Mucous gland stained by the immunoperoxidase method using an antiserum to lysozyme. The serous demilunes show the dark reaction product (×400).

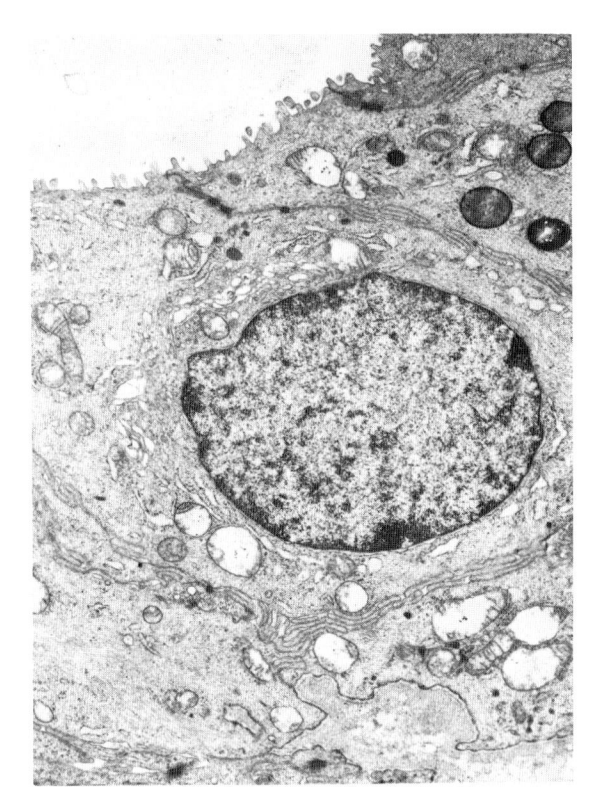

Figure 2–13. Epithelial cell lining the collecting duct of a mucous gland. The luminal surface has a few microvilli. The cell has a relatively large supranuclear Golgi apparatus but no secretory granules. The granules in the cell at the top right have the appearance of lysosomes (×8000).

Neuroendocrine Cells

With the use of special argyrophilic stains or electron microscopy, it is possible to demonstrate a class of cells containing large numbers of cytoplasmic granules 0.1 to 0.2 μm in diameter.[47] These cells have been variously named Feyrter cells, Kultschitzsky (K) cells, amine precursor uptake and decarboxylation (APUD) cells, and "small-granule" cells. These cells are more numerous in fetal than adult tissues and are most plentiful in small airways (bronchioles), although they also can be found in large airways and in ducts of mucous glands.[48–52] They occur in two anatomic forms (Fig. 2–14). Solitary endocrine cells are found near the basal lamina between columnar cells. These endocrine cells are flask shaped and send out an apical extension between the columnar cells to the bronchial lumen, where they have a small exposed surface. Organized or corpuscular collections of endocrine-type cells occur near bronchial branch points. The organized clusters, called neuroepithelial bodies by Lauweryns, are innervated by both afferent and efferent nerves and are associated with capillaries of the fenestrated type in the underlying lamina propria.[53–55]

The histochemical properties of the solitary endocrine cells and the cells of neuroepithelial bodies are similar but not identical. Cells of both types are argyrophilic and show formaldehyde-induced fluorescence with a fluorescent spectrum characteristic of 5-hydroxytryptamine. If lung slices are incubated in vitro with L-3,4-dihydroxyphenylalanine (DOPA) or 5-hydroxytryptophane, the number of fluorescent cells and their intensity increase, indicating the capacity to take up and decarboxylate amine precursers,[56] the defining characteristic for cells of the so-called APUD system.[57] By immunohistochemistry several peptide hormones have been localized to cells of this class,[58,59] and it is by no means certain that the list is complete. Table 2–2 summarizes the results of one such study.[59] In the fetus, bombesin-containing cells were present at all levels of the developing tracheobronchial tree, whereas in adults, they were confined to the peripheral airways. Leucine-enkephalin-containing cells were infrequent and were not present in neuroepithelial bodies. Although it was uncertain whether bombesin, calcitonin, and leu-enkephalin occur in the same or separate cells, it is notable that Hage[60] has distinguished three types of endocrine cells in human fetuses based on granule morphology.

The functions of neuroendocrine cells are unknown. Their prominence in fetal lung suggests that they may have a more important function in utero than during postnatal life. Lauweryns and colleagues[61,62] have proposed the hypothesis that neuroepithelial bodies are chemoreceptors sensitive to hypoxia. They found that

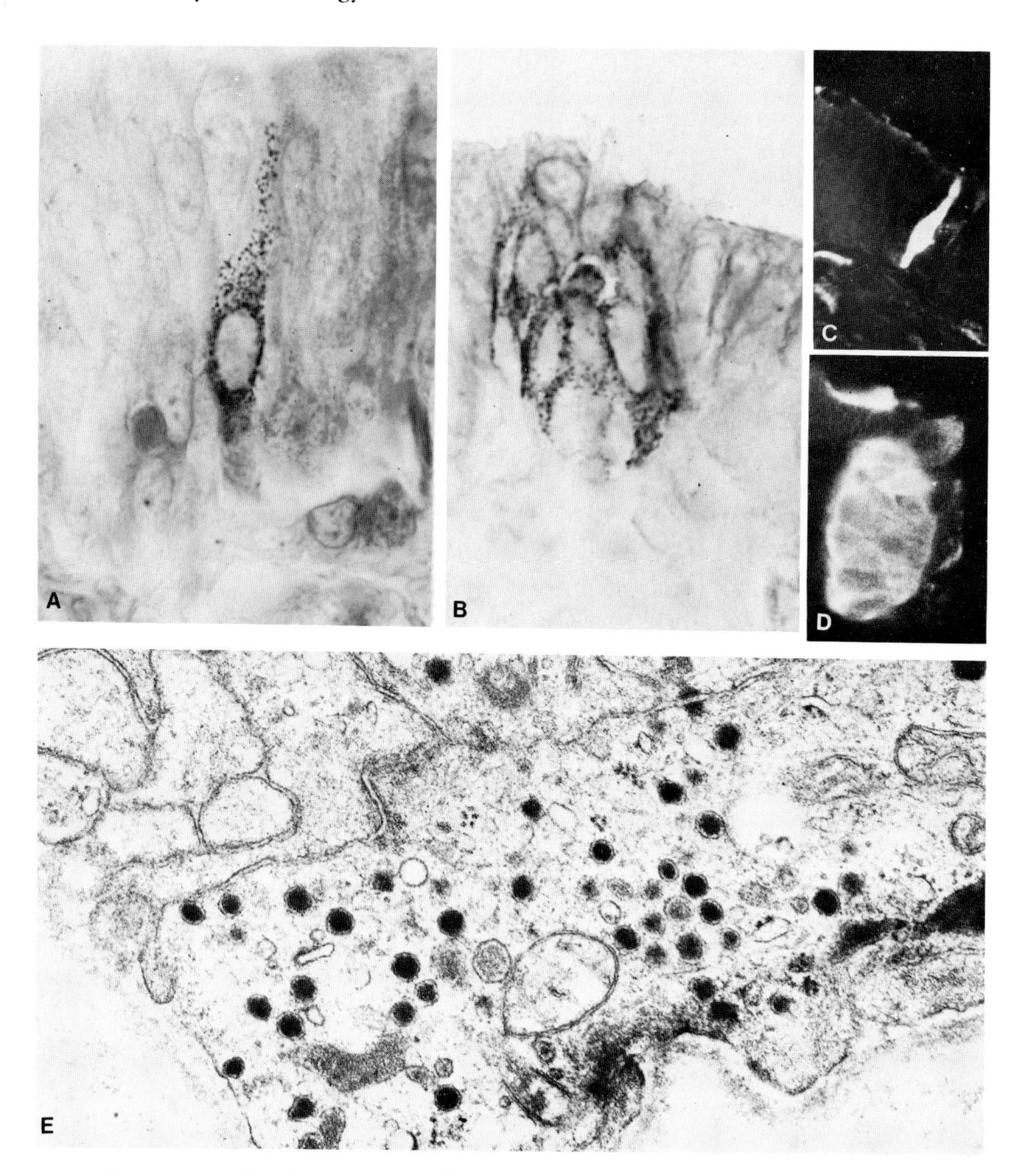

Figure 2–14. Bronchial endocrine cells. A. Solitary endocrine cell in a human bronchus (Grimelius argyrophilic stain, ×1100). B. Neuroepithelial body in a human bronchus (Grimelius stain, ×1100). C. Solitary endocrine cell in a rabbit bronchiole (formaldehyde-induced fluorescence, ×400). D. Neuroepithelial body in a rabbit lung (formaldehyde-induced fluorescence, ×400). E. Granules in an endocrine cell of a human neuroepithelial body (×32,000). A through D from Cutz: Exp Lung Res 3:185–208, 1982. Used with permission of Elsevier Science Publishing Co.

they degranulated when exposed to acute hypoxia, but not when perfused by hypoxemic blood.[63] Thus they are candidates for receptors mediating hypoxic vasoconstriction.[64] Consistent with this hypothesis, animals raised at high altitude have increased numbers of both single neuroendocrine cells and neuroepithelial bodies. Changes in granule morphology are similar to the changes in the granule-containing cells of carotid body under comparable conditions of hypoxia.[65]

Bronchioles

The walls of the airways less than 1 mm in diameter lack cartilage and consist of smooth muscle enclosed in a thin

Table 2–2. Immunohistochemistry of Bronchial Endocrine Cells[a]

	Solitary Cells	Neuroendocrine Bodies
Bombesin	+++	+++
Calcitonin	++	+
Leu-enkephalin	+	—

[a] Based on the results of Cutz et al.[59] The plus signs indicate the relative abundance of cells staining for the antigen in question, with +++ the most numerous and − the least. No neuroendocrine bodies stained for leu-enkephalin.

connective tissue space. The appearance of the bronchioles varies considerably, depending on the degree of expansion of the lung. In unexpanded lung, the mucosa is thrown into longitudinal ridges that appear papillary in cross-section, whereas in the fully expanded lung, the mucosa is thin with a smooth circular outline. The mucosa is of a simple columnar type. Basal cells are absent, and without the use of special stains for endocrine cells, only two types of cells can be identified—ciliated cells and nonciliated secretory cells, the so-called Clara cells.[66] Mucous cells are not normally found, but may be present in a variety of diseases and are common in lung exposed to chronic respiratory irritants such as tobacco smoke.[67]

The nonciliated cells of membranous bronchioles are columnar cells with a basal nucleus, a well-developed rough endoplasmic reticulum, Golgi apparatus, numerous mitochondria, and secretory granules in the apical cytoplasm (Fig. 2–15). The apical cytoplasm often projects as a dome above the level of the apices of the more numerous ciliated cells and hence can be readily identified in the scanning electron microscope (Figure 2–16). The secretory granules of human nonciliated bronchiolar cells are 0.3 to 0.8 μm in diameter, membrane-limited, and nonuniform in electron density with electron-dense condensations against a more lucent background matrix. The granules are not stained with the usual light or electron microscopic stains for mucin and consist predominantly of basic protein.[68,69] In respiratory bronchioles, the proportion of ciliated cells decreases, and in distal respiratory bronchioles, ciliated cells often disappear completely. The nonciliated cells become cuboidal, and their granules have a homogenous electron-dense matrix[70] (Fig. 2–17).

One function of the nonciliated bronchiolar cells is the secretion of bronchiolar lining fluid. The bronchioles are lined by a fluid which consists of a hypophase covered by a surface film of surfactant[69,71–73] which presumably is produced in the alveoli and is transported to the bronchioles. Little is known of the other components of the bronchiolar lining material, but histochemical and autoradiographic data favor the hypothesis that it is a proteinaceous fluid.[68,69,74] Singh and coworkers[75] have developed antisera to Clara cell secretions and have shown that they react with at least two antigenically distinct proteins. Since there is considerable physiologic evidence that bronchioles close at low lung volume, it is not surprising that their lining should be a proteinaceous fluid and not mucus, which being sticky would impede their reopening.

Nonciliated bronchiolar cells also serve as stem cells in the repair of bronchiolar injury and can proliferate and differentiate into ciliated cells following necrosis of bronchiolar epithelium.[76] Nonciliated bronchiolar cells in rodents are a rich source of mixed function oxidases and are important in the metabolism of a variety of simple organic chemicals, some of which are transformed to toxic intermediates which selectively damage the nonciliated cells.[77–81] Rodent nonciliated bronchiolar cells possess an extensive smooth endoplasmic reticulum, the presumed site of mixed function oxidases, whereas human nonciliated bronchiolar have mainly rough endoplasmic reticulum.[9] Because of this difference, it may not be valid to extrapolate the rodent experiments to humans.

The Acini

General Organization

Acini are units of lung supplied by a single terminal bronchiole. All the air passages comprising an acinus partake to some extent in gas exchange—all have alveoli. The components are respiratory bronchioles, alveolar ducts, and alveolar sacs (Figs. 2–18, 2–19). Respiratory bronchioles are air passages composed in part of muscular bronchiolar wall covered with cuboidal epithelium and in part by alveoli. Alveolar ducts are conducting structures lined entirely by alveoli and lead to a final generation of alveolus-lined spaces that end blindly, the alveolar sacs. Three-dimensional reconstruction of acinar structure is exceedingly time-consuming, and only a few acini have been analyzed completely. Boyden[82] spent 3 years reconstructing a single acinus from the lung of a 6-year-old child by serial sectioning. Others[83–85] have carefully analyzed and dissected casts (Fig. 2–20), although in casts of air space lumens, it is often impossible to distinguish respiratory bronchioles from alveolar ducts.

Acini vary considerably in their detailed structure, depending on the space to be filled. Some abut the pleura or perilobular septa, some occupy the niches between bifurcations of bronchi or vessels, and some are entirely enclosed by lung parenchyma. The number of generations of respiratory air passages from terminal bronchiole to alveolar sac is variable even within a given acinus, ranging from four to ten. The first-generation respiratory bronchiole is usually mainly bronchiolar in structure, with an average of only three alveoli; subsequent generations of respiratory bronchioles consist mainly of alveoli with cuboidal bronchiolar type of lining limited to one side where the accompanying artery runs. Usually after two or three generations of respiratory bronchioles, the passages become fully alveolated alveolar ducts. There are from two to six generations of alveolar ducts, the final generation in a given pathway giving rise to as many as six alveolar sacs. Individual respiratory bronchioles or alveolar ducts vary in length,

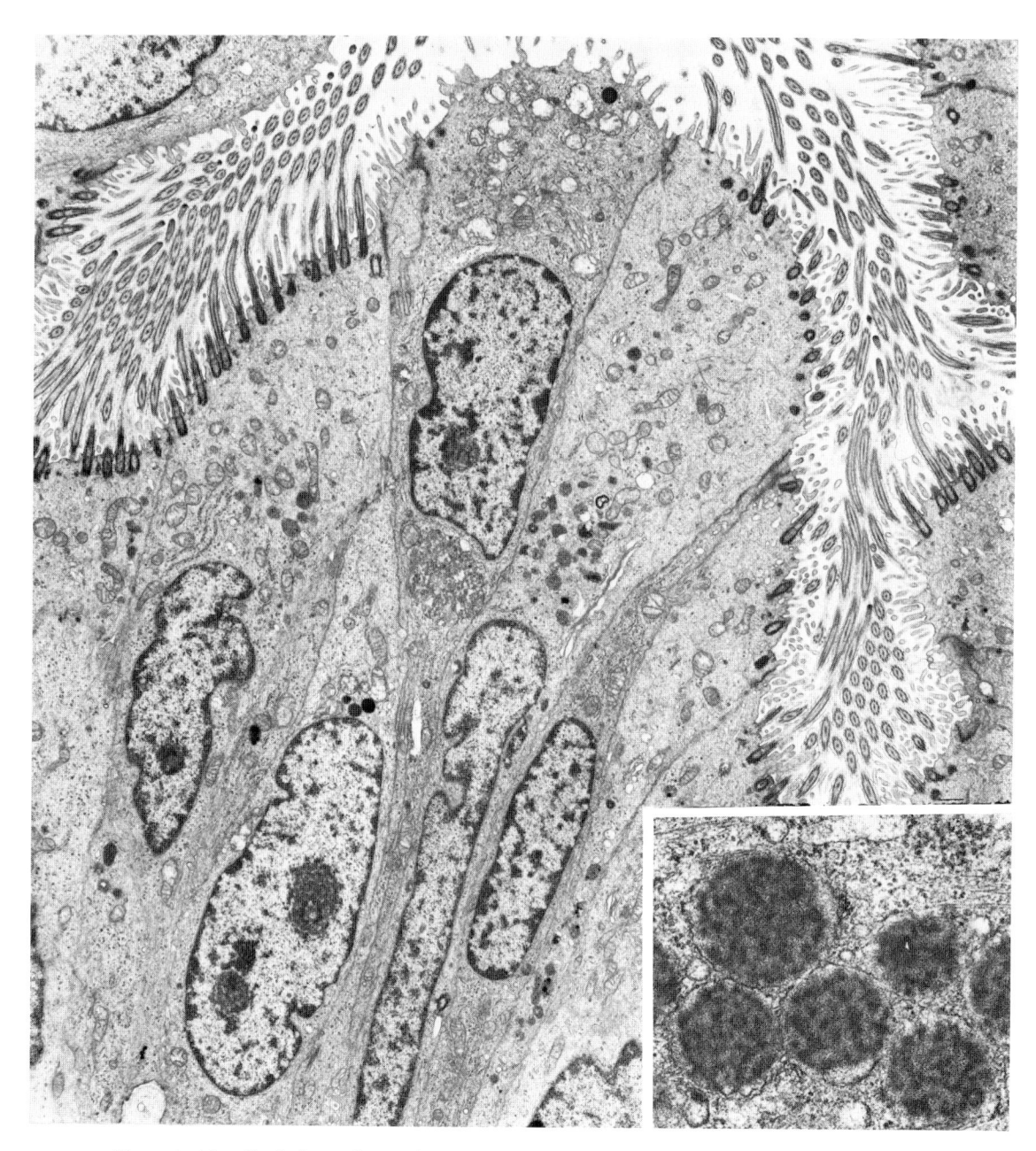

Figure 2–15. Epithelium of a membranous bronchiole. A Clara cell with a few secretory granules just beneath the apical membrane is sandwiched among several ciliated cells (×5000). Inset, The granules of a Clara cell have a flocculent texture (×31,000).

number of alveoli, and angle and pattern of branching. Although dichotomous branching predominates, trichotomy and greater degrees of branching are often encountered.

The Blood Supply to the Acinus

The pulmonary arteries accompany the bronchi and bronchioles, usually sharing a common connective tissue sheath. The muscular arteries are only slightly smaller than the bronchioles they accompany. Within the acinus, the diameter of the arteries decreases more rapidly than the air passages, so that in the periphery of the lung, the diameters of the arterial branches are much smaller than those of the respiratory bronchioles or alveolar ducts they accompany. Some muscular pulmonary arteries do not branch with the bronchial tree but arise as sidebranches; these vessels have been termed supernumerary.

The muscular arteries give rise to precapillary vessels, which in turn feed the rich capillary network that forms

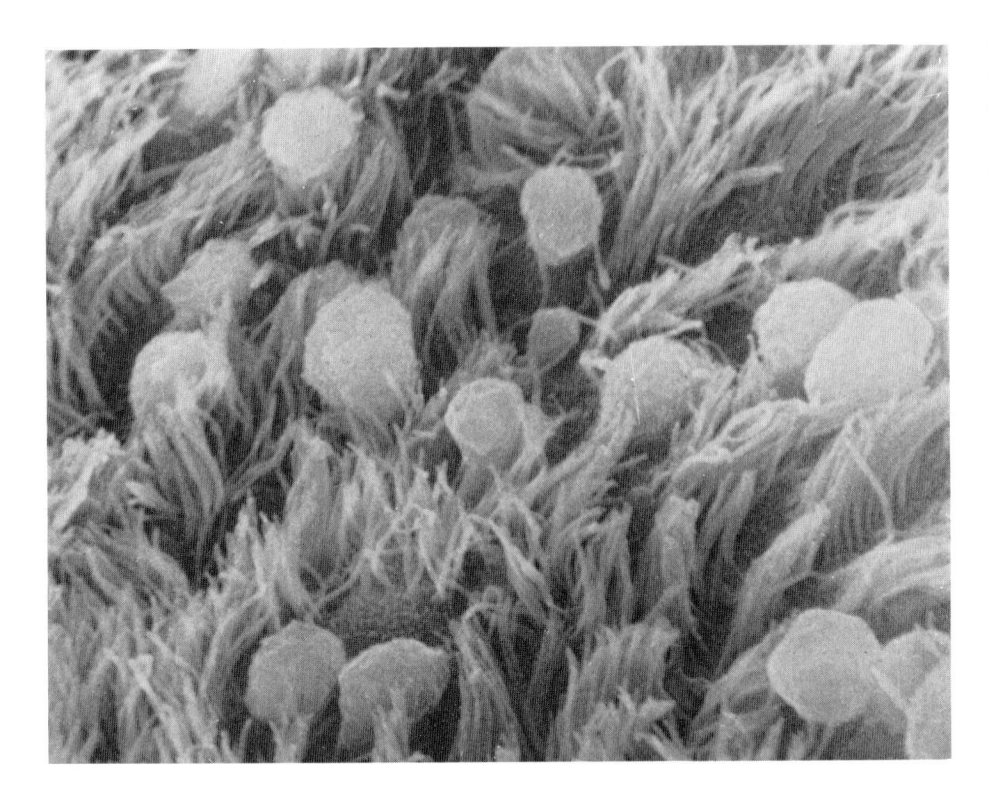

Figure 2–16. Mucosal lining of a bronchiole from a child's lung. The Clara cells protrude above the level of the cilia (scanning electron micrograph, ×4000).

the major part of the alveolar walls. The capillaries are collected into venules which drain into veins at the periphery of the acini, receiving blood from two or three contiguous acini. Where the interlobular septa are well formed, the veins lie within the septa (see Figure 2–19). Thus the blood enters the acini along the bronchioles, is distributed through the alveolar walls, and is collected into veins at the periphery and remote from the bronchioles.[4]

Alveolar Ducts

The organization of the alveolar ducts has been the subject of several studies[86–88] since it is critical to the process of ventilation. The alveoli, which evaginate from the alveolar ducts, vary in size and shape but are on the average hexagonal in outline and 150 to 200 μm in diameter in the fully distended lung. In ordinary histologic sections, the free tips of the interalveolar septa are enlarged and contain smooth muscle and connective tissue fibers. These enlargements are the wall of the alveolar duct proper. Studies using thick or serial sections show that the smooth muscle and accompanying bundles of collagen and elastic fibers spiral down the alveolar duct like a spring. Alveoli are arranged in tiers between the thick spiral fiber bundle, with thinner rings of collagen and elastic fibers at their mouths (Fig. 2–21). The elongation and enlargement of the alveolar ducts during inspiration take place in part by axial elongation of the connective tissue fiber bundles but also in part by uncoiling of the spring.[86,87]

Alveoli evaginating from adjacent alveolar ducts or sacs are packed in an interdigitating manner similar to the packing of soap bubbles so that the junctions of alveoli are always formed of three alveolar walls.[88]

The walls separating adjacent alveoli are composed of interwoven networks of connective tissue and capillaries covered by a thin layer of epithelium. The alveolar capillaries are arranged in a net or grid-like pattern (Fig. 2–22), the mesh of which is tightest where the wall separates two air spaces and somewhat more open where an air space abuts the pleura, interlobular septum, or bronchovascular sheath.[4] An analysis of the organization of the capillary net by Sobin and associates[89] indicates that the blood flow through the lung is approximated by a laminar flow model in which the blood is spread into a thin film percolating between "posts" (the spaces between capillaries) rather than the more usual model of flow through tubes.

The interstitial connective tissue of the air space walls contains types I, III, and V collagen and elastic fibers.[90,91] Generally, the collagen and elastic fibers run together in bundles which are interwoven through the capillary net (Fig. 2–23) so that in most planes of section, the connective tissue and capillary appear side by side. Thus in cross-section, the capillary has a thin blood-air barrier on one side, where there is no connective tissue bundle, and a thick blood-air barrier on the opposite side, where the connective tissue bundle is found (Fig. 2–24). This organization provides support for the alveolar wall while minimizing the barrier to diffusion.[92,93]

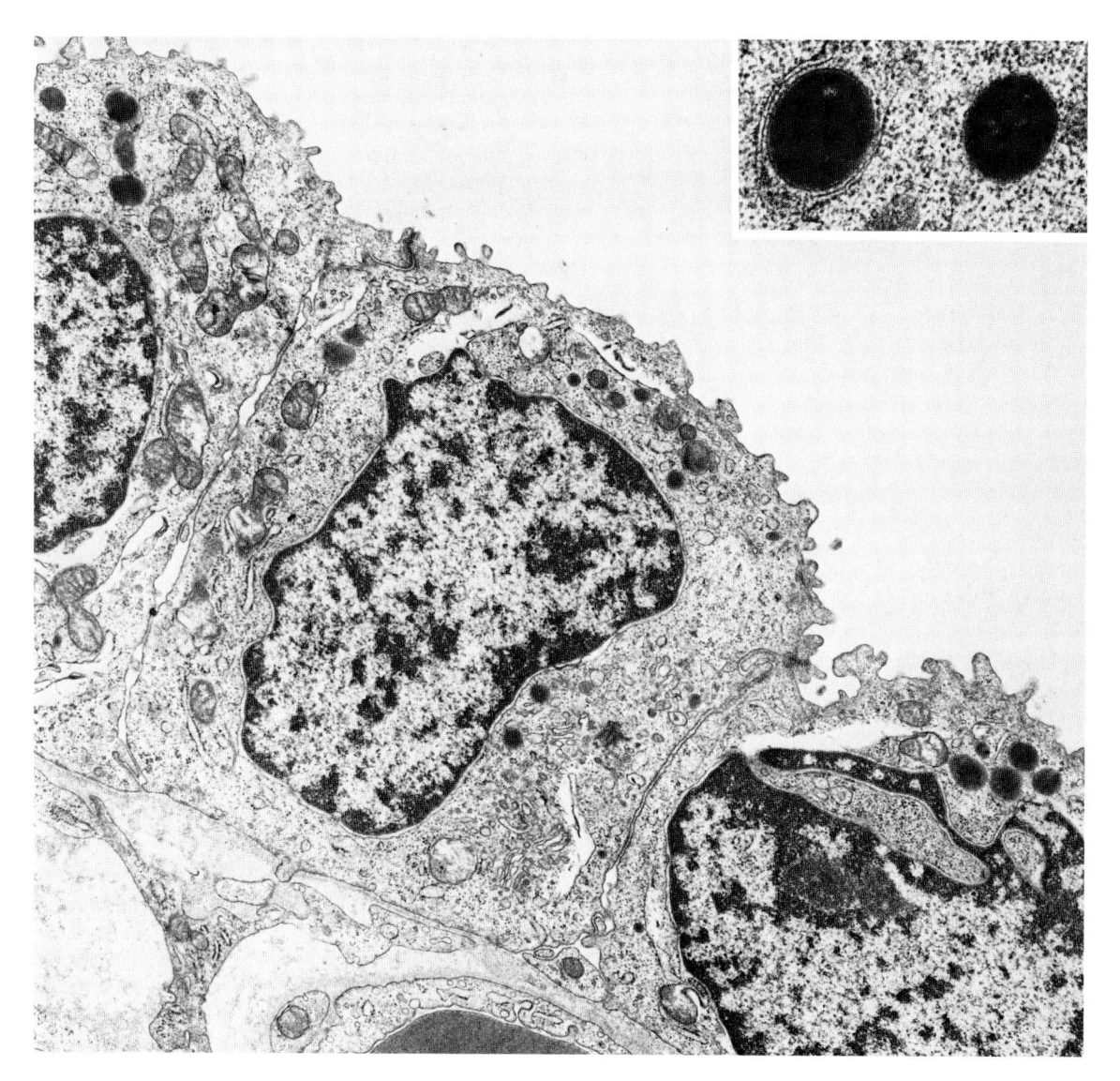

Figure 2–17. Epithelium of a respiratory bronchiole. The epithelial cells are cuboidal and the secretory granules are solid, differing in texture from those in the more proximal bronchiole in Figure 2–15 (×9000). Inset, granules at greater magnification (×28,000).

Alveolar Walls

The principal cells composing the walls of the interalveolar septa are the alveolar epithelium, endothelium, and interstitial cells.[94] There are nearly equal numbers of endothelial cells and interstitial cells, and both types are more plentiful than epithelial cells (Fig. 2–25). The epithelial cells, which cover the alveolar septa, are of two types. One, commonly called the type I epithelial cell or membranous pneumonocyte,[95] is a simple squamous epithelial cell which is thickened in the region of the nucleus with an extensive thin sheet of cytoplasm approximately 0.1 to 0.2 μm thick which extends out to cover most of the air space walls. These cytoplasmic extensions of the type I cells are too thin to be consistently resolved by light microscopy, which accounts for the long-standing controversy whether the alveolar capillaries are naked or covered by epithelium, which was finally resolved when electron microscopy was applied to the lung.[96] The type I cell cytoplasm contains some mitochondria and endoplasmic reticulum, mainly but not exclusively confined to the perinuclear region. Organelles are sparse in the thin cytoplasmic extensions except for variable numbers of pinocytic vesicles.

The second type of epithelial cell, the type II cell or granular pneumonocyte, is a cuboidal cell with microvilli on its apical surface. In many mammals, the type II cells are recessed in niches in the alveolar septa, but human type II cells often protrude into the alveolar space. In the light-microscope, they can be recognized by their content of cytoplasmic vacuoles 1 to 2 μm in diameter. In the electron microscope, type II cells have a fairly large Golgi

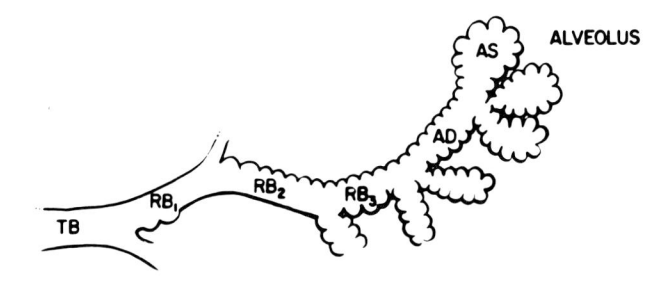

Figure 2–18. Schematic diagram of the components of an acinus. AD—alveolar duct, AS—alveolar sac, RB—respiratory bronchiole, TB—, terminal bronchiole. From Thurlbeck.[234]

apparatus, conspicuous mitochondria, and characteristic secretory granules known as lamellar bodies, which are composed of closely packed whorled lamellae of osmiophilic membrane-like material, the alveolar surfactant (Fig. 2–26). These inclusions are extracted by lipid solvents, leaving the empty vacuoles which characterize type II cells in paraffin sections. Type II epithelial cells are more numerous than type I cells, but only cover a tiny fraction of the alveolar surface (2.5 percent in the rat), the great majority being covered by the attenuated cytoplasmic cytoplasm of type I cells.[97] Often the cytoplasm of the type I cell even extends as a flap covering part of the type II cell, leaving only a portion exposed to the alveolus (Fig. 2–26). The intercellular junctions between type I and II epithelial cells are low-permeability tight junctions with three to five junctional strands in electron micrographs of freeze-fracture replicas.

Type II cells have two established functions: secretion of surfactant[98–100] and repair in alveolar injury.[101,102] The air spaces of the lung are lined by a layer of fluid which was first detected by Terry[103] using the technique of micropuncture. Having a fluid lining, the alveoli are subject to the forces that act at the air-fluid interface. These forces produce a fine modeling of the alveolar walls in the air-filled lung and also are responsible for a major part of the elastic recoil of the lung.[104]

The alveoli of the air-filled lung are not polygonal, but have smoothly curved surfaces. With the resolution of the electron microscope, the smoothing of the alveolar contour can be seen to be produced in part by pleating of the alveolar capillary membrane with folds projecting into the capillaries (Fig. 2–27) and in part by the filling of

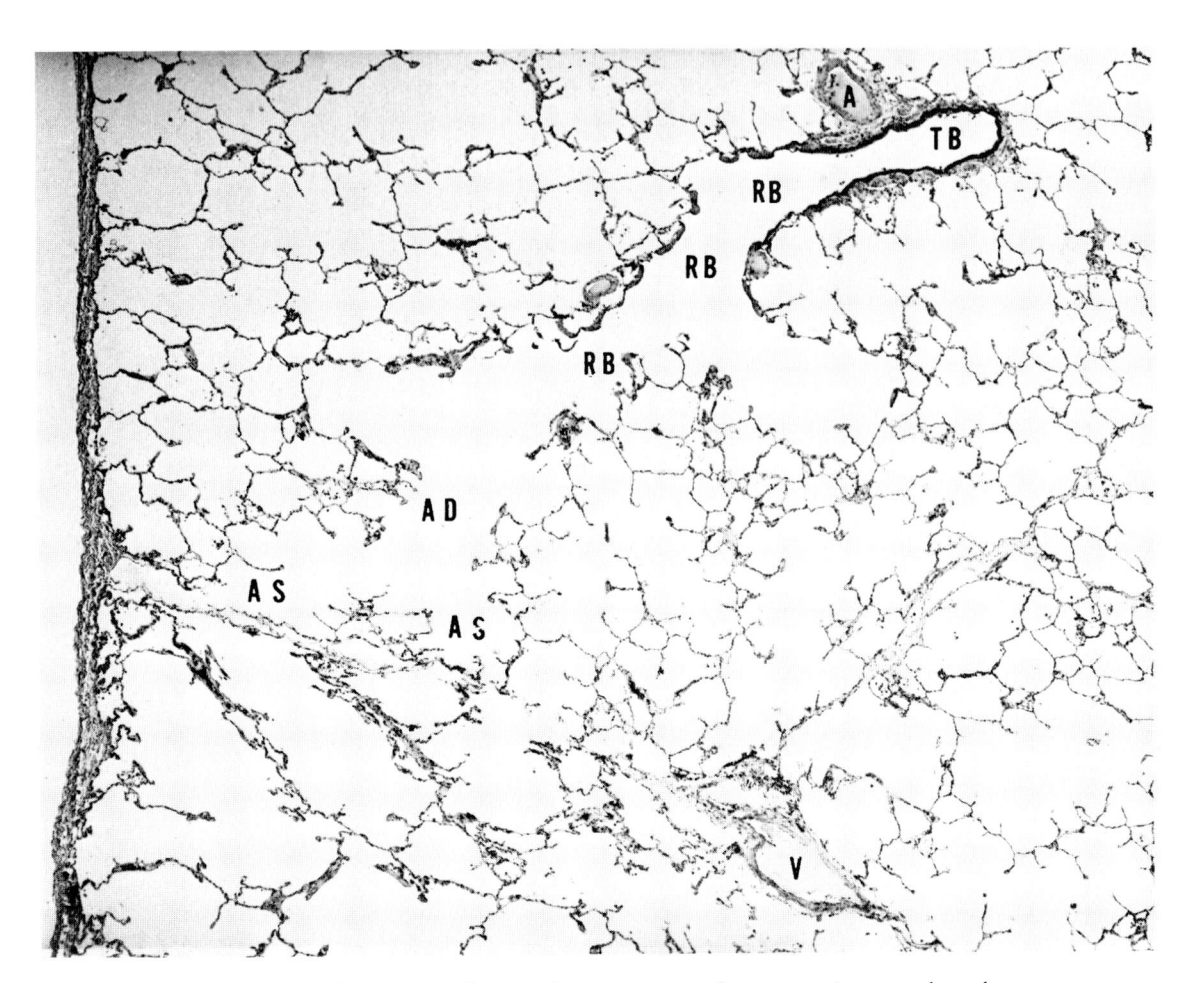

Figure 2–19. Histologic section showing the components of an acinus. A—muscular pulmonary artery, V—vein. The remaining abbreviation are listed in Figure 2–18.

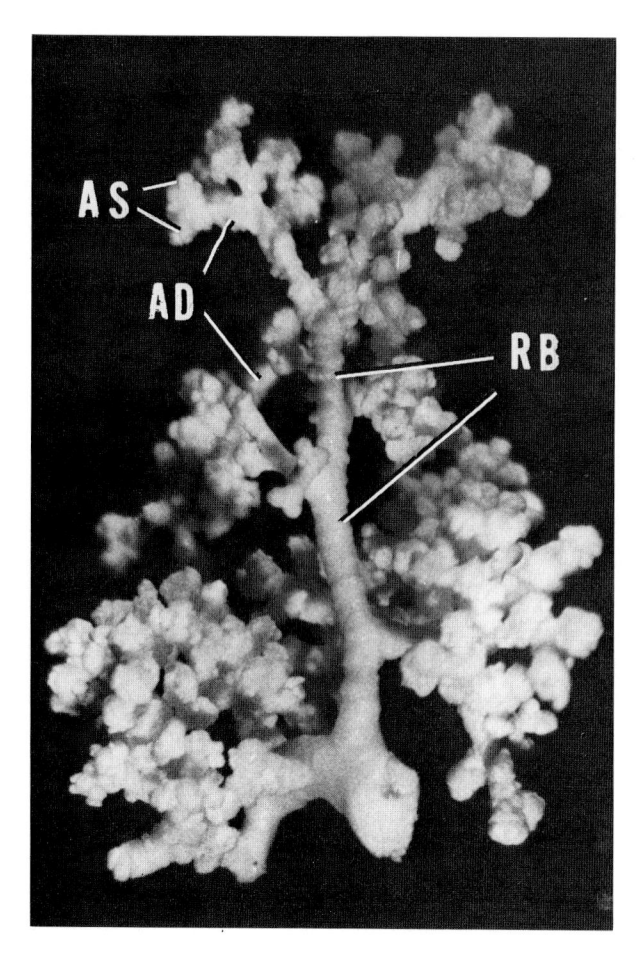

Figure 2–20. Partially filled cast of an acinus to demonstrate the variability and complexity of branching. Abbreviations are listed in Figure 2–18.

irregular depressions in the alveolar wall by the fluid of the lining layer.[105] The changes in alveolar volume that occur with ventilation are accompanied by an unfolding of the pleats in the alveolar wall which project more deeply into the capillaries at low lung volume and become shallow as the lung is expanded.[106] One suggested function of the so-called alveolar surfactant is to facilitate the pulling apart of the folds.[107]

The other function is the stabilization of lung volume. This function of surfactant can be understood if one assumes the air spaces to be spherical. La Place's law relates the pressure in a gas bubble to its radius:

$$P = \frac{2\gamma}{R}$$

in which P is the pressure, γ the surface tension, and R the radius. If surface tension in the lung lining fluid were constant, the pressure in spherical air spaces of smallest radius (alveoli) would be higher than that in larger air spaces (alveolar ducts), and the alveoli would tend to collapse and alveolar ducts dilate. The alveolar surfactant has the property of lowering surface tension γ as the area decreases. Hence, as alveoli decrease in volume and R falls, γ also falls, which tends to prevent alveolar collapse. In reality, of course, air spaces are not spherical and the actual mathematical relationships are more complicated.[93,108]

The alveolar surfactant consists of approximately 15 percent protein; the remainder is lipid. The principal lipid is phosphatidylcholine which is remarkable for its high degree of saturation, but surfactant also contains 10 percent phosphatidylglycerol, a relatively rare phospholipid in mammalian cells.[109,110]

The surfactant is synthesized in type II cells and stored in lamellar bodies.[99,111–113] The lamellar bodies are discharged into the alveolar space by exocytosis (Fig. 2–28) in response to a number of stimuli, including ventilation, prostaglandin E, and adrenergic agonists.[114]

The reparative function of type II cells is manifest in a variety of forms of lung injury. The type I cells, with 50 times as much exposed surface as type II cells, are easily damaged and their thin cytoplasmic extensions disintegrate. Type I cells appear unable to divide, but Evans and associates[102] have shown that type II cells proliferate and can differentiate into type I cells.

Both the alveolar epithelium and the capillary endothelium rest on basal lamina which they probably secrete. The capillary and alveolar basal laminae remain distinct and separate on the thick side of the blood-air barrier, but appear to fuse on the thin side, so that the blood-air barrier on the thin side of the septum consists only of alveolar lining fluid, epithelium, shared basal lamina, and endothelium, a total thickness of approximately 0.4 μm (see Fig. 2–24). Biochemically the alveolar and capillary basal laminae differ somewhat. Both probably contain type IV collagens, laminin, and fibronectin, but the proteoglycan of the alveolar basal lamina is heparan sulfate, whereas the capillary basal lamina has sparser proteoglycan particles containing chondroitin sulfate.[115] The fused basal lamina of the thin blood-air barrier retains a demonstrable contribution from each structure.[116]

The space between the alveolar and capillary basal laminae is the interstitial compartment of the septum. The principal cell of the interstitium is a mesenchymal cell which resembles a fibroblast, particularly a cultured fibroblast with stress fibers (bundles of contractile filaments that insert at points of attachment to its substrate). The interstitial cells are highly irregular in outline, with long slender projections of cytoplasm which extend into the interstitial space. They are commonly closely associated with collagen and elastin fibers of which they are almost certainly the source. As Kapanci and associates[117] noted in the rat, they have distinct bundles of contractile filaments which suggest that they have a contractile function. The cytoplasmic processes of different interstitial cells make contact via gap or nexus-type junctions[118] which function in the electrophysiologic coupling of cells, so that if indeed the interstitial cells are contractile, several cells may contract as a functional syncytium. Kapanci and colleagues have suggested that these cells may help in the matching of ventilation to perfusion, but

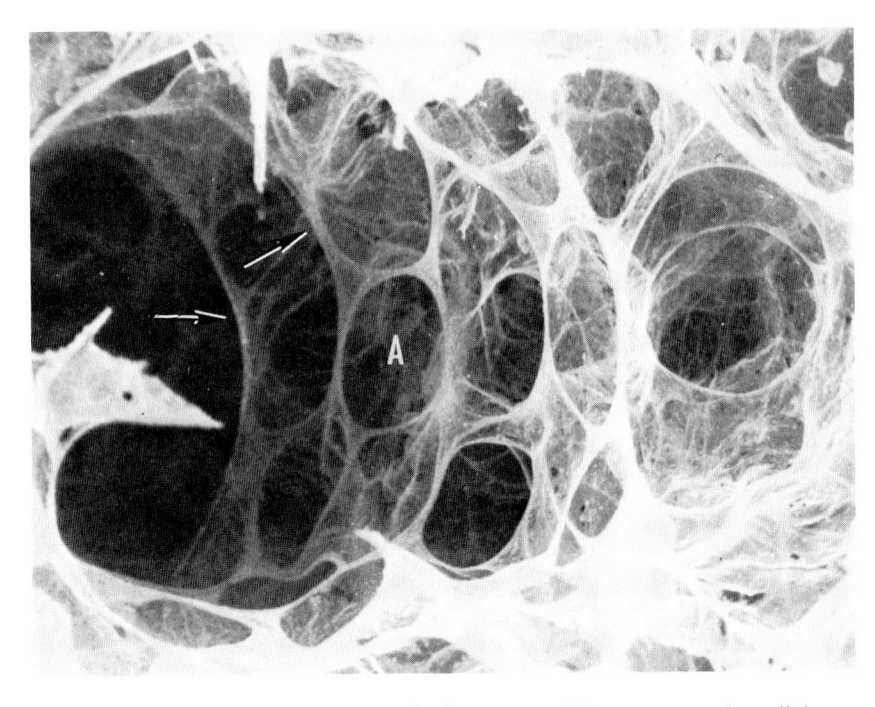

Figure 2–21. Connective tissue skeleton of a lung prepared by extracting the cellular protein with NaOH. The lung was then dried fully inflated and prepared for scanning electron-microscopy. Heavy ridges of connective tissue wind down the alveolar duct (arrows). Rings of connective tissue outline the mouths of alveoli (A). Fine fiber bundles can be seen crossing alveolar walls (×120).

further work is needed to establish the validity of this intriguing suggestion.

The capillary endothelial cells are nonfenestrated and form a continuous lining of the alveolar capillaries. The individual cells are joined by tight junctions which physiologic studies have shown to be more permeable to macromolecules than are the junctions between epithelial cells. In freeze-fracture replicas, endothelial junctions have from one to three junctional strands and occasional discontinuities in the strands, which contrast with the three to five strands in the junctions between epithelial cells.[119] The morphology and metabolic functions of endothelial cells are discussed in greater detail in the section on the pulmonary circulation (see p. 36) as well as in review by Ryan.[120]

Pericytes are uncommon in the normal pulmonary capillaries. They lie within the capillary basal lamina and send long slender processes along the capillary. Their cytoplasm contains relatively few organelles but has bundles of contractile microfilaments. They increase in number in fibrotic lungs.

Interalveolar Pores (of Kohn)

In all mammalian species so far examined, there are openings called pores of Kohn penetrating the interalveolar septa, the number varying considerably among species.[121] Pores are generally absent at birth, but they appear early in life and are established in human lungs by 1 year of age. They are round to oval, varying in diameter with the degree of lung inflation. In humans at total lung volume, they range from 2.5 μm to an upper limit of normal taken somewhat arbitrarily at 12 to 15 μm. Takaro and associates[122] found 5.3 μm to be the average diameter. Since electron-microscopy has invariably shown them to be lined by alveolar epithelium, they are probably not an artifact.[122–124]

The presence of openings between alveoli offers an obvious pathway for collateral ventilation. The actual importance of the pores of Kohn for collateral ventilation remains uncertain. As discussed by Macklem,[121] the diameter of the pores in vivo at tidal lung volumes will depend on surface forces influenced by their detailed geometry and relationship to the alveolar lining fluid. Takaro[122] demonstrated that only a minority of pores are patent. The majority of pores are filled with alveolar lining fluid, and surface tension acts across the diameter to constrict them. The minority that are open are larger, suggesting that surface tension acting on the margins of open pores tends to stretch them.

It has been controversial for over one hundred years whether the pores of Kohn are to be regarded as anatomic structures or a pathologic condition. In adult animals, they do not appear to increase with age,[125] but Pump[126] reported that in humans they do increase in number with age. He considered them acquired lesions, the earliest form of emphysema. Certainly in a statistical sense, the presence of pores is normal. In this regard, it is notable that resistance to collateral ventilation in human adults does not demonstrably decrease with age.[127]

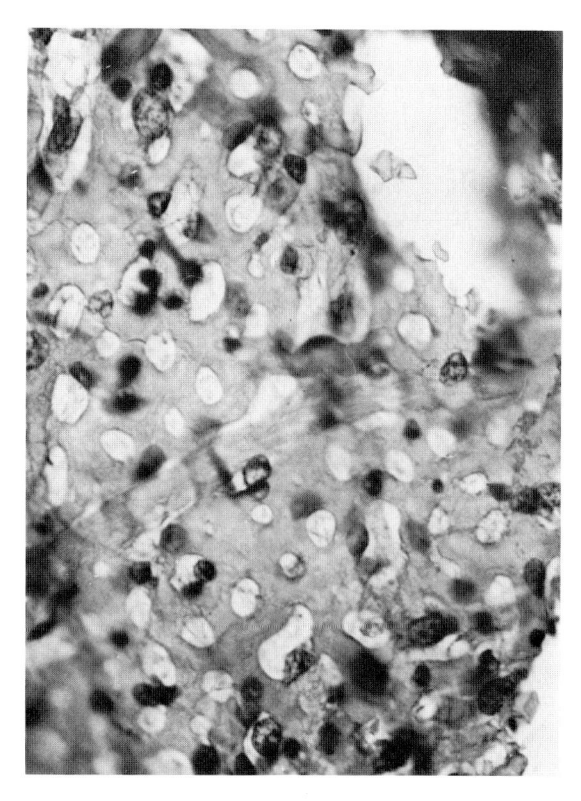

Figure 2–22. En face view of an alveolar wall in a 50 μm thick histologic section showing that the capillaries form a grid-like network rather than a series of tubes (×1500).

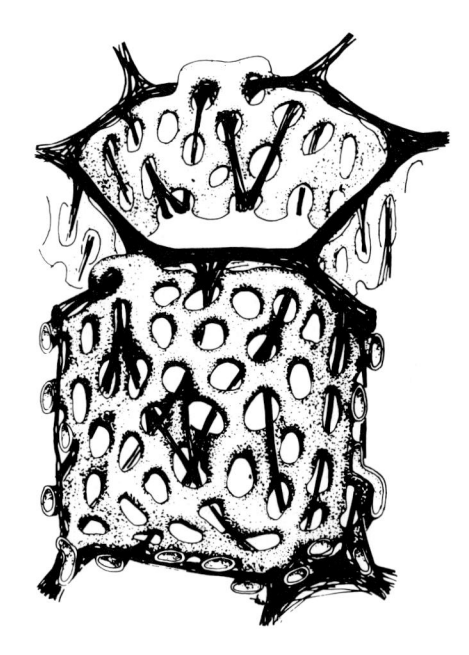

Figure 2–23. Diagram of the interweaving of the capillary network and bundles of connective tissue fibers in alveolar walls From Weibel and Gil in West (ed): *Bioengineering Aspects of the Lung*, 1977, pp. 1–81. Used with permission of Marcel Dekker Publishing Co.

Macrophages

Under normal conditions, less than 10 percent of the cells in the acinar zone of the lung are alveolar macrophages, mononuclear phagocytes that are found spread on the surface of the alveolar epithelial cells partially immersed in the alveolar lining fluid. In routine histologic preparations, the alveolar macrophages are floated off their moorings on the alveolar wall and appear free in the air spaces. Other macrophages are normally spread on the bronchial epithelium or located in various interstitial sites, including small numbers in the alveolar interstitium, in the mucosa of airways, and in the loose connective tissue around blood vessels. Still other pulmonary macrophages are found in the organized pulmonary lymphoid deposits.

The macrophages of the alveolar spaces and airways are easily obtained from humans or animals by bronchoalveolar lavage, and far more is known about them than about the interstitial macrophages.[128] The alveolar macrophages are relatively large cells, averaging 25 μm in diameter, with an eccentric oval or reniform nucleus. They have a prominent cytocenter containing a centriole and large Golgi apparatus surrounded by a zone of large lysosomal granules of varied size, shape, and content (Fig. 2–29). Intermediate filaments are often prominent in the central zone of the cytoplasm. The periphery of the cell is thrown into leaf-like folds and pseudopods, which usually contain few organelles except for a cortical gel of fine contractile filaments.

Metabolically, the alveolar macrophages differ from other mononuclear phagocytes. They are larger and have many features suggesting that they are more highly activated than other resident macrophages, including a more abundant cytoplasm containing high levels of lysosomal enzyme activity, high levels of secretion of certain neutral proteases, and high levels of oxygen consumption.[129,130] They are specifically adapted to function in the high oxygen tensions that exist in the alveoli by having higher levels of superoxide dismutase and of the enzymes involved in the electron transport chain and lower levels of glycolytic enzymes than peritoneal macrophages or monocytes.[131–133]

Macrophages are continuously removed from the alveoli and transported to the oropharynx by mucociliary clearance. Masse and colleagues[134] have estimated the rate of removal at 3.5 percent of the resident population daily. This rate of removal requires continuous replacement. In addition, in response to irritants, infectious agents, or even relatively inert dusts, the macrophage population can expand rapidly. Much controversy has been generated concerning the immediate source of alveolar macrophages. The three suggested sources are: (1) the bone marrow via the circulating monocytes; (2) the interstitial macrophage pool in the lung; and (3) proliferation of macrophages within the alveolar spaces. If total body irradiation is given to eliminate endogenous sources and syngeneic bone marrow transplanted, re-

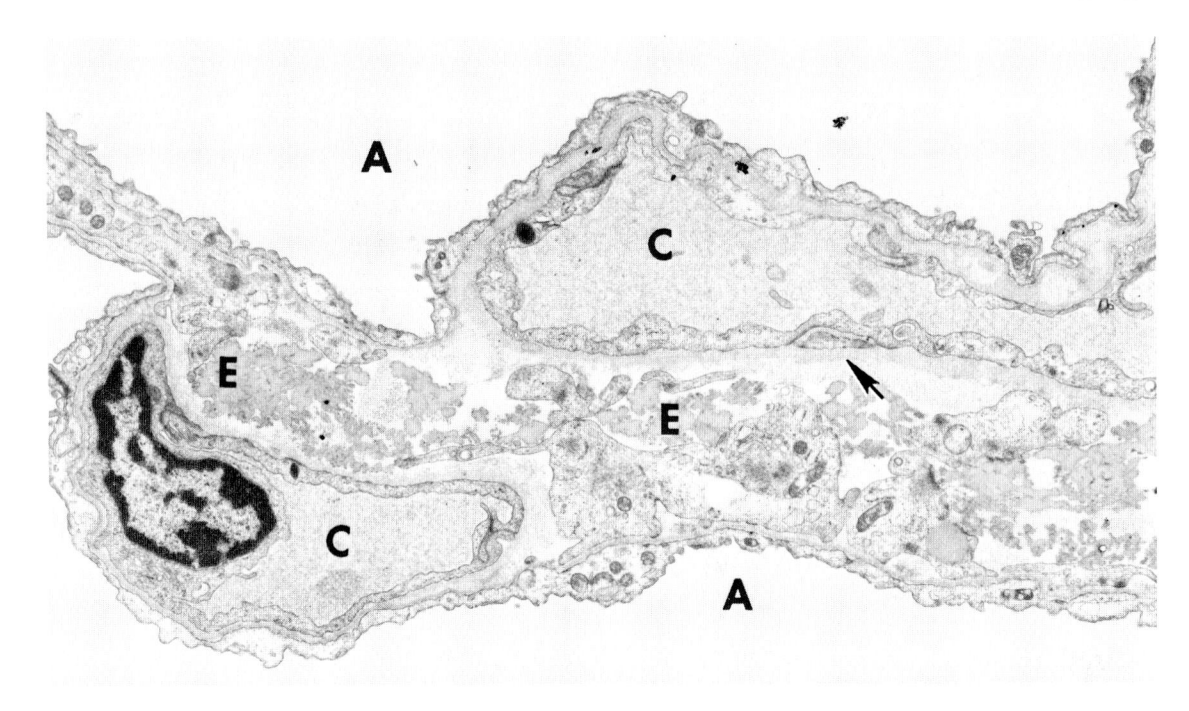

Figure 2–24. Cross-section through an alveolar septum. A connective tissue bundle containing elastic fibers (E) passes through a gap between two capillaries (C). The capillaries and connective tissue space appear side by side, so that on one side each capillary is separated from the alveolar space (A) only by a thin barrier consisting of epithelium, endothelium, and a shared basal lamina, whereas on the opposite side, the barrier is thick owing to the presence of the connective tissue between epithelial and endothelial basal laminae. The arrow indicates the cytoplasm of a pericyte associated with the capillary (×8000).

placement of alveolar macrophages comes from the donor marrow.[135–137] In patients with aplastic anemia or leukemia or in animals treated with corticosteroids, the blood monocytes can disappear from the circulation but only a minor if any reduction of alveolar macrophages occurs.[138,139] Under these conditions, local sources in the lung can maintain the population. Thymidine labeling indicates that, under some experimental conditions, interstitial macrophages are an important local source.[140,141] The alveolar macrophages have receptors for macrophage growth factor and can proliferate extensively in vitro.[142,143] Although few free alveolar macrophages are in cycle in the resting lung, in inflammatory states, intra-alveolar mitoses occur.[144] Thus, under specific experimental conditions, each of the three sites can provide replacement of macrophages. Thymidine labeling under normal steady state conditions indicates that the bone marrow is the more important source.[145,146] Two-thirds to three-fourths of the replacement macrophages come from the circulating monocytes, the lung receiving approximately 15 percent of the total output of monocytes by the marrow.[145] There is always a low level of labeling of macrophages in the lung as well, however.

The function of alveolar macrophages as professional phagocytes is well known. They are a major defense against inhaled bacteria and dust.[147] They have the capacity to process antigens and present them to T lymphocytes, which then proliferate and may participate in specific immune reactions.[148] The anatomic pathways involved in bringing together the macrophages and lymphocytes in vivo to produce such immune reactions are not well understood. Macrophages also produce a wide variety of secretory products, some of which are listed in Table 2–3. The products include enzymes, protease inhibitors, complement components, interfer-

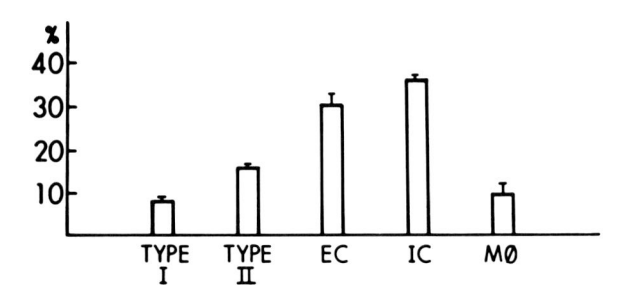

Figure 2–25. The relative numbers of different types of cells in the alveolar walls as a percentage of the total, from data by Crapo and associates[94] Type I and type II—alveolar epithelial cells, EC—endothelial cells, IC—interstitial cells, Mϕ—macrophages.

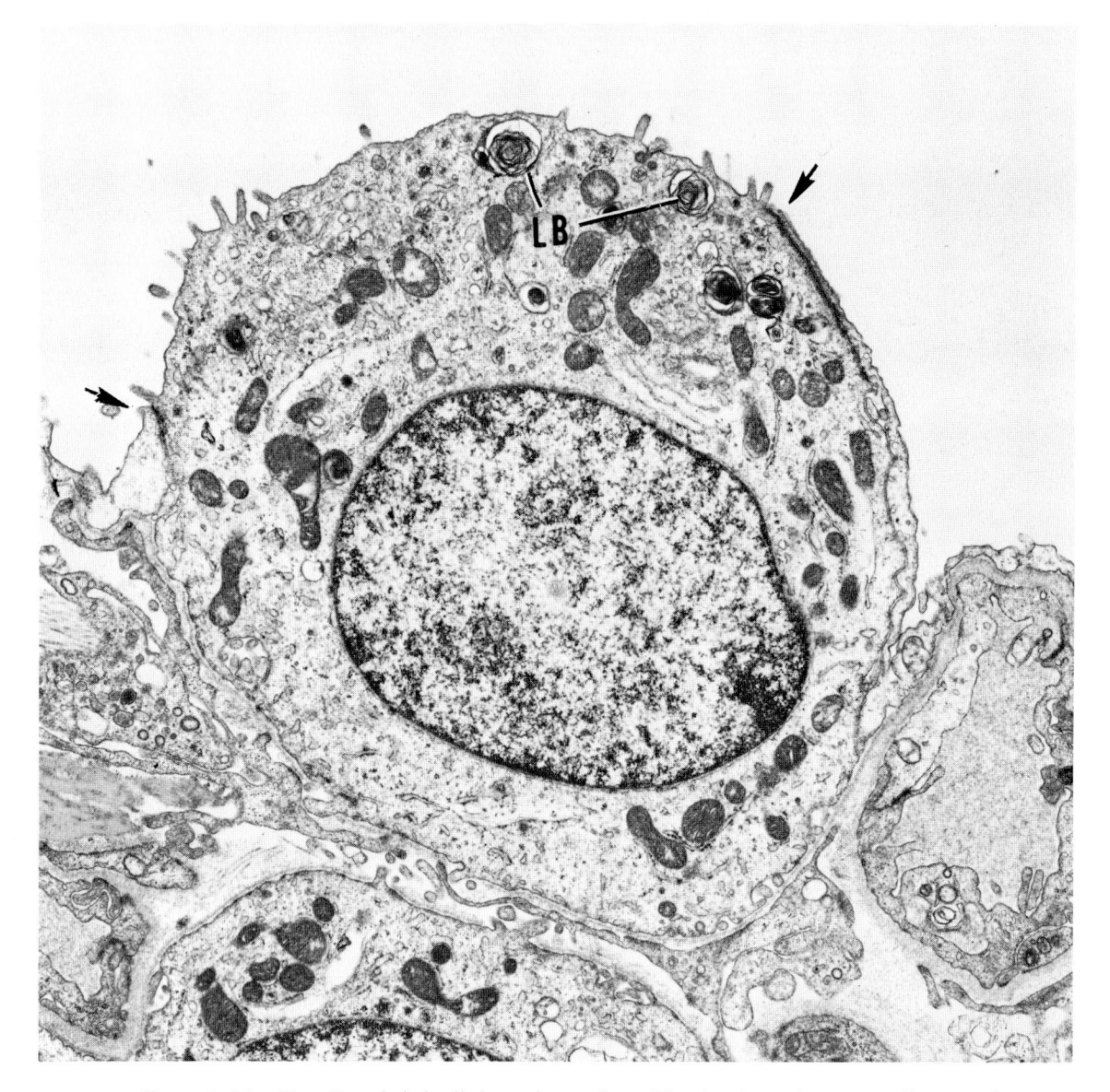

Figure 2–26. Type II epithelial cells from a human lung. The alveolar surface is partially covered by flaps of cytoplasm from type I epithelial cells up to the intercellular junctions at the arrows. There are several lamellar bodies (LB) in the apical cytoplasm. Microvilli are present on the exposed apical surface (×19,000).

ons, nonimmunologic opsonins such as fibronectin, and a variety of factors that influence the behavior of other cells, including chemotactic factors, mitogens, and other modulators of activity acting on neutrophils, fibroblasts, endothelial cells, and lymphocytes.[149]

The Circulatory System

The lung receives blood through both the bronchial and pulmonary arteries. The former carries blood at systemic pressure and has thicker, more muscular walls than the pulmonary arteries which carry blood under one-sixth as much pressure. The microscopic appearance of the pulmonary blood vessels is strongly influenced by the technique of fixation. The tunica media appears thinner when the lung is fully distended than when it is collapsed. Elastic stains are a great aid in the study of vascular structure, and Brenner's classification of pulmonary arteries (used in the following section) is based on the pattern of the elastic tissue.[125]

Histology

Elastic Pulmonary Arteries

The pulmonary trunk and pulmonary arteries larger than 500 or 1000 μm in diameter are designated elastic

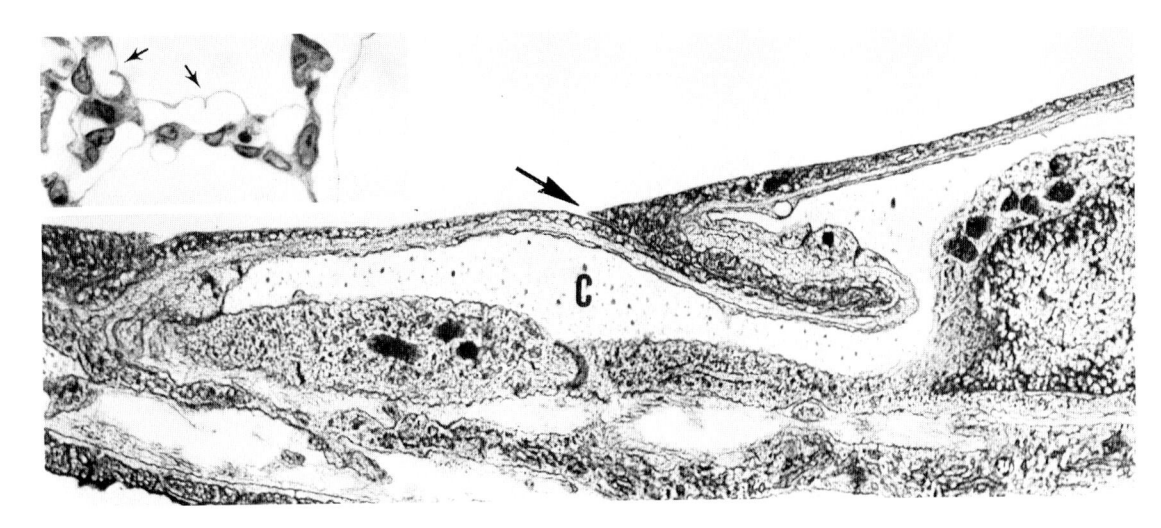

Figure 2–27. Electron micrograph of a hamster lung prepared by rapid freezing in situ in order to fix the tissue without disrupting the various physical forces which act in vivo. The alveolar surface is smoothly curved; the alveolar capillary membrane is folded on itself at the arrow, projecting into the capillary lumen (C). The depth of the folds decreases and increases with inflation and deflation of the lung (×8000). Inset, Lung fixed by perfusion through the arterial system. The capillaries are empty as a result of perfusion. This technique also achieves fixation while surface forces at the alveolar surface are maintained. Again the alveolar capillary-membrane folds into the capillaries (arrows) (×1400).

pulmonary arteries. Their media consists of multiple concentric elastic laminae separated by smooth muscle, collagen, and ground substance containing proteoglycan (Fig. 2–30). At birth the pulmonary trunk is equal in thickness to the aorta, and both have a similar configuration of elastic fibers. The laminae in the pulmonary trunk are somewhat fewer in number than those in the aorta, but tend to be thicker and more variable. During the first few months of life, the laminae become fragmented and relatively reduced in density. By the age of 2 years, the adult pattern is achieved. By then the thickness of the pulmonary trunk is only 40 to 70 percent of that of the aorta, and the elastic tissue is sparser, consisting of short fibrils separated by numerous slender wisps of elastin which branch in all directions.

The elastic tissue of the intrapulmonary arteries does not show the widely separated irregular elastic fibrils of the pulmonary trunk, but instead takes the form of concentric laminae. The number of laminae varies from 16 or 20 in the central arteries to three to four in arteries of 1000 μm in diameter or less. A thin intima containing collagenous fibers separates the endothelium from the innermost elastic lamina.

Muscular Pulmonary Arteries

The arteries that accompany the distal membranous and respiratory bronchioles range from 500 μm to 100 μm and are muscular in structure. They have a tunica media of circularly oriented smooth muscle sandwiched between distinct internal and external elastic laminae of nearly equal thickness (Fig. 2–31). The media is much thinner than that of typical systemic arteries. Medial thickness of muscular pulmonary arteries expressed as a percentage of the external diameter of the vessel ranges from 2.8 to 6.8 percent in lungs fully distended with fixative[176] and averages 4.4 percent.[177,178] In young adults, no intima is discernable in muscular arteries and the endothelial basal lamina abuts the internal elastic lamina. Intimal fibrosis is usual with advancing age. This form of intimal proliferation is due to myofibroblasts which tend to differentiate into mature smooth muscle in pulmonary arteries where they are exposed to pulsation. In pulmonary veins, in contrast, they tend to differentiate into mature fibroblasts.

Muscular pulmonary arteries lie close to the bronchioles, respiratory bronchioles, and alveolar ducts, and they branch with the bronchial tree. The diameter of the arteries decreases more rapidly than the air passages they accompany, so that the diameters of the arterial branches in the periphery of the lung are much smaller than those of adjacent bronchioles they accompany. Some muscular pulmonary arteries do not branch with the bronchial tree but arise as side-branches. These vessels have been termed supernumerary.[179]

Bronchial Arteries

The lung receives a dual blood supply, for the bronchial tree is supplied by blood via the bronchial arteries. On leaving the aorta, the bronchial arteries have a coat of circularly oriented smooth muscle and a thick internal elastic lamina. Once they enter the lung, the bronchial arteries lie in the walls of bronchi where they are subjected to the stimulus of repeated longitudinal stress. In response, they sometimes develop a characteristic

Figure 2–28. Secretion by a type II cell from hamster lung. Two lamellar bodies can be seen in the process of exocytosis from secretory vacuoles that have fused with the plasma membrane (arrows). Two more open vacuoles at the bottom are surrounded by pouting rims of cytoplasm (×16,800). From Farrell (ed): *Lung Development: Biological and Clinical Perspectives*, vol 1, 1982, p. 44. Used with permission of Academic Press, Inc.

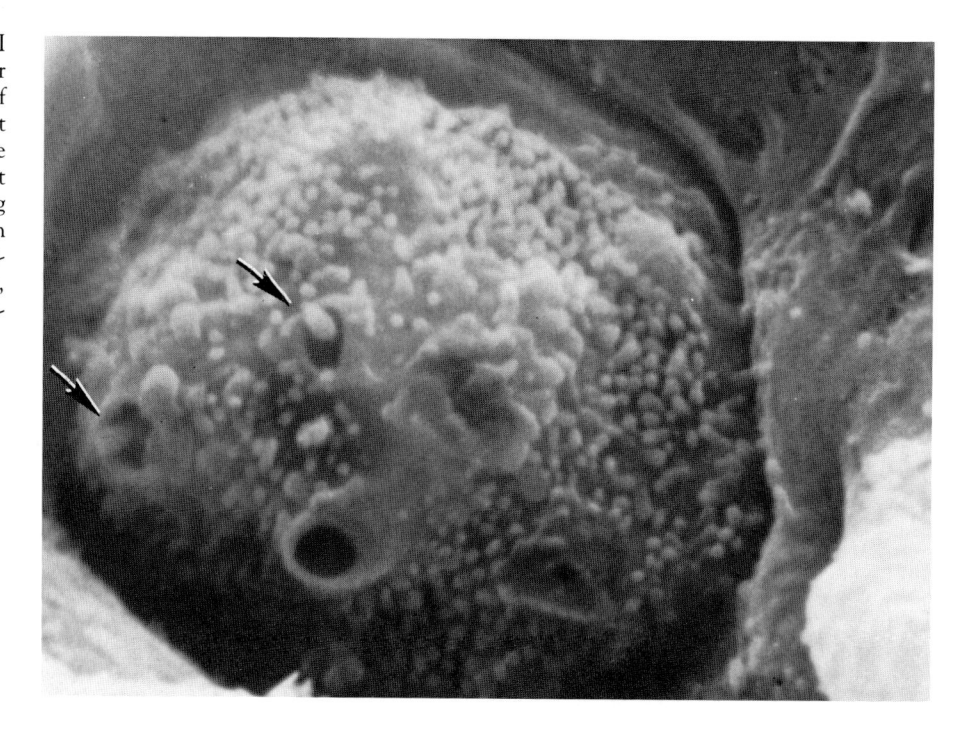

layer of longitudinally oriented smooth muscle. The muscle fibers in this layer are often separated by elastic fibrils (Fig. 2–32). The internal elastic lamina is well developed, but the external elastic lamina is thin or even absent. The bronchial arterioles are typical of the systemic vasculature with a thick media of circular smooth muscle. Bronchopulmonary anastomoses are found in the normal lung of the neonate and infant and probably are of functional significance. On the other hand, the presence of such anastomoses in the adult lung is doubtful. Bronchial arteries show age changes in the form of deposition of collagen in the intimal layer, and they may appear to be occluded by such fibrotic changes.

Pulmonary Arterioles

These vessels arise as terminations or side-branches of parent muscular pulmonary arteries. The muscle coat of the parent vessel extends for a short distance in the wall of the arteriole. The diameter at which the arteriole loses its coat is not 100 μm as originally defined[175] but approximately 70 μm.[180] The muscle coat of the parent muscular pulmonary artery is lost gradually, running as a spiral in the wall so that there is a transitional zone of the arteriole for a variable length before completely disappearing. In the spiral segment, cross-sections through the arteriole show muscularized segments alternating with segments devoid of muscle (Fig. 2–33). Thus, the histologic appearance of a pulmonary arteriole varies depending on the level of section. The proximal part has a complete media, the intermediate an interrupted media, and the distal portion is devoid of muscle (Fig. 2–34).

Arterioles have a lining of endothelial cells resting on a basement membrane.

Muscular evaginations are also a common feature in pulmonary blood vessels, especially in veins.[181] There is no internal elastic lamina in these vessels to prevent their formation. They project from the innermost layer of muscle through the basal lamina to the endothelium, which may be displaced toward the lumen as a result. They are less common in muscular pulmonary arteries, but they can sometimes be found projecting into the adventitia, or more rarely, herniating through small gaps in the internal elastic lamina. Evaginations in normal pulmonary blood vessels are caused by contraction of the vessels during preparation, since they are abolished if the lungs are fixed in a state of distension.[181,182] When active vasoconstriction has occurred during life, however, muscular evagination becomes pronounced and is not reversed by distending the lung. Thus, administration of the pyrrolizidine alkaloids fulvine[182] and monocrotaline[183] to rats or subjecting them to hypoxia[184,185] induces an intense evagination of the vascular smooth muscle. So far these observations are confined to animal experiments and require verification in human pulmonary blood vessels.

Pulmonary Capillaries

The pulmonary arterioles give rise to precapillaries, which then branch to form a rich capillary network in the walls of the alveolar ducts and alveoli. Electron microscopy shows that the pulmonary capillaries are lined with endothelial cells which lack fenestrae but do have numerous caveolae cellulares.

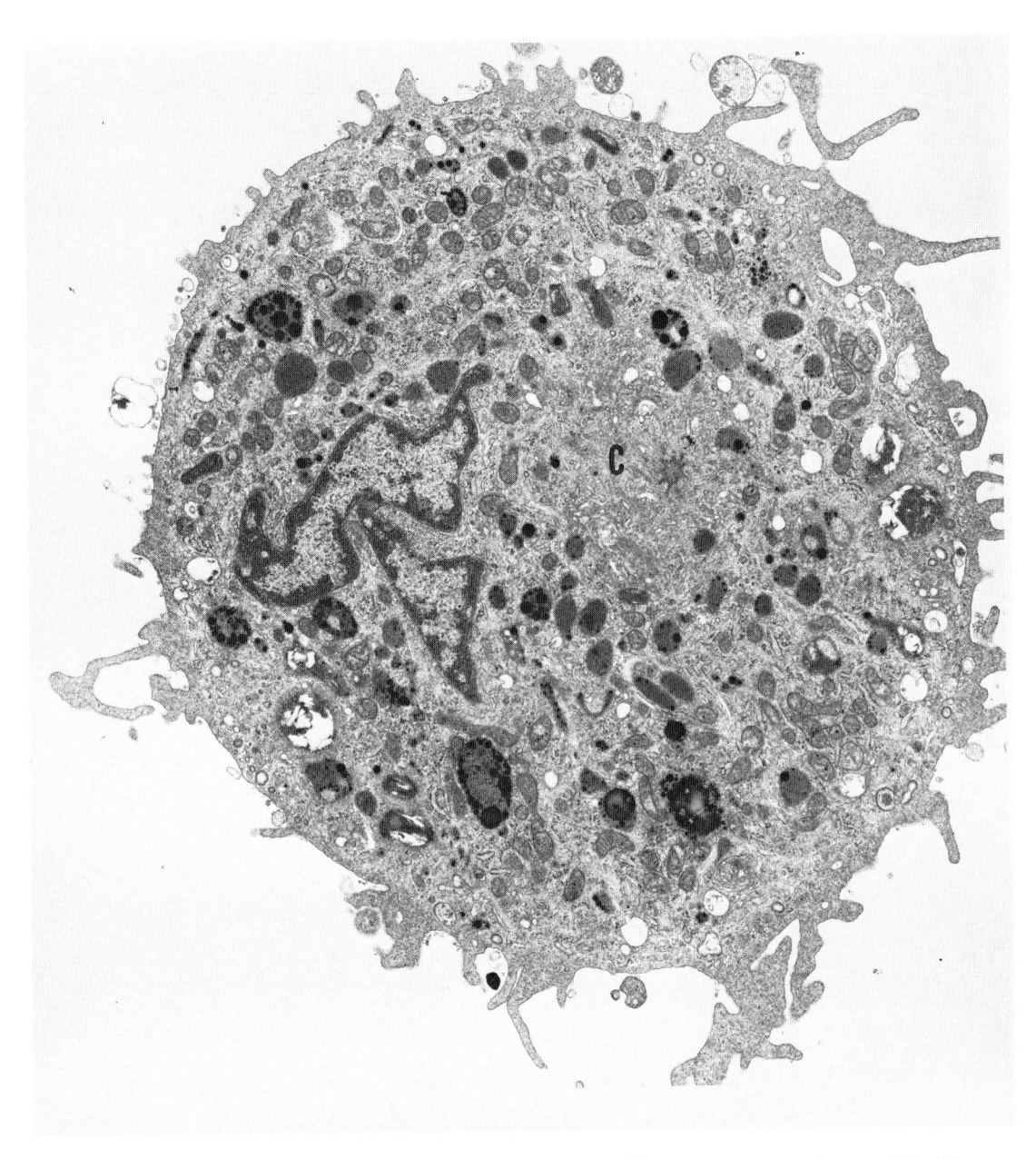

Figure 2–29. Alveolar macrophage. The cytocenter (C) contains a centriole and Golgi apparatus. The cytoplasm contains many mitochondria and lysosomes of varied content. The periphery of the cell projects as irregularly shaped pseudopodia (×10,000).

Pulmonary Venules and Veins

The smallest tributaries of pulmonary veins are indistinguishable histologically from the pulmonary arterioles except by tracing their origin and drainage. Thus, the venules have a wall consisting of a single elastic lamina, gradually acquiring a muscular media downstream. Formed near bronchioles, they pass through successive generations to drain into muscular veins in the connective tissue septa between secondary lobules. In young people, the intima of the veins is thin, composed mainly of collagen and a few myofibroblasts, but it gradually thickens with age (Fig. 2–35). The tunica media is slightly irregular in thickness consisting of bundles of obliquely and circularly arranged smooth muscle fibers and collagen. Irregular elastic fibrils occur in both the media and the adventitia, and the boundary between these two coats is frequently ill defined (Fig. 2–36). There is usually a distinct internal elastic lamina. The adventitia includes mainly longitudinally oriented elastic fibers and bundles of muscle. There is some extension of cardiac muscle from the left atrium along the walls of the major pulmonary veins at the hilus, but this is not as prominent as in the lungs of rodents. There are no valves in pulmonary veins.

Table 2–3. Some Secretory Products of Macrophages

Enzymes
    Lysosomal enzymes[149]
    Lysozyme[149]
    Plasminogen activator[149]
    Collagenase[150–152]
    Elastase[153,154]
Inhibitors
    Alpha$_1$-protease inhibitor[155]
    Alpha$_2$-macroglobulin[156,157]
Modulators of cell activity
    Fibroblast growth factor(s)[158,159]
    Fibroblast inhibitor(s)[160]
    Angiogenesis factor[149]
    Colony-stimulating factor[161]
    Interleukin I (lymphocyte-activating factor)[162]
    Chemotactic factors[163]
    Prostaglandins[164,165]
    Leukotrienes[166,167]
Other
    Complement proteins[149]
    Interferons[168]
    Fibronectin[169,170]
    Oxidants (H_2O_2, O_2, HO, etc.)[171–174]

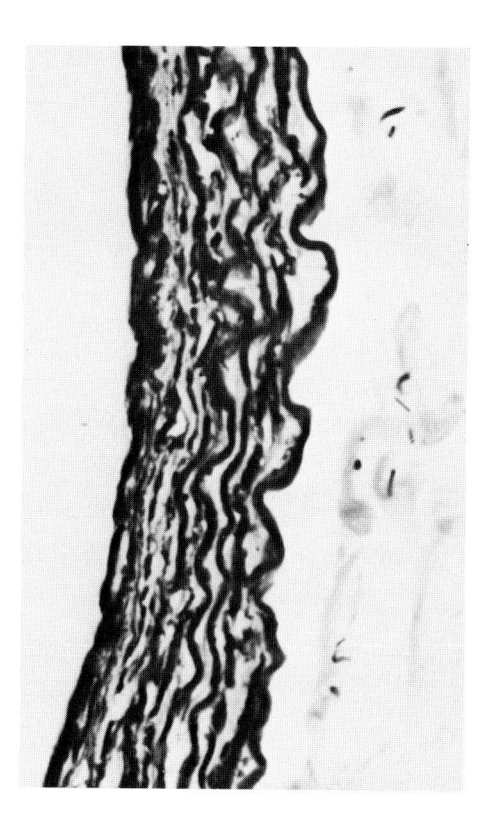

Figure 2–30. Part of an intrapulmonary elastic pulmonary artery showing the parallel arrangement of elastic laminae alternating with bands of smooth muscle (elastic van Gieson [EVG], ×600).

Endothelial Specialization

In routine histologic material, the details of endothelial morphology cannot be resolved. Using techniques with greater resolving power, it is clear that there are differences in structure between the endothelium of the capillaries and larger vessels (Table 2–4) and indeed between different segments of the arterial and venous systems. These differences include size and shape of the cells, their surface configuration, intercellular junctions, and organelle content. Undoubtedly, these differences reflect differences in endothelial function.

The endothelial surface can be studied by scanning electron microscopy. The endothelium of the pulmonary arteries is covered with microvilli, whereas capillary endothelium is flat.[186] The intercellular junctions between arterial endothelial cells are complex structures. They consist of tight junctions formed of two to six interconnecting rows of particles. There are large gap junctions between the rows of tight junction particles (Fig. 2–37). In the capillaries, the rows of tight junction particles are fewer. At the arterial end of the capillary bed, there are two to six rows, but at the venous end of the range there are one to three rows, often with discontinuities in the rows. Only few small gap junctions are present at the arterial end of the capillary bed and none at the venous end. In the pulmonary veins, the junctions consist of several rows of sparsely interconnecting tight junction particles. Gap junctions are fewer than in the arteries and tend to be more numerous in small veins than in large veins.[187] The pattern of tight junctions suggests that large vessel endothelium is less permeable than capillary endothelium and that at the arterial end of the capillary, microcirculation is less permeable than at the venous end.

Arterial and venous endothelia also contain organized bundles of contractile filaments.[188] The presence of filament bundles along with gap junctions, a specialization commonly associated with electrophysiologic or metabolic coupling of cells, suggests that these endothelia may contract as a functional unit, contributing to the maintenance of vascular tone. In the capillaries, in contrast, microfilaments are few, mainly associated with the junctions, and are not organized into distinct bundles.

Weibel-Palade granules (Fig. 2–38) are elongated, electron-dense granules containing von Willebrand's factor which are found only in endothelium.[189] They vary in number from cell to cell, but can be found in both arterial and venous endothelium. They are lacking in capillaries.

Pulmonary Endothelial Pavement Patterns

In the description of the pulmonary endothelium presented so far, the cells have been considered from the point of view of conventional transverse sections examined by transmission electron-microscopy. Revealing as

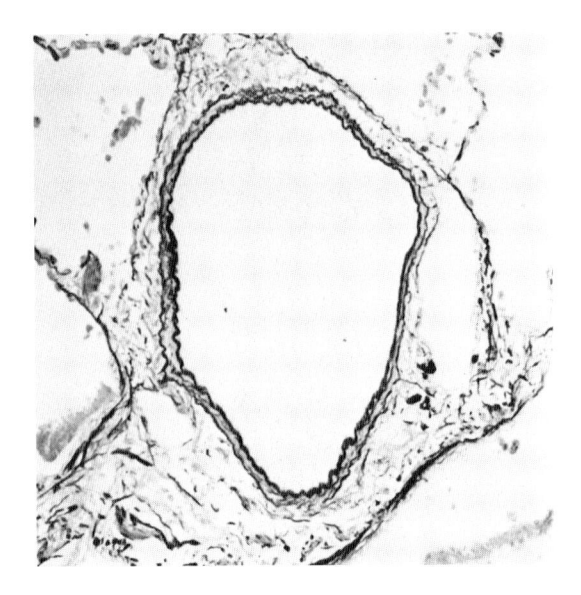

Figure 2–31. Transverse section of a muscular pulmonary artery consisting of a thin media of circularly oriented smooth muscle sandwiched between internal and external elastic laminae (EVG, ×165).

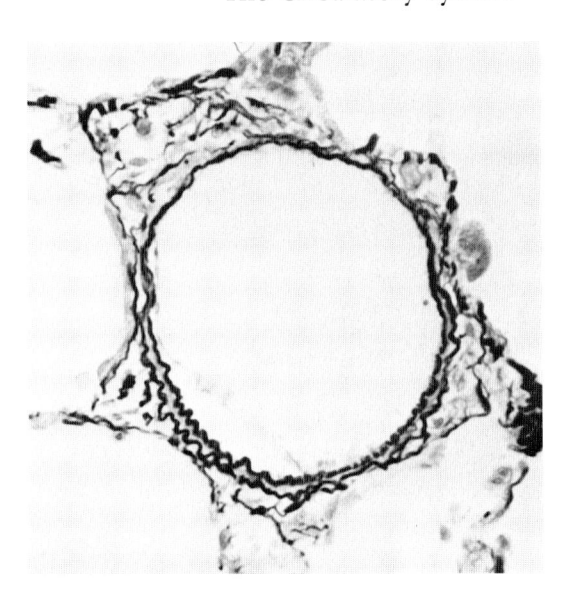

Figure 2–33. Transverse section of a pulmonary arteriole near its origin from a muscular pulmonary artery. Half of the circumference of the vessel has a muscular media, but the remainder consists merely of a single elastic lamina (EVG, ×420).

such sections are, they tell us nothing about the shape and size of the endothelial cells when viewed from the surface. The scanning electron microscope can provide this information, but it is an expensive and time-consuming instrument to use for the routine study of the surface of endothelial cells. A much simpler but equally

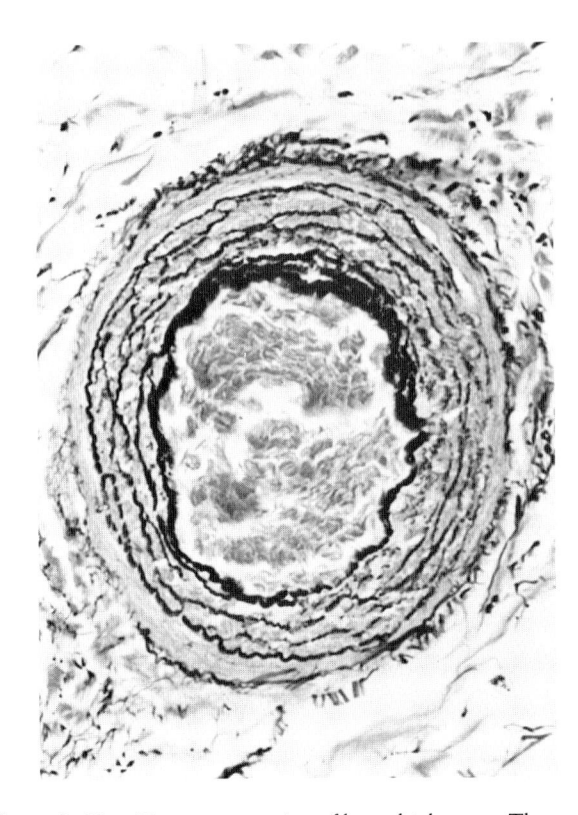

Figure 2–32. Transverse section of bronchial artery. The vessel consists of a clearly defined internal elastic lamina, a media of circularly oriented smooth muscle, and a discontinuous, poorly defined external elastic lamina. The intima contains numerous, small fasciculi of longitudinally oriented smooth muscle separated by anastomosing elastic fibers (EVG, ×425).

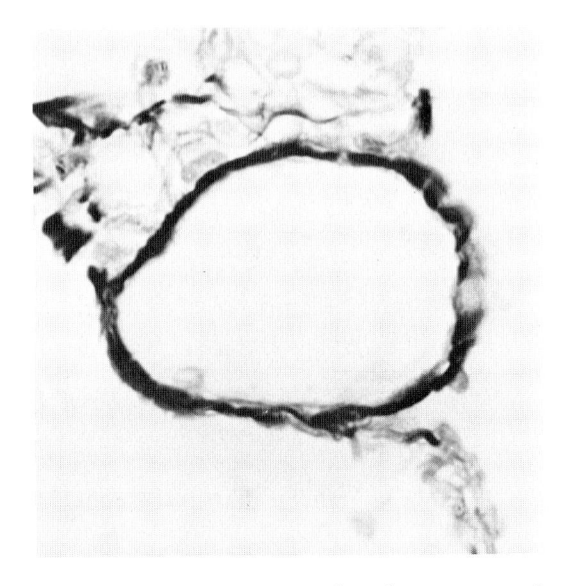

Figure 2–34. Transverse section of a pulmonary arteriole consisting of a single elastic lamina lined by endothelium. Such vessels are indistinguishable from pulmonary venules, and serial sections may be required to demonstrate their origin from muscular pulmonary arteries (EVG, ×660).

38 Normal Anatomy and Histology

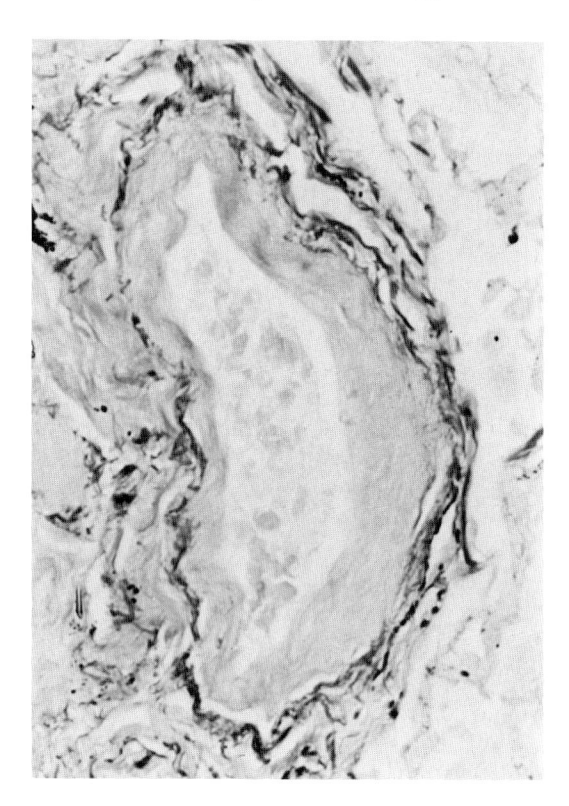

Figure 2–35. Oblique section of a small pulmonary vein from a 55-year-old man in which the intima shows a proliferation of acellular collagenous tissue. This is typical of age-change intimal fibrosis (EVG, ×412).

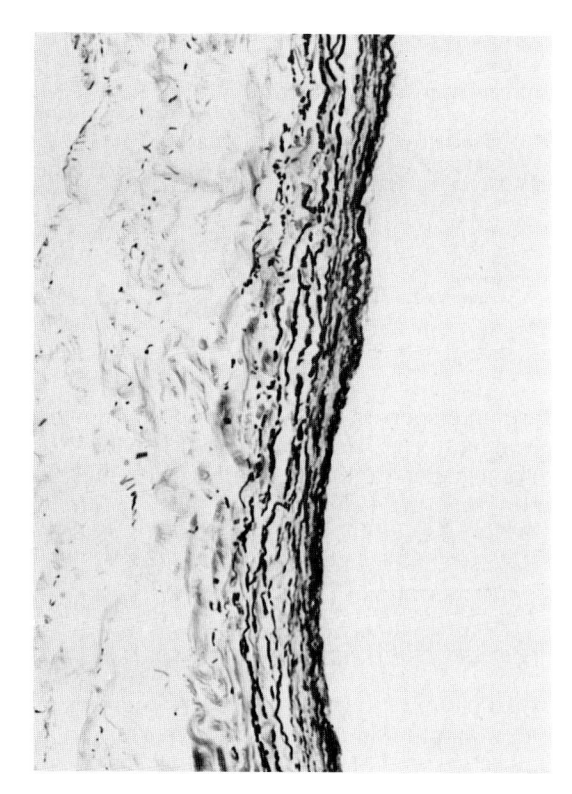

Figure 2–36. Part of a transverse section of a large pulmonary vein. The media consists of circularly oriented smooth muscle cells interspersed with short, irregular elastic fibers. The internal elastic lamina is broad and continuous, but the distinction between the media and the adventitia is poorly defined (EVG, ×165).

effective technique which has been used for many years is silver staining.[190–193] A modified and improved technique[194] involves staining the endothelium with silver nitrate solution, causing a precipitate of metallic silver to collect between the cells. The silver deposit accurately and clearly delineates the boundary of the endothelial cells so that they can be viewed en face with the light microscope.

Using this technique, it has been found that the size and shape of endothelial cells in the rat are not constant throughout the cardiovascular system. Indeed each vessel has its own characteristic endothelial pavement pattern.[195] Thus, whereas the endothelial cells of the aorta are fusiform in shape, those of the pulmonary trunk are polygonal with finely tesselated borders. In the inferior vena cava, the cells are larger and, although elongated, have truncated ends. Occasionally Y-shaped forms are seen. The largest cells are found in the pulmonary veins and, like those of the pulmonary trunk, they are polygonal.

The pavement pattern in the pulmonary trunk changes when pulmonary arterial hypertension is induced in rats by feeding them on pyrrolizidine alkaloids contained in the seeds of the plant *Crotalaria spectabilis*.[195] The average surface area of the cells increases, probably due to distension of the vessel by the increased pulmonary arterial blood pressure. However, there is also a loss of uniformity of cell size and shape, so that many of the cells become fusiform like those in the aorta. Although some of the cells are larger than normal, many are very small, giving the pavement pattern an irregular, heterogeneous appearance.

If the endothelium is stained with hematoxylin, many of the larger cells are found to be binucleated, a feature rarely encountered in the controls. These observations strongly suggest that pulmonary arterial hypertension stimulates endothelial cells in the pulmonary trunk to proliferate and some of them to adopt a fusiform shape. If pulmonary hypertension is induced by exposing the rats to hypoxia for 4 to 5 weeks, the endothelial cells of the pulmonary trunk show a striking change in which they are virtually all fusiform so that the pavement pattern cannot be distinguished from that of the aorta.[196]

It is not known whether a similar change occurs in the human pulmonary trunk. Investigations are hampered by the fact that endothelial cells in arterial vessels of human adults have a pleomorphic pavement pattern.[197,198] Thus, within a single segment of vessel, fusiform and polygonal cells are intermixed and have surface areas ranging from 500 to 7000 μm^2. Occasional multinucleated giant cells are found with surface areas anywhere between 10,000 and 130,000 μm^2. Most endothelial cells in the pulmonary trunk are polygonal in shape but of variable size.

Table 2–4. Morphologic Features of Endothelium from Different Vessels

Type of Vessel	Surface Microvilli	Contractile Filaments	Gap Junctions	Weibel-Palade Granules
Artery	Many	Yes	Many	Yes
Capillary	None	Few	Rare	No
Vein	Few	Yes	Moderate	Yes

They are interspersed with foci of fusiform cells or irregular giant cells. This pleomorphism is probably a feature of aging, since the pattern becomes more disorganized when there is intimal thickening or atherosclerosis.[198] Also the pattern is more uniform in younger subjects[197]; in the fetus, the pavement pattern is uniform except in the vicinity of lateral branches.[199]

Metabolic Functions of Endothelium

The endothelium of the pulmonary circulation has functions other than serving as a conduit for respiratory gas exchange and fluid filtration. It also acts as a sort of biochemical filter because of its efficient and highly selective metabolic machinery. This machinery enables endothelium to degrade many physiologically active compounds that are generated in peripheral tissues to serve local functions and ensures that they do not spill over into the systemic circulation. Other compounds, often closely related to the compounds that are destroyed, are passed unchanged to exert hormonal effects on distant targets or are even activated to greater physiologic potency (Table 2–5). Although many of the metabolic capabilities of pulmonary endothelium are shared by endothelial cells in other locations, the physiologic impact is probably greater in the case of pulmonary endothelium, since the lung receives the entire cardiac output and the pulmonary capillary net spreads the blood into a thin film ensuring close contact with the endothelial cells.

There are two patterns of endothelial metabolism: some compounds are metabolized in the vascular lumen by enzyme systems that are located in the plasma membrane of the endothelial cell, whereas other compounds are taken into the cytoplasm. The adenine nucleotides and the vasoactive peptides angiotensin and bradykinin are of the first type. Histochemically the adenine nucleotidases have been localized selectively to the caveolae intracellulares, whereas the enzyme angiotensin-converting enzyme has been found along the entire luminal surface of the endothelial cell.[200] Angiotensin-converting enzyme, or kininase II, converts the inactive decapeptide angiotensin I to the octapeptide angiotensin II, a vasoconstrictor, and inactivates the vasodilator bradykinin. Both reactions involve the cleavage of a dipeptide from the carboxy terminal end of the molecule.

The other metabolic transformations enumerated in Table 2–5 depend on uptake by the endothelium. For some compounds, such as serotonin and norepinephrine, there is evidence that the metabolism takes place within the endothelium.[201,202] For others the site of catabolism is unknown, but transport by the endothelial cell is a necessary step.

The Lymphoid System

The lung's lymphatic drainage is commonly divided into two systems: the superficial or pleural lymphatics and the deep lymphatics, consisting of the septal perivenous

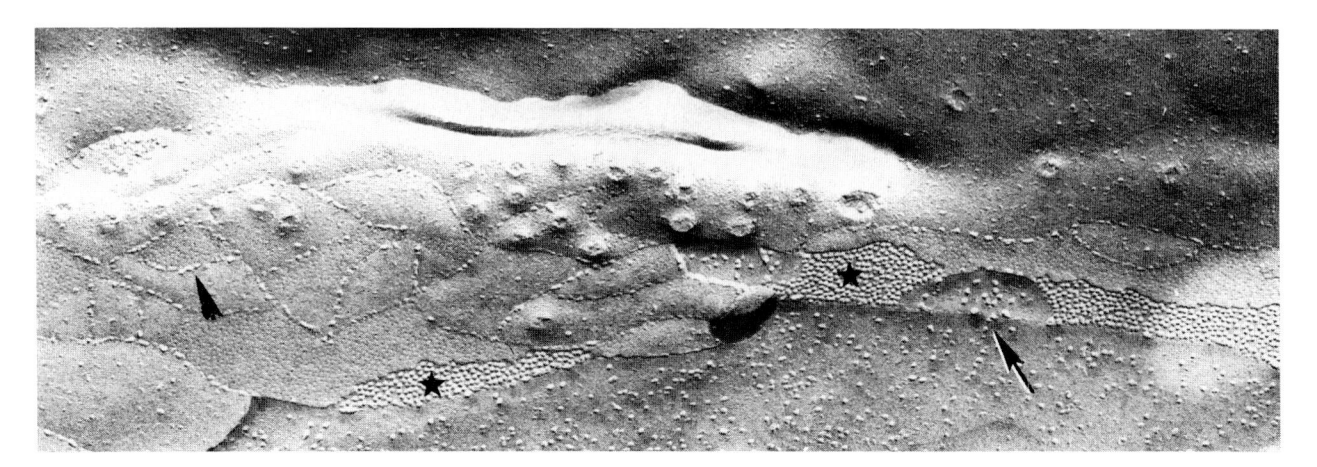

Figure 2–37. Freeze-fracture replica of an intercellular junction from a pulmonary artery in a rat lung. On the extracellular face, rows of tight junction particles are situated in shallow grooves (arrowhead). On the protoplasmic face, the tight junction is a low ridge with few attached particles (arrow). The tightly packed arrays of particles (*) are gap junctions between the meshes of tight junction (×75,000). From Schneeberger Circ Res 49:1102–1111, 1981. Used with permission of the American Heart Association.

Figure 2–38. An endothelial cell from a muscular pulmonary artery of a rat. Except for a thin basal lamina, the cell rests directly on the internal elastic lamina (el). The cell contains mitochondria (m), rough and smooth endoplasmic reticulum, and the characteristic Weibel-Palade bodies (arrow) (electron micrograph, ×25,000). Insert, Weibel-Palade granule showing characteristic tubular content in cross-section (×140,000).

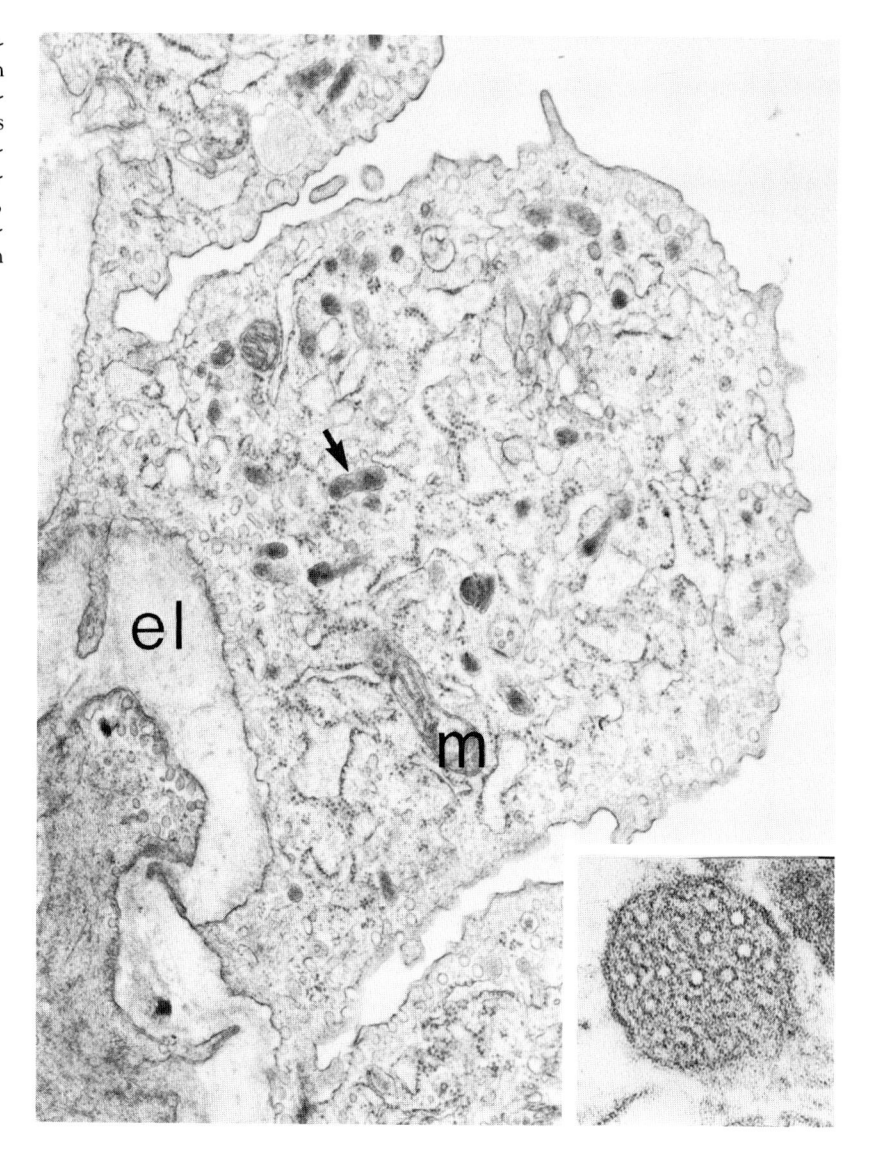

lymphatic plexuses and the bronchoarterial plexuses.[4,203–205] The pleural lymphatic plexus consists of lymphatic trunks mainly located at the junctions of the interlobular septa with the pleura, fed by fine lymphatic capillaries crossing the polygonal spaces enclosed by the larger lymphatic trunks. Lateral channels off the smaller lymphatics end blindly. The pleural lymphatics are larger in the lower zones of the lung than the upper zones,[203,204] presumably because the vertical gradient in hydrostatic pressure favors greater lymph formation at the bases. The deep lymphatics run in the loose connective tissue of the interlobular septa and surrounding the vessels and conducting airways. The major lymphatic trunks course longitudinally along the major vessels and airways with an extensive plexus of tributaries surrounding the vessels and airways. In the interlobular septa, the septal and perivenous lymphatics anastomose, forming a common plexus. Since the bronchi and arteries run together and often share a common connective tissue sheath, their lymphatics also anastomose extensively. The bronchoarterial lymphatics begin at the level of respiratory bronchioles; there are no lymphatic capillaries in the interalveolar septa or in the walls of alveolar ducts. However, when tracers such as labeled albumin, horseradish peroxidase, or ferritin are injected into the air spaces, they are cleared in part by the lymphatic system.[206] Lauweryns[204–206] has pointed out that many of the lymphatic capillaries have a close relationship to the alveolar spaces although they occupy adventitial connective tissue spaces (Fig. 2–39). He calls them juxta-alveolar lymphatics and has suggested that they contribute to the removal of fluid from the alveoli.

The structure of the pulmonary lymphatics is similar to that of lymphatics in other tissues. The smallest lymphatic channels (lymphatic capillaries) are essentially tubes of endothelial cells which rest on the connective tissue with only a few discontinuous patches of basement membrane material as support. The basal surface of the endothelial

Table 2–5. Metabolic Specificity of Endothelium

Class of Compound	Metabolized	Not Metabolized
Adenine nucleotides	Adenosine menophosphate	
	Adenosine diphosphate	
	Adenosine triphosphage	
Vasoactive amines	Serotonin	Histamine
	Norepinephrine	Epinephrine
Prostaglandins	PGE_2	PGA
	$PGF_{2\#}$	PGI_2
Vasoactive peptides	Angiotensin I	Vasopressin
	Bradykinin	Vasoactive intestinal peptide
Lipoproteins	Very-low-density Lipoprotein	Low-density liproprotein

Abbreviatlion: PG, prostaglandin.

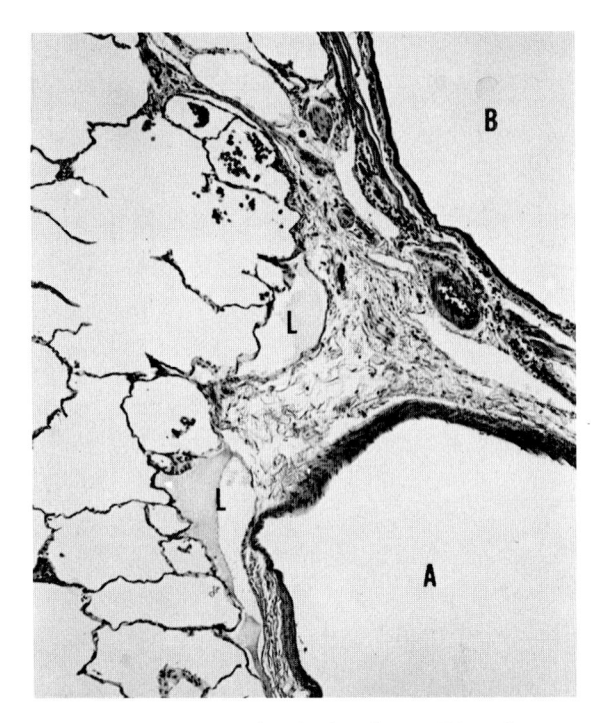

Figure 2–39. Two juxta-alveolar lymphatics (L) in the connective tissue sheath enclosing a bronchiole (B) and pulmonary artery (A). The lymphatics are closely associated with the alveolar walls and may drain alveolar as well as interstitial fluid.

cells dips into the connective tissue in a series of projections, each projection attached to or enmeshed in bundles of 10-nm filaments, the so-called lymphatic anchoring filaments. The contacts between neighboring endothelial cells are often patent, overlapping without forming specialized attachment structures. The endothelial cytoplasm contains both intermediate and actin filaments and pinocytic vesicles and occasionally lysosomes.[205,207] Lauweryns' tracer studies[206] indicate that the main route of uptake into the lymphatics is through the intercellular junctions. The predominant direction of pinocytosis seemed to be back from lumen into the cytoplasm.

The lymphatic-collecting vessels have a less open structure. The endothelial cells are joined by tight junctions and rest on a basal lamina. There is a muscular media one to two cells thick.

The valves present in the lymphatic trunks consist of a delicate core of connective tissue covered by endothelial cells which are joined by tight junctions.[205] Most observers have considered that the valves are bicuspid, although Lauweryns[205] concluded that the large majority of those which he studied by serial sections had only a single conical cusp. The few lymphatic valves that the writer has observed in the scanning electron microscope have been bicuspid, however.

Organized collections of lymphoid cells are associated with the lymphatic vessels at several points.[4,208] Nodules of lymphocytes are often found at the bifurcations of small bronchioles or respiratory bronchioles where they lie in the connective tissue between the bronchioles and artery. They are usually closely associated with an efferent lymphatic, but have neither a true capsule nor a subcapsular sinus (Fig. 2–40). Nodules of lymphocytes are also found associated with the lymphatics at the periphery of the acini, both in the pleura and in the interlobular septa. They vary in extent of development from nodules to structures partially enclosed by a subcapsular sinus (Fig. 2–40). Trapnell[209] found fully formed lymph nodes with a complete subcapsular sinus in the periphery of 7 percent of lungs.

Miller[4] inferred from the direction of the valves that the drainage of the pleural lymphatics was through the superficial plexus over the surface of the lung to the lymph nodes of the hilus, whereas the deep lymphatics drained centripetally along the airways and vessels. Injection studies[203,204] indicate, however, that some of the drainage of the costal pleura passes directly via the septal and venous plexuses and even occasionally through anastomoses to the bronchoarterial portion of the deep lymphatic system to the hilar lymph nodes.

The hilar lymph nodes, which are encountered within the lung at the bifurcations of large bronchi, are complete nodes with a subcapsular sinus and follicles. From the hilar nodes, the lymph drains via extensively anastomosing channels through tracheobronchial lymph nodes clustered alongside the main stem bronchi, beneath the carina, and along the course of the trachea. In the mediastinum, the pulmonary lymph is joined by lymph from the trachea, heart, esophagus, diaphragm, and chest wall before emptying into the venous system. On the right side, the thoracic lymphatics enter the subclavian vein at its confluence with the jugular vein, either via a separate duct or after joining the lymphatic trunks from the arm, head, and neck to form a common duct. On the left, the mediastinal lymphatics may join the

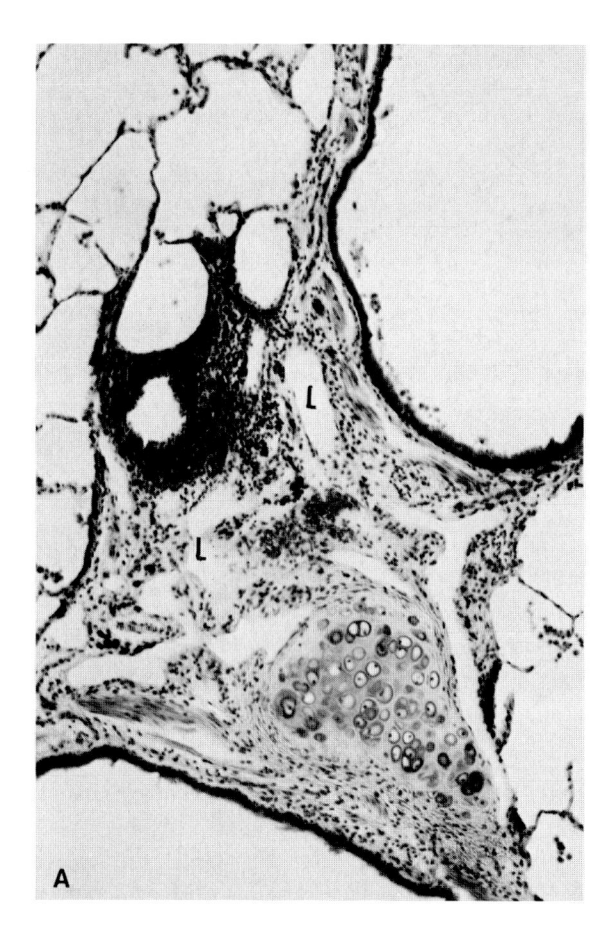

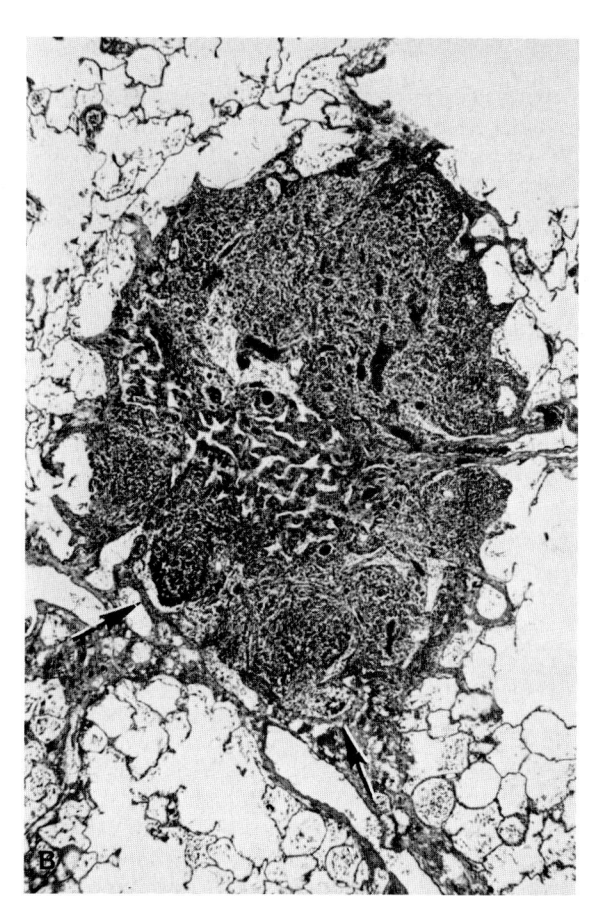

Figure 2–40. Lymphoid tissue in the lung. A. Lymphoid nodule in the tissue surrounding a small bronchus. The nodule has no nodal structure, but there are lymphatics (L) adjacent to it (×200). B. Lymphoid tissue associated with a perilobular septum. The nodule has partial nodal architecture. Sinusoids are present in the center of the nodule, and a subcapsular sinus is present along side the septum (arrow), but not where the nodule abuts the alveoli (×75).

thoracic duct or empty into the subclavian vein independently.

Nerves

General Organization

The lung receives its major sensory and motor innervation from the tenth cranial (vagus) nerve. Postganglionic fibers from the thoracic sympathetic plexus mingle with the vagal fibers as they enter the lung at the hilus, and the combined nerves break up into plexuses which accompany the ramifications of the arteries, bronchi, and veins.[4,210] According to Larsell,[211] the nerves to the bronchi form two plexuses, a large plexus external to the cartilages and a smaller plexus deep to the cartilage. Beyond the termination of the cartilages, the two plexuses merge and continue distally to the respiratory bronchioles. Ganglia are present within the larger nerves of the extrachondral plexus along the proximal three bronchial generations becoming rare farther distally.[211]

The periarterial plexus lies in the adventitia of the arteries, and its bundles anastomose with those of the extrachondral bronchial plexus. Fibers from the arterial plexus enter the media with the vasa vasorum and supply its outermost portion. The plexus continues distally as far as the arterioles.

The perivenous plexus accompanies the veins into the perilobular septa and even reaches the visceral pleura to supply the subpleural alveolar walls. Spencer and Leof[212] have described twigs of the venous plexus reaching and ramifying in the subendothelial space of the veins. A few ganglia are present in the perivenous plexus near the hilus.

Tiny unmyelinated nerve fibers have been identified by electron microscopy in the walls of alveoli, not only in animals (Fig. 2–41) but recently in humans.[213] They are distinctly rare. According to some estimates,[214] there are only 104 fibers for the 300×10^6 alveoli per lung. It is not clear whether the source of these fibers is the bronchial or perivascular plexuses or both.

Sensory Receptors

Most sensory (afferent) fibers travel with the vagus nerves along myelinated axons of neurons located in the nodose ganglion. Other sensory fibers may travel through the thoracic sympathetic plexus. Physiologists have identified receptors of several types in the walls of airways.[215,216] In the main bronchi are the receptors, which when stimulated initiate the cough reflex. In smaller airways, irritant receptors respond to inert dusts, mechanical stimuli, and irritant gases. Stimulation of the irritant receptors produces reflex bronchoconstriction and hyperventilation as well as a sensation of chest discomfort. Classic neural stains and electron microscopy have shown the presence of delicate nerve endings from the subchondral plexus ramifying between epithelial cells of the bronchial mucosa. They probably correspond to the irritant receptors since no motor endings have been detected in the epithelium either by electron microscopy or by histochemical techniques. Substance P, in all probability a sensory neurotransmitter, has been localized within nerves associated with the bronchial epithelium.[217]

The receptors responsible for the Hering-Breuer reflex are mechanoreceptors located deep in the airway walls. They fire off with increasing frequency as the lung is expanded and progressively inhibit the inspiratory center. Nerve endings associated with the smooth muscle of the bronchial wall are believed to account for the mechanoreception, although ultrastructural detail is still scant.[216] Substance P also occurs in nerves in the smooth muscle.[217]

The unmyelinated fibers identified in the alveolar walls may be the J- (juxtacapillary) receptors. In animals these receptors respond to interstitial fluid pressure as well as certain chemicals; they cause transitory reflex apnea followed by rapid shallow respiration.[215]

Chemoreceptor tissue similar in structure to the carotid and aortic bodies is found constantly in the adventitia of the posterior wall of the pulmonary trunk, just caudal to its bifurcation.[218] Other microscopic glomera have been described in the soft tissue surrounding the major pulmonary arteries near the hilus and within the lung.[219] The physiologic role of these structures is unclear, since there is little physiologic evidence that the pH or partial pressure of oxygen or carbon dioxide in pulmonary blood plays a role in the regulation of ventilation or perfusion.[220,221] It is controversial whether the pulmonary glomus receives its blood from the pulmonary or bronchial circulation.[218,220]

Motor Innervation

The main motor innervation of the lung is cholinergic. Stimulation of the nerves to the lung produces bronchoconstriction and secretion of mucus which can be blocked by atropine. The parasympathetic fibers carried in the vagus nerve synapse with the ganglion cells in the bronchial walls. Unmyelinated postganglionic cholinergic fibers enter the subchondral plexus to end in close

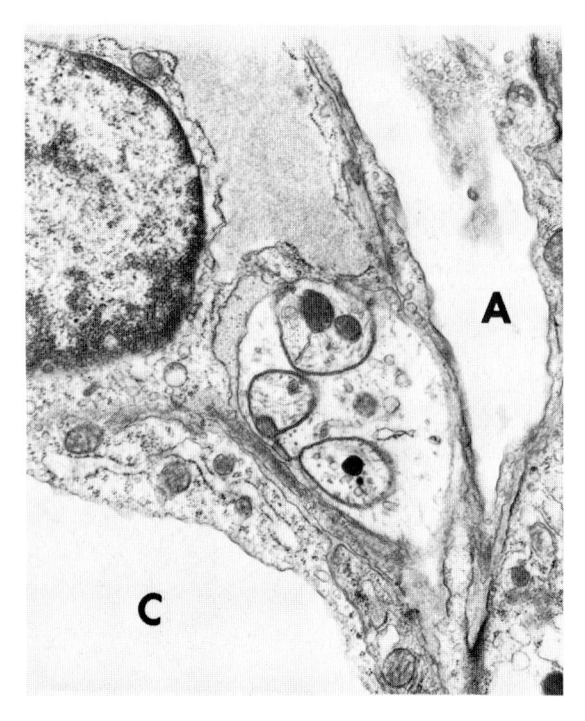

Figure 2–41. Unmyelinated nerve in an alveolar wall of a rat lung. A Schwann cell containing three axones. A—alveolar space, C—capillary. The cell with its nucleus included in the micrograph is an interstitial cell (×17,000).

association with the mucous glands and bronchial smooth muscle.[222]

Inhibitory neural control of bronchial muscle can only be demonstrated in the presence of atropine blockade of cholinergic efferents and when end-organ tone is stimulated by noncholinergic means, for example by histamine. Under these conditions, field stimulation of pulmonary nerves relaxes bronchoconstriction.[223–225] Although it has been known for many years (and applied clinically) that β-adrenergic agonists have bronchodilator activity, adrenergic blockers have no effect on the inhibition of bronchoconstriction produced by electric stimulation of pulmonary nerves. Fluorescent techniques for the demonstration of catecholamines, which show catecholamine-containing nerve endings associated with the blood vessels and ganglion cells, show none with bronchial glands or smooth muscle.[225] Electron microscopy shows motor nerve endings close to bronchial glands and smooth muscle which are not characteristic of cholinergic or adrenergic endings. Motor nerve endings are replete with electron-dense neuroendocrine granules, but the granule matrix nearly fills the membrane and is thus distinguishable from typical adrenergic granules, which have an eccentric matrix with a wide gap between the matrix and membrane.[216,224] Thus, results with inhibitors, fluorescence microscopy, and electron microscopy all point to the conclusion that the inhibitory nerves to the bronchi are nonadrenergic. The mediator of the inhibitory effect is not established at present and might be either a purine nucleotide or a polypeptide. A likely

Normal Anatomy and Histology

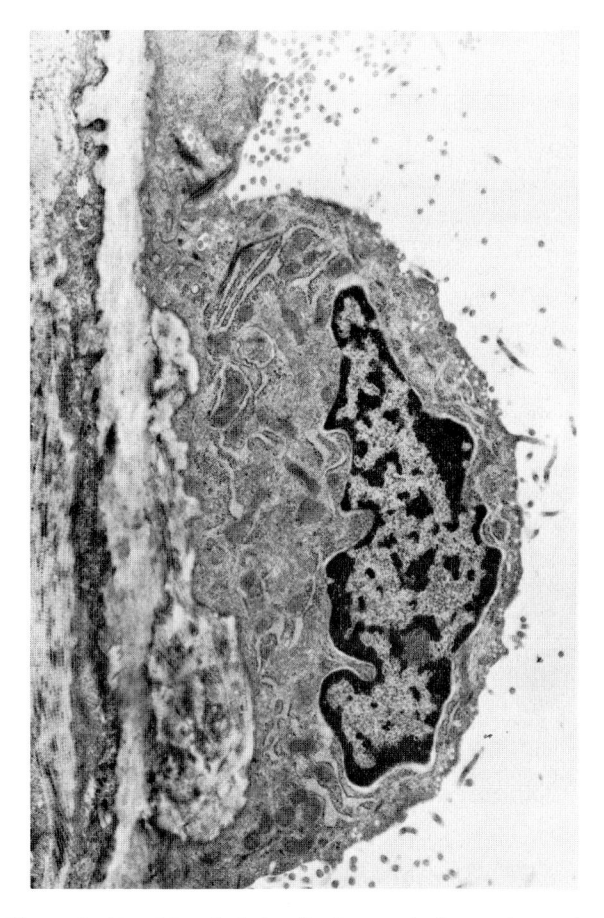

Figure 2–42. Mesothelial cell of visceral pleura of a rat lung. The characteristic long microvilli are seen here mostly in cross-section. The well-developed endoplasm suggests that this cell has a major biosynthetic function and is not merely a passive lining cell (×9000).

candidate is the so-called vasoactive intestinal peptide as it relaxes airway and vascular smooth muscle and is found in neurons of the peribronchial ganglia and in axons terminating close to bronchial glands and smooth muscle.[221,226] In the absence of adrenergic nerves, the adrenergic receptors on the smooth muscle cells must respond to circulating catecholamines.

Despite a great deal of interest among physiologists in the control of blood flow through the lung, the role of neural factors in regulating human pulmonary circulation is poorly understood. Recent anatomic studies have shown that there are cholinergic, catecholamine-containing, and vasoactive intestinal peptide–containing endings on vascular smooth muscle of both arteries and veins.[225–227]

Pleura

The pleural investment of the lung is a serous membrane that continues over the lung root and pulmonary ligament to cover the mediastinal, diaphragmatic, and costal surfaces of the thoracic cavity. It consists of connective tissue covered by simple squamous epithelium known as the mesothelium, which is composed by polygonal cells 15 to 30 μm in thickness in the region of the nucleus and thinning toward the periphery.[228] These cells are joined by terminal bar complexes with tight and gap junctions and desmosomes. The nucleus lies in the center of the cell surrounded by mitochondria, short lamellae of endoplasmic reticulum, and a well-developed Golgi apparatus (Fig. 2–42). The thinner peripheral portions of the cell have fewer mitochondria, but have cisterns of endoplasmic reticulum and small vesicles, both free in the cytoplasm and in contact with apical and basal plasma membranes. The most conspicuous feature of the mesothelium is the presence of long sinuous microvilli 0.1 μm in diameter and up to 3 μm in length covered by a thick glycocalyx. The density of the microvilli varies in different regions of the pleura, but is generally higher on the visceral pleura and over the inferior portions of the mediastinal pleura than on the costal and phrenic surfaces of the parietal pleura.[229] Occasionally a cell thrusts a single cilium into the pleural space. These are probably nonfunctional cilia arising from the centriole and lacking a central pair complex.

The well-developed microvilli may function in two ways. The pleural fluid is similar in composition to a plasma filtrate but not identical. In particular the bicarbonate concentration is 20 to 50 percent higher than that of plasma; sodium and chloride concentrations are somewhat lower.[230] This implies selective ion transport by the mesothelium, which might be one function of the microvilli. Agostini and colleagues[231] studied the thickness of the pleural fluid layer in animals by rapidly freezing the lung in situ. They observed that the thickness of the pleural fluid was only 5 to 10 μm at functional residual capacity and even less at higher lung volumes; it did not vary from the superior to the most dependent portions of the lung. One explanation for the failure of the fluid to follow a gravitational gradient could be that it is bound to the mesothelium, for example, as water of hydration of the thick glycocalyx covering the microvilli.

The mesothelium rests on a basal lamina covering a superficial layer of coarse connective tissue fibers. In the visceral pleura, the connective tissue includes one or two layers of thick elastic fibers beneath the mesothelium. Below this layer is a zone mainly of collagenous fibers with a few fine elastic fibers, blood vessels, and lymphatics. Where the pleura abuts the alveoli, there is an additional layer of elastic fibers which is properly part of the elastic network of the alveoli. The deep connective tissue layers of the pleura extended into the parenchyma as the interlobular septa containing collagen, a lymphatic plexus, and the pulmonary veins. The elastic network of the alveoli delimits the outer edge of the interlobular septa.[4]

The structure of the parietal pleura is generally similar to that of the visceral pleura.[228] The parietal mesothelium rests on a connective tissue layer, the fibers of which merge with those of the endothoracic fascia. Elastic fibers are absent. The parietal pleura possesses a rich lymphatic plexus which communicates directly with the pleural cavity through special stomata up to 5 μm in diameter.[232,233] At the stomata, the lymphatic endothelium is continuous with the pleural mesothelium. Pinchon and associates[233] have suggested that flaps of endothelium behave as valves directing flow away from the pleural cavity. These stomata are of sufficient size to permit the uptake of particles the size of erythrocytes from the pleural cavity. The parietal pleural lymphatics drain to the internal mammary, para-aortic, and diaphragmatic lymph node groups.

Acknowledgment. The section on the pulmonary circulation was taken from a manuscript kindly provided by Prof. Donald Heath and Dr. Paul Smith who also provided Figures 2–30 through 2–36 and 2–38. The author is also indebted to Drs. Ernest Cutz, John Heuser, Eveline Schneeberger, and Ursula Goodenough who generously provided illustrations from their work.

References

1. Murray JF: *The Normal Lung. The Basis for Diagnosis and Treatment of Pulmonary Disease*. Philadelphia: WB Saunders, 1976.
2. Whimster WF, MacFarlane AJ: Normal lung weights in a white population. Am Rev Respir Dis 110:478–483, 1974.
3. Boyden EA: *Segmental Anatomy of the Lungs. A study of the patterns of the segmental bronchi and related pulmonary vessels*. New York: McGraw Hill, 1955.
4. Miller WS: *The Lung*, 2nd ed. Springfield, IL: Charles C Thomas, 1947.
5. Hayward J, Reid LM: The cartilage of the intrapulmonary bronchi in normal lungs, in bronchiectasis, and in massive collapse. Thorax 7:98, 1952.
6. Horsefield K: The relation between structure and function in the airways of the lung. Br J Dis Chest 68:145–160, 1974.
7. Brinkman GL, Brooks N, Bryant V: The ultrastructure of the lamina propria of the human bronchus. Am Rev Respir Dis 99:219–228, 1969.
8. McCarter JH, Vazquez JJ: The bronchial basement membrane in asthma. Immunohistochemical and ultrastructural observations. Arch Pathol 82:328, 1966.
9. Breeze RB, Wheeldon EB: The cells of the pulmonary airways. Am Rev Respir Dis 116:705–777, 1977.
10. Wanner A: Clinical aspects of mucociliary transport. Am Rev Respir Dis 116:73–125, 1977.
11. Luchtel DL: The mucus layer of the trachea and major bronchi in the rat. Scan Electron Microsc 2:1089–1099, 1978.
12. Sturgess JM: The mucous lining of major bronchi in the rabbit lung. Am Rev Respir Dis 115:819–827, 1977.
13. Yeager H: Tracheobronchial secretions. Am J Med 50:493–509, 1971.
14. Hochstrasser K: The acid stable proteinase inhibitors of the respiratory tract. Chemistry and function. Clin Respir Physiol 16(Suppl):223–230, 1980.
15. Watson JHL, Brinkman GL: Electron microscopy of the epithelial cells of normal and bronchitic human bronchus. Am Rev Respir Dis 90:851–866, 1964.
16. Kaufman DG, Baker MS, Harris CC, et al.: Coordinated biochemical and morphologic examination of hamster tracheal epithelium. J Natl Cancer Inst 49:783, 1972.
17. Gibbons IR: Cilia and flagella of eucaryotes. J Cell Biol 91:1075–1245, 1981.
18. Warner FD, Satir P: The substructure of ciliary microtubules. J Cell Sci 12:313–326, 1973.
19. Gibbons IR: Studies on the protein components of cilia from tetrahymena pyriformis. Proc Natl Acad Sci USA 50:1002–1010, 1963.
20. Goodenough UW, Heuser JE: The substructure of the outer dynein arm. J Cell Biol 95:798–815, 1982.
21. Warner FD, Satir P: The structural basis of ciliary bend formation. Radial spoke positional changes accompanying microtubule sliding. J Cell Biol 63:35–63, 1974.
22. Jeffery PK, Reid L: New observations of rat airway epithelium: A quantitative and electron microscopic study. J Anat 120:295–320, 1975.
23. Kuhn C, Engleman W: The structure of the tips of mammalian respiratory cilia. Cell Tissue Res 186:491–498, 1978.
24. Anderson RGW, Hein CE: Distribution of anionic sites on the oviduct ciliary membrane. J Cell Biol 72:482–492, 1977.
25. Gilula NB, Satir P: The ciliary necklace. A ciliary membrane specialization. J Cell Biol 53:494–509, 1972.
26. Anderson RGW: The three dimensional structure of the basal body from the rhesus monkey oviduct. J Cell Biol 54:243–265, 1972.
27. Sanderson MJ, Sleigh MA. Ciliary activity of cultured rabbit tracheal epithelium: Beat pattern and metachrony. J Cell Sci 47:331–347, 1981.
28. Blum JJ, Hayes A, Jamieson GA, Vanaman TC: Calmodulin confers calcium sensitivity on ciliary dynein ATPase. J Cell Biol 87:386–397, 1980.
29. Brokaw CF: Flagellar movement. A sliding filament model. Science 178:455, 1972.
30. Summers KE, Gibbons IR: Adenosine triphosphate-induced sliding of tubules in trypsin-treated flagellae of sea urchin sperm. Proc Natl Acad Sci USA 68:3092–3096, 1971.
31. Satir P: Studies on cilia. III. Further studies on the cilium tip and a "sliding filament" model of ciliary motility. J Cell Biol 39:77–94, 1968.
32. Summers KE, Gibbons IR: Effects of trypsin on flagellar structures and their relation to motility. J Cell Biol 58:618–629, 1973.
33. Nadel JA, Davis B, Phipps RJ: Control of mucus secretion and ion transport in airways. Annu Rev Physiol 41:369–381, 1979.
34. McDowell EM, Barrett LA, Glavin F, et al.: The respiratory epithelium, human bronchus. J Natl Cancer Inst 61:539–545, 1978.
35. Meyrick B, Sturgess J, Reid L: A reconstruction of the duct system and secretory tubules of the human bronchial submucosal glands. Thorax 24:729–736, 1969.
36. Lamb D, Reid L: Histochemical and autoradiographic investigation of the serous cells of the human bronchial glands. J Pathol 100:127–138, 1970.
37. Spicer SS, Chakrin LW, Wardell JR, Kendrick W: Histochemistry of mucosubstances in the canine and human respiratory tract. Lab Invest 25:483–490, 1971.
38. Mason DY, Taylor CR: The distribution of muramidase (lysozyme) in human tissues. J Clin Pathol 28:124–132, 1975.
39. Klockars M, Reitamo S: Tissue distribution of lysozyme in man. J Histochem Cytochem 23:932–940, 1975.
40. Bowes D, Corrin B: Ultrastructural immunocytochemical localization of lysozyme in human bronchial glands. Thorax 32:163–170, 1977.
41. Mooren HWD, Meyer CJL, Kramps JA, et al.: Ultrastructural localization of the low molecular weight protease inhibitor in

human bronchial glands. J Histochem Cytochem 30:1130–1134, 1982.
42. Tourville DR, Adler RH, Bienenstock J, et al.: The human secretory immunoglobulin system, immunohistological localization of γA, secretory "piece" and lactoferrin in normal human tissues. J Exp Med 129:411–429, 1969.
43. Meyrick B, Reid L: Ultrastructure of the cells in the human submucosal glands. J Anat 167:281–299, 1970.
44. Matsuba K, Takizawa T, Thurlbeck WM: Oncocytes in human bronchial mucous glands. Thorax 27:181–184, 1972.
45. Martinez-Tello FJ, Braun DG, Blanc WA: Immunoglobulin production in bronchial mucosa and lymph nodes particularly in cystic fibrosis of the pancreas. J Immunol 101:989–1003, 1968.
46. Goodman MR, Link DW, Brown WR, Nakane PK: Ultrastructural evidence of transport of secretory IgA across bronchial epithelium. Am Rev Respir Dis 123:115–119, 1981.
47. Cutz E: Neuroendocrine cells of the lung. An overview of morphologic characteristics and development. Exp Lung Res 3:185–208, 1982.
48. Tateishi R: Distribution of argyrophil cells in adult human lungs. Arch Pathol 96:196 200, 1973.
49. Gmelich JT, Bensch KG, Liebow AA: Cells of Kultschitzky type in bronchioles and their relation to the origin of peripheral carcinoid tumor. Lab Invest 17:88–98, 1967.
50. Hage E: The morphological development of the pulmonary epithelium of human fetuses studied by light and electron microscopy. Z Anat Entwicklungs Gesch 140:271–279, 1973.
51. Hage E, Hage J, Juel G: Endocrine-like cells of the pulmonary epithelium of the human adult lung. Cell Tissue Res 178:39–48, 1977.
52. Bensch KG, Gordon GB, Miller LR: Studies on the bronchial counterpart of the Kultschitzky (Argentaffin) cell and innervation of bronchial glands. J Ultrastruct Res 12:668–686, 1965.
53. Lauweryns JM, Goddeoris P: Neuroepithelial bodies in the human child and adult lung. Am Rev Respir Dis 111:469–476, 1975.
54. Lauweryns JM, Cokelaere M, Theunynck P: Serotonin producing neuroepithelial bodies in rabbit respiratory mucosa. Science 180:410, 1973.
55. Hung K, Hertweck MS, Hardy JD, Loosli GH: Ultrastructure of nerves and associated cells in bronchiolar epithelium of the mouse lung. J Ultrastruct Res 43:426–437, 1973.
56. Hage E: Amine handling properties of APUD cells in the bronchial epithelium of human foetuses and in the epithelium of the main bronchi of human adults. Acta Pathol Microbiol Scand [A] 81:64, 1973.
57. Pearse AGE: The cytochemistry and ultrastructure of polypeptide-hormone-producing cells of the APUD series and the embryologic, physiologic and pathologic implications of the concept. J Histochem Cytochem 17:303, 1969.
58. Becker KL, Monaghan KG, Silva DL: Immunocytochemical localization of calcitonin in Kulchitscky cells of human lung. Arch Pathol Lab Med 104:196–198, 1980.
59. Cutz E, Chan W, Track NS: Bombesin, calcitonin and leuenkephalin immunoreactivity in endocrine cells of human lung. Experientia 37:765–767, 1981.
60. Hage E: Electron microscopic identification of several types of endocrine cells in the bronchial epithelium of human fetuses. Z Zellforsch 141:401–412, 1973.
61. Lauweryns JM, Cokelaere M: Hypoxia sensitive neuroepithelial bodies: Intrapulmonary secretory neuroreceptors modulated by the CNS. Z Zellforsch 145:521–540, 1973.
62. Lauweryns JM, Cokelaere M, Deleersnyder M, Liebens M: Intrapulmonary neuroepithelial bodies in newborn rabbits. Influence of hypoxia, hyperoxia, hypercapnea, nicotine, reserpine, L-DOPA and 5-HTP. Cell Tissue Res 182:425–440, 1977.
63. Lauweryns JM, Cokelaere M, Lerut T, Theunynck P: Cross-circulation studies on the influence of hypoxia and hypoxemia on neuroepithelial bodies in young rabbits. Cell Tissue Res 193:373–386, 1978.
64. Fishman AP: Hypoxia on the pulmonary circulation. How and where it acts. Circ Res 38:221–231, 1976.
65. Moosavi H, Smith P, Heath D: The Feyrter cell in hypoxia. Thorax 28:729–741, 1973.
66. Clara M: Zur Histobiologie des Bronchialepithels. Z Mikrosk Anat Forsch 41:321–347, 1937.
67. Ebert RV, Terracio MJ: The bronchiolar epithelium in cigarette smokers. Observations with the scanning electron microscope. Am Rev Respir Dis 111:4, 1975.
68. Cutz E, Conen PE: Ultrastructure and cytochemistry of Clara cells. Am J Pathol 62:127–134, 1971.
69. Kuhn C, Callaway LA, Askin FB: The formation of granules in the bronchiolar Clara cells of the rat. 1. Electron microscopy. J Ultrastruct Res 49:387–400, 1974.
70. Basset F, Poirier J, LeCrom M, Turiaf J: Elude ultrastructurale de l'epithelium bronchiolaire humain. Z Zellforsch 116:425, 1971.
71. Macklem PT, Proctor DF, Hogg JC: The stability of peripheral airways. Respir Physiol 8:191–203, 1970.
72. Gil J, Weibel ER: Extracellular lining of bronchioles after perfusion fixation of rat lung for electron microscopy. Anat Rec 169:185–199, 1971.
73. Ebert RV, Terracio MG: Observations of the secretion on the surface of the bronchioles with the scanning electron microscope. Am Rev Respir Dis 112:491–496, 1975.
74. Ebert RV, Kronenberg RS, Terracio MJ: Study of the surface secretion of the bronchiole using autoradiography. Am Rev Respir Dis 114:567–574, 1976.
75. Singh G, Katyal SL, Ward SM, et al.: Secretory proteins of the lung in rodents. J Histochem Cytochem 33:564–568, 1985.
76. Evans MJ, Cabral-Anderson LJ, Freeman G: The role of the Clara cell in renewal of the bronchiolar epithelium. Lab Invest 38:648–653, 1978.
77. Reid WD, Ilett KF, Glick JM, Krisha G: Metabolism and binding of aromatic hydrocarbons in the lung. Relationship to experimental bronchiolar necrosis. Am Rev Respir Dis 107:539–551, 1973.
78. Mahvi D, Bank H, Harley R: Morphology of a naphthalene-induced bronchiolar lesion. Am J Pathol 86:559–572, 1977.
79. Serabjit-Singh CJ, Wolf CR, Philpot RM, Plopper CG: Cytochrome P-450: Localization in rabbit lung. Science 207:1469–1470, 1980.
80. Boyd MR, Statham CN, Longo NS: The pulmonary Clara cell as a target for toxic chemicals requiring metabolic activation. Studies with carbon tetrachloride. J Pharmacol Exp Ther 212:109–114, 1980.
81. Devereux TR, Jones KG, Bend JR, et al.: In vitro metabolic activation of the pulmonary toxin 4-ipomeanol in non-ciliated bronchiolar epithelial (Clara) cells and alveolar type II cells isolated from rabbit lung. J Pharmacol Exp Ther 220:223–227, 1982.
82. Boyden EA: The structure of the pulmonary acinus in a child of six years and eight months. Am J Anat 132:275–300, 1971.

83. Pump KK: Morphology of the acinus of the human lung. Dis Chest 56:126–134, 1969.

84. Schreider JP, Raabe OG: Structure of the human respiratory acinus. Am J Anat 162:221–232, 1981.

85. Parker H, Horsefield K, Cumming G: Morphology of distal airways in the human lung. J Appl Physiol 31:386–391, 1971.

86. Pierce JA, Ebert RV: Fibrous network of the lung and its change with age. Thorax 20:469–476, 1965.

87. Whimster WF: The microanatomy of the alveolar duct system. Thorax 25:141–149, 1975.

88. Young CD, Moore CW, Hutchins GM: Connective tissue arrangement in respiratory airways. Anat Rec 198:245–254, 1980.

89. Sobin SS, Tremer HM, Fung YC: Morphometric basis of the sheet-flow concept of the pulmonary alveolar microcirculation in the cat. Circ Res 26:397–414, 1970.

90. Bateman E, Turner-Warwick M, Adelmann-Grill BC: Immunohistochemical study of collagen types in human foetal lung and fibrotic lung disease. Thorax 36:645–653, 1981.

91. Konomi H, Hori H, Sano J, et al.: Immunohistochemical localization of type I, II, III and IV collagens in the lung. Acta Pathol Jpn 31:601–610, 1981.

92. Weibel ER, Knight BW: A morphometric study on the thickness of the pulmonary air-blood barrier. J Cell Biol 21:367, 1964.

93. Weibel ER, Gil J: Structure-function relationships at the alveolar level. In West JB (ed): *Bioengineering Aspects of the Lung*. New York: Marcel Dekker, 1977, pp 1–81.

94. Crapo JD, Barry BE, Gehr P, et al.: Cell number and cell characteristics of the normal human lung. Am Rev Respir Dis 126:332–337, 1982.

95. Macklin CC: The pulmonary alveolar mucoid film and the pneumonocytes. Lancet 266:1099, 1954.

96. Low FN: The pulmonary alveolar epithelium of laboratory mammals and man. Anat Rec 117:241, 1953.

97. Haies DW, Gil J, Weibel ER: Morphometric study of rat lung cells. 1. Numerical and dimensional characteristics of parenchymal cell populations. Am Rev Respir Dis 123:533–541, 1981.

98. Askin FB, Kuhn C: The cellular origin of pulmonary surfactant. Lab Invest 25:260–268, 1971.

99. Kikkawa Y, Yoneda K, Smith F, et al.: The type II epithelial cells of the lung. II. Chemical composition and phospholipid synthesis. Lab Invest 32:295–302, 1975.

100. Mason RJ, Dobbs LG, Greenleaf RD, Williams MC: Alveolar type II cells. Fed Proc 36:2697–2702, 1977.

101. Evans MJ, Cabral LJ, Stephens RJ, Freeman G: Renewal of alveolar epithelium in the rat following exposure to NO_2. Am J Pathol 70:175, 1973.

102. Evans MJ, Cabral LJ, Stephens RJ, Freeman G: Transformation of alveolar type 2 cells into type 1 cells following exposure to NO_2. Exp Mol Pathol 22:142–150, 1975.

103. Terry RJ: On the presence of fluid in the pulmonary alveoli. J Mo State Med Assoc 17:40–41, 1920.

104. Von Neergaard K: Neue Auffassungen uber einen Grundbegriff der Atemtechnik. Die Retraktionskraft der Lunge, abhangig von der Oberfachensspannung in der Alveolen. Z Gesampte Exp Med 66:373–394, 1929.

105. Kuhn C, Finke EH: The topography of the pulmonary alveolus: Scanning electron microscopy using different fixations. J Ultrastruct Res 38:161–173, 1972.

106. Assimacopoulos A, Guggenheim R, Kapanci Y: Changes in alveolar capillary configuration at different levels of lung inflation in the rat. An ultrastructural and morphometric study. Lab Invest 34:10–22, 1976.

107. Sanderson RJ, Paul GW, Vatter AE, Filley GF: Morphological and physical basis for lung surfactant action. Respir Physiol 27:379–392, 1976.

108. Clements JA, Hustead RF, Johnson RP, Gribetz I: Pulmonary surface tension and alveolar stability. J Appl Physiol 16:444–450, 1961.

109. King RJ, Clements JA: Surface active materials from dog lung. II. Composition and physiological correlates. Am J Physiol 223:715–726, 1972.

110. Van Golde LMG: Metabolism of phospholipids in the lung. Am Rev Respir Dis 114:977–1000, 1976.

111. Gil J, Reiss OK: Isolation and characterization of lamellar bodies and tubular myelin from rat lung homogenates. J Cell Biol 58:152–171, 1973.

112. Mason RJ, Dobbs LG: Synthesis of phosphatidylcholine and phosphatidylglycerol by alveolar type II cells in primary culture. J Biol Chem 255:5101–5107, 1980.

113. Williams MC, Benson BJ: Immunocytochemical localization and identification of the major surfactant protein in adult rat lung. J Histochem Cytochem 29:291–305, 1981.

114. Oyarzum MG, Clements JA: Control of lung surfactant by ventilation adrenergic mediators and prostaglandins in the rabbit. Am Rev Respir Dis 117:879–891, 1978.

115. Vaccaro CA, Brody JS: Structural features of alveolar wall basement membrane in the adult rat lung. J Cell Biol 91:427–437, 1981.

116. Huang TW: Composite epithelial and endothelial basal laminas in human lungs. Am J Pathol 93:681–692, 1978.

117. Kapanci Y, Assimacopoulos A, Irle C, et al.: Contractile interstitial cells in pulmonary alveolar septa: A possible regulator of ventilation-perfusion ratio. Ultrastructural, immunofluorescence and in vitro studies. J Cell Biol 60:375–392, 1974.

118. Bartels H: Freeze fracture demonstration of communicating junctions between interstitial cells of the pulmonary alveolar septa. Am J Anat 155:125–129, 1979.

119. Inoue S, Michel RP, Hogg JC: Zonulae occludentes in alveolar epithelium and capillary endothelium of dog lungs studied with the freeze-fracture technique. J Ultrastruct Res 56:215–225, 1976.

120. Ryan US: Structural bases for metabolic activity. Annu Rev Physiol 44:223–239, 1982.

121. Macklem PT: Airway obstruction and collateral ventilation. Physiol Rev 51:368–436, 1971.

122. Takaro T, Price HP, Parra SC, Gaddy LR: Ultrastructural studies of apertures in the interalveolar septum of the adult human lung. Am Rev Respir Dis 119:425–434, 1979.

123. Cordingly JL: Pores of Kohn. Thorax 27:433–441, 1972.

124. Weibel ER: The mystery of "non-nucleated plates" in the alveolar epithelium of the lung explained. Acta Anat 78:425–443, 1971.

125. Martin HB: The effect of aging on the alveolar pores of Kohn in the dog. Am Rev Respir Dis 88:773–778, 1963.

126. Pump KK: Emphysema and its relation to age. Am Rev Respir Dis 114:5–13, 1976.

127. Terry PB, Traystman RJ, Newball HH, et al.: Collateral ventilation in man. N Engl J Med 298:10–15, 1978.

128. Hocking WG, Golde DW: Pulmonary alveolar macrophage. N Engl J Med 301:580, 638, 1979.

129. Dannenberg AM, Burstone MS, Walter PC, Kinsley JW: A histochemical study of phagocytic and enzymatic functions of rabbit mononuclear and polymorphonuclear exudate cells and

alveolar macrophages. 1. Survey and quantitation of enzymes and states of cellular activation. J Cell Biol 17:465–486, 1963.

130. Oren R, Farnham AE, Saito K, et al.: Metabolic patterns in three types of phagocytizing cells. J Cell Biol 17:487–501, 1963.

131. Liu J, Simon LM, Phillips JR, Robins ED: Superoxide dismutase (SOD) activity in hypoxic mammalian systems. J Appl Physiol 42:107–110, 1977.

132. Rister M, Baehner RL: A comparative study of superoxide dismutase activity in polymorphonuclear leukocytes, monocytes, and alveolar macrophages of the guinea pig. J Cell Physiol 87:345–356, 1976.

133. Simon LM, Robin ED, Phillips JR, et al.: Enzymatic basis for bioenergetic differences of alveolar versus peritoneal macrophages and enzyme regulation by molecular O_2. J Clin Invest 59:443–448, 1977.

134. Masse R, Fritsch P, Nolibe D, Sedaghat B: Evaluation quantitative et homeostasie de la population des macrophages alveolaires. Pathol Biol 23:464–469, 1975.

135. Pinkett MO, Cowdrey CR, Nowell PC: Mixed hematopoietic and pulmonary origin of alveolar macrophages as demonstrated by chromosome markers. Am J Pathol 48:859–867, 1966.

136. Brunstetter M-A, Hardie JA, Schiff R, et al.: The origin of pulmonary alveolar macrophages. Arch Intern Med 127:1064, 1971.

137. Godleski JJ, Brain JD: The origin of alveolar macrophages in mouse radiation chimeras. J Exp Med 136:630, 1972.

138. Golde DW, Finley TN, Cline MJ: The pulmonary macrophages in acute leukemia. N Engl J Med 290:875–878, 1974.

139. Lin H-S, Kuhn C, Chen DM: Effects of hydrocortisone acetate on pulmonary alveolar macrophage colony-forming cells. Am Rev Respir Dis 125:712–715, 1982.

140. Bowden DH, Adamson IYR, Grantham WG, Wyatt JP: Origin of the lung macrophage evidence derived from radiation injury. Arch Pathol 88:540, 1969.

141. Bowden DH, Adamson YR: The alveolar macrophage delivery system kinetic studies in cultured explants of murine lung. Am J Pathol 83:123, 1976.

142. Lin HS, Kuhn C, Kuo TT: Clonal growth of hamster free alveolar cells in soft agar. J Exp Med 142:877–886, 1975.

143. Byrne PV, Guilbert LS, Stanley ER: Distribution of cells bearing receptors for a colony stimulating factor (CSF-1) in murine tissues. J Cell Biol 91:848–853, 1981.

144. Evans MJ, Cabral LJ, Stephens RJ, Freeman G: Cell division of alveolar macrophages in rat lung following exposure to NO_2. Am J Pathol 70:119, 1973.

145. Van Oud Ablas AB, Van Furth R: Origin, kinetics and characteristics of pulmonary macrophages in the normal steady states. J Exp Med 149:1504–1518, 1979.

146. Bowden DH, Adamson IYR: The role of monocytes and interstitial cells in the generation of alveolar macrophages. I. Kinetic studies in normal mice. Lab Invest 42:511–517, 1980.

147. Green GM, Kass EH: The role of the alveolar macrophage in the clearance of bacteria from the lung. J Exp Med 119:167, 1964.

148. Lipscomb MF, Toews GB, Lyons CR, Uhr JW: Antigen presentation by guinea pig alveolar macrophages. J Immunol 126:286–291, 1981.

149. Unanue ER: Secretory function of mononuclear phagocytes. Am J Pathol 83:396–417, 1976.

150. Horowitz AL, Crystal RG: Collagenase from rabbit pulmonary alveolar macrophages. Biochem Biophys Res Commun 69:296–303, 1976.

151. Horowitz AL, Kelman JA, Crystal RG: Activation of alveolar macrophage collagenase by a neutral protease secreted by the same cell. Nature 264:772–774, 1976.

152. Marom Z, Weinberg KS, Fanburg BL: Effect of bleomycin on collagenolytic activity of the rat alveolar macrophage. Am Rev Respir Dis 121:859–867, 1980.

153. White RR, Lin HS, Kuhn C: Elastase secretion by mouse peritoneal exudative and alveolar macrophages. J Exp Med 146:802–807, 1977.

154. Green MR, Lin JG, Berman LB, et al.: Elastolytic activity of alveolar macrophages in normal dogs and human subjects. J Lab Clin Med 94:549–562, 1979.

155. White R, Lee D, Habicht GS, Janoff A: Secretion of alpha-1-proteinase inhibitor by cultured rat alveolar macrophages. Am Rev Respir Dis 123:447–449, 1981.

156. White R, Janoff A, Godfrey HP: Secretion of alpha 2 macroglobulin by human alveolar macrophages. Lung 158:9, 1980.

157. White R, Habicht GS, Godfrey HP, et al.: Secretion of elastase and alpha-2-macroglobulin by cultured peritoneal exudative macrophages. J Lab Clin Med 97:718–729, 1981.

158. Leibovich SJ: Production of macrophage dependent fibroblast stimulating activity (M-FSA) by murine macrophages. Exp Cell Res 113:47–56, 1978.

159. Bitterman PB, Rennard SI, Hunninghake GW, Crystal RG: Human alveolar macrophage growth factor for fibroblasts. Regulation and partial characterization. J Clin Invest 70:806–822, 1982.

160. Clark JG, Kostal KM, Marino BA: Bleomycin induced pulmonary fibrosis in hamsters. An alveolar macrophage product increases fibroblast prostaglandin E_2 and cyclic adenosine monophosphate and suppresses fibroblast proliferation and collagen production. J Clin Invest 72:2082–2091, 1983.

161. Golde DW, Finley TN, Cline MJ: Production of colony stimulating factor by human macrophages. Lancet 2:1397, 1972.

162. Unanue ER, Beller DI, Calderon J, et al.: Regulation of immunity and inflammation by mediators from macrophages. Am J Pathol 85:465, 1976.

163. Merrill WW, Naegel GP, Matthay RA, Reynolds HY: Alveolar macrophage-derived chemotactic factor. J Clin Invest 65:268–276, 1980.

164. Hsueh W, Kuhn C, Needleman P: Relationship of prostaglandin secretion by rabbit alveolar macrophages to phagocytosis and enzyme release. Biochem J 184:345–354, 1979.

165. Scott WA, Pawlowski NA, Murray HW, et al.: Regulation of arachidonic acid metabolism by macrophage activation. J Exp Med 155:1148–1160, 1982.

166. Rouzer CA, Scott WA, Hamill AL, Cohn ZA: Dynamics of leukotriene production by macrophages. J Exp Med 152:1236–1247, 1980.

167. Hsueh W, Sun FF: Leukotriene B_4 biosynthesis by alveolar macrophages. Biochem Biophys Res Commun 106:1085–1091, 1982.

168. Kolot FB, Baron S, Yeager H, Schwartz SL: Comparative production of interferon by explanted lymphoreticular tissue and alveolar macrophages from rabbits and humans. Infect Immun 13:63–68, 1976.

169. Villiger B, Kelley DG, Engleman W, et al.: Human alveolar macrophage fibronectin: Synthesis secretion and ultrastructural localization during gelatin latex binding. J Cell Biol 90:711–720, 1981.

170. Rennard SI, Hunninghake GW, Bitterman PB, Crystal RG: Production of fibronectin by the human alveolar macrophage: Mechanism for the recruitment of fibroblasts to sites of tissue

injury in interstitial lung diseases. Proc Natl Acad Sci USA 78:7147–7151, 1981.

171. Drath DR, Karnovsky ML: Superoxide production by phagocytic leukocytes. J Exp Med 141:257–262, 1975.

172. Hoidal JR, Beall GD, Repine JE: Production of hydroxyl radical by human alveolar macrophages. Infect Immun 26:1088–1092, 1979.

173. Hoidal JR, Fov RB, LeMarbe PA, et al.: Oxidative metabolism of alveolar macrophages from young asymptomatic cigarette smokers. Increased superoxide anion release and its potential consequences. Chest 77:2705, 1980.

174. Jackett PS, Andrew PW, Aber VR, Lowrie DB: Hydrogen peroxide and superoxide release by alveolar macrophages from normal and BCG vaccinated guinea pigs after intravenous challenge with mycobacterium tuberculosis. Br J Exp Pathol 62:419–428, 1981.

175. Brenner O: Pathology of the vessels of the pulmonary circulation. Arch Intern Med 56:211–237, 1935.

176. Heath D, Best PV: The tunica media of the arteries of the lung in pulmonary hypertension. J Pathol Bacteriol 76:165–74, 1959.

177. Granston AS: Morphologic alterations of the pulmonary arteries in congenital heart disease. Proc Inst Med Chic 22:116–117, 1958.

178. Wagenvoort CA: Vasoconstriction and medial hypertrophy in pulmonary hypertension. Circulation 22:535–546, 1960.

179. Elliott FM, Reid L: Some new facts about the pulmonary artery and its branching pattern. Clin Radiol 16:193–198, 1965.

180. Wagenvoort CA, Wagenvoort N: *Pathology of Pulmonary Hypertension*. New York: John Wiley & Sons, 1977.

181. Smith P, Heath D, Mooi W: Observations on some ultrastructural features of normal pulmonary blood vessels in collapsed and distended lungs. J Anat 128:85–96, 1978.

182. Dingemans KP, Wagenvoort CA: Ultrastructural study of contraction of pulmonary vascular smooth muscle cells. Lab Invest 35:205–212, 1976.

183. Smith P, Heath D: Evagination of vascular smooth muscle cells during the early stages of Crotalaria pulmonary hypertension. J Pathol 124:177–183, 1978.

184. Mooi W, Smith P, Heath D: The ultrastructural effects of acute decompression on the lung of rats: The influence of frusemide. J Pathol 126:189–196, 1978.

185. Smith P, Heath D, Padula F: Evagination of smooth muscle cells in the hypoxic pulmonary trunk. Thorax 33:31–42, 1978.

186. Smith U, Ryan JW, Mitchie DD, Smith DS: Endothelial projections as revealed by scanning electron microscopy. Science 173:925–926, 1971.

187. Schneeberger EE: Segmental differentiation of endothelial intercellular junctions in the intraacinar arteries and veins of the rat lung. Circ Res 49:1102–1111, 1981.

188. Beusch KG, Gordon GB, Miller L: Fibrillar structures resembling leiomyfibrils in endothelial cells of mammalian pulmonary blood vessels. Z Zellforsch 63:759–766, 1964.

189. Weibel ER, Palade GE: New cytoplasmic components in arterial endothelia. J Cell Biol 23:101–112, 1964.

190. O'Neill JF: The effects on venous endothelium of alterations in blood flow through vessels in vein walls and the possible relation to thrombosis. Ann Surg 126:270–288, 1947.

191. Samuels PB, Samuels BM, Webster DR: New techniques in the study of venous endothelium. Lab Invest 1:50–60, 1952.

192. Lautsch EV, McMillan GC, Duff GL: Techniques for the study of the normal and atherosclerotic arterial intima from its endothelial surface. Lab Invest 2:397–407, 1953.

193. McGovern VJ: Reactions to injury of vascular endothelium with special reference to the problem of thrombosis. J Pathol Bacteriol 283–293, 1955.

194. Poole JCF, Saunders AG, Florey HW: The regeneration of aortic endothelium. J Pathol Bacteriol 75:133–143, 1958.

195. Kibria G, Heath D, Smith P, Biggar R: Pulmonary endothelial pavement patterns. Thorax 35:186–191, 1980.

196. Kombe AH, Smith P, Heath D, Biggar R: Endothelial pavement pattern in the pulmonary trunk in rats in chronic hypoxia. Br J Dis Chest 74:362–368, 1980.

197. Cotton R, Wartman WB: Endothelial patterns in human arteries. Arch Pathol 71:3–12, 1961.

198. Helliwell T, Smith P, Heath D: Endothelial pavement patterns in human arteries. J Pathol 136:227–240, 1982.

199. Gau GS, Ryder TA, MacKenzie ML: The effect of blood flow on the surface morphology of the human endothelium. J Pathol 131:55–64, 1980.

200. Ryan US: Structural bases for metabolic activity. Annu Rev Physiol 44:223–239, 1982.

201. Strum JM, Junod AF: Radioautographic demonstration of 5-hydroxytryptamine-^{3}H uptake by pulmonary endothelial cells. J Cell Biol 54:456–467, 1972.

202. Nicholas TE, Strum JM, Angelo LS, Junod AF: Site and mechanism of uptake of ^{3}H-1-norepinephrine by isolated perfused rat lungs. Circ Res 35:670–680, 1974.

203. Trapnell DH: The peripheral lymphatics of the lung. Br J Radiol 36:660–672, 1963.

204. Lauweryns JM: The blood and lymphatic microcirculation of the lung. Pathol Annu 6:365–415, 1971.

205. Lauweryns JM, Baert JH: Alveolar clearance and the role of the pulmonary lymphatics. Am Rev Respir Dis 115:625–683, 1977.

206. Lauweryns JM, Baert JH: The role of the pulmonary lymphatics in the defenses of the distal lung. Morphological and experimental studies of the transport mechanisms of intratracheally instillated particles. Ann NY Acad Sci 221:244–275, 1974.

207. Lauweryns JM, Baert J, DeLoecker W: Fine filaments in lymphatic endothelial cells. J Cell Biol 68:163–167, 1976.

208. Emery JL, Dinsdale F: The postnatal development of lymphoreticular aggregates and lymph nodes in infant's lungs. J Clin Pathol 26:539–545, 1973.

209. Trapnell DH: Recognition and incidence of intrapulmonary lymph nodes. Thorax 19:44–50, 1964.

210. Richardson JB: Nerve supply to the lungs. Am Rev Respir Dis 119:785–802, 1979.

211. Larsell O: The ganglia, plexuses and nerve terminations of the mammalian lung and pleura pulmonalis. J Comp Neurol 35:97–132, 1922.

212. Spencer H, Leof D: The innervation of the human lung. J Anat 98:599–609, 1964.

213. Fox B, Bull TB, Guz A: Innervation of alveolar walls in the human lung: An electron microscopic study. J Anat 131:683, 1980.

214. Sant'Ambrogio G: Information arising from the tracheobronchial tree of mammals. Physiol Rev 62:531–569, 1982.

215. Fillenz M, Widdicome JG: Receptors of the lungs and airways. In Neil E (ed): *Handbook of Sensory Physiology*, vol. 3. New York: Springer Verlag, 1972, p 81.

216. Jeffery PK: The innervation of bronchial mucosa. In Cumming G, Bonsignore G (eds): *Cellular Biology of the Lung*. New York: Plenum, 1982, pp 1–32.

217. Polak JM, Bloom SR: Regulatory peptides and neuron-

specific enolase in the respiratory tract of man and other mammals. Exp Lung Res 3:313–328, 1982.

218. Krahl VE: The glomus pulmonale: Its location and microscopic anatomy. In de Reuck AVS, O'Connor M (eds): *Ciba Foundation Symposium on Pulmonary Structure and Function*. Boston: Little, Brown, 1962, pp 53–69.

219. Blessing MH, Hora BI: Glomera in der Lunge des Menschen. Z Zellforsch 87:562–570, 1968.

220. Coleridge H, Coleridge JCG, Howe A: A search for pulmonary arterial chemoreceptors in the cat, with a comparison of the blood supply of the aortic bodies in the newborn and adult animal. J Physiol 191:353–374, 1967.

221. Uddman R, Alumets J, Densert R, et al.: Occurrence and distribution of VIP nerves in the nasal mucosa and tracheobronchial wall. Acta Otolaryngol 86:443–448, 1978.

222. El-Bermani Al-WI, Grant M: Acetyl cholinesterase positive nerves of the rhesus monkey bronchial tree. Thorax 30:162–170, 1975.

223. Richardson J, Beland J: Nonadrenergic inhibitory nervous system in human airways. J Appl Physiol 41:764–771, 1976.

224. Richardson JB: The innervation of the lung. Eur J Respir Dis 63(Suppl):14–31, 1982.

225. Doidge JM, Satchell DG: Adrenergic and non-adrenergic inhibitory nerves in mammalian airways. J Auton Nerv Syst 5:83–99, 1982.

226. Dey RD, Shannon WA, Said SI: Localization of VIP-immunoreactive nerves in airways and pulmonary vessels of dogs, cats, and human subjects. Cell Tissue Res 220:231–238, 1981.

227. Amenta F, Cavallotti C, Ferrante F, Tonelli F: Cholinergic innervation of the human pulmonary circulation. Acta Anat 117:58–64, 1983.

228. Legrand M, Pariente R, Andre J, et al.: Ultrastructure de la plèvre parietale humaine. Presse Med 79:2515–2520, 1970.

229. Wang NS: The regional difference of mesothelial cells in the pleural cavity of the rabbit. Am Rev Respir Dis 107:1115, 1973.

230. Miserocchi G, Agostoni E: Contents of the pleural space. J Appl Physiol 30:208–213, 1971.

231. Agostoni E, D'Angelo E, Roncoroni G: The thickness of the pleural liquid. Respir Physiol 5:1–13, 1968.

232. Wang NS: The performed stomas connecting the pleural cavity and the lymphatics in the parietal pleura. Am Rev Respir Dis 111:12–20, 1975.

233. Pinchon MC, Bernandin JF, Bignon J: Pleural permeability in the rat. 1. Ultrastructural basis. Biol Cell 37:269–272, 1980.

234. Thurlbeck WM: Chronic obstructive lung disease. In Sommers SC (ed): *Pathology Annual*. New York: Appleton-Century-Crofts, 1968, p 377.

235. Farrell PM (ed): *Lung Development: Biological and Clinical Perspectives*, vol 1. New York: Academic Press, 1982, p 44.

Additional Readings

De Water R, Willems LNA, VanMuijen GNP, et al.: Ultrastructural localization of bronchial antileukoprotease in central and peripheral human airways by a gold-labelling technique using monoclonal antibodies. Am Rev Respir Dis 133:882–890, 1986.

Fels AOF, Cohn ZA: The alveolar macrophage. J Appl Physiol 60:353–369, 1986.

Gail DB, Lenfant CJM: State of the art: Cells of the lung: Biology and clinical implications. Am Rev Respir Dis 127:366–387, 1983.

Nadel JA, Barnes PJ: Autonomic regulation of the airways. Annu Rev Med 35:451–468, 1984.

Pack RJ, Widdicombe JG: Amine-containing cells of the lung. Eur J. Respir. Dis. 65:559–578, 1984.

Ryan US, Ryan JW: Cell biology of pulmonary endothelium. Circulation 70(suppl III):42–46, 1984.

Uddman R, Lutz A, Sundler F: Occurrence and distribution of calcitonin-gene-related peptide in the mammalian respiratory tract and middle ear. Cell Tissue Res 241:551–555, 1985.

Uddman R, Moghimzadeh E, Sundler F: Occurrence and distribution of GRP-immunoreactive nerve fibers in the respiratory tract. Arch Otorhinolaryngol 239:145–151, 1984.

Weibel ER: *The Pathway for Oxygen*. Cambridge, MA: Harvard University Press, 1984.

Widdicombe JG, Pack RJ: The Clara cell. Eur J Respir Dis 63:202–220, 1982.

3 Quantitative Anatomy of the Lung

William M. Thurlbeck

Introduction

The quantitative structure of the lung is better known than that of any other internal organ, mainly because Weibel was primarily interested in it, and wrote a classic monograph on the subject.[1] Considerable information is available concerning the quantitative anatomy of the lung in many animal species, but this information has no relevance to this book and will not be covered here. Instead, this chapter summarizes the findings in the human lung that are relevant to the understanding of its structure and function. Readers interested in morphometric techniques are referred to the two standard monographs.[2,3]

The data from eight normal human lungs from six adult males and two females between 10 and 40 years of age[4] are shown in Table 3–1. The following should be noted concerning the data in that table. Total lung volumes are considerably (50 to 60 percent) smaller than would be predicted from total lung capacity plus volume of tissue, in life. In part, this is because fixed distended lung volumes are on the average about 10 percent less than the maximum volumes inside the chest in living subjects and about 30 percent smaller than fresh, excised lungs maximally inflated.[5] These factors cannot account for this large discrepancy and it is not clear why the volumes are so small in this particular study. Thus the absolute dimensions that are quoted are probably underestimates with the exception of the measurements of alveolar surface area which were recorded using an electron microscope. These values are roughly double the values of alveolar surface area using light microscopy.[6] The light microscope measurements may be the more relevant ones. As indicated in Chapter 2, alveoli are lined by surfactant and a hypophase and these render the surface of the alveoli smooth. Much of the increase in surface area as assessed electron microscopically is due to surface irregularities.

Airways

Conceptually, airways can be divided into three categories:

1. The conducting zone, in which there is no gas exchange. This consists of bronchi and (membranous) bronchioles (see Chapter 2) that have no gas exchanging epithelium (alveoli).
2. The transitional zone that both conducts air and exchanges gas. These airways have both gas exchanging and non-gas-exchanging epithelium in their walls, and consist of respiratory bronchioles.
3. The gas exchanging zone that consists of the alveolated airways (alveolar ducts and sacs).

The precise dimensions of these structures are not known, but reasonable estimates can be made. Until the great thrust of applied pulmonary physiology of the 1950s and 1960s, the details did not seem important and Weibel's work was largely stimulated by the need for such data for structure-functional correlative studies. Another reason for the relative paucity of data is the extreme difficulty of obtaining accurate data. For example, the most useful data on airway dimensions and branching came from an investigation lasting several years, using the cast of one lung.[7]

Conducting Airways

The conducting airways have to reach a compromise between two conflicting requirements. Low resistance to flow has a mechanical advantage and is best achieved by short, large-caliber airways, but a small dead space is

Table 3–1. Morphometric Data from Eight Normal Human Lungs[a]

Body weight	74 kg
Height	177 cm
Total lung volume	4,341 ml
Alveolar surface area	143 m²
Capillary surface area	126 m²
Capillary blood volume	213 ml
Air blood thickness	
Arithmetic mean	2.2 µm
Harmonic mean	0.62 µm

[a] Based on the results of Gehr et al.[4]

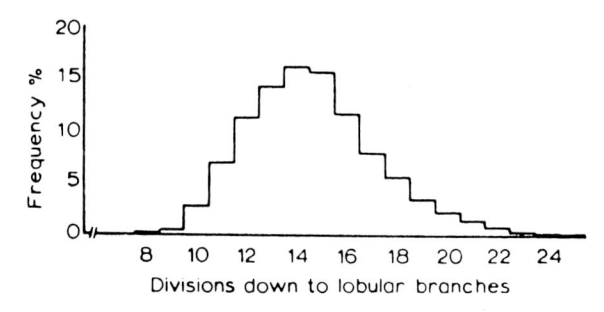

Figure 3–2. The number of generations "down" from the trachea to lobular bronchiole varies from 8 to 23 (from Horsfield and Cumming.[7])

required for better gas exchange and this requires that conducting airways have minimum volume. (Biologic requirements may be assisted by angular branching, cellular activity, and flexibility which protect the lung from the environment, and allow the lung to adapt to it.)

The most widely used model of airways is Weibel's model A of symmetric dichotomy[1] because of its simplicity and ease of use. However, this model has little to do with the real world, and the striking feature of human airways in most of the conducting zone is their striking asymmetry. Horsfield and Cumming have described a widely quoted and useful model.[7] They studied a cast of the airways, and defined the lobular bronchiole as the first airway less than 0.7 mm in diameter (in a lung with a volume of 5 L). They then counted "up" to the trachea from the lobular bronchiole in "orders" as well as "down" from the trachea in "generations" as is the usual custom. This distinction is not explicitly stated in their study but it is essential to grasp the concept of the difference between counting up and down. The term orders and generations are useful in this regard. When counting down, the trachea is generation 0, and the lobar bronchi generation 1. When counting up the lobular bronchiole is order 0, and the first order beyond it toward the trachea (up) is order 1. When airways of different orders meet, the next order gets its value from the higher of the order of the joining airways (e.g., if an order 2 airway meets an order 1, the succeeding order would be order 3). Horsfield and Cumming found that the number of airways of any given order could be calculated from the formula $n = 1.38^{25-u}$ where n is the number of airways of order u. If airways branch by symmetric dichotomy the number of airways would be predicted by the equation $n = 2^{25-u}$. The difference in n between the two equations represents the effect of asymmetric branching, and is large. For example, order 10 has 32,768 members by symmetric dichotomy; 125 by the Horsfield and Cumming equation. Because of asymmetric branching there is an enormous variation in distance and number of branches from carina to the lobular bronchiole (hence to the acinus). The longest distance, which is found in axial pathways, where the route to the acinus is closest to a straight line, was about 22 cm and there were 25 generations to the lobular bronchiole (Figs. 3–1 and 3–2). A lateral or spiral pathway is the shortest pathway to the acinus and, as the term indicates, the pathway, tends to be via angled airways branching toward the hilum. The shortest pathway from the carina to the lobular bronchiole was 7.7 cm, and it had seven generations (see Figs. 3–1 and 3–2).

The dimensions of conducting airways derived from the Horsfield and Cumming equations and other standard anatomic data are shown in Fig. 3–3. It should be noted that the length and cross-sectional area of *each* set of airways are drawn on a logarithmic scale. Some simplifications are, of course, necessary. The longest single pathway is the upper airway. The cross-sectional area of the trachea is 2 to 3 cm², but the narrowest part of the cross-sectional area of the airways is at about the level of segmental bronchi.[1] The increase in total cross-sectional area in the figure is not nearly as rapid as in the Weibel model and at order 0, at the proximal end of the lobular bronchiole, it is only 14 cm² as opposed to approximately 100 cm² in the Weibel model. Since there is symmetric dichotomy from the lobular bronchiole to the terminal bronchiole, there is a more rapid increase in cross-sectional area so that at the terminal bronchiole the cross-sectional area of the airways totals about 80 cm².

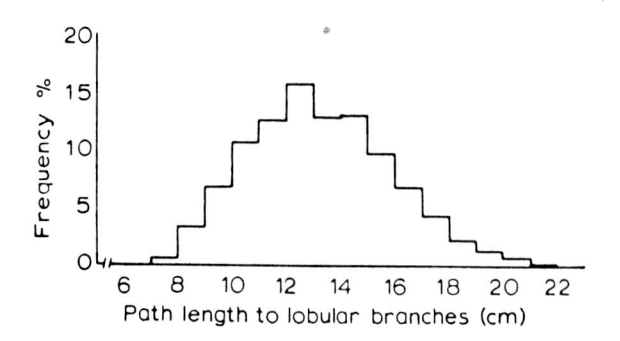

Figure 3–1. The distance from trachea to lobular bronchiole (the first membranous bronchiole less than 0.7 mm in diameter) varies from 7 to 21 cm. From Horsfield and Cumming.[7]

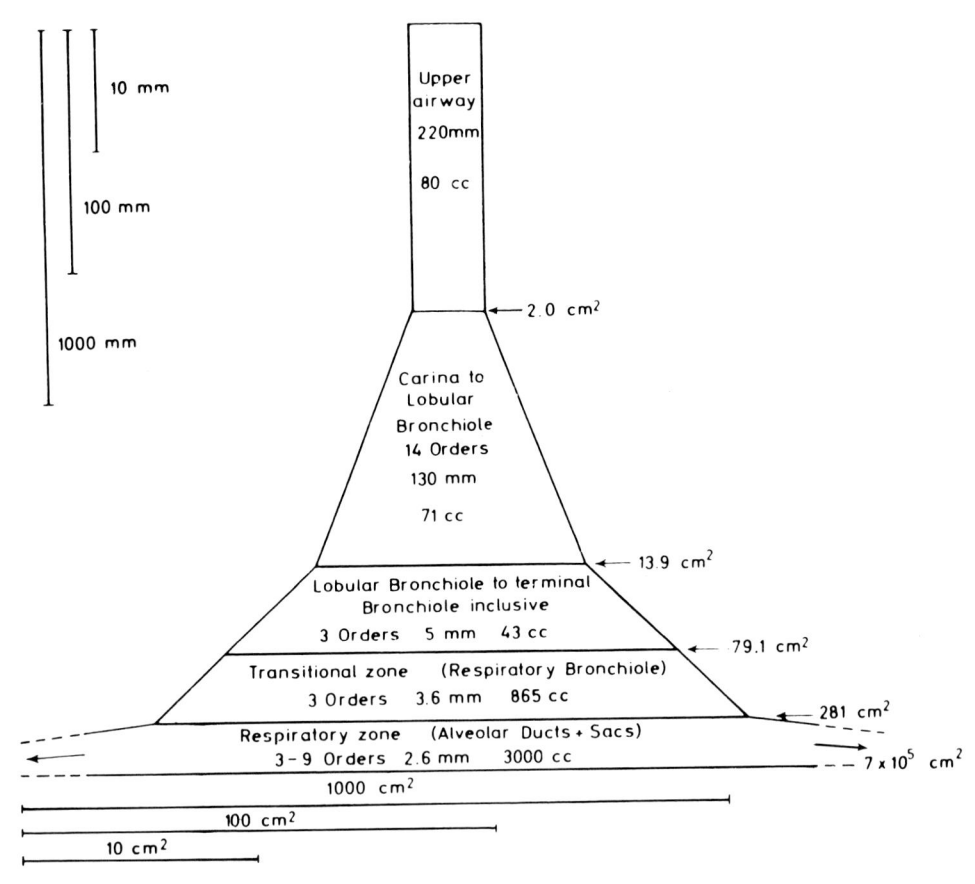

Figure 3–3. Dimensions of the airways in the lung as estimated from available data are illustrated in the diagram. From Thurlbeck.[21]

The Transitional Zone

This consists of respiratory bronchioles, or the proximal part of the acinus. Although there is no complete agreement between those who have reconstructed respiratory bronchioles,[8–12] the description of symmetric dichotomy of the three generations of respiratory bronchioles is generally accepted. With this model, the transition zone, though less than 4 mm long, has a volume of almost a liter. Thus it is in this zone that the "front" of inspired gas meets alveolar gas. For gas exchange to occur, gas must be transported in the conducting airways and then gas is exchanged by mixing beyond the front.

Respiratory Zone

This zone is the most difficult to study since the units are small and closely applied to each other. Thus, casts are hard to interpret. Serial sections of the lung are difficult to superimpose on each other so that completely accurate reconstructions are not possible. It is generally agreed that irregular dichotomy is the rule and it would appear that alveolar ducts and spaces fill up lung tissue as best they can during the phase of alveolar multiplication (see p. 7, Chapter 1). The described observations concerning this zone are quite similar.[8–12] Parker and co-workers found that alveolar sacs were three to eight generations beyond the most distal respiratory bronchiole.[12] The most notable feature of this zone is its short average length (3 mm), large number of units (23×10^6) and its large lung volume of about 3 L.

As indicated previously, estimates of alveolar surface area differ depending on whether they have been measured using light or electron microscopy. There is a wide variation in alveolar surface area as measured by light microscopy, with a range of 40 to 100 m^2 and an average of about 70 m^2.[6] Alveolar surface area is directly related to stature; the largest figure was that in the lung of a 188-cm male and the smallest figure in a 140-cm female.[6] Estimates of the total number of alveoli vary considerably, particularly in the older literature.[1] More recently a constant value of 300×10^6 has been suggested.[1] In our hands, however, the total number of alveoli has been extremely variable, with a range of 200 to 600×10^6, with an average of about 375×10^6. Like surface area, the total number of alveoli was directly related to stature.[13]

Number of Acini

As described in Chapter 2, acini are the unit gas exchanging structures of the lung, or the units distal to terminal bronchioles. Horsfield and Cumming calculated that there were 27,992 terminal bronchioles.[7] Radiologically the average acinus is 7.4 mm in diameter and approximately spherical, and thus there would be about 25,000 acini in a lung with a volume of 5.25 L.[14] Calculations from the number of bronchioles produced a similar number of acini.[15] It is not clear whether the number of acini varies with stature, but an indirect estimate of acinar number from bronchiolar count[15] suggested that the number of acini was constant and thus taller people with larger lungs would have larger acini. However, more recently we have shown that the radial count of Mithal and Emery (Chapter 7) is not related to stature in children,[16] suggesting that taller people with larger lungs have more acini.

Other Changes with Stature, Sex, and Age

Besides the changes described above, the dimensions of major and segmental bronchi are directly related to stature.[17] The number of bronchioles is thought to be the same in the lungs of different sizes so that this suggests that these airways also increase in size with stature.[15] The observation that dead space is related to stature would also suggest that all the conducting airways would be stature related.[18]

No study has been made of sex-related differences in adults. Since men have larger lungs than women for a given stature, this suggests that men have either more structures or larger structures per unit body length. Studies in children suggest that boys have more alveoli rather than larger alveoli when compared to girls of similar stature,[19] and the same may be true of men compared to women.

As discussed in Chapter 21, changes occur with age and these result in diminished surface area, increasing alveolar and alveolar duct size, and diminished alveolar number with age.

Pulmonary Arteries

Quantitation of the pulmonary arterial system is much more complex than of the airways, for several reasons. The smallest units, even excluding capillaries, are much smaller in arteries compared to airways. This makes arteries much more numerous and difficult to recognize. Also, pulmonary arteries have numerous lateral or accessory branches (see Chapter 2) that complicate analysis. Nonetheless a description has been made by Singhal and colleagues[20] using a cast of the pulmonary artery of a single subject, utilizing similar techniques to that used in the airways. In the arterial system it was only feasable to use orders to count "up" to the main pulmonary artery. They divided their cast and analysis into three zones—proximal, from the main pulmonary artery to the first branch less than 0.8 mm in diameter; intermediate, between 0.8 and 0.1 mm in diameter; distal, less than 0.1 mm in diameter. Reasonably complete data were obtained concerning the first, only a small sample of the second could be analyzed, and the data concerning the third were mostly conjectural. However, interesting information was produced. There were eight orders in the proximal zone, four in the intermediate, and five in the distal zone. The number of arteries in the lowest order of the distal zone (the smallest vessels) was 300×10^6; this figure was 1.57×10^5 in the lowest order of the intermediate zone, and 2.23×10^3 in the lowest order of the proximal zone. It is of interest to note that the total number of the smallest vessels was close to the total number of alveoli, suggesting that a single vessel supplied each alveolus. The total cross-sectional area of the arteries had some resemblance to that of the airways. In the main pulmonary artery, this was 7.07 cm^2 and then narrowed slightly at the subsegmental level. There was then a slight and gradual increase in cross-sectional area going "down" the orders beyond this. A very sudden increase of 43.85 to 398.2 cm^2 occurred between orders 2 and 1 in the peripheral zone. The functional significance of these measurements is related to the computed velocity; at the specific sites mentioned above this was 11.32 cm/s in the main pulmonary artery, 1.82 cm/s in order 2, and 0.20 cm/s in order 1. The huge cross-sectional area in the most distal arteries and the slow flow explain the facility for gas exchange in the lung.

The capillary network of the lung is most dense in the body and capillaries are best thought of as short cylinders that interconnect with each other to form hexagonal structures that share one or two common sides.[1] The number of segments is enormous, estimated at about 280×10^9,[1] and there are thus approximately one thousand segments per alveolus. Each segment has a length of about 12 μm and a diameter of about 8.5 μm. Consequences of these were shown in Table 3–1—capillary surface area is enormous and there is a large capillary blood volume. With the thin air-blood barrier, diffusion of gas from blood to air is rapid. It should be noted that the capillary dimensions represent the maximum possible. During life a relatively small proportion are open and may also be narrower. This accounts for the much greater morphologically determined diffusing capacity than that found by physiologic techniques.

References

1. Weibel ER: Morphometry of the Human Lung. New York: Academic Press, 1963.

2. Weibel ER: *Stereological Methods*. Volume 1, Practical Methods for Biological Morphometry, 1st ed., London: Academic Press, 1979.

3. Aherne WA, Dunnill MS: *Morphometry*, 1st ed. London: 1982.

4. Gehr P, Bachofen M, Weibel ER: The normal lung: Ultrastructure and morphometric estimation of diffusion capacity. Respir Physiol 32:121–140, 1978.

5. Berend N, Skoog C, Waszkiewicz E, Thurlbeck WM: Maxi-

mum volumes in excised human lungs: Effects of age, emphysema and formalin inflation. Thorax 35:859–864, 1980.

6. Thurlbeck WM: The internal surface area of nonemphysematous lungs. Am Rev Respir Dis 95:765, 1967.

7. Horsfield K, Cumming G: Morphology of the bronchial tree in man. J Appl Physiol 24:373–383, 1968.

8. Ogawa C: The finer ramifications of the human lung. Am J Anat 27:315–332, 1920.

9. Willson HG: The terminals of the human bronchiole. Am J Anat 30:267–295, 1922.

10. Pump KK: Morphology of the acinus of the human lung. Dis Chest 56:126–134, 1969.

11. Boyden EA: The structure of the pulmonary acinus in a child of six years and eight months. Am J Anat 132:275–299, 1972.

12. Parker H, Horsfield K, Cumming G: Morphology of distal airways in the human lung. J Appl Physiol 31:386–391, 1972.

13. Angus GE, Thurlbeck WM: Number of alveoli in the human lung. J Appl Physiol 32:483–485, 1972.

14. Gamsu G, Thurlbeck WM, Macklem PT, Fraser RG: Roentgenographic appearance of the human pulmonary acinus. Invest Radiol 6:171–175, 1971.

15. Matsuba K, Thurlbeck WM: The number and dimensions of small airways in nonemphysematous lungs. Am Rev Respir Dis 104:516–524, 1971.

16. Cooney TP, Thurlbeck WM: The radial alveolar count method of Emery and Mithal: A reappraisal I—Postnatal lung growth. Thorax 37:572–579, 1982.

17. Thurlbeck WM, Haines JR: Bronchial dimensions and stature. Annu Rev Respir Dis 112:142–145, 1975.

18. Radford E: Ventilation standards for use in artificial respiration. J Appl Physiol 7:451–460, 1955.

19. Thurlbeck WM: Postnatal human lung growth. Thorax 37:564–571, 1982.

20. Singhal S, Henderson R, Horsfield K, Harding K, et al: Morphology of the human pulmonary arterial tree. Circ Res 33:190–197, 1973.

21. Thurlbeck WM: The structure of the lungs. In Widdicombe JG (ed): *Physiology Series 1*, vol 2. *Respiratory Physiology*. London and Baltimore: Butterworths, University Park Press, 1974, pp 1–30.

4 Pulmonary Defense Mechanisms

James C. Hogg

Adult human beings breathe approximately 10,000 to 20,000 L of air daily in order to obtain the oxygen needed for their metabolic requirements. As this air can be contaminated with toxic gases and particles that may contain infectious agents, allergens, or other noxious material, it is imperative that the ventilatory system have efficient methods of defense.

Protection from Gaseous Injury

The purpose of ventilation is to obtain oxygen from the air to carry out the vital process of cellular respiration. During the course of evolution the gradual change from anaerobic to microaerophilic and then aerobic organisms was associated with a rise in the oxygen content of the atmosphere.[1] These changes made it possible for the organism to obtain the increased energy provided by oxidation but also made it mandatory to develop the biochemical defense mechanisms that allow the toxic intermediates of oxygen metabolism to be destroyed.[2,3] Although these defense mechanisms are adequate at sea level where the inspired PO_2 is on the order of 150 mmHg, they become quite inadequate when the inspired PO_2 rises to 760 mmHg or even higher in pressurized environments.[4] The oxygen molecules normally interact with cytachrome C oxidase which produces the transfer of four electrons during the utilization of oxygen by aerobic cells. However, biologic oxidation may also involve the transfer of a single electron from an O_2 molecule to produce the superoxide anion O_2^-.[3] The superoxide anion can alter the structure of DNA, induce lipid peroxidation, damage membranes, and kill cells. However, it is thought that the superoxide anion is normally compartmentalized near the reaction that produces it and is destroyed so rapidly by superoxide dismutase that these adverse reactions have little likelihood of occurring. In addition to its own toxicity, the superoxide anion can react with hydrogen peroxide to generate the hydroxyl radical which is extremely toxic and capable of attacking virtually any type of organic molecule.[3] This means that free radical formation must be inhibited by the organism if tissue injury is to be prevented. The major defense mechanism against free radical generation is the enzyme superoxide dismutase[5] which catalyzes the dismutation of a superoxide anion to hydrogen peroxide and water.

Free radicals can also be generated in the photochemical reactions of air pollutants. It has been estimated that 90 percent of the oxidants in smog are due to ozone[6,7] and most of the remaining 10 percent are due to nitrogen dioxide and other oxides of nitrogen.[8] The normal concentration of ozone in air increases with altitude ranging from 0.01 ppm at sea level to 10 ppm in the upper atmosphere. While ozone occasionally reaches toxic concentration in commercial airplanes flying above 30,000 feet, this is usually prevented by loss that occurs when ozone is heated or contacts metal surfaces. Ozone can also be generated by high-voltage electrical equipment, inert gas-shielded arc welding devices, and ozone-generating devices for air and water purification.[9] Nitrogen dioxide is a common pollutant arising from emissions of automobile exhaust and other internal combustion engines and occurs in association with arc welding, combustion of explosives, exhaust of underground diesel equipment, and hay stacked in silos.[9]

Both ozone and the oxides of nitrogen have free radical potential because they contain unpaired electrons. Nitrogen dioxide is more soluble in tissue fluids than ozone so there is a tendency for nitrogen oxide to be absorbed more readily in the central airways. This may account for the propensity of nitrogen dioxide to produce bronchitis and for ozone to cause peripheral lung injury. It is also probable that ozone has a tendency to damage the superficial epithelium whereas nitrogen dioxide may pass into the interstitium to produce deeper injury.[10] In any case, the ability of the tissue to combat free radicals generated when these gases are breathed in is a very important defense mechanism. A more complete description of situations where free radical injury are thought to damage the lung can be found in Chapter 23 and in Autor.[2]

Protection from Inhaled Particles

The nature of the pathology produced by an inhaled particle depends on the content of the particle. If the particle is a water droplet containing an infectious agent, the response will be quite different than if it is an organic or inorganic dust. The defense against inhaled particles begins after the particles are deposited, therefore the nature of particle deposition in the lung will be presented before we discuss defense mechanisms. When a gas is inhaled at a constant flow rate, the velocity of the gas at each point in the respiratory tract depends on the cross-sectional area at that point. This means that at the same flow rate the gas velocity will be high in the upper airways, larynx, and central conducting airways and low at the level of the terminal bronchioles.

General Features of Particle Deposition

When an airstream containing aerosol particles is moving at a certain velocity and makes a sudden change in direction at a branch point in the airways, the particles tend not to change from their path because of their momentum.[11] As momentum (m) is proportional to density and velocity ($m = \frac{1}{2} \rho v^2$ where ρ = density and v = velocity) the tendency is for large, fast-moving particles to leave the airstream and be deposited on the airway wall. This means that larger particles tend to get filtered out of the airstream in the upper airways larynx and major bronchi because these airways may have branch points and a narrow cross-section so that velocities are high.[12]

Particles with a density greater than that of air also experience a downward force due to gravity. These particles are accelerated downward by the force of gravity until their velocity has increased to a point where the retarding force, due to its motion through the air, balances their weight. If the particle is spherical then Stoke's law can be used to predict the retarding force. For unit density particles, Stoke's law has been found to be valid within 10 percent for particles ranging from 1 to 40 μm in diameter.[11] Many particles that are small enough not to be deposited in the central airways reach the lung parenchyma where they can settle to the surface if there is sufficient time. Those that do not have time to reach the surface are removed by exhalation.

The constant random motion of gas molecules with small aerosol particles pushes them around and about in an irregular fashion called Brownian movement.[11] This means that even in the absence of gravity a particle will move around in the air in a random fashion where it has the probability of moving in all three dimensions. This displacement increases as particle size decreases and is independent of density. For unit density particles, settling it much more important than Brownian motion for deposition of particles down to about 0.5 μm in diameter. In particles below 0.5 μm in diameter, Brownian motion becomes a more important factor than settling.

While the surfaces of the respiratory tract are uncharged, they are electrically conducting.[11] This means that when an electrically charged particle approaches the surface it induces an image charge of opposite polarity on the surface and is attracted toward it. This electrostatic force becomes stronger as the particle approaches the surface so that the deposition of charge particles may be much greater than that of neutral ones. Similarly, if all of the aerosol particles have charges of the same polarity, they will repel each other and potentially enhance their deposition. Unfortunately the quantity of charge on particles is difficult to measure or predict.

Protection Provided by the Upper Airway

The upper respiratory tract is constructed so that swallowing can occur without contamination of the lungs and inspired air can be modified before it enters the trachea.[12] The main airstream travels upward from the nostril in a curved path along the middle meatus and backward to a sharp downward turn at the nasal pharynx. The air in the olfactory area in the upper nose and along the floor of the nose is thought to be relatively stationary.[12] The nasal and oral cavities are separated by the palate and base of the tongue which makes it possible to breathe through the nose even when the mouth is full.

The nose provides a ready filter for particles present in the airstream because it has a complex cross-sectional area that is narrow enough to make flow through it turbulent in nature. It also has a large surface area with a good blood supply so that gases may be readily absorbed into nasal tissue. The function of the nasal tissue is to warm and humidify the air but it can also cause water droplets that are present in the air to grow so that they can be more readily filtered. In experiments using radioactive particles it has been shown that the normal nasal mucosa moves particles from an anterior to posterior direction in the nose so that they collect on the palate where they are scraped off by a sucking motion and swallowed.[13] Many experiments using radioactive aerosols have confirmed the filtering function of the nose and pharynx and the rapid progression from these sites to the esophagus and stomach.

The closure of the larynx during swallowing is accomplished by strong adduction of the true vocal chords, closure of the false vocal chords, approximation of the ariepiglottic folds, and movements of the epiglottis backward and downward.[12] The epiglottis does not appear to be an essential part of this valvular mechanism because swallowing can occur normally even when the epiglottis has been destroyed by disease.[12] The glottis closes reflexly during vomiting or gagging and more or less involuntarily during micturition, defecation, and parturition. Closure of the glottis is also a very important feature of coughing and sneezing.[12]

Lower Respiratory Tract

Figure 4–1 shows the branching pattern of the human tracheobronchial tree. If the pathways are followed individually, it is clear that it is possible to get to the terminal branches of the airway by traversing either a great many branch points (that is, to the basal segments of the lower lobes) or relatively few number of branch points (that is, to the apical segments of the lower lobes). This means that the human tracheobronchial tree does not branch in a simple dichotomous fashion because it is possible (see Fig. 4–1B) to get from the alveolated surface of the lung in as few as 8 or as many as 20 branches.[14] Figure 4–1C shows that the airways narrow at different rates depending on the pathway followed so that it is possible to reach 2-mm airways by the 4th to the 14th generation of branching depending on the pathway taken.[15] Both physiologic and morphologic (see Fig. 4–1D) studies suggest that the total cross-sectional area of the airways increases greatly toward the periphery of the lung and it has been estimated that the cross-sectional area of the airways increases by several logs from the trachea to the terminal airways.[15] While this estimate was made assuming a dichotomous branching system,[15] other studies that did not make this assumption reached similar conclusions.[14]

The anatomic facts shown in Figure 4–2 are of great importance in relation to aerosol deposition. As the central airways are relatively narrow, the velocity of flow in these airways will be high so that inertial impaction at branch points is maximized. Toward the periphery of the lung, deposition is governed largely by settling so that the particles deposit in relation to their settling times. From these arguments one would predict that large particles would be deposited in the central airway and smaller particles in the peripheral airways. Recent studies by Gerrity and colleagues[16] (Fig. 4–3) have confirmed these predictions by showing that radioactive particles 5 to 10 μm in diameter were deposited largely in generations 0 to 12 whereas those from 1 to 3 μm in diameter were deposited largely in generations 14 to 20.

Particle Clearance

The clearance of particles from the airway involves several mechanisms—these include the sneeze to clear the upper airway and the cough to clear the lower airways. Just prior to the cough or sneeze the glottis opens widely to permit a quick, deep inspiration and it then closes firmly during a subsequent expiratory maneuver. When a high intrathoracic pressure has been reached, the glottis opens wide to permit an explosive outflow of air to occur through either the nose (sneeze) or lower airway (cough). As persons with healthy airways do not habitually cough or sneeze, effective clearance of the airways must occur without these maneuvers. The mucociliary escalator is the most important mechanism for clearing the central airways and the alveolar macrophages are primarily responsible for clearing the more peripheral airways. Absorption of foreign material through the epithelium by blood and lymph occurs in both bronchi and alveoli but these are of much less importance.

Mucociliary Clearance

The mucociliary system protects the conducting airways by trapping inhaled particles and sweeping them back up the airway and through the glottis where they are swallowed. The system is two-layered,[17,18] and consists of a nonviscid, serous fluid which surrounds the cilia and an upper layer of mucus which is viscoelastic and propelled by the cilial beat. The cilia[19] conduct their power stroke while they are fully extended and attached to the surface layer of mucus. The recovery stroke takes place by a bending motion which allows them to remain in the nonviscous periciliary fluid. This is analogous to swimming where the body is propelled through the water with the fully extended arm that recovers by a bending motion through the less-viscous air. The mean linear velocity of the mucus layer is influenced by the ciliary beat frequency, the viscosity and depth of the serous fluid, and the nature of the mucoid material. One might expect that the clearance would be optimal when the serous fluid depth was approximately equal to that of the outstretched cilium. However, it has been reported that mucus depth is unimportant to clearance by mucociliary transport until it is greater than 20 μm. At this depth airflow and gravity become important in the movement of the mucous layer so that the mucus flow will alter its direction in relation to these factors. The cilia are made up of microtubules which are arranged in nine doublets around a central pair. The central microtubules are surrounded by a sheath and each of the nine doublets are connected to the sheath by a radial spoke.[19] The individual doublets are attached to one another by arms. The cilia are capable of beating independently of the underlying cell and have been shown to continue to beat after separation from the cell by laser beams.[19] Their beat is accomplished by a sliding motion of the microtubules over one another without shortening individual microtubules. This has been beautifully illustrated by Satir and colleagues who have shown crowding and spreading of the doublets as the cilia moves from side to side.[19] It has been suggested that chronic infectious processes of the lung may be associated with abnormal ciliary function.[20] This has been established for the bronchiectasis present in Kartagener's syndrome[21] and may be important in other forms of chronic bronchiectasis.[22] However, not all observers agree that the syndrome can be diagnosed morphologically.[23]

Several authors[17-23] have suggested that the ratio of viscosity to elasticity of the mucous layer is an important determinant of clearance so that mucus that is either too rigid or too watery is transported with less than optimal frequency. In diseases where hypersecretion of mucus

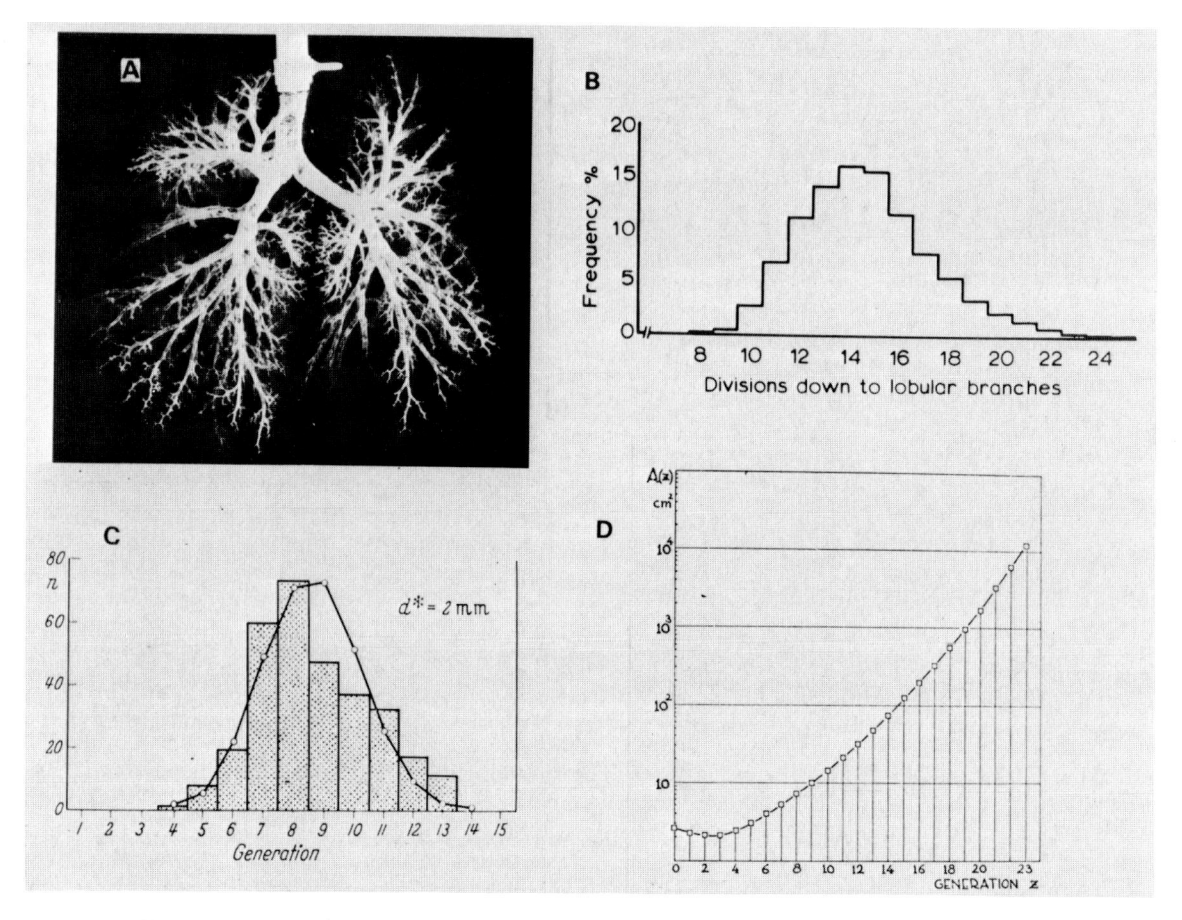

Figure 4-1. A. Normal bronchogram from a human lung. B. Data from Horsfield and Cumming[14] showing the number of divisions to the lobular (and gas-exchanging) airways varies from as few as 8 to as many as 23 depending on the pathway taken in A. C. Graph from Wiebel[15] showing the distribution of 2-mm airways from the 4th to the 14th generation. D. Diagram from Wiebel[15] showing that the cross-sectional area increases substantially beyond the 2-mm airways (that is, beyond generation 14).

occurs, the range of sputum viscoelastic properties is extended and suboptimal transport can be expected.

Because the surface area of the peripheral airways is much greater than that of the trachea, it follows that the speed of clearance must be greater in the trachea or else the mucus would pile up in this airway and drown the lung. Morrow and associates[24] have estimated that the half-time of clearance in the trachea is 2.7 minutes as compared to 80 to 300 minutes in the lower bronchi. Computed velocity of mucus clearance in centimeters per minute is therefore 1.4 cm/min in the trachea as compared to approximately 0.06 cm/min in the smaller bronchi.

Clearance from Nonciliated Airways

The mucociliary escalator can only clear the central ciliated airways. Clearance from the more peripheral parts of the lung that do not have ciliated cells must depend on other mechanisms. While the primary mechanism of clearance from the alveolar surface is thought to be the alveolar macrophage, clearance from the intermediate zone between the alveolated surface and ciliated airways is less well understood. Movement between these two regions might be accomplished by differences in the surface tension of the lining fluid which might cause movement from surfactant to mucus-covered areas or an actual flow of fluid up the airways.

The Alveolar Macrophage

The alveolar macrophage is part of the mononuclear phagocyte system. The cells of this system originate from precursor cells in the bone marrow,[25,26] are transported in the blood as monocytes, and eventually become tissue macrophages.[27,28] As there are differences in morphologic, metabolic, and functional characteristics between the blood monocyte and the alveolar macrophage, several authors have suggested that a maturation process occurs in these cells before the macrophage reaches the

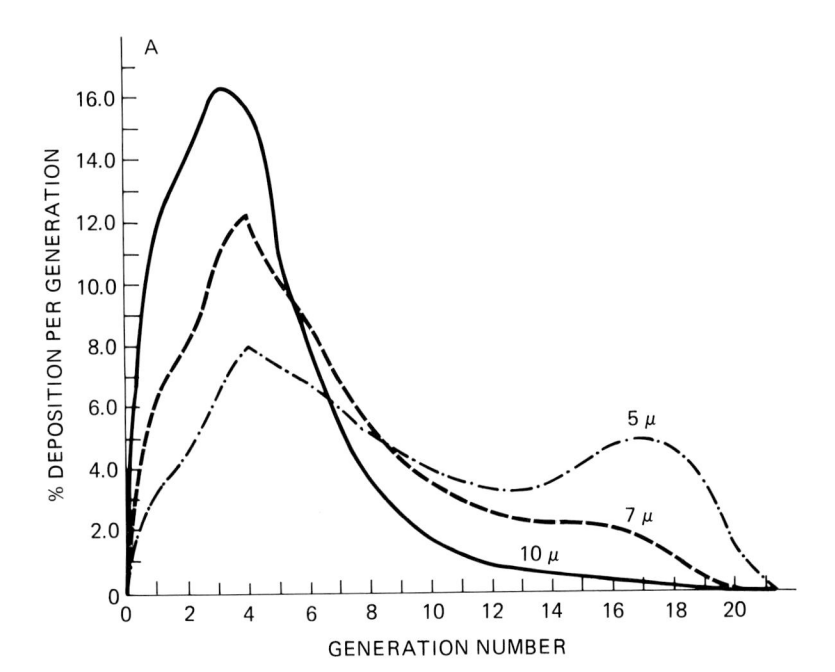

Figure 4–2. These graphs show that (A) large particles (5–10 μm) deposit in the central airways while (B) small particles (1–3 μm) deposit in peripheral airways From Gerrity et al.[16]

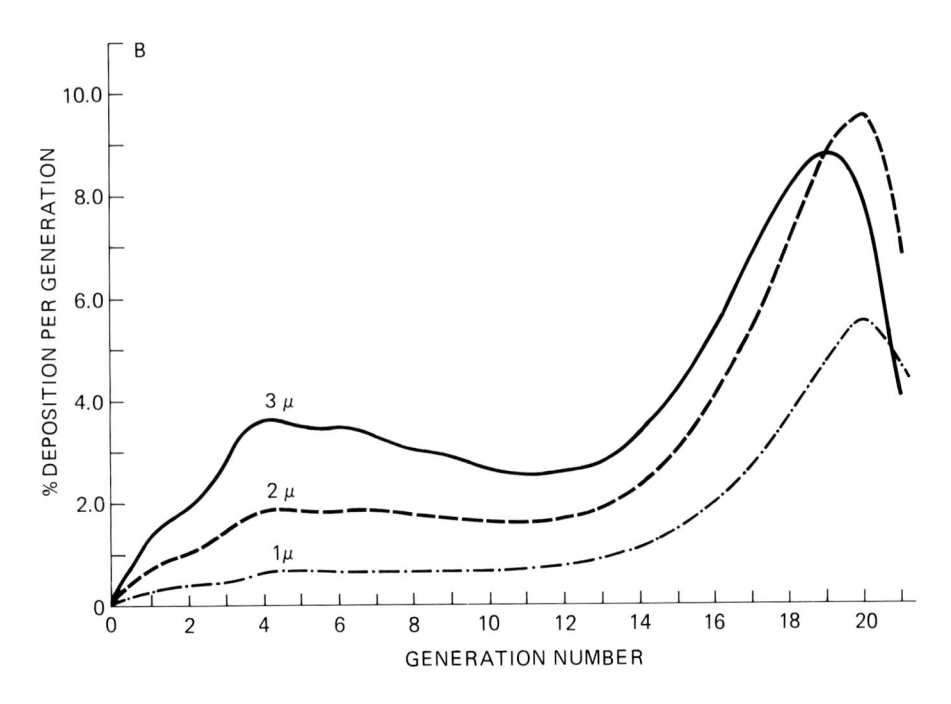

air space. Bowden and Adamson[29] have suggested that there is an interstitial compartment of cells intermediate between the blood monocyte and the free alveolar macrophages. In studies using whole-body radiation to suppress circulating monocytes and organ cultures, these investigators found that cell division occurred in the interstitial cells of the explant but not in the cells in the alveoli. They suggested that a normal steady state exists where macrophage loss in the mucociliary escalator is balanced by cell production in the interstitial compartment.

The alveolar macrophages have been calculated to cover less than 5 percent of the total alveolar surface.

Studies of the clearance of iron particles from the lung by Brain and associates[28] suggest that these cells are actively motile and capable of cleaning up the surface after it has been covered by foreign particles. However, it is less clear what happens to the cells after they have ingested the particles. The majority probably make their way to the mucociliary escalator and are cleared in the airways but it remains controversial whether any of the cells migrate back through the epithelium to the interstitium. While particulate material inhaled in the air can be found in regional lymph nodes and some of it is found within macrophages, Brain and colleagues have argued that this is a result of the free particles penetrating the epithelium

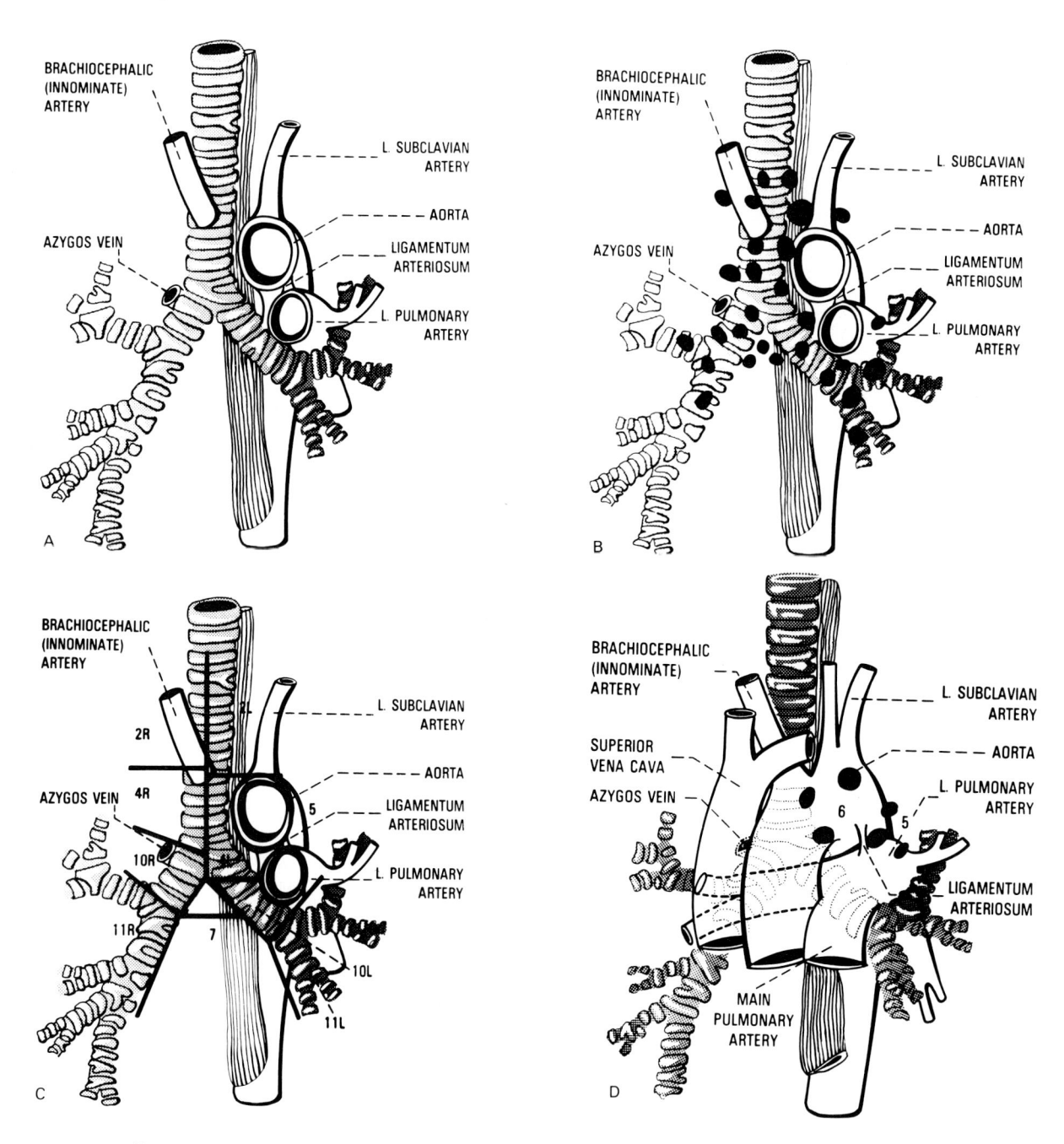

Figure 4–3. Diagrams from the American Thoracic Society system showing: A. landmarks that are used to describe nodes; B. position of nodes; C. overlay that allows nodes to be placed in certain regions; D. drainage to regions 5 and 6 which are anterior to the aorta and drain the right upper lobe (from American Thoracic Society).[40]

and being picked up by macrophages on the other side. However, Corry and associates[30] have suggested that the cells may penetrate the epithelium and make their way to the lymph nodes.

Clearance by Blood and Lymph

The epithelial surfaces of the airways are quite impermeable to large molecules.[31] Radiolabeled compounds and other tracers such as horseradish peroxidase are cleared from these surfaces into the blood at a rate per hour that is less than 1 percent of the total deposited dose.[32,33] In experiments where all of the lung lymph has been collected, the relative clearance into the blood has been estimated to be five times greater than clearance into the lymph.[34] However, as the lymphatic drainage is important in disease, it will be considered in some detail.

The lung lymphatics consist of loose collections of lymphoid cells in the peripheral portions of the lung which gradually become better organized as the hilum is approached.[35] True intrapulmonary lymph nodes with a marginal sinus, germinal center, and an efferent lymph vessel can be found in relation to segmental and lobar airways. Miller[38] concluded that the peripheral lymphoid tissues were related to both the bronchi in blood vessels in normal lungs and that those found underlying the pleura were principally related to pulmonary veins. Miller believed that the intrapulmonary lymphoid tissues proliferated on stimulation by anthracotic deposits. The bronchial-associated lymphoid tissue (BALT) is much more conspicuous in some species than in others but is present in humans and increases with irritant stimuli.[39] Their surface lining layer is somewhat different than that covering the surrounding airway. Bronchial-associated lymphoid tissues are thought to be capable of absorbing solid particles including bacteria and transporting them via lymphatics to the regional nodes.

The classification of the bronchopulmonary, peribronchial, hilar, and mediastinal lymph nodes is a confusing subject and the American Thoracic Society has proposed a system for identifying these nodes.[40] This system is particularly helpful in the staging of lung cancer but it also provides insights into the pathways of lung clearance. The American Thoracic Society proposal provides landmarks that are identifiable to both radiologist and surgeon to describe the regional nodes (see Fig. 4–3A, B) and has tried to avoid the confusion that results when nodes are named by strict anatomic definitions. In this classification there are four groups of paratracheal nodes (right and left, upper and lower). A fifth group called the aortopulmonary nodes are located lateral to the ligamentum arteriosum (see Fig. 4–3D). The sixth group lie in the anterior mediastinum anterior to the ascending aorta and innominate artery. The seventh group lie in the subcarinal area, the eighth group are the paraesophageal nodes, and the ninth group are found in relation to the right and left pulmonary ligaments. The tenth group or tracheobronchial nodes extend from the midline of the trachea to the origin of the right upper lobe bronchus while on the left they extend from the midline of the trachea from the carina to the left upper lobe bronchus. The American Thoracic Society provides a simple diagram with an overlay to assist in naming these nodes and also indicates the criteria for locating them by means of computed tomography (Fig. 4–4).

The following account of the nature of the lymph drainage from the lung to the regional nodes is based on the work of Nohl[41] which has been modified by the author and which I have tried to integrate with the studies of Nagashi.[35] Beginning with the right lung, the lymph drains from the upper lobe through its intrapulmonary nodes to regional 11R and 4R. The 11R area represents the so-called sump region of the right lung where all three lobes of the right lung drain. These classic studies of the involvement of lymph nodes in lung cancer suggest that lesions from the upper lobe can be cleared completely by removing the lobe and these nodes. The middle lobe bronchus is surrounded by lymph nodes that can enlarge to cause a collapse of the middle lobe to produce the so-called middle lobe syndrome. The lower lobe, on the other hand, also drains through the pulmonary ligament to group 9L.

The left upper lobe drains both to the sump region 11 and then to region 5 which takes a course over the aorta to the paratracheal nodes. The left lower lobe, on the other hand, drains to regions 11 to 10 to 4. The sump region on the left side is confined to region 11 but there is more cross-over from the upper to the lower because there is no intermediate stem bronchus. The prognosis of right upper lobe cancer may be better than that of left upper lobe cancer because few right upper lobe lesions metastasize below the sump region while many left upper lobe lesions do.

Immunologic Defense

The deposition of foreign material on the surface of the respiratory tract, its entry into the tissue, and its clearance by macrophages, blood, and lymph provides ample opportunity for the body's immune system to mount a defensive response. This response is partially determined by the genetic makeup of the host. The immune response genes of experimental animals are thought to be closely located on chromosome 6, and are thought to be respon-

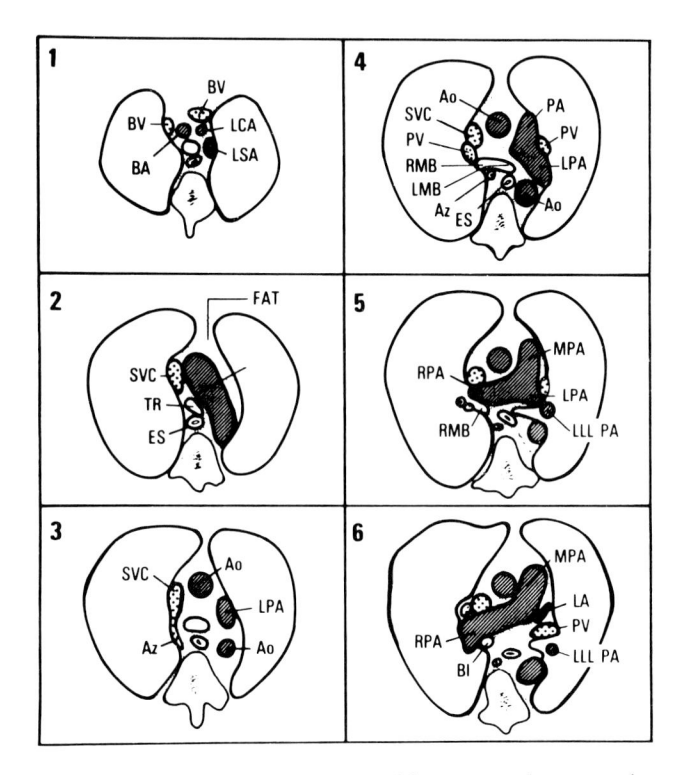

Figure 4–4. Cross-sections obtained by computed tomography showing the anatomy landmarks needed to assign nodes to different areas (see text, Clearance by Blood and Lymph, for further explanation). (*Abbreviations:* Ao, aorta; AZ, azygos vein; BA, brachiocephalic artery; BI, bronchus intermedius; ES, esophagus; LBV, left brachiocephalic vein; LCA, left common carotid artery; LSA, left subclavian artery; LLL, left lower lobe; MB, mainstem bronchus; PA, pulmonary artery; PV, pulmonary vein; RBV, right brachiocephalic vein; SVC, superior vena cava; TR, trachea.)

sible for formation of the human leukocyte–associated (HLA) antigens.[42] The close association between HLA antigens and the immune response genes is leading to a rapidly accumulating literature on HLA typing and immunologically determined lung disease.[43,44] It is to be hoped that a complete understanding of how the genes control the response to antigen will provide clearer insights into individual susceptibility to disease.

Respiratory Immunoglobulins

Local humoral immunity plays an important role in respiratory tract defense. Immunoglobulin G and IgM are produced from cells within the germinal follicles of the regional lymph nodes whereas IgE is produced in the lymphoid tissue in the upper respiratory tract, particularly in the tonsils.[45] Immunoglobulin A is formed in the regional lymph nodes as well but can also be produced in plasma cells lining the respiratory mucosa, especially in the neighborhood of the bronchial glands.[46]

The IgA found in secretions has several distinctive structural, immunologic, and biologic differences from the IgA found in the serum.[46] In the sputum it occurs mainly as dimers linked to two types of small-molecular-weight junctional pieces. The first to be described was the secretory T-piece or secretory component that is believed to link IgA molecules through their FC portions.[46] This component is probably formed in the mucosal glands and epithelial cells, and immunofluorescent studies have demonstrated secretory component IgA within mucosal cells. The major function of IgA appears to be blocking of adherence of organisms to the mucosal surfaces.[48] This probably accounts for the experimental observations that showed that virus infections could be more readily prevented by intranasal instillation rather than by parenteral injection of a vaccine. It has now been amply confirmed that the protective immunity following intranasal immunization is more closely related to levels of secretory IgA than to serum levels of either IgA or IgG. In summary, IgA provides the first line of defense against surface invaders that deposit on the airway mucosa. The antibodies in the serum provide a backup defense against the organisms that penetrate the mucosal barrier into the interstitial tissue.

When an individual meets an infecting agent for the first time, specific IgM is the first immunoglobulin to increase and is detectable within 3 to 4 days.[45] Its production tends to be transient, and increases indicate recent infection. It is characteristic of blood group isoagglutinins, cold agglutinins, and some bacterial antibodies. Immunoglobulin G increases more slowly, beginning at about 10 days and peaking at 3 weeks. With reinfection the IgG response is accelerated and reaches a much higher level at about 3 weeks. Immunoglobulin G occurs in the greatest amount in the serum and is the major specific antibody against bacteria, viruses, and other organisms.

Immunoglobulin E has a short half-life of 2 to 3 days in serum but survives in tissue where it is linked to the surfaces of basophils and mast cells.[47] It is formed in the lymphoid tissue and plasma cells of the upper respiratory tract and tonsils, and to a lesser extent in the trachea and main bronchi.[45] Salvaggio and Laskowitz[48] showed that the intranasal administration of a variety of antigens stimulated production of circulating skin-sensitizing antibodies in atopic individuals whereas no such response was observed in control subjects. In contrast, parenteral administration of the antigen primarily showed IgG antibody production. Very low levels of IgE are found in the neonate and this level begins to rise by about 6 weeks and reaches adult values at about 5 years.[45] Immunoglobulin E increases during the pollen season in allergic subjects, and excessively high IgE values are found in patients with parasitic infestations. Antigen interaction with IgE on the surface of mast cells causes the release of mediators that modulate the inflammatory response to the inhaled antigen.[46]

Cell-Mediated Immunity

A group of immune reactions are mediated by sensitized T lymphocytes. This cell-mediated immune reaction has been best studied as the response to bacterial antigens such as those of the tubercle bacillus. It is now recognized that cell-mediated immunity is a complex reaction that is expressed in a variety of biologic events. In experimental studies it is best induced by proteins or other chemical determinants conjugated to proteins. In some cases the chemical may be quite simple (haptene) but the cell-mediated response appears to be directed against both haptene and protein. This differs from the antibody response which can be directed against either the haptene or the protein.[49]

Another important feature of the cell-mediated immune response is the route of antigen introduction. Sometimes intravenous injection of large amounts of soluble antigen will be unable to induce cell-mediated immunity. However, small amounts of particulate or adjuvant-associated antigen introduced into an area with appropriate lymphocyte drainage is followed by cellular sensitization at that site and in the draining lymph nodes.[50,51] While the T cells are recognized as the instruments of cell-mediated immunity, the way they interact with antigen has been a much-debated issue. The general consensus appears to be that the antigen is presented to the T cell by the macrophage. The T cell then differentiates to a blast form and begins to divide. The sensitized T cell provides the basis of immunologic memory and the expanse of this clone of cells increases the intensity of the response.[52] The observation by Tada[53] that an intact thymus was required to shut off the IgE response in skin sensitized rats after antigen challenge led to the discovery of the T-suppressor cell. The control of antibody synthesis by helper and suppressor T cells is now a well-recognized concept. Indeed, the failure to produce thymic suppressor cells has been postulated to be responsible for the over-production of antibody and appearance of multiple auto-antibodies in systemic lupus erythematosis. Similarly, vigorous suppressor T-cell activity has been postulated as a cause of one form of hypogamma globulinemia. The important fact is that every immune response is controlled by positive and negative influences and failure to shut down a response may be a significant cause of disease.

The nature of the histologic changes in the cell-mediated immune response are characteristic but not specific and depend on the tissue site, species, and the method of exposure to antigen. The lymphocytes that are responsible for the reaction make up a small proportion of the cells present in the expression of the reaction.[52] This appears to be possible because the sensitized T cell is able to release factors that control the inflammatory response. Some of these factors have been reasonably well characterized and include (1) migratory inhibitory factor which modulates the accumulation of inflammatory cells, (2) interlukins which induce cell proliferation, (3) cytotoxins which damage other cells, and (4) a rapidly growing list of other less well-characterized factors.[52]

Granulomatous Inflammation

The difference in the histologic appearance of the delayed hypersensitivity reaction seen following the injection of tuberculin in the skin and the granulomatous inflammation associated with tuberculous inflammation in all tissue, has been a confusing issue.[54] Until 1950 granulomatous inflammation was thought to be a nonspecific response to lipids and other foreign material. Recently the importance of granuloma formation in the delayed hypersensitivity reaction induced by particulate antigens has been better appreciated. The formation of granuloma in response to mycobacterial infection has been shown to be suppressed in animals that lack functional T lymphocytes and it has also been shown that granuloma formation can be suppressed by measures directed against T lymphocytes.[54] The fact that the T cell recognizes macrophage-associated antigens probably best explains why cell-mediated reactions are stimulated by the residue of intracellular parasites. Indeed, this could account for the fact that intracellular parasites such as the organisms of tuberculosis, leprosy, and brucellosis as well as a variety of viral, chlamydial, and fungal organisms cause granulomatous inflammation.[54,55] However, not all granulomas form as part of a clearly defined immunologic response and some granulomata that form in response to inorganic particles such as silica are not associated with cell-mediated immunity.

Summary

The lung is protected by several mechanisms that include filtration mucociliary clearance, drainage through blood and lymph, and the inflammatory response. These defense mechanisms allow the respiratory tract to carry out its functions of exchanging gas with the environment in a wide variety of unfavorable circumstances. It is not surprising that they are occasionally overpowered or that the response is some patients is so exuberant that it contributes to the progress of disease.

References

1. Schopf JW: The evolution of the earliest cells. Sci Amer 239:110–140, 1978.
2. Autor AP (ed): *The Pathology of Oxygen*. New York: Academic Press, 1982.
3. Fridovich I: Oxygen radicals in hydrogen peroxide and oxygen toxicity, In Prior WA (ed): *Free Radicals in Biology*, vol 1. New York: Academic Press, 1976, p 239.
4. Clark JM, Lambertson CJ: Pulmonary oxygen toxicity: A review. Pharmacol Rev 23:37–133, 1971.
5. Fridovich I: Superoxide dismutases. Annu Rev Biochem 44:147–159, 1975.
6. Nasr ANM: Biochemical aspects of ozone intoxication: A review. J Occup Med 9:589, 1967.
7. Menzel BD: Toxicity of ozone oxygen and radiation. Annu Rev Pharmacol 10:379–394, 1970.
8. Perry WH, Tabor EC: National air sampling network: Measurement of sulphur dioxide and nitrogen dioxide. Arch Environ Health 4:254–264, 1962.
9. Evans MJ, Cabrell LJ, Stevens RJ, Freeman G: Renewal of alveolar epithelium in the rat following exposure to nitrogen dioxide. Am J Pathol 70:175–798, 1973.
10. Mustafa MG, Tierney DF: Biochemical and metabolic changes in the lung with oxygen, ozone and nitrogen dioxide toxicity: State of the art. Am Rev Respir Dis 118:1061–1090SA, 1978.
11. Brain JD, Valberg PA: Deposition of aerosol in the respiratory tract: State of the art. Am Rev Respir Dis 120:1325–1373, 1979.
12. Proctor DF: Physiology of the upper airway. In Fenn WO, Raun H (eds): *Handbook of Physiology*, vol 1. Washington: American Physiological Society, 1964.
13. Proctor DF: The upper airways. I. Nasal physiology and defense of the lungs. State of the art. Am Rev Respir Dis 115:97–129SA.
14. Horsfield K, Cumming G: Morphology of the bronchial tree in man. J Appl Physiol 24:373–383, 1968.
15. Weibel E: *Morphometry of the Human Lung*. New York: Academic Press, 1963.
16. Gerrity TR, Lee TS, Haas FJ, et al.: Calculated deposition of inhaled particles in the airway generations of normal subjects. J Appl Physiol 47:867–873, 1979.
17. Sturgess JM: The mucus lining of major bronchi in the rabbit lung. Am Rev Respir Dis 115:819–827, 1977.
18. Hulbert WC, Forster BB, Laird W, et al.: An improved method for fixation of the respiratory epithelial surface with mucus and surfactant layers. Lab Invest 47:354–363, 1982.
19. Satir P: How cilia move. Sci Am 231:44–63, 1974.
20. Eliason R, Mosberg B, Cammer P, Afzelius BA: Immobile cilia, chronic airway infection and male sterility. N Engl J Med 277:1–6, 1977.
21. Afzelius BA: A human syndrome caused by immobile cilia. Science 193:317–319, 1976.
22. Warte D, Steele R, Ross I, Wakefield J, McKay J, Wallace J. Cilia and sperm tail abnormalities in Polynesian bronchiectatics. Lancet 2:132–133, 1978.
23. Fox B, Bull TB, Makay AR, Rawbone R: Significance of ultrastructural abnormalities in human cilia. Chest 80(6)(suppl): 796–799, 1981.
24. Morrow PE, Gibb ER, Gazioglu KM: A study of particulate clearance from human lungs. Am Rev Respir Dis 96:1209–1221, 1967.

25. Brunstetter M, Hardy JA, Schiff R, et al.: The origin of the pulmonary alveolar macrophage. Arch Intern Med 127:1064–1068, 1971.

26. Godleski JJ, Brain JD: The origin of the alveolar macrophage in mouse radiation shimmers. J Exp Med 136:630–643, 1972.

27. Roser B: The origin, kinetics and fate of macrophage population. J Reticuloendothel Soc 8:139–161, 1970.

28. Brain JD, Godleski JJ, Syroken SP: Quantification, origin and fate of pulmonary macrophages. In Lenfent C (ed): *Respiratory Defense Mechanisms*, part II. New York: Marcel Dekker, 1977, pp 849–889.

29. Bowden DH, Adamson IYR: Pulmonary interstitial cell as an immediate precursor of the alveolar macrophage. Am J Pathol 68:521–536, 1972.

30. Corry D, Padmakar K, Lipscomb MF: The migration of macrophages into hilar lymph nodes. Am J Pathol 115:321–329, 1984.

31. Simami AS, Inoue S, Hogg JC: The penetration of respiratory epithelium of guinea pigs following exposure to cigarette smoke. Lab Invest 31:75–81, 1974.

32. Hulbert WC, Walker DC, Jackson A, Hogg JC: Airway permeability to horseradish peroxidase in guinea pigs: The repair phase after injury by cigarette smoke. Am Rev Respir Dis 123:320–326, 1981.

33. Huchon GJ, Little JW, Murray JF: Assessment of alveolar capillary membrane permeability in dogs. J Appl Physiol 51:955–962, 1981.

34. Meyer EC, Dominquez EAM, Bensch CG: Pulmonary lymphatic and blood absorption of albumin from alveoli. A quantitative comparison. Lab Invest 20:1–8, 1969.

35. Nagashi C: *Functional Anatomy and Histology of the Lung*. Baltimore and London: University Park Press, 1972.

38. Miller WS: The distribution of lymphoid tissue in the lung. Anat Rec 5:99, 1911.

39. Bienenstock J, Johnson M, Perry DYW: Bronchial lymphoid tissue. Lab Invest 28:686–692, 693–698, 1973.

40. American Thoracic Society: Official Statement on Clinical Staging of Lung Cancer. Ad hoc committee chaired by Tisi GM. Am Rev Respir Dis 127:659–664, 1983.

41. Nohl HC: An investigation into lymphatic and vascular spread of carcinoma of the bronchus. Thorax 11:172–185, 1956.

42. Levine BB, Stember RH, Fotino M: Ragweed hayfever, genetic control and linkage to HLA haptotypes. Science 178:1201, 1972.

43. Thorsby E, Enges ETA, Lie SO: HLA antigens and susceptibility to diseases. Tissue Antigens 1:147, 1971.

44. Blumenthal MN, Bach FH: Immunogenetics of atopic disease. In Elliot M Jr, Reed CE, Ellis EF (eds): *Allergy: Principles and Practice*. St. Louis and Toronto: CV Mosby, 1983, pp 11–17.

45. Turner-Warwick M: Immunology of the lung. In Turk J (ed): *Current Topics in Immunology*. London: Edward Arnold, 1978.

46. McDermott MR, Befus AD, Bienenstock J: The structural basis of immunity in the respiratory tract. Int Rev Exp Pathol 23:47–112, 1982.

47. Ishizaka K, Ishizaka T: Biological function of gamma E antibodies and mechanism of reagenic hypersensitivity. Clin Exp Immunol 6:25–42, 1970.

48. Salvaggio JE, Laskowitz S: The comparison of immunological responses of normal and atopic individuals to potential precipitated protein antigen. Int Arch Allergy Appl Immunol 26:264–268, 1965.

49. Greene MI, Benacerraf B: Studies on antigen specific cell immunity and suppression. Immunol Rev 50:163–186, 1980.

50. Bach BA, Sherman L, Banaseraf B, Greene MI: Mechanisms of regulation of cell mediated immunity: II. Induction and suppression of a delayed-type hypersensitivity by azobenzene-arsonate-coupled syngeneic cells. J Immunol 127:1460–1468, 1978.

51. Clayman HN, Miller SD, Suy M, Moorehead JW: Suppressive mechanisms involving sensitization and tolerance in contact allergy. Immunol Rev 50:105, 1980.

52. Zweiman B, Levinson AI: Cell-mediated immunity. In Elliot M Jr, Reed CE, Ellis EF (eds): *Allergy: Principles and Practice*. St. Louis and Toronto: CV Mosby, 1983, pp 75–102.

53. Tada T: Regulation of reagenic antibody formation in animals. Prog Allergy 19:122, 1975.

54. Borros DL: Hypersensitivity granulomas. In Elliot M Jr, Reed CE, Ellis EF (eds): *Allergy: Principles and Practice*. St. Louis and Toronto: CV Mosby, 1983, pp 103–118.

55. Borros DL: Granulomatous inflammation. Prog Allergy 24:183, 1978.

5 Lung Biopsy: Handling and Diagnostic Limitations

Andrew Churg

Introduction

Over the last 10 years, lung biopsies have become increasingly common specimens in many pathology laboratories. This phenomenon reflects in part the development and popularization of the transbronchial biopsy[1] and the extensive use of open lung biopsy.[2] However, there is still a lack of recognition among both pathologists and clinicians of the diagnostic limitations inherent in different types of lung biopsy.

This chapter reviews two general topics: handling of biopsy specimens and the application of different types of biopsy to different disease processes. Most of the processes are discussed in other chapters in this book; the emphasis here will be on why certain types of diagnosis may or may not be possible from transbronchial and open biopsies. Trephine needle biopsy is not discussed because the procedure is rarely used in North America, but the interested reader can find commentary and references on the subject in Gaensler's review of lung biopsy,[2] which also considers complication rates for all types of biopsies. (Cytologic techniques are covered in Chapter 9 and pleural biopsies in Chapter 26.)

The importance of correlating pathologic features with clinical findings for the proper interpretation of lung biopsies cannot be overemphasized. Many pulmonary processes as seen on biopsy have relatively nonspecific (and sometimes misleading) pathologic features; in such instances, the correct diagnosis can only be made by the addition of clinical information. It is critical to know, for example, whether there is radiographic evidence of a mass lesion or a diffuse infiltrate, whether there is evidence of functional impairment, or whether the patient is immunocompromised. The clinical significance of honeycombing, for instance, may vary from none, if a biopsy has chanced upon a localized old scar, to end-stage lung disease (for example, as shown in Fig. 5–3). Even something as "simple" as a carcinoma may be a metastasis rather than a primary. The pathologist should develop the habit of inquiring not only about radiographic and functional changes, but also about the clinical differential diagnosis before rendering a final reading on any lung biopsy.

Open Lung Biopsy

Handling

As a general rule, open lung biopsies should be fixed in inflation. Alveolar walls behave somewhat like rubber bands: if stretched they become thinner, and if allowed to contract, thicker. Additionally, in uninflated specimens, the alveolar walls tend to collapse on each other. Both of these processes can produce a false impression of interstitial fibrosis and inflammation (Fig. 5–1). Some notion of whether interstitial disease is actually present may be obtained by finding an area of the biopsy which is definitely normal and tracing the alveolar walls into the apparently abnormal areas. If the individual walls can be clearly followed and do not appear to change, the biopsy is probably normal. Reticulum or elastic tissue strains may be of some help in this situation if they demonstrate that several independent juxtaposed alveolar walls are present. However, it is often difficult and sometimes impossible to determine whether interstitial disease is actually present in uninflated biopsies, and other processes may occasionally be hidden in the mass of collapsed parenchyma.

There are two basic methods for achieving fixation in inflation. One is to have the surgeon clamp the inflated lung at the time of biopsy[2–4] and immediately drop the resected piece, still held in inflation by clamps, into fixative. Unfortunately, this technique requires a close

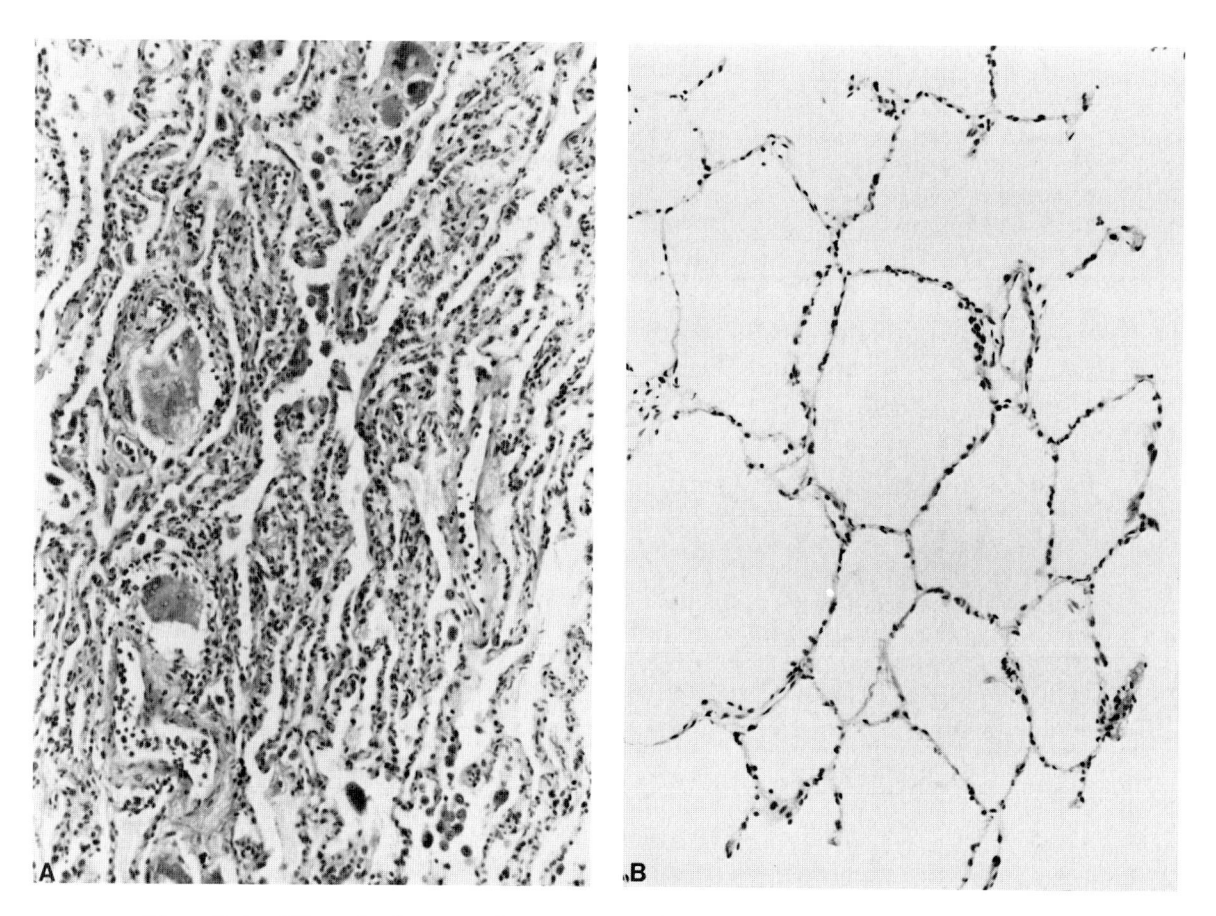

Figure 5–1. Effect of inflation on the appearance of open biopsy specimens. A portion of this biopsy was inflated and a portion was processed as it was received from the operating room. A. The uninflated portion mimics a chronic interstitial pneumonia; there are also some giant cells present surrounding asbestos fibers. B. The inflated specimen shows that the parenchyma is completely normal. The biopsy was performed to rule out asbestosis; such a diagnosis might have been incorrectly made on the uninflated specimen (H&E, both ×160).

cooperation among surgeons, operating room nurses, and pathologists that is rarely achieved in practice.

An alternate procedure is to inflate the resected specimen with fixative in the laboratory. The technique is simple and quick: a small (approximately 25-gauge) needle attached to a fixative-filled syringe is inserted into the parenchyma through the pleura or through a cut surface; fixative is *gently* instilled until the lung is expanded.[5] Once the lung has been expanded, the specimen is put into formalin for 30 to 60 minutes, then cut and blocked to give the largest possible faces for histologic examination. The procedure sometimes produces a degree of edema in the interlobular septa, particularly if the specimen is overinflated, but this artifact does not interfere with interpretation and is worth accepting, given the far superior ease of interpretation of the important parts of the biopsy (*see* Fig. 5–1). (More details of the method are provided in Churg.[5])

Unless one is dealing with a known malignancy, lung biopsies must always be cultured for aerobic and anaerobic bacilli, mycobacteria, fungi, and viruses. This is best performed in the operating room, but if necessary, a piece of the edge of the specimen can be taken for culture when it is received in the surgical pathology laboratory. Additional pieces can be removed for electron microscopy and/or immunohistochemistry, as well as for frozen section. The remainder is then inflated with the syringe technique. However, the author does not agree with the suggestion of Katzenstein and Askin[6] that a frozen section should be performed on all open lung biopsies; frozen sections of open biopsies invariably are collapsed, and subtle features are uninterpretable. Unless the clinical situation demands an immediate answer, for example, when dealing with pulmonary disease in immunocompromised patients, far better results are obtained from paraffin-embedded material.

Unfortunately, the syringe inflation technique does not work on partially fixed specimens; unless one is sure that the surgeon will inflate and cut the lung properly, it is probably best to insist that all lung biopsies immediately be brought fresh to the surgical pathology laboratory. The specimen must be accompanied by a good clinical history and some indication of the nature of the functional and radiograhic abnormalities.

An open lung biopsy samples a very small portion of peripheral lung, and problems of sampling error are made worse by taking very small biopsies. The pathologist should ordinarily expect a wedge at least 2 cm on a side. Sampling error can be greatly reduced by taking two or three biopsies from different areas.

The stains which are required for a given type of biopsy vary with the underlying disease; for diffuse disease in the nonimmunosuppressed patient, the author routinely prepares hematoxylin and eosin and elastic stains; the latter permits evaluation of vascular abnormalities. For specimens from immunosuppressed patients, all of the usual stains for organisms (Gram, acid-fast, methenamine-silver) are added (see Chapter 15).

It is difficult to provide general guidelines for electron-microscopic and immunohistochemical examination of lung biopsies. Electron-microscopy in particular has relatively few routine uses, but is of value in classifying tumors (especially the diagnosis of small-cell carcinoma), in detecting immune complex deposits (particularly in pulmonary hemorrhage), in finding Langerhans' granules in questionable cases of eosinophilic granuloma, and sometimes in demonstrating the presence of viral particles. Electron-microscopic examination is also useful for detecting ciliary abnormalities in bronchial or tracheal biopsies (see Chapter 21, and the recent review by Wang[7]).

Immunohistochemical examination is potentially applicable to many of the areas just mentioned and is often superior to electron-microscopy, either because of the ability to examine large areas (for example, to detect viral particles or to find the few tumor cells that produce some specific marker) or to detect substances that have no specific structure by electron-microscopy (for example, Goodpasture's syndrome, in which linear immunohistochemical staining for immunoglobulin is present, but no deposits are seen by electron microscopy). However, currently neither electron-microscopic nor immunohistochemical examination is required as a routine diagnostic tool for most biopsies.

Electron optical techniques are also useful for the demonstration of mineral particles in suspected occupational or environmental exposures. In some instances, ordinary tissue sections can be employed for qualitative analysis using scanning electron microscopy[7]; techniques for the quantitation of asbestos fibers and other mineral particles by transmission electron-microscopy have been described by Churg.[8]

Site of Biopsy

The site of biopsy is just as important as the handling of the specimen. Where the biopsy should be performed varies with the nature of the lesion. Obviously biopsies should be taken directly from mass lesions. However, many surgeons apply this same principle to lungs with diffuse interstitial disease and biopsy the area that feels or looks worst. Frequently such a biopsy will yield only nonspecific honeycombing (see Nonspecific or Unreliable Diagnoses, below), a finding that renders the biopsy worthless. In this situation, the best area to biopsy is one that is intermediately between worst and best or, alternately, to take more than one biopsy. Dahlquen and Oberholzer[9] suggest biopsying the zone where normal parenchyma gives way to abnormal.

Biopsies should not be taken from the tips of the lobes, particularly the lingula and right middle lobe tips. These dependent areas may show pathologic features completely different from those seen in the rest of the lung, especially vascular abnormalities and interstitial fibrosis and inflammation (Fig. 5–2), even when the rest of the lobe is completely normal.[10,11] If presented with such a biopsy, the pathologist should be extremely cautious in making a diagnosis of any type of acute or chronic diffuse interstitial pneumonia or vascular disease.

Specific and Nonspecific Diagnoses

Compared with transbronchial biopsy, open biopsy allows the physician to examine a large area at low power and to find a low-power pattern that is potentially either diagnostic despite the lack of any one specific feature [for example, in usual interstitial pneumonia (UIP)] or specific, but has widely or irregularly scattered features (for example, the lesions of eosinophilic granuloma).

Given a biopsy that appears to show a pathologic abnormality, three broad diagnostic possibilities exist see (see Table 5–1):

1. The histopathologic features provide a reasonably high morphologic specificity. Obvious examples are malignancies, eosinophilic granuloma, and sarcoidosis. (These diseases are considered in detail in other chapters.)
2. The histologic features are nonspecific, unreliable, or misleading. Emphysema and honeycombing fall into this category.
3. The morphologic features are considerably less specific than category 1, and their significance depends almost entirely on the clinical, functional, and radiographic setting. Examples are chronic interstitial pneumonias (and, to some extent, pneumoconioses such as asbestosis that resemble chronic interstitial pneumonias), diffuse alveolar damage, and bronchiolitis obliterans with organizing pneumonia

Nonspecific or Unreliable Diagnoses

Diagnosis of emphysema requires the inflated whole lung or lobe. Accurate assessment of the presence and type of emphysema may not be possible on the basis of a lung biopsy, and certainly no judgment of its severity is possible on such evidence.[12] If only emphysema is present in an open biopsy, it is likely that the biopsy has missed the lesion of importance.

Honeycombing is a term used by both radiologists and pathologists to refer to end-stage lung disease (see Chapter 20 for definitions and descriptions). Histologically it is easy to decide that honeycombing is present in a biopsy. However, honeycombing is a common end stage

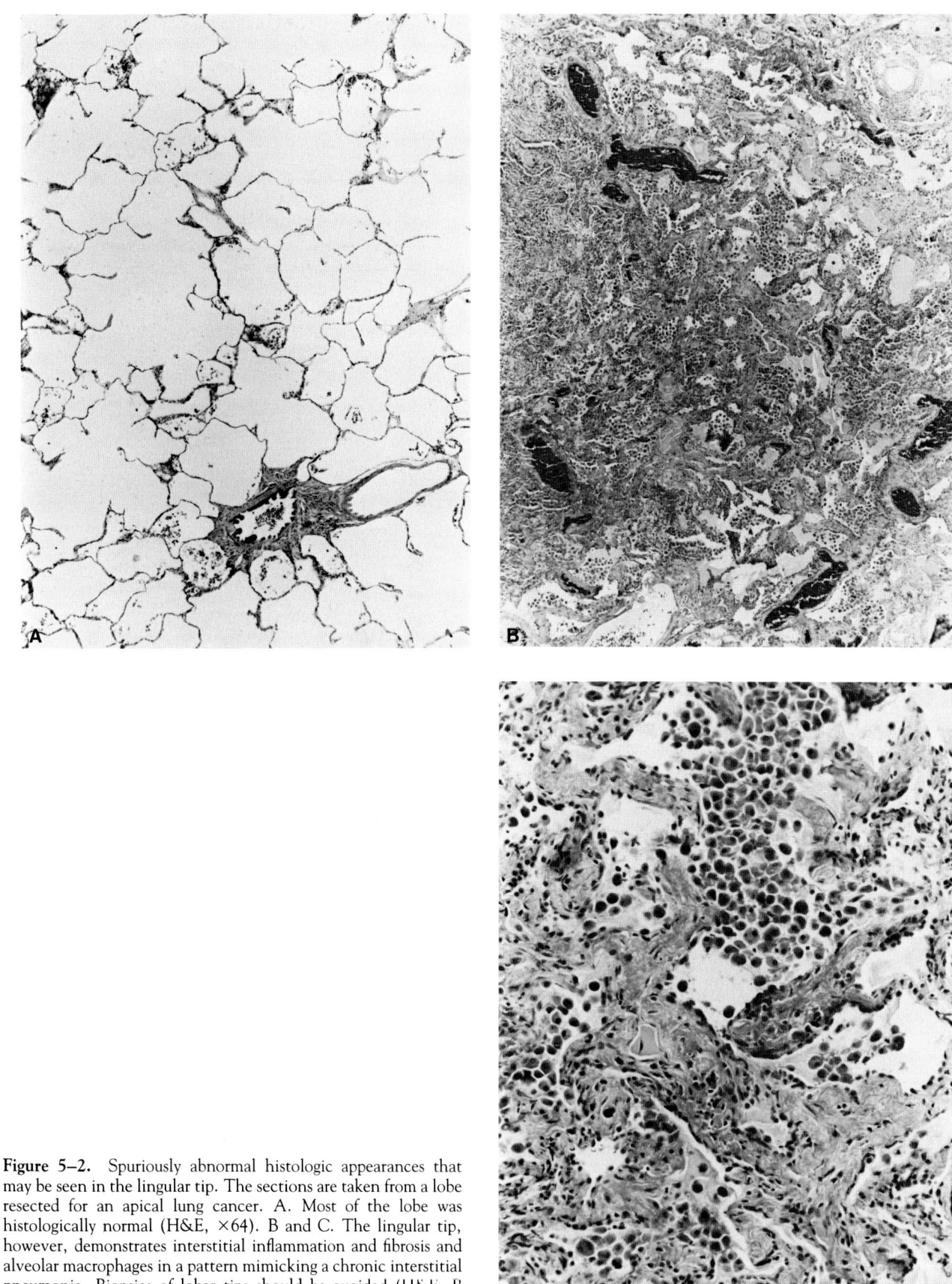

Figure 5–2. Spuriously abnormal histologic appearances that may be seen in the lingular tip. The sections are taken from a lobe resected for an apical lung cancer. A. Most of the lobe was histologically normal (H&E, ×64). B and C. The lingular tip, however, demonstrates interstitial inflammation and fibrosis and alveolar macrophages in a pattern mimicking a chronic interstitial pneumonia. Biopsies of lobar tips should be avoided (H&E, B ×40, C ×60).

Table 5–1. Diagnostic Possibilities for Open Biopsy Specimens

Morphologic High Specificity
    Eosinophilic pneumonia
    Eosinophilic granuloma
    Lymphocytic interstitial pneumonia
    Some pneumoconioses
    Extrinsic allergic alveolitis
    Alveolar proteinosis
    Lymphangioleiomyomatosis
    Sarcoidois
    Infections
    Noninfectious granulomas (Wegener's, etc.)
    Vascular changes associated with pulmonary hypertension
    Neoplasms

Morphologic Specificity Depends Entirely on Clinical and Pathologic Setting
    Chronic interstitial pneumonias (UIP/DIP) and pneumoconioses such as asbestosis that resemble chronic interstitial pneumonias
    Bronchiolitis obliterans with organizing pneumonia
    Diffuse alveolar damage

Morphologic Findings Nonspecific or Unreliable
    Emphysema
    Honeycombing

Abbreviations: DIP, desquamative interstitial pneumonia; UIP, usual interstitial pneumonia.

of many processes (*see* Chapter 20 and Fig. 5–3). In addition to specific diffuse diseases, localized scars of many causes can appear as honeycombed lung (*see* Fig. 5–3C). Therefore, if an open lung biopsy shows only honeycomb lung, it is impossible to determine what the underlying disease (if any) might be; hence, the biopsy yields no useful information concerning either treatment or prognosis.

Diagnoses Specific Only in the Proper Clinical Context

The most common diseases in this category are chronic interstitial pneumonias (*see* Chapter 20). A nonspecific morphologic picture identical to usual UIP or desquamative interstitial pneumonia (DIP) can be found in association with honeycombed areas of any origin, old scars, and around mass lesions such as tumors and lesions of eosinophilic granuloma. The diagnosis therefore requires functional and radiographic changes compatible with a diffuse interstitial process and the lack of evidence of localized lesions.

Diffuse alveolar damage may or may not be a specific diagnosis, depending on the clinical setting. In nonimmunosuppressed patients, biopsy is sometimes performed to attempt to establish a cause for a process that appears clinically as the adult respiratory distress syndrome or to the extent of irreversible fibrosis.[13] The etiologies of diffuse alveolar damage are numerous[14] (*see* Chapter 16), and it is uncommon that biopsy actually does provide an cause. In this situation, diffuse alveolar damage is an acceptable pathologic diagnosis, and etiology must be based on the clinical history.

By contrast, in the immunocompromised patient, the problem is usually not one of finding an etiologic agent but of excluding the numerous possibilities. Typically such patients have been treated with radiation or a variety of immunosuppressive/antineoplastic agents and have more or less widespread pulmonary infiltrates on chest radiograph and diffuse alveolar damage histologically. In this circumstance, etiology includes infections, neoplasms, drug toxicity, radiation, hemorrhage, and oxygen toxicity.[15–17] As a consequence, diffuse alveolar damage in the immunocompromised patient, whether found by open or transbronchial biopsy, is a nonspecific diagnosis from the clinical management point of view. Indeed, the finding of this histologic pattern is no guarantee that another well-defined process such as an infection has not been missed,[16] and special stains should always be performed. One should be extremely cautious in labeling such reactions "drug lung" or "radiation pneumonitis" because the patient may be treated with steroids, thus potentiating an infection.

Proliferating granulation tissue in air spaces has been variably referred to as organizing pneumonia, bronchiolitis obliterans, or sometimes bronchiolitis obliterans with organizing pneumonia[18,19] (*see* Chapter 20). Lesions of this type are particularly common in biopsies of immunosuppressed patients in whom they often appear to be an organizing phase of diffuse alveolar damage,[17] and the same extensive etiologies, especially infectious causes, apply. In nonimmunocompromised patients, bronchiolitis obliterans with organizing pneumonia-type reactions can be seen at the edge of mass lesions of any type, behind obstructing lesions such as tumors, and in some specific diseases such as extrinsic allergic alveolitis. However, there is no doubt that this histologic pattern also occurs without other associated diseases,[18] and in this setting, the diagnosis of bronchiolitis obliterans with organizing pneumonia is a reasonable one if other causes have been ruled out.

Yield of Open Biopsy

Definitive estimates of the expected yield of open biopsy are difficult to make, because it is not easy to determine just what pathologic diagnoses or combinations of pathologic diagnoses and clinical situations are considered diagnostic in most published series. For example, Ray and associates[20] considered 122 of 416 biopsies (29 percent) nonspecific, but it is not clear what their nonspecific categories of nonspecific interstitial pulmonary fibrosis (? = honeycombing), nonspecific granuloma, and pneumonitis might mean. Nonetheless, the yield appears to be high: Gaensler[2] has tabulated the results of 15 biopsy series totaling 2290 cases. A "diagnostic" result was reported overall for 94 percent of biopsies, with individual series ranging from 72 to 100 pecent.

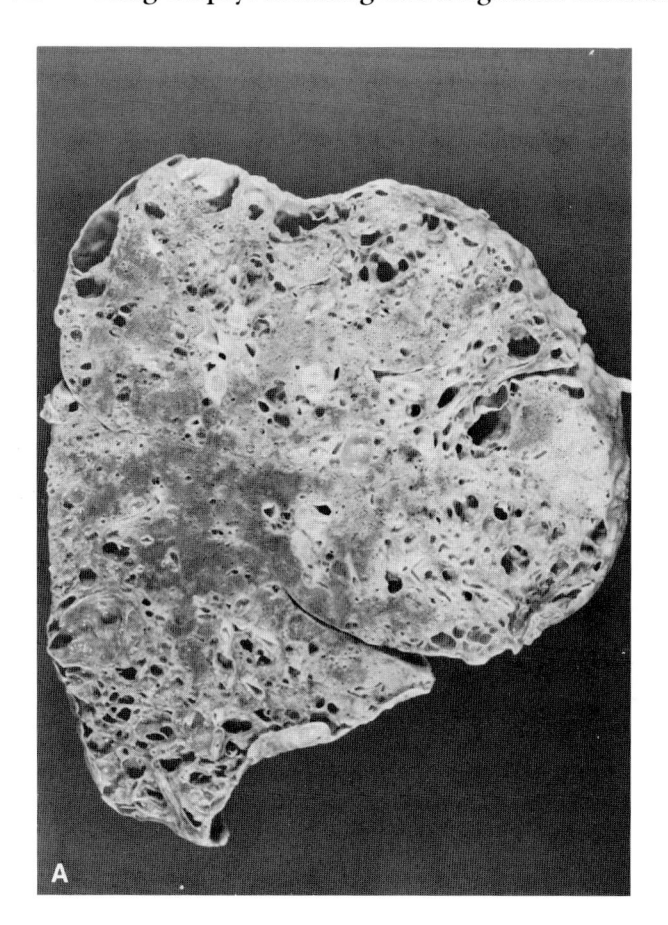

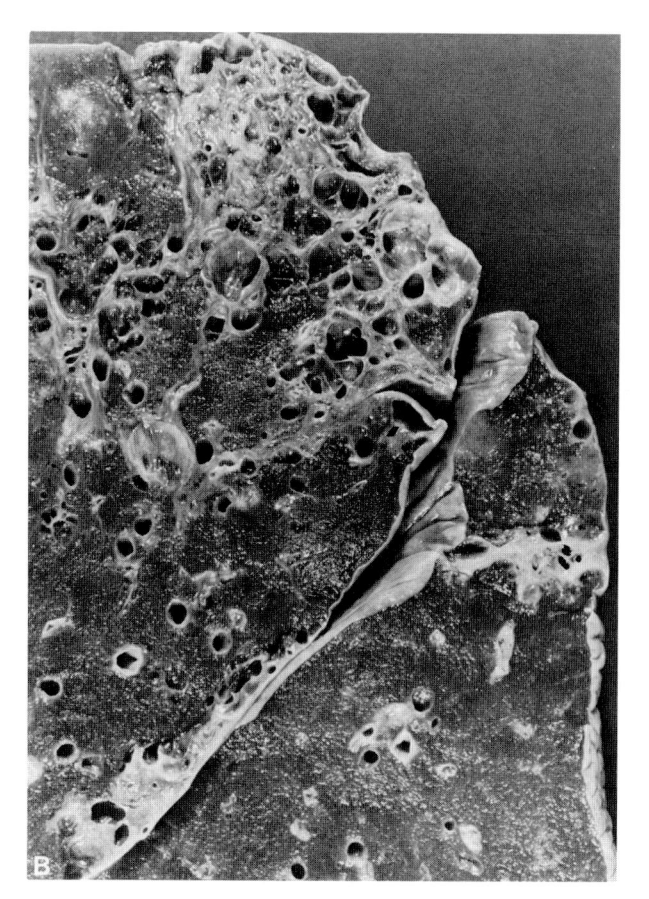

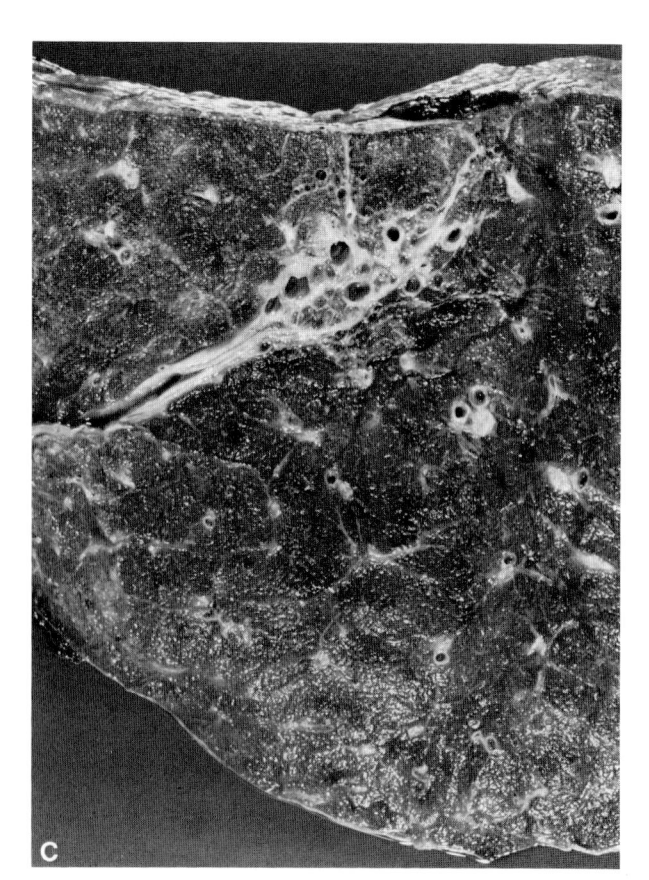

72 Lung Biopsy: Handling and Diagnostic Limitations

Figure 5–3. Three different diseases that may produce honeycombing. A. Pattern of usual interstitial pneumonia (UIP) with honeycombing from a patient with rheumatoid arthritis. B. Upper lobe honeycombing from a patient with old eosinophilic granuloma. C. Nonspecific honeycomb scar found incidentally at autopsy. A biopsy of any of these lesions would probably be identical to Figure 5–5A.

Table 5–2. Diagnostic Possibilities for Transbronchial Biopsy Specimens

Specific Diagnoses	Nonspecific or Unreliable Diagnoses
High Morphologic Yield	Chronic interstitial pneumonias (UIP, DIP)
Most malignancies (including some high-grade lymphomas)	Pneumoconioses resembling chronic interstitial pneumonias
Sarcoidosis	Extrinsic allergic alveolitis
Many infections	Most lymphoid proliferations
Low Morphologic Yield	Diffuse alveolar damage
Eosinophilic granuloma	Bronchiolitis obliterans with organizing pneumonia
Alveolar proteinosis	
Lymphangioleiomyomatosis	
Chronic eosinophilic pneumonia	
Other conditions in which a small microscopic feature is diagnostic	

Transbronchial Biopsy

Handling

Provided that samples have been obtained for culture, all fragments from a transbronchial biopsy are usually embedded and serial sections are prepared. Since the specimens are small, it is often a good idea initially to leave alternate slides unstained, so that sufficient tissue will be available when special stains are needed. Because of the nature of the biopsy procedure, transbronchial biopsies usually show considerable crush artifact, and this is not reversed by techniques such as immersion in a carbon dioxide–containing medium.[2] The use of large biopsy forceps alleviates this problem to a variable but almost never complete degree.

Specific Diagnosis Categories

As is true for open biopsies, transbronchial biopsies can produce specific and nonspecific diagnoses (Table 5–2). Because of the size of transbronchial biopsies, diseases falling into the specific diagnosis categories are generally those in which a small structure or a specific feature defines the diagnosis. Empirically, only three conditions—sarcoidosis, malignancies, and infections—appear to produce relatively high yields in large series of transbronchial biopsies.

Malignancies

Transbronchial biopsy has been used extensively for the diagnosis of malignancies, and yields in the range of 60 percent for peripheral lesions have been reported in some series[21,22]; the yield is increased by the use of multiple biopsies[22] and is higher for larger lesions. However, transbronchial biopsy is probably inferior to fine needle aspiration biopsy for the diagnosis of malignant peripheral lesions.[23] The diagnosis of malignancy from transbronchial biopsies is based to a large extent on cytologic features; the pattern is frequently difficult to discern. Hence, one may be in the position of deciding that a pulmonary mass is a malignant neoplasm and that it appears to be a carcinoma, but exactly what type of carcinoma is unclear. Another common finding is that the lesion in question is not a small cell carcinoma of the lung, but whether it is a squamous or adeno- or large cell carcinoma cannot be resolved. Since the distinction between small-cell and non-small-cell carcinoma is the only critical one for the treatment of primary lung cancers, this problem is not serious. Transbronchial biopsy also appears to be excellent for detecting lymphangitic carcinoma,[24] in large part because the pulmonary lymphatics surround the bronchial tree. Fechner and colleagues[25] emphasize that multiple levels may need to be examined to find small foci of tumor.

In contrast to carcinoma, the diagnosis of lymphoma by transbronchial biopsy is often difficult. Lymphoid cells are fragile and are easily distorted by the crushing associated with the biopsy process. Since transbronchial biopsy yields virtually no information about tissue pattern, lymphomas that are cytologically bland (for example, well-differentiated lymphocytic lymphoma) cannot be diagnosed by this procedure. Even when cytologically malignant cells are present, transbronchial biopsy should not be used to define a previously undiagnosed lymphoma.

Sarcoidosis

Sarcoid granulomas also tend to follow the lymphatic distribution in the lung,[26] and it is probably for this reason that transbronchial biopsy has such a high success rate in this condition. Some authors[9] claim that sarcoidosis is the only non-neoplastic disease for which transbronchial biopsy is useful. A positive diagnosis has been achieved in 60 to 90 percent of cases[27,28]; the yield is higher in those stages in which parenchymal changes are visible radiographically,[27,28] and it is also increased by taking multiple biopsies.[27] The obvious differential diagnosis of granulomas must be considered, and appropriate special stains performed. A negative biopsy in a patient thought to have sarcoidosis is in no way exclusionary; for example, in the series of Wall and associates[29] (discussed in Nonspecific or Unreliable Diagnosis Categories, below), sarcoidosis was missed by transbronchial biopsy and subsequently found by open biopsy in six of 30 patients.

Infections

Infections can also be diagnosed reliably and with relatively high yield by transbronchial biopsy, particularly when results are combined with microbiologic studies of brushings and washings taken at the same time. Transbronchial biopsy is particularly useful for this type of diagnosis in the immunocompromised patient. In a collected series of 240 transbronchial biopsies from immunocompromised patients,[16,30–36] a diagnosis of infection was made in 64 (27 percent); one-third of these 64 patients had pneumocystis pneumonia. By comparison, in this same series, recurrent neoplasm was diagnosed in 20 cases (8 percent; see Chapter 19).

Transbronchial biopsy is specific but provides a relatively low yield in a variety of other conditions which are characterized by a morphologically distinctive feature, but in which the feature of interest is either unevenly distributed or widely scattered within the pulmonary parenchyma. Examples of the first instance are lymphangioleiomyomatosis[37] and pulmonary alveolar proteinosis; eosinophilic granuloma is typical of the second. Pneumoconioses such as asbestosis that resemble chronic interstitial pneumonias cannot be diagnosed by this technique.

Nonspecific or Unreliable Diagnosis Categories

Transbronchial biopsy is unsuited for the diagnosis of diseases that requires histologic evaluation of a fairly nonspecific pattern over a large area, rather than any specific cytologic or histologic finding. This problem is particularly apparent with four different disease groups: (1) diffuse alveolar damage; (2) bronchiolitis obliterans with organizing pneumonia. These two categories have already been considered; the only difference between open and transbronchial biopsy in this situation is that the latter is considerably more likely to miss another lesion; (3) chronic interstitial pneumonias and morphologically similar conditions such as extrinsic alveolitis and some pneumoconioses; and (4) lymphoid proliferations. Attempts to diagnose any of these conditions on the basis of a transbronchial biopsy not only are likely to be wrong but are often dangerous to the patient, since incorrect and potentially toxic therapy may be instituted.

The attempt to diagnose chronic interstitial pneumonias (UIP, and DIP) and morphologically similar conditions has probably been the area of greatest controversy regarding transbronchial biopsy. Several reports have considered the correlation between transbronchial and open biopsy diagnoses for these conditions[29,38,39]; the most thorough study has been that of Wall and associates.[29] They compared transbronchial and open biopsy results in a series of patients who had evidence of diffuse infiltrative lung disease found by physical examination, pulmonary function tests, and chest radiograph. These patients first underwent a transbronchial biopsy; if sarcoidosis, malignancy, or infection was not observed, an open biopsy was then performed. Their data are summarized in Table 5–3. Of 21 patients thought to have either normal lung or a nonspecific pattern of interstitial inflammation and fibrosis by transbronchial biopsy, 9 were found to have a chronic interstitial pneumonia by open biopsy. Of the nine patients whose transbronchial biopsies showed a pattern of fibrosis and inflammation thought consistent with chronic interstitial pneumonia,

Table 5–3. Comparison of Transbronchial and Open Biopsy in the Same Patients[a]

Transbronchial Biopsy (No. of Patients)	Open Biopsy		
	Chronic Interstitial Pneumonia	Sarcoid/EGL	Miscellaneous
Normal lung (10)	4	5	1
Nonspecific fibrosis or inflammation (11)	5	3	3
Chronic interstitial pneumonia or interstitial fibrosis (9)	2	1	6

[a] Modified from Wall et al.[29]

Abbreviation: EGL, eoginophilic granuloma of lung.

the diagnosis was confirmed in only two (22 percent). The transbronchial biopsy missed lesions of eosinophilic granuloma or sarcoidosis in 9 of these 30 patients (30 percent).

The presence of interstitial fibrosis and inflammation in a transbronchial biopsy is therefore a poor predictor of chronic interstitial pneumonia in an open biopsy; conversely, the absence of this pattern in a transbronchial biopsy does not reliably indicate the absence of chronic interstitial pneumonia. This conclusion is supported by the clinical study of Wilson and colleagues.[40] They showed that, in the face of a diagnosis of chronic interstitial inflammation and fibrosis by transbronchial biopsy, the disease process either regressed or stabilized in 22 of 24 (91 percent) of patients with a localized infiltrate on chest radiograph and in 12 of 16 (75 percent) of patients with a diffuse infiltrate. This outcome is clearly contrary to the usual clinical progression seen with chronic interstitial pneumonias.

These comments concerning chronic interstitial pneumonias of unknown origin also apply to pneumoconioses such as asbestosis or talcosis, which are histologically similar; in particular, the combination of asbestos bodies, interstitial fibrosis, and interstitial inflammation in a transbronchial biopsy does not permit the diagnosis of asbestosis.[41]

The reasons why the diagnosis of chronic interstitial pneumonia is not feasible by transbronchial biopsy are not entirely evident, but a number of factors are important:

1. As noted, uninflated lung tissue tends to produce a false impression of interstitial inflammation and fibrosis, even when the tissue is completely normal (Figs. 5–1, 5–4).
2. Inflammation and fibrosis in many of the chronic interstitial pneumonias are characteristically patchy. Thus, a single transbronchial biopsy may reveal only honycombing or only normal lung in a patient who really does have a chronic interstitial pneumonia (Fig. 5–5). This problem is apparently not solved by taking multiple biopsies.

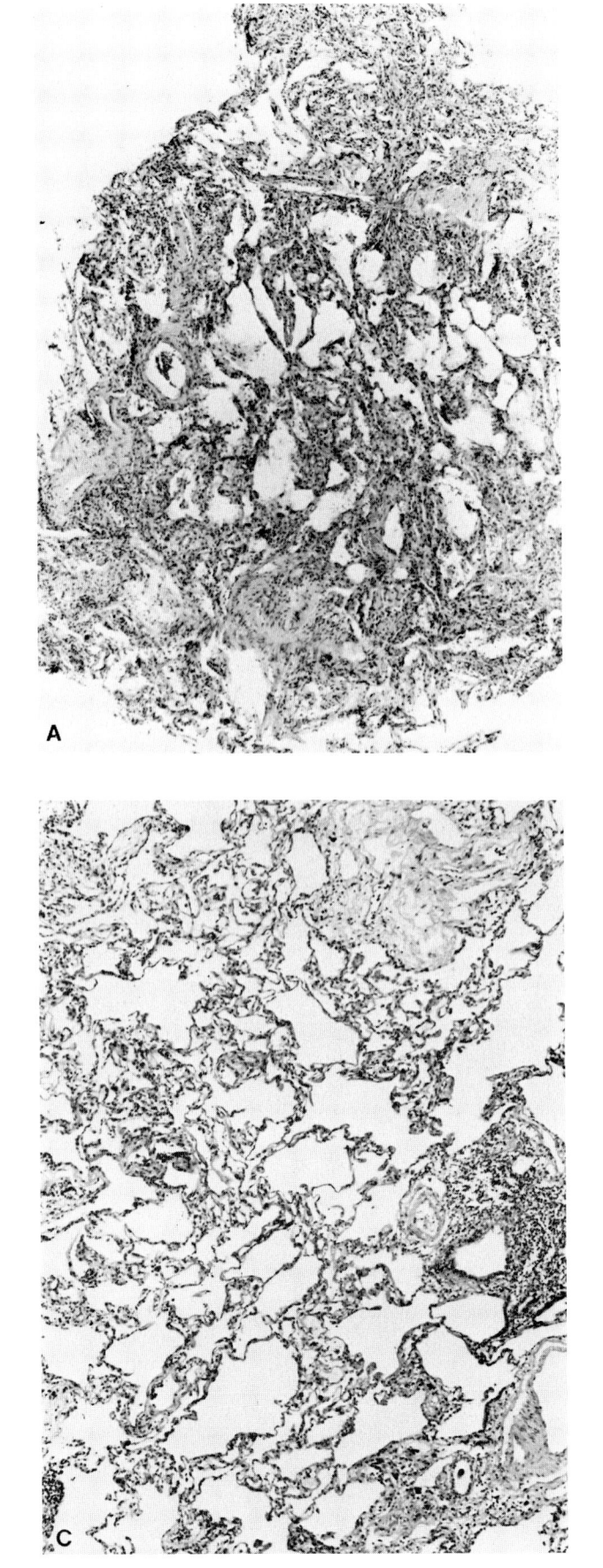

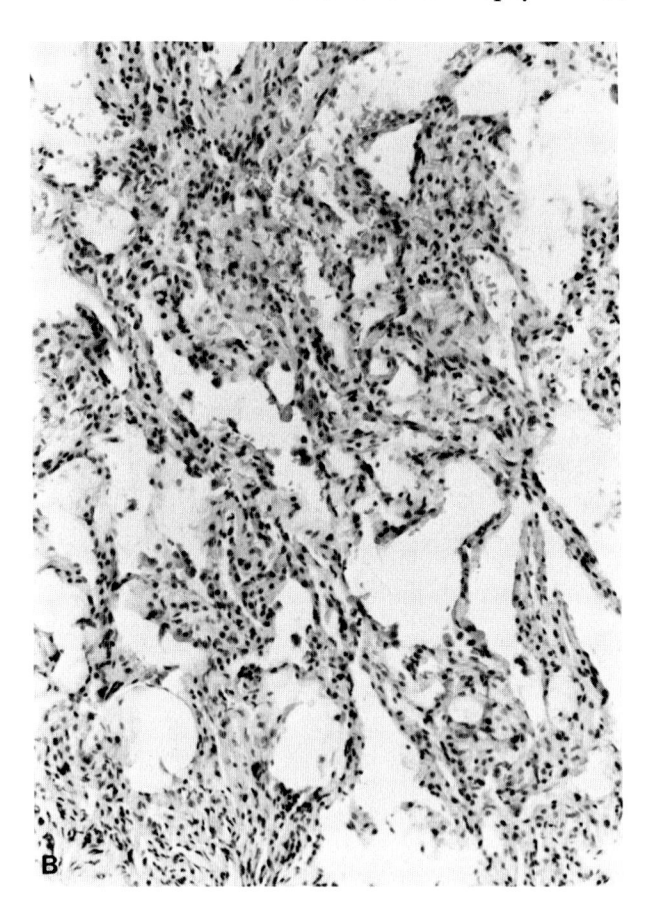

Figure 5–4. False appearance of interstitial inflammation and fibrosis in a transbronchial biopsy. A. The whole biopsy at low power appears to have a thickened interstitium (H&E, ×64). B. This appearance persists at higher power, but in reality is produced by collapse of alveolar walls on each other (H&E, ×160). C. A subsequent open biopsy from this patient demonstrating that in fact the parenchyma is normal (H&E, ×40).

76   Lung Biopsy: Handling and Diagnostic Limitations

Figure 5–5. Three transbronchial biopsy size fields all taken from the same slide from a patient with UIP, illustrating how a transbronchial biopsy might pick up any pattern in a patient who actually does have a chronic interstitial pneumonia. A. Marked honeycombing (H&E, ×64). B. A rather typical pattern of UIP (H&E, ×64). C. Normal lung (H&E, ×64).

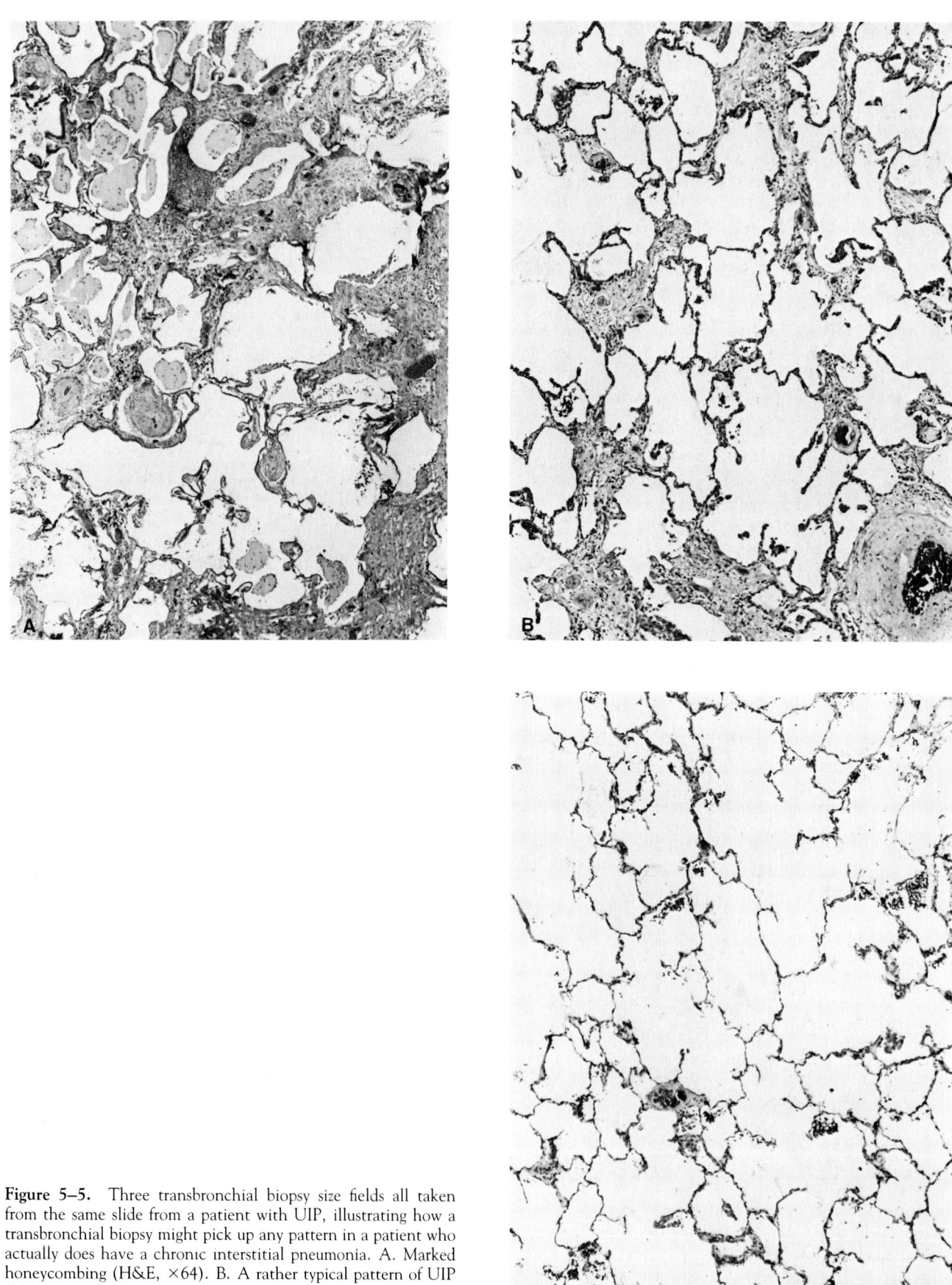

3. Even if present, chronic interstitial inflammation and fibrosis are a nonspecific reaction pattern which may be found around airway walls, particularly in smokers, and adjacent to a variety of other processes in the lung, including tumors and lesions of eosinophilic granuloma (see Chapter 20).

The conclusion to be drawn from these clinical and pathologic observations is that chronic interstitial inflammation and fibrosis in a transbronchial biopsy are nonspecific findings that do not confirm or rule out any disease process. This fact should be emphasized in the diagnosis rendered on such a biopsy.

A similar conclusion applies to most lymphoid proliferations. Even when obviously malignant lymphoid cells are present, the crushing effect of the biopsy may render exact classification impossible. Cytologically bland lymphoid proliferations may represent tumor, chronic interstitial pneumonia or hypersensitivity reaction (extrinsic allergic alveolitis), normal lymphoid aggregates, or nonspecific reactions to other processes such as tumors or cigarette smoke. Diagnoses such as lymphocytic interstitial pneumonia, extrinsic allergic alveolitis, pseudolymphoma, and well-differentiated lymphocytic lymphoma cannot be further sorted out without resort to the large-area, low-power pattern which by definition is not available in transbronchial biopsies. Indeed, in conditions such as well-differentiated lymphocytic lymphoma or angioimmunoblastic lymphadenopathy involving the lung, the low-power pattern may provide the major clue to the diagnosis.[42]

Given these problems, what yield should the pathologist expect from transbronchial biopsy? Obviously this depends on the nature of the patient population and the frequency with which physicians will biopsy in a given clinical setting. However, the initial claims for "specific" diagnoses in the range of 60 to 85 percent[1] are unrealistic.[2] If, for example, one takes Anderson's[1] data on 939 biopsies with a claimed yield (excluding 21 percent inadequate tissue and about 4 percent normal lung) of about 75 percent, and also excludes the nondiagnostic categories of chronic interstitial pneumonitis and fibrosis (39 percent), collagen disease (3 percent, presumably the same as the previous category), lipoid pneumonitis (0.5 percent), acute or subsiding pneumonitis (1.5 percent), and drug-induced fibrosis (0.5 percent), the actual specific yield is reduced to 31 percent. Gaensler[2] has similarly tabulated 1289 biopsies from eight series in the literature; the claimed diagnostic yield was 72.1 percent, but excluding just those cases listed as fibrosis and those with normal lung, the overall yield was 30.3 percent.

References

1. Anderson HA: Transbronchoscopic lung biopsy for diffuse pulmonary diseases. Chest 73:734–736, 1978.
2. Gaensler EA: Open and closed lung biopsy. In Sackner MA (ed): *Diagnostic techniques in Pulmonary Disease*, part II. New York: Marcel Dekker, 1980, pp 579–622.
3. Carrington CB, Gaensler EA: Clinical-pathologic approach to diffuse infiltrative lung disease. In Thurlbeck WM, Abell MR (eds): *The Lung*. Baltimore: Williams & Wilkins, 1978, pp 58–87.
4. Stockinger VL, Hofler H: Praparations und Fixationsabhangigkeit der Alveloarstrukturen. Anat Anz 127:200–209, 1976.
5. Churg A: An inflation technique for open lung biopsies. Am J Surg Pathol 7:69–71, 1983.
6. Katzenstein ALA, Askin FB: *Surgical Pathology of Nonneoplastic Lung Disease*. Philadelphia: WB Saunders, 1982.
7. Wang N-S: Applications of electron microscopy to diagnostic pulmonary pathology. Hum Pathol 14:888–900, 1983.
8. Churg A: Fiber counting and analysis in the diagnosis of asbestos-related disease. Hum Pathol 14:381–392, 1982.
9. Dahlquen P, Oberholzer M: Lung biopsy: Methods, value, complications, timing, and indications. Pathol Res Pract 164:95–103, 1979.
10. Gaensler EA, Carrington CB: Open biopsy for chronic diffuse infiltrative lung disease: Clinical, roentgenographic, and physiologic correlations in 502 patients. Ann Thorac Surg 30:411–425, 1980.
11. Newman SL, Michel RP, Wang NS: Open lung biopsy: is the lingula representative? Lab Invest 52:48A, 1985.
12. Gaensler EA, Carrington CB, Coutu RE, et al.: Pathological, physiological, and radiological correlations in the pneumoconioses. Ann NY Acad Sci 200:574–607, 1972.
13. Pratt PC: Pathology of adult respiratory distress syndrome. In Thurlbeck WM, Abell MR (eds): *The Lung*. Baltimore: Williams & Wilkins, 1978, pp 43–57.
14. Hopewell PC, Murray JF: The adult respiratory distress syndrome. Annu Rev Med 27:343–353, 1976.
15. Churg A: Pulmonary disease in the immunocompromised host. In Thurlbeck WM (ed): *Pathology of the Lung*. New York: Thieme, 1987.
16. Katzenstein ALA, Askin FB: Interpretation and significance of pathologic findings in transbronchial lung biopsy. Am J Surg Pathol 4:223–234, 1980.
17. Nash G: Pathologic features of the lung in the immunocompromised host. Hum Pathol 13:841–858, 1982.
18. Epler GR, Colby TV: The spectrum of bronchiolitis obliterans. Chest 83:161–162, 1983.
19. Epler GR, Colby TV, McLoud TC, et al.: Idiopathic bronchiolitis obliterans with organizing pneumonia. Am Rev Respir Dis 127(part 2): 91, 1983.
20. Ray JF, Lawton BR, Myers WO, et al.: Open pulmonary biopsy: Nineteen year experience with 416 consecutive operations. Chest 69:43–47, 1976.
21. Mitchell DM, Emerson CJ, Collins JV, Stableforth DE: Transbronchial lung biopsy with the fibreoptic bronchoscope: Analysis of results in 433 patients. Br J Dis Chest 75:258–262, 1981.
22. Radke JR, Conway WA, Eyler WR, Kvale PA: Diagnostic accuracy in peripheral lung lesions. Factors predicting success with flexible fiberoptic bronchoscopy. Chest 76:176–179, 1979.
23. Frable WJ: *Thin Needle Aspiration Biopsy*. Philadelphia: WB Saunders, 1983, p 186.
24. Aranda C, Sidhu G, Sasso LA, Adams FV: Transbronchial lung biopsy in the diagnosis of lymphangitic carcinomatosis. Cancer 42:1995–1998, 1978.
25. Fechner RE, Greenberg SD, Wilson RK, Stevens PM: Evaluation of transbronchial biopsy of the lung. Am J Clin Pathol 68:17–20, 1977.
26. Carrington CB, Gaensler EA, Mikus JP, et al.: Structure and function in sarcoidosis. Ann NY Acad Sci 278:265–283, 1976.
27. Gilman MJ, Wang KP: Transbronchial lung biopsy in sarcoidosis. An approach to determine the optimal number of biopsies. Am Rev Respir Dis 122:721–724, 1980.

28. Whitcomb ME, Domby WR, Hawley PC, Kataria YP: The role of fiberoptic bronchoscopy in the diagnosis of sarcoidosis. Chest 74:205–208, 1978.

29. Wall CP, Gaensler EA, Carrington CB, Hayes JA: Comparison of transbronchial and open biopsies in chronic infiltrative lung diseases. Am Rev Respir Dis 123:280–285, 1981.

30. Cunningham JH, Zavala DC, Corry RJ, Keim LW: Trephine air drill, bronchial brush, and fiberoptic transbronchial lung biopsies in immunosuppressed patients. Am Rev Respir Dis 115:213–220, 1977.

31. Feldman NT, Pennington JE, Ehrie MG: Transbronchial lung biopsy in the compromised host. JAMA 238:1377–1379, 1977.

32. Jaffe JP, Make DG: Lung biopsy in immunocompromised patients: One institution's experience and an approach to management of pulmonary disease in the compromised host. Cancer 48:1144–1153, 1981.

33. Matthay RA, Farmer WC, Odero D: Diagnostic fiberoptic bronchoscopy in the immunocompromised host with pulmonary infiltrates. Thorax 32:539–545, 1977.

34. Poe RH, Utell MJ, Hall WJ, Eshleman JD: Sensitivity and specificity of the nonspecific transbronchial lung biopsy. Am Rev Respir Dis 119:25–31, 1979.

35. Springmeyer SC, Silvestri RC, Sale GE, et al.: The role of transbronchial biopsy for the diagnosis of diffuse pneumonias in immunocompromised marrow transplant recipients. Am Rev Respir Dis 126:763–765, 1982.

36. Toledo-Pereyra LH, DeMeester TR, Kinealey A, et al.: The benefits of open lung biopsy in patients with previous nondiagnostic transbronchial biopsy. Chest 77:647–650, 1980.

37. Carrington CB, Cugell DW, Gaensler EA, et al.: Lymphangioleiomyomatosis. Physiologic-pathologic-radiologic correlations. Am Rev Respir Dis 116:977–994, 1977.

38. Ellis JH: Transbronchial lung biopsy via the fiberoptic bronchoscope. Chest 68:524–532, 1975.

39. Levin DC, Wicks AB, Ellis JH: Transbronchial lung biopsy via the fiberoptic bronchoscope. Am Rev Respir Dis 110:4–12, 1974.

40. Wilson RK, Fechner RE, Greenberg SD, et al.: Clinical implications of a "nonspecific" transbronchial biopsy. Am J Med 65:252–256, 1978.

41. Craighead J, Abraham J, Churg A, et al.: Pathology standards for the diagnosis of asbestos-related diseases. Arch Pathol Lab Med 106:543–597, 1982.

42. Turner RR, Colby TV, Doggett RS: Well-differentiated lymphocytic lymphoma. A study of 47 patients with primary manifestations in the lung. Cancer 54:2088–2096, 1984.

6 Gross Examination of Lung Resection Specimens

Roberta R. Miller
Bill Nelems

The vast majority of segmental, lobe, and whole-lung resections are performed for proven or suspected neoplasms. The specimen should be received in the fresh state as soon as possible after resection. At that time, there should be communication between pathologist and surgeon regarding the need for frozen sections (see Indications for Frozen Section in Lung Resection Cases below) and relating to any special or unusual surgical, clinical, or radiologic findings in the case. Such special or unusual features include, for example, suspected coexistent interstitial disease, occupational exposures, previous surgery or radiation, absense of definitive preoperative diagnosis, en bloc resection of parietal pleura, presence of preoperative lobar atelectasis, and so forth.

Superior results are obtained from examination of all lung specimens if they are fixed in the inflated state. By convention, resection specimens are inflated endobronchially with formalin. If endobronchial inflation is impossible due to an obstructing tumor, satisfactory results are obtained by syringe inflation. A large-bore needle is introduced into each segment transpleurally and fixative is *gently* infused with a 50-ml syringe. Tying or clamping of the bronchus has been recommended to prevent escape of the fixative. This procedure should be avoided. Clamping can be easily accomplished only in a left pneumonectomy specimen, since the bronchial stump in most other resection specimens is quite short. Furthermore, tying or clamping introduces crushing artifact at the closure site. Much better results are obtained by gently plugging the bronchial lumen with soft gauze following inflation. Fixative leakage is not a problem in specimens handled in this fashion.

The conventional formalin fixative may be substituted with Bouin's fixative or glutaraldehyde if special studies, such as neuroendocrine investigations or electron microscopy are desired.

The specimen is allowed to fix in the inflated state for several hours or overnight. The specimen is then sectioned at 1-cm intervals with a large sharp knife. By convention, the plane of sectioning is sagittal from lateral to medial to correspond to a lateral chest film. This plane may be substituted by coronal slicing to correspond to a posteroanterior chest film, or horizontal slicing to correspond to a computed tomography scan. The choice of the plane of section depends to some extent on the radiologic findings and interest in the case.

Staging of Lung Cancer

The tumor, nodes, and metastases (TNM) staging system is widely in use, and it is important that resection specimens be handled and reported in such a way that tumor and nodal status is apparent so that accurate staging can be achieved. For many years, the definitions of TNM categories as set forth by the American Joint Committee for Cancer Staging and End Results Reporting (AJC) and as adopted by the American Thoracic Society[1] have been as follows:

Primary Tumor (T)

- *TX:* Tumor proved by the presence of malignant cells in secretions, but not visualized radiographically or bronchoscopically, or any tumor that cannot be assessed.
- *T0:* No evidence of primary tumor.
- *TIS:* Carcinoma in situ.
- *T1:* Tumor is 3.0 cm or less in greatest diameter, surrounded by lung or visceral pleura, and there is no evidence of invasion proximal to a lobar bronchus.
- *T2:* Tumor is more than 3.0 cm in greatest diameter; or tumor of any size that has invaded the visceral pleura; or tumor of any size associated with

atelectasis or obstructive pneumonia that extends to the hilar region, but that involves less than the entire lung; *and* that is not associated with a pleural effusion; *and* the proximal extent of demonstrable tumor must be within a lobar bronchus or at least 2.0 cm distal to the tracheal carina.
- *T3:* Tumor of any size with direct extension into an adjacent structure such as the parietal pleura, chest wall, diaphragm, or mediastinum; *or* tumor involving a main bronchus less than 2.0 cm distal to the tracheal carina; *or* tumor associated with atelectasis or obstructive pneumonia of an entire lung; *or* tumor associated with a pleural effusion.

Nodal Involvement (N)

- *N0:* No demonstrable metastasis to regional lymph nodes.
- *N1:* Metastasis or direct extension to lymph nodes in the ipsilateral peribronchial or hilar region.

MEDIASTINAL

#1 Superior mediastinal or highest mediastinal
#2 Paratracheal
#3 Pretracheal, retrotracheal or posterior mediastinal (#3p) and anterior mediastinal (#3a)
#4 Tracheobronchial
#5 Subaortic or Botallo's
#6 Paraaortic (ascending aorta)

#7 SUBCARINAL

MEDIASTINAL

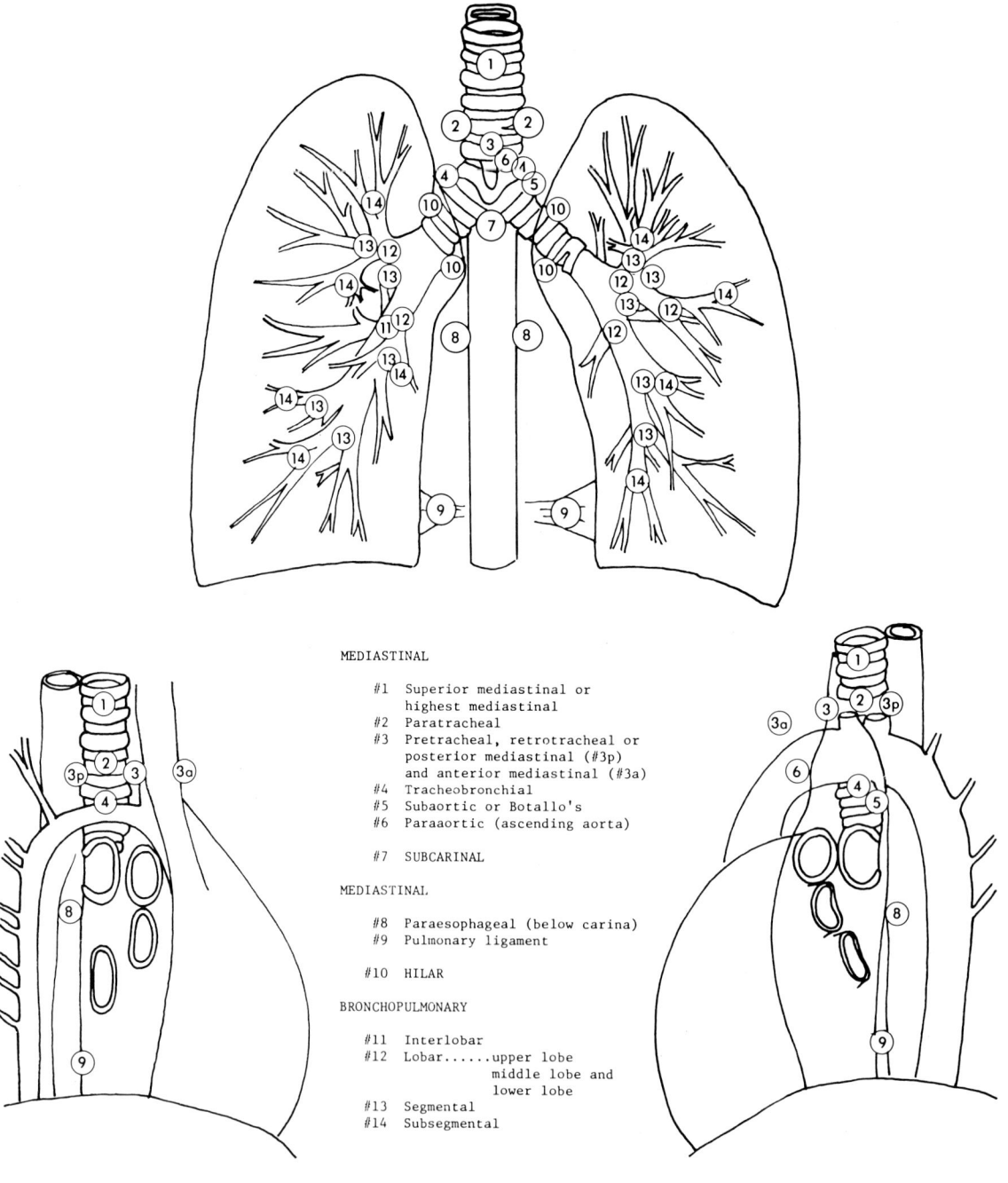

#8 Paraesophageal (below carina)
#9 Pulmonary ligament

#10 HILAR

BRONCHOPULMONARY

#11 Interlobar
#12 Lobar......upper lobe
      middle lobe and
      lower lobe
#13 Segmental
#14 Subsegmental

Figure 6–1. Lung Cancer Study Group modification of the Naruke node mapping diagrams.[5] It is useful if copies of these diagrams are visible in the operating room and pathologist's room, and if lymph node specimens are labeled according to position number.

Staging of Lung Cancer   81

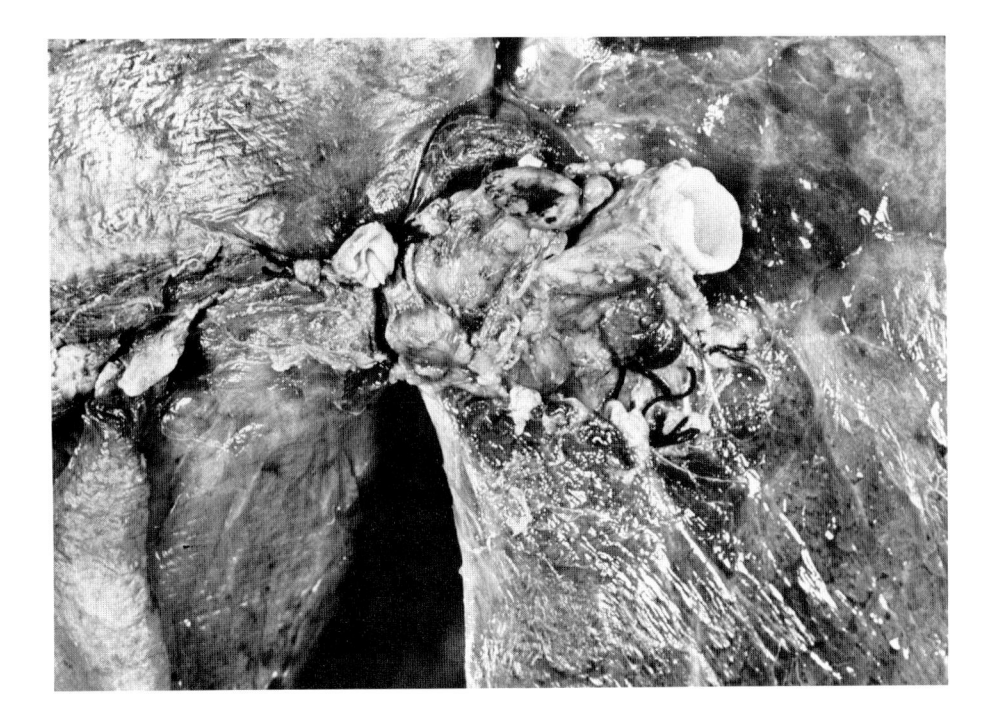

Figure 6–2. Hilum of left pneumonectomy. Lymph nodes that can be removed from around the main bronchus without entering the pleural envelope are N2 nodes.

- *N2:* Metastasis to lymph nodes in the mediastinum.

The National Cancer Institute (NCI) Lung Cancer Study Group uses the level at which the main bronchus penetrates the pleural envelope at the lung hilum as the separation between N1 and N2 nodes (Figs. 6–1, 6–2).

Distant Metastasis (M)

- *MX:* Not assessed.
- *M0:* No known distant metastasis.
- *M1:* Distant metastasis present.

It is helpful if the final pathologic diagnosis specifies the cell type, site (peripheral or central, segment or bronchus), size, status of nodes, pleura, and resection margin and actually gives the TN status (Fig. 6–3).

Two separate staging protocols have been used based on the TNM characteristics of a tumor. The American Thoracic Society has traditionally used the following stage grouping:

- *Occult carcinoma:* TX N0 M0.
- *Stage I:* TIS N0 M0; T1 N0 M0; T1 N1 M0; T2 N0 M0.
- *Stage II:* T2 N1 M0.
- *Stage III:* T3 any N any M; any T N2 any M; any T any N M1.

The Union Internationale Contre Cancer (UICC) has used a different stage grouping as follows:

Left pneumonectomy specimen showing

1. Moderately differentiated squamous cell carcinoma, left main bronchus, 1.4 cm, with transbronchial invasion of mediastinal soft tissue and metastases to hilar and lobar nodes (T3N2)
2. Bronchial resection margin, visceral pleura, and separately submitted mediastinal lymph nodes negative for malignancy.

Right lower lobectomy specimen showing

1. Poorly differentiated adenosquamous carcinoma, peripheral anterior basilar segment, 2.5 cm, with metastases to segmental and lobar lymph nodes (T1N1).
2. Bronchial resection margin, visceral pleura and separately submitted mediastinal lymph nodes negative for malignancy.

Right lower lobectomy specimen showing

1. Poorly differentiated adenocarcinoma, peripheral superior segment, 1.8 cm, with visceral pleural invasion (T2N0).
2. Bronchial resection margin and all lymph nodes negative for malignancy.

Figure 6–3. Examples of recommended format for resection diagnoses. The final diagnosis should answer the questions, "What is it?", "Where is it?", "How big is it", "What is it doing to lymph nodes, pleura and resection margins?", and "What is the pathologic stage?" Other physicians should be able to schematically diagram the extent of the tumor from the final pathologic diagnosis.

Figure 6–4. Double primary tumors in a right pneumonectomy. The larger tumor is a T2 poorly differentiated adenocarcinoma, the smaller tumor is a T1 well-differentiated adenocarcinoma.

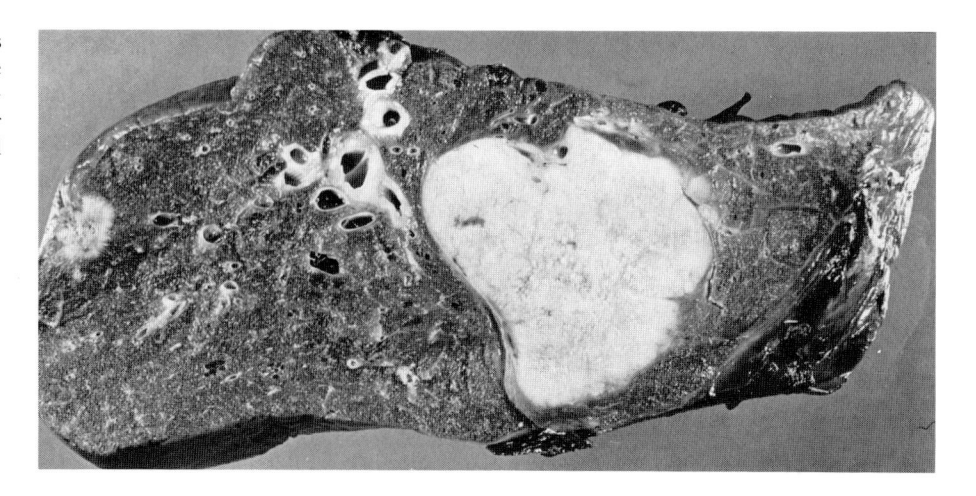

- *Occult carcinoma:* TX N0 M0.
- *Stage Ia:* T1 N0 M0; T2 N0 M0.
- *Stage Ib:* T0 N1 M0; T1 N1 M0.
- *Stage II:* T2 N1 M0.
- *Stage III:* T3 any N M0; any T N2 M0.
- *Stage IV:* Any T any N M1.

Recently, the AJC and UICC have agreed to accept a new staging system for lung cancer.[4] This new proposal has been accepted by the NCI Lung Cancer Study Group and it is likely to be even more widely adopted in the near future. Its definitions are as follows:

Primary Tumor (T)

- *TX:* Unchanged.
- *T0:* Unchanged.
- *TIS:* Unchanged.
- *T1:* Tumor is 3.0 cm or less in greatest diameter, surrounded by lung or visceral pleura, *and* there is no evidence of extrabronchial invasion proximal to a lobar bronchus.
- *T2:* Unchanged except that benign pleural effusion is acceptable.
- *T3:* Tumor of any size with direct extension into chest wall, diaphragm, mediastinal pleura, or pericardium; *and* no invasion of the heart, great vessels, trachea, esophagus, or vertebral body; *or* tumor involving a main bronchus less than 2.0 cm distal to the tracheal carina but not involving the tracheal carina.
- *T4:* Tumor of any size that invades the mediastinum, heart, great vessels, trachea, esophagus, or vertebral body; *or* tumor associated with a malignant pleural effusion.

In addition to the modifications indicated above, one point should be emphasized. Any pleural effusion must be shown to be malignant before it assumes staging significance. A pleural effusion that is considered to be benign does not alter the T assessment of the tumor.

Figure 6–5. Three clinically occult, but grossly apparent, foci of bronchoalveolar carcinoma are present in a lobectomy for a 2.5-cm tumor (not shown in this photograph). Microscopic sections of grossly normal lung in cases like this will show innumerable separate foci of tumor cell proliferation. Case of Dr. K. G. Evans.

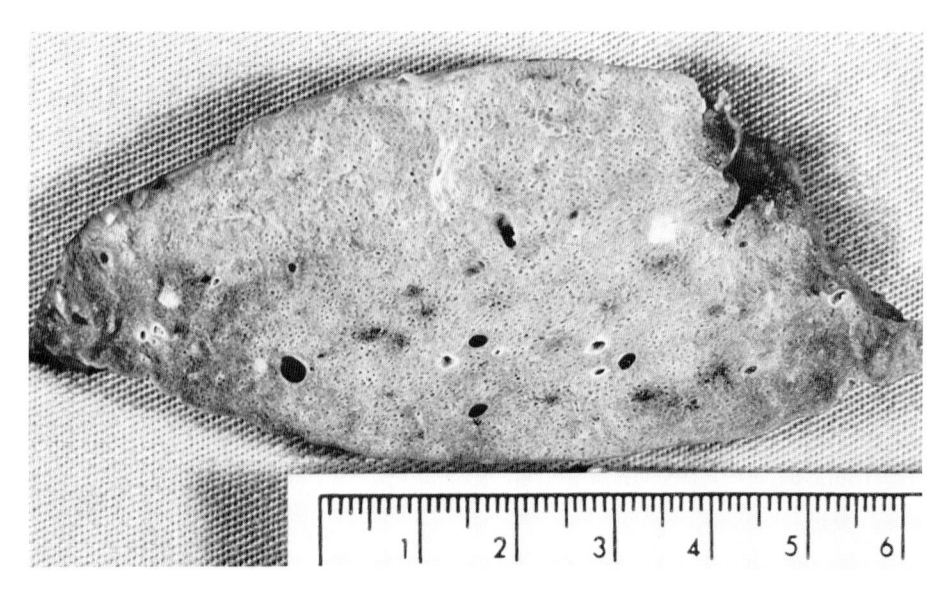

Nodal Involvement (N)

- *N0:* Unchanged.
- *N1:* Unchanged.
- *N2:* Metastasis to ipsilateral mediastinal or subcarinal lymph nodes.
- *N3:* Metastasis to contralateral mediastinal or hilar lymph nodes or to scalene or supraclavicular lymph nodes.

Distant Metastasis (M)

- *MX:* Unchanged.
- *M0:* Unchanged.
- *M1:* Unchanged.

The suggested stage grouping based on these TNM characteristics are as follows:

- *Occult carcinoma:* TX N0 M0.
- *Stage 0:* TIS N0 M0.
- *Stage I:* T1 N0 M0; T2 N0 M0.
- *Stage II:* T1 N1 M0; T2 N1 M0.
- *Stage IIIa:* T3 N0–1 M0; T1–3 N2 M0.
- *Stage IIIb:* Any T N3 M0; T4 Any N M0.
- *Stage IV:* Any T Any N M1.

This stage grouping recognizes the unfavorable sign of any nodal disease including N1, and more importantly distinguishes a stage IIIa tumor as potentially resectable in contrast to stage IIIb. Stage IV is a new addition to the AJC classification.

Problems in T and N Pathologic Staging

While the T and N staging categories are straightforward and readily applied to lung resection specimens in general, some cases present particular difficulties in assessment.

Multicentricity

Occasionally, a resection specimen will contain, in addition to the dominant tumor for which the surgery was performed, a second small, clinically inapparent tumor. Adequate resection of two synchronous primary tumors may be curative. Each tumor should receive independent T assessment (Fig. 6–4).

Rarely a resection specimen will contain innumerable tiny, microscopically similar tumors in addition to the dominant lesion (Fig. 6–5). These cases are almost invariably well-differentiated adenocarcinomas or bronchoalveolar tumors confined to the lung at the time of diagnosis. This type of multicentric malignancy is considered to be incurable disease due to the likelihood of additional foci of tumor in the remaining lung. The T status of these tumors is thus indeterminant (TX).

Carcinoma In Situ

Rarely a resection specimen will contain squamous carcinoma in situ which may extend for several centimeters down the bronchial tree (Fig. 6–6). Extension into the submucosal glands may mimic microinvasion and if this extension is deep enough to involve bronchial associated lymphoid tissue, the lesion may mimic nodal metastases (*see* Fig. 6–6). Squamous carcinoma in situ is considered TIS disease, even if it is several centimeters in length. If a focus of microinvasion is clearly present, the tumor is considered T1 even if the length of the in situ component exceeds 3 cm.

Visceral Pleural Invasion

The normal visceral pleura is composed of submesothelial connective tissue containing fibroblast-like cells covered by a surface layer of mesothelial cells with many epithelial characteristics. A thin elastic lamina is demonstrable in the superficial aspects of the submesothelial connective tissue layer (Fig. 6–7). As a result of injury, whether by obstruction, tumor invasion, or coexistent, but not directly related, pleuropulmonary abnormalities, the architecture of the visceral pleura may be altered by fibrous thickening of the submesothelium, mesothelial hyperplasia, or adhesions (Fig. 6–8). When a tumor abuts on abnormal pleura, the evaluation for actual pleural invasion can be difficult, and involves the following considerations.

1. Is the mesothelial connective tissue layer invaded? This evaluation can be quite difficult if there is fibrous pleural thickening over a tumor. The best marker of the visceral pleural connective tissue is its elastic layer. Tumor involvement of that layer indicates visceral pleural invasion and therefore T2 status. Fragmentation of the elastic fibers or fibrous pleural adhesions in the area of tumor may complicate pleural assessment. In these cases, the elastic layer is at least partly maintained and elastin staining can be useful (Figs. 6–9, 6–10). Pleural puckering alone is not diagnostic of pleural invasion.
2. Is the mesothelial surface layer invaded? If perforation of pleura is present, visceral pleural invasion has obviously occurred (Fig. 6–11). Free pleural perforation is uncommon in a resection specimen and is an unfavorable prognostic sign probably more ominous than simple pleural invasion.
3. Is there a pleural effusion? By the new staging proposal, any tumor associated with a malignant pleural effusion is considered to be a T4 tumor. Rarely, a tumor that would otherwise be operable is associated with a pleural effusion which by cytologic examination is negative for malignant cells. These lesions would be classified according to the tumor without further consideration of the effusion. Needless to say, the presence of a pleural effusion is detected clinically or radiographically rather than by examination of a resection specimen.

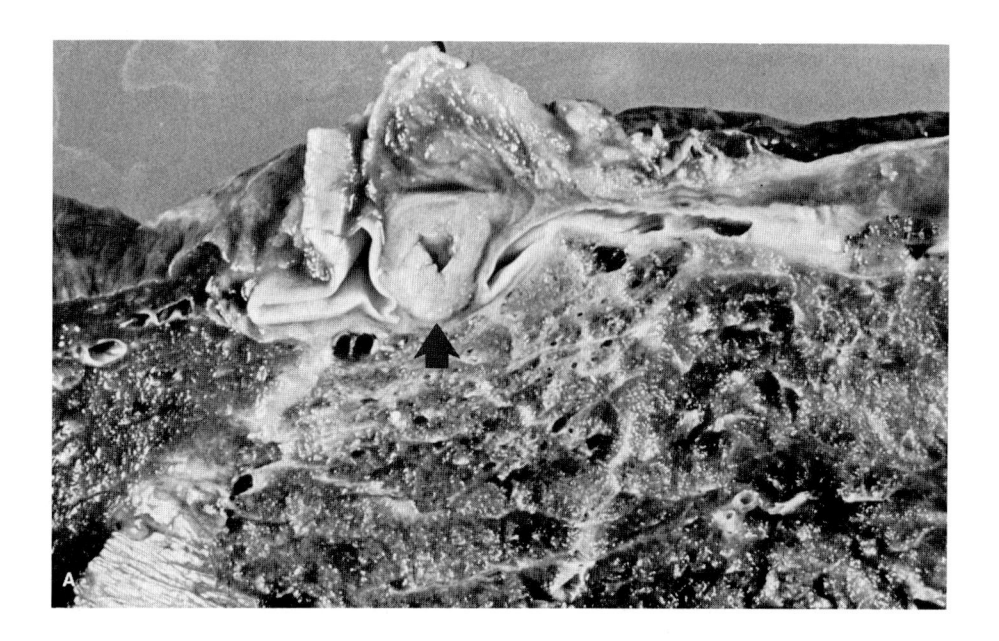

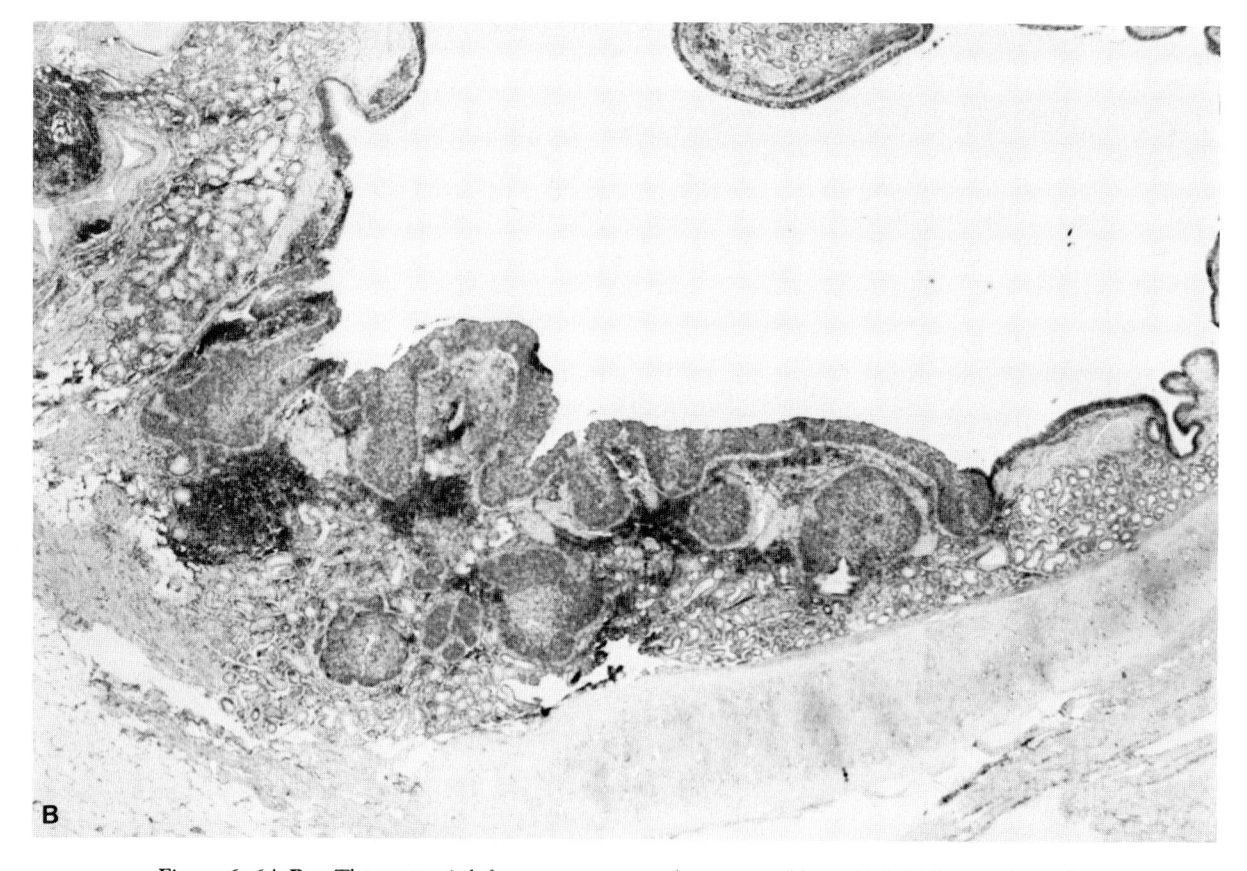

Figure 6–6A,B. This patient's left pneumonectomy demonstrated bronchial thickening (arrow) of the distal main bronchus (A) which extended into the upper lobe bronchus and apical posterior segmental bronchus for a total length of approximately 4 cm. (total length of involvement not shown). Microscopic examination (B) showed partial mucosal replacement by squamous carcinoma in situ with considerable involvement of submucosal glands (H&E, ×25).

Problems in T and N Pathologic Staging 85

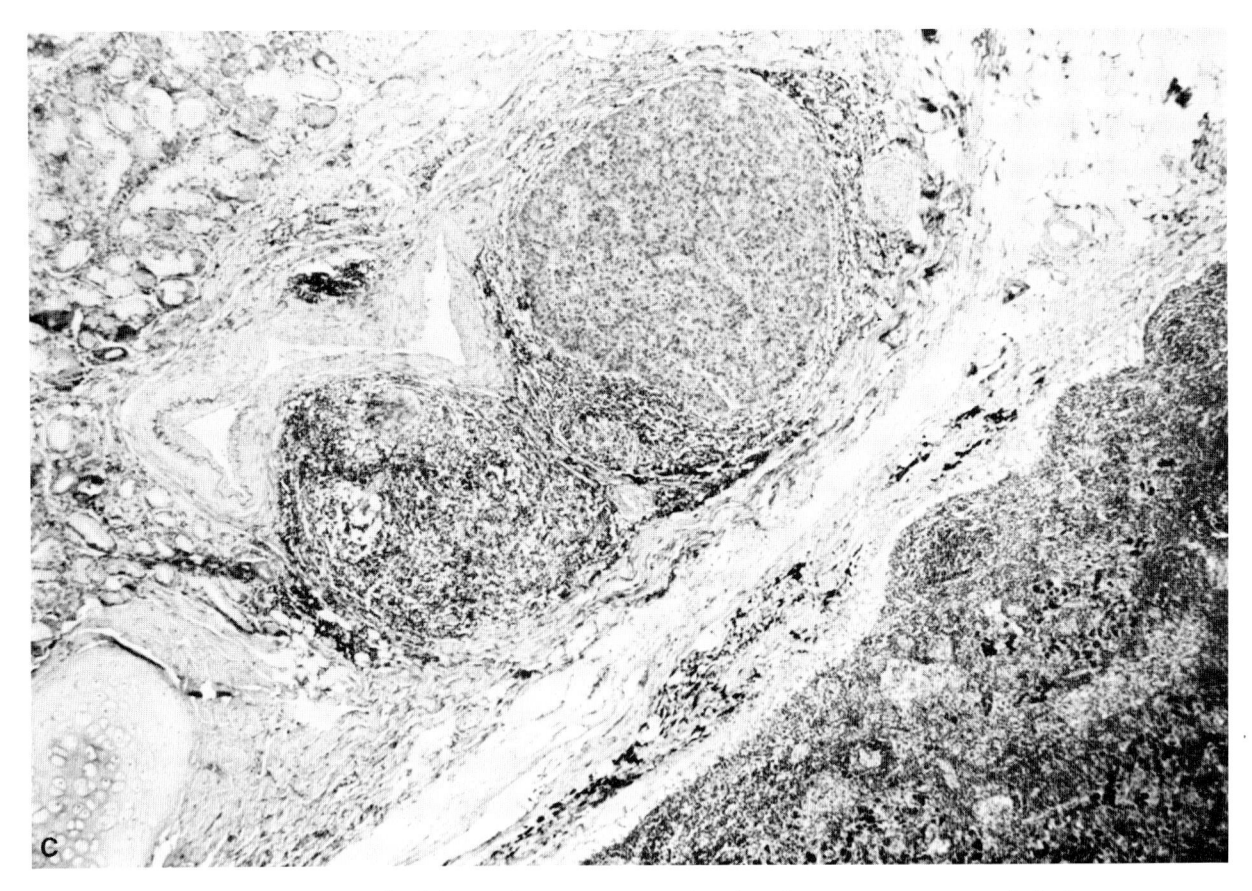

Figure 6-6C. Deep glandular involvement next to a lymph node requires assessment of whether or not nodal metastasis has occurred (H&E, ×63). Case of Dr. K. G. Evans.

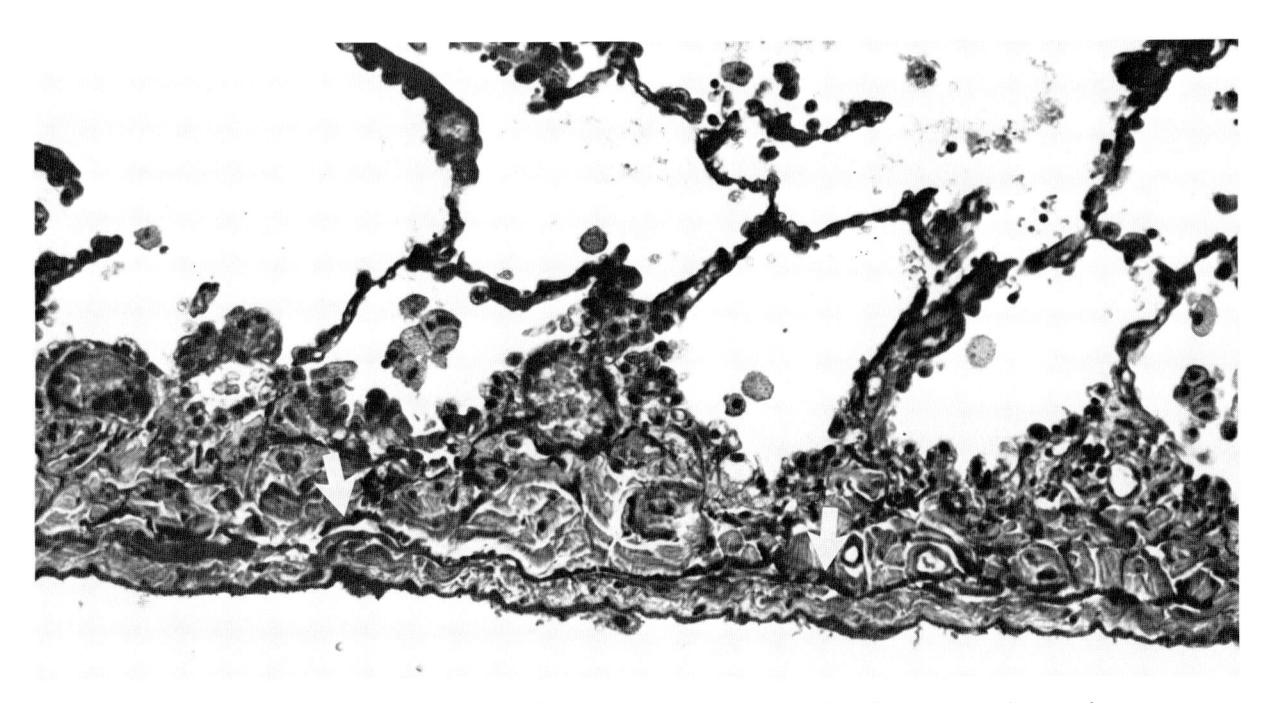

Figure 6–7. Relationship of elastic lamina (arrow) to mesothelial surface in normal visceral pleura. (VVG, ×265).

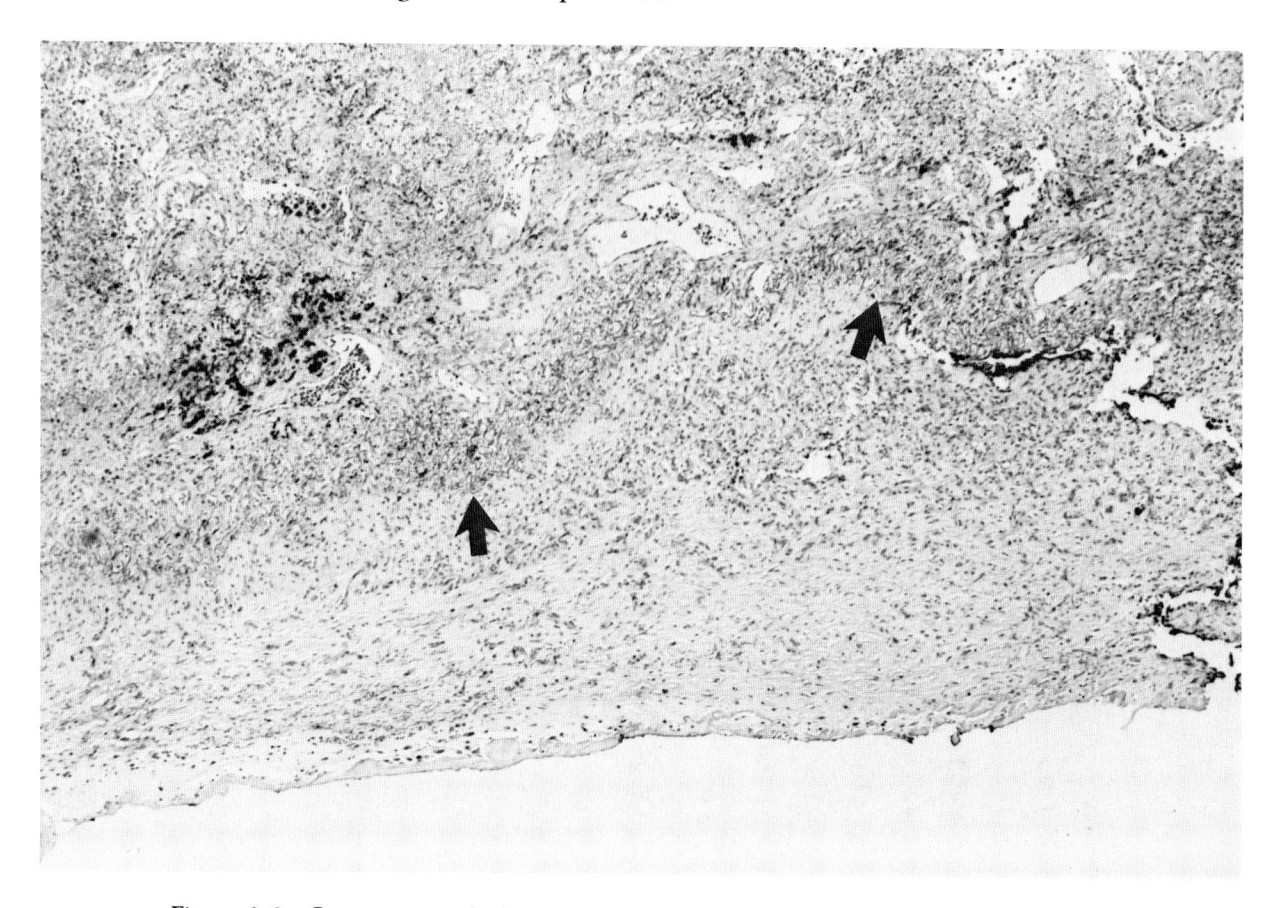

Figure 6–8. Reactive visceral pleural thickening over an organizing infarct. Elastic lamina (arrows) is apparent deep to the granulation tissue and fibrinous exudate, and represents the true pleural marker (H&E, ×63).

4. Is the parietal pleura invaded? In cases requiring sharp dissection of the tumor from the parietal pleura, the adherent parietal pleura may show only reactive changes or may show actual tumor invasion. In the latter instance, the tumor is T3, even if the tumor invasion is only microscopic. One microscopic marker of parietal pleura overlying adhesions is fat (Fig. 6–12).
5. Is the chest wall invaded? Skeltal muscle infiltration is a reliable marker of T3 chest wall invasion (Fig. 6–13).

Obstruction

Lobar obstruction indicates a T2 tumor regardless of the tumor size. The application of this criterion is straightforward for tumors of the right lung. For purposes of T2 staging, the apical posterior and anterior segments are considered to be the proper left upper lobe and the lingula is considered to be the "left middle lobe." Thus, obstruction of either the lingula only or the proper left upper lobe only each constitute T2 tumors because they each produce atelectasis that extends to the hilar region. Most commonly, however, tumors in the area obstruct both lobes together (Fig. 6–14).

Mediastinal Invasion

Invasion of the mediastinum by tumor indicates an unresectable T4 lesion. Mediastinal soft tissue invasion may be mimicked by perinodal tumor extension from metastatic disease in mediastinal nodes. Contiguous spread from the primary tumor into the mediastinum must be demonstrated to fulfill this criterion (Fig. 6–15).

Nodal Status

In a lobectomy specimen, all intraspecimen lymph nodes are in the N1 group. In a pneumonectomy specimen, one may find lymph nodes around the main bronchus that are outside the hilar pleural envelope (*see* Fig. 6–2) and these nodes are regarded as N2 nodes. Separate peribronchial nodes may be submitted for assessment and it is essential that the surgeon identify the location of these nodes with reference to the pleural envelope. The actual node count is not so important in staging as the simple presence of metastases (Fig. 6–16). Thus, all grossly negative nodes must be entirely blocked and examined even if several sections of the same node are required to do so.

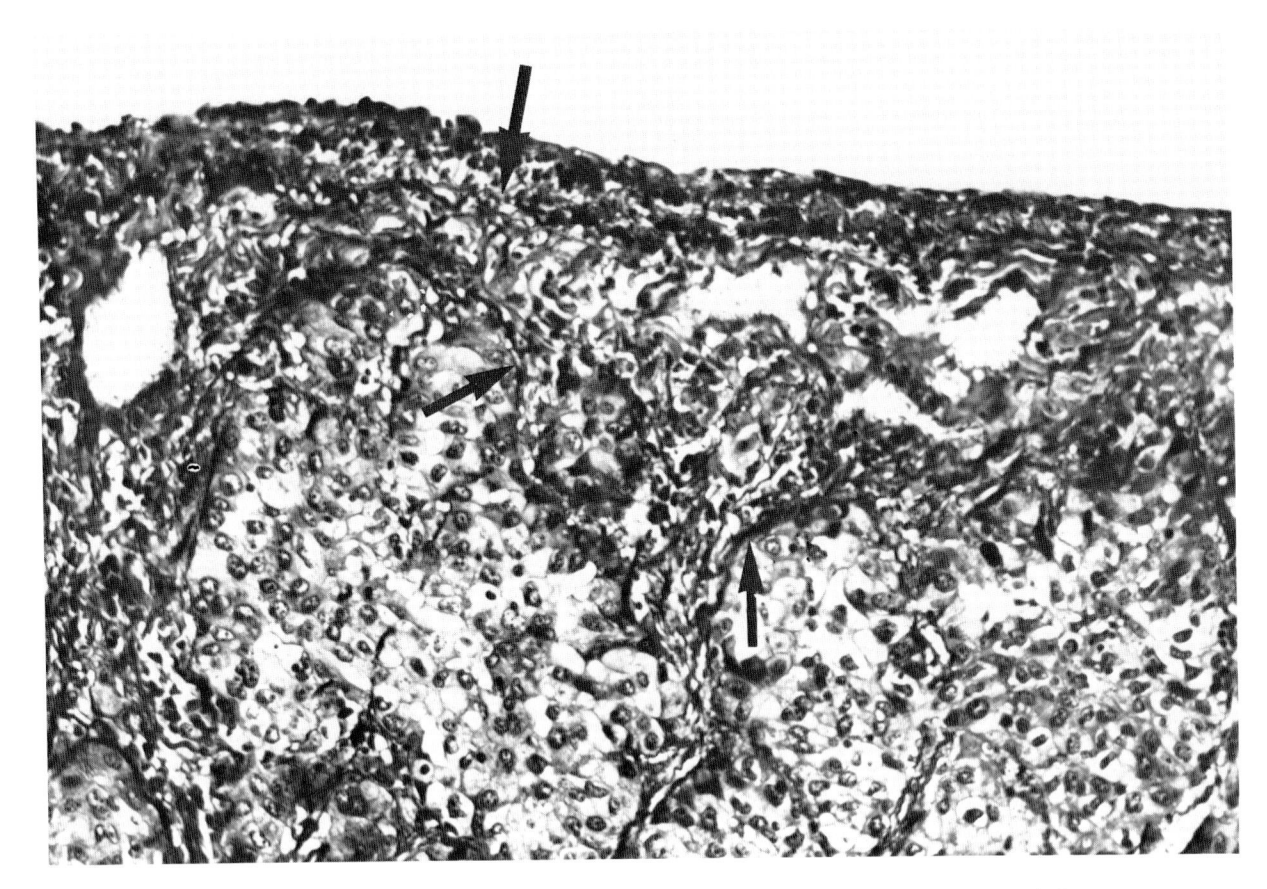

Figure 6-9. Tumor cells (small arrows) pushing against pleura without transgression of elastic lamina (large arrows). Pleural invasion has not occurred and, if less than 3 cm in diameter, this lesion is T1 (VVG, ×265).

Indications for Frozen Section in Lung Resection Cases

Four separate situations may require frozen section interpretation in potential lung resection cases.

Mediastinoscopy

Mediastinoscopy is performed to determine the status of most N2 and N3 lymph nodes. If high paratracheal or contralateral N3 lymph nodes contain metastatic tumor, the patient is considered inoperable. Low ipsilateral or subcarinal N2 metastasis may come to radical resection with postoperative adjuvant therapy. Ideally, mediastinoscopy is performed at least 2 days prior to the planned resection operation so that the surgeon will have the results well before the planned operation. If the mediastinoscopy shows gross tumor involvement, frozen section may be performed to confirm the diagnosis and to avoid delay in beginning therapy. Occasionally, the surgeon may schedule thoracotomy to follow mediastinoscopy immediately and in these patients, frozen section of nodal biopsies will be requested. At times, frozen section of grossly negative lymph nodes will be requested to assist in scheduling of operating room time. The manner in which these requests are handled depends on the surgeon and pathologist involved.

Intraoperative Lymph Node Sampling

If grossly suspicious N2 or N3 lymph nodes are discovered intraoperatively, frozen section should be performed since the result will often determine resectability. Frozen section of interlobar lymph nodes may be requested to determine if a planned lobectomy should be extended to a pneumonectomy. Finally, frozen section of grossly normal lobar N1 lymph nodes at the planned resection margin may be requested.

Resection Margins

Request for frozen section of the bronchial margin of a resection specimen depends to a great extent on the surgeon. The most common policy is to request a frozen

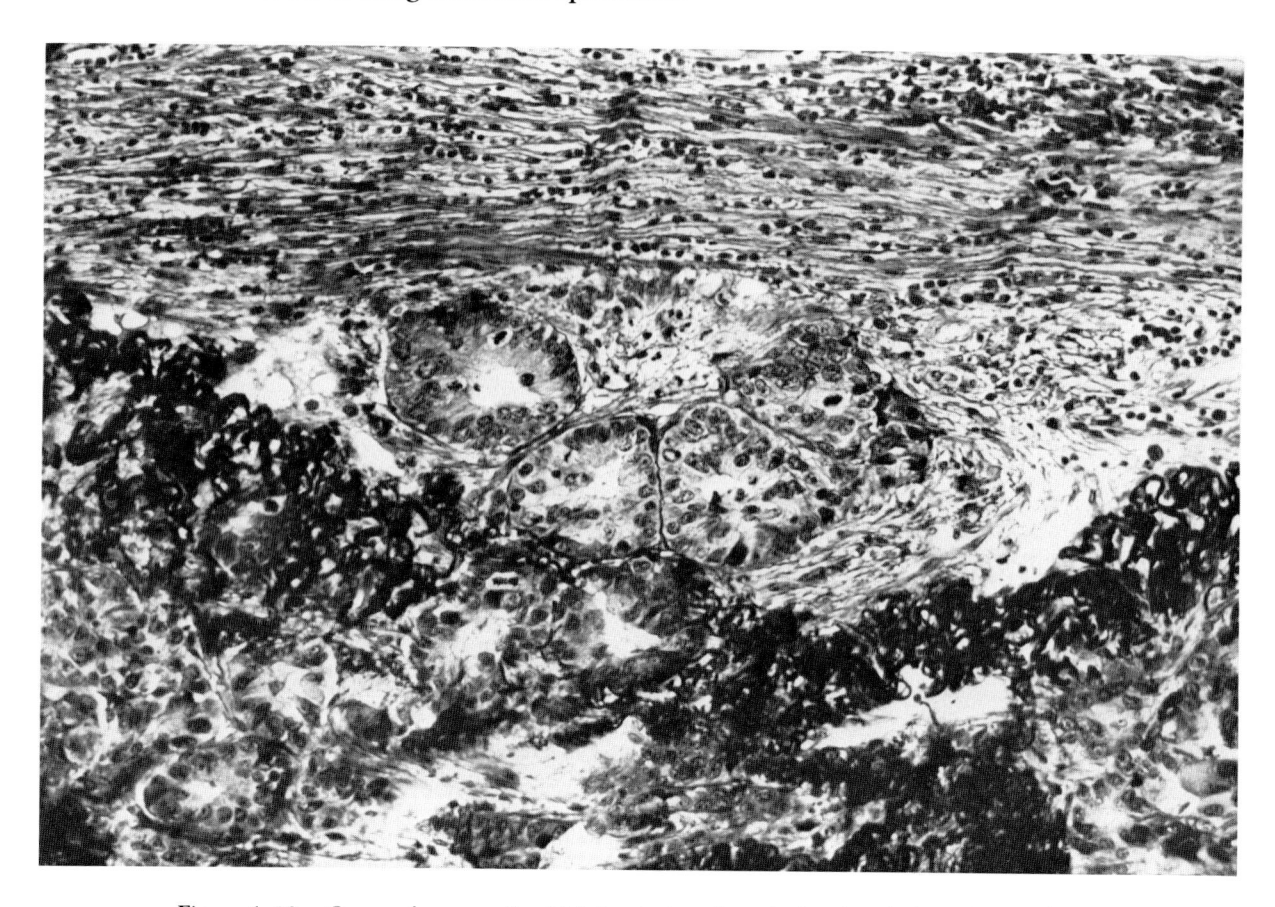

Figure 6–10. Group of tumor cells which has broken through the pleural elastic lamina. Note pleural reaction with remarkable elastic lamina thickening in the area of invasion (VVG, ×265).

section on any case where an endobronchial tumor was visible by bronchoscopy, and not necessarily to request frozen section in cases of peripheral tumors. Frozen section is not performed in the occasional patients where additional bronchus cannot technically be obtained. When parietal pleura has been dissected overlying a peripheral tumor, the margins of the parietal pleural patch should be immediately assessed. This assessment is often best made by careful gross examination.

Peripheral Nodule Without Definitive Diagnosis

In cases of a peripheral nodule located so closely to the pleura that the lesion can be wedge-resected or enucleated, frozen section must be performed. If the lesion is benign, no further surgery will be performed. If the lesion is malignant, formal definitive resection will be carried out. If the nodule is too deep in the lobe to be wedge-resected, a full lobar or segmental resection may be performed. Pneumonectomy is contraindicated without a tissue diagnosis of malignancy.

Gross Room Procedure—Lung Resection for Neoplasm

The following section is intended to be used as a guide to the actual handling of a resection specimen from the time of its receipt from the operating room.

1. The specimen weight is noted.
2. Complete transections of the bronchial and vascular resection margins are taken.
3. Lymph nodes present around the bronchus are removed and sectioned. In a pneumonectomy specimen, N1 and N2 nodes must be sampled separately as discussed above.
4. The specimen is palpated for the tumor. The pleural surface overlying the tumor is first painted with ink, the tumor is then incised, and small samples of tumor are fixed in glutaraldehyde for possible electron-microscopy. This incision is made lateral to the tumor and the tumor is sampled deeply to avoid artifactual disruption of the pleural relationships.
5. The specimen is inflated with fixative and the specimen is allowed to fix in the inflated state for several hours or overnight.
6. The fixed specimen is sectioned in the desired plane

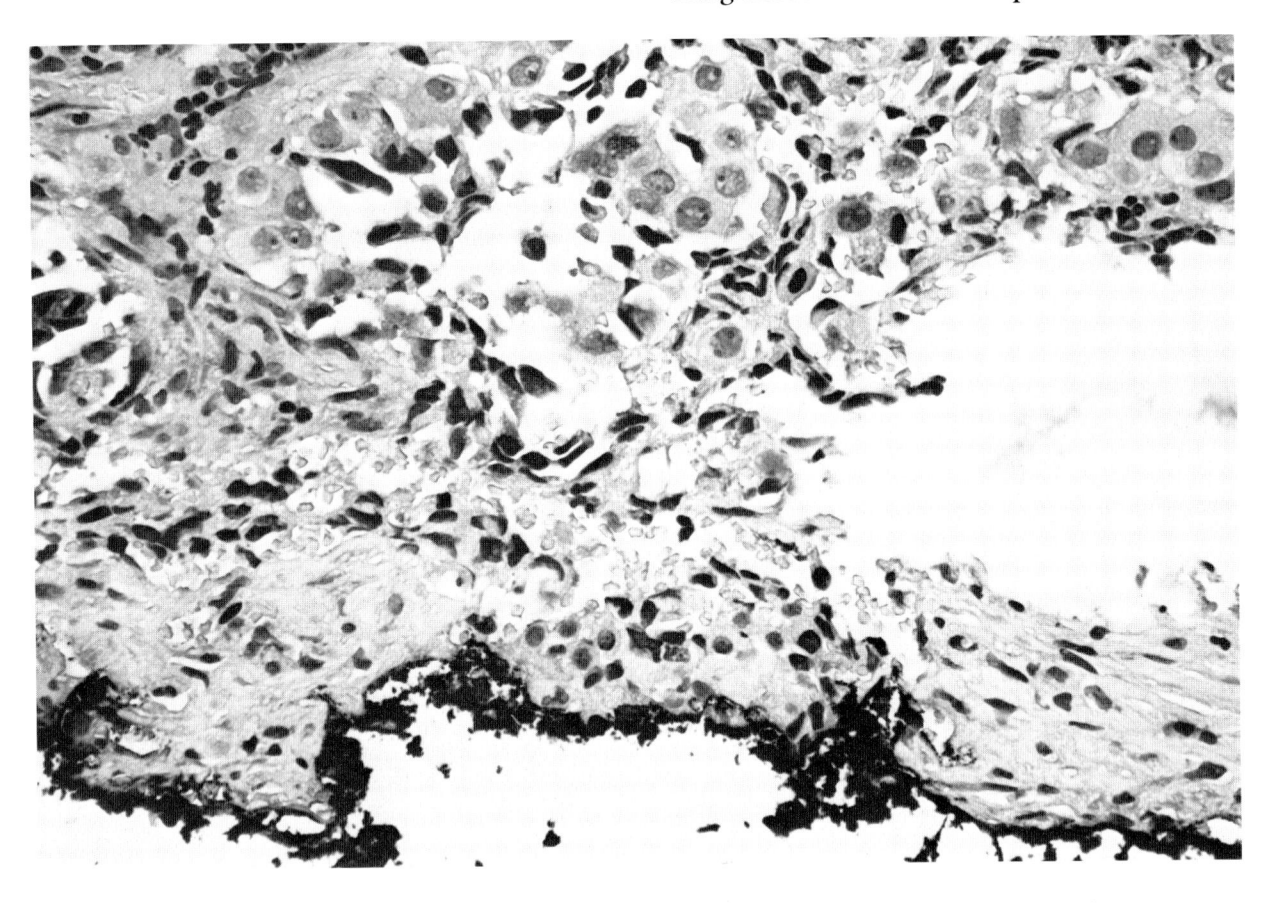

Figure 6–11. Virtual pleural perforation by tumor cells. Pleural surface has been painted with ink (H&E, ×400).

with a large sharp knife at approximately 1-cm intervals.

7. If the tumor is a peripheral nodule, its segmental location and its distance from the pleura or fissure is noted. If adherent parietal pleura has been removed en bloc, it is important to carefully assess this tissue, since parietal pleural invasion indicates a T3 lesion. If the tumor is present in a major bronchus in the medial aspect of the specimen, the involved bronchus, the gross depth of invasion, the degree of lumenal occlusion, and the distance from the bronchial margin are all noted. Assessment of the relationship between a tumor, its parent bronchus, and the proximal bronchial stump often is facilitated by gentle probing of the lobar and segmental bronchi.
8. Further gross description should include (a) size of tumor, (b) presence of necrosis, cavitation, or hemorrhage in the tumor, (c) presence and extent of obstructive pneumonia or bronchiectasis distal to the lesion, (d) presence and appearance of lymph nodes within the specimen, (e) presence and nature of any pleural abnormalities, (f) appearance of noninvolved parenchyma with respect to emphysema, fibrosis, and so forth.
9. In addition to sections of bronchovascular margins and proximal lymph nodes, sections are taken as follows: (a) at least three or four sections of tumor including its relationship to pleura or major bronchus (for relatively small peripheral tumors that are clearly abutting on the visceral pleura, it is often useful to submit the entire pleural-tumor interface); (b) at least one section of parenchyma and pleura distal to the tumor (if possible); (c) any lymph nodes found within the specimen; (d) at least one or two representative sections of grossly uninvolved lung parenchyma; and (e) at least two or three sections of grossly uninvolved major bronchi, particularly if the tumor arose in a major bronchus.

Lung Resection for Nonneoplastic Disease

Occasionally, lung resection is performed for nonneoplastic diseases such as bronchiectasis, tuberculosis, echinococcal cyst, and so on. In these cases, the gross room procedure is simpler. As before, the following section is intended to be used as a guide to the handling of such specimens. The reader will note many points of overlap with the procedure recommended for lung tumor specimens.

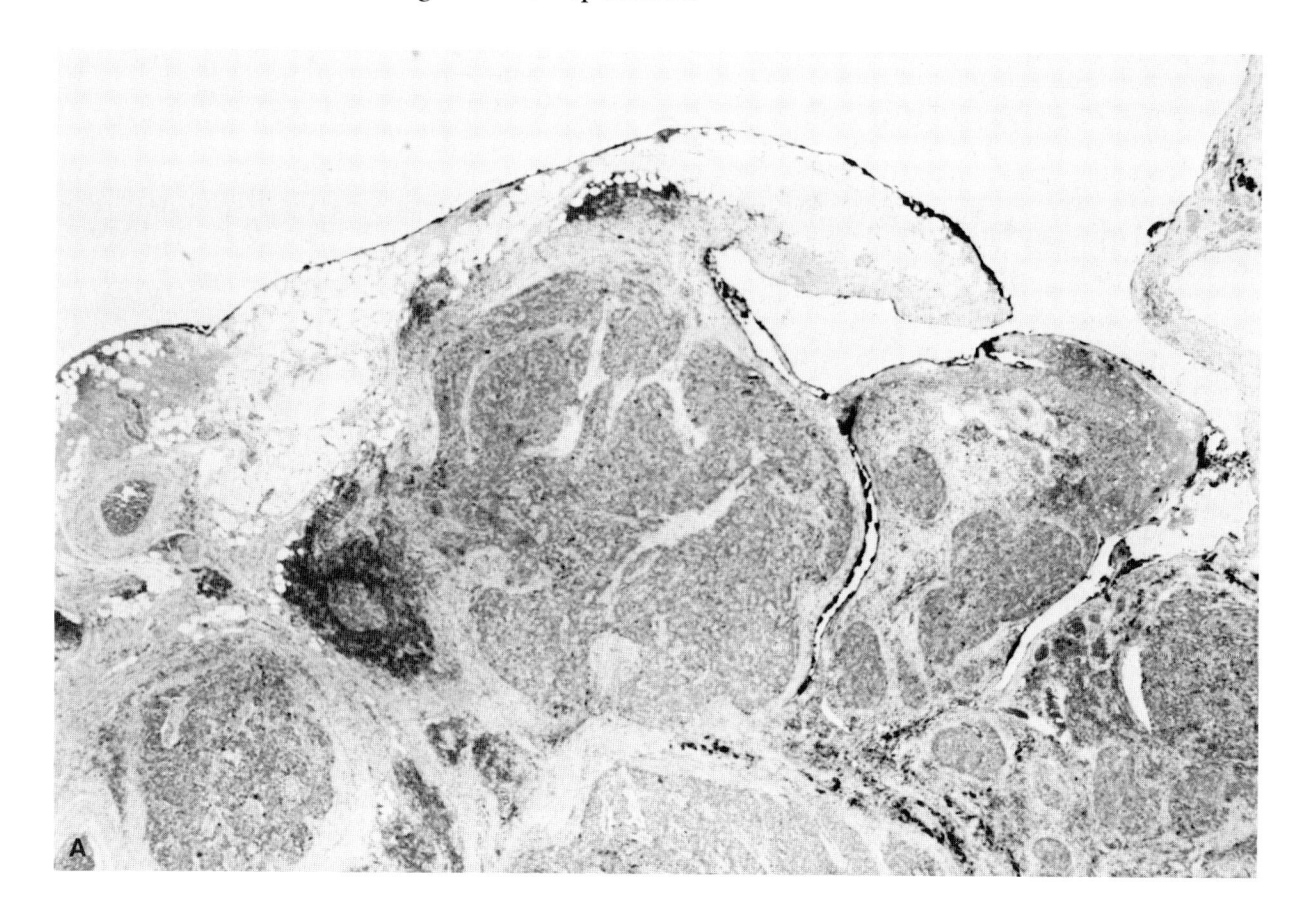

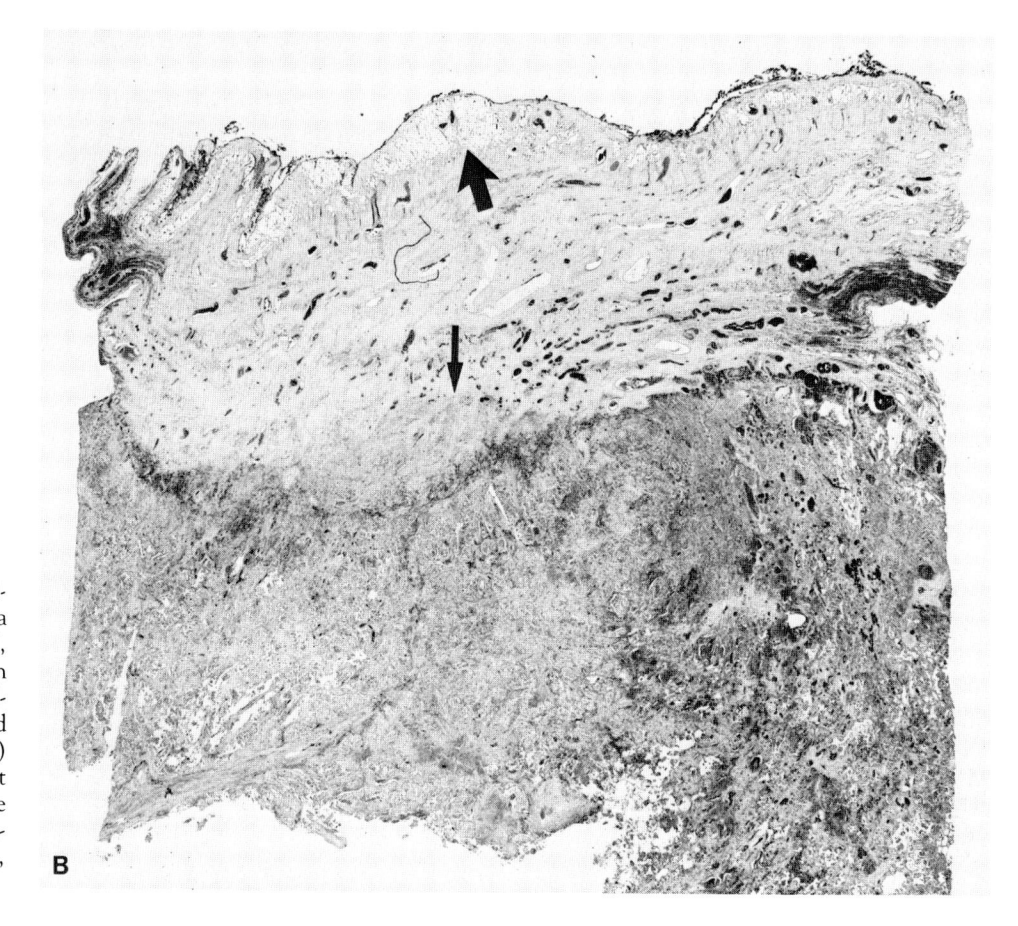

Figure 6–12. A. Tumor infiltration into fat of parietal pleura indicates a T3 tumor (H&E, ×25). B. Resection specimen with visceral-parietal pleural adhesions. The tumor has invaded the visceral pleura (small arrow) and involves the adhesions but has not reached the fat of the parietal pleura (large arrow), indicating a T2 lesion (H&E, ×6.3).

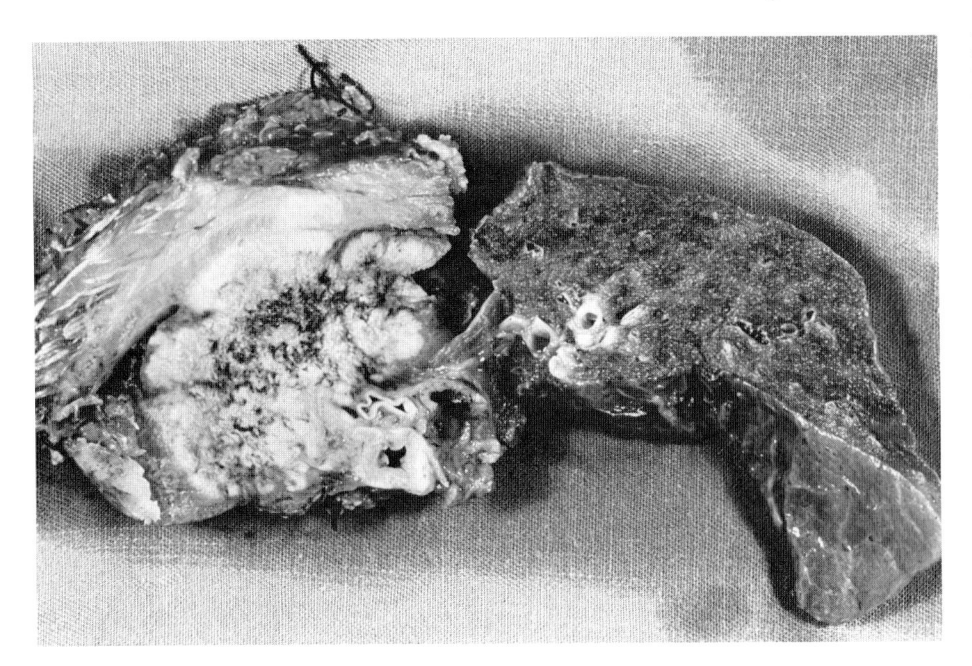

Figure 6–13. Extended pneumonectomy with obvious chest wall invasion. Case of Dr. K. G. Evans.

Gross Room Procedure—Lung Resection for Nonneoplastic Disease

1. If appropriate, cultures are obtained at once in the gross room provided the surgical team has not already done so.
2. The specimen weight is noted.
3. The specimen is inflated with fixative and allowed to fix in the inflated state for several hours. (Fixation with formalin for 48 hours is recommended in suspected active tuberculosis cases.)
4. The fixed specimen is sectioned in the desired plane with a large sharp knife at approximately 1-cm intervals.
5. The lesion is described to include size, apparent nature, site and relationship to pleura or fissure, bronchi, and vessels.
6. Further description should include (a) presence and appearance of lymph nodes within the specimen, (b) presence and nature of any pleural abnormalities, and (c) appearance of noninvolved parenchyma.
7. Sections are taken as follows: (a) at least three sections

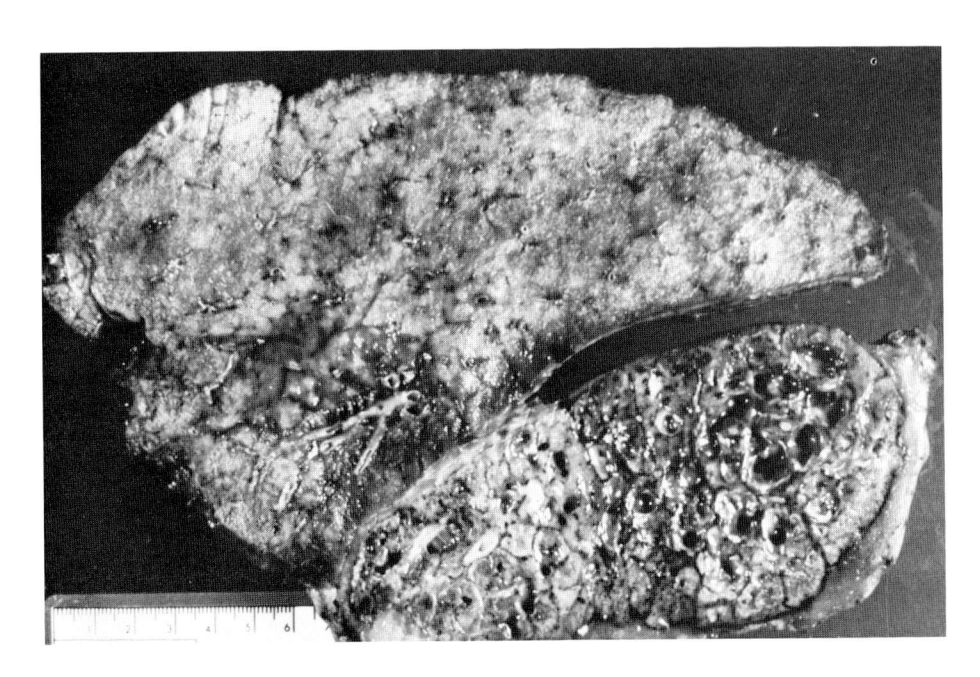

Figure 6–14. Left pneumonectomy with total upper lobe obstructive pneumonitis. The tumor was a 2-cm squamous cell carcinoma of the upper lobe bronchus (tumor not shown) but the pattern of upper lobe and lingular obstruction indicates a T2 lesion.

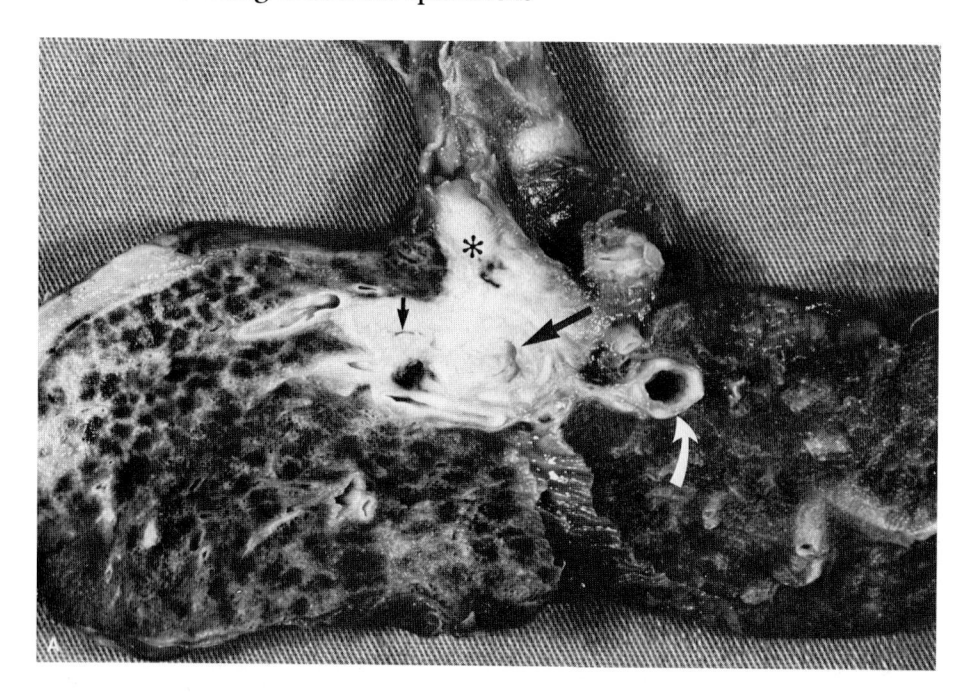

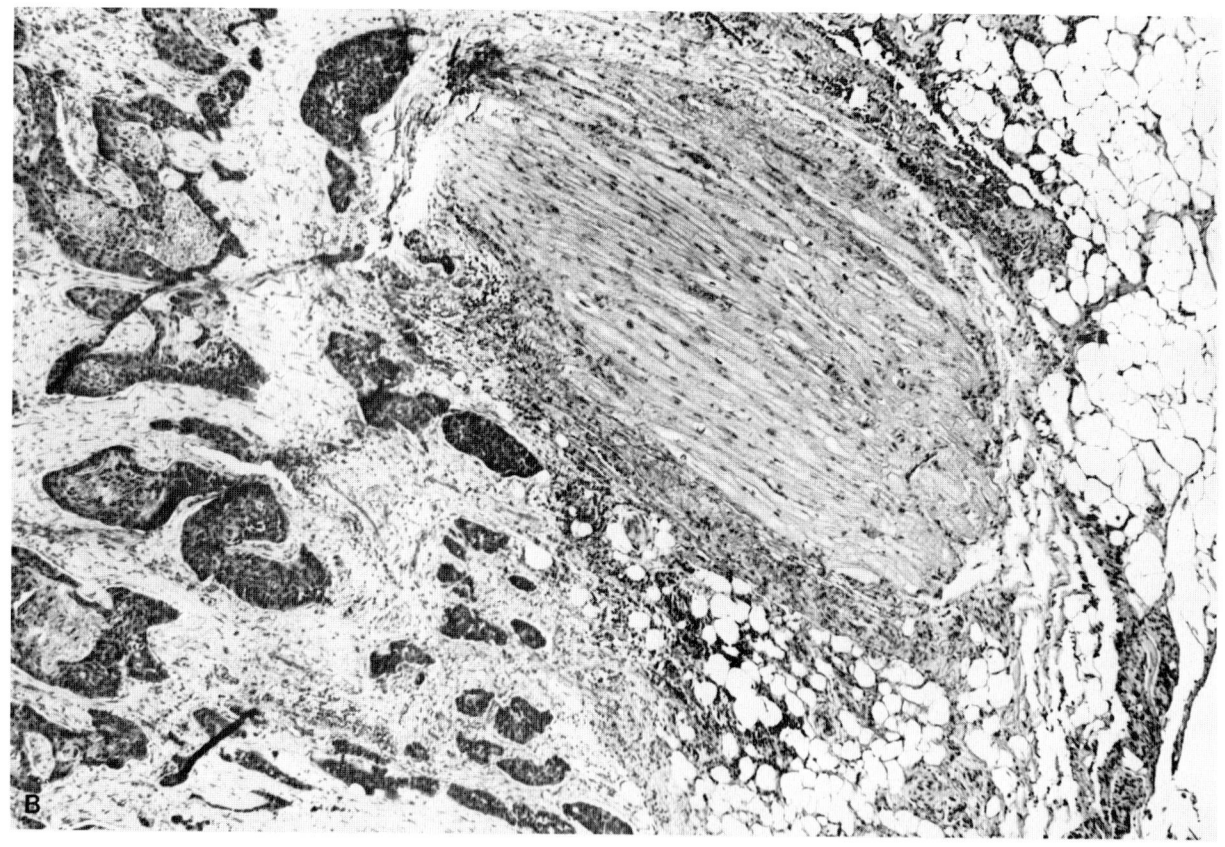

Figure 6–15. A. Left pneumonectomy with a central squamous cell carcinoma of the lower lobe bronchus. The specimen was cut horizontally in the orientation of a computed tomography scan. The superior segment bronchus (small arrow), main bronchus to the basilar segments (large arrow), and middle lobe bronchus (curved arrow) are all seen. Note extension into the soft tissue around the main bronchus and an entrapped anthracotic lymph node (asterisk). B. Tumor infiltrating cardiac-type muscle of the pulmonary vein indicates a T4 tumor (H&E, ×63).

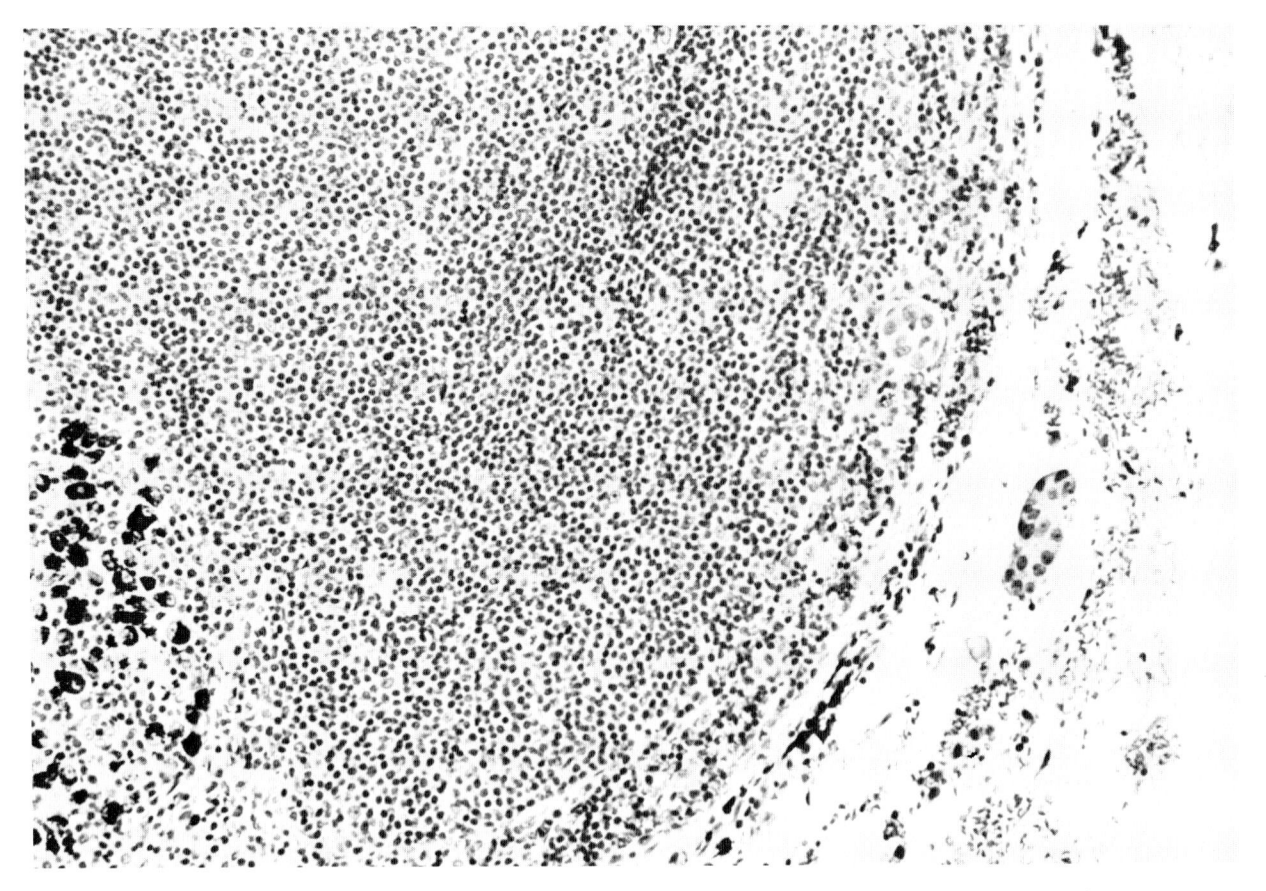

Figure 6–16. Micrometastasis in an N2 lymph node. Complete sampling of grossly benign lymph nodes is essential (H&E, ×160).

of the lesion, (b) one or more sections as appropriate of grossly uninvolved parenchyma, bronchovascular tree, and lymph nodes.

The handling of the specimen for microbiologic diagnosis is described in Chapter 8.

References

1. Tisi GM, Friedman PJ, Peters RM, et al.: Clinical staging of primary lung cancer. Am Rev Respir Dis 127:659–664, 1983.
2. Feld R, Rubinstein LV, Weisenberger TH, Lung Cancer Study Group: Site of recurrence in resected stage I non-small-cell lung cancer: A guide for future studies. J Clin Oncol 2:1352–1358, 1984.
3. Gail MH, Eagan RT, Feld R, et al.: Prognostic factors in patients with resected stage I non-small cell lung cancer. A report from the Lung Cancer Study Group. Cancer 54:1802–1813, 1984.
4. Mountain CF: A new international staging system for lung cancer. Chest 89(suppl):225S–233S, 1986.
5. Naruke T, Suemasu K, Ishikawa S: Lymph node mapping and curability at various levels of metastasis in resected lung cancer. J Thorac Cardiovasc Surg 76:832–839, 1978.

7 Examination of the Lung: Autopsy

William M. Thurlbeck

It is doubtful whether any organ is usually as incompletely examined at autopsy as the lung is. This is because of inherent difficulties—it is the largest organ of the body and consists of airways, arterial and venous systems, as well as parenchyma, and each of these requires examination and recognition. Furthermore, diseases are characteristically distributed irregularly through the lung.

At least one lung should be inflated at autopsy, and frequently both. Inflation has the major advantages that the lung can be more thoroughly examined since it is possible to look at multiple slices and thus a large surface area of the lung. Also, inflation of the lung is essential if emphysema is to be recognized. Inflation has the disadvantage that it obscures edema, may displace material in the airways, notably pus, to the alveoli, and may make bacteriologic examination impossible. It also makes examination of the airways and vessels more difficult since it is not possible to open these structure longitudinally all the way to the periphery. Nothing can be done about mild edema but moderately severe and severe edema can still be recognized. In any event, lung weight is probably a better way of recognizing mild edema and formalin (as opposed to alcohol-based fixative), and fixation of uninflated lung may also obscure edema. Displacement of intra-airway material has been shown to diminish the amount of intra-airway mucus[1] and it seems likely that mild degrees of bronchopneumonia may be partially obscured.

Distention of the lung can be accomplished simply by distending the lung intrabronchially in a sink from a large container of fixative raised at least 30 cm and preferably 1 m above the lung. Formalin is the most convenient and inexpensive fixative, but glutaraldehyde can be used if electron-microscopy, especially scanning microscopy, is intended. It is important to leave the bronchus as long as possible and this is most effectively done by cutting the left main bronchus at right angles to the direction of the bronchus immediately across its origin. This leaves the entire right main bronchus, which is shorter, attached to the trachea. The plastic tube from the fixative should be fitted with a variable-diameter plastic connector so that the connector fits snugly into the bronchus. The lung should then be distended until it appears fully inflated. The bronchus is usually clamped or tied but this maneuver is not important. The lung loses about 25 percent of its volume even with the bronchus clamped and tied and not much more is lost without clamping.[2] Clamping or tying has the disadvantage that the main bronchi get damaged and this may render histology inadequate. Following distention the lung should be placed in a large tank containing the same fixative and covered with a moist cloth and left until it can be cut at a convenient time. Fixation is rapid since the formalin comes into close proximity to all structures in the lung following inflation and lungs can be cut 2 hours after distention.

The lung is then cut into slices, sagittal slices being the most useful since these leave the hilar structures and main vessels and airways intact. A mid-coronal slice through the trachea and main bronchi may be used to display the airways to advantage for demonstration purposes. If correlations are needed for correlation with computed tomography, then horizontal slices are in order. Slicing can be done with a commercial meat slicer but often thick (2-cm) slices cannot be obtained and it is cheaper and just as efficient to use a slicing board with two sturdy parallel plastic runners about 3 cm high along the long edge. Parallel slots 1 and 2 cm above the surface of the board should be cut through most of the runner. A sharp—and sharpness is critical—flat knife is placed at one end of the slots to cut the desired thickness (usually 1 cm) of lung slices. The lung is then placed lateral surface downward and cut into slices. It is useful to cut the mid-sagittal slice 2 cm thick if a paper-mounted whole-lung section[3] is to be made (*see* Paper-Mounted Whole Lung Sections, below). The slices should then be examined and generally they can be washed in running water before further examination or dissection.

Many modifications of the slicing can be made. If it is desired to make a dissection of the airways and vessels, then the lung can be cut in the mid-sagittal plane. The bronchi and arteries can then be traced to at least three divisions beyond the segmental bronchus or vessel from the medial half. If an area of infection is suspected, the pleural surface over it can be seared, incised, and cultured before fixation. An additional leak will not hamper inflation but a clamp or ligature can be placed over the incision. A swab can also be put down a bronchus before fixation and this procedure should be done if grossly purulent material is seen in a bronchus. Caution is required in interpreting material in pulmonary arteries. Postmortem clots become firm after formalin fixation and anything other than classical thromboemboli should be sampled for histology. (In any event these should be sampled; it may be necessary to sample more possible thromboemboli in formalin-fixed lungs than in fresh ones.) Pneumonia is usually easy to recognize and has a reddish-brown or grey color. Often an area of apparent poor fixation turns out to be pneumonia. Presumably formalin has difficult access to the consolidated region which remains red from congestion.

A wide variety of methods have been described for inflating the lung; these have been reviewed elsewhere.[4]

The fresh lung can be handled in a similar way, though slicing is more difficult and only three, and often two, slices can be made. Dissection of bronchi and pulmonary artery branches is easier and absolute indications for examining the lung fresh *may* be a suspected diagnosis of multiple recurrent pulmonary emboli and of a very small bronchogenic carcinoma. Suspected pulmonary edema is another indication and it may be essential to examine the lung fresh for medicolegal purposes if a cause of death must be given immediately and this is thought to be in the lung.

Diagrams are essential for recording lesions and it is remarkable how easily—and often—anterior is confused with posterior, superior with inferior, medial with lateral, and even right with left. Real and suspected gross lesions should be sampled. A convenient way of identifying lobes is to code them by shape, such as triangular for the upper lobe, square for the middle lobe and lingula, and oblong for the lower lobe. A main stem bronchus should always be taken for histology.

Extreme caution should be excised in interpreting bacteriologic specimens obtained from the lung at autopsy, and interpretation should only be based on sampling obviously infected lesions, and obtaining cultures consistent with the autopsy and clinical findings. Routine culture of the lungs or bronchi produces information that is generally not useful.

Examination for Emphysema

Inflation of the lung was first introduced by Laennec in the early 19th century and enabled him to make the first adequate description of emphysema. Lung inflation then more or less ceased until the 1940s and 1950s when it was primarily reintroduced to study the morphology of emphysema. Inflation itself is not a guarantee that emphysema can be recognized adequately. Severe emphysema is easily and more accurately recognized from a slice of inflated lung as described above, than from uninflated lung. Mild to moderate degrees of panacinar emphysema cannot be recognized with facility even on slices from inflated lung and can be suspected as the lung parenchyma "falls away" and airways, vessels, and lobular septa are raised above the surface of the slice. Mild centrilobular emphysema can usually be recognized because of associated pigment, but the mildest degree of centilobular emphysema may require the use of a hand lens. For this reason different techniques have been developed. One is the paper-mounted whole lung-section technique (see Paper-Mounted Whole-Lung Sections, below) and the other is the barium sulfate impregnation technique described by Heard,[5] followed by examination with a dissecting microscope of the slice immersed in water. All of the ingredients and equipment for the latter technique are cheap and readily available. Two photographic developing pans (or two baking pans) are filled with 7.5 percent barium nitrate and 10 percent sodium sulfate, respectively. The slice is immersed first in one solution, gently squeezed, and left for about 0.5 minutes. It is then transferred to the other pan and treated similarly. This is repeated about three times and the slice washed in running water, with some squeezing, for about 5 minutes. It is then transferred to a new tray, washed further, and the pan filled with water. The slice is then held beneath the surface using a rectangular frame of either heavy plastic or steel that has transparent fishing thread extending diagonally across from the four corners and from one side to the other at the center of the sides of the frame. A frame size of 12 inches × 10 inches will accommodate most lungs, and a 14 inch × 12 inch-frame will accommodate all but the most emphysematous lungs. Bubbles can be a nuisance depending on water supply. Under these circumstances a drop or two of caprylic alcohol (octanoic acid) will usually suffice, or recently distilled water can be used. The lung is then examined with a hand lens or preferably with a dissecting microscope with a long arm. The results are highly pleasing and the three-dimensional structure of the lung is clearly seen and mild lesions are readily recognized (see Figs. 19, 24–26, 28, 29, and 36 in Chapter 21).

Special Procedures

A variety of special procedures can be applied to the lung at postmortem examination. Many of them are likely to be used primarily for research and for that purpose investigators need to have a full knowledge of the literature and have some trial and error experience with the technique involved. A detailed description of these techniques is therefore inappropriate, but a brief and general reference will be made to several techniques.

Electron Microscopy

Fixative with a marker dye can be injected into the lung in situ as soon as autopsy permission is obtained and the injection site identified and sampled at a later time.[6] The lung appears to be quite remarkably resistant to postmortem autolysis, and relatively well-preserved normal lung has been described 8 hours postmortem.[6]

Even fresh lungs not specially prepared, formalin-fixed after long periods of time, and lung tissue in paraffin blocks may provide useful information. Typically, virus particles and tumor markers can be identified from such tissues. Ferguson and Richardson have shown a quite startling return to normal ultrastructural appearance following treatment of the autolyzed lung with a modified Krebs-Henseleit solution and 95 percent oxygen and 5 percent carbon dioxide.[7]

Quantitation of Lung Structure

If absolute measurements, such as alveolar volumes or surface area, are required then the lung needs to be fixed at a standard distending pressure. A variety of techniques have been described and have been reviewed in some detail.[4] The simplest technique is a modification of that described by Heard.[5] A constant distending pressure of 25 or 30 cm is usually used. A tank can be built from sturdy plastic for less than $200 and immersion pumps can be quite cheap. Fixative is recirculated from the tank holding the lungs to a reservoir that has an outflow into the main tank, and the level of the overflow determines the distending pressure. Conduits from the reservoir lead from the plastic tube into the bronchi of the lungs to be distended and are tied in place using variable diameter plastic connectors. Tanks are best placed in a well-ventilated place, a standard fume-hood, a small portable hood, or custom-built hood. It is important that the lungs be leak-free and this is best achieved by tying the major arteries and veins before removing the lungs from the heart. Special care needs to be taken when removing the lungs from the cadaver and a towel placed over the cut ends of the ribs is useful in preventing lacerations. The lungs should first be distended rapidly to apparent full distention, as described above, with fixative and then attached to the constant inflation device. This is necessary because fixation proceeds as distention occurs and large lungs may not reach full inflation. During the transfer of apparently fully distended lung, formalin will escape from the bronchus so that the fear of overinflation is groundless. Lungs inflated in this way are smaller than the volume predicted from life and considerably smaller than air-filled lungs at comparable pressures,[8] but close to lung volumes assessed radiologically.[9] No purpose is served by correcting to predicted total lung capacity (TLC) in individual patients since observed and predicted TLCs vary by ± 20% in individual patients. It may be appropriate to correct to air-distended lung volumes but this requires an additional procedure and there is no guarantee that it is the appropriate reference volume. The advantage of a standard pressure of fixative is that it is standard, and thus observers using this technique can refer to the results of others using it. Lung volumes are easily and accurately measured by water displacement.[10] This is best accomplished using a bottom-loading balance and a maximum of 10 kg is necessary for adult lungs.

An extensive literature exists concerning sampling of tissue, correction for shrinkage, and stereologic techniques,[11–15] particularly of the lung.[11–13] One of the problems is that several of the descriptions are hard to follow, and hide the fact that the major techniques—point counting, measurements of intercepts, mean linear intercept, and counting structures per unit area—are simple in concept and application. Significant errors result from ignoring such basics as measuring shrinkage accurately (which is easy to do) and sampling inappropriately.

A simple technique that has much to recommend it is the radial count of Emery and Mithal,[16] although many stereologists find it hard to take seriously. In this method, using standard histologic sections a line is dropped at right angles from the most distal respiratory bronchiole to the closest margin of the acinus, preferably a lobular septum or vein, but bronchi and arteries also suffice. The number of alveoli that have been intercepted along that line are then counted. We have made a formal study of this method[17] and indicated that a standard technique must be used if between- and within-observer variation are to be minimized.

It should be noted that inflated lungs produce a higher value than that of Emery and Mithal.[16,17] The major application of this technique is in assessing hypoplasia of the lung. As indicated (see Chapter 1), it is an assessment of the complexity of the acinus and alveolar development. It is easy and quick to do, and is an integral part of the assessment of lung hypoplasia.

Bronchograms

Bronchograms can be performed postmortem using usual clinical contrast media, lead,[18] or tantalum.[19] The second of these is toxic and the third potentially explosive.

Arteriograms (and Venograms)

Reid and associates have the most experience with this technique and have published extensively about normal and abnormal appearance of the pulmonary arterial tree in children and adults.[20] The particular feature of the technique is that it is advisable that the postmortem interval be long and freezing and warming may be advantageous to obviate arterial reactivity. In addition, unphysiologic pressures (120 mmHg) is advisable so as that full distention of vessels is obtained in all cases. A major problem with this technique is the presence of postmortem clots and saline lavage or detergent lavage may obviate this to some extent. The easiest contrast medium to use is that described by Schlesinger.[21] It is not necessary to add formalin to the injection mass since

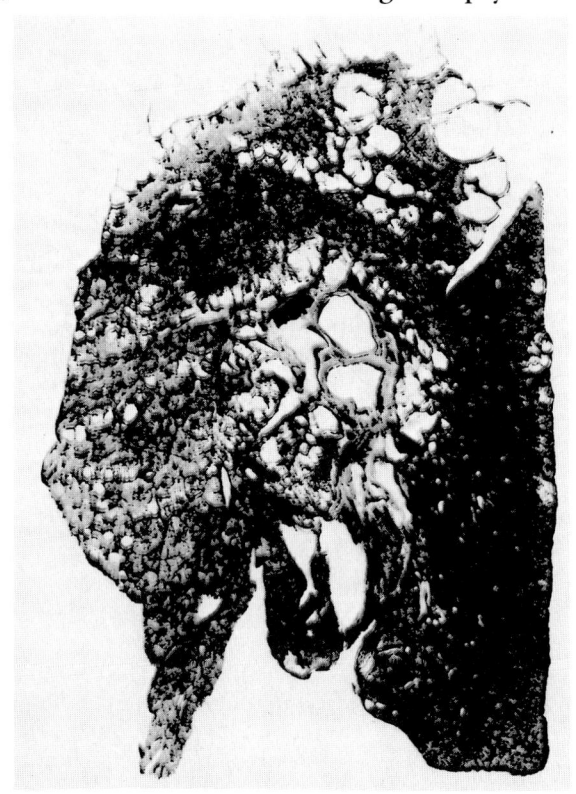

Figure 7–1. Paper-mounted whole lung section of an emphysematous lung prepared by Marlyce George.

subsequent intrabronchial formalin fixation will harden it. The standard injection technique is that of Short.[22]

Casts of Airways and Vessels

The two major exponents of casting techniques were Liebow[23] and Thompsett.[24] The resin used by the latter is not available in North America because of hazards in transportation. Large numbers of other resins are available.

Paper-Mounted Whole-Lung Sections

This technique, described by Gough and Wentworth,[3] was responsible for a major breakthrough in the pathology and pathophysiology of emphysema and pneumoconiosis. The original technique[3] and a modification that obviates the necessity of a special microtome[25] have been well described. We have extensive experience with this technique and have modified the procedure over the years. The best paper-mounted whole-lung sections that I have seen have been those prepared by Marlyce George at the Webb-Waring Institute in Denver, CO (Fig. 7-1). Her modifications are recorded in the Appendix at the end of this chapter.

The major advantages of this technique are that it keeps a compact record of the lung and that it provides excellent teaching specimens. Its disadvantages compared to the Heard technique is that milder grades of emphysema are hard to see and impossible to confirm (with the Heard technique a histologic section can be taken from the area in question), and expense (our present estimate is approximately $100 per patient). A special microtome is needed, and the MSE microtome that was originally used is now no longer on the market. Of the presently available alternative microtomes the one we use is considerably more expensive ($5,500) than the MSE device and requires a specially made guard to prevent possible accidents.

Appendix: Procedure for Paper-Mounted Lung Sections

Marlyce George, Webb-Waring Lung Institute, Denver, CO

Perfusion and Fixation

An excised right or left lung, with no tears or holes preferably, is cannulated through the main stem bronchus. The lung is then placed in a large tank filled with 1.7% isotonic buffered glutaraldehyde (IBG). The cannula is connected to a large, elevated reservoir of IBG adjacent to the fixation tank and the lung is fully distended. The cannula is then connected to a tube inside the tank that has IBG recirculating at a constant pressure of 25 cm of water pressure. The lung is covered with a piece of IBG-soaked cheesecloth so all surfaces remain moist.

The formula for the 1.7% isotonic buffered glutaraldehyde is:

- Potassium phosphate monobasic   68 g
- Sodium hydroxide   17.2 g
- Glutaraldehyde (25% in water)   680 ml
- Distilled water   9320 ml

The lung is perfused in this manner for 6 to 7 days.

Obtaining a Proper Specimen

The lung is clamped off at the cannula to maintain distention and removed to a cutting board. One-centimeter sagittal slices are taken from the surface most distal to the hilum and set aside, then a 2-cm slice from the mid-sagittal region is taken for paper-mounted sections. The 2-cm slice, at this point, can be placed in a large, flat container of IBG so it floats freely until ready to continue processing. To prepare for processing, the slice is placed in running water and gently washed for 2 to 3 days to remove IBG.

Infiltration

On the day processing is to continue, early in the day make up the following solution:

- Gelatin (Hormel Co.—250 mesh)   250 g
- Cellosolve (ethylene glycol monoethyl ether)   40 ml
- Caprylic alcohol   2.5 ml
- Tap water   850 ml

To make this solution easily use a hot-plate stirrer. Place magnetic stirrer and water in a container and put on the hot plate to stir and heat; add cellosolve and caprylic alcohol. When solution is warm, slowly add gelatin, stirring and heating constantly; continue stirring and heating until steam rises. Place in a 35°C oven for about 30 to 45 minutes to allow all the gelatin to dissolve.

Remove the lung slice from running water and carefully squeeze as much water from the slice as possible. Place the slice in a Teflon-coated pan slightly larger than the slice. Place the side to be cut on the bottom of the pan. Put identification number on the outside of the pan with a wax pencil. Add enough gelatin to completely cover the slice. Weights must be placed on top of the slice to keep it submerged. Place the pan with the slice in a vacuum oven heated to 60°C with the pressure to 20 pounds per square inch. This helps the gelatin to displace the air in the slice. Leave under decreased pressure 1 hour. Release pressure. Repeat this step at least two more times. Remove from vacuum oven and transfer to an incubator at 35°C for 24 hours or overnight.

Embedding

The next day remove weights and pour excess gelatin into a large container, and reserve. Place the pan containing the slice with a small amount of gelatin in the freezer long enough for gelatin to set. If possible, leave the pan in the freezer while slowly adding the reserve gelatin back to the pan. Be careful not to disturb the lung slice. Completely cover the slice and add about 1/4 inch more to form a good base. This should remain in the freezer until gelatin is completely set, and shows signs of starting to freeze around the edges. Remove the pan from the freezer and run hot water on the bottom of the pan to help release gelatin block. Place the block holder for the microtome under running hot water with the surface for mounting the gelatin block facing down. This will heat the blockholder enough to melt the 1/4-inch layer of gelatin so it will adhere to the blockholder. While the blockholder is warming, trim excess gelatin from the block to within 1/2 inch of the specimen. Place the gelatin block on the blockholder with the surface to be cut facing up. With hands, apply pressure so all areas of the gelatin block are in contact with the surface of the blockholder and melted gelatin can be seen around all edges of the block. Place the identification number on the end of the blockholder. Place blockholder with the specimen back in the freezer until completely frozen or overnight.

The blockholder needs to be kept level so there is a need for some type of support. Thick cardboard tubes or wooden squares, long enough and with a center opening large enough to accommodate the shank of the blockholder, work well. Anything that will hold the base plate of the holder in a level position will do.

Cutting Sections

Place blockholder with the specimen on the microtome. Allow the gelatin block to start thawing. As soon as the gelatin around the edge of the specimen has thawed enough, cut the gelatin away on a bevel. Cut sections as the block thaws; a warm cloth rubbed on the cutting surface speeds thawing. Cut the sections at 400 µm.

Place the sections in a 10 percent formalin-acetate solution for 24 to 48 hours. They may be kept longer if refrigerated. The formula for the 10 percent formalin-acetate solution is:

- Formaldehyde (37 to 40 percent)   100 ml
- Sodium acetate   40 g
- Tap water   To 1000 ml

This will harden gelatin.

Mounting Sections

To mount the sections on paper gently wash in cold water for 1 to 2 hours to remove excess formalin. Make a *fresh* solution of the following:

- Gelatin   37.5 g
- Glycerin   35 ml
- Cellosolve   20 ml
- Water   402.5 ml

Prepare on hot-plate stirrer. Keep in 35°C oven until ready to use.

1. Place one slice on a wet surface such as a piece of plastic and trim any gelatin from the edges and anywhere else that will not compromise the structure of the slice.
2. Pour about a 4-inch-diameter pool of the above-mentioned solution on to a clean sheet of acrylic resin, that is, plastic. Spread to accommodate the size of the lung slice. Place the trimmed slice on top of the solution and cover with an 8 1/2 × 11-inch sheet of Whatman number 1 filter paper.
3. Using hands gently smooth out the paper to remove the excess gelatin and all the bubbles. Stand the plastic sheet on edge and remove the excess gelatin from around the paper with hand.
4. Place the plastic sheet on edge in the drying stand. (The stand is made of wood measuring 3 feet × 4 inches. There are grooves cut into the board at 4-inch intervals at about a 25 degree angle.) Allow the plates to thoroughly air-dry at room temperature.
5. Remove paper section from the plastic by lightly running a sharp blade around the edge of the paper; lift one corner and peel off.
6. The sections are then laminated by placing the paper section in a 9 × 12-inch pouch of laminating plastic, placed inside two carriers and laminated on a Laminex PAK 1X.

References

1. Matsuba K, Thurlbeck WM: Disease of the small airways in chronic bronchitis. Am Rev Respir Dis 107:552–558, 1973.

2. Thurlbeck WM: The incidence of pulmonary emphysema: With observations on the relative incidence in spacial distribution of various types of emphysema. Am Rev Respir Dis 87:206–215, 1963.

3. Gough J, Wentworth JE: Thin sections of entire organs mounted on paper. Harvey Lect 53:182–185, 1957–1958, 1958.

4. Thurlbeck WM: *Chronic Airflow Obstruction in Lung Disease*. Philadelphia, London, and Toronto: WB Saunders, 1976.

5. Heard BE: Pathology of emphysema: Methods of study. Am Rev Respir Dis 82:792–799, 1960.

6. Bachofen M, Weibel ER, Roos B: Postmortem fixation of human lungs for electron microscopy. Am Rev Respir Dis 111:247–256, 1975.

7. Ferguson CC, Richardson JB: A simple technique for the utilisation of postmortem tracheal and bronchial tissues for ultarstructural studies. Hum Pathol 9:463–470, 1978.

8. Berend N, Skoog C, Waszkiewicz L, Thurlbeck WM: Maximum volumes in excised human lungs: effects of age, emphysema and formalin inflation. Thorax 35:859–864, 1980.

9. Thurlbeck WM: Post mortem lung volumes. Thorax 34:735–739, 1979.

10. Scherle W: A simple method for volumetry of organs in quantitative stereology. Mikroskopie 26:57–60, 1970.

11. Dunnill MS: Quantitative methods in the study of pulmonary pathology. Thorax 17:320–328, 1962.

12. Thurlbeck WM: Measurement of pulmonary emphysema. Am Rev Respir Dis 95:752–764, 1967.

13. Weibel ER: *Morphometry of the Human Lung*. New York: Academic Press, 1963.

14. Weibel ER: *Stereologic Methods*, vol. 1. *Practical Methods for Biological Morphometry*. London, New York, Toronto, Sydney, and San Francisco: Academic Press, 1979.

15. Aherne W, Dunnill MS: *Morphometry*. London: Edward Arnold, 1982.

16. Emery JL, Mithal A: The number of alveoli in the terminal respiratory unit of man during late intrauterine life in childhood. Arch Dis Child 35:544–547, 1960.

17. Cooney TP, Thurlbeck WM: The radial alveolar count method of Emery and Mithal: A reappraisal 1-Postnatal lung growth. Thorax 37:527–579, 1982.

18. Leopold JG, Gough J: Post-mortem bronchography in the study of bronchitis and emphysema. Thorax 18:172–177, 1963.

19. Nadel JA, Wolff WG, Graf PD: Powdered tantalum as a medium for bronchography in canine and human lungs. Invest Radiol. 3:229–235, 1968.

20. Reid LM: The Pulmonary circulation: Remodelling in growth and disease. The 1978 J. Burns Amberson Lecture. Am Rev Respir Dis 119:531–546, 1979.

21. Schlesinger MJ: New radioopaque mass for vascular injection. Lab Invest. 6:1–11, 1957.

22. Short DS: Post-mortem pulmonary arteriography with special reference to the study of pulmonary hypertension. J Facul Radiol 8:118–124, 1956.

23. Liebow AA, Hales MR, Lindskog GE, Bloomer WE: Plastic demonstrations of pulmonary pathology. Bull Int A Med Museums 27:116–127, 1947.

24. Thompsett DH: *Anatomical Techniques*. Edinburgh: E & S Livingstone, 1956.

25. Whimster WF: Techniques for the examination of excised lungs. Hum Pathol 1:305–314, 1970.

8 *Microbiologic Diagnosis*

Anna-Luise A. Katzenstein

The importance of cultures and special stains in diagnosing lung diseases cannot be overemphasized. Cultures should be taken whenever infection is suspected either because of the gross or histologic appearance of the lesion or because of the clinical history, as in immunocompromised patients. Likewise, special stains should be performed on similar patients and should be examined carefully even in patients with pending cultures. Special stains and cultures are frequently complementary in identifying organisms. Although negative cultures usually signify absence of infection, there are occasions when special stains will demonstrate organisms when cultures are negative (*see* Special Stains, below). Techniques for culturing surgical and autopsy specimens, recommended special stains, and helpful diagnostic criteria in specific situations will be discussed in the following sections.

Cultures in Surgical and Autopsy Specimens

A representative piece of tissue should always be cultured rather than a swab touched to the tissue. In selecting a portion of tissue for culture, care should be taken to sample areas that appear grossly abnormal. Open lung biopsy specimens should be serially sectioned using sterile instruments, and areas with induration, necrosis, hemorrhage, or purulent material chosen for culture. The pathologist rather than the surgeon should choose the area for culture, since if this procedure is left to the surgeon, appropriate involved areas may not be selected, or they may be completely removed for culture, leaving no diagnostic tissue for microscopic examination.

In autopsy specimens, the lung should be palpated externally and indurated areas chosen. Alternatively, areas known to be abnormal from antemortem chest radiographs can be selected. The pleural surface should be briefly heated with a hot spatula to sterilize it, and the lung incised with a sterile knife. Tissue deep to the surface is sent for culture.

The usefulness of postmortem cultures has been questioned.[1] Routine cultures of postmortem lungs are likely to be contaminated with gram-negative enteric bacteria. However, cultures from areas of grossly infected lung can be productive and should be performed. This is especially true, for example, in cases of tuberculous and fungal infections, since antibiotics are used in the culture media and will generally suppress the growth of bacterial contaminants. Cultures are not so useful in cases of bacterial pneumonia either because of contamination problems, or because antemortem antibiotic therapy may inhibit growth. Also, organisms in these patients usually have been identified before death and therefore this information is not that important clinically. Print cultures have been advocated to obviate problems with bacterial contamination.[1]

Of course, the ideal specimen for culture is the open lung biopsy that arrives in the surgical pathology laboratory in a sterile container and is handled from the beginning with sterile technique. However, more frequently specimens are obtained that are not sterile, but are suspected of harboring an infection, for example, after frozen section examination or after gross inspection. Although it is not feasible to culture such specimens for routine bacteria, they can and should be cultured for acid-fast bacilli and fungi, since antibiotics to suppress bacterial contaminants are used in the culture media for these organisms.

Special Stains

The special stains available for identifying organisms are fairly standard.[2] The Brown-Brenn or Brown-Hopps stains are the most commonly used tissue gram stains to identify bacteria. They also outline actinomyces and nocardia. They are less helpful in cases of Legionnaire's disease where the Brown-Brenn stain is usually negative and the Brown-Hopps stain is infrequently positive. The Dieterle stain has been widely recommended to stain the organisms in Legionnaire's disease. We have found this stain to be unreliable and difficult to interpret due to nonspecific background staining, and therefore we no longer utilize it in our laboratory. However, laboratories that have more experience with it and use it more consistently might find it useful. We prefer to use immunoperoxidase or immunofluorescent techniques with antibodies to Legionella species to identify the organisms.[3]

Either of two techniques may be used in identifying acid-fast bacteria. The Ziehl-Neelsen acid-fast stain is very reliable and colors the organisms red against a light-blue background. Equally useful is the auramine-rhodamine stain.[4] This stain must be viewed in a fluorescent microscope, but has the advantage of brightly staining the organisms against a dark background. Some investigators prefer this method since the organisms are thought to stand out better against the background. The disadvantage is that the underlying tissue reaction is not well visualized, and therefore, it is difficult to judge whether a presumed organism is really part of the inflammatory reaction or a contaminant. In our judgment, either technique is equally productive, and the choice of one over the other depends on the individual pathologist's experience with them rather than on real differences in effectiveness.

A variety of stains will outline fungi, including Gomori methenamine-silver (GMS), periodic acid-Schiff (PAS), and modified PAS stains such as the PAS-Gridley. We recommend the GMS stain to screen for fungi, since the organisms are colored black and contrast sharply with the light green background. This stain is also excellent for identifying Pneumocystis. We believe that the GMS stain is superior to the PAS stain because the latter may not adequately differentiate the organisms from the background. This is especially true in necrotizing granulomas where both organisms and necrotic debris stain pink, and also occurs in cases of Pneumocystis pneumonia where organisms and surrounding exudate appear eosinophilic. Modifications of the PAS stain such as the PAS-Gridley are available that better differentiate organisms from background and are almost as good as GMS stain. In the PAS-Gridley stain, the organisms appear purple to lavender against a yellow background. The PAS stain and its modifications have the advantage of outlining the internal structure of fungi, whereas this is obscured in the GMS stain. Therefore, while the PAS stain is not as reliable in screening for organisms for the reasons mentioned, it is useful in examining the morphology of the organisms and aiding in their classification. Another useful stain for fungi and Pneumocystis is the Cresyl-Echt violet stain.[5] This stain has the advantage of being rapid (approximately 30 minutes) and simple to perform, and therefore is especially useful in frozen sections from immunocompromised patients. A rapid GMS stain has also been developed that depends on heating the ingredients, and it is equally reliable for frozen section diagnosis.[6]

Immunofluorescent and Immunoperoxidase Techniques

Antibodies are now available commercially against a variety of microorganisms, including herpes virus, aspergillus species, Legionella species, and various other organisms. Direct or indirect immunofluorescence or immunoperoxidase techniques can be used in the staining, although the indirect methods are more sensitive. This is a reliable method for identifying organisms, although there may be cross-reactions among some of the fungal and bacterial antibodies. For most antibodies, routine formalin-fixed, paraffin-embedded sections can be used, and special modes of fixation are not necessary. As more and more antibodies become available commercially, this technique may surpass routine special stains in usefulness.

Granulomatous Infections

As already mentioned, a representative portion of all necrotizing granulomas should be cultured for acid-fast bacilli and fungi, and an acid-fast stain as well as a GMS stain should be performed. It has been shown that examination of two tissue blocks will identify the organism in over 90 percent of patients, provided that the blocks contain necrotic zones.[7] The pathologist will save time if he begins the search for organisms within the central most necrotic areas of the granuloma, rather than randomly scanning the slides, since the organisms will almost always be found in this location. In cases of solitary lung granulomas, special stains frequently will demonstrate the organism when cultures are negative. This is particularly true for granulomas containing histoplasma but may also occur in tuberculosis. There are several explanations for this observation. Histoplasma is notoriously difficult to culture from necrotizing granulomas, most likely because the organism is not viable. However, this is not the entire explanation, since other fungi and tuberculous organisms may not grow in culture either. The technique of culturing may be another factor, that is, whether a swab or a piece of tissue is taken and how quickly it is sent to the microbiology laboratory. In any case, the important role of the pathologist in addition to the microbiology laboratory in diagnosis of infection needs to be emphasized.

Smears, Touch Preparations, and Bronchoalveolar Lavage Specimens

Some individuals advocate the usefulness of smears and touch preparations from open lung biopsies to identify organisms, especially in immunocompromised patients. We have found no advantage of this technique over frozen sections. Its disadvantage, as in all techniques utilizing fluid or smears, is that the organisms may be difficult to distinguish from artifacts since the background inflammatory reaction that would be present in tissue sections is absent.

Bronchoalveolar lavage has been recently advocated in diagnosing infection, especially in immunocompromised patients.[8] This technique suffers from the same disadvantage as described above for smears and touch preparations. Routine special stains, including Gram, acid-fast, and GMS stains should be performed on all smear or fluid preparations.

References

1. duMoulin G, Paterson D: Clinical relevance of postmortem microbiologic examination: A review. Hum Pathol 16:539, 1985.

2. Luna L: *Manual of Histologic Staining Methods of the Armed Forces Institute of Pathology*, 3rd ed. New York; McGraw-Hill, 1968.

3. Lowry B, Vega F, Hedlund K: Localization of Legionella pneumophilia in tissue using FITC-conjugated specific antibody and a background stain. Am J Clin Pathol 77:601, 1982.

4. Kommareddi S, Abramowsky C, Swinehart G, Hrabak L: Nontuberculous mycobacterial infections: Comparison of the fluorescent auramine-O and Ziehl-Neelsen techniques in tissue diagnosis. Hum Pathol 15:1085, 1984.

5. Bowling M, Smith M, Wescott S: A rapid staining procedure for Pneumocystis carinii. Am J Med Technol 39:267, 1973.

6. Maham C, Sale G: Rapid methenamine silver stain for Pneumocystis and fungi. Arch Pathol Lab Med 102:351, 1978.

7. Ulbright T, Katzenstein A: Solitary necrotizing granulomas of the lung. Differentiating features and etiology. Am J Surg Pathol 4:13, 1980.

8. Hartman B, Koss M, Hui A, et al.: Pneumocystis carinii pneumonia in the acquired immunodeficiency syndrome (AIDS). Diagnosis with bronchial brushings, biopsy and bronchoalveolar lavage. Chest 87:603, 1985.

9 Diagnostic Cytology Techniques Including Fine Needle Aspirations: Practical Considerations

Linda Ferrell
Geno Saccommono

Introduction

Pulmonary cytology for the diagnosis of lung cancer has evolved over the last 40 years into a frequently used diagnostic tool. Gynecologic cytology, in comparison to pulmonary cytology, is relatively simple since few tumor types develop in the uterus. Unfortunately, it has taken many years for pathologists and cytotechnologists to realize that pulmonary cytology is much more complex because of the variety of tumors and reactive inflammatory diseases of the lung. Initially technology was inadequate and added to the difficulties of recognizing cell types and cell concentrations. Pulmonary cytology now adds significantly to the diagnosis and the better understanding of reactive inflammatory and degenerative diseases of the lung, but much is still to be learned in this field.

Approximately 30 different tumors, both benign and malignant, occur in the lung. Each is cytologically different, particularly in the early stages of development. Inflammatory diseases of the lung are numerous, and the cytology shed by the diseased parenchyma may indicate these. Viral diseases modify the metaplastic squamous cells and tall columnar cells so that they are easily confused with neoplastic cells. With the gradual recognition of these diagnostic problems, lung cancer can now be diagnosed readily in most cases, particularly when the lesions involve the larynx, trachea, and bronchi. Only the peripheral lesions, which arise in scars or small bronchioles which became obstructed early in the development of tumor, are difficult or impossible to diagnose by use of exfoliative or brush cytology.

Examination of sputum samples is performed primarily for the diagnosis of cancer, but it should be recognized that differences exist from sample to sample and patient to patient. Some samples abound with histiocytes, others with acute inflammatory cells, and others with lymphocytes. Therefore, a variety of specimens must be examined depending on such factors as presence or absence of neoplasia on radiographs (including size and position of the suspected lesion), clinical findings, and history.

Techniques in Exfoliative Lung Cytology

Sputum Collection for Cytologic Study

The object of sputum collection is to obtain a satisfactory amount of sputum of pulmonary origin. The patient not only should be informed of the need to produce an adequate amount of sputum, but should also be given some information on the physiology and anatomy of the respiratory system, with detailed instructions that the sputum collected must come from "deep in the lung." One must explain that nasal aspirates and tongue scrapings are inadequate since they are not of pulmonary origin. The patient must be at ease with the person explaining the impending procedure; it has been the authors' experience that patients are frequently so worried that they hear little of the instructions. It is sometimes worthwhile to ask patients direct questions to confirm that they understood the instructions. Once the patient knows what is desired, the specimen can be collected either at home after first rising from bed or by use of an aerosol.

Patients with diagnostic lung problems are usually cigarette smokers and, after discussion about the type of sputum sample desired, understand exactly what is needed. They will readily admit that on rising from bed, they cough up material from deep in the lungs. Rarely even a cigarette smoker will not be able to produce sufficient cough material for study, but 90 percent of all patients will yield a satisfactory specimen spontaneously. The remaining 10 percent must have aerosol administered.

Collection and Preservation of Early Morning Specimens

When the sputum is collected at home, the patient is given three wide-mouth specimen bottles each containing 50 ml of fixative, consisting of 48 ml of 50 percent ethyl alcohol (ETOH) diluted from 95 percent ethyl alcohol (do not use absolute alcohol) to which has been added 1 ml of 50 percent polyethylene glycol (Carbowax 1540, Union Carbide Corp., New York, NY) and 1 ml of ethyl alcohol containing 3 mg of rifampin (Dow Chemical Co., Midland, MI). The patient must understand that this is not a potable alcohol and must be used for fixation only; a stain, such as eosin or methylene blue, may be added to prevent drinking of the fixative. The patient is instructed to use one collection container each morning, adding no more than 15 to 20 ml (or the equivalent of 4 or 5 tablespoons) of sputum. The patient should first rinse the mouth with water on rising. After coughing, the patient should spit into the bottle, firmly tighten the lid, and shake vigorously for a few seconds. The procedure is repeated until approximately 4 to 5 tablespoons of sputum are collected one each of three consecutive mornings. These three separate specimens are delivered to the laboratory where they are pooled for processing.

Noncoughing patients are administered an aerosol. Various aerosol instruments are available; the authors prefer the one manufactured by DeVilbiss (Toledo, OH), but the Monaghan Ultrasonic Nebulizer (Pueblo, CO) is also satisfactory. Aerosolization introduces a significant amount of water into the lungs. Irritants or mucolytic agents can be added, but the authors' experience with these has demonstrated no improvement over tap water. Again, it is important to explain the procedure and the expected result to the patient. After 20 to 30 minutes of aerosol inspiration, the patient should take at least four deep breaths, and on the fifth breath attempt to cough forcefully. This procedure should be repeated with reasonable rest periods between attempts. Sometimes, if an adequate sample cannot be produced using an aerosol, the patient will have a productive cough within the next 24 hours. Therefore, the patient should be given a collection bottle containing fixative and instructions for collecting a sputum sample during this period of time. The sputum specimen should always be collected after the patient rinses the mouth with water.

The fixative described here (50 percent ETOH plus Carbowax) adequately sterilizes the specimens. However, the authors add 1 ml of 50 percent ETOH containing 3 mg of rifampin to the fixative in each bottle prior to collection and again upon arrival of the specimen in the laboratory. The specimen is processed after 24 hours. The blending should be done in a negative-pressure hood if available. These added precautions should be observed, particularly if the specimens are from populations showing a high incidence of tuberculosis. In areas of high incidence of pathogenic fungi, amphotericin B probably should be added to the fixative before it is processed.

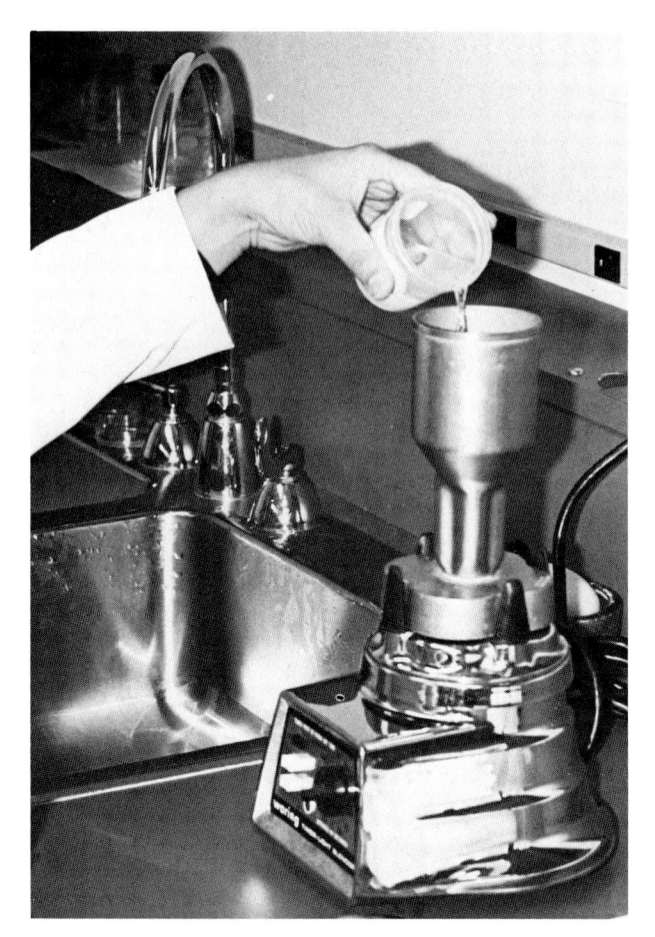

Figure 9–1. Transfer of sputum specimen to blender.

Processing of Fixed Sputum Samples

The specimen bottle lid is removed, and the sample is visually inspected to note color, coarseness, and presence of large mucous blobs, which are important criteria in assessing the length of blending time. If the material is pale and cloudy, the blending time is minimal; if large mucous blobs or thick masses of brown material are noted, blending time must be longer. Blending at 22,000 rpm does not fragment cells but does create currents that liquify most of the fine mucous fibers and partly dissolve the larger fibers, although some are only cut and will be seen as segments of mucous fibers on the smear.

The bottle containing the sputum is emptied into the blending vessel (Fig. 9–1) which is covered and attached to the blender. Blending for 3 to 4 seconds should be adequate for most specimens. When the lid is removed, visual examination of the specimen will reveal a homog-

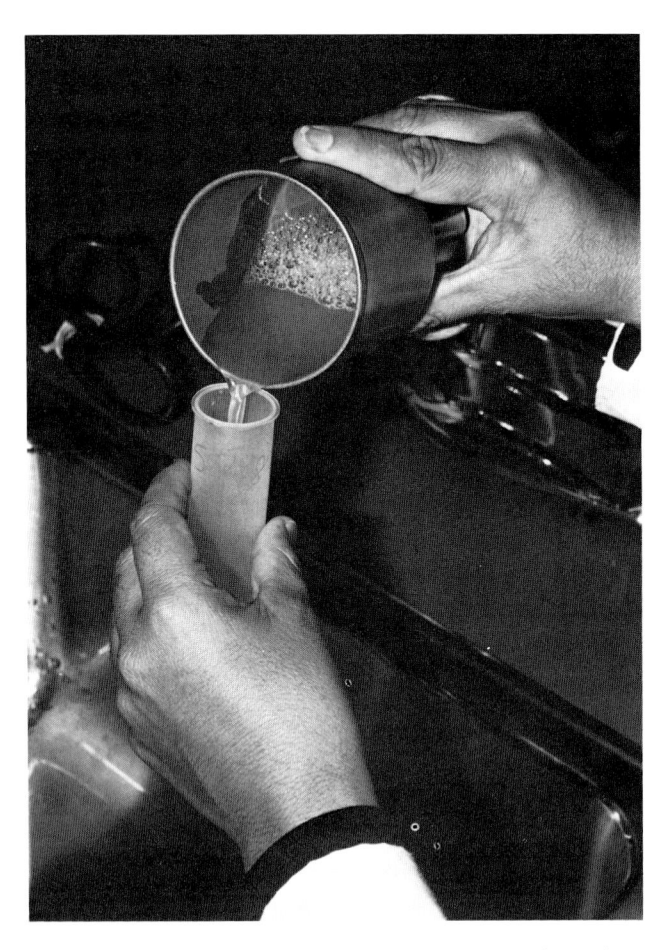

Figure 9–2. Transfer of blended specimen to centrifuge tube.

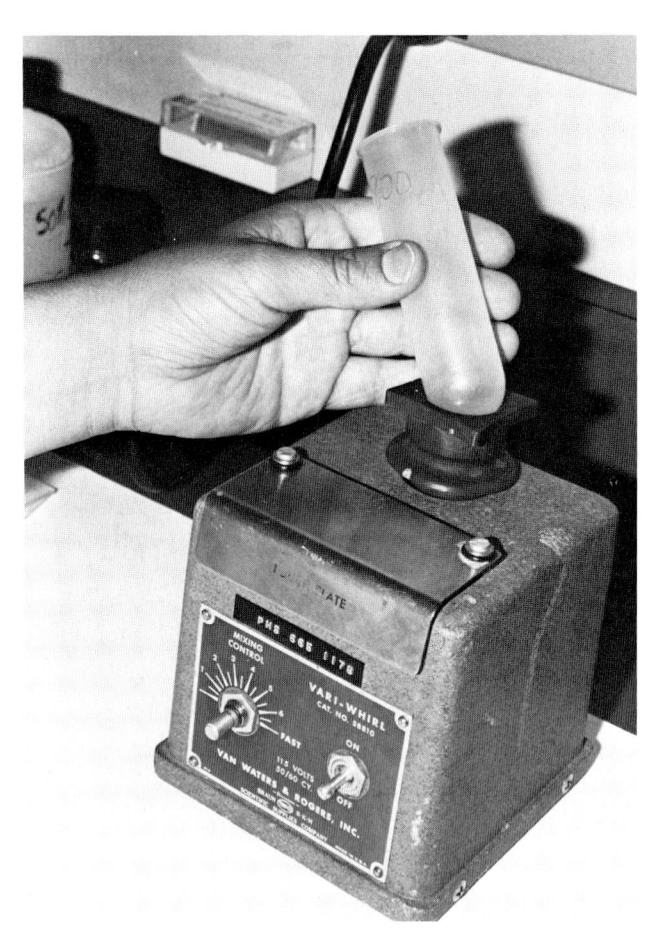

Figure 9–3. Vibration of ventrifuge tube to resuspend centrifugate.

enous, cloudy liquid. If coarse particles are noted, the specimen should be blended for another two or three seconds. The blended sputum is then poured into 50-ml plastic or glass test tubes (10 cm in length and 22 to 26 mm in diameter) for centrifugation (Fig. 9–2).

The blender chamber is washed between specimens with hot running water until foam no longer forms. Because the chamber has a smooth surface, no carryover cells have been found experimentally. The specimens are then centrifuged at 1500 rpm for 15 minutes, and the supernatant material is decanted. This step is critical because if the centrifugate is abundant, less fluid should be decanted than if a small amount of centrifugate is noted. Enough fluid should remain in the test tube so that after vibrating the tube (Fig. 9–3), sufficient supernatant liquid is present to allow the centrifugate to be resuspended. Too much fluid will result in a very thin smear, and too little will result in a thick slide preparation. The tube is vibrated for only a few seconds. If a vibrator is not available, the tubes can be agitated by snapping the side of the tube with a flip of one's finger.

Once the specimen has been vibrated, an aspirator pipette may be used to withdraw two drops of the suspension, or the tube can be everted allowing about two drops to fall on a properly labeled slide. Another slide is placed over the specimen; the two slides are worked in a sliding manner until the material appears to be distributed uniformly into a thin film on the slides. The slides are separated along the long axis and allowed to dry for at least 1 hour before staining. These slides can be kept at this stage for no longer than 2 to 3 days before staining; excessive drying can cause cell shrinkage. It is thought that the Carbowax forms a cellular coating which prevents cellular shrinkage. After fixation for 10 minutes in 95 percent ETOH, followed by a 5-minute wash in running tap water, the slides are stained with Papanicolaou's (PAP) stain (Table 9–1). Three control slides are checked daily for stain quality.

Alternative preparations are possible. If the sputum specimen can be transported to the laboratory in less than 1 hour, the specimen can be collected in a clean container that can be sealed tightly. Once the specimen arrives in the laboratory, the ETOH/Carbowax/rifampin solution is added, and the specimen is processed as previously described. A direct smear of the sample can be made without adding the solution. The direct smears are fixed in ethanol until stained by PAP technique.

108 Diagnostic Cytology: Practical Considerations

Table 9–1. Staining Procedure for Sputum Smears

1. Postfix sputum smear in 95 percent ETOH for 10 minutes.
2. Rinse in running tap water for 5 minutes.
3. Stain with hematoxylin for 1 minute.
4. Rinse under running tap water until the water is clear.
5. Immerse in 95 percent ETOH two times for 1 minute each.
6. Stain with OG-6 (Ortho Pharmaceutical Corp., Raritan, NJ) for 2½ minutes.
7. Agitate in 95 percent ETOH three times for 1 minute each.
8. Stain with EA-36 or EA-50 (Ortho Pharmaceutical Corp.) for 1½ minutes.
9. Agitate in 95 percent ETOH three times for 1 minute each.
10. Rinse in absolute alcohol two times for 1 minute each.
11. Clear in xylene, three changes (5 minutes minimum), until specimen is ready for cover glass.

ETOH, ethyl alcohol.

Bronchial Brushings

Disposable brushes yield an excellent sample if all of the cells are recovered. The authors have devised a brush-wash system that allows total recovery of all the cells, immediate fixation, and monolayer smears (Fig. 9–4). When the disposable brush is withdrawn by the fiberoptic bronchoscopist, it is given to the person responsible for the preparation, preferably a cytotechnologist who will be reading the slides. The brush is inserted in the brush-wash tube and worked back and forth very rapidly eight or ten times through the crimped area of the tube. The brush is discarded or, if the cytotechnologist on visual examination believes that the cells are not totally removed, he or she should reinsert the brush and cut the wire, leaving about 2 inches. The specimen is then taken to the laboratory where the process of working the brush in the tube can be repeated. Meanwhile, the cells are fixed with fixative, and smears can be prepared in the usual manner.

Filter preparations can be made of the brushing specimen instead of using the centrifugation and smearing technique. Some think filter preparation allows for better concentration of the specimen with little or no loss of cellular material. The specimen, suspended in 95 percent ETOH or normal saline solution, is filtered using a standard glass or porcelain vacuum filter apparatus onto circular millipore filter paper. The filter paper is halved, and each half is carefully placed sample side up onto a glass slide. The filter is held in place by a paperclip during staining.

Bronchial Lavages and Washes

These procedures involve the use of a normal saline solution to wash or dislodge cells from the bronchial structures and alveoli. This solution is collected by the bronchoscopist in a clean, sealed container by suction through the bronchoscope. The containers with the suspended cell sample are then sent to the cytology laboratory where it is centrifuged, the supernatant discarded, and the remaining pellet then smeared onto clean, dry slides using the pipette method as previously described, except that the slides are immediately fixed in 95 percent ETOH rather than air-dried.

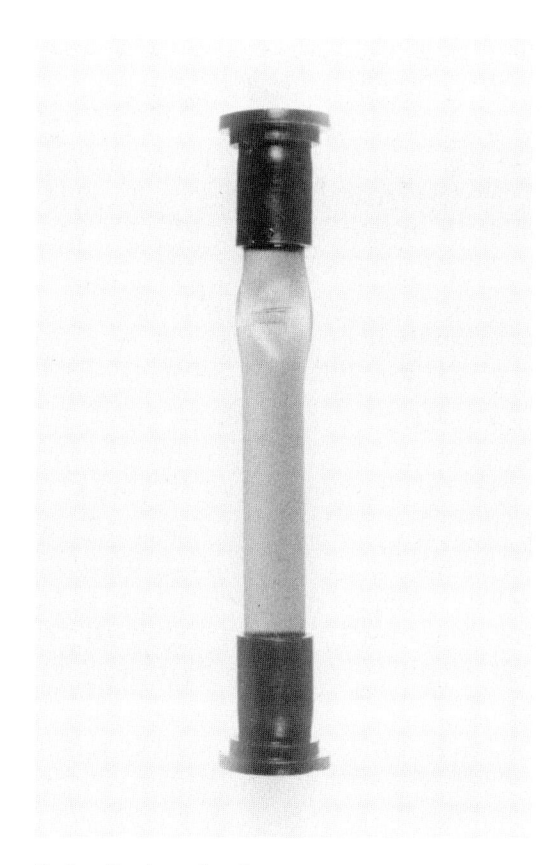

Figure 9–4. Brush-wash tube.

Use of Bronchoalveolar Lavage in Non-Neoplastic Disease

Interest in bronchoalveolar lavage has increased recently because it collects cells from terminal airways and alveoli. This method of collection and examination of respiratory cells, including alveolar macrophages and lymphocytes, has proven to be a useful research tool. The definitive use of bronchoalveolar lavage for diagnosis, however, has certain limitations.

Bronchoalveolar lavage appears to be a good method for the diagnosis of Pneumocystis pneumonia. The lavage washes the foamy exudate containing the organisms out of the alveoli. This exudate in turn can be identified on PAP stain and confirmed by restaining with silver-methenamine. Diagnosis using lavage specimens are just as accurate (and possibly more so) for pneumocystis as transbronchial biopsies. Likewise, this procedure can be used to identify viral inclusions or fungal organisms, although one must be aware that Candida from the oral cavity can contaminate the specimen.

The use of bronchoalveolar lavage for diagnosis of interstitial lung disease is less conclusive.[1-3] Specific diagnoses can occasionally be suggested on the basis of bronchoalveolar lavage findings, given the proper clinical setting. For example, macrophages for electron microscopic examination can be collected to make a diagnosis of histiocytosis X. Numerous macrophages containing erythrocytes and hemosiderin suggest intra-alveolar hemorrhage or pulmonary hemosiderosis. Pulmonary alveolar proteinosis produces a thick, proteinaceous material within alveoli that can also be demonstrated on lavage specimens.

Other interstitial lung diseases, such as idiopathic pulmonary fibrosis, sarcoidosis, hypersensitivity pneumonitis, and fibrosis associated with collagen vascular diseases, have even less clear-cut features. Thus, the use of lavage for these diseases now seems to center around determination of inflammatory activity and response to therapy as a means to determine prognosis. This is done by doing cell differential counts to determine the percentages of lymphocytes, neutrophils, eosinophils, and macrophages. For example, with idiopathic pulmonary fibrosis, a greater percentage of neutrophils means more active disease or worse prognosis. In contrast, a specimen with very few neutrophils or lymphocytes suggests the disease is in a quiescent phase. In addition, patients with active interstitial disease have increased levels of immunoglobulin G-secreting bronchoalveolar mononuclear cells.[4] Response to corticosteroid therapy can also be suggested by cell counts. If lymphocytes total more than 11 percent of the cell population, a favorable response to corticosteroid therapy might be expected. However, if the eosinophils or neutrophils (or both) are greater than normal (5 percent) without an increase in lymphocytes, response may be poor.[5] For sarcoidosis, patients who have greater than 28 percent T lymphocytes (plus a positive gallium scan of the lung parenchyma) may do poorly clinically.[6] One must remember, however, that the use of cell differentials in the evaluation of interstitial lung disease still remains somewhat controversial.

Needle Aspiration

Needle aspiration of the lung is a much older procedure than commonly realized. Early studies by Leyden[7] and Menetrier[8] cited the use of needle aspiration for the diagnosis of pneumonia and cancer, respectively. The first "modern" use of lung aspirates was done by Martin and Ellis[9] in the 1930s. They used large needles (16- to 18-gauge) and had considerable complications, such as hemorrhage and pneumothorax. However, probably because of the complications and the fear of spreading the tumor along the needle track, needle aspiration biopsy of the lung was infrequently used until the Scandinavians established the use of smaller needles (20 to 23 gauge). Dahlgren and Nordenstrom[10] reported that this reduced the complication rate considerably. With the development of computed tomography (CT) and refined fluoroscopy techniques, the demand for fine needle aspiration biopsy has increased dramatically.

In spite of a push for less-invasive techniques to obtain diagnostic information and to lower medical costs, use of fine needle aspiration biopsy for diagnosis has met with some resistance by many physicians, especially in the United States. Fox[11] has suggested several reasons for this, including: (1) unavailability of appropriately trained personnel to perform the biopsy and to interpret the material obtained; (2) fears that the technique is not as good in obtaining an accurate and specific diagnosis as other methods; (3) fears that the tumor will be spread along the needle track; and (4) anxiety over lawsuits. All of these reasons relate to use of fine needle aspiration biopsy in general, not specifically to the lung. In the last 2 or 3 years, more data have become available on the relative safety and diagnostic accuracy of the procedure. More pathologists are learning how to interpret the smears, and radiologists are becoming more experienced in obtaining the specimens. Koss[12] stated that the greatest dangers in the use of the procedure lie in the inexperience of the personnel involved. Thus, with time and adequately trained individuals performing and interpreting the test, this method should become even more popular and useful in obtaining diagnostic material quickly and safely, and most of the diagnostic pitfalls can be avoided.

Techniques

Discussion of the radiographic localization of lesions under fluoroscopy or CT guidance, patient preparation, and needle approach to lesions are beyond the scope of this chapter, but this methodology is well covered by Bonfiglio,[13] Lalli and colleagues,[14] Sinner,[15] and Green.[16] It is recommended that a pathologist or cytotechnologist trained in the proper handling and rapid interpretation of the smears assist the radiologist during the procedure.

Various needle types and aspiration techniques have been used in order to collect adequate cytology samples. In recent years, the use of 18- to 23-gauge needles of both the beveled (Chiba needle) and screw type (Rotex needle) has dominated.[13-15,17-22] The use of these thin needles has considerably reduced the complication rate without losing diagnostic accuracy. The beveled-tip needles are similar to those used for fine needle aspiration biopsy of superficial sites in the body and are the type used originally in Sweden. This type of needle is probably used most frequently as it obtains a sample that can be easily sprayed and smeared onto slides for quick processing.[13,15,20] The screw-tip needle, as described by Nordenstrom,[18] has gained popularity,[17,19,21,22] especially for use in small, peripheral lesions of a benign or fibrotic, firm nature. The screw tip acts as an anchor in such lesions, and it is better able to extract the connective tissue elements.

Once the needle has been placed by the radiologist, aspiration is a fairly straightforward procedure. With the Chiba-type needles, the stylet is first partially withdrawn,

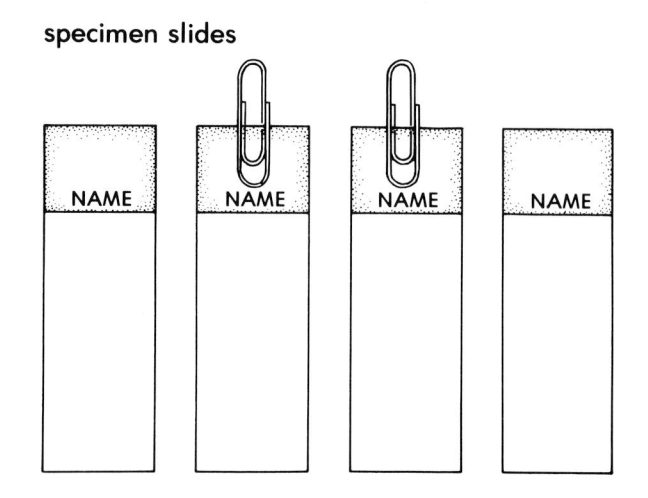

110   Diagnostic Cytology: Practical Considerations

Figure 9–5. Arrangement of slides prior to receiving specimen.

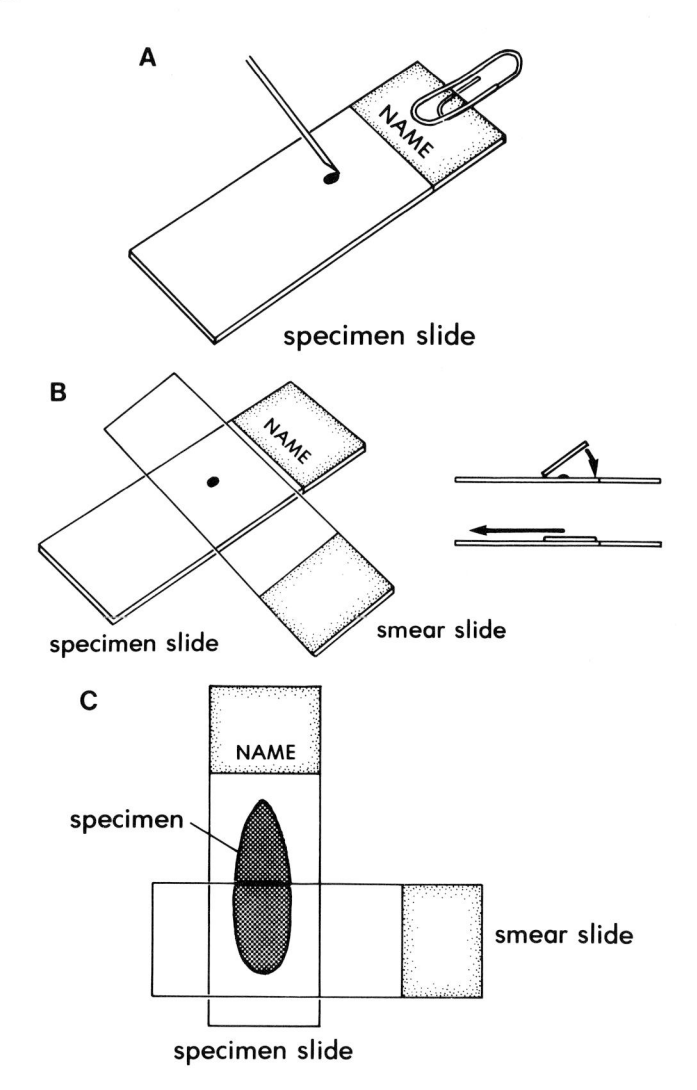

Figure 9–6. Standard one-drop smearing technique. A. Place one drop of sample onto specimen slide. B. Place smearer slide onto specimen slide and rotate slide down and along specimen slide. C. Final appearance.

and the cutting needle is rotated back and forth twice to help free the cells. The patients are then asked to hold their breath, the stylet is completely removed, a 10- to 20-cc syringe is attached to the needle, and a vacuum is applied by pulling back on the syringe handle. Once the suction is begun, the needle is moved quickly back and forth with rotation within the lesion several times for a period of no less than 5 seconds or until blood appears in the syringe hub. These passes should be at about 1 cm in depth, but can be more or less depending on the size of the lesion so that the needle remains within the lesion at all times. The suction is released, and the needle and syringe are removed still attached together. The sample is given immediately to the pathologist for preparation of the smears.

Prior to receiving the specimen, the pathologist prepares the necessary slides and other materials. It is most convenient to have the necessary supplies stored in radiology; however, if this is not possible, a portable cart or even a small box containing the equipment should be taken to the radiology suite by the pathologist at the time of the biopsy. The materials needed include a box of clean glass slides, preferably those with one frosted end to facilitate proper labeling with the patient's name or other identifying number; a lead pencil for labeling slides; appropriately sized containers of 95 percent ETOH for fixation of the smears; and paperclips. At least 1 to 2 feet of countertop space should be available for the pathologist to use to place the slides and to prepare the smears. In addition, if a rapid interpretation of the sample is needed, it is preferable that the pathologist do the stain and interpret it in the radiology suite. If so, the staining materials including appropriate dyes, coverslips, and a microscope should be available.

Before receiving the specimen, the pathologist sets out several clean, dry slides in a row on the countertop (Fig. 9–5). Extra slides should be readily available. In addition, one or two containers of 95 percent ETOH should be open and close at hand for immediate fixation of the smears. Paperclips should be placed at the frosted end of the slides; these will keep the slides from sticking together once placed in fixative.

The pathologist removes the collected sample from the needle shaft by first removing the needle from the hub of the syringe. He or she then draws air into the syringe, reattaches the needle to the syringe hub, and uses this air to blow the sample out of the needle onto clean, dry glass slides near the frosted label (Fig. 9–6 A). Care should be taken that no more than one drop of specimen be placed on each slide, otherwise there will be too much material on the slide to smear correctly. The pathologist then picks up the slide with the specimen with the left hand (right hand if left-handed), holding it steady with the thumb and forefinger at the frosted end (the end distant from the pathologist) and resting the opposite end on the remaining fingertips (the end closest to the pathologist). With the right hand, the pathologist picks up another clean, dry slide (the smearing slide) and holds it above the specimen, perpendicular in axis to the specimen slide (Fig. 9–6 B). The pathologist then lowers the front edge of the smearing slide onto the specimen slide in front of the sample (*see* Fig. 9–6 B). The smearing slide is gently rotated down onto the specimen until it barely touches the sample and begins to spread it. The smear slide is gently brought forward toward the pathologist in a quick motion, leaving the sample smeared in an oval pattern (Fig. 9–6 C). Within a second or two after the smear is prepared, the slides for PAP staining should be immersed in the 95 percent ETOH. This should be done quickly to insure that no air drying occurs on these smears.

At this point, an ETOH-fixed smear can be immediately stained using fast hematoxylin and eosin, PAP,[13,17] or toluidine blue wet preparation techniques. The latter is the fastest and simplest method and is done by applying one drop of 0.1 percent toluidine blue solution (0.1 g toluidine blue, 20 ml 95 percent ETOH, 80 ml water) directly on the smeared specimen on the ETOH-fixed slide. A coverslip is placed over the sample, and the material is examined immediately under a microscope. This fast technique allows for the evaluation of adequacy of the sample so that rebiopsy can be done quickly if needed. This same smear is then placed back in 95 percent ETOH and restained at a later time by PAP technique. Thus, this same smear can be used in making the permanent final diagnosis.

The use of the Rotex screw-type needle requires a slightly different biopsy and smearing technique. The radiologist places the needle with surrounding cannula in the edge of the lesion. The screw needle is then rotated and pushed downward into the mass. The cannula is advanced over the screw tip, and both are removed together. The slides are prepared by either rubbing and rolling the needle directly onto the slide or by using another slide to scrape the material off the needle. The latter technique involves holding the screw tip of the needle on the specimen slide that is lying on the countertop. The short edge of another slide is then placed onto the crevices of the screw tip and the needle is then circularly rotated so that the edge of the smearing slide scrapes the sample off the needle and on to the specimen slide (Fig. 9–7). The sample can then be smeared as previously described.

A combination of screw needle biopsy and aspiration can also be used. The screw-tip needle is removed first, leaving the cannula in place for a subsequent aspiration biopsy (as described).

Most believe that the dry aspiration technique is preferable to a specimen collected in saline[13–15,19] and prepared as a filter or cell button. The dry technique allows for concentration of the specimen, which in turn allows for rapid analysis and easier final processing. However, cell buttons can be helpful for the final interpretation, especially when the rapid stain is not diagnostic or suggests that the lesion may be somewhat unusual. In such cases an additional sample can be collected in saline or extruded from the needle into a small amount of formalin or saline. The tissue fragments collected can be centrifuged into a pellet and processed by routine paraffin-embedded techniques. This allows for the examination of certain architectural features, such as glandular or papillary configurations, that may be helpful in the diagnosis. Such specimens can even be placed into standard glutaraldehyde solutions for possible electron microscopic examination.

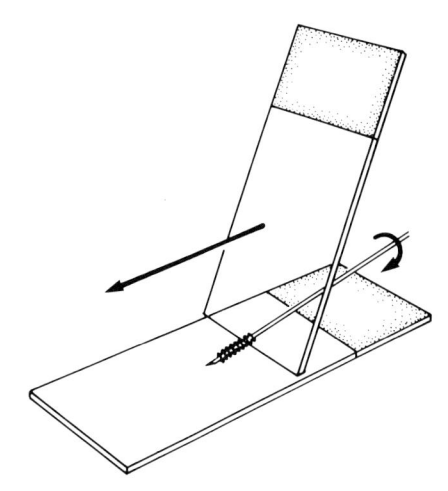

Figure 9–7. Technique for smear preparation using screw-type needle.

Air-dried smears stained by Wright-Giemsa technique can also be helpful for the final interpretation. Such smears are especially useful for any tumors or lesions with hematopoeitic or lymphoid elements, since most pathologists are most familiar with observing these cell types using Wright-Giemsa stains on routine bone marrow aspirates. Air-dried smears also allow extremely good evaluation of nuclear size, especially in relation to any erythrocytes or leukocytes also present on the smear. Nuclear shapes are also well preserved, and these two features are helpful for diagnosis of well-differentiated tumors. Finally, certain tumors contain connective tissue elements that stain metachromatically with Wright-Giemsa preparations. Such characteristic findings of this type can often be diagnostic for a particular tumor.

Indications

Before any biopsy is performed, one should determine whether the lesion can be localized well enough by radiographic techniques to ensure that a representative biopsy will be obtained. The lesion should be well visualized, localized to a particular lobe, and it should be established that the mass is of a permanent and ominous nature, as opposed to being a focus of organizing pneumonia or old burned out granulomatous disease. There should probably be an initial "wait-and-see" period of 1 to 2 weeks from the initial discovery of a small peripheral lung mass. A repeat study after this waiting period may prove or disprove the transient nature of a lesion and save the patient from an invasive procedure.

If a lesion has been found suitable for biopsy, indications for the use of fine needle aspiration over other biopsy techniques are as follows:

1. To obtain diagnostic material when routine methods have not been adequate.
2. To obtain diagnostic material in patients of high surgical risk, such as those with severe cardiac disease, or in generally debilitated patients.

There are other important indications for fine needle aspiration that because of its low complication rate and high diagnostic accuracy make the procedure preferable to thoracotomy and even bronchoscopy. Such indications include:

1. Diagnosis in patients with metastatic cancers and inoperable tumors of unknown cell type, which would require irradiation or chemotherapy.
2. Determining the nature of a small, peripheral "coin" lesion, since many of these are benign. Thoracotomy can be avoided, and bronchoscopy will most likely not be successful in obtaining diagnostic material.
3. Determining whether a "new" lesion represents a new primary or a metastasis from a previous carcinoma from any site.
4. Determining the nature of multiple pulmonary nodules or diffuse lung lesions in immunocompromised patients, including cancer and leukemia patients, in order to identify opportunistic infections such as abscesses or pneumonia as opposed to metastatic, leukemic, or recurrent disease. Many of these patients are debilitated and thus are poor surgical risks.
5. Providing a diagnosis of tumors for which preoperative radiation is preferred.
6. Diagnosis of small (oat) cell carcinoma of the lung, preventing surgery and permitting early chemotherapy and radiation. This tumor can often be more reliably diagnosed on good cytology specimens than on the typically crushed and distorted biopsies obtained by bronchoscopy or mediastinoscopy.

Less tangible reasons for the use of fine needle aspiration relate to (1) allaying the patient's anxiety about a mass in the lung by providing quick identification of the nature of the lesion without waiting to see growth of the lesion or proceeding immediately to thoracotomy; (2) offering an alternative to the patients who would prefer a diagnosis of cancer before proceeding to surgery; and (3) in the cases of an unknown mass, ensuring prompt identification and early resection of operable malignancies and preventing unnecessary surgery for benign lesions.[13,14,16]

Contraindications

Because of the decreased risk of fine needle aspiration compared with thoracotomy, the contraindications usually relate to how necessary proper histologic diagnosis is for proper therapy. Such instances when fine needle aspiration may not be the safest method include the following.[13,14,16,23]

1. An uncooperative patient who cannot or will not stop breathing in order to allow appropriate sampling.
2. Significant respiratory disease in which a pneumothorax could be critical. Patients with severe emphysema are especially susceptible to pneumothoraces and do not tolerate them well. These patients are often also operative risks, so precautions should be taken for immediate insertion of a chest tube if pneumothorax occurs.
3. Bleeding diathesis, coagulation disorders, or anticoagulant therapy can result in severe hemorrhage following the procedure, but this is a relative risk, since these patients are also prone to hemorrhage following other means of biopsy.
4. Pulmonary hypertension increases the risk of hemorrhage, so smaller needles should be used if biopsy is necessary.

Fine needle aspiration is probably contraindicated in:

5. Echinococcal cysts.
6. Known vascular lesions, although aspiration of aortic aneurysms, aortic valve malformation, and normal vessels in general are well tolerated.
7. Patients on positive pressure mechanical ventilation because of increased risk of air embolism.[16]

Complications

Pneumothorax is the most frequent complication of transthoracic fine needle aspiration biopsies, occurring in about 25 to 30 percent of patients[14,15,19–22,24–27] as seen on routine chest radiograph done within 3 to 4 hours following the biopsy procedure. However, only about one in four or five patients is symptomatic or has pneumothorax large enough to require placement of a chest tube or direct aspiration of the air. Tension pneumothorax has been reported as a cause of death.[28] The incidence of pneumothorax increases with larger-bore needles[24] (again emphasizing the value of using 21- to 23-gauge needles) and with the number of passes through the pleura. In addition, patients with central lesions or emphysema often have a more severe pneumothoraces requiring tube placement.[21,27] The incidence decreases considerably as the operator becomes more experienced.[24]

Hemorrhage is probably the next most common complication, with clinically insignificant amounts occurring in 3 to 4 percent of patients. Severe hemorrhage with loss of blood leading to transfusion or death is extremely rare,[29,30] but is probably the most common cause of demise following the procedure.[13] Again, the smaller-bore needles cause less hemorrhage.

Implantation of tumor cells is very rare,[31] with many large series of cases citing no examples.[14,15,17,19–22,26] This does not seem to be a significant problem, similar to fine needle aspiration biopsies at other sites.

Air embolism is a very rare, but potentially dangerous complication.[13,32,33] Care should be taken that once the needle is in the lung it should remain plugged by the stylet, finger, or syringe and no passes be made when the patient is coughing or inhaling.

The overall mortality rate is low, less than 0.2 percent.[13–15]

Diagnostic Accuracy

Most studies[15,19–21,25,26,35–37] show fine needle aspiration biopsies to be accurate in the diagnosis of malignancy in more than 90 percent of the cases, with most recent studies[17,19,26] showing accuracy of 87 to 99 percent. The sensitivity (true positive rate) is approximately 90 percent. The specificity (true negative rate) is also approximately 90 percent. One must remember that accurate interpretation and diagnosis is dependent on obtaining adequate clinical correlation with the history (history of chemotherapy, irradiation, and so on) and radiographic findings, receiving an adequate and representative sample, and proper fixation and staining of the specimens.

False negatives are most commonly due to incorrect placement of the needle, especially in small lesions (less than 1 to 1.5 cm in diameter). Other factors, such as extensive tumor necrosis or fibrosis can result in scant or acellular specimens. Large tumors are often centrally necrotic; biopsy of the growing peripheral portions of the large tumors may yield positive results if an attempt to obtain material from the lesion's center is unsuccessful. At least one attempt to biopsy the center is recommended in order to avoid missing the diagnosis of an abscess or other inflammatory lesions (see false positives, below). Poor aspiration technique can also result in unsatisfactory specimens. With experienced personnel, repeat biopsies (up to three aspirations) can result in adequate cytologic material in more than 95 percent of patients. The false-negative rate usually is 5 to 10 percent in most series.[15,19,20,21,26]

False positives are usually due to misinterpretation of reactive, inflammatory, or reparative changes mistaken for malignant changes. Processes that can cause problems in this area include irradiation, chemotherapy, granulomatous inflammation, abscesses, pneumonia, pulmonary infarct, bronchiectasis, and chronic obstructive pulmonary disease. Any or all of these conditions can result in atypical changes of the alveolar lining cells, bronchiolar epithelium, and macrophages that can be quite numerous on aspirate specimens. A biopsy of the periphery of an abscess (or other inflammatory process) without sampling the center could lead to a false-positive diagnosis of carcinoma. Thus, the clinical history is very important, and adequate sampling of the entire lesion is essential. False-positive rate is still usually less than 2 percent in most studies.[15,17,19,21,25]

Diagnostic accuracy of nonneoplastic lesions is not as good since findings are often nonspecific,[25] especially in cases of a granulomatous or fibrotic process. However, specific fungal, parasitic, viral, acid-fast, or other bacterial organisms can often be identified on the direct smears of the aspirates or by culture.

Comparison of this technique to bronchoscopic biopsy[38] shows that fine needle aspiration biopsy is at least as accurate and safe and is better for small, peripheral, or upper lobe lesions. The same applies for comparisons to bronchial brushing,[39,40] except that brushing has a somewhat lower complication rate. Comparison of fine needle aspiration biopsy to sputum cytology[41] showed 93 percent diagnostic rate compared with 64 percent by sputum. Others[42] have reported up to 80 percent accuracy with sputum.

Histologic correlation to specific tumor types has also been evaluated. Most studies[15,17,19,26,35,36,43] show more than 90 percent accuracy in diagnosis of small cell carcinomas, 70 to 80 percent for adenocarcinoma, 70 to 100 percent for squamous carcinoma, and 60 to 70 percent for large cell carcinoma. Almost all of the missed diagnoses occurred among the poorly differentiated adenocarcinomas, poorly differentiated squamous carcinomas, and large-cell undifferentiated carcinoma. Clinically, this is not a significant problem since all of these tumor types are treated similarly. Small-cell carcinoma, however, is important to type accurately because of the different therapies involved.

References

1. Gee JBL, Fick RB: Bronchoalveolar lavage. Thorax 35:1–8, 1980.
2. Smith LJ: Bronchoalveolar lavage today. Chest 80:251, 1981.
3. Fulmer JD: Bronchoalveolar lavage. Am Rev Respir Dis 126:961–963, 1982.
4. Lawrence EC, Martin RR, Blaese RM, et al.: Increased bronchoalveolar IgG-secreting cells in interstitial disease. N Engl J Med 302:1186–1188, 1980.
5. Haslam PL, Turton CWG, Lukoszek A, et al.: Bronchoalveolar lavage fluid cell counts in cryptogenic fibrosing aveolitis and their relation to therapy. Thorax 35:328–329, 1980.
6. Keogh B, Hunninghake G, Line B, et al.: Therapy decisions in sarcoidosis: Prospective use of bronchoalveolar lavage and gallium-67 scanning. Am Rev Respir Dis 121(suppl):155, 1980.
7. Leyden E: Uber infectious Pneumonie. Dtsch Med Wochenshr 9:52–54, 1883.
8. Menetrier P: Cancer primitif du poumon. Bull Soc Anat 11:643–647, 1886.
9. Martin HE, Ellis EB: Biopsy by needle puncture and aspiration. Ann Surg 22:169–181, 1930.
10. Dahlgren SE, Nordenstrom B: *Transthoracic Needle Biopsy.* Chicago: Year Book, 1966.
11. Fox C: Innovation in medical diagnosis—the Scandinavian curiosity. Lancet 1:1387–1388, 1979.
12. Koss LG: Thin needle aspiration biopsy. Acta Cytol 24:1–3, 1979.
13. Bonfiglio TA: *Cytopathologic Interpretation of Transthoracic Fine-Needle Biopsies.* New York: Masson, 1983.
14. Lalli AF, McCormack LJ, Zelch M, et al.: Aspiration biopsies of chest lesions. Radiology 127:35–40, 1978.
15. Sinner WN: Transthoracic needle biopsy of small peripheral malignant lung lesions. Invest Radiol 8:305–314, 1973.
16. Green R: The chest. In Athanasoulis CA (ed): *Interventional Radiology.* Philadelphia: WB Saunders, 1982.
17. Mitchell ML, King DE, Bonfiglio TA, Patten SF: Pulmonary fine needle aspiration cytology. A five-year correlation study. Acta Cytol 28:72–76, 1984.
18. Nordenstrom B: New instruments for biopsy. Radiology 117:474–475, 1975.

19. Poe RH, Tobin RE: Sensitivity and specificity of needle biopsy in lung malignancy. Am Rev Respir Dis 122:725–729, 1980.

20. Meyer JE, Gandbhir LH, Milner LB, McLaughlin MM: Percutaneous aspiration biopsy of nodular lung lesions. J Thorac Cardiovasc Surg 73:787–791, 1977.

21. House AJS, Thomson KR: Evaluation of a new transthoracic needle biopsy of benign and malignant lung lesions. Am J Roentgenol 129:215–220, 1977.

22. Hayata Y, Oho K, Ichiba M, et al.: Percutaneous pulmonary puncture for cytologic diagnosis—its diagnostic value for small peripheral pulmonary carcinoma. Acta Cytol 17:469–475, 1973.

23. Fennessey JJ: Bronchographic criteria of inflammatory disease and radiologic lung biopsy techniques. Radiol Clin North Am 11:371, 1973.

24. Sinner WN: Complications of percutaneous transthoracic needle aspiration biopsy. Acta Radiol [Diagn] (Stockh) 17:813–828, 1976.

25. Greenberg SD: Recent advances in pulmonary cytopathology. Hum Pathol 14:901–912, 1983.

26. Zavala DC, Schoell JE: Ultrathin needle aspiration of the lung in infectious and malignant disease. Am Rev Respir Dis 123:125–131, 1981.

27. Landman S, Burgener FA, Lim GHK: Comparison of bronchial brushing and percutaneous needle aspiration biopsy in the diagnosis of malignant lung lesions. Radiology 115:275–278, 1975.

28. Lauby VW, Burnett WE, Rosemond GP, et al.: Value and risk of biopsy of pulmonary lesions by needle aspiration: Twenty-one years of experience. J Thorac Cardiovasc Surg 49:159–175, 1965.

29. Pearce JG, Patt NL: Fatal pulmonary hemorrhage after percutaneous aspiration lung biopsy. Am Rev Respir Dis 220:346–349, 1975.

30. Meyer JE, Ferrucci JT, Janower MC: Fatal complications of percutaneous lung biopsy. Radiology 96:47–48, 1970.

31. Sinner WN, Zajicek J: Implantation metastasis after percutaneous transthoracic needle aspiration biopsy. Acta Radiol [Diagn] (Stockh) 17:473–480, 1976.

32. Westcott JL: An embolism complicating percutaneous needle biopsy of the lung. Chest 63:108–110, 1973.

33. Woolf CR: Application of aspiration biopsy with review of the literature. Dis Chest 25:286–300, 1954.

34. Herman PG, Hessel SJ: The diagnostic accuracy and complications of closed lung biopsies. Radiology 125:11–14, 1977.

35. Francis D: Transthoracic aspiration biopsy. Acta Pathol Microbiol Scand 85:535–538, 1977.

36. King EB, Russell WM: Needle aspirations biopsy of the lung – Technique and cytologic morphology. Acta Cytol 11:319–324, 1967.

37. Caya JG, Clowry LJ, Wollenberg BS, Tieu TM: Transthoracic fine needle aspiration cytology. Am J Clin Pathol 82:100–103, 1984.

38. Dahlgren E, Lind B: Transthoracic needle biopsy or bronchoscopic biopsy? Scand J Respir Dis 50:265–272, 1969.

39. Landman S, Burgener FA, Lim GHK: Comparison of bronchial brushing and percutaneous needle aspiration biopsy in the diagnosis of malignant lung lesions. Radiology 115:275–278, 1975.

40. Janower ML, Land RE: Lung biopsy: Bronchial brushing and percutaneous puncture. Radiol Clin North Am 9:73–83, 1971.

41. Dahlgren E, Lind B: Comparison between diagnostic results obtained by transthoracic needle biopsy and by sputum cytology. Acta Cytol 16:53–58, 1971.

42. Russell WO, Nerhardt HW, Mountain CF, et al.: Cytodiagnosis of lung cancer. Acta Cytol 7:1–44, 1963.

43. Thornbury JR, Burke DP, Naylor B: Transthoracic needle aspiration biopsy: Accuracy of cytologic typing of malignant neoplasms. Am J Radiol 136:719–724, 1981.

10 Pulmonary Disorders in the Neonate Infant and Child

Frederic B. Askin

This chapter is devoted to a discussion of those disorders encountered most specifically in the pediatric age group.[1–9] Congenital anomalies, while not the sole provenance of children, are detailed here as are disorders of the transition between intra- and extrauterine life. In addition, specific infections affect the lungs of neonates and infants.

Congenital Anomalies of the Lower Respiratory Tract

Congenital absence of the lung may be bilateral or unilateral.[10–15] In either instance the affected lung(s) may be completely absent or may be represented by a rudimentary bronchus. As part of this spectrum there may also be a dysplastic mass of pulmonary tissue, occasionally containing striated muscle (see Rhabdomyomatous Dysplasia). Bilateral agenesis is quite rare and may be associated with a wider spectrum of anomalies involving tracheal and esophageal atresia.[10,11] Unilateral absence of the lung is a more common entity and may be compatible with essentially normal life.[12–14] Absence of the left lung appears to occur more frequently and in fact the prognosis is generally regarded as worse for patients with agenesis on the right. The excess morbidity in the latter case may be associated with tracheal or bronchial compression by a deviated aorta (Fig. 10–1); severe mediastinal shift may also occur. Unilateral pulmonary agenesis may be associated with a variety of distal skeletal (thumb) and chest wall anomalies.[15] Morphometric analysis of the single lung in one case of unilateral agenesis revealed an increased volume with an increased number of smaller than normal alveoli.[16] The number of bronchial branches was reduced.

Isolated absence of one or more lobes is a very rare occurrence[17] and should not be confused with the "bilateral left lungs" seen in association with cardiac defects (see below).[6]

Congenital bronchial anomalies include the bronchial isomerism syndromes ("bilateral" right or left lungs) associated with anisosplenia or polysplenia and various associated cardiac defects.[6,18] True supernumerary bronchi[19] are rare and at least one reported case may actually be more closely related to extralobar sequestration or bronchogenic cyst.[20] Displaced bronchi are encountered, however, with some frequency.[6,21] The tracheal bronchus[6,22,23] connects a segment of the upper lobe usually, but not always, the right to the trachea or, less often, a mainstem bronchus. Both displaced and supernumerary bronchi have been included in this category. These lesions often produce no symptoms but recurrent infection, sublobar overinflation of the lung or associated upper respiratory tract anomalies may give rise to clinical problems. The so-called "bridging" bronchus connects the left lung to the right lower lobe by coursing across the mediastinum.[24] Other anomalous bronchi include the accessory cardiac bronchus arising from the intermediate bronchus[6]; origin of the anterior segmental upper lobe bronchus from the middle lobe bronchus ("posteparterial bronchus"),[25] and a variety of minor variations. Congenital intrinsic stenosis of a mainstem bronchus has been reported, associated with atelectasis.[26] The lesion is vanishingly rare as compared to extrinsic partial obstruction or with segmental atresia associated with overinflation (see Chapter 21). Bronchobiliary fistula is a rare anomaly which may be associated with the production of green sputum. A variety of biliary tract abnormalities has been reported in association with the lesion.[27,28]

Abnormal pulmonary fissures, usually absent or incomplete, but also supernumerary, are extremely common[6,21] and Landing and Dixon stress that the number of external lobes should not be taken to indicate the number of lobar bronchi.[6] Horseshoe lung, fused behind

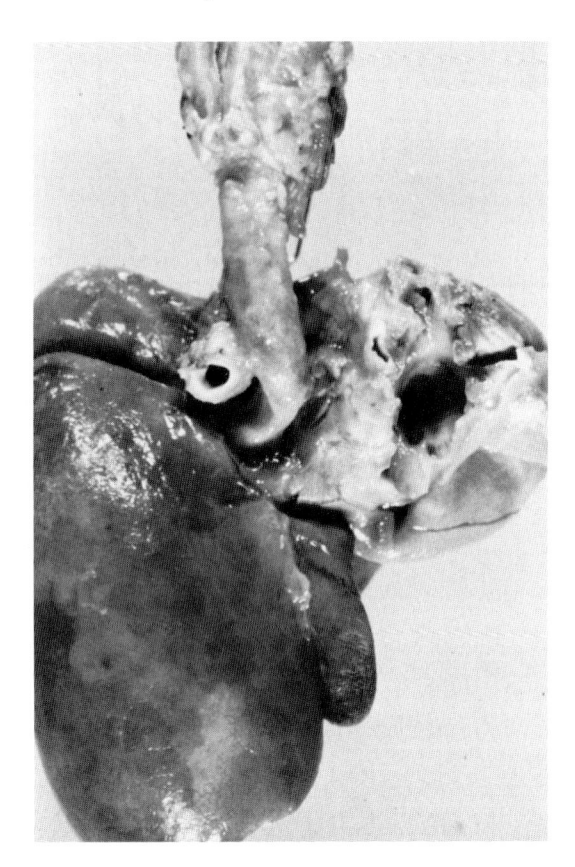

Figure 10–1. Agenesis of the right lung, posterior view. Note the prominent aortic indentation in the left mainstem bronchus. This patient had clinical and laboratory evidence of airflow obstruction.

Table 10–1. Etiology of Bilateral Pulmonary Hypoplasia

Category	Example and References
Unexplained	Idiopathic (sporadic or familial) Down's syndrome
Compression of lungs Inadequate or abnormal thoracic space	Diaphragmatic hernia, scoliosis, thoracic mass lesions, thoracic dystrophy, various types of dwarfism, other causes of abnormal shape or development of bony thorax
Large extrathoracic mass	Polycystic kidneys, urethral valves with resultant large bladder, abdominal masses
Decreased fetal respiratory movement or loss of lung fluid	Amniotic fluid deficit (renal agenesis/dysplasia, amniotic fluid leak), neuromuscular disorders affecting diaphragm and other respiratory muscles, anencephaly, ?polyhydramnios
Metabolic defect	Renal agenesis, anencephaly, RH incompatibility
Decreased bloow flow	Congenital pulmonic valve stenosis

the heart but anterior to the esophagus, is a rare entity[6,29,30]; the lesion has been associated with anomalous pulmonary veins and arteries including variants of the "scimitar syndrome."

Segmental bronchomalacia has been reported in the left mainstem bronchus. Functionally there is narrowing and partial collapse of the airway with exhalation. The pathologic features are poorly documented but include abnormal and abnormally spaced cartilaginous rings. The etiology of the disorder is unknown.[6] Congenital bronchiectasis (Campbell-Williams syndrome) *tracheobronchiomegaly* (Mounier-Kuhn syndrome) and bronchiectasis associated with structurally abnormal cilia are discussed in Chapter 21.

Pulmonary *hypoplasia* implies an abnormal reduction in the weight or volume of the lung without the absence of any of its lobes.[31–34] A number of age-related standards have been proposed.[3,35–39] Page and Stocker[38] found that a lung weight/body weight ratio of 0.010 identified pulmonary hypoplasia in most instances. Wigglesworth and associates[3,39] indicated that a ratio of 0.015 was useful until 28 weeks' gestation and that after that time 0.012 was a more useful figure. Cooney and Thurlbeck[36,37] employed the radial alveolar counting technique originally devised by Emery and Mithal and provided a set of normal standards for gestational age 18 weeks (1.5) through age 18 years (12). According to their figures the count at term birth should be approximately 5. As another approach the number of bronchial branches can be determined by bronchography or use of the dissecting microscope.[32]

Hypoplasia represents the end result of many different and not necessarily related phenomena (*see* Chapter 1).[3,31–42] Structurally, decreased lung weight and volume could result from a decreased number of bronchial branches, reduced number of alveoli, decreased alveolar size, or from any combination of the three. Bilateral pulmonary hypoplasia is usually associated with conditions that can be grouped into several major categories (Table 10–1) as related to chest wall deformities,[32,43] lung compression, reduced pulmonary blood flow,[44] or to a combination of decreased fetal respiratory motion and loss of the fluid that normally distends the developing lung.[3,45–48] A reduced volume of amniotic fluid, or oligohydramnios, appears to cause a net loss of lung fluid into the amniotic cavity resulting in reduced lung distention and loss of respiratory movement-features required for normal lung development.[3,33,45–48] Polyhydramnios may also affect lung motion but some of the disorders associated with excess amniotic fluid may affect lung growth via immune-mediated mechanisms.[32,33] The etiology of pulmonary hypoplasia in Down's syndrome is not clear although the morphologic defect is known to be a reduced number of alveoli in each acinar unit.[49] In many of the disorders associated with reduced lung size, multiple factors may be operant. For example, renal agenesis produces a reduced amniotic fluid volume but may also interfere with collagen metabolism.[6,34] Primary or idiopathic hypoplasia may be sporadic or familial and has been reported in association with several malformation syndromes.[6,41,46,49] Diaphragmatic hernia (*see* p. 138) is almost uniformally associated with hypoplasia of the ipsilateral and, to a lesser extent contralateral lung (Fig.

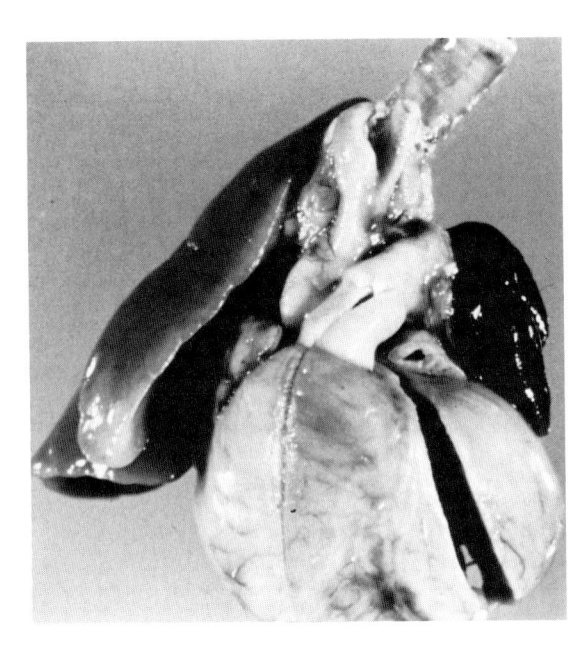

Figure 10–2. Hypoplasia of the left lung in patient with a postero-lateral (Bochdalek's) hernia. Anterior view. The number of airways and the total alveolar number are decreased markedly on the left but the right lung is also affected.

10–2). Unilateral hypoplasia of the lung appears to involve a more limited differential diagnosis in terms of etiology. Idiopathic hypoplasia, pulmonary artery anomalies (usually absence), anomalous venous return, and diaphragmatic hernia or accessory diaphragm (see p. 140) were the main causes of unilateral hypoplasia in one recent series.[50] *Heterotopic* tissues have been reported in the lung and include adrenal cortex,[51] striated muscle ("rhabdomyomatous dysplasia"),[52,53] and glial tissue.[54] Glial heterotopia is usually found in the lung parenchyma of anencephalic infants and must be separated from traumatic emboli of central nervous system tissue to the pulmonary arteries.[9]

Congenital alveolar capillary dysplasia (Fig. 10–3) is rare developmental anomaly in which there is a profound absence of capillaries in the alveolar wall.[55] Extrauterine oxygenation of the lung is essentially too poor to support life although in one reported case the affected infant survived for 30 hours with pulmonary hypertension thought to be related to reduced of cross-sectional area of the pulmonary vasculature.[56]

Pulmonary Vascular Anomalies

Arterial anomalies (see also p. 136) include origin of one or both pulmonary arteries from the aorta its branches or the ductus arteriosus.[6,57–59] Origin of the left pulmonary from the right ("vascular sling") represents one of multiple vascular anomalies that can cause respiratory distress via compression of the trachea.[60–63]

The so-called absent or occult pulmonary artery actually represents interruption of the proximal portion of the vessel; the intrapulmonary branches of the vessel are usually present and complete.[64] Hislop and associates reported three unusual cases of absent or hypoplastic pulmonary artery associated with mesenchymal dysplasia in the ipsilateral lung.[65] Diffuse hypoplasia of the pulmonary arterial system is described as a consequence of intrauterine rubella.[66] Goldstein and co-workers reported several other unusual cases in which the affected infant had hypoplastic pulmonary artery branches in association with abnormal pulmonary venous connections and partial systemic arterial supply to both lungs.[67] Segmental stenosis in the pulmonary arterial system appears to represent a broad spectrum of disorders (see Fig. 10–5).[68–70] The stenosis may be single or multiple and peripheral or central. In some instances cardiac anomalies may be present as well. Children with the Alagille's syndrome of cholestasis, paucity of intrahepatic bile ducts, and a peculiar facies often have peripheral stenotic lesions in the pulmonary arteries.[6] Peripheral stenosis has been also described in association with Down's syndrome, Ehlers-Danlos syndrome, cutis laxa, the "LEOPARD" syndrome of multiple lentigenes, and in association with café-au-lait spots possibly representing a form of von Recklinghausen's disease.[6,70,71]

Haworth and Reid studied the intrapulmonary vessels in cases of pulmonary valvular atresia and found a reduced number of intrapulmonary arteries.[72] The arteries that were present had thin muscular walls and an abnormally small diameter.

Arteriovenous malformations (fistulas) occur in the lung either as an isolated entity or as part of the Osler-Weber-Rendu syndrome. The lesions can be acquired on the basis of trauma as well.[73,74] The blood supply of the fistula is usually derived from the pulmonary artery but may arise from systemic vessels. Abe and associates reported direct connection of the right pulmonary artery to the left atrium.[75] We have seen a similar lesion involving a segmental pulmonary artery. Complicated vascular malformations involving anastomosis of chest wall vessels to the lung have also been described.[76] Rarely an infant's lung may be infiltrated by a diffuse capillary hemangioma (Fig. 10–4) with the clinical result of a large arteriovenous shunt.[77] It is not clear whether or not this diffuse hemangioma is related to capillary hemangiomatosis as described in the adult. The lesion in children seems to lack a component of veno-occlusion.

Pulmonary venous abnormalities include anomalous venous return, either total or partial.[78,79] In total anomalous return all of the four main pulmonary veins converge and then drain into the innominate vein, coronary veins, or right atrium. They may also run below the diaphragm and enter the inferior vena cava or portal vein. Lymphangiectasis may be prominent in the pulmonary parenchyma. Partial forms of anomalous venous return also occur; one such lesion is the so-called "scimitar" syndrome in which a large anomalous pulmonary vein drains one lung, usually the right, into the inferior vena cava.[80,81] The broad roentgenographic shadow of this vein forms the scimitar. The ipsilateral lung is hypoplastic has complete or at least partial systemic arterial blood supply and may have abnormal

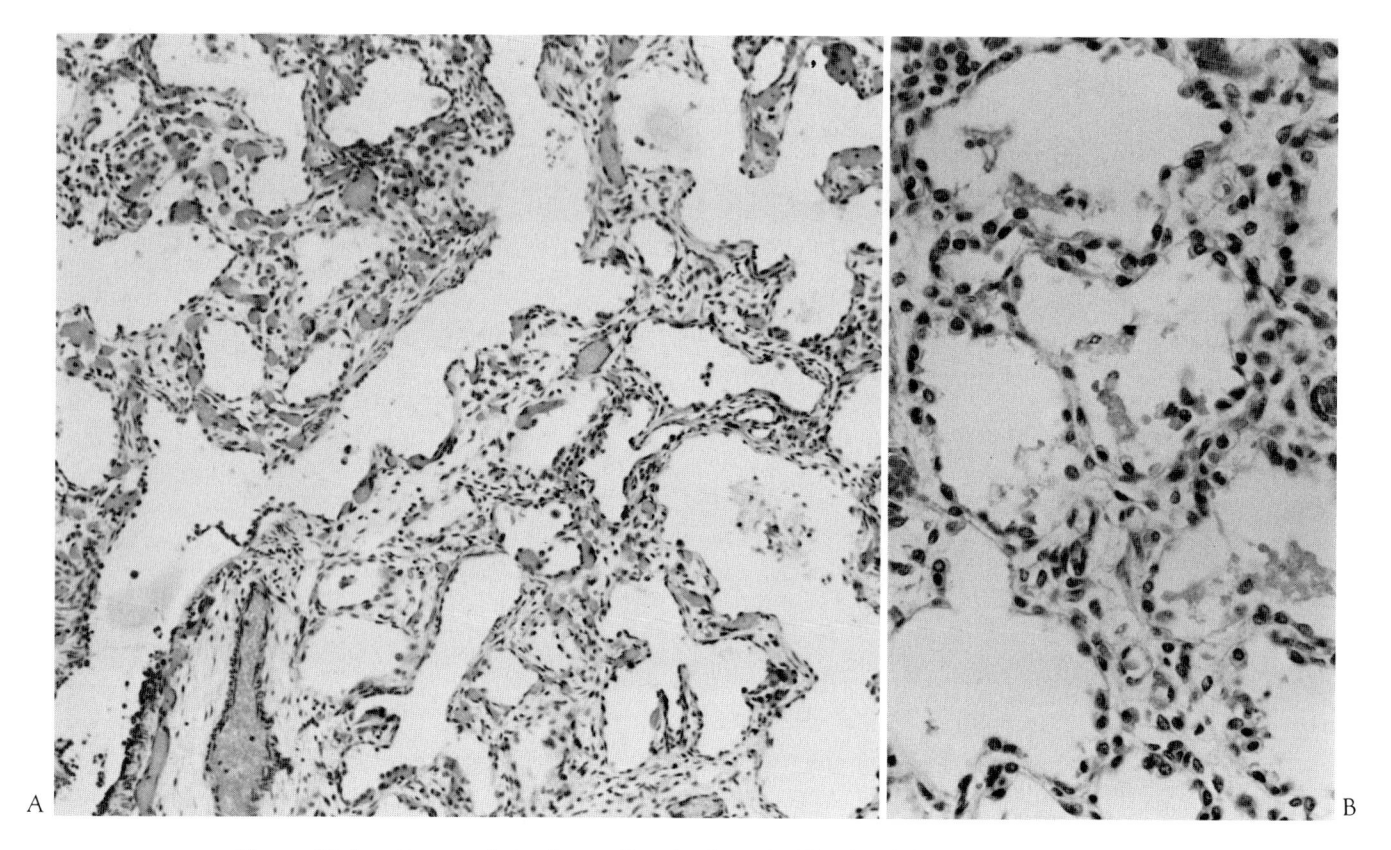

Figure 10–3. Congenital alveolar capillary dysplasia. A. The alveoli have thickened septa with central vascular cores. B. At higher magnification the paucity of capillaries in the alveolar wall can be seen.

lobation. This complicated syndrome may overlap with horseshoe lung or bronchopulmonary sequestration.[6,82]

Isolated or multiple areas of stenosis or atresia may be found in the pulmonary veins.[83–85] These lesions are associated with diffuse or localized lymphangiectasis (see p. 123) or hemorrhage and hemosiderin deposition in the lung. Unilateral venous stenosis in association with ventricular septal defect may cause pulmonary hypertension very early in infancy.[86] Dilated, nonobstructed pulmonary veins ("varices") are usually found in adults but have been described in children and even infants.[87]

Bronchopulmonary Sequestration

Sequestration of pulmonary lobes or segments implies (1) absence of a normal connection to the airway system of the surrounding lung and (2) blood supply to the sequestered areas via systemic vessels arising from the aorta or its branches either above or below the diaphragm. Savic and associates and other authors have produced extensive reviews of the subject.[88–92] Two major types of sequestration occur: intralobar and extralobar. Rarely, both types of lesions occur in the same patient.[6,91]

Intralobar sequestrations (ILS) are incorporated within the pleural investment of a pulmonary lobe (Fig. 10–5). The lesion occurs with almost equal frequency in children and adults.[6,88] The usual, but not invariable, location is in the posterior segment of the left lower lobe.[6,88] Upper lobe and even bilateral examples of ILS have been reported.[6,88,91,92] One or more elastic arteries supply the area and the usual venous drainage is through the pulmonary system to the left atrium. The lesion is often discovered during the investigation of recurrent localized pneumonia or as a mass lesion seen on a routine chest radiograph.[94,95] Pathologically the features are those of chronic pneumonitis and bronchiectasis (Fig. 10–6). On gross examination the lesion may be solid or cystic depending on the degree of inflammatory change and infection.[6,88,93] The elastic arteries supplying the lesion often show extensive atherosclerotic change, especially in adults.

Extralobar sequestrations (ELS, accessory lobes) are completely separate from the pleural covering of the normal lung.[6,91,96] The usual location of the lesion is in the left lower hemithorax but ELS may be found in the mediastinum, near the esophagus or even within or below the diaphragm.[88] Both the arterial supply and the venous drainage are usually of systemic origin. In contrast to ILS, the extralobar lesion is found predominantly in infants and may be associated with coexisting malformations, especially diaphragmatic hernia and pectus excavatum.[6,88,91,96] Again in contrast to ILS, secondary

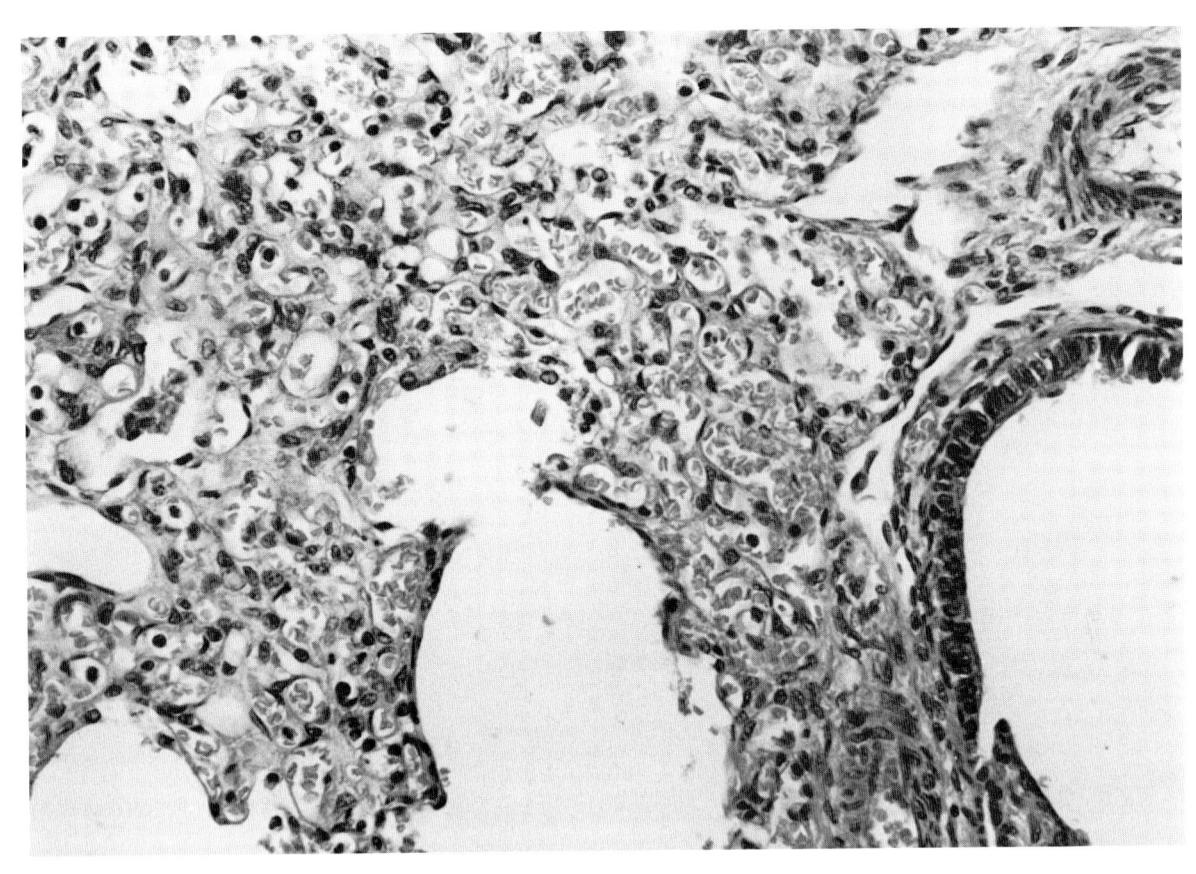

Figure 10–4. Diffuse capillary hemangioma in the lung of a neonate. Thin-walled vessels ramify in the septa and in the bronchovascular bundles. The infant developed heart failure. Courtesy of Dr. Beverly Dahms, Cleveland, OH.

infection and obstructive changes are not common features. On gross examination the lesion has a spongy character (Fig. 10–7) and the basic microscopic architecture (Fig. 10–8) often resembles that of immature lung or may resemble certain types of adenomatoid malformation.[96] Striated muscle may be found within the parenchyma of an ELS.[96] Lymphatic dilation is common in ELS and several cases of massive pleural effusion and hypoplasia of the ipsilateral lung have been reported.[97]

The origin of pulmonary sequestration has provided fertile ground for both debate and imagination.[6,88,89,98,99] A practical classification is presented in Table 10–2. It seems certain that extralobar sequestration represents an accessory lung bud from the foregut. Some intralobar sequestrations may represent an accessory lung bud, presumably occuring later in embryogenesis than that associated with ELS. It has become increasing clear that other forms of ILS are, in fact, acquired lesions resulting from recurrent localized inflammation.[99,100] Aspirated foreign bodies could produce such a lesion.[99] There is subsequent enlargement of the small systemic arteries normally present in the pulmonary ligament.[100] Presumably these recently demonstrated arteries play a role in the blood supply of ELS as well.

Reported complications of sequestration include a variety of problems such as clinically significant arteriovenous shunts (ELS or ILS),[88,101] infarction of an ELS,[102] aneurysmal dilatation of the systemic artery and resultant hemoptysis (ILS),[103] and respiratory distress in a newborn related to a mediastinal mass (ELS).[104]

In some instances, with either ELS or ILS, the lung bud connection to the foregut may persist and connect the sequestered lobe or area to the esophagus or stomach ("bronchopulmonary foregut malformation").[105–107] Pancreatic tissue has been found in several ILS, presumably as part of this spectrum.[108,109] Not surprisingly, sequestration may occur in association with tracheoesophageal fistula (see discussion of total sequestration, below) and with duplication of portions of the gastrointestinal tract.[110–113]

Certain vascular anomalies may mimic or even belong in the spectrum of sequestion. Isolated systemic arterial supply of an otherwise normal lobe can occur and may produce a large shunt.[114,115] In a very young infant without recurrent infection in the lung, it might be difficult to separate this lesion from ILS without a presurgical or specimen bronchogram. A variety of anomalous patterns of venous return have been noted in associated with ELS or ILS[116] and the "scimitar syndrome" may in fact, be related to sequestration. The term total sequestration (pulmonary ectoplasia) appears in the literature, usually in reference to a malformed lung with

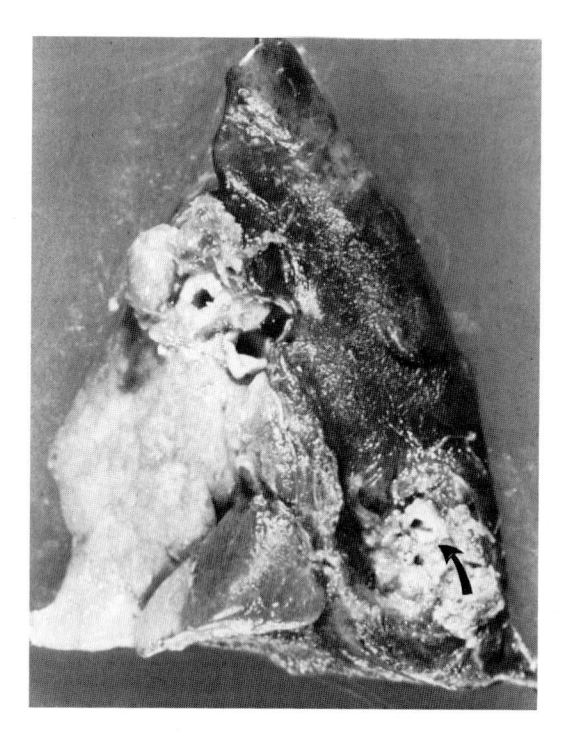

Figure 10-5. Intralobar sequestration. Medial view. The abnormal elastic artery (arrow) arose from the thoracic aorta just above the diaphragm.

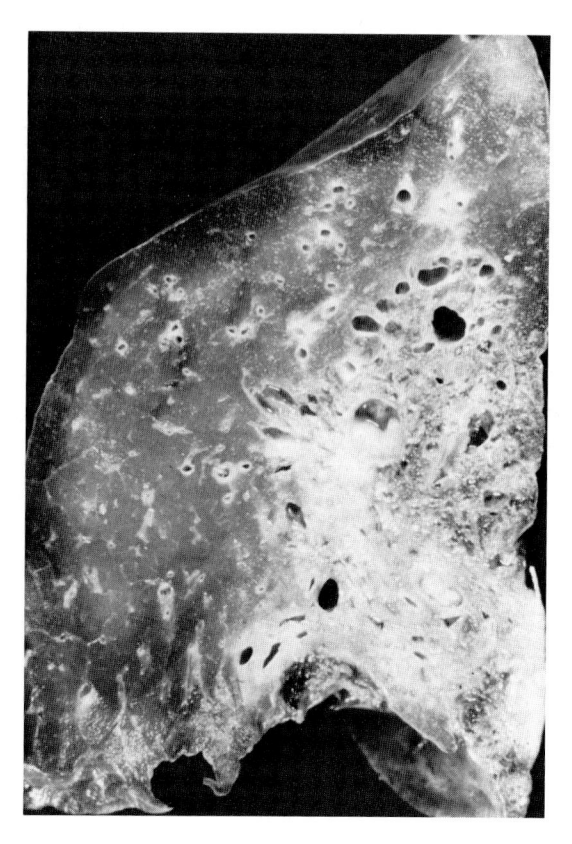

Figure 10-6. Intralobar sequestration. The cut surface shows bronchiectasis, mucus plugs, and organizing pneumonia in the posterior basal segment of this lobe.

systemic arterial supply and its main bronchial connection to the esophagus.[111,117]

Bronchogenic and Other Cysts

Bronchogenic cysts also arise from accessory lung buds from the foregut.[106,119–121] In rare instances there may be a peripheral rim of poorly developed pulmonary tissue[106] but ordinarily these cysts are characterized by a muscular or fibrous wall with a lining of bronchial epithelium. Cartilage is present in the wall (Fig. 10-9) but may be difficult to find without multiple sections. Bronchogenic cysts are usually found in the anterior mediastinum but may appear within the lung substance as well.[119] Rare connections to the gut have been described, similar to sequestration.[122] A similar lesion has also been described in skin of the neck or anterior chest wall.[123] The cysts are unilocular and may contain mucus, watery fluid, or even pus. In the mediastinum they must be separated from *enteric cysts*, which are lined by gastric epithelium and usually occur in the posterior compartment.[124,125] Within the lung, bronchogenic cysts may be confused with lung abscesses. The abscess however, should have multiple bronchi communicating with the lesion whereas the bronchogenic cyst will not. The nature of the epithelial lining may not be of help.[126] Bronchiectasis in infants has been described, mistakenly, in the past as a specific type of congenital cystic disease of the lung. *Pneumatoceles* are also cystic foci in the lung.[6] They probably result from areas of necrosis of broncho-

pulmonary tissue during infection, with subsequent escape of air into the interstitium. Staphylococcal pneumonia is the common antecedent but viral infection or kerosene aspiration have also been impicated.[1,2]

Lymphangiectasis (*see* p. 123) and pulmonary interstitial emphysema (PIE) may also form grossly visible, but

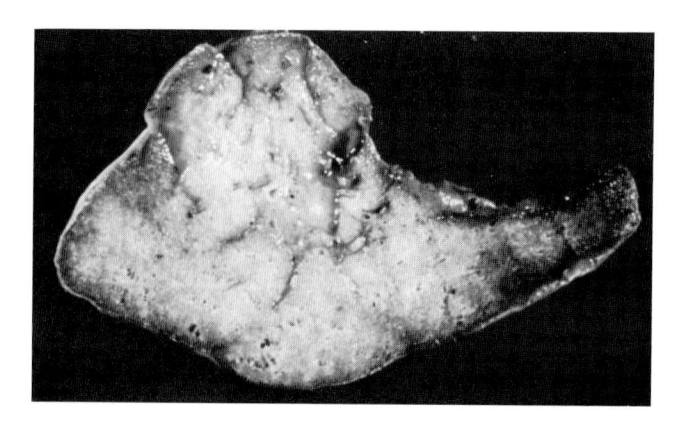

Figure 10-7. Extralobar sequestration. The cut surface shows spongy tissue but no fibrosis or inflammatory changes. The lesion was located just above the diaphragm and received its blood supply from an intercostal artery.

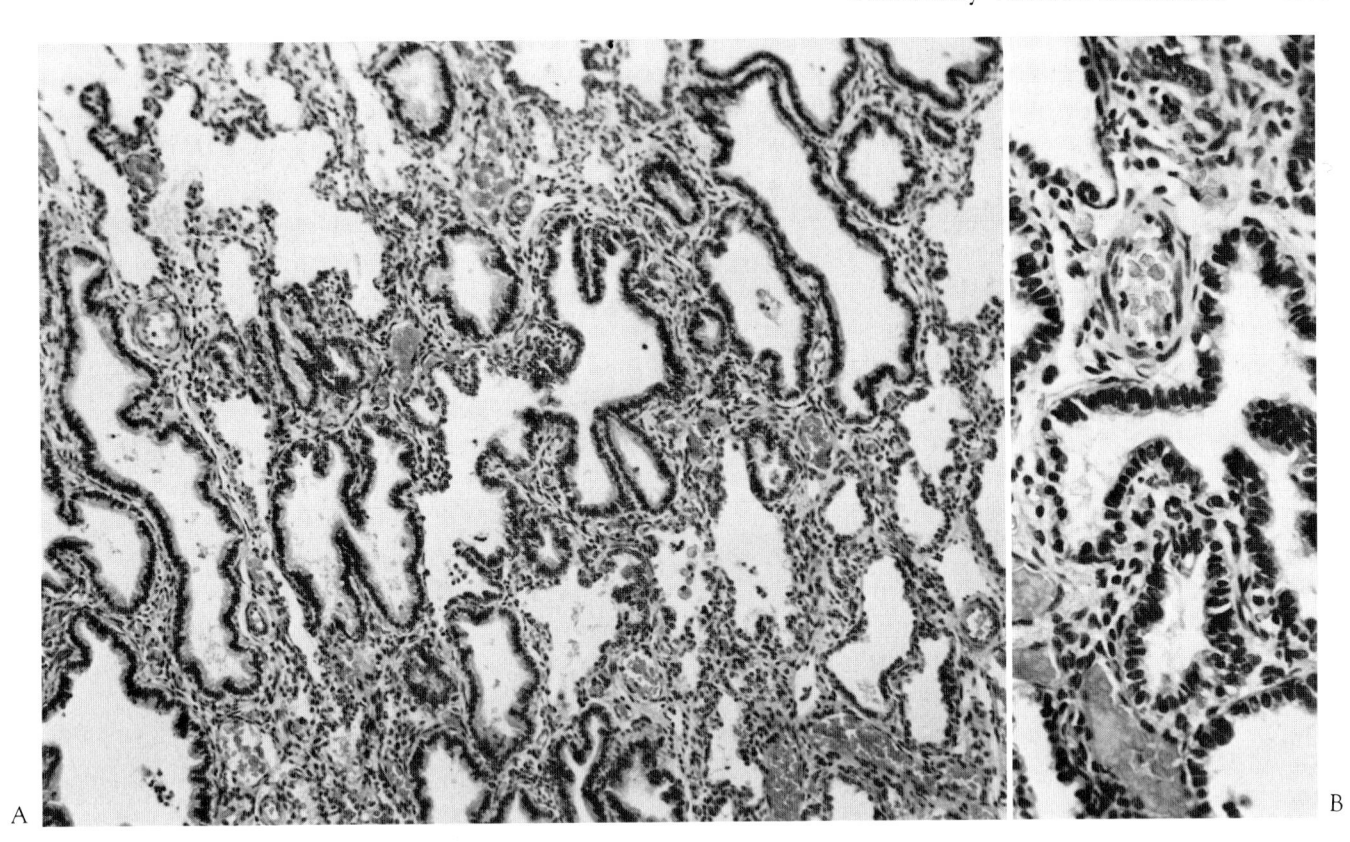

Figure 10–8. Extralobar sequestration (ELS). A. Microscopically this lesion shows branching airways and apparent alveoli lined by low cuboidal epithelium. B. The cuboidal epithelium resembles that of immature bronchioles and the overall picture of this particular lesions resembles that of some congenital adenomatoid malformations (see Fig. 10–13). Other examples of ELS may resemble normal lung parenchyma.

thin-walled, cysts in the lung parenchyma, as may the end stages of bronchopulmonary dysplasia. True congenital cysts of the lung are extremely rare and are not well documented. Weinberg and Zumwalt described a patient with multiple lung cysts and bilateral nephromegaly.[127]

Table 10–2. Practical Classification of Pulmonary Sequestration

True sequestration
   Intralobar
   Extralobar
Bronchopulmonary-foregut malformation
   Intra- or extralobar sequestration with communication to esophagus or stomach
Pseudosequestration
   Inflammatory intrabronchial mass or foreign body. Recurrent infection with engorgement of normal pulmonary ligament arteries[a]
Vascular anomalies
   Systemic arterial supply to otherwise normal lung
   "Scimitar" syndrome

[a] See Stocker and Malczak.[100]

Congenital Adenomatoid Malformation

Congenital adenomatoid malformation (CAM) is an unusual lesion combining features of hamartoma, dysplastic growth, or even neoplasia.[128–144] Congenital adenomatoid malformation is usually found in newborns or very young children, although cases have been reported in adults.[139] Antenatal diagnosis has been described.[140,142,143] The lesion usually is restricted to a single lobe and presents as an expanding mass which causes respiratory distress and even death. The patient may have any of a variety of clinical presentations and the affected lung may have a gross appearance that ranges from solid to that of a large multiloculated cyst (Figs. 10–10 to 10–12). Fetal anasarca and stillbirth are not uncommon in infants with the solid variants of adenomatoid malformation.[128,138] Maternal polyhydramnios may be present.[142] Pneumothorax is a rare presenting feature.[133] Anomalous (systemic) arterial blood supply is distinctly rare but has been reported.[138,141]

In general, the CAM lacks bronchi but does appear to communicate in many instances with the normal tracheobronchial tree, a feature that allows air-trapping

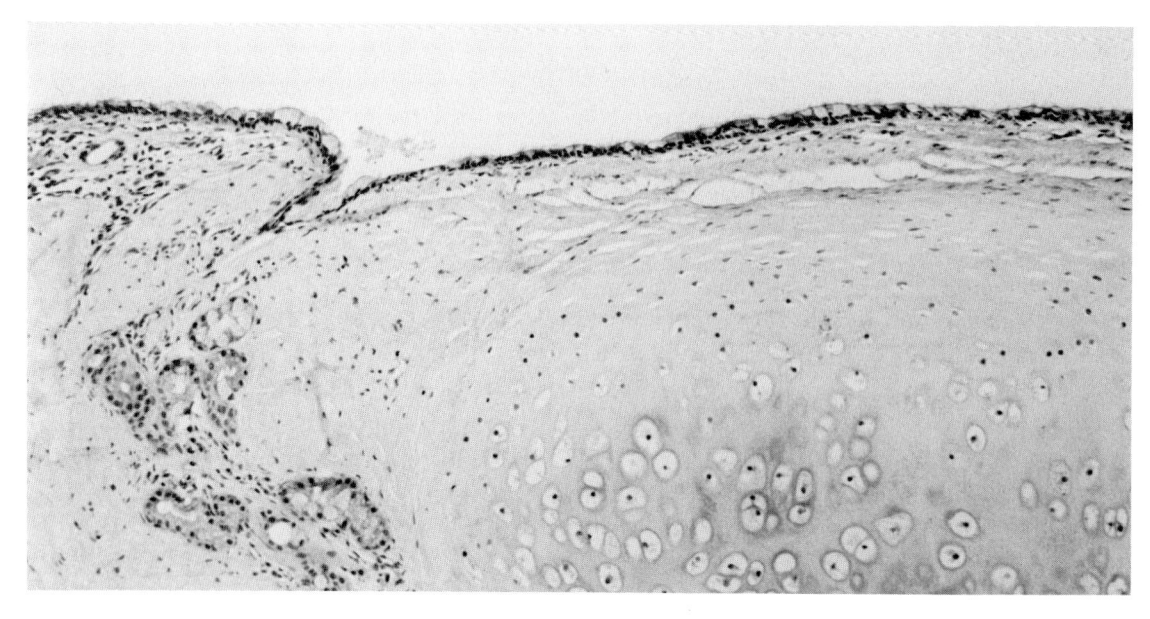

Figure 10–9. Bronchogenic cyst. Cuboidal epithelium and submucosal glands are seen next to a small fragment of cartilage.

and expansion to occur after birth. In a smaller number of cases bronchial atresia has been found in association with the lesion.[145] Whether solid or cystic, CAM is usually surrounded by a partial or complete peripheral rim of normal lung.[135]

The microscopic appearance of CAM varies with that of the gross appearance.[128,138] Solid lesions are composed of multiple curved, branched structures that resemble immature or dysplastic bronchioles (Fig. 10–13). Lesions

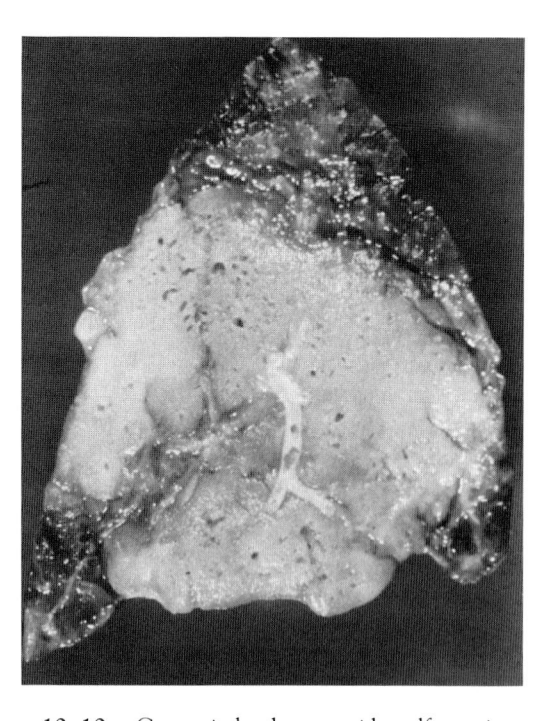

Figure 10–10. Congenital adenomatoid malformation, solid type. The lesion was surrounded by a rim of normal lung.

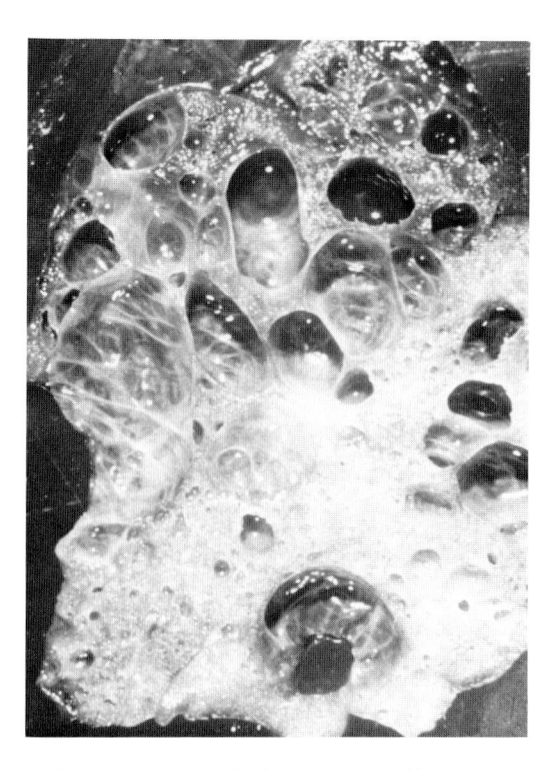

Figure 10–11. Congenital adenomatoid malformation (CAM) small cyst type. The largest cysts were 2 cm in diameter. In one series[128] this type of CAM was associated with renal and other anomalies.

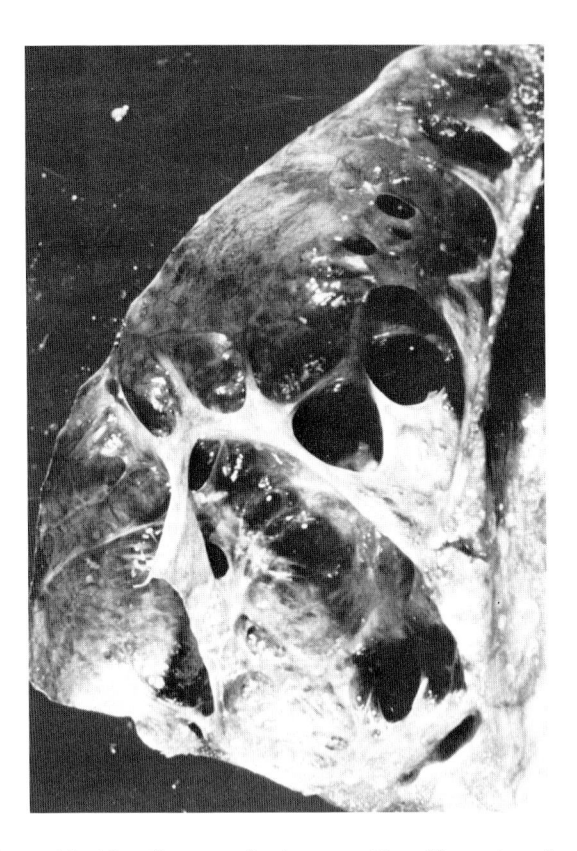

Figure 10–12. Congenital adenomatoid malformation, large-cyst type. This patient developed mediastinal shift and respiratory distress because of air-trapping and subsequent enlargement of this lesion in the right lower lobe.

with cysts of intermediate or large size contain similar areas of bronchiole-like structures interspersed between normal areas of lung. Electron-microscopic study of the cuboidal cells lining the bronchiolar areas in either solid or cystic lesions has suggested a resemblance to the cells of fetal airways.[130] All types of CAM, but especially the cystic lesions, may have prominent collections or tufts of "mucigenic cells" interspersed along thin septa (Fig. 10–14).[129] Fisher and associates reported a peculiar variant of CAM with papillary features [144] and we and others have seen a diffuse cartilaginous malformation that may be related to CAM.[137]

The pathogenesis of the adenomatoid malformation is unknown. Overgrowth of bronchioles with suppression of alveolar differentiation has been suggested as the basic defect.[128,138] The microscopic resemblance of some ELS to CAM is interesting but unexplained. A classification of CAM based on a combination of cyst size and microscopic features has been proposed and justified because of an apparent association of extrapulmonary anomalies with the small-cyst lesion.[128] Other investigators have not found a specific association of anomalies and prefer to separate only the cystic and the solid lesions.[137,138] There does appear to be an association of CAM with all forms with renal dysgenesis.[6,128]

Embryonic malignant neoplasms including pulmonary blastoma and embryonal rhabdomyosarcoma have been reported to arise in congenital lung cysts; some of these were CAM and others were bronchogenic cysts.[146,147]

Congenital Pulmonary Lymphangiectasis

Congenital distention of the pulmonary lymphatics is a rare lesion with a number of separate etiologies (Table 10–3).[148–153] The disorder is characterized by a marked dilatation of the subpleural and septal lymphatics giving the lung a cobblestone appearance (Fig. 10–15). Lymphangiectasis most frequently occurs in the clinical setting of congenital heart disease with or without pulmonary venous obstruction (total anomalous venous return, atresia of large pulmonary veins).[78,83–86] Rarely, the disorder may be primary in the lung or it may be part of a systemic disorder with chylous effusions, lymphangiectasis, and lymphangiomas in many organs and with "vanishing bones."[153] Most cases of lymphangiectasis occur in infants but localized cases with late onset in young adults have been described.[154]

Lymphangiectasis involves dilatation of normal structures (see Fig. 10–15), a feature that helps to separate it from the destructive lesions seen with pulmonary interstitial air ("emphysema").

Congenital lobar overinflation ("emphysema")[155] and segmental bronchial atresia with sublobar overinflation[155] are discussed in Chapter 21. An acquired form of lobar overinflation has been reported in infants with antecedent respiratory disease and described as related to partial bronchial obstruction by granulation tissue or polypoid areas of fibrosis.[155,156] These lesions were secondary to injury from repeated suctioning during the neonatal period. Complete bronchial stenosis with lobar collapse has been described in the same population of infants.[157]

Segmental overinflation may occur in the presence of a tracheal bronchus[158] and that condition should not be confused with segmental bronchial atresia as described in Chapter 21. Unilateral hyperlucent lung (Swyer-James or McLeod's syndrome) (see Chapter 21) is an acquired form of pulmonary overinflation related to diffuse bronchiolitis obliterans, presumably postinfectious in origin.[159] Gastroesophageal reflux may also be a cause of obliterative bronchiolitis in infants although apneic spells and asthma-like symptoms are more common.[160] A related but more advanced variant of the postinfectious disorder is associated with bronchitis obliterans and consequent lobar collapse (Fig. 10–16).[161]

Disorders of the Transition to Extrauterine Life

The lung in utero is distended by fluid secreted through the respiratory epithelium. Because of fetal respiratory movement this liquid has opportunity to mix to a limited extent with amniotic fluid and its particulates and it is not

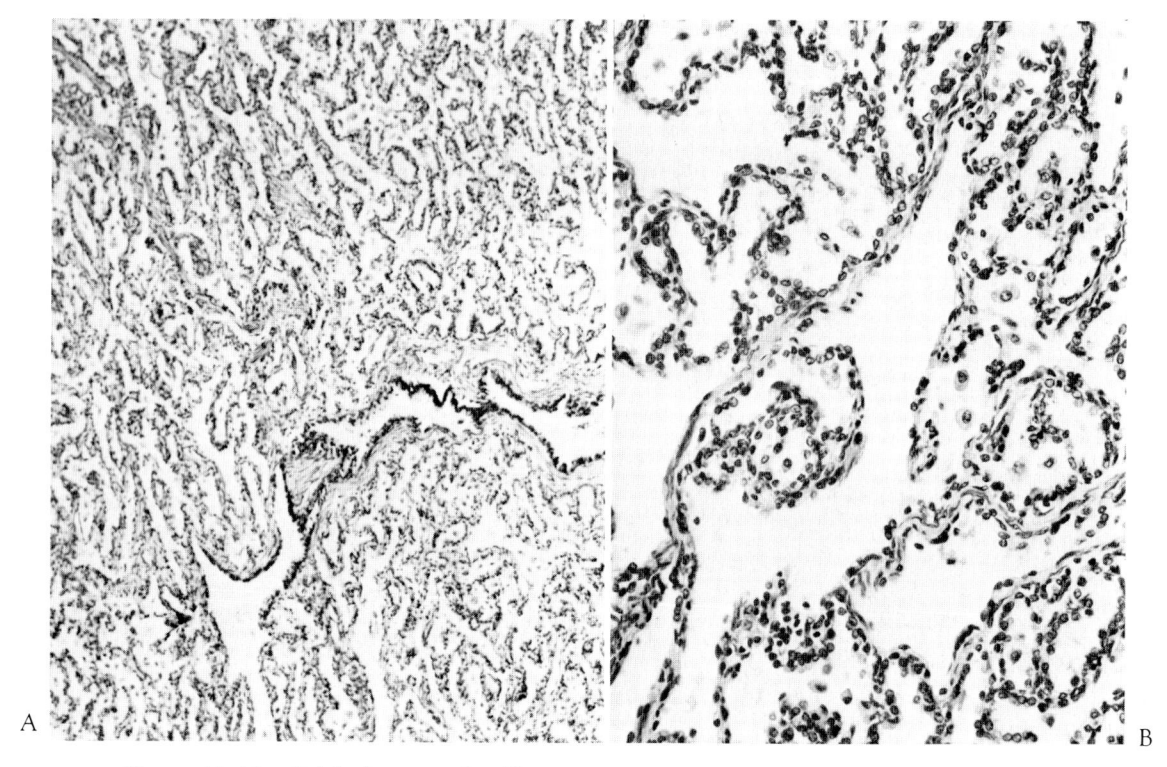

Figure 10–13. Solid adenomatoid malformation. A. Multiple irregularly curved and branching spaces are seen in the mass. B. At higher magnification cuboidal epithelium can be seen lining the adjacent lung parenchyma.

uncommon to find fetal squames in the airspaces of an infant that is either stillborn or dies soon after birth.

The transition from intrauterine life to the air-breathing state requires removal of lung liquid, inflation of the lung with air, and development of sufficient lung stability to provide a pulmonary residual volume.[4,162–167] Surface tension forces in the lung account for a majority of the collapsing pressure and lung stability therefore depends to a great extent on the secretion of "surfactant" into the alveolar space and its subsequent coating of alveolar and small airway walls as well. This surface active material is composed of a mixture of active ingredients including phosphatidylcholine and phosphatidylglycerol.[162–167] A protein moiety is present as well. The presence of surfactant in alveoli of the newborn depends on biochemical maturity of enzyme systems involved in phospholipid synthesis and on the release of adequate amounts of this material from the alveolar type II cells in which surfactant components are synthesized. Environmental and hormonal factors that accelerate or impede surfactant production are reviewed elsewhere but include perinatal stress and steroid production.[4,165–167] Insulin appears to impede functional maturation of type II cells, explaining in part the susceptibility of infants of diabetic mothers to respiratory distress syndrome (RDS).[4,165–167] Since fetal lung liquid is in communication with the amniotic fluid the presence of surface active material in the amniotic fluid can be detected and used in a variety of methods as an index of the biochemical readiness of the fetal lung for extrauterine life.[166] Functional immaturity of the newborn lung may lead to a variety of complications, many iatrogenic, which result in further respiratory impairment. These disorders, hyaline membrane disease (HMD), bronchopulmonary dysplasia (BPD), and pulmonary interstitial air ("emphysema") constitute the major disorders of the "transition" period. Aspiration of meconium, pulmonary hemorrhage, and perinatal pneumonia are other life-threatening disorders seen in neonates. Disorders of lung structure such as hypoplasia and functional disorders such as persistent unexplained pulmonary hypertension in the newborn ("persistent fetal circulation") constitute the other major disorders of the immediate neonatal period.

Transient tachypnea of the newborn ("neonatal wet lung") is a mild disorder caused by delayed clearance of fetal lung liquid.[4] The infants are mildely tachypneic and have an alveolar filling pattern on chest radiographs. The disorder usually remits in 24 to 48 hours and no pathologic description exists. Retention of lung liquid within cysts or other congenital lesions may, however produce unusual and confusing radiographic pictures until the fluid is resolved.

Hyaline membrane disease (idiopathic RDS) is a disorder related to deficiency of pulmonary surfactant.[4,166,167] The most usual cause of the deficit is biochemical immaturity of the lung but it is clearly possible for multiple types of insult to damage the delicate enzyme systems involved in surfactant produc-

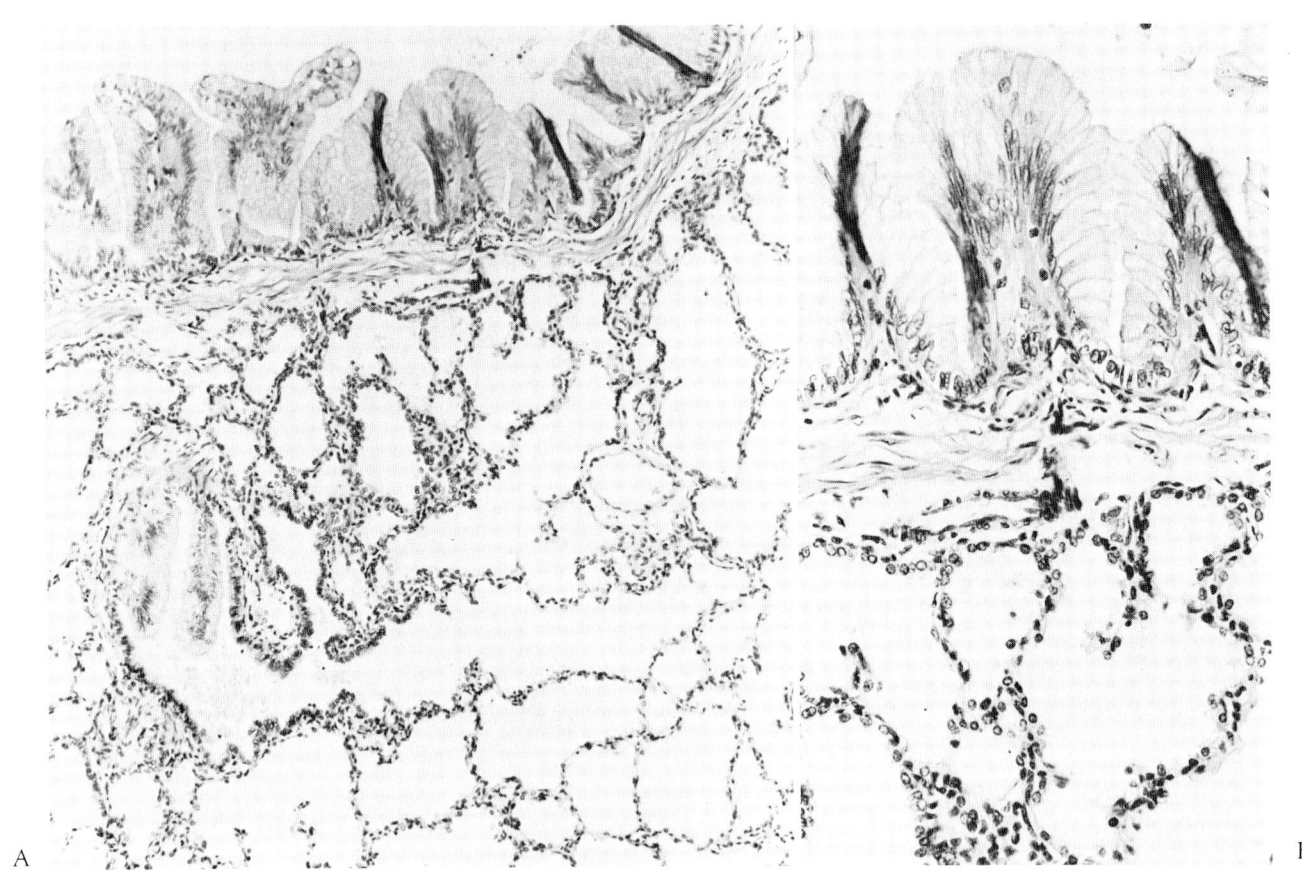

Figure 10–14. Adenomatoid malformation, large-cyst type. A. Fronds and papillae of mucinous cells line airways and cyst walls. B. The "mucigenic" cells have clear cytoplasm and basal nuclei.

tion. The end result is high alveolar surface forces with production of an injury essentially comparable to diffuse alveolar damage. Hyaline membrane disease occurs in a rather specific population of infants: premature white males, appropriate in size for their gestation age. Other predisposing factors include maternal diabetes, twins, and birth by Ceasarean section without a trial of labor.[4]

Female and nonwhite infants appear to be relatively protected as are infants with a variety of prenatal stresses including amniotic fluid infection and growth retardation.[4] Hyaline membrane disease has been described in term infants but any deviation from occurrence in the usual population should be the cause for intense scrutiny before a diagnosis of HMD is made.

Clinically, the affected infant develops respiratory distress at or soon after birth. The radiograph shows ground glass opacification of the lung fields and "air bronchograms" are seen.[4,7,8,166,167] On gross examination the lungs have a solid or liver-like consistency. Microscopically the most important feature is uniform alveolar collapse.[168,171] The distal airways are dilated and lined by the characteristic eosinophilic membranes (Fig. 10–17). The septal lymphatics are often prominently dilated and focal hemorrhages and alveolar edema fluid may be seen. These features correlate with the radiographic appearance of the chest film in HMD and to physiologic features of ventilation-perfusion inequity and decreased pulmonary compliance. The histologic features may be altered by the fixative employed (mercury- or chromate-based solutions show the edema fluid more prominently),[171] the time between death and autopsy,[168] and the method of fixation of the lung. Fixative perfusion of the lung through the airways removes the air-liquid interface and obscures the morphologic effect of abnormally high surface tension on the lung. Under most circumstances it is best to perfuse one lung with fixative through the bronchial tree and to at least sample the other lung without prior perfusion. In this way both the expansion

Table 10–3. Classification of Pulmonary Lymphangiectasis

Cardiac
   Mechanical or functional obstruction of large pulmonary veins
   Noonan's syndrome, asplenia, other defects without venous obstruction
Generalized
   Multiple lymphangiomas, chylous effusions, "vanishing bones"
Primary
   Isolated to the lung. No cardiac or venous anomalies.

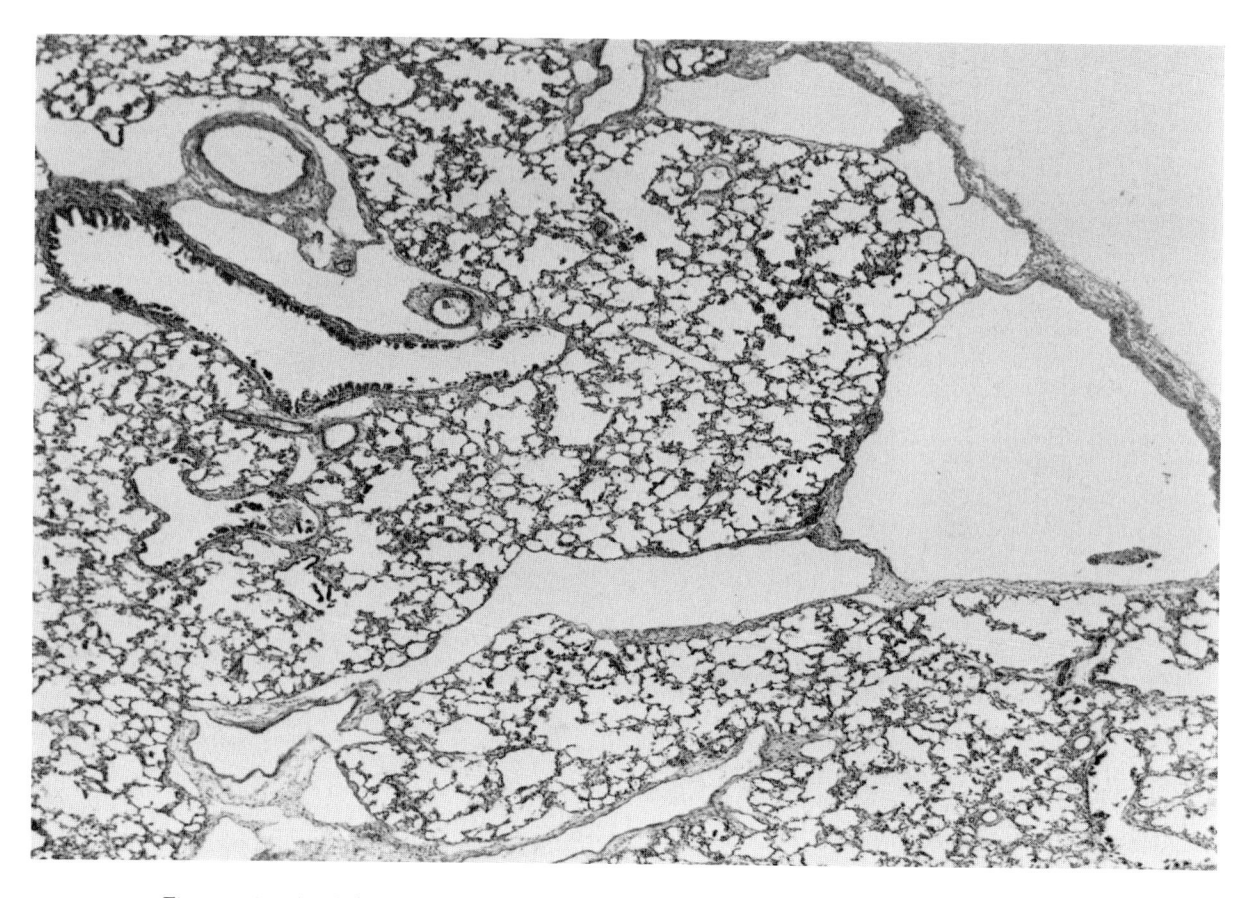

Figure 10–15. Pulmonary lymphangiectasis. Dilated lymphatic channels are seen beneath the pleura (right), along septa, and around bronchovascular bundles.

pattern and the interstitium of the lung can be examined. Hyaline membranes per se are not diagnostic of primary surfactant deficiency and the histologic patterns seen in HMD can be mimicked by infection. In most other entities, however, the alveolar collapse pattern is not as striking nor as diffuse as that seen in HMD.

Morphologic variations of HMD include a peculiar rounded pattern of dilated airways alternating with collapsed alveoli and described by Gruenwald as "exaggerated atelectasis"[172]; yellow-staining of the hyaline membranes, apparently by bilirubin[173]; and sloughing of bronchial or alveolar epithelium to form a pseudoglandular pattern (Fig. 10–18). The diagnosis of HMD in very small infants may be difficult histologically because the infants expire before the membranes form or because the immature lung may not be able to collapse in the characteristic pattern. Since most infants with HMD who die have been treated with oxygen, the histologic features of resolving HMD are not clearly separable from BPD (see below) but it appears that an influx of macrophages, repair of alveolar walls, and proliferation of type II lining cells are major features.[174] The long-term prognosis of survivors of HMD is difficult to separate from that of premature birth per se and from BPD. Prior to the advent of mechanical ventilation most affected infants either died or recovered by 72 hours after birth.[4]

Hyaline membrane disease (surfactant deficiency) in the neonate is associated with a variety of complications, often iatrongenic but closely related to therapeutic measures necessary to preserve life. Patent ductus arteriosus, BPD, and pulmonary interstitial air are the most common problems.

Persistent patency of the ductus arteriosus (PDA) as a complication of HMD has assumed an increasing role as a complication that parallels the increased survival of small neonates with HMD.[175–182] An overall 21 percent incidence of PDA in of all newborns weighing less than 2500 g was reported from one institution. Several studies have suggested that histologic examination can identify a specific feature, the subendothelial elastic lamina, associated with permanent patency.[175]

Clinical and physiologic symptoms related to the open ductus may vary from infants with minor problems to those with an acute, severe left to right shunt. A third group of patients with predominant respiratory symptoms such as BPD (see below) have patent ductus as part of their clinical and pathologic picture. The exact role that the ductus plays in the production of pulmonary disease in neonates is not clear although Jacob and associates have produced evidence that HMD in low-

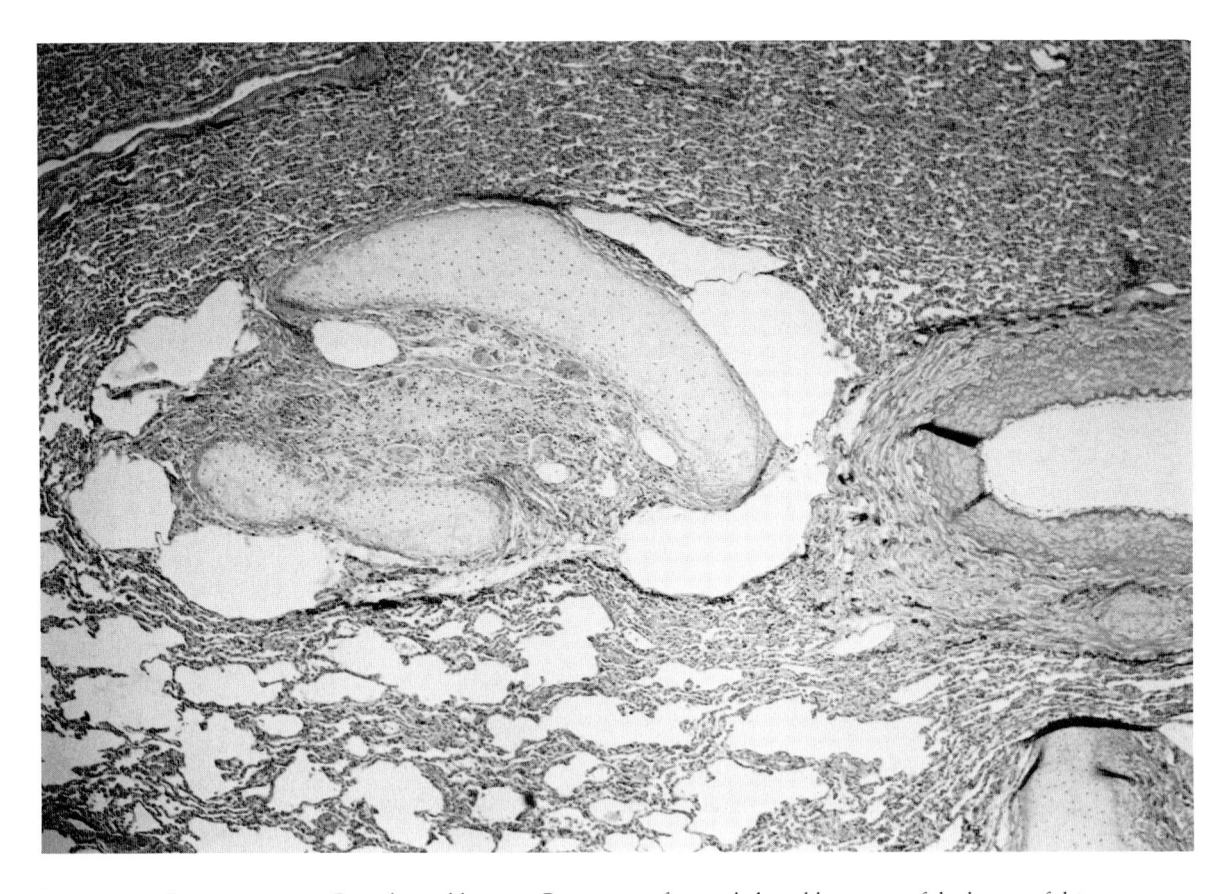

Figure 10–16. Bronchitis obliterans. Recurrent infection led to obliteration of the lumen of this cartilaginous airway. In contrast to the picture in bronchiolitis obliterans, the chest radiograph showed lobar collapse.

weight newborns may be more a manifestation of ductal patency than of surfactant deficiency.[179]

Factors promoting patency of the ductus are multiple and include hypoxia, prostaglandins of the E type, and perhaps the naturally deficient musculature of the distal fetal pulmonary arteries.[178] In one study treatment with the diuretic furosemide was associated with ductal patency.[178] Both surgical and phamacologic closure of the ductus have been effective.[176,178]

Just as antenatal stress appears to reduce the incidence of HMD, there is morphologic evidence that "maturation" and accelerated closure of the ductus may occur in preterm infants exposed to chronic intrauterine stress.[177] Other reported complications involving the ductus include necrosis[181] and aneurysm formation.[182]

Bronchopulmonary dysplasia is a complex, multistage, structural, and physiologic alteration of the lungs which occurs as a prolonged response to acute injury in the neonatal period.[170,183–201] The acute insult was originally considered to be mechanical ventilation and high concentration of inspired oxygen in infants treated for HMD. Further studies have expanded the syndrome and it has been suggested that oxygen alone and that mechanical ventilation without high oxygen concentration can produce BPD.[186,187] Furthermore, it appears that BPD can occur as a response to lung injury other than that associated with HMD.[186,187]

The typical infant with BPD is premature, has developed HMD, and has required prolonged ventilatory support.[4,186,187] The incidence of BPD varies with the birth weight of the population studied, ranging from 10 percent in infants over 2500 g to 40 percent or even higher as birth weight declines toward 1000 g.[4,186,187] The original histologic description of the evolution of BPD by Rosan and co-workers is pertinent[4,170] but has been refined somewhat in the classification proposed by Anderson and Engel[184] (Table 10–4). All of the stages and histologic features are based on infants studied at autopsy so that it is difficult if not impossible to know whether one is observing a orderly progression of disease or whether different tissue responses of individual patients or different degrees of injury account for the histologic differences seen in patients dying early or late in the course of BPD. Furthermore, the relevance of lesions seen at autopsy to possible lung disease in survivors is not yet known. Diffuse alveolar damage and possibly reversible bronchiolar obstruction characterize the early phase of disease, while interstitial fibrosis is the predominant and probably irreversible feature of late-stage disease.[170,184,185] The histologic changes seen in infants dying early in the course of BPD (1 to 2 weeks) are those

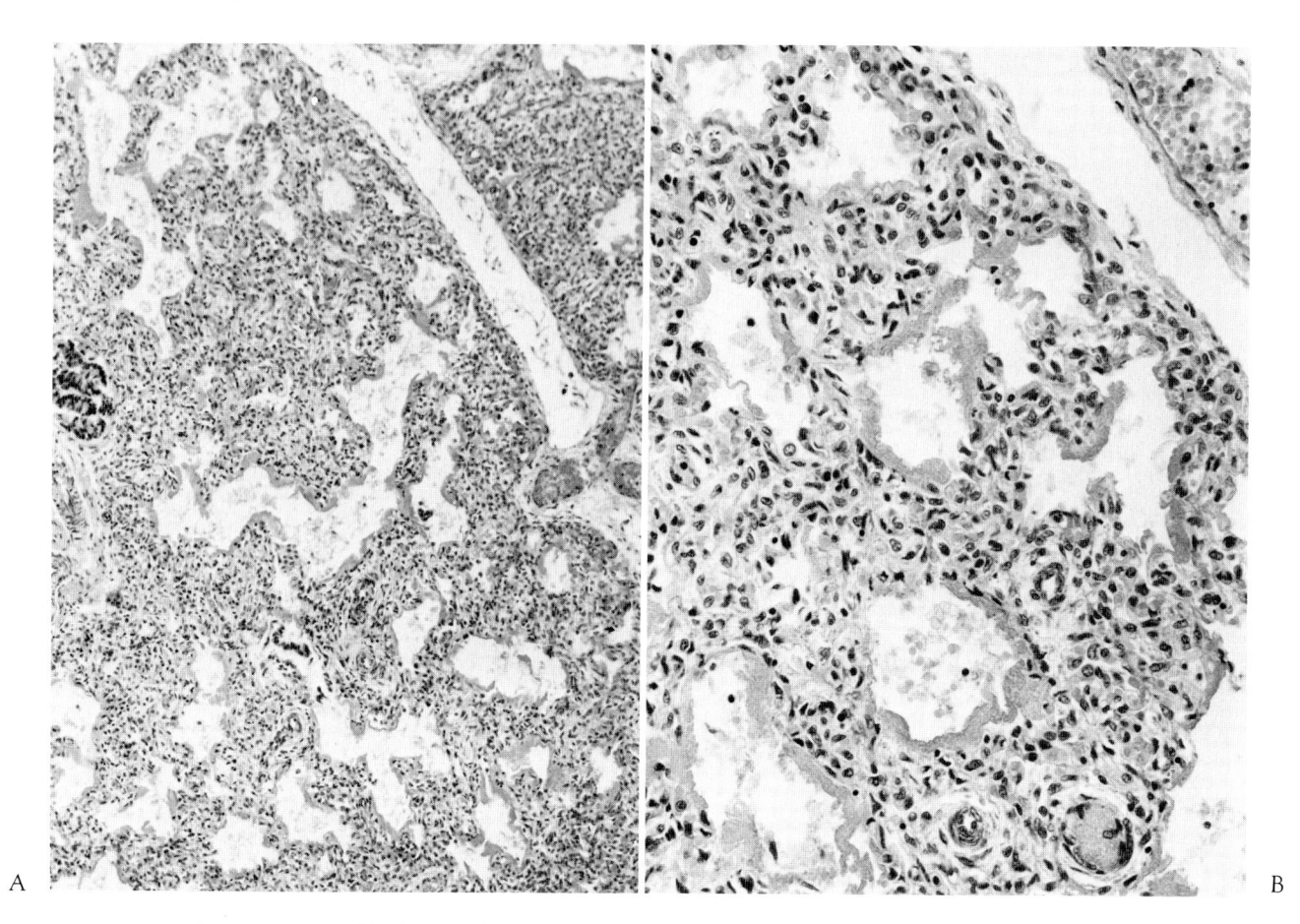

Figure 10–17. Hyaline membrane disease. A. Alveoli are collapsed and the dilated spaces seen here are alveolar ducts and small bronchioles. Note the dilated septal lymphatic in the upper right. B. Hyaline membranes line small airways.

of HMD disease on which has been engrafted bronchiolar necrosis and obliterative, reparative bronchiolitis (Fig. 10–19). In some cases fibrous obliteration of the bronchiolar lumen may lead to erroneous interpretation of the tubular structure as an artery. Elastic tissue stains showing the single submucosal fenestrated elastic lamina of the airway will resolve the question. Cystic dilatation of alveolar ducts and bronchioles may be prominent feature.[184] The ductus arteriosus is often patent at this stage.

Infants dying from 2 to 4 weeks after the onset of BPD show a subacute fibroproliferative stage of the disease.[183–185] Interstitial and perialveolar duct fibrosis supervenes (Fig. 10–20). Reactive alveolar type II pneumocytes line the restructured airspaces and there is proliferation of interstitial capillaries (Fig. 10–21). Small round cells in the alveolar wall interstitium may appear to be inflammatory cells but can often be identified as smooth muscle or myofibroblasts by electron-microscopy. The prominent restructuring of distal lung parenchyma is clearly analogous to the honeycombing and interstitial fibrosis that occur in the adult lung as a response to diffuse alveolar damage.

Table 10–4. Bronchopulmonary Dysplasia: Evolution[a]

Stage	Pathologic Features
Exudative, early reparative	Hyaline membranes, bronchial necrosis
	Bronchiolitis obliterans, bronchiolectasis
	Early septal fibrosis
Subacute, fibroproliferative	Bronchiolitis obliterans, bronchiolectasis
	Rare residual hyaline membranes
	Type II cell hyperplasia/regeneration
	Perialveolar duct fibrosis
	Increasing interstitial fibrosis, smooth muscle proliferation
	Overexpanded/collapsed acini
Chronic, fibroproliferative	Interstitial fibrosis, smooth muscle proliferation
	Honeycomb lung
	Vascular wall thickening
	No bronchiolitis obliterans or bronchiolectasis

[a] Based on the results of Anderson and Engel.[184]

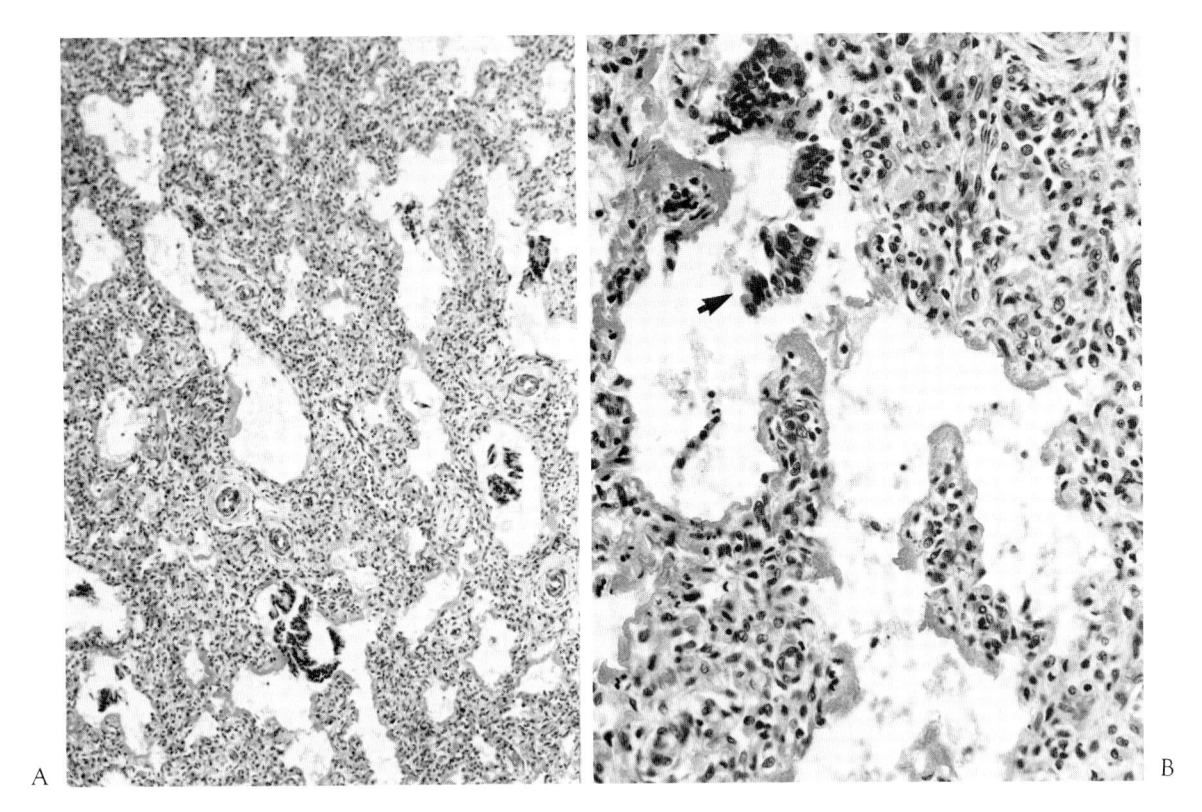

Figure 10–18. Hyaline membrane disease. A. The characteristic collapse pattern of alveoli is present. Small clusters of bronchial epithelium have been artifactually dislodged from the wall of the airway and should not be interpreted as a part of a cystic malformation. B. At higher power the clusters (arrow) are identifiable as bronchial epithelium.

The chronic fibroproliferative stage of BPD is seen in infants dying several to many months after the onset of disease.[184] Hyaline membranes are no longer seen. Interstitial fibrosis is prominent and smooth muscle hyperplasia may be seen in the septal wall. Alternating areas of overexpanded and collapsed airspaces are present. The origin of this phenomenon is not clear. Air-trapping, true destructive emphysema, and honeycomb change may all play a role.[184,186,187] It is logical to suggest that loss of small airways may contribute to overexpansion, but in one morphometric study of a single case this hypothesis could not be confirmed.[189] In contrast to the early stages of BPD, bronchiolitis obliterans is no longer seen, although squamous metaplasia may be found in the bronchial epithelium. Morphologic evidence of pulmonary hypertension is often present (medial hyperplasia and intimal thickening of small arteries) and cor pulmonale may supervene.

There is, in general, only broad radiographic correlation with the pathologic stage[190-192] and several studies have suggested a role for cytologic evaluation of lung washings in the detection of early stages of BPD.[193] Early lung opacity is replaced by hyperinflation and a variety of radiographic "bubbles" in the lung parenchyma.[191] In all stages of BPD, pulmonary interstitial air (see below) and pneumothorax and its complications may be an added clinical and pathologic feature. Lobar overinflation or collapse may occur in relation to bronchial trauma with resultant granulation tissue and fibrosis causing either partial or complete obstruction.

Autopsy studies and the availability of open lung biopsy material has begun to show what is probably a variant or modified pattern of BPD in infants dying 3 or more months after birth.[194-196] The patients are small premature infants who may have had either acute respiratory distress or the insidious onset of respiratory insufficiency. The chest radiograph shows both overexpanded and collapsed areas in the lung and the infants may have a prominent component of carbon dioxide retention. Microscopically there are restructured, coalescent airspaces, areas of overexpanded lung, and areas of collapse (Figs. 10–22, 10–23). Fibrosis in the interstitium may be minimal. It is possible that this variant pattern may be an endstage of BPD analogous to honeycomb lung in the lung with adult respiratory distress syndrome (ARDS) but the clinical course suggests that the evolution may be slower and less fibroblastic than the acute disease originally described and is perhaps more related to altered maturation and development of the premature infants lung than to damage

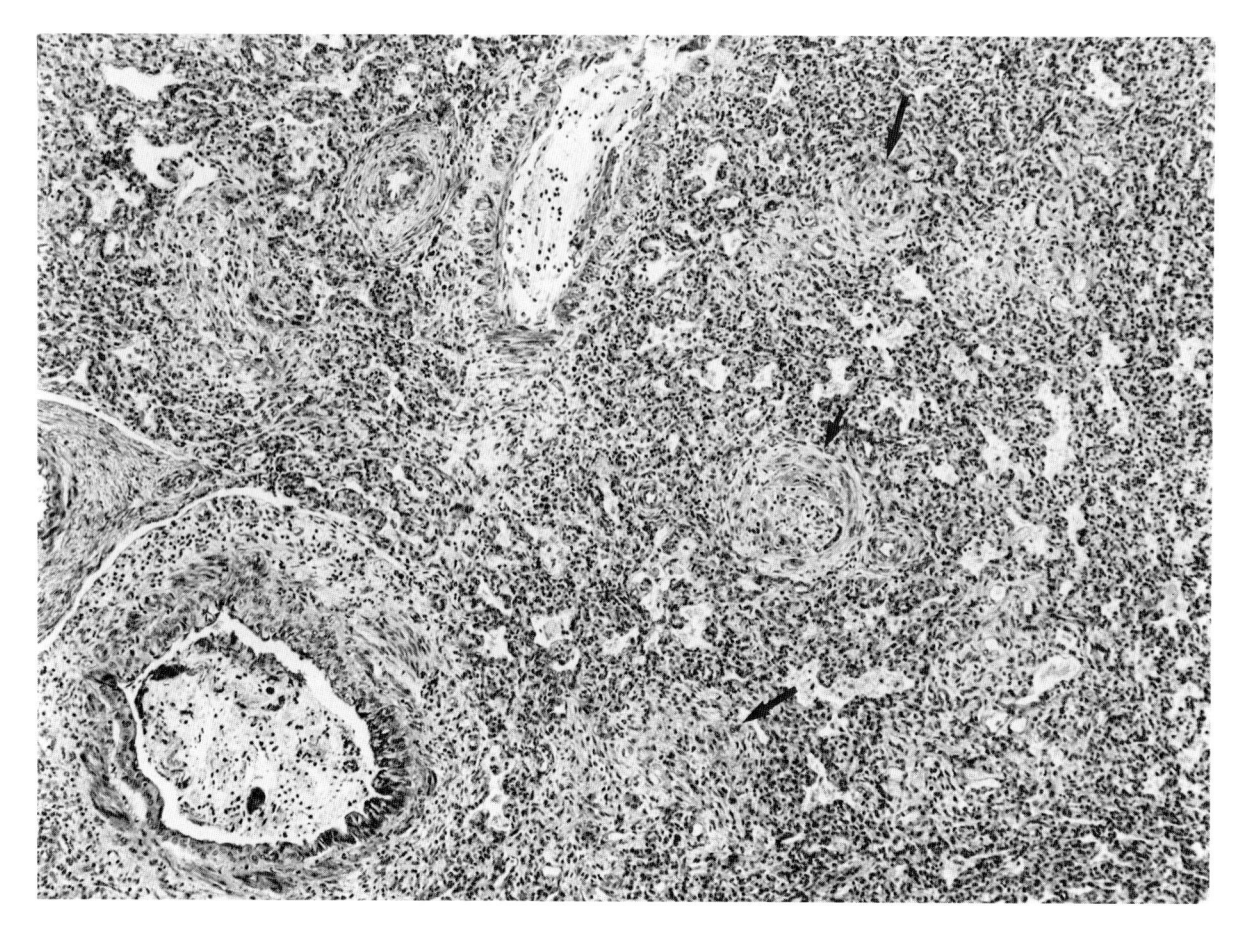

Figure 10–19. Bronchopulmonary dysplasia. Acute phase with necrotizing bronchiolitis and reparative bronchiolitis obliterans (arrows). Loss of bronchial epithelium may cause bronchioles (top center) to be interpreted as arteries.

oxygen and barotrauma. Histologic comparison and the slow clinical evolution of disease suggest that this variant pattern is the same entity as that described as the Wilson-Mikity syndrome.[195]

The etiology of BPD is complex and unclear. Oxygen toxicity and barotrauma are obvious suspects but antioxidant deficiency, increased pulmonary epithelial permeability, and blood flow through a patent ductus have been implicated as well.[186,187] Prematurity per se, with abnormal development of alveoli and small airways, may be a factor in the production of chronic effects of BPD.[196] Furthermore, infants with a family history of asthma seem to have an increased susceptibility to BPD, a phenomenon suggesting a genetically determined decreased tolerance to lung damage.[186,187] There is experimental evidence that oxygen toxicity may be more responsible for bronchiolar necrosis than for fibrosis and restructuring of the distal lung parenchyma.[197]

Pathophysiologic alterations in BPD include hypoxia, carbon dioxide retention, decreased lung compliance, airflow obstruction, and ventilation-perfusion inequity in variable combination depending on the pathologic stage of disease.[186,187]

Many complications of BPD (Table 10–5) occur in relation to therapy but are not directly related to the lower respiratory trace.[186,187,198–201] Tracheal scarring and stenosis may result from intubation. Spells of apnea and of unexplained cyanosis are not uncommon. Feeding difficulties including aspiration, gastroesophageal reflux, and rumination occur frequently. Fat emboli may result from intravenous hyperalimentation.[198] Growth failure is common and osteopenia with multiple fractures may also occur. Long-term complications of BPD include[198–201] ramifications of psychosocial family trauma, recurrent respiratory problems with a distinct risk of respiratory failure during viral infection, and an increased risk for the sudden infant death syndrome.[200] Central nervous system deficits may be demonstrable. Studies on 5- or 10-year survivors of BPD are not complete, but there is good evidence for small airway dysfunction and bronchial hyperreactivity[201] and there is some suggestion that children with BPD may be at risk for chronic airflow obstruction in adult life.[186,187]

Pulmonary interstitial air (PIE; persistent interstitial pulmonary interstitial emphysema, PIPE) and resultant pneumothorax may occur spontaneously in neonates, but are usually a complication of HMD, BPD, or meconium aspiration in that population.[202–212] Infants with pulmo-

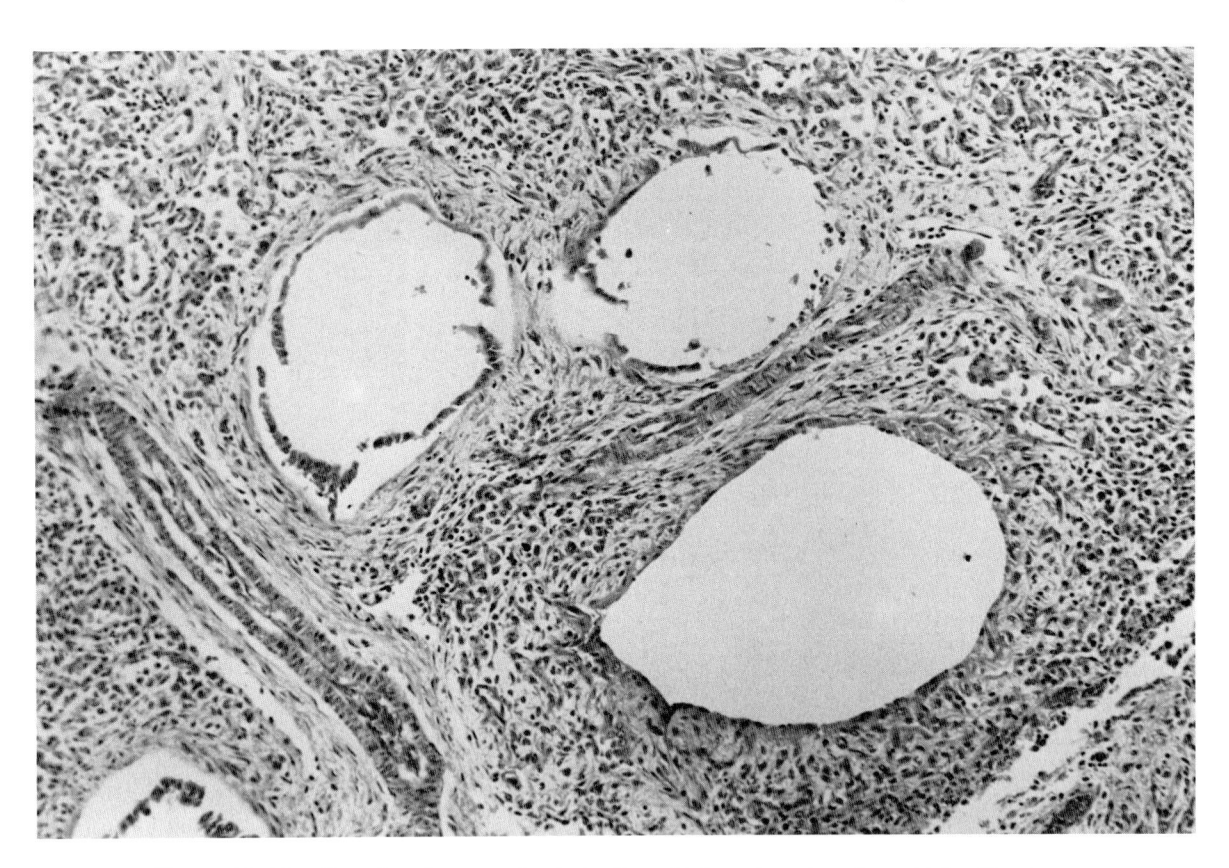

Figure 10–20. Bronchopulmonary dysplasia. Bronchiolectasis and peribronchiolar fibrosis are characteristic features of the subacute stage of disease.

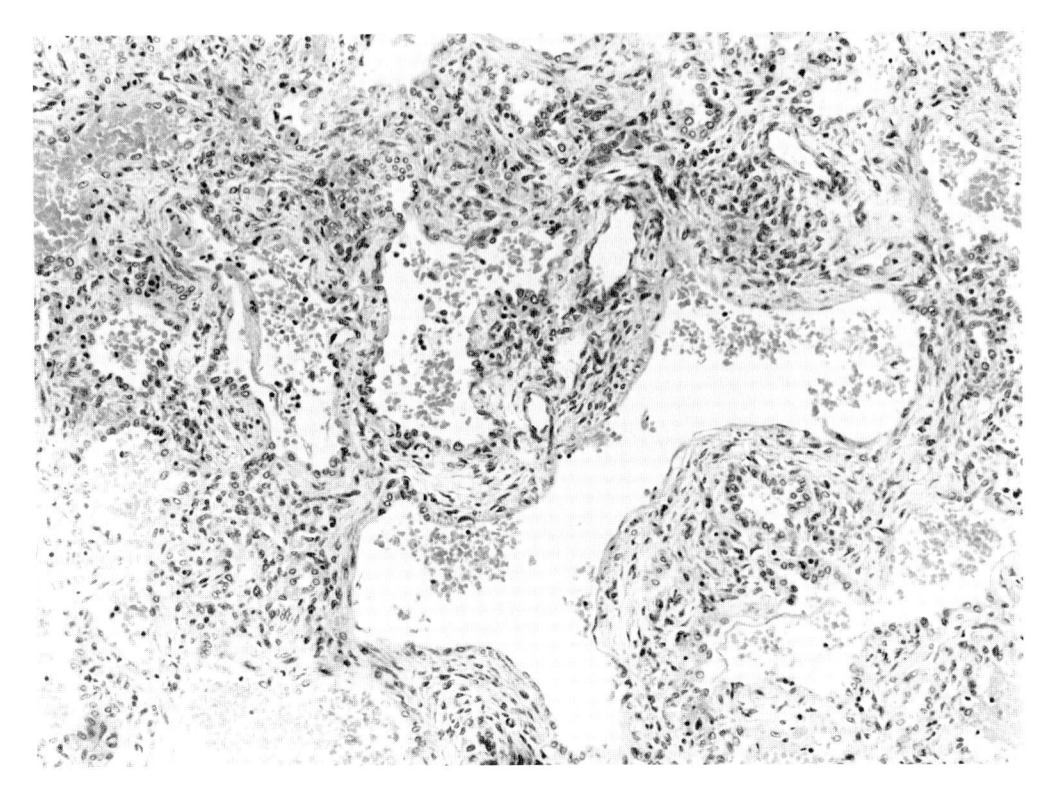

Figure 10–21. Bronchopulmonary dysplasia. Interstitial fibrosis and restructuring of the lung architecture have occurred. A few interstitial inflammatory cells are present but most of the small round cells in the interstitium are smooth muscle or myofibroblasts.

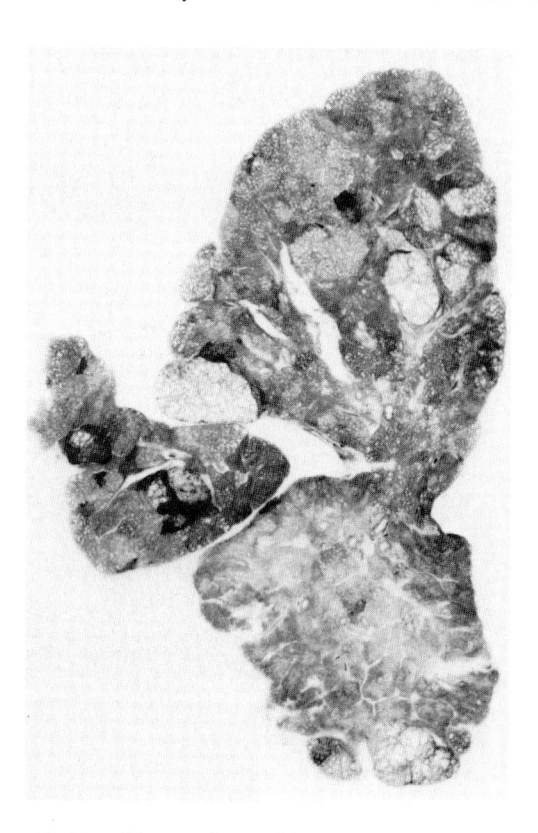

Figure 10–22. Variant form of bronchopulmonary dysplasia. This Gough paper section shows the alternating areas of collapsed and overinflated lung. Courtesy of Drs. Charles Carrington and Averill Liebow.

nary hypoplasia are also at risk for PIE. Dissection of air into the connective tissue of bronchovascular bundles or interlobular septa may be followed by pneumothorax, pneumomediastinum, or pneumopericardium.[209]

In rare instances pneumoperitoneum may occur but that complication is much more likely to be a consequence of perforation of the stomach or of neonatal necrotizing enterocolitis. The radiographic appearance of PIE is that of course, linear cysts or bubbles that may coalesce to form large subpleural air collections ("pseudocysts").[212]

Several forms of persistent (present for several days) PIE are seen clinically.[203] The most common is that of diffuse, multilobar involvement, but localized, unilobar, or at least exaggerated involvement of a single lobe may also occur.[210,211] In the latter instance the major physiologic effect is that of an expanding mass lesion in the thorax. Surgical therapy may be necessary. "Air block" is a rare phenomenon in which the hilar vascular structures are occluded by the dissecting air.[207]

The pathogenesis of these pulmonary air leak syndromes in the neonate is that of alveolar rupture with escape of air into the interstitium.[207,209] In contrast to older children and adults, neonatal air leak is rather commonly associated with dissection of air into the septal lymphatics and even veins. Endolymphatic air may then produce systemic emboli in the brain and other organs.[208]

The characteristic gross pathologic feature of diffuse pulmonary interstitial air is the presence of linear sausage-shaped spaces following septa or airways (Fig. 10–24). Subpleural blebs may also be seen. In lobar PIE the spaces may be so large and round as to suggest a congenital "cystic" anomaly of the lung (Fig. 10–25). Microscopically the air-filled spaces are variable in size and shape, and are often associated with destruction of adjacent lung parenchyma (Fig. 10–26). In persistent PIE a prominent giant-cell foreign body reaction may be seen lining the wall of whatever space the air has invaded (Fig. 10–27).

The differential diagnosis of PIE includes pulmonary lymphangiectasis as the most common cause of confusion. Cystic forms of adenomatoid malformation may be suggested when interstitial air is localized. Postinfarction subpleural cysts are discussed on p. 138.

Pulmonary Hemorrhage

Focal intraalveolar or interstitial hemorrhage is a frequent histologic finding in the lungs of infants with hyaline membrane disease, BPD, or other neonatal lung disorders.[213] Massive bleeding into airways and, to some extent, the interstitium is a distinct clinical and pathologic entity.[213–217] The affected infants are predominantly male, premature, small for gestational age infants who have suffered birth asphyxia or some other perinatal stress.[217] Both still and live-born infants manifest the lesion. Clinically the affected infant collapses suddenly, usually in the first week of life, with blood-stained fluid pouring from the trachea and nose.

Microscopically these are confluent areas of hemorrhage with blood filling alveoli and dissecting into the interstitium as well.[213,215] The presence of other pathologic lesions such as HMD or BPD does not exlude the diagnosis of massive pulmonary hemorrhage.

The etiology of this disorder, other than a relationship to perinatal stress and asphyxia, is unkown. Multiple theories have been proposed, including a reaction to cold, to increased spinal fluid pressure, or to increased pulmonary blood flow and pressure. Capillary fragility and coagulation abnormalities have been suggested as well.[214–216]

Meconium Aspiration

A wide variety of types of intrauterine perinatal stress cause the infant to pass meconium into the amniotic fluid and, concomitantly, to make a deep respiratory movement.[218–222] Symptomatic aspiration of meconium is usually seen at delivery in term infants of appropriate gestational size. Tenacious, mucoid, green meconium may coat the infant and placenta and can be seen in the larynx and trachea as well. Radiographically, patchy areas of infiltrate are seen and there may be pulmonary interstitial air and pneumothorax—features related to air-trapping distal behind partially obstructed air-

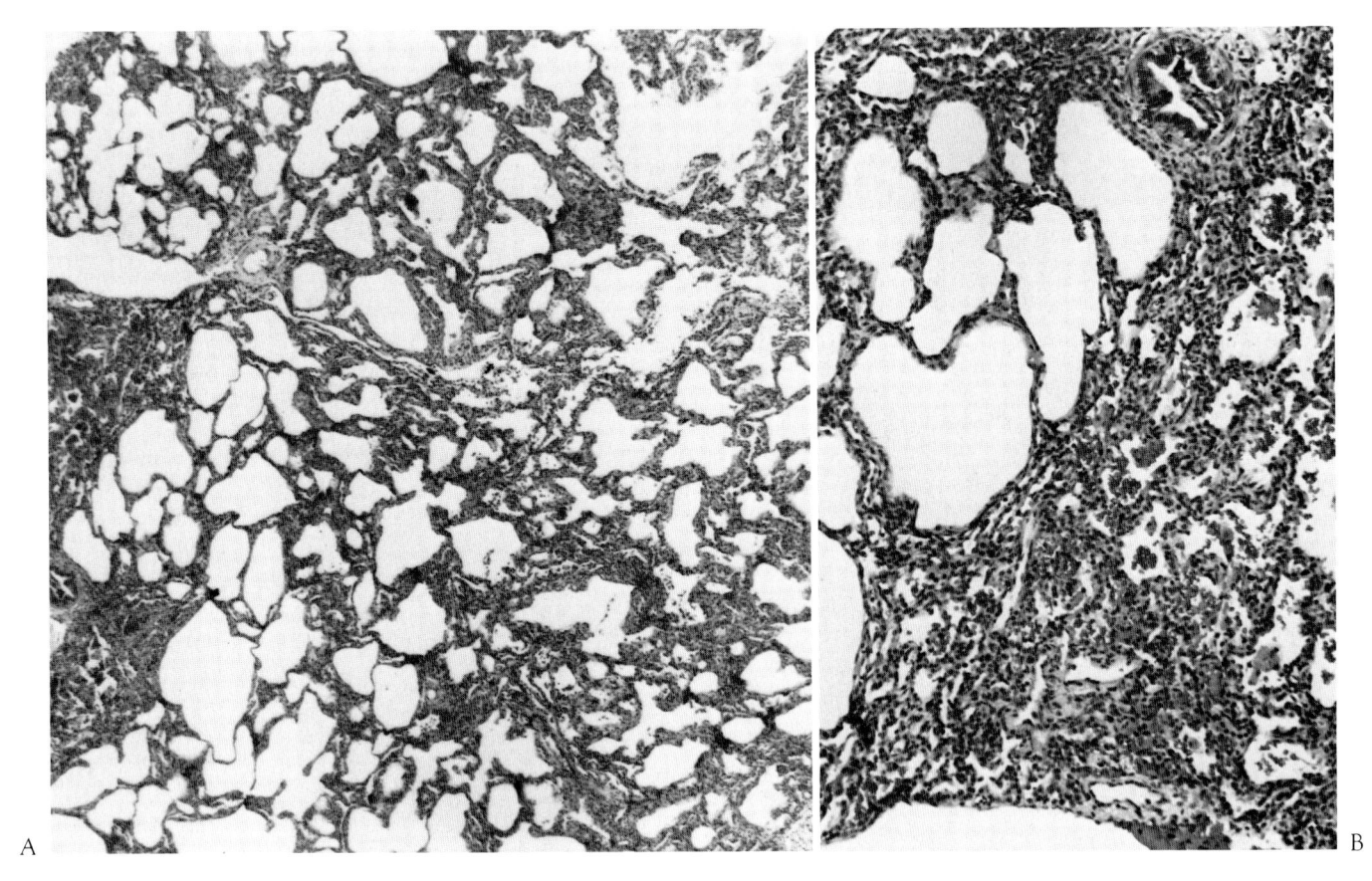

Figure 10–23. Variant bronchopulmonary dysplasia. A. Alternating areas of collapse and of overexpansion. B. Interstitial fibrosis is not a prominent feature. The overexpanded areas probably represent a mixture of overinflation and destructive emphysema.

ways.[8,219] The mortality of severe meconium aspiration is still high.[218] At autopsy in infants dying soon after aspiration, the lungs often have a silvery-green discoloration and sticky meconium can be seen in the airways as well. Microscopically airways are obstructed not only by masses of fetal squamous cells but also by aggregated mucus (Fig. 10–28). Bacterial infection and chemical pneumonitis associated with the components of meconium may supervene and in infants dying later in the course, mucus and even squames may not be obvious. At least one subset of infants with the meconium aspiration syndrome has morphologic evidence of pulmonary hypertension manifested microscopically by abnormally muscularized small pulmonary arteries.[222] As noted above, pulmonary interstitial air may be seen as well.

The presence of isolated foci of fetal squames in the alveoli is not unusual in any infant dying in the perinatal period and squames alone do not prove that meconium aspiration has occurred. Aspiration of vernix caseosa has been reported as a rare entity that may produce a similar clinical but not microscopic picture.[223]

Table 10–5. Bronchopulmonary Dysplasia: Complications and Long-term Prognosis[a]

Early
  Pulmonary interstitial emphysema, pneumothorax
  Honeycomb lung
  Patent ductus
  Necrotizing enterocolitis
  Gastroesophageal—reflux, aspiration
  Complications of hyperalimentation
  Growth failure, osteopenia
  Transient systemic hypertension
Late
  Tracheal stenosis
  Apneic spells, sudden infant death syndrome
  Respiratory failure during viral infection
  Small airway disease
  Bronchial hyperreactivity
  ? Chronic airflow obstruction in adults?

[a] Based on the results of Nickerson[186] and O'Brodovich and Mellins.[187]

Perinatal Pneumonia

Infectious diseases in the lung are discussed in detail in Chapters 11–14 but certain general principles and a few specific disorders need to be considered in relation to the lungs of the newborn.

Pulmonary infection is a common finding in neonatal necropsies.[3,224,225] Pneumonia as primary or complicating

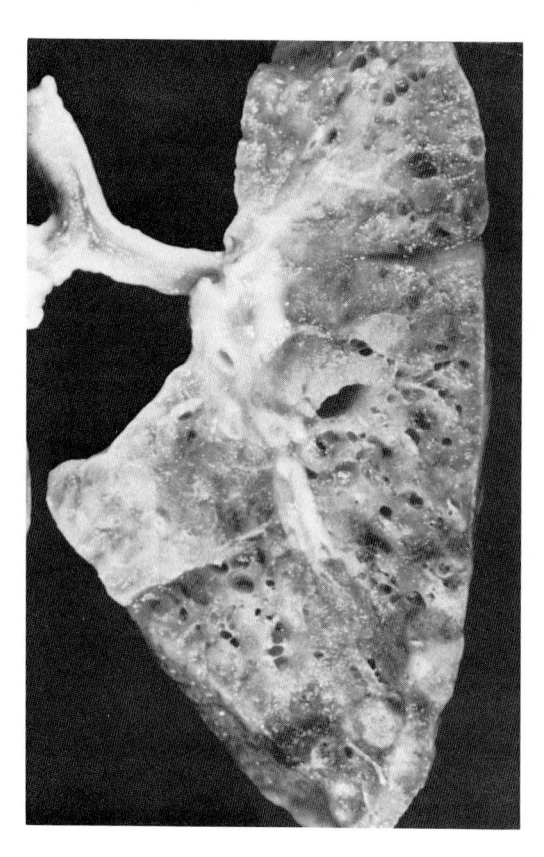

Figure 10–24. Diffuse pulmonary interstitial emphysema. Round, linear, and sausage-shaped spaces are seen in the interlobular septa. The spaces in lymphangiectasis would be much more uniform.

phenomenon was found in 36 percent of cases in the British Perinatal Mortality Survey and, including the "amniotic fluid infection syndrome," accounted for approximately 20 percent of neonatal deaths in the U.S. Collaborative Perinatal Project.[224] The organisms and pathologic manifestations vary with the clinical features. Pneumonias in the perinatal period can be classified on the basis of time of appearance of the lesion and how it was acquired (Table 10–6).[3]

Congenital (intrauterine) pneumonia is essentially a form of aspiration pneumonia and usually accompanies ascending infection of the amniotic fluid from a vaginal source. Both gram-positive and gram-negative organisms may be involved. Clusters of polymorphonuclear cells are found in bronchi and alveoli and concomitantly the placental membranes are inflamed. These membranes may have ruptured prematurely but it is not clear whether infection is the result or cause of the amniotic fluid infection.[224] The presence of pulmonary vessels filled with polymorphonuclear cells has been used as a microscopic feature to differentiation infants with "true" pulmonary infection from those who "drowned in pus" from aspirated infected amniotic fluid. Basically, however, the lung findings represent different portions of the spectrum of the same disease.

Pneumonia acquired during birth usually represents a reaction to organisms acquired from the birth canal.[3] Group B streptococcal infection (GBS) has attracted major attention as an example of this phenomenon because of its rapidly fatal course and the histologic feature, in some cases, of hyaline membranes which may be interpreted as a manifestion of surfactant deficiency and thus obscure the true diagnosis of infection.[226–228] When present the hyaline membranes often contain rows of gram positive cocci (Fig. 10–29) and there may in fact, be an alveolar collapse pattern suggesting HMD. In other cases, cocci, polys, and edema fluid may fill the alveoli and in rare cases there may be a paucity of polymorphonuclear cells in the lung and in the circulating blood.[226,227] A late-onset form of the disease with sepsis and meningitis may also be seen.[228] Group B streptococcal infection may also be acquired prior to delivery as a congenital pneumonia related to infected amniotic fluid.[3] Other causes of postnatal early-onset pneumonia are coliform organisms. Hemophilus infection may produce a clinical and pathologic disease that mimics group B streptococcal disease.[3]

Although many viral pneumonias are acquired transplacentally, herpes infection may occur as a result of delivery of the infant through a vagina with active herpetic lesions.[3,225] Chlamydial pneumonitis is a distinctive pneumonitis in the neonate. The disease usually presents around 3 weeks of age with tachypnea and a "stacatto" cough. Conjunctivitis may be seen in up to 50 percent of affected infants and an absolute blood eosinophilia is not uncommon.[3,225] Open lung biopsy in one reported case showed bronchiolitis and an associated interstitial lymphocytic and plasma cell infiltrate in the pulmonary interstitium (see Fig. 10–30).

Late-onset pneumonia represents a reaction to organisms acquired from human or environmental contacts and includes infection caused by staphylococci, coliform organisms, and Pseudomonas among others.[3,225]

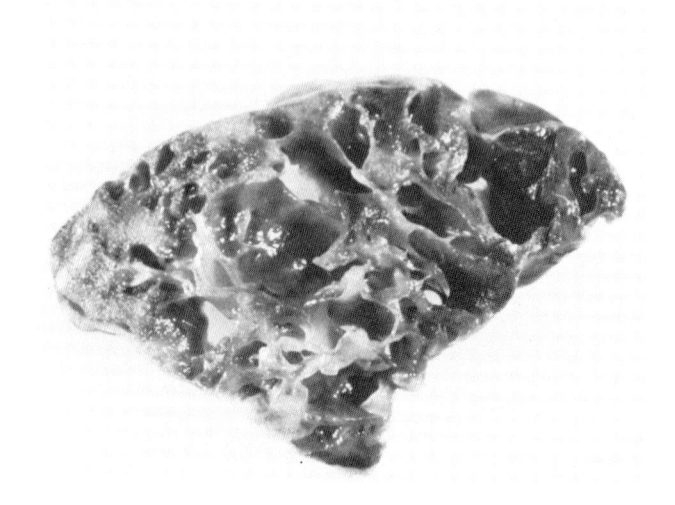

Figure 10–25. Localized pulmonary interstitial emphysema. This patient with hyaline membrane disease developed an enlarging mass in the left upper lobe. Mediastinal shift ensued and a lobectomy was performed. Courtesy of Drs. R. C. Rosan and J. Blair.

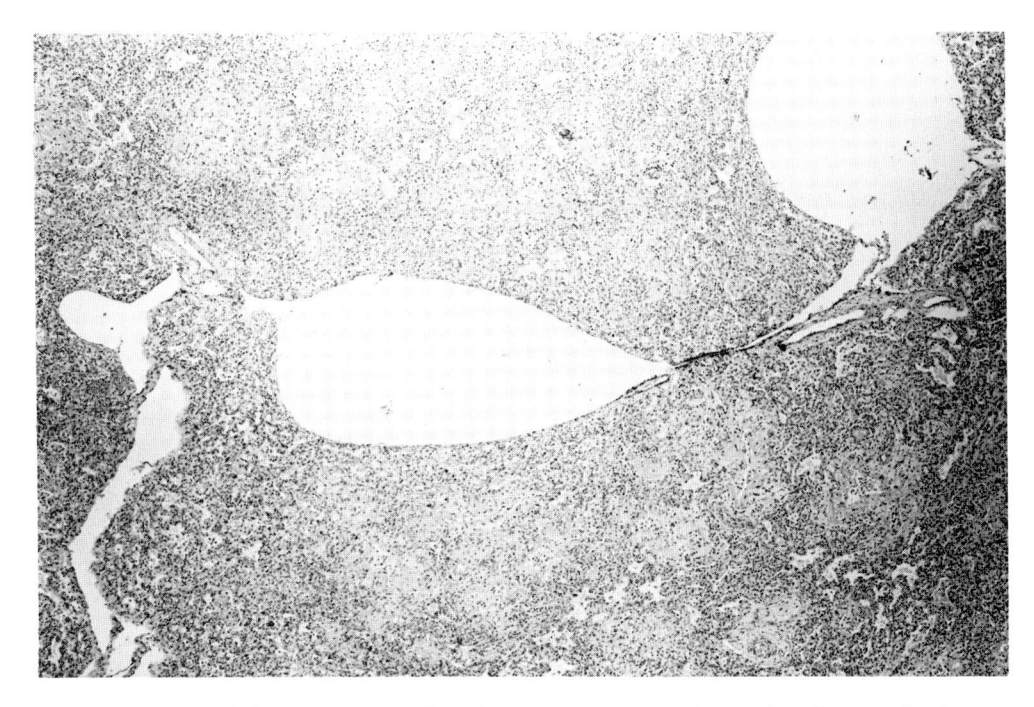

Figure 10–26. Pulmonary interstitial emphysema in a patient with bronchopulmonary dysplasia. The clear spaces represent dissection of air along interlobular septa.

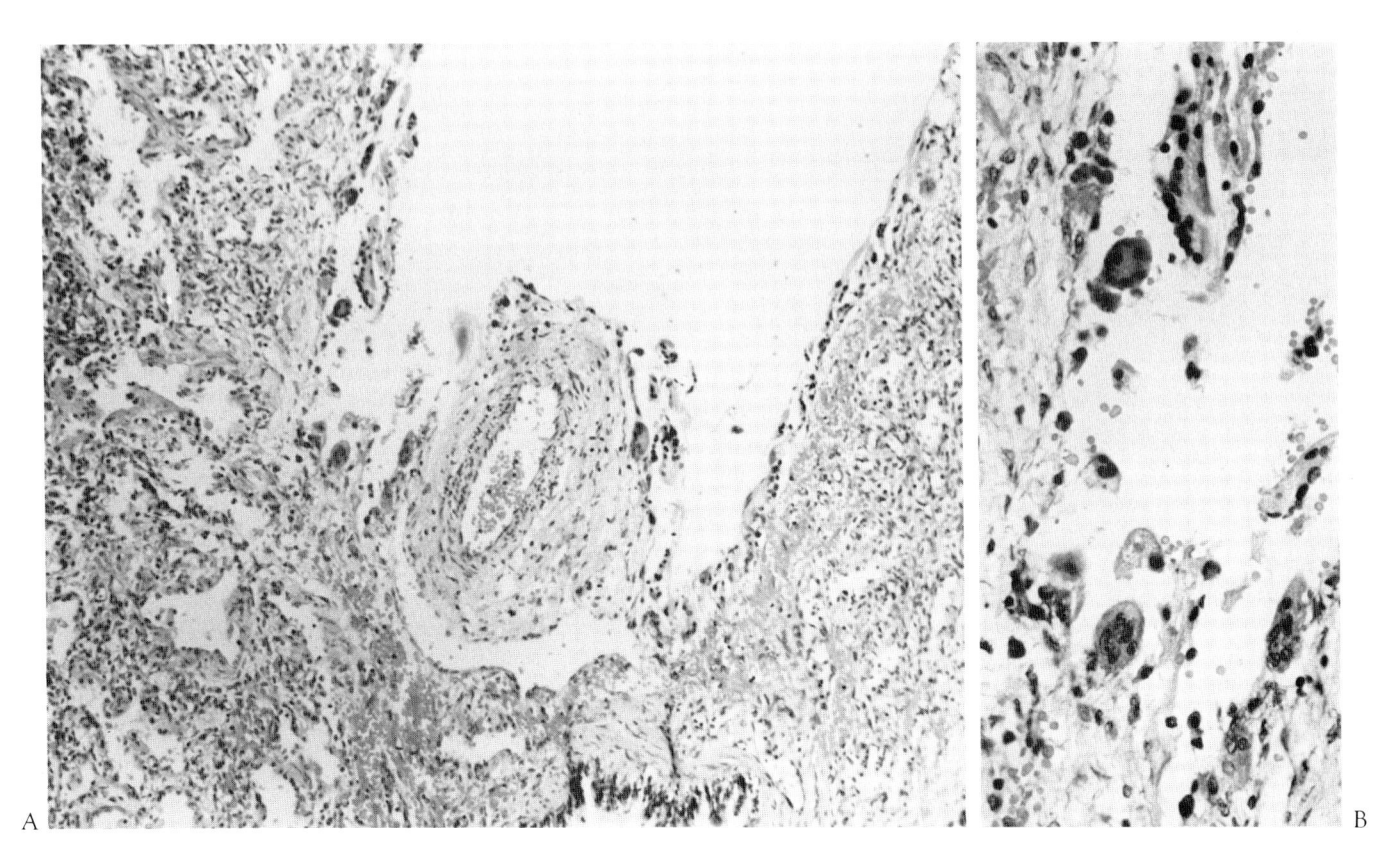

Figure 10–27. Persistent interstitial pulmonary emphysema. A. Dissection of air in the loose connective tissue around a bronchovascular bundle has produced a foreign body reaction. B. Multinucleated giant cells line the spaces.

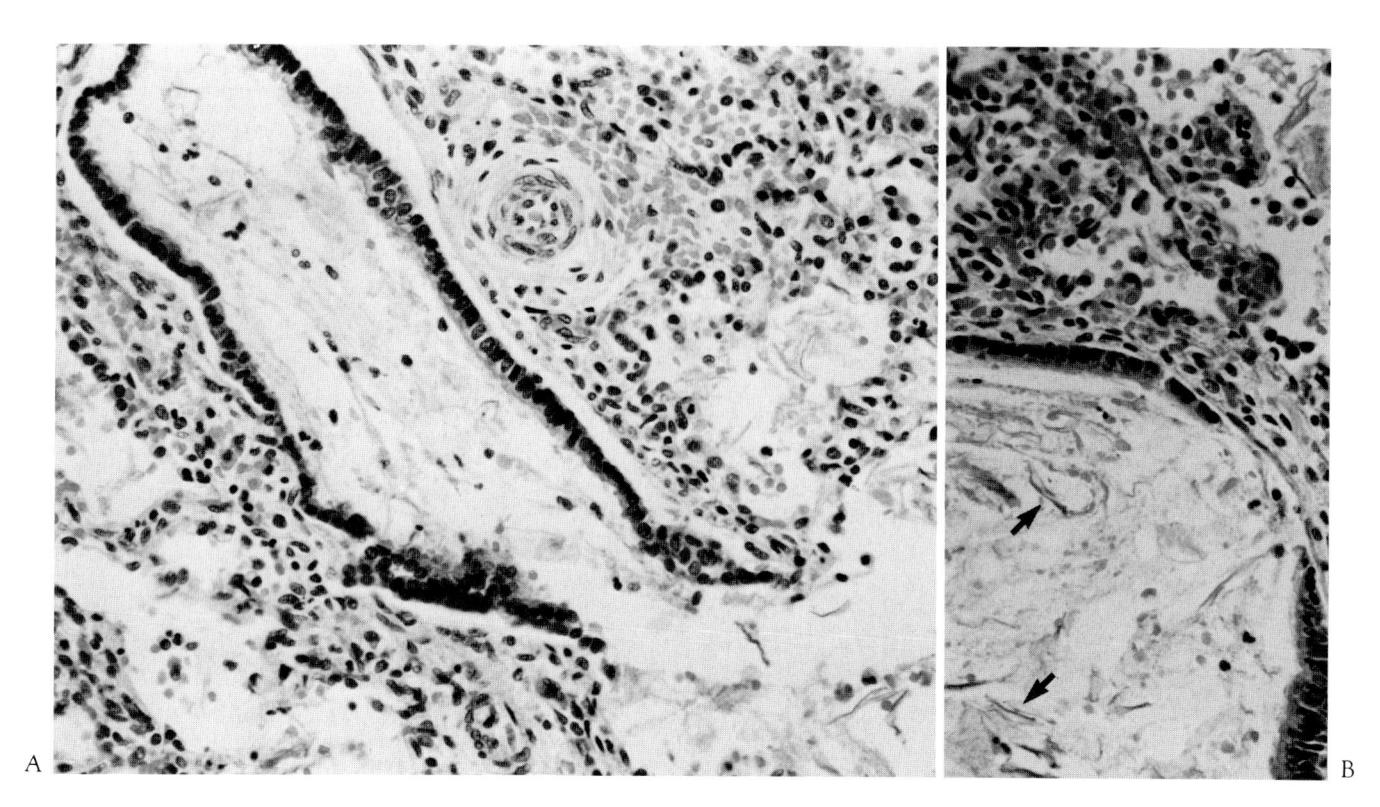

Figure 10–28. Meconium aspiration. A. Aspirated mucus and fetal squames fill a bronchiole. B. Higher magnification shows wispy strands of mucin and plate-like fetal squames (arrows).

Pulmonary Vascular Disorders in the Newborn

Pulmonary hypertension, in regard to pathophysiology, pathologic features, and causes is covered in Chapter 24. There do appear to be histologic differences in the clinicopathologic grading of plexogenic pulmonary hypertension in children as opposed to adults.[229–233] The anatomic differences in muscle distribution between the pulmonary arteries of infants and adults have led to studies which suggest that the classical Heath-Edwards grading system for cardiac-associated pulmonary hypertension may need to be supplemented, in infants, by a grading system that includes muscle distribution.[232,233]

Persistent pulmonary hypertension of the newborn (PPHN, persistent "fetal" circulation) is, however, an important cause of mortality in the neonate and is discussed here. The syndrome consists of many disorders that cause persistent high vascular resistance in the lung after birth, but the term persistent pulmonary hypertension of the newborn is often used in reference to the idiopathic form of the disorder.[234–238] The classification proposed by Rudolph divides the etiologies of PPHN into several disparate categories (Table 10–7).[238] The infants present with cyanosis, respiratory distress, and evidence of right-to-left shunt with elevated pulmonary artery pressure. By definition, cardiac anomalies causing pulmonary hypertension could be considered as part of the syndrome of PPHN, but most authors consider that etiology separately. Patients with pulmonary hypoplasia and with diaphragmatic hernia (see below) commonly have PPHN, presumably as a consequence of reduced cross-sectional area of the pulmonary vascular bed.[237,238] In the idiopathic form a variety of perinatal stresses such czs fetal hypoxia and premature closure of the ductus arteriosus have been postulated as responsible for increased pulmonary vascular smooth muscle development.[239] Leukotrienes have been suggested as a cause of

Table 10–6. Perinatal Pneumonia

Transplacental
  Part of a systemic congenital infection, usually of maternal origin
Intrauterine
  Present at birth; a form of aspiration pneumonia associated with infected amniotic fluid; usually due to organisms in the maternal vagina
Acquired during birth
  Signs appear in the first week of life; usually associated with maternal vaginal infection
Acquired after birth
  Appears in the first month of life, organisms acquired from the environment

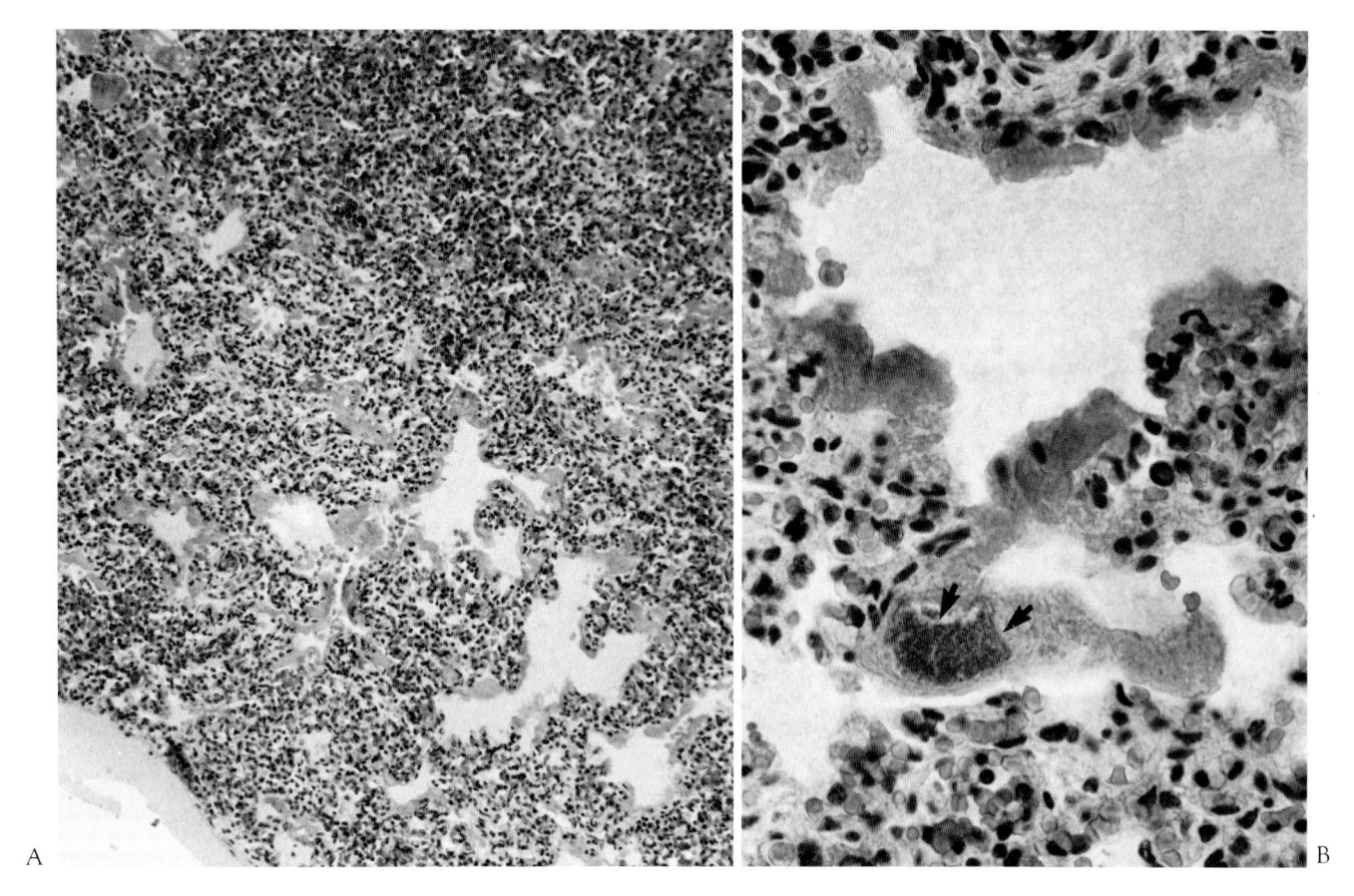

Figure 10–29. Group B streptococcal infection mimicking hyaline membrane disease. A. Note the collapse pattern resembling that of hyaline membrane disease. B. The hyaline membranes here are filled with cocci (arrows). The lack of a polymorphonuclear cell response is not unusual.

pulmonary artery constriction. Obstruction of an anatomically normal pulmonary arterial bed might occur in the presence of hyperviscosity of the neonate's blood or, as frequently seen in PPHN, in association with thrombi, either in situ or as emboli from a pulmonary valve affected by nonbacterial endocarditis.[240,241]

Table 10–7. Anatomic and Functional Causes of Persistent Pulmonary Hypertension in the Newborn (PPHN)[a]

Failure of postnatal decrease in pulmonary vascular resistance (implies normal anatomic prenatal development)
  Increased blood viscosity
  Large unrestricted VSD
  ?hypoxia
Excessive prenatal muscularization of the distal pulmonary vasculature
  Idiopathic PPHN
  Meconium aspiration
  Congenital heart disease
Developmental decrease in cross-sectional area of the distal pulmonary vasculature
  Pulmonary hypoplasia
  Congenital diaphragmatic hernia
  Alveolar capillary dysplasia

[a] Modified from Rudolph[238] and from Geggel and Reid.[236]

Microscopically, the idiopathic form of PPHN is characterized by a distinctive alteration of the normal muscular pattern of small pulmonary arteries.[236] In the normal term fetus and the neonate, the intra-acinar pulmonary arteries distal to the level of the terminal bronchiole lack a muscular media coat.[236] A muscular wall is ordinarily not well developed in these arteries until adolescence. In infants with idiopathic PPHN there is abnormal extension of muscle into small intra-acinar arteries with resultant compromise of the lumen (Fig. 10–31). In addition, there is proliferation of connective tissue in the adventia of these vessels.[236] This remodeling is considered to represent the development of new muscle as opposed to persistence of fetal musculature or constriction of normal arteries. The nature of the lesion suggests that it occurs before birth, probably in response to intrauterine stress. As noted above, intravascular thrombi and nonbacterial endocarditis are frequently associated with the other histologic findings described for idiopathic PPHN.

Pulmonary emboli are not uncommon in the lungs of infants dying in the neonatal period. Often foreign material, presumably fragments of catheters or other material used in life support can be seen in association with a thrombus.[3,9] Nonbacterial thrombotic endocarditis may be the source of multiple thromboemboli in the lung.[241]

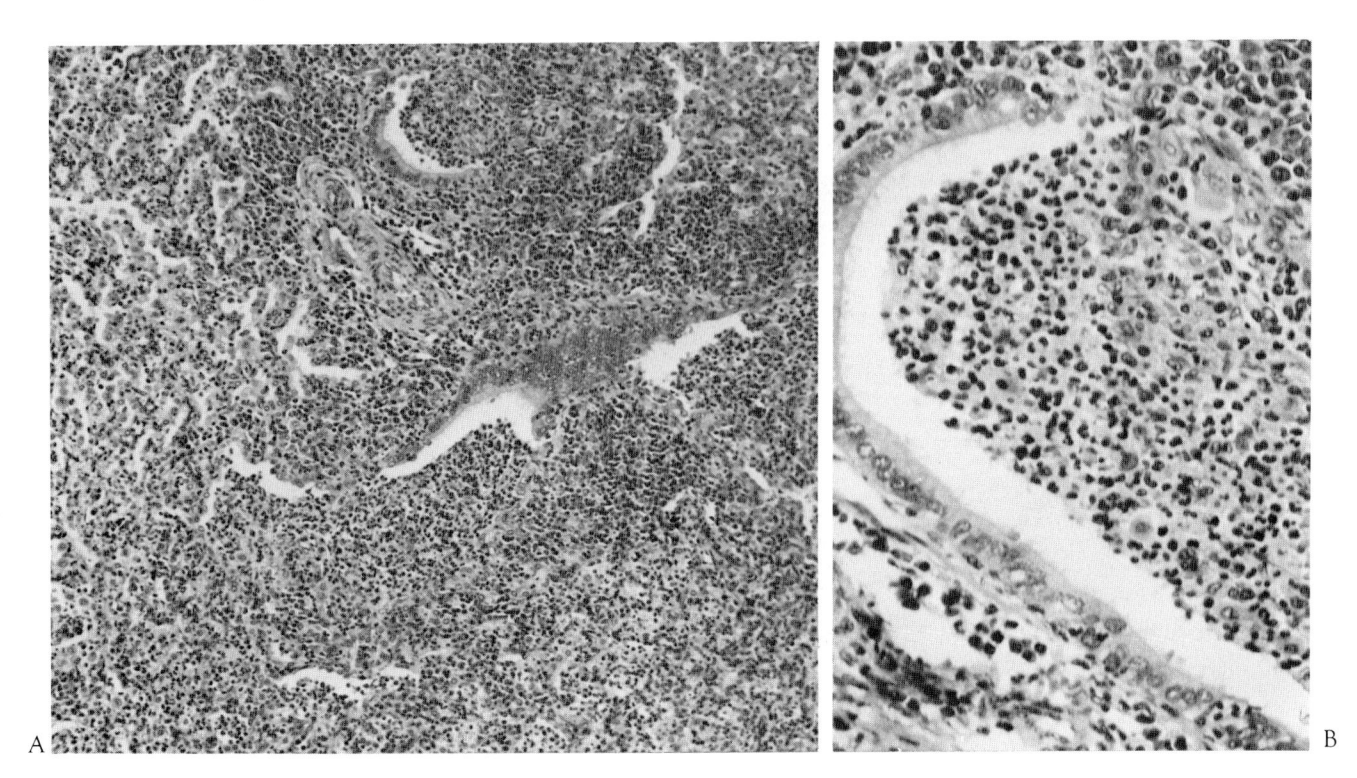

Figure 10–30. Chlamydial pneumonitis. A. Lymphoplasmacytic bronchiolitis and focal interstitial inflammation are seen. B. The bronchiole is filled with lymphocytes, macrophages, and necrotic polymorphonuclear cells. Courtesy of Dr. Barbara Von Schmidt. This case was published in J Pediatr 93:447–449, 1978.

Stocker and associates reported several infants with peripheral subpleural lung cysts thought to be related to pulmonary artery occlusions and lung infarction.[242]

Rendas and associates described the development of progressive pulmonary hypertension and the ultimate death of a small premature infant.[243] There was extreme hypoplasia of the pulmonary vascular bed. The clinical circumstances suggested that this infant had a disorder that was different from PPHN and that was, perhaps, related to disturbances in lung growth.

Disorders of the Diaphragm

Congenital posterolateral diaphragmatic (Bochdalek's) hernia occurs in from 1 in 2000 to 1 in 5000 live births.[244–250] The incidence appears to be higher in stillborn infants and abortuses. Left-sided hernia is much more common than right at birth but the incidence of right-sided hernia rises in older children.[250] The incidence of associated anomalies may be as high as 20 percent overall but infants surviving over 1 hour after birth rarely have other significant malformations.[244,251] There appears to be a notable association of pulmonary extralobar sequestrations with diaphragmatic hernia.[6]

The etiology of the defect is unknown. A small number of familial cases have been reported.[252]

Affected infants present with cyanosis, respiratory distress, and bowel sounds in the chest. Most patients develop signs and symptoms at or shortly after birth but delayed onset of clinical problems may occur.[247,250] Antenatal, ultrasonic, diagnosis has been reported. Interposition of the colon between the liver and diaphragm (Chilaiditi's syndrome) may mimic a right-sided hernia.[253] One of the major complications of congenital diaphragmatic hernia is development of persistent pulmonary hypertension (see p. 136) in the newborn period—either directly at birth or after a "honeymoon" period of normal vascular resistance.[254–256]

Morphologic features of congenital diaphragmatic hernia include gross reduction in size of the ipsilateral lung (Fig. 10–32). The contralateral lung shows a varying degree of hypoplasia as well. Morphometric study has shown a reduction in bronchial branches and in pulmonary arteries. The number of alveoli per acinus is normal but total alveolar number is reduced because there are fewer acinar units.[32,33] These changes are most marked in the ipsilateral lung but, again, occur in the contralateral lung as well. Reduction in cross-sectional area of the vascular bed produces pulmonary hypertension. In addition, recent studies have shown that infants who have no "honeymoon period" have excessive muscularization of the distal (intra-acinar) pulmonary arteries and increased medial thickness of preacinar arteries as compared to those infants with diaphragmatic hernia who do have an early period of normotensive pulmonary vascular flow.[256]

The reported mortality of infants with congenital diaphragmatic hernia varies from 25 to 75 percent with the

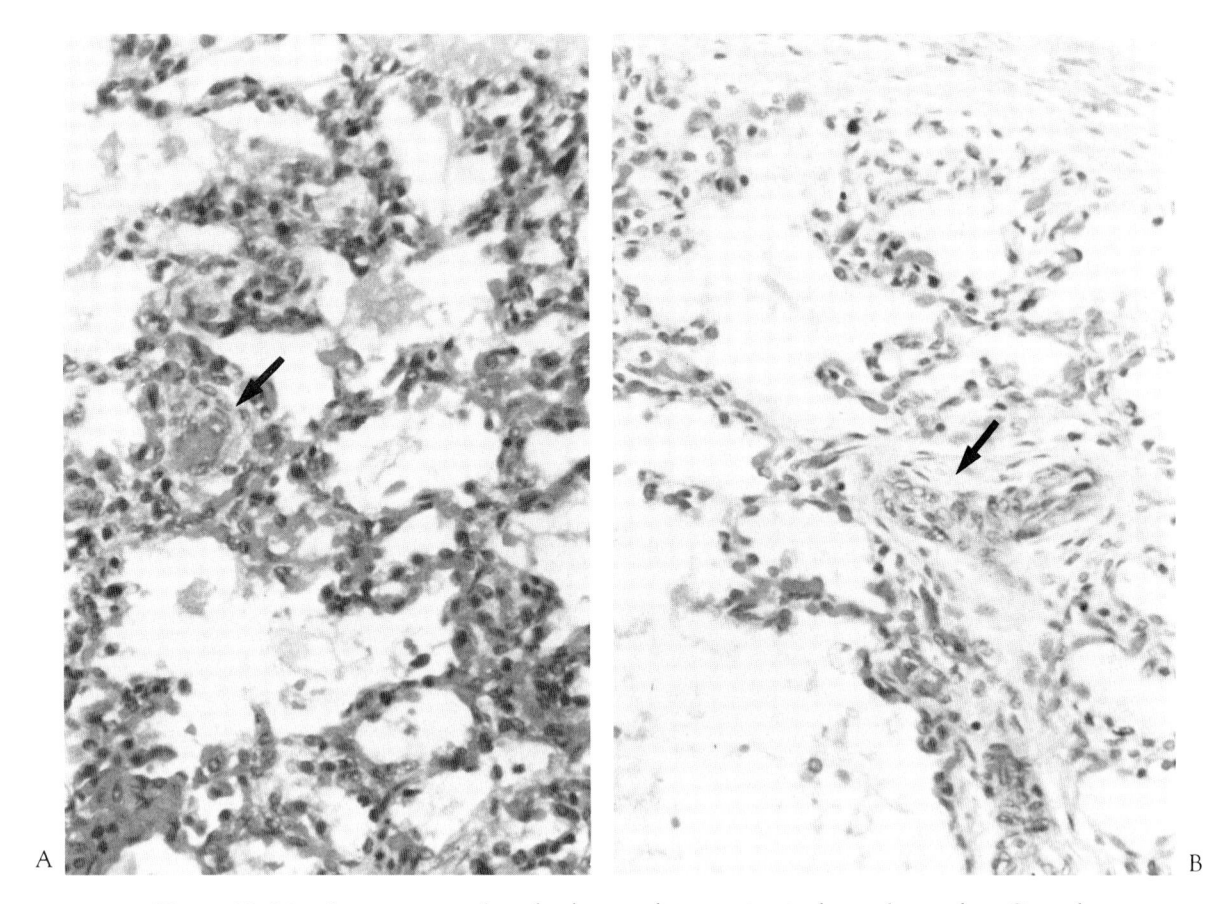

Figure 10–31. Persistent unexplained pulmonary hypertension in the newborn infant. Control pulmonary artery (A) has a thin wall but the vessel in the same location (B) from an infant with PPHN shows a complete muscular coat. Both vessels were located in similar peripheral areas of the lung acinus (distal to the bronchioles).

worst outcome in infants symptomatic at or soon after birth.[244] In survivors after surgical repair pneumothorax and pulmonary hypertension are early causes of mortality. Long-term survivors after surgical repair show a reduction in forced expiratory volume in 1 second (FEV_1), and evidence of significant air-trapping. Diminished flow of blood to the ipsilateral lung is demonstrable and, as might be expected, there is diminished diaphragmatic movement on the effected side.[257] Morphologic study in a few survivors shows destructive emphysema and diminished alveolar and bronchiolar number in the ipsilateral lung. There is a suggestion that compensatory alveolar multiplication may occur on the contralateral side.[257]

Accessory diaphragm is a rare congenital anomaly in which a fibrous membrane divides the hemithorax into two compartments.[258] Most cases involve the right side and the entrapped pulmonary lobe or lobes may be hypoplastic. In some examples a lower lobe is divided into two parts by the membrane. Associated malformations such as anomalous venous return or aberrant systemic arterial supply to the lung are frequent, as are cardiac defects. The disorder is usually diagnosed in adults and is ordinarily not fatal.

Chest wall anomalies may restrict lung growth but other than as a feature of dwarfism or "short-rib" syndromes are more likely to be a problem in adolescents or young adults.[6] Apical pneumatoceles, however, do occur in children. In this entity weakness in or absence of Sibson's fascia is associated with a cervical bulge represented as herniation.[259]

Cystic Fibrosis

Cystic fibrosis is a complex, inherited systemic disorder of exocrine glands with prominent involvement of the respiratory tract.[260–268]

The disorder classically affects infants and children but milder forms of the disease are being diagnosed with increasing frequency in adults.[266,267] Recurrent pulmonary infection by staphylococcal organisms and various strains of pseudomonas is a prominent feature. Viral infection may also be a major cause of deterioration in pulmonary function.[268] Mucoid impaction, areas of atelectasis and of overinflation, bronchiectasis, and necrotizing pneumonia are other features of respiratory tract involvement in cystic fibrosis.[264] Allergic bronchopulmonary aspergillosis may also complicate the picture.[264]

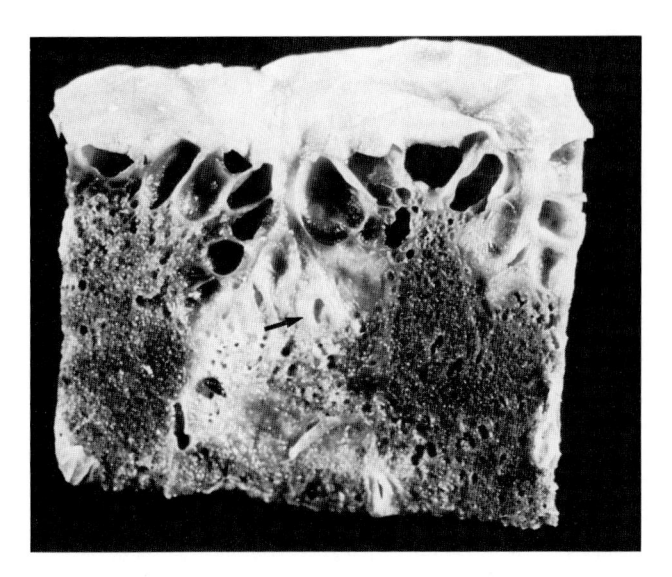

Figure 10-32. Postinfarction subpleural cysts. Stocker and associates[242] propose that occlusion of a pulmonary artery (arrow) produces these cysts and that they may then be a cause of spontaneous pneumothorax. Courtesy of Dr. J. T. Stocker.

Pneumothorax is a common occurrence and studies have implicated not only pulmonary interstitial "emphysema" but also emphysematous subpleural bullae and postinfectious bronchiectatic cysts in the pathogenesis of pleural air leaks.[262]

The basic defect in cystic fibrosis is unknown. There is evidence that the thick tenacious mucus characteristic of cystic fibrosis and putatively responsible for airway obstruction and subsequent infection, may be caused by abnormal electrolyte transport through respiratory and bronchial gland epithelium.[261]

References

1. Kendig EL Jr, Chernick V (eds): *Disorders of the Respiratory Tract in Children*, 4th ed. Philadelphia: WB Saunders, 1983.
2. Gerbeaux J, Couvreur J, Tournier G (eds): *Pediatric Respiratory Disease*, 2nd ed. New York: John Wiley & Sons, 1982.
3. Wigglesworth JS: Perinatal Pathology. Philadelphia, WB Saunders, 1984.
4. Avery ME, Fletcher BD, Williams RG: The Lung and its Disorders in the Newborn Infant, 4th ed. Philadelphia: WB Saunders, 1981.
5. Cox JN: Respiratory system. In Berry Cl, (ed): *Paediatric Pathology*. New York: Springer-Verlag, 1981, pp 299–394.
6. Landing BH, Dixon LG: Congenital malformations and genetic disorders of the respiratory tract (larynx, trachea, bronchi and lungs). Am Rev Respir Dis 120:151–185, 1979.
7. Stern L (ed): *Diagnosis and Management of Respiratory Disorders in the Newborn*. Menlo Park, CA: Addison-Wesley, 1983.
8. Swischuk LE: Respiratory system. In *Radiology of the Newborn and Young Infant*, 2nd ed. Baltimore: Williams & Wilkins, 1980, pp 1–190.
9. Valdes-Dapena M: Iatrogenic disease in the perinatal period as seen by the pathologist. In Naeye RL, Kissane JM, Kaufman N (eds): *Perinatal Disorders*. Baltimore, Williams & Wilkins, 1981, pp 382–418.
10. Ostor AG, Stillwell R, Fortune DW: Bilateral pulmonary agenesis. Pathology 10:243–248, 1978.
11. Brereton RJ, Rickwood AMK: Esophageal atresia with pulmonary agenesis. J Pediatr Surg 18:618–620, 1983.
12. Mygrind H, Paulsen SM: Agenesis of the right lung. Arch Pathol Lab Med 104:444, 1980.
13. Maltz DL, Nadas AS: Agenesis of the lung. Presentation of eight new cases and review of the literature. Pediatrics 42:175–188, 1960.
14. Booth JB, Berry Cl: Unilateral pulmonary agenesis. Arch Dis Child 2:361–373, 1967.
15. Mardini MK, Nyhan WL: Agenesis of the lung. Report of four patients with unusual anomalies. Chest 87:522–527, 1985.
16. Ryland D, Reid L: Pulmonary aplasia—a quantitative analysis of the development of the single lung. Thorax 26:602–609, 1971.
17. Storey CF, Marrangoni AG: Lobar agenesis of the lung. J Thorac Surg 28:536–543, 1954.
18. Landing GH: Syndromes of congenital heart disease with tracheobronchial anomalies. Amer J Roentgenol Rad Ther Nucl Med 123:679–686, 1975.
19. Maesen FPV, Santana B, Lamers J, Brekel B: A supernumerary bronchus of the right upper lobe. Eur J Respir Dis 64:473–476, 1983.
20. Lesbros D, Ferran J-L, Rieu D, Jean D: Stenose tracheale congenitale et bronche surnumeraire. Arch Franc Pediatr 36:703–708, 1979.
21. Foster-Carter AF: Bronchopulmonary abnormalities. Br J Tuberc Dis Chest 40:111–124, 1946.
22. Siegel MJ, Shackelford DG, Francis RS, McAlister WH: Tracheal bronchus. Radiology 130:353–355, 1979.
23. Remy J, Smith M, Marache P, Nuyts JP: La bronche "tracheale" gauche pathogène. Revue de la littérature à propos de 4 observations. J Radiol 58:621–630, 1977.
24. Starshak RJ, Sty JR, Woods G, Keitzer FV. Bridging bronchus: A rare airway anomaly. Radiology 140:95–96, 1981.
25. Odell J: Anomalous origin of the anterior segmental bronchus of the right upper lobe. Thorax 35:213–214, 1980.
26. Chang N, Hertzler JH, Gregg RH, et al.: Congenital stenosis of the right mainstem bronchus. A case report. Pediatrics 41:739–742, 1968.
27. Kalayoglu M, Olcay I: Congenital bronchobiliary fistula associated with esophageal atresia and tracheo-esophageal fistula. J Pediatr Surg 11:463–464, 1976.
28. Chan YT, Ng WD, Tymak WP, et al.: Congenital bronchobiliary fistula associated with biliary atresia. Br J Surg 73:240–241, 1984.
29. Freedom RM, Burrows PE, Moes CAG: "Horseshoe" lung: Report of five new cases. AJR 146:211–215, 1986.
30. Frank JL, Poole CA, Rasas G: Horseshoe lung: Clinical, pathologic and radiologic features and a new plain film finding. AJR 146:217–226, 1986.
31. Langston C, Kida K, Reed M, Thurlbeck WM: Human lung growth in late gestation and in the neonate. Amer Rev Respir Dis 129:607–613, 1984.
32. Reid L: Lung growth in health and disease. Br J Dis Chest 78:113–134, 1984.
33. Langston C, Thurlbeck WM: Lung growth and development

in late gestation and early postnatal life. Perspect Pediatr Pathol 1982; 7:203–235.

34. Thurlbeck WM: Postnatal human lung growth. Thorax 37:564–571, 1982.

35. Askenazi SS, Perlman M: Pulmonary hypoplasia: Lung weight and radial alveolar count as criteria of diagnosis. Arch Dis Child 54:614–618, 1979.

36. Cooney TP, Thurlbeck WM: The radial alveolar count method of Emery and Mithal: A reappraisal 1—postnatal lung growth. Thorax 37:572–579, 1982.

37. Cooney TP, Thurlbeck WM: The radial alveolar count method of Emery and Mithal a reappraisal 2—intrauterine and early postnatal lung growth. Thorax 37:580–583, 1982.

38. Page DV, Stocker JT: Anomalies associated with pulmonary hypoplasia. Am Rev Respir Dis 125:216–221, 1982.

39. Wigglesworth JS, Desai R, Guerrini P: Fetal lung hypoplasia: Biochemical and structural variations and their possible significance. Arch Dis Child 56:606–615, 1981.

40. Boulley AM, Imbert MC, Dehan M, et al.: Hypoplasie pulmonaire bilateral du nouveau-né. Etude clinique et anatomo-pathologique. A propos de 17 case. Arch Fr Pediatr 125:216–221, 1982.

41. Swischuck LE, Richardson CJ, Nichols MM, Ingman MJ: Bilateral pulmonary hypoplasia in the neonate. AJR 133:1057–1063, 1979.

42. Wigglesworth JS, Desai R: Is fetal respiratory function a major determinant of perinatal survival? Lancet 1:264–267, 1982.

43. Davies G, Reid L: Effect of scoliosis on growth of alveoli and pulmonary arteries and on right ventricle. Arch Dis Child 46:623–632, 1971.

44. DeTroyer A, Yernault J-C, Englert M: Lung hypoplasia in congenital pulmonary valve stenosis. Circulation 56:647–651, 1977.

45. Hislop A, Hey E, Reid L: The lungs in congenital bilateral renal agenesis and dysplasia. Arch Dis Child 54:32–38, 1979.

46. Elias S, Boelen L, Simpson JL: Syndrome of camptodactly, multiple ankylosis, facial anomalies and pulmonary hypoplasia. Birth Defects Orig Art Ser 14(6B):243–251, 1978.

47. Fewell JE, Hislop AA, Kitterman JA, Johnson P: Effect of tracheostomy on lung development in fetal lambs. J Appl Physiol: Respir Environ Exercise Physiol 55:1103–1108, 1983.

48. Nakayama DK, Glick PL, Harrison MR, et al. Experimental pulmonary hypoplasia due to oligohydramnios and its reversal by relieving thoracic compression. J Pediatr Surg 18:347–353, 1983.

49. Cooney TP, Thurlbeck WM: Pulmonary hypoplasia in Down's Syndrome. N Engl J Med 307:1170–1173, 1982.

50. Currarino G, Williams B: Causes of congenital unilateral pulmonary hypoplasia: A study of 33 cases. Pediatr Radiol 15:15–24, 1985.

51. Bozic C: Ectopic fetal adrenal cortex in the lung of a newborn. Virchows Arch [A] 363:371–374, 1974.

52. Remberger K, Hubner G: Rhabdomyomatous dysplasia of the lung. Virchows Arch [A] 363:363–369, 1974.

53. Chi JG, Shong Y-K: Diffuse striated muscle heteroplasia of the lung. An autopsy case. Arch Pathol Lab Med 106:641–644, 1982.

54. Campo E, Bombi JA: Central nervous system heterotopia in the lung of a fetus with cranial malformations. Virchows Arch [A] 391:117–122, 1981.

55. Janny CG, Askin FB, Kuhn CK III: Congenital alveolar dysplasia—an unusual cause of respiratory distress in the newborn. Am J Clin Pathol 76:722–727, 1981.

56. Khorsand J, Tennant R, Gillies C, Phillipps AF: Congenital alveolar capillary dysplasia: A developmental vascular anomaly causing persistent pulmonary hypertension of the newborn. Pediatr Pathol 3:299–306, 1985.

57. Keith JD, Rowe RD, Vlad P: *Heart Disease in Infancy and Childhood*, 3rd ed. New York: Macmillan, 1978.

58. Freedom RM, Culhan JAG, Moes CAF: *Angiocardiography of Congenital Heart Disease*. New York: Macmillan, 1984.

59. Penkoske PA, Castaneda AR, Fyler DC, Van Praagh R: Origin of pulmonary artery branch from ascending aorta. Primary surgical repair in infancy. J Thorac Cardiovasc Surg 85:537–545, 1983.

60. Tesler UF, Balsara RH, Niguidula FN: Aberrant left pulmonary artery (vascular sling): Report of five cases. Chest 66:402–407, 1974.

61. Grover FL, Norton JB Jr, Webb GE, Trinkle JK: Pulmonary sling. J Thorac Cardiovasc Surg 69:295–300, 1975

62. Grote WR, Tenholder MF: Pulmonary artery malformation syndrome. South Med J 77:1139–1143, 1984.

63. Berdon WE, Baker DH: Vascular anomalies and the infant lung: Rings, slings and other things. Semin Roentgenol 7:39–64, 1972.

64. Presbitero P, Bull C, Haworth SG, deLaval MR: Absent or occult pulmonary artery. Br Heart J 52:178–185, 1984.

65. Hislop A, Sanderson M, Reid L: Unilateral congenital dysplasia of lung associated with vascular anomalies. Thorax 28:435–441, 1973.

66. Tang JS, Kauffman SL, Lynfield J: Hypoplasia of the pulmonary arteries in infants with congenital rubella. Am J Cardiol 27:491–496, 1971.

67. Goldstein JD, Rabinovitch M, Van Praagh R, Reid L: Unusual vascular anomalies causing persistent pulmonary hypertension in a newborn. Am J Cardiol 43:962–968, 1979.

68. Kamio A, Fukushima K, Takebayashi S, Toshima H: Isolated stenosis of the pulmonary artery branches—an autopsy case with review of the literatures. Jpn Circ J 42:1289–1296, 1978.

69. Loser H, Osswald P, Apitz J, Schmalta AA: Periphere pulmonalstenosen: Mogliche ursachen und syndromale zusammenhange. Klin Padiatr 189:137–145, 1977.

70. McCue CM, Robertson LW, Lester RG, Mauck JP Jr: Pulmonary artery coarctations. A report of 20 cases with review of 319 cases from the literature. J Pediatr 67:222–238, 1965.

71. Pernot C, Deschamps J-P, Didier F: Stenose de l'artère pulmonaire, taches cutaneés pigmentaires et anomalies du squelette. Quatre observations. Arch Franc Pediatr 28:593–603, 1979.

72. Haworth SG, Reid L: Quantitative structural study of pulmonary circulation in the newborn with pulmonary atresia. Thorax 32:129–133, 1977.

73. Dines DE, Seward JB, Bernatz PE: Pulmonary arteriovenous fistulas. Mayo Clin Proc 58:176–181, 1983.

74. Pryzbojewski JZ, Maritz F: Pulmonary arteriovenous fistulas. A case presentation and review of the literature. S Afr Med J 57:366–372, 1980.

75. Abe T, Kuribayashi R, Sato M, Nieda S: Direct communication of the right pulmonary artery with the left atrium. J Thorac Cardiovasc Surg 64:38–44, 1972.

76. Brundage BH, Gomez AC, Cheitlin MD, Gmelich JT: Systemic artery to pulmonary vessel fistulas. Report of two cases and a review of the literature. Chest 62:19–23, 1972.

77. Utzon F, Brandrup F: Pulmonary arteriovenous fistulas in children. A review with special reference to the disperse

telangiectatic type illustrated by report of a case. Acta Paediatr Scand 62:422–432, 1973.

78. Lucas RV Jr: Anomalous venous connections, pulmonary and systemic. In Adams FH, Emmanouilides GC (eds): *Moss' Heart Disease in Infants, Children and Adolescents*, 3rd ed. Baltimore: Williams & Wilkins, 1983, pp 458–500.

79. Haworth SG, Reid L: Structural study of pulmonary circulation and of heart in total anomalous pulmonary venous return in early infancy. Br Heart J 39:80–92, 1977.

80. Mardini MK, Sakati NA, Lewall DB, et al.: Scimitar syndrome. Clin Pediatr 21:350–354, 1982.

81. Mathey J, Galey JS, Logeais Y, et al.: Anomalous pulmonary venous return into inferior vena cava and associated bronchovascular anomalies (The scimitar syndrome). Report of three cases and review of the literature. Thorax 23:298–407, 1968.

82. Alivizatos P, Cheatle T, deLaval M, Stark J: Pulmonary sequestration complicated by anomalies of pulmonary venous return. J Pediatr Surg 20:76–79, 1985.

83. Sade RM, Freed MD, Matthews EC, Castaneda AR: Stenosis of individual pulmonary veins. Review of the literature and report of a surgical case. J Thorac Cardiovasc Surg 67:953–962, 1974.

84. Swischuk LE, L'Heureux P: Unilateral pulmonary vein atresia. AJR 135:667–672, 1980.

85. Hawker RE, Celermajer, Gengos DC, et al.: Common pulmonary vein atresia. Premortem diagnosis in two infants. Circulation 46:368–374, 1972.

86. Presibitero P, Bull C, MaCartney FJ: Stenosis of pulmonary veins with ventricular septal defect. A cause of premature pulmonary hypertension in infancy. Br Heart J 49:600–603, 1983.

87. Perelman R, Gauthier N, Nathanson M, et al.: Varice pulmonaire chez l'enfant. A propos d'un cas. Revue de la litterature. Ann Pediatr 22:411–420, 1975.

88. Savic B, Birtel FJ, Knoche R, et al.: Pulmonary sequestration. Ergebn Kinderheilk 43:58–92, 1979.

89. O'Mara CS, Baker RR, Jeyasingham K: Pulmonary sequestration. Surg Gynecol Obstet 147:609–616, 1978.

90. Telander RL, Lennox C, Sieber W: Sequestration of the lung in children. Mayo Clin Proc 51:578–584, 1976.

91. Stocker JT, Drake RM, Madewell JE: Cystic and congenital lung disease in the newborn. Perspect Pediatr Pathol 4:93–154, 1978.

92. Karp W: Bilateral sequestration of the lung. AJR 513–515, 1977.

93. Takahashi M, Ohno M, Mihara K, et al.: Intralobar pulmonary sequestration. With special emphasis on bronchial communication. Radiology 114:543–549, 1975.

94. Hopkins RL, Levine SO, Waring WW: Intralobar sequestration. Demonstration of collateral ventilation by nuclear lung scan. Chest 82:192–193, 1982.

95. Case records of the Massachusetts General Hospital (case 18-1981). N Engl J Med 304:1090–1096, 1981.

96. Stocker JT, Kagan-Hallet K: Extralobar pulmonary sequestration. Analysis of 15 cases. Am J Clin Pathol 72:917–925, 1979.

97. Lucaya J, Carcia-Conesa JA, Bernado L: Pulmonary sequestration associated with unilateral pulmonary hypoplasia and massive pleural effusion. A case report and review of the literature. Pediatr Radiol 14:228–229, 1984.

98. Iwai K, Shindo G, Hajikano H, et al.: Intralobar pulmonary sequestration, with special reference to developmental pathology. Am Rev Respir Res 167:911–920, 1973.

99. Case records of the Massachusetts General Hospital (case 48-1983)

100. Stocker JT, Malczak HT: A study of pulmonary ligament arteries. Relationship to intralobar pulmonary sequestration. Chest 86:611–615, 1984.

101. Goldblatt E, Vimpani G, Brown JH: Extralobar pulmonary sequestration. Presentation as an arteriovenous aneurysm with cardiac failure in infancy. Am J Cardiol 29:100–103, 1972.

102. Maull KI, McElvein RB: Infarcted extralobar pulmonary sequestration. Chest 68:98–99, 1975.

103. Shuman RL, Libby G, Riker J: Pulmonary sequestration with aneurysmal anomalous systemic artery. Vasc Surg 17:183–188, 1983.

104. Werthammer JW, Hatten HP Jr, Blake WB Jr: Upper thoracic extralobar pulmonary sequestration presenting with respiratory distress in a newborn. Pediatr Radiol 9:116–117, 1980.

105. Graves VB, Dahl DD, Power HW: Congenital bronchopulmonary foregut malformation with anomalous pulmonary artery. Radiology 114:423–424, 1975.

106. Heithoff KB, Sane SM, Williams HJ, et al.: Bronchopulmonary foregut malformations. A unifying etiological concept. AJR 126:46–55, 1976.

107. Leithiser RE Jr, Capitanio MA, Macpherson RI, Wood BP: "Communicating" bronchopulmonary foregut malformations. AJR 146:227–231, 1986.

108. Beskin CA: Intralobar enteric sequestration of the lung containing aberrant pancreas. J Thorac Cardiovasc Surg 41:314–317, 1961.

109. Corrin B, Danel C, Allaway A, et al.: Intralobar pulmonary sequestration of ectopic pancreatic tissue with gastropancreatic duplications. Thorax 40:637–638, 1985.

110. Lewis JE, Murray RE: Pulmonary sequestration with bronchoesophageal fistula. J Pediatr Surg 3:575–579, 1968.

111. Benson JE, Olsen MM, Fletcher BD: A spectrum of bronchopulmonary anomalies associated with tracheoesophageal malformations. Pediatr Radiol 15:377–380, 1985.

112. Flye MW, Izant RJ: Extralobar pulmonary sequestration with esophageal communication and complete duplication of the colon. Surgery 71:744–752, 1972.

113. Thornhill BA, Cho KC, Morehouse HT: Gastric duplication associated with pulmonary sequestration: CT manifestations. AJR 138:1168–1171, 1982.

114. Gabrielle OF: Arterial supply to the lung via the celiac axis. Am J Roentgenol Rad Ther Nucl Med 169:522–527, 1970.

115. Yabek SM, Burstein J, Berman W Jr, Dillon T: Aberrant systemic arterial supply to the left lung with congestive heart failure. Chest 80:636–637, 1981.

116. Thilenius OG, Ruschaput DG, Replogle RL, et al.: Spectrum of pulmonary sequestration: Association with anomalous pulmonary venous drainage in infants. Pediatr Cardiol 4:97–103, 1983.

117. Masaoka A, Maeda M, Monden Y, et al.: Total lung ectoplasia with systemic arterial supply. Ann Thorac Surg 27:76–79, 1979.

118. Allain O, Montagne JP, Balquet P, et al.: Les manifestations radiologiques des kystes bronchogeniques de la carène chez l'enfant. A propos de 5 observations. Arch Fr Pediatr 39:803–806, 1982.

119. Ramenofsky ML, Leape LL, McCauley RGK. Bronchogenic cyst. J Pediatr Surg 14:219–224, 1979.

120. Snyder ME, Luck SR, Hernandez R, et al.: Diagnostic dilemmas of mediastinal cysts. J Pediatr Surg 20:810–815, 1985.

121. Case records of the Massachusetts General Hospital (case 1-1984). N Engl J Med 310:36–41, 1984.

122. Amendola MA, Shirazi KK, Brooks J, et al.: Transdiaphragmatic bronchopulmonary foregut anomaly: "Dumbell" bronchogenic cyst. AJR 138:1165–1167, 1982.

123. Dubois P, Belanger R, Wellington JL: Bronchogenic cyst presenting as a supraclavicular mass. Can J Surg 24:530–531, 1981.

124. Reed JC, Sobonya RE: Morphologic analysis of foregut cysts in the thorax. AJR 120:851–860, 1974.

125. Salyer DC, Salyer WR, Eggleston JC: Benign developmental cysts of the mediastinum. Arch Pathol Lab Med 101:136–139, 1977.

126. Pryce DM: The lining of healed but persistent abscess cavities in the lung with epithelium of the ciliated columnar type. J Pathol Bacteriol 60:259–265, 1948.

127. Weinberg AG, Zumwalt RE: Bilateral nephromegaly and multiple pulmonary cysts. Am J Clin Pathol 67:284–288, 1977.

128. Stocker JT, Madewell JE, Drake RM: Congenital adenomatoid malformation of the lung: Classification and morphologic spectrum. Hum Pathol 8:155–171, 1977.

129. Daroca PJ Jr: Mucogenic cells of congenital adenomatoid malformation of lung. Arch Pathol Lab Med 103:258–260, 1979.

130. Alt B, Shikes RH, Stanford RE, Silverberg S: Ultrastructure of congenital cystic adenomatoid malformation of lung. Ultrastr Pathol 3:217–228, 1982.

131. Madewell JE, Stocker JT, Korsower JM: Cystic adenomatoid malformation of the lung. Morphologic analysis. Am J Roentgenol Rad Ther Nucl Med 124:436–448, 1975.

132. Tucker TT, Smith WL, Smith JA: Fluid-filled cystic adenomatoid malformation. AJR 129:323–325, 1977.

133. Gaisie G, Oh KS: Spontaneous pneumothorax in cystic adenomatoid malformation. Pediatr Radiol 13:281–283, 1983.

134. Nishibayashi SW, Andrassy RJ, Woolley MM: Congenital cystic adenomatoid malformation: A 30-year experience. J Pediatr Surg 16:704–706, 1981.

135. Craig JM, Kirkpatrick J, Neuhauser EBD: Congenital cystic adenomatoid malformation of the lung in infants. Am J Roentgenol Rad Ther Nucl Med 76:516–526, 1956.

136. Halloran LG, Silverberg SG, Salzberg AM: Congenital cystic adenomatoid malformation of the lung. A surgical emergency. Arch Surg 104:715–719, 1972.

137. Bale PM: Congenital cystic malformation of the lung. A form of congenital bronchiolar ("adenomatoid") malformation. Am J Clin Pathol 71:411–420, 1979.

138. Miller RK, Sieber WK, Yunis EJ: Congenital adenomatoid malformation of the lung. A report of 17 cases and review of the literature. Pathol Annu 15(prt 1):387–407, 1980.

139. Avitabile AM, Greco MA, Hulnick DH, Feiner HD: Congenital cystic adenomatoid malformation of the lung in adults. J Surg Pathol 8:193–202, 1984.

140. Stauffer UG, Savoldelli G, Muth D: Antenatal ultrasound diagnosis in cystic adenomatoid malformation of the lung—case report. J Pediatr Surg 19:141–142, 1984.

141. Hutchin P, Friedman PJ, Saltzstein SL: Congenital cystic adenomatoid malformation with anomalous blood supply. J Thorac Cardiovasc Surg 62:220–225, 1974.

142. Glaves J, Baker JC: Spontaneous resolution of maternal hydramnios in congenital cystic adenomatoid malformation of the lung. Antenatal ultrasound features. Case report. Br J Obstet Gynaecol 90:1065–1068, 1983.

143. Adzick NS, Harrison MR, Glick PL: Fetal cystic adenomatoid malformation: Prenatal diagnosis and natural history. J Pediatr Surg 20:483–488, 1985.

144. Fisher JE, Nelson SJ, Allen JE, Holzman RS: Congenital cystic adenomatoid malformation of the lung. A unique variant. Am J Dis Child 136:1071–1074, 1982.

145. Cachia R, Sobonya RE: Congenital cystic adenomatoid malformation of the lung with bronchial atresia. Hum Pathol 12:947–950, 1981.

146. Krous HF, Sexauer CL: Embryonal rhabdomyosarcoma arising within a congenital bronchogenic cyst in a child. J Pediatr Surg 16:506–508, 1981.

147. Holland-Moritz RM, Heyn RM: Pulmonary blastoma associated with cystic lesions in children. Med Pediatr Oncol 12:85–88, 1984.

148. Shannon MP, Grantmyre EB, Reid WD, Wotherspoon AS: Congenital pulmonary lymphangiectasis. Report of two cases. Pediatr Radiol 2:235–240, 1974.

149. Case records of the Massachusetts General Hospital (case 30-1980). N Engl J Med 303:270–276, 1980.

150. Baltaxe HA, Lee JG, Ehlers KH, Engle MA: Pulmonary lymphangiectasis demonstrated by lymphangiography in two patients with Noonan's syndrome. Radiology 115:149–153, 1975.

151. Gardner TW, Domm AC, Brock CE, Pruitt AW: Congenital pulmonary lymphangiectasis. A case complicated by chylothorax. Clin Pediatr 22:75–78, 1983.

152. Hernandez RJ, Stern AM, Rosentahl A: Pulmonary lymphangiectasis in Noonan syndrome. AJR 134:75–80, 1980.

153. Bhatti MAK, Ferrante JW, Gielchinsky I, Norman JC: Pleuropulmonary and skeletal lymphangiomatosis with chylothorax and chylopericardium. Ann Thorac Surg 40:398–401, 1985.

154. Wagenaar SS, Swierenga J, Wagenvoort CA: Late presentation of primary pulmonary lymphangiectasis. Thorax 33:791–795, 1978.

155. Katzenstein A-LA, Askin FB: *Surgical Pathology of Nonneoplastic Lung Disease.* Philadelphia: WB Saunders, 1982.

156. Miller KE, Edwards DK, Hilton S, et al.: Acquired lobar emphysema in premature infants with bronchopulmonary dysplasia: An iatrogenic disease? Radiology 138:589–592, 1981.

157. Nagaraj HS, Shott R, Fellows R, Yacoub U: Recurrent lobar atelectasis due to acquired bronchial stenosis in neonates. J Pediatr Surg 15:411–415, 1980.

158. Iancu T, Boyanover Y, Eilam N, et al.: Infantile sub-lobar emphysema and tracheal bronchus. Acta Paediatr Scand 64:551–554, 1975.

159. Daniel T, Woodring JH, Vandiviere HM, Wilson HD: Swyer-James syndrome—unilateral hyperlucent lung syndrome. A case report and review. Clin Pediatr 23:393–397, 1984.

160. Allen CI, Newhouse MT: Gastroesophageal reflux and chronic respiratory disease. Am Rev Resp Dis 129:645–647, 1984.

161. Azizirad H, Polgar G, Bonns PR: Bronchiolitis obliterans. Clin Pediatr 14:572, 1975.

162. Hallman M: Fetal development of surfactant: Considerations of phosphatidylcholine, phosphatidylinositol and phosphatidyl-glycerol formation. Prog Resp Res 15:27–40, 1981.

163. Comroe JH Jr: Premature science and immature lungs (parts I–III). Am Rev Respir Dis 116:127–135, 311–323, 497–518. 1977.

164. Perelman RH, Engle MJ, Farrell PM: Perspectives on fetal lung development. Lung 159:53–80, 1981.

165. Rooney SA: The surfactant system and lung phospholipid biochemistry. Am Rev Respir Dis 131:439–460, 1985.

166. Raivo KO, Hallman N, Kowalainer K, Valimaki I (eds): *Respiratory Distress Syndrome.* London: Academic Press, 1984.

167. Nelson GH (ed): *Pulmonary development. Transition from Intrauterine to Extrauterine Life.* New York: Marcel Dekker, 1985.

168. Lauweryns JM: "Hyaline membrane disease" in newborn infants. Macroscopic, radiographic and light and electron microscopic studies. Hum Pathol 175–204, 1970.

169. Robertson B, Ivemark BI: The association between trabecular rarefaction in the costochondral junction and the idiopathic respiratory distress syndrome. Biol Neonate 16:342–353, 1970.

170. Rosan RC: Hyaline membrane disease and a related spectrum of neonatal pneumonopathies. Perspect Pediatr Pathol 2:15–60, 1975.

171. Shanklin DR: Criteria for diagnosis of hyaline membrane disease. Arch Pathol 99:345–346, 1975.

172. Gruenwald P: Exaggerated atelectasis of prematurity. A complication of recovery from the respiratory distress syndrome. Arch Pathol 86:81–85, 1968.

173. Doshi N, Klionsky B, Kanbour A: Yellow hyaline membrane disease in neonates: Clinical diagnosis by tracheal aspiration cytology. Pediatr Pathol 1:193–198, 1983.

174. Boss JH, Craig JM: Reparative phenomena in lungs of neonates with hyaline membranes. Pediatrics 29:890–898, 1962.

175. Gittenberger-de Groot AC, vanErtbruggen I, Moulaert AJMG, Harinck E: The ductus arteriosus in the preterm infant: Histologic and clinical observations. J Pediatr 96:88–93, 1980.

176. Smith ORS, Cook DH, Izukawa T, et al.: Surgical management of patent ductus arteriosus in newborn infants of low birthweights. Arch Dis Child 56:436–439, 1981.

177. King DT, Emmanouilides GC, Andrews JC, Hirose FM: Morphologic evidence of accelerated closure of the ductus arteriosus in preterm infants. Pediatrics 65:872–880, 1980.

178. Green TP, Thompson RT, Johnson DE, Lock JE: Furosemide promotes patent ductus arteriosus in premature infants with the respiratory-distress syndrome. N Engl J Med 208:743–748, 1983.

179. Jacob J, Gluck L, DiSessa T, et al.: The contribution of PDA in the neonate with severe RDS. J Pediatr 96:79–87, 1980.

180. Oh KS, Bowe AD, Park SC, et al.: Patent ductus arteriosus. Its occurrence with unequal pulmonary vascularity and hyperlucent left lung. Am J Dis Child 135:637–639, 1981.

181. Benjamin DR, Wiegenstein L: Necrosis of the ductus arteriosus in premature infants. Arch Pathol 94:340–342, 1972.

182. Kirks DR, McCook TA, Serwer GA, Oldham HN Jr: Aneurysm of the ductus arteriosus in the neonate. AJR 134:573–576, 1980.

183. Ahlstrom H, Mortenson W, Robertson B: Alveolar lesions in bronchopulmonary dysplasia. OPMEAR 29:102–105, 1984.

184. Anderson WR, Engel RR: Cardiopulmonary sequelae of reparative stages of bronchopulmonary dysplasia. Arch Pathol Lab Med 107:603–608, 1983.

185. Bonikos DS, Bensch KG, Northway WH Jr, Edwards DK: Bronchopulmonary dysplasia: The pulmonary pathologic sequel of necrotizing bronchiolitis and pulmonary fibrosis. Hum Pathol 7:643–666, 1976.

186. Nickerson BG: Bronchopulmonary dysplasia. Chronic pulmonary disease following neonatal respiratory failure. Chest 87:528–535, 1984.

187. O'Brodovich HM, Mellins RB: Bronchopulmonary dysplasia. Unresolved neonatal acute lung injury. Am Rev Respir Dis 132:694–709, 1985.

188. Vodovar M, Voyer M, Belloy C, et al.: Dysplasie bronchopulmonaire. Semin Hop Paris 59:2759–2768, 1983.

189. Sobonya RE, Logvinoff MM, Taussig LM, Theriault A: Morphometric analysis of the lung in prolonged bronchopulmonary dysplasia. Pediatr Res 16:969–972, 1982.

190. Oppermann HC, Wille L, Bleyl U, Obladen M: Bronchopulmonary dysplasia in premature infants. A radiological and pathological correlation. Pediatr Radiol 5:137–141, 1977.

191. Swischuk LE: Bubbles in hyaline membrane disease. Radiology 122:417–426, 1977.

192. Tou SS, Farrell PM, Leavitt LA, et al.: Clinical and roentgenographic scoring systems for assessing bronchopulmonary dysplasia. Am J Dis Child 138:581–585, 1984.

193. Merritt TA, Puccia JM, Stuard ID: Cytologic evaluation of pulmonary effluent in neonates with respiratory distress syndrome and bronchopulmonary dysplasia. Acta Cytol 25:631–639, 1981.

194. McKay CA Jr, Faulkner CS II, Edwards WH: Unusual pulmonary reaction to respiratory therapy in a premature newborn. Hum Pathol 16:629–631, 1985.

195. Hodgman JE, Mikity VG, Tatter D, Cleland RS: Chronic respiratory distress in the premature infant. Wilson-Mikity syndrome. Pediatrics 44:179–195, 1969.

196. Edwards DK, Jacob J, Gluck L: The immature lung: Radiographic appearance course and complications. AJR 135:659–666, 1980.

197. O'Bara H, Pappas CT, Northway WH Jr, Beusch KG: Comparison of the effect of two and six week exposure to 80% and 100% oxygen on the lung of the newborn mouse: a quantitative SEM and TEM correlative study. Int J Radiation Oncol Biol Phys 11:285–298, 1985.

198. Levine MI, Batisti O, Wigglesworth JS, et al.: A prospective study of intrapulmonary fat accumulation in the newborn lung following intralipid infusion. Acta Paediatr Scand 73:454–460, 1984.

199. Koops BL, Abman SH, Accurso FJ: Outpatient management and follow-up of bronchopulmonary dysplasia. Clin Perinatol 11:101–122, 1984

200. Werthammer J, Brown ER, Neff RK, Taeusch HW Jr: Sudden infant death syndrome in infants with bronchopulmonary dysplasia. Pediatrics 69:301–304, 1982.

201. Bertrand J-M, Riley SP, Popkin J, Coates AL: The long-term pulmonary sequelae of prematurity: The role of familial airway hyperreactivity and the respiratory distress syndrome. N Engl J Med 312:742–745, 1985.

202. Mayo P, Saha SP: Spontaneous pneumothorax in the newborn. Am Surg 49:192–195, 1983.

203. Stocker JT, Madewell JE: Persistent interstitial pulmonary emphysema: Another complication of the respiratory distress syndrome. Pediatrics 59:847–852, 1977.

204. Smith TH, Currarino G, Rutledge JC: Spontaneous occurrence of localized pulmonary interstitial and endolymphatic emphysema in infancy. Pediatr Radiol 14:142–145, 1984.

205. Wood BP, Anderson VM, Mauk JE, Merritt TA: Pulmonary lymphatic air: Locating "pulmonary interstitial emphysema" of the premature infant. AJR 138:809–814, 1982.

206. Zimmermann H: Progressive interstitial pulmonary lobar emphysema. Eur J Pediatr 138:258–262, 1982.

207. Madansky DL, Lawson EE, Chernick V, Taeusch HW Jr.: Pneumothorax and other forms of pulmonary air leak in newborns. Am Rev Respir Dis 120:729–737, 1979.

208. Oppermann HC, Wille L, Obladen M, Richter E: Systemic air embolism in the respiratory distress syndrome of the newborn. Pediatr Radiol 8:139–145, 1979.

209. Plenat F, Vert P, Didier F, Andre M: Pulmonary interstitial emphysema. Clin Perinatol 5:351–375, 1978.

210. Bauer CR, Brennan MJ, Coyle C, Poole CA: Surgical resection for pulmonary interstitial emphysema in the newborn infants. J Pediatr 93:656–661, 1978.
211. Levine DH, Trump DS, Waterkotte G: Unilateral pulmonary interstitial emphysema: A surgical approach to treatment. Pediatrics 68:510–514, 1981.
212. Clarke TA, Edwards DK: Pulmonary pseudocysts in newborn infants with respiratory distress syndrome. AJR 133:417–421, 1979.
213. Esterly JR, Oppenheimer EH: Massive pulmonary hemorrhage in the newborn. I. Pathologic considerations. J Pediatr 69:3–11, 1966.
214. Trompeter R, Yu VYH, Aynsley-Green A, Roberton NRC: Massive pulmonary haemorrhage in the newborn infant. Arch Dis Child 50:123–127, 1975.
215. Castile RG, Kleinberg F: The pathogenesis and management of massive pulmonary hemorrhage in the neonate. Case report of a normal survivor. Mayo Clin Proc 51:155–158, 1976.
216. Kotas RV, Wells TJ, Mims LC, et al.: A new model for neonatal pulmonary hemorrhage research. Pediatr Res 9:161–165, 1975.
217. Fedrick J, Butler NR: Certain causes of neonatal death. Massive pulmonary haemorrhage. Biol Neonate 18:243–262, 1971.
218. Bacsik RD: Meconium aspiration syndrome. Pediatr Clin N Am 24:463–479, 1977.
219. Hoffman RR Jr, Campbell RE, Decker JP: Fetal aspiration syndrome. Clinical, roentgenologic and pathologic features. AJR 122:90–96, 1974.
220. Jose JH, Schreiner RL, Lemons JA, et al.: The effect of amniotic fluid aspiration on pulmonary function in the adult and newborn rabbit. Pediatr Res 17:976–981, 1983.
221. Manning FA, Schreiber J, Turkel SB: Fatal meconium aspiration "in utero": A case report. Am J Obstet Gynecol 132:111–113, 1978.
222. Murphy JD, Vawter GF, Reid LM: Pulmonary vascular disease in fatal meconium aspiration. J Pediatr 104:758–762, 1984.
223. Ohlsson A, Cumming WA, Najjar H: Neonatal aspiration syndrome due to vernix caseosa. Pediatr Radiol 15:193–195, 1985.
224. Naeye RL, Tafari N: *Risk Factors in Pregnancy and Diseases of the Fetus and Newborn.* Baltimore: Williams & Wilkins, 1983.
225. Remington JS, Klein JO, (eds): *Infectious Diseases of the Fetus and Newborn Infant*, 2nd ed. Philadelphia: WB Saunders, 1983.
226. Craig JM: Group B beta hemolytic streptococcal sepsis in the newborn. Perspect Pediatr Pathol 6:139, 1982.
227. Gilbert GL, Garland SM: Perinatal Group B streptococcal infections. Med J Aust 1:566, 1983.
228. Baker C: Group B streptococcal infections. Adv Intern Med 25:475, 1980.
229. Yamaki S, Wagenvoort CA: Comparison of primary plexogenic arteriopathy in adults and children. A morphometric study in 40 patients. Br Heart J 54:428–434, 1985.
230. Perkin RM, Anas NG: Pulmonary hypertension in pediatric patients. J Pediatr 105:511–522, 1984.
231. Haworth SG: Pulmonary vascular disease in different types of congenital heart disease. Implications for interpretation of lung biopsy findings in early childhood. Br Heart J 52:551–571, 1984.
232. Rabinovitch M, Keane JF, Norwood WI, et al.: Vascular structure in lung tissue obtained at biopsy correlated with pulmonary hemodynamic findings after repair of congenital heart defects. Circulation 69:655–667, 1984.
233. Haworth SG: Primary and secondary pulmonary hypertension in childhood: A clinicopathological reappraisal. Curr Top Pathol 73:92–152, 1983.
234. Fox WW, Duara S: Persistent pulmonary hypertension in the neonate: diagnosis and management. J Pediatr 103:505–514, 1983.
235. Murphy JD, Rabinovitch M, Goldstein JD, Reid LM: The structural basis of persistent pulmonary hypertension of the newborn infant. J Pediatr 98:962–967, 1981.
236. Geggel RL, Reid LM: The structural basis of PPHN. Clin Perinatol 11:525–549, 1984.
237. Levine DL: Primary pulmonary hypoplasia. J Pediatr 95:550–551, 1979. (This article really is about pulmonary hypertension.)
238. Rudolph AM: High pulmonary vascular resistance after birth. 1. Pathophysiologic considerations and etiologic classification. Clin Pediatr 19:585–590, 1980.
239. Stenmark KR, James SL, Voelkel NF, et al.: Leukotrienes C_4 and D_4 in neonates with hypoxia and pulmonary hypertension. N Engl J Med 309:77–80, 1983.
240. Levin DL, Weinberg AG, Perkin RM: Pulmonary microthrombi syndrome in newborn infants with unresponsive pulmonary hypertension. J Pediatr 102:299–303, 1983.
241. Morrow WR, Haas JE, Benjamin DR: Nonbacterial endocardial thrombosis in neonates: Relationship to persistent fetal circulation. J Pediatr 100:117–122, 1982.
242. Stocker JT, McGill LC, Orsini EN: Post-infarction peripheral cysts of the lung in pediatric patients: A possible cause of idiopathic spontaneous pneumothorax. Pediatr Pulmonol 1:7–18, 1985.
243. Rendas A, Brown ER, Avery ME, Reid LM: Prematurity, hypoplasia of the pulmonary vascular bed, and hypertension: Fatal outcome in a ten-month-old infant. Am Rev Respir Dis 121:873–880, 1980.
244. Cullen ML, Klein MD, Philippart AI: Congenital diaphramatic hernia. Surg Clin North Am 65:1115–1138, 1985.
245. Woolley MM: Congenital posterolateral diaphragmatic hernia. Surg Clin North Amer 56:317–327, 1976.
246. Paris F, Blasco E, Canto KA, et al.: Diaphragmatic eventration in infants. Thorax 28:66–72, 1973.
247. Siegel MJ, Shackelford GD, McAlister WH: Left-sided congenital diaphragmatic hernia: delayed presentation. AJR 137:43–46, 1981.
248. Stahl GE, Warren WS, Rosenberg H, et al.: Congenital right diaphragmatic hernia. A case report and review of the literature. Clin Pediatr 20:422–425, 1981.
249. Srousi M, Buck B, Downes JJ: Congenital diaphragmatic hernia: Deleterious effects of pulmonary interstitial emphysema and tension extrapulmonary air. J Pediatr Surg 16:45–54, 1981.
250. Booker DD, Meerstadt PWD, Bush GH: Congenital diaphragmatic hernia in the older child. Arch Dis Child 56:253–257, 1981.
251. Puri P, Gorman F: Lethal nonpulmonary anomalies associated with congenital diaphragmatic hernia: Implications for early intrauterine surgery. J Pediatr Surg 19:29–32, 1984.
252. Wolff G: Familial congenital diaphragmatic defect: Review and conclusions. Hum Genet 54:1–5, 1980.

253. Gillot F, Quezede J, Sellah A: L'interposition hepato-diaphragmatique du colon chez l'enfant. Syndrome de Chilaiditi. Arch Franc Pediatr 34:248–257, 1977.

254. Cloutier R, Rournier L, Levasseur L: Reversion to fetal circulation in congenital diaphragmatic hernia: A preventable postoperative complication. J Pediatr Surg 18:551–554, 1983.

255. Harrison MR, Adzick NS, Nakayana DK, de Lorimer AA: Fetal diaphragmatic hernia: Fatal but fixable. Semin Perinatol 9:103–112, 1985.

256. Geggel RL, Murphy JD, Langleben D, et al.: Congenital diaphragmatic hernia: Arterial structural changes and persistent pulmonary hypertension after surgical repair. J Pediatr 107:457–464, 1985.

257. Thurlbeck WM, Kida K, Langston C, et al.: Postnatal lung growth after repair of diaphragmatic hernia. Thorax 34:338–343, 1979.

258. Hart JC, Cohen IT, Ballantine TVN, Varrano LF: Accessory diaphragm in an infant. J Pediatr Surg 16:947–949, 1981.

259. Devgan BK, Brodeur AE: Apical pneumatocele. Arch Otolaryngol 102:121–123, 1976.

260. Oppenheimer EH, Esterly JR: Pathology of cystic fibrosis Review of the literature and comparison with 146 autopsied cases. Perspect Pediatr Pathol 2:241–278, 1975.

261. Boucher RC, Knowles MR, Stutts MJ, Gatzy JT: Epithelial dysfunction in cystic fibrosis lung disease. Lung 161:1–17, 1983.

262. Tomashefski JF, Bruce M, Stern RC, et al.: Pulmonary air cysts in cystic fibrosis: Relation of pathologic features to radiologic findings and history of pneumothorax. Hum Pathol 16:253–261, 1985.

263. Littlefield JW: Research on cystic fibrosis (editorial). N Engl J Med 304:44–45, 1981.

264. Wood RE, Boat TF, Doershuk CF: Cystic fibrosis. Am Rev Respir Dis 113:833–878, 1976.

265. Marmon L, Schidlow D, Palmer J, et al.: Pulmonary resection for complications of cystic fibrosis. J Pediatr Surg 18:811–815, 1983.

266. Case records of the Massachusetts General Hospital (case 6-1984). N Engl J Med 310:375–383, 1984.

267. Freidman PJ, Harwood IR, Ellenbogen PH: Pulmonary cystic fibrosis in the adult: Early and late radiologic findings with pathologic correlation. AJR 1131–1144, 1981.

268. Wang EEL, Prober CG, Manson B, et al.: Association of respiratory viral infections with pulmonary deterioration in patients with cystic fibrosis. N Engl J Med 311:1653–1658, 1984.

11 Viral Infections of the Respiratory Tract

Roberta R. Miller

Introduction

Viral respiratory tract infections are common causes of morbidity in patients of all age groups, and important causes of mortality, particularly in infants, elderly individuals, and immunocompromised patients.

While different viruses characteristically damage different areas of the respiratory tract (Table 11–1), there is sufficient overlap to make clinical and anatomic patterns of involvement not particularly useful as a classification scheme. An upper respiratory tract illness is defined[1] as any combination of nasal obstruction, nasal catarrh, sneezing, sinusitis, sinus pain, sore or scratchy throat, and hoarseness or loss of voice. A lower respiratory tract illness is defined as cough with purulent sputum, shortness of breath, and wheezing that are either new or increased over the usual level. Since laryngitis produces upper respiratory tract symptoms and tracheobronchitis produces lower respiratory tract symptoms, a logical anatomic point of division between the upper and lower respiratory tracts is the inferior aspect of the cricoid cartilage or first tracheal ring.

Four clinical syndromes have been described in association with viral infection of the respiratory tract.[1a] A "cold" includes tonsillopharyngitis, pharyngitis, sinusitis, otitis media, and epiglottitis and is characterized by upper respiratory tract symptoms as defined above. The "influenza syndrome" includes abrupt fever, headache, myalgia, and malaise. Lower respiratory tract symptoms are found in only about 10 percent of cases, and most of the patients with this complication are elderly or chronically ill. The "influenza syndrome" does not necessarily imply influenza virus etiology. The "acute bronchitis" syndrome refers to productive cough without radiographic or clinical pneumonia. The "pneumonia" syndrome refers to diffuse interstitial infiltrates radiologically with or without cough and dyspnea. These symptoms correlate poorly with any specific viral etiologic agent.

In a review[2] of radiologic findings in lower respiratory tract viral infections, patterns of involvement are divided into four groups. Bronchial and perihilar shadows were found in most patients, 3- to 6-mm lobular parenchymal infiltrates were found in over half of patients, 7- to 10-mm coalescent parenchymal infiltrates were occasionally found, and 40 percent of patients had 1- to 2-mm nodular shadows, but there was no correlation between pattern of involvement and the responsible viral agent. Indeed, the radiographic pattern of involvement cannot reliably distinguish between bacterial and viral pneumonia in all cases.[3]

The "gold standard" for identification of viruses is culture of the agent from secretions or tissue, although this technique is not available in all hospitals, and may give false-negative results if not employed early in the course of the disease. For these reasons, a variety of other laboratory techniques for viral diagnosis have been developed and are described in detail in reviews.[4,5] These techniques include serologic diagnosis, microscopy, detection of structural or enzymatic viral protein, and detection of viral nucleic acid.

Serologic diagnosis in general requires paired acute and convalescent sera to demonstrate a rise in virus-specific antibody titers.

Several microscopic techniques are available for viral diagnosis. Demonstration of viral antigen in nasopharyngeal secretions by fluorescent antibody techniques has been shown to be reliable in the diagnosis of infection with respiratory syncytial virus (RSV), parainfluenza, influenza, adenovirus, and measles.[6] In fact, in some cases of parainfluenza, influenza A, and RSV infection, viral antigen may be detected in cells by immunofluorescence even after the agent can no longer be cultured.[7,8] The greater sensitivity of immunofluorescent techniques over culture occurs relatively late in the

148 Viral Infections of the Respiratory Tract

Table 11–1. Morphologic Patterns of Reaction to Viral Infections

Agent	Upper Respiratory Tract Infection	Laryngo-tracheo-bronchitis	Bronchiolitis	Diffuse Alveolar Damage	Hemorrhagic Necrotic Nodules	Inclusions
Influenza	+[a]	+	+	+	−	−
Measles	−	+	+	+[d]	−	+
Parainfluenza	+[b]	+[a]	Occasional	Occasional[d]	−	−
Respiratory syncytial virus	+[b]	+	+[c]	Occasional	−	Occasional
Picornaviridae and Coronaviridae	+	Occasional	Rare	Rare	−	−
Adenovirus	+	+	+	+	−	+
Herpes simplex	−	+[d]	+[d]	Occasional[d]	+[d]	+
Varicella-zoster	−	Rare[d]	+[b,d]	+	+[b,d]	r
Cytomegalovirus	−	−	Rare	+[d]	+[d]	+

[a] Especially in children.
[b] Especially in adults.
[c] Especially in infants.
[d] Especially in immunocompromised patients.

course of viral infection, and reflects the fact that only a small amount of viral protein and nucleic acid synthesized in infected cells actually gets assembled into virions, and a minority of newly assembled virions are actually infectious.[5] Fluorescent antibody testing on touch preparations or frozen sections of lung tissue might theoretically be useful, but the technique presents difficulties in interpretation, particularly due to autofluorescence of lung tissue, and is not widely practiced. Attempts to demonstrate viral antigen in formalin-fixed, paraffin-embedded tissue by immunoperoxidase reactions have given disappointing, difficult to interpret results.[5]

A major criterion used to make a microscopic diagnosis of respiratory tract viral infection in tissue sections is the presence of characteristic inclusion bodies. The various inclusions will be discussed under the specific viruses, but it should be stated at the outset that not all cases of proven viral respiratory tract infections have recognizable inclusions (false negatives), and that pseudoinclusions such as particularly prominent nucleoli may lead to erroneous diagnoses as well (false positives).[9] Formalin fixation is poor for preserving the light-microscopic appearance of viral inclusions, and in cases of suspected viral infection, Bouin's fixative provides superior results.

Electron microscopy may be useful in confirming the presence of viral particles, and the electron-microscopic appearance of the various respiratory tract viruses will also be discussed in detail below. Viral particles may be identified in negatively stained preparations from exudates or secretions, or in thin sections of tissue routinely prepared for electron microscopy. The latter technique is particulary useful in that autopsy tissue, formalin-fixed tissue, paraffin-embedded tissue and even 6-μm hematoxylin and eosin–stained tissue on glass slides may be successfully reprocessed for electron-microscopy. Explanations of preparation techniques are beyond the scope of this discussion but are available elsewhere.[10,11] However, there are serious drawbacks in the use of routine electron-microscopy to diagnose viral diseases. "Pseudoviral particles" and preparation artifacts may lead to falsely-positive diagnoses, particularly in poorly preserved material. Related viruses, such as the various members of the Herpetoviridae group, are ultrastructurally indistinguishable. Prolonged search may be required to exclude viral agents with relative assurance.

Detection of viral protein can be accomplished by radioimmmuoassay or enzyme-linked immunospecific assay (ELISA). Finally, detection of viral genome may be

Table 11–2. Common Viral Pathogens of the Respiratory Tract

Virus Family	Viral Agent
RNA Viruses	
Orthomyxoviridae	Influenza A, B, C
Paramyxoviridae	Measles
	Parainfluenza 1–4
	Respiratory syncytial virus
Picornaviridae	Rhinovirus
	Enterovirus
	Coxsackie B
	Echovirus
Coronaviridae	Coronavirus
DNA Viruses	
Adenoviridae	Adenovirus
Herpetoviridae	Herpes simplex 1 and 2
	Varicella-zoster
	Cytomegalovirus

accomplished by nucleic acid sandwich hybridization. This technique has been applied to demonstrate adenovirus,[12] herpes simplex virus (HSV),[5] herpes varicella-zoster (V-Z),[13] and cytomegalovirus (CMV),[14] and sensitivity appears to be comparable to or better than culture. Unfortunately, RNA viruses are more difficult to demonstrate by this technique since their RNA is altered in preparation.[5] However, this obstacle may be overcome by synthesizing complementary DNA from the viral RNA by means of reverse transcriptase.[14a]

The most typical histologic appearance of viral pneumonia is diffuse alveolar damage, often with bronchitis and bronchiolitis. In the earliest stages, there is capillary congestion and edema; hyaline membranes and an interstitial mononuclear cell infiltrate become apparent over the course of a few days. Subsequently, there is proliferation of alveolar epithelial type II cells and these often have enlarged nuclei and prominent eosinophilic nucleoli which may simulate viral inclusions. As discussed elsewhere (*see* Chapter 16), diffuse alveolar damage is a nonspecific pulmonary reaction to many types of injury, but in the appropriate setting, its presence should alert one to the possibility of viral infection.

Table 11–2 classifies the most common respiratory tract viral pathogens.

Influenza

In nonimmunocompromised adults, the overwhelming majority of cases of lower respiratory tract viral infections are caused by influenza.[15] There are three epidemiologic forms of influenza outbreaks: pandemic, regional epidemic, and local sporadic, the latter occurring essentially yearly. All three forms tend to occur during the winter months, the outbreaks are relatively short-lived (2 to 4 weeks), and the clinicopathologic features are similar from outbreak to outbreak.[16]

The epidemiologic patterns of influenza are related to the characteristics of the viruses themselves.[17] Types A, B, and C are antigenically different with respect to the hemagglutinin (H) and neuraminidase (N) antigens. Hemagglutinin antigen is responsible for attaching to the host cell and initiating infection, N antigen is responsible for release of mature virions from infected cells. Influenza A shows continuous changes in the H and N antigens to a much greater degree than types B and C, a

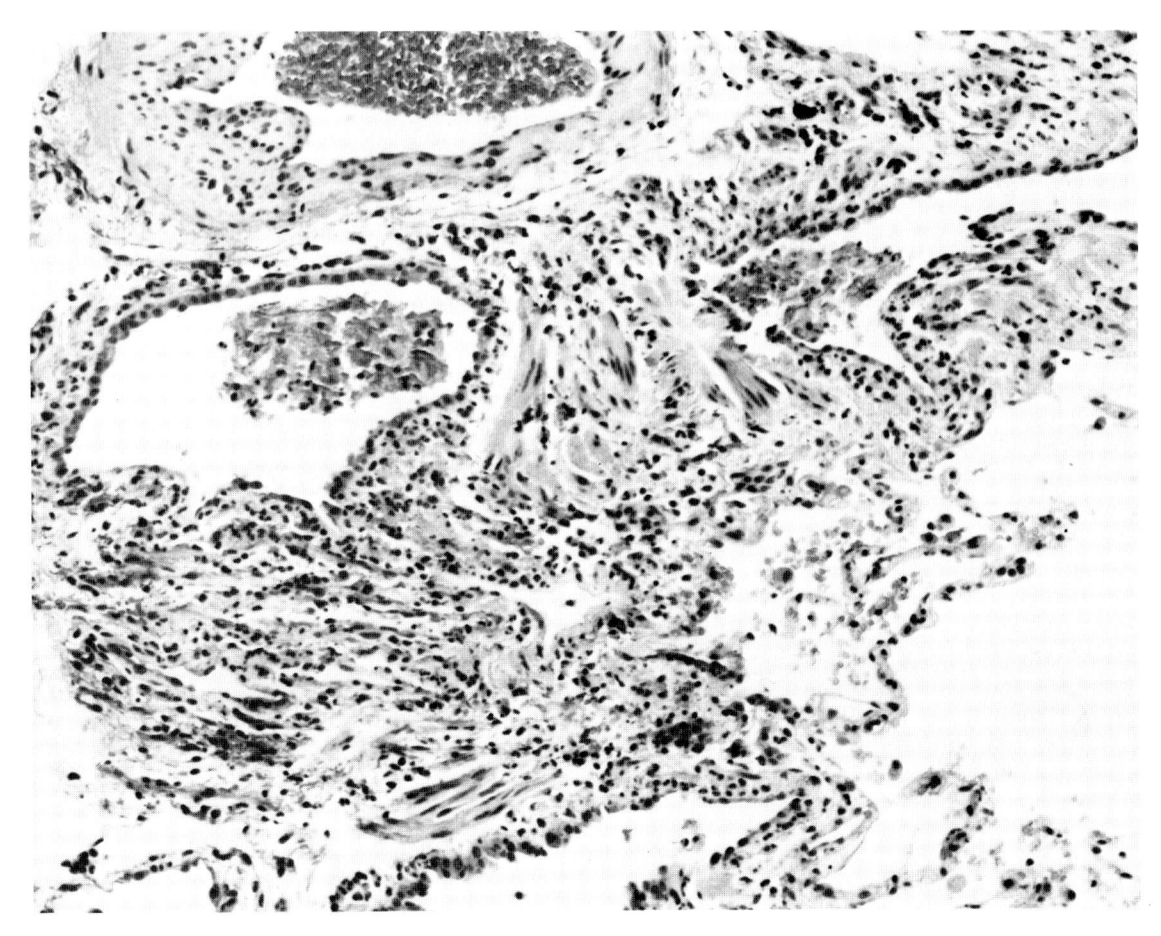

Figure 11–1. Early influenza showing necrotizing bronchiolitis with intralumenal debris (H&E ×180).

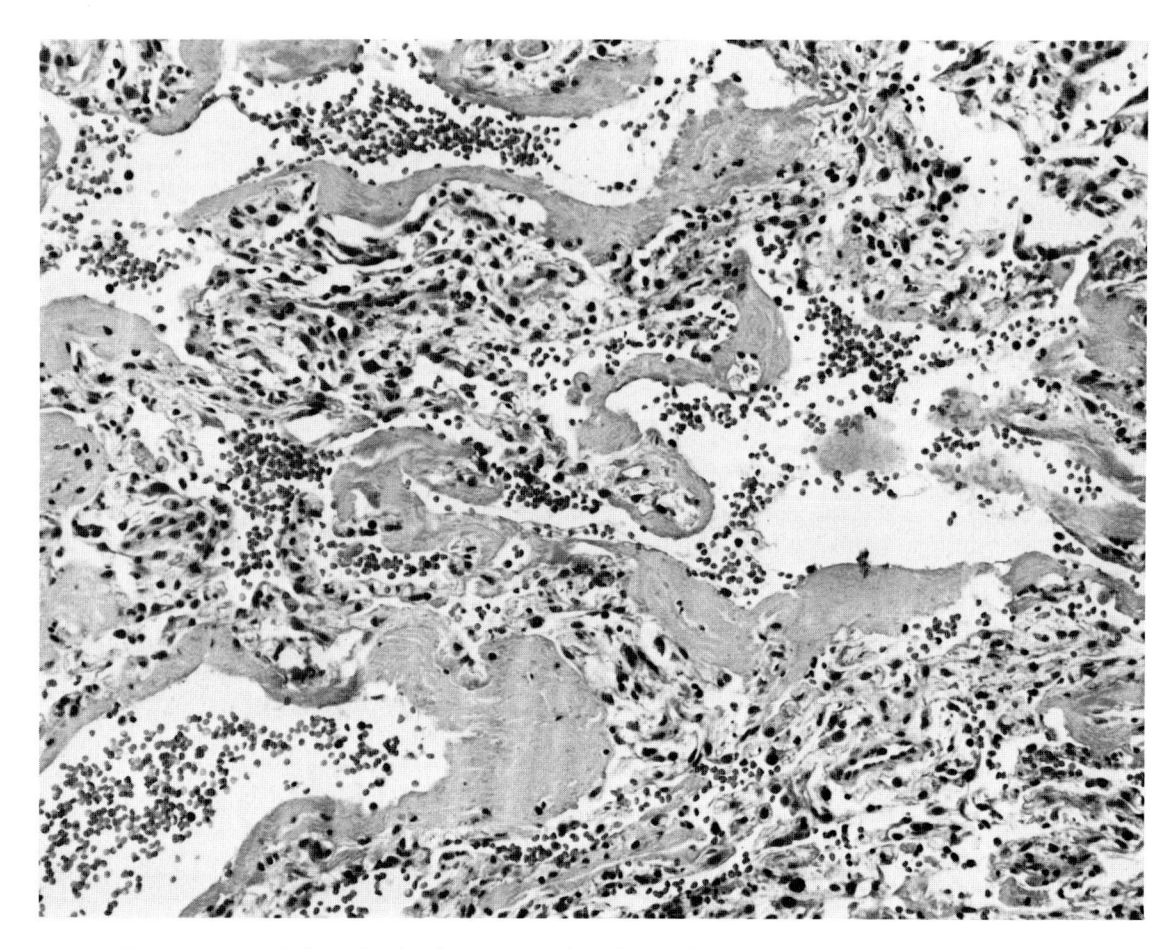

Figure 11–2. Diffuse alveolar damage in early influenza showing extensive hyaline membrane formation (H&E, ×130).

phenomenon referred to as "antigenic drift" which is responsible for epidemics every few years. Influenza A is also capable of undergoing abrupt major "antigenic shifts" which allow for pandemics every 10 to 15 years.

Influenza B illness is not as common as influenza A, but may cause clinically similar disease. In general, influenza C causes only mild upper respiratory tract infections, is considered to be of neglible public health importance[16] and will not be discussed further.

While influenza infection is somewhat unusual in neonates, presumably due to protection by maternal antibodies, older children have a higher incidence of influenza infection than adults, but usually have milder disease with fewer and milder pulmonary symptoms.[15] Disease limited to the upper respiratory tract is not uncommon in childhood influenza[18] and in fact, approximately 40 percent of children requiring hospitalization for influenza infection present with convulsions rather than specific respiratory complaints.[18] Occasional childhood influenza cases may lead to serious postinfection sequelae such as bronchiolitis obliterans,[19] but these complications are uncommon.

Otherwise healthy adults ordinarily recover from influenza lower respiratory tract infection, but there is a serious risk of fatality in the elderly, particularly those with underlying chronic cardiovascular or respiratory diseases, this risk being equal in epidemic and nonepidemic situations.[20]

Morphology

The gross appearance of the lung in influenza pneumonia is nonspecific, as is the case for all viral pneumonias. In fatal cases, the lungs are heavy, edematous, and hemorrhagic, often with increased firmness, and often with obvious tracheobronchitis on gross examination.

Patterns of lower respiratory tract involvement have been divided into three goups[15]: influenza pneumonia followed by bacterial superinfection, concurrent influenza and bacterial pneumonia, and rapidly progressive "pure" viral pneumonia. The first two types account for 80 percent of hospitalized patients, but the third type has the highest mortality rate.

If biopsy or autopsy is performed early in the course of the disease (4 to 10 days), there is conspicuous damage to the conducting airways, with necrotizing bronchitis and bronchiolitis[21,22] (Fig. 11–1), as well as exudative

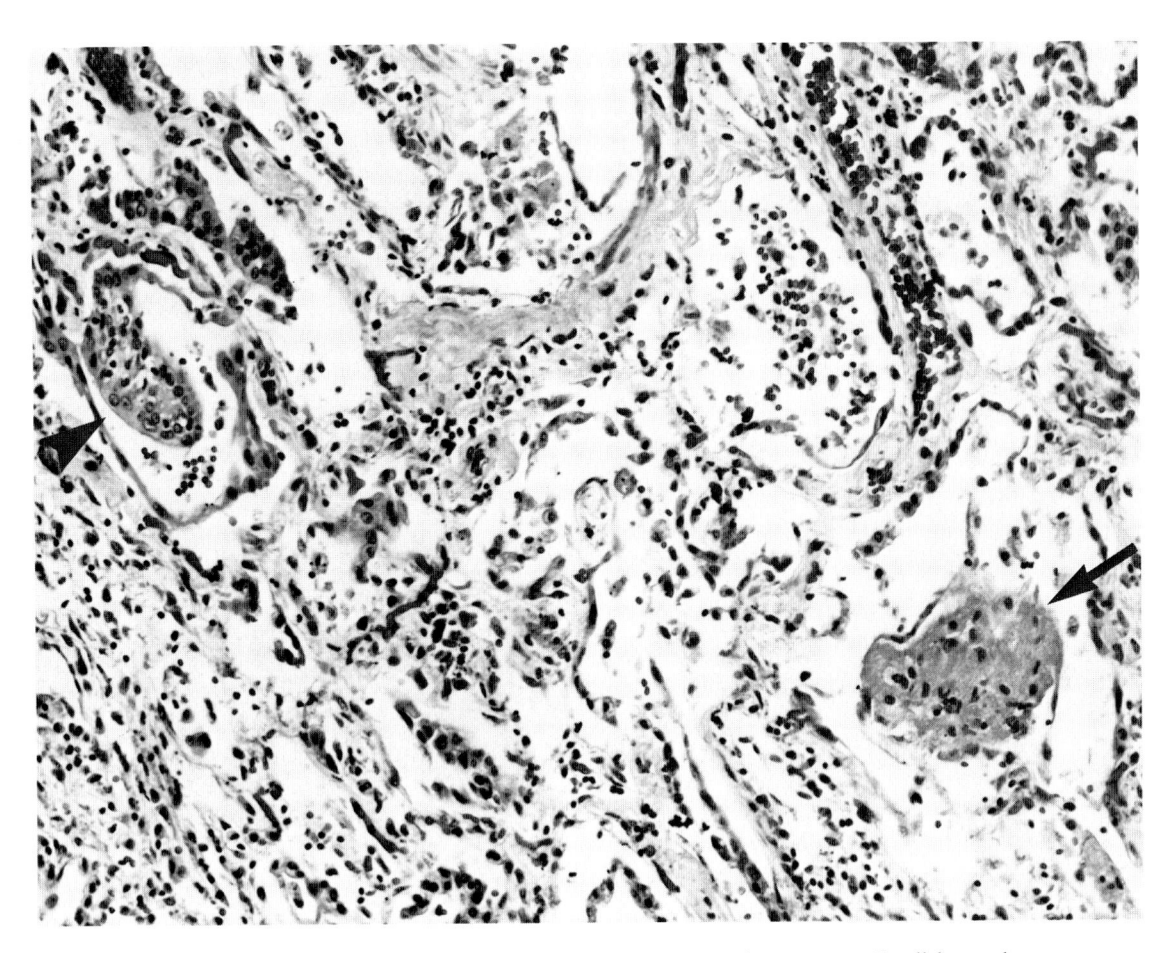

Figure 11–3. Influenza pneumonia of 2 to 3 weeks duration showing type II cell hyperplasia, organizing hyaline membranes (arrow) and squamous metaplasia (arrowhead) (H&E, ×130).

diffuse alveolar damage with hyaline membranes (Fig. 11–2). By 2 to 3 weeks, the conducting airways show organization of the necrotic epithelial and inflammatory debris, and reparative changes, chiefly squamous metaplasia (Figs. 11–3, 11–4). The parenchyma by this time shows organizing diffuse alveolar damage with type II cell proliferation. The lesions may ultimately heal as nonspecific interstitial fibrosis resembling usual interstitial pneumonitis.[22-24]

In some cases of influenza pneumonia, one may be able to discern that damage to conducting airways is worse proximally than distally.[21] This observation correlates with an experimental model of influenza A infection[25,26] in which, in general, less-virulent strains remain confined to the upper respiratory tract, whereas more virulent strains spread down the trachea to produce bronchial and bronchiolar epithelial necrosis in hilar zones worse than mid-zones, and mid-zones worse than peripheral zones, with relative sparing of alveolar epithelial cells.

Light-microscopy of bronchial epithelial cells infected with influenza virus may show intracytoplasmic basophilic "inclusions" but their presence or absence is not diagnostically helpful due to their nonspecific appearance. Negatively stained electron-microscopic preparations of intact viral particles show generally rounded, sometimes pleomorphic particles 80 to 120 nm in diameter with surface projections of H and N antigens.[11] In thin sections for transmission electron microscopy, filamentous nucleocapsid material measuring approximately 10 nm in diameter may be seen in the cytoplasm.

Measles

Asymptomatic chest film changes, both parenchymal and hilar, are frequently seen in otherwise uncomplicated cases of measles (rubeola).[15,27] Pneumonia is the most common complication of measles infection in immunologically competent patients, although the cited incidence varies widely from less than 5 percent to nearly 40 percent.[27,28] Life-threatening or fatal measles pneumonia occurs rarely in children[29] and adults[28] without any apparent background immunologic abnormality, but serious measles pneumonia is much more commonly seen in immunocompromised children.[29-31] The clinical course of complicated measles is quite variable, with respiratory complaints of a few days to several weeks duration. The radiographic appearance is one of diffuse fine nodules 1 to 3 mm in size early in the disease course,

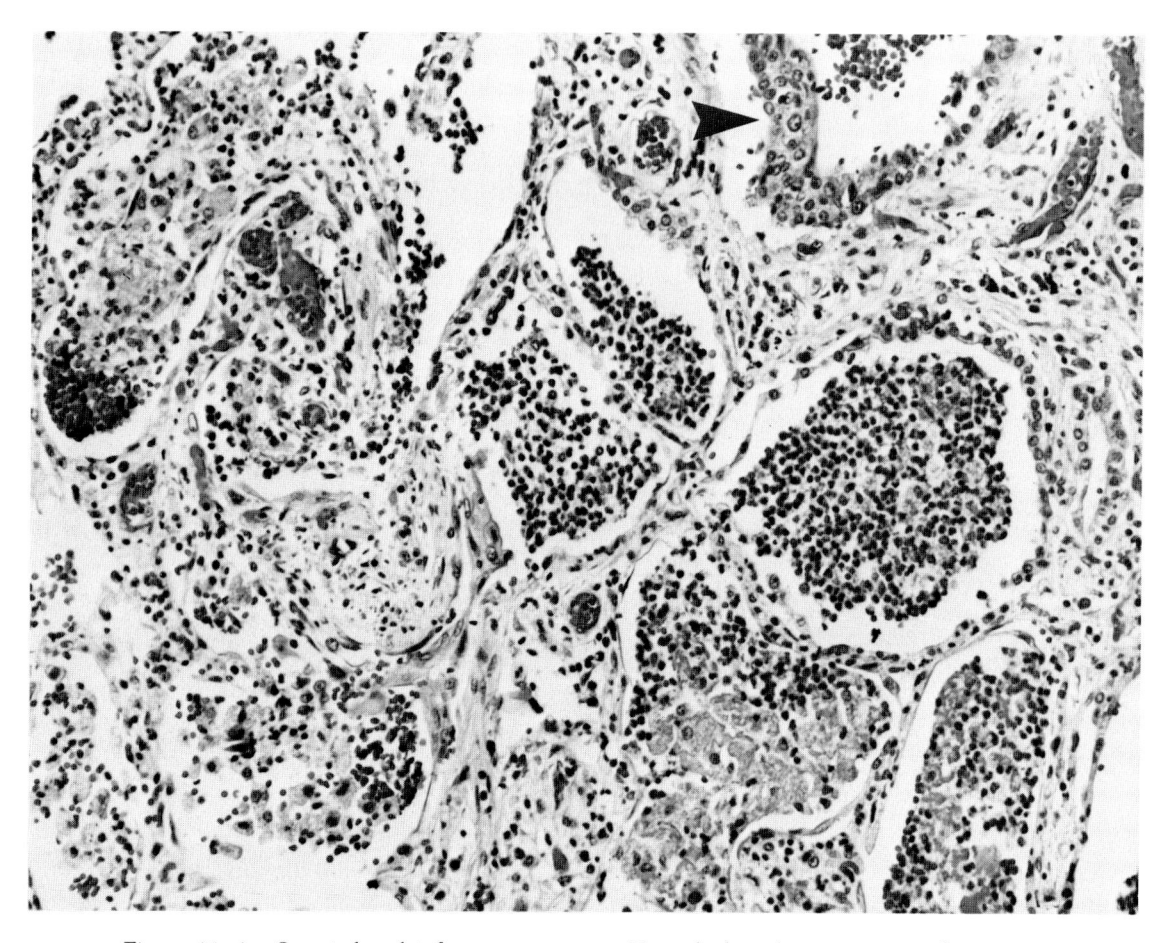

Figure 11-4. Superinfected influenza pneumonia. Note thickened interstitium and squamous metaplasia (arrowhead) (H&E, ×130).

but these become confluent with time and may eventually result in diffuse opacification.[29]

In immunologically competent measles patients, inclusion-bearing giant cells may be seen in epithelia of a variety of organ systems including the upper and lower respiratory tract during the prodromal stages, but these disappear as the characteristic rash develops.[30] There is a relationship between development of rash, presence of tissue giant cells, presence of culturable or immunohistologically identifiable virus in tissue, and antibody response. The development of the rash is thought to be an expression of intact cellular immunity, and in general, the better developed the rash, the fewer the number of giant cells in tissue.[29] Absent or slowly developing rash, persistence of tissue giant cells, persistence of culturable virus, and poor antibody response are all indicators of inadequate reaction to virus and subsequent poor prognosis, and one or more of these factors are characteristically found in fatal cases. The persistence of tissue giant cells in fatal cases is of historical interest, since cases morphologically similar to Hecht's giant cell pneumonia[32] were subsequently proven to be due to measles infection in immune-compromised patients without the typical rash.[33]

Morphology

The gross appearance ranges from essentially normal, to fine nodularity, to a diffusely edematous and hemorrhagic pattern similar to influenza.

Microscopically, one finds epithelial hyperplasia, squamous metaplasia, and occasional inclusions in the trachea and major bronchi, often with a striking extension of this process into the submucosal glands (Fig. 11-5). The terminal and respiratory bronchioles show particularly exuberant hyperplastic and metaplastic changes which extend into the nearby alveoli, provoking a fibroblastic response and giving rise to the nodular quality of the early lesions[29] (Fig. 11-6). The remainder of the parenchyma often shows diffuse alveolar damage with multinucleate giant cells of alveolar epithelial derivation containing intranuclear and intracytoplasmic inclusions (Fig. 11-7; Plate 1).

Intracytoplasmic inclusions precede the development of intranuclear inclusions, and they are often more difficult to identify.[9] They develop in a perinuclear location, then enlarge and acquire an eosinophilic, hyalinized appearance. Intranuclear inclusions begin as tiny eosinophilic bodies which coalesce to a single, relatively

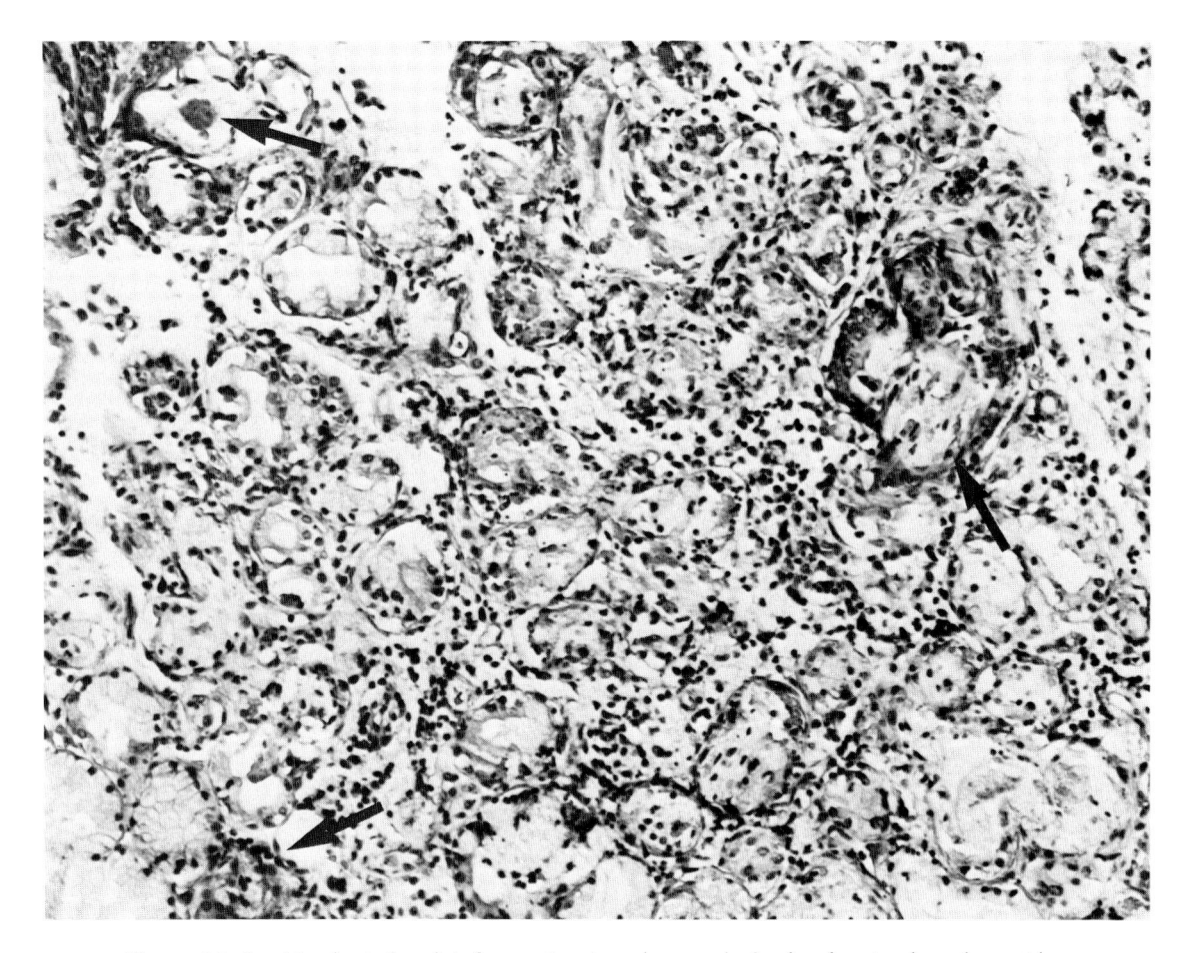

Figure 11–5. Measles-induced inflammation in submucosal glands of major bronchus with scattered multinucleate giant cells (arrows) (H&E, ×118).

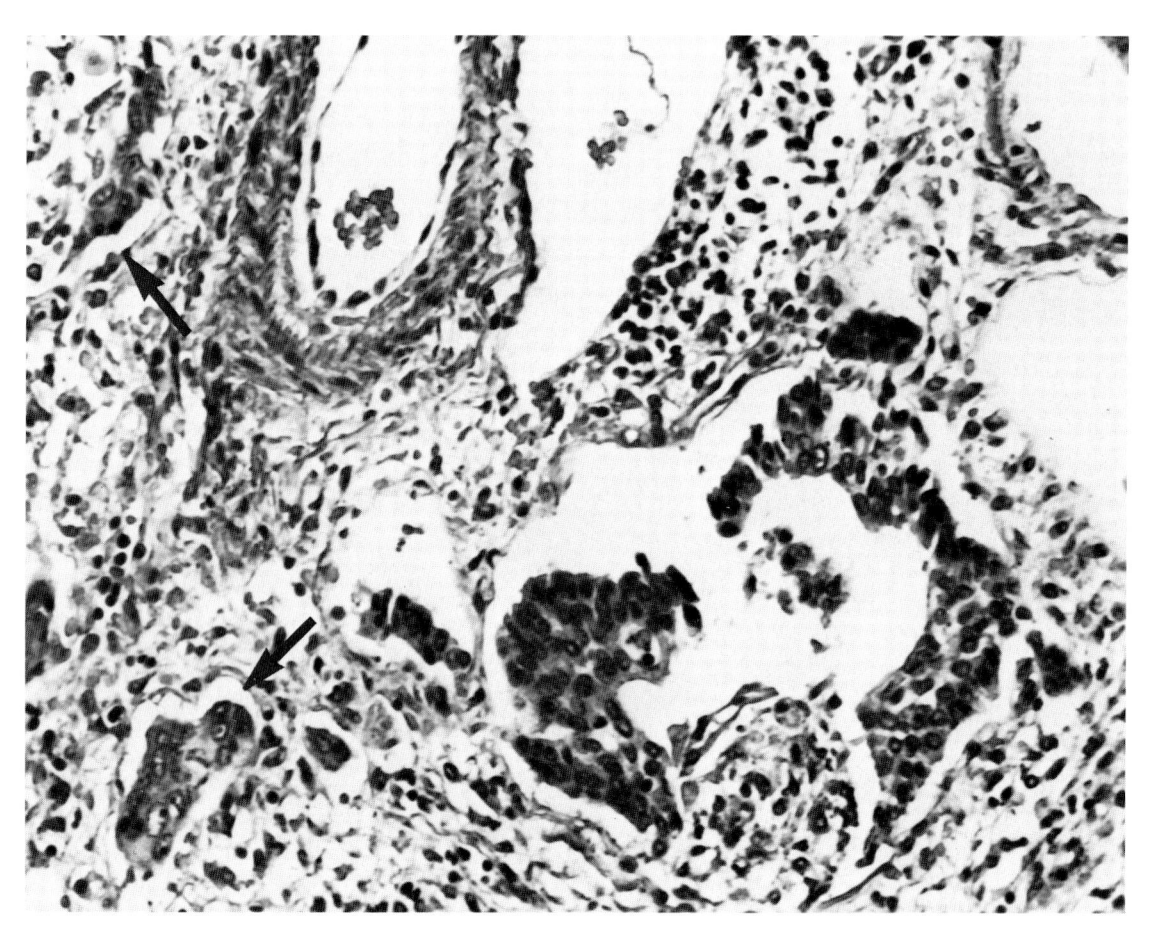

Figure 11–6. Hyperplastic epithelial changes in respiratory bronchiole in measles. Note multinucleated giant cells (arrow) (H&E, ×198).

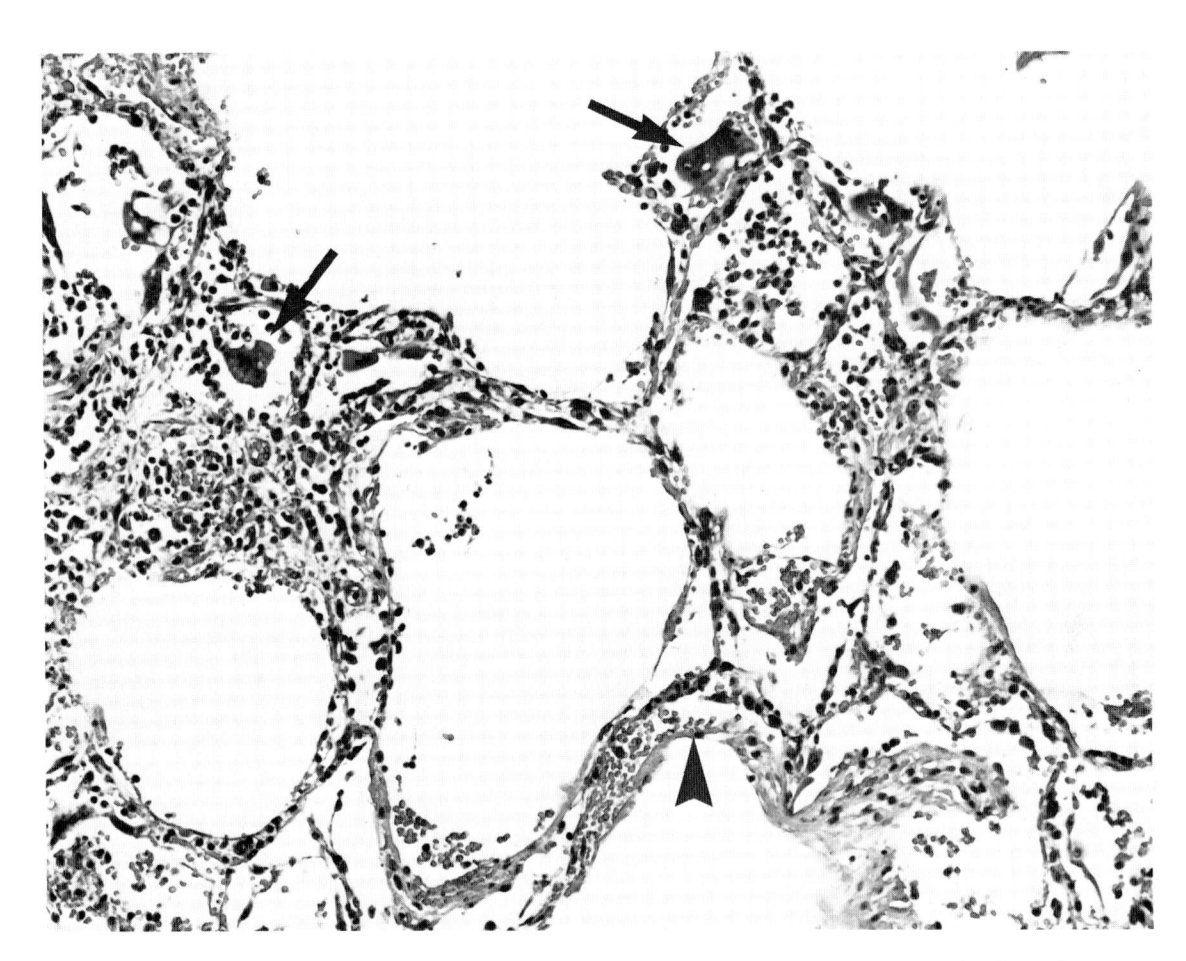

Figure 11–7. Diffuse alveolar damage in measles with hyaline membranes (arrowheads) and multinucleate giant cells (arrows) (H&E, ×115).

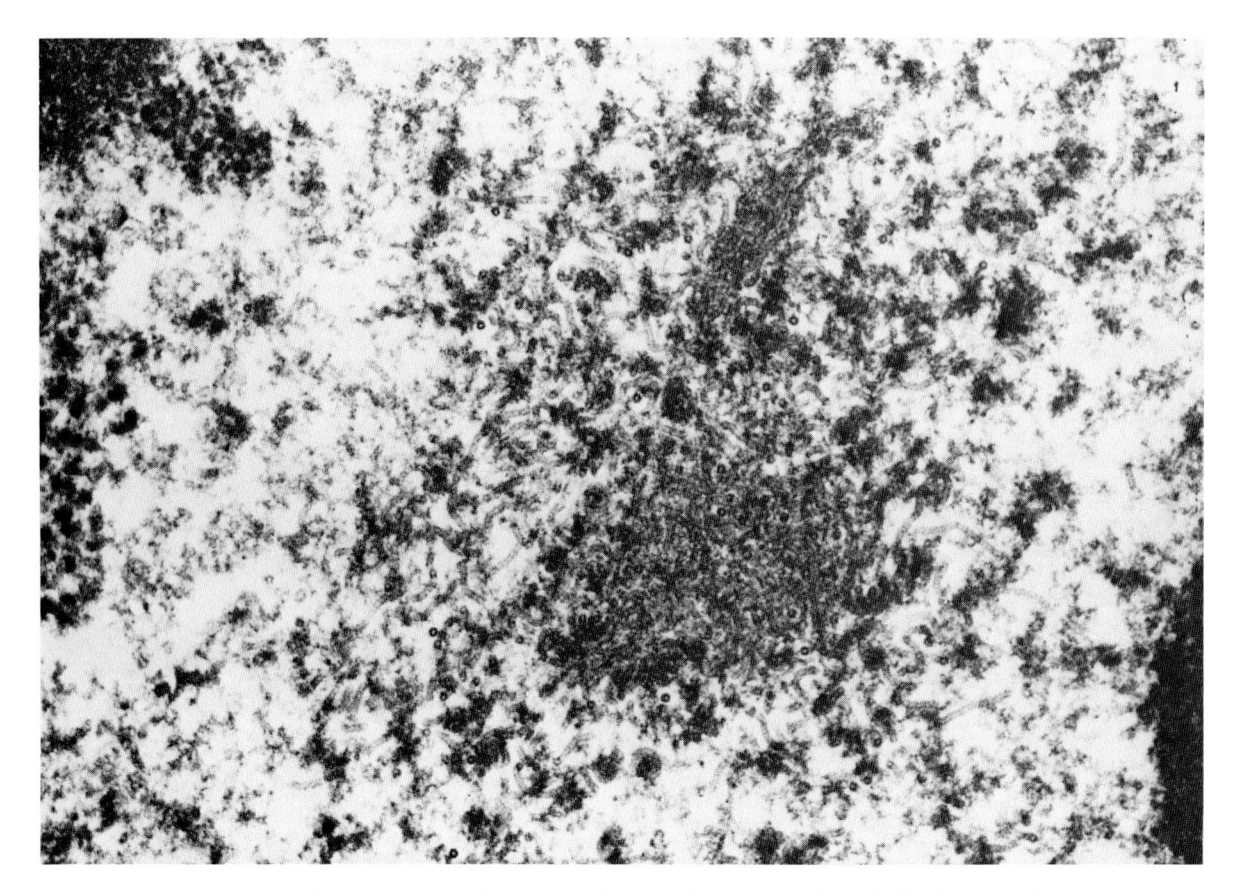

Figure 11–8. Electron micrograph of intranuclear measles inclusion (×61,700). Courtesy of Dr. F. E. Cuppage, Kansas University Medical Center.

small eosinophilic inclusion surrounded by a inconspicuous halo and minimally marginated chromatin. While multinucleated giant cells with inclusions are suggestive of measles etiology, they are not absolutely specific and can be mimicked by other RNA viruses (see below).

Negatively stained particles are generally rounded with pleomorphic forms, measuring 100 to 300 nm in diameter. In thin sections, tubular nucleocapsid material may be found in the nucleus or cytoplasm, the tubules measuring 15 to 20 nm in diameter[11] (Fig. 11–8).

Atypical measles is a syndrome that occurs in patients who are exposed to wild measles virus years after immunization with killed measles vaccine[34,35] which was in use from 1962 to 1968. The illness is characterized by fever, myalgias, cough, headache, an atypical rash, and extremely high measles hemagglutination inhibition antibody titers. The chest film shows patchy alveolar infiltrates with confluence, and these infiltrates may form nodules which simulate metastatic disease. Rapid clinical recovery is the rule, but the radiologic nodules may persist for several months. The histologic appearance of these nodules is presumably nonspecific, but no descriptions of them are available, since awareness of the syndrome obviates biopsy of these lesions.

Parainfluenza

Parainfluenza types I to IV are all respiratory pathogens in humans and are second in frequency only to RSV in causing viral respiratory illness in children.[15] Parainfluenza type III infection may occur in infants since [like Respiratory Syncytial Virus (RSV) infection] maternal antibody affords relatively little protection against infection. Other types of parainfluenza-related illness usually occur in a slightly older population, with most cases being seen in the 6-month to 4- to 5-year age group.[36] In older children and adults, parainfluenza virus ordinarily causes only a mild upper respiratory infection,[37] although exceptionally parainfluenza may cause pneumonia in adults.[38] The incidence of respiratory tract infection due to parainfluenza virus is no higher for immunocompromised patients than for immunologically normal people, but once infected. immune-compromised hosts have more difficulty limiting infection and destroying the virus.[39]

There is a range of illnesses caused by parainfluenza including, most commonly, laryngotracheobronchitis (croup), but also bronchiolitis and pneumonia,[17] with a slight tendency to occur in the fall, winter, and early

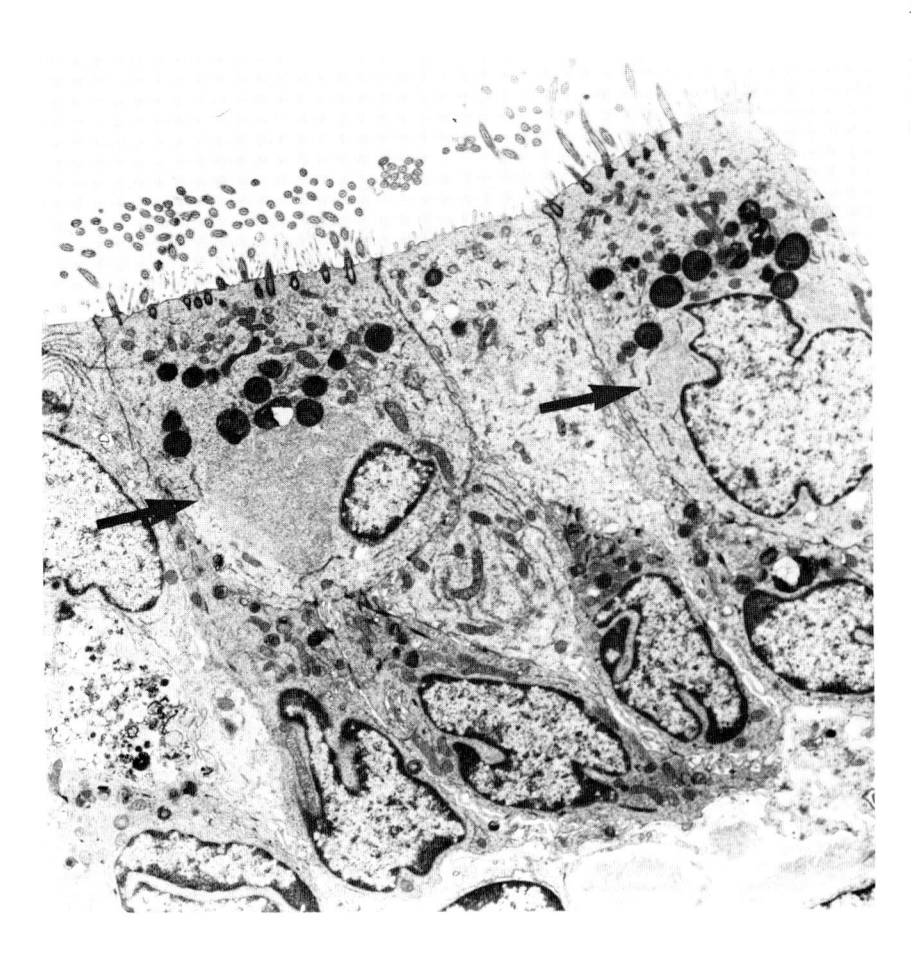

Figure 11-9. Parainfluenza in bronchial epithelium; note perinuclear cytoplasmic inclusions (arrows) (×4200).

summer months. Antibody responses are not always detectable, and immunofluorescence or culture of nasopharyngeal secretions are often necessary for the diagnosis to be made.[7] Antibody production and immunity are transient so that reinfection is common[37] although subsequent infections are usually milder and limited to the upper respiratory tract.[36]

Type III virus is most often responsible for lower respiratory tract parainfluenza infection. Parainfluenza pneumonia may occasionally be fatal, particularly in immunocompromised infants[7,40] and in these cases, there may be prolonged viral shedding for several weeks.

Morphology

Death from parainfluenza pneumonia is quite uncommon, and in the above-mentioned immunocompromised infants, the appearance of the lungs was that of a diffuse alveolar damage type of pneumonia similar to that found in influenza.[40] Exceptionally, interstitial pneumonia with multinucleate giant cells containing intracytoplasmic inclusions mimicking measles may be found.[41] Pathologic examination of parainfluenza type II pneumonia in dogs ("kennel cough") shows denudation of terminal bronchiolar epithelium with a mononuclear cell infiltrate but minimal parenchymal changes.[42] No well-defined inclusions are seen by light-microscopy; the ultrastructural characteristics are similar to measles virus (Figs. 11-9, 11-10) except that virus particles are found in the cytoplasm and not in the nucleus.

Respiratory Syncytial Virus

Respiratory syncytial virus is the major cause of serious lower respiratory tract infections in children under 1 year of age, and is particularly prevalent in infants less than 6 months of age, with a tendency to occur in the winter and early spring months.

The epidemiologic and immunologic characteristics of RSV are peculiar. In spite of the fact that there is no multiplicity of antigenic types, anti-RSV antibody added to cell cultures does not prevent infection in vitro.[43] Maternally acquired anti-RSV antibody is generally thought to have no notable effect on the incidence or severity of RSV infection in infants[43,44] although studies suggest some degree of maternal antibody protection.[45] Attempts to immunize infants with killed RSV vaccine have been unsuccessful, these infants developing more severe disease when later exposed to wild virus.[43] Prolonged viral shedding is common, leading to a substantial risk of nosocomial spread.[46] Reinfection is also common, although secondary infections are usually milder[18,47] and eventually result in the production of natural anti-RSV antibodies, the latter being quite prevalent in the adult population. Even in immune adults, however, RSV may cause protracted upper respiratory tract infections, espe-

Figure 11–10. Tubular parainfluenza cytoplasmic inclusion (×72,000).

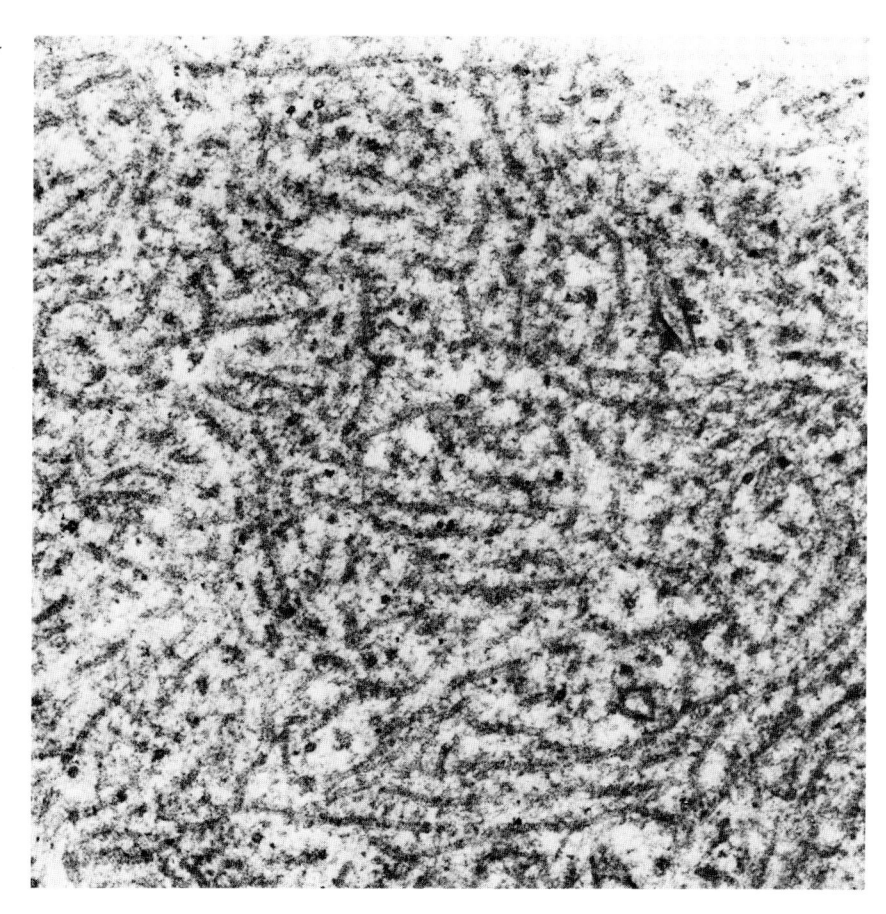

cially in adults working closely with infants during the winter months.[48,49] Occasionally, the virus may cause life-threatening or fatal pneumonia in adults, particularly the elderly.[48,50–52] The poor correlation between humoral or cellular immunity and the clinical course of RSV infection implies that an as yet uncharacterized local immune mechanism must play a major role in response to infection.[53]

The clinical and radiologic patterns of RSV-related respiratory tract disease in infants are variable. The most common, and classic, pattern is bronchiolitis, characterized by dyspnea, wheezing, and chest film evidence of air-trapping. Other patterns include croup,[54] bronchitis with radiographic bronchial wall thickening and linear perihilar infiltrates, and pneumonia with rales and radiographic consolidation.[15] In children ages 0 to 5, approximately one-third of RSV infections are clinically apparent.[53] Respiratory disease sufficiently severe to require hospitalization has been estimated at 1 to 2 percent of infections, and of hospitalized patients, approximately 1 percent are fatal,[43] although a higher fatality rate has been noted for infants with cardiac disease.[46] Respiratory syncytial virus bronchiolitis has been associated with long-term pulmonary function abnormalities[43] (see Relationship of Viral Infections to Chronic Airflow Obstruction, below).

In addition to respiratory symptoms, a significant number of infants with RSV infection present with apnea,[55,56] this symptom being particularly frequent in premature infants or infants younger than 2 months of age, and not necessarily being accompanied by appreciable degrees of pulmonary inflammation.[57] These children are at high risk for sudden ("cot") death[58] and recommendations have been made to hospitalize very young or premature infants with RSV bronchiolitis[56] and infants with RSV-associated apnea.[55]

Morphology

The classic histologic appearance is characterized by bronchiolar epithelial cell necrosis, purulent intralumenal exudate, and peribronchiolar mononuclear infiltrates (Figs. 11–11, 11–12). The bronchiolar epithelium in the later stages of infection may have a disorganized appearance which has been described as "pleomorphic undifferentiated"[59] and which possibly reflects reparative processes altered by virus. One may find a mononuclear inflammatory infiltrate in the alveolar walls around involved bronchioles. Exceptionally, RSV may cause a fulminant diffuse alveolar damage type of reaction superimposed on bronchiolitis[59], or giant cell pneumonia mimicking measles.[59a]

Respiratory syncytial virus may produce intracytoplasmic inclusions in bronchial, bronchiolar, and alveolar epithelial cells, although inclusions cannot be found in all cases, and if present, tend to occur early in the course of the disease[9] (Plate 2). The inclusions are rounded,

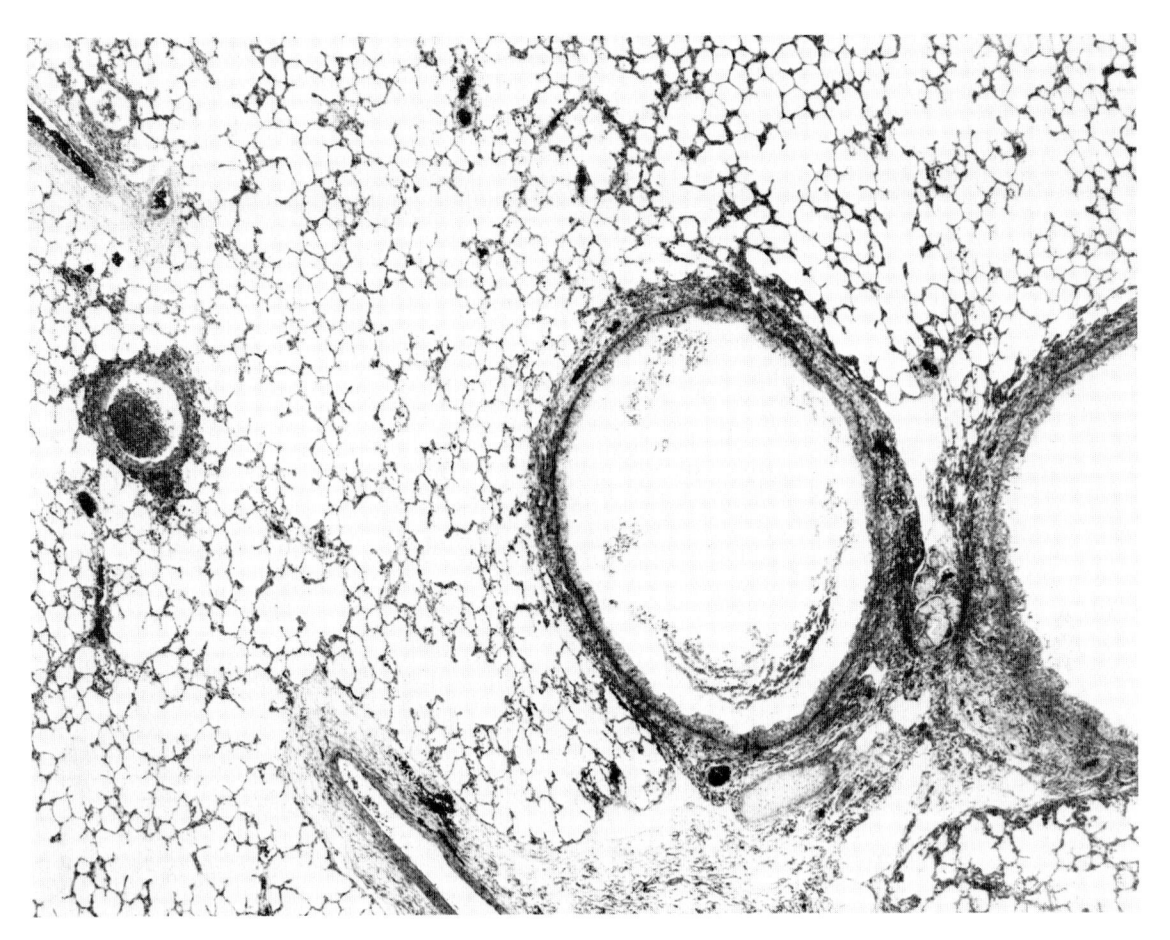

Figure 11–11. Respiratory syncytial virus (RSV) bronchiolitis. Note conspicuous involvement of bronchi and bronchioles with sparing of alveoli (H&E, ×30).

eosinophilic, and may stain positively with Giemsa stain. They are quite difficult to identify with certainty, and immunofluorescence techniques have been used to confirm the diagnosis.[59,60]

Electron-microscopy of thin sections of RSV-infected cells show an appearance similar to other paramyxoviruses, but the nucleocapsid tubules are slightly smaller (12 to 15 nm in diameter)[11] (Figs. 11–13, 11–14).

Picornaviruses, Coronavirus

The various specific viruses of the Picornaviridae and Coronaviridae families are common causes of upper respiratory tract infections, and have limited pathogenicity to the lower respiratory tract.[61] Occasional cases of bronchiolitis and pneumonia,[44,54] and rare cases of fatal infections[62] have been described with these agents.

Adenovirus

At least 41 species of adenovirus have been found at the time of this writing, and several of these have been associated with lung disease in a variety of epidemiologic patterns. Adenovirus infection is an important cause of lower respiratory tract disease in infants and young children occuring slightly more commonly in winter months, and causing occasional epidemics. Coassociation of measles and adenovirus pneumonia in children has been described.[63] Native Canadian Indian children,[64] aboriginal New Zealand children,[65,66] and black South African children[63] have an apparent predilection for adenovirus pneumonia. Adenovirus pneumonia occurs sporadically in immunocompromised patients,[67–70] rarely in normal adults,[71] and has a peculiar predilection to occur in military recruits.[15]

The typical clinical presentation is that of an acute systemic illness with fever, malaise, cough, and wheezing. Severe hypoxemia is found in some cases. The acute radiographic changes are nonspecific and include bronchial thickening, peribronchial infiltrates, patchy or confluent parenchymal infiltrates, and air-trapping.[64,66] Adenovirus pneumonia in children carries a high risk of long-term pulmonary abnormalities, with over half of survivors having some clinical, functional, or radiographic abnormalities in most series.[43,64–66,72–74] Clinical abnormalities include cough, dyspnea, cyanosis, club-

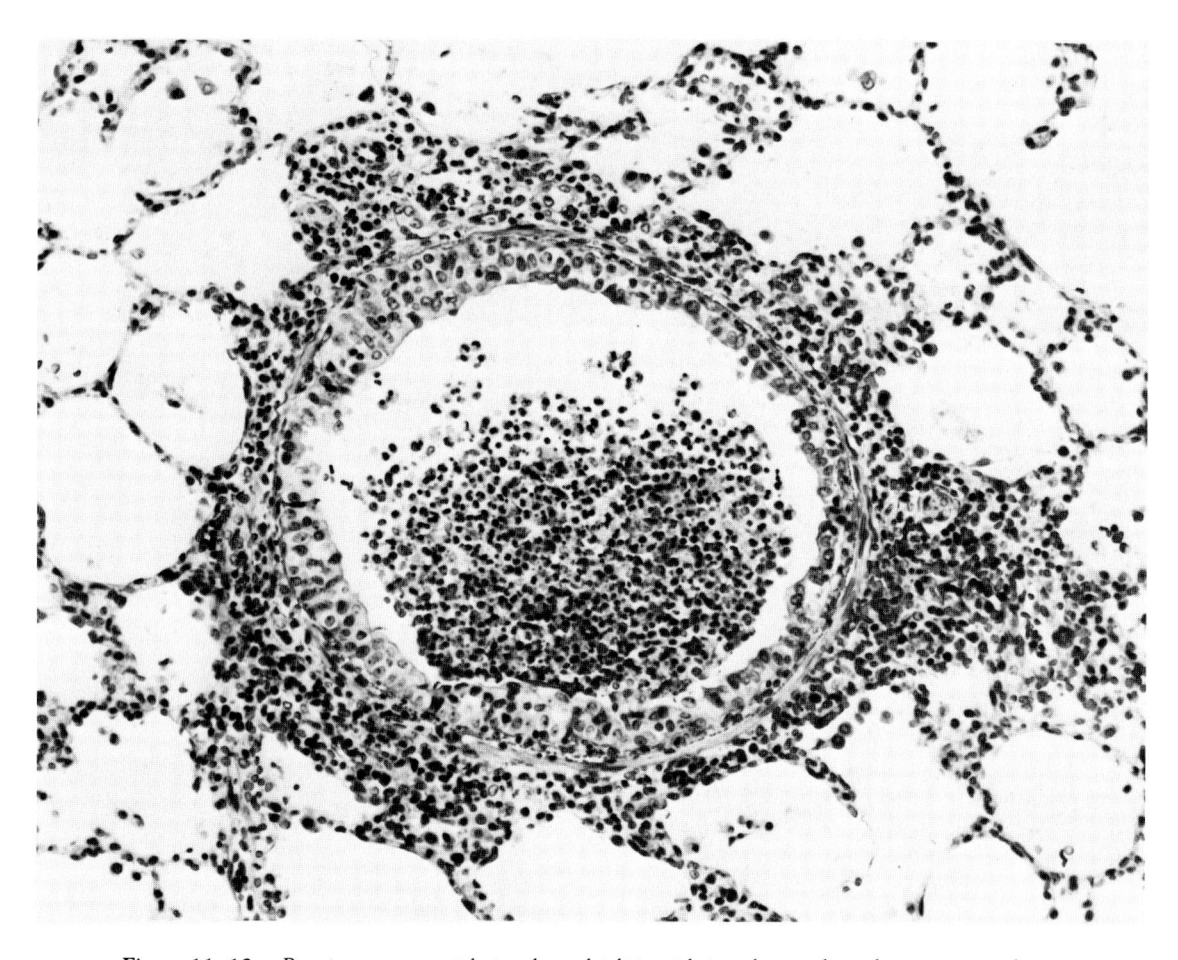

Figure 11–12. Respiratory syncytial virus bronchiolitis with intralumenal exudate, mononuclear peribronchiolar infiltrate, and disordered epithelium (H&E, ×188).

Adenovirus 161

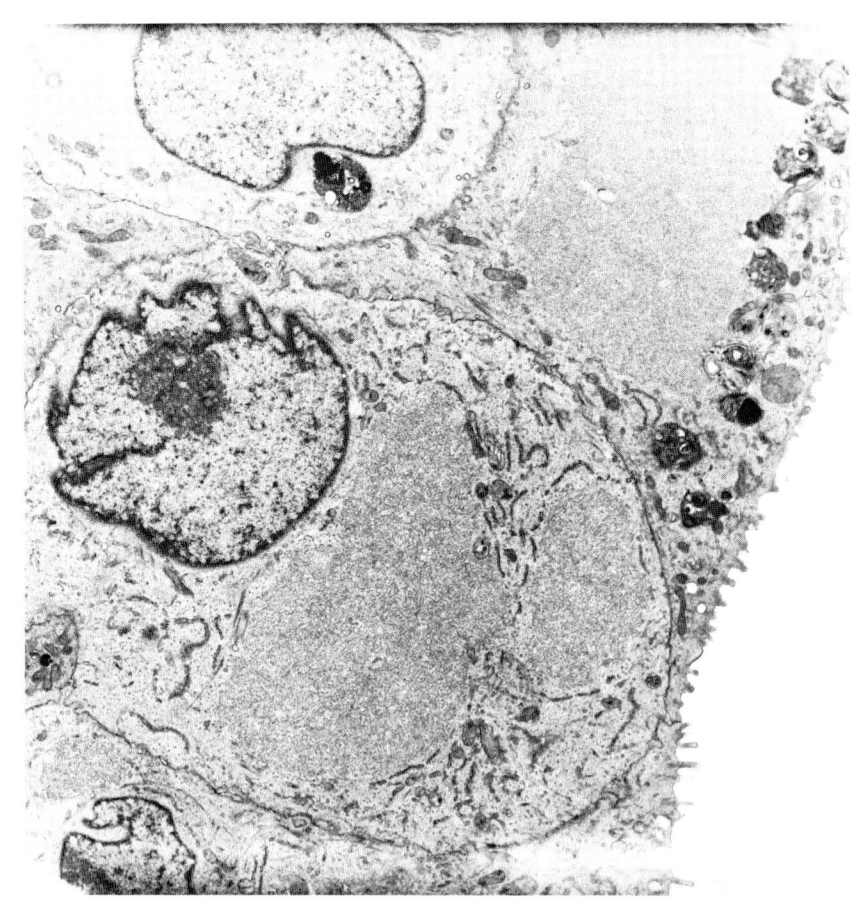

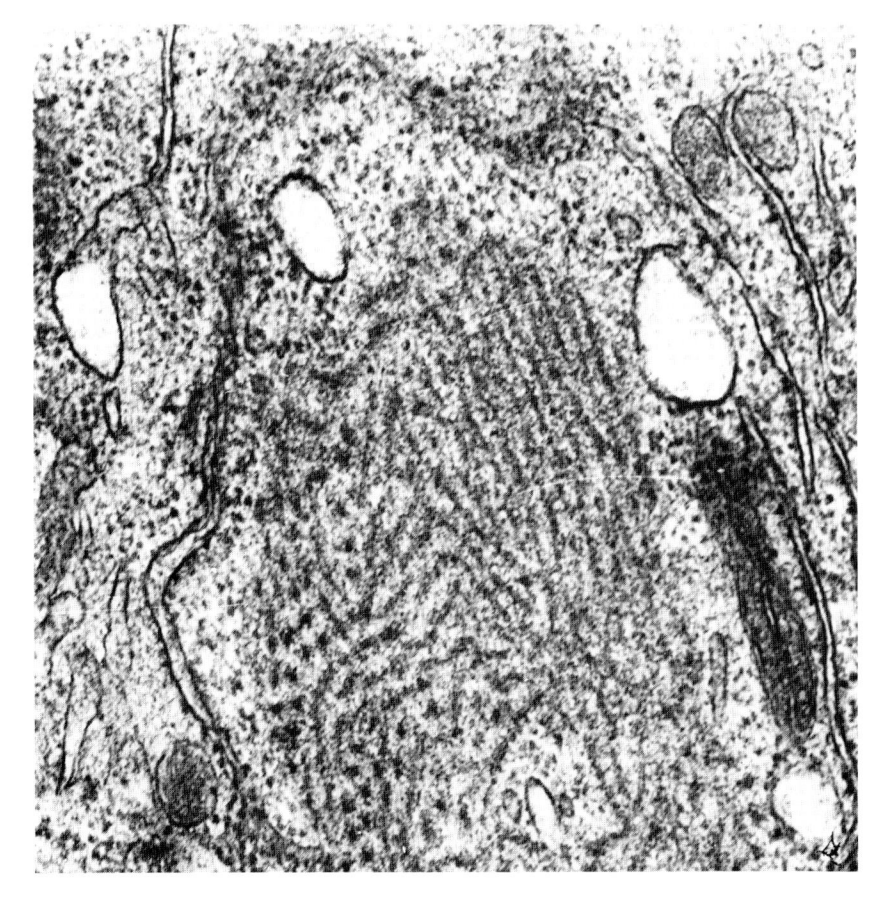

Figure 11–13. Electron micrographs of RSV-infected respiratory epithelium with cytoplasmic tubular inclusions (×5600).

Figure 11–14. Tubular intracytoplasmic RSV particles (×56,000).

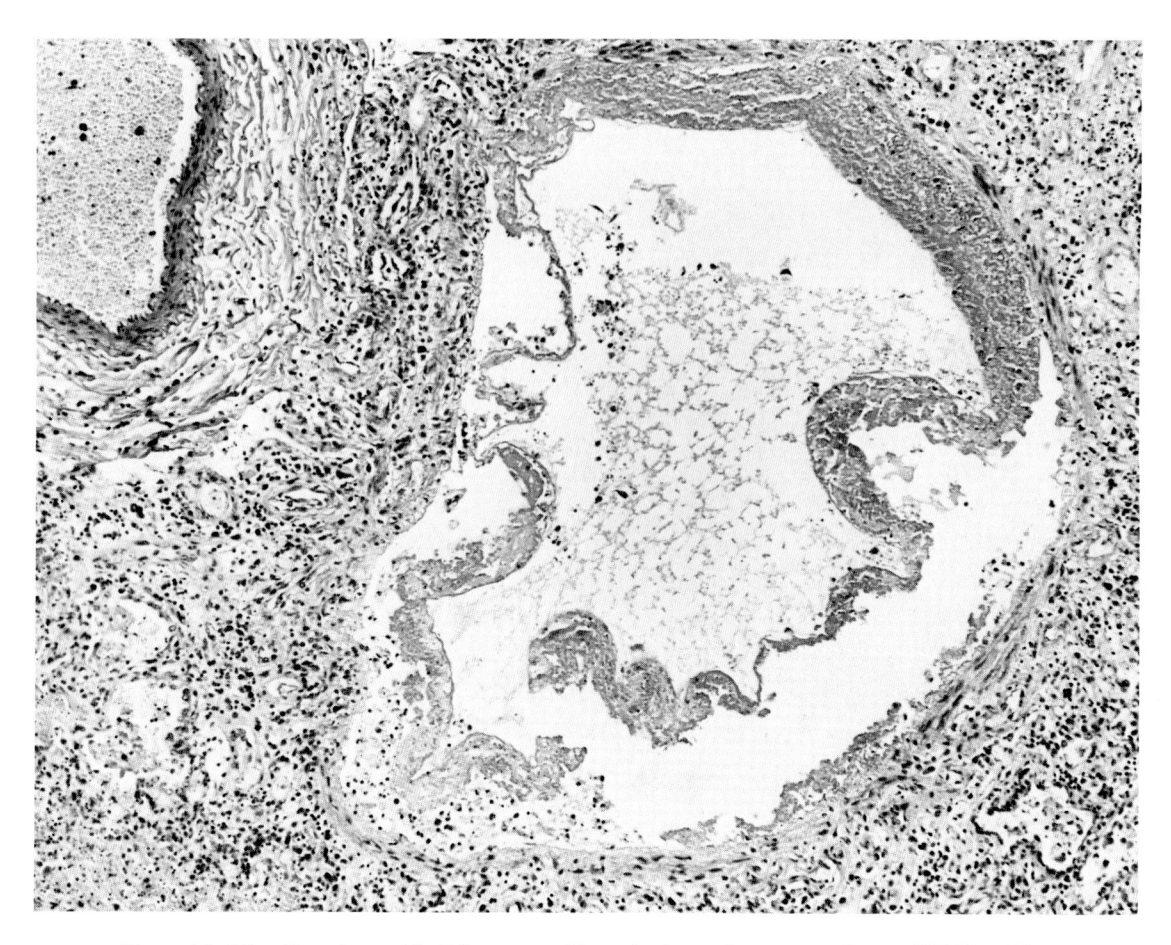

Figure 11–15. Complete epithelial necrosis of bronchiole in adenovirus infection (H&E, ×98).

bing,[73] wheezing, and recurrent infections.[43] The most notable anatomic sequelae are bronchiectasis and bronchiolitis obliterans[43,72,74] in at least one-quarter of patients.

Morphology

The upper respiratory tract usually shows no specific abnormalities. There is a necrotizing bronchitis with ulcers covered by inclusion-bearing, degenerate epithelial cells and debris; this process may extend into the submucosal glands to a striking degree.[75] Bronchioles similarly show necrotizing inflammation with epithelial inclusions, the process being more severe proximally than distally (Fig. 11–15). Diffuse alveolar damage with hyaline membranes may be found either in a peribronchiolar distribution or more diffusely; inclusions are also identified in sloughed alveolar epithelial cells (Figs. 11–16, 11–17).

Characteristically, the bronchial, bronchiolar, and peribronchiolar changes are more severe than the parenchymal changes,[75] suggesting that inhalation is the route of infection. However, instances of apparent hematogenous infection in the immunocompromised host have been described in which bronchiolar changes are minimal and parenchymal changes are quite severe.[67]

Chronically damaged lung tissue examined months to years after the acute episode show combinations of nonspecific scarring, bronchiectasis, and obliterative bronchiolitis which is most severe at the level of the terminal bronchioles.[72] No inclusions remain in these specimens.

There are two distinctive types of inclusions caused by adenovirus (see Fig. 11–17; Plate 3). The smaller, and usually less numerous inclusion is an irregular, granular, eosinophilic intranuclear inclusion surrounded by a small, often incomplete halo. This type of inclusion, by itself, could be misinterpreted as herpes. The other inclusion, termed "smudge cell," is larger and more conspicuous; the entire cell appears deeply basophilic with no halo. It is believed that the halo inclusion represents an earlier, more lightly infected cell, and the smudge cell is heavily and perhaps lethally infected.[9,75] Thin-section electron microscopy of adenovirus shows intranuclear crystalline arrays of virions measuring 60 to 90 nm in diameter (Fig. 11–18).

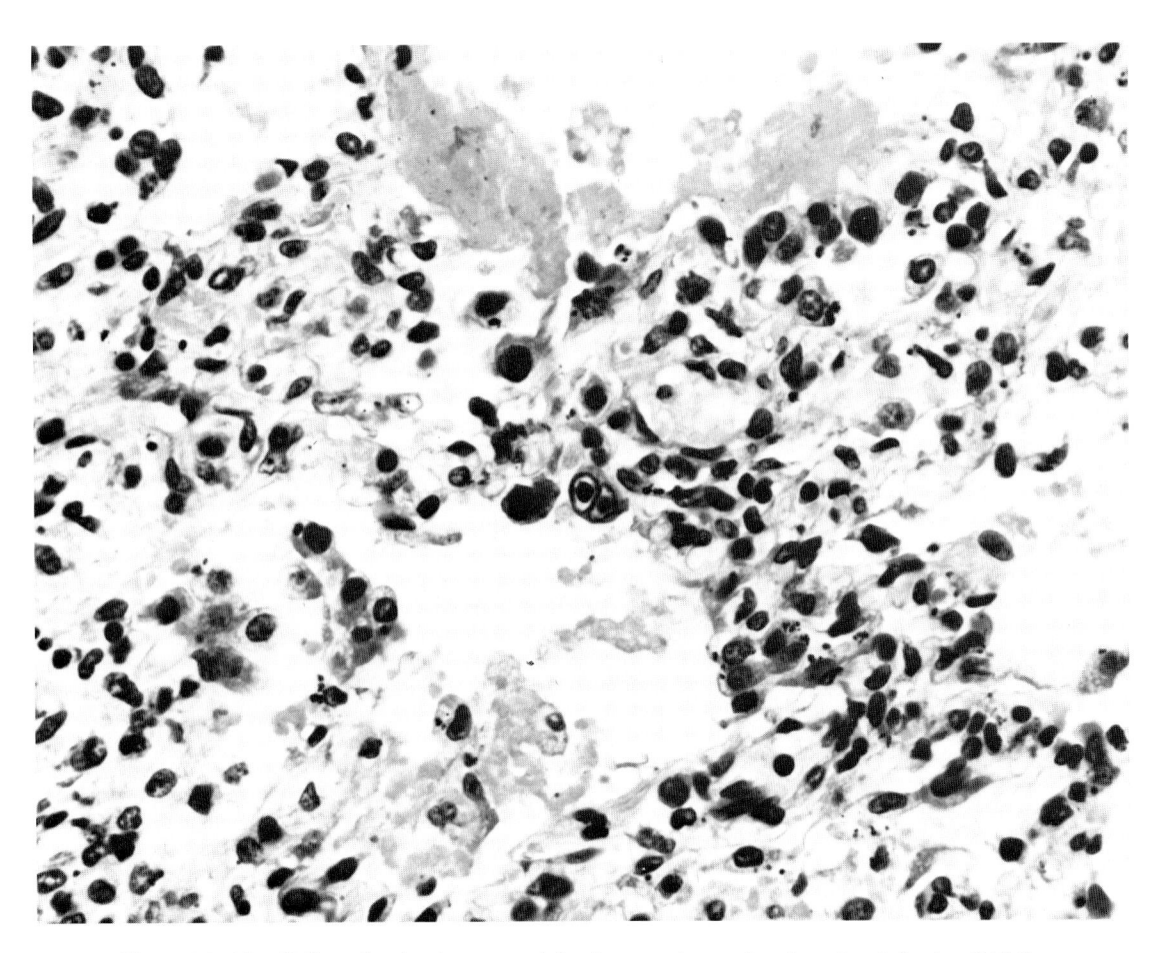

Figure 11–16. Diffuse alveolar damage with hyaline membranes in adenovirus infection (H&E, ×460).

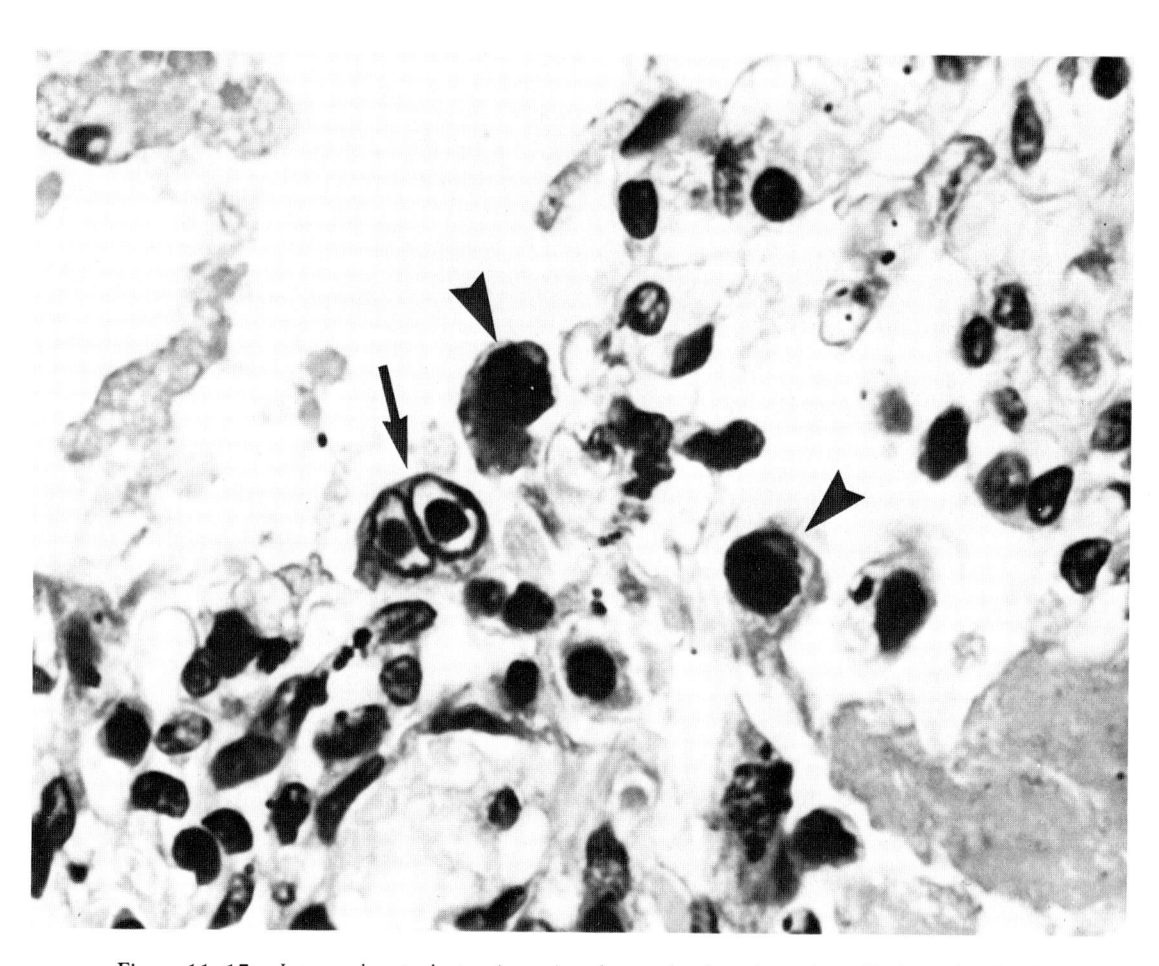

Figure 11–17. Intranuclear inclusion (arrow) and several enlarged smudge cells (arrowhead) of alveolar epithelial origin (H&E, ×860).

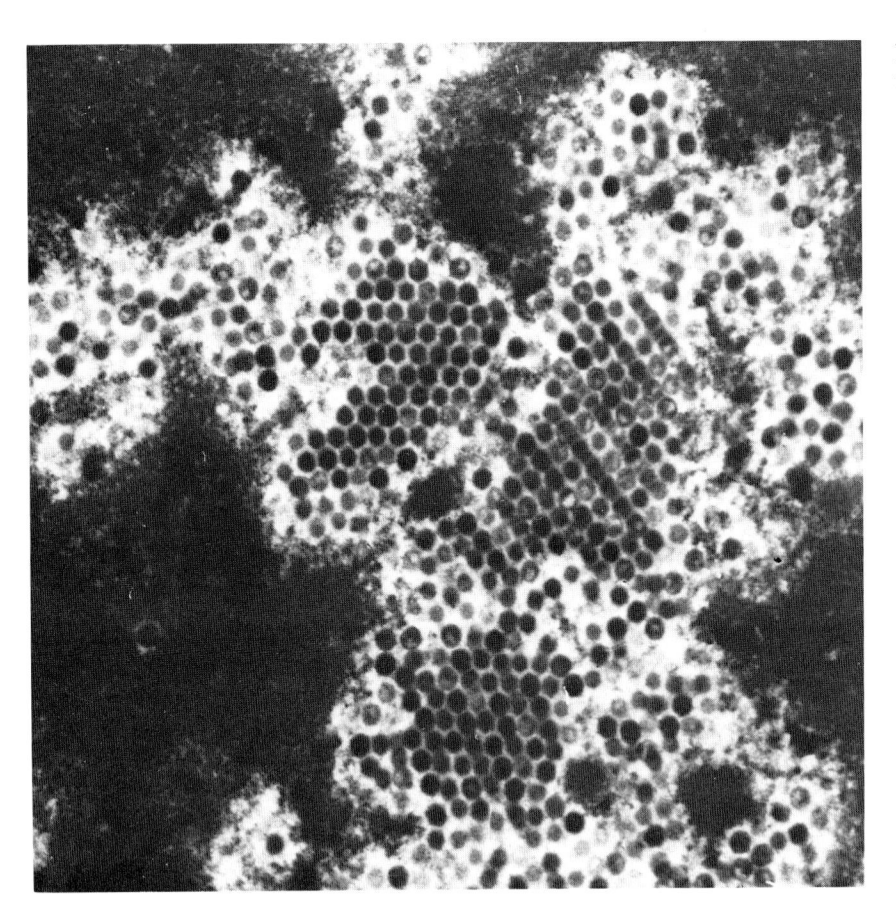

Figure 11–18. Electron-micrograph of intranuclear adenovirus (×42,000).

Herpes Simplex

Herpes simplex virus pneumonitis occurs primarily in immunosuppressed patients, patients with a variety of serious underlying chronic diseases,[76] patients with burns,[77] and alcoholics.[78] Herpes simplex virus tracheobronchitis with or without parenchymal involvement has also been found in a large proportion of patients with adult respiratory distress syndrome of various etiologies,[79] in a small proportion of unselected cases in a consecutive autopsy series,[80] and rarely in otherwise normal adults.[76,81] The immunologic response to HSV involves both humoral and cellular immunity, although it is thought that the latter is most important in prevention of recurrent infections.[76] Anti-HSV antibodies are not diagnostically useful since naturally acquired antibodies do not protect against recurrent infection, however, they are prognostically useful in that patients without an antibody titer rise in response to reinfection are more likely to have a fatal outcome. The prognosis in general is related to the underlying health of the patient.

Typically, HSV respiratory tract infection begins with lesions in the upper airway, and may spread contiguously to the bronchi, bronchioles, and parenchyma. This pattern of involvement is thought by some to be related to tracheal trauma (i.e., intubation[70]), however, other investigators have failed to confirm this possible association.[79] Less commonly, and primarily in the immunosuppressed population, the pattern of involvement is one of miliary nonbronchial-related parenchymal nodules and multiorgan involvement, implying hematogenous dissemination.[70,82] Both patterns of involvement may be caused by either HSV type I or type II although type I is more common. The majority of cases of HSV respiratory tract infection are believed to be due to reactivation rather than primary infection.[79,82]

Morphology

Herpes simplex virus lesions of the tracheobronchial tree are characterized by necrotic ulcers covered with a fibrinopurulent exudate (Fig. 11–19). Characteristic inclusion-bearing epithelial cells (see below) are found primarily at the viable ulcer margins, and may also be found in the submucosal glands.

The parenchymal reaction is characterized by nodular foci of necrosis and hemorrhage with inclusions in alveolar epithelial cells and alveolar macrophages. Proteinaceous exudate with a variable inflammatory reaction, and hyaline membranes are also found (Figs. 11–20, 11–21). In cases of contiguous spread, the parenchymal changes are peribronchiolar; in cases of hematogenous spread, the parenchymal changes are more randomly distributed.

There are two types of HSV nuclear alterations that are presumed to represent stages of infection.[9] The earliest alteration is characterized by slight nuclear enlargement with a basophilic to amphophilic "ground-glass" appear-

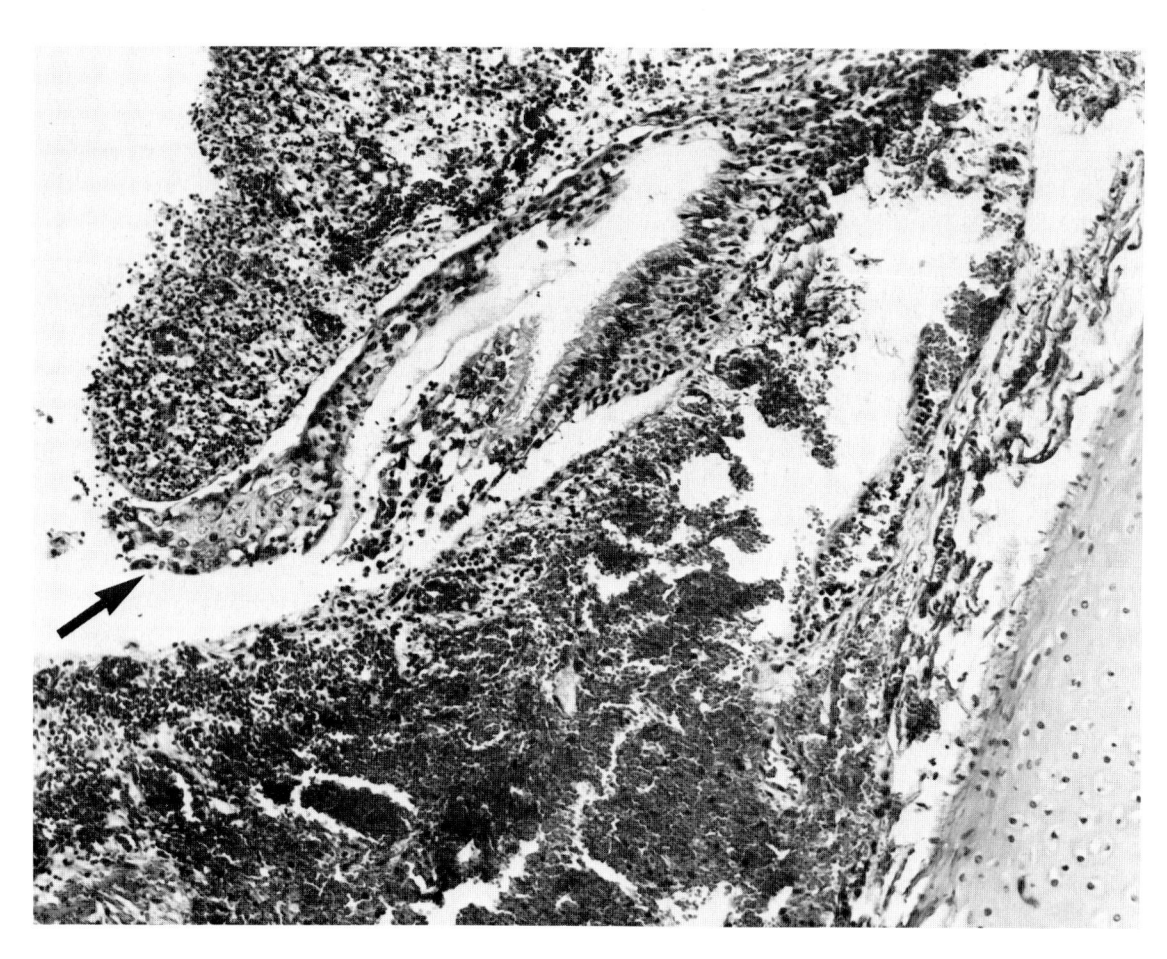

Figure 11–19. Two adjacent ulcers of trachea due to herpes simplex virus. Central strip of viable mucosa shows focal squamous metaplasia with herpetic inclusions (arrow) (H&E, ×100).

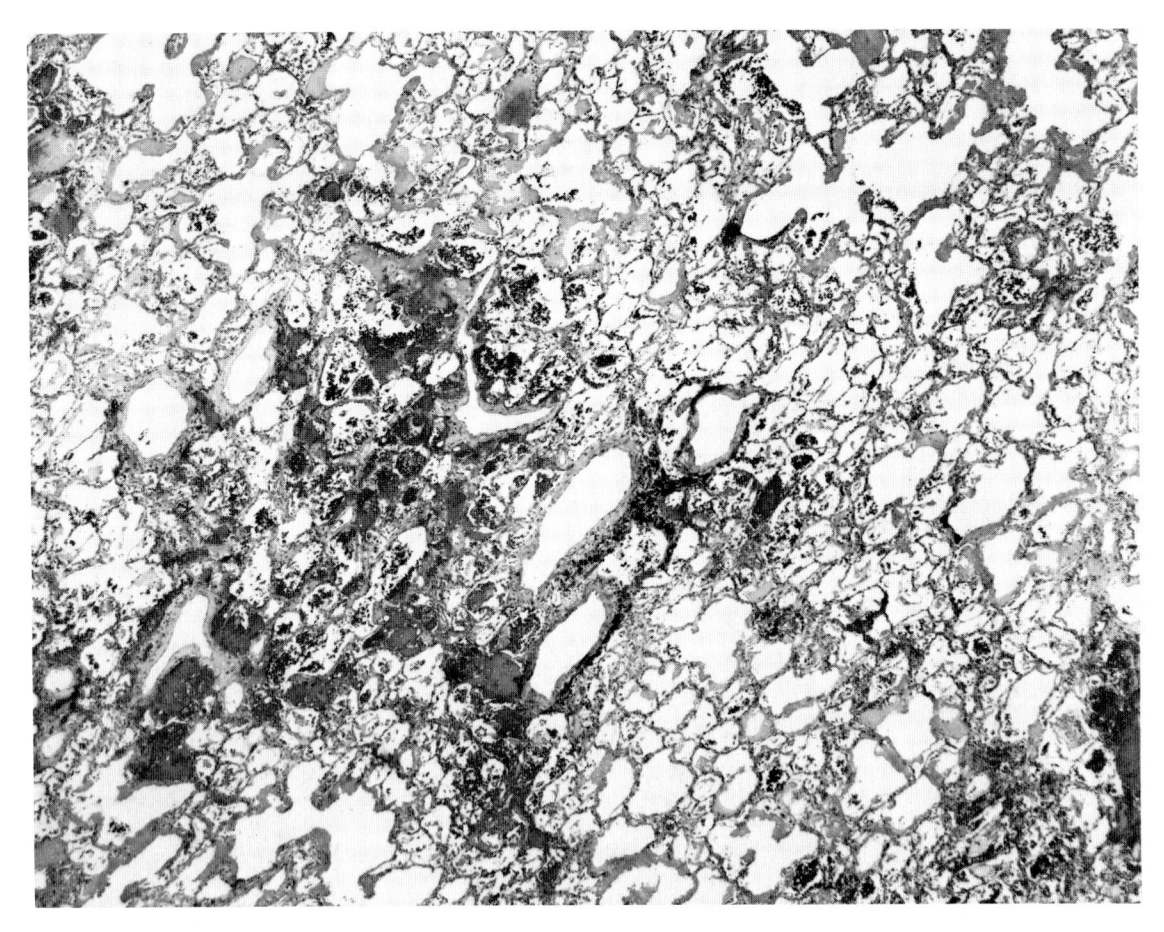

Figure 11–20. Periphery of nodule of hemorrhagic necrosis showing diffuse alveolar damage with hyaline membranes (H&E, ×30).

ance of the nucleoplasm (Fig. 11–22). Subsequently, the intranuclear material coalesces into a single, eosinophilic, hyalinized ("Cowdry A") inclusion surrounded by a well-defined clear halo (Plate 4). The chromatin is marginated at the nuclear membrane and the nucleolus is not apparent. Multinucleate inclusion-bearing cells are unusual in HSV respiratory tract infection. There are several potential pitfalls in the identification of herpetic inclusions. Inclusions are most numerous early in infection, and in later stages, they may simply be overlooked without a careful search and a high index of suspicion. One type of adenovirus inclusion resembles HSV, and the inclusions of V-Z are identical to HSV. There is a potential for misinterpretation of especially prominent nucleoli as viral inclusions. These sources of error may be circumvented by HSV-specific immunofluorescense, by immunoperoxidase staining, or by confirmation of the presence of viral particles by electron-microscopy.[83] Inspection of HSV by transmission electron-microscopy reveals particles of nucleocapsid surrounded by a lipid-containing envelope, which measures 150 to 200 nm in diameter (Fig. 11–23).

Varicella-Zoster

Infection with the herpes V-Z virus causes two relatively distinct clinical forms of illness: (primary) varicella ("chickenpox") and (recurrent) zoster ("shingles").

Varicella ordinarily occurs in childhood and is characterized by superficial vesicles primarily involving the skin of the trunk, and to a lesser degree, the face and scalp. In otherwise healthy immunologically normal patients, new vesicles cease to form after 3 to 4 days and start to scab over by 7 days. Primary infection is a systemic illness and results in the development of antibodies that are present in the vast majority of adults. Pulmonary complications of varicella in normal children occur in less than 1 percent of patients, but when primary varicella occurs in adults, radiographic pneumonitis is considerably more common, occurring in approximately 15 percent of patients.[84,85] The radiographic abnormalities are nonspecific and are characterized by perihilar, bilateral fine nodularity; the nodules usually measure less than 5 mm, but may become confluent.[85] Hilar lymph nodes and pleura usually appear normal. Pulmonary symptoms be-

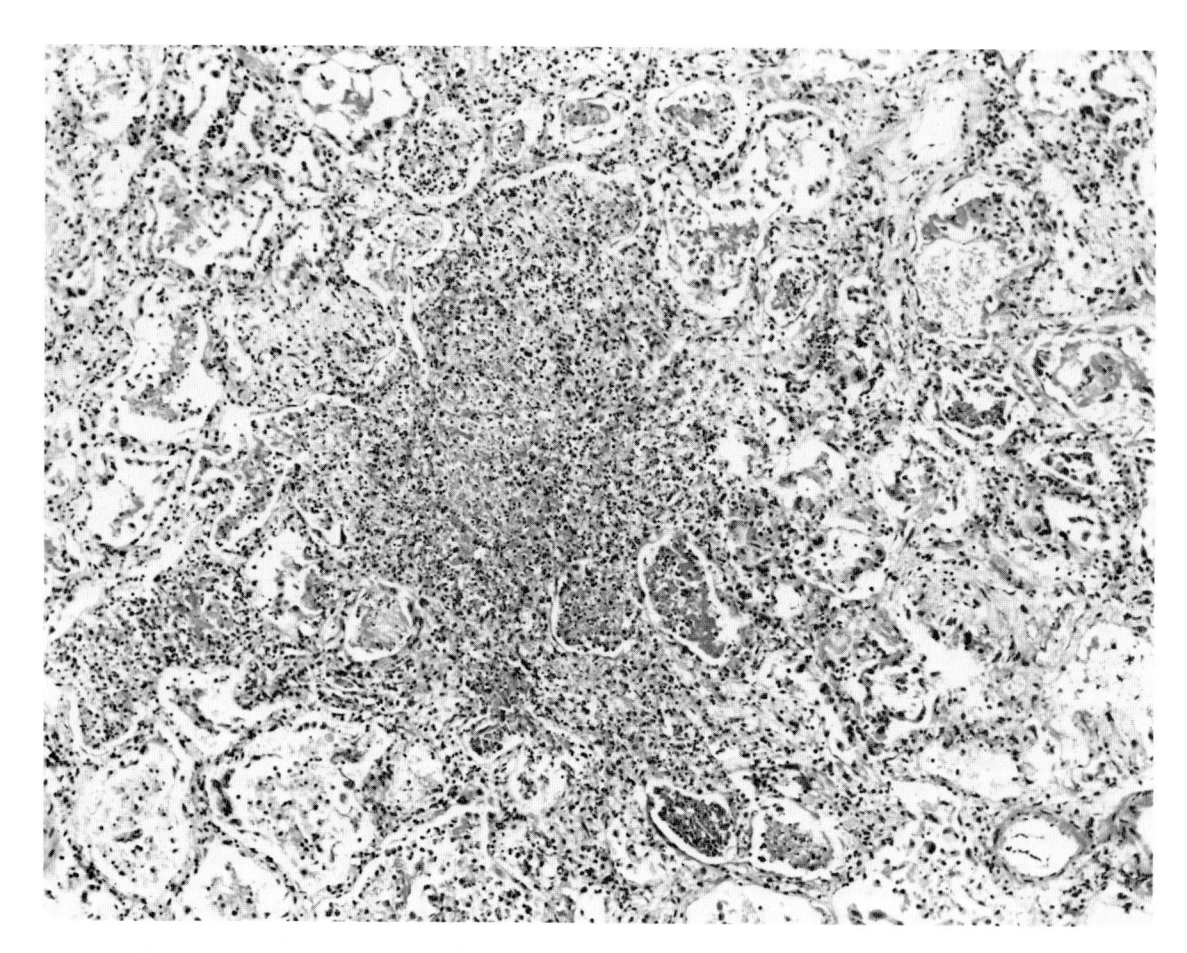

Figure 11–21. Herpetic parenchymal nodule of necrosis with polymorphonuclear leukocyte reaction and nuclear dust (H&E, ×100).

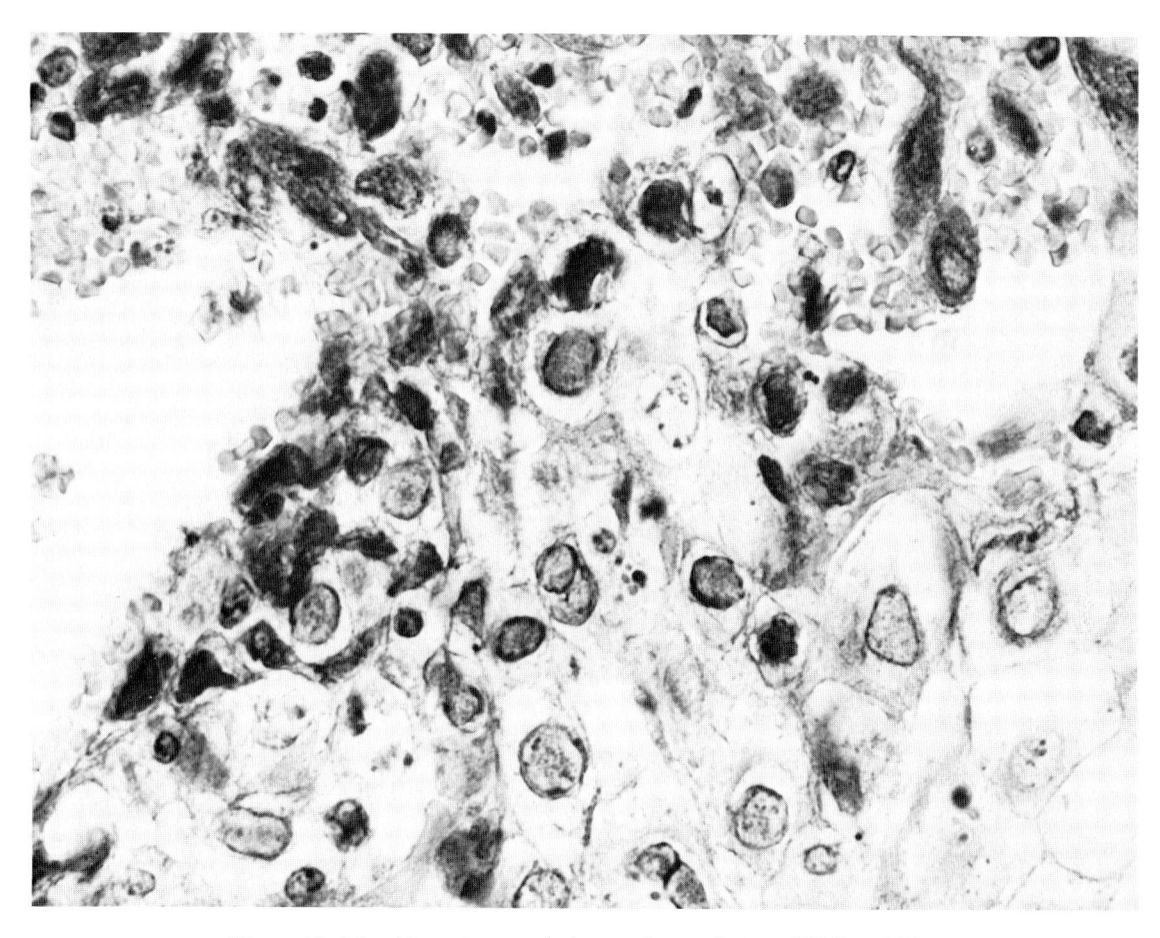

Figure 11–22. Herpetic ground-glass nuclear inclusions (H&E, ×460).

Figure 11–23. Electron micrograph of cytoplasmic herpetic virion (×150,000).

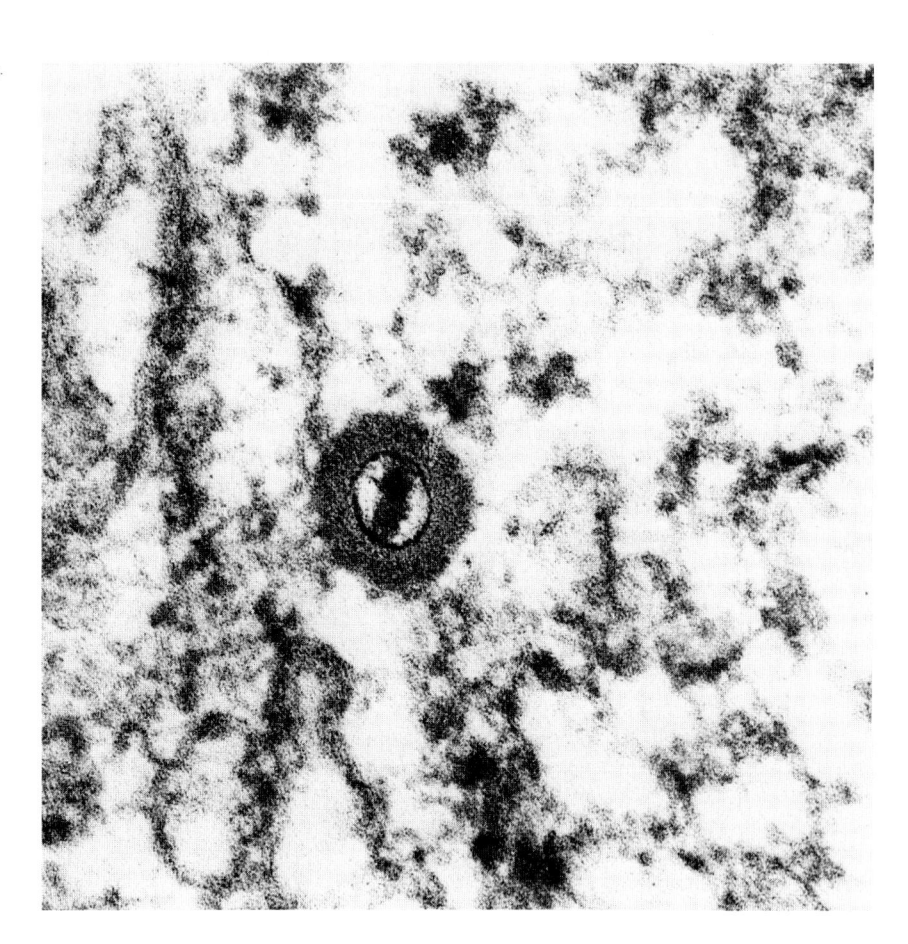

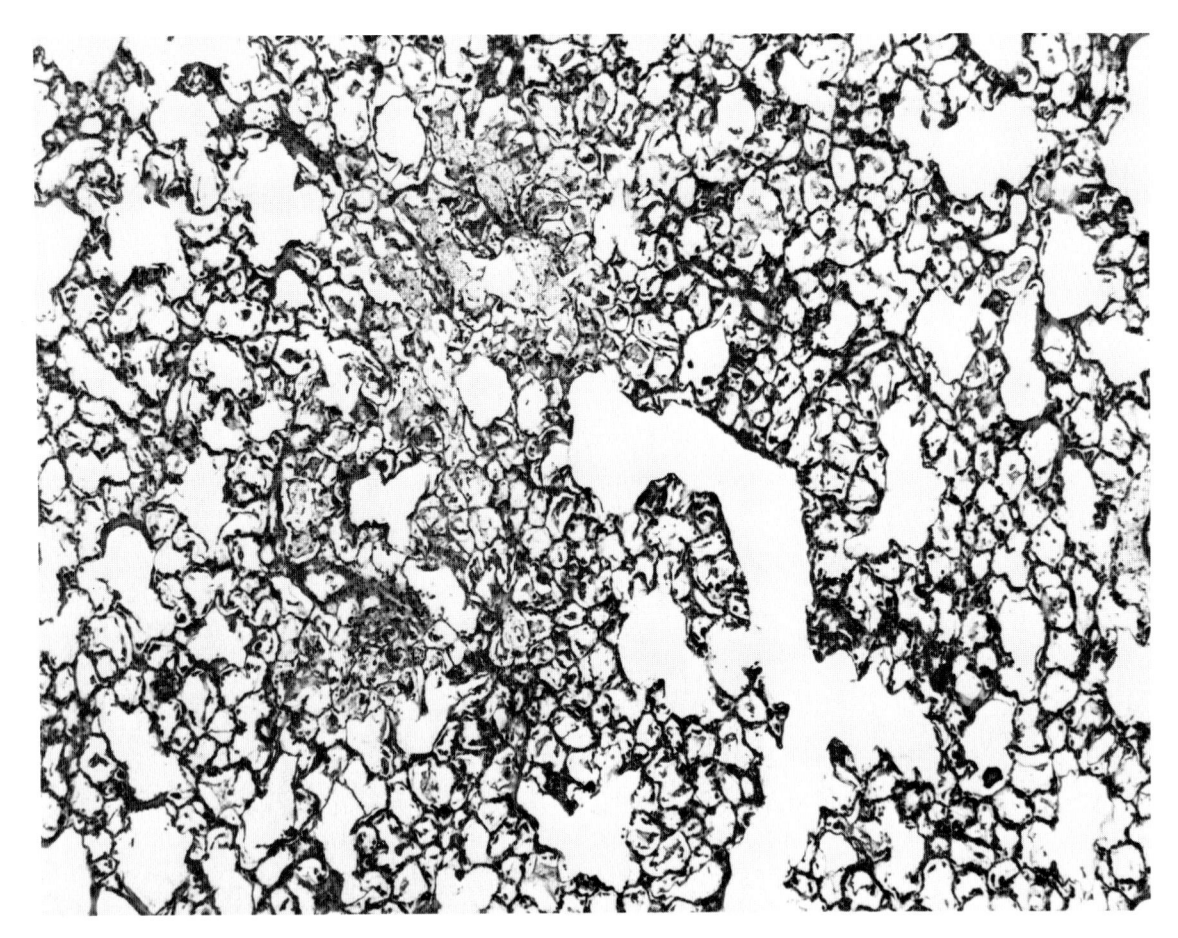

Figure 11–24. Varicella pneumonia. Note hemorrhagic, necrotic nodules surrounded by diffuse alveolar damage (H&E, ×35).

gin a few days after the rash appears and range from almost none, to cough, dyspnea, and chest pain, to severe respiratory distress. Adults, and in particular pregnant women, with varicella pneumonia are at risk for sudden death,[86] this event being heralded by rapidly progressive dyspnea and tachycardia. While most cases of varicella pneumonia in adults also have the typical rash, rare cases without skin changes have been reported,[87] and in this instance serology and culture are critical for the diagnosis. Some adult cases of varicella pneumonia heal as numerous bilateral small calcified nodules which are radiographically impressive but clinically benign.[88]

Following recovery from primary varicella infection, the V-Z virus is thought to reside in latent form in nerve cells. If reactivation of V-Z virus occurs, it occurs in the form of zoster, which is a painful vesicular rash in a dermatome distribution. In elderly patients, zoster disseminates to some extent in approximately one-third of cases.[89] Recurrence in the form of varicella is exceedingly rare.[4] Like HSV infection, there is both a humoral and cellular immune response to infection, but the latter is considerably more important in prevention of recurrence.

In immunocompromised patients, primary varicella presents as skin vesicles which may be larger, more numerous, and more persistent than usual, and are associated with multiorgan involvement.[90] Varicella-zoster virus reactivation in this population still takes the form of zoster, but there may be cutaneous dissemination, defined as vesicular lesions in at least two noncontiguous dermatomes, or multiorgan dissemination.[4] Disseminated varicella and disseminated zoster merge as a morphologic entity.[90–92]

Morphology

Varicella zoster pneumonia is similar in immunocompetent[85,86] and immunocompromised patients, and the parenchymal findings are similar to herpes simplex pneumonia (see above).[70,92] The trachea and major bronchi are less often involved in V-Z infection than HSV infection. The parenchyma shows foci of hemorrhagic, necrotizing inflammation-containing inclusion bodies in alveolar macrophages and alveolar epithelial cells, as well as areas of diffuse alveolar damage with hyaline membranes (Figs. 11–24, 11–25). The inclusions

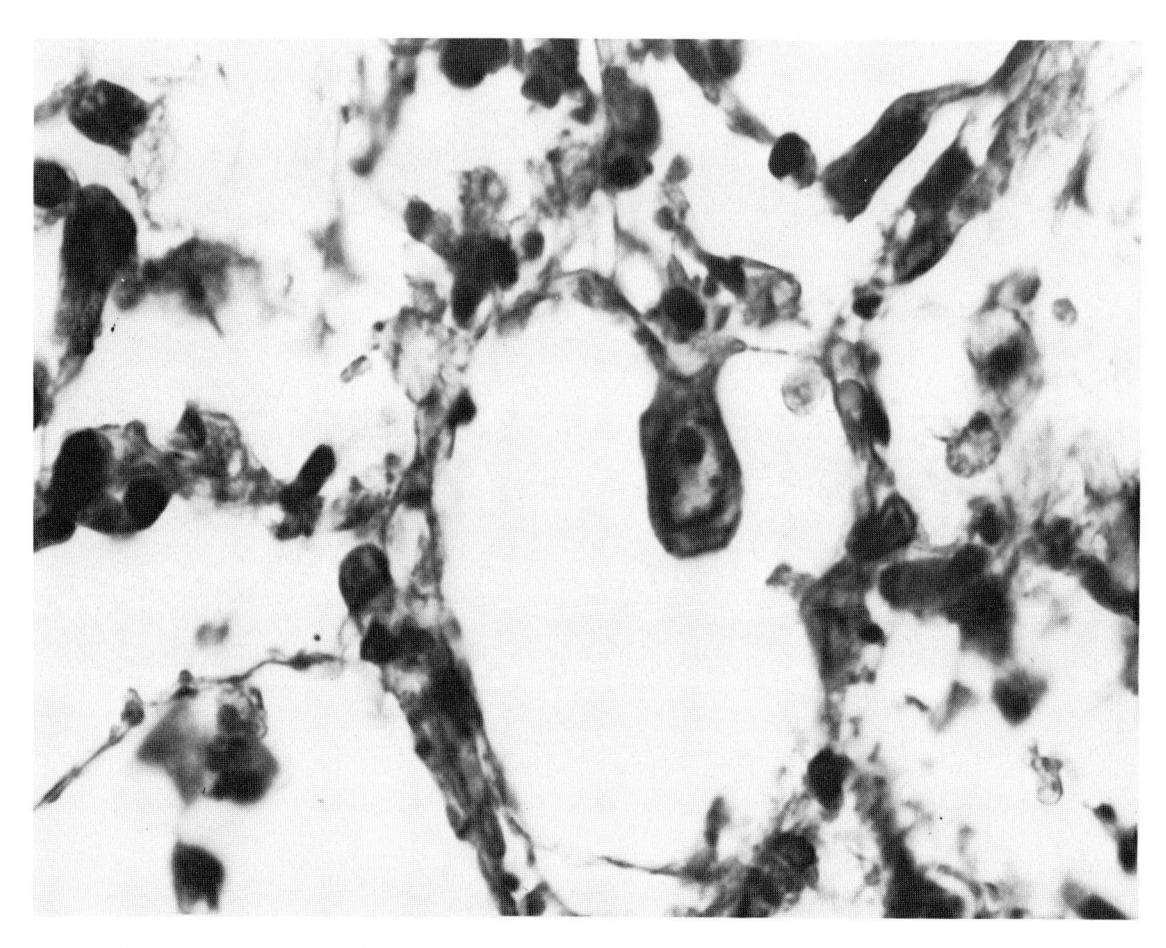

Figure 11–25. Intranuclear inclusion in alveolar epithelial cell in varicella pneumonia (H&E, ×830).

are solely intranuclear and are identical by light- and electron-microscopy to HSV.

The nodules of healed adult varicella pneumonitis consist of rounded fibrous scars with central calcification, peripheral fibroblasts, and occasional multinucleated giant cells. No inclusions are found in these lesions.[88]

Cytomegalovirus

Cytomegalovirus infection can be classified into five groups, based on the patient population involved and the clinical behavior.[92a] In immunologically competent children and adults, the majority of primary CMV infections are asymptomatic. These infections are detected serologically.

Symptomatic illness in nonimmunocompromised children and adults is characterized by fever, malaise, hepatosplenomegaly, and atypical lymphocytosis, the "heterophil-negative infectious mononucleosis syndrome."[93] Clinical or radiographic evidence of pulmonary disease in this setting is distinctly unusual, but is described.[92a,94] Pneumonia in this population is rarely life-threatening.

Cytomegalovirus may be acquired in children and adults from transfusions. Approximately one-third of patients infected in this way become symptomatic, but respiratory tract symptoms are not a prominent feature of their illness.

Classic CMV disease in infants is congenitally (transplacentally) acquired although the mother ordinarily is asymptomatic and the pregnancy is not a clinically complicated one. Cytomegalovirus disease in infants may also be acquired from the birth canal, breast milk, or transfusions. In either of these settings, lung involvement is a part of multiorgan system disease, and is not usually responsible for major morbidity. Cytomegalovirus may also cause relatively mild cases of pneumonia in infants in the absense of apparent multiorgan involvement.[95]

Most cases of symptomatic pulmonary CMV inclusion disease are seen in debilitated or immunocompromised hosts, renal transplant patients being the most extensively studied group. Prospective series indicate that roughly one-half of these patients develop CMV infection, usually in the second or third postoperative month.[96–98] There are significant differences between patients with primary CMV infection (seronegative before transplant) and reactivation CMV (seropositive before transplant).[97,98] Reacti-

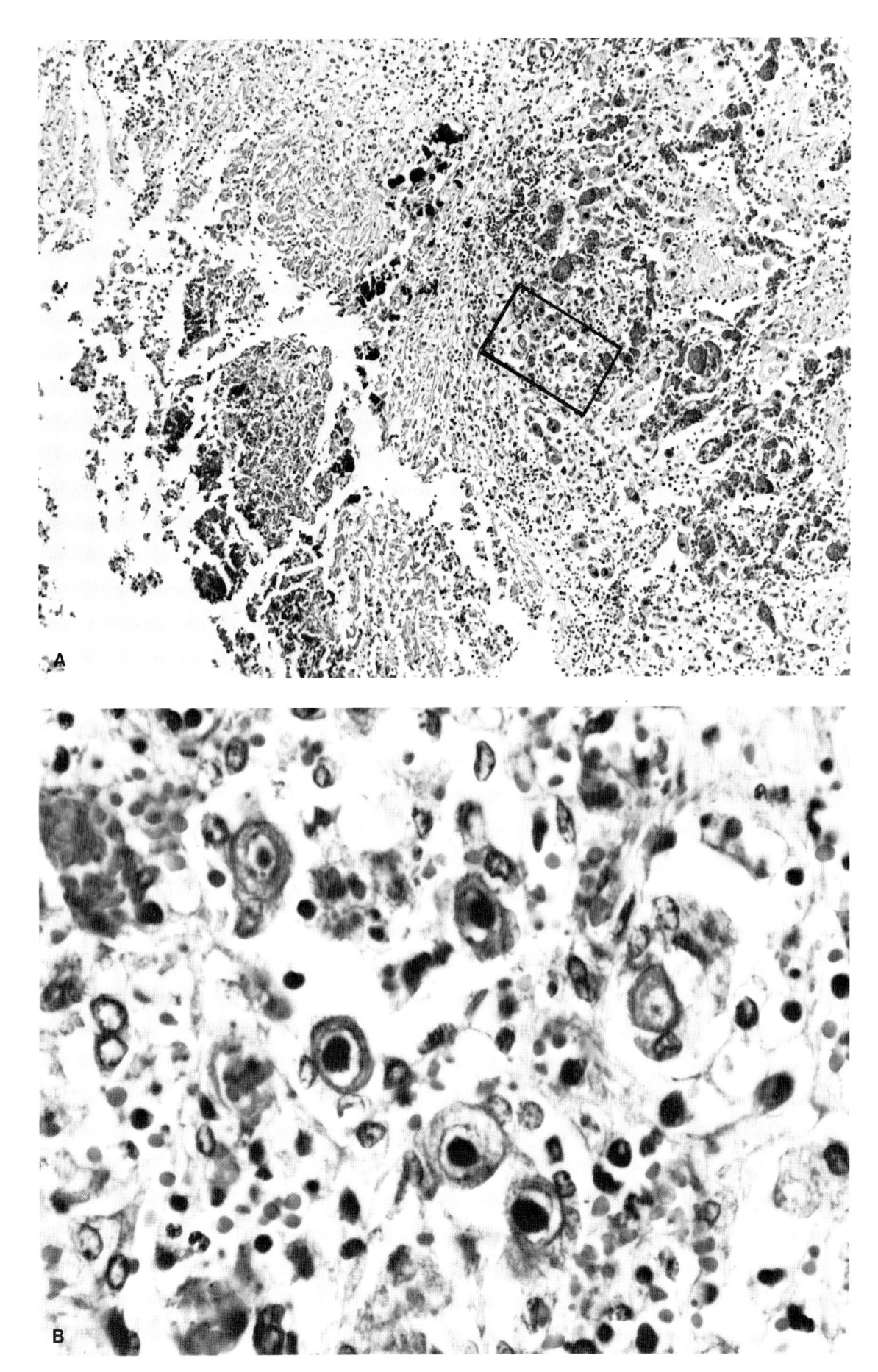

Figure 11–26. A. Edge of a lung abscess containing cytomegalic inclusions (box) (H&E, ×100). B. Higher-power view of enclosed area from A (H&E, ×500).

vation is considerably more common but is often asymptomatic in spite of culture-positive viremia. Primary infection is symptomatic in the vast majority of patients, causing malaise, fever, leukopenia, thrombocytopenia, and respiratory tract disease. The donor kidney is presumed to be the usual source of primary CMV infection, and the suggestion has been made that seronegative recipients should receive kidneys only from seronegative donors.[97]

Cytomegalovirus infection probably is not a factor in most instances of graft rejection, although there is some controversy on this issue. Mortality related to CMV infection in renal transplant patients appears to be relatively uncommon (less than 20 percent).[99] Failure to mount an antibody response to CMV infection is a bad prognostic sign, associated with increased mortality.[78,100]

Bone marrow transplant patients are also remarkably susceptible to CMV infection, which occurs in over half of these patients and is associated with CMV viremia which may be prolonged.[101] Cytomegalovirus pneumonia occurs in 15 to 20 percent of bone marrow transplant patients and, in contrast to renal transplant recipients, has a mortality rate in excess of 80 percent.[102,103] Cytomegalovirus viremia and pneumonitis is also commonly found in patients with the acquired immunodeficiency syndrome.[104]

In a number of immunocompromised patients with CMV pneumonia, coexistent infection with *Pneumocystis carinii* has been identified.[105-107] While this coexistence may simply be a reflection of the host's immunologic weakness, the possibility of a truly symbiotic relationship has been suggested with ultrastructural evidence of CMV virions residing inside Pneumocystis trophozooites.[105,107]

Morphology

The hallmark of CMV infection is the characteristic inclusion which may be seen in macrophages, endothelial cells, and epithelial cells (Plate 5). The involved cell is enormously enlarged up to 40 μm, with a large prominent nucleus. The chromatin is marginated to the nuclear membrane, and the center of the nucleus is occupied by a slightly granular, variably staining, extremely prominent inclusion surrounded by a clear halo. Cytoplasmic inclusions may develop after the nuclear inclusion has become established; these consist of basophilic specks beginning in the perinuclear zone and extending peripherally toward the cytoplasmic border.

The pattern of lung involvement in CMV infection is variable.[103,108] Some cases contain inclusions in scattered macrophages with no inflammatory reaction. Some cases show small miliary nodules with numerous inclusions, hemorrhagic necrosis, and a polymorphonuclear leukocyte response reminiscent of herpes simplex pneumonia; these patients often die with CMV viremia. Some cases show typical diffuse alveolar damage with inclusions in bronchiolar and alveolar epithelial cells, and on occasion one may find a localized nodule of CMV-related interstitial pneumonitis which can grossly or radiologically simulate a neoplasm.[109] Furthermore, CMV inclusions may occur in areas of active cellular reduplication such as ulcers, granulation tissue, or nonviral pneumonia[96] (Fig. 11–26); an important implication is that the presence of occasional CMV inclusions in an immunocompromised host does not exclude the possibility that another organism such as *Pneumocystis carinii* is the prime offender. It is most unusual to find CMV-induced ulcers or CMV inclusions in the trachea or main bronchi, suggesting that inhalation is an uncommon route of infection for this virus. There is some evidence that in most cases, CMV is carried to the lung by monocytes that are capable of crossing the endothelium, entering the interstitium, and infecting epithelial cells secondarily.[96]

The varying morphologic patterns do not correlate well with viral load, severity of infection, or type of infection, that is, primary vs. reactivation.[108] Furthermore, there are many instances of culture-positive, inclusion-negative CMV pneumonia.[108,110] DNA hybridization studies indicate that viral products may be present in tissues that are both inclusion-negative and culture-negative.[14]

Electron-microscopy of CMV-infected cells [111] shows central filamentous nuclear material, a relatively electron lucent halo, and scattered noncoated intranuclear round viral particles approximately 100 nm in diameter. The cytoplasmic inclusions consist of aggregates of virions mostly in membrane-bound packets. Most of the individual virions have acquired an outer coat, presumably from nuclear or cytoplasmic membranes, measure approximately 140 nm, and have a configuration similar to herpes simplex (Fig. 11–27).

Relationship of Viral Infections to Chronic Airflow Obstruction

As mentioned previously, the development of bronchiolitis obliterans after adenovirus infection is a well-established pathogenetic sequence. More subtle relationships between viral infection and chronic bronchitis, asthma, and functional obstruction are suspected but are not as firmly established.

Adult patients with chronic bronchitis probably are not at increased risk to acquire respiratory viral infections over the general population,[112] but viral infections are a major cause of acute respiratory illness in chronic bronchitis and there is excessive mortality in this patient population during influenza epidemics.[113] Patients with cystic fibrosis are also not apparently at increased risk to acquire viral infection of the respiratory tract, but viral infection exacerbates deterioration of pulmonary function.[114]

The relationship between lower respiratory tract infection in infancy, atopy, and obstructive airway dysfunction is a complicated and unresolved issue which has been the subject of numerous retrospective studies, prospective studies, and reviews.[115-117] Children who have been hospitalized for RSV infection in infancy have an increase incidence of long-term episodic wheezing.[118] It is uncertain whether atopic children are more likely to develop symptomatic viral respiratory tract infection or whether

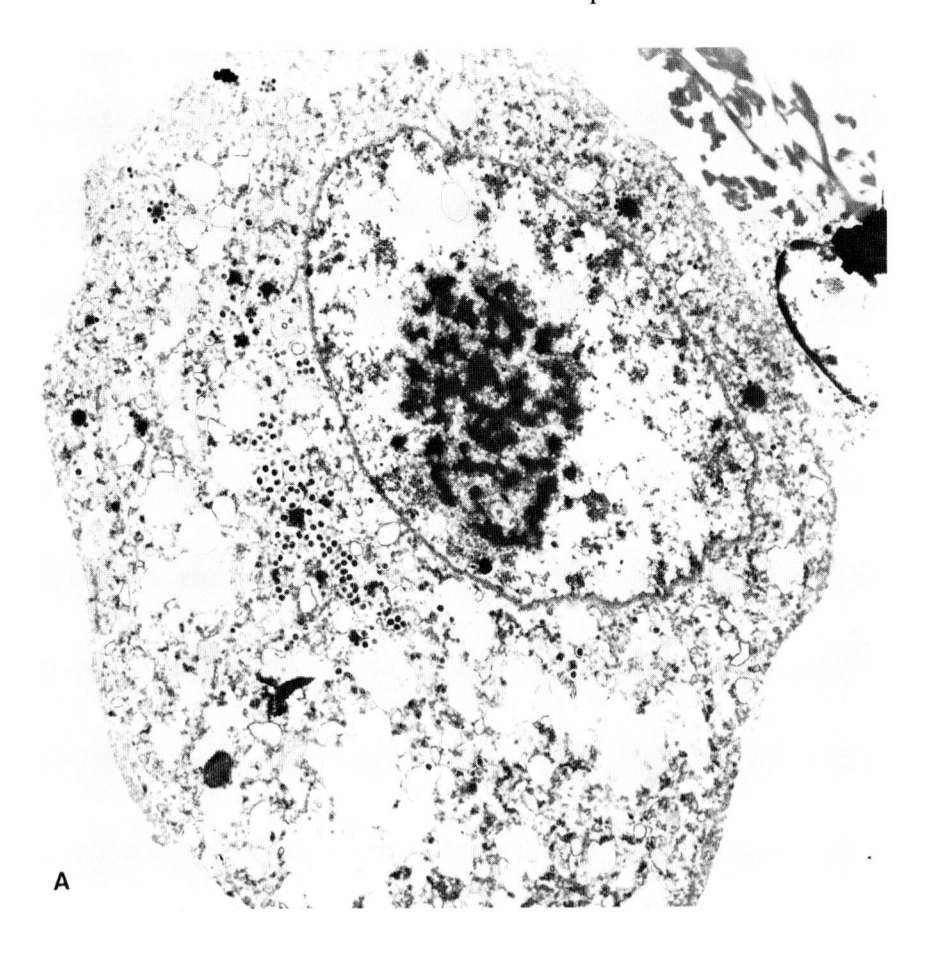

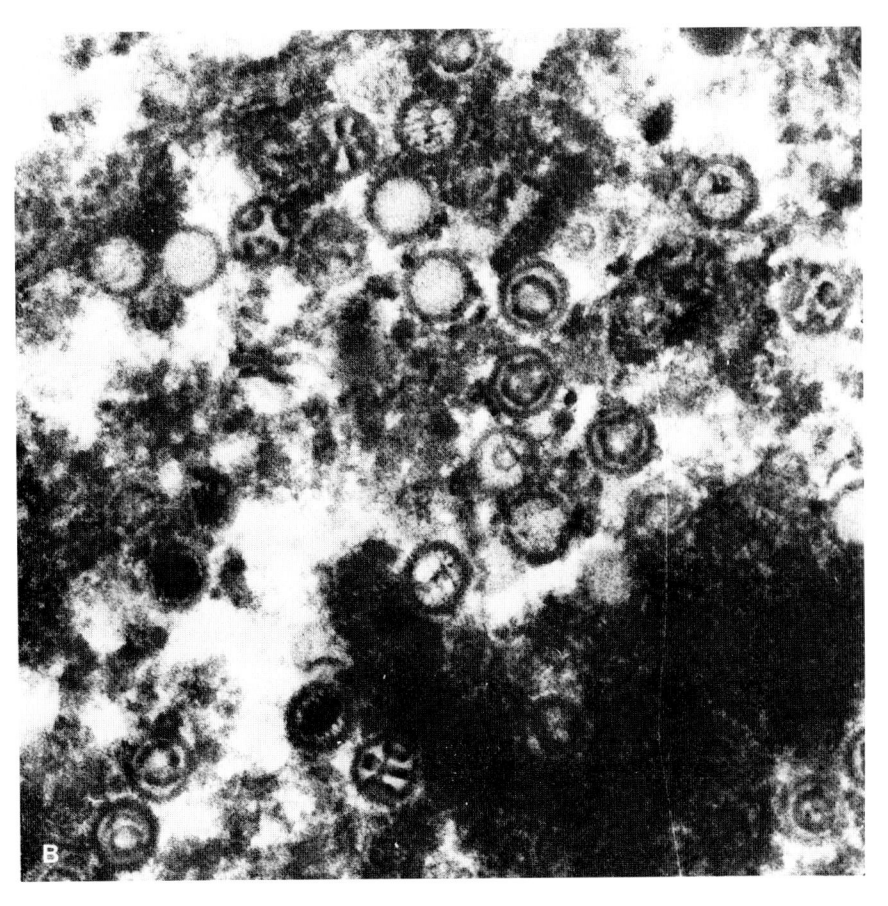

Figure 11–27. A. Electron micrograph of autopsy case of cytomegalovirus. Note prominent nuclear inclusion and membrane-bound cytoplasmic virions (×5600). B. Nuclear viral particles enmeshed in electron-dense inclusion (×96,000). See part C on following page.

Figure 11–27. C. Cytoplasmic-coated virions in membrane-bound vesicles (×72,000).

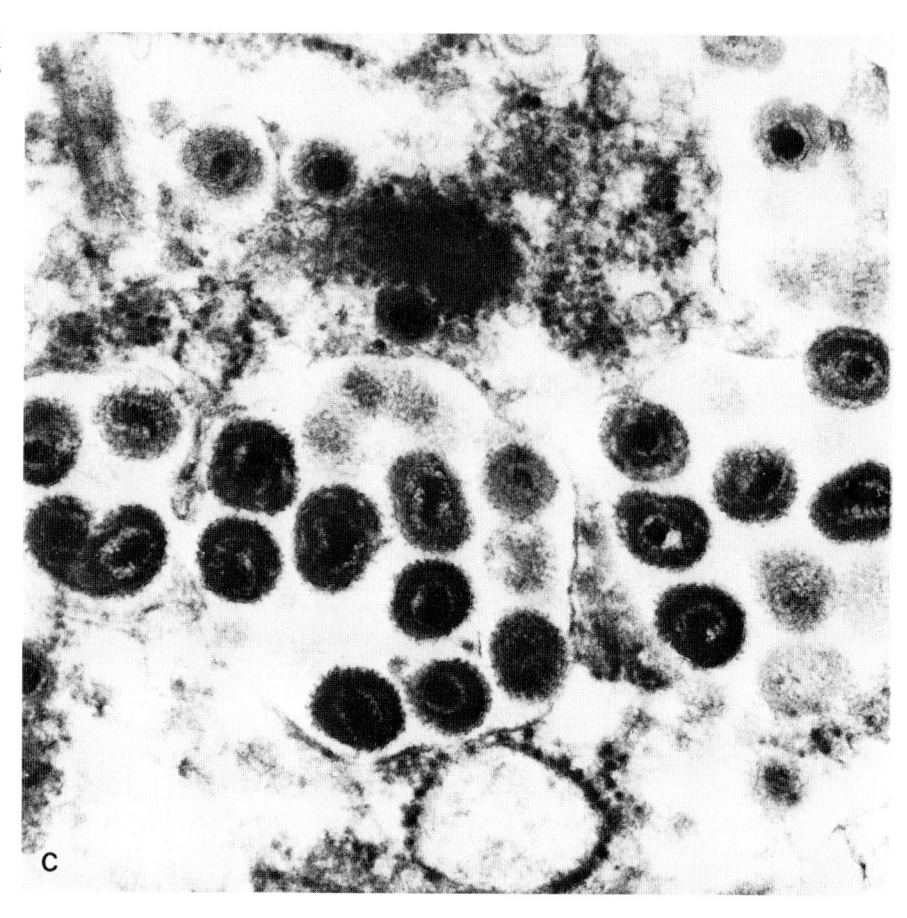

viral infection at an early age injures the respiratory tract in such a way that these patients develop atopic symptoms. Welliver and co-workers[119–121] have presented data suggesting that an immunologic abnormality, that is, atopy, is of primary importance in the viral infection-asthma relationship, whereby atopic children have a more severe and more "wheezy" response to viral infection. In patients with established childhood asthma, viral respiratory tract infection often results in exacerbation of asthmatic symptoms.[122,123] There is also evidence, albeit inconclusive, that childhood viral respiratory infections predispose to obstructive dysfunction later in life, either alone or in conjunction with other respiratory toxins.[116,117,124–126]

References

1. Kanner RE, Renzetti AD, Klauber MR, et al.: Variables associated with changes in spirometry in patients with obstructive lung diseases. Am J Med 67:44–50, 1979.

1a. Anderson LJ, Patriarca PA, Hierholzer JC, Noble GR: Viral respiratory illnesses. Med Clin North Am 67:1009–1030, 1983.

2. Osborne D: Radiologic appearance of viral disease of the lower respiratory tract in infants and children. AJR 130:29–33, 1978.

3. Tew J, Calenoff L, Berlin BS: Bacterial or nonbacterial pneumonia: Accuracy of radiographic diagnosis. Radiology 124:607–612, 1977.

4. Peterson LR, Balfour HH Jr: Advances in clinical virology. Prog Clin Pathol 8:239–267, 1981.

5. Richman DD, Cleveland PH, Redfield DC, et al.: Rapid viral diagnosis. J Infect Dis 149:298–310, 1984.

6. Uren E, Elsum R, Jack I: A comparative study of the diagnosis of respiratory virus infections by immunofluorescence and viral isolation in children. Aust Pediatr J 13:282–286, 1977.

7. Downham MAPS, McQuillin J, Gardner PS: Diagnosis and clinical significance of parainfluenza virus infections in children. Arch Dis Child 49:8–15, 1974.

8. Lauer BA: Comparison of virus culturing and immunofluorescence for rapid detection of respiratory syncytial virus in nasopharyngeal secretions: Sensitivity and specificity. J Clin Microbiol 16:411–412, 1982.

9. Strano AJ: Light microscopy of selected viral diseases (morphology of viral inclusion bodies). Pathol Annu 53–75, 1976.

10. Yunis EJ, Hashida Y, Haas JE: The role of electron microscopy in the identification of viruses in human disease. Pathol Annu (part I) 311–330, 1977.

11. Yunis EJ, Agostini RM Jr, Atchison RW: An atlas of viral particles from human specimens. Perspect Pediatr Pathol 4:387–429, 1978.

12. Virtanen M, Palva A, Laaksonen M, et al.: Novel test for

rapid viral diagnosis: Detection of adenovirus in nasopharyngeal mucus aspirates by means of nucleic-acid sandwich hybridisation. Lancet 1(8321):381–383, 1983.

13. Seidlin M, Takiff HE, Smith HA, et al.: Detection of varicella-zoster virus by dot-blot hybridization using a molecularly cloned viral DNA probe. J Med Virol 13:53–61, 1984.

14. Myerson D, Hackman RC, Nelson JA, et al.: Widespread presence of histologically occult cytomegalovirus. Hum Pathol 15:430–439, 1984.

14a. Kulski JK, Norval M: Nucleic acid probes in diagnosis of viral diseases of man; Brief review. Arch Virol 83:3–15, 1985.

Influenza

15. Reichman RC, Dolin R: Viral pneumonias. Med Clin North Am 64:491–506, 1980.

16. Gregg MB: The epidemiology of influenza in humans. Ann NY Acad Sci 353:45–53, 1980.

17. Lennette EH: Viral respiratory diseases: vaccines and antivirals. Bull WHO 59:305–324, 1981.

18. Caul EO, Waller DK, Clarke SKR: A comparison of influenza and respiratory syncytial virus infections among infants admitted to hospital with acute respiratory infections. J Hyg 77:383–392, 1976.

19. Laraya-Cuasay LR, DeForest A, Huff D, et al.: Chronic pulmonary complications of early influenza virus infection in children. Am Rev Respir Dis 116:617–625, 1977.

20. Barker WH, Mullooly JP: Pneumonia and influenza deaths during epidemics; implications for prevention. Arch Intern Med 142:85–89, 1982.

21. Noble RL, Lillington GA, Kempson RL: Fatal diffuse influenzal pneumonia: Premortem diagnosis by lung biopsy. Chest 63:644–647, 1973.

22. Finckh ES, Bader L: Pulmonary damage from Hong Kong influenza. Aust N Z J Med 4:16–22, 1974.

23. Pinsker KL, Schneyer B, Becker N, Kamholz SL: Usual interstitial pneumonia following Texas A2 influenza infection. Chest 80:123–126, 1981.

24. Jakab GJ, Astry CL, Warr GA: Alveolitis induced by influenza virus. Am Rev Respir Dis 128:730–739, 1983.

25. Sweet C, Macartney JC, Bird RA, et al.: Differential distribution of virus and histological damage in the lower respiratory tract of ferrets infected with influenza viruses of differing virulence. J Gen Virol 54:103–114, 1981.

26. Husseini RH, Sweet C, Bird RA, et al.: Distribution of viral antigen within the lower respiratory tract of ferrets infected with a virulent influenza virus: Production and release of virus from corresponding organ cultures. J Gen Virol 64:589–598, 1983.

Measles

27. Fawcitt J, Parry HE: Lung changes in pertussis and measles in childhood. A review of 1894 cases with a follow-up study of the pulmonary complications. Br J Radiol 30:76–82, 1957.

28. Sobonya RE, Hiller C, Pingleton W, Watanabe I: Fatal measles (rubeola) pneumonia in adults. Arch Pathol Lab Med 102:366–371, 1978.

29. Becroft DMO, Osborne DRS: The lungs in fatal measles infection in childhood: Pathological, radiological and immunological correlations. Histopathology 4:401–412, 1980.

30. Breitfeld V, Hashida Y, Sherman FE, et al.: Fatal measles infection in children with leukemia. Lab Invest 28:279–291, 1973.

31. Young LW: Radiological case of the month. Am J Dis Child 134:511–512, 1980.

32. Hecht V: Die Riesenzellenpneumonie im Kindesalter, eine historische-experimentelle Studie. Beitrage zur pathologischen Anatomie und zer allemeinen Pathologie 48:262–310, 1910.

33. Enders JF, McCarthy K, Mitus A, Cheatham WJ: Isolation of measles virus at autopsy in cases of giant-cell pneumonia without rash. N Engl J Med 261:875–881, 1959.

34. Margolin Fr, Gandy TK: Pneumonia of atypical measles. Radiology 131:653, 1979.

35. Frey HM, Krugman S: Atypical measles syndrome: Unusual hepatic, pulmonary and immunologic aspects. Am J Med Sci 281:51–55, 1981.

Parainfluenza

36. Viral respiratory diseases. WHO Tech Rep Ser (642):1–63, 1980.

37. Welliver R, Wong DT, Choi T-S, Ogra PL: Natural history of parainfluenza virus infection in childhood. J Pediatrics 101:180–187, 1982.

38. Wenzel RP, McCormick DP, Beam WE Jr: Parainfluenza pneumonia in adults. JAMA 221:294–295, 1972.

39. Wong DT, Ogra PL: Viral infections in immunocompromised patients. Med Clin North Am 67:1075–1092, 1983.

40. Jarvis WR, Middleton PJ, Gelfand EW: Parainfluenza pneumonia in severe combined immunodeficiency disease. J Pediatr 94:423–425, 1979.

41. Delage G, Brochu P, Pelletier M, et al.: Giant cell pneumonia caused by parainfluenza virus. J Pediatr 94:426–429, 1979.

42. Wagener JS, Minnich L, Sobonya R, et al.: Parainfluenza type II infection in dogs, a model for viral lower respiratory tract infection in humans. Am Rev Respir Dis 127:771–775, 1983.

Respiratory Syncytial Virus

43. Wohl MEB, Chernick V: Bronchiolitis. Am Rev Respir Dis 118:759–781, 1978.

44. Jacobs JW, Peacock DB, Corner BD, et al.: Respiratory syncytial and other viruses associated with respiratory disease in infants. Lancet 1:871–876, 1971.

45. Glezen WP, Paredes A, Allison JE, et al.: Risk of respiratory syncytial virus infection for infants from low-income families in relationship to age, sex, ethnic group, and maternal antibody level. J Pediatr 98:708–715, 1981.

46. Hall CB: Nosocomial viral respiratory infections: Perennial weeds on pediatric wards. Am J Med 70:670–676, 1981.

47. Henderson FW, Collier AM, Clyde WA Jr, Denny FW: Respiratory syncytial virus infections, reinfections and immunity; a prospective, longitudinal study in young children. N Engl J Med 300:530–534, 1979.

48. Hall WJ, Hall CB, Speers DM: Respiratory syncytial virus infection in adults. Ann Intern Med 88:203–205, 1978.

49. Mathur U, Bentley DW, Hall CB: Concurrent respiratory syncytial virus and influenza A infections in the institutionalized elderly and chronically ill. Ann Intern Med 93:49–52, 1980.

50. Respiratory syncytial virus infection in the elderly 1976–82. Br Med J 287:1618–1619, 1983.

51. Spelman DW, Stanley PA: Respiratory syncytial virus pneumonitis in adults. Med J Aust 1:430–431, 1983.

52. Capewell A, Inglis JM, Williamson J: Respiratory syncytial virus infection in the elderly. Br Med J 288:235–236, 1984.

53. Tyeryar FJ: National Institute of Allergy and Infectious Diseases News: Report of a workshop on respiratory syncytial virus and parainfluenza viruses. J Infect Dis 148:588–598, 1983.

54. Glezen WP, Loda FA, Clyde WA Jr, et al.: Epidemiologic patterns of acute lower respiratory disease of children in a pediatric group practice. J Pediatr 78:397–406, 1971.

55. Anas N, Boettrich C, Hall CB, Brooks JG: The association of apnea and respiratory syncytial virus infection in infants. J Pediatr 101:65–68, 1982.

56. Colditz PB, Henry RL, DeSilva LM: Apnoea and bronchiolitis due to respiratory syncytial virus. Aust Pediatr J 18:53–54, 1982.

57. Scott DJ, Gardner PS, McQuillin J, et al.: Respiratory viruses and cot death. Br Med J 2:12–13, 1978.

58. Hall CB, Kopelman AE, Douglas RG Jr, et al.: Neonatal respiratory syncytial virus infection. N Engl J Med 300:393–396, 1979.

59. Aherne W, Bird T, Court SDM, et al.: Pathological changes in virus infections of the lower respiratory tract in children. J Clin Pathol 23:7–18, 1970.

59a. Delage G, Brochu P, Robillard L, et al.: Giant pneumonia due to respiratory syncytial virus, Occurrence in severe combined immunodeficiency syndrome. Arch Pathol Lab Med 108:623–625, 1984.

60. Garner PS: How etiologic, pathologic, and clinical diagnoses can be made in a correlated fashion. Pediatr Res 11:254–261, 1977.

Miscellaneous RNA Viruses

61. Halperin SA, Eggleston PA, Hendley JO, et al.: Pathogenesis of lower respiratory tract symptoms in experimental rhinovirus infection. Am Rev Respir Dis 128:806–810, 1983.

62. Cheeseman SH, Hirsch MS, Keller EW, Keim DE: Fatal neonatal pneumonia caused by Echovirus type 9. Am J Dis Child 131:1169, 1977.

Adenoviruses

63. Schonland M, Strong ML, Wesley A: Fatal adenovirus pneumonia; clinical and pathological features. S Afr Med J 50:1748–1751, 1976.

64. Wenman WW, Pagtakhan RD, Reed MH, et al.: Adenovirus bronchiolitis in Manitoba. Chest 81:605–609, 1982.

65. Lang WR, Howden CW, Laws J, Burton JF: Bronchopneumonia with serious sequelae in children with evidence of adenovirus type 21 infection. Br Med J 1:73–79, 1969.

66. Osborne D, White P: Radiology of epidemic adenovirus 21 infection of the lower respiratory tract in infants and young children. AJR 133:397–400, 1979.

67. Myerowitz RL, Stalder H, Oxman MN, et al.: Fatal disseminated adenovirus infection in a renal transplant recipient. Am J Med 59:591–598, 1975.

68. Zahradnik JM, Spencer MJ, Porter DD: Adenovirus infection in the immunocompromised patient. Am J Med 68:725–732, 1980.

69. Siegal FP, Dikman SH, Arayata RB, Bottone EJ: Fatal disseminated adenovirus 11 pneumonia in an agammaglobulinemic patient. Am J Med 71:1062–1067, 1981.

70. Nash G: Pathologic features of the lung in the immunocompromised host. Hum Pathol 13:841–858, 1982.

71. Case Records of the Massachusetts General Hospital, case 6-1979. N Engl J Med 300:301–309, 1979.

72. Becroft DMO: Bronchiolitis obliterans, bronchiectasis, and other sequelae of adenovirus type 21 infection in young children. J Clin Pathol 24:72–82, 1971.

73. James AG, Lang WR, Liang AY, et al.: Adenovirus type 21 bronchopneumonia in infants and young children. J Pediatr 95:530–533, 1979.

74. Simila S, Linna O, Lanning P, et al.: Chronic lung damage caused by adenovirus type 7: A ten year follow-up study. Chest 80:127–131, 1981.

75. Becroft DMO: Histopathology of fatal adenovirus infection of the respiratory tract in young children. J Clin Pathol 20:561–569, 1967.

Herpes Simplex

76. Graham BS, Snell JD Jr. Herpes simplex virus infection of the adult lower respiratory tract. Medicine 62:384–393, 1983.

77. Nash G, Foley FD: Herpetic infection of the middle and lower respiratory tract. Am J Clin Pathol 54:857–863, 1970.

78. Williams DM, Krick JA, Remington JS: Pulmonary infection in the compromised host. Am Rev Respir Dis 114:593–627, 1976.

79. Tuxen DV, Cade JF, McDonald MI, et al.: Herpes simplex virus from the lower respiratory tract in adult respiratory distress syndrome. Am Rev Respir Dis 126:416–419, 1982.

80. Nash G: Necrotizing tracheobronchitis and bronchopneumonia consistent with herpetic infection. Hum Pathol 3:283–291, 1972.

81. Vernon SE: Cytologic features of nonfatal herpes-virus tracheobronchitis. Acta Cytol 26:237–242, 1982.

82. Ramsey PG, Fife KH, Hackman RC, et al.: Herpes simplex virus pneumonia; Clinical, virologic, and pathologic features in 20 patients. Ann Intern Med 97:813–820, 1982.

83. White CL III, Taxy JB: Early morphologic diagnosis of herpes simplex virus encephalitis: Advantages of electron microscopy and immunoperoxidase staining. Hum Pathol 14:135–139, 1983.

Varicella-Zoster

84. Weber DM, Pellecchia JA: Varicella pneumonia; study of prevalence in adult men. JAMA 192:572–573, 1965.

85. Triebwasser JH, Harris RE, Bryant RE, Rhoades ER: Varicella pneumonia in adults. Medicine 46:409–423, 1967.

86. Burton GG, Sayer WJ, Lillington GA: Varicella pneumonitis in adults; frequency of sudden death. Dis Chest 50:179–185, 1966.

87. Nikki P, Meretoja W, Valtonen V, et al.: Severe bronchiolitis probably caused by varicella-zoster virus. Crit Care Med 10:344–346, 1982.

88. Raider L: Calcification in chickenpox pneumonia. Chest 60:504–507, 1971.

89. Weller TH: Varicella and herpes zoster. Changing concepts of the natural history, control, and importance of a not-so-benign virus (first of two parts). N Engl J Med 309:1362–1368, 1983.

90. Miliauskas JR, Webber BL: Disseminated varicella at autopsy in children with cancer. Cancer 53:1518–1525, 1984.

91. Pek S, Gikas PW: Pneumonia due to herpes zoster; report

of a case and review of the literature. Ann Intern Med 62:350–358, 1965.

92. Rosen P, Hajdu SI: Visceral herpesvirus infections in patients with cancer. Am J Clin Pathol 56:459–465, 1971.

Cytomegalovirus

92a. Cohen JI, Corey GR: Cytomegalovirus infection in the normal host. Medicine 64:100–114, 1985.

93. Betts RF: Cytomegalovirus infection epidemiology and biology in adults. Semin Perinatol 7:22–30, 1983.

94. Idell S, Johnson M, Beauregard L, Learner N: Pneumonia associated with rising cytomegalovirus antibody titers in a healthy adult. Thorax 38:957–958, 1983.

95. Stagno S, Brasfield DM, Brown MB, et al.: Infant pneumonitis associated with cytomegalovirus, chlamydia, pneumocystis, and ureaplasma: A prospective study. Pediatrics 68:322–329, 1981.

96. Craighead JE: Cytomegalovirus pulmonary disease. Pathobiol Annu 5:197–220, 1975.

97. Suwansirikul S, Rao N, Dowling JN, Ho M: Primary and secondary cytomegalovirus infection; Clinical manifestations after renal transplantation. Arch Intern Med 137:1026–1029, 1977.

98. Walker DP, Longson M, Mallick NP, Johnson RWG: A prospective study of cytomegalovirus and herpes simplex virus disease in renal transplant recipients. J Clin Pathol 35:1190–1193, 1982.

99. Marker SC, Howard RJ, Simmons RL, et al.: Cytomegalovirus infection: A quantitative prospective study of three hundred twenty consecutive renal transplants. Surgery 89:660–671, 1981.

100. Rifkind D, Goodman N, Hill RB: The clinical significance of cytomegalovirus infection in renal transplant recipients. Ann Intern Med 66:1116–1128, 1967.

101. Zaia JA, Forman SJ, Gallagher MT, et al.: Prolonged human cytomegalovirus viremia following bone marrow transplantation. Transplantation 37:315–317, 1984.

102. Neiman PE, Reeves W, Ray G, et al.: A prospective analysis of interstitial pneumonia and opportunistic viral infection among recipients of allogeneic bone marrow grafts. J Infect Dis 136:754–767, 1977.

103. Beschorner WE, Hutchins GM, Burns WH, et al.: Cytomegalovirus pneumonia in bone marrow transplant recipients: Miliary and diffuse patterns. Am Rev Respir Dis 122:107–114, 1980.

104. Hui AN, Koss MN, Meyer PR: Necropsy findings in acquired immunodeficiency syndrome: A comparison of premortem diagnoses with postmortem findings. Hum Pathol 15:670–676, 1984.

105. Wang N-S, Huang S-N, Thurlbeck WM: Combined pneumocystis carinii and cytomegalovirus infection. Arch Pathol 90:529–535, 1970.

106. Abdallah PS, Mark JBD, Merigan TC: Diagnosis of cytomegalovirus pneumonia in compromised hosts. Am J Med 61:326–332, 1976.

107. Ernst P, Chen M-F, Wang N-S, Cosio M: Symbiosis of pneumocystis carinii and cytomegalovirus in a case of fatal pneumonia. Can Med Assoc J 128:1089–1092, 1983.

108. Craighead JE: Pulmonary cytomegalovirus infection in the adult. Am J Pathol 63:487–504, 1971.

109. Ravin CE, Smith GW, Ahern MJ, et al.: Cytomegaloviral infection presenting as a solitary pulmonary nodule. Chest 71:220–222, 1977.

110. Volpi A, Whitley RJ, Ceballos R, et al.: Rapid diagnosis of pneumonia due to cytomegalovirus with specific monoclonal antibodies. J Infect Dis 147:1119–1120, 1983.

111. Kasnic G Jr, Sayeed A, Azar HA: Nuclear and cytoplasmic inclusions in disseminated human cytomegalovirus infection. Ultrastruct Pathol 3:229–235, 1982.

Relationship of Viral Infections to Chronic Airflow Obstruction

112. Smith CB, Golden CA, Kanner RE, Renzetti AD Jr: Association of viral and mycoplasma pneumoniae infections with acute respiratory illness in patients with chronic obstructive pulmonary diseases. Am Rev Respir Dis 121:225–232, 1980.

113. Blackwelder WC, Alling DW, Stuart-Harris CH: Association of excess mortality from chronic nonspecific lung disease with epidemics of influenza. Am Rev Respir Dis 125:511–516, 1982.

114. Wang EEL, Prober CG, Manson B, et al.: Association of respiratory viral infections with pulmonary deterioration in patients with cystic fibrosis. N Engl J Med 311:1653–1658, 1984.

115. Burrows B, Taussig LM: As the twig is bent, the tree inclines (perhaps). Editorial. Am Rev Respir Dis 122:813–816, 1980.

116. Samet JM, Tager IB, Speizer FE: The relationship between respiratory illness in childhood and chronic airflowobstruction in adulthood. Am Rev Respir Dis 127:508–523, 1983.

117. Welliver RC: Viral infections and obstructive airway disease in early life. Pediatr Clin North Am 30:819–828, 1983.

118. Pullan CR, Hey EN: Wheezing, asthma, and pulmonary dysfunction 10 years after infection with respiratory syncytial virus in infancy. Br Med J 284:1665–1669, 1982.

119. Welliver RC, Kaul TN, Ogra PL: The appearance of cell-bound IgE in respiratory-tract epithelium after respiratory-syncytial-virus infection. N Engl J Med 303:1198–1202, 1980.

120. Welliver RC, Wong DT, Sun M, et al.: The development of respiratory syncytial virus-specific IgE and the release of histamine in nasopharyngeal secretions after infection. N Engl J Med 305:841–846, 1981.

121. Welliver RC, Wong DT, Middleton E Jr, et al.: Role of parainfluenza virus-specific IgE in pathogenesis of croup and wheezing subsequent to infection. J Pediatr 101:889–896, 1982.

122. Roldaan AC, Masural N: Viral respiratory infections in asthmatic children staying in a mountain resort. Eur J Respir Dis 63:140–150, 1982.

123. Carlsen KH, Orstavik I, Leegaard J, Hoeg H: Respiratory virus infections and aeroallergens in acute bronchial asthma. Arch Dis Child 59:310–315, 1984.

124. Burrows B, Knudson RJ, Lebowitz MD: The relationship of childhood respiratory illness to adult obstructive airway disease. Am Rev Respir Dis 115:751–760, 1977.

125. Mok JYQ, Simpson H: Outcome for acute bronchitis, bronchiolitis, and pneumonia in infancy. Arch Dis Child 59:306–309, 1984.

126. Hall CB, Hall WJ, Gala CL, et al.: Long-term prospective study in children after respiratory syncytial virus infection. J Pediatr 105:358–364, 1984.

12 Mycoplasma, Chlamydia, and Coxiella Infections of the Respiratory Tract

Roberta R. Miller

In the 1930s and 1940s, the term primary atypical pneumonia was coined to refer to a syndrome distinct from "typical" lobar pneumonia. The features of this syndrome included fever, patchy infiltrates on chest radiographs, and a minimally productive cough without a predominant organism identified by Gram stain of sputum. No conventional bacteria could be cultured from blood, sputum, or pleural fluid from these cases. Leukocytosis tended to be less pronounced than in typical lobar pneumonia and the onset of disease was often less abrupt. Since that time, a variety of organisms have been found to be responsible for the atypical pneumonia syndrome, including *Mycoplasma pneumoniae*, Chlamydia, Coxiella, Legionella, and viruses. The latter two groups of agents are discussed elsewhere (*see* Chapters 11 and 13). The former three are the subject of this chapter.

Mycoplasma pneumoniae

The *Mycoplasma pneumoniae* organism is a bacterium lacking a cell wall. Its shape and size is thus variable although it usually assumes a tubular shape 200 nm × 10 nm. It is capable of extracellular replication but grows slowly with a doubling time up to 20 times longer than the more conventional bacteria, and also requires a more complex media for successful culture.[1] The organism attaches itself to the ciliated respiratory epithelial cells via a specialized terminal filament which can be seen ultrastructurally in experimental models and occasionally in clinical material.[2] Replication occurs in this site, with the organism being shed in secretions as long as a week prior to development of symptoms.

M. pneumoniae infection is typically a disease of otherwise healthy adolescents and young adults, and is estimated to be a common pathogen in this population.[3] Approximately 20 percent of infections are asymptomatic. The majority of symptomatic infections are either mild upper respiratory tract infections or tracheobronchitis, but approximately 5 to 10 percent of infections result in actual pneumonia.[3,4] The portal of entry and site of primary infection for *M. pneumoniae* is the respiratory tract. Contagion within families or closed populations is common, leading to miniepidemics of the disease.[3,5–8] While *M. pneumoniae* tends to affect patients under the age of 40 years, approximately 25 percent of cases are seen in older age groups[8] and there is some evidence that this population has a higher frequency of complicated infection.[1] *M. pneumoniae* is estimated to cause approximately 15 percent of cases of pneumonia in patients over 40 years of age,[4] and may exacerbate symptoms of underlying asthma or chronic obstructive lung disease.[7,9] It can occasionally cause serious respiratory disease in immunocompromised patients[1,10,11] but is not generally regarded as a typical opportunistic organism in that unfortunate population.

The usual clinical symptoms of *M. pneumoniae* infection include cough which is productive of purulent sputum in approximately 30 percent of cases[7] and is worse at night.[8] Nonspecific complaints of fever, chills, headache, and malaise are frequent. Often the actual clinical signs are disproportionately small compared to the symptoms. Less-constant symptoms include chest pain, high fever,[11] hemoptysis,[7] and a variety of extrapulmonary symptoms seen in up to 40 percent of patients[9] and discussed in more detail below.

The abnormalities seen on chest radiographs in *M. pneumoniae* pneumonia are highly variable. The "classic" radiographic abnormality is unilateral, lower lobar, segmental consolidation. However, bilateral changes are seen in 40 to 50 percent of cases,[9,11,12] upper lobe infiltrates are seen in approximately 20 percent of cases,[9,11] diffuse reticular interstitial infiltrates are seen in 10 to 20 percent of cases,[8,9,11] and central, perihilar bilateral infiltrates are seen in up to 40 percent of cases.[7] Pleural effusions occur in approximately 20 percent of cases and these are usually small and unilateral.[7,11,12] Hilar adenopathy is seen in approximately 20 percent of cases.[12] This marked variability in radiographic changes is likely to be at least partly related to variability of changes with time in any given patient.[11]

Three unusual laboratory features may be found at the time of presentation. The first is that the total white blood cell count is normal in 75 to 90 percent of cases of *M. pneumoniae* infection[4] although there may be a mild elevation of absolute neutrophil count.[5] Even in cases of actual pneumonia, the white count, if elevated, is usually only modestly so. Second, Gram strain of sputum may show numerous polymorphonuclear leukocytes but no predominant bacteria.[4] Third, abnormal cold hemagglutinins are seen in many patients, the estimates ranging from 33 to 76 percent.[4,7] These hemagglutinins have anti-I specificity, are detectable within 1 to 2 weeks of infection and persist up to 6 weeks.[3] They may be associated with a detectable hemolytic anemia. While these cold agglutinins are neither highly sensitive nor highly specific, the syndrome of pneumonia and anti-I specific hemolytic anemia is quite suggestive of *M. pneumoniae* infection.[9]

The definitive diagnosis of *M. pneumoniae* infection is made by either culture or serology. As mentioned previously, the organism is a slowly growing bacterium which requires complex media and as long as 10 days incubation time for successful culture.[1,4] The usual serologic test is complement fixation. With paired acute and convalescent sera, a fourfold or greater titer rise indicates infection. With convalescent sera only, a titer of 1:64 or greater is highly suggestive of infection. Titer elevations begin approximately 1 week after infection, peak from 1 to 4 months following infection, then slowly fall.[4]

The course of uncomplicated *M. pneumoniae* infection is one of resolution of most of the symptoms in 1 to 2 weeks, with persistence of the cough, and to a lesser extent the radiographic abnormalities, for several weeks after clinical improvement. Antibiotic therapy (tetracyclines, erythromycin) accelerates resolution of clinical illness and radiologic abnormalities. However, it often takes a few days for the response to begin, and relapses in the face of appropriate antibiotic therapy do occur.[4] In addition to the hemolytic anemia mentioned above, a wide variety of extrapulmonary manifestations may occur with *M. pneumoniae* infection. These include gastroenteritis, arthralgias or arthritis, myocarditis, pericarditis, meningitis, encephalitis, and peripheral neuropathies.[4,7,9] Another extrapulmonary manifestation that can cause serious long-term sequelae is erythema multiforme of skin and mucosa (Stevens-Johnson syndrome).[4] These extrapulmonary changes usually occur in patients with clinically evident respiratory tract disease and develop within the first 2 weeks of the illness. They resolve with variable speed and do not seem to be influenced by antibiotic therapy.[4]

Infection with *M. pneumoniae* does not result in long-lasting immunity.[11]

The histopathology of *M. pneumoniae* pneumonia is elusive for two reasons. The first reason is that few patients with the disease come to biopsy or autopsy early in its course. The second reason is that the findings are nonspecific and can be mimicked by various other bacterial and viral agents. Thus, the diagnosis rests with serology and culture, and not with the histopathologic findings.

In a recent series of six lung biopsies in *M. pneumoniae* pneumonia,[13] the predominant abnormality was acute bronchiolitis, in which there was purulent intraluminal material, eroded or metaplastic bronchiolar epithelial cells, and a lymphoplasmacytic infiltrate in the bronchiolar walls. The alveoli immediately around involved bronchioles contained a mononuclear cell interstitial infiltrate with alveolar type II cell enlargement but no hyaline membranes. Two of the six cases contained a notable monocyte infiltrate in the subpleural or paraseptal areas, and one had a truly diffuse mononuclear cell interstitial infiltrate in addition to the bronchiolitis.

In the rare instance of fatal pneumonia, various abnormalities have been described.[6] Necrotizing tracheobronchitis with purulent intraluminal material and a mononuclear cell infiltrate in the walls may been seen. Peribronchiolar abscesses may be seen. Either a diffuse interstitial mononuclear cell infiltrate in alveolar walls, or a more ordinary bronchopneumonia-type appearance may be seen in the mid- and peripheral zones of the lobules. A diffuse alveolar damage type of reaction pattern with hyaline membranes is apparently uncommon.[1,7] Large pleural effusions are uncommon and superinfection by other bacterial organisms are uncommon.[4]

A hamster model for *M. pneumoniae* pneumonia is described[2] in which the animals have a self-limited infection similar to that seen in humans. These animals develop patchy bronchiolitis with a mononuclear infiltrate in the walls and polymorphonuclear leukocytes in the lumen, and relative sparing of alveolar walls. Presumably if there is a typical histologic reaction to *M. pneumoniae* infection, it appears in this fashion.

A most unusual reaction to *M. pneumoniae* infection has also been described, namely, caseating granulomas simulating tuberculosis.[14]

Chlamydia

The Chlamydia genus has two species, *C. psittaci* and *C. trachomatis*. While the general characteristics of the two are similar in terms of life cycle,[14,15] each causes a different clinical type of lung disease. The bacterial nature of the organisms is confirmed by the presence of both DNA and RNA, by the presence of a cell wall, by their susceptibility to antibiotics, and by replication by binary fission. The major peculiarities of the organisms are that they have separate intracellular and extracellular forms and that they depend on the host cell for adenosine triphosphate (ATP) and other metabolites. The extracellular form, termed the "elementary body," has a rigid cell wall and is metabolically inactive. It is the infective particle and is the form that attaches to and is taken in by the host cell. Within a few hours, the elementary body develops into the metabolically active intracellular form, termed the "reticulate" or "initial" body. This form is an obligate intracellular organism without a cell wall and is the replicative form. In 1 to 2 days following infection, the initial bodies revert to elementary bodies and are released by cell lysis. Prior to cell lysis, the newly formed elementary bodies may be recognized in cultures as intracytoplasmic inclusions. These inclusions can occasionally be recognized in lung issue by specific immunofluorescence.[17,18]

Chlamydia psittaci

The natural host for *C. psittaci* are birds and domestic poultry, and thus the alternate term for "psittacosis" (psittacus = parrot) is "ornithosis" (ornis = bird). In the vast majority of cases, the human patient acquires the disease from a bird, either an overtly sick animal or a carrier, and the relevant history can be elicited in approximately 90 percent of cases.[18] Human to human transmission and infection in the laboratory has been rarely documented.[20]

Following an incubation time of 1 to 2 weeks, the presentation is usually that of a nonspecific "flu-like" illness, with fever, headache, and cough which may or may not be productive.[21,22] On occasion, patients may present with life-threatening generalized toxemia or respiratory failure.[17,18,23]

Chest radiographs are abnormal in approximately 75 percent of cases seen clinically[21,22] although, like *M. pneumoniae* pneumonia, the patterns of radiographic abnormalities are highly variable.[12] Most often, the changes are unilateral, are located in the lower lobes, and are patchy or segmental, but bilateral disease and lobar consolidation are also seen. Small pleural effusions are described in approximately 20 percent of cases.[12] Typically, the radiologic abnormalities are more dramatic than the findings by physical examination.

The presenting laboratory findings in psittacosis are not useful. The total white blood cell count and differential are usually normal. Sputum examination tends to be noncontributory. The definitive diagnosis is made serologically. Culture is possible but is potentially dangerous to laboratory personnel.[7]

The course of the respiratory disease is resolution of clinical symptoms with persistence of radiologic changes for a few weeks following clinical recovery. Various extrapulmonary manifestations are seen occasionally, including myocarditis, encephalitis, cold agglutinin-negative hemolytic anemia, and hepatosplenomegaly.[7,20]

The histopathology of psittacosis is similar to viral bronchiolitis. Edema and polymorphonuclear leukocyte reaction is transient and the usual reaction is a mononuclear cell infiltrate in the walls of the respiratory bronchioles and adjacent alveoli.[7,20] Proliferation of type II alveolar epithelial cells may be seen but diffuse alveolar damage is not really a feature of this disease. Positive specific immunofluorescence in lung tissue has been described.[17,18]

Chlamydia trachomatis

C. trachomatis is known to be a common infection of the genitourinary tract in adults. In 1977, Beem and Saxon described a respiratory tract syndrome in 20 infants,[24] characterized by recovery of *C. trachomatis* from the nasopharynx, IgG and IgM anti-*C. trachomatis* antibodies, and diffuse lung disease. The course in all of these infants was benign and afebrile but chronic, with cough, tachypnea, and radiologic abnormalities persisting for over a month. Additional studies[16,25] have provided further details on this syndrome. The infection is acquired intrapartum with a transmission rate of approximately 50 percent. The pneumonia syndrome develops in 10 to 20 percent of infected babies. The syndrome is not life-threatening therefore no autopsy studies are available, however, a few infants have had open lung biopsy.[16,24,26] The usual pattern of reaction is a diffuse interstitial mononuclear cell infiltrate without hyaline membranes but bronchiolitis and a more intra-alveolar than interstitial reaction has also been described.[26] An animal model is available[27] with features very similar to the disease in humans.

Since the appearance of descriptions of the *C. trachomatis* infantile pneumonia syndrome, several cases of *C. trachomatis* pneumonia in immunocompromised adults have been reported.[28–30] Most of these cases were diagnosed by a positive culture rather than serology, which is important because of the relatively high prevalence of positive serology in adults due to genitourinary tract infections. Several of the patients were coinfected with cytomegalovirus. The reaction pattern is described as interstitial and intra-alveolar infiltrates, primarily composed of mononuclear inflammatory cells together with a variable degree of bronchiolitis, and no inclusions or other specific features.

Coxiella burneti

This form of atypical pneumonia was first described in Australia in 1937 following an outbreak of fever at a meat packing plant.[31] It was termed Q fever, the "Q" being an abbreviation for "query." The "answer" is *Coxiella burneti*, an obligate intracellular organism, whose usual hosts are farm animals such as goats, sheep, and cattle. Thus, the human population at risk for developing the disease are farm workers and in the largest series of cases of Q fever,[31] a history of appropriate exposure could be elicited in over 90 percent of patients. Nevertheless, exceptional cases of infections in immunocompromised patients without obvious exposure have been described.[32] The usual presentation is nonspecific with fever, headache, and myalgias as the most impressive symptoms following an incubation period of 2 to 4 weeks. Pneumonia occurs only in a minority of patients.[7,31] Chest radiograph abnormalities, if present, are entirely nonspecific. The leukocyte count is usually normal. The diagnosis is established serologically. Culture is possible but, as is the case for psittacosis, it is dangerous to laboratory personnel.[7]

The course of Q fever is generally one of resolution in 2 to 3 weeks, although in a significant proportion of patients[31] some symptoms may persist for up to 10 weeks. Likewise, the radiologic changes in cases of Q fever usually resolve in 2 to 3 weeks but occasionally can persist as rounded densities simulating neoplasms.[33]

A variety of extrapulmonary manifestations of Q fever may occur including excephalitis,[34] hepatitis, pericarditis, and endomyocarditis.[7]

Fatality from Q fever is most unusual and descriptions of pulmonary histopathology at biopsy or autopsy are sparse. Lobar consolidation with a mononuclear inflammatory cell reaction is said to occur.[7]

References

1. Case records of the Massachusetts General Hospital #39-1983. N Engl J Med 309:782–789, 1983.

2. Collier AM, Clyde WA: Appearance of *Mycoplasma pneumoniae* in lungs of experimentally infected hamsters and sputum from patients with natural disease. Am Rev Respir Dis 110:765–773, 1974.

3. Clyde WA Jr: *Mycoplasma pneumoniae* respiratory disease symposium: Summation and significance. Yale J Biol Med 56:523–527, 1983.

4. Murray HW, Masur H, Senterfit LB, Roberts RB: The protean manifestations of *Mycoplasma pneumoniae* infection in adults. Am J Med 58:229–242, 1975.

5. Stevens D, Swift PGF, Johnston PGB, et al.: *Mycoplasma pneumoniae* infections in children. Arch Dis Child 53:38–42, 1978

6. Koletsky RJ, Weinstein AJ: Fulminant *Mycoplasma pneumoniae* infection; report of a fatal case and a review of the literature. Am Rev Respir Dis 122:491–496, 1980.

7. Murray HW, Tuazon C: Atypical pneumonias. Med Clin North Am 64:507–527, 1980.

8. Izumikawa K, Hara K: Clinical features of mycoplasmal pneumonia in adults. Yale J Biol Med 56:505–510, 1983.

9. Linz DH, Tolle SW, Elliot DL: *Mycoplasma pneumoniae* pneumonia. Experience at a referral center. West J Med 140:895–900, 1984.

10. Foy HM, Ochs H, Davis SD, et al.: *Mycoplasma pneumoniae* infections in patients with immunodeficiency syndromes: Report of four cases. J Infect Dis 127:388–393, 1973

11. Dean NL: Mycoplasma pneumonias in the community hospital. The "unusual" manifestations become common. Clin Chest Med 2:121–131, 1981.

12. MacFarlane JT, Miller AC, Roderick-Smith WH, et al.: Comparative radiographic features of community acquired legionnaires' disease, pneumococcal pneumonia, mycoplasma pneumonia, and psittacosis. Thorax 39:28–33, 1984.

13. Rollins S, Colby T, Clayton F: Open lung biopsy in *Mycoplasma pneumoniae* pneumonia. Arch Pathol Lab Med 110:34–41, 1986

14. Linz D, Kessler S, Kane J: Pulmonary caseating granulomas associated with *Mycoplasma pneumoniae* pneumonia. South Med J 76:1429–1432, 1983.

15. Schachter J. Chlamydial infections. N Engl J Med 298:428–435, 1978.

16. Hammerschlag MR: Chlamydial lung disease: No longer a curiosity. J Respir Dis 5:81–93, 1984.

17. Byrom NP, Walls J, Mair HJ: Fulminant psittacosis. Lancet 1:353–356, 1979.

18. van Berkel M, Dik H, van der Meer JWM, Versteeg J: Acute respiratory insufficiency from psittacosis. Br Med J 290:1503–1504, 1985

19. File TM Jr, Tan JS, Murphy DP: Atypical pneumonia syndrome. Primary Care 8:673–694, 1981.

20. MacFarlane JT, MacRae AD: Psittacosis. Br Med Bull 39:163–167, 1983.

21. Kuritsky JN, Schmid GP, Potter ME, et al.: Psittacosis, a diagnostic challenge. J Occup Med 26:731–733, 1984

22. Coutts II, Mackenzie S, White RJ: Clinical and radiographic features of psittacosis infection. Thorax 40:530–532, 1985.

23. Wheatley T, Park GR: Acute respiratory insufficiency from psittacosis (letter). Br Med J 291:53–54, 1985.

24. Beem MO, Saxon EM: Respiratory tract colonization and a distinctive pneumonia syndrome in infants infected with *Chlamydia trachomatis*. N Engl J Med 296:306–310, 1977.

25. Harrison HR, English MG, Lee CK, Alexander ER: *Chlamydia trachomatis* infant pneumonitis. N Engl J Med 298:702–708, 1978.

26. Arth C, Von Schmidt B, Grossman M, Schachter J: Chlamydial pneumonitis. J Pediatr 93:447–449, 1978.

27. Harrison HR, Lee SM, Lucas DO: *Chlamydia trachomatis* pneumonitis in the C57BL/KsJ mouse: Pathologic and immunologic features. J Lab Clin Med 100:953–962, 1982.

28. Tack KJ, Peterson PK, Rasp FL, et al.: Isolation of *Chlamydia trachomatis* from the lower respiratory tract of adults. Lancet 1:116–120, 1980.

29. Ito JI Jr, Comess KA, Alexander ER, et al.: Pneumonia due to *Chlamydia trachomatis* in an immunocompromised adult. N Engl J Med 307:95–98, 1982,

30. Meyers JD, Hackman RC, Stamm WE: *Chlamydia trachomatis* infection as a cause of pneumonia after human marrow transplantation. Transplantation 36:130–134, 1983.

31. Spelman DW: Q fever. A study of 111 consecutive cases. Med J Aust 1:547–553, 1982.

32. Heard SR, Ronalds CJ, Heath RB: *Coxiella burnetii* infection in immunocompromised patients. J Infect 11:15–18, 1985.

33. Janigan DT, Marrie TJ: An inflammatory pseudotumor of the lung in Q fever pneumonia. N Engl J Med 308:86–88, 1983.

34. Marrie TJ: Pneumonia and meningoencephalitis due to *Coxiella burnetii*. J Infect 11:59–61, 1985.

13 Bacterial Infections

Charles Kuhn III

Routes of Infection

The majority of pulmonary infections result from organisms that reach the lung through the airways, either by inhalation of infected aerosols or by aspiration from the upper air passages. Bacteria can also infect the lung through the bloodstream, spread from contiguous tissues or traumatic implantation. Aerosol spread occurs either from environmental sources, as in the transmission of anthrax spores from contaminated wool, the spread of Legionella from air conditioner cooling towers, or the inadvertent dissemination of Pseudomonas with contaminated respiratory therapy equipment, or from person to person by the formation of droplet nuclei from infected secretions. Droplet nuclei form when coughing, sneezing, speaking, or singing generate airborne droplets bearing organisms. Evaporation of water from the surface of the droplets leaves the solutes and organisms in the form of tiny particles 1 to 3 μm in diameter that remain suspended by air currents for hours and are efficiently retained by the lung.[1] Droplet nuclei are the most important route of spread of many of the classic infections such as tuberculosis, diphtheria, and whooping cough, as well as a number of viruses.

Most sporadic bacterial infections in the lung result from aspiration of organisms from the upper respiratory tract. Infection by this route is promoted by conditions that favor colonization of upper airways by pathogens, increase the likelihood of aspiration, and depress host defenses. Recent studies have demonstrated some of the factors that determine the flora of the upper respiratory tract. Colonization of the pharynx by gram-negative bacilli is increased in chronic pulmonary disease, diabetes, alcoholism,[2] acute viral infections,[3] and hospitalization for acute serious illness.[4-6] Tracheostomy promotes colonization of the trachea, often by different organisms from those in the pharynx.[7]

Two factors that influence the colonization process are bacterial interference and the ability of bacteria to adhere to mucosal surfaces. The normal pharyngeal flora contains bacteria such as the alpha-hemolytic streptococci, which suppress the growth of other bacteria. Sprunt and Redman[8] showed that treatment with antibiotics to which the streptococci are sensitive favors the overgrowth of gram-negative bacilli.

The ability of certain bacteria to adhere to epithelial cells prevents their removal by the cleansing action of mucosal secretion and permits them to colonize. Thus, virulent strains of *Bordetella pertussis* adhere to tracheal epithelium and resist ciliary clearance which removes avirulent strains.[9] It appears that specific adhesion is one of the major determinants of the composition of the normal bacterial flora and accounts for its strict site specificity. In the oral cavity, for example, the dorsum of the tongue, tooth surface, gingival margins, and buccal mucosa each has its own specific flora related to its bacterial adhesive properties.[10] In the case of Gram-negative bacilli, adhesion to epithelial surfaces is mediated by the proteins which form thread-like structures called pili that are attached to the bacterial membrane through the cell wall. Changes in the binding specificity of mucosal surfaces are accompanied by changes in the composition of the flora. Johanson and colleagues[11] showed that an increase in the ability of pharyngeal epithelial cells to bind Gram-negative rods was associated with greatly increased probability of colonization by these organisms. These investigators[12] obtained evidence that a variety of severe illnesses increased the protease activity in the oropharyngeal secretions and that this in turn produced alterations in the cell surfaces that enhanced their ability to bind Gram-negative bacilli.

Aspiration of pharyngeal secretions permits the colonizing flora to reach the lung. Huxley and colleagues[13] found that nearly half of the normal subjects whom they tested aspirated a bolus of radiolabeled tracer from the pharynx into the lung during sleep. These investigators believed that 50 percent was only a minimum figure for the frequency of aspiration since many of those who did not aspirate slept fitfully under the conditions of the experiment. Patients with depressed consciousness aspirated more commonly than did normal subjects.

Once bacteria reach the acini, their ability to cause progressive infection depends on their growth rate and on the efficiency of local defenses. In experimental systems, it has been demonstrated that physical removal of bacteria from the lower respiratory tract is relatively slow, and that the initial control of bacteria deposited in the alveoli is due to phagocytosis and killing within phagocytes.[14] The alveolar lining fluid may play a role in this process. Lavage fluid from peripheral lung contains immunoglobulin (mainly IgG), complement components, and fibronectin, a nonimmunologic opsonin for certain Gram-positive cocci. Alveolar lining material is required for efficient killing of *Staphylococcus aureus* by macrophages following phagocytosis,[15] and some of the lysophosphatides associated with surfactant have direct bactericidal activity themselves.[16]

Species of bacteria differ in their growth rates in the lung and in their susceptibility to killing by phagocytes. In mice, for example, *S. aureus* is readily killed within macrophages, whereas Klebsiella and Pseudomonas require neutrophils as well.[17]

A number of clinically relevant conditions have been shown experimentally to depress phagocyte function, including hypoxia, alcohol, corticosteroids, nephrectomy, tobacco smoke, and viral infection.[18] When mixed bacterial contamination of the lower respiratory tract occurs, suppressive agents can exert a differential effect on phagocytic defenses leading to selective overgrowth of a single more resistant species.

Bacterial Infections of the Airways

Acute Tracheobronchitis

Although most cases of acute bronchitis are probably due to viruses and mycoplasma, some are due to bacteria, especially pneumococci. Bacteria are commonly implicated in acute exacerbations in patients with chronically impaired airway defenses such as the immotile cilia syndrome, agammaglobulinemia, cystic fibrosis, or chronic bronchitis. For reasons that are not understood, there is a tendency for particular organisms to occur in specific settings, for example, *Hemophilus influenzae* in chronic bronchitis or *Staph. aureus* and mucoid strains of *Pseudomonas aeruginosa* in cystic fibrosis.

Acute bacterial tracheitis in young children is a potentially life-threatening form of infection most often caused by *Staph. aureus* or type b *H. influenzae*.[19,20] Clinically, the disorder can be mistaken for croup (acute viral laryngotracheobronchitis), but the larynx is spared and the infection is limited to the subglottic region. Symptoms develop acutely with stridor, high fever, toxicity, and purulent sputum. Because of the small caliber of the trachea in young children, it can become obstructed by edema and purulent exudate, requiring tracheotomy or intubation.

Diphtheria

Diphtheria is a localized infection usually involving the tonsil or oropharynx. It can involve the larynx, trachea, and bronchi either primarily or by contiguous spread. The infection is accompanied by systemic manifestations which are a consequence of the absorption of toxin; the organisms remain localized to the mucosal site.

The causative organism, *Corynebacterium diphtheriae* (Klebs-Loeffler bacillus), belongs to the genus Corynebacteria, a group of pleomorphic, Gram-positive, nonmotile bacilli related to the Nocardia and mycobacteria. Characteristically the Corynebacteria vary in size, but they have a club-shaped enlargement at one end and display metachromatic granules when stained with alkaline methylene blue. *C. diphtheriae* cannot be reliably distinguished by its morphology from the diphtheroids, nonpathogenic Corynebacteria that are commonly isolated from the throat or upper respiratory tract of normal subjects. The distinction is made using cultural characteristics and biochemical reactions.

The ability to produce toxin is not an inherent property of the bacterium. The gene encoding the toxin is introduced into the Corynebacterium by a bacteriophage and can be expressed during either a lytic infection of the bacterium or a lysogenic infection in which a viral prophage is incorporated into the bacterial nucleoid and carried from one generation to the next. Toxigenic strains of bacteria, then, are those carrying the lysogenic phage.

The toxin is a single polypeptide chain weighing 62,000 daltons and bearing two intramolecular sulfhydryl cross-links.[21,22] Limited tryptic digestion followed by reduction of the sulfhydryl bridges releases two peptides, a 21,000-dalton fragment (A) corresponding to the aminoterminal portion of the molecule and a 39,000-dalton fragment (B) from the carboxyterminus. Fragment B by itself lacks toxic activity, but binds to membrane receptors on susceptible cells and presumably promotes uptake in the intact toxin. Fragment A, the active toxin, is an enzyme that inhibits protein synthesis by blocking translation. It acts by transferring adenosine diphosphate ribose (ADPR) from nicotinamide adenine dinucleotide (NAD) to "elongation factor 2" (EF2), an enzyme that moves ribosomes bearing nascent polypeptide chains from one codon to the next along the mRNA message:

$$NAD^+ + EF2 \longrightarrow ADPR\text{-}EF2 + \text{nicotinamide} + H^+$$

The ADP-ribosylated elongation factor is devoid of enzymatic activity, although it retains the capacity to bind to ribosomes. Studies[22] in which liposomes or erythrocyte ghosts were used to introduce known doses of toxin fragment A into cells indicate that internalization of only a single molecule of toxin is sufficient to kill a cell.

Although diphtheria has become rare where vaccina-

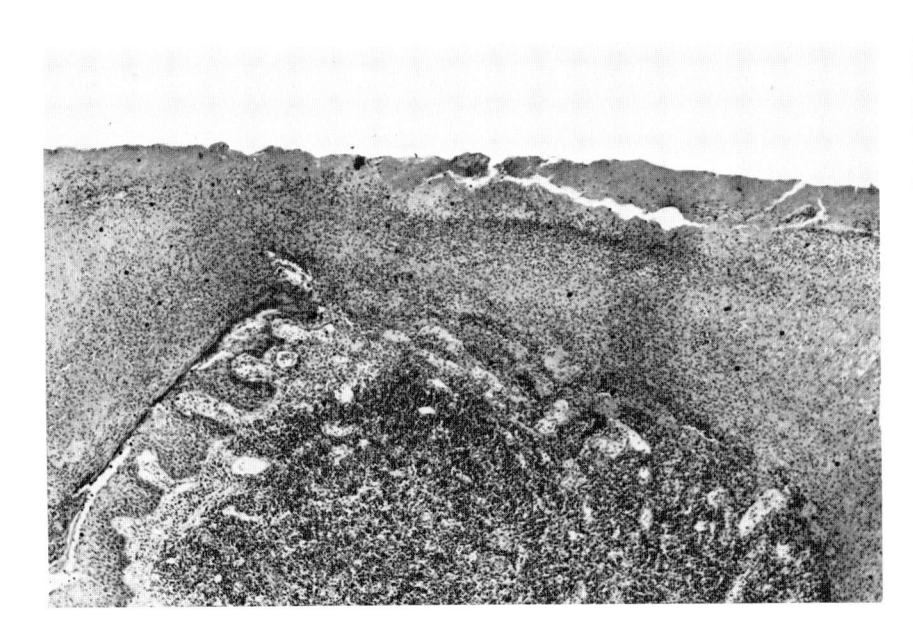

Figure 13–1. Diphtheritic pseudomembrane on a tonsil. The squamous epithelium is preserved on the left but has undergone necrosis on the remainder of the surface. A membrane of fibrin, imflammatory cells, and necrotic epithelium covers the luminal surface (×50).

tion is prevalent, it remains common in many parts of the world. The disease mainly affects children younger than age 15 years but older than 6 months when passively acquired immunity disappears. The incidence has a peak around age three to four years. The bacteria are spread from person to person by those with current infection or by asymptomatic carriers—persons who are either convalescing from infection or have been immunized with toxoid and thus have no symptoms despite being colonized by toxigenic strains.

The organisms are deposited on the epithelium of the upper or lower respiratory tract where they grow and produce toxin which causes necrosis of the superficial layers of epithelium. Conditions in the necrotic epithelium favor further growth resulting in continued spread of the process. The inflammatory response in the adjacent tissue produces capillary dilation and transudation of fibrin which becomes mixed with the necrotic epithelium, inflammary neutrophils, and organisms to give rise to grey patches on the affected mucosa, the characteristic diphtheritic pseudomembranes[23,24] (Fig. 13–1). During the next several days, the pseudomembranes grow in thickness, coalesce, and may change from grey to yellow, brown, or black depending on the amount of hemorrhage. They adhere tightly to the underlying tissue and strip away with difficulty, leaving multiple small bleeding points. The absorption of toxin locally produces soft tissue swelling and lymphadenopathy (bullneck), while systemically it produces fever, tachycardia, and mild leukocytosis. Lesions usually begin on the fauces or posterior pharynx, where they either remain localized or spread to involve the uvula, nasopharynx, nose, larynx, trachea, or bronchi. Less commonly the process begins in the larynx, trachea, or nose.

In the second week of illness, systemic manifestations become prominent. Myocarditis develops in 50 percent of patients and can cause arrhythmias, cardiac failure, or cardiogenic shock. Histologically the heart shows interstitial edema, fatty change, or granular degeneration of myocardial fibers; in some instances, there is an interstitial mononuclear inflammatory infiltrate. A segmental demyelinating neuropathy is seen in a small proportion of cases beginning late in the course, sometimes even weeks after the local mucosal lesions subside.

The respiratory tract lesions are similar to those seen in the fauces. The mucosa is erythematous and covered with a shaggy pseudomembrane, which separates from the underlying stroma more easily than the pseudomembrane in the throat, owing to the thinner type of epithelium (Fig. 13–2). Rarely a complete cast of the tracheobronchial tree is formed. More often segments of membrane slough leading to obstruction of the airways with air trapping or foci of collapse. Respiration can be further impaired by paralysis of the palate or weakness of the accessory respiratory muscles due to neuropathy.

The severity and clinical pattern of diphtheria vary in any individual case depending on the amount of toxin produced by the particular strain of organism involved, the immune status of the patient, and the site of infection. Overall the mortality is approximately 10 percent, and is higher for patients younger than 5 years of age.[25] The most common cause of death is respiratory tract disease.

Whooping Cough

In the opening decade of this century, Bordet first detected the bacillus now called *Bordetella pertussis* in his own children during attacks of whooping cough. Nevertheless, it was still possible for Rich[26] to argue in 1932 that whooping cough was caused by a virus and that the Bordet-Gengou bacillus was a secondary invader. The following year, an intrepid medical couple demonstrated that *B. pertussis* could cause whooping cough, transmitting the disease to their own children.[27] Although whooping cough is a clinical syndrome that can sometimes be

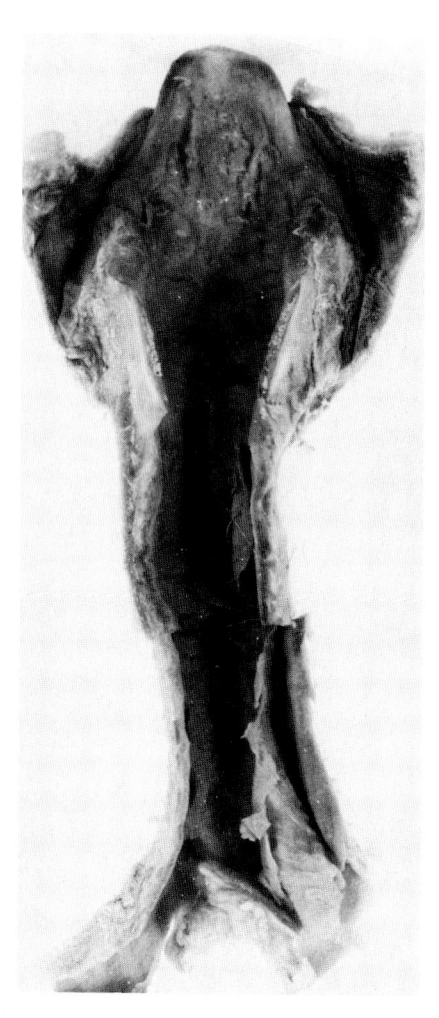

Figure 13–2. Diphtheria of the larynx, trachea, and bronchi. The pseudomembrane is loosely adherent on the trachea and bronchi. From the Pathological Museum of the University of Manchester, UK.

caused by a virus or combined infection,[28–30] the success of vaccination against *B. pertussis* in controlling this illness leaves no doubt that *B. pertussis* is its principal cause. In some populations, particularly in eastern Europe, the closely related organism, *B. parapertussis* is responsible for up to 30 percent of cases.[31] The third member of the genus Bordetella, *B. bronchiseptica*, is a cause of chronic respiratory disease in animals but rarely infects humans.

When vaccination to *B. pertussis* was introduced in the 1940s, the incidence of whooping cough declined dramatically. Even when children who fail to complete the full course of immunization become infected, their illness is milder than in the completely unvaccinated child. The bacillus remains endemic, and with relaxation of immunization requirements, the disease can break out anew. In Britain immunization rates in children declined markedly, from 80 percent in 1974 to 30 percent in 1978 as the result of widespread publicity given to the rare serious side effects of vaccination. In 1977 the incidence of whooping cough began to climb. In the years 1977–1979, more than 100,000 cases were reported to the authorities, and in the first 9 months of 1982, there were more than 47,000 cases.[32] For comparison, in the United States where no comparable decline in vaccination took place, 1227 cases were reported for 1979 through 1981.[33]

Whooping cough is mainly a disease of children less than 5 or 6 years of age, although older children and even adults can be affected. The illness is more serious in children less than one year old in whom the mortality can be as much as 17-fold greater than for patients of all ages combined. The disease is both endemic and epidemic. When *B. pertussis* is newly introduced into nonimmune populations, attack rates approach 100 percent.

Clinical illness passes through three phases.[27] The prodromal or catarrhal phase lasts between 6 days and 3 weeks. During this time, the patient's symptoms are nonspecific, consisting of mild cough, runny nose, sneezing, and lacrimation accompanied by at most a mild fever. The second stage of the illness is marked by the appearance of the characteristic paroxysms, sudden violent fits of coughing that may terminate in a characteristic inspiratory whoop, leaving the patient exhausted. Frequently the paroxysms are followed by retching, or more rarely by coma or convulsions (encephalopathy). The peripheral blood demonstrates an absolute lymphocytosis unaccompanied by adenopathy. The paroxysmal phase can last from 1 to 6 weeks. During the final or convalescent phase, symptoms gradually subside. Occasionally a secondary bacterial pneumonia develops, caused by *H. influenzae* or one of the Gram-positive cocci. Pneumonia due to *B. pertussis* itself is decidedly rare.[34] Table 13–1 summarizes the frequency of various clinical features as they are observed at the present time.[33]

During the catarrhal phase, patients are highly infectious, and their coughing and sneezing spread the organisms on droplet nuclei. When organisms are deposited in the airways of nonimmune individuals, they attach to ciliated epithelial cells by their pili and proliferate among the cilia. The tropism of the organism for ciliated cells is quite specific. In tracheal organ culture, Muse and colleagues[35] showed by scanning electron microscopy that organisms grow only on ciliated cells and fail to attach to secretory cells. The only site other than airways in which experimental infection is readily produced is in the

Table 13–1. Frequency of Major Manifestations of Pertussis[a]

Whoop	72%
Apnea	41%
Pneumonia	29%
Seizures	4%
Encephalopathy	0.4%
Death	0.5%

[a] U.S. experience, 1979–1981.[33]

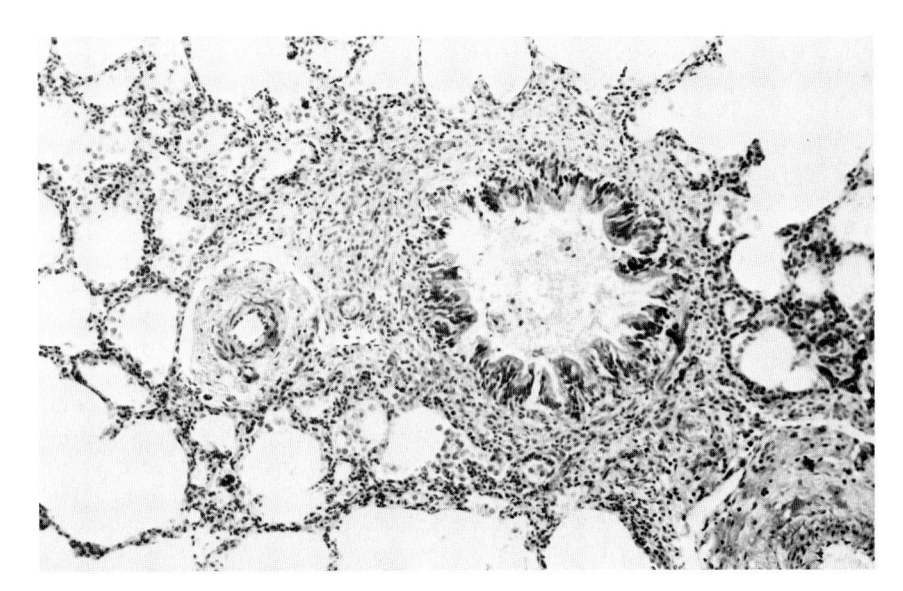

Figure 13–3. Pertussis. Inflammation mainly limited to the bronchiole (H&E ×150).

ventricles of the brain where the organisms grow attached to ciliated ependymal cells.

Infection is noninvasive. The organisms remain localized on the epithelial surface where they can be demonstrated with bacterial stains.[36] In tracheal explants, the colonized cells degenerate and slough to lie free on the epithelial surface.[35]

In humans the histopathologic lesions are bronchitis and bronchiolitis accompanied by only slight extension of the interstitial inflammatory infiltrate into the walls of neighboring alveoli. The bronchial lumens fill with mucus and cellular debris which leads to air trapping or patches of alveolar collapse. Bronchial walls are infiltrated by mononuclear inflammatory cells (Fig. 13–3). Neutrophils characteristically infiltrate in the region of the junction between the epithelium and the lamina propria and cluster about sloughing and degenerating epithelial cells (Fig. 13–4). Severe sloughing can leave sections of bronchial wall denuded of epithelium, and regeneration can result in squamous metaplasia.[34]

The pathogenesis of the disease is related to the production of toxins by the bacteria. The three principal toxins are the heat labile toxin, lipopolysaccharide endotoxin, and pertussigen or pertussis toxin.[37,38]

Toxic factors associated with pertussis culture filtrates have long been known by the various activities used to detect them: "histamine-sensitizing factor," "lymphocytosis-promoting factor," and "islet-activating protein." All of these activities probably reside in the pertussigen molecule, a protein with a molecular weight of approximately 77,000 daltons composed of multiple subunits whose detailed structure is still unknown. This toxin is responsible for the characteristic lymphocytosis, which it causes by blocking lymphocyte recirculation through the high endothelial venules in the lymphoid tissues. This causes the accumulation of long-lived lymphocytes in the circulating pool. Hypoglycemia has only infrequently been noted in patients, but is a well-known effect of pertussis

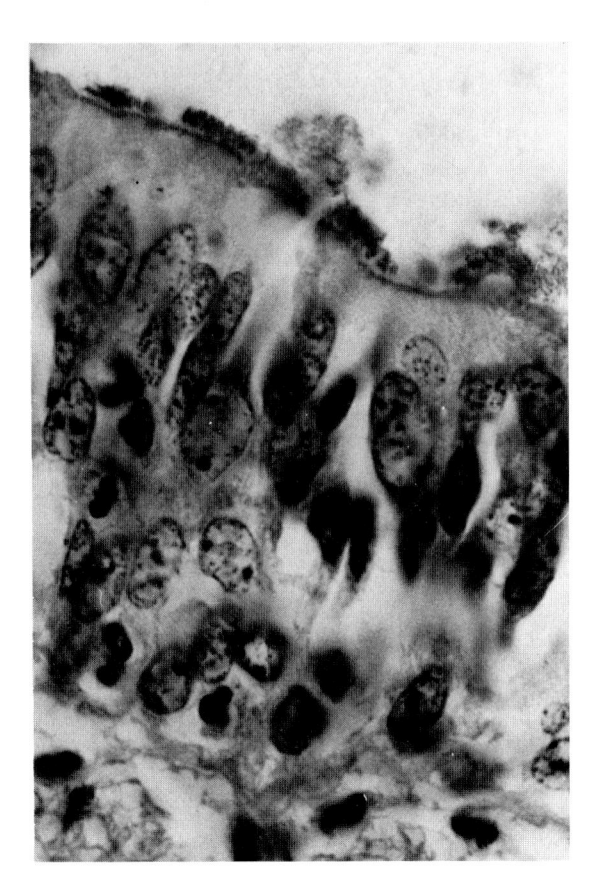

Figure 13–4. Pertussis. Darkly stained bacteria are visible on the luminal surface of ciliated cells. Several ciliated cells are undergoing necrosis and have pyknotic nuclei. A few neutrophils have invaded the basal region of the epithelium on the left (Goodpasture's bacterial stain, ×1250).

toxin in animals. Normally stimulation of β-cells in pancreatic islets by hyperglycemia produces a rise in cyclic adenosine monophosphate (cAMP) which in turn is coupled to insulin secretion. In animals treated with pertussigen, the insulin response to hyperglycemia is exaggerated, apparently due to an abnormally large rise or delayed decay of cAMP.

B. pertussis has an enzyme, adenyl cyclase, in its cell envelope that can be shed in soluble form. In old cultures, approximately 20 percent of the adenyl cyclase is extracellular.[39] This adenyl cyclase is taken up by alveolar macrophages and neutrophils, where it produces unregulated synthesis of intracellular cAMP from ATP, which suppresses the chemotactic, phagocytic, and bactericidal activity of the neutrophils and macrophages. This ability to suppress phagocyte defenses may account for the long persistence of organisms in the airways of patients with this disease and contribute to the development of secondary infections.[40]

After recovery from pertussis, patients remain immune for several years, much as they do after vaccination, but immunity gradually wanes. The immunity can be conferred by antibodies directed to either the pilar antigens involved in bacterial adherence or to the pertussigen toxin.[41] Antibodies also are produced to other components of the bacterium but play little role in protection. Formerly bronchiectasis was a recognized sequela of pertussis. Recent follow-up of children who recovered from pertussis infection gave little evidence of permanent lung damage. Although an excess of respiratory symptoms was found, pulmonary function was normal.[42] Patients who develop pertussis encephalopathy may have permanent neurologic damage. This is commonly attributed to hypoxic brain damage and small hemorrhages during paroxysms of coughing. As Olson pointed out,[27] hypoglycemia could also contribute.

Pneumonia Caused by Gram-Positive Cocci

Pneumococcal Infection

Streptococcus pneumoniae, known familiarly as the pneumococcus accounts for 40 to 80 percent of cases of bacterial pneumonia acquired outside the hospital.[43-46] It is also responsible for approximately 5 percent of cases of nosocomial pneumonia. The very old and very young are particularly susceptible to pneumococcal pneumonia and often present an atypical clinical picture. Persons with chronic pulmonary disease, alcoholism, cirrhosis, splenectomy, sickle cell disease, or multiple myeloma are at particular risk.

Properties of the Organism

Streptococcus pneumoniae is gram-positive and grows in tissue as pairs or short chains of lancet-shaped organisms. When cultured on blood agar, it produces alpha-hemolysis. Organisms in the center of older colonies tend to lyse spontaneously. Lysis can also be induced in suspensions of the organism by the addition of bile salts such as deoxycholate, a property used to identify the organism in the bile solubility test. On lysis, the pneumococcus releases a hemolysin that is related antigenically to streptolysin O but is not known to have any major role in the production of disease.

Despite a vast amount of research, the details of how the pneumococcus produces disease remain unknown. Toxins seem to play little part. Extracellular growth of the organism appears to be the critical process, and once organisms are phagocytosed, they are rapidly destroyed and their disease-producing potential is abolished. Pneumococci are protected from phagocytosis by a polysaccharide capsule or slime coat which is one of the many determinants of their virulence.

More than 80 different serotypes of pneumococcus can be distinguished on a basis of antigenic and biochemical differences in their capular polysaccharide. The majority of cases of pneumonia are caused by types I through VIII. Formerly types I and II predominated,[47] but more recently types VIII and VI were reported to be the most common.[48] Type III is the most destructive owing to its production of a large quantity of capsule that protects it from phagocytosis and provides an excess of soluble antigen to absorb opsonizing antibodies.[49]

The phagocytosis of pneumococci takes place by two mechanisms. In surface phagocytosis, the organisms are immobilized against a surface enabling the leukocyte to engulf them.[50] This mechanism facilitates uptake in the fully developed inflammatory response when the alveoli are tightly packed with leukocytes and fibrin. The second mechanism is phagocytosis, mediated by receptors either for the Fc portion of immunoglobulin or C3b component of complement. Capsular polysaccharides of some strains directly fix C3 by the alternate pathway of complement activation, enabling them to be opsonized in the absence of specific antibody. Other strains are only opsonized in the presence of antibody. Strains of the latter type produce the majority of pneumonias, suggesting that immediate opsonization by the alternate pathway is protective for the host.[51]

Pathology

Pneumococci can produce either lobar pneumonia, in which the process spreads rapidly from a single focus to involve an entire lobe homogeneously, or bronchopneumonia (lobular pneumonia), in which focal lesions form in multiple lobules centered on the terminal bronchioles. Even in the preantibiotic era, one-third to one-half of pneumonias caused by the pneumococcus were "atypical," that is, not lobar, and more recent reports[52] put the proportion of bronchopneumonias at two-thirds. Both host factors and organism influence the morphologic pattern of pneumonia. Bronchopneumonias are more common in the very young, the elderly, and those with underlying disease. Certain serotypes, notably types I and II, almost always produce a lobar distribution, whereas other serotypes are unpredictable.[47]

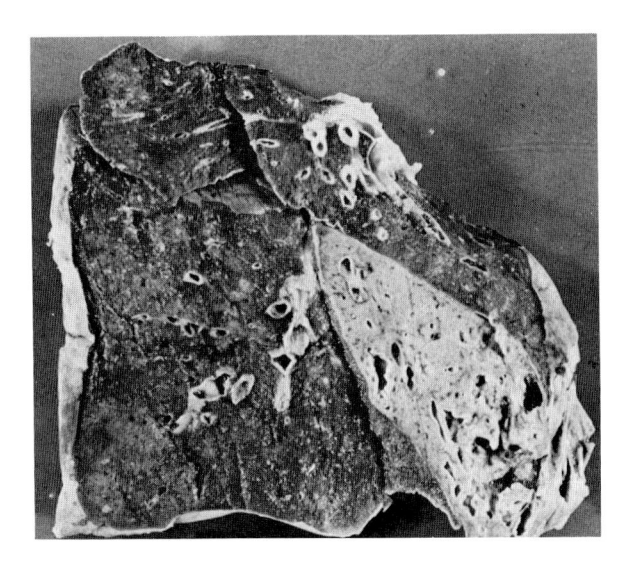

Figure 13–5. Pneumococcal lobar pneumonia. The middle lobe is in the stage of grey hepatization, and there is early abscess formation. Reproduced with permission from Kissane JM (ed): *Anderson's Pathology*. St. Louis: CV Mosby, 1984.

and the lobe changes to rusty brown, then grey. At this time, the term grey hepatization describes the gross appearance of the lobe (see Fig. 13–5). Bacteria are now few and in the normal course of events, recovery begins between 5 and 10 days after onset.

The lesions of pneumococcal lobar pneumonia can either resolve and the lobe returns to normal, or they can organize. Since the exudation in lobar pneumonia is intra-alveolar, the interstitium is relatively normal, and alveolar walls are usually intact and free of necrosis, complete restoration of normal lung architecture is possible. The intra-alveolar exudate is removed partly by expectoration and partly through the activity of macrophages. The process has been described in detail by Robertson.[55]

Monocytes begin to appear in the alveolar exudates within 48 hours, becoming more numerous, differentiating into macrophages as time passes. By the second week of infection, they become the predominant type of inflammatory cell. The neutrophils degenerate, and the fibrin network dissolves under the influence of proteases released from the neutrophil granules and plasminogen activator secreted by the macrophages. As the debris is engulfed by the macrophages, empty space appears in

In lobar pneumonia, one or more lobes are involved nearly completely and uniformly (Fig. 13–5). The process spreads through the affected lobe with such rapidity that the histology is quite uniform early in the process. The right lung is involved twice as often as the left. In fatal cases, one, two, or three lobes are involved with almost equal frequency.[53]

Colonization of the upper respiratory tract by pneumococci can be demonstrated in 5 to 70 percent of normal people depending on the population studied.[54] The organisms from the upper respiratory tract reach the lung by aspiration, commonly following a viral infection when the abundant watery secretions and damage to the ciliated epithelium pave the way. The initial response in the lung is an outpouring of edema, which spreads the organisms throughout the lobe via small bronchi and pores of Kohn and at the same time provides a nutrient-rich medium for bacterial growth. Grossly the affected lobe appears purple and moist; frothy fluid exudes from the sectioned surface. In microscopic sections, the alveolar septa are congested, the air spaces filled with proteinaceous fluid, erythrocytes, and innumerable bacteria (Fig. 13–6). During the next few hours, more and more fibrin and neutrophils enter the air spaces. Phagocytosis of pneumococci begins, and by 24 or 48 hours, the majority of organisms are intracellular. The involved lobe becomes firmer and drier as the air spaces fill with fibrin and cells, giving it a liver-like consistency. The congested capillaries combined with focal hemorrhages still present in the alveolar exudate give the lobe a red color (Fig. 13–7). Hence the term red hepatization is classically used to describe the lobe at this stage. With the progressive accumulation of more fibrin and inflammatory cells in the next few days, the capillaries become compressed and ischemic, the hemorrhages break down,

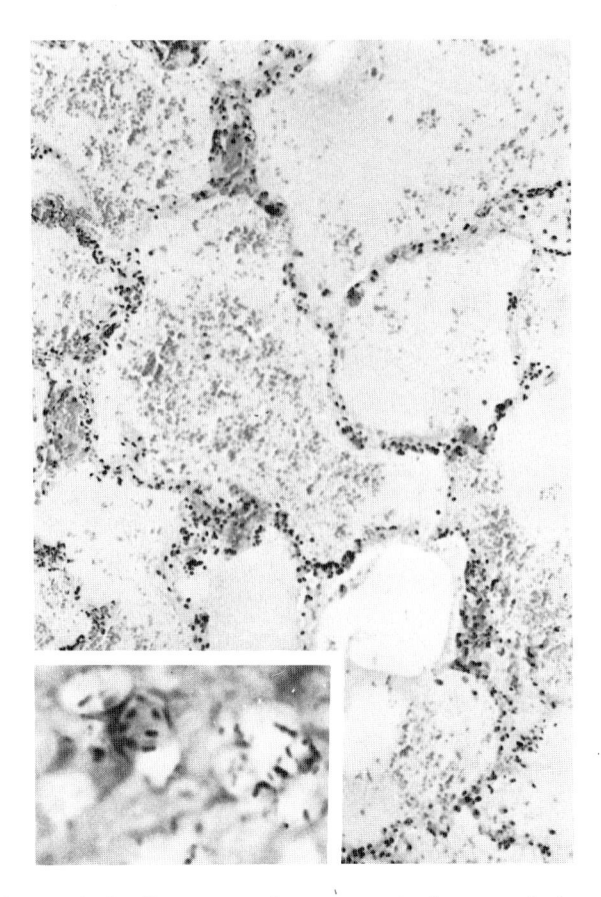

Figure 13–6. Pneumococcal pneumonia in the stage of edema. Air spaces filled with edema and hemorrhage with few leukocytes (×300). Inset, The edema fluid teems with bacteria (Gram's stain, ×2000).

Figure 13–7. Pneumococcal pneumonia, red hepatization. The alveolar septa are congested but well preserved. The alveoli are filled with leukocytes and some erythrocytes (×600).

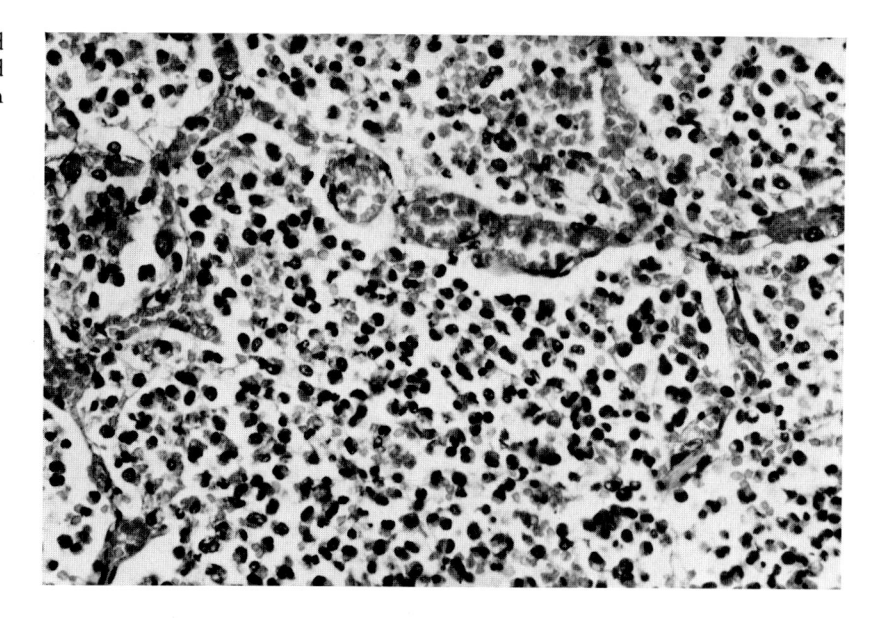

the alveolar exudate, becoming progressively more abundant as the debris is cleared or expectorated.

Although resolution is the rule, sometimes a lobe or a portion thereof may organize, leading to permanent fibrosis. Fibroblasts from the alveolar septa invade incompletely lysed fibrin and gradually convert it to connective tissue. Initially the fibrin is replaced by edematous-appearing weakly basophilic matrix rich in proteoglycan (Fig. 13–8). Subsequently the matrix becomes more eosinophilic as progressively more collagen is deposited. At times the outlines of normal alveolar walls remain clearly marked by alveolar capillaries and elastic fibers, and the air spaces fill with fibrous tissue that can take the form of characteristic polypoid fibrous buds known as Masson bodies. Where there has been necrosis of alveolar septa, the pattern of scarring will be more disorganized.

The factors that lead to fibrosis and failure of resolution include obstruction of a bronchus or necrosis of alveolar tissue. It has been reported [56] that organizing pneumonia became more frequent after the introduction of antibiotics. This observation has two possible explanations: patients with more severe pneumonia are now surviving and their more extensively damaged lungs organize, or if the organisms are killed before the full development of the inflammatory cell response, the protease content of the alveoli will not be sufficient to break down all the fibrin which consequently organizes.

Pneumococcal lobular or bronchopneumonia is often bilateral. Morphologically it is not distinctive, beginning as multiple foci of neutrophil-rich intra-alveolar exudate grouped on terminal airways. With time, they may focally become confluent.

Complications

The pleura is commonly involved in pneumonococcal pneumonia. Two-thirds of patients develop fibrinous pleuritis which may be accompanied by a parapneumonic effusion. In a small number of patients, the pleural space becomes infected and empyema develops. The pleural surface of the lung becomes encased in shaggy white layers of fibrin and neutrophils, the fluid becomes turbid, then purulent, and as organization begins, loculated pockets of pus form. The organization of an enpyema can lead to encasement of the lung by a thick rind of fibrous tissue several millimeters thick which can restrict lung expansion and require surgical decortication.

Bacteremia is a serious complication that develops in 20 to 35 percent of patients with lobar pneumonia. Its frequency is lower in pneumococcal bronchopneumonia. The mortality rate of 20 to 30 percent has not changed substantially since the introduction of antibiotics.[57] Bacteremia may lead to serious metastatic infections including meningitis, septic arthritis, bacterial endocarditis, and pericarditis.

Lung abscess is rare in pneumococcal pneumonia. Type III pneumococcus produces this complication more often than other serotypes, a property usually attributed to its relative resistence to phagocytosis.[58]

Beta-Hemolytic Streptococcal Pneumonia

Pneumonia caused by beta-hemolytic streptococci has become rare. Formerly Lancefield's group A (*Streptococcus pyogenes*) was responsible for most pneumonia, but recently the group B streptococci (*Streptococcus agalactia*) have been gaining in importance both as a cause of pneumonia and other infections. Group A streptococcal pneumonia often affects older children and young adults, usually as a complication of a viral infection such as influenza or one of the common childhood illnesses.[59,60] Group B streptococci colonize the upper

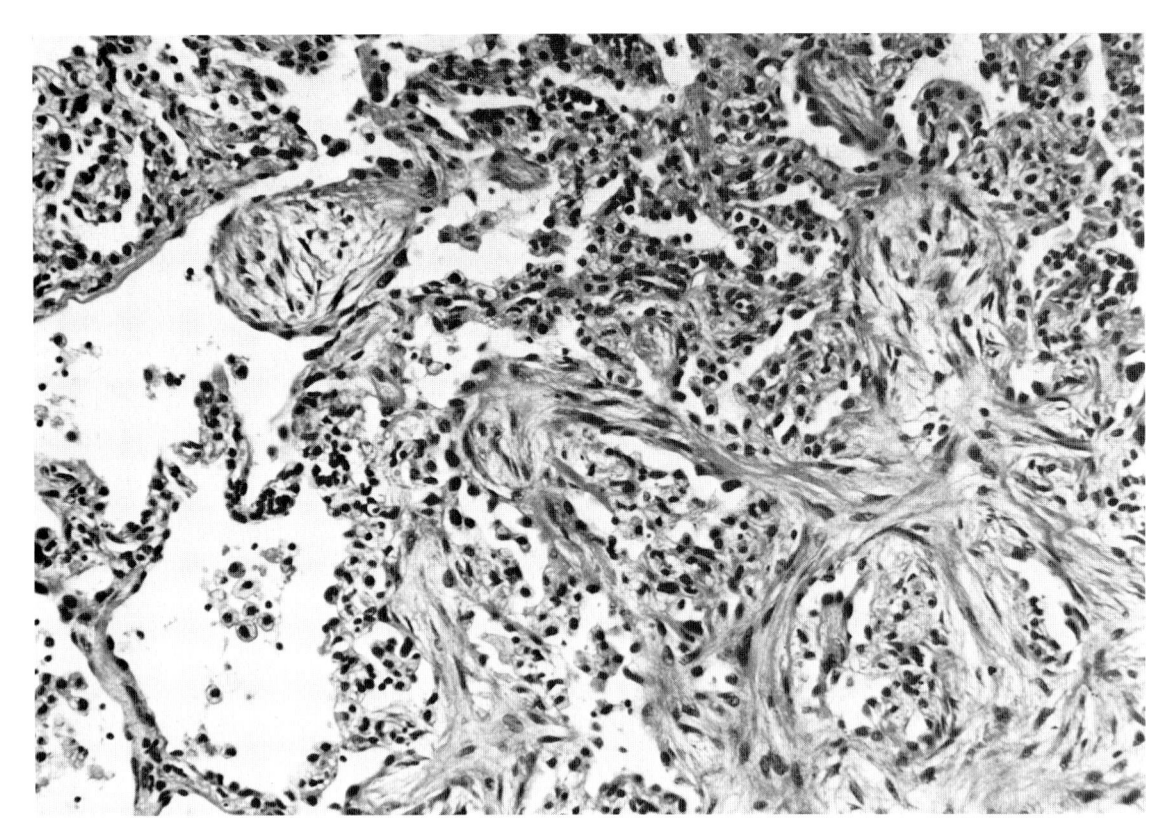

Figure 13–8. Organizing pneumonia. Air spaces are filled with elongated fibroblasts in a proteoglycan-rich matrix. At the upper left, the fibrous tissue forms a polypoid structure (Masson body) protruding into an alveolar duct (×500).

airways, but in pregnant women, they can also colonize the genital tract. Consequently group B streptococcal pneumonia affects two populations: newborns who acquire the organism during delivery[61,62] and elderly debilitated adults including diabetics.[63,64] Group A streptococci usually reach the lung by aspiration either from asymptomatic colonization of the upper respiratory tract or from an associated pharyngitis. Symptoms of pneumonia strike abruptly with high fever, prostration, myalgias, cough, tachypnea, and pleuritic chest pain. Pleural effusion develops rapidly in the majority of patients and soon evolves into an empyema.[60,65]

The lesions of Group A streptococcal pneumonia have been well described by MacCallum.[66] In most cases, there is a lobular (broncho-) pneumonia that is most severe in the dependent portions of the lung. The airways appear thickened and contain bloody or purulent exudate. Microscopically there is greater interstitial involvement than is found with other acute bacterial pneumonias. The bronchiolar epithelium undergoes necrosis, and the walls of the bronchioles become infiltrated by a exudate of neutrophils and mononuclear cells. The interstitial inflammation fans out into the walls of adjacent alveoli. There is edema in the alveoli surrounding the lesions. The perilobular and peribronchial connective tissue septa are swollen with edema, and the lymphatics are distended and often occluded by fibrin. The lymphatic obstruction may play a role in the rapid spread of the infection to the pleura that is so characteristic with this organism.

Less often the group A streptococci produce abscesses centered on terminal airways.

Acute complications of streptococcal pneumonia are mainly related to the high incidence of pleural involvement and include pneumothorax, bronchopleural fistula, and spread to the pericardium. Organization of an empyema can lead to alter development of a trapped lung. Nonsuppurative complications include acute glomerulonephritis but not acute rheumatic fever.[60,65]

The histopathology of pneumonia caused by group B streptococci has not been described in any detail. This type of pneumonia can be highly destructive and coalesce to give large zones of abscess.[64]

Staphylococcal Pneumonia

The species of Staphylococcus responsible for most serious infections is *Staphylococcus aureus*, a name now applied to all coagulase-positive staphylococci irrespective of the color of their colonies.[67] *S. aureus* colonizes the nose and throat of 15 to 40 percent of normal adults and the skin of somewhat fewer. In newborn infants, colonization of the upper respiratory tract is extremely

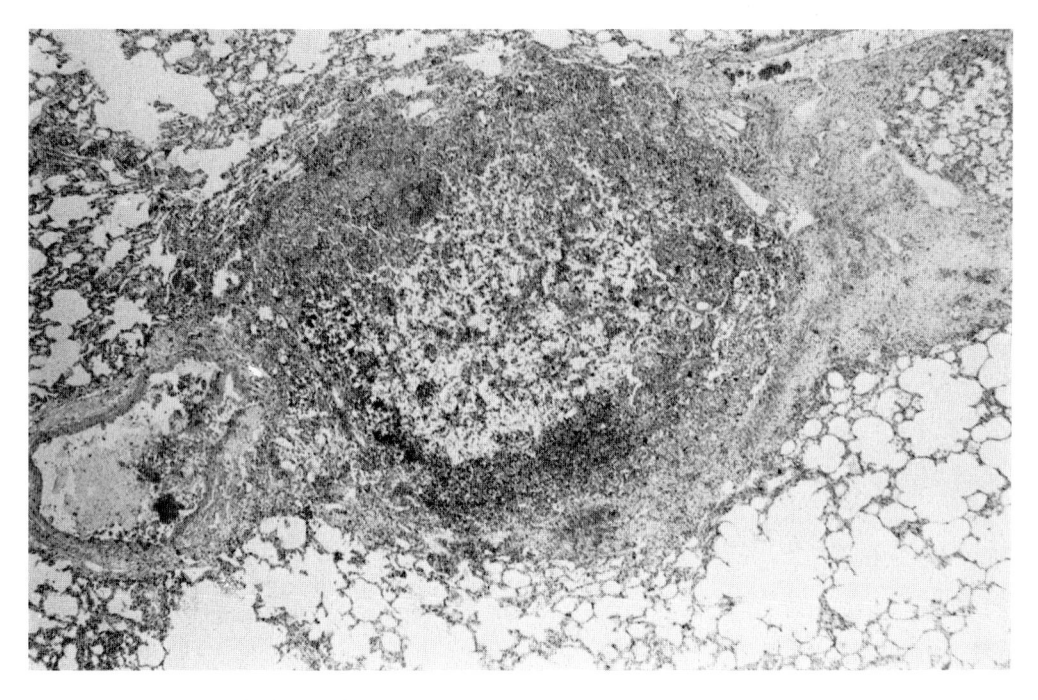

Figure 13–9. Staphylococcal pneumonia. Abscess centered on a bronchiole which is only identifiable by its accompanying artery (×37).

prevalent, reaching rates of 90 percent at a few days of age and then declining gradually. *S. epidermidis* is a coagulase-negative staphylococcus that normally inhabits the skin. Although of low virulence, it is potentially pathogenic, particularly in those with impaired defenses. It is notable for its propensity to infect prosthetic materials[68] whence it gains access to the circulation.

Staphylococcal pneumonia can develop as a result of either aspiration of organisms from the upper respiratory tract or seeding of the lung during bacteremia. Spread down the airways is especially prone to occur in debilitated patients, as a complication of influenza[69,70] or in children with cystic fibrosis. The clinical onset of staphylococcal pneumonia is often insidious, but it may be acute with chills, fever, and prostration.[71] Patients developing bacterial pneumonia as a complication of influenza usually appear to be recovering uneventfully from an ordinary bout of influenza when they abruptly relapse with high fever, cough, and pleuritic chest pain.[70] Chest roentgenogram may show local areas of consolidation. The course of staphylococcal pneumonia is highly variable and may be fulminant or protracted.

In acute fatal cases, the pleura is dark, mottled, and usually free of exudate, although some degree of pleural effusion is common.[72] The bronchi are filled with purulent exudate, and their mucosa is hemorrhagic. The lung parenchyma is dark and edematous with small grey patches of consolidation centered on terminal airways. In sections at the earliest stages, the bronchioles are necrotic with only a few neutrophils and monocytes in their walls and small numbers of cells spilling out into alveoli.[72] The alveolar capillaries are thrombosed, but focal hemorrhages are present in the alveoli. Colonies of bacteria are easily found. In cases of longer duration, the bronchopneumonia progresses to abscesses (Fig. 13–9). The amount of cellular exudate increases, alveolar walls undergo necrosis and dissolution, leaving a central cavity surrounded by pneumonia with intact alveolar walls. The abscesses can erode through the bronchial walls into the adjacent arteries, permitting organisms to seed downstream and set up new foci within the acinus.[73]

In patients who survive a week or longer, the lung is fibrotic and abscess cavities of varying size are enclosed within the fibrous tissue. The pleural space is adherent to the chest wall, and the bronchi are bronchiectatic.[72]

Hematogenous staphylococcal pneumonia develops in the presence of peripheral source of staphylococcal septicemia, such as a soft tissue infection, an infected dialysis shunt, or intravenous line.[74–76] In intravenous drug abusers, septic thrombophlebitis or right-sided bacterial endocarditis are common.[77] In many patients, the clinical picture is dominated by the primary source of sepsis. Cough and pleuritic chest pain are the most common local manifestations of pneumonia.

Hematogenous lesions predominate in the lower lobes and tend to be located subpleurally. Lesions begin as a localized area of hemorrhage which acquires a pale necrotic center, grows soft, and cavitates. Microscopically the lesions often center on a necrotic artery (Fig. 13–10). Frank septic infarcts can develop in relation to macroscopic thromboemboli. They initially preserve the pleural-based triangular outline of infarcts but rapidly acquire a grey-yellow purulent appearance and undergo cavitation (Fig. 13–11). Complications include empyema and pneumothorax.

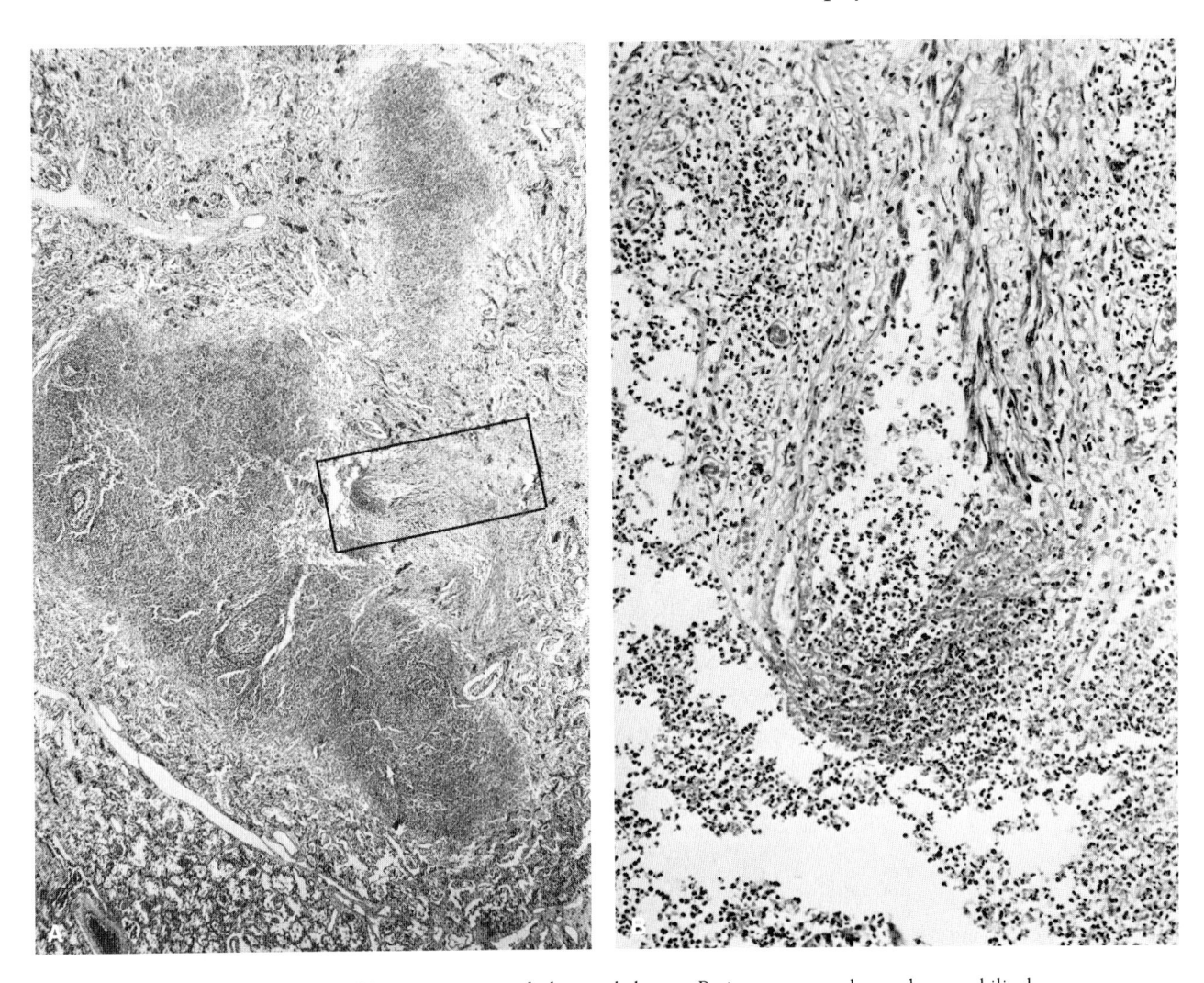

Figure 13–10. A. Hematogenous staphylococcal abscess. Patient was a newborn whose umbilical vein catheter became infected with S. *epidermidis* (×50). B. Higher-power view of the artery shown in the box in A to show purulent arteritis (×150).

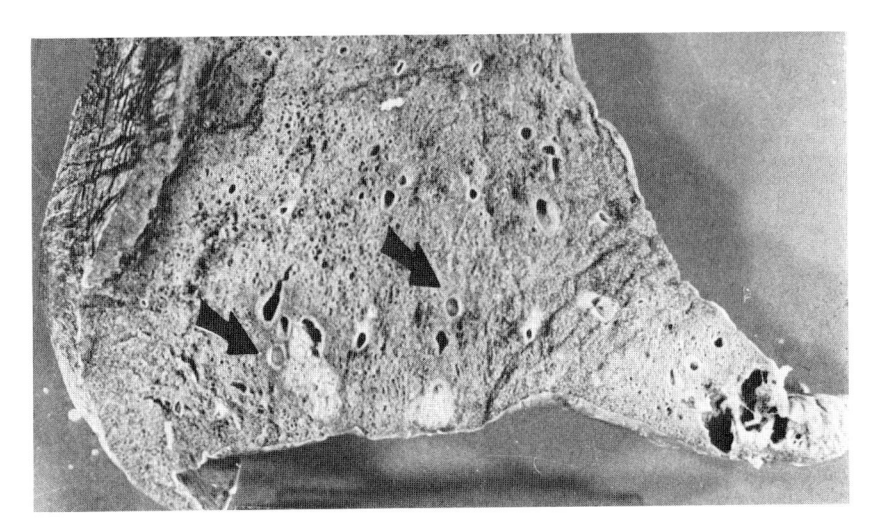

Figure 13–11. Septic infarcts in an intravenous drug abuser. The arrows identify septic emboli.

In children staphylococcal pneumonia usually occurs before the age of 6 months.[78] This age distribution is probably as much a consequence of the high nasal carriage rates in small children as of the immaturity of immunologic defenses in the very young. Two notable features of staphylococcal pneumonia in infants are a high frequency of pleural involvement and a tendency to develop pneumatoceles.[78–80] Well known to radiologists, pneumatoceles are smooth, round, air-containing radiolucencies seen within areas of pneumonia. They enlarge rapidly and resolve over several weeks.[80] Although not specific for staphylococcal pneumonia, having been described in chemical, viral, and bacterial pneumonias,[81] they are nonetheless characteristic. Few have been studied pathologically. It is not likely that they are simply abscesses because they are thin walled and usually disappear completely. Radiologists attribute their rapid growth to air trapping distal to a partially obstructed bronchus which acts as a check valve.[80] Some have been clearly shown to be foci of interstitial emphysema within the pleura which probably formed when air dissected through the interlobular septa and collected within the pleura forming a bleb visible radiographically.[82] Others may arise by acute distension of a necrotic cavity.[83]

Pneumonia Caused by Gram-Negative Aerobic Bacteria

Pneumonia caused by Gram-negative aerobic bacteria was uncommon in the preantibiotic era, accounting for less than 5 percent of pneumonias. Today between 5 and 30 percent of community-acquired pneumonias and 30 to 50 percent of hospital-acquired pneumonias are due to this group of organisms.[84–89] Despite the availability of a range of antibiotics, the mortality of Gram-negative pneumonia hovers around 50 percent.[86,87] Most gram-negative pneumonias occur in subjects with chronic underlying illness, a feature that contributes to their high mortality.[86–89] The bacteria reach the lung by various routes. Often a period of colonization of the upper airways precedes the onset of the pneumonia which is triggered by aspiration.[4] *Escherichia coli*, Enterobacter, and Pseudomonas often reach the lung by hematogenous spread from an abdominal source. Some hospital epidemics have been traced to contamination of inhalation therapy equipment,[90–93] but improved technique and the development of ethylene gas sterilization have greatly mitigated the problem. Home whirlpool baths can also transmit gram-negative organisms.

Klebsiella Pneumoniae

In the preantibiotic era, *Klebsiella pneumoniae*, the Friedlander's bacillus, was responsible for less than 1 percent of pneumonias, but was notable for its high mortality.[94,95] Like other Gram-negative organisms, it is probably increasing in incidence, and its mortality is still far from negligible (50 percent).[86] Pneumonia caused by Klebsiella is a disease of those past middle age, 80 to 90 percent being men. Alcoholism is the most common predisposing factor, but diabetes, chronic pulmonary disease, and malignancy also are common.

K. pneumoniae is a common inhabitant of the oral cavity and tonsils. In most instances, it gains access to the lung by aspiration which accounts for its predilection for the upper and lower lobes of the right lung, sites that are dependent in supine subjects.[96] Symptoms usually begin with sudden chills, fever, tachypnea, cyanosis, and cough. Gelatinous, bloody sputum is considered characteristic, but is noted in only one-third of cases. Leukocytosis may be present, but leukopenia is more common. Although lobar consolidation is often present, serial radiographs indicate that the lesions probably begin as a bronchopneumonia which rapidly progresses to confluence and then abscess formation.[97] At autopsy the involved lobe is large and bulging, with a film of purulent exudate on the pleura. The lobe is massively consolidated and varies from red to dark brown to grey-yellow depending on the duration of the pneumonia. The sectioned surface appears less dry and granular than that of pneumococcal pneumonia. A gelatinous slimy fluid exudes from the cut surface. When the exudate is scraped off the surface, the remnants of the early lobular pattern of pneumonia can be recognized as focal elevation of the consolidated tissue in the centers of the lobules. In cases of more than a few days' duration, abscesses are found.[94,95,97,98]

In sections of early pneumonia, the alveolar septa are congested, and the air spaces are filled with a cellular exudate that is relatively poor in fibrin. The exudate contains both neutrophils and macrophages, but usually the latter predominate. In untreated cases, organisms are abundant, both free and within phagocytes (Fig. 13–12). Necrosis of alveolar walls begins within a day or two, and by 4 to 5 days, granulation tissue appears at the margins of the resulting abscesses. A few cases of *K. pneumoniae* run a chronic course. The involved tissue shows bronchiectasis, fibrosis, and focally cavities blending into areas of acute pneumonia. At times the gross appearance may suggest tuberculosis.[98]

In the acute phase of the infection, bacteremia is not uncommon, but it rarely leads to the establishment of infection at distant sites. Nevertheless, the mortality is higher in bacteremic pneumonia than in patients without bacteremia.[94,95]

Proteus

Proteus is an uncommon cause of pneumonia with many features similar to Klebsiella. It affects men of middle age or older, usually alcoholics with other underlying diseases, including chronic pulmonary disease and diabetes. The onset often follows an episode of alcoholic stupor or delerium tremens. After several days of mild cough, symptoms suddenly worsen with the appearance of chills, fever, and dyspnea. The consolidation usually involves the dependent segments and produces multiple abscesses. The alveoli are filled with a mixed mononuclear and neutrophil exudate with focal hemorrhages and

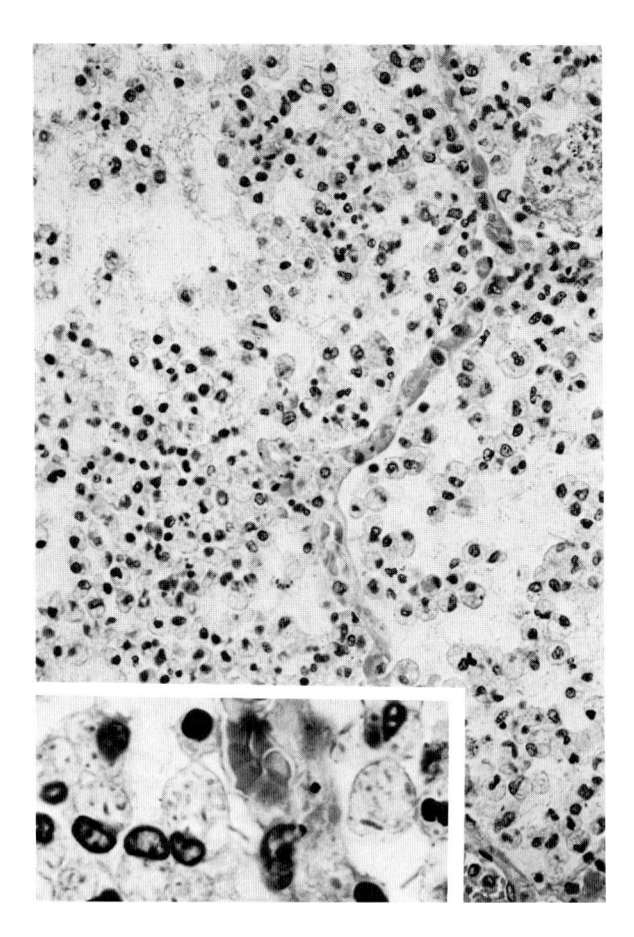

Figure 13–12. *Klebsiella pneumoniae.* The predominant inflammatory cells in this instance are macrophages (×750). Inset, Encapsulated bacilli mainly within macrophages (×2500).

necrosis of alveolar walls (Fig. 13–13). As a rule, the pleura is spared. The mortality is relatively low, and healing occurs with closure of the abscesses, leaving little fibrosis.[99]

Escherichia coli

In contrast to the preceding organisms, *E. coli* usually reaches the lung via the circulation from an infection of the urinary tract, gastrointestinal tract, biliary system, or peritoneum. Urinary tract infection is the most common predisposing illness, but diabetes, heart disease, and chronic lung disease are also common.[100] The symptoms do not differ from those of the other Gram-negative pneumonias.

E. coli produces a bilateral patchy or lobular lower lobe pneumonia. In patients who die in the first 2 days, there is no pleural fluid. The air spaces fill with edema and hemorrhage accompanied by a scanty, predominantly mononuclear inflammatory exudate. In patients who survive longer, the alveolar walls become slightly thickened due to engorgement of the capillaries and infiltration with mononuclear cells. The mononuclear inflammatory exudate in the alveolar spaces becomes pronounced, and there is focal hyperplasia of the epithelium lining the alveoli. In patients surviving a week or more, empyema is common, and typical abscesses form in the parenchyma with breakdown of alveolar walls and purulent exudate.[100]

In the series reported by Tillotson and Lerner,[100] in which community-acquired cases were the majority, the mortality was 60 percent. In more recent series [101,102] with predominantly nosocomial and bacteremic cases, the mortality was even higher, although one group [103] achieved 70 percent survival.

Hemophilus Influenzae

H. influenzae is a Gram-negative aerobic coccobacillus that is found in the upper respiratory passages of many normal individuals. It is relatively fastidious in its nutrition and requires both hematin as a source of preformed tetrapyrrole and exogenous nicotinamide dinucleotide in order to grow in culture. Consequently it is a true parasite unable to survive in the general environment. Six serotypes, designated A through F, are distinguished based on their capsular antigens.[104] In addition, there are unencapsulated strains that can not be typed.

In children the encapsulated strains of *H. influenzae*, in particular type B, are important pathogens responsible for meningitis, conjunctivitis, otitis, arthritis, and epiglottitis as well as pneumonia. The incidence of infection is greatest at age one year[105] and declines rapidly thereafter as children acquire protective antibodies to the capsular polysaccharide. In adults there is some evidence that *H. influenzae* infections are increasing. This may be in part an artifact of improved culture techniques,[106] but there is also evidence for diminishing immunity in the adult population.[106]

H. influenzae frequently colonizes the lower respiratory tract of those patients with chronic bronchitis or bronchiectasis. The colonizing organisms are usually unencapsulated strains of low virulence. Their role in acute exacerbations of bronchitis is still in question.[107,108] In some studies, either the proportion of patients with *H. influenzae* in their sputum or the number of organisms per unit volume of sputum has increased during exacerbations, but other observers have been unable to confirm this. Hers and Mulder[109] were able to study the bronchial morphology of nine subjects with acute bronchitis and untypeable strains either at autopsy or in resected bronchiectatic lobes. The bronchial epithelium was intact but was infiltrated with neutrophils. There were lymphocytes and neutrophils in the lamina propria as well. Bacteria were present among the epithelial cells and beneath the basement membrane.

Since *H. influenzae* is found in sputum in the absence of disease, most authors have required the isolation of the organism from blood or pleural fluid for inclusion of cases in published series. Consequently published series have a high proportion of bacteremic patients and undoubtedly underestimate the true incidence of pneumonia by this organism.

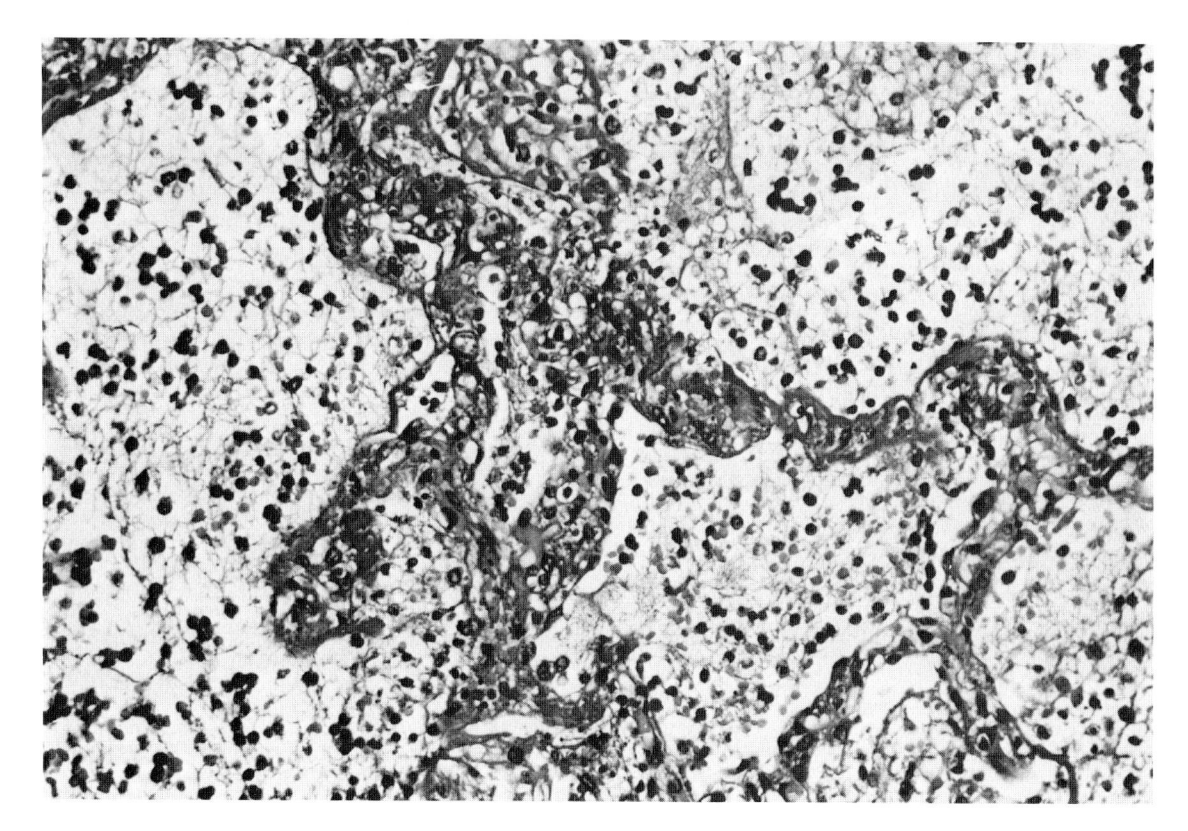

Figure 13–13. Pneumonia caused by *Proteus morgagni* showing necrosis and fibrin deposition in alveolar septa.

Patients with *H. pneumoniae* are typically either small children [110,111] or adults 50 years or older.[106,108,112–114] Risk factors in adults are chronic pulmonary disease and alcoholism. The pneumonia is preceded by a viral infection in 30 to 50 percent of patients. Fever, cough, increased sputum production, and myalgias are present in the majority of patients. Tillotson and Lerner[112] described two roentgenographic patterns: lobar or segmental consolidation, which is associated with bacteremia, and a diffuse miliary mottling, which occurs in patients with chronic lung disease without bacteremia. Cavitation, pleural effusion, or empyema may develop, particularly in the lobar type. The prognosis is relatively good, with usual mortality rates less than 10 percent unless meningitis is also present. Mortalities can be higher for bacteremic cases.[114]

Pseudomonas aeruginosa

Once rare, infections with *P. aeruginosa* have become a bane of the hospital environment. Although Pseudomonas produces only 1 to 2 percent of community-acquired bacterial pneumonias, it accounts for 20 to 50 percent of nosocomial pneumonias. Pseudomonal pneumonia appears to be increasing in incidence because of several factors, including selection of antibiotics to which the organism is relatively insensitive, the growing use of immunosuppressive therapies, and increased survival of critically ill patients who seem to be particularly prone to colonization of their upper airways by this organism. Some hospital epidemics have been traced to a specific common source, such as a contaminated aerosol generator,[90] but the major increase is probably related to general attributes of current hospital populations and patterns of medical practice.[115] Almost all patients developing pseudomonal pneumonia have an underlying disease, notably chronic lung disease, diabetes, and heart disease,[116] solid or hematologic malignancy especially if accompanied by leukopenia,[117,118] or severe burns.[119]

There are two relatively distinct patterns of pseudomonal pneumonia that differ in pathogenesis, morphology, and prognosis. One type results from spread of Pseudomonas by colonization of the upper airways and subsequent aspiration into the lung.[116] This type of spread is common in subjects with chronic lung disease and critically ill patients in intensive care units. In the latter group, the frequency of colonization increases with duration of hospitalization and severity of illness.[4] The pneumonia produced by airway spread of Pseudomonas is a bronchopneumonia which can become confluent (Fig. 13–14), or lead to the development of multiple abscesses. Pleural effusions are usually small and empyemas infrequent. The histology is not distinctive. The air spaces are filled with an exudate of fibrin neutrophils and mononuclear phagocytes, and focally hematologic malignancy.[117,118] The lesions are distinctive foci of hemorrhagic necrosis, most numerous subpleurally and in the lower lobes.[120,121] They begin as small foci of hemorrhage that develop into firm grey nodules of necrosis. With time they grow more yellow and enlarge to produce yellow nodules several centimeters in diameter surrounded by a rim hemorrhage (Fig. 13–15). Under the microscope, the nodules consist of coagulative necrosis in which the alveoli are filled with eosinophilic debris, and the outlines of the underlying tissue remain. Many arteries and veins within the area of necrosis teem with bacteria which form a pale-blue haze in the wall of the vessel as seen in hematoxylin and eosin (H & E)–stained sections (Fig. 13–16, 13–17). Inflammatory cells are rare.

Although the quality of the necrosis resembles that of infarcts, the vessels that are the site of bacterial invasion often remain patent with intact erythrocytes in their lumen. Although ischemia may contribute to the necrosis, *P. aeruginosa* produces a number of toxic extracellular products,[122] and it is these that are mainly responsible. The toxic products include exotoxin A, an inhibitor of protein synthesis similar to diphtheria toxin

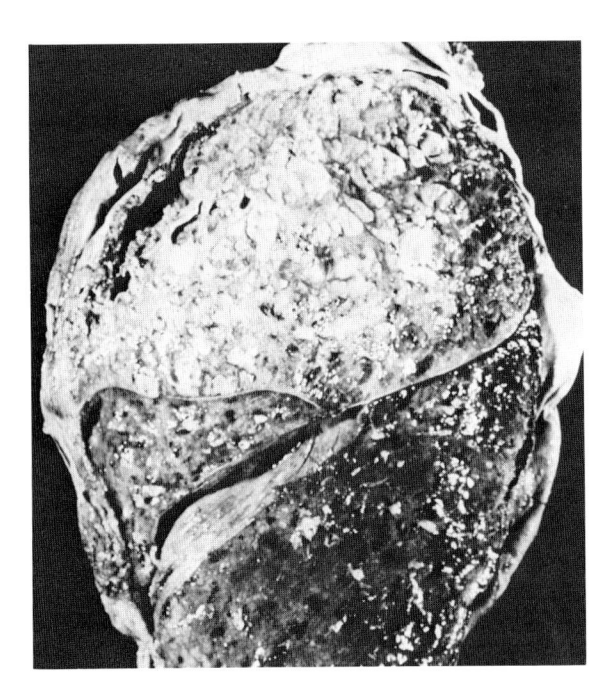

Figure 13–14. The upper lobe of this lung is involved by confluent bronchopneumonia caused by *Pseudomonas aeruginosa*. The patient had spent several weeks on mechanical ventilation following an automobile accident in which he fractured several ribs.

there is hemorrhage and necrosis of alveolar walls. Secondary bacteremia is common.

Pneumonia caused by bacteremic spread of Pseudomonas is common in patients with burns [119] or

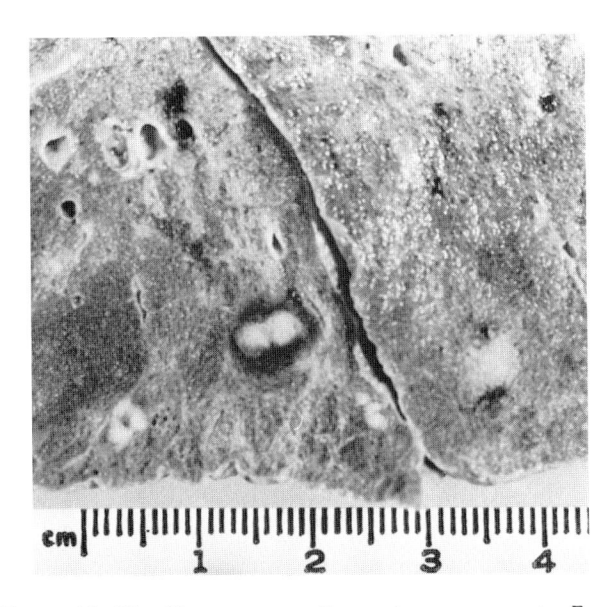

Figure 13–15. Hematogenous *P. aeruginosa* pneumonia. Focal subpleural nodules of necrosis. The one in the center is rimmed by hemorrhage.

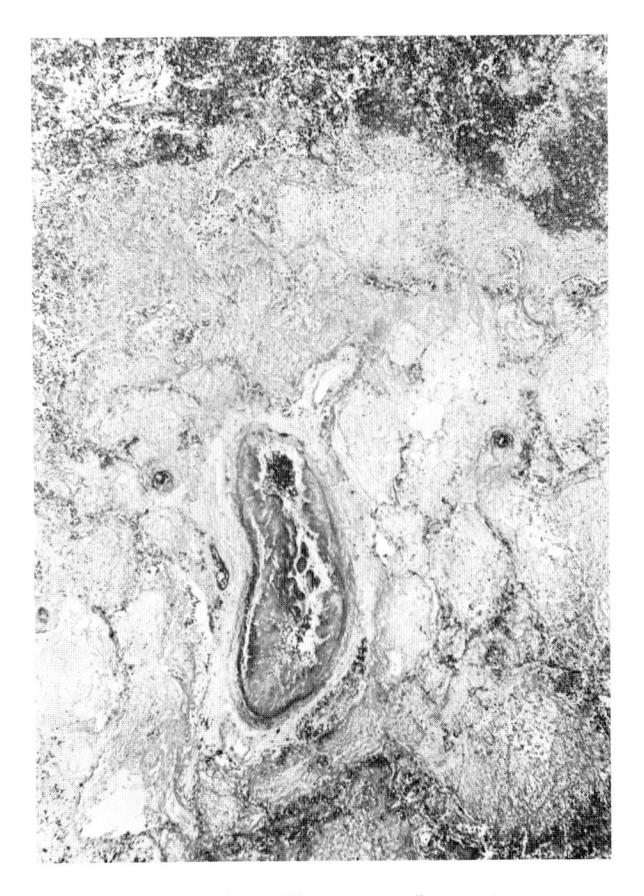

Figure 13–16. Histology of bacteremic. *P. aeruginosa* pneumonia. An area of coagulative necrosis surrounded by hemorrhage. The vessel in the center of the necrosis has basophilic staining of its wall owing to the presence of bacteria (×100). Reproduced with permission from Kissane JM (ed): *Anderson's Pathology*. St. Louis: CV Mosby, 1984.

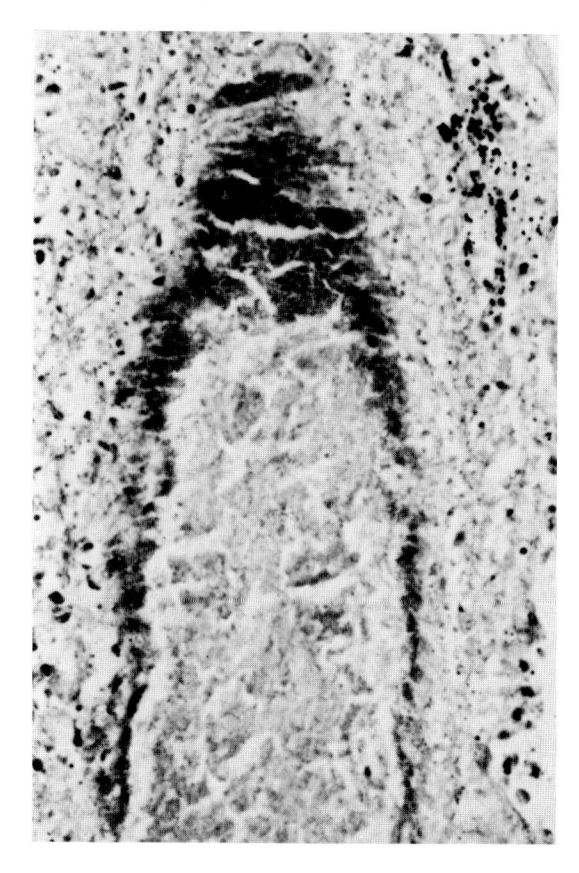

Figure 13-17. Bacterial strain of an artery in septicemia pseudomonal pneumonia. Darkly stained bacteria outline the vessel wall (Goodpasture's stain, ×1000).

in its mechanism of action,[123] a hemolysin, a phospholipase, and a powerful protease, elastase.

The prognosis of pseudomonal pneumonia is grim, and the introduction of new antibiotics in the past 20 years has had almost no effect.[124] The mortality of airborne pseudomonal pneumonia was reported to be 70 percent in 1966[86] and remains in the 70 to 80 percent range. The mortality of bacteremic pseudomonal pneumonia is higher still.[102,125-127]

Melioidosis

Melioidosis is a geographically restricted pseudomonal infection of extraordinarily varied manifestations. Although it was first described by Whitmore in drug addicts in Rangoon, it does not appear to have a particular predilection for debilitated subjects. The disease is endemic in a zone 20 degrees on either side of the equator that extends from Madagascar in the west to Guam in the east and includes southeast Asia, portions of Australia, New Guinea, and the Philippines. Few cases have been reported that were acquired outside this zone, including two from the western hemisphere. The engagement of large numbers of French and later American troops in southeast Asia again brought the disease to the attention of western physicians.

The infection is caused by *P. pseudomallei*, an unencapsulated gram-negative rod that is closely related to the causative organism of glanders (*P. mallei*) from which it differs in that it is motile due to its polar flagellae. *P. pseudomallei* grows readily on simple media, and colonies more than 72 hours old have a distinctive furrowed morphology.

The usual manner of transmission of the infection is not yet conclusively established. The organism grows readily in moist soil or stagnant water, such as that of rice paddies, and most infections are probably acquired by contamination of skin abrasions from these sources. The disease can also be acquired by the inhalation of contaminated dusts and aerosols. Many types of animals are susceptible to experimental infection; mosquitoes and fleas have been used to transmit the organism in the laboratory, but there is little evidence from field studies that this is an important mechanism in nature. The ingestion of bacteria and penetration of the conjunctiva round out the list of possible routes.

Three types of infection are recognized.[128-130] First is an asymptomatic infection that has been deduced from the presence of positive hemagglutinating or complement fixing antibodies in 5 to 15 percent of the population in some endemic areas. The second is an acute form of the disease that is either a fulminant septicemia or a pneumonic illness of explosive onset.[128,129] Acute melioidosis leads to death in 24 hours to a few weeks in the majority of instances. Occasionally the onset may be somewhat more gradual with diarrhea or pustular skin lesions for several days before the appearance of severe septicemic symptoms. The third type is a chronic form of the disease that is usually localized to one or a few organs.[129,130] It can affect any organ or tissue but most often involves the lung. The patients have unilateral upper lobe lesions that appear nodular or cavitary in the chest roentgenogram and closely mimic tuberculosis. Organisms can usually be cultured from sputum or tissue but not from blood.

The basis for the extremely varied expression of the infection is not well understood. Presumably the virulence of the infecting strain, the dose of organisms, and the immunologic history and competence of the host each plays a role. A noteworthy property of the organism is its ability to lie dormant for months or years, only to be activated by the stress of some unrelated illness.[131]

The acute form of the infection will usually be encountered by the pathologist at autopsy. Disseminated abscesses may be found in any organ. The lungs, liver, and spleen are the organs most often involved. When the lungs are involved, the bronchi are hyperemic and may contain little or much exudate. As a rule, the amount of bronchial exudate is greater when parenchymal abscesses are large and confluent. Yellow hemorrhagic nodules in the lung may be visible through the pleura. The lung parenchyma either appears diffusely consolidated or shows discrete abscesses.[132] On microscopic examination, the most characteristic finding is multiple discrete abscesses one or a few millimeters in size often surrounded by hemorrhage. Both neutrophils and monocytes are present in the exudate. Giant cells resembling megakaryocytes are often present.[132,133] As the lesions grow and coalesce to form larger abscesses, the exudate comes to consist entirely of neutrophils.[133] In patients who survive several weeks, lymphocytes and monocytes appear at the periphery of the abscesses.[134] Chronic melioidosis is rarely fatal, but the lesions may be encountered in resected tissue. In this form of the disease, the lesions are granulomatous. Usually the center of small lesions consists of an irregularly shaped or stellate collection of purulent exudate enclosed by a zone of epithelioid cells. Giant cells of either Langerhans or foreign body type may be present. This type of granuloma resembles those of cat-scratch disease or lymphogranuloma venereum. Sometimes the center of the granulomas consists of a caseous type of necrosis, in which case the lesions are indistinguishable morphologically from tuberculosis.[133] When cavities are resected after extensive antibiotic treatment, active granulomatous inflammation may no longer be present and sections show only a fibrous wall with nonspecific chronic inflammatory cells.[130]

Organisms are usually abundant in the acute abscesses. Piggott and Hochholzer[133] recommend Giemsa stains and the Brown and Hopps modification of the Gram stain as the most suitable. In the chronic granulomatous form of infection, stains fail to show organisms, although cultures usually will confirm their presence. Fluorescent antibodies can be used for the rapid and specific identification of organisms when they are present in sufficient numbers.

Legionella

The Legionellaceae owe their name to the circumstances that led to their identification as a distinct genus of bacteria. In the summer of 1976, a pneumonic illness broke out among visitors attending an American Legion convention in Philadelphia. One hundred and eighty-two individuals became ill and 29 died. Investigation into the cause of this mysterious illness lead to the isolation of a hitherto unrecognized bacterium, now known as *Legionella pneumophila*.[135] *L. pneumophila* is not an uncommon cause of pneumonia, but it had escaped detection owing to its poor staining by Gram's technique and its fastidious growth requirements in the laboratory. Currently nine different species of Legionella are known that differ antigenically and share less than 30 percent DNA homology (Table 12–2). However, all are motile rods with a single flagellum and a high content of branched-chain fatty acids, and all can be grown on buffered charcoal yeast extract agar. There are at least eight serotypes of *L. pneumophila*, and one other Legionella, *L. longbeachae*, also has two serotypes (see Table 12–2).[136]

L. pneumophila produces two distinct types of epidemic illness: Pontiac fever, an acute febrile illness with a very high attack rate, an incubation period of 24 to 48 hours, and no mortality,[137,138] and Legionnaire's disease,

Table 13–2. The Legionellae

Species	Serotypes
Legionella pneumophila	8
Legionella micdadei	1
Legionella bozemanii	1
Legionella dumofii	1
Legionella gormanii	1
Legionella longbeachae	2
Legionella oakridgensis	1
Legionella jordanis	1
Legionella wadsworthii	1

a pneumonia with a relatively low attack rate, an incubation period of 2 to 10, days, and significant mortality.[136] *L. pneumophila* is also a cause of sporadic pneumonias both in the community and among hospitalized patients.[139–141] Instances of wound infection by *L. pneumophila* have been reported.[142] Of the other Legionellae, *L. micdadei* is a fairly frequent cause of nosocomial pneumonia, especially in the immunosuppressed patient.[143,144] Only a few infections with the other Legionellae have been reported.[145]

In both epidemic and sporadic infections, Legionella is acquired from environmental sources. Many infections have been traced to aerosols of contaminated water, from shower heads, air conditioning cooling towers, and evaporative condensors; other epidemics have been associated with construction sites.[136,146–149] Person to person spread is unknown. Impaired host defenses also play a role. Patients are usually older than age 50, and in the original epidemic, most were smokers. Nosocomial infections have occurred in those with chronic illness, particularly those with malignant tumors, renal transplants, or those receiving corticosteroids. Members of the hospital staff exposed to the same environment have not been affected.

Pneumonia caused by *L. pneumophila* varies considerably in severity.[136,150] Typically the onset is gradual, and systemic symptoms predominate at first. The illness begins with fever, malaise, and myalgias accompanied by diarrhea, mild cough, headache, and confusion. The white blood count may either be elevated or depressed, and hyponatremia and abnormal liver function tests are common. The cause of the systemic symptoms is not yet clear. The organism produces endotoxins, hemolysin, and extracellular enzymes which might be absorbed systemically, but the occurrence of bacteremia has also been documented.

Typical features of pneumonia, such as dyspnea, sputum production, and signs of consolidation, may not appear until as long as a week after the onset of symptoms. Patchy infiltrates will be seen radiographically and usually continue to progress, especially if therapy consists of beta-lactam and aminoglycoside antibiotics to which the organisms are usually insensitive. The course

Figure 13–18. Legionnaires' disease. There is necrosis of the intraalveolar exudate, but the alveolar walls remain intact (×750).

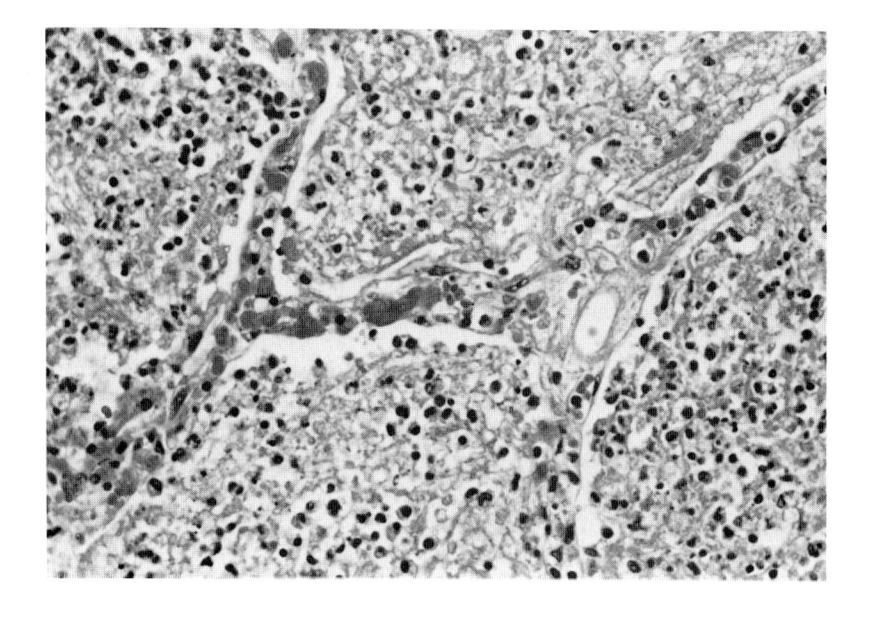

is protracted, most cases resolving, some healing with fibrosis. The mortality is approximately 15 to 20 percent.

At autopsy[145,151-153] there may be a small amount of serosanguineous pleural fluid. Multiple lobes are involved by a patchy lobular pneumonia with large areas of confluence. Occasionally entire lobes may be consolidated by confluence of smaller foci. Rarely discrete round lesions or abscesses may be seen grossly.

The microscopic appearance is that of a fibrinopurulent pneumonia. Alveoli are filled by an exudate of fibrin and inflammatory cells. Either neutrophils or macrophages may predominate, and extensive degeneration and breakdown of the phagocytes (leukocytoclasis) are common (Fig. 13–18). The alveolar walls usually remain intact, showing only congestion and focal epithelial hyperplasia. Thrombosis of vessels, septic vasculitis, or necrosis of alveolar walls, when present, are only rarely sufficiently severe to produce macroscopic cavities.[145] In cases of several weeks' duration, fibrous organization of the intra-alveolar exudate occurs.

Organisms are usually abundant, mainly within phagocytes but also extracellularly. The most satisfactory stain for showing the organisms is Dieterle's silver stain[154] (Fig. 13–19). Gram's stain and its variants are usually negative on tissue sections, although Gram's stain may work on imprints. Gimenez stain and Wolbach's modification of the Giemsa stain have been reported to give satisfactory results on sections.[145] None of these stains is specific, and positive identification of the organism requires either immunohistochemistry or culture.

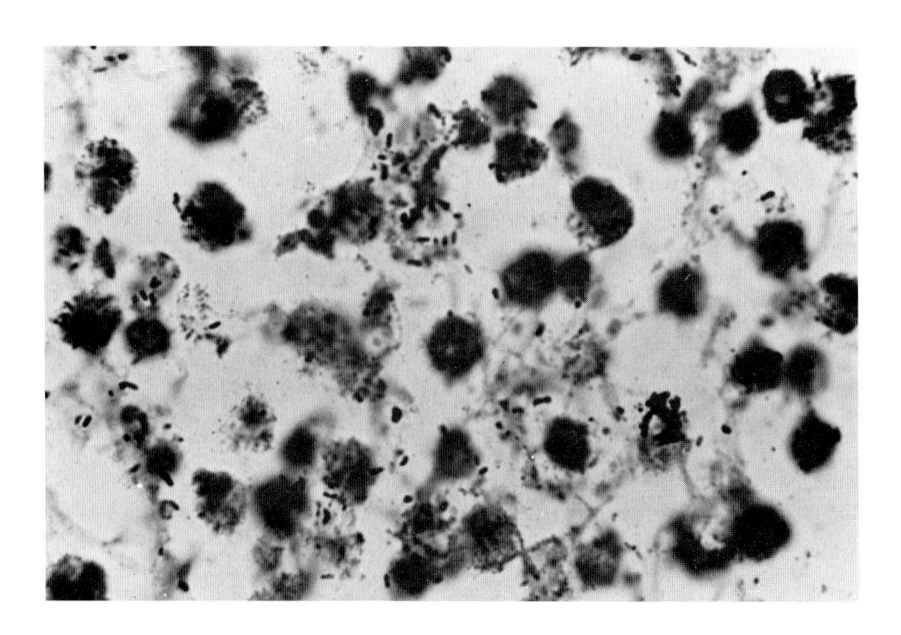

Figure 13–19. Legionnaires' disease. Bacteria are mainly intracellular (Dieterle's silver stain, ×2500).

The antigens are stable to formalin fixation and paraffin embedding, and routinely processed tissue is usually adequate for either direct immunofluorescene or for immunoenzymatic staining.[155] However, type-specific antisera are required. A polyvalent antiserum to types I–IV is available for screening, but the remaining types must be stained individually.

Immunity to Legionella depends more on cellular than humoral immunity. In vitro studies show that the organisms are intracellular parasites that can proliferate within cytoplasmic vacuoles of mononuclear phagocytes. Antibodies and complement promote uptake by monocytes but do not enhance bacterial killing. Antibiotics such as erythromycin or rifampin at concentrations that are lethal to extracellular organisms suppress the growth of intracellular organisms without killing them.[156] Thus, phagocytized bacteria are paradoxically protected from antibiotics, and premature discontinuance of antibiotics can lead to recrudescence of disease. Intracellular mechanisms will slowly lead to elimination of organisms, and activation of the phagocytes accelerates the process.

L. micdadei, also known as Pittsburgh pneumonia agent and *Tatlockia micdadei*, has also been responsible for a number of cases nosocomial pneumonia, especially in chronically ill, debilitated, or immunosuppressed patients.[143,144,157] The clinical and pathologic features are similar to those of pneumonia caused by *L. pneumophila*. The organisms are weakly acid-fast and can be colored by variants of the acid-fast stain, such as Fite's or Putt's stains, that substitute 1 percent sulfuric acid decolorization for the standard ethanolic HCl.[143,145,157] The small size of the organisms as well as the histologic character of the lesions should enable them to be distinguished from mycobacteria.

Anaerobic Infections

Anaerobic bacteria are normal inhabitants on many mucosal surfaces. They are plentiful in the gastrointestinal tract, genital tract, certain areas of skin, and the oral cavity. In the mouth, they particularly thrive in specific sites such as the gingivodental sulcus and the tonsilar crypts where the redox potential is low.[158] The lower respiratory tract is normally free of anaerobes. They often colonize bronchiectatic bronchi, however.[159]

Anaerobic infections of the lower respiratory tract give rise to three overlaping types of lesions—pneumonitis, lung abscess, and necrotizing pneumonia—which usually share a common pathogenesis, aspiration occurring outside the hospital in a setting of impaired consciousness or disordered swallowing.[160,161] Common predisposing factors include alcoholism, general anesthesia, seizures, and neurologic or esophageal disease. Formerly tonsillectomy was attended by substantial risk, but this has largely been eliminated by the use of cuffed endotracheal tubes during anesthesia. Periodental infections, which increase the anaerobic bacterial burden in the oral cavity, also play a major role. In the absence of a cause for aspiration, the main predisposing conditions are bronchogenic carcinoma or an extrathoracic source for bacteremia such as a gynecologic infection or a perforation of the gastrointestinal tract.[162]

Aspiration introduces a mixed innoculum into the lung. Although the host response, local environment, and therapy can all modify this population, most anaerobic infections remain polymicrobial. The predominant organisms reflect the oral flora: Peptostreptococci, Peptococcus, *Fusobacterium nucleatum*, and *Bacteroides melaninogenicus*. In roughly one-third of cases, there are aerobic as well as anaerobic bacteria.[160]

The localization of anaerobic lesions reflects their pathogenesis. The right lung is involved more commonly than the left owing to the more direct course of the right main bronchus. The most frequent sites are the posterior segments of the upper and lower lobes, which are dependent in the supine position, followed by the basilar segment of the right lower lobe, which is dependent if the subject is erect. The pneumonia secondary to *Bacteroides bacteremia* preferentially involves the lower lobes.

Anaerobic pneumonitis initially is difficult to distinguish from other forms of pneumonia. It begins as a febrile illness with cough and radiographic infiltrate. Chills and rigors do not occur, but the sputum infrequently has the characteristic fetid odor of anaerobes.[163] If therapy is instituted at this stage, the response is rapid, most patients will heal, and the mortality is low unless the predisposing illness is lethal. Untreated or poorly responsive pneumonitis can evolve into either lung abscess or the more severe necrotizing pneumonia.

Abscesses resulting from aspiration are commonly called primary lung abscesses to distinguish them from abscesses secondary to bronchial obstruction or spread from an extrathoracic infection. Although serial radiographs indicate that primary lung abscesses usually evolve over several weeks from an area of pneumonitis, they present clinically as relatively indolent lesions accompanied by fever, anemia, and weight loss.[160] Fetor of the sputum is present in half of cases. Although some clinical studies arbitrarily require that a large cavity be visible radiographically for the diagnosis to be made, pathologically abscesses can be seen that do not communicate with major bronchus and thus will not have an air-containing cavity (Fig. 13–20). Generally primary lung abscesses are well-circumscribed lesions varying from grey-green to dirty brown. The center may be occupied by pasty necrotic material (*see* Fig. 13–20), fluid pus or an air-filled cavity (Fig. 13–21); the lining may be trabeculated or smooth. The margins may be thin, merge with an area of chronic pneumonia, or have a well-developed fibrous capsule.

Microscopically corresponding variations may be found. The cavity usually contains necrotic sloughed lung tissue and degenerated purulent exudate in varied proportions (Fig. 13–22). A pyogenic membrane lines the cavity in active cases. The cavity may be surrounded by pneumonic lung, granulation tissue, or, in long-standing cases, a well-developed fibrous capsule. Reepithelialization of the cavity occurs by ingrowth of squamous epithelium in most cases. Eventually in healed lesions, the squamous epithelium may revert to a ciliated type. Large arteries and veins in the abscess wall usually show

Figure 13–20. Lung abscesses in a patient with esophageal diverticulum. The cavities are filled with necrotic slough.

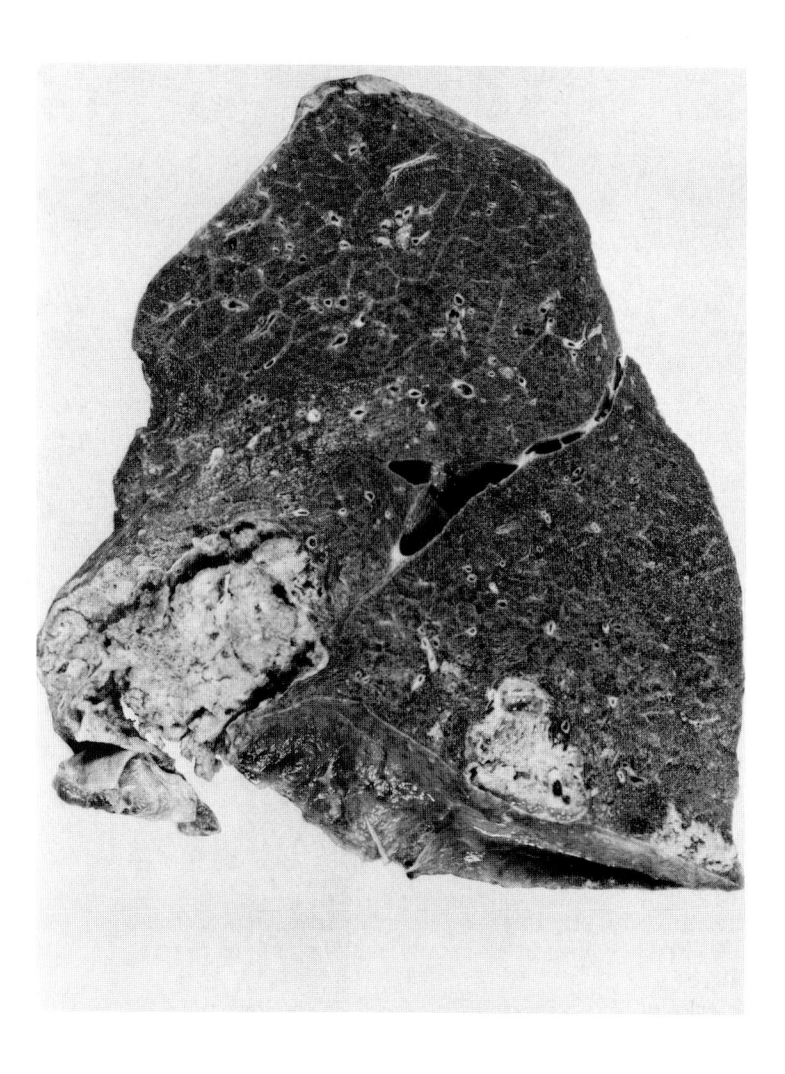

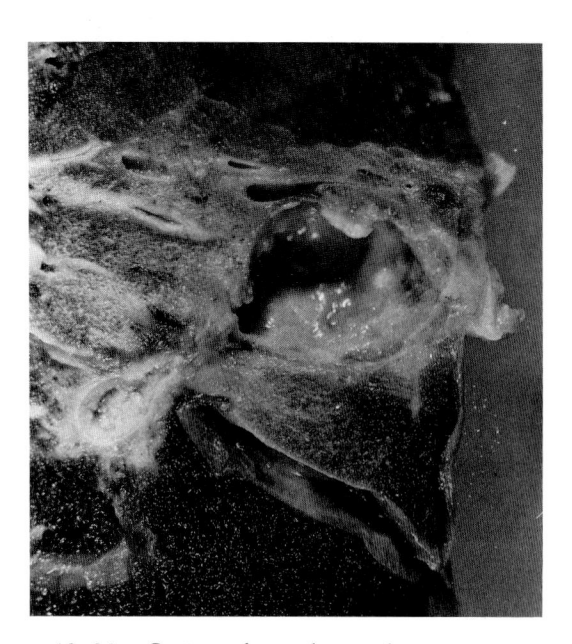

Figure 13–21. Cavitary lung abscess due to aspiration of microaerophilic streptococci. The cavity is surrounded by pneumonitis.

marked intimal fibrosis, often to the point of complete obliteration of the lumen.

Treatment with antibiotics is successful for most primary lung abscesses. Although healing is gradual and may require months, closure of the abscess occurs in most cases.[164–166] Mortality rates are in the 1 to 2 percent range. Deaths are either a consequence of sudden massive hemoptysis[167] or extrathoracic spread of the infection. In secondary lung abscess, the prognosis is closely tied to that of the underlying disease, and the mortality is higher than for primary lung abscess.

Necrotizing pneumonia (chronic destructive pneumonia) is a more severe type of infection that also probably develops from untreated anaerobic pneumonitis. As with other forms of anaerobic infection, patients often have poor dental hygiene.[168] The spectrum of organisms recovered is similar to that cultured from aspiration pneumonitis and lung abscess; the factors that lead to this more severe type of evolution are not understood.

The course of necrotizing pneumonia is extremely variable.[160,168] Some patients are minimally symptomatic; some have a smoldering chronic disease with fever, anemia, and weight loss; others have a fulminant pneumonia. Sputum has the characteristic fetid odor, and

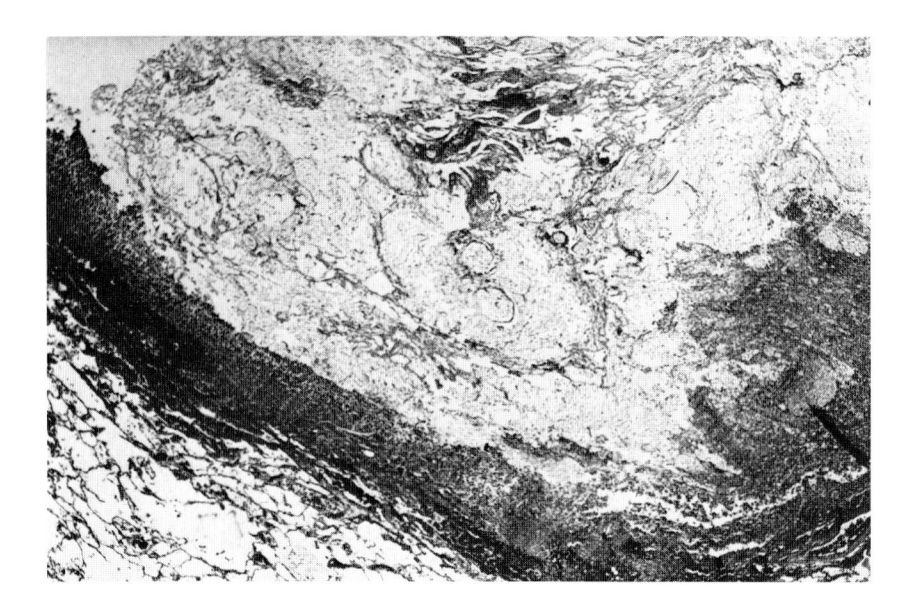

Figure 13–22. Histology of the abscesses illustrated in Figure 13–20 showing well-developed capsule and cavity filled with slough (×50).

hemoptysis is common. Roentgenograms show circumscribed areas of consolidation with multiple small areas of cavitation less than 1 cm in diameter. The response to treatment is slow; Bartlett and Finegold[160] reported a mean time to cure of 2 months in successfully treated cases. The mortality is 8 to 18 percent.

At autopsy or in resected specimens, the process usually involves more than one lobe. The involved tissue is grey and airless and encased in thickened pleura. The interlobular septa may be fibrotic, or the process may march through the lung obliterating septa and fissures. Bronchi are thickened and usually bronchiectatic; the parenchyma contains multiple cavities containing pus or necrotic tissue (Fig. 13–23). The microscopic picture is variable even within the same lung, with areas of fibrosis and organizing pneumonia interspersed with areas of necrosis and suppuration.[168]

Empyema can complicate each of the foregoing types of anaerobic pulmonary parenchymal infection. In the experience reported by Bartlett and Finegold,[160] about one-third of patients with each type of infection developed empyema. In some patients, empyema is associated with subphrenic abscess rather than pneumonia, presumably the result of spread of organisms across the diaphragm.

Plague

History

Whether or not one agrees with one authority[169] that the fourth great pandemic of plague is now in progress, plague certainly has not disappeared. The disease has infected man for thousands of years. Its original home is in dispute, and the central Asiatic plateau and central Africa each has its champions.[169,170] The first well-documented pandemic began in Egypt in the 15th year of Justinian's reign (542 A.D.) and spread through Constantinople into Europe, skipping from seaport to seaport and spreading inland. The pandemic that came to be known as the Black Death began in central Asia whence it spread to China, India, and Asia Minor. The Crimean ports became infected in 1346; a year later, it

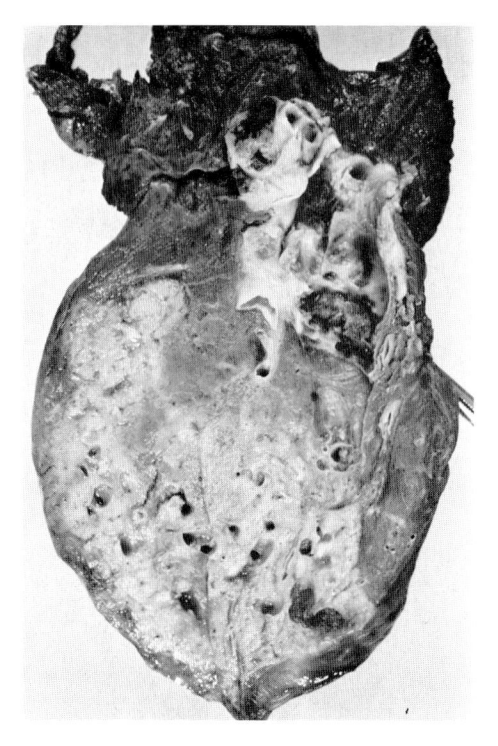

Figure 13–23. Resected lobe showing necrotizing pneumonia. Most of the holes seen on the cut surface are bronchiectatic bronchi.

spread through Italy into Europe where it is estimated to have claimed the life of one inhabitant in three. The third pandemic waxed and waned in Europe, continuing to claim lives from the 15th century into the 17th. In the first half of the 19th century, the infection again seeped out of central Asia and became established in northeast Burma and Yunnan province, China. Spread by a rebellion of the Moslems in 1855 with its attendant troop movements and refugees, the infection reached the provincial capital, Kunming, in 1866 and extended slowly to the Chinese coast, striking Canton and Hong Kong in 1894. From there it was carried by ships to India, the Philippines, Japan, Hawaii, Brazil, and San Francisco. At present the plague bacillus is established worldwide. In the 1970s, cases of plague were identified in South America, Libya, sub Saharan Africa, and Southeast Asia. In the United States, the bacillus is enzootic in sylvatic rodent populations from the eastern slope of the Rocky Mountains to the Pacific littoral.[171] Although the disease is rare in the United States, the incidence is on the rise. Only 45 cases were reported in the 20 years between 1949 and 1969, but 105 cases were reported between 1970 and 1979, the largest number in any decade since the 1920s. All the U.S. cases were acquired in eight western states, over half (56 percent) in New Mexico, where there have been a number of cases among children living on Indian reservations.[172]

Pathogenesis

Plague is caused by *Yersinia pestis*, a small Gram-negative nonmotile and non-spore-forming bacillus which typically demonstrates bipolar staining. The reservoir for the organism can be domestic rats and mice or, as in the American west, wild rodents such as chipmunks, ground squirrels, and prairie dogs.[170] The organism is transmitted among rodents by fleas and other blood-sucking insects; humans ordinarily become infected incidently when bitten by a rodent flea. Following ingestion by the flea, organisms proliferate in the flea's gut, achieving great numbers which occlude its proventriculus. When the flea attempts to ingest a blood meal from a new host, blood contaminated with bacteria is regurgitated from the blocked proventriculus and inoculated into the skin. The disease can also be transmitted to humans by dogs and cats, or be spread person to person by infected secretions.

The properties of the bacteria that determine virulence have been studied in some detail. Virulent strains have metabolic pathways which enable the organisms to fulfill their nutritional requirements in vivo, such as the ability to synthesize purines and form pigment. Virulent strains also produce a capsular antigen, fraction 1, which protects the organism from phagocytosis, apparently by virtue of its anticomplementary activity. This antigen is produced at 37°C, but not at temperatures below 27°C. As the organisms emerge from the flea, they usually lack fraction 1 and are phagocytosed by neutrophils and monocytes. Those bacteria that are ingested by neutrophils are killed. Monocytes are less efficient than neutrophils, however, and the organisms can divide within their cytoplasm. After a few cycles of division in the monocyte at body temperature, the organisms have acquired fraction 1 antigen; when they are released from the monocyte, they are resistant to further phagocytosis and proliferate rapidly.[173]

The clinical illness is the result both the hugh number of organisms in the body and the toxins that they produce. The uncontrolled growth of the organism results in large tissue burdens. By the time of death in lethally infected animals, there may be 10^8 or 10^9 organisms per gram of tissue.[169] The two major toxins produced by *Y. pestis* are a lipopolysaccharide endotoxin similar to that found in other enterobacteriaceae and a protein toxin derived from the cell envelope and known as the murine toxin.[174] Endotoxin has been demonstrated in the circulation of infected human subjects and may be responsible for the shock, disseminated intravascular coagulation (DIC), and widespread tissue hemorrhages which are so characteristic of the disease. The murine toxin is composed of at least two distinct proteins, designated toxins A and B, which occur as aggregates of molecular weights 240,000 and 120,000, respectively. The murine toxin, as the name implies, is highly toxic to mice but less so to other species. It functions as a beta-adrenergic blocking agent producing several metabolic aberrations, such as impaired epinephrine-induced mobilization of glucose from the liver and free fatty acid mobilization from peripheral tissues.[174]

In the bubonic and septicemic forms of plague, the lung becomes involved hematogenously (secondary pneumonia). Organisms that are either implanted by the bite of a flea or that penetrate a small abrasion or skin wound are carried to the regional lymph nodes where they proliferate and give rise after a few days or a week to the characteristic buboes of the bubonic plague—large edematous and necrotic lymph node groups usually in the groin or axilla but occasionally in other sites. Bacteria released from the nodes reach the bloodstream from which they can give rise to metastatic foci in the liver, spleen, meninges, and lung. In septicemic plague, the passage of organisms through the regional lymph nodes to the blood stream is accompanied by relatively minor lymphadenopathy, and clinical illness is dominated by the early appearance of septicemia. In either form, pulmonary involvement occurs later, heralded by the appearance of cough, dyspnea, and bloody or frothy sputum.

Patients with plague pneumonia are highly infectious and can spread the disease in its most rapidly lethal form: pneumonic plague, a primary pneumonia resulting from the inhalation of droplets of infected secretions.

Pathology

In cases of plague without pneumonia, the lung can show edema, hyaline membranes, and fibrin thrombi in small blood vessels.[175] These changes are probably the consequences of endotoxemia, shock, and DIC. They may

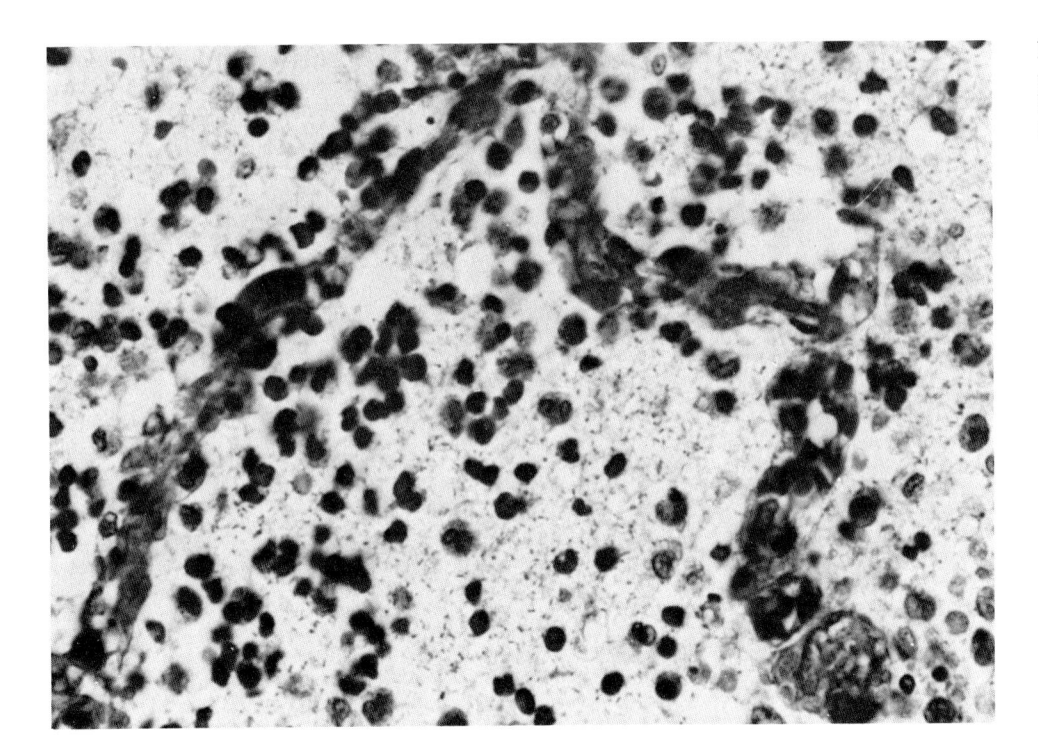

Figure 13–24. Plague pneumonia. Note the enormous number of extracellular bacteria (Goodpasture's stain, ×1500).

account for the rapidly reversible diffuse infiltrates seen radiographically.[176]

Plague pneumonia is usually bilateral and may be accompanied by hilar lymph node enlargement and pleural effusion. The lung is deeply congested and hemorrhagic, with patchy grey foci of consolidation which may become confluent. Alveoli in the consolidated areas contain fibrin, erythrocytes, neutrophils, and monocytes. Enormous numbers of extracellular baccili are present in the alveolar exudate and within the alveolar walls (Fig. 13–24). The diagnosis can be made either by culture of the organisms or fluorescent antibody staining.

Tularemia

Epidemiology

Tularemia is a zoonosis caused by the gram-negative bacillus *Francisella tularensis*. The organism is an intracellular parasite which produces an infection lasting weeks or months unless treated. The infection can be acquired from contact with blood or tissues of infected mammals; from the bites of blood sucking arthropods such as ticks, deerflies, or mosquitoes; or from water or dusts contaminated by the excreta of infected animals. Over one hundred different species of mammals have been reported to be susceptible to the organism. The hunting and dressing of rabbits are still sources of human infection but are outranked by transmission via the bites of ticks and deerflies, currently the leading cause of infection in the United States.[177] A number of epidemics have also occurred among laboratory personnel working with the organism.

Arthropods probably provide the reservoir for the survival of the organism. Ticks, for example, can pass the organism from one generation to the next transovarially. Mammals are not a true reservoir. When infected they become ill and either die of the infection or become immune and eliminate the bacteria.

The disease is found in a broad zone of the northern hemisphere between 30 and 70° north latitude including North America and many parts of Europe, Russia, and Japan. The seasonal distribution of cases varies in different parts of the world. In the United States, there are two distinct peaks of incidence, one in early summer corresponding to the height of the tick and deerfly season and one in winter during the season for rabbit hunting. The incidence in the United States has fallen sharply since the 1940s, but the disease is by no means rare.[177]

Pathogenesis

Organisms are introduced into the body through a break in the skin or penetrate a mucous membrane. They are carried by the lymphatics to the regional lymph nodes and then to the bloodstream where a transient septicemia results. Bacteria are picked up by the reticuloendothelial system and survive for extended periods within phagocytes giving rise to distant lesions, most frequently in the liver, spleen, peripheral lymph nodes, and lung.

Usually an erythematous papule appears at the site of primary inoculation during the first 48 hours, followed rapidly by enlargement of the draining lymph nodes. The primary lesion undergoes necrosis and sloughs leaving an indolent ulcer in its place. This, the most common type of clinical presentation, is classically called the ulceroglandular type. The hand or face is the most frequent site for the primary lesion. In a few cases, the organism penetrates the conjunctiva and spreads from there to the lymph nodes producing the oculoglandular type of tularemia. In instances in which the organism is inhaled or ingested so that the primary lesion is inapparent, or in the few cases in which the cutaneous site and regional nodes fail to develop the characteristic lesions, the illness is ushered in by systemic symptoms, the so-called typhoidal type of tularemia.

Involvement of the lung is common in the early septicemic phase of the disease, and some 90 percent of patients are reported to have mild transient radiographic changes. Clinical pneumonia is less common, occurring in 10 to 15 percent of those with the ulceroglandular or oculoglandular type and 50 to 75 percent of those with the typhoidal type.[178–180] The lung is involved in 62 to 73 percent of autopsied cases of tularemia.[180,181]

Pathology

The pathology of the pulmonary lesions has been reviewed by several authors.[180–182] Tularemia produces a nodular pneumonia which may involve one or several lobes. Lesions may undergo confluence to give an appearance similar to lobar pneumonia, but more typically there are multiple discrete areas of yellow-grey consolidation from one to several centimeters in diameter. Cavitation is unusual, but when it occurs, the lesions may resemble tuberculosis. Microscopic sections show alveoli filled with an exudate of mononuclear phagocytes, caseous necrotic debris, fibrin, and erythrocytes admixed in varying proportions. Even in early lesions, the predominant cell is a macrophage (Fig. 13–25); in later lesions, these cells are often laden with nuclear debris. Although a few neutrophils may be present, large numbers of neutrophils suggest superinfection with a pyogenic organism.[182] The alveolar septa may show mild thickening and infiltration with mononuclear cells or may be necrotic with thrombosed capillaries. In contrast to the scanty cellular infiltration of alveolar walls, the interstitial connective tissue of the perilobular septa and bronchovascular sheaths may be heavily infiltrated by lymphocytes, plasma cells, and mononuclear phagocytes (Fig. 13–26). Granulomas and giant cells are not ordinarily seen in the lung parenchyma.

Involvement of the hilar lymph nodes is present in two-thirds of cases radiographically.[183] At autopsy, involved nodes appear bound together and contain discrete foci of pasty yellow necrosis.[182] Microscopically there is caseous necrosis often with a mantle of macrophages. Epithelioid cells and giant cells may be present. The pleura is also involved in approximately two-thirds of patients with pneumonia. The type of involvement varies from serous effusion to fibrinous exudate to necrotic pleural nodules.

Organisms are few and difficult to find in tissue sections using ordinary stains, but can be identified using fluorescent antibodies. The bacteria can be cultured from infected tissue or transmitted to guinea pigs, but this is not ordinarily done by hospital laboratories because of the hazard of infection. Clinical diagnosis is usually made by serology, and heart blood can be obtained at necropsy for this purpose.

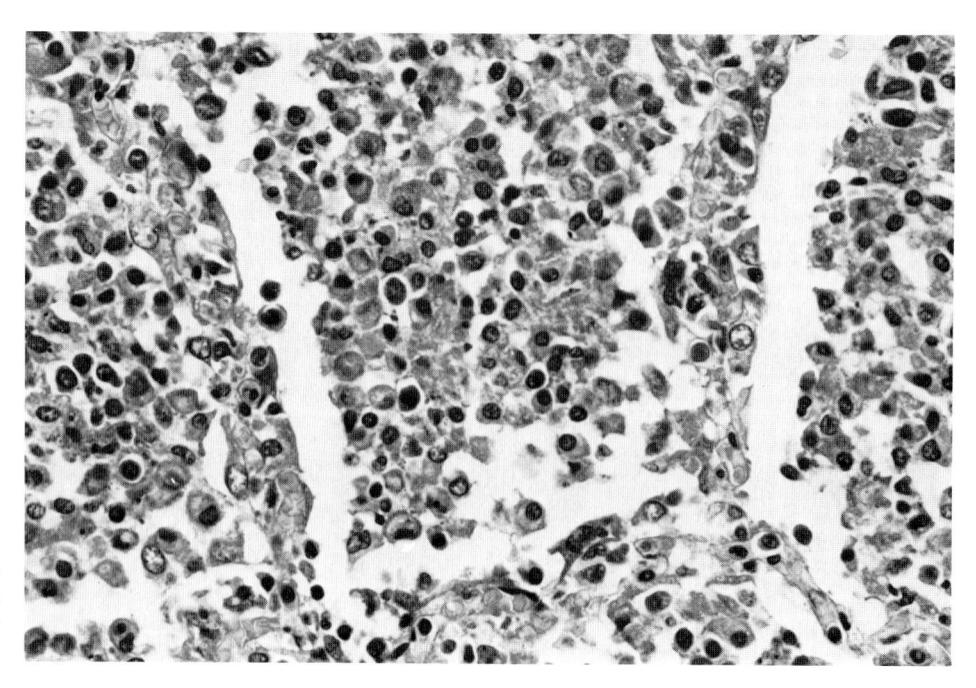

Figure 13–25. Tularemic pneumonia. The alveolar exudate is almost entirely mononuclear (×1000).

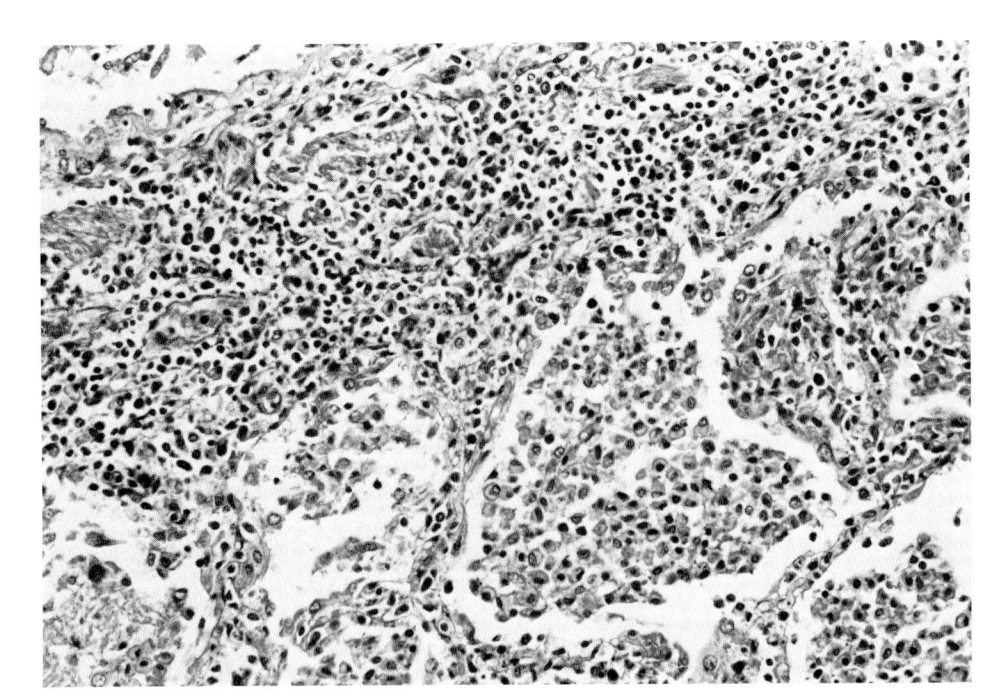

Figure 13–26. Tularemic pneumonia. The upper half of the field is occupied by the wall of a bronchus whose lumen is at the upper left corner. The bronchial epithelium has sloughed. The bronchial wall is heavily infiltrated with mononuclear cells. The alveolar septa below also have some interstitital infiltrate (×700).

Natural History

Although humans are easily infected by *F. tularensis*, they are relatively resistant to the lethal effects of the organism. The overall mortality of untreated cases is 6 to 7 percent. Pneumonia is a particularly serious manifestation, but 70 percent survive with only symptomatic treatment.[184] With modern antibiotic therapy, the mortality is less than 1 percent. Pneumonic lesions can resolve, undergo fibrosis, or calcify.[183]

Recovered patients or animals are immune to reinfection. During infections in humans, the skin test becomes positive toward the end of the first week, and antibodies appear later, usually in the second week. Animal experiments indicate that cell-mediated reactions are more important than antibodies in resistance to the infection. Resistance can be transfered with lymph node cells, but not serum. Immunity is induced by recognition of the specific antigen but expressed as a nonspecific enhancement of the ability of the macrophages to kill not only *F. tularensis* but other intracellular bacteria as well.[185]

Brucellosis

Three of the six known species of Brucella produce most human infections: *B. abortus* from cattle, *B. melitensis* from goats, and *B. suis* from swine. The Brucellae are facultative intracellular parasites that produce a low-grade chronic infection in domestic animals. The infection is disseminated by the bloodstream and settles particularly in the reticuloendothelial organs, the reproductive organs, and mammary glands. Transplacental infection in gravid female animals results in epidemic abortion. Humans acquire the infection either by the ingestion of raw milk products or by direct contact with infected animals. Occupations at particular risk include abattoir workers, farmers, ranchers, and veterinarians. Most cases in the United States are due to *B. abortus*, although in other parts of the world *B. melitensis* predominates.[186]

The organisms penetrate the gastrointestinal tract or skin, are engulfed by neutrophils and macrophages, and are transported to the regional lymph nodes where they continue to proliferate and from which they reach the circulation. Hematogenous dissemination leads to involvement of liver, spleen, bone marrow, and other organs.

Clinical manifestations are extraordinarily varied, ranging from asymptomatic seroconversion to fulminant illness to chronic debility simulating neurosis.[186] Commonly the illness is classified into three types: acute, relapsing, and chronic localized. The acute form usually occurs after a clear-cut occupational exposure. Following an incubation period of 1 week to 1 month, the patient develops malaise, fever often accompanied by chills, drenching afternoon sweats, backache, headache, and sometimes local or generalized lymphadenopathy. Blood cultures are often positive. Treated patients can relapse up to several months after the initial acute episode. Localized brucellosis most often affects the lung, bones and joints, nervous system, genitourinary system, or the valves of the heart.

In patients dying in the acute phase, the involved organs show a combination of diffuse mononuclear cell infiltration and epithelioid granulomas, some with collections of neutrophils or necrosis in the center.[187] Organisms are difficult to find, and the diagnosis is usually made by culture or serologically.

Respiratory tract involvement is not rare in brucellosis. The most common clinical manifestation is bronchitis. Some 12 to 25 percent of patients with acute or relapsing brucellosis complain of cough with sputum production. Most have normal chest roentgenograms, but some have hilar adenopathy or peribronchial infiltrates.[188–191] Organisms generally cannot be cultured from the sputum, and the pathology is not well documented. A laryngeal biopsy from a patient with cough and peribronchial infiltrates showed normal epithelium, hyperemia, edema, and lymphocytic infiltration of the lamina propria.[189] Nodular parenchymal infiltrates are seen radiographically in a small fraction of patients, but their pathologic anatomy has not generally been reported.[191,192] Following recovery from brucellosis, the chest roentgenogram may show miliary calcifications.[191]

Weed and associates[193] have shown that chronic localized pulmonary brucellosis is one of the lesions responsible for a solitary nodule detected radiographically. Cultures of the sputum were negative in their three cases, and surgery was required to exclude carcinoma. In each case *B. suis* was cultured from the resected tissue. Morphologically the nodules were not distinguishable from tubercular granulomas. Grossly they were spherical nodules of necrosis enclosed by a thin fibrous capsule. A central zone of caseous necrosis was enclosed by a zone of palisading epithelioid histiocytes with occasional giant cells. Lymphocytes and plasma cells infiltrated the periphery of the lesions.

Anthrax

Anthrax refers to infection resulting from the introduction into the tissues of the spores of a large gram-positive bacillus, *Bacillus anthracis*. The name derives from the black eschar which is characteristic of the cutaneous lesions that are produced when the skin is the portal of entry. The disease is an uncommon occupational infection of those who work with hides, hair, or bone meal from animals imported from countries in which the infection is still prevalent. The bacillus survives in the soil by sporulating when conditions are dry. The spores can remain viable for years until ingested by grazing sheep or cattle when they germinate giving rise to the vegetative form of the bacillus. Herbivores are highly susceptible, and the infection resulting from ingestion of spores can be so fulminant as to produce death almost before clinical signs are seen. Contamination of the soil by fluids from the dead animal completes the soil-animal-soil cycle.[194]

In humans, cutaneous anthrax is fortunately much more common than infection by inhalation. If introduced into a skin abrasion, the spores germinate, and the bacilli produce a "pimple" which enlarges and forms a black eschar surrounded by vesicles. Ordinarily purulence is not a feature of the lesions. With antibiotics the cutaneous lesions heal and only rarely lead to septicemia. In the 19th century, epidemics of inhalation anthrax or woolsorters' disease were frequent. With improvements in dust control and vaccination of animals, the disease has become rare, although a small outbreak occurred in a textile mill in Manchester, NH in 1957,[195] and sporadic cases continue to occur mainly associated with the use of bone meal. Although the portal of entry for the spores in inhalation anthrax is the lung, the disease is septicemic and typical pneumonia is not observed even pathologically. The events that occur have been well studied in experimental animals including guinea pigs[196] and monkeys.[197,198] Spores are inhaled into the alveoli where they are rapidly ingested by macrophages and to some extent by alveolar epithelial cells.[196] During the next several hours, they are transported by the lymphatics to the regional lymph nodes where the spores germinate and the vegetative bacilli rapidly proliferate in the sinusoids of the node. Flecks of necrosis appear in the germinal centers, and the nodes swell due to edema and hemorrhage which eventually engulf the node. Organisms spill into the efferent lymph reaching the blood on the second or third day, producing septicemia with massive growth of organisms in the circulation and secondary infection mainly in the spleen and meninges.

Autopsies of humans show changes similar to those in experimental animals.[199] The striking findings are massive edema of the soft tissue of the mediastinum, swelling edema, and hemorrhagic necrosis of the hilar and mediastinal lymph nodes. The mucosa of the trachea and bronchi is erythematous, and there may be hemorrhages in the airway walls. The lungs are congested and edematous but show little in the way of cellular exudate. The pulmonary vessels teem with bacilli. Bacilli are also found in association with hemorrhages in the alveoli.

Clinically inhalation anthrax evolves in two phases. The initial phase lasting 3 to 4 days is a mild febrile illness with cough, malaise, myalgia, and sometimes a sense of fullness in the chest. The second phase, corresponding to the massive septicemia, is characterized by severe toxicity, dyspnea, hypotension, cyanosis, and death within 24 hours. Stridor due to tracheal compression by the mediastinal edema can be severe. The lethal effects of infection result from a toxin produced by the bacilli that causes severe vascular injury, thrombosis, and shock.[200] Whether the toxin also has a direct toxic action on the central nervous system is controversial.

Pneumonias Caused by Higher Bacteria

Actinomycosis

The "ray fungi," actinomyces, are now classified among the higher bacteria and are related to the mycobacteria and diphtheroids rather than to fungi. These anaerobic, gram-positive, nonmotile, branching rods are normal inhabitants of the oral cavity and gastrointestinal tract but sometimes produce chronic suppurative infections. The species responsible for the majority of human infections is *Actinomyces israelii*, but other actinomycetes, notably *A. naeslundii*, *A. odontolyticus*, *A. viscosus*, *Arachnia*

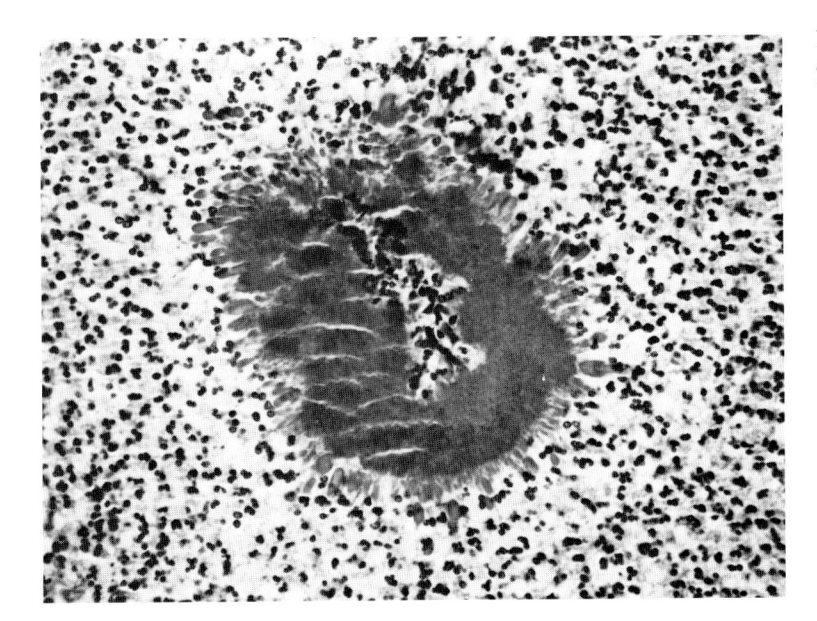

Figure 13–27. Actinomycosis. A sulfur granule in the center of an abscess consists of a center composed of the bacterial colony and radiating peripheral clubs (×800).

propionica, and *Bifidobacterium adolescentis*, have also been reported to cause infection.

A. israelii is commonly found in dental plaque and tonsilar crypts as well as in the flora of the lower gastrointestinal tract. Infections result from penetration of tissue by the endogenous flora. Person to person transmission is unknown, and environmental sources are unimportant. *A. israelii* is an opportunist in the sense that infection usually occurs in tissue damaged by disease or surgical trauma, but it is not one of the organisms that characteristically infects immunosuppressed individuals. Indeed it may be decreasing in incidence, despite the increasing use of immunosuppressive therapies.[201]

Infection can occur at any age, but most cases are in adults. Men outnumber women nearly 3:1. Any tissue can be involved, but the most frequent sites are the cervicofacial, thoracic, and abdominal regions. Clinical diagnosis can be difficult, and symptoms are often present for months before the nature of the illness is recognized. Manifestations are local pain and swelling. The tendency to form draining fistulas is well known and occurs in about one-third of patients. Fever and leukocytosis are usually mild, but in chronic cases, weight loss can be severe.[201,202]

The lungs and mediastinum are involved in 15 to 35 percent of cases. Usually the route of infection is aspiration from the oral cavity, but in some instances the thoracic structures become involved secondarily following septicemia or penetration from adjacent structures, for example through the diaphragm from an abdominal focus.

On gross inspection, the involved lung is extensively fibrotic and may be tightly adherent to the chest wall or mediastinum. Abscess cavities and irregular sinus tracts burrow within the fibrous mass. Drainage from the tracts or purulent contents of the cavities may contain hard yellow granules rarely exceeding 1 mm in diameter.

These are the characteristic "sulfur granules" whose presence should alert one to the correct diagnosis.

The histologic appearance of the lesions is that of purulent abscesses encapsulated by granulation tissue containing lymphocytes and plasma cells. Giant cells are present infrequently and usually indicate aspiration. Sulfur granules vary in number and may be difficult to find. In 25 percent of the cases at the Armed Forces Institute of Pathology, only a single sulfur granule was found, and in another 4 percent, the organisms were cultured but no sulfur granules found.[203]

The sulfur granules are actually colonies of bacteria consisting of a granular basophilic center surrounded by a radiating zone of eosinophilic, hyaline, club-shaped projections (Fig. 13–27). The basophilic center is composed of matted branching Gram-positive rods. Bacterial hyphae projecting from the periphery of the colony become coated with a layer of glycoprotein as much as 5 μm thick which is responsible for the characteristic eosinophilic clubs. Brown[203] has speculated that this coating protects the organisms from phagocytes, antibiotics, and oxygen.

Organisms other than Actinomyces can form colonies in abscesses which can be mistaken for sulfur granules. Staphylococci and true fungi can be distinguished by their morphology in appropriate stains. Nocardia and Streptomyces are aerobic actinomycetes that closely resemble Actinomyces. Generally the colonies of Nocardia and Streptomyces are looser than the sulfur granules of actinomycosis and lack the peripheral mantle of clubs. In addition, Nocardia often is acid-fast. Thus the appearance of actinomycosis in a biopsy is sufficiently characteristic to justify beginning therapy while waiting for cultures to grow out.

Cultures of typical lesions of actinomycosis often show the presence of aerobic bacteria accompanying the Actinomyces. Perhaps this is not surprising in view of the propensity of Actinomyces to infect damaged tissues and the ease with which fistulas can become superinfected. The accompanying aerobic bacteria may help establish infection by the anaerobic Actinomyces by consuming oxygen and creating conditions suitable for the growth of the latter.

The tendency of actinomycosis to spread by penetrating through tissue planes is well known. Although pulmonary actinomycosis can remain localized for many months, it may extend into the pericardium, vertebral bone, or form fistulas through the chest wall. Most cases of disseminated actinomycosis probably begin in the lungs.[203] The brain, liver, skin, and subcutaneous tissue are common sites of spread.[203,204]

Nocardia

The Nocardia are aerobic members of the order Actinomycetaceae, and like the anerobic actinomycetes, they grow as branching, Gram-positive, beaded filaments or hyphae. The Nocardia are widespread in the environment and have been cultured from soil in many parts of the world. Three species of Nocardia produce infections in humans. *N. asteroides* is responsible for the majority of cases of pneumonia and disseminated nocardiosis. *N. brasiliensis* and *N. caviae* usually produce localized subcutaneous infections known as mycetomas and only rarely involve the lung.

Nocardial infection is associated with underlying disease in 59 percent of cases, often with steroid therapy and other causes of immunosuppression.[205-208] Organisms probably reach the lung by inhalation from environmental sources. It is uncertain whether Nocardia can colonize without causing disease.

The lesions of nocardial pneumonia are abscesses which vary from one or a few large cavitating lesions to a miliary appearance (Fig. 13–28). Usually they produce less fibrosis than actinomycosis but share the same propensity to burrow and form sinus tracts. In some immunosuppressed patients, necrosis can be severe.[209]

The organisms within the abscesses are invisible in H&E-stained sections, but can be demonstrated with Gomori's methenamine silver or Gram's stains as long branching filaments, which may fragment into cocci and rods of varying length (Fig. 13–29). Many strains of Nocardia are acid-fast, particularly if a mild decolorizing solution such as 1 percent aqueous sulfuric acid is substituted for the acid alcohol of the standard Ziel-Nielsen stain.[210] Although acid-fastness under controlled conditions of staining is helpful for distinguishing Nocardia from related organisms, other stains, especially methenamine silver, are more sensitive.

The course of nocardial pneumonia can be acute or chronic. Not unexpectedly, the acute form occurs particularly in the immunosuppressed.[209] In nearly half of patients, the infection becomes disseminated, frequently to the central nervous system.[207,211] If therapy is started in a timely fashion, the infection can be controlled even in immunosuppressed patients.

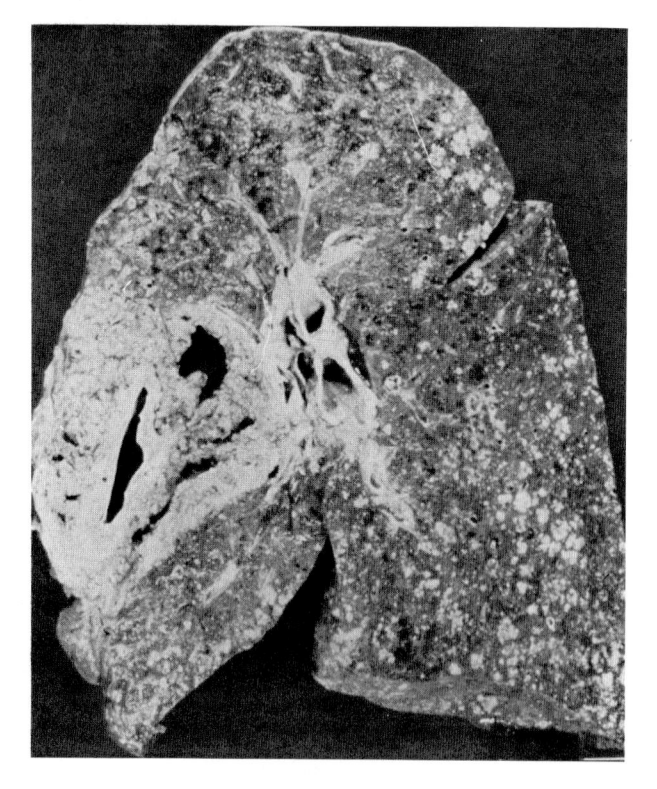

Figure 13–28. Nocardiosis. One large cavitary abscess and innumerable miliary abscesses.

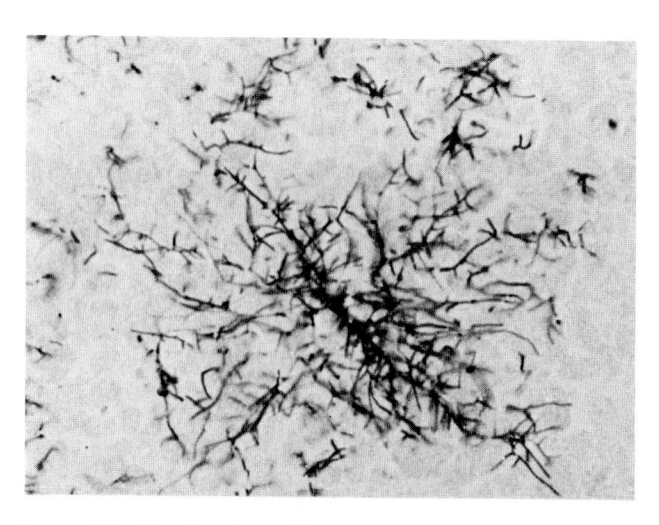

Figure 13–29. Nocardia. The organisms take the form of branching filaments, long or short rods (Gomori's silver methenamine stain, ×1500).

Syphilis

Syphilis in its secondary and tertiary stages is a generalized infection with the potential to involve the respiratory tract. The mucous patches of secondary syphilis can involve the bronchi as well as other mucous membranes

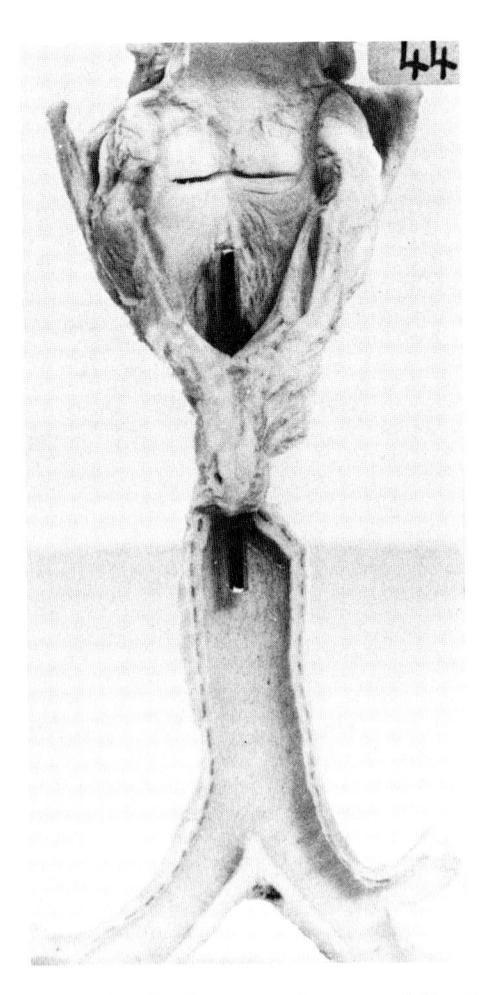

Figure 13–30. Tracheal stenosis due to syphilis. From the Pathological Museum of the University of Manchester, UK.

and have been seen by bronchoscopy.[212] Clinical involvement of the respiratory tract was usually a manifestation of the tertiary stage; as late syphilis has become rare, pulmonary syphilis has virtually disappeared from medical practice. Even when syphilis was prevalent, nonspecific obstructive pneumonia secondary to bronchial compression by an aortic aneurysm was more common than specific infection of the respiratory tract.

The manifestations of syphilis in the lung were comprehensively reviewed by McIntyre in 1931;[213] clinical and pathologic diagnostic criteria were discussed more recently by Morgan and colleagues.[214] A variety of classifications have been proposed for the pulmonary lesions in adults, but essentially the active lesions fall into three types: tracheobronchial syphilis, luetic pneumonia, and gummas.[213–216]

Tracheobronchial syphilis affects a circumscribed segment of one or more airways. Initially the epithelium is hyperplastic, and the lamina propria is infiltrated with lymphocytes and plasma cells. If healing takes place at this stage, there are no residua. If the reaction is more intense and sustained, the airway ulcerates and the mucosa is replaced by a focal zone of granulation tissue infiltrated with lymphocytes and plasma cells. Healing by fibrosis results in severe distortion of the bronchus and adjacent lung, with the production of either an aneurysm-like dilation of the bronchus or an annular region of stenosis (Fig. 13–30).[213]

The pneumonia of syphilis is a chronic pneumonia involving both the interstitium and the air spaces. The involved area appears grossly as a zone of grey gelatinous consolidation fanning out from the hilum to the periphery. Microscopically there is a heavy inflammatory infiltrate composed of histiocytes, plasma cells, and lymphocytes particularly in the interstitial connective tissue ensheathing the bronchi and arteries and forming the interlobular septa. The bronchial and bronchiolar epithelium is preserved. The alveolar spaces are filled by fibrin, debris, and cellular exudate of plasma cells and histiocytes. The alveolar walls show minor thickening by an infiltrate of similar cells. Small foci of necrosis may appear which are thought to be the forerunners of gummas (miliary gummata).[215,216]

Gummas vary in size from less than a few millimeters to several centimeters and are often multiple. They consist of a center of pale grey to yellow dry necrosis encased by a fibrous capsule from which irregular bands of scar extend into and distort the surrounding tissue. If gummas erode a bronchus, they can cavitate. The microscopic appearance of the necrosis can resemble caseation, but typically the outlines of the underlying tissue structure can still be discerned; if elastic stains are used, the elastic network of the lung remains intact. The junction between the necrosis and fibrous capsule is usually quite abrupt, and epithelioid cells are few and giant cells exceptional. A mantle of lymphocytes, plasma cells, and histiocytes surrounds the capsule. Arteries and arterioles may show syphilitic endarteritis, but this change is often absent.

Since Spirochaeta are rarely demonstrable by staining in tertiary syphilis, an unambiguous pathologic diagnosis of gumma is often impossible. Nevertheless several authors[214,216] have outlined criteria which help to distinguish gummas from tuberculous granulomas, particularly when supported by compatible serologic tests:

1. Gummas tend to be subpleural and to occur in the middle and lower lung zones. They do not show the predilection for the subapical region that is so typical of tuberculosis.
2. The fibrosis accompanying gummas is usually pearly white and does not show the same propensity to accumulate anthracotic pigment as tuberculous scarring.
3. Absence of typical caseation and preservation of elastic tissue are characteristic of gummatous necrosis.
4. The circumference of the zone of necrosis in gummas is irregular and jagged, rather than round as in a tubercle.
5. Epithelioid and giant cells are rarely present in gummas.
6. Calcification is rare in gummas.
7. The adventitia of blood vessels is commonly involved in syphilis.

The healing of gummas leads to dense hyaline scarring of the lung. The pattern of scarring is relatively characteristic. Healing of peribronchial and perivascular inflammation leads to a radiating pattern of fibrous bands from the hila. Scars extending from the fibrous remnants of the gummas intersect the radiating bands irregularly producing a coarsely distorted lung termed pulmo lobatum.[217]

In addition to the parenchymal lung involvement, the pulmonary artery may be the site of luetic arteritis. Histologically, the arteritis produces destruction of the medial elastic tissue like that seen in aortitis and, as with the aorta, results in the formation of aneurysms.[217]

Pneumonia alba, the white lung of congenital syphilis, is encountered both in stillborn infants and in neonates dying shortly after birth. In stillborn infants, the lungs were enlarged, pale and heavy, sinking in water. In babies who had breathed, McIntyre[213] described "bleached islands that stand out vividly against the red color of the normal part of the lung". The amount of collagen and elastic fibers was increased in the perilobular and perivascular connective tissue and in the interalveolar septa. Fibroblasts appeared active with hypertrophied cytoplasm. Lymphocytes and plasma cells were present cuffing blood vessels and aggregated into compact islands (microgummas). The air spaces contained macrophages and fat. Spirochaeta were invariably present within macrophages and often free in the fibrous tissue.[213]

Since the development of techniques for cultivating *Treponema pallidum* in vitro is very recent,[218] understanding of the pathogenesis of syphilis, particularly late syphilis, is rudimentary. *T. pallidum* produces no toxin and is toxic to cultured eukaryotic cells only when high concentrations of viable organisms are used.[219] In light of the paucity of organisms in the late lesions of syphilis, it is likely that tissue damage is a consequence of the host response. The immune response to *T. pallidum* results in both the production of antibodies and the sensitization of T lymphocytes. Antibody is not protective by itself but does promote phagocytosis of organisms by macrophages. Activation of macrophages by lymphokines enhances their ability to dispose of the organisms. Sell's suggestion is attractive, that during the long latent phase of syphilis, a few organisms survive this two-pronged attack in some immunologically sheltered compartment. With the waning of immunity with age, the organisms slowly increase in number until sufficient numbers are present to stimulate a new tissue response.[219,220]

Unusual Variants of Lung Abscess

Pulmonary Gangrene

Gangrene of the lung refers to ischemic necrosis of all or part of a lobe of the lung, usually occurring in one of three settings: trauma, torsion of the lung, or infection. Traumatic gangrene follows mechanical damage to the arteries and veins to a lobe or lung. Torsion of an accessory lobe can occur spontaneously, but normally developed lobes undergo torsion only when surgical procedures such as ipsilateral lobectomy or repair of an hiatal hernia leave sufficient space in the hemithorax.[221,222] In the context of lung infections, gangrene refers to the development of necrotic sloughs of all or a major portion of a lobe during the course of pneumonia. The evolution of the process produces a highly characteristic sequence roentgenographically. It begins as an area of lobar consolidation with convex bulging fissures. In following days, small foci of cavitation appear and coalesce into a large cavity. Often a crescent-shaped area of lucency marks the beginning of the separation of the necrotic slough from the cavity wall. In the fully developed lesion, a large mass occupies the cavity and is completely separated from the cavity wall so that it shifts position between decubitus and upright films.[223,224] The clinical manifestations can also be striking. Some patients expectorate fragments of necrotic lung tissue in their sputum.[223] Even more dramatically, spontaneous lobectomy has been described in patients undergoing operation for open drainage of their lung abscess. As much as an entire necrotic lobe was extruded through the drainage wound during or after the procedure.[225,226]

The appearance of the lobes at resection or necropsy varies. Often there is a large ragged cavity filled with dry, coagulated yellow-brown tissue.[224,228] At the other extreme, the lobe can be liquified, a sac of visceral pleura filled with brown, foul-smelling fluid with pieces of necrotic lung floating in it.[223,227] In the necrotic slough, the outlines of the tissue structure remain recognizable in histologic sections. The underlying pathologic process is obliteration of the blood supply to the affected tissue. Specific pathologic lesions include acute thrombosis,[223,224,227] septic vasculitis,[224] and obliterative endarteritis involving large and small vessels.[228,229] Several reports have specifically mentioned that bronchial as well as pulmonary vessels were occluded.[228]

Gangrene can complicate pneumonia caused by a number of organisms, of which *K. pneumoniae* has been reported most commonly.[224–227] Others include *P. aeruginosa*,[277,230] *E. coli*,[228,229] anaerobes,[229] and perhaps fungi.[229] Pneumococcal pneumonia has been reported to precede several cases of lung gangrene.[223,231] Leatherman and co-workers[231] observed that the sputum may turn fetid with the appearance of the diagnostic roentgenographic changes. Since necrosis is not ordinarily a feature of pneumococcal pneumonia and the two patients that they saw with pneumococcal pneumonia and gangrene were alcoholics with poor dental hygiene, they suggested that concomitant anaerobic infection offers a logical explanation for the gangrene.

Botryomycosis

Occasionally in chronic indolent suppurative infections, colonies of bacteria become enclosed within a hyaline coating and resemble the sulfur granules of actinomycosis. The terms botryomycosis or bacterial pseudomycosis are used to describe this state. Botryomycosis was first described in horses in 1870 and is not rare in animals. In humans it usually involves the skin and subcutaneous tissues with or without osteomyelitis.[232] Visceral botryomycosis is distinctly rare, but lung involvement has been reported in sporadic lung abscesses in those who are immunologically intact[233–235] and in children with cystic fibrosis (CF).[236] It occurs in less than 1 percent of patients, with CF producing atypical manifestations: lobar consolidation or extension of pulmonary infection into the mediastinum or bone.[236]

The histologic reaction to the infection may be granulomatous or suppurative. In some cases, the organisms have been found in epithelioid granulomas with giant cells, in others in abscesses filled with purulent exudate enclosed by granulation tissue or fibrosis. In CF the lesions are always within the tissue proper. Granules are not found within the pus filling the lumina of bronchiectatic airways.[236]

The feature that is diagnostic of botryomycosis is the presence of colonies of bacteria coated with a shell of hyaline refractile eosinophilic material. The coating or shell may be smooth, fan-like, or project in radiating clubs or spikes. The causative organisms include *Staphy. aureus*,[233,236] Proteus[232] *P. aeruginosa*,[234,236] and microaerophilic Streptococci.[235] The granules average 150 μm in diameter but can be large enough to detect grossly. They are slightly softer and less cohesive than the sulfur granules of actinomycosis which they otherwise resemble. They can, however, be recovered intact from pus by saline washing.[236] The nature and pathogenesis of the coating is not known, but it has long been believed to reflect a delicate balance between host and parasite.

Acknowledgments. The author is indebted to Dr. Washington Winn for sections of Legionnaire's pneumonia, Dr. Liselotte Hochholzer for sections of plague pneumonia, and Prof. Peter Yates for permission to photograph specimens in the Pathological Museum of the University of Manchester.

References

1. Riley RL: Airborne infection. Am J Med 57:466–475, 1974.
2. Mackowick PA, Martin RM, Jones SR, Smith JW: Pharyngeal colonization by Gram negative bacilli in aspiration-prone persons. Arch Intern Med 138:1224–1227, 1978.
3. Ramirez-Ronder CH, Luxench-Lopez Z, Nevarez M: Increased pharyngeal bacterial colonization during viral illness. Arch Intern Med 141:1599–1603, 1981.
4. Johanson WG Jr, Pierce AK, Sanford JP, Thomas GD: Nosocomial respiratory infections with Gram-negative bacilli. The significance of colonization of the respiratory tract. Ann Intern Med 77:701–706, 1972.
5. LaForce FM: Hospital-acquired Gram-negative rod pneumonias: An overview. Am J Med 70:664–669, 1981.
6. Garibaldi RA, Britt MR, Coleman ML, et al: Risk factors for postoperative pneumonia. Am J Med 70:677–680, 1981.
7. Niederman MS, Ferranti RD, Ziegler A, et al.: Respiratory infection complicating long-term tracheostomy. Chest 85:39–44, 1984.
8. Sprunt K, Redman W: Evidence suggesting importance of role of interbacterial inhibition in maintaining balance of normal flora. Ann Intern Med 68:579–590, 1968.
9. Matsuyama T: Resistance of *Bordetella pertussis* phase I to mucociliary clearance by rabbit tracheal mucous membrane. J Infect Dis 136:609–616, 1977.
10. Higuchi JH, Johanson WG: Colonization and bronchopulmonary infection. Clin Chest Med 3:133–141, 1982.
11. Johanson WG, Higuchi JR, Chaudhuri TR, et al.: Bacterial adherence to epithelial cells in bacillary colonization of the respiratory tract. Am Rev Respir Dis 121:55–63, 1980.
12. Woods DE, Straus DC, Johanson WG, Bass JA: Role of salivary protease activity in adherence of Gram negative bacilli to mammalian buccal epithelial cells in vivo. J Clin Invest 68:1435–1440, 1981.
13. Huxley EJ, Viroslav J, Gray WR, Pierce AK: Pharyngeal aspiration in normal adults and patients with depressed consciousness. Am J Med 64:564–568, 1978.
14. Green GM, Kass EH: The role of the alveolar macrophage in the clearance of bacteria from the lung. J Exp Med 119:167–176, 1964.
15. Juero JA, Rogers RM, McCurdy JB, Cook WW: Enhancement of bactericidal capacity of alveolar macrophages by human alveolar lining material. J Clin Invest 58:271–275, 1976.
16. Coonrod JD, Yoneda K: Detection and partial characterization of antibacterial factor(s) in alveolar lining material of rats. J Clin Invest 71:129–141, 1983.
17. Rehm SR, Gross GN, Pierce AK: Early bacterial clearance from murine lungs. Species-dependent phagocyte response. J Clin Invest 66:194–199, 1980.
18. Kass EH, Green GM, Goldstein E: Mechanisms of antibacterial action in the respiratory system. Bacteriol Rev 30:488–496, 1966.
19. Jones R, Santos JI, Overall JC: Bacterial tracheitis. JAMA 242:721–726, 1979.
20. Sofer S, Duncan P, Chernick V: Bacterial tracheitis: An old disease rediscovered. Clin Pediatr 22:407–411, 1983.
21. Pappenheimer AM: Diphtheria toxin. Annu Rev Biochem 46:69–94, 1977.
22. Uchida T: Diphtheria toxin. Pharmacol Ther 19:107–122, 1983.
23. Mallory FB: The pathology of diphtheria. In Nuttall GHF, Graham-Smith GS (eds): The *Bacteriology of Diphtheria*. Cambridge, England Cambridge University Press, 1908, pp 82–121.
24. McLeod JW, Orr JW, Woodcock HE: The morbid anatomy of gravis, intermedius and mitis diphtheria. J Pathol Bacteriol 48:99–123, 1939.
25. Munford RS, Ory HW, Brooks GF, Feldman RA: Diphtheria deaths in the United States 1959–1970. JAMA 229:1890–1893, 1974.
26. Rich AR: On the etiology and pathogenesis of whooping cough. Bull Johns Hopkins Hosp 51:346–359, 1932.
27. Olson LC: Pertussis. Medicine 54:427–469, 1975.
28. Pereira MS: Association of viruses with clinical pertussis. J Hyg 69:399–403, 1971.
29. Keller MA, Aflandelians R, Conner JD: Etiology of pertussis syndrome. Pediatrics 66:50–55, 1980.
30. Klenk EL, Gaultney JF, Bass JM: Bacteriologically proved pertussis and adenovirus infection. Am J Dis Child 124:203–207, 1972.
31. Linnerman CC, Perry EB: *Bordetella parapertussis*. Recent experience and review of the literature. Am J Dis Child 131:560–563, 1970.

32. Pertussis—England and Wales. MMWR 31:629–632, 1982.

33. Pertussis surveillance, 1979–81. MMWR 31:333–336, 1982.

34. Smith LW: The pathologic anatomy of pertussis with special reference to pneumonia caused by the pertussis bacillus. Arch Pathol 4:732–742, 1927.

35. Muse KE, Collier AM, Baseman JB: Scanning electron microscopic study of hamster tracheal organ culture infected with *Bordetella pertussis*. J Infect Dis 136:768–777, 1977.

36. Mallory FB: The pathologic lesions of whooping cough. Boston Med Surg J 169:575, 1913.

37. Morse SI: Biologically active components and properties of *Bordetella pertussis*. Adv Appl Microbiol 20:9–26, 1976.

38. Wardlow AC, Parton R: *Bordetella pertussis* toxins. Pharmacol Ther 19:1–53, 1983.

39. Hewlett EL, Urban MA, Manclark CR, Walff J: Extracytoplasmic adenylate cyclase of *Bordetella pertussis*. Proc Natl Acad Sci USA 73:1926–1930, 1976.

40. Confer DL, Eaton JW: Phagocyte impotence caused by invasive bacterial adenylate cyclase. Science 217:948–950, 1982.

41. Pittman M: Pertussis toxin: The cause of the harmful effects and prolonged immunity of whooping cough. A hypothesis. Rev Infect Dis 1:401–412, 1979.

42. Johnston IDA, Anderson HR, Lambert HP, Patel S: Respiratory morbidity and lung function after whooping cough. Lancet 2:1104–1108, 1983.

43. Fekety RF, Caldwell J, Gumps D, et al.: Bacteria viruses and mycoplasmas in acute pneumonia in adults. Am Rev Respir Dis 104:499–507, 1971.

44. Sullivan RJ, Dowdle WR, Marine WM, Hierholzer JC: Adult pneumonia in a general hospital. Arch Intern Med 129:935, 1972.

45. White RJ, Blainey AD, Harrison, KJ, Clarke SKR: Causes of pneumonia presenting to a district general hospital. Thorax 36:566–570, 1981.

46. Macfarlane JT, Finch RG, Ward MJ, et al.: Hospital study of adult community acquired pneumonia. Lancet 2:255–258, 1982.

47. Finland M, Brown JW, Ruesegger JM: Anatomic and bacteriologic findings in infections with specific types of pneumococci including types I to XXXII. Arch Pathol 23:801–820, 1937.

48. Mufson MA, Krass DM, Wasil RE, Metzger WI: Capsular types and outcome of bacteremic pneumococcal disease in the antibiotic era. Arch Intern Med 134:505–510, 1974.

49. Finland M, Sutliff WD: Infections with pneumococcus type III and type VIII. Arch Intern Med 53:481, 1934.

50. Wood WB: Studies on the cellular immunology of acute bacterial infections. Harvey Lect 1951–1952, 47:72–98, 1953.

51. Fine DP: Pneumococcal type-associated variability in alternate complement pathway activation. Infect Immun 12:772–778, 1975.

52. Ort S, Ryan JL, Burden G, D'Esopo N: Pneumococcal pneumonia in hospitalized patients. Clinical and radiological presentations. JAMA 249:214–218, 1983.

53. Berry FB: Lobar pneumonia analysis of 400 autopsies. Med Clin North Am 4:571–581, 1920.

54. Tuazon CU: Gram positive pneumonias. Med Clin North Am 64:343, 1980.

55. Robertson OH, Uhley CG: Changes occurring in the macrophage system of the lungs in pneumococcus lobar pneumonia. J Clin Invest 15:115–130, 1936.

56. Auerback SH, Mims OM, Goodpasture EW: Pulmonary fibrosis secondary to pneumonia. Am J Pathol 28:69–81, 1952.

57. Austrian R, Gold J: Pneumococcal bacteremia with special reference to bacteremic pneumococcal pneumonia. Ann Intern Med 60:759–776, 1964.

58. Yangco BG, Deresinski SC: Necrotizing or cavitating pneumonia due to streptococcus pneumoniae. Medicine 59:449–457, 1980.

59. Kevy S, Low BA: Streptococcal pneumonia and empyema in childhood. N Engl J Med 264:738–743, 1961.

60. Molteni RA: Group A β-hemolytic streptococcal pneumonia. Am J Dis Child 131:1366–1371, 1977.

61. Eickhoff TC, Klein JO, Daly AK, et al.: Neonatal sepsis and other infections due to group B beta-hemolytic streptococci. N Engl J Med 271:1221–1228, 1964.

62. Barker CJ, Barett FF: Transmission of group B streptococci among parturient women and their neonates. J Pediatr 83:919, 1973.

63. Bayer AS, Chow AW, Anthony BF, Guze LB: Serious infections in adults due to group B streptococci. Am J Med 61:498–503, 1976.

64. Verghese A, Berk SL, Boelen LN, Smith JK: Group B streptococcal pneumonia in the elderly. Arch Intern Med 142:1642 1645, 1982.

65. Burmeister RW, Overholt EL: Pneumonia caused by hemolytic streptococcus. Arch Intern Med 111:367–375, 1963.

66. MacCallum WG: The pathology of the pneumonia in the United States army camps during the winter of 1917–18. Monogr Rockefeller Inst Med Res No. 10, 1919.

67. Sheagren JN: *Staph. aureus*. the persistent pathogen. N Engl J Med 310:1368–1313, 1984.

68. Lowy FD, Hammer SM: Staphylococcus epidermidis infections. Ann Intern Med 99:834–839, 1983.

69. Hers JF, Masurel N, Mulder J: Bacteriology and histopathology of the respiratory tract and lungs in fatal Asian influenza. Lancet 2:1141–1143, 1958.

70. Louria DB, Blumenfeld HL, Ellis JT, et al.: Studies on influenza in the pandemic of 1957–1958. II. Pulmonary complications of influenza. J Clin Invest 38:213–265, 1959.

71. Finland M: *Staphylococcus aureus* pneumonia. Oxford Med 4:886(55)–886(71), 1943.

72. Wollenman OJ, Finland M: Pathology of staphylococcal pneumonia complicating clinical influenza. Am J Pathol 19:23–41, 1943.

73. Miller WR, Jay AR: Staphylococcal pneumonia in influenza. 5 cases. Arch Intern Med 109:76–86, 1962.

74. Naraqi S, McDonnell G: Hematogenous staphylococcal pneumonia secondary to soft tissue infection. Chest 79:173–175, 1981.

75. Hay DR: Pulmonary manifestations of staphylococcal pyaemia. Thorax 15:82–88, 1960.

76. Nolan CM, Beaty HN: *Staphylococcus aureus* bacteremia. Current clinical patterns. Am J Med 60:495–500, 1976.

77. Louria DB, Hensle T, Rose J: The major medical complications of heroin addiction. Ann Intern Med 67:1–22, 1967.

78. Slim MS, Firzli SS, Melhem RE: Staphylococcic pneumonia in infants under the age of 6 months. Dis Chest 48:6–10, 1965.

79. Highman JH: Staphylococcal pneumonia and empyema in childhood. Am J Roentgenol 106:103–108, 1969.

80. Dines DE: Diagnostic significance of pneumatocele of the lung. JAMA 204:1169–1172, 1968.

81. Amitai I, Mogie P, Godfrey S, Aviad I: Pneumatocele in infants and children. Clin Pediatr 22:420–425, 1983.

82. Boisset GF: Subpleural emphysema complicating staphylococcal and other pneumonias. J Pediatr 81:259–266, 1972.

83. Victoria MS, Steiner P, Rao M: Persistent post pneumonic pneumatoceles in children. Chest 79:359–361, 1981.

84. Pierce AK, Sanford JP: Aerobic Gram-negative bacillary pneumonias. Am Rev Respir Dis 110:647–657, 1974.

85. Reyes MP: The aerobic Gram-negative bacillary pneumonias. Med Clin North Am 64:363–383, 1980.

86. Tillotson JR, Lerner AM: Pneumonias caused by Gram negative bacilli. Medicine 45:65–76, 1966.

87. Graybill JR, Marshall LW, Charache P, et al.: Nosocomial pneumonia. A continuing major problem. Am Rev Respir Dis 108:1130–1140, 1973.

88. Steven RM, Teres D, Skillman JJ, Feingold DS: Pneumonia in an intensive care unit. Arch Intern Med 134:106–111, 1974.

89. Valdivieso M, Gil-Extremera B, Zornosa J, et al.: Gram-negative bacillary pneumonia in the compromised host. Medicine 56:241–254, 1977.

90. Grieble HG, Colton R, Bird TJ, et al.: Fine particle humidifiers: Source of *Pseudomonas aeruginosa* infections in a respiratory disease unit. N Engl J Med 282:531–535, 1970.

91. Sanders CV, Luby JP, Johanson WG, et al.: *Serratia marcescens* infection from inhalation therapy medications: Nosocomial outbreak. Ann Intern Med 73:15–21, 1970.

92. Pierce AK, Edmondson EB, McGee G, et al.: An analysis of factors predisposing to Gram-negative bacillary necrotizing pneumonia. Am Rev Respir Dis 94:309–315, 1966.

93. Cross AS, Roup B: Role of respiratory assistance devices in endemic nosocomial pneumonia. Am J Med 70:681–685, 1981.

94. Bullowa JG, Chess J, Friedman NB: Pneumonia due to bacillus Friedlanderi. Arch Intern Med 60:735–752, 1937.

95. Hyde L, Hyde B: Primary Friedlander pneumonia. Am J Med Sci 205:660–657, 1943.

96. Erasmus LD: Friedlander bacillus infection of the lung with special reference to classification and pathogenesis. QJ Med 25:507–521, 1956.

97. Collius LH, Kornbum K: Chronic pulmonary infection due to the Friedlander bacillus. Arch Intern Med 43:351–362, 1929.

98. Sweany HC, Stadnichenko A, Henrichsen KJ: Multiple pulmonary abscesses simulating tuberculosis caused by the Friedlander bacillus. Arch Intern Med 47:565–582, 1931.

99. Tillotson JR, Lerner AM: Characteristics of pneumonia caused by *Bacillus proteus*. Ann Intern Med 68:287–294, 1968.

100. Tillotson JR, Lerner AM: Characteristics of pneumonias caused by *Escherichia coli*. N Engl J Med 277:115–122, 1967.

101. Jonas M, Cunha BA: Bacteremic *Escherichia coli* pneumonia. Arch Intern Med 142:2157–2159, 1982.

102. Phair JP, Bassaris HP, Williams JE, Metzger E: Bacteremic pneumonia due to gram negative bacilli. Arch Intern Med 143:2147–2149, 1983.

103. Berk SL, Newmann P, Holtsclaw S, Smith JK: *Escherichia coli* pneumonia in the elderly. Am J Med 72:899–902, 1982.

104. Pittman M: Variation and type specificity in the bacterial species *Hemophilus influenzae*. J Exp Med 53:471–495, 1931.

105. Redmond SR, Pichichero ME. *Hemophilus influenzae* type b disease. An epidemiologic study with special reference to day-care centers. JAMA 252:2581–2584, 1984.

106. Wallace RJ, Musher DM, Martin RR: *Hemophilus influenzae* pneumonia in adults. Am J Med 64:87–93, 1978.

107. Tager I, Speizer FE: Role of infection in chronic bronchitis. N Engl J Med 292:562–571, 1975.

108. Hirschman JV, Everett ED: *Hemophilus influenzae* infections in adults. Report of nine cases and a review of the literature. Medicine 58:80–94, 1979.

109. Hers JFP, Mulder J: The mucosal epithelium of the respiratory tract in muco-purulent bronchitis caused by *Hemophilus influenzae*. J Pathol Bacteriol 66:103–108, 1953.

110. Jacobs NM, Harris VJ: Acute hemophilus pneumonia in childhood. Am J Dis Child 133:603–605, 1979.

111. Horing PJ, Pasquariello PS, Stool SS: *H. influenzae* pneumonia in infants and children. J Pediatr 83:215–219, 1973.

112. Tillotson JR, Lerner AM: *Hemophilus influenzae* bronchopneumonia in adults. Arch Intern Med 121:428–432, 1968.

113. Quintiliani R, Hyamo PJ: The association of bactermic *Hemophilus influenzae* pneumonia in adults with typeable strains. Am J Med 50:781–786, 1971.

114. Levin DC, Schwartz MI, Matthay RA, LaForce FM: Bacteremic *Hemophilus influenzae* pneumonia in adults. Am J Med 62:219–224, 1977.

115. Morrison A, Wenzel RP: Epidemiology of infections due to *Pseudomonas aeruginosa*. Rev Infect Dis 6(Suppl): S627–S642, 1984.

116. Tillotson JR, Lerner AM: Characteristics of nonbacteremic pseudomonas pneumonia. Ann Intern Med 68:295–307, 1968.

117. Forkner CE, Frei E, Edgcomb JH, Utz JP: *Pseudomonas septicemia*. Observations on twenty-three cases. Am J Med 25:877–889, 1958.

118. McHenry MC, Baggenstoss AR, Martin WJ: Bacteremia due to Gram-negative bacilli. Clinical and autopsy findings in 33 cases. Am J Pathol 59:160–173, 1968.

119. Rabin ER, Graber CD, Vogel EH, et al.: Fatal Pseudomonas infection in burned patients. A clinical, bacteriologic and anatomic study. N Engl J Med 265:1225–1231, 1961.

120. Fetzer AE, Werner AS, Hagstrom JWC: Pathologic features of pseudomonal pneumonia. Am Rev Respir Dis 96:1121–1130, 1967.

121. Renner RR, Coccaro AP, Heitzman ER, et al.: *Pseudomonas pneumonia*: A prototype of hospital-based infection. Radiology 105:555–562, 1972.

122. Pollack M: The virulence of *Pseudomonas aeruginosa*. Rev Infect Dis 6(Suppl):3S617–S626, 1984.

123. Iglewski BH, Kabat D: NAD-dependent inhibition of protein synthesis by *Pseudomonas aeruginosa* toxin. Proc Natl Acad Sci USA 72:2284–2288, 1975.

124. Andriole VT: *Pseudomonas bacteremia*: Can antibiotic therapy improve survival? J Lab Clin Med 94:196–200, 1979.

125. Pennington JE, Reynolds HY, Carbone PP: *Pseudomonas pneumonia*. A retrospective study of 36 cases. Am J Med 55:155–160, 1973.

126. Flick MR, Cluff LE: *Pseudomonas bacteremia*. Review of 108 cases. Am J Med 60:501–508, 1976.

127. Verghese A, Berk SL: Bacterial pneumonia in the elderly. Medicine 52:271–285, 1983.

128. James AE, Dixon GD, Johnson HG: Melioidosis: A correlation of the radiologic and pathologic findings. Radiology 89:230–235, 1967.

129. Weber DR, Douglass LE, Brundage WG, Stallkamp TC: Acute varieties of melioidosis occurring in US soldiers in Vietnam. Am J Med 46:234–244, 1969.

130. Everett ED, Nelson RA: Pulmonary melioidosis. Observations in thirty-nine cases. Am Rev Respir Dis 112:331–340, 1975.

131. Mackowiak PA, Smith JW: Septicemic melioidosis. Occurrence following acute influenza A six years after exposure in Vietnam. JAMA 240:764–766, 1978.

132. Greenwald KA, Nash G, Foley FD: Acute systemic melioidosis. Autopsy findings in four patients. Am J Clin Pathol 52:188–198, 1969.

133. Piggott JA, Hochholzer L: Human melioidosis. A histopathologic study of acute and chronic melioidosis. Arch Pathol 90:101–111, 1970.

134. Baumann BB, Morita ET: Systemic melioidosis presenting as myocardial infarct. Ann Intern Med 67:836–842, 1967.

135. Fraser DW, Tsai TR, Orenstein W, et al.: Legionnaires' disease. Description of an epidemic of pneumonia. N Engl J Med 297:1189–1197, 1977.

136. Blackmon JA, Chandler FW, Cherry WB, et al.: Review article: Legionellosis. Am J Pathol 103:428–465, 1981.

137. Glick TH, Gregg MB, Berman B, et al.: Pontiac fever: An epidemic of unknown etiology in a health department. 1. Clinical and epidemiological aspects. Am J Epidemiol 107:149–160, 1978.

138. Kaufmann AF, McDade JE, Patton CM, et al.: Pontiac fever: Isolation of the etiologic agent (Legionella pneumophila) and demonstration of its mode of transmission. Am J Epidemiol 114:337–347, 1981.

139. England AC, Fraser DW, Plikaytis BD, et al.: Sporadic Legionellosis in the United States. The first thousand cases. Ann Intern Med 94:164 170, 1981.

140. Kirby BD, Snyder KM, Meyer RD, Finegold SM: Legionnaires' disease: Report of sixty-five nosocomially acquired cases and review of the literature. Medicine 59:188, 1980.

141. Yu VL, Kroboth FJ, Shonnard J, et al.: Legionnaires' disease: New clinical perspective from a prospective pneumonia study. Am J Med 73:357–361, 1982.

142. Brabander W, Hinthorn DR, Asher M, et al.: *Legionella pneumophila* wound infection. JAMA 250:3091–3092, 1983.

143. Meyerowitz RL, Pasculle AW, Dowling JN, et al.: Opportunistic lung infection due to "Pittsburgh pneumonia agent." N Engl J Med 301:953–958, 1979.

144. Muder RR, Yu VL, Zuravleff JJ: Pneumonia due to the Pittsburgh pneumonia agent: New clinical perspective with a review of the literature. Medicine 62:120, 1983.

145. Winn WC, Meyerowtiz RL: The pathology of the Legionella pneumonias. A review of 74 cases and the literature. Hum Pathol 12:401–421, 1981.

146. Band JD, LaVenture M, Davis JP, et al.: Epidemic Legionnaires disease. Airborne transmission down a chimney. JAMA 245:2404–2407, 1981.

147. Helms CM, Massanari RM, Zeitler R, et al.: Legionnaires' disease associated with a hospital water system: A cluster of 24 nosocomial cases. Ann Intern Med 99:172–178, 1983.

148. Shands KN, Ho JL, Meyer RD, et al.: Potable water as a source of Legionnaires' disease. JAMA 253:1412–1416, 1985.

149. Meyer RD: Legionella infections: A review of five years of research. Rev Infect Dis 5:258–278, 1983.

150. Swartz MN: Clinical aspects of Legionnaires' disease. Ann Intern Med 90:492–495, 1979.

151. Blackmon JA, Hicklin MD, Chandler FW: Legionnaires' disease. Pathologic and historical aspects of a "new" disease. Arch Pathol Lab Med 102:337–343, 1978.

152. Boyd JF, Buchanan WM, MacLeod TIF, et al.: Pathology of five Scottish deaths from pneumonic illnesses acquired in Spain due to Legionnaires' disease agent. J Clin Pathol 31:809–816, 1978.

153. Winn WC, Glavin FL, Perl DP, et al.: The pathology of Legionnaires' disease. Arch Pathol Lab Med 102:344–350, 1978.

154. Chandler FW, Hicklin MD, Blackmon JA: Demonstration of the agent of Legionnaires' disease in tissue. N Engl J Med 297:1218–1220, 1977.

155. Suffin SC, Kaufmann AF, Whitaker B, et al.: *Legionella pneumophila*. Identification in tissue sections by a new immunoenzymatic procedure. Arch Pathol Lab Med 104:283–286, 1980.

156. Horrowitz MA, Silverstein SC: Intracellular multiplication of Legionnaires' disease bacteria (*Legionella pneumophila*) in human monocytes is reversibly inhibited by erythromycin and rifampicin. J Clin Invest 71:15, 1983.

157. Rogers BH, Donowitz GR, Walker GK, et al.: Opportunistic pneumonia. N Engl J Med 301:959–961, 1979.

158. Johanson WG Jr, Harris GD: Aspiration pneumonia, anaerobic infections and lung abscess. Med Clin North Am 64:385–394, 1980.

159. Rytel MW, Conner GH, Welch CC, et al.: Infectious agents associated with cylindrical bronchiectasis. Dis Chest 46:23–27, 1964.

160. Bartlett JG, Finegold SM: Anaerobic infections of the lung and pleural space. Am Rev Respir Dis 110:56–77, 1974.

161. Lorber B, Swenson RM: Bacteriology of aspiration pneumonia. A prospective study of community- and hospital-acquired cases. Ann Intern Med 81:329–331, 1974.

162. Tillotson JR, Lerner AM: Bacterioides pneumonias: Characteristics of cases with empyema. Ann Intern Med 68:308–317, 1968.

163. Bartlett JG: Anaerobic bacterial pneumonitis. Am Rev Respir Dis 119:19–23, 1979.

164. Schweppe IH, Knowles JH, Kane L: Lung abscess: An analysis of the Massachusetts General Hospital cases from 1943 through 1956. N Engl J Med 265:1039–1043, 1961.

165. Safron RD, Tate CF: Lung abscesses, a five year evaluation. Dis Chest 53:12–18, 1968.

166. Perlman LV, Lerner E, D' Esopo N: Clinical classification and analysis of 97 cases of lung abscess. Am Rev Respir Dis 99:390–397, 1969.

167. Thomas NW, Wilson RF, Puro HE, Arbulu A: Life-threatening hemoptysis in primary lung abscess. Ann Thorac Surg 14:347–358, 1972.

168. Cameron EWJ, Appelbaum PC, Pucifin D, et al.: Characteristics and management of chronic destructive pneumonia. Thorax 35:340–346, 1980.

169. Butler T: *Plague and Other Yersinia Infections.* New York: Plenum, 1983.

170. Pollitzer R: *Plague*. Monograph series No. 225. Geneva: World Health Organization, 1954.

171. Kaufmann AF, Boyce JM, Martone WJ: Trends in human plague in the United States. J Infect Dis 141:522–524, 1980.

172. Human plague—United States, 1981. MMWR 31:74–76, 1982.

173. Cavanaugh DC, Randall R: The role of multiplication of *Pasteurella pestis* in mononuclear phagocytes. J Immunol 83:348–363, 1959.

174. Monte TC: Properties and pharmacological action of plague murine toxin. Pharmacol Ther 12:491–499, 1981.

175. Finegold MJ: Pathogenesis of plague. A review of plague deaths in the United States during the last decade. Am J Med 45:549–554, 1968.

176. Alsofrom DJ, Mettler FA, Mann JM: Radiographic manifestations of plague in New Mexico, 1975–1980. Radiology 139:561–565, 1981.

177. Boyce JM: Recent trends in the epidemiology of Tularemia in the United States. J Infec Dis 131:197–199, 1975.

178. Forshay L: Tularemia: A summary of certain aspects of the disease including methods for early diagnosis and the results of serum treatment in 600 patients. Medicine 19:1–84, 1940.

179. Pullen RL, Stuart BM: Tularemia analysis of 225 cases. JAMA 129:495–500, 1945.
180. Blackford SD, Casey CJ: Pleuropulmonary tularemia. Arch Intern Med 67:43–71, 1941.
181. Stuart BM, Pullen RL: Tularemic pneumonia. Review of American literature and report of 15 additional cases. Am J Med Sci 210:223–236, 1945.
182. Lillie RD, Francis E: The pathology of Tularemia in man (Homo sapiens). Natl Inst Health Bull 10–24, 1936.
183. Mille RP, Bates JH: Pleuropulmonary tularemia. A review of 29 patients. Am Rev Respir Dis 99:31–41, 1969.
184. Forshay L: Cause of death in Tularemia. Arch Intern Med 60:22–38, 1937.
185. Kostiala AAI, McGregor DD, Logie PS: Tularemia in the rat. The cellular basis of host resistance to infection. Immunology 28:855–869, 1975.
186. Smith IM: Brucella species (Brucellosis). In Mandell GL, Douglas RG, Bennett JE (eds) *Principles and Practice of Infectious Diseases*. New York: John Wiley & Sons, 1979, pp 1772–1784.
187. Hunt AC, Bothwell PW: Histological findings in human brucellosis. J Clin Pathol 20:267–272, 1967.
188. Buchanan TM, Faber LC, Feldman RA: Brucellosis in the United States 1960–1972. An abbatoir-associated disease. Part 1. Clinical features and therapy. Medicine 53:403–413, 1974.
189. Haden RL, Kyger ER: Pulmonary manifestations of brucellosis. Cleve Clin Q 13:220–227, 1946.
190. Pfischner WCE, Ishak KG, Neptune EM, et al.: Brucellosis in Egypt. A review of experience with 228 patients. Am J Med 22:915–929, 1957.
191. Greer AE: Pulmonary brucellosis. Dis Chest 29:508–519, 1956.
192. Harvey WA: Pulmonary brucellosis. Ann Intern Med 28:768–781, 1948.
193. Weed LA, Sloss PT, Clagett OT: Chronic localized pulmonary brucellosis. JAMA 161:1044–1047, 1956.
194. Smith IM: A brief review of anthrax in domestic animals. Postgrad Med J 49:571–572, 1973.
195. Plotkin SA, Brachman PS, Utell M, et al.: An epidemic of inhalation anthrax, the first in the twentieth century. I. Clinical features. Am J Med 29:992–1001, 1960.
196. Ross JM: The pathogenesis of anthrax following the administration of spores by the respiratory route. J Pathol Bacteriol 73:485–494, 1957.
197. Dalldorf FG, Kaufmann AF, Brachman PS: Wool sorters disease. An experimental model. Arch Pathol 92:418–426, 1971.
198. Albrink WS, Goodlow RJ: Experimental inhalation anthrax in the chimpanzee. Am J Pathol 35:1055–1063, 1959.
199. Albrink WS, Brooks SM, Biron RE, Kopel M: Human inhalation anthrax. A report of three fatal cases. Am J Pathol 36:457–471, 1960.
200. Stephen J: Anthrax toxin. Pharmacol Ther 12:501–513, 1981.
201. Slade PR, Slesser BV, Southgate J: Thoracic actinomycosis. Thorax 28:73–85, 1973.
202. Weese WC, Smith IM: A study of 57 cases of actinomycosis over a 36 year period. A diagnostic "failure" with good prognosis after treatment. Arch Intern Med 135:1562–1568, 1975.
203. Brown JR: Human actinomycosis. A study of 181 subjects. Hum Pathol 4:319–330, 1973.
204. Varkey B, Landis FB, Tang TT, Rose HD: Thoracic actinomycosis. Dissemination to skin, subcutaneous tissue, and muscle. Arch Intern Med 134:689–693, 1974.
205. Cross RM, Binford CH: Is nocardia asteroides an opportunist? Lab Invest 11:1103–1109, 1962.
206. Saltzman HA, Chick EW, Conant NF: Nocardiosis as a complication of other diseases. Lab Invest 11:1110–1117, 1962.
207. Palmer DL, Harvey RL, Wheeler JK: Diagnostic and therapeutic considerations in nocardia asteroides infection. Medicine 53:391–401, 1974.
208. Gorevic PD, Katler EI, Agus B: pulmonary nocardiosis. Occurrence in men with systemic lupus erythemalosus. Arch Intern Med 140:361–363, 1980.
209. Neu HC, Silva M, Hajen E: Necrotizing nocardial pneumonitis. Ann Intern Med 66:274–284, 1967.
210. Robboy SJ, Vickery AJ: Tinctorial and morphologic properties distinguishing actinomycosis and nocardiosis. N Engl J Med 282:593–596, 1970.
211. Curry WA: Human nocardiosis. A clinical review with selected case reports. Arch Intern Med 140:818–826, 1980.
212. Ornstein GG: Pulmonary syphilis. Med Clin North Am 9:357–370, 1926.
213. McIntyre MC: Pulmonary syphilis. Its frequency, pathology and roentgenologic appearance. Arch Pathol 11:258–280, 1931.
214. Morgan AD, Lloyd WE, Price-Thomas C: Tertiary syphilis of the lung and its diagnosis. Thorax 7:125–133, 1952.
215. Wilson JM: Acquired syphilis of the lung. Report of a case with autopsy findings and demonstration of spirochetes. Ann Intern Med 25:134–146, 1946.
216. Pearson RS, DeNavasquez S: Syphilis of the lung. Guy's Hosp Rep 88:1–21, 1938.
217. DeNavasquez S: Aneurysm of the pulmonary artery and fibrosis of the lungs due to syphilis. J Pathol Bacteriol 54:315–319, 1942.
218. Fieldsteel AH, Cox DL, Moeckli R: Cultivation of virulent *Treponema pallidum* in tissue culture. Infect Immunol 32:908–915, 1981.
219. Schell RF, Musher DM (eds): *Pathogenesis and Immunology of Treponemal Infection*. New York: Marcel Dekker, 1983.
220. Sell S, Norris SJ: The biology pathology and immunopathology of syphilis. Int Rev Exp Pathol 24:203–276, 1983.
221. Kirsh MM, Rotman H, Behrendt DM, et al.: Complications of pulmonary resection. Ann Thorax Surg 20:215–236, 1975.
222. Kelly MV, Kyger ER, Miller WC: Postoperative lobar torsion and gangrene. Thorax 32:501–504, 1977.
223. Danner PK, McFarland DR, Felson B: Massive pulmonary gangrene. Am J Roentgenol Rad Ther Nucl Med 103:548–554, 1968.
224. Knight L, Fraser RG, Robson HG: Massive pulmonary gangrene: A severe complication of *Klebsiella pneumonia*. Can Med Assoc J 112:196–198, 1975.
225. Taylor JW: Spontaneous lobectomy. Br Med J 2:500–501, 1944.
226. Humphreys DR: Spontaneous lobectomy. Br Med J 2:185–186, 1945.
227. Proctor RJ, Griffin JP, Eastridge CE: Massive pulmonary gangrene. South Med J 70:1144–1146, 1977.
228. Gutman E, Pongdee O, Park YS: Massive pulmonary gangrene. Radiology 107:293–294, 1973.
229. Gutman E, Rao KV, Park YS: Pulmonary gangrene with vascular occlusion. South Med J 71:772–775, 1978.
230. Young JN, Samson PC: *Pseudomonas aeruginosa* septicemia with gangrene of the lung and empyema. Ann Thorac Surg 29:254–257, 1980.
231. Leatherman JW, Iber C, Davies SF: Cavitation in bacteremic pneumococcal pneumonia. Causal role of mixed infection with

anaerobic bacteria. Am Rev Respir Dis 129:317–321, 1984.

232. Winslow DJ: Botryomycosis. Am J Pathol 35:153–167, 1959.

233. Fink AA: Staphylococcic actinophytotic (Botryomycotic) abscess of the liver with pulmonary involvement. Arch Pathol 31:103–107, 1941.

234. Winslow DJ, Chamblin SA: Disseminated visceral botryomycosis. Report of a fatal case probably caused by *Pseudomonas aeruginosa*. Am J Clin Pathol 33:43–47, 1960.

235. Greenblatt M, Heredia R, Rubenstein L, Alpert S: Bacterial pseudomycosis ("Botryomycosis"). Am J Clin Pathol 41:188–193, 1964.

236. Katzenelson D, Vawter GF, Foley GE, Schwachman H: Botryomycosis. A complication in cystic fibrosis. Report of 7 cases. J Pediatr 65:525–539, 1964.

Additional Readings

Bartlett JG, O'Keefe P, Tally FP, et al.: Bacteriology of hospital-acquired pneumonia. Arch Intern Med 146:868–871, 1986.

Lipsky BA, Boyko EJ, Inui TS, et al.: Risk factors for acquiring pneumococcal infections. Arch Intern Med 146:2179–2185, 1986.

Mills EL: Viral infections predisposing to bacterial infections. Annu Rev Med 34:469–480, 1984.

Myerowitz RL: *The Pathology of Opportunistic Infections with Pathogenetic, Diagnostic and Clinical Correlations*. New York: Raven Press, 1983.

Pennington JE (ed): *Respiratory Infections: Diagnosis and Management*. New York: Raven Press, 1983.

14 Mycobacterial Infections and Fungal and Protozoal Disease

Anna-Luise A. Katzenstein

Tuberculosis

Despite the development of effective chemotherapeutic agents, tuberculosis remains an important cause of pulmonary disease. The clinical and radiographic manifestations of this infection have changed considerably since the introduction of antituberculous drugs, and diagnosis in some cases may be delayed or even obscured until postmortem examination.[1,2] Although the radiographic findings combined with the results of tuberculous skin test reactivity and microbiologic cultures are usually sufficient to establish the diagnosis, in some cases biopsy specimens will be necessary. They are especially useful in miliary tuberculosis, because organisms can be scant and cultures are often negative. The lung is frequently involved in such cases and both transbronchial and open lung biopsies are productive in obtaining diagnostic tissue.[3,4] Some examples of chronic pulmonary tuberculosis present as radiographically discrete nodular densities that may resemble malignant neoplasms. Since sputum cultures are frequently negative in such cases, they are usually excised for diagnosis. It is, therefore, not unusual for the pathologist to initially suggest the diagnosis of tuberculosis in infected individuals, either from biopsy specimens or at postmortem examination. In the following discussion, the classification of pulmonary tuberculosis is briefly reviewed, and its pathology is discussed in detail. Methods of culturing the tissue and the choice of special stains have been reviewed in Chapter 8.

Classification of Tuberculosis

The lung is the portal of entry for most infections caused by *Mycobacterium tuberculosis*. Pulmonary involvement may occur as a primary infection in patients with no previous exposure to the organism, or it may be a secondary infection in a patient who has been exposed in the past.[5] Hematogenous spread of the disease throughout the lungs and to multiple other organs (miliary tuberculosis) may occur in both primary and secondary forms of the disease. A classification of tuberculosis based on various detailed reviews,[1,5,6–13] is outlined in Table 14–1.

Primary Pulmonary Tuberculosis

Primary pulmonary tuberculosis usually occurs in the lower lobes or anterior segments of the upper lobes. The organisms multiply within the parenchyma at these sites and as well as within the regional lymph nodes. The associated inflammatory reaction occurring in the lung and draining lymph nodes is known as the primary complex or Ghon's focus (Fig. 14–1). Patients with primary tuberculosis are usually asymptomatic or have only mild symptoms. In over 90% of individuals the infection is contained and tuberculin sensitivity manifest by positive skin test reactivity develops within 4 to 8 weeks. This tuberculin reactivity and immunity is retained for life in the majority of patients. The primary focus eventually heals by fibrosis and calcification, often leaving a calcified scar which may be visible radiographically.

Progressive Primary Tuberculosis

In a small number of individuals, acquired immunity is not sufficient to contain the primary infection and the disease may spread into the adjacent parenchyma, causing areas of consolidation (tuberculous pneumonia). Occasionally cavitary lesions may develop in the apices. The latter appearance is indistinguishable from chronic tuberculosis (*see* the following section) and is recognized only if a recent PPD conversion is noted. Progressive primary tuberculosis occurs predominantly in infants and young children or in immunocompromised individuals, although otherwise apparently healthy adults may also be affected.[13]

Chronic (Secondary, Postprimary) Tuberculosis

Chronic tuberculosis occurs in individuals previously sensitized to the tubercle bacillus, and it may develop many years after the primary infection. The apices are the most common portions of the lungs that are involved. Progressive destruction of the upper lobes may occur, or the process may be walled-off and confined by the inflammatory reaction (tuberculoma). Symptoms are variable. A few patients are asymptomatic, especially when the lung lesions are small and limited. With larger lesions patients frequently have fever, malaise, weight loss, cough, and night sweats. Most cases (90% percent) of chronic tuberculosis are considered to represent reactivation of a previously dormant focus of infection, although there is evidence that reinfection by the organism may occur in a few cases.

Generalized (Miliary) Tuberculosis

Generalized tuberculosis results from the hematogenous spread of organisms to multiple organs. The spleen, liver, lungs, and bone marrow are most frequently involved.[1,11] Hematogenous spread may occur either early (during primary tuberculosis) or late (during secondary tuberculosis). Early generalized tuberculosis may heal by fibrosis and calcification and be relatively asymptomatic, or it may be progressive and accompanied by an acute, life-threatening illness. Late generalized tuberculosis can present as a similar acute illness, or it may be more insidious or even episodic. In the preantibiotic era generalized tuberculosis occurred predominantly in young adults, but in recent years this form of tuberculosis more often affects elderly individuals, many of whom have other chronic diseases. The diagnosis can be difficult to establish premortem since symptoms can be absent or obscured by other diseases, chest radiographs can be negative, and patients may be anergic.

Table 14-1. Classification of Tuberculosis

Primary pulmonary tuberculosis
Progressive primary tuberculosis
Chronic (secondary, postprimary) pulmonary tuberculosis
    Reactivation tuberculosis
    Reinfection tuberculosis
Generalized (miliary) tuberculosis
    Primary (abortive or acute)
    Secondary (acute, chronic, or episodic)

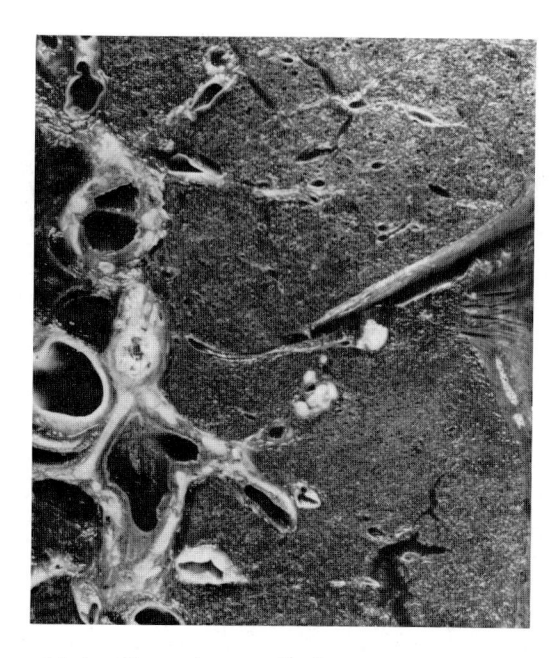

Figure 14-1. Gross photograph of a primary complex (Ghon's focus) in tuberculosis. Two caseating granulomas are seen in the parenchyma of the left lower lobe and one hilar lymph node is replaced by caseating granulomas.

Histopathologic Features of Tuberculosis

Gross Pathology

The usual tissue reaction in tuberculosis is caseating granulomatous inflammation. The granulomas may vary considerably in size. In miliary tuberculosis they appear as numerous tiny, 2- to 3-mm-diameter, white to yellow nodules (Fig. 14-2). The term "miliary" is derived from the resemblance of these tiny nodules to millet seeds. In other forms of tuberculosis the granulomas can become quite large and widely destroy the lung parenchyma. In those cases the central caseation is more obvious grossly than in miliary tuberculosis, and appears yellow with a soft cheesy consistency (Fig. 14-3). The caseous areas may be iregularly shaped with little surrounding fibrosis, or they may be surrounded by discrete fibrous capsules with the formation of rounded tuberculomas. As the lesions heal they become replaced by fibrous tissue and may be accompanied by parenchymal shrinkage. Calcification is common.

Histopathology

The predominant histologic finding in tuberculosis is necrotizing granulomatous inflammation (Fig. 14-4). The necrotic cores of the granulomas may be composed of amorphous, granular eosinophilic debris (caseous necrosis) or they may contain shadows of residual lung structures. We described partly caseous necrosis when remnants of vessels or bronchioles are identifiable in the

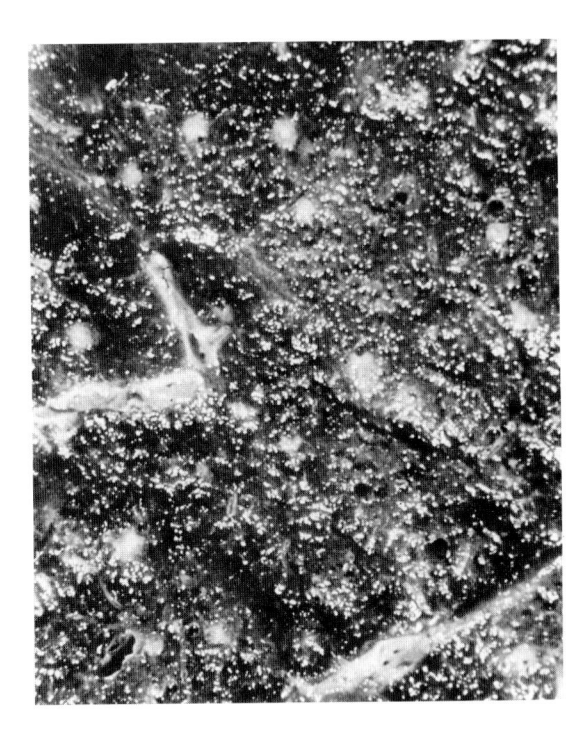

Figure 14–2. Gross photograph of miliary tuberculosis. There are numerous 2- to 3-mm-diameter white nodules (caseating granulomas) scattered throughout the lung.

mycobacteria.[6,10] The most important human pathogens are group I (*M. kansasii*) or group IV (*M. intracellulare/M. avium*) organisms, although rare infections with other atypical mycobacteria have been reported.[15] These organisms tend to be especially virulent and respond poorly to standard antituberculous therapies. They frequently occur in persons who have serious underlying lung diseases or who are otherwise debilitated.[10,16]

Atypical mycobacterial infections in the lung cannot be distinguished from tuberculosis by clinical or radiographic means, and the tissue response of these two diseases is also identical.[6,9,10,17] Although reliable identification of the organisms requires microbiologic cultures, some atypical mycobacteria have been described as larger, thicker, and more curved than *M. tuberculosis*.[18]

Bacillus-Calmette Guérin Infection. Granulomas have been reported in the lungs of a few patients receiving bacillus Calmette-Guérin (BCG) immunotherapy for malignancy.[19–21] The lesions appeared radiographically as solitary nodules or as diffuse reticulonodular infiltrates. Microscopically there were both caseating and noncaseating granulomas, but acid-fast bacilli could not be identified.

necrotic zones and infarct-like necrosis when there are shadows of alveolar septa resembling an ordinary thromboembolic infarct.[14] Epithelioid histiocytes are present around the necrotic zones and frequently are arranged in a palisading pattern. Small noncaseating granulomas may be seen within the adjacent parenchyma as well. Bronchioles can be surrounded and destroyed by the granulomatous reaction. Inflammation of blood vessel walls near the granulomatous area is common.[14] This vasculitis is characterized by edema and transmural infiltration by lymphocytes and plasma cells. Occasionally hystiocytes or even small granulomas may be present within vessel walls, but significant vascular necrosis does not occur.

The organisms are best demonstrated by means of the Ziehl-Neelsen acid-fast stain or the auramine-rhodamine fluorescent stain (*see* Chapter 8). They are almost always found within the most central necrotic portion of the granulomas, and are only rarely found within histiocytes or noncaseating granulomas.[14] The search for the bacteria, therefore, should begin within the necrotic zones. In most cases examination of sections from two blocks containing necrotizing granulomas will be sufficient to identify the bacilli, although occasionally more sections will be needed to find them. The morphology of mycobacteria in the Ziehl-Neelsen stain is distinct. The organisms are thin, bright red, often slightly curved bacilli, with a prominent beaded appearance.

Atypical mycobacterial infection. A small number of mycobacterial lung infections are caused by atypical

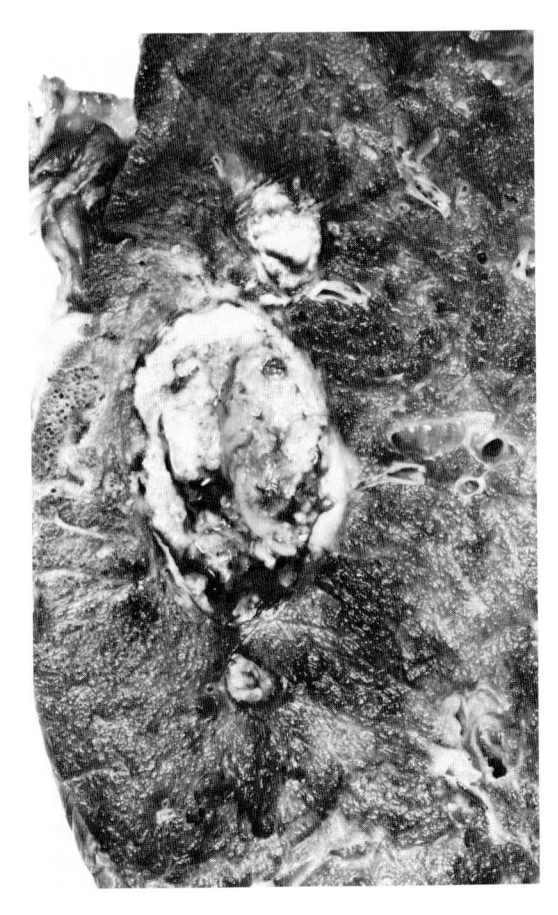

Figure 14–3. Caseating granuloma from a case of chronic tuberculosis. There is a central cavitating nodule containing caseous debris. Two satellite granulomas are also present.

Figure 14-4. Photomicrograph of typical necrotizing granulomatous inflammation in tuberculosis. There are large, irregularly shaped necrotic zones bounded by palisading histiocytes and numerous multinucleated giant cells (H&E, ×90).

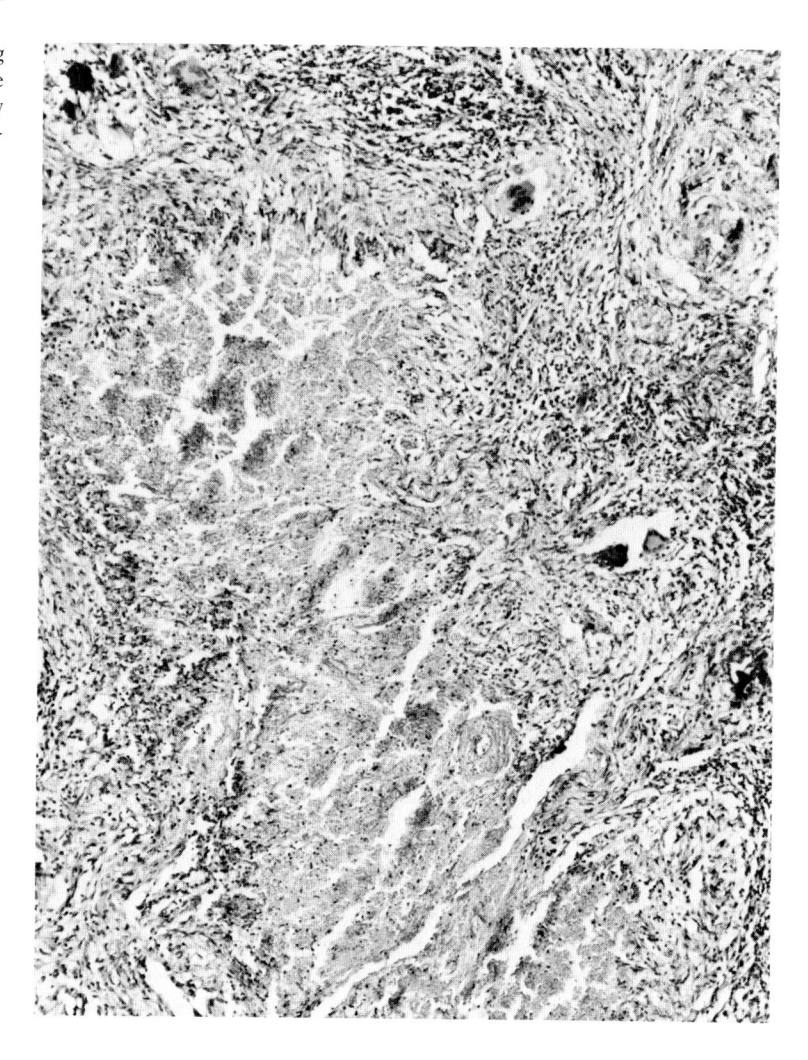

Granulomatous Fungal Infections

Histoplasmosis

Histoplasma capsulatum, the agent of histoplasmosis, is a widespread fungus whose natural habitat is the soil. Infection results from inhalation of airborne spores, a mechanism similar to that responsible for tuberculous first infections. Histoplasmosis is most heavily endemic in the central United States, but is widely distributed throughout temperate zones of the world.

Like tuberculosis, histoplasmosis can be subclassified into several distinct forms depending on the clinical circumstances. It is not possible, however, to accurately classify histoplasmosis on the basis of primary, reactivation, or reinfection types as is done for tuberculosis. Goodwin and co-workers[22] have emphasized that the primary infection in histoplasmosis, in contrast to primary tuberculosis, is usually not followed by life-long immunity to the organism, and therefore, the term "primary" histoplasmosis does not have the same implications as primary tuberculosis. Furthermore, reinfection (rather than reactivation) is common in histoplasmosis, unlike tuberculosis, and may even occur on multiple occasions during an individual's lifetime.

Goodwin and co-workers,[22] therefore, have proposed a classification in which they divide histoplasmosis into three separate categories: (1) acute pulmonary histoplasmosis, (2) disseminated histoplasmosis, and (3) chronic histoplasmosis. In this schema acute pulmonary histoplasmosis is a broad category that includes so-called primary histoplasmosis, reinfection histoplasmosis, and epidemic histoplasmosis. Since many of the latter terms are utilized in the literature about histoplasmosis, and since they do have distinct clinical implications, we utilize a classification that encompasses all these various entities. It is a modification of other published classifications[22-27] and is summarized in Table 14-2.

Acute Pulmonary Histoplasmosis

The majority of first infections by histoplasma are asymptomatic and self-limited (asymptomatic primary histoplasmosis).[22-24] Primary histoplasmosis, like primary tuberculosis, heals by fibrosis and calcification. Cases can be detected by means of positive skin reactivity to histoplasma or less often by the presence of radiographic

Table 14–2. Classification of Histoplasmosis

> Acute pulmonary histoplasmosis
>   Primary histoplasmosis
>   Asymptomatic
>   Symptomatic
>   Epidemic histoplasmosis
>   Primary
>   Reinfection
> Histoplasmoma
> Chronic histoplasmosis
> Disseminated histoplasmosis

changes such as infiltrates or punctate calcification. Asymptomatic reinfection probably occurs frequently and is difficult to document.

Symptomatic infection by histoplasma is uncommon and can occur under circumstances related to both the immune status of the patient and the quantity of spores inhaled. Symptomatic primary histoplasmosis affects predominantly infants and children.[22,24] These patients usually present with fever and cough accompanied by hilar lymph node enlargement and patchy lung infiltrates. The illness is generally self-contained, although dissemination (*see* Disseminated Histoplasmosis, below) occurs in a small number of individuals. An immature immune system is thought to predispose these young children to symptomatic infection and may also be pathogenetic in subsequent dissemination.[26]

Epidemic histoplasmosis is the term applied to symptomatic infection by histoplasma that is related to the inhalation of large numbers of spores.[24] It is characterized clinically by influenza-like symptoms and radiographically by patchy chest infiltrates or nodules. Epidemic histoplasmosis may occur as a primary infection in patients without prior exposure to histoplasma or it may represent a type of reinfection in individuals previously exposed to the organism. Generally, the illness is more severe in patients without prior exposure, although it is self-limited in both groups.

Histoplasmoma

Histoplasmomas are discrete, spherical masses that are composed of necrotizing granulomatous inflammation surrounded by dense fibrosis.[27] The lesions may slowly enlarge due to fibroblastic proliferation and collagen deposition around their periphery. They are thought to result from an abnormal healing process surrounding a focus of primary histoplasmosis. They are frequently excised because of their radiographic resemblance to a neoplasm.[28] Patients are usually asymptomatic.

A fibrosing process similar to that seen in histoplasmomas may occur around granulomatous mediastinal lymph nodes in histoplasmosis.[24,28] This condition is characterized by widespread mediastinal fibrosis (fibrosing or sclerosing mediastinitis).

Chronic Histoplasmosis

Chronic histoplasmosis occurs in patients with underlying chronic lung disease, especially severe emphysema, and for this reason it is considered a type of opportunistic infection.[25] The organisms in this form of the disease infect abnormal air spaces, causing the formation of multiple small nodules on chest radiographs, or larger cavitary densities if bullae are infected. Segmental or subsegmental areas of consolidation may also occur (pneumonic form), presumably due to bronchial spread of the contents of an infected bulla or cavity. Patients usually have mild to moderate symptoms, including cough, chest pain, malaise, low-grade fever, and weight loss. A few individuals are asymptomatic. The natural history of chronic histoplasmosis is uncertain since many patients are treated with amphotericin and in others the severity of the underlying chronic lung disease overshadows the histoplasmosis. It appears, however, that cavitary chronic histoplasmosis is slowly progressive. Treatment with amphotericin B will eradicate the cavities in most individuals, although it is not clear that amphotericin therapy significantly improves long-term survival. Pneumonic infiltrates of chronic histoplasmosis apparently resolve without therapy within several weeks, although adjacent airspaces and bullae may remain infected.

Disseminated Histoplasmosis

Young infants, especially those under 1 year old, seem especially susceptible to disseminated histoplasmosis, although the disease can occur at any age.[26] Individuals with known immunologic defects are no more frequently affected than apparently normal individuals.[29] The symptomatology varies from an acute life-threatening illness (usually in infants or immunocompromised patients) to a mild nonspecific illness (usually in adults) with localizing manifestations related to focal lesions. Constitutional symptoms may or may not be present in the latter cases.

Multiple organs are involved in disseminated histoplasmosis, but the lung and bone marrow are clinically the most important. Radiographically, evidence of interstitial pneumonia is common, and hematologic abnormalities may result from the bone marrow involvement. Other organs are also frequently affected, including liver, spleen, lymph nodes, kidney, and adrenals, but generally the clinical consequences of their involvement are not significant.

Amphotericin B is the therapy of choice for disseminated histoplasmosis. Most cases can be cured if treatment is instituted promptly and full doses are administered.[26]

Pathologic Features of Histoplasmosis

All forms of histoplasmosis except for disseminated histoplasmosis (*see* below) are characterized by necrotizing granulomatous inflammation which is identical to the tissue response in tuberculosis and in certain other fungal diseases.[24,30–32] The histoplasmoma grossly is a solitary spherical lesion composed of a necrotic

Figure 14–5. Gross photograph of a histoplasmoma. There is a well-circumscribed caseating granuloma with prominent concentric laminations. From Katzenstein A, Askin F: *Surgical Pathology of Non-Neoplastic Lung Disease. Major Problems in Pathology*, vol 13, Philadelphia: WB Saunders, 1982.

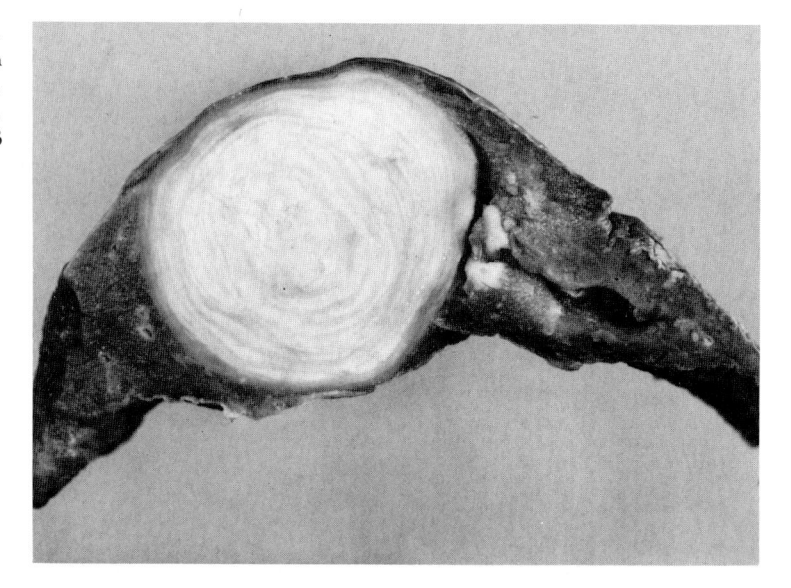

yellow core surrounded by fibrosis (Fig. 14–5). Concentric rings of fibrosis are often seen within the lesion and although they are characteristic of histoplasmomas they may also be seen in tuberculomas and solitary granulomas due to various other fungi. In chronic histoplasmosis the characteristic gross findings are thick or thin-walled cavities containing necrosis in a setting of severe bullous emphysema.

Disseminated histoplasmosis differs from the other forms of histoplasmosis in that there is parasitization of the mononuclear phagocyte system in multiple organs.[26] In the lung an infiltrate of macrophages containing numerous organisms is present within the interstitium. Caseating granulomas are generally not seen in this form of the disease.

Identification of Organisms

Histoplasma capsulatum is a dimorphic fungus that exists in the mycelial form in nature, but occurs as a yeast in tissue. The yeast form is oval-shaped and uniform, measuring 3 to 5 μm in diameter. Budding forms are not numerous. The organism is best demonstrated in tissues by means of a silver stain [Gomori's methenamine silver (GMS)] or a modified periodic acid-Schiff (PAS) stain (PAS-Gridley) (Fig. 14–6).[14] When the yeasts are located intracellularly, as in disseminated histoplasmosis, they can be visualized in hematoxylin and eosin (H&E) stains (Fig. 14–7). In such cases they appear as thick-walled ovoid structures containing a central nucleus surrounded by a clear space. When the more common caseating granulomatous reaction is present, however, the organisms can not be seen with H&E stains. The yeasts in these cases are located within the central caseous necrosis and are not present within surrounding histiocytes. They tend to blend in with the background necrosis and thus cannot be seen unless a special stain is used. The PAS stain, without a counterstain, may similarly

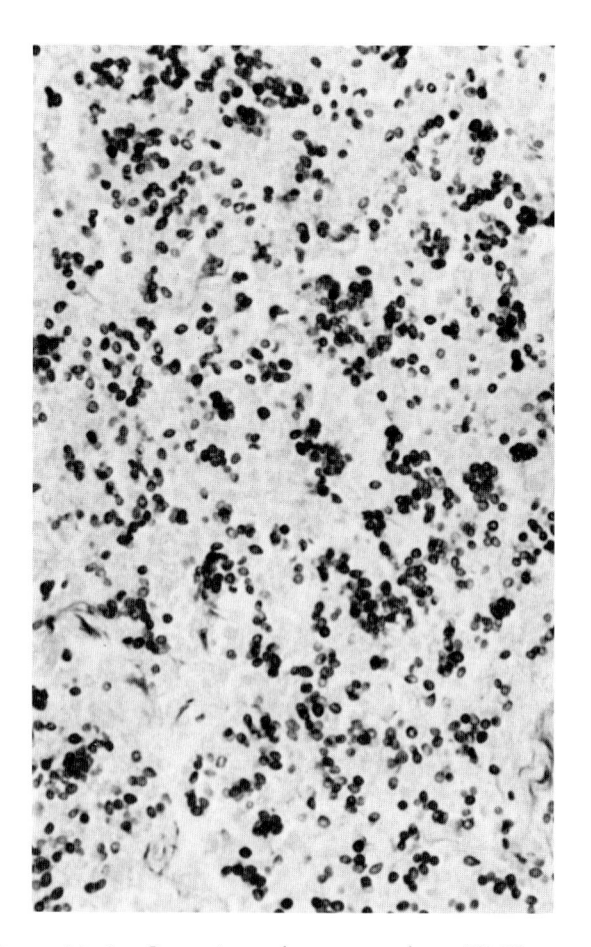

Figure 14–6. Gomori's methenamine silver (GMS)–stained sections showing *Histoplasma capsulatum*. The organisms are small, uniform, oval-shaped yeasts. Budding forms are not easily identified (×450).

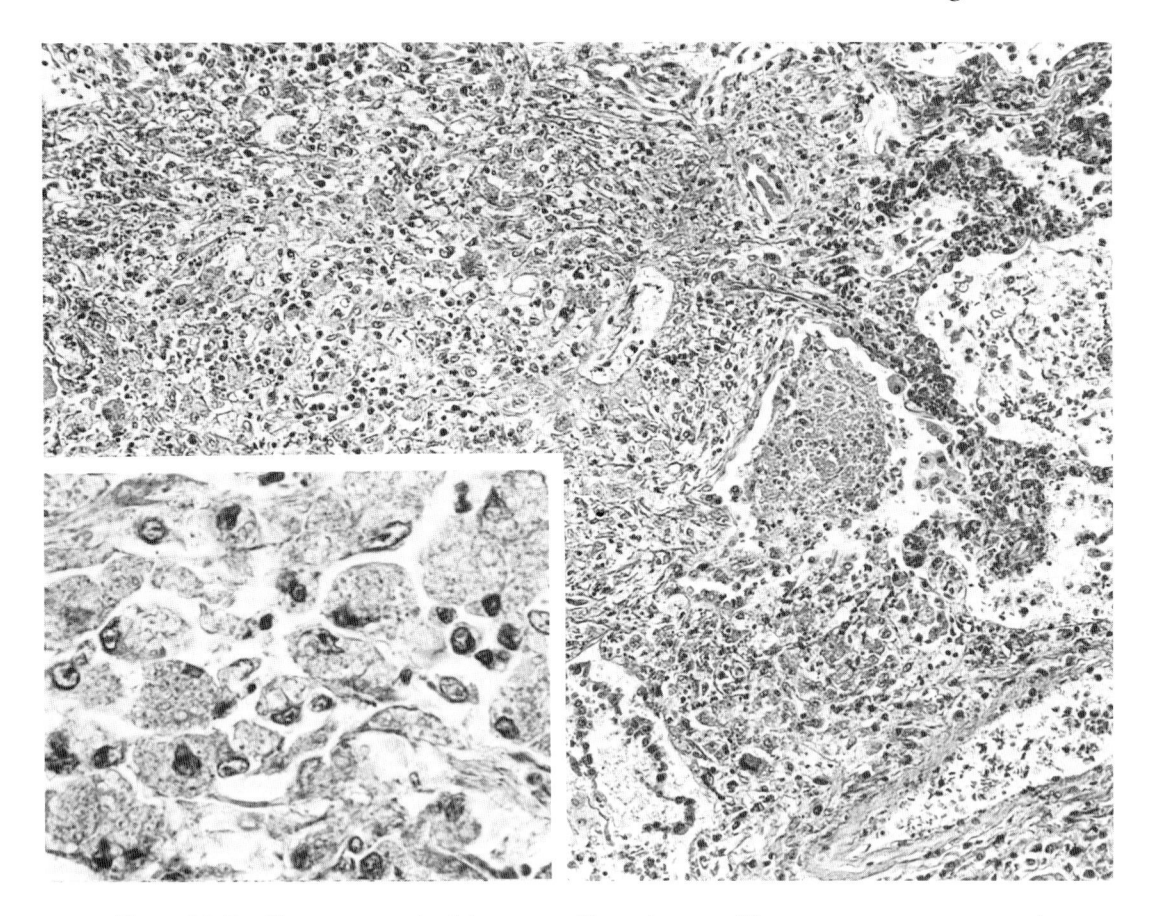

Figure 14–7. Photomicrograph of disseminated histoplasmosis. There is a prominent interstitial histiocytic infiltrate. At higher magnification (inset) organisms can be seen within the histiocyte cytoplasm, imparting a granular appearance (H&E, ×150; inset, ×600).

fail to delineate the organisms in such cases, since it stains both the organism and the background necrosis the same color.

Coccidioidomycosis

Coccidioides imitis is a dimorphic saprophytic fungus that is restricted to the Western hemisphere. It occurs naturally in the soil and is highly endemic in the arid southwestern United States. In nature and on artificial media it grows as a mold, but in tissues it forms characteristic spherules and reproduces by endosporulation. The lung is the portal of entry for almost all coccidioidal infections. A variety of clinical syndromes can be caused by the organism, including primary pulmonary coccidioidomycosis, persistent primary coccidioidomycosis, and disseminated coccidioidomycosis (Table 14–3).[33–38] Diagnosis is usually based on microbiologic cultures, skin test reactivity, serologic tests, and occasionally biopsy.

Primary Pulmonary Coccidioidomycosis

Most cases of primary pulmonary coccidioidomycosis are asymptomatic and are detected by skin test conversion. Symptoms occur in approximately 40 percent of individuals and range from mild, nonspecific complaints to manifestations of an acute, febrile, pneumonic illness.[33,35] In a few patients there may be prominent skin lesions such as erythema nodosum or erythema multiforme combined with evidence of polyserositis. This symptom complex is known as *acute valley fever* and occurs predominantly in young women. Nonspecific, patchy, or hazy chest infiltrates that may resemble atypical pneumonia, are seen radiographically in primary coccidioidomycosis. Hilar lymph node enlargement and pleural effusion are occasional accompanying features that may

Table 14–3. Clinical Forms of Coccidioidomycosis

Primary pulmonary coccidioidomycosis
Persistent primary coccidioidomycosis
Persistent coccidioidal pneumonia
Chronic progressive pneumonia
Miliary pulmonary coccidioidomycosis
Nodules (coccidioidoma)
Disseminated coccidioidomycosis

help distinguish coccidioidomycosis from atypical pneumonias.³³ In the majority of cases primary coccidioidomycosis is self-limited and clears within 6 to 8 weeks.

Persistent Primary Coccidioidomycosis

Persistent disease, in which the primary infection fails to clear after 6 to 8 weeks, occurs in approximately 5 percent of infected individuals and may have several different manifestations.³³,³⁵ In persistent coccidioidal pneumonia, patients are quite ill with fever, chest pain, cough, hemoptysis, and large pulmonary infiltrates. The course is usually indolent in immunologically intact individuals, with resolution occurring after many months. In immunocompromised patients, however, a rapidly fatal outcome may occur. Amphotericin B therapy is usually recommended for patients with persistent coccidioidal pneumonia, especially if they are immunocompromised. Chronic progressive pneumonia is an uncommon form of persistent primary coccidioidomycosis.³⁴,³⁷ Clinically and radiographically it mimics pulmonary tuberculosis and is characterized by low-grade fever, cough, and weight loss associated with biapical, fibronodular, and often cavitary chest infiltrates. The disease is distinguished from chronic tuberculosis by the finding of positive sputum cultures for *C. immitis*. Serology is usually helpful as well, since complement fixation antibody titers to *C. immitis* are generally high.

In a small number of patients miliary pulmonary infiltrates occur in coccidioidomycosis.³³,³⁵ These individuals have mild chest symptoms, although a severe rapidly progressive disease with respiratory failure may occur in immunocompromised patients. Response to amphotericin B therapy is generally favorable.

Well-circumscribed, spherical densities (coccidioidal nodule or coccidioidoma) can occasionally evolve from an area of pneumonic infiltration and some nodules have central cavitation.³³,³⁵,³⁸

Patients are usually asymptomatic or only mildly symptomatic, although hemoptysis is common in cavitary lesions. Because cultures are frequently negative in such cases, biopsy may be necessary for diagnosis because of their radiographic resemblance to malignant neoplasms.

Disseminated Coccidioidomycosis

Extrapulmonary dissemination is an infrequent complication of coccidioidomycosis.³⁵ Immunocompromised individuals, pregnant women, Mexicans, blacks, and Filipinos seem to be predisposed to this condition. Dissemination can occur many months after a primary pulmonary infection, at which time evidence of the pulmonary infection may no longer be present. Any organ of the body can be involved, although skin, bones, meninges, and genitourinary system are most frequently affected. The clinical course may be acute or chronic, episodic or progressive.

Histopathologic Features of Coccidioidomycosis

The usual tissue reaction to *C. immitis* is necrotizing granulomatous inflammation.¹⁴,³⁵,³⁶,³⁹ Early in the course of the infection, suppuration can be seen in the center of the granulomas. In later stages of the disease, the granulomas usually contain amorphous or partially caseous necrosis without suppuration. It is thought that the endospores elicit an acute inflammatory reaction while the spherules stimulate granuloma formation.³⁵ As healing progresses in the later stages of the disease only empty spherules remain and hence the acute inflammation wanes.

The histologic diagnosis depends on finding spherules within the tissue (Figs. 14–8, 14–9). These structures can usually be visualized in H&E-stained sections. They range from 30 to 60 μm in diameter and are composed of a thick, somewhat refractile cell wall surrounding numerous 2- to 5-μm-diameter basophilic endospores. Special stains such as the GMS, PAS, or PAS-Gridley stains can facilitate identification of the organisms, especially when they are not numerous. Also, the natural history of a spherule is characterized by rupture and release of its endospores and the empty spherule and free endospores may be difficult to recognize in H&E-stained sections. Mycelial forms are uncommon in tissue, but can occasionally be found in addition to the more typical elements.³⁹,³⁶

Cryptococcosis

Cryptococcus neoformans in a ubiquitous yeast with a worldwide distribution. Its natural habitat is the soil, especially that containing pigeon or other avian excreta.

Clinical Forms of Disease

Pulmonary cryptococcosis can occur at any age, although it is most common in the fourth to sixth decades. White men are affected more often than blacks or women. Clinical manifestations are variable.⁴⁰⁻⁴⁷ Approximately one-third of patients are asymptomatic, while in the rest symptoms range from mild cough and low-grade fever to an acute, febrile, life-threatening illness. Radiographically, single or multiple, well-circumscribed nodular densities are the most common findings.⁴⁵,⁴⁸ Cavitation occurs in 10 to 15 percent of cases and calcification is usually absent.⁴⁰,⁴⁴ Segmental pneumonic infiltrates and miliary densities are seen less commonly and pleural effusions occur rarely.⁴⁹ A primary complex analogous to the primary (Ghon) complex of tuberculosis has been demonstrated in a few cases.⁵⁰,⁵¹ Saprophytic colonization of the tracheobronchial tree without tissue invasion may also occur, especially in patients with preexisting lung disease.⁴⁷,⁵²

Approximately 10 percent of patients with pulmonary cryptococcosis have an underlying disease that compromises their immune system.⁴⁰ Of patients with cryptococ-

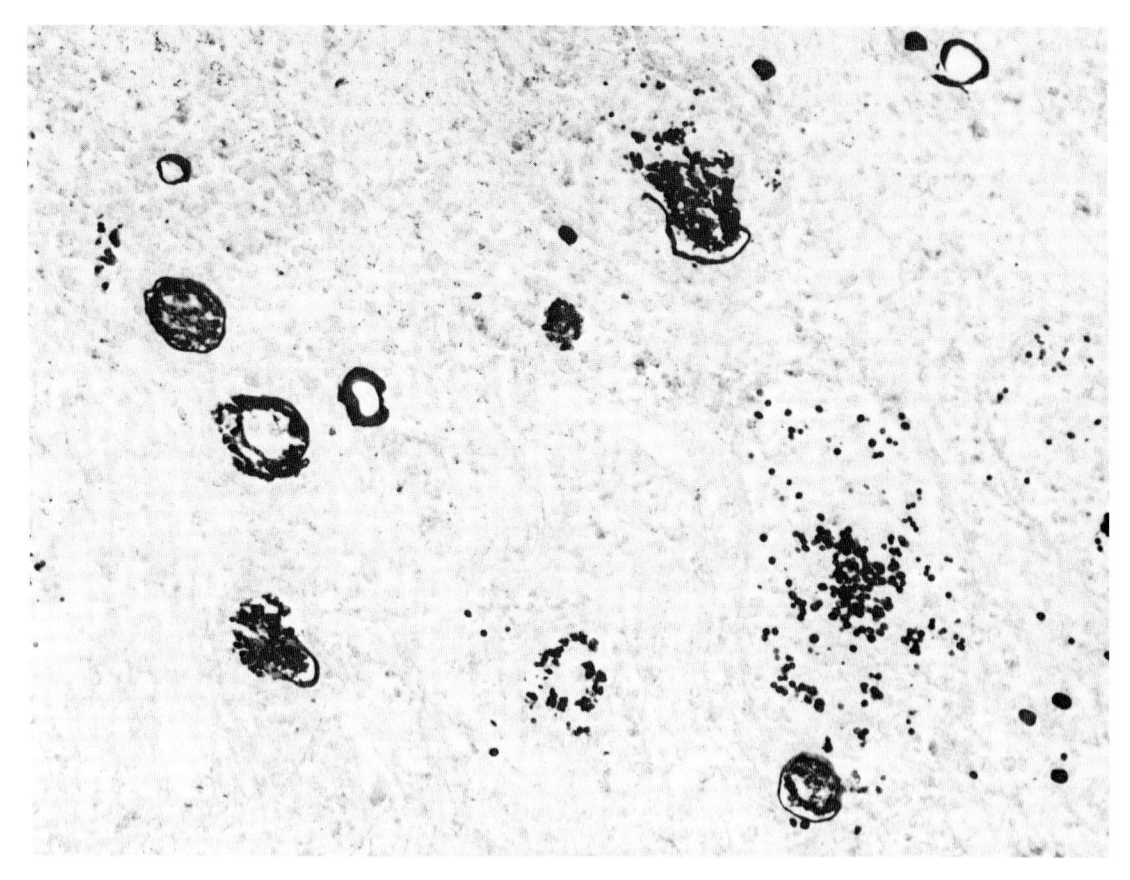

Figure 14–8. Gomori's methenamine silver–stained section of coccidioidal pneumonia showing the organism in various stages of development. On the left there are intact mature spherules, at top right a rupturing spherule is seen, and at bottom right there is a group of free endospores (×180).

cal meningitis, in contrast, a larger percentage (approximately 50 percent) are immunocompromised. The immunocompromised patients differ from the immunologically intact individuals both in the tissue response to the organism (see Histopathologic Features, below) and in the course of the disease. The disease can spread rapidly throughout the lungs and disseminate to extrapulmonary sites, especially the meninges in immunocompromised individuals. In contrast, it is more usual in immunologically intact individuals for the infection to be localized to one area of the lung. Amphotericin B therapy is usually indicated when the infection occurs in immunocompromised patients, when lesions progress or cannot be resected, or when there is evidence of dissemination.[41,43,45]

Histopathologic Features

The tissue reaction in pulmonary cryptococcosis varies depending partly on the status of the patient's immune system. In immunologically intact individuals a granulomatous response is seen.[14,42,44,50,53,54] This reaction may consist of numerous noncaseating granulomas (Fig. 14–10), or there may be extensive caseation similar to that seen with tuberculosis and other fungal diseases discussed in this chapter. In immunocompromised patients little, if any, inflammatory reaction occurs around the organisms.[55] Instead, intact alveolar spaces become filled with the yeasts, and the affected area often has a mucoid gross appearance due to the thick mucinous capsule that is usually present around the organisms (Fig. 14–11).

Identification of Cryptococci in Tissue

C. neoformans can be visualized within H&E-stained sections although they are best demonstrated with the GMS, PAS, or PAS-Gridley stains. They also can be seen in Papanicolaou-stained cytologic preparations.[56] The organisms are round, budding yeasts averaging 4 to 7 μm in diameter (range, 2 to 15 μm). They appear grey to light blue with little internal structure in H&E-stained sections and are often surrounded by a clear space (Fig. 14–12). The latter feature is a processing artefact due to the shrinkage of the thick mucinous capsule that usually covers the surface of organism. Cryptococci are frequently severely fragmented in tissue and may vary considerably in size (Fig. 14–13). These features are best

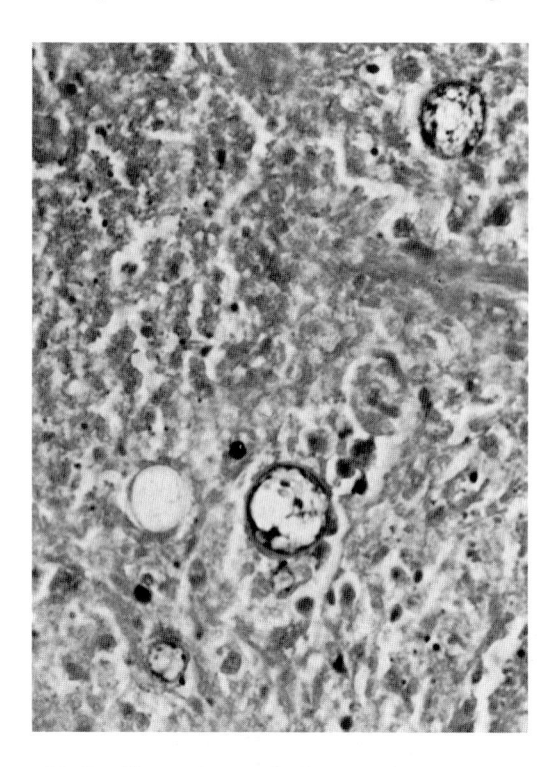

Figure 14–9. Photomicrograph showing characteristic appearance of coccidioidal spherule in an H&E-stained section. Note the well-defined, thick wall surrounding a granular, basophilic internal structure (endospores) (×450).

demonstrated by means of the above-mentioned special stains. The mucinous capsule stains brightly with the mucicarmine stain and this feature, when present, is considered diagnostic of *C. neoformans*. Examples of unencapsulated cryptococcus have been described, however, and they may be confused histologically with other fungi, especially histoplasma.[54,57,58] Cultures may be needed in such cases for definitive diagnosis.

Cryptococci can be found both within the necrotic centers of granulomas and within multinucleated histiocytes. When present intracellularly they impart a characteristic bubbly apearance to the cell cytoplasm.

North American Blastomycosis

Blastomyces dermatitidis is a dimorphic fungus that grows as a mycelium at room temperature and converts to the yeast phase at 37°C. The yeast forms are usually found in infected tissues although mycelia can rarely occur as well.

The soil is generally considered to be the natural habitat of *B. dermatitidis*, although the organism has only occasionally been cultured from soil samples. Epidemiologic studies of blastomycosis have been incomplete both because of difficulties in isolating the organism from nature and also because skin and serologic tests are unreliable. Endemic areas, therefore, have been defined

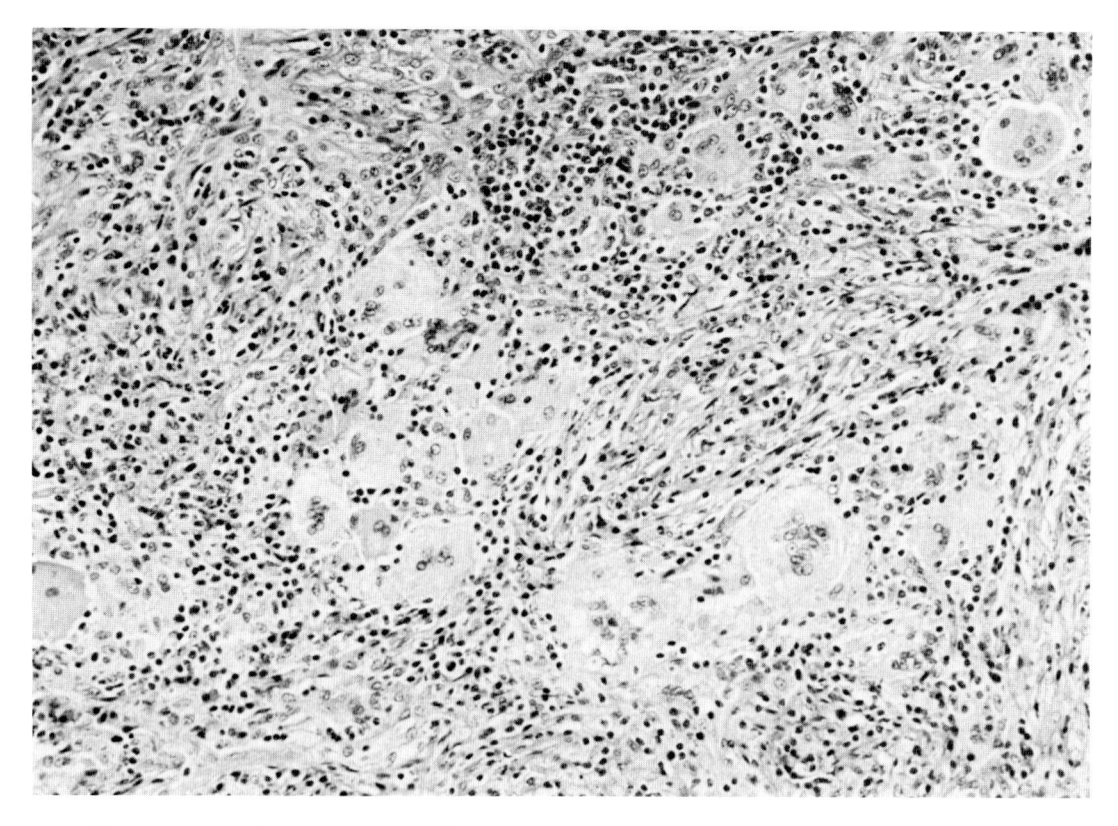

Figure 14–10. Noncaseating granulomatous reaction in cryptococcosis. The bubbly appearance of histiocyte cytoplasm due to the presence of intracellular organisms can be appreciated at even this low magnification (H&E, ×180).

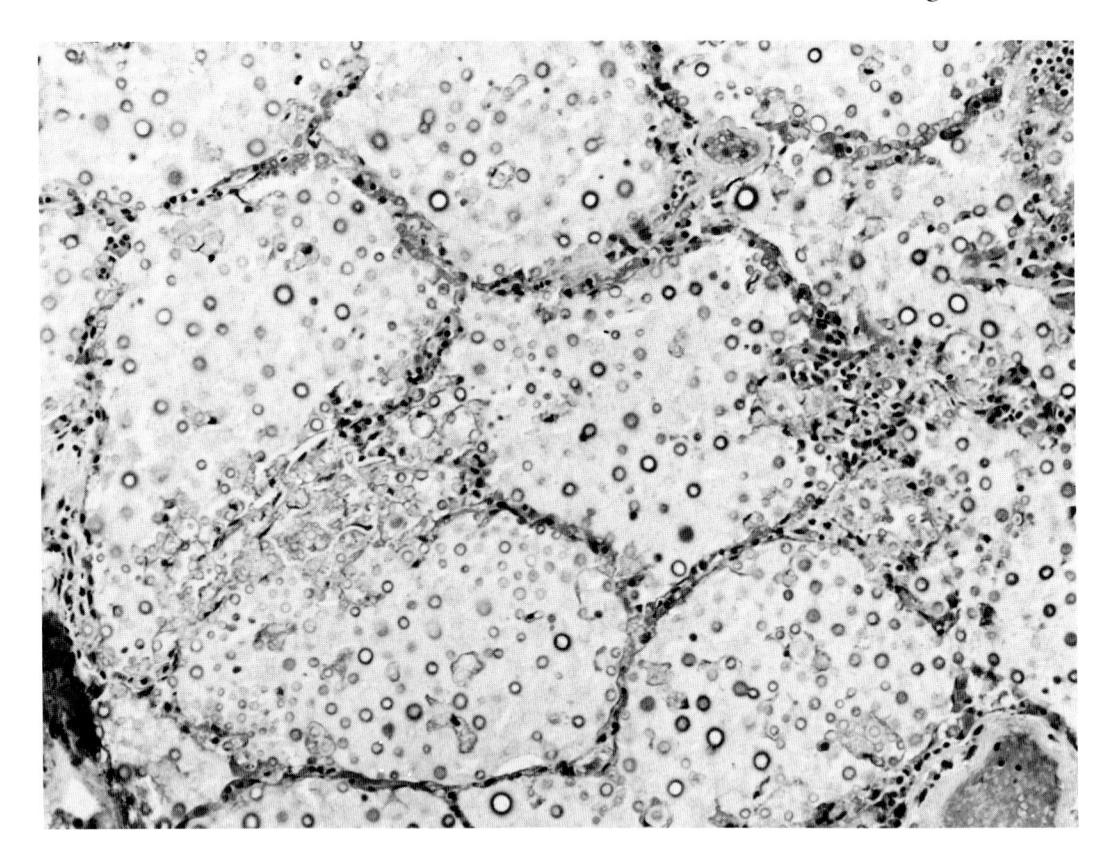

Figure 14–11. Cryptococcosis in an immunocompromised patient. Masses of organisms fill the alveolar spaces, but there is no host cellular reaction (mucicarmine, ×180).

only by case finding. They include the south, southcentral, and Great Lakes areas of the United States and Canada. Cases can occur well outside of these areas, however, and have been reported as far away as Africa and South America.[59]

Clinical Manifestations

Blastomycosis usually occurs in young to middle-aged adults, and men are affected more often than women. Several different clinical syndromes can occur (Table 14–4).[59,60–64] On initial exposure to the organism, an acute pneumonia develops. Most of these patients manifest high fever, chills and cough accompanied by patchy chest infiltrates. This form of the disease is generally self-limited and patients recover within several weeks. Asymptomatic or subclinical acute pneumonia, analogous to asymptomatic primary histoplasmosis or coccidioidomycosis, has also been documented in a few cases from local epidemics. Most investigators believe that asymptomatic infection by *B. dermatitidis* is more common that currently appreciated and that as soon as more reliable immunologic tests are available the frequent occurrence of this form of the disease will be documented. In a few patients with acute pneumonia, the infection cannot be controlled and there is rapid spread throughout both lungs (progressive pulmonary blastomycosis). Extrapulmonary involvement may occur as well in this form of the disease and mortality is high.

Chronic (recurrent or reactivation) blastomycosis occurs months to years following an episode of symptomatic acute pneumonia which appeared to have resolved. In some patients, a previous acute pneumonia is not documented and the initial infection is assumed to have been asymptomatic or subclinical.[59,65,66]

Chronic blastomycosis may be confined to the lung or it may involve extrapulmonary organs or both. When it disseminates, the skin is the most frequent extrapulmonary site of involvement.

Histopathologic Features

The usual tissue response in the lung to *B. dermatitidis* infection is necrotizing granulomatous inflammation.[63,67,68] The granulomas characteristically are composed of a core of necrotic neutrophils surrounded by epithelioid, often palisading, histiocytes (Fig. 14–14). True caseation is usually not present. Noncaseating granulomas may be found in the surrounding parenchyma and in a few reported cases, noncaseating granulomas have been the only tissue reaction.[63]

The organisms can be found intermingled with the necrotic neutrophils at the center of the granulomas or they may be present within the surrounding histiocytes.

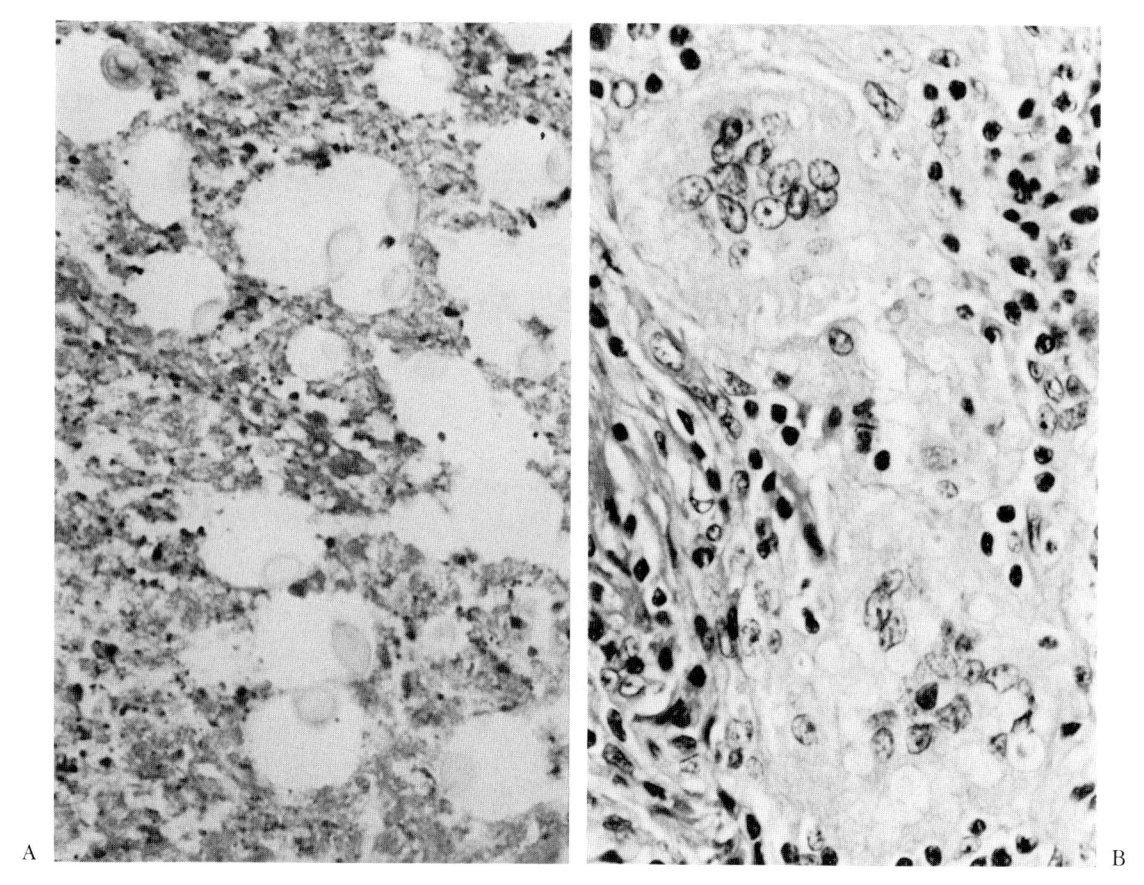

Figure 14–12. Higher-magnification photomicrographs showing the typical appearance of *Cryptococcus neoformans* in H&E-stained sections. A. *C. neoformans* in a necrotic area showing the characteristic clear halos surrounding the organisms (×720). B. Intracellular apearance of *C. neoformans* (×450).

They are round, budding yeasts which average 8 to 15 μm in diameter and may range up to 30 μm. They are easily visualized in H&E-stained sections where a thick, somewhat refractile cell wall can be seen surrounding multiple, basophilic nuclei (Fig. 14–15). As with other fungi, special stains (GMS, PAS, PAS-Gridley) facilitate their identification. Mycelial forms are rarely encountered in tissue.[69]

Other Granulomatous Fungal Diseases

In rare cases the lung is infected with *Sporothrix schenckii*, the agent of cutaneous sporotrichosis.[70–73] This organism causes necrotizing granulomas containing central suppuration. The fungus can be visualized with special stains where it appears as either a 2- to 3-μm-diameter round yeast or as an elongated 1- to 2-μm × 4- to 5-μm cigar-shaped form. Sometimes spicules of amorphous proteinaceous material are deposited around the yeast forming star-shaped eosinophilic structures which are known as asteroid bodies.

Paracoccidioides brasiliensis, the agent of South American blastomycosis, can occasionally produce lung infection in North America.[74] This organism is a budding yeast that differs morphologically from *Blastomyces dermatitides* in that it contains multiple thin-necked buds, in contrast to the single, wide-necked bud of the latter organism. *Alternaria* is another fungus that rarely causes lung granulomas.[75]

Invasive Fungal Diseases

Aspergillosis

Infection with aspergillus species is classically divided into three types, saprophytic, allergic, and invasive, depending on the host response and the degree of tissue invasion.[76–79] Recently a semi-invasive type has also been described (*see* Semi-Invasive Aspergillosis, below).[80] In the saprophytic form of aspergillosis the organism inhabits abnormal lung spaces, often producing a mycetoma (*see* Clinical Features, below). Tissue invasion by the fungus is usually absent. In allergic aspergillosis significant tissue invasion also does not occur, but there is a

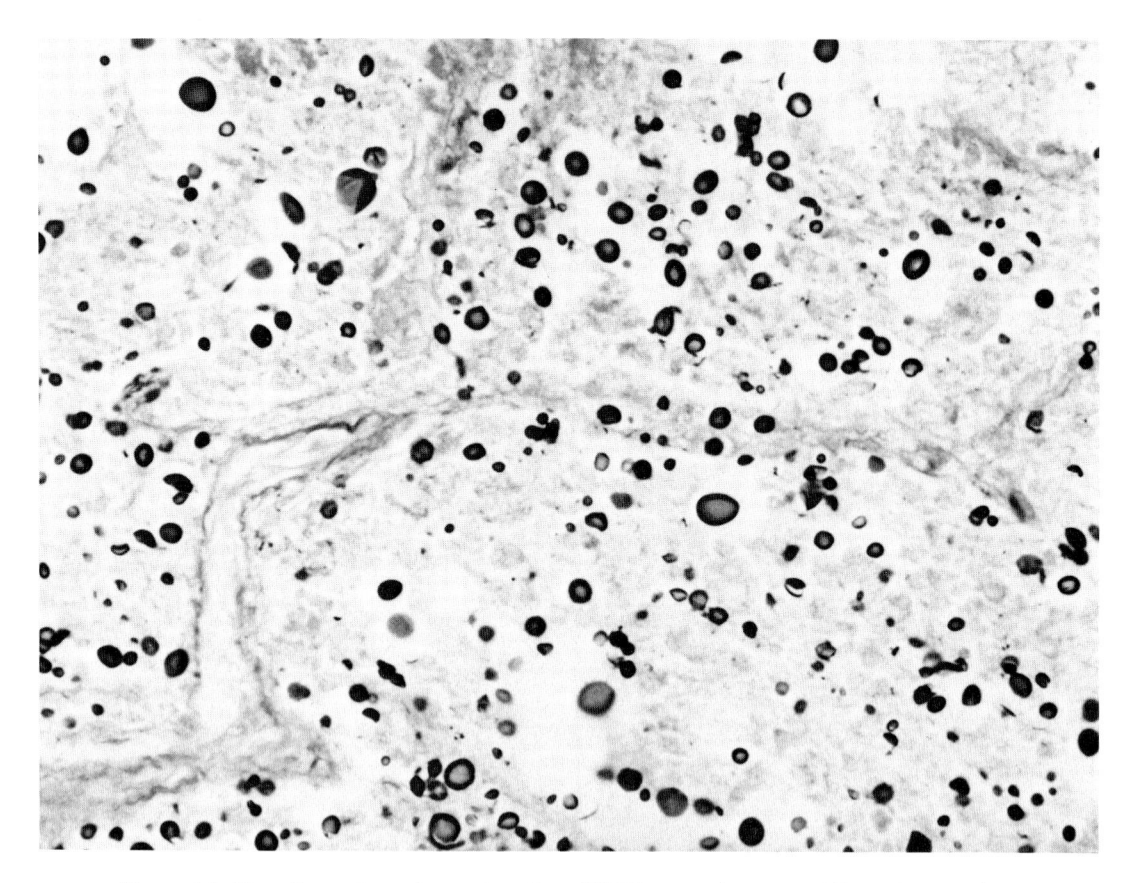

Figure 14–13. Gomori's methenamine silver (GMS)–stained section of C. *neoformans* showing characteristic variation in size of the organism and numerous fragmented forms (×720).

characteristic inflammatory response containing numerous eosinophils. This form of the disease is responsive to corticosteroid therapy. Invasive aspergillosis, as the name implies, is associated with extensive tissue invasion and destruction by the organism. It will be discussed in detail in the following section.

Invasive Aspergillosis

Invasive aspergillosis occurs almost exclusively in immunocompromised individuals, although there are rare reports of this condition in apparently healthy persons.[78,81–83] Patients with underlying acute leukemia and severe granulocytopenia are especially susceptible, but the infection can occur in individuals with a variety of other malignant or debilitating diseases, or in persons who are receiving immunosuppressive drugs.[78,82a–86] The lung is the primary site of infection in all cases and inhalation of air-borne spores is thought to be the cause.[82,86] *Aspergillus fumigatus*, *A. niger*, and *A. flavus* are the usual species involved and they may be admixed with various other organisms.[83,87] Rare examples of invasive infection involving the pleura have been described in nonimmunocompromised patients with previously damaged pleura.[90a]

Clinical Features

Patients with invasive aspergillosis generally present with high fever, dyspnea, and nonproductive cough.[79,83,87,88] Pleuritic chest pain and hemoptysis are occasional associated features.[78,89] Radiographically, rounded infiltrates with irregular margins are the most common initial finding.[87,90] They may be solitary or multiple. These lesions can evolve into pleural-based consolidations resembling hemorrhagic infarcts, or they may progress to a nonspecific bronchopneumonic pattern involving an entire lobe. Cavitation occurs in some cases, and occasionally mycetomas develop in an area of previous infiltration (*see* Mycetomas, below). Rarely, the initial finding is a miliary pattern. The prognosis in invasive aspergillosis is

Table 14–4. Classification of North American Blastomycosis

Acute pneumonia (symptomatic or asymptomatic)
Progressive pulmonary blastomycosis
Chronic (recurrent or reactivation) blastomycosis
    Pulmonary
    Extrapulmonary

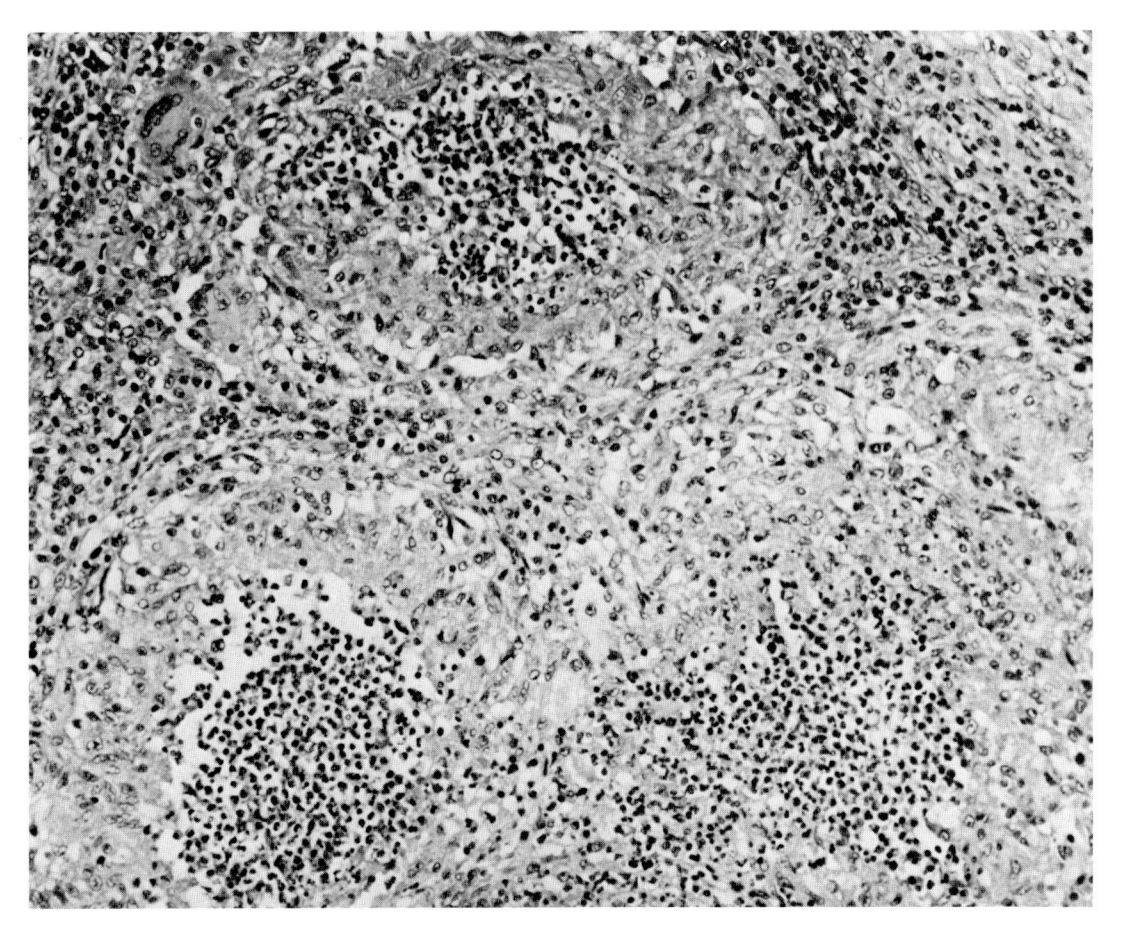

Figure 14–14. Photomicrograph showing granulomatous inflammation in blastomycosis. Plump, palisading histiocytes surround a central core of necrotic neutrophils (H&E, ×180).

very poor, although cures can be attained in some cases if therapy with amphotericin B is begun early.[82a,85,90a]

A lung biopsy is usually necessary for the diagnosis of invasive aspergillosis for two reasons.[87,90a,91] First, sputum cultures are generally negative, probably because the organism cannot be expectorated. Second, since aspergillus is a ubiquitous fungus and is frequently present as a saprophyte in normal individuals, its significance when present in sputum from patients with infiltrates is difficult to assess.

Histopathology

Aspergillus infection is thought to begin with invasion by the organisms through the bronchial wall and into the adjacent lung parenchyma. Arterial invasion with resultant thrombosis is characteristic and the most common tissue reaction is a hemorrhagic infarct secondary to the vascular occlusion (Fig. 14–16).[79,83,87] Organisms can be seen invading the alveolar septa and other interstitial structures of the lung as well as the blood vessels. The amount of associated acute inflammation depends upon the state of available bone marrow stores. Sparse inflammation is the usual finding and is seen in patients with severe granulocytopenia. As acute bronchopneumonia, however, can be seen in individuals who have sufficient available neutrophils. The areas of bronchopneumonia in such cases frequently have a characteristic gross appearance described as a "target lesion" by Orr and associates.[87] This lesion is typified by a round, yellow-grey center surrounded by a hemorrhagic rim.

Aspergillus is easily recognized within the tissue in H&E and in specially stained (GMS, PAS) sections. Slender, septate mycelia that average 4 μm in diameter and have dichotomous, 45 degree angle branch points are characteristic (Fig. 14–17). They appear uniform and are often oriented in a parallel arrangement.

Semi-Invasive Aspergillosis

Gefter and co-workers[80] have suggested that the classification of aspergillosis into saprophytic, allergic, and invasive may be an oversimplification. They describe five cases of a chronic, often progressive, cavitary infiltrate due to aspergillus infection. Their patients were only mildly immunosuppressed or had an underlying lung disease. Lung destruction occurred, but there was no

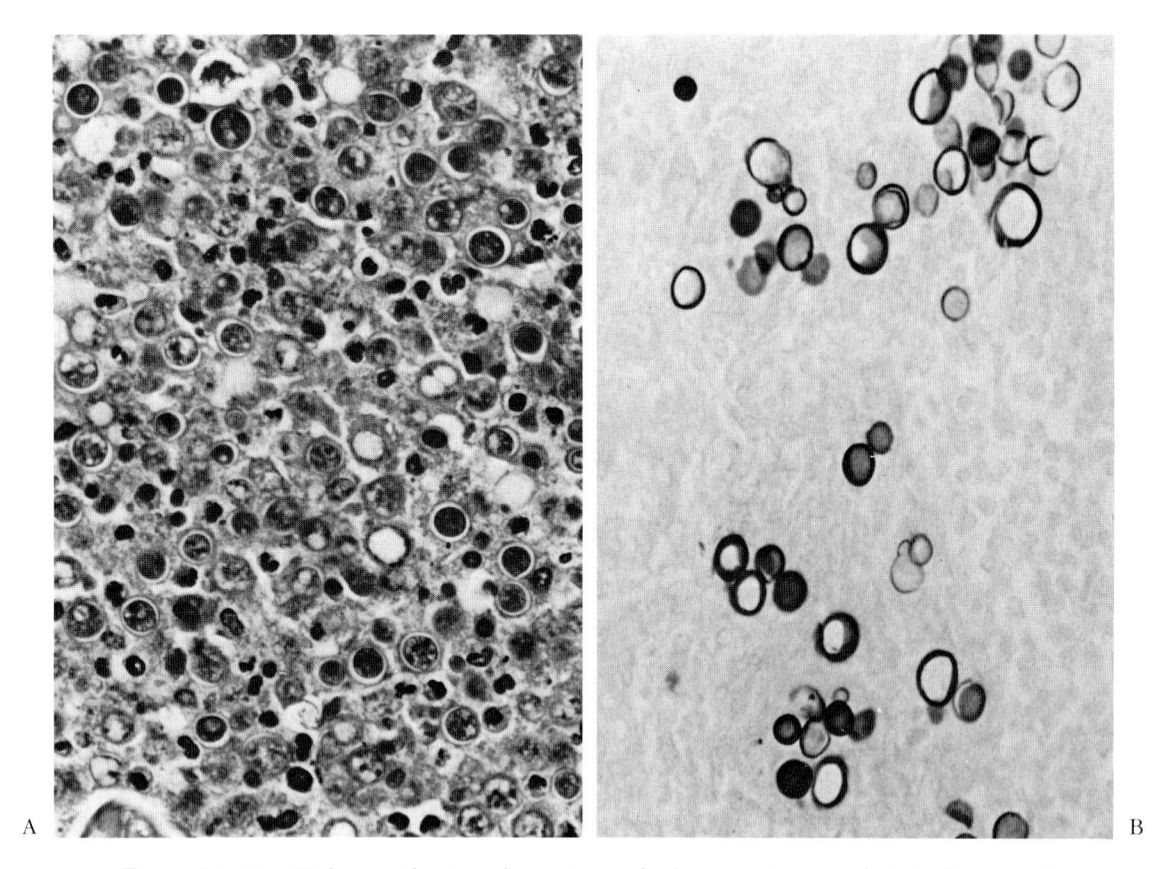

Figure 14–15. High-magnification photomicrograph demonstrating morphologic features of *Blastomyces dermatides*. A. H&E-stained section showing uniform, round yeast with granular basophilic internal structure surrounded by a prominent cell wall. B. Gomori's methenamine silver–stained section showing well-defined outline of organisms, but loss of internal structural detail (A and B, ×450).

evidence of vascular invasion and the fulminant course characteristic of invasive aspergillosis was not seen.

Mucormycosis (Phycomycosis)

Pulmonary infection can be caused by several genera of the family Mucoraceae, most commonly *Rhizopus*, *Absidia*, and *Mucor*. Invasive mucormycosis shares many clinical, radiographic and pathologic characteristics with invasive aspergillosis. It occurs almost exclusively in immunocompromised patients or in patients with underlying debilitating diseases, especially leukemia, lymphoma, and diabetes mellitus.[92–97] It has also been reported in acutely ill but previously healthy individuals who were receiving corticosteroids and broad-spectrum antibiotics.[98] Fever and chest pain are the usual clinical findings and hemoptysis occurs in occasional patients. Rounded pneumonic infiltrates, hemorrhagic infarcts, or large consolidated areas are seen radiographically.[90,94] Sputum cultures are rarely positive and direct cultures of infected tissue are also frequently negative. The disease can be rapidly progressive and is associated with a high mortality rate.

Histopathology

The histopathologic changes in mucormycosis are very similar to those in invasive aspergillosis. The usual finding is hemorrhagic infarction with sparse, if any, associated inflammatory reaction.[92,95,99] The organisms can be seen invading the blood vessels and interstitial tissues of the lung. Extensive vascular occlusion is common.

The mycelia of Mucor are easily visualized as basophilic structures in H&E-stained sections (Fig. 14–18). They are considerably wider than Aspergillus species, measuring 10 to 15 μm in diameter, and lack septa. They are frequently fragmented, appearing less uniform than Aspergillus and they have haphazardly arranged branch points usually oriented at a 90 degree angle.

Candidiasis

Candida species are a common cause of infection in patients who are immunocompromised, either due to an underlying malignancy or because they are receiving

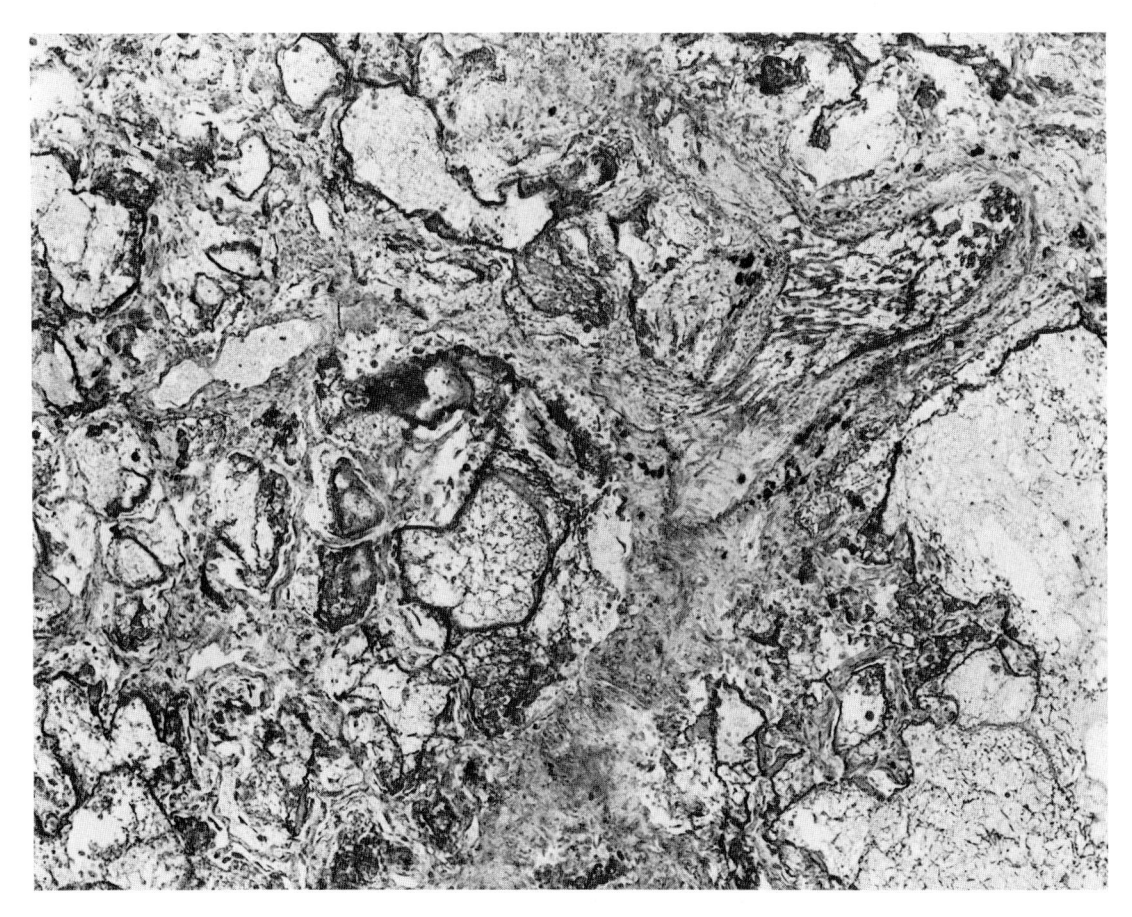

Figure 14–16. Low-magnification photomicrograph showing hemorrhagic infarct in aspergillosis. Note the pulmonary artery (right) that is occluded by fungal hyphae (H&E, ×45).

cytotoxic therapy. Indwelling venous catheters, prolonged antibiotic therapy, severe burns, and abdominal surgery also predispose persons to infection by this organism.[91,100–103] *Candida albicans* or *C. tropicalis* are the most frequent species isolated.[91,104,105] Infection by these organisms can be either superficial or deep. Superficial infections involve mucosal surfaces and are very common, especially in the oral cavity. In deep, disseminated infection, there is hematogenous spread to multiple organs and the prognosis is grave.

The lung is frequently involved in disseminated candidiasis, but clinically significant lung involvement is very uncommon.[104,106,106a,107] Moreover, there are no specific clinical or radiographic features of pulmonary candidiasis.[106a] Positive sputum cultures are not helpful since the organism is a common saprophyte in the oral cavity, skin, and respiratory tree. The diagnosis can be made with certainty, therefore, only by identifying the organism within the tissue.

Histopathologic Features

Two distinct patterns of pulmonary infection by Candida species occur, depending on whether the infection results from hematogenous spread or by aspiration.[104,106,108,109]

In the hematogenous variant of pulmonary candidiasis, the lung is one of multiple organs affected. This form of candidiasis is characterized by multiple miliary (2- to 4-mm) nodules which are spread randomly throughout the lung parenchyma. The nodules consist of central necrosis with varying amounts of acute inflammation, depending on whether or not the patient is neutropenic. Clusters of pseudohyphae and yeasts are present within the necrotic zones. They can be visualized with H&E in addition to PAS and GMS and they are weakly gram positive (Fig. 14–19). The pseudohyphae are composed of elongated blastospheres attached to each other in a chain-like fashion resembling sausage links. The yeasts are uniform, round to oval structures that range from 3 to 6 μm in diameter. Although occasional organisms can be found within blood vessels,[106] the extensive vascular invasion and tissue infarction characteristic of invasive aspergillosis and mucormycosis are not seen.

Pulmonary candidiasis secondary to aspiration usually occurs in moribund patients and is of little clinical significance. It is generally found in individuals who have associated candidiasis involving the oral cavity, esophagus, larynx, or trachea. This form of the disease is

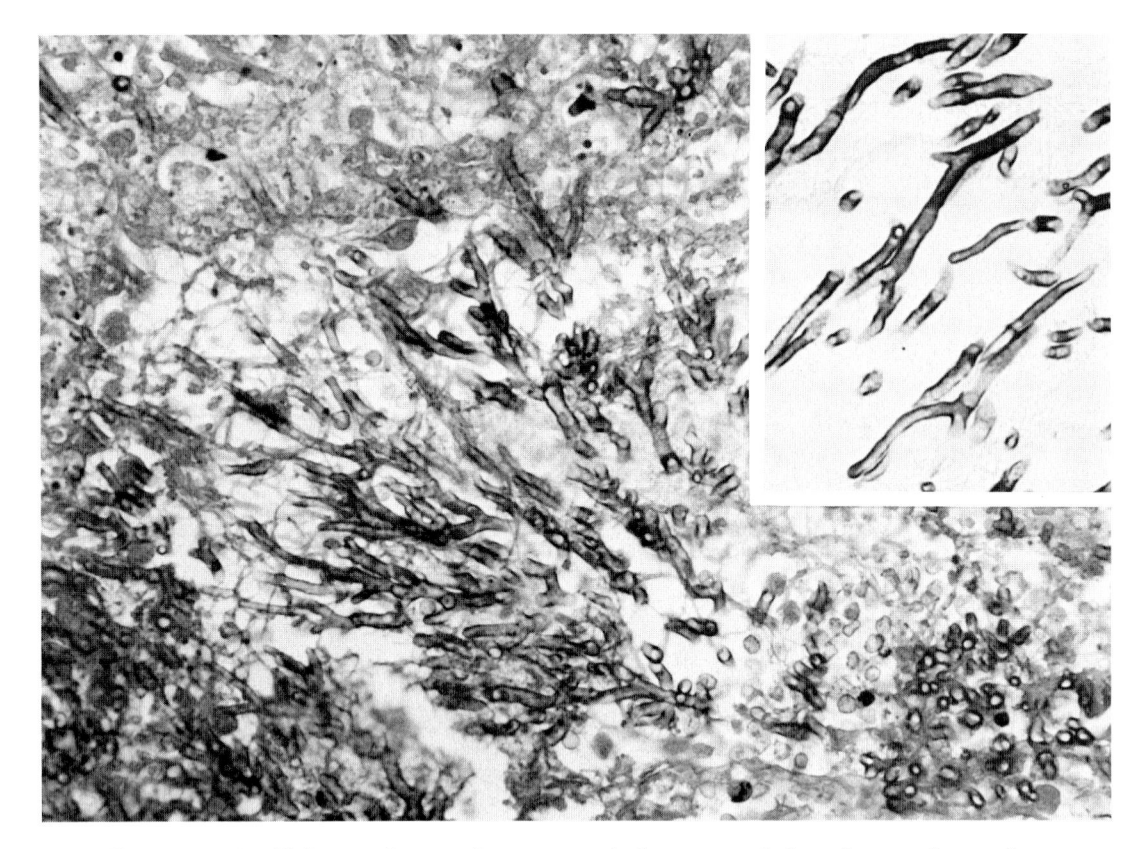

Figure 14–17. High-magnification photomicrograph showing morphologic features of aspergillus species. The organisms are thin, uniform in size, and show dichotomous branching. They are arranged in parallel and appear to be oriented in one direction (H&E, ×450). Inset: typical cross-septations can be identified in the hyphae (H&E, ×450).

characterized by foci of acute bronchopneumonia which often contain food particles as evidence of aspiration. Abscess formation may also occur. These lesions further differ from hematogenous candidiasis in that they are distributed predominantly around bronchioles rather than randomly throughout the parenchyma. In cases of preterminal aspiration, clusters of organisms are seen in the air spaces without any associated inflammatory reaction.

Other Invasive Fungi

Torulopsis glabrata

Torulopsis glabrata is a saprophytic yeast which may cause either fungemia or deep infection in immunocompromised patients.[110–112] It is not to be confused with *Torula* which is another name for *Cryptococcus neoformans*. Lung involvement generally occurs secondary to widely disseminated disease, although primary pneumonia has been reported. The usual tissue response to this organism is necrosis with a varying amount of associated acute and chronic inflammation. Microabscesses may also occur. The organisms are small, round to oval, budding yeasts that average 2 to 4 μm in diameter.[112,113] They resemble Candida species, except that they are smaller and do not form pseudohyphae.

Allescheria boydii

Allescheria boydii, the usual agent of maduromycosis, has been rarely reported to cause pneumonia in immunocompromised or otherwise debilitated individuals.[114–116] The usual tissue reaction to the fungus is acute inflammation and necrosis. The organisms can be visualized within the necrotic zones where they appear as broad, septate hyphae with rounded ends and measure 2 to 5 μm in diameter. They have a characteristic disorganized growth pattern and are often aggregated into dense clusters. In some cases it may be difficult to distinguish *A. boydii* from Aspergillus species morphologically and cultures may be necessary for definite diagnosis.

Mycetomas

Pulmonary mycetomas or fungus balls usually represent saprophytic growths of fungi within preexisting lung cavities.[67,77,82a,117] A variety of chronic lung disorders may have produced the cavities, including chronic obstructive

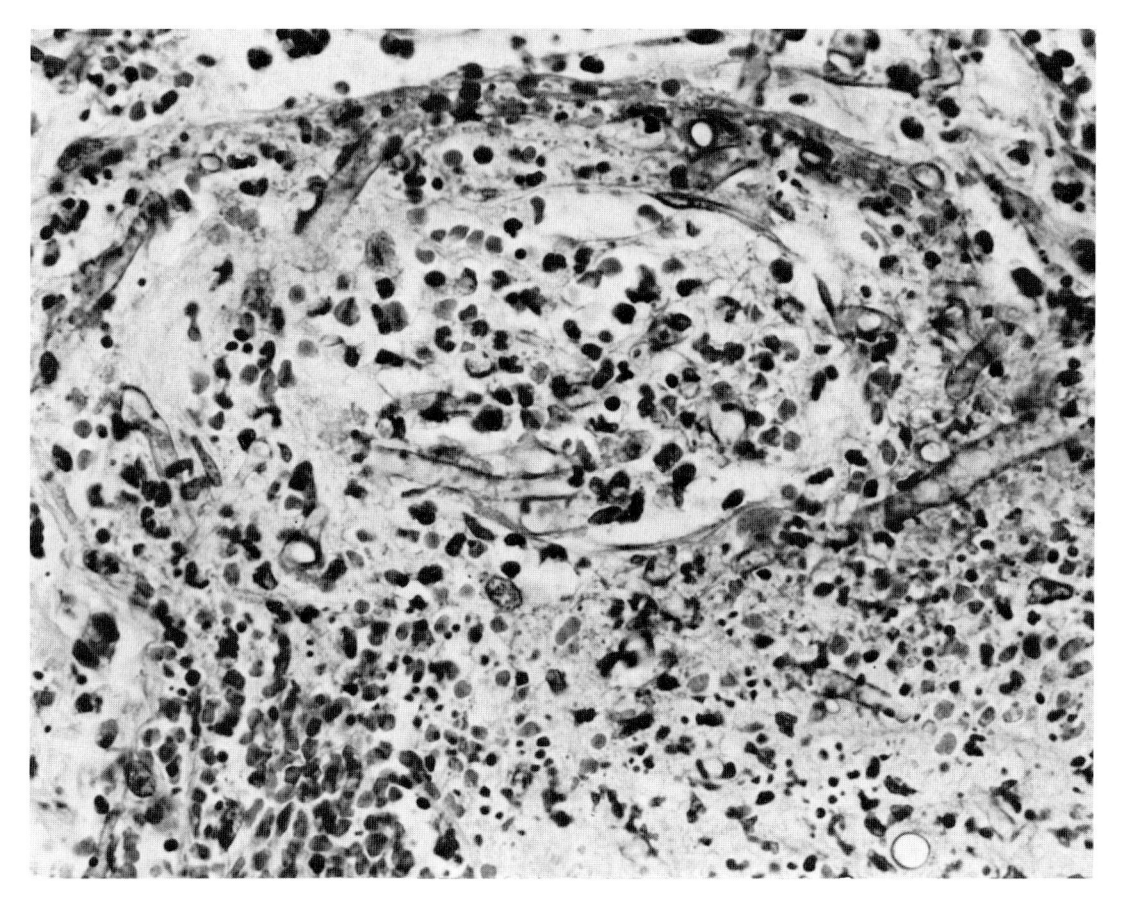

Figure 14–18. Photomicrograph showing organisms of mucormycosis. The hyphae are wide and irregular in size and orientation. They are present within a blood vessel (H&E, ×450).

lung disease, healed tuberculosis, bronchiectasis, sarcoidosis, healed infarcts, and cancers. There is a suggestion that patients with ankylosing spondylitis have an increased incidence of mycetomas.[67,117] In a few patients without underlying lung disease mycetomas can develop from areas of previous infiltration due to invasive aspergillosis or mucormycosis.[67,73,80] Most mycetomas are caused by Aspergillus species, but other fungi have also been identified, including various phycomycetes,[118,119] *Allescheria boydii*,[120,121] *Coccidioides immitis*,[122] *Cladosporium cladosporioides*,[123] and *Nocardia asteroides*.[124]

Clinical Manifestations

Many mycetomas are unassociated with clinical symptoms and are found on routine chest radiographs. In symptomatic patients hemoptysis is the most common complaint, and may vary from minor bloodstreaking of sputum to massive, even fatal blood loss.[77,82,177] A few patients present with chronic cough and weight loss. The radiographic appearance is characteristic and consists of a thick-walled cavity containing a central density that is separated from the surrounding wall superiorly by a semicircular space. The central density can be seen to move when the patient changes position.

Amphotericin B therapy is generally considered to be ineffectual in treating mycetomas. Since many lesions remain stable for years and some even regress without treatment[82,125] the role for surgical intervention vs. close medical follow-up is controversial. Most investigators advocate surgery only in patients with life-threatening hemoptysis.[82,117]

Pathologic Features

Grossly, mycetomas are composed of a core of soft, friable, tan-brown material surrounded by a firm, fibrous capsule (Fig. 14–20). Microscopically, the central core consists of a tangled mass of mycelia admixed with necrotic cellular debris and the surrounding wall is composed of fibrosis and chronic inflammation. Granulomatous inflammation is usually not seen. Although the fungi can occasionally superficially invade the fibrous wall, the vascular occlusion and tissue necrosis characteristic of invasive fungal diseases are not seen in mycetomas. Occasionally, in cases containing Aspergillus species, birifringent calcium oxalate crystals are deposited on the edge of the cavity.[126–128]

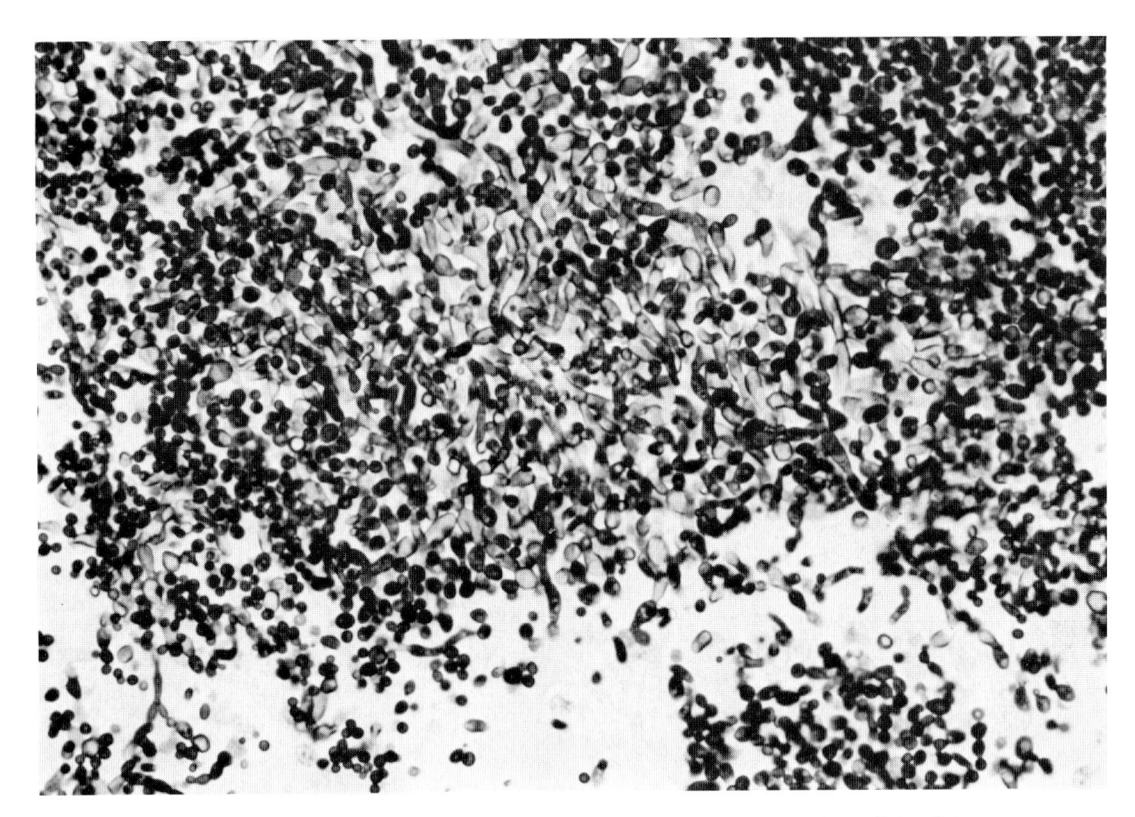

Figure 14–19. Photomicrograph showing typical yeasts and pseudohyphae of Candida species (GMS, ×450).

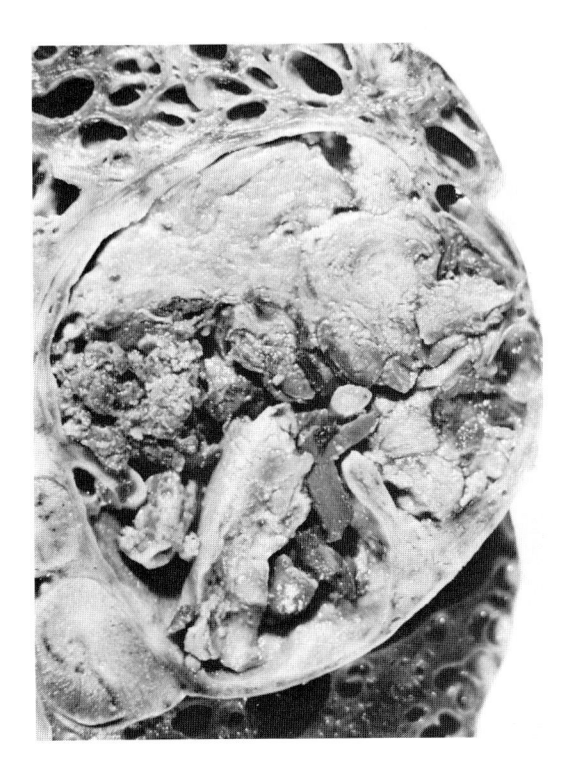

Figure 14–20. Gross appearance of a fungus ball (mycetoma). This mycetoma developed in an area of honeycombing (top) due to long-standing sarcoidosis. Soft, friable, tan-white material fills the cavity and is surrounded by a fibrous capsule.

Protozoal Infections

Pneumocystis Pneumonia

In Europe in the 1940s epidemics of *Pneumocystis carinii* pneumonia were common in debilitated, malnourished infants. The disease was known as interstitial plasma cell pneumonitis because the most prominent pathologic change was a marked interstitial infiltrate of plasma cells.[129–132] Mortality rates were high.

The epidemiology and also the histopathology, of Pneumocystis infection has changed dramatically in recent years.[132,133] Although interstitial plasma cell pneumonitis is still seen in some underdeveloped parts of the world, this epidemic form of the disease is almost never seen any more in Europe or the United States. Currently, in developed areas of the world, Pneumocystis pneumonia occurs almost exclusively as a sporadic infection in immunocompromised patients, with no particular preference for children or adults. It is this sporadic form of the disease that will be discussed in detail in the following sections.

Clinical Features

The incidence of pneumocystis infection in immunocompromised individuals has been increasing in recent years. Patients with hematologic malignancy are most susceptible to this disease, although other malignant diseases, immunosuppressive therapy for organ transplantation, and collagen vascular diseases are also predisposing factors.[129–135]

Recently, pneumocystis pneumonia has been described as a common cause of pneumonia in patients with AIDS.[136,136a,136b] These individuals are also frequently infected with other organisms as well, especially cytomegalovirus, and they have an increased incidence of Kaposi's sarcoma.

Patients with Pneumocystis pneumonia are usually acutely ill with fever, dry cough, and dyspnea although a more insidious onset may be seen in some cases. Bilateral, diffuse interstitial and alveolar infiltrates are the usual radiographic findings, although rare examples of localized infiltrates have been reported.[131,138] Rapid progression to respiratory failure can occur if treatment is not instituted quickly.

The diagnosis of Pneumocystis pneumonia requires a lung biopsy in most cases, since the organisms are only rarely found in sputum samples, and they can be identified only occasionally in transtracheal aspirates or bronchial washings. Open lung biopsy is generally considered the most reliable method for making the diagnosis, although success has been reported with a variety of less-invasive procedures such as transbronchial or percutaneous biopsies.[129,133,139] Recently bronchial washings and bronchoalveolar lavage have been advocated to diagnose pneumocystis in patients with AIDS.[150a,150b]

Histopathology

The classically described pathologic finding Pneumocystis pneumonia is the presence within alveolar spaces of an eosinophilic foamy, frothy, or honeycomb exudate associated with a moderate interstitial pneumonia. (Fig. 14–21).[129,135,140] Plasma cells are not numerous in the sporadic form of the disease. The presence of intra-alveolar froth is pathognomonic of Pneumocystis pneumonia, but it has been our experience,[141] as well as that of other investigators,[129,138,142] that the froth is frequently absent or difficult to find. A more common, but little emphasized, feature of Pneumocystis pneumonia is the presence within alveolar spaces of hyaline membranes associated with an intra-alveolar fibrinous exudate admixed with alveolar macrophages and cellular debris

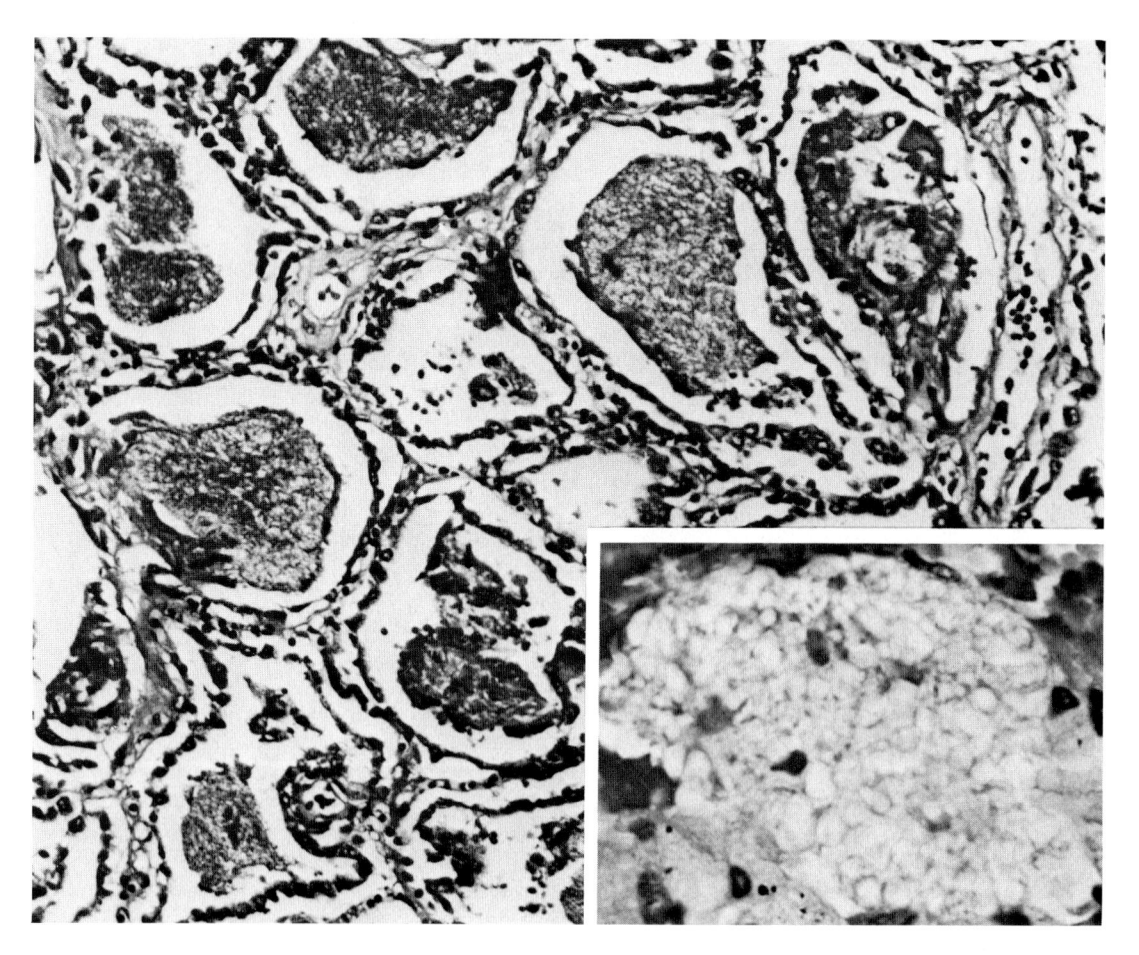

Figure 14–21. Photomicrograph of Pneumocystis pneumonia. A frothy exudate is seen in alveolar spaces and there is associated mild interstitial thickening (H&E, ×180). Inset shows intra-alveolar forth at higher magnification (H&E, ×720).

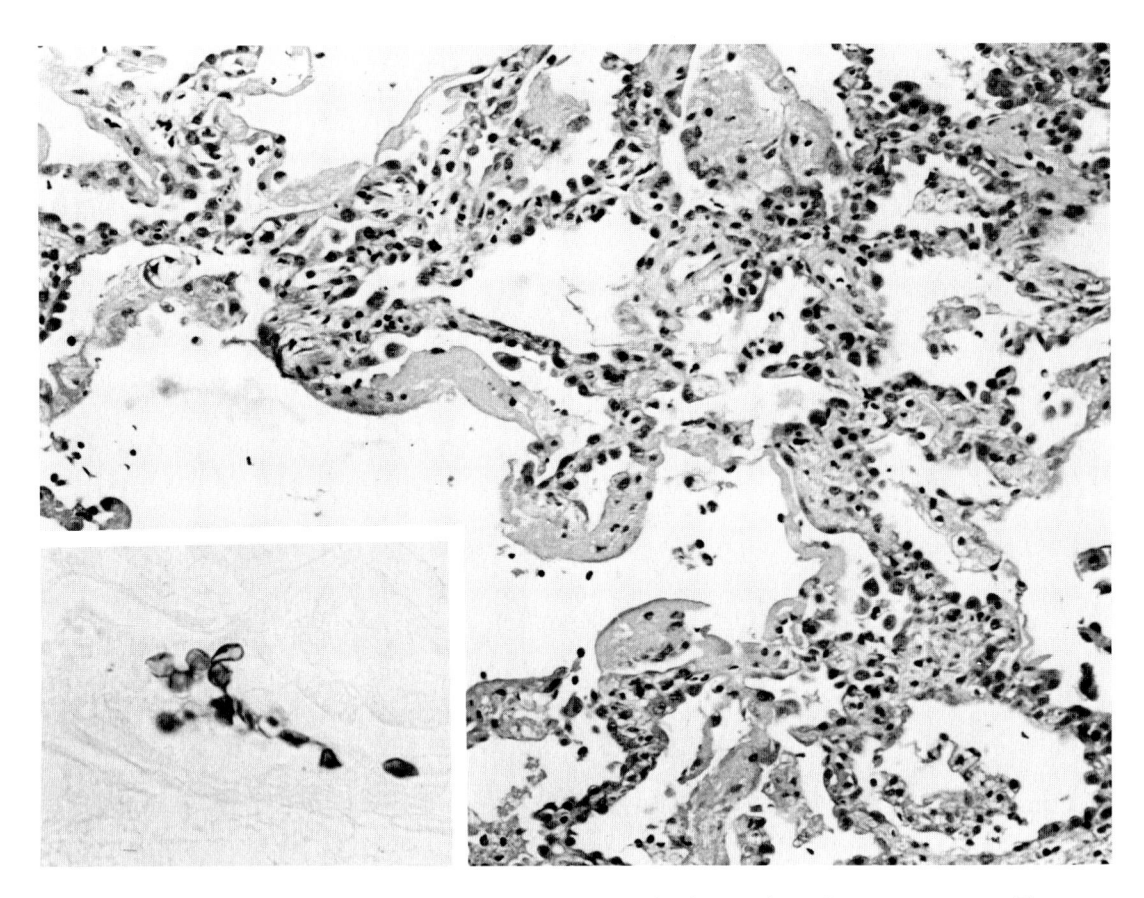

Figure 14–22. Photomicrograph showing diffuse alveolar damage due to *Pneumocystis carinii*. The classically described alveolar froth is absent in this case (H&E, ×180). Inset shows a GMS stain outlining organisms within a hyaline membrane (×72).

(Fig. 14–22). These findings are identical to diffuse alveolar damage (DAD) due to a variety of other causes (*see* Chapter 16), and the diagnosis of Pneumocystis in such cases can be made only by examining special stains for organisms. A variety of less-typical reactions to Pneumocystis have also been described, including multinucleated giant cell formation, granulomatous inflammation, interstitial fibrosis, and calcification.[142–144] *Pneumocystis carinii* has also been identified in lungs without any significant tissue reaction.[137]

Identification of the Organism

Although the characteristics intra-alveolar froth which is easily visualized in H&E-stained sections contains numerous organisms, the individual cysts cannot be visualized with this stain. The cysts are best demonstrated by the GMS stain which outlines their wall although obscuring their internal structure. A known Pneumocystis infection should be used as a positive control for the GMS stain in order to avoid false-negative results.[145] In this stain the organisms appear as round, often indented or helmet-shaped, nonbudding structures which measure 4 to 6 μm in diameter (Fig. 14–23). They are located within the alveolar spaces. Other stains, such as Cresyl-echt violet and toluidine blue O can also be used to outline the cysts and they have the advantage of being less time consuming and, therefore, are useful in staining frozen section material.[146,147] A rapid-acting GMS stain is also available.[137,148] The PAS stain is not recommended since it fails to distinguish the organisms from the background exudate, although the Gridley modification of the PAS stain is adequate.

The mature cysts are shown by electron microscopy to consist of a thick wall surrounding multiple intracystic forms (sporozoites).[129,139,149,150] Certain histologic stains, such as Giemsa or polychrome methylene blue, will color the sporozoites.[133,135] These stains are not recommended as routine screening techniques, however, because they do not outline the cyst wall well and the tiny sporozoites may be difficult to distinguish from cellular debris.

Dirofilariasis (Dog Heartworm Disease)

The dog heartworm (*Dirofilaria immitis*) is an uncommon cause of lung granulomas in humans. Most individuals are asymptomatic and the lesions are detected on a

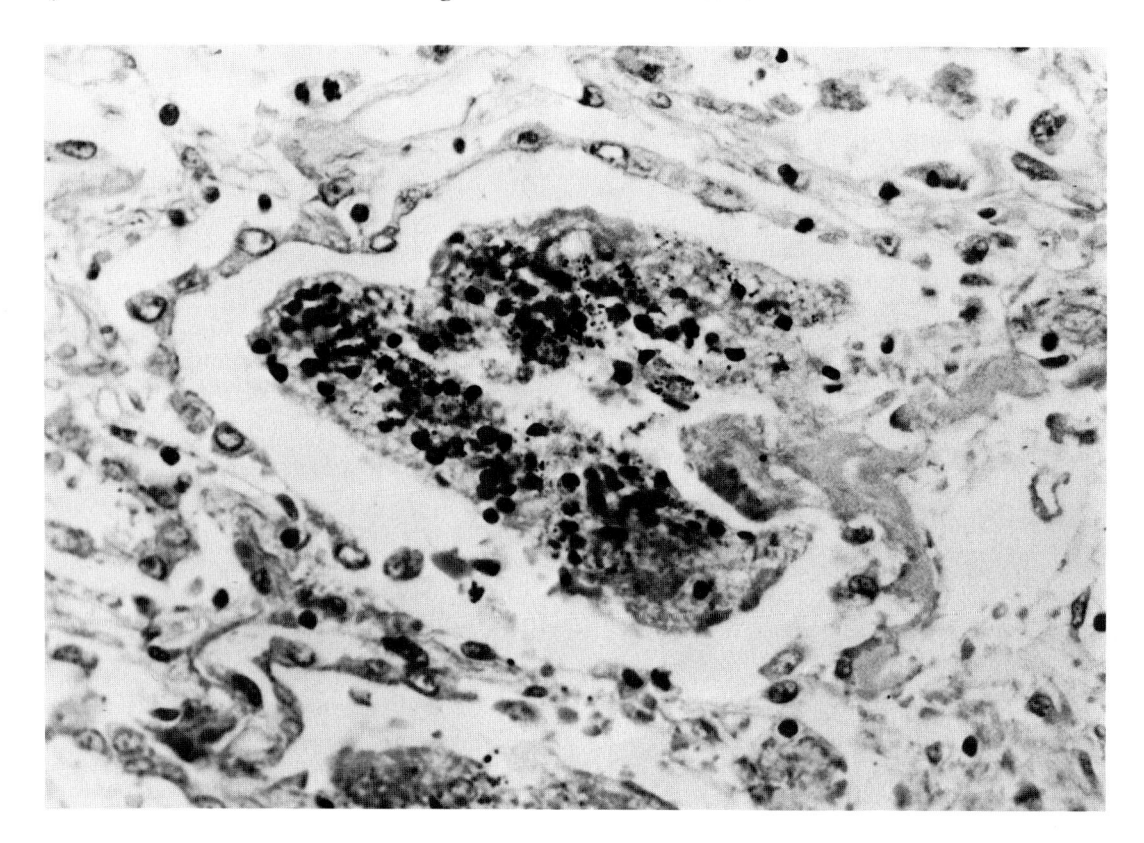

Figure 14–23. Photomicrograph showing a cluster of *P. carinii* cysts within the alveolar exudate. The organisms are round, uniform, and sometimes indented. Budding forms are not seen (GMS, ×450).

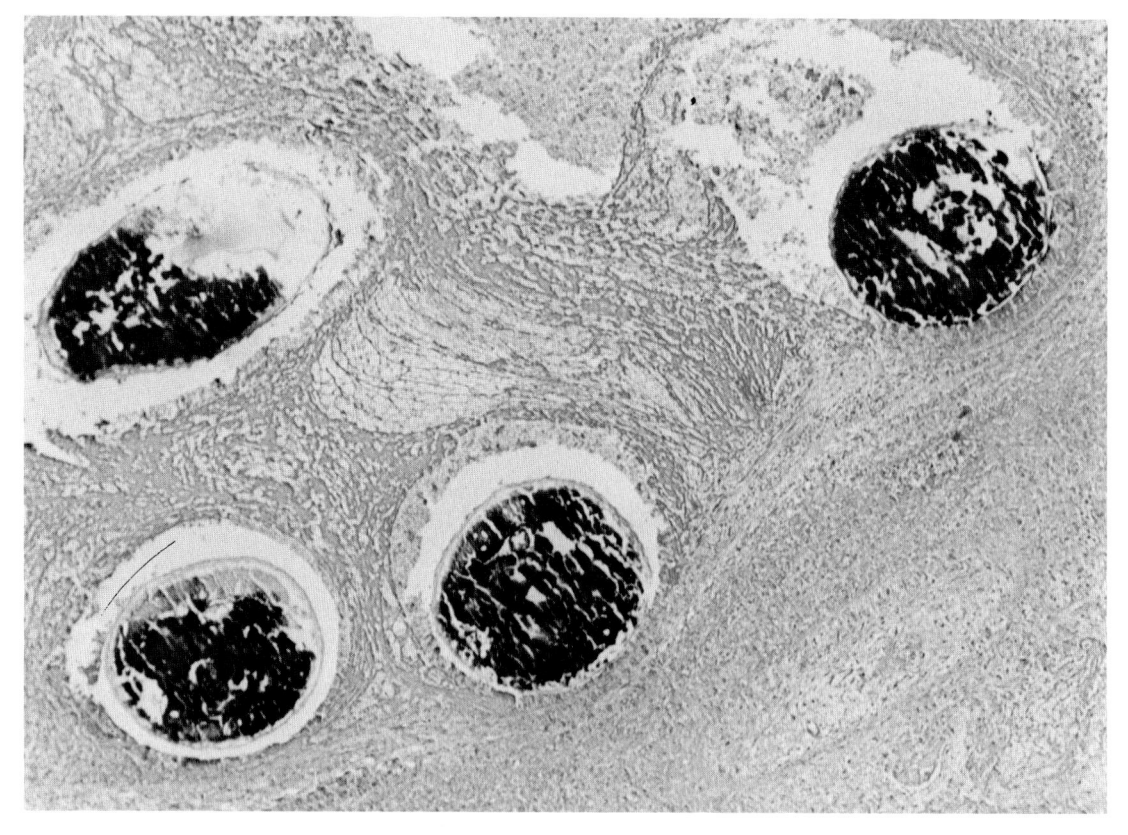

Figure 14–24. Photomicrograph of *Dirifilaria imitis* within a lung granuloma. Note the remnant of artery wall (right) surrounding the organisms which are partially calcified (H&E, ×70).

routine chest radiograph.[151–153] They usually appear as solitary, spherical densities resembling neoplasms radiographically.[154–156] Rarely, multiple lesions occur. Occasional patients present with various minor symptoms, including fever, cough, hemoptysis, or chest pain. Blood eosinophilia is found in a few cases.[151–153]

Distribution of D. immitis

The endemic area of dirofilarial infestation in dogs currently includes the entire Eastern Seaboard, south along the Gulf of Mexico to Texas, up the Mississippi River Valley, and into the southern Great Lake States.[152,153,157–159] Some cases have been reported from adjacent Midwestern states and from Canada as well. The disease appears both to be spreading in geographic distribution and also to be increasing in incidence. It is likely, therefore, that lesions in humans will become an increasingly important problem.

Life Cycle of D. immitis

Dogs and certain other mammals, including cats and foxes, are natural hosts for *D. immitis*.[152,153,157–159] The mature worm resides in the right ventricle and sheds numerous microfilaria into the bloodstream. The infection is spread by mosquitoes, which take up the microfilaria during a bite and deposit them in the skin of another host during a second bite. The microfilaria migrate into the subcutaneous tissues where they mature over a period of 3 to 4 months. They then enter the venous circulation and reach the right ventricle where they become adult forms and start the cycle over again. The human being is a dead-end host and the few forms that reach the right ventricle die. Pulmonary lesions result from the embolization of dead organisms to the lungs.

Pathologic Changes

The lung lesions in man are necrotizing granulomas containing extensive central necrosis surrounded by epithelioid, often palisading, histiocytes.[154,157,158,160–162] Chronic inflammation and fibrosis are seen in the adjacent parenchyma. Eosinophils are numerous in some cases, but are not always present. The organisms are located within the central necrosis and can usually be identified within remnants of a pulmonary artery. They are large, round structures ranging from 100 to 350 µm (average 200 µm) in diameter and have a characteristic multilayered cuticle containing transverse striations (Fig. 14–24). Sometimes they undergo calcification which can obscure their internal structure, but they can still be recognized because of their large size and intravascular location.

References

1. Slavin R, Walsh T, Pollack A: Late generalized tuberculosis: A clinical pathologic analysis and comparison of 100 cases in the preantibiotic and antibiotic eras. Medicine 59:352, 1980.

2. Steer A: Histogenesis of tuberculous pulmonary lesions. A study of reticulum patterns. Am Rev Respir Dis 95:200, 209, 1967.

3. Sahn S, Levin D: Diagnosis of miliary tuberculosis by transbronchial biopsy. Br Med J 2:667, 1975.

4. Wallace J, Deutsch A, Harrell J, Moser K: Bronchoscopy and transbronchial biopsy in evaluation of patients with suspected active tuberculosis. Am J Med 70:1189, 1981.

5. Geppert E, Leff A: The pathogenesis of pulmonary and miliary tuberculosis. Arch Intern Med 139:1391, 1979.

6. Glenn W, Liebow A, Lindskog G: *Thoracic and Cardiovascular Surgery with Replated Pathology*, 3rd ed. New York: Appleton-Century-Crofts, 1975, pp 204–225, 262–309.

7. Auerbach O: Acute generalized miliary tuberculosis. Med Clin North Am 43:239, 1959.

8. Medlar G: The behavior of pulmonary tuberculous lesions. A pathological study. Am Rev Tuberc 71(suppl) 1, 1955.

9. Nayak N, Sabharwal B, Bhathena D: The pulmonary tuberculous lesion in North India. I. Incidence, nature and evolution. Am Rev Respir Dis 101:1, 1970.

10. Ortbals D, Marr J: A comparative study of tuberculosis and other mycobacterial infections and their association with malignancy. Am Rev Respir Dis 117:39, 1978.

11. Sahn S, Neff I: Miliary tuberculosis. Am J Med 56:495, 1974.

12. Stead W: Pathogenesis of the sporadic case of tuberculosis. N Engl J Med 277:1008, 1967.

13. Stead W, Kerby G, Schlueter D, et al.: The clinical spectrum of primary tuberculosis in adults. Ann Intern Med 68:731, 1968.

14. Ulbright T, Katzenstein A: Solitary necrotizing granulomas of the lung. Differentiating features and etiology. Am J Surg Pathol 4:13, 1980.

15. Costrini A, Mahler D, Gross W, et al.: Clinical and roentgenographic features of nosocomial pulmonary disease due to *Mycobacterium xenopeni*. Am Rev Respir Dis 123:104, 1981.

16. Engbaek H, Vergmann B, and Bentzon M: Lung disease caused by *Mycobacterium avium/Mycobacterium intracellulare*. An analysis of Danish patients during the period 1962–1976. Eur J Respir Dis 62:72, 1981.

17. Christensen G, Dietz G, Ahn C, et al.: Pulmonary manifestations of *Mycobacterium intracellularis*. AJR 133:59, 1979.

18. Snijder J. Histopathology of pulmonary lesions caused by atypical mycobacteria. J Pathol Bacteriol 90:65, 1965.

19. Au F, Webber B, Rosenberg S: Pulmonary granulomas induced by BCG. Cancer 41:2209, 1978.

20. Quesada J, Libshitz H, Hersh E, Gutterman J: Pulmonary abnormalities in patients intravenously receiving the methanol extraction residue (MER) of bacillus Calmette-Guerin. Cancer 45:1340, 1980.

21. Voith M, Lichtenfeld K, Schimpff S, Wiernik P: Systemic complications of MER immunotherapy of cancer. Pulmonary granulomatosis and rash. Cancer 43:500, 1979.

22. Goodwin R, Loyd J, Des Prez R: Histoplasmosis in normal hosts. Medicine 60:231, 1981.

23. Goodwin R Jr, Des Prez R: Pathogenesis and clinical spectrum of histoplasmosis. South Med J 66:13, 1973.

24. Goodwin R Jr, Des Prez R: Histoplasmosis. Am Rev Respir Dis 117:929, 1978.

25. Goodwin R Jr, Owens F, Snell J, et al.: Chronic pulmonary histoplasmosis. Medicine 55:413, 1976.

26. Goodwin R, Shapiro J, Thurman G, et al.: Disseminated histoplasmosis: Clinical and pathologic correlations. Medicine 59:1, 1980.

27. Goodwin R Jr, Snell J: The enlarging histoplasmoma. Concept of a tumor-like phenomenon encompassing the

tuberculoma and coccidioidoma. Am Rev Respir Dis 100:1, 1969.

28. Prager R, Burney P, Waterhouse G, Bender H Jr: Pulmonary, mediastinal and cardiac presentations of histoplasmosis. Ann Thorac Surg 30:385, 1980.

29. Kauffman C, Israel K, Smith J et al.: Histoplasmosis in immuno-suppressed patients. Am J Med 64:923, 1978.

30. Binford C: Histoplasmosis. Tissue reactions and morphologic variations of the fungus. Am J Clin Pathol 25:25, 1955.

31. Puckett T: Pulmonary histoplasmosis. A study of twenty-two cases with identification of *H. capsulatum* in resected lesions. Am Rev Tuberc 67:453, 1953.

32. Straub M, Schwarz J: Histoplasmosis, coccidioidomycosis and tuberculosis. A comparative pathological study. Pathol Microbiol 25:421, 1962.

33. Bayer A: Fungal pneumonias: Pulmonary coccidioidal syndromes (Part I). Primary and progressive primary coccidioidal pneumonias—diagnostic, therapeutic and prognostic considerations. (Part II). Miliary, nodular and cavitary pulmonary coccidioidomycosis. Chemotherapeutic and surgical considerations. Chest 79:575, 686, 1981.

34. Bayer A, Yoshikawa T, Guze L: Chronic progressive coccidioidal pneumonitis. Report of six cases with clinical, roentgenographic, serologic and therapeutic features. Arch Intern Med 139:536, 1979.

35. Drutz D, Catanzaro A: Coccidioidomycosis. Am Rev Respir Dis 117:559, 727, 1978.

36. Fiese M: *Coccidioidomycosis*. Springfield, IL, Charles C Thomas, 1958.

37. Sarosi G, Parker J, Doto I: Chronic pulmonary coccidioidomycosis. N Engl J Med 283:325, 1970.

38. Winn W: A long term study of 300 patients with cavitary-abscess lesions of the lung of coccidioidal origin. An analytical study with special reference to treatment. Dis Chest 54:12, 1968.

39. Deppisch L, Donowho E: Pulmonary coccidioidomycosis. Am J Clin Pathol 58:489, 1972.

40. Campbell G: Primary pulmonary cryptococcosis. Am Rev Respir Dis 94:236, 1966.

41. Hammerman K, Powell K, Christianson C, et al.: Pulmonary cryptococcosis: Clinical forms and treatment. Am Rev Respir Dis 108:1116, 1973.

42. Hatcher C Jr, Sehdeva J, Waters W III et al.: Primary pulmonary cryptococcosis. J Thorac Cardiovasc Surg 61:39, 1971.

43. Kerkering T, Duma R, Shadomy S: The evolution of pulmonary cryptococcosis. Clinical implications from a study of 41 patients with and without compromising host factors. Ann Intern Med 94:611, 1981.

44. Littman M, Walter J: Cryptococcosis: Current status. Am J Med 45:922, 1968.

45. Smith F, Gibson P, Nicholls T, Simpson J: Pulmonary resection for localized lesions of cryptococcosis (torulosis): A review of eight cases. Thorax 31:121, 1976.

46. Taylor E: Pulmonary cryptococcosis. Analysis of 15 cases from the Columbia area. Ann Thorac Surg 10:309, 1970.

47. Warr W, Bates J, Stone A: The spectrum of pulmonary cryptococcosis. Ann Intern Med 69:1109, 1968.

48. Gordonson J, Birnbaum W, Jacobson G, Sargent E: Pulmonary cryptococcosis. Radiology 112:556, 1974.

49. Young E, Hirsch D, Fainstein V, Williams T: Pleural effusions due to Cryptococcus neoformans: A review of the literature and report of two cases with cryptococcal antigen determinations. Am Rev Respir Dis 121:743, 1980.

50. Baker R: The primary pulmonary lymph node complex of Cryptococcus. Am J Clin Pathol 65:83, 1976.

51. Salyer W, Salyer D, Baker R: Primary complex of Cryptococcus and pulmonary lymph nodes. J Infect Dis 130:74, 1974.

52. Tynes B, Mason K, Jennings A, Bennett J: Variant forms of pulmonary cryptococcosis. Ann Intern Med 69:1117, 1968.

53. Clinicopathologic conference, case 37-1978. N Engl J Med 299:644, 1978.

54. Farmer S, Komorowski R: Histologic response to capsule-deficient Crptococcus neoformans. Arch Pathol 96:383, 1973.

55. Kent T, Layton J: Massive pulmonary cryptococcosis. Am J Clin Pathol 38:596, 1962.

56. Gleason T, Hammar S, Barthas M, et al. Cytological diagnosis of pulmonary cryptococcosis. Arch Pathol Lab Med 104:384, 1980.

57. Gutierrez F, Fu Y, Lurie H: Cryptococcosis histologically resembling Histoplasmosis. A light and electron microscopic study. Arch Pathol 99:347, 1975.

58. Harding S, Scheld W, Feldman P, Sande M: Pulmonary infection with capsule-deficient Cryptococcus neoformans. Virchows Arch Pathol Anat 382, 113, 1979.

59. Sarosi G, Davies S: Blastomycosis. Am Rev Respir Dis 120:901, 1979.

60. Cush R, Light R, George R: Clinical and roentgenographic manifestations of acute and chronic blastomycosis. Chest 69:345, 1976.

61. O'Neill R, Penman R: Clinical aspects of blastomycosis. Thorax 25:708, 1970.

62. Rabinowitz J, Busch J, Buttram W: Pulmonary manifestations of blastomycosis. Radiological support of a new concept. Radiology 120:25, 1976.

63. Schwarz J, Salfelder K: Blastomycosis. A review of 152 cases. Curr Top Pathol 65:165, 1977.

64. Witorsch P, Utz J: North American blastomycosis. A study of 40 patients. Medicine 47:169, 1968.

65. Laskey W, Sarosi G: Endogenous activation in blastomycosis. Ann Intern Med 88:50, 1978.

66. Sarosi G, Hammerman K, Tosh F, Kronenberg R: Clinical features of acute pulmonary blastomycosis. N Engl J Med 290:540, 1974.

67. Vanek J, Schwarz J, Hakim S: North American blastomycosis. A study of ten cases. Am J Clin Pathol 54:384, 1970.

68. Weed I. North American blastomycosis. Am J Clin Pathol 25:37, 1955.

69. Hardin H, Scott D: Blastomycosis. Occurrence of filamentous forms in vivo. Am J Clin Pathol 60:104, 1974.

70. Berson S, Brandt F: Primary pulmonary sporotrichosis with unusual fungal mrphology. Thorax 32:505, 1977.

71. Jay S, Platt J, Reynolds R: Primary pulmonary sporotrichosis. Am Rev Respir Dis 115:1051, 1977.

72. Mohr J, Griffiths W, Long H: Pulmonary sporotrichosis in Oklahoma and susceptibilities in vitro. Am Rev Respir Dis 119:961, 1979.

73. Smith A, Morgan W, Hornick R, Funk A: Chronic pulmonary sporotrichosis: Report of a case, including morphologic and mycologic studies. Am J Clin Pathol 54:401, 1970.

74. Agia G, Hurst D, Rogers W: Paracoccidioidomycosis presenting as a cavitating pulmonary mass. Chest 78:650, 1980.

75. Lobritz R, Roberts T, Marraro R, et al. Granulomatous pulmonary disease secondary to Alternaria. JAMA 241:596, 1979.

76. Aslam P, Eastridge C, Hughes F Jr: Aspergillosis of the lung. An eighteen year experinece. Chest 59:28, 1971.

77. Hinson K, Moon A, Plummer N: Broncho-pulmonary as-

pergillosis. A review and a report of eight new cases. Thorax 7:317, 1952.

78. Pennington J: Aspergillus lung disease. Med Clin North Am 64:475, 1980.

79. Young R, Bennett J, Vogel C, et al.: Aspergillosis. The spectrum of the disease in 98 patients. Medicine 49:147, 1970.

80. Gefter W, Weingrad T, Epstein D, et al.: "Semi-invasive" pulmonary aspergillosis. A new look at the spectrum of *Aspergillus* infections of the lung. Radiology 140:313, 1981.

81. Brown E, Freedman S, Arbeit R, Come S: Invasive pulmonary aspergillosis in an aparently nonimmunocompromised host. Am J Med 69:624, 1980.

82. Cooper J, Weinbaum D, Aldrich T, Mandell G: Invasive aspergillosis of the lung and pericardium in a nonimmunocompromised 33 year old man. Am J Med 71:903, 1981.

82a. Burton J, Zachery J, Bessin R, et al.: Aspergillosis in four renal transplant recipients. Diagnosis and effective treatment wih amphotericin B. Ann Intern Med 77:383, 1972.

83. Emmons R, Able E, Tenenberg D, Schachter J: Fatal pulmonary psittacosis and aspergillosis. Case report of dual infection. Arch Intern Med 140:697, 1980.

84. Mirsky H, Cuttner J: Fungal infection in acute leukemia. Cancer 30:348, 1972.

85. Pennington J: Aspergillus pneumonia in hematologic malignancy. Improvements in diagnosis and therapy. Arch Intern Med 137:769, 1977.

86. Rose H, Varkey B: Deep mycotic infection in the hsopitalized adult. A study of 123 patients. Medicine 54:499, 1975.

87. Orr D, Myerowtiz R, Dubois P: Pathoradiologic correlation of invasive pulmonary aspergillosis in the compromised host. Cancer 41:2028, 1978.

88. Sinclair A, Rossof A, Coltman C Jr: Recognition and successful management in pulmonary aspergillosis in leukemia. Cancer 42:2019, 1978.

89. Borkin M, Arena F, Brown A, Armstrong D: Invasive aspergillosis with massive fatal hemoptysis in patients with neoplastic disease. Chest 78:835, 1980.

90. Libshitz H, Pagani J: Aspergillosis and mucormycosis. Two types of opportunistic fungal pneumonia. Radiology 140:301, 1981.

90a. Fisher B, Armstrong D, Yu B, Gold S: Invasive aspergillosis. Progress in early diagnosis and treatment. Am J Med 71:571, 1981.

91. Cho S, Choi H: Opportunistic fungal infection among cancer patients. An autopsy study. Am J Clin Pathol 72-617, 1979.

92. Bartrum R Jr, Watnick M, Herman P: Roentgenographic findings in pulmonary mucormycosis. Am J Roentgenol Radium Ther Nucl Med 117:810, 1973.

93. Brown J, Gottlieb L, McCormick R: Pulmonary and rhinocerebral mucormycosis. Successful outcome with amphotericin B and griseofulvin therapy. Arch Intern Med 137:936, 1977.

94. Lehrer R, Howard D, Sypherd P, et al.: Mucormycosis. Ann Intern Med 93 (part 1): 93, 1980.

95. Meyer R, Rosen P, Armstrong D: Phycomycosis complicating leukemia and lymphoma. Ann Intern Med 77:871, 1972.

96. Murray H: Pulmonary mucormycosis with massive fatal hemoptysis. Chest 68:65, 1975.

97. Record N Jr, Ginder D: Pulmonary phycomycosis without obvious predisposing factors. JAMA, 235:1256, 1976.

98. Agger W, Maki D: Mucormycosis. A complication of critical care. Arch Intern Med 138:925, 1978.

99. Straatsma B, Zimmerman L, Gass J: Phycomycosis. A clinicopathologic study of fifty-one cases. Lab. Invest 11:963, 1962.

100. Gaines J, Remington J: Disseminated candidiasis in the surgical patient. Surgery 72:730, 1972.

101. Law E, Kim O, Stieritz D, McMillan B: Experience with systemic candidiasis in the burned patient. J Trauma 12:543, 1972.

102. Myerowitz R, Pazin G, Allen C: Disseminated candidiasis. Changes in incidence, underlying diseases and pathology. Am J Clin Pathol 68:29, 1977.

103. Parker J Jr, McCloskey J, Knauer K: Pathobiologic features of human candidiasis. A common deep mycosis of the brain, heart and kidney in the altered host. Am J Clin Pathol 65:991, 1976.

104. Masur H, Rosen P, Armstrong D: pulmonary disease caused by Candida species. Am J Med 63:914, 1977.

105. Wingard J, Merz W, Saral R: Candida tropicalis: A major pathogen in immunocompromised patients. Ann Intern Med 91:539, 1979.

106. Dubois P, Myerowitz R, Allen C: Pathoradiologic correlation of pulmonary candidiasis in immunosuppressed patients. Cancer 40:1026, 1977.

106a. Kassner E, Kauffman S Yoon J, et al.: Pulmonary candidiasis in infants: Clinical, radiologic and pathologic features. AJR 137:707, 1981.

107. Ramirez G, Shuster M, Kozub W, Pribor H: Fatal acute Candida albicans bronchopneumonia. Report of a case. JAMA 199:118, 1967.

108. Louria D, Stiff D, Bennett B: Disseminated moniliasis in the adult. Medicine 41:307, 1962.

109. Rose H, Sheth N: Pulmonary candidiasis. A clinical and pathological correlation. Ann Intern Med 138:964, 1978.

110. Aisner J, Schimpff, Sutherland J, et al.: Torulopsis glabrata infections in patients with cancer. Increasing incidence and relationship to colonization. Am J Med 61:23, 1976.

111. Aisner J, Sickles E, Schimpff S: Torulopsis glabrata pneumonitis in patients with cancer. Report of three cases. JAMA 230:584, 1974.

112. Valdivieso M, Luna M, Bodey G, et al.: Fungemia due to torulopsis glabrata in the compromised host. Cancer 38:1750, 1976.

113. Grimley P, Wright L, Jennings A: Torulopsis glabrata infection in man. Am J Clin Pathol 43:216, 1965.

114. Alture-Werber E, Edberg S, Singer J: Pulmonary infection with *Allescheria boydii*. Am J Clin Pathol 66:1019, 1976.

115. Walker D, Adamec T, Krigman M: Disseminated petriellidosis (allescheriosis). Arch Pathol Lab Med 102:158, 1978.

116. Winston D, Jordan M, Rhodes J: *Allescheria boydii* infections in the immunosuppressed host. Am J Med 63:830, 1977.

117. Varkey B, Rose H: Pulmonary aspergilloma. A rational approach to treatment. Am J Med 61:626, 1976.

118. Cohen M, Brook C, Naylor B, et al.: Pulmonary phycomycetoma in a patient with diabetes mellitus. Am Rev Respir Dis 116:519, 1977.

119. Kirkpatrick M, Pollock H, Wimberley N: An intracavitary fungus ball composed of Syncephalastrum. Am Rev Respir Dis 120:843, 1979.

120. Arnett J, Hatch H Jr: Pulmonary allescheriasis. Report of a case and review of the literature. Arch Intern Med 135:1250, 1975.

121. Bakerspigel A, Wood T, Burke S: pulmonary allescheriasis. Report of a case from Ontario, Canada. Am J Pathol 68:299, 1977.

122. Putnam J, Harper W, Greene J Jr, et al.: *Coccidioides immitis*. A rare cause of pulmonary mycetoma. Am Rev Respir Dis 112:733, 1975.

123. Kwon-Chung K, Schwartz I, Rybak B: A pulmonary fungus

ball produced by *Cladosporium cladosporioides*. Am J Clin Pathol 64:564, 1975.

124. Wilhite J, Cole F: Invasion of pulmonary cavities by *Nocardia asteroides*. Report of five cases. Am Surg 32:107, 1966.

125. Fahey P, Utell M, Hyde R: Spontaneous lysis of mycetomas after acute cavitating lung disease. Am Rev Respir Dis 123:336, 1981.

126. Chaplin A: Histopathologic occurrence and characterization of calcium oxalate: A review. J Clin Pathol 30:800, 1977.

127. Kurrein F, Green G, Rowles S: Localized deposition of calcium oxalate around a pulmonary Aspergillus niger fungus ball. Am J Clin Pathol 64:556, 1975.

128. Nime F, Hutchins G: Oxalosis caused by Aspergillus infection. Johns Hopkins Med J 133:183, 1973.

129. Burke B, Good R: *Pneumocystis carinii* infection. Medicine 52:23, 1973.

130. Dutz W: *Pneumocystis carinii* pneumonia. Pathol Annu, 5:309, 1970.

131. Robbins J, DeVita V Jr, Dutz W (eds): Symposium on *Pneumocystis carinii* infection. Natl Cancer Inst Monogr 43:1, 1976.

132. Walzer P: *Pneumocystis carinii* infection. South Med J 70:1330, 1977.

133. Hughes W: Pneumocystis pneumonia: A plague of the immunosuppressed. Johns Hopkins Med J 143:184, 1978.

134. Fossieck B Jr, Spagnolo S: *Pneumocystis carinii* pneumonitis in patients with lung cancer. Chest 78:721, 1980.

135. Price R, Hughes W: Histopathology of *Pneumocystis carinii* infestation and infection in malignant disease in childhood. Hum Pathol 5:737, 1974.

136. Center for Disease Control Morbidity and Mortality Weekly Report. Kaposi's sarcoma and *Pneumocystis* pneumonia among homosexual men—New York City and California, vol. 30, 1981, p 305.

136a. Murray J, Felton C, Garay S, et al.: Pulmonary complications of the acquired immunodeficiency syndrome. New Engl J. Med 310:1682, 1984.

136b. Marchevsky A, Rosen M, Chrystal G, Kleinerman J: Pulmonary complications of the acquired immunodeficiency syndrome: A clinicopathologic study of 70 cases. Hum Pathol 16:659, 1985.

137. Mahan C, Sale G: Rapid methenamine silver stain for Pneumocystis and fungi. Arch Pathol Lab Med 102:351, 1978.

138. Dee P, Winn W, McKee K: *Pneumocystis carinii* infection of the lung: Radiologic and pathologic correlation. AJR 132:741, 1979.

139. Huang S, and Marshall K. *Pneumocystis carinii* infection. A cytologic, histologic and electron microscopic study of the organism. Am Rev Respir Dis 102:623, 1970.

140. Binford C, Connor D (eds): *Pathology of Tropical and Extraordinary Diseases*. Washington DC: Armed Forces Institute of Pathology, 1976.

141. Askin F, Katzenstein A: Pneumocystis infection masquerading as diffuse alveolar damage: A potential source of diagnostic error. Chest 79:420, 1981.

142. Weber W, Askin F, Dehner L: Lung biopsy in *Pneumocystis carinii* pneumonia. Am J Clin Pathol 67:11, 1977.

143. Cruickshank B: Pulmonary granulomatous pneumocystosis following renal transplantation. Report of a case. Am J Clin Pathol 63:384, 1975.

144. LeGolvan D, Heidelberger J: Disseminated granulomatous *Pneumocystis carinii* pneumonia. Arch Pathol 95:344, 1973.

145. Demicco W, Stein A, Urbanetti J, Fanburg B: False negative biopsy of *Pneumocystis carinii* pneumonia. Chest 75:389, 1979.

146. Bowling M, Smith M, Wescott S: A rapid staining procedure for *Pneumocystis carinii*. Am J Med Techol 39:267, 1973.

147. Cameron R, Watts J, Kasten B: *Pneumocystis carinii* pneumonia. An approach to rapid laboratory diagnosis. Am J Clin Pathol 72:90, 1979.

148. Pintozzi R: Modified Grocott's methenamine silver nitrate method for quick staining of *Pneumocystis carinii*. J Clin Pathol 31:803, 1978.

149. Campbell W Jr: Ultrastructure of pneumocystis in human lung. Life cycle in human pneumocystosis. Arch Pathol 93:312, 1972.

150. Sueishi K, Hisano S, Sumiyoshi A, Tanaka K: Scanning and transmission electron microscopic study of pulmonary pneumocystosis. Chest 72:213, 1977.

150a. Golden J, Hollander H, Stulbarg M, Gamsu G: Bronchoalveolar lavage as the exclusive diagnostic modality for Pneumocystis carinii pneumonia. Chest 90:18, 1986.

150b. Tuazon C, Delaney M., Simon G, Witorsch P, Varma V: Utility of Gallium^{67} scintigraphy and bronchial washings in the diagnosis and treatment of pneumocystis carinii pneumonia in patients with the Acquired Immunodeficiency Syndrome. Am Rev Resp Dis 132:1087, 1985.

151. Larrieu A, Wiener I, Gomez L, Williams E: Human pulmonary dirofilariasis presenting as a solitary pulmonary nodule. Chest 75:511, 1979.

152. Prioleau W, Parker E, Bradham R, Gregorie H Jr: *Dirofilaria immitis* (dog heartworm) as a pulmonary lesion in humans. Ann Thorac Surg 21:382, 1976.

153. Robinson N, Chavez C, Conn J: Pulmonary dirofilariasis in man. J Thorac Cardiovasc Surg 74:403, 1977.

154. Awe R, Mattox K, Alvarez A, et al.: Solitary and bilateral pulmonary nodules due to *Dirofilaria immitis*. Am Rev Respir Dis 112:445, 1975.

155. Levinson E, Ziter F Jr, Westcott J: Pulmonary lesions due to *Dirofilaria immitis* (dog heartworm). Radiology 131:305, 1979.

156. Navarret-Reyna A, Noon G: Pulmonary dirofilariasis manifested as a coin lesion. Arch Pathol 85:266, 1968.

157. Case records of the Massachusetts General Hospital, case 13-1979. N Engl J Med 300:723, 1979.

158. Harrison G, Thompson J Jr: Dirofilariasis of human lung. Am J Clin Pathol 43:224, 1965.

159. Merrill J, Otis J, Logan W Jr, Dvais M: The dog heartworm (*Dirofilaria immitis*) in man. An epidemic pending or in progress? JAMA 243:1066, 1980.

160. Dayal Y, Neafie R: Human pulmonary dirofilariasis. A case report and review of the literature. Am Rev Respir Dis 112:437, 1975.

161. Leonardi H, Lapey J, Ellis F Jr: Pulmonary dirofilariasis: Report of a human case. Thorax 32:612, 1977.

162. Neafie R, Piggott J: Human pulmonary dirofilariasis. Arch Pathol 92:342, 1971.

General Reading

Baker R. *Human Infection with Fungi, Actinomycetes and Algae*. New York, Springer-Verlag, 1971.

Katzenstein A. The histologic spectrum and differential diagnosis of necrotizing granulomatous inflammation in the lung. In Fenoglio C, Wolff M (eds): *Progress In Surgical Pathology*, vol 2. New York, Masson, 1980, pp 41–70.

Putnam J, Tuazon C (eds): Symposium on infectious lung diseases. Med Clin North Am 64:317, 1980.

15 Pulmonary Disease in the Immunocompromised Host

Andrew Churg

Over the last 10 to 15 years, pulmonary disease in patients who are immunocompromised because of disease or therapy for disease has become a major problem in large medical centers. Most occurrences have been in those patients with underlying malignancy, especially a hematopoietic or lymphoreticular malignancy, those receiving cytotoxic therapy for a malignancy, those with organ transplants, and, less commonly, those with collagen disease treated with high doses of steroids.[1-12] The significance of pulmonary disease in this group can be appreciated from the experience at the National Cancer Institute, where 43 percent of deaths in a large series of lymphoma and leukemia patients were caused by pneumonia.[1] In renal transplant patients, the incidence of pneumonia is less common (10 to 20 percent),[4,5] but half of those affected die of their pulmonary disease. The problem is complicated by the fact that many infections are caused by unusual organisms requiring specialized and often potentially toxic treatment, for example, the antifungal agent amphotericin B. Although infection remains the most common cause of pulmonary infiltrates in this group of patients (accounting for 75 percent of cases in a series of 151 cancer and transplant patients at the Massachusetts General Hospital),[6] a variety of other processes may be seen as well, as noted in Table 15–1. These include drug and radiation reactions, recurrent tumor, emboli, hemorrhage, and edema, and most require their own specific therapy.

In the last 6 years, another form of immunosuppression, the acquired immunodeficiency syndrome (AIDS), has become a common disease in some areas. The disease is characterized in its full blown state by the appearance of opportunistic infections such as pneumocystis or cytomegalovirus pneumonia and/or a fulminant variety of Kaposi's sarcoma in patients with no apparent predisposing cause for immunologic abnormalities. These patients have profound immunodepression with leukopenia, anergy, and poor T-cell responsiveness to a variety of mitogens. Reversal of the T-helper/suppressor cell ratio is common.[13-20] About 75 percent of cases have been seen in homosexuals, another 13 percent in intravenous drug abusers, and the remainder in hemophiliacs who have received blood products, apparently otherwise normal Haitians, contacts of patients with the syndrome, and rarely in persons who do not fit into any of the above groups.[17] Mortality has been greater than 40 percent and may in fact be 100 percent, since no long-term cures have been reported. The disease is caused by a human T-cell leukemia virus.[21] From a diagnostic viewpoint, much of the pulmonary disease seen in this group is similar to that seen in the traditional type of immunocompromised patient, and the descriptions in this chapter apply to both groups, except as noted.

There is an extensive literature dealing with the clinical aspects of disease in immunocompromised patients,[1-12] and various clinical and radiographic schemes have been devised to attempt an etiologic diagnosis without resort to biopsy. In a proportion of cases, particularly bacterial pneumonias,[1] the process resolves before biopsy is required. In many others, however, standard antibiotic treatment, examinations, and cultures based on sputum or transtracheal aspirates are unrevealing, and biopsy is performed in an attempt to define an etiology for the infiltrate. (Detailed descriptions of pathologic processes associated with the various infective agents seen in these patients can be found in Chapters 11–14). This chapter considers three areas: (1) types of reaction patterns seen in the lungs of immunocompromised patients; (2) results of various types of biopsy procedures; and (3) handling of biopsies from such patients.

Pathologic Reaction Patterns

A variety of different pathologic reaction patterns can be seen in biopsies from immunocompromised patients

Table 15-1. Causes of Pulmonary Infiltrates in Immunocompromised Patients

Infections
  Bacterial
  Fungal
  Viral
  Chlamydial
  Protozoal
  Mycoplasma
  Helminthic
Pulmonary edema
Pulmonary hemorrhage
Embolism
Infarction
  From Emboli
  From fungal vascular occlusion
Radiation
Drug toxicity
Transfusion reactions
Neoplasms
Underlying collagen disease
Synergistic reactions

Table 15-2. Pathologic Reaction Patterns in Immunocompromised Patients

Diffuse alveolar damage/chronic interstitial pneumonia/organizing pneumonia
  Infections
    Viral
    Fungal
    Bacterial
    Pneumocystis
  Radiation
  Drug reactions
  Oxygen therapy
  Collagen disease
  Combinations of above
Usual interstitial pneumonia
  Underlying collagen disease
Interstitial pneumonia with foamy alveolar infiltrates penumocystis
  Alveolar proteinosis
  ? Mycobacteria
  ? Drugs
Acute pneumonia
  Non-necrotizing
    Bacteria
  Necrotizing
    Mycobacteria
    Fungi
    Gram-negative bacteria
    Viruses
    Nocardia
  Infarct-like or nodular
    Fungi
    Viruses
Granulomas
  Non-necrotzing
    Drug reactions
    Pneumocystis
    Reactions to tumor
  Necrotizing
    Mycobacteria
    Fungi
Necrotizing tracheobronchitis/bronchiolitis
  Viruses
  Chlamydia
Diffuse alveolar hemorrhage
Tumors

(Table 15-2). The following discussion, which is based partly on the scheme proposed by Nash,[22] tries to correlate etiologic agents with reaction patterns; however, there is a great deal of variation from case to case, and because these patients react poorly to many infectious agents, the patterns seen are often atypical for the given agent. An important conclusion from this observation is that special stains must always be performed, even if there is no morphologic reason to believe a given organism is present. A second conclusion is that culture for all types of agents is a critical part of the biopsy process. Culture results should always be checked before rendering a negative or nonspecific report. Multiple processes (for example, two infections or infection plus tumor) are not unusual in this type of patient; finding one infective agent on the first stain examined does not obviate the need to examine the rest.

Diffuse Alveolar Damage/Chronic Organizing or Chronic Interstitial Pneumonia

In collected series (see below), some 30 to 40 percent of open biopsies and a larger portion of transbronchial biopsies show a pattern that appears as diffuse alveolar damage with various degrees of chronicity and organization, or as a chronic interstitial pneumonia, which is probably derived from organization of diffuse alveolar damage. Histologically the typical pattern of diffuse alveolar damage with hyaline membranes in alveolar ducts and collapse of alveolar parenchyma is usually obvious. Superimposed on this may be variable amounts of interstitial inflammation and fibrosis as well as air space filling by proliferating granulation tissue (Fig. 15-1). Hyperplastic alveolar epithelium and metaplastic bronchiolar epithelium are commonly present, as are hyperchromatic and enlarged alveolar lining cells. In some instances, hyaline membranes are sparse or not present, and one finds what appears to be an active interstitial pneumonia (see Fig. 15-1). Much less commonly, there is marked diffuse interstitial fibrosis with little air space reaction. In most instances, the pathologic process is diffuse and bilateral, or, in radiation pneumonia, follows the radiation port. However, occasionally a similar process is seen pathologically when the radiographic picture is that of localized, even nodular lesions.[23,24]

The range of agents that can produce this picture is remarkably large (Tables 15-2, 15-3) and includes

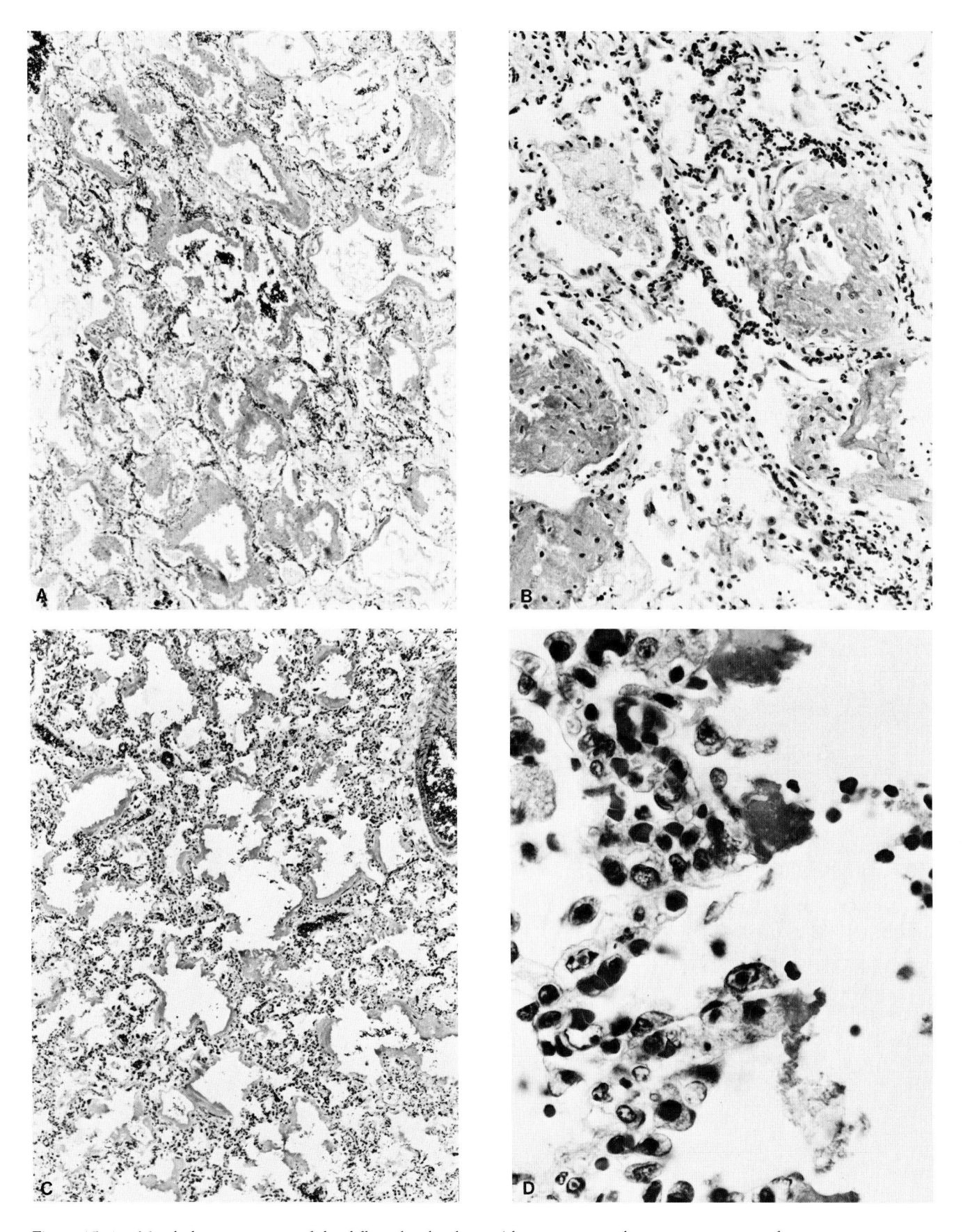

Figure 15–1. Morphologic variations of the diffuse alveolar damage/chronic interstitial pneumonia pattern of reaction seen in many biopsies from immunosuppressed patients. A and B. Acute diffuse alveolar damage characterized by many hyaline membranes and an interstitial inflammatory infiltrate in a patient with lymphoma who has received multiple chemotherapeutic agents. This appearance is nonspecific and has many different possible causes (1A ×20, B ×160). C and D. Diffuse alveolar damage of specific etiology; in this instance, varicella pneumonia in a patient with acute myelogenous leukemia. Numerous inclusions can be seen in the higher-power view. Such well-defined causes of diffuse alveolar damage are relatively uncommon in this group of patients (C ×20, D ×400).

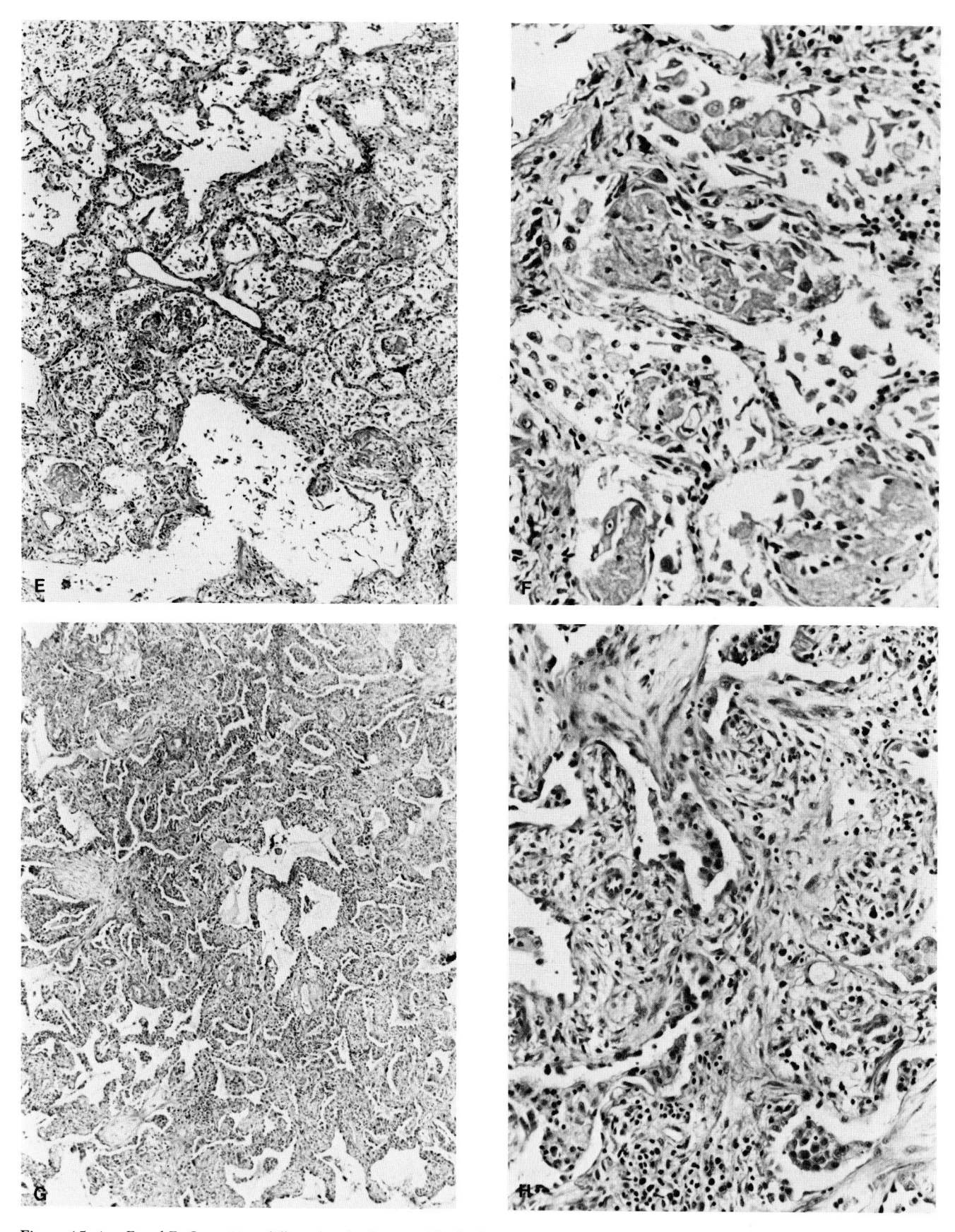

Figure 15–1. E and F. Organizing diffuse alveolar damage. The higher-power view shows the growth of the pulmonary epithelium over the fragmented hyaline membranes that will eventually be incorporated into the interstitium. From a patient with lymphoma treated with multiple chemotherapeutic agents (E ×20, F ×160). G and H. Another variant of this process in which the appearance is that of a relatively diffuse and homogenous of a chronic interstitial pneumonia. Note the extensive air space organization visible particularly in the higher-power view. Most of the fibrous tissue is clearly of recent origin. This appearance should not be confused with the common type of usual interstitial pneumonia, since it most likely represents a subacute or organizing form of diffuse alveolar damage. From a renal transplant patient (G ×20, H ×160).

Table 15–3. Cytoxic Drugs Reported to Produce Diffuse Alveolar Damage/Interstitial Pneumonia[a]

Bulsulfan	Chlorambucil
Cyclophosphamide	Melphalan
Uracil mustard	Bleomycin
Mitomycin	Zinostatin
6-Mercaptopurine	Methotrexate
Procarbazine	Carmustine (BCNU)
Semustine	

[a] Based on the results of Weiss and Muggia.[30]

cytotoxic drugs, radiation, oxygen therapy, bacterial sepsis, and bacterial, fungal, viral, and pneumocystis pneumonias.[22, 25–31] There is also evidence that some of these agents, particularly the combinations of oxygen and cytotoxic drugs[32] or drugs and radiation,[32] act synergistically. Careful histologic examination to define an infective agent is critical, and, as mentioned previously, so are examination of special stains and culture results. Inclusions of cytomegalovirus or a herpes virus, for example, may be easily found or may only be demonstrable on culture[26]; adenovirus inclusions are often extremely difficult to detect by light microscopy, and influenza and respiratory syncytial virus rarely produce visible inclusions. Special stains sometimes demonstrate a totally unexpected agent, for example, *Pneumocystis carinii* pneumonia appeared histologically as diffuse alveolar damage in 9 of 17 cases reported by Askin and Katzenstein.[25]

Radiation is another agent that produces diffuse alveolar damage and chronic interstitial pneumonia. There is little evidence to support the claim of distinctive vascular changes in radiation pneumonia; in fact the microscopic features are generally not distinguishable from those caused by drugs or infectious agents.[32] More helpful is the gross or radiographic finding of disease sharply limited to the radiation port.

In the absence of a documented infectious cause, there is a tendency to report this type of histologic pattern as a drug-induced injury, particularly when enlarged alveolar lining cells are present.[27, 28] However, enlarged hyperchromatic alveolar lining cells are not specific to any type of drug, with the possible exception of the bizarre cells seen after busulfan therapy,[22] and in the author's experience, may be seen following drugs, radiation, or oxygen. Any of the cytotoxic agents listed in Table 15–3 can produce the same picture, and the majority of patients have been treated with more than one drug.

Nash[22] has equated this histologic picture with usual interstitial pneumonia (UIP), but in most instances, the disease seen in immunocompromised patients is much more active and much more evenly and diffusely spread than is the case in UIP. In addition, in immunocompromised patients, organization and fibrosis are "recent" (the pattern is that of granulation tissue rather than dense fibrosis) and frequently involves air space as well as interstitium, whereas in UIP, as a rule, the process appears much older and predominantly involves the interstitium. This rule is not invariable, and intermediate histologic features may be seen. Some immunocompromised patients will show a UIP picture, particularly those with an underlying collagen disease or those with old radiation or drug injury. In this circumstance, a knowledge of the clinical situation is extremely helpful in making the diagnosis. If the history is one of gradually increasing dyspnea/infiltrates over weeks to months, a diagnosis of UIP-like reaction on the basis of drugs, radiation, and so forth is reasonable. If the current process is acute, a histologic background of UIP probably does not explain the acute episode and another diagnosis must be sought.

The nonspecificity of this process must be emphasized, and this is even more true of transbronchial biopsies than open biopsies (see later). The latter type of biopsy can easily miss a few viral inclusions or a few air spaces with foamy infiltrate of pneumocystis that might be found on an open biopsy. Cultures of the biopsy should always be checked before rendering a diagnosis when this pattern is found. If nothing appears on culture or special stains, this author usually renders a purely descriptive diagnosis and does not attempt to ascribe etiology unless the patient falls into one on the narrowly restrictive categories just described.

Interstitial Pneumonia with Foamy Exudate

Diffuse interstitial pneumonia accompanied by a foamy alveolar infiltrate is the pattern classically described for infection by *Pneumocystis carinii*[25, 29, 33] (Fig. 15–2A, B). In practice, an entirely typical picture is the exception rather than the rule with this organism. Weber and colleagues[29] found atypical histologic features in 69 percent of cases; in 47 percent foamy exduate was not present at all, and 33 percent had only interstitial fibrosis and inflammation. Even when foamy exudate is present, it may be extremely focal, and careful examination of the entire biopsy with hematoxylin and eosin (H&E) and silver stains is critical for the diagnosis. Pneumocystis may also produce a granulomatous or giant cell reaction[29] or diffuse alveolar damage.[25] Figure 15–2C shows a case in which another process is present, and pneumocystis is identified without any accompanying reaction. Whether the organism is the actual pathogen in such instances is not clear.

In general the histologic picture of foamy exudate is readily recognized, but occasionally there may be confusion with alveolar proteinosis.

Alveolar Proteinosis

Although pulmonary alveolar proteinosis most often occurs in patients with normal immune systems, it may be seen in immonocompromised patients.[34] The most common association has been with mycobacterial infections, particularly in leukemic patients, but other infective agents and underlying diseases have been reported as well. The histologic picture in such cases is similar to that in nonimmunosuppressed patients, but staining with

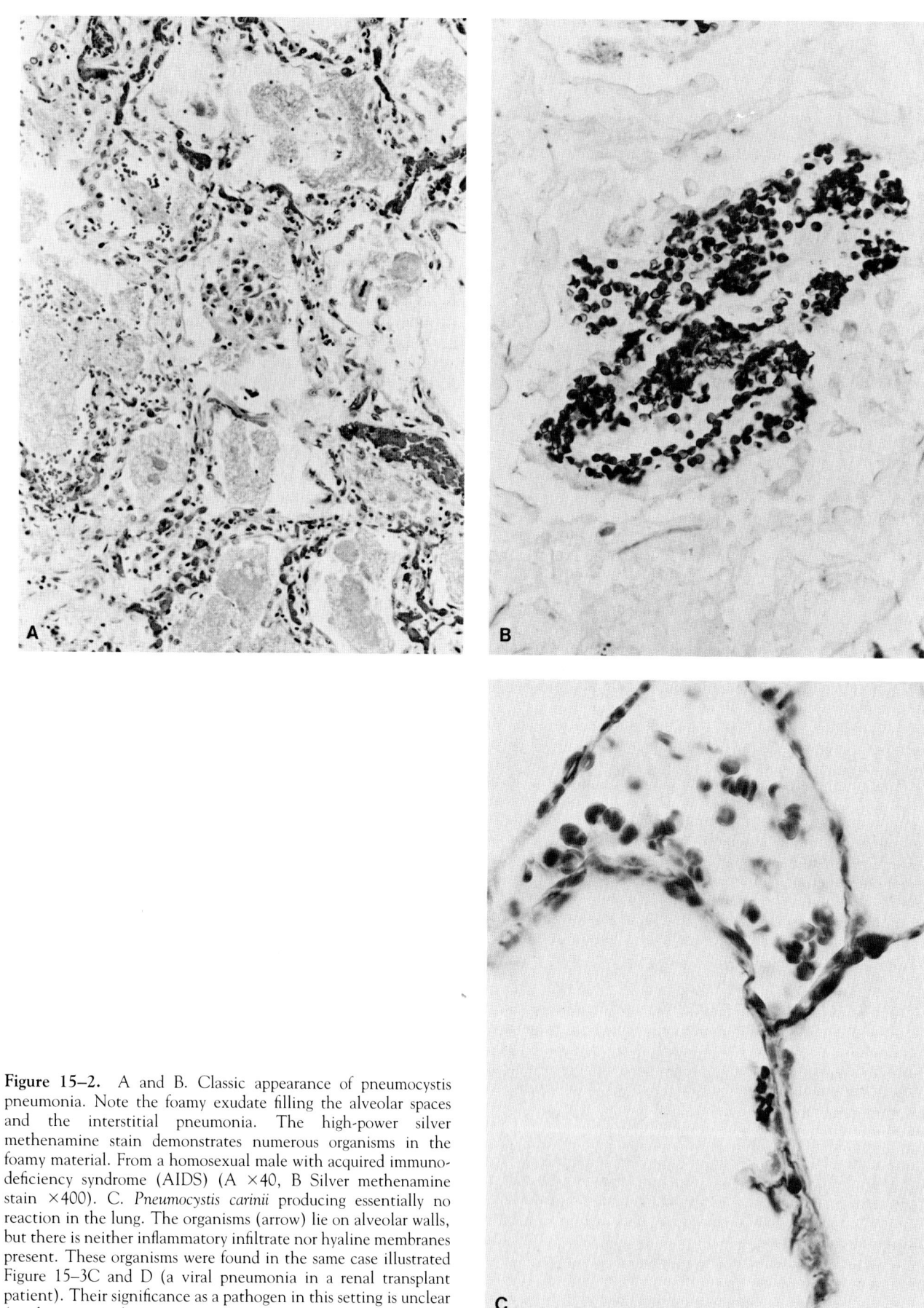

Figure 15–2. A and B. Classic appearance of pneumocystis pneumonia. Note the foamy exudate filling the alveolar spaces and the interstitial pneumonia. The high-power silver methenamine stain demonstrates numerous organisms in the foamy material. From a homosexual male with acquired immunodeficiency syndrome (AIDS) (A ×40, B Silver methenamine stain ×400). C. *Pneumocystis carinii* producing essentially no reaction in the lung. The organisms (arrow) lie on alveolar walls, but there is neither inflammatory infiltrate nor hyaline membranes present. These organisms were found in the same case illustrated Figure 15–3C and D (a viral pneumonia in a renal transplant patient). Their significance as a pathogen in this setting is unclear (methenamine silver stain, ×400).

antibody to surfactant apoprotein may fail to demonstrate the immunoreactive material seen in the air spaces in ordinary proteinosis.[35] Singh and associates[35] suggested that this situation, which they termed secondary alveolar proteinosis, is actually a different process than the "primary" form in which alveoli are filled with material which does stain for surfactant. It is commonly supposed that proteinosis in this setting is caused by infection or by impaired alveolar clearance,[34] but in fact infection may be secondary, and, given the numerous drugs (either cytotoxic or antimicrobial) with which these patients are treated, the primary process may actually be a toxic drug reaction.

Non-Necrotizing Pneumonias

Judging by responses to antibiotic therapy, bacterial pneumonia caused by ordinary pathogens is one of the most common infective processes in immunocompromised patients. These cases come to biopsy relatively infrequently and histologically are no different from the usual bacterial pneumonia.

Necrotizing Pneumonias

Many different types of organisms including ordinary bacteria, Nocardia, fungi, viruses, protozoa such as *Toxoplasma gondii*, and helminths such as *Strongyloides stercoralis* can produce necrotizing lesions. In the usual bacterial or nocardial pneumonia, polymorphonuclear leukocytes are generally present in large numbers, but this may not be true in granulocytopenic patients. A common example is the necrosis and perivascular growth of organisms seen in pneumonia caused by Pseudomonas. Legionella is another bacterium which tends to produce a necrotizing pneumonia.[36] Fungi such as Aspergillus, Mucor, and Candida may evoke a marked neutrophilic response, but they are particularly common in granulocytopenic leukemic patients and may produce only extensive necrosis. Fungal disease as a whole is frequent in leukemic patients: in the series of DeGregorio and associates,[37] 27 percent of patients had an invasive fungal infection. Cytomegalovirus and Herpes simplex or zoster infections may produce necrotizing nodules, either few or many in a miliary pattern[22] (Fig. 15–3A, B). The polymorphonuclear leukocyte reaction in such nodules is often characterized by extensive karyorrhexis, a phenomenon which is not specific but can be an indicator that virus may be present (Fig. 15–3C, D). The difficulties of demonstrating inclusions in such cases have been noted previously. Electron microscopy may be of value in adenoviral pneumonias, in which the organisms are widespread even when not apparent by light microscopy; however, "blind" cutting of electron microscopic sections will almost never reveal Herpes or cytomegalovirus inclusions unless large numbers can be found by light microscopy.

Mycobacterial infections in immunocompromised patients may show a wide range of reactions, from classic granulomas to extensive necrosis with virtually no cellular reaction.[38–40] Stains for acid-fast organisms will often demonstrate huge numbers of organisms in this setting (Fig. 15–4). Severe disseminated infection with atypical myobacteria and reactionless acellular necrosis is apparently frequent in patients with AIDS.[39, 49]

Necrotizing Pneumonia with Infarction

Aspergillus, Mucor species, and *Petrillidium boydii*[41] show a distinct propensity to invade vessels, resulting in both hematogenous spread of the organisms and infarction of tissue. Fungal infarcts of this type are as a rule not subpleural and wedge-shaped, but are distinctly spherical and on cut section may show a peculiar hemorrhagic targetting pattern.[42] The latter is also sometimes seen with viral pneumonias. Prezyjemski and Mattli[43] and Sinclair and colleagues[44] have shown that, if the patient recovers enough immunologic function to contain the organism, this type of fungal infarct will be converted to a walled-off fungus ball.

Necrotizing Granulomatous Reactions

Necrotizing granulomas may be seen with mycobacterial infection or with a variety of fungi, including *Histoplasma capsulatum*, *Coccidiodes immitis*, and *Cryptococcus neoformans*, and Helminths. The extent to which the granulomas are well-defined structures varies with the immune status of the patients, and extensive necrosis without giant cells or epithelioid histiocytes may predominant. *Cryptococcus neoformans* may evoke only a minimal macrophage response.

Non-Necrotizing Granulomas

Poorly formed, non-necrotizing granulomas are not common but have been reported with pneumocystis[29] and as a probable drug reaction, particularly in patients treated with cyclophosphamide.[27, 28] In the latter situation, the granulomas are usually seen in conjunction with the pattern of diffuse alveolar damage/organizing pneumonia. Granulomas may also be seen as a response to tumors, especially Hodgkin's disease (Fig 15–5). In the author's experience, this reaction is less common in the lung than in hilar lymph nodes.

Tracheobronchitis/Bronchiolitis

Tracheobronchitis/bronchiolitis is a common pattern of response to viral infection.[22] The process may be severe with extensive necrosis of the airway epithelium, and a surrounding karyorrhexic polymorphonuclear leukocyte infiltrate (Fig. 15–6). In other instances, there is only focal loss of epithelium, and atypical regenerative forms may be present. Diagnosis requires either the finding of inclusions or culture evidence of the organism. Ito and

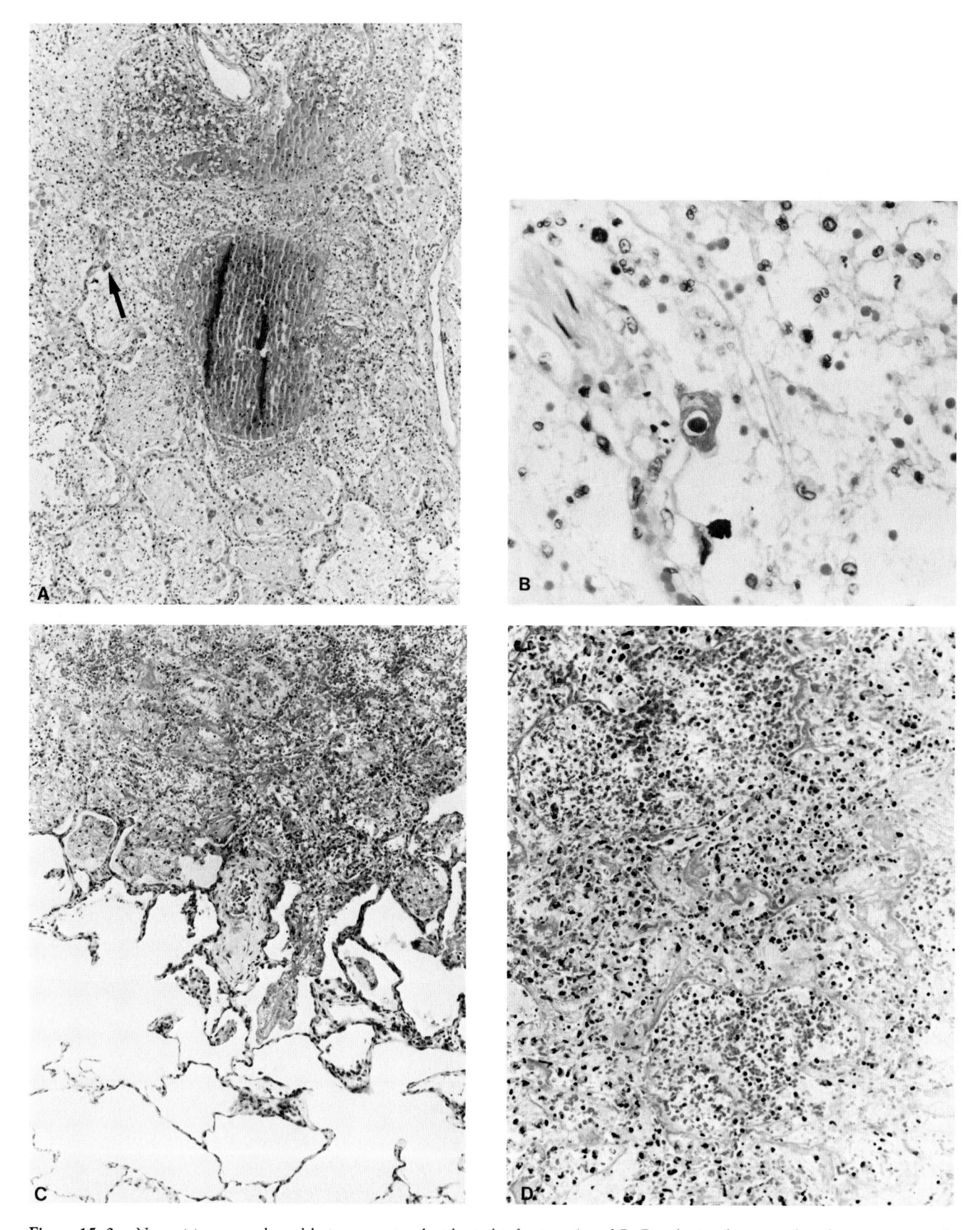

Figure 15–3. Necrotizing parenchymal lesions associated with viral infections A and B. Developing focus in a lymphoma patient with cytomegalovirus infection. An inclusion can be seen in the low-power view (arrow) and is illustrated more clearly in the high-power view (A ×20, B ×400). C and D. One of many necrotizing nodules seen in the lung of a renal transplant patient with clinical evidence of Herpes zoster infection. Although no viral inclusions were seen by microscopy, Herpes was grown from a culture of the biopsy. Note the numerous karyorrhexic fragments in the higher power view, which suggest the possibility of viral pneumonia. Necrotizing foci are seen with many infectious agents in this patient group; when no organism can be found by light microscopic examination, viral infection should be considered. Note also the surrounding pulmonary parenchyma: this apparently normal lung tissue harbored the Pneumocystis organisms shown in Figure 15–2C (C ×40, D ×160).

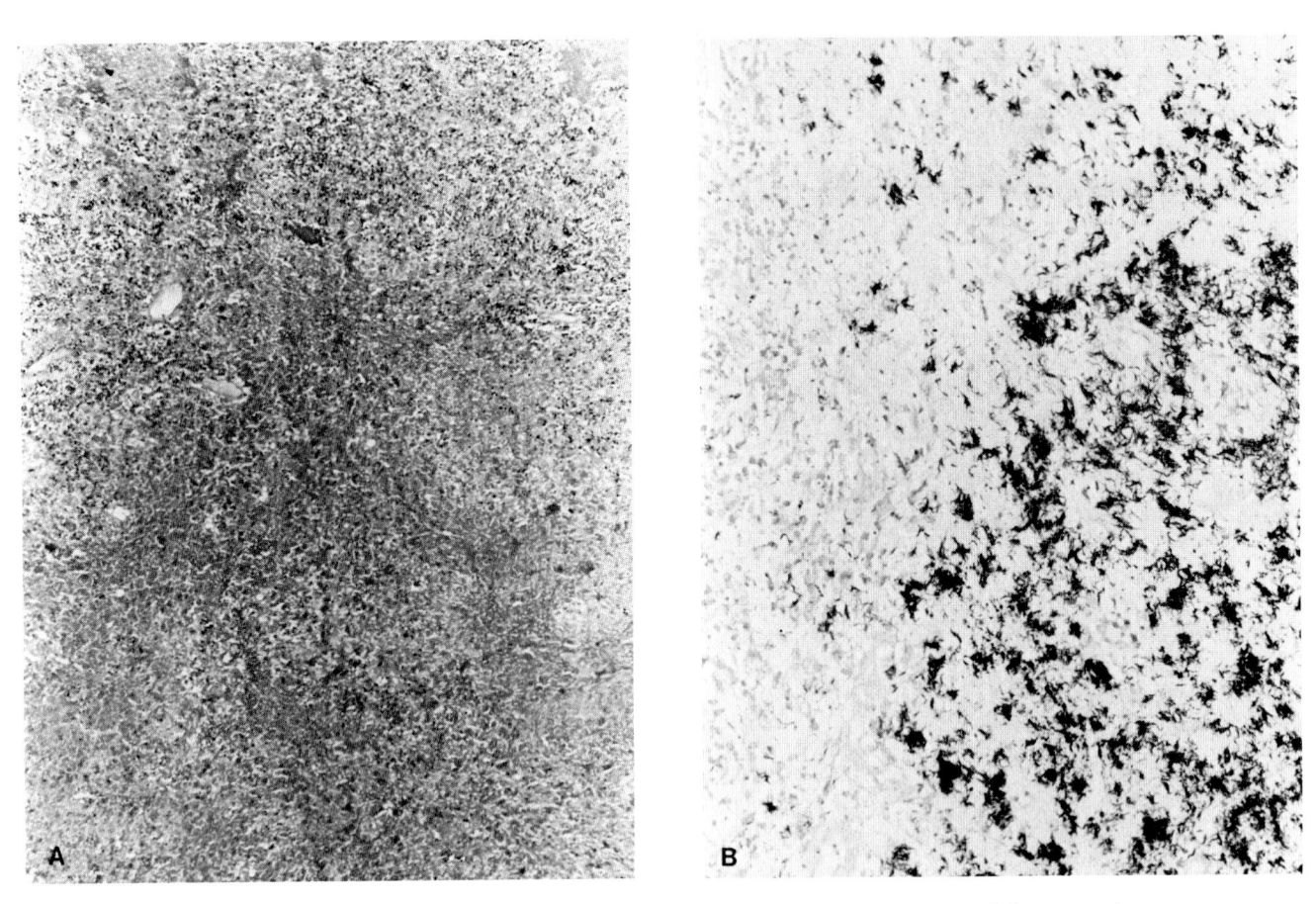

Figure 15–4. A and B. Necrotizing nongranulomatous inflammation caused by atypical mycobacteria in a patient with hairy cell leukemia. Note the numerous organisms visible in B (A ×10, B Ziehl-Nielson, ×160).

associates[45] have reported a bronchiolocentric reaction pattern in a patient with chlamydial pneumonia; the diagnosis was obtained by culture and serologic evidence of infection.

Diffuse Pulmonary Hemorrhage (Chapter 18)

Diffuse hemorrhage without any other abnormality visible by light microscopic examination is common as a cause of fever and radiographic infiltrates in immunocompromised patients. The majority of cases are seen in individuals with low platelet counts. Another category of hemorrhage is that seen in patients with systemic lupus. In this setting, hemorrhage may be acute and life threatening. The light microscopic picture is not distinctive, but electron microscopy or immunohistochemical examination will reveal granular immune complex deposits[46] (Fig. 15–7). This finding is of value since some of these patients will respond to steroids or immunosuppressive agents.

Tumors

In general the diagnosis of recurrent or new neoplasm is straightforward; it should not be forgotten that tumors, particularly lymphomas, may develop in transplant patients and in patients with AIDS.[47–49] Transbronchial biopsies are adequate when the neoplastic cells are cytologically malignant and the presence of only a few such cells confirms the diagnosis. However, the diagnosis of conditions in which cytologic changes are minimal and evaluation of the low-power pattern is required—for example, chronic lymphocytic leukemia or well-differentiated lymphocytic lymphoma—is usually impossible by transbronchial biopsy. Kaposi's sarcoma (Fig. 15–8) may also be difficult to confirm by this means if only relatively bland proliferating fibroblast-like cells are seen. A survey of histologic appearances of this tumor is provided by Enzinger and Weiss.[50]

Diagnostic Yield and Long-Term Consequences of Various Biopsy Procedures

This section tabulates results from some of the many different reported series of biopsies in immunocompromised patients in order to provide some idea of the efficacy of various biopsy procedures in obtaining a diagnosis. This task is not entirely straightforward, since they underlying disease proportions vary from series to series and, in some instances, are based on transplant patients rather than patients with underlying neoplasm. Some interpretation has been necessary to squeeze these data into the same format, and there may be small differences from the apparent original numbers. Tables 15–4 through 15–9 and Figure 15–9 also include data on a series of 106 patients who underwent open lung biopsy at Stanford between 1970 and 1978 and who were followed for 6 months or more. Of this group, 96 had an underlying malignancy and 10 were transplant or collagen disease cases. About half of these cases were included in the series of Rossiter and associates.[51]

A variety of invasive procedures have been used to attempt a specific diagnosis in patients with pulmonary infiltrates. The two in common use are transbronchial biopsy and open lung biopsy. Cutting needle biopsy has been occasionally employed and returns a reasonably high yield (specific diagnosis in 46 percent of cutting needle biopsies in the series of Greenman and colleagues[52]; 65 percent in the series of Cunningham and colleagues[53]), but produces serious pneumothorax in a large number of instances[53, 54] and is not widely employed. Fine needle aspiration and bronchial brushing

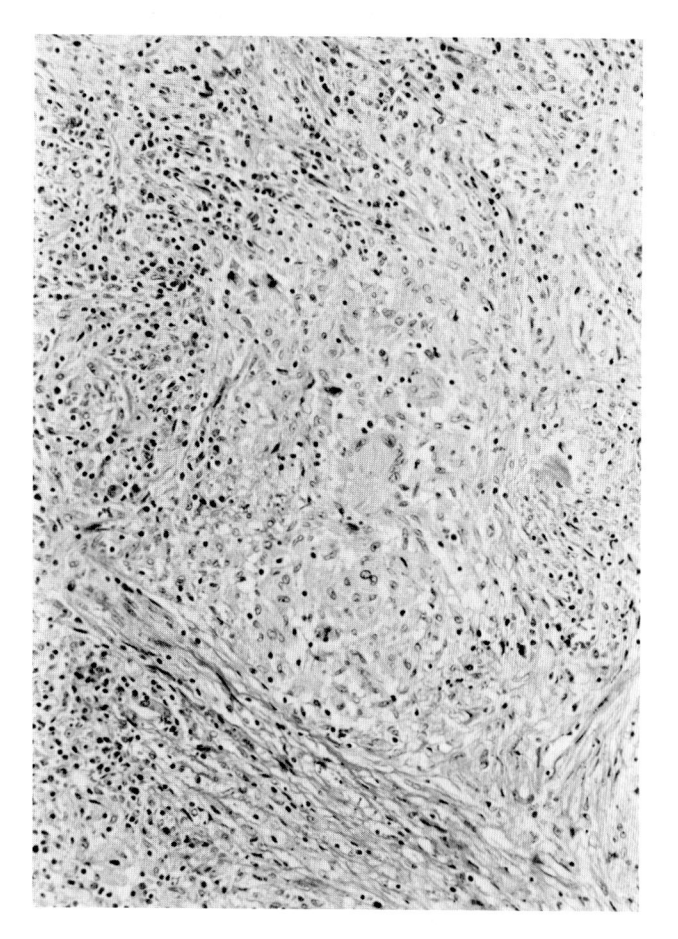

Figure 15–5. Noncaseating granuloma occurring in the lung of a patient with Hodgkin's disease. Tumor was present elsewhere in the lung (×160).

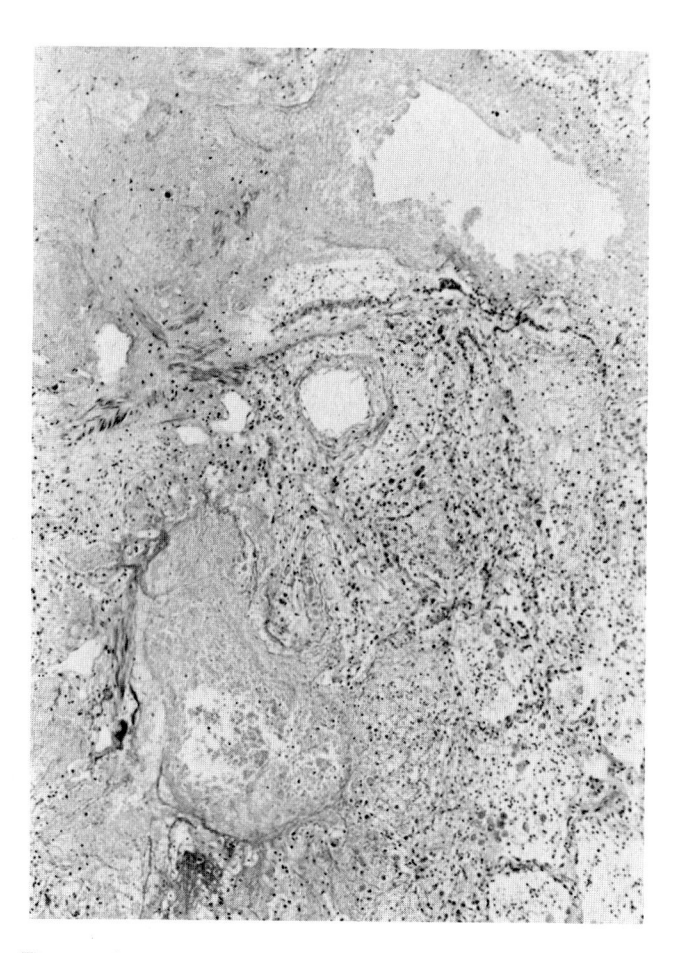

Figure 15–6. Necrotizing bronchiolitis, another typical viral infection pattern, produced in this instance by cytomegalovirus (same case as Figure 15–3A and B). A small amount of respiratory epithelium is still present in the upper portion of the field, and the lumen of the affected bronchiole is still partially patent. This pattern can be produced by a wide variety of viruses. (×20).

are also used[52, 53, 55] in some institutions, but the resulting material most commonly is used for microbiologic rather than pathologic examination.

Tables 15–4 through 15–7 show the results obtained in 240 transbronchial biopsies and almost 350 open biopsies. Transbronchial biopsy produced a specific diagnosis in 35 percent of cases, whereas open lung biopsy produced a specific diagnosis in 61 percent of cases. Despite some variation, there is remarkably good uniformity of these values from report to report. Infection accounted for the largest proportion of specific diagnosis: 27 percent of all diagnoses and 75 percent of specific diagnoses obtained by transbronchial biopsy were infectious; similarly 39 percent of all diagnoses and 64 percent of specific diagnoses obtained by open biopsy were infectious. By far the largest single contributor to these numbers was infection by *Pneumocystis carinii*, which accounted for 39 percent of infectious diagnoses obtained by transbronchial biopsy and 57 percent of infectious diagnoses obtained by open lung biopsy.

Most of the remaining specific diagnoses were neo-

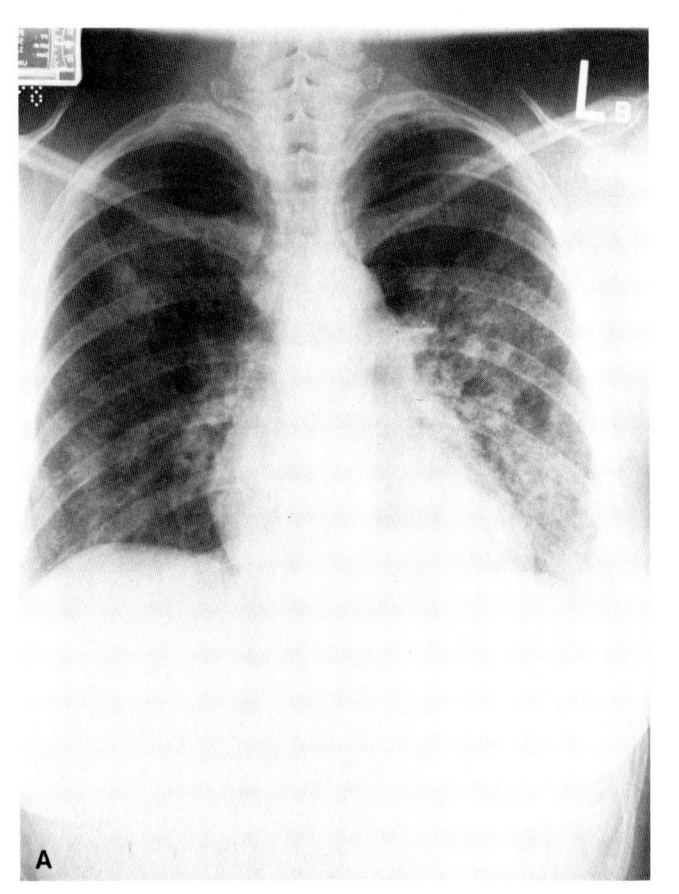

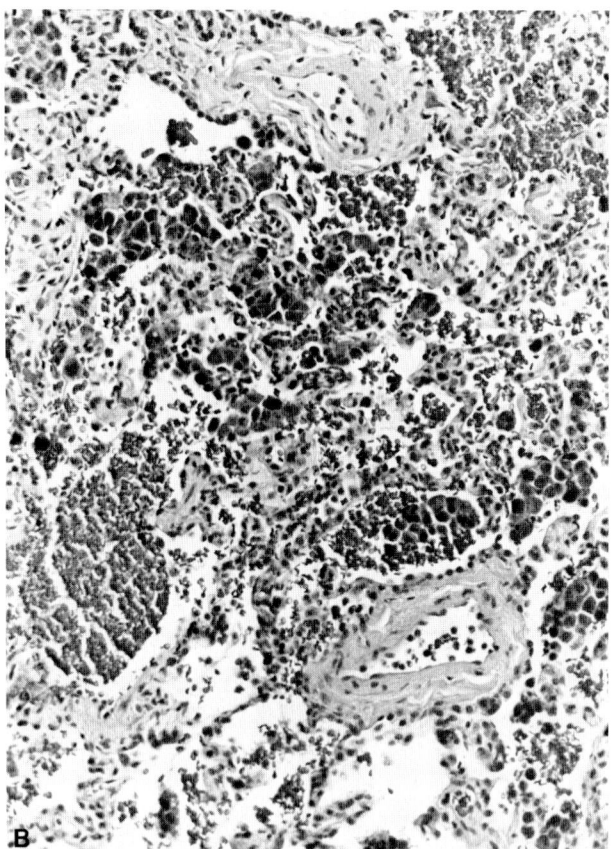

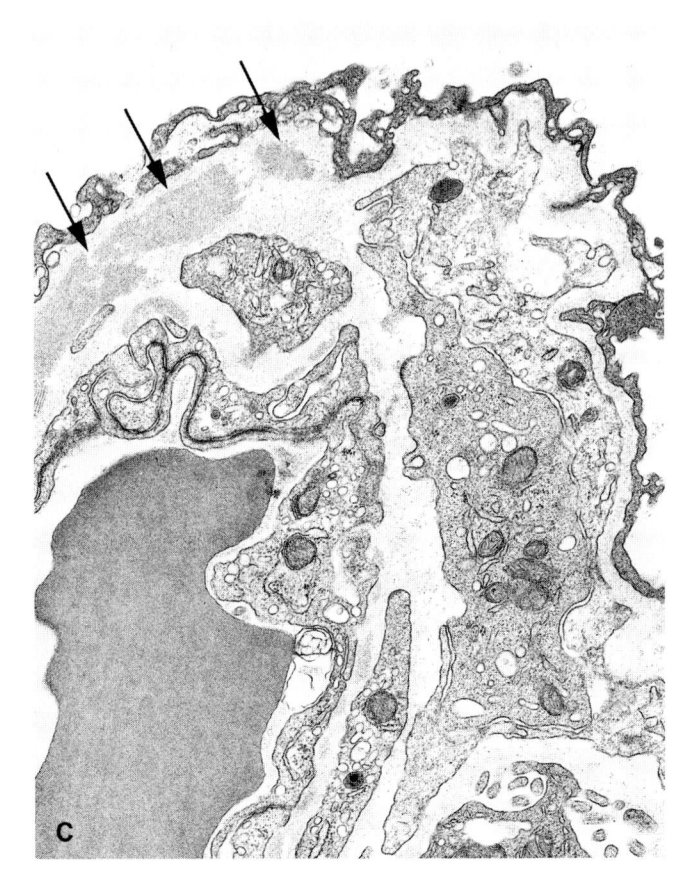

Figure 15–7. Immune complex-induced hemorrhage in a patient with systemic lupus. The patient presented with fevers and hemoptysis. A. Chest radiograph showed the alveolar infiltrates. B. Open biopsy demonstrated only diffuse hemorrhage (×160). C. However, immune complex deposits (arrows) were visible by electron microscopy and by immunofluorescence examination in alveolar walls. (C ×1200, from Churg A et al.: Arch Pathol Lab Med 104:388, 1980).

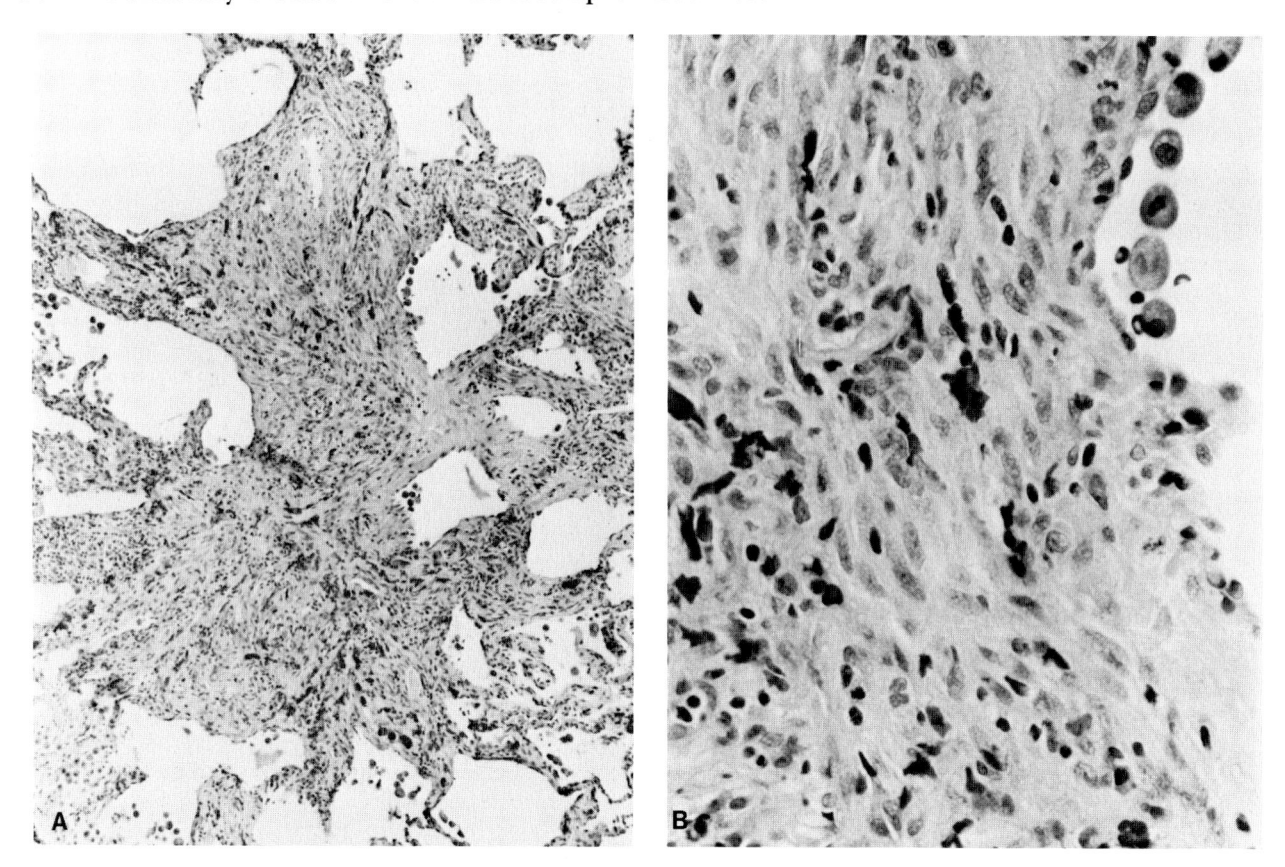

Figure 15–8. Low- and high-power views of Kaposi's sarcoma in the lung of a homosexual man with AIDS. Note the spindled cells and red blood cells in slit-like spaces. The cytologically bland appearance of this tumor can make diagnosis difficult, particularly on transbronchial biopsy (A ×64, B ×400).

plasms, accounting for 23 percent of specific diagnoses by transbronchial biopsy and 30 percent of specific diagnoses by open biopsy. Other specific diagnoses were seen in only 3 to 5 percent of cases. The conclusions from these data are straightforward: a nonspecific diagnosis can be expected in 30 to 50 percent of open biopsies, and in 50 to 80 percent of transbronchial biopsies. Not surprisingly, transbronchial biopsies are more useful for detecting infections and open biopsies for detecting neoplasms. However, these data do not support the claim of Poe and associates[59] that a negative transbronchial biopsy virtually excludes a treatable opportunistic infec-

Table 15–4. Results of Transbronchial Biopsy in Immunocompromised Patients

Series	Number Biopsies	Specific Diagnosis	Nonspecific Diagnosis
Katzenstein and Askin[56]	50	18 (36%)	32 (64%)
Feldman et al.[57]	38	10 (26%)	28 (74%)
Cunningham et al.[53]	31	13 (42%)	18 (58%)
Matthay et al.[58]	25	18 (72%)	7 (26%)
Poe et al.[59]	35	14 (40%)	21 (60%)
Jaffe and Maki[60]	22	7 (32%)	15 (68%)
Springmeyer et al.[61]	19	4 (21%)	15 (79%)
Toledo-Pereyra et al.[62]	20	1 (5%)	19 (95%)
Total	240	85 (35%)	155 (65%)

Table 15–5. Breakdown of Specific Diagnoses Obtained by Transbronchial Biopsy

Series	Infection	Pneumocystis	Neoplasm
Katzenstein and Askin[56]	12/50	6/12	6/50
Feldman et al.[57]	10/38	—	0/38
Cunningham et al.[53]	12/31	6/12	1/31
Matthay et al.[58]	14/25	1/14	3/25
Poe et al.[59]	7/35	4/7	7/35
Jaffe and Maki[60]	4/22	0/4	3/22
Springmeyer et al.[61]	4/19	3/4	0/19
Toledo-Pereyra et al.[62]	1/20	1/1	0/20
Proportion of all diagnoses	64/240 (27%)	21/240 (9%)	20/240 (8%)
Proportion of specific diagnoses	64/85[a] (75%)	21/54 (39%)[b]	20/85 (23%)

[a] Total number of specific diagnoses from Table 15–4.
[b] Proportion of all infection.

Table 15-6. Results of Open Lung Biopsies in Immunocompromised Patients

Series	Number Cases	Specific Diagnosis	Nonspecific Diagnosis
Jaffe and Maki[60]	26	19 (73%)	7 (27%)
Springmeyer et al.[61][a]	24	11 (46%)	13 (54%)
Toledo-Pereyra et al.[62]	13	10 (77%)	3 (23%)
Leight and Michaelis[63]	42	30 (71%)	12 (29%)
Singer et al.[64]	44	27 (61%)	17 (39%)
Hiatt et al.[65]	68	25 (37%)	43 (63%)
Waltzer et al.[66][b]	23	17 (74%)	6 (26%)
Present report	106	71 (67%)	35 (33%)
Total	346	210 (61%)	136 (39%)

[a] Bone marrow transplant patients.
[b] Renal transplant patients.

tion; in fact the recent report of Springmeyer and colleagues,[61] in which transbronchial biopsy detected only 4 of 11 infections found on open biopsy, and the study of Toledo-Pereyra and colleagues,[62] in which transbronchial biopsy missed 4 infections subsequently found on open biopsy, distinctly contradict Poe and associates.[59]

Open biopsy is always assumed to be the gold standard, but it is unclear whether even open biopsy results are always to be believed in this context. Hiatt and associates[65] compared biopsy and autopsy results in 28 patients; in ten cases, there was a major discrepancy between the two results, most often the finding of a specific treatable condition in the autopsy specimen had not been present in the biopsy. Seven of 19 patients with treatable conditions at autopsy had not been receiving appropriate therapy. This report must, however, be viewed with caution, since the interval between biopsy and autopsy apparently was long in many instances and the pathologic picture in the lung could have changed in

Table 15-7. Breakdown of Specific Diagnoses from Open Biopsy

Series	Infection	Pneumocystis	Neoplasm
Jaffe and Maki[60]	13/26	6/13	4/26
Springmeyer et al.[61]	11/24	5/11	0/24[a]
Toledo-Pereyra et al.[62]	4/13	3/4	6/13
Leight and Michaelis[63]	21/42	10/21	1/42
Singer et al.[64]	21/44	17/21	6/44
Hiatt et al.[65]	14/65	4/14	8/65
Waltzer et al[66]	17/23	3/17	0/23[b]
Present report	34/106	29/34	37/106
Proportion of all diagnoses	135/343 (39%)	77/343 (22%)	62/343 (18%)
Proportion of specific diagnoses	135/210[c] (64%)	77/135 (57%)[d]	62/210 (30%)

[a] Bone marrow transplantation patients.
[b] Renal transplant patients.
[c] Total number of specific diagnoses from Table 15-6.
[d] Proportion of all infections.

Table 15-8. Autopsy versus Open Biopsy Diagnosis in Patients who Died within Two Weeks of Biopsy[a]

Open Biopsy Diagnosis	Autopsy Diagnosis
Nonspecific findings: 8	Nonspecific: 6
	Infection: 2
Infection: 6	Infection: 2
	Neoplasm: 4

[a] See text for details of these patients.

the interval. The author examined the correlation between biopsy and autopsy in 14 patients of the 106 described previously who died within 2 weeks of biopsy (Table 15-8). For eight patients with an initial nonspecific diagnosis (usually diffuse alveolar damage/chronic interstitial pneumonia), the diagnosis was confirmed in six, but two others had infections. Of six patients with infectious diagnoses on open biopsy, the diagnosis was confirmed in two, but four others had evidence of neoplastic disease, Again, the time interval in several of these cases is sufficiently long that a new infection may have developed or a previous infection may have disappeared as a consequence of treatment, but the conclusion still remains that even open biopsy probably misses a sizable fraction of specific diagnoses in this situation.

One naturally tends to assume that a specific biopsy diagnosis will result in improved survival, but it is by no means clear that this assumption is correct. Greenman and associates[52] claimed that 70 percent of those with specific diagnoses recovered, compared with 25 percent of those with nonspecific diagnoses, but in fact 38 of their 78 patients (49%) died during hospitalization, 22 of them with 1 week of biopsy. As shown on Table 15-9, three subsequent reports have failed to demonstrate any significant difference in survival between those with specific and those with nonspecific diagnoses. There are little data on the effects of different diagnoses or of change in therapy, but what data exist are not encouraging. Hiatt and associates[65] found that 56 percent of patients with a treatable disease on biopsy never left the hospital. In the 106 patients mentioned, the survival curves for those with a change of therapy as a result of biopsy and those with

Table 15-9. Mortality in Immunocompromised Patients Undergoing Lung Biopsy

Series	Time Period (months)	With Specific Diagnosis (%)	With Nonspecific Diagnosis (%)
Greenman et al.[52]	?	30	75
Katzenstein and Askin[56]	2	39	35
Cunningham et al.[53]	2	44	39
Present report	1	30	28
	6	49	56

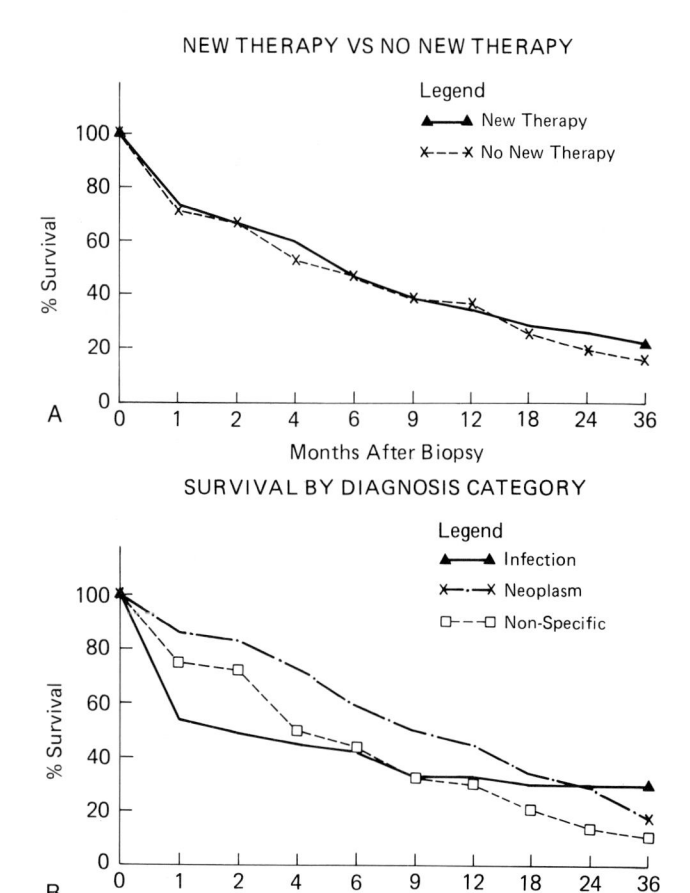

Figure 15–9. Survival data for the group of 106 immunosuppressed patients undergoing lung biopsy as described in the text. A. Survival plotted against time after biopsy for those with a change of therapy made on the basis of the biopsy versus those with no change of therapy. B. Survival as a function of the diagnosis of neoplasm, infection, or nonspecific process.

no change were identical (Fig. 15–9A). In this group, patients with infection fared worse initially than those with neoplasms or nonspecific diagnoses (Fig. 15–9B), but by 6 months, the differences were not statistically significant and the 6-month mortality was approximately 50 percent. Whether these findings indicate that biopsy is allowing adjustment to optimal therapy in a group of patients with a poor prognosis (if they have an underlying malignancy), or whether they imply that blind antimicrobial therapy might in many instances be just as effective, is a question that needs to be considered. It is worth noting that pneumocystis pneumonia accounted for 40 to 60 percent of infectious diagnoses in the collected series listed previously. Most of these date from the period before the widespread prophylactic use of Septra[67,68]; assuming that current therapy greatly decreases the incidence of pneumocystis pneumonia, the specific yield from biopsy is likely to drop sharply in the future.

Handling of Lung Biopsies from Immunocompromised Patients

In general these biopsies are handled much the same way as biopsies from nonimmunocompromised patients (*see* Chapter 5). Appropriate culture is of course critical, and the pathologist's first duty should be to ensure that cultures for routine and unusual bacteria, fungi, mycobacteria, and viruses have been taken. Similarly, every specimen must be stained for fungi and acid-fast organisms and with a Gram's stain, even if a specific agent or diagnosis may be apparent on H&E stain. If Legionnaires' disease is suspected, the Dieterle silver stain or a specific immunohistochemical stain can be added.[69,70] *Toxoplasma gondii* is more easily seen with period acid-Schiff stain. The auramine/rhodamine fluorescent stain provides a quick and efficient screen for acid-fast bacilli.

If no frozen section is desired, open biopsies should always be inflated; a simple technique has been published.[71] In the author's experience, touch preparations stained with methenamine silver are just as effective as frozen sections in demonstrating *Pneumocystis carinii* and do not suffer from the tendency of frozen sections to fall off the slide in hot staining baths; however, they are disadvantageous because one does not get to examine tissue reaction pattern. Rosen and colleagues[72] have advocated use of a Wright-Giemsa staining for detecting pneumocystis, but many pathologists (personal communication) find this difficult to interpret even on touch preparations and virtually useless for tissue. Several rapid variants of the traditional 3-hour methenamine silver stain have been developed.[73,74]

Electron microscopy generally has little role in the diagnosis of lung disease in the immunocompromised. A limited role exists for the demonstration of some types of viral inclusion, but, as noted previously, not for the demonstration of herpes or cytomegalovirus. Electron microscopy is useful in detecting immune complexes in patients with lupus and pulmonary hemorrhage.

Immunohistochemical techniques are also of limited but definite usefulness. One application is the diagnosis of Legionnaires' disease. Another is the demonstration of immune complex deposits in patients with pulmonary hemorrhage. Immunohistochemical staining is also useful for demonstrating viral infection where good quality specific antisera are available.

Except for the issue of time course, the specific clinical features in a given case provide relatively little aid to the pathologist. However, one should still be sure that the pathologic findings correlate with the general setting of a febrile patient with more or less widespread radiographic infiltrates. For example, the pattern of diffuse alveolar damage/chronic interstitial pneumonia fits this setting. However, the finding of small isolated granulomas with no other reaction and no staining for organisms is of no clinical help, even though these granulomas might in fact represent a drug or tumor reaction. This principle should not be overused: the finding of a few penumocystis organisms and otherwise little change may indicate that a widespread pneumocystis infection is present and that the biopsy has missed the major lesions; care should be exercised in rendering interpretations in this setting.

References

1. Fanta CH, Pennington JE: Fever and new lung infiltrates in the immunocompromised host. Clin Chest Med 2:19, 1981.

2. Mattson K, Edgren J, Kuhlback B: Pulmonary infections after renal transplantation. Ann Clin Res 11:63, 1979.

3. Pennington JE, Feldman NT: Pulmonary infiltrates and fever in patients with hematologic malignancy: Assessment of transbronchial biopsy. Am J Med 62:581, 1977.

4. Rubin RH: The cancer patient with fever and pulmonary infiltrates: Etiology and diagnostic approach. In Remington JS, Swartz MN (eds): *Current Clinical Topics in Infectious Disease,* vol 1. New York: McGraw-Hill, 1980, pp 288–303.

5. Rubin RH, Greene R: The immunocompromised patient with fever and pulmonary infiltrates. In Rubin RH, Young LS (eds): *A Clinical Approach To Infection in the Compromised Host.* New York: Plenum, 1981, pp 269–334.

6. Rubin RH: Pneumonia in the immunocompromised host. In Fishman AP (ed): *Update: Pulmonary Diseases and Disorders.* 1982, pp 1–25.

7. Singer C, Turnbull AD: Diffuse interstitial pneumonia in immunocompromised hosts. pp 58–65.

8. Tenholder MF, Hooper RG: Pulmonary infiltrates in leukemia. Chest 78:468, 1980.

9. Williams DM, Krick JA, Remington JS: Pulmonary infection in the compromised host (part 1). Am Rev Respir Dis 114:359, 1976.

10. Williams DM, Krick JA, Remington JS: Pulmonary infection in the compromised host (part 2). Am Rev Respir Dis 114:593, 1976.

11. Wolff LJ, Bartlett MS, Baehner RL, et al.: The causes of interstitial pneumonitis in immunocompromised children: An aggressive systematic approach to diagnosis. Pediatrics 60:41, 1977.

12. Levine AS, Schmipff SC, Graw RG, Young RC: Hematologic malignancies and other marrow failure states: Progress in the management of complicating infections. Semin Hematol 11:141, 1974.

13. Small CB, Klein RS, Friedland GH, et al.: Community-acquired opportunistic infections and defective cellular immunity in heterosexual drug abusers and homosexual men. Am J Med 74:433, 1983.

14. Stahl RE, Friedman-Kien A, Dubin R, et al.: Immunologic abnormalities in homosexual men: Relationship to Kaposi's syndrome. Am J Med 73:171, 1982.

15. Drew WL, Miner RC, Ziegler JL, et al.: Cytomegalovirus and Kaposi's sarcoma in young homosexual men. Lancet 1:125, 1982.

16. Editorial: Immunocompromised homosexuals. Lancet 1:1325, 1981.

17. Editorial: Acquired immunodeficiency syndrome. Lancet 1:162, 1983.

18. Freeman ML, Talbot GH: Nongranulomatous mycobacterial lymphadenitis in homosexual patients. Lab Invest 48:27A, 1983.

19. Green JB, Sidhu GS, Lewin S, et al.: Mycobacterium avium-intracellulare: A cause of disseminated life-threatening infection in homosexuals and drug abusers. Ann Intern Med 97:539, 1982.

20. Masur H, Michelis MA, Wormser GP, et al.: Opportunistic infection in previously healthy women: Initial manifestations of a community-acquired cellular immunodeficiency. Ann Intern Med 97:533, 1982.

21. Gallo RC, Sarin PS, Gelmann EP, et al.: Isolation of human T-cell leukemia virus in acquired immune deficiency syndrome (AIDS). Science 220:865, 1983.

22. Nash G: Pathologic features of the lung in the immunocompromised host. Hum Pathol 13:841, 1982.

23. Bellot PA, Valdiserri RO: Multiple pulmonary lesions in a patient treated with BCNU (1,3-bis-(2-chloroethyl)-1-nitrosourea) for glioblastoma multiforme. Cancer 43:46, 1979.

24. McCrea ES, Diaconis JN, Wade JC, Johnston CA: Bleomycin toxicity simulating metastatic nodules to the lungs. Cancer 48:1096, 1981.

25. Askin FB, Katzenstein ALA: Pneumocystis infection masquerading as diffuse alveolar damage: A potential source of diagnostic error. Chest 79:420, 1981.

26. Craighead JE: Pulmonary cytomegalovirus infection in the adult. Am J Pathol 63:487, 1971.

27. Sostman HD, Matthay RA, Putman CE: Cytotoxic drug-induced lung disease. Am J Med 62:608, 1977.

28. Schein PS, Winokur SH: Immunosuppressive and cytotoxic chemotherapy: Long-term complications. Ann Intern Med 82:84, 1975.

29. Weber WR, Askin FB, Dehner LP: Lung biopsy in *Pneumocystis carinii* pneumonia: A histopathologic study of typical and atypical features. Am J Clin Pathol 67:11, 1977.

30. Weiss RB, Muggia FM: Cytotoxic drug-induced pulmonary disease: Update 1980. Am J Med 68:259, 1980.

31. Witschi HR, Haschek WM, Klein-Szanto AJP, Hakkinen PJ: Potentiation of diffuse lung damage by oxygen: Determining variables. Am Rev Respir Dis 123:98, 1981.

32. Fajardo LF, Berthong M: Radiation injury in surgical pathology I. Am J Surg Pathol 2:159, 1978.

33. Burke BA, Good RA: *Pneumocystis carinii* infection. Medicine 52:23, 1973.

34. Bedrossian CWM, Luna MA, Conklin RG, Miller WC: Alveolar proteinosis as a consequence of immunosuppression. Hum Pathol 11(suppl):527, 1980.

35. Singh G, Katyal SL, Bedrossian CWM, Rogers RM: Pulmonary alveolar proteinosis: Staining for surfactant apoprotein in alveolar proteinosis and in conditions simulating it. Chest 1:82, 1983.

36. Winn WC, Myerowitz RL: The pathology of the Legionella pneumonias. Hum Pathol 12:401, 1981.

37. Degregorio MW, Lee MWF, Linker CA, et al.: Fungal infections in patients with acute leukemia. Am J Med 73:543, 1982.

38. Freeman ML, Talbot GH: Nongranulomatous mycobacterial lymphadenitis in homosexual patients. Lab Invest 48:27A, 1983.

39. Marchevsky A, Damsker B, Gribetz A, et al.: The spectrum of pathology of nontuberculous mycobacterial infections in open-lung biopsy specimens. Am J Clin Pathol 78:695, 1982.

40. Miller WT: Tuberculosis in the immunosuppressed patient. Semin Roentgenol 14:249, 1979.

41. Walker DH, Adamec T, Krigman M: Disseminated petriellidosis (allescheriosis). Arch Pathol Lab Med 102:158, 1978.

42. Orr DP, Myerowitz RL, Dubois PJ: Patho-radiologic correlation of invasive pulmonary aspergillosis in the compromised host. Cancer 41:2028, 1978.

43. Przyjemski C, Mattii R: The formation of pulmonary mycetomata. Cancer 46:1701, 1980.

44. Sinclair AJ, Rossof AH, Coltman CA: Recognition and successful management in pulmonary aspergillosis in leukemia. Cancer 42:2019, 1978.

45. Ito JI, Comess KA, Alexander ER, et al.: Pneumonia due to Chlamydia trachomatis in an immunocompromised adult. N Engl J Med 307:95, 1982.

46. Eagen JW, Memoli VA, Roberts JL, et al.: Pulmonary hemorrhage in systemic lupus erythematosus. Medicine 57:545, 1978.

47. Frenandez R, Moudradian J, Moore A, Asch A: Malignant lymphoma with central nervous system involvement in six homosexual men with acquired immunodeficiency syndrome. Lab Invest 48:25A, 1983.

48. Thiru S, Calne RY, Nagington J: Lymphoma in renal allograft patients treated with cyclosporin-A as one of the immunosuppressive agents. Transplant Proc 13:359, 1981.

49. Ziegler JL, Miner RC, Rosenbaum E, et al.: Outbreak of Burkitt's-like lymphoma in homosexual men. Lancet 2:631, 1982.

50. Enzinger FE, Weiss SW: *Soft Tissue Tumors.* St Louis: CV Mosby, 1983.

51. Rossiter SJ, Miller DC, Churg AM, et al.: Open lung biopsy in the immunosuppressed patient. J Thorac Cardiovasc Surg. 77:338, 1979.

52. Greenman RL, Goodall PT, King D: Lung biopsy in immunocompromised hosts. Am J Med 59:488, 1975.

53. Cunningham JH, Zavala DC, Corry RJ, Keim LW.: Trephine air drill, bronchial brush, and fiberoptic transbronchial lung biopsies in immunosuppressed patients. Am Rev Respir Dis 115:213, 1977.

54. Gaensler EA: Open and closed lung biopsy. In Sackner MA (ed): *Diagnostic Techniques in* Pulmonary Disease Part II. New York, Marcel Decker, 1980, pp. 579-622. II. 1980, pp 579–622.

55. Zavala DC, Schoell JE: Ultrathin needle aspiration of the lung in infectious and malignant disease. Am Rev Respir Dis 123:125, 1981.

56. Katzenstein ALA, Askin FB: Interpretation and significance of pathologic findings in transbronchial lung biopsy. Am J Surg Pathol 4:223, 1980.

57. Feldman NT, Pennington JE, Ehrie MG: Transbronchial lung biopsy in the compromised host. JAMA 238:1377, 1977.

58. Matthay RA, Farmer WC, Odero D: Diagnostic fibreoptic bronchoscopy in the immunocompromised host with pulmonary infiltrates. Thorax 32:539, 1977.

59. Poe RH, Utell MJ, Israel RH, et al.: Sensitivity and specificity of the nonspecific transbronchial lung biopsy. Am Rev Respir Dis 119:25, 1979.

60. Jaffe JP, Maki DG: Lung biopsy in immunocompromised patients: One institution's experience and an approach to management of pulmonary disease in the compromised host. Cancer 48:1144, 1981.

61. Springmeyer SC, Silvestri RC, Sale GE, et al.: The role of transbronchial biopsy for the diagnosis of diffuse pneumonias in immunocompromised marrow transplant recipients. Am Rev Respir Dis 126:763, 1982.

62. Toledo-Pereyra LH, DeMeester TR, Kinealey A, et al.: The benefits of open lung biopsy in patients with previous nondiagnostic transbronchial lung biopsy: A guide to appropriate therapy. Chest 77:647, 1980.

63. Leight GS, Michaelis LL: Open lung biopsy for the diagnosis of acute, diffuse pulmonary infiltrates in the immunosuppressed patient. Chest 73:477, 1978.

64. Singer C, Armstrong D, Rosen PP, et al.: Diffuse pulmonary infiltrates in immunosuppressed patients: Prospective study of 80 cases. Am J Med 66:110, 1979.

65. Hiatt JR, Gong H, Mulder DG, Ramming KP: The value of open lung biopsy in the immunosuppressed patient. Surgery 82:285, 1982.

66. Waltzer WC, Sterioff S, Zincke H, et al.: Open-lung biopsy in the renal transplant recipient. Surgery 88:601, 1980.

67. Hughes WT, Kuhn S, Chaudhary S, et al.: Successful chemoprophylaxis for *Pneumocystis carinii* pnemonitis. N Engl J Med 297:1419, 1977.

68. Winston DJ, Lau WK, Gale RP, Young LS: Trimethoprim-sulfamethoxazole for the treatment of *Pneumocystis carinii* pneumonia. Ann Intern Med 92:762, 1980.

69. Chandler FW, Hicklin MD, Blackmon JA: Demonstration of the agent of Legionnaires' disease in tissue. N Engl J Med 297:1218, 1977.

70. Saravolatz LD, Russell G, Cvitkovich D: Direct immunofluorescence in the diagnosis of Legionnaires' disease. Chest 79:566, 1981.

71. Churg A: An inflation procedure for open lung biopsies. Am J Surg Pathol 7:69, 1983.

72. Rosen PP, Martin N, Armstrong D: *Pneumocystis carinii* pneumonia: Diagnosis by lung biopsy. Am J Med 58:794, 1975.

73. Mahan CT, Sale GE: Rapid methenamine silver stain for Pneumocystis and fungi. Arch Pathol Lab Med 102:351, 1978.

74. Musto L, Flanigan M, Elbadawi A: Ten-minute silver stain for *Pneumocystis carinii* and fungi in tissue sections. Arch Pathol Lab Med 106:292, 1982.

16 Pulmonary Edema and Diffuse Alveolar Injury

James C. Hogg
Anna-Luise A. Katzenstein

Introduction

The lung becomes edematous when the amount of extravascular water present in its exceeds 4 to 5 ml/g of dry blood-free tissue.[1] This can occur either by increasing the pressure across the pulmonary microvasculature (high-pressure edema) or damaging the capillaries so that they leak (increased permeability edema) or by some combination of these two mechanisms. The sequence of events in these two basic forms of edema have some similarities[2] but also important differences. For example, high-pressure edema can usually be reversed quickly when the factor responsible for increasing the pressure is removed. Edema that follows capillary injury, on the other hand, tends to be more prolonged and has a much greater tendency toward organization and progression to acute and chronic interstitial lung disease. In discussing these two forms of edema, we will begin with a description of the microvascular and interstitial spaces and then describe how these change with various disease processes. Because of the very large number of causes of increased permeability edema, we will begin this section with a description of adult respiratory distress syndrome (ARDS) which is the clinical syndrome associated with diffuse alveolar injury in the lung.

The Pulmonary Microvasculature

In general, the term microvascular is preferable to capillary when speaking of the vessels involved in fluid exchange because pulmonary arterioles and venules as well as capillaries can participate in this process.[3] Arterioles that are less than 100 μm in external diameter are normally devoid of muscle and consist of a single elastic lamina lined by endothelium.[4] Pulmonary venules, less than 100 μm in external diameter, have an identical structure and can be separated from arterioles only by their position in the lobule.[4] The capillary density is somewhat variable between species, but in the dog there are approximately 80 capillaries per 100 μm of alveolar septum[5] and there is still controversy as to whether they dilate or are recruited when pulmonary blood flow is increased.[6] The pulmonary capillaries are located both in the flat part of the alveolar wall and in the corners where three alveoli meet (Fig. 16–1). The function of the capillaries at these different locations is of interest in that those at the corners are thought to remain open while the capillaries in the flat portion of the wall collapse when alveolar pressure is higher than pulmonary artery pressure.[6]

The lining of the entire microvasculature consists of flat endothelial cells which are joined by tight junctions.[7] Fluid and solute exchange is thought to take place through "pores" between these cells. These "pores" have been difficult to define anatomically because the total area required for fluid and solute exchange across this endothelial membrane accounts for approximately 10^{-6} of 1 percent of the available endothelial surface area.[8] Because the pores have been so difficult to visualize, their exact location and whether or not they can be stretched by elevating hydrostatic pressure are matters of considerable controversy.[3]

The Interstitial Space

Alveolar Wall Interstitial Space

The alveolar wall interstitial space lies between the basement lamina of the alveolar epithelial and capillary endothelial cells on the thick side of the alveolar wall (see Chapter 2).[9] On the thin side the basal lamina of the

Figure 16–1A. Appearance of alveolar wall when the capillary bed is fully recruited under zone III conditions.

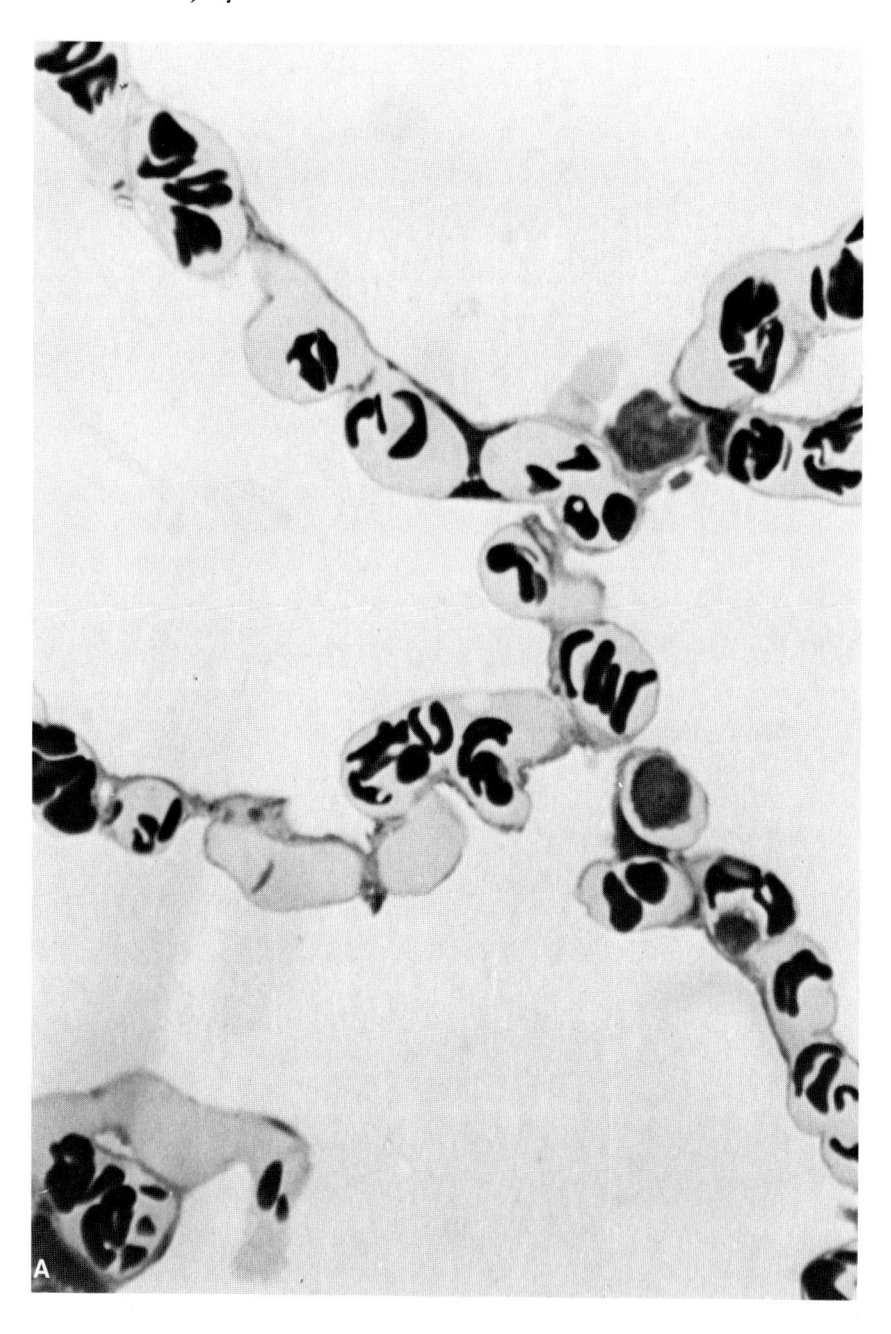

alveolar lining cell and of the capillary endothelial cells fuse, leaving a space estimated at 30 to 50 nm in width. On the thick side the basement membrane of the endothelium and epithelium separate leaving a space that is estimated at about 1 μm in diameter. This tiny space normally contains fluid, elastin and collagen fibrils, proteoglycans, fibroblasts, and macrophages but no lymphatics. This means that fluid leaving the capillaries must traverse the alveolar wall interstitial space to gain access to the lymphatics in the extra-alveolar interstitial space.

Extra-Alveolar Interstitial Space

The interstitial space of the alveolar wall and the extra-alveolar portions of the lung are continuous. The extra-alveolar space surrounds the corner capillaries (see Fig. 16–1) and communicates centrally with the space formed by the connective tissue around the bronchovascular bundle. It also communicates with the space formed by the connective tissue that surrounds the pulmonary lobules. The space contains the lymphatic vessels, which differ from venous capillaries in that they have valves that provide a capability of moving lymphatic fluid to larger lymphatics. The lymph is eventually collected and returned to the vascular compartment by both the right and left lymphatic ducts which drain into systemic veins. The size of the extra-alveolar interstitial space is difficult to estimate but is known to increase as lung volume is increased.[10] Under normal circumstances, this volume is taken up by expansion of the extra-alveolar vessels, but when excess extravascular fluid is present it tends to

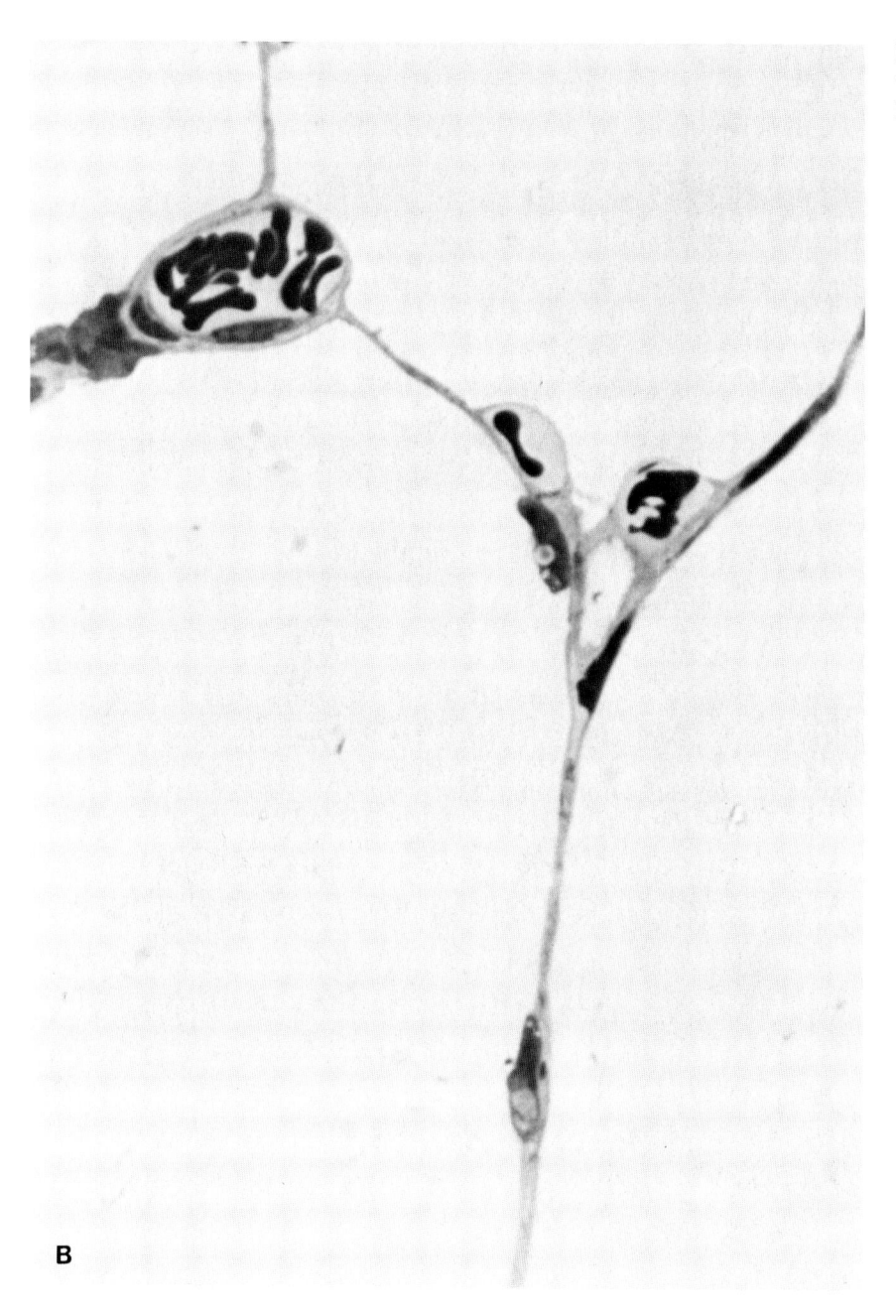

Figure 16–1B. Appearance of the alveolar wall under zone I condition where the most prominent vessels appear at the corners.

collect in this space first.[2] The external surfaces of the lymphatic capillaries are anchored to the connective tissue boundary of the interstitial space,[13] so that they also dilate and provide better drainage of the space when it becomes expanded by fluid.

Fluid Movement Across the Microvasculature

Flow through the "pores" in the microvascular wall is governed by Poiseuille equation[1] where the resistance offered by the pore in the membrane must be overcome by the pressure drop from the capillary lumen to the interstitial space.

$$\text{Flow} = \frac{\text{Pressure}}{\text{Resistance}} \quad (1)$$

It is usual to express resistance as its reciprocal or conductance K so that the equation becomes

$$\text{Flow} = K \times \Delta P \quad (2)$$

The value of K is complex because it must account for both the surface area and the permeability of the pores in the membrane. The four pressures that account for the pressure drop across the capillary wall were first delineated by Starling.[11] These include two hydrostatic pressures, one in the microvascular lumen and the other in the interstitial space, and two oncotic pressures, one in

Figure 16–1C. High-power of corner vessel showing red blood cells, polymorphonuclear leukocytes and platelets. Courtesy of Dr. W. Hulbert.

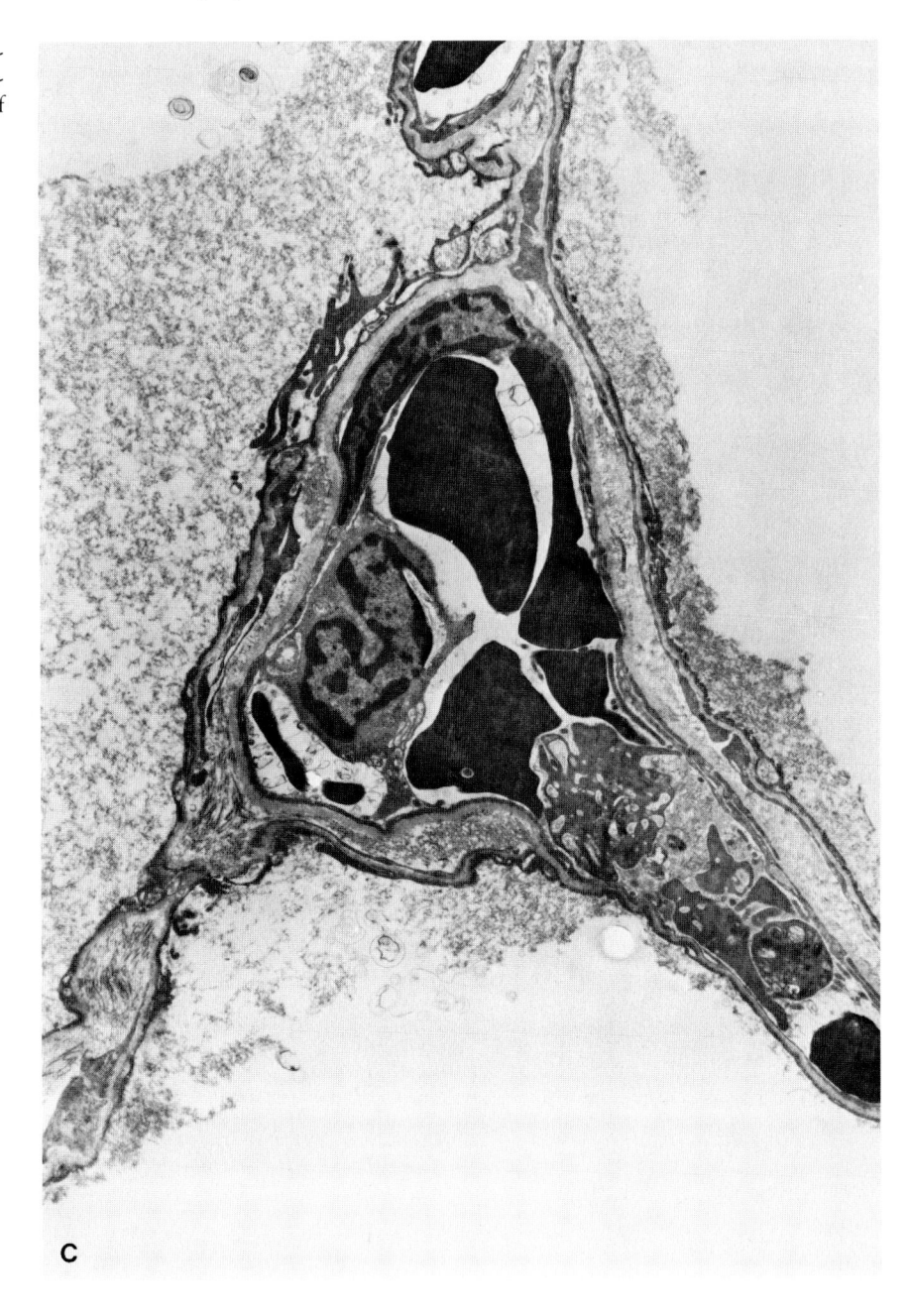

the microvascular lumen and the other in the interstitial space.

The most important of these four pressures is the microvascular hydrostatic pressure which results from the action of the heart. When the heart stops, all of the pressures across the microvascular membrane equilibrate so that ΔP becomes 0. The value of the interstitial hydrostatic pressure surrounding the microvasculature has been a controversial issue. Staub[3] has argued that the pressure in the alveolar wall interstitial space is the same as alveolar pressure. Guyton and associates,[12] on the other hand, have stressed the difference between the surface pressure and interstitial liquid and contact pressure. Their argument is that when the pressure at the surface is 0, the pressure in the wall is made up of a combination pressure that tends to be negative and the pressure at contact points between the solid elements that tends to be positive. These two pressures sum to the appropriate surface pressure. The important feature of this relationship is that the surface pressure is the appropriate pressure to consider when determining the compliance of the transmural pressure the microvasculature, whereas the more negative liquid pressure is the important determinant of fluid and exchange.

The oncotic pressure in the microvasculature and the interstitial space depends on the protein concentration in these two locations. As the smaller molecules are not restricted by the pores and can equilibrate across the microvascular membrane, they do not contribute to the difference in osmotic pressure across the membrane. It follows that as fluid moves through the microvascular pores to the interstitial space and the larger protein molecules are restricted, the protein osmotic pressure will be greater in the microvasculature than in the interstitial space. The difference in protein osmotic pressure that develops across the membrane will depend on the relative size of the protein molecule to the pore in the membrane. This is usually expressed as a reflection coefficient (σ) which varies between 0 and 1 depending on whether the molecule is restricted by the pore ($\sigma = 1$) or able to pass freely through the pore ($\sigma = 0$). An expansion of the fluid balance equation to take all four pressures into account as well as the reflection coefficient of the membrane is shown in Equation 3.

$$\text{Fluid movement} = K\left[(PMv - PIs) - \sigma(\pi Mv - \pi Is)\right] \quad (3)$$

where Mv and Is refer to the microvascular and interstitial space, P and π refer to hydrostatic and oncotic pressures, and σ is the reflection coefficient of the membrane.

Fluid Movement in the Alveolar Wall Interstitial Space

As there are no lymphatics in the alveolar wall, the fluid that moves across the alveolar capillaries must be moved to the extra-alveolar interstitial space if it is to be cleared by the lymphatics. The exact mechanism by which this occurs is controversial.[3] In our opinion it seems that the most probable explanation is that the compliance of the alveolar wall interstitial space is low so that fluid entering it will cause the pressure in the space to rise and provide the force necessary to move the fluid from the alveolar wall to the extra-alveolar interstitial space.

Fluid Movement in the Extra-Alveolar Interstitial Space

Fluid collects in the extra-alveolar space first in most forms of edema and is drained back into the systemic venous system via the lymphatics. The collection of fluid in this space lowers the resistance to flow through the lymphatics because they are tethered to the walls of interstitial space,[13] so that they dilate as the space expands. It has been shown that once the space is filled the resistance of the lymphatics may be so low that the fluid entering this compartment appears to drain into the lymphatics preferentially.

Air Space Flooding

The exact site where fluid enters the air space is not clear. Some investigators believe that the fluid moves across the alveolar wall epithelium and others that it may leak near bronchoalveolar junctions.[3] Once excess fluid begins to accumulate in the air space, it collects first at alveolar corners and then spreads over the free surface. The radius of curvature of the free surface of the fluid gradually decreases as the fluid accumulates. The relationship between the transpulmonary pressure holding the alveolus open and the forces tending to close it are governed by the Laplace relationship

$$P = \frac{2T}{R} \quad (4)$$

where P = pressure, T = surface tension, and R = radius. As the alveoli flood the surface tension increases as the surfactant is replaced by edema fluid and the radius narrows so that a much greater pressure is required to keep the alveolus open. When this pressure can no longer be generated, the alveoli collapse.

Safety Factors that Prevent Pulmonary Edema

A number of features act as safety factors to prevent pulmonary edema. For example, a rise in capillary hydrostatic pressure causes fluid to move across the microvasculature and as protein is restricted by the pores, protein osmotic pressure increases in the microvasculature and decreases in the interstitial space so that the net difference in osmotic pressure across the membrane is restored to normal. Similarly, as fluid moves into the interstitial space the hydrostatic pressure in that space tends to rise and restore the difference in hydrostatic pressure to its previous value. Thirdly, the lymphatics act to remove the excess fluid and return it to the vascular space. Finally the lung volume can be increased so that the interstitial space expands and the storage capacity for extravascular fluid is increased.

Classification of Pulmonary Edema

On the basis of the arguments presented above it is clear that pulmonary edema can be classified into those causes that increase the pressure across the microvasculature and others that increase net filtration by damaging the capillaries[14,15] (Table 16–1).

Edema Due to Increased Microvascular Pressure

Cardiogenic pulmonary edema occurs when left atrial pressure increases and causes the capillary hydrostatic pressure to rise. This occurs with myocardial failure from any cause. It can also occur with mitral valve disease or rarer disorders such as atrial myxomas that occlude the mitral orifice. While noncardiogenic causes such as pulmonary veno-occlusive disease, fibrosing mediastinitis, and a variety of mediastinal masses can produce pulmonary edema, these causes are relatively rare. A common cause of pulmonary edema in hospitalized patients with

Table 16–1. Classification of Pulmonary Edema

Edema Produced by Increased Pressure Across the Microvasculature
    Hydrostatic microvascular pressure becomes more positive
        Left heart failure
        Mitral stenosis
        Expansion of the microvascular space by overtransfusion
        Obliteration of pulmonary veins
    Hydrostatic interstital pressure becomes more negative
        Acute atelectasis (drowned lung)
        Rapid reexpansion of hydro-or pneumothorax
    Microvascular colloid osmotic pressure decreased
        Overtransfusion with crystalloid
        Hypoalbuminemia due to liver or renal disease
        Starvation
    Interstitial colloid osmotic pressure increased
        Obstructed lymphatics
Edema Due to a Damaged Microvascular Membrane (Endothelium or Epithelium)
    Infectious agents
        Viruses, mycoplasma, other (especially in innumocompromised patients)
    Inhaled substances
        Gases: Oxygen, nitrogen dioxide, sulfur dioxide, smoke, other noxious gases and fumes
        Liquid aspiration: gastric contents, salt and fresh water drowning
    Ingestants
        Chemotherapeutic agents: azathioprine, BCNU, bleomycin, bulsufan, chlorambucil, cytosine arabinoside, cytoxan, melphalan, methotrexate, mitomycin
        Other medications: amphotericin B, colchicine, gold, hexamothonium, hydrochlorothiazide, nitrofurantoin, placidyl, practolol, salicylate, penicillamine, phenylbutazone
        Other: heroin, kerosene, paraquat
    Shock, trauma, and sepsis
    Radiation
    Miscellaneous
        Acute pancreatitis, cardiopulmonary bypass, fat or air embolism, uremia, heat, molar pregnancy, systemic lupus erythematosus, postlymphangiography
Edema due to Undetermined Origin
    High altitude
    Neurogenic

Abbreviations: BCNU = 1, 3 Bis [2 Chlorethyl]-1 Nitrosourea

---

normal cardiac function is overexpansion of the vascular space by excessive intravenous therapy, particularly in patients with compromised renal function.

Edema Due to Lowered Interstitial Hydrostatic Pressure

In a small number of conditions the pressure drop across the microvascular membrane can increase because the interstitial hydrostatic pressure becomes more negative.[16, 17] Acute atelectasis has been thought to be associated with pulmonary edema and is often referred to as the "drowned lung syndrome." In this situation the collapse of a lobe results in a more negative interstitial pressure so that the pressure across the microvasculature is thought to increase. However, when acute atelectasis has been produced in dogs in an attempt to reproduce this clinical syndrome, it has been difficult to show that there is an actual increase in the amount of extravascular fluid in the lung.[18] On the other hand, convincing cases of acute pulmonary edema have been reported in association with rapid reexpansion of a lung or lobe following a hydro- or pneumothorax.[16, 17] This form of edema usually clears rapidly when the lung is fully expanded.

Edema Due to Low Plasma Oncotic Pressure

Guyton and Lindsey[19] showed that acute reduction in plasma oncotic pressure from 25 to 15 torr produced measurable pulmonary edema at capillary hydrostatic pressures that were only modestly elevated. It follows that patients with reduced plasma protein concentrations may develop edema with modest fluid overload in the absence of overt left heart failure. Such situations may occur with hypoalbuminemia associated with liver and renal disease and is a theoretical possibility with starvation. However, the oncotic pressure is more commonly lowered by the overtransfusion of crystalloid materials.

Edema Due to Elevated Interstitial Oncotic Pressure

As the lymphatics clear the protein out of the interstitial space, obstruction of the lymphatics should be associated with a raised interstitial protein concentration. In experimental animals partial ligation of pulmonary lymphatics has resulted in impressive pulmonary edema when left atrial pressure is elevated.[20] It is also said that patients with silicosis are predisposed to the development of pulmonary edema with raised left atrial pressure because of partial obstruction of the lymphatics by the reaction of silica.[21] As the lymphatics represent a major protective feature against edema by removing fluid and protein from the interstitial space and are known to be able to dilate substantially with disease, it follows that interference with this mechanism could be an important predisposition to pulmonary edema.

Edema Due to Microvascular Damage

As indicated in Table 16–1, edema due to microvascular damage can occur under a very wide variety of circumstances. However, as the consequences of the injury are fairly stereotyped, it is practical to describe the syndrome associated with these various injuries before dealing with any of the specific examples.

The Adult Respiratory Distress Syndrome

Adult respiratory distress syndrome is the name given to the clinical syndrome that results from damage to the alveolar capillary membrane. It therefore represents an extremely heterogeneous group of disorders that have widely differing etiologies but a reasonably similar final common pathway. It is a major cause of morbidity and mortality in critically ill patients and affects more than 150,000 persons each year in the United States and approximately 15,000 persons in Canada.* It is often a particularly tragic disorder because it affects persons who are quite healthy prior to the onset of this devastating form of respiratory failure. Ashbaugh and associates[22] were the first to draw attention to this disorder where patients with no prior history of lung disease or left-sided heart failure suddenly present with severe dyspnea, tachypnea, hypoxemia, decreased lung compliance, and diffuse pulmonary infiltrates on the chest film. The precipitating factors can include any of the disorders listed in Table 16–1 but are most often associated with trauma and sepsis, although a very wide variety of other causes have been identified. In centers experienced in dealing with ARDS, the mortality rate ranges from 20 to 60 percent with the higher rates associated with patients having superimposed problems such as renal failure and myocardial infarction.

Pathophysiology. It is useful to consider ARDS by dividing it into the preclinical and clinical events. There is substantial evidence that the microvascular injury develops during a preclinical phase of the syndrome when there is no evidence of respiratory failure. The clinical phase of the syndrome becomes apparent with the development of hypoxemic respiratory failure associated with diffuse pulmonary infiltrates which often cause a diffuse increase in density of the chest radiograph or "white out." Finally, there is a late phase of the injury where the patients gradually develop stiffer and stiffer lungs due to the deposition of connective tissue. The pathologic features of the preclinical state have been largely elucidated in the animal laboratory while the description of the lesions in the clinical phase has been described by the term diffuse alveolar damage (DAD).

The Preclinical Phase of Adult Respiratory Distress Syndrome. It is clear that this form of pulmonary edema often develops after a quiescent period following a severe insult to the body that may not involve the lungs. This period is much easier to characterize in experimental animals. Studies have shown that the pulmonary capillaries leak following the injection of endotoxin,[24] Pseudomonas bacteria,[25] hemorrhagic shock,[8] and microembolism[26] without there necessarily being either an increase in extravascular lung water or hypoxemic respiratory failure. The capillary leak is thought to be realated to endothelial and epithelial damage produced by polymorphonuclear leukocytes[27,28] after they have become activated via the complement cascade.[29] Polymorphonuclear leukocytes damage the endothelium either by release of their lysosomal enzymes or by the generation of oxygen-free radicals which can damage the membrane or inactivate the inhibitors of the lysosomal enzymes so that the alveolar-capillary membrane is severely damaged.[30] The evidence that the polymorphonuclear cells are important comes from several sources. First, insults such as air embolization,[27] or glass bead[28] or endotoxin injection which damage the microvascular membrane can be prevented by depleting the animal of polymorphonuclear leukocyte before administering the insult.[31] Second, the polymorphonuclear leukocyte is known to be well endowed with lysosomal enzymes and can generate oxygen-free radicals when stimulated by C5A.[32] Third, the administration of xanthene plus xanthene oxidase to generate oxygen-free radicals[32] can produce similar damage.

Histologic studies of hemorrhagic shock have shown that the alveolar capillary membrane appears normal when the increased permeability first occurs.[33] This seems likely to be due to the fact that the injury to the capillary membrane involves such a small part of the total capillary surface area so that it is difficult to demonstrate.

The Clinical Phase of Adult Respiratory Distress Syndrome. The clinical phase of the syndrome begins with flooding of the alveolar spaces and obvious hypoxemic respiratory failure.[22] The hypoxemia is due primarily to the fact that a shunt develops because the blood passing through edematous areas is unable to take part in gas exchange. As the total ventilation remains adequate to remove the carbon dioxide, the respiratory failure is not associated with carbon dioxide retention.

The pathologic features of the lung at this stage are covered by the descriptive term diffuse alveolar damage (DAD)[34] which can be divided into two fairly discrete but overlapping stages. The early, acute or exudative stage occurs within the first week following lung injury, while the later, organizing or proliferative stage is seen 2 or more weeks after injury.

Grossly, the lungs in the acute exudative phase are heavy, congested, and airless. Fluid frequently exudes from the cut surface.[35] The earliest recognizable histologic change results from microvascular damage and results in hemorrhagic pulmonary edema. The alveolar septa are thickened by interstitial edema and the alveolar spaces contain proteinous fluid often admixed with hemorrhage. Electron microscopy at this stage demonstrates degenerative changes such as cytoplasmic swelling and bleb formation in alveolar lining cells and capillary endothelium. It is thought that the damage to the capillary endothelium causes leakage of fluid from the vascular space into the interstitium and alveolar spaces. Increased vascular permeability has also been demonstrated by means of radioisotope studies in patients with ARDS.

The histologic hallmark of the early clinical stage is hyaline membrane formation (Fig. 16–2). This occurs 24 to 48 hours after the onset of edema and is accompanied by fibrinous exudates and cellular debris within alveolar spaces. These changes are most prominent 3 to 4 days following injury and begin to disappear after about 1 week following injury.[36] By light microscopy the hyaline membranes appear as homogeneous eosinophilic structures that are arranged in a layer along the alveolar septa (*see* Fig. 16–2). By electron microscopy, however, they

---

* Estimate provided by Statistics Canada, Ottawa, Canada.

Figure 16–2A. Low power view of the acute stage of diffuse alveolar damage. This shows thickened edematous alveolar walls with exudate in the airspaces. Hyaline membranes are prominent.

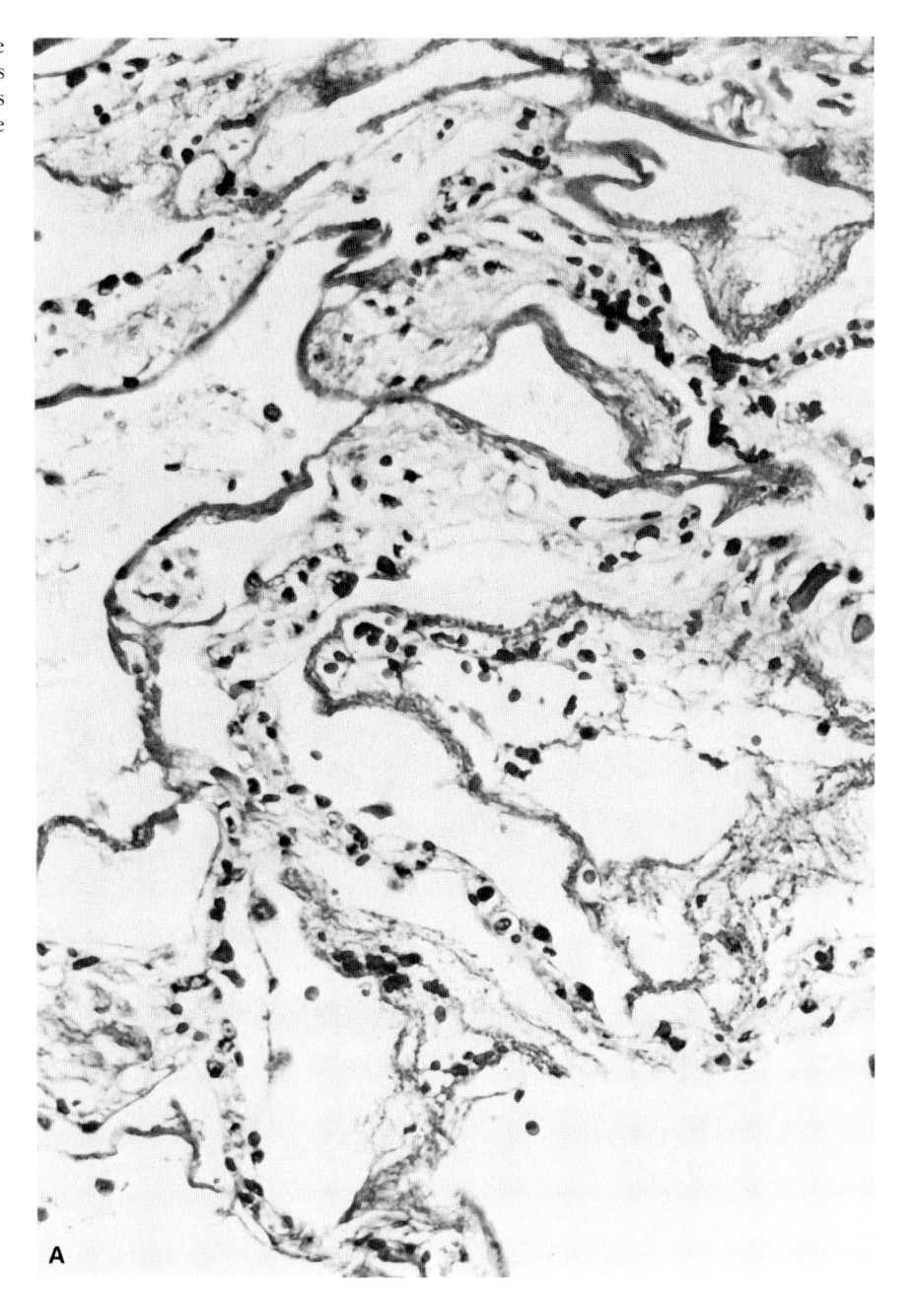

have been shown to consist of a heterogenous mixture of debris from necrotic cells, proteinaceous material, and small amounts of fibrin (Fig. 16–3). Erythrocytes, fibrin, and a proteinaceous exudate often accompany the hyaline membranes within the alveolar spaces. The alveolar septa themselves are thickened by a combination of edema, a scant chronic inflammatory cell infiltrate, and increasing numbers of fibroblasts (Fig. 16–5). Alveolar lining cells and capillary endothelial cells can become completely sloughed leaving their respective basement membranes denuded of cells. Microthrombi are common within the capillaries in acute DAD, and probably form around damaged or sloughed endothelial cells. Damage to bronchial mucosa can also occur, but it is usually not as prominent as alveolar lining cell injury.

Several days to a week following the onset of the exudative phase of the injury the proliferation of type II-pneumocytes begins. This finding bridges the acute and organizing stages of injury.[34–36] The proliferating type II cells replace the sloughed type I cells and reline the denuded epithelial basement membrane. This is an attempt at repair, since the type II cells have been shown, at least experimentally, to have a capacity to differentiate into type I cells.[37] The newly formed type II cells tend to be closely spaced, forming a row along the alveolar septa. They often have large nuclei that project in a hobnail configuration into the alveolar lumen (Fig. 16–4). Mitotic figures are frequent and the cells may appear quite

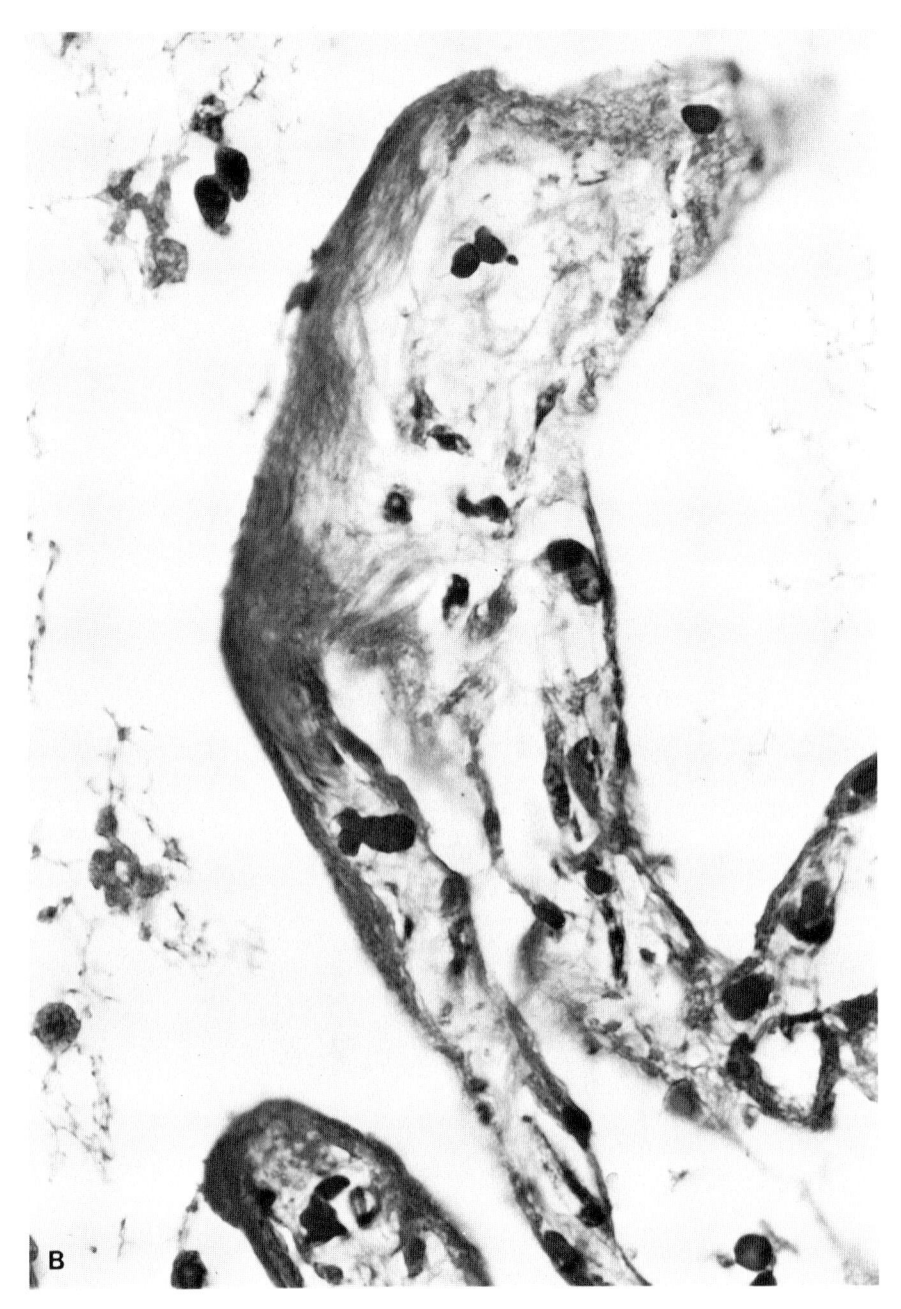

Figure 16–2B. Higher power view of hyaline membrane.

atypical with prominent nucleoli, clumped chromatin, and variation in size. Hyaline change resembling alcoholic hyaline seen in hepatocytes, and vacuolar lipid deposits have been noted within their cytoplasm.[38] Abnormalities can be seen by electron microscopy, including dilatation of rough endoplasmic reticulum, intracytoplasmic edema, and a change in the number and size of lamellar bodies.

As its name implies, the organizing stage of this lung injury is analogous to the organization of a pneumonia, except that most of the fibrosis occurs within the interstitium rather than within alveolar spaces. Although connective tissue deposition can be seen as early as 3 to 4 days following injury, it is not usually prominent until after about 2 weeks.[36] Grossly, the lungs are firm and airless, and may have a grey appearance.[36] The alveolar septa become thickened by proliferating fibroblasts combined with residual edema and scattered chronic inflammatory cells (see Fig. 16–4). Hyperplastic type II pneumocytes remain prominent along the alveolar wall (see Fig. 16–4). By electron microscopy bundles of collagen and elastin are present within alveolar septa along with occasional histiocytes, plasma cells, lymphocytes, and scattered mast cells. Fibrosis is not limited to the alveolar septa, and can be seen to a smaller extent within air spaces, especially the alveolar ducts, and around alveolar ducts and small bronchioles. The latter finding may explain the obstructive defects noted in

Figure 16–2C. Appearance of type 2 cells show beginning of the alveolar repair phase.

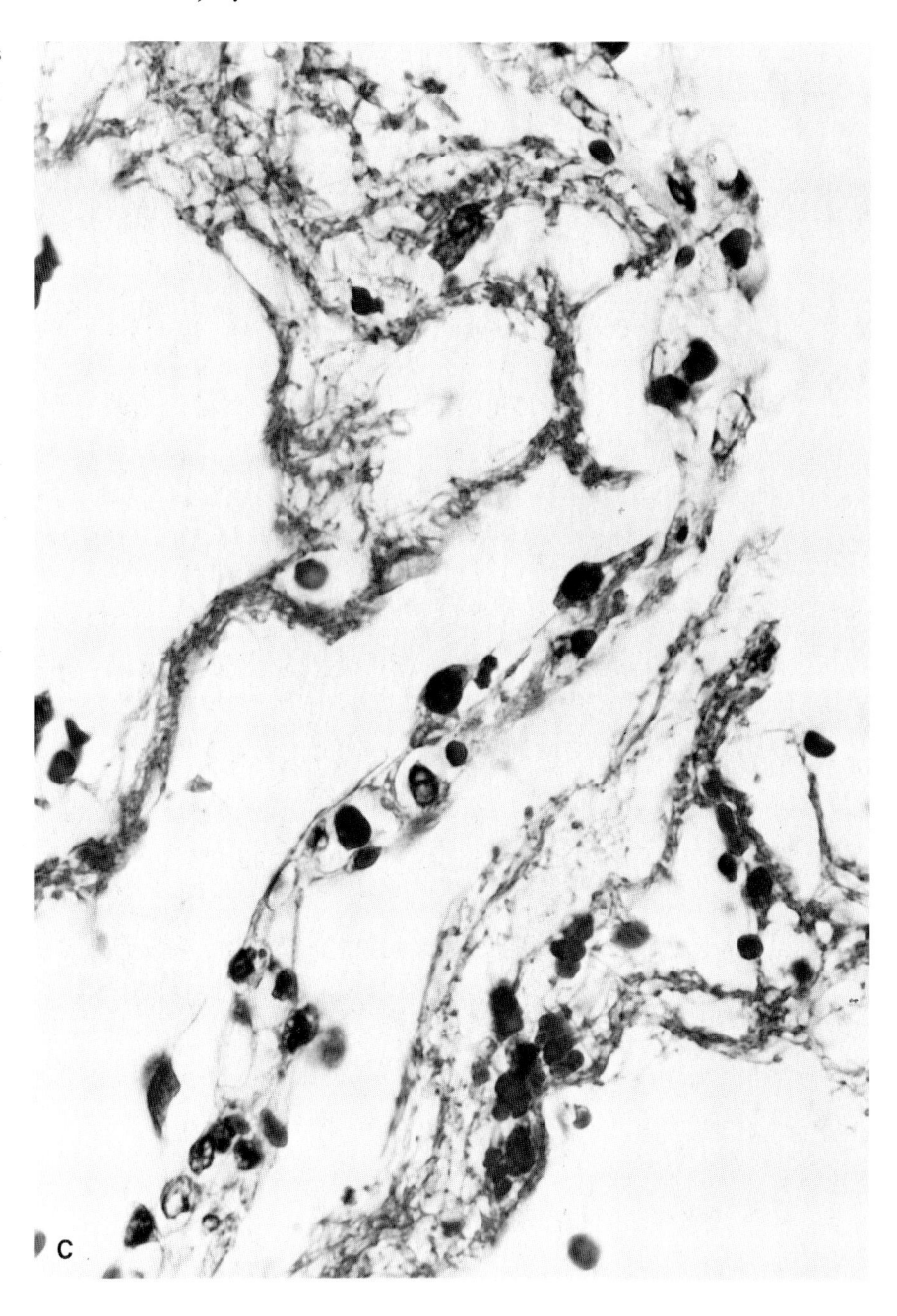

some patients with ARDS.[39] Remnants of hyaline membranes and proteinaceous exudates can still be found within alveolar spaces at this stage. They may be phagocytosed by alveolar macrophages, and frequently they are incorporated into the thickened alveolar septa by the fibrosis. The bronchiolar mucosa may undergo squamous metaplasia (see Fig. 16–5) that can appear very atypical. This squamous tissue or even the normal-appearing bronchial mucosa can extend along the pores of Kohn to line nearby alveolar walls.

Diffuse alveolar damage can sometimes progress to end-stage interstitial fibrosis or honeycomb lung in 10 days to 2 weeks.[40] This change can also be characterized by a restructuring of the distal lung parenchyma such that there are cyst-like spaces with fibrotic walls lined by II pneumocytes or bronchiolar epithelium. Normal sized alveolar spaces may also remain, but they contain fibrotic walls lined by type II pneumocytes. The nature of the large cystic structures which are a common feature of end-stage or honeycomb lung and a less frequent feature of end-stage ARDS is obscure. One possibility[40] is that the increased surface tension caused by exudate covering the surface causes the alveoli to collapse on the alveolar duct. The reorganization of the interstitium by fibroblast proliferation, deposition of collagen, incorporation of hyaline membranes, and regeneration of epithelium could then result in the multiple cysts that cause the lung to have a honeycomb appearance.

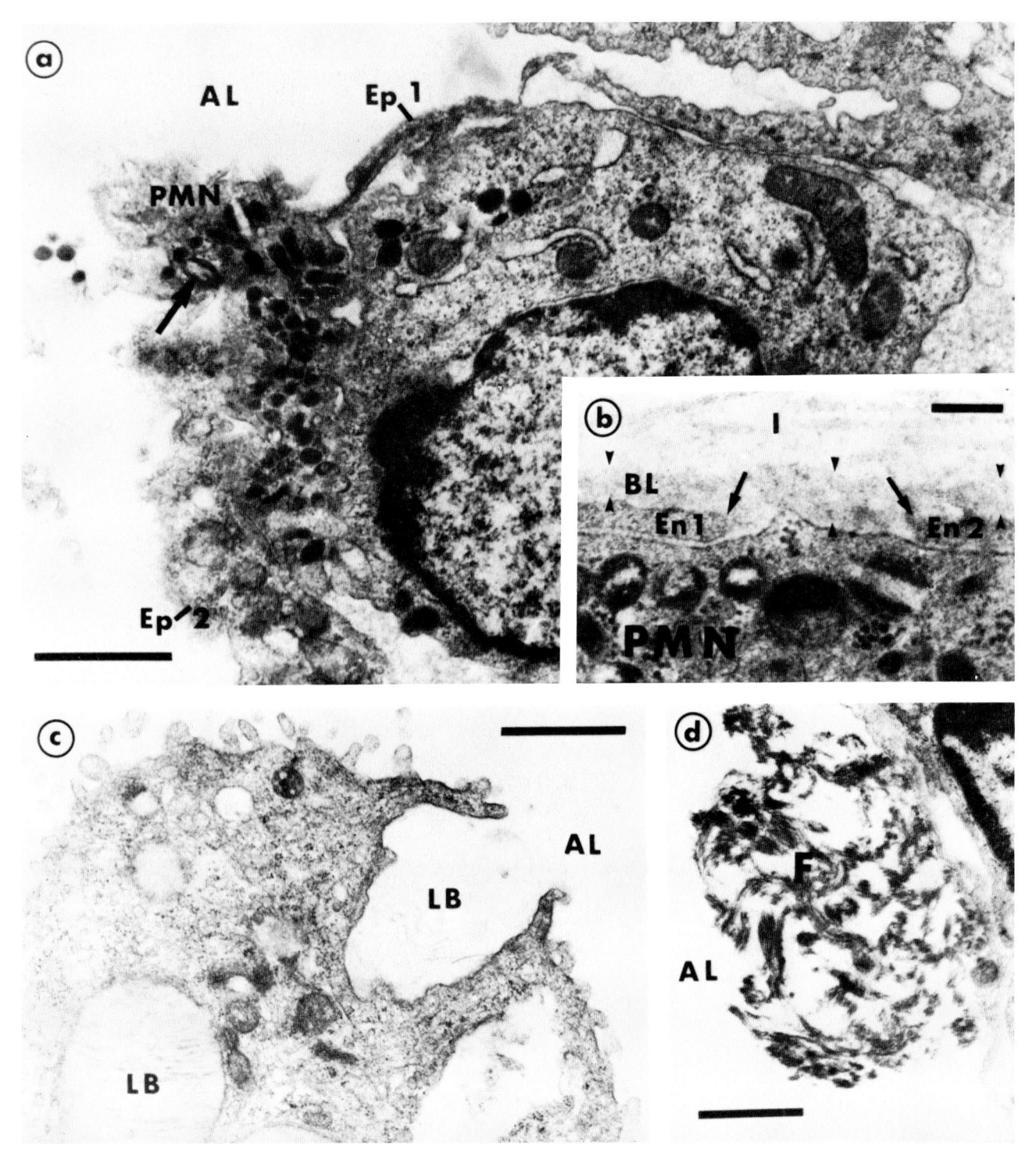

Figure 16–3. An example of experimentally induced diffuse alveolar injury in a dog lung (oleic acid IV 0.08 mg/kg). (a) Polymorphonuclear leukocyte (PMN) entering the airspace (AL) between two epithelial cells. (b) PMN entering gap between two endothelial cells. (c) Spaces which lamellar body (LB) of type 2 cell emptied into the alveolar space. (d) Fibrin on the alveolar surface. Courtesy of Dr. David Walker.

Figure 16–4. The proliferative phase of diffuse alveolar damage where type 2 cells cover the alveolar surface. These have the capacity to differentiate to type 1 cells and restore the normal alveolar architecture.

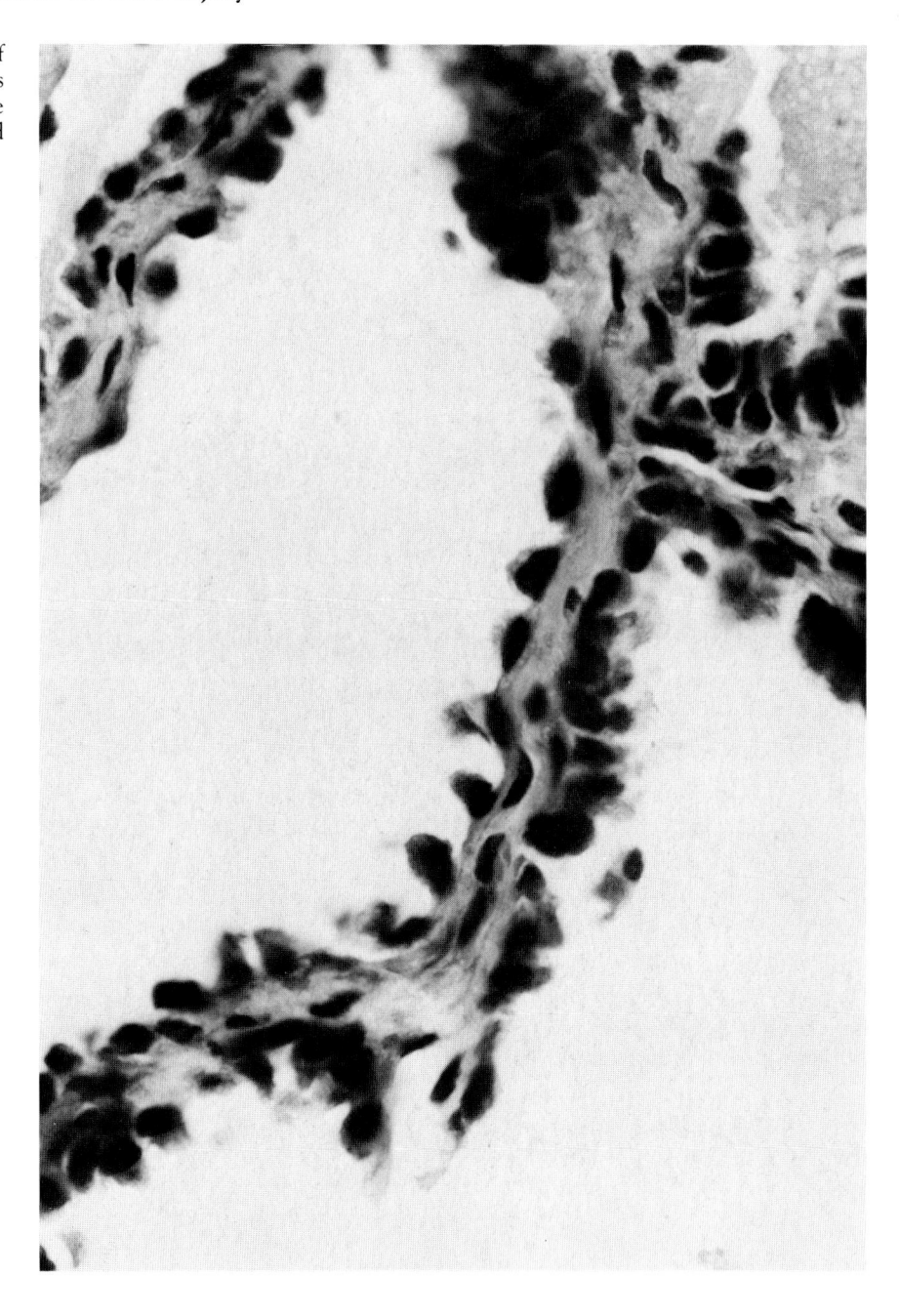

In some ways organizing diffuse alveolar damage resembles usual interstitial pneumonia (UIP) and bronchopulmonary dysplasia in infants (see Chapter 10): the interstitial inflammation and fibrosis with type II pneumocyte proliferation are similar in both conditions. Because of these features Leibow[41] believed that UIP was a type of diffuse alveolar injury that followed a prolonged course. To be correct, this theory would have to explain why DAD is characterized by an acute onset and a rapid clinical course, with normal pulmonary function if recovery occurs, while UIP has an insidious onset, and a slowly progressive downhill course with death occurring in the majority of patients after 5 or more years. The difference between the two conditions might be reconciled by studies of Gibson and Pride[42] that suggest subtraction of units in parallel in chronic fibrosing alveolitis. This would mean that UIP would progress slowly because small areas of the lung are sequentially subtracted by a series of focal injuries over the course of years while ARDS results from the same injury to greater areas of lung. Organizing DAD and UIP may be difficult to distinguish on a single biopsy, although organizing remnants of hyaline membranes and proteinaceous exudates are more usual with DAD. The interstitial fibrosis in organizing DAD is more cellular and immature than in UIP and contains numerous fibroblasts compared to the less cellular more dense collagen deposition in UIP. In difficult cases the clinical history should help establish

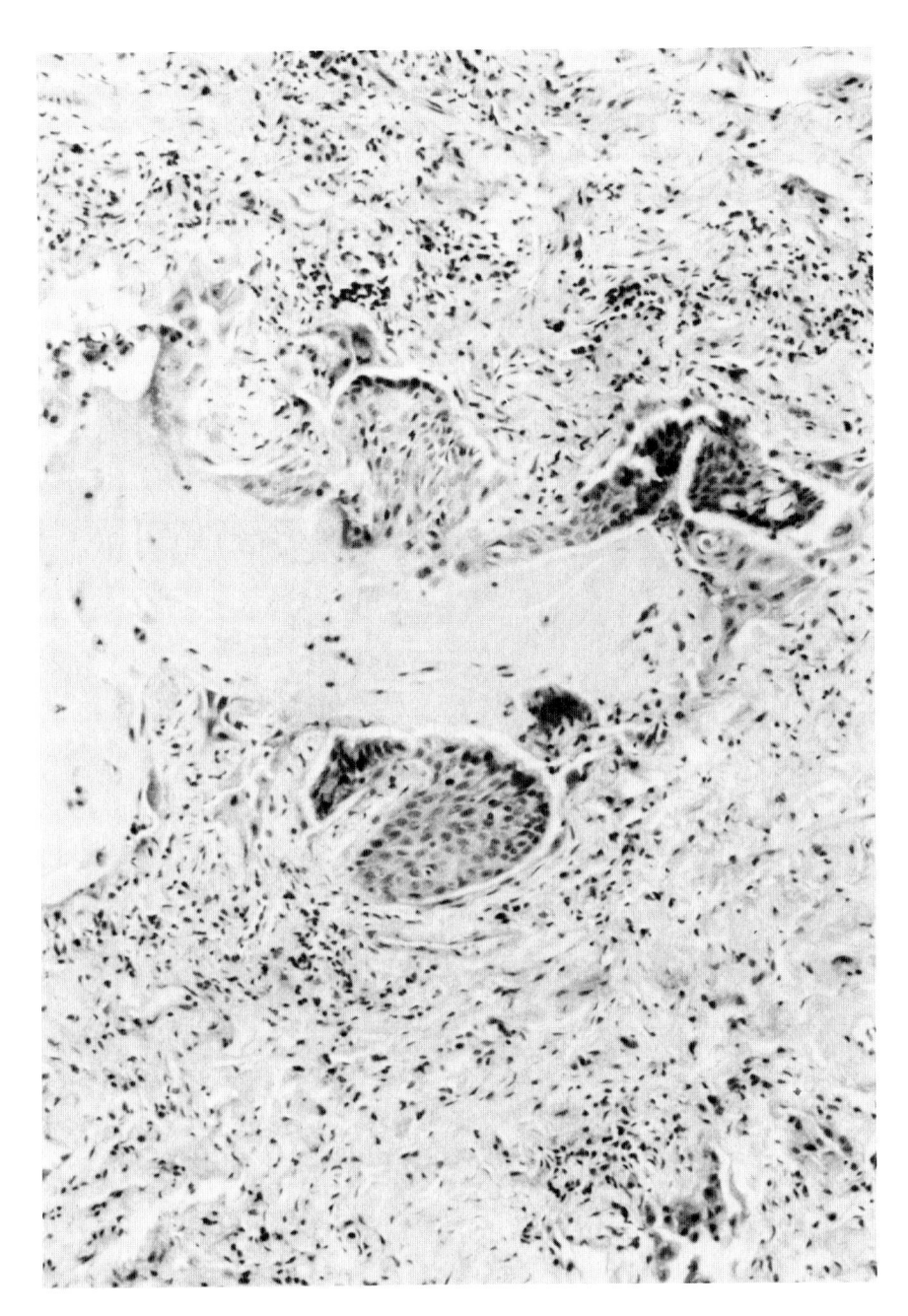

Figure 16–5. Squamous metaplasia is present in an area of diffuse alveolar damage.

the correct diagnosis.

The separation of DAD into acute and organizing stages is useful as a concept for understanding the variable histologic patterns that may be seen in this condition. The two stages should not be considered distinct since considerable overlap may occur. Foci of acute DAD frequently are seen superimposed on otherwise typical organizing DAD. This finding may occur because the treatment for ARDS (that is, oxygen) can itself induce DAD, or because complications that can cause DAD (that is, sepsis, shock, disseminated intravascular coagulation, and so on) may arise sequentially in very ill patients.

The Etiology of Diffuse Alveolar Injury

Having reviewed some of the general pathologic and clinical features of microvascular injury under the heading of ARDS, we now propose to review some specific examples of this syndrome.

Table 16–2 shows the distribution of a group of patients admitted to the St. Paul's Hospital Intensive Care Unit (Vancouver, B.C., Canada) because there was a high risk of ARDS. Only 10 of the 140 patients actually developed ARDS and 7 of these 10 had either trauma or sepsis as the major problem. The additional three pa-

Table 16–2. Distribution of Adult Respiratory Distress Syndrome

	No. Patients	M	F	Age (Mean ± SD)
Trauma				
ARDS	4	3	1	31 ± 19
No ARDS	12	11	1	35 ± 16
Sepsis				
ARDS	3	2	1	75 ± 4
No ARDS	9	6	3	54 ± 21
Miscellaneous				
ARDS	3	3	0	38 ± 15
No ARDS	9	8	1	56 ± 17
Total	40	33	7	

tients that developed ARDS consisted of one with acute pancreatitis and two who aspirated gastric contents. Additional frequent causes are viral infections and a variety of infections in the immunocompromised host. As these topics are covered in detail in Chapters 11 and 15 of this book, we will only discuss the noninfectious causes of the syndrome here.

Liquid Aspiration. The aspiration of stomach contents in the unconscious patient is a common example of diffuse alveolar damage that can result in hypoxemic respiratory failure (*see* Chapter 25). The severity of the injury depends on the pH of the liquid aspirated, and hydrochloric acid has been shown to cause a particularly florid form of edema accumulation.[43] Drowning[44–46] is associated with the filling of the lungs with liquid. As the epithelium acts as a semipermeable membrane, fresh water drowning is thought to cause a movement of water into the interstitial and the vascular compartment where it lowers the osmotic pressure and produced hemolysis. Sea water drowning, on the other hand may actually cause fluid to move from the vascular and interstitial compartment into the air spaces. The fact that drowning victims frequently show edema with a very high protein concentration suggests that the fluid in the air spaces damages the pulmonary capillaries to allow protein to leak out.[45] It has been recognized that near-drowning in fresh water can be associated with a late onset of pulmonary edema which is referred to as "secondary" drowning.[46,47] This late onset of edema probably occurs because the osmotic damage to the alveolar capillary membrane causes it to leak. It seems likely that if this leak is relatively small, the protective mechanisms described above (*see* Safety Factors that Prevent Pulmonary Edema, above) prevent the formation of edema so that its onset is delayed enough to be referred to as secondary drowning.

Inhalation of Noxious Gases and Fumes
Oxygen. The adverse effects of breathing 100 percent oxygen for prolonged periods of time have been known for many years.[48,49] Morphologic changes have been documented in numerous animal species following exposure to high concentrations of oxygen. A marked variation in susceptibility has been noted from species to species and also in young animals as compared to old animals. Mild symptoms occur in normal humans after 6 to 12 hours of exposure, but there are no associated functional or radiographic abnormalities after this amount of time.[50,51] Slight decreases in pulmonary function have been reported with longer exposures, but morphologic alterations have not been documented.[50] Two prospective studies have examined the effects of breathing high concentrations of oxygen in patients. Barber and co-workers[51] treated five patients who had irreversible brain damage with 100 percent oxygen for 31 to 72 hours. Although functional abnormalities were found after 40 hours, no changes in lung structure were noted between the study group and a control group of nonexposed patients. Singer[50] administered 100 percent oxygen to one group of patients recovering from cardiac surgery and minimal oxygen (less than 42 percent) to maintain tissue oxygenation to a second group. No differences between the two groups were noted, although maximum exposure was only 48 hours. Two additional patients received 100 percent oxygen for 5 to 7 days, respectively; the former recovered completely, while the latter died of pulmonary hemorrhage due to a clotting defect. One histologic section of the lung from the last-mentioned individual showed evidence of interstitial pneumonia with hyaline membranes. Recently, Hasleton and associates[52] studied the lungs of seven men who died 3 to 13 days following a mine explosion. All were severely burned and had received multiple injuries. Despite mechanical ventilation with 30 to 100 percent inspired oxygen, evidence of diffuse alveolar injury was seen in only one patient, and was a focal change in that individual.

Despite the difficulties in demonstrating unequivocal pathologic abnormalities in prospective studies of normal individuals or of patients without prior lung disease who were exposed to 100 percent oxygen, for many years it has been known that characteristic pathologic lesions result from treating seriously ill patients with 100 percent oxygen. This apparent contradiction can be explained in two ways. First, in humans it is likely that some other factor in addition to oxygen is necessary for significant lesions to occur. That is, the lung must be already damaged for oxygen toxicity to develop, and that damage may result from any number of toxic agents including sepsis, shock, intravascular coagulation, infection, and so on. Second, it may be that in the absence of prior lung damage, longer exposure times to pure oxygen than were reported by Barber and associates[51] or Singer and colleagues[50] are required to produce changes. For example, in Hyde and Rawson's[53] study of five patients with respiratory insufficiency due to muscular weakness, chest infiltrates developed only after 4 to 10 days of therapy with inspired oxygen ranging from 83 to 91 percent. The concentration of inspired oxygen that is safe in patients is not definitely known so that the usual practice is to use the lowest inspired PO_2 that will adequately oxygenate the arterial blood.

Pratt[48,49] was the first to suggest that certain lung changes noted at autopsy were due to oxygen toxicity. He described alveolar septal thickening and prominent congested capillaries in patients receiving 100 percent inspired oxygen. Subsequently, numerous additional investigators described hyaline membranes and other features of DAD in patients receiving oxygen. Nash and associates[35] presented the first detailed pathologic study of this lesion in a classic article. They correlated the pathologic changes with both the length of exposure and the concentration of inspired oxygen, and on this basis were able to divide the lesions into typical exudative and proliferative stages.

Similar changes have also been described in neonates who received oxygen therapy for the respiratory distress syndrome[54-56]; these changes are frequently termed bronchopulmonary dysplasia.[57]

The mechanism of cell injury by oxygen is thought to result from the formation of free radicals or other toxic products during oxygen metabolism.[58-60] The most important cytotoxic substances formed by this mechanism include the superoxide anion (O_2^-), hydrogen peroxide (H_2O_2), the hydroxyl radical ($OH^·$), and singlet oxygen (O_2^-). These substances act by inactivating sulphydryl enzymes, disrupting DNA, and destroying cell membrane integrity. There are certain intrinsic defence mechanisms that can protect the cell from oxygen damage: enzymes such as superoxide dismutase, catalase, and glutathione peroxidase; intracellular compounds such as glutathione, cysteine, and ascorbate; and vitamin E, a lipid membrane component. The amounts of these various protective agents within cells may vary among individuals, and may account for differences in individual susceptibility to oxygen toxicity. The possibility of increasing the intracellular concentration of these substances may prove to be an important therapeutic modality in counteracting the adverse effects of oxygen.

Oxides of Nitrogen. Nitrogen forms a series of gaseous oxides of which nitric acid (NO) and nitrogen dioxide (NO_2 and N_2O_4) are the most likely to cause damage to human lungs. Perhaps the best example of this injury is that found in silo fillers' disease.[62-63] When corn is harvested before it is fully grown, the young plants have a high nitrate content. During storage, anaerobic fermentation of potassium nitrate liberates nitrates which form oxides of nitrogen as the temperature rises with fermentation. Lethal concentrations can be reached within about 8 to 10 days and because the gas is heavier than air, it usually fills the depression in the silage *at the top of the silo*. Workers entering this depression can be overcome with the gas and those who do not immediately succumb, suffer a diffuse lung injury from inhaling the oxides of nitrogen. The outcome depends on the concentration of the nitrogen dioxide and the length and frequency of exposure. Maximum safe industrial exposures are usually thought to be about 10 parts per million of air. The oxides of nitrogen are readily soluble in water and are rapidly absorbed by the respiratory epithelium. This leads to diffuse alveolar damage with massive edema at high concentration, but chronic sublethal doses can result in bronchopneumonia with bronchiolitis obliterans.

Nitric acid is also a by-product of the production of sulfuric, chromic, and picric acid and can be a problem in copper, brass, and silver industries. The slow combustion of nitrocellulose in the plastics industry is also an important source, as may be burning x-ray film files. Oxides of nitrogen are also a by-product of metropolitan automobile pollution and in certain circumstances values of up to 0.8 parts per million have been recorded[64] in particularly dense smogs.

Ozone. The exposure to ozone occurs as a result of the effect of sunlight on hydrocarbons from automobile exhaust fumes and ultraviolet radiation. This is partially responsible for the lung injury resulting from smog in cities such as Los Angeles where the concentration may exceed 0.7 parts per million for periods of an hour. Recent work by Golden and associates[65] has shown that breathing even low concentrations during exercise may result in high tissue exposures and resultant airways inflammation and increased airways reactivity.[66] In much higher concentrations it leads to diffuse pulmonary injury similar to that seen in ARDS.[67] As the oxides of nitrogen tend to be more soluble than ozone, it is much more common for the oxides of nitrogen to damage the airways and the ozone to damage the more peripheral portions of the lung.

Smoke Inhalation. Smoke inhalation is a well known cause of pulmonary edema and the edema can occasionally have a delayed onset. A very high incidence of late onset pulmonary edema has been reported following some fires with the best reported example being the Cleveland Clinic fire[68] where the inhalation of smoke from burning nitrocellulose film produced large amounts of oxides of nitrogen. The reason for the delayed onset is uncertain but probably reflects the time taken to overcome the protective factors that keep the alveoli dry.

Chemical Ingestion. A large number of drugs have been implicated in the etiology of diffuse alveolar injury. As the lung lesions may be reversible upon discontinuation of the drug, a careful history of possible ingestants should be taken in all cases of DAD. Several excellent reviews of pulmonary drug toxicity have been published.[69-74]

Chemotherapeutic Agents. Chemotherapeutic agents are the most common drugs associated with the development of DAD and the list of individual agents that can produce it is long and continually growing. Clinically, chemotherapy-associated DAD is characterized by an acute onset of dyspnea, cough diffuse chest infiltrates, and often fever. The differential diagnosis includes infection, recurrence of the underlying malignant disease, radiation pneumonitis, and drug toxicity. The usual histologic lesion in all these conditions is DAD at various stages of evolution. Unless an infectious agent is found in the tissue, these entities cannot be distinguished by light or electron microscopy. The diagnosis of drug toxicity is one of exclusion and can be made only by carefully evaluating the possibility of other causes. It may be extremely difficult to implicate a single drug as causing lung toxicity since the patients frequently receive several drugs sometimes in combination with radiation. In addition, the course of these individuals is often complicated by sepsis, hypotension, or disseminated intravascular coagulation, all factors that in themselves can cause DAD.

The prognosis of lung disease produced by chemotherapy is generally poor. In most cases there is rapid progression of the pulmonary lesion to interstitial fibrosis, and the mortality rate is high. One exception is methotrexate toxicity in which a good response to withdrawal of the drug and corticosteroid therapy has been described. Although DAD has been reported due to methotrexate,[75] this drug more commonly produces a granulomatous interstitial pneumonia that histologically resembles hypersensitivity pneumonia.[76, 77] It may be that the reversible cases are the ones with the latter lesion, while those cases with DAD have a poor prognosis.

There are not specific histologic features to definitely implicate a drug in the etiology of DAD or to distinguish one drug reaction from another. However, there are a few characteristic, although nonspecific, features that have been described with certain drugs. Cytologically highly atypical alveolar lining cells have been noted in busulfan and bleomycin toxicity.[78-84] Similar changes are common in radiation but may also be seen with a variety of other toxic agents. By electron microscopy, unusual tubular structures have been found in the nuclei of type II pneumocytes from patients receiving bleomycin and busulfan.[82] These structures are probably not specific for drug toxicity. We have seen similar ones in usual interstitial pneumonia and they have been reported in certain lung tumors.

The exact mechanism of the pulmonary damage from chemotherapeutic agents is unknown. The toxicity of certain drugs appears to be dose related. Busulfan toxicity, for example, usually occurs after 3 to 10 years of therapy[78, 79, 85], and bleomycin toxicity is seen mainly after doses larger than 400 mg.[80, 81] The effects of certain toxic agents appear to be additive. For example, lung lesions have been reported with smaller doses of bleomycin in patients who had prior radiation or were receiving other potentially toxic drugs.[83] In BCNU toxicity other factors in addition to total dose are important in producing lung lesions, including duration of therapy and the presence of serious underlying lung disease.[84] The production of lung injury by other drugs is assumed to represent an idiosyncratic reaction, although in many of these examples sufficient cases are not available to adequately assess alternative mechanisms.

Other Drugs. Nitrofurantoin is an important cause of pulmonary toxicity. This drug causes two distinct syndromes, one *acute* and one *chronic*.[81-89] The acute reaction is characterized by the sudden onset of fever, dyspnea, and blood eosinophilia occurring several hours to several days after ingestion of the drug. Areas of consolidation are seen radiographically, and there is often an associated pleural effusion. This lesion is usually not biopsied since it resolves when the drug is discontinued. Most cases are assumed to represent examples of eosinophilic pneumonia, although acute DAD has been reported in one case.[86]

The chronic reaction to nitrofurantoin is characterized by an insidious onset of dyspnea and diffuse interstitial lung infiltrates. The disease may begin after many months or seven years of chronic nitrofurantoin therapy. The usual histologic findings is a chronic interstitial pneumonia with features resembling organizing DAD. Changes suggestive of desquamative interstitial pneumonia (DIP; *see* Chapter 20) have been described in two cases.[90]

There are scattered reports of chronic reactions to other drugs including gold,[91-96] practolol,[97, 98] hexamethonium,[99] and penicillamine.[100, 101] Acute DAD has been reported from hydrochlorothiazide[102] and from overdoses of colchicine[103] and placidyl.[104] The pulmonary edema that occasionally follows intravenous heroin administration[105-108] as well as that characteristic of salicylate intoxication[109] probably represent other examples of acute DAD.

Paraquat Lung. Paraquat is a potent herbicide that is sold in several forms: solid, granular material (Weedol, containing 2.5 percent paraquat), aqueous solutions with different concentrations [Gramoxine (20 percent), Ortho paraquat (29% percent), and Orthodual paraquat (42 percent)] and aerosol spray [Ortho spot weed and grass killer (0.44 percent].[110-116] Ingestion of even tiny amounts of these substances is frequently fatal.

The initial reaction to paraquat ingestion includes burning of the mouth and throat followed by nausea, vomiting, and diarrhea. Dyspnea, hypoxemia, and diffuse chest infiltrates develop several days to a week later and in most cases there is rapid progression to diffuse fibrosis and death. The most common finding in lung biopsies or autopsies is organizing DAD and honeycomb lung, athough acute DAD is seen if the patients are biopsied early in the course.[113, 116] An unusual type of intraalveolar fibrosis has been reported with fatal paraquat poisoning.[117] The toxic effects of paraquat[110-115] are thought to be mediated by the formation of free radicals.

Shock. While microvascular injury is often associated with hemorrhagic shock, the exact relationship between the low circulatory blood volume and subsequent changes is unclear. In the experimental situation this has been shown to increase microvascular permeability but not to produce edema.[8, 33] Septic shock on the other hand, is much more frequently associated with diffuse alveolar injury and ARDS.[23] In this situation it seems likely that the PMN are activated by endotoxin to produce the alveolar injury.[24]

Radiation. Radiation pneumonitis is a well-described complication of therapeutic radiation to the lungs, mediastinum, breast, and esophagus.[116, 118-125] It may be present as an acute or a chronic syndrome. Acute radiation pneumonitis is characterized clinically by fever, dyspnea, and cough that develop from 1 to 6 months after radiation therapy. Chest infiltrates conform to the region of the previous radiation portal. Favorable responses have been reported with corticosteroid therapy. Diffuse alveolar injury is the usual finding seen following acute radiation injury. In addition there is often severe atypia of hyperplastic alveolar lining cells which appear enlarged and are sometimes multinucleated. They frequently contain hyperchromatic nuclei with prominent nucleoli. Foam cells can occasionally be found in vascular intima and media, and when present are highly suggestive of prior radiation.

Chronic radiation pneumonitis is generally considered to represent a late stage of acute radiation pneumonitis. Although most patients with the acute lesion recover clinically, interstitial fibrosis eventually develops in the affected area. In a few patients with chronic radiation pneumonitis is clinically apparent acute stage is not documented. The usual histologic finding in chronic radiation pneumonitis is interstitial fibrosis. The atypical, hyperplastic alveolar lining cells seen in the acute stage are still present. Deposition of foam cells within vascular walls tends to be more prominent, and blood vessels may appear hyalinized.

The development of radiation pneumonitis is dependent on many factors including individual susceptibility, amount of radiation, duration of therapy, and volume of lung irradiated.[123,124] Additional factors may increase the toxicity of the radiation, including certain chemotherapeutic agents, infection, and prior irradiation.[118–120] The toxic effects of radiation are thought to result from injury to capillary endothelium and alveolar epithelium, as are the toxic effects of most of the other agents described in this chapter.

Pulmonary Edema of Uncertain Etiology

High Altitude

Perhaps the greatest enigma in the study of pulmonary edema is that produced at high altitude.[126,127] The mechanism of this edema has been extensively studied but remains obscure. Most studies have shown pulmonary arterial hypertension with normal or nearly normal pulmonary wedge pressure so that it is difficult to attribute it to left ventricular failure.[128] Similarly, allowing animals to breathe low concentrations of oxygen for long periods of time has not resulted in pulmonary edema so that the hypoxia itself does not seem to damage the pulmonary microvasculature.[129] Whayne and Severinghaus[130] suggested that the edema developed because of rupture of arterial walls proximal to the hypoxemically constricted pulmonary arterioles but at present no single mechanisms seem to satisfactorily explain the pathogenesis of high-altitude pulmonary edema.

Neurogenic Pulmonary Edema

Neurogenic pulmonary edema can be produced experimentally by injecting fibrin into the fourth ventricle[131] and occurs clinically in patients who have suffered head injury[132] or intracerebral hemorrhage.[133] Recent studies as to its mechanism have shown that while it is related to a massive sympathetic discharge,[134] it is not necessarily related to either systemic hypertension or left ventricular failure. Indeed, one recent study showed that when left atrial pressure was kept within normal limits neurogenic pulmonary edema still developed.[135] The nature of the fluid and protein leak suggests that in the early stages the edema is due to markedly raised pulmonary vascular pressures. The occasional case report[136] has documented increase left atrial pressures which do not remain elevated for a long time. Robin[137] has suggested that capillary pores become stretched during these brief elevations of pulmonary vascular pressure and that normal pressure pulmonary edema with high protein concentration occurs following this stretched pore phenomenon.

Miscellaneous Pulmonary Edema

Pulmonary edema can also occur during a wide variety of seemingly unrelated conditions where the mechanism is unknown. These include eclampsia, cardioversion, cardiopulmonary bypass, and following pulmonary embolism, cardioversion, cardiopulmonary bypass, and following pulmonary embolism. It is impossible to classify any of these forms of edema simply under the mechanism of high-pressure edema or damaged capillaries and their precise mechanism awaits future investigation.

References

1. Muir AL, Hall DL, Despas P, Hogg JC: Distribution of blood flow in the lungs in acute pulmonary edema in dogs. J Appl Physiol 33:763–769, 1972.

2. Staub NC, Nagano H, Pearce ML: Pulmonary edema in dogs especially the sequence of fluid accumulation in the lungs. J Appl Physiol 22:227–240, 1967.

3. Staub NC: Pulmonary edema. Physiol Rev 54:678–811, 1974.

4. Michel RP: Arteries and veins of the normal dog lung: Qualitative and quantitative structural differences. Am J Anat 164:227–241, 1982.

5. Muir AL, Hogg JC, Naimark A, et al.: Effect of alveolar liquid on distribution of blood flow in dog lungs. J Appl Physiol 39:885–890, 1975.

6. Glazier JB, Hughes JMB, Maloney JE, West JB: Measurements of capillary dimensions and blood volume in rapidly frozen lungs. J Appl Physiol 26:65–76, 1969.

7. Schneeberger-Keley EE, Karnovsky MJ: The ultrastructural basis of alveolar capillary membrane permeability to peroxidase used as tracer. J Cell Biol 37:781–793, 1968.

8. Tood TRJ, Baile EM, Hogg JC: Pulmonary capillary permeability during hemorrhagic shock. J Appl Physiol 45:298–306, 1978.

9. Weibel ER: Fleischner Lecture: Looking into the lung: What can it tell us? AJR 133:1021–1031, 1979.

10. Permutt S, Howell JBL, Procter DF, Riley RL: Effect of lung inflation on static pressure-volume characteristics of pulmonary vessels. J Appl Physiol 16:64–70, 1971.

11. Starling EH: On the absorption of fluids from the connective tissue. J Physiol (Lond) 19:312–326, 1896.

12. Guyton AC, Granger HJ, Taylor AE: Interstitial fluid pressure. Physiol Rev 51:527–563, 1971.

13. Leak LV, Burke JF: Ultrastructural studies of the lymphatic anchoring filaments. J Cell Biol 36:129–149, 1968.

14. Robin ED, Cross CE, Zelis R: Pulmonary edema — Part I. N Engl J Med 288:239–246, 1973.

15. Robin ED, Cross CE, Zelis R. Pulmonary edmea — Part II. N Engl J Med 288:292–304, 1973.

16. Ziskind MM, Wiell H, George RA: Acute pulmonary edema following the treatment of spontaneous pneumothorax with excessive negative intrapleural pressure. Am Rev Respir Dis 92:632–636, 1965.

17. Trapnell DH, Thurston JT: Unilateral pulmonary edema after pleural aspiration. Lancet 1:1367–1369, 1970.

18. Stein LA, Vidal JJ, Hogg JC, Fraser RG: Acute lobar collapse in canine lungs. Invest Radiol 11:518–517, 1976.

19. Guyton AC, Lindsey AW: Effect of elevated left atrial pressure and decreased plasma protein concentration on the development of pulmonary edema. Circ Res 7:649–657, 1959.

20. Rusznyak J, Foldi M, Szabo G: Lymphatics and Lymph Circulation: Physiology and Pathology. Youlten L (ed) 2nd English ed. Oxford and New York: Pergamon Press, 1967.

21. Cross CR, Shaver JA, Wilson RJ, Robin ED: Mitral stenosis and pulmonary fibrosis: Special reference to pulmonary edema and lung lymphatic function. Arch Intern Med 125:248–254, 1970.

22. Ashbaugh DG, Bigelow DB, Petty TL, Levine BE: Acute respiratory distress in adults. Lancet 2:319–323, 1967.

23. Pepe PE, Potkin RT, Reus DH, Hudson LD, Carrico CJ: Clinical predictors of the adult respiratory distress syndrome. Am J Surg 144:124–130, 1982.

24. Brigham KL, Bowers RE, Hanes J: Increased sheep lung vascular permeability caused by *Escherichia coli* endotoxin. Circ Res 45:292–297, 1979.

25. Brigham KL, Woolverton WC, Staub NC: Reversible increase in pulmonary vascular permeability after *Pseudomonas aeruginosa* bacteremia in unanesthetized sheep. Chest 65 (suppl) 51S–54S, 1974.

26. Malik AB, Van der Zee H: Mechanisms of pulmonary edema produced by microembolization. Cir Res 42:72–79, 1979.

27. Flick MR, Perel A, Staub NC: Leukocytes are required for increased lung microvascular permeability after micro-embolization in sheep. Circ Res 48:344–351, 1981.

28. Johnson A, Malik AB: Effect of granulocytopenia on extravascular lung water content after micro-embolization. Am Rev Respir Dis 122:561–566, 1980.

29. Larsen GL, Mitchell BC, Henson PM. The pulmonary response of C5 sufficient and deficient mice to immune complexes. Am Rev Respir Dis 123:434–439, 1981.

30. Meyrik B, Brigham KL: Acute effects of *Escherichia coli* endotoxin on the pulmonary microcirculation of anesthetized sheep structure-function relationships. Lab Invest 48:458–470, 1983.

31. Heflin AC, Brigham KL: Prevention by granulocyte depletion of increased vascular permeability of sheep lung following endotoxemia. J Clin Invest 68:1253–1260, 1981.

32. Fantone JC, Ward PA: Role of oxygen-derived free radicals and metabolites in leukocyte-dependent inflammatory reactions. Am J Pathol 107:397–418, 1982.

33. Michel RP, Laforte M, Hogg JC: Physiology and morphology of pulmonary microvascular injury during shock and reinfusion. J Appl Physiol 50:1227–1235, 1981.

34. Katzenstein AA, Bloor CM, Leibow AA: Diffuse alveolar damage: the role of oxygen, shock and related factors. Am J Pathol 85:210–228, 1976.

35. Nash G, Blennerhassett JB, Pontoppidan H. Pulmonary lesions associated with oxygen therapy and artificial ventilation. N Engl J Med 276:368–374, 1967.

36. Pratt PC, Vollmer RT, Shelburne JD, Crapo JD: Pulmonary morphology in the multihospital collaborative extracorporeal membrane oxygenation project. Am J Pathol 95:191–214, 1979.

37. Adamson IYR, Bowden DH: The type 2 cell as progenitor of alveolar epithelial regeneration: A cytodynamic study in mice after exposure to oxygen. Lab Invest 30:35–42, 1974.

38. Warnock ML, Press M, Churg A: Further observations on cytoplasmic hyaline in the lung. Hum Pathol 11:59–65, 1980.

39. Simpson DL, Goodman M, Spector SL, Petty TL: Long-term follow-up in bronchial reactivity testing in survivors of the adult respiratory distress syndrome. Am Rev Respir Dis 117:449–454, 1978.

40. Churg A, Golden J, Fligiel S, Hogg JC: Bronchopulmonary dysplasia in the adult. Am Rev Respir Dis 127:117–120, 1983.

41. Leibow AA: Definition and classification of interstitial pneumonias in human pathology. Prog Respir Res 8:1–33, 1975.

42. Gibson GJ, Pride NB: Pulmonary mechanics in fibrosing alveolitis. Am Rev Respir Dis 116:637–647, 1977.

43. Ribaudo CA, Grace WJ: Pulmonary aspiration. Am J Med 50:510–520, 1971.

44. Cahill JM: Drowning: The problem of non-fatal submersion and the unconscious patient. Surg Clin North Am 48:423–430, 1968.

45. Modell JH, Graves SA, Ketover A: Clinical course of 91 consecutive near-drowning victims. Chest 70(2):231–238, 1976.

46. Swann HG, Spafford NR. Body salt and water changes during fresh and sea water drowning. Tex Respir Biol Med 9:356–382, 1951.

47. Sladen A, Zauder HL: Methylprednisolone therapy for pulmonary edema following near-drowning. JAMA 215:1793–1795, 1971.

48. Pratt PC: Pulmonary capillary proliferation induced by oxygen inhalation. Am J Pathol 34:1033–1049, 1958.

49. Pratt PC: Pathology of pulmonary oxygen toxicity. Am Rev Respir Dis 110:51–57, 1974.

50. Singer MM, Wright F, Stanley L, et al.: Oxygen toxicity in man: A prospective study in patients after open-heart surgery. N Engl J Med 283:1473–1478, 1970.

51. Barber RE, Lee J, Hamilton WK: Oxygen toxicity in man: A prospective study in patients with irreversible brain damage. N Engl J Med 283:1478–1484, 1970.

52. Hasleton PS, Penna P, Torry J: Effect of oxygen on the lungs after blast injury and burns. J Clin Pathol 34:1147–1154, 1981.

53. Hyde RW, Rawson AJ: Unintentional iatrogenic oxygen pneumonitis—response to therapy. Ann Intern Med 71:517–531, 1969.

54. Anderson WR, Strickland MB: Pulmonary complications of oxygen therapy in the neonate: Postmortem study of bronchopulmonary dysplasia with emphasis of fibroproliferative obliterative bronchitis and bronchiolitis. Arch Pathol 91:506–514, 1971.

55. Anderson WR, Strickland MB, Tsai SH, Haglin JT: Light microscopic and ultrastructural study of the adverse effects of oxygen therapy on the neonate lung. Am J Pathol 73:327–348, 1973.

56. Banerjee CK, Girling DJ, Wigglesworth JS. Pulmonary fibroplasia in newborn babies treated with oxygen and artificial ventilation. Arch Dis Child 47:509–518, 1972.

57. Bonikos DS, Bench KG, Northway WH, Edwards DK. Bronchopulmonary dysplasia: The pulmonary pathologic sequel of necrotizing bronchiolitis and pulmonary fibrosis. Hum Pathol 7:643–666, 1976.

58. Deneke SM, Fanburg BL. Normobaric oxygen toxicity of the lung. N Engl J Med 303:76–86, 1980.

59. Frank L, Massaro D. Oxygen toxicity. Am J Med 69:117–126, 1980.

60. Fridovich I. Superoxide dismutase in biology and medicine. In Autor AP (ed): *Pathology of Oxygen*. New York: Academic Press, 1982, pp 1–19.

61. Hayhurst ER, Scott E: Four cases of sudden death in a silo. JAMA 63:1570–1572, 1914.

62. Delaney LT, Schmidt HW, Stroebel CF: "Silo-filler's disease." Proc Mayo Clin 31:189–198, 1956.

63. Moskowitz RL, Lyons HA, Cottell HR: Silo filler's disease: Clinical, physiologic and pathologic study of a patient. Am J Med 36:457–462, 1964.

64. Hamming WJ, MacBeth WT, Chass RL: The photochemical air pollution syndrome. Arch Environ Health 14:137–149, 1967.

65. Golden JA, Nadel JA, Boushey HA: Bronchial hyperirritability in healthy subjects after exposure to ozone. Am Rev Respir Dis 118:287–294, 1978.

66. Holtzman MJ, Fabbri LM, O'Byrne PM, et al.: Importance of airway inflammation for hyperresponsiveness induced by ozone. Am Rev Respir Dis 127:686–690, 1983.

67. Bils RF: Ultrastructural alterations of alveolar tissue of mice. III. Ozone. Arch Environ Health 20:468–480, 1970.

68. Nichols BH: Clinical effects of the inhalation of nitrogen dioxide. AJR 23:516–520, 1930.

69. Lippman M: Pulmonary reaction to drugs. Med Clin North Am 61:1353–1367, 1977.

70. Morrison DA, Goldman AL: Radiologic patterns of drug-induced lung diseases. Radiology 131:299–304, 1979.

71. Rosenow E III: The spectrum of drug-induced pulmonary disease. Ann Intern Med 77:977–991, 1972.

72. Sostman HD, Matthay RA, Putman CE: Cytotoxic drug-induced lung disease. Am J Med 62:608–615, 1977.

73. Sostman HD, Putnam CE, Gamsu G: Review: Diagnosis of chemotherapy lung. AJR 136:33–40, 1981.

74. Weiss RB, Muggia FM: Cytotoxic drug-induced pulmonary disease: Up-date 1980. Am J Med 68:259–266, 1980.

75. Lascari AD, Strano AJ, Johnson WW, Collins G: Methotrexate-induced sudden fatal pulmonary reaction. Cancer 40:1393–1397, 1977.

76. Hill JD, Ratliffe JL, Parrott J, et al.: Pulmonary pathology in acute respiratory insufficiency: Lung biopsy as a diagnostic tool. J Thorac Cardiovasc Surg 71:64–71, 1976.

77. Bedrossian CWM, Miller WC, Luna MA: Methotrexate-induced diffuse interstitial pulmonary fibrosis. South Med J 72:313–318, 1979.

78. Kirschner RH, Esterly JR: Pulmonary lesions associated with busulphan therapy of chronic myelogenous leukemia. Cancer 27:1074–1080, 1971.

79. Littler WA, Kay JM, Hasleton PS, Heath D: Busulphan lung. Thorax 24:639–655, 1969.

80. Luna MA, Bedrossian CWM, Lichtiger B, Salem PA: Interstitial pneumonitis associated with bleomycin therapy. Am J Clin Pathol 58:501–510, 1972.

81. Pearl M: Busulphan lung. Am J Dis Child 131:650–652, 1977.

82. Gyorkey F, Gyorkey P, Sinkovics JG: Origin and significance of intranuclear tubular inclusions in type II pulmonary alveolar epithelial cells of patients with bleomycin and busulphan toxicity. Ultrastruct Pathol 1:211–221, 1980.

83. Iacovino JR, Leitner J, Abbas AK, et al.: Fatal pulmonary reaction from low doses of bleomycin: An idiosyncratic tissue response. JAMA 235:1253–1255, 1976.

84. Aronin PA, Mahaley MS, Rudnick SA, et al.: Prediciton of BCNU pulmonary toxicity in patients with malignant gliomas: An assessment of risk factors. N Engl J Med 303:183–188, 1980.

85. Heard BE, Cook RA: Busulphan lung. Thorax 23:187–193, 1968.

86. Geller M, Dickie HA, Kass DA, et al.: The histopathology of acute nitrofurantoin-associated pneumonitis. Ann Allergy 37:275–279, 1976.

87. Holmberg L, Boman G, Bottiger LE, et al.: Adverse reactions to nitrofurantoin: Analysis of 921 reports. Am J Med 69:733–738, 1980.

88. Israel KS, Brashnear RE, Sharma HM, et al.: Pulmonary fibrosis and nitrofurantoin. Am Rev Respir Dis 108:353–356, 1973.

89. Rosenow EC III, DeRemee RA, Dines DE: Chronic nitrofurantoin pulmonary reaction: Report of 5 cases. N Engl J Med 279:1258–1262, 1968.

90. Bone RC, Wolfe J, Sobonya RE, et al.: Desquamative interstitial pneumonia following long-term nitrofurantoin therapy. Am J Med 60:697–701, 1976.

91. James DW, Whimster WF, Hamilton EB: Gold lung. Br Med J 1:1523–1524, 1978.

92. Geddes DM, Brostoff J: Pulmonary fibrosis associated with hypersensitivity to gold salts. Br Med J 1:1444, 1976.

93. Gould PW, McCormack PL, Palmer DG: Pulmonary damage associated with sodium aurothiomalate therapy. J Rheumatol 4:252–260, 1977.

94. McCormick J, Cole S, Lahirir B, et al.: Pneumonitis caused by gold salt therapy: Evidence for the role of cell-mediated immunity in its pathogenesis. Am Rev Respir Dis 122:145–151, 1980.

95. Scott DL, Bradby GV, Aitman TJ, et al.: Relationship of gold and penicillamine therapy to diffuse interstitial lung disease. Ann Rheum Dis 40:136–141, 1981.

96. Smith W, Ball GV: Lung injury due to gold treatment. Arthritis Rheum 23:351–354, 1980.

97. Winterbauer RH, Wilske KR, Wheelis RF: Diffuse pulmonary injury associated with gold treatment. N Engl J Med 294:919–921, 1976.

98. Erwteman TM, Braat MC, van Aken WG: Interstitial pulmonary fibrosis: A new side effect of practolol. Br Med J 2:297–298, 1977.

99. Marshall AJ, Eltringham WK, Barritt DW, et al.: Respiratory disease associated with practolol therapy. Lancet 2:1254–1257, 1977.

100. Heard BE: Fibrous healing of old iatrogenic pulmonary edema (hexamenonium lung). J Pathol Bacteriol 83:159–164, 1962.

101. Eastmond CJ: Diffuse alveolitis as a complication of penicillamine treatment for rheumatoid arthritis. Br Med J 1:1506, 1976.

102. Dorn MR, Walker BK: Noncardiogenic pulmonary edema associated with hydroclorothiazide therapy. Chest 79:482–483, 1981.

103. Hill RS, Spragg RG, Wedel MK, Moser KM. Adult respiratory distress syndrome associated with colchicine intoxication. Ann Intern Med 83:523–524, 1975.

104. Glauser FL, Smith WR, Caldwell A, et al.: Etchlorvynol (placidyl)-induced pulmonary edema. Ann Intern Med 84:46–48, 1976.

105. Byers J, Soin JS, Fisher RS, Hutchins G: Acute pulmonary alveolitis in narcotics abuse. Arch Pathol 99:273–277, 1975.

106. Siegel H: Human pulmonary pathology associated with narcotic and other addictive drugs. Hum Pathol 3:55–66, 1972.

107. Smith WR, Glauser FL, Dearden LC, et al.: Deposits of immunoglobulin and complement in the pulmonary tissue of patients with 'heroin lung'. Chest 73:471–476, 1978.

108. Steinberg AD, Karliner JS: The clinical spectrum of heroin pulmonary edema. Arch Intern Med 122:122–127, 1968.

109. Heffner J, Sahn SA: Salicylate-induced pulmonary edema; clinical features and prognosis. Ann Intern Med 95:405–409, 1981.

110. Dearden LC, Fairshter RD, McRae DM, et al.: Pulmonary ultrastructure of the late aspects of human paraquat poisoning. Am J Pathol 93:667–680, 1978.

111. Harley JB, Grinspan S, Root RK: Paraquat suicide in a young woman: Results of therapy directed against the superoxide radical. Yale J Biol Med 50:481–488, 1977.

112. Higenbottam T, Crome P, Parkinson C, Nunn J: Further clinical observations on the pulmonary effects of paraquat ingestion. Thorax 34:161–165, 1979.

113. Rebello G, Mason JK: Pulmonary histological appearances in fatal paraquat poisoning. Histopathology 2:53–66, 1978.

114. Spector D, Whorton D, Zarchary J, Slavin R. Fatal paraquat poisoning: tissue concentrations and implications for treatment. Johns Hopkins Med J 142:110–113, 1978.

115. Toner PG, Vetters JM, Spilg WG, Harland W: Fine structure of the lung lesion in a case of paraquat poisoning. J Pathol 102:182–185, 1970.

116. Bennett DE, Million RR, Ackerman LV: Bilateral radiation pneumonitis; a complication of the radiotherapy of bronchogenic carcinoma (report and analysis of seven case with autopsy). Cancer 23:1001–1018, 1969.

117. Copland GM, Kolin A, Shulman HS: Fatal pulmonary intra-alveolar fibrosis after paraquat ingestion. N Engl J Med 291:290–291, 1974.

118. Braun SR, doPico A, Olson CE, Caldwell W: Low-dose radiation pneumonitis. Cancer 35:1322–1324, 1974.

119. Castellino RA, Glatstein E, Turbow MM, et al.: Latent radiation injury of lungs or heart activated by steroid withdrawal. Ann Intern Med 80:593–599, 1974.

120. Einhorn L, Krause M, Hornback N, Furnas B: Enhanced pulmonary toxicity with bleomycin and radiotherapy in oat-cell lung cancer. Cancer 37:2414–2416, 1976.

121. Fajardo LF, Berthrong M: Radiation injury in surgical pathology, Part 1. Am J Surg Pathol 2:159–199, 1978.

122. Gross NJ: Pulmonary effects of radiation therapy. Ann Intern Med 86:81–92, 1977.

123. Gross NJ: The pathogenesis of radiation-induced lung damage. Lung 159:115–125, 1981.

124. Littman P, Davis LW, Nash J, et al.: The hazard of acute radiation pneumonitis in children receiving mediastinal radiation. Cancer 33:1520–1525, 1974.

125. Roswit B, White DC: Severe radiation injuries of the lung. AJR 129:127–136, 1977.

126. Hultgren HN, Grover RF: Circulatory adaption to high altitude. Ann Rev Med 19:119–152, 1968.

127. Hultgren HN, Lopez CE, Lundberg E, Miller H: Physiologic studies of pulmonary edema at high altitude. Circulation 29:393–408, 1964.

128. Nicholoff DM, Ballin HM, Visscher MB: Hypoxia and edema of the perfused isolated canine lung. Proc Soc Exp Biol Med 131:22–26, 1969.

129. Fisher AB, Hyde RW, Reif J: Insensitivity of the alveolar septum to local hypoxia. Am J Physiol 23:770–776, 1972.

130. Whayne TF Jr, Severinghaus JW: Experimental hypoxia pulmonary edema in the rat. J Appl Physiol 25:729–732, 1968.

131. Sarnoff SJ, Sarnoff LC: Neurohemodynamics of pulmonary edema. II. Role of sympathetic pathways in the elevation of pulmonary and systemic vascular pressures following intercisternal injection of fibrin. Circulation 6:52–62, 1952.

132. Mickersie RC, Christensen JM, Lawrence H, et al.: Pulmonary extravascular fluid accumulation following intracranial injury. J Trauma 23:968–975, 1983.

133. Fein IA, Racknow EC: Neurogenic pulmonary edema. Chest 81:318–320, 1982.

134. Hoff JT, Nishimura M, Garcia-Uria J, Miranda S: Experimental neurogenia pulmonary edema. Part I: The role of systemic hypertension. J Neurosurg 54:627–631, 1981.

135. Garcia-Urcia J, Hoff JT, Miranda S, Nishimura M: Experimental neurogenia pulmonary edema. Part II: The role of cardiopulmonary pressure change. J Neurosurg 54:632–636, 1981.

136. Carlson RW, Schaeffer RC, Michaels SG, Wiel MN: Pulmonary edema following intracranial hemorrhage. Chest 75:731–734, 1979.

137. Robin ED: Permeability pulmonary edema. In Fishman A, Renkin EM, (eds): *Pulmonary Edema*. Baltimore: Williams & Wilkins, 1979, pp 217–228.

17 Pulmonary Angiitis and Granulomatosis

Anna-Luise A. Katzenstein

Introduction

Liebow was the first investigator to define and classify the pulmonary angiitides and granulomatoses.[1] He divided these diseases into four categories: Wegener's granulomatosis, necrotizing sarcoid granulomatosis, lymphomatoid granulomatosis, and bronchocentric granulomatosis. Liebow was also the first to describe the latter three entities which, although probably not new diseases, were previously lumped under the diagnosis of Wegener's granulomatosis. The classification of pulmonary angiitis and granulomatosis that we utilize is summarized in Table 17–1.[2, 3] It is identical to that proposed by Liebow except that allergic angiitis and granulomatosis is included in addition to the other entities.

As the term angiitis and granulomatosis implies, the diseases constituting this group all manifest inflammation or cellular infiltration of vessel walls combined with destruction and necrosis of the pulmonary parenchyma. Liebow believed that vascular inflammation was the primary, initiating event in all the diseases except for bronchocentric granulomatosis, in which the process begins around small bronchi and bronchioles. Although this concept may be true for Wegener's granulomatosis, allergic angiitis and granulomatosis, and possibly necrotizing sarcoid granulomatosis, most investigators believe that the vascular lesion in lymphomatoid granulomatosis is a secondary event related to an aggressive cellular infiltrate. This disease also differs from the other angiitides and granulomatoses in that while it is characterized by a lymphohistiocytic infiltrate and necrosis, true granulomatous inflammation is not seen. Lymphomatoid granulomatosis is currently considered by most investigators to belong to the lymphoproliferative diseases, and its infiltrate is felt to be more neoplastic than inflammatory.[2, 3] Despite these observations, we prefer to continue classifying lymphomatoid granulomatosis with the angiitides and granulomatoses rather than with lymphoproliferative diseases, since it so commonly enters the differential diagnosis of the former entities.

Pulmonary angiitis and granulomatosis should not be considered to represent a spectrum of similar diseases having only minor differences in clinical or pathologic features.[1–8] Rather, each disorder is a distinct clinicopathologic entity, and each likely has different etiologies and pathogeneses.[9] For example, Wegener's granulomatosis is thought to be a primary vasculitis of unknown etiology, lymphomatoid granulomatosis a lymphoproliferative disease, and bronchocentric granulomatosis represents, in many cases, a hypersensitivity reaction to Aspergillus. The correct differentiation of these diseases is especially important because both prognosis and therapy differ for each. Wegener's granulomatosis, a lethal disease if untreated or inappropriately treated, responds dramatically to a combination of cyclophosphamide and corticosteroids. The same therapy would be unnecessary and even dangerous in necrotizing sarcoid granulomatosis or bronchocentric granulomatosis, two diseases that have excellent prognoses. In lymphomatoid granulomatosis mortality rates are very high, and the optimal therapy is not well defined. The contrasting clinical and pathologic features of pulmonary angiitis and granulomatosis are summarized in Tables 17–2 and 17–3.

Mycobacterial or fungal infections are major lesions in the differential diagnosis of the pulmonary angiitides and granulomatoses, especially when signs of extrapulmonary involvement are absent.[2] The handling and interpretation of suspected infectious granulomas have been discussed in detail elsewhere.[2, 10] Briefly, a portion of all such lesions should be cultured at the time of excision and appropriate special stains for organisms examined before the diagnosis of a pulmonary angiitis and granulomatosis is considered.

Table 17–1. Pulmonary Angiitis and Granulomatosis

Wegener's granulomatosis
Allergic angiitis and granulomatosis
Necrotizing sarcoid granulomatosis
Lymphomatoid granulomatosis
Bronchocentric granulomatosis

Wegener's Granulomatosis

Wegener's granulomatosis is characterized by necrotizing vasculitis and granulomatous inflammation involving primarily the lungs but also other organs.[1, 11–14] A triad of involvement, including the upper respiratory tract, lungs, and kidney is classically described in this disease. It has been shown, however, that a single or any combination of these three major sites can be involved, and other sites, especially skin, nervous system, and heart are occasionally affected as well. Liebow subdivided Wegener's granulomatosis into a classical and a limited or localized form.[1] According to this nomenclature, classical Wegener's granulomatosis is characterized by lung lesions along with involvement in one or both of the other sites from the classically described triad. Additionally more widespread organs may also be affected. Limited Wegener's granulomatosis is characterized by lung involvement in the absence of upper respiratory tract and kidney lesions, although occasionally other organs, especially the skin, may be involved.[1, 15–18] Although the histologic features of classical and limited Wegener's granulomatosis are identical, the clinical course is less fulminant and the prognosis better in the limited form. DeRemee and associates[19] consider the two forms to represent a continuum of disease in which any single or combination of anatomic sites can be involved. They prefer to more specifically classify Wegener's granulomatosis by the site of involvement, using the mnemonic ELK (upper respiratory tract, lung, kidney).

Clinical Features

Middle-aged adults are affected most often by Wegener's granulomatosis, although the disease can occur at any age.[1, 11, 14, 20] Cases have even been reported in children.[21, 22] The presenting clinical manifestations depend on the major site of involvement. With upper respiratory tract lesions, the most common findings are mucosal ulcerations in the nose or nasopharynx, destruction of nasal cartilages, or evidence of sinusitis. These patients may have a bloody or purulent discharge from the affected area and frequently complain of pain. With lung involvement a variety of nonspecific chest complaints are common, including cough, occasionally with hemoptysis, chest pain, and fever. Multiple, often bilateral mass-like nodular densities, are the most common chest radiographic findings, although solitary lesions can also occur.[1, 11, 13, 14, 17, 20] Cavitation is common. Less-frequent patterns of lung involvement include parenchymal consolidation or a reticulonodular pattern. Involvement of the airways has also been described and may produce bronchial narrowing or an endobronchial mass. Pleural thickening or pleural effusion are other less-common findings.[23] In patients with renal involvement renal failure can develop, or evidence of glomerulonephritis may be found on urinalysis.

A variety of other less-common manifestations may also occur with Wegener's granulomatosis, including serous otitis media, conjunctivitis, uveitis, proptosis,[24] signs of nervous system involvement,[25, 26] and skin lesions.[27, 28] Rare patients may present with joint involvement mimicking rheumatoid arthritis.[29] The disease has been reported in association with ulcerative colitis.[30]

Table 17–2. Pulmonary Angiitides and Granulomatoses: Contrasting Clinical Features[a]

		Extra-pulmonary Involvement				
	Chest Radiograph	Glomerulonephritis	Other[b]	Asthma/Eosinophilia	Treatment	Prognosis
Wegener's granulomatosis	Usually multiple nodules	Common	Upper respiratory tract, skin	No/no	Cyclophosphamide, steroids	Good
Allergic Angiitis and granulomatosis	Infiltrates, often transient	Occasional	Heart, skin, nervous system	Yes/yes	Steroids	Good
Necrotizing sarcoid, granulomatosis	Solitary or multiple nodules	No	No	No/no	None/?steroids	Good
Lymphomatoid granulomatosis	Usually multiple nodules	No	Skin, nervous system	No/no	?Chemotherapy, ?steroids	Poor
Bronchocentric granulomatosis	Consolidation	No	No	Frequent/frequent	None/steroids	Good

[a] Based on the results of Katzenstein.[2]
[b] These include only the most common clinically apparent extrapulmonary manifestations; other sites may be less frequently involved.

Table 17–3. Pulmonary Angiitides and Granulomatoses: Contrasting Histologic Features[a]

	Topography	Atypical Lymphoreticular Cells	Eosinophils	Palisading Histiocytes	Sarcoid-like Granulomas
Wegener's granulomatosis	Angiocentric	No	±	Yes	±
Allergic angiitis and granulomatosis	Angiocentric	No	Many	Yes	±
Necrotizing sarcoid granulomatosis	Angiocentric	No	No	±	Extensive
Lymphomatoid granulomatosis	Angiocentric	Yes	No	No	No
Bronchocentric granulomatosis	Bronchocentric	No	Many[b]	Yes	±

[a] Based on the results of Katzenstein.[2]
[b] In nonasthmatic patients with bronchocentric granulomatosis, eosinophils are not always prominent.

Treatment

Without appropriate therapy, classical Wegener's granulomatosis follows a fulminant course. Approximately 90 percent of patients die within 2 years if untreated. Although limited Wegener's granulomatosis has a somewhat better prognosis, death is still common in this form of the disease. Cyclophosphamide is currently the mainstay of treatment for Wegener's granulomatosis and in extremely ill patients corticosteroids are

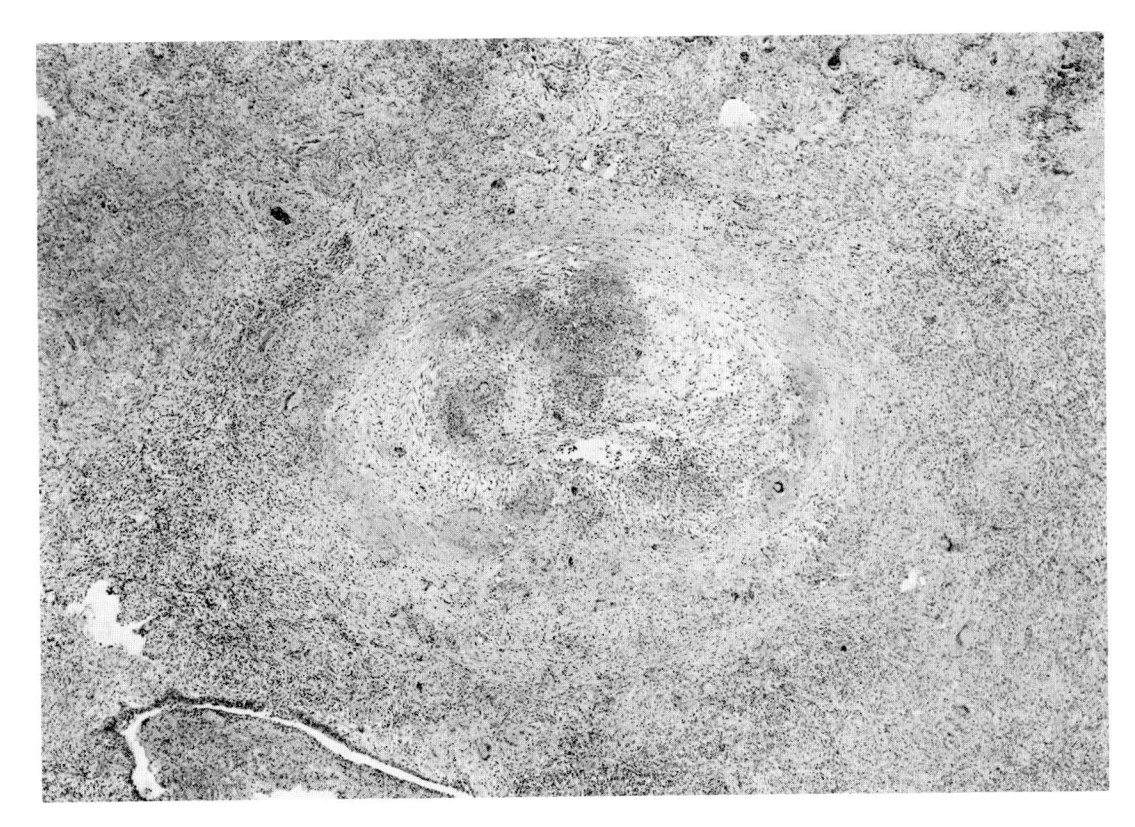

Figure 17–1. Low-magnification photomicrograph showing necrotizing vasculitis in Wegener's granulomatosis. In this example there are large areas of necrosis within the vessel wall accompanied by a chronic inflammatory cell infiltrate containing numerous multinucleated giant cells. Extensive necrosis and a similar cellular infiltrate are present in the surrounding parenchyma. (H&E, ×40).

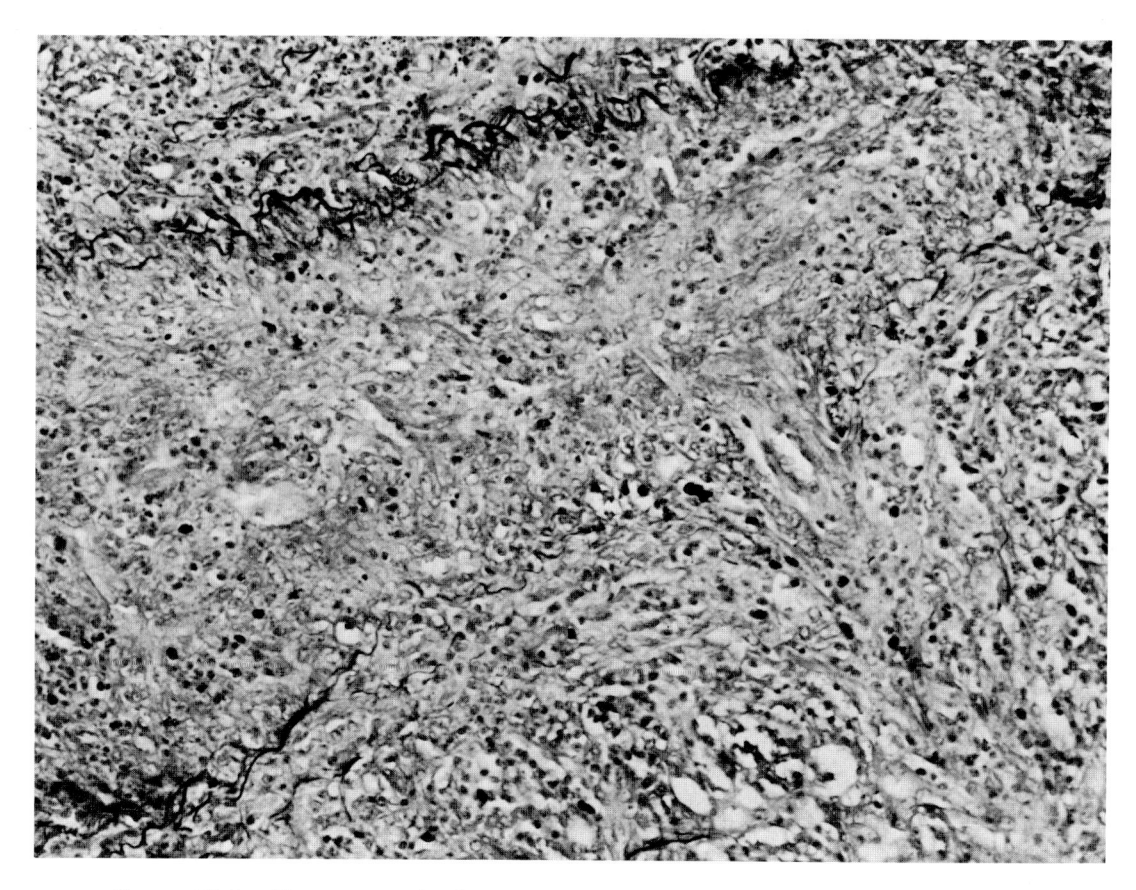

Figure 17–2. Photomicrograph showing vasculitis involving a small vein in Wegener's granulomatosis. A transmural chronic inflammatory cell infiltrate has severely fragmented the elastic lamina of the vein and has almost completely occluded the lumen (Verhoeff van Gieson's stain, ×180).

also added to the regimen.[4, 20–31] With this therapy, dramatic remissions are now achieved in over 90 percent of patients, although recurrences can occur even after many years. Whether chemotherapy is necessary for solitary lung lesions that have been totally resected is controversial. Some investigators advocate careful follow-up and chemotherapy only if new lesions develop in this situation.

Pathologic Features

Grossly, the characteristic lung lesions of Wegener's granulomatosis are discrete, firm hemorrhagic to yellow-grey, spherical masses. They are randomly distributed in the lung, and are usually multiple and often bilateral. They show varying degrees of central necrosis, and may superficially resemble caseating granulomas or necrotic tumors. Some examples have a characteristic friable, meaty, rather than caseous, internal appearance. Occasionally a grossly visible necrotic blood vessel can be identified entering the mass.

Microscopically, the most characteristic feature is a necrotizing vasculitis that is accompanied by necrotizing granulomatous inflammation in the surrounding parenchyma.[1, 12–17] The vasculitis involves both arteries and veins and can be recognized by the presence of two distinct features: (1) transmural infiltration of vessel walls by inflammatory cells, and (2) necrosis either of the vessel wall itself or of the infiltrating inflammatory cells (Figs. 17–1, 17–2. The inflammatory cells can be either acute or chronic, and variously include neutrophils, lymphocytes, plasma cells, histiocytes, and multinucleated giant cells. A particularly characteristic appearance is a small collection of pyknotic neutrophils associated with focal necrosis of the arterial media (Fig. 17–3). Sometimes the media is replaced by histiocytes arranged in a palisading pattern around the central lumen. The presence of the vasculitis in an area of otherwise uninflamed lung parenchyma is considered pathognomonic of Wegener's granulomatosis (Fig. 17–4) This finding, however, is rare. More commonly the vasculitis is found in inflamed parenchyma adjacent to necrotic areas. In these cases the pathologist must be careful to exclude an infection before diagnosing Wegener's granulomatosis, since vasculitis can occur in infections and affects vessels in a similar location (see Differentiation from Infection, below). The vasculitis associated with infections differs, however, from that of Wegener's granulomatosis in that it is rarely necrotizing.

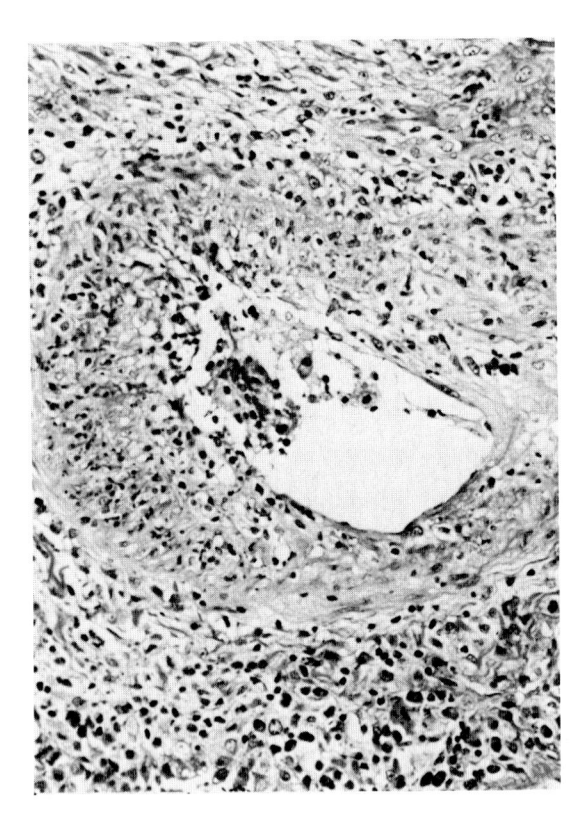

Figure 17-3. Necrotizing vasculitis in Wegener's granulomatosis. The media of this artery is infiltrated by acute inflammatory cells (left). There is extensive individual cell necrosis (H&E, ×180).

In most cases the lung parenchyma is extensively destroyed by necrotizing granulomatous inflammation which can vary in appearance from case to case. There are usually large zones of necrosis which may consist of amorphous eosinophilic debris or necrotic neutrophils and nuclear dust, or may contain remnants of recognizable lung parenchyma resembling an infarct. The necrotic regions are often irregularly or geographically shaped, and may be bordered by palisading histiocytes (Fig. 17-5). Multinucleated giant cells, containing many peripherally arranged and often pyknotic nuclei, frequently surround the necrotic zone (Fig. 17-6). Noncaseating granulomas can be found as well, but are usually not prominent. Numerous chronic inflammatory cells and fibroblasts are present, but eosinophils are not abundant. Randomly scattered smaller foci of necrosis, often containing a central purulent core and surrounded by multinucleated histiocytes and other chronic inflammatory cells, are also common.

Electron microscopy has been reported in one example of Wegener's granulomatosis of the lung.[38] It showed endothelial damage presumably due to intravascular lysis of leukocytes and occlusion of vessels. We have done electron microscopy and immunofluorescence in similar cases and have found neither dense deposits nor immune complex deposits in vascular basement membranes. Recently granular deposition of IgG and complement has been reported in alveolar septa and small blood vessels.[39]

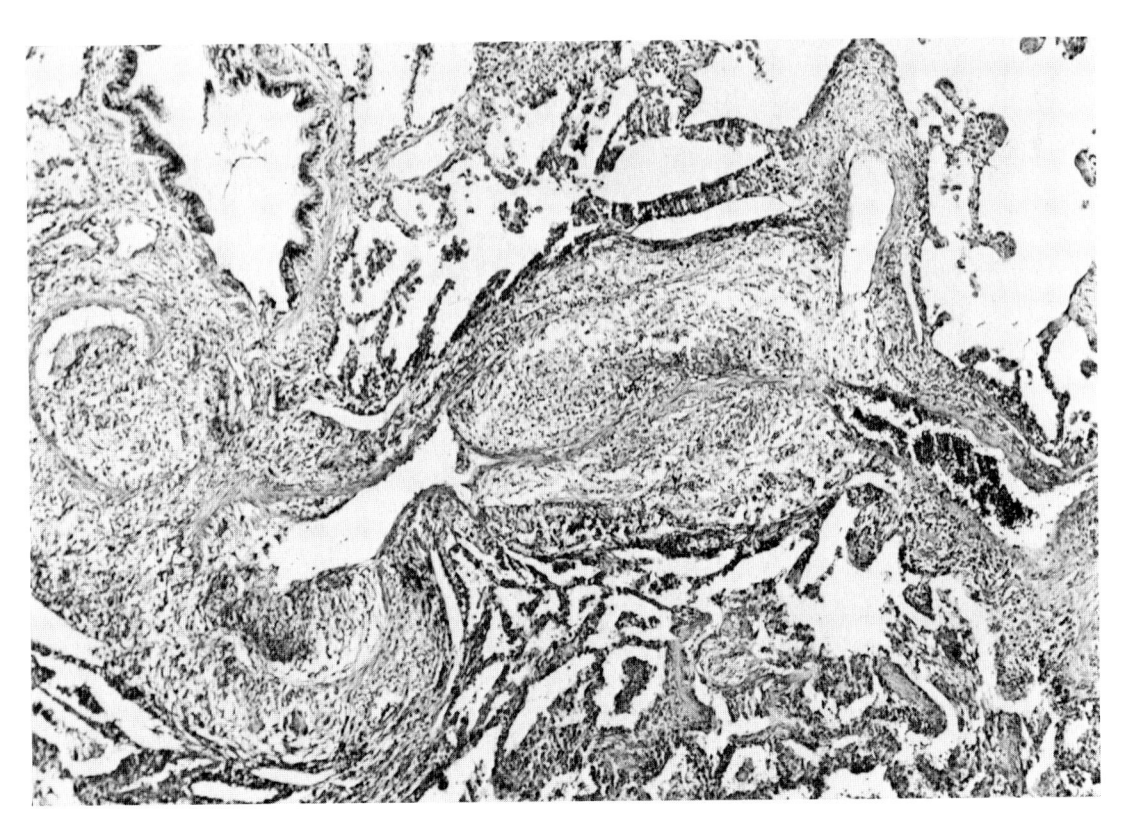

Figure 17-4. Necrotizing vasculitis in Wegener's granulomatosis occurring in relatively normal, uninflamed parenchyma (H&E, ×70).

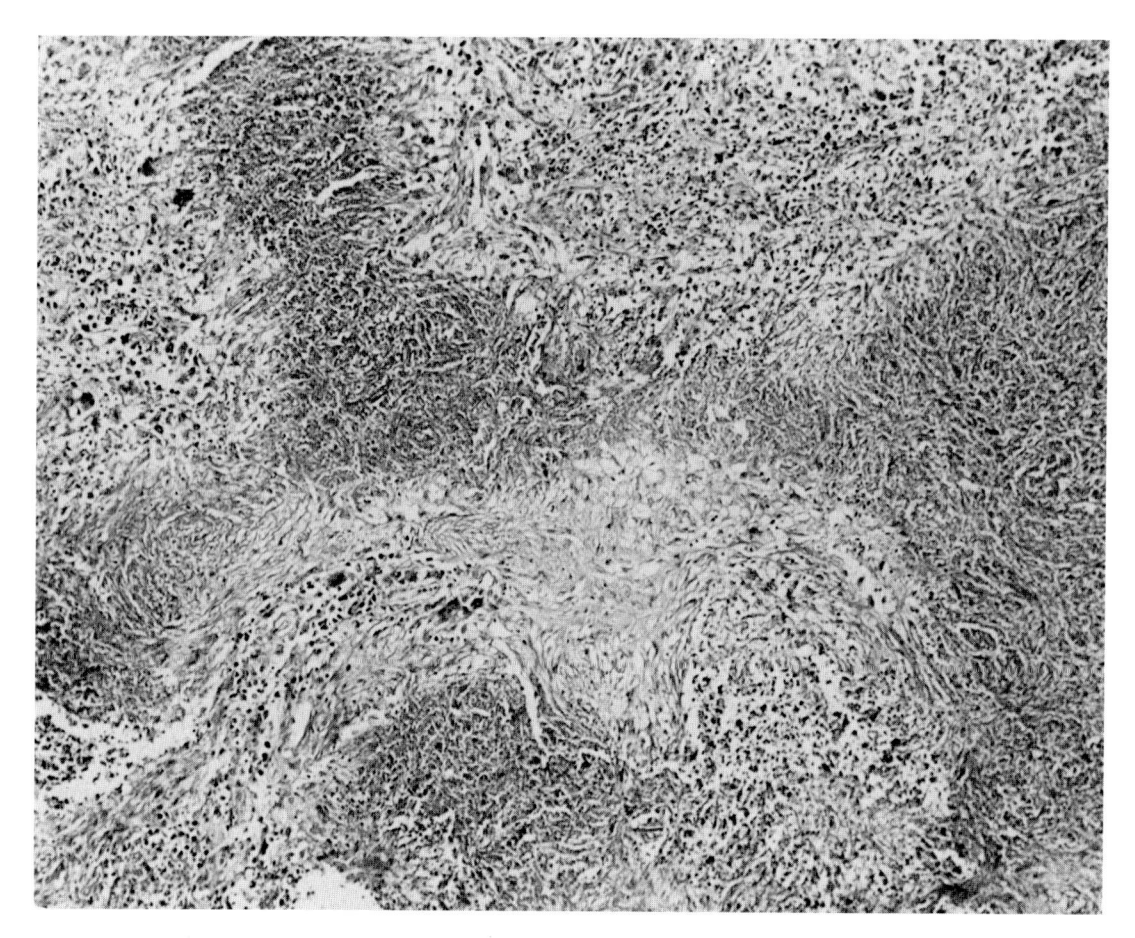

Figure 17–5. Geographically shaped necrotic zone in Wegener's granulomatosis. Palisading histiocytes are arranged around the area of necrosis in this case (H&E, ×70).

Differentiation from Infection

Granulomatous infection is perhaps the most important lesion in the differential diagnosis of Wegener's granulomatosis. Both fungal and tuberculous lung infections share many histologic features with Wegener's granulomatosis.[2,3,10] They are characterized by necrotizing granulomatous inflammation which can contain remnants of necrotic cells or shadows of lung structures and may show a geographic shape. Vasculitis is also common in infection, but it is usually found only in vessels within inflamed parenchyma. It is generally non-necrotizing and is characterized by chronic inflammation and edema of vessel walls. Foci of acute inflammation and necrosis of vascular media are not seen. The difference between granulomatous infections in the lung and Wegener's granulomatous, therefore, is more relative than absolute. All such cases should be cultured and examined carefully using special stains before diagnosing Wegener's granulomatosis.

The clinical manifestations may also help in differentiating Wegener's granulomatosis from infections. The presence of extrapulmonary involvement, especially of the nasopharynx, paranasal sinuses, or kidneys would favor Wegener's granulomatosis. Biopsy specimens from these sites or from other accessible areas such as skin can also help to confirm the diagnosis. In these areas necrotizing granulomatous inflammation and vasculitis similar to that in the lung lesions should be found, although the usual finding in the kidney in Wegener's granulomatosis is a necrotizing glomerulonephritis.

Pathogenesis

The etiology and pathogenesis of Wegener's granulomatosis are unknown. Various immunologic abnormalities have been reported, including elevated serum levels of IgE, IgA, and C3, circulating immune complexes, and defects in chemotaxis and certain aspects of cellular immunity.[40-43] The significance of these findings is unclear. The morphologic similarity of the lesions in Wegener's granulomatosis and granulomatous infections suggests that Wegener's granulomatosis may represent an abnormal or uncontrolled cell-mediated immunologic reaction which may have begun as a normal response to an infection.

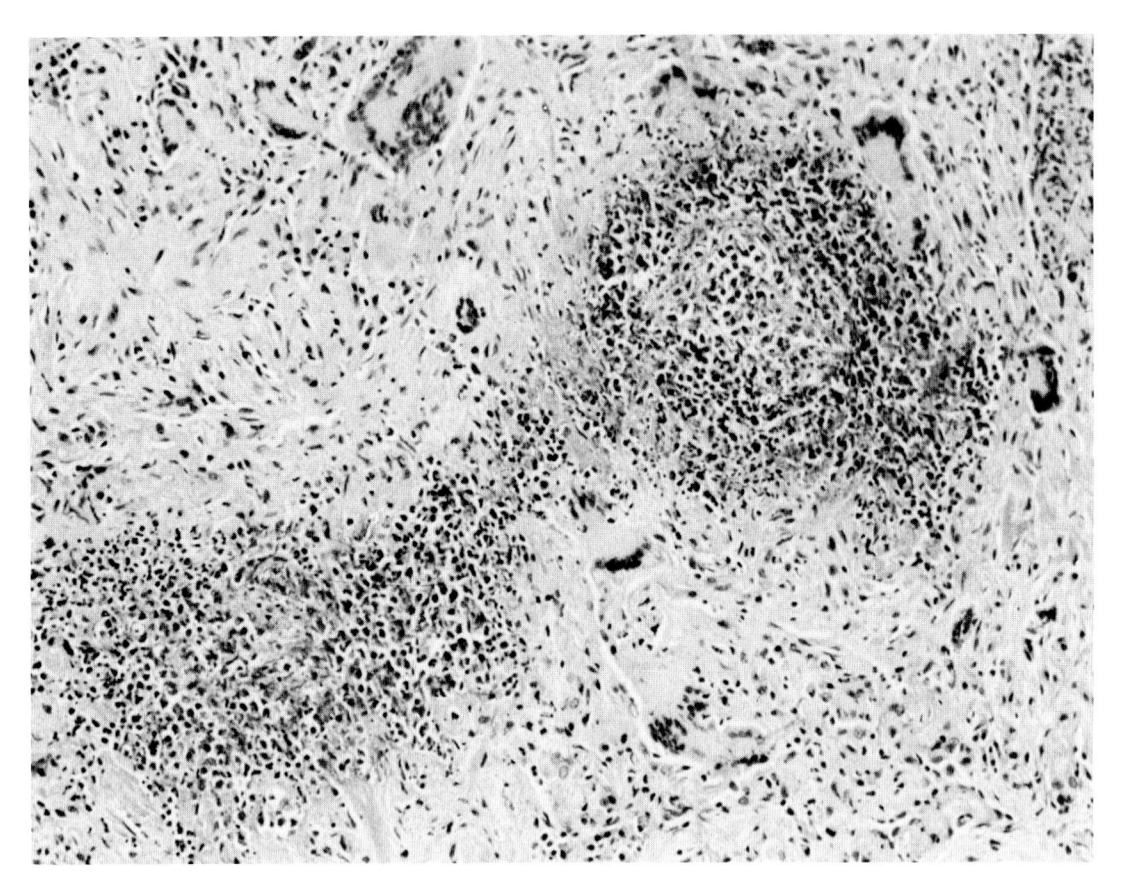

Figure 17–6. Necrotic zone in Wegener's granulomatosis surrounded by characteristic, darkly staining, multinucleated giant cells. The necrotic area in this case contains abundant cellular and nuclear debris (H&E, ×180).

Most investigators consider the vascular lesion to be the primary event in Wegener's granulomatosis and the parenchymal necrosis to be related to vascular destruction. Fienberg[27] has proposed that necrosis of both blood vessels and parenchyma occurs independently, and that one may occur without the other. Until the underlying immunologic mechanisms in this disease are better understood, these questions cannot be adequately answered.

Allergic Angiitis and Granulomatosis (Churg-Strauss Syndrome)

Allergic angiitis and granulomatosis is a rare disorder, which can involve multiple organs and is characterized pathologically by vasculitis, necrotizing granulomatous inflammation, and tissue eosinophilia. Some cases have been reported as examples of polyarteritis nodosa involving the lung.[44] It may occur at any age and affects persons of both sexes equally.[45–51] Almost all individuals with this illness have a history of chronic asthma, or they develop asthma at the time of presentation. Allergic rhinitis is a common accompanying feature. Peripheral blood eosinophilia, which can be quite high, is a constant finding, and fever is usually present at some time during the course of the disease.

Sites of Involvement

The lung is a common site of involvement in allergic angiitis and granulomatosis. Radiographically, pneumonic infiltrates are usually seen.[45, 47, 52] They may appear as patchy or dense areas of the lung or may spontaneously resolve and reappear. Other less-common radiographic patterns include nodular densities and interstitial infiltrates.

Other organs, of which the skin is probably the most common, are frequently affected in allergic angiitis and granulomatosis.[44, 45, 47, 53] Nodular subcutaneous lesions, petechiae or purpuric areas are the usual skin manifestations. Nervous system involvement is also frequent, and often presents as mononeuritis multiplex or other peripheral neuropathy. Cerebral vascular accidents, convulsions, disorientation, and coma can also occur. Evidence of gastrointestinal involvement is common, especially abdominal pain and diarrhea that may be bloody. Con-

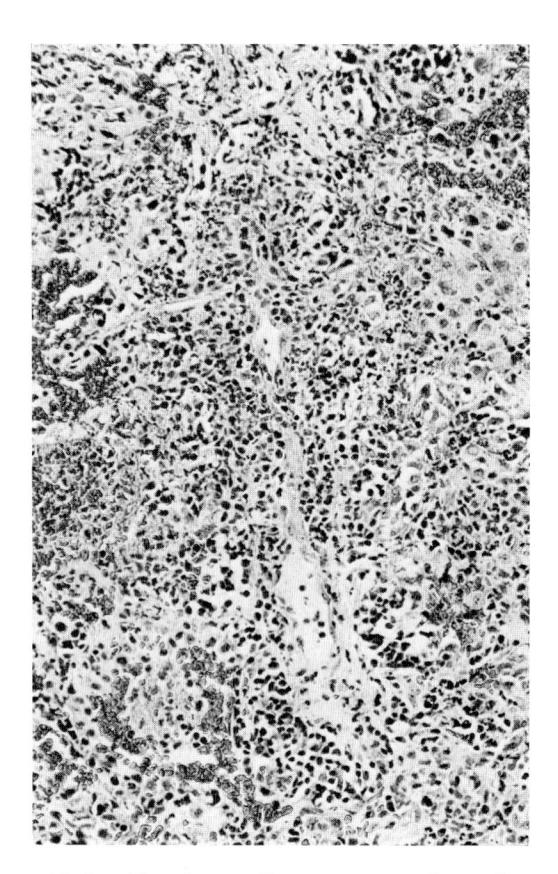

Figure 17–7. Vasculitis in allergic angiitis and granulomatosis. The media of the venule in the center of the photomicrograph is infiltrated by eosinophils admixed with a few lymphocytes and plasma cells (H&E, ×150).

gestive heart failure due to myocardial damage is a well-documented complication. Microscopic hematuria occurs in a minority of patients, but renal failure is extremely rare. A focal glomerulonephritis has been described in a few biopsied or autopsied patients, but evidence of immune complex deposition has not been found. The lower urinary tract in males is another uncommon site of involvement.[54, 55] Destructive upper respiratory tract lesions like those seen in Wegener's granulomatosis do not occur.

Treatment and Prognosis

The prognosis of untreated allergic angiitis and granulomatosis is poor. The majority of reported patients in Rose and Spencer's review were dead within a year following the onset.[44] Improved prognosis has been achieved by means of corticosteroid therapy, and some refractory cases have also responded to cytotoxic agents.[48] A 62 percent 5-year survival rate was reported by Chumbley and colleagues.[45] The major cause of death is related to heart involvement. Lung involvement and renal failure are less-common causes of death.

Histopathologic Features

The lung findings in allergic angiitis and granulomatosis are characterized by vasculitis, necrotizing granulomatous inflammation, and numerous eosinophils.[44, 46, 51, 52, 56] The vasculitis involves both arteries and veins. It may appear granulomatous, containing numerous multinucleated giant cells, or there may be a mixture of chronic inflammatory cells, especially eosinophils, within vessel walls (Fig. 17–7). In our experience, the vasculitis in allergic angiitis and granulomatosis is less necrotizing than that in Wegener's granulomatosis. Large areas of parenchyma are usually destroyed by irregularly shaped necrotic zones, often bounded by a characteristic layer of palisading, spindled histiocytes (Figs. 17–8, 17–9). Necrotic eosinophils, loose eosinophil granules, and Charcot-Leyden crystals can be identified within the necrotic foci. Eosinophils are numerous within the cellular infiltrate surrounding the necrotic granulomas, and they may fill alveolar spaces, producing an appearance identical to eosinophilic pneumonia. Airways elsewhere in the lung frequently show morphologic evidence of chronic asthma.

Differentiation from Polyarteritis Nodosa

A major lesion in the differential diagnosis of allergic angiitis and granulomatosis is polyarteritis nodosa. Patients with this condition often have chronic asthma, and there is usually associated tissue and blood eosinophilia. Beyond these similarities, however, polyarteritis nodosa differs in several major ways from allergic angiitis and granulomatosis. First, pulmonary involvement is rare in polyarteritis nodosa.[44, 57] Most cases reported by Rose and Spencer[44] as polyarteritis nodosa with pulmonary involvement would probably now be classified as allergic angiitis and granulomatosis. Histologically, polyarteritis nodosa is characterized by a vasculitis involving medium-sized arteries, but not veins, and extravascular granulomatous lesions are not a feature. When polyarteritis does involve the lung, it is predominantly the bronchial arteries that are affected.

Necrotizing Sarcoid Granulomatosis

Necrotizing sarcoid granulomatosis was first described by Liebow in 1973.[1] Although this disease shares with the other angiitides and granulomatoses the presence of lung necrosis and vasculitis, it possesses other unique clinical and pathologic features which allow for its recognition as a distinct entity.

Clinical Features

Necrotizing sarcoid granulomatosis occurs predominantly in young to middle-age adults, although the re-

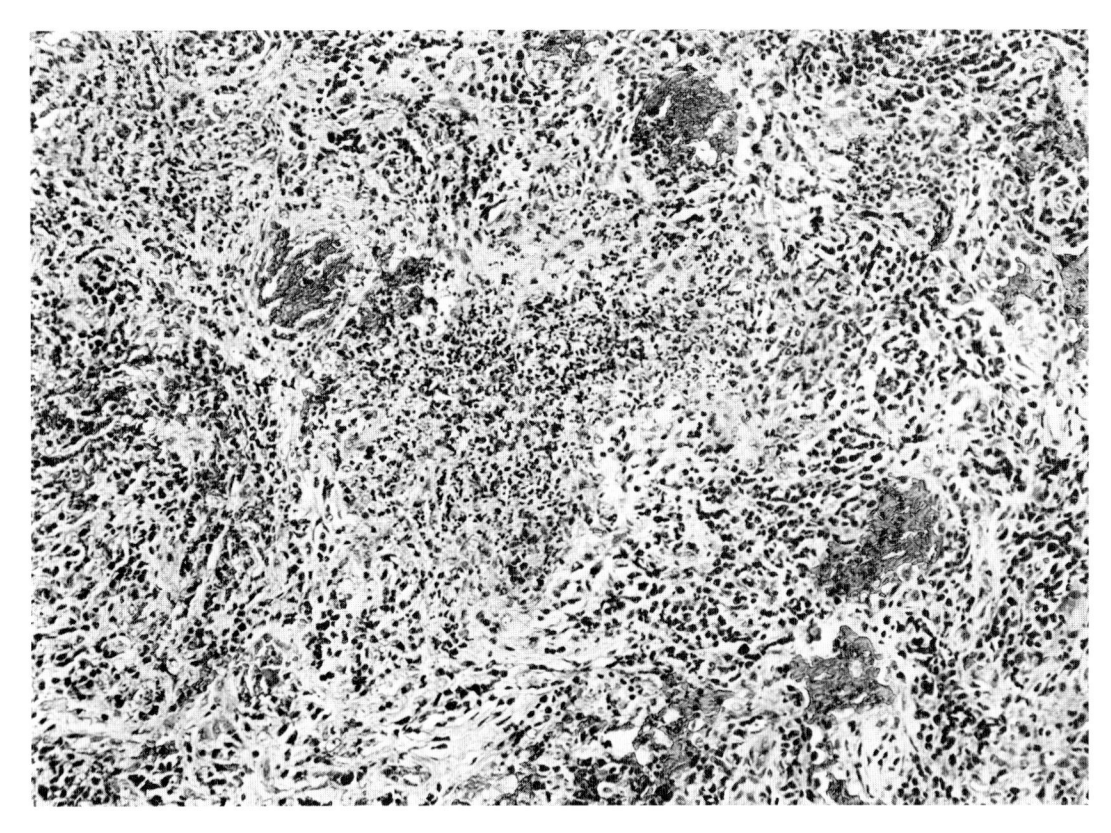

Figure 17–8. Necrotic zone bounded by epithelioid histiocytes from the same case of allergic angiitis and granulomatosis shown in Figure 17–7. Eosinophils predominate in the surrounding cellular infiltrate (H&E, ×150).

ported age range varies from 23 to 75. A female preponderance was reported in two series,[58,59] while an equal sex distribution was originally described by Liebow.[1] Patients generally present with nonspecific chest complaints such as cough, dyspnea, chest pain, and occasionally hemoptysis. Fever is a frequent accompanying finding. A few patients are asymptomatic and their chest lesions are found on a routine chest radiograph.

The most common radiographic findings are multiple, bilateral nodular densities.[1,58,59] Solitary, discrete masses or infiltrates occur less frequently and finely nodular or miliary infiltrates have been described occasionally. Hilar lymph node enlargement was noted in over half of the 12 patients reported by Churg and colleagues,[58] but in only 2 of 25 patients reported by others.[1,59,60]

The prognosis of necrotizing sarcoid granulomatosis is excellent. Unlike many of the other pulmonary angiitides and granulomatoses, extrapulmonary involvement (other than hilar lymph nodes) usually does not occur, although uveitis has been described in two patients by Churg and co-workers.[58] In the one reported patient with neurologic involvement,[61] the diagnosis of necrotizing sarcoid granulomatosis rather than Wegener's granulomatosis was not convincingly established. Patients with solitary, surgically resected lesions require no further therapy. Multiple lesions generally respond to corticosteroid therapy.

Histopathologic Features

The main histologic finding the distinguishes necrotizing sarcoid granulomatosis from the other angiitides and granulomatoses is the replacement of extensive portions of lung parenchyma by masses of noncaseating or sarcoid-like granulomas (Fig. 17–10).[1,58–60] The granulomas are distinct and well-circumscribed, and are often surrounded by a thin rim of small lymphocytes and fibroblasts. They are closely packed in clusters to form large aggregates. Necrosis is common within the coalescent masses of granulomas, but central necrosis within individual granulomas is usually not seen (Fig. 17–11). The necrotic zones bounded by noncaseating granulomas destroy the lung in a cross-country, irregular fashion.

The presence of a vasculitis involving both arteries and veins is also central to the diagnosis of necrotizing sarcoid granulomatosis. This vasculitis, which can occur in parenchyma away from maximally inflamed areas, differs somewhat in appearance from case to case. In its most characteristic form, noncaseating granulomas infiltrate the intima and media of blood vessels, and may cause narrowing or occlusion of vascular lumens (Fig. 17–12). Necrosis of vessel walls is not a prominent feature. In other cases vessel walls are infiltrated by mixed chronic inflammatory cells containing

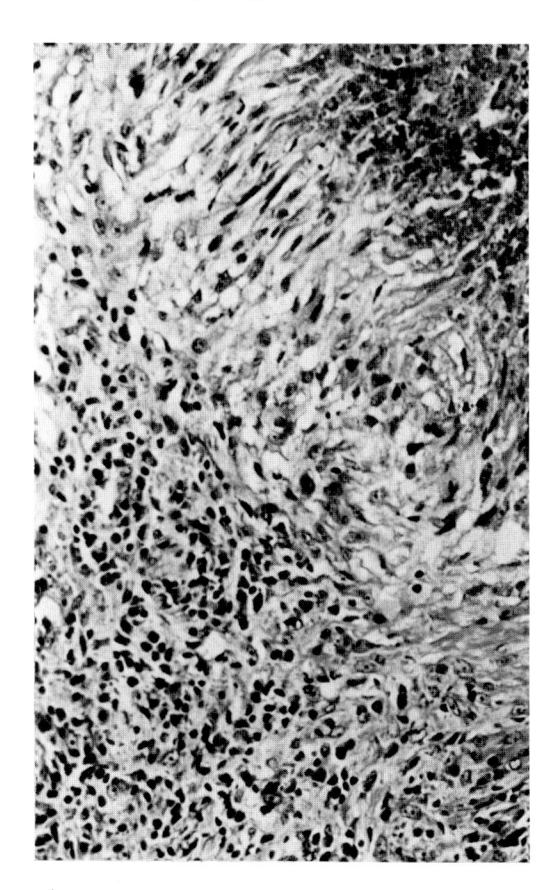

Figure 17-9. Palisading histiocytes surrounding a necrotic zone from a case of allergic angiitis and granulomatosis. Numerous eosinophils are present external to the layer of histiocytes (H&E, ×180).

numeroushistiocytes and multinucleated giant cells (Fig. 17-13). This appearance may resemble that seen in giant cell or temporal arteritis. The third form of vasculitis is characterized by a mixture of lymphocytes and plasma cells within vessel walls, without granuloma formation or giant cells.

In all cases it is extremely important to carefully examine special stains for organisms, since both tuberculosis and various fungal diseases can have a similar appearance.

Relationship to Sarcoidosis

As the name necrotizing sarcoid granulomatosis implies, this disease shares features with both Wegener's granulomatosis (necrosis, vasculitis) and sarcoidosis (noncaseating granulomas). Whether this disorder would best be considered a variant of sarcoidosis rather than a separate angiitis and granulomatosis is not completely resolved at this time. We believe, however, that several features favor its present classification as a different entity from sarcoidosis: (1) The histologic findings of extensive vasculitis and necrosis would be unusual in sarcoidosis. Although vascular invasion is common in sarcoid, it occurs within the area of maximum granuloma concentration, and appears to result from extension of the parenchymal granulomas into adjacent vessels.[62] (2) The radiographic appearance of rounded, mass-like densities would be unusual for sarcoid. Also, hilar lymph node enlargement which is common in sarcoid is found in only a minority of reported cases of necrotizing sarcoid granulomatosis. (3) Other common extrapulmonary manifestations of sarcoidosis, such as erythema nodosum or uveitis are rarely found in necrotizing sarcoid granulomatosis. Additional studies, such as determining serum angiotensin-converting enzyme, may help to elucidate these questions.

Lymphomatoid Granulomatosis

Lymphomatoid granulomatosis was first described by Liebow and co-workers in a classic article in 1972.[63] This disease differs from the other angiitides and granulomatoses in that true granulomatous inflammation is absent. Instead there is an aggressive, mixed cellular infiltrate of lymphocytes, plasma cells, and histiocytes that destroys the lung parenchyma. Lymphomatoid granulomatosis can thus be considered to represent a type of lymphoproliferative disease rather than an abnormal inflammatory reaction. Several reviews of this disease have been published.[64-66]

Clinical Features

Lymphomatoid granulomatosis affects middle-aged adults predominantly, but it can occur at any age.[7, 8, 63-71] There is a slight male preponderance of cases. The most common presenting complaints are related to chest involvement and include cough, shortness of breath, and chest pain. Systemic symptoms such as fever, malaise, and weight loss are also common. Some individuals present with symptoms related to involved extrapulmonary sites, especially the skin and nervous system (see Extrapulmonary Involvement, below). In exceptional instances, patients are asymptomatic. A few individuals with lymphomatoid granulomatosis have evidence of an impaired immune system either because of underlying malignancy or other debilitating disease, or because of organ transplantation.[65, 72-75]

The most common radiographic manifestations are multiple, bilateral nodular densities.[65] The nodules are usually well defined and discrete, and may measure several centimeters in diameter. They are often interpreted radiographically as representing so-called cannonball lesions suggestive of metastatic cancer. Solitary masses or areas of consolidation can be seen in a small number of patients. Fluffy alveolar infiltrates and diffuse reticulonodular markings have been described occasionally, and cavitation occurs in a few cases. Hilar lymph node enlargement is usually not present.

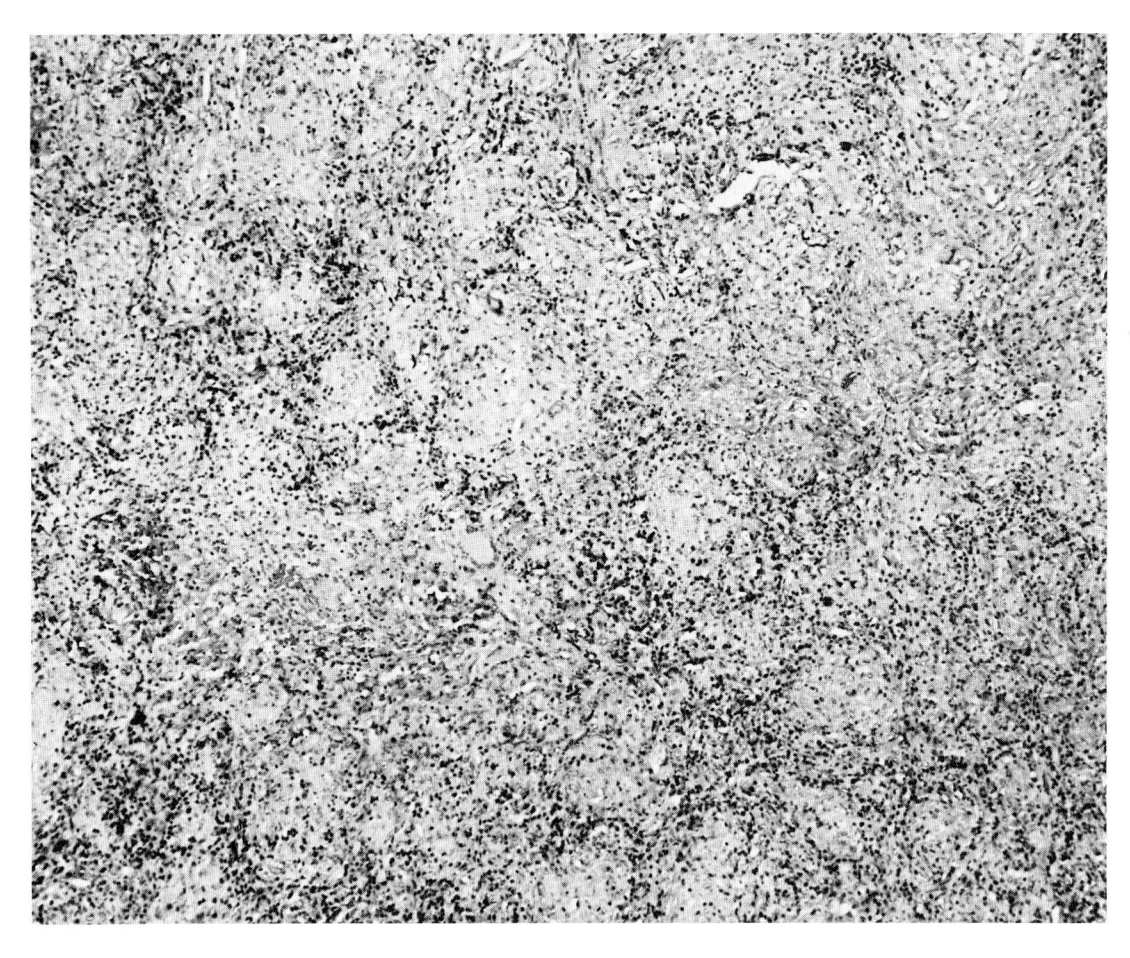

Figure 17–10. Extensive noncaseating granulomatous inflammation replacing large areas of lung from a case of necrotizing sarcoid granulomatosis (H&E, ×90).

Extrapulmonary Involvement

Lymphomatoid granulomatosis may affect a number of extrapulmonary sites, especially skin, nervous system, and kidney.[65] Skin involvement occurs in approximately 40 percent of patients, and may precede, coincide with, or follow the development of lung infiltrates.[65, 75, 77] Subcutaneous or dermal nodules are the most common skin manifestations, while maculopapular rashes or macular erythema are seen less often. The nervous system, both central and peripheral, is affected in almost one-third of cases. Evidence of cranial or peripheral nerve involvement is common, and may present as Bell's palsy, diplopia, deafness, vertigo, or paresthesias. Less frequently there are signs of brain involvement including confusion, ataxia, convulsions, and hemiparesis.

The kidney is involved in approximately one-third of cases at autopsy, but renal lesions are generally not apparent clinically since they consist of interstitial and perivascular infiltrates rather than glomerulonephritis. Renal function tests tend to be normal, therefore, and renal failure does not occur. Occasionally involvement of the upper respiratory tract develops with destructive lesions occurring in the nasopharynx, palate, or paranasal sinuses. In the absence of lung lesions such cases have been termed *polymorphic reticulosis* or *malignant midline reticulosis*, although most investigators believe that the latter entities and lymphomatoid granulomatosis likely represent variations of the same disease.[78–80] Hepatomegaly, splenomegaly, and lymphadenopathy have been reported in a small number of individuals with lymphomatoid granulomatosis. We now believe, however, that the presence of this type of organomegaly should suggest that the process has evolved into malignant lymphoma (see Differentiation from Malignant Lymphoma, below). Adrenal glands, heart, gastrointestinal tract, and multiple other organs have also been reported to be involved in rare cases.

Prognosis and Treatment

Mortality rates are high in lymphomatoid granulomatosis. Over 60 percent of patients in our series died, and their median survival was only 14 months.[65] A number of different treatment regimens have been attempted in this disease, including corticosteroids, a variety of cytotoxic

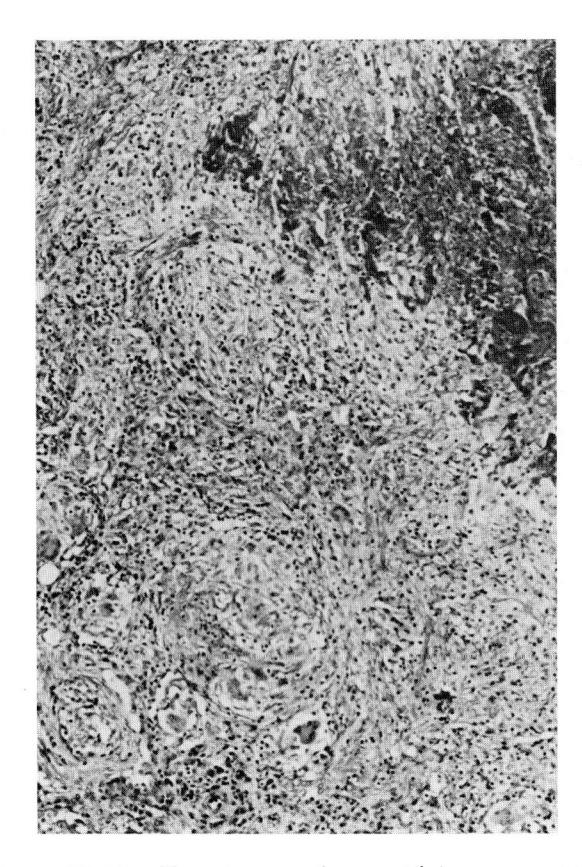

Figure 17-11. Necrotic zone (upper right) in necrotizing sarcoid granulomatosis surrounded by clusters of noncaseating granulomas (H&E, ×70).

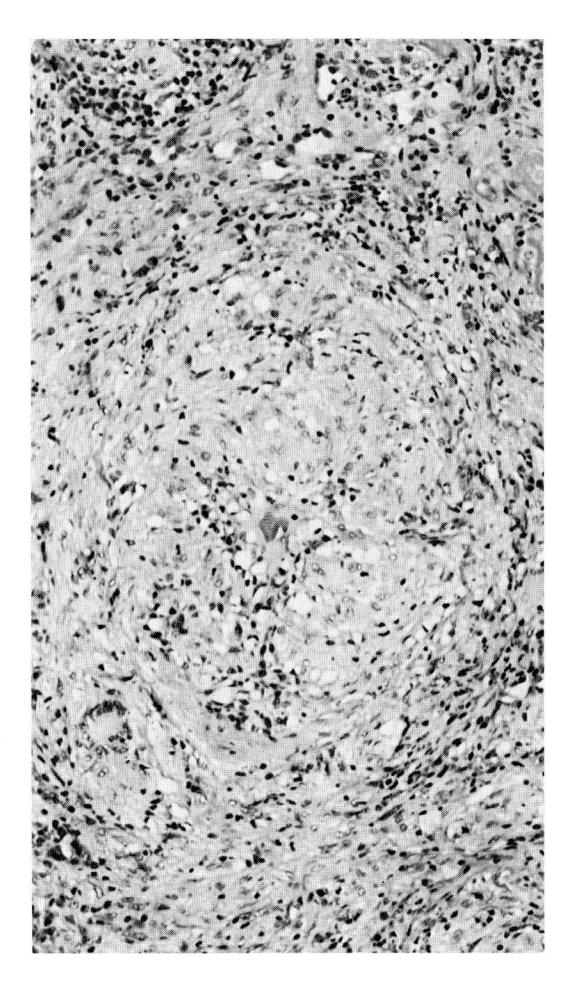

Figure 17-12. Vasculitis in necrotizing sarcoid granulomatosis. The media of this artery is infiltrated by noncaseating granulomas and the lumen is almost completely occluded (H&E, ×150).

chemotherapeutic agents, and many combinations of both. In retrospective studies no single regimen has proven to be more efficaceous than any other, although some investigators favor high-dose corticosteroids.[7,65] In the only published prospective study, Fauci and co-workers[81] advocate prompt treatment with cyclophosphamide and prednisone. However, their conclusions are based on only 13 patients and there was no control group treated with other regimens for comparison. Furthermore, many of their patients had atypical clinical features, including young age at presentation and prominent lymphadenopathy. In addition, malignant lymphoma developed in an unusually large number of patients (almost 50 percent). There is some evidence that irradiation to localized areas of involvement is useful.[82,83]

Certain prognostic features have been identified in lymphomatoid granulomatosis.[65] The presence of unilateral chest disease imparts a better prognosis, while nervous system or liver involvement is associated with a grave prognosis. Histologically, the presence the large numbers of atypical lymphoid cells in the pulmonary infiltrate is associated with a higher mortality, while numerous small lymphocytes and normal histiocytes are associated with lower mortality rates.

Histopathology

Lymphomatoid granulomatosis is characterized by a mixed mononuclear cell infiltrate that destroys the lung parenchyma and has a propensity for blood vessel invasion.[63] The usual gross appearance is the presence of multiple, discrete, firm white to yellow nodular masses in the lung. They may contain prominent central necrosis.

Microscopically, a dense infiltrate of small lymphocytes, histiocytes, plasma cells, and atypical lymphoreticular cells is present around areas of necrosis (Fig. 17-14). These cells occur in varying proportions, but always the infiltrate always maintains a polymorphous, heterogeneous appearance (Fig. 17-15). The so-called atypical lymphoreticular cells are larger mononuclear cells that contain abundant amphophilic cytoplasm and often possess an eccentric nucleus with multiple nucleoli. They resemble transformed lymphocytes and would probably be termed immunoblasts in current nomenclature. Electron microscopy has confirmed the spectrum of mononuclear cells noted by light microscopy,[77,84] and

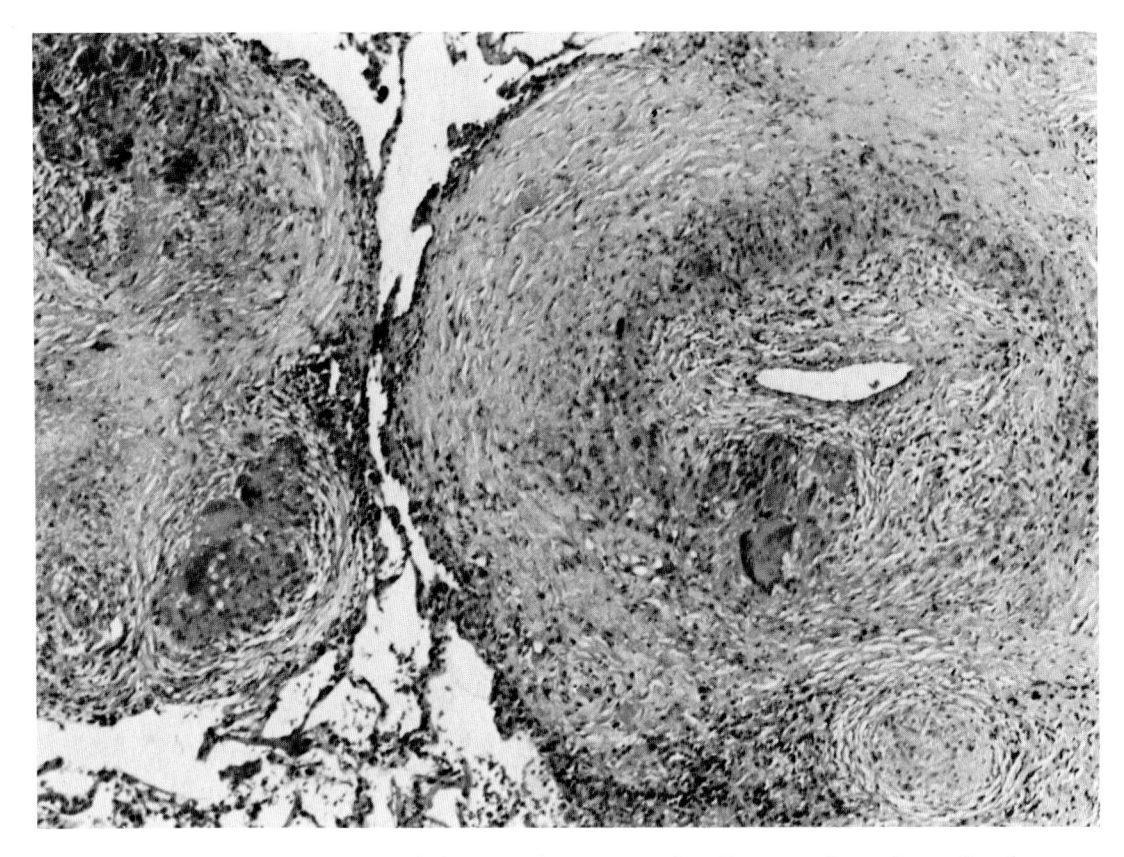

Figure 17–13. Histiocytic and chronic inflammatory cell infiltrate involving the media of a pulmonary artery in necrotizing sarcoid granulomatosis. Noncaseating granulomas with surrounding fibrosis are seen in the parenchyma to the left of the vessel (H&E, ×70).

immunoperoxidase staining has demonstrated the presence of polyclonal immunoglobulins within the cells.[85]

The amount of necrosis varies from case to case. In most examples, necrosis is prominent, and there is extensive cross-country destruction of the parenchyma. Rarely, necrotic foci are difficult to find or even absent, and in such cases one must be certain that other more typical features of lymphomatoid granulomatosis are present. True granulomatous inflammation, consisting either of well-formed, noncaseating granulomas or organized epithelioid histiocytes surrounding necrotic foci, is not found. Likewise, multinucleated giant cells are not features of this disease, and eosinophils are usually not prominent in the cellular infiltrate.

Vascular involvement in lymphomatoid granulomatosis is extensive and is characterized by invasion of all layers of vessel walls by the mixed mononuclear cell infiltrate described above (Fig. 17–16). The intima is often markedly thickened by the infiltrate and the vascular lumens can be narrowed or even occluded (Fig. 17–17). Unlike the vasculitis in Wegener's granulomatosis, however, there is relatively little necrosis of the vessel wall itself, especially considering the density of the cellular infiltrate.

Differentiation from Malignant Lymphoma

The differentiation of lymphomatoid granulomatosis from malignant lymphoma can be difficult, especially when atypical lymphoreticular cells are numerous within the infiltrate. Colby and Carrington[86] have emphasized that malignant lymphomas in the lung may demonstrate prominent vascular infiltration and they may be accompanied by extensive necrosis. Therefore the nature of the cellular infiltrate must be carefully examined in all patients. We use criteria in the lung that are similar to those utilized in lymph nodes to distinguish between atypical hyperplasia and malignant lymphoma: a uniform or monomorphous infiltrate of abnormal or immature lymphoid cells is diagnostic of lymphoma, while a heterogeneous mixture of lymphoid and plasma cells or histiocytes favors hyperplasia.[87] Difficulties can arise since a monomorphous infiltrate of abnormal lymphoid cells may occur as a small focus in the background of an otherwise typical mixed cellular infiltrate. Such an example would be considered to represent a malignant lymphoma arising in lymphomatoid granulomatosis, and underscores the need to carefully examine multiplesec-

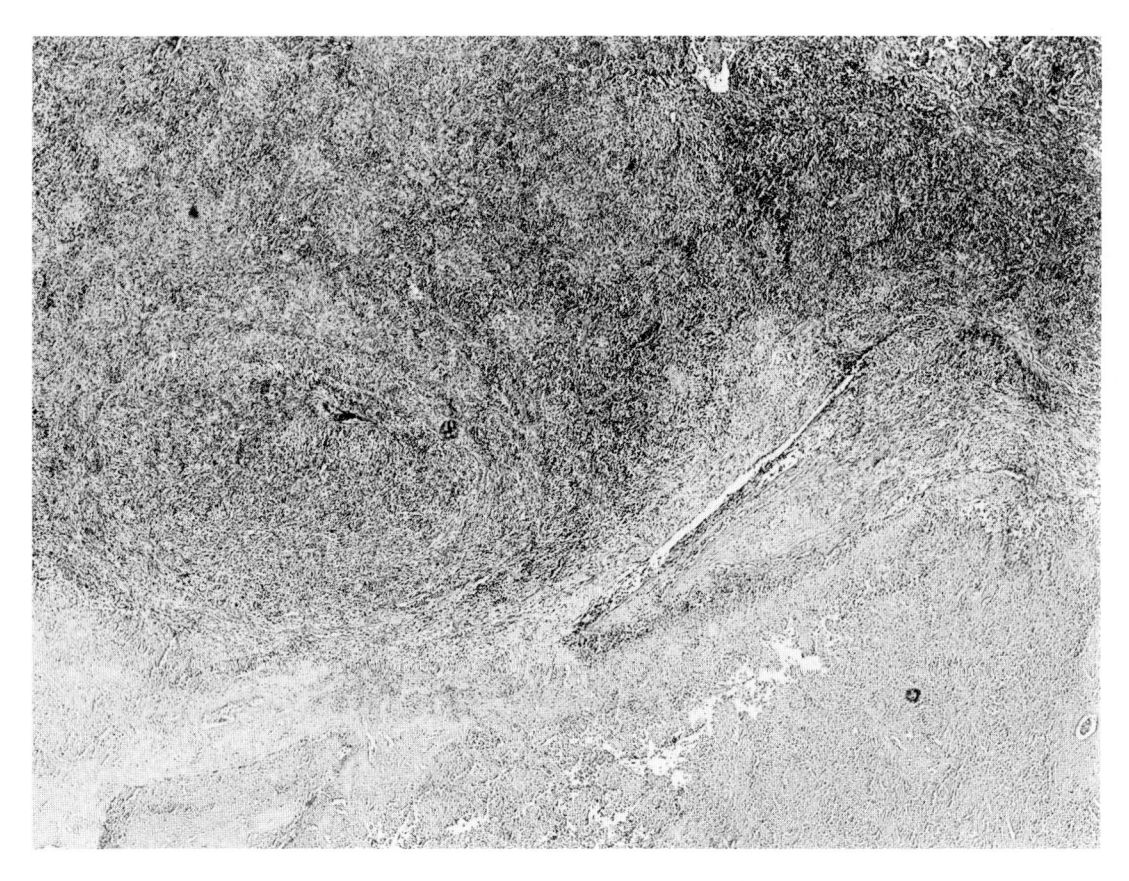

Figure 17–14. Necrotic zone (bottom) in lymphomatoid granulomatosis surrounded by a dense mononuclear cell infiltrate. Remnants of a vessel (left) can be seen with a transmural infiltrate and severely narrowed lumen (H&E, ×40).

tions for the possibility of identifying early lymphoma. Small foci of lymphoma may be more easily recognized by using immunoperoxidase staining for immunoglobulins.[85] The lymphomatous foci in this technique can often be shown to contain a single, monoclonal immunoglobulin in contrast to polyclonal immunoglobulin staining in typical areas of lymphomatoid granulomatosis.

The presence of certain clinical features may also help to distinguish malignant lymphoma from lymphomatoid granulomatosis. Hilar and mediastinal lymph node enlargement is very unusual in lymphomatoid granulomatosis and should raise the suspicion of lymphoma. Similarly, hepatomegaly, splenomegaly, and peripheral lymphadenopathy favor lymphoma.

Malignant lymphoma has been reported to develop in 10 to 15 percent of patients with lymphomatoid granulomatosis.[65, 71, 72, 88] The lymphoma in these cases most often resembles a large-cell, "histiocytic," or immunoblastic lymphoma.

Bronchocentric Granulomatosis

Bronchocentric granulomatosis differs from the other angiitides and granulomatoses in that the characteristic tissue reaction involves predominantly the bronchi and bronchioles, although it may extend somewhat into the surrounding parenchyma as well. This condition, further differs from the others in that the pathogenesis has been well documented, at least for some examples, to result from hypersensitivity to Aspergillus antigens.

Clinical Features

Almost half of the first 23 patients described with this disease had a history of chronic asthma,[89] although asthma was a less-frequent finding in a subsequently published smaller series of patients.[90] The clinical features of the asthmatic and nonasthmatic patients were somewhat different. As a group, the asthmatic patients were younger (average age, 20) than the nonasthmatics (average age, 50). The asthmatics were usually acutely ill, and commonly complained of exacerbation of asthmatic symptoms, fever, chest pain, cough, or shortness of breath. The nonasthmatics more often were only mildly symptomatic, with nonspecific complaints, such as an upper respiratory tract infection, mild cough, or malaise. Occasional individuals were asymptomatic. Peripheral blood eosinophilia was usually present in asthmatics, but was uncommon in nonasthmatics.

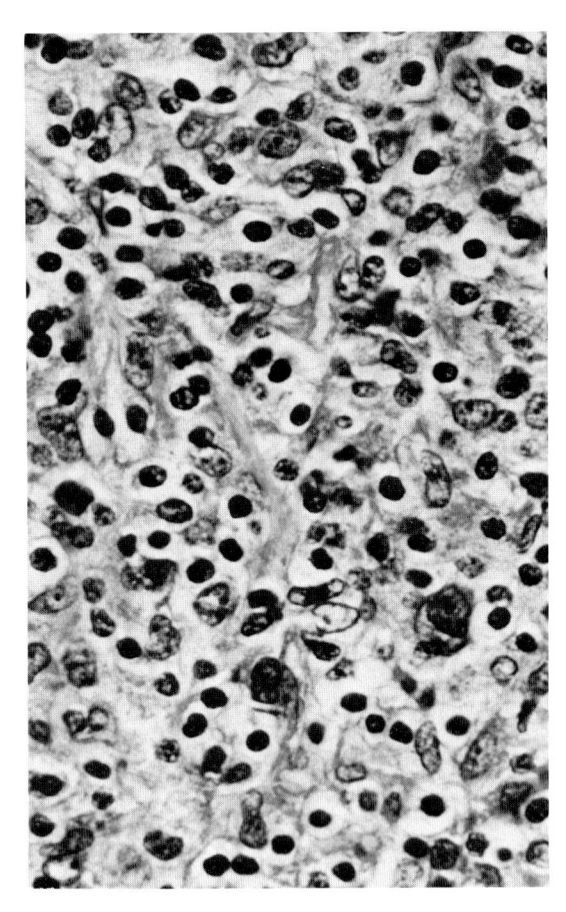

Figure 17–15. High-magnification photomicrograph of the cellular infiltrate in lymphomatoid granulomatosis showing the typical polymorphous mixture of mononuclear cells (H&E, ×450).

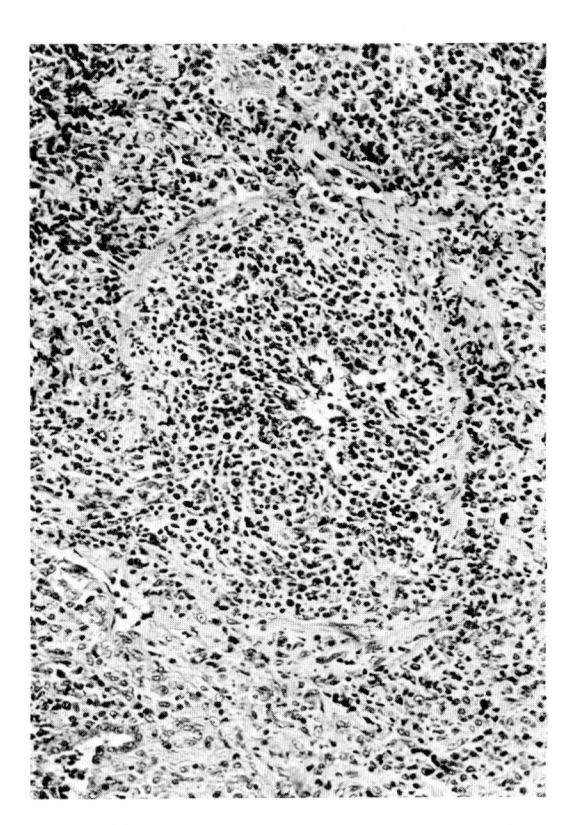

Figure 17–16. Vascular infiltration in lymphomatoid granulomatosis. The intima of this artery is markedly thickened, and the lumen compressed, by a dense mixed mononuclear cell infiltrate (H&E, ×150).

Histopathologic Features

The diagnostic pathologic changes in this condition are found in the conducting airways, most often the distal bronchioles.[89] The earliest change is the replacement of branchiolar mucosa by a layer of palisading histiocytes (Fig. 17–18). Eventually the entire bronchiolar wall is destroyed and the lesion resembles an ordinary necrotizing granuloma with prominent palisading histiocytes. At this stage the reaction is inferred to be bronchocentric because of its location adjacent to a pulmonary artery (Fig. 17–19). The gross appearance can also be helpful, since caseous necrosis can be found that follows the linear, branching distribution of bronchioles. Special stains for elastic tissue are helpful because they may outline remnants of the typical interrupted elastic layer of the destroyed bronchiole, and they can confirm that the adjacent blood vessel is a pulmonary artery because pulmonary arteries possess two elastic layers (Fig. 17–20). The necrotic centers of the granulomas may contain degenerated neutrophils or structureless eosinophilic material. Numerous eosinophils admixed with other chronic inflammatory cells usually surround the layer of palisading histiocytes, although eosinophils may be inconspicuous in nonasthmatic individuals. Occasionally, multinucleated giant cells are found engulfing amorphous eosinophilic material that is thought to represent remnants of necrotic eosinophils. Special stains for fungi have demonstrated scattered fungal hyphae within the granulomas in the asthmatic patients. The fungi are present only in the necrotic centers of the granulomas, and there is no evidence of true tissue invasion.

Although the typical inflammatory reaction predominantly involves the bronchioles, the surrounding parenchyma is not totally spared of changes. Frequently the adjacent pulmonary arteries are infiltrated by inflammatory cells extending from the bronchioles. Necrosis of vessel walls is not found, however, and evidence of vasculitis remote from the immediate peribronchiolar areas is not found.

The major bronchi can also be involved in this condition, but the changes are somewhat different from those in the bronchioles. A common finding, especially in asthmatic patients, is mucoid impaction of bronchi.[89, 91] In this condition the bronchi are markedly dilated and their lumens are packed with firm grey-tan, often laminated-appearing material. Microscopically, this luminal material is composed of a mixture of mucus, necrotic

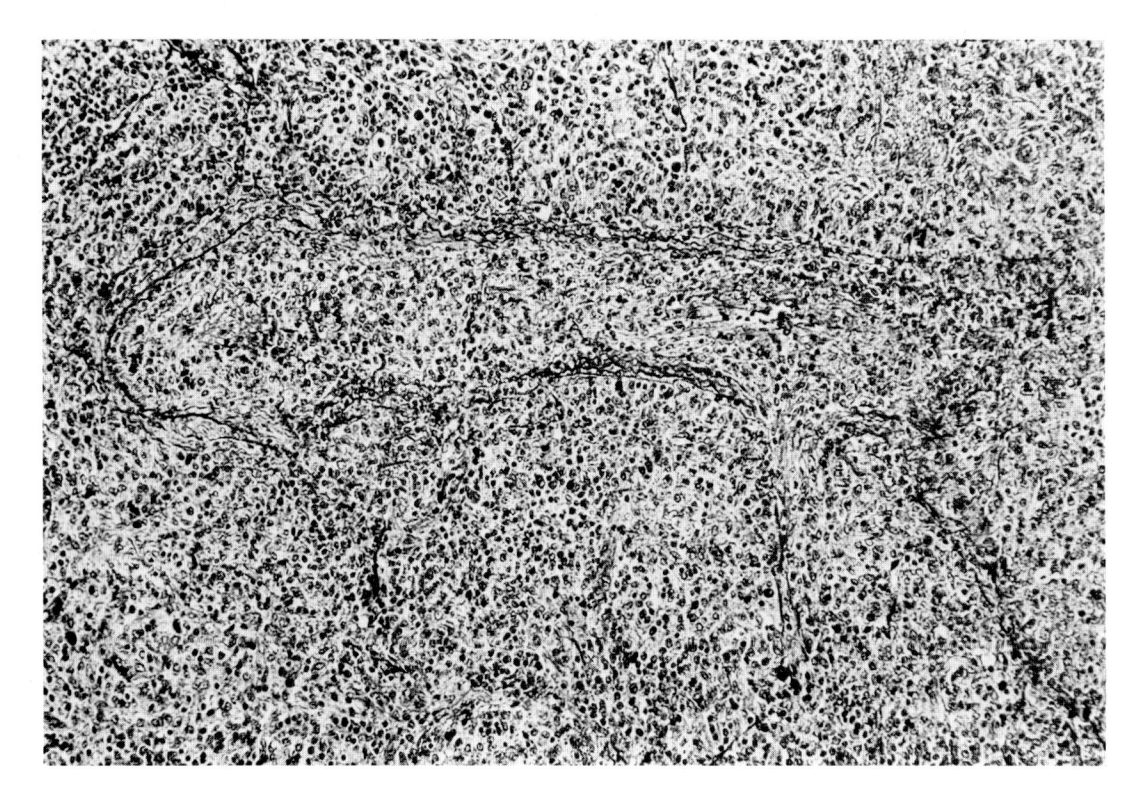

Figure 17–17. Occlusion of a vein lumen by a cellular infiltrate in lymphomatoid granulomatosis (Verhoeff van Gieson's stain, ×150).

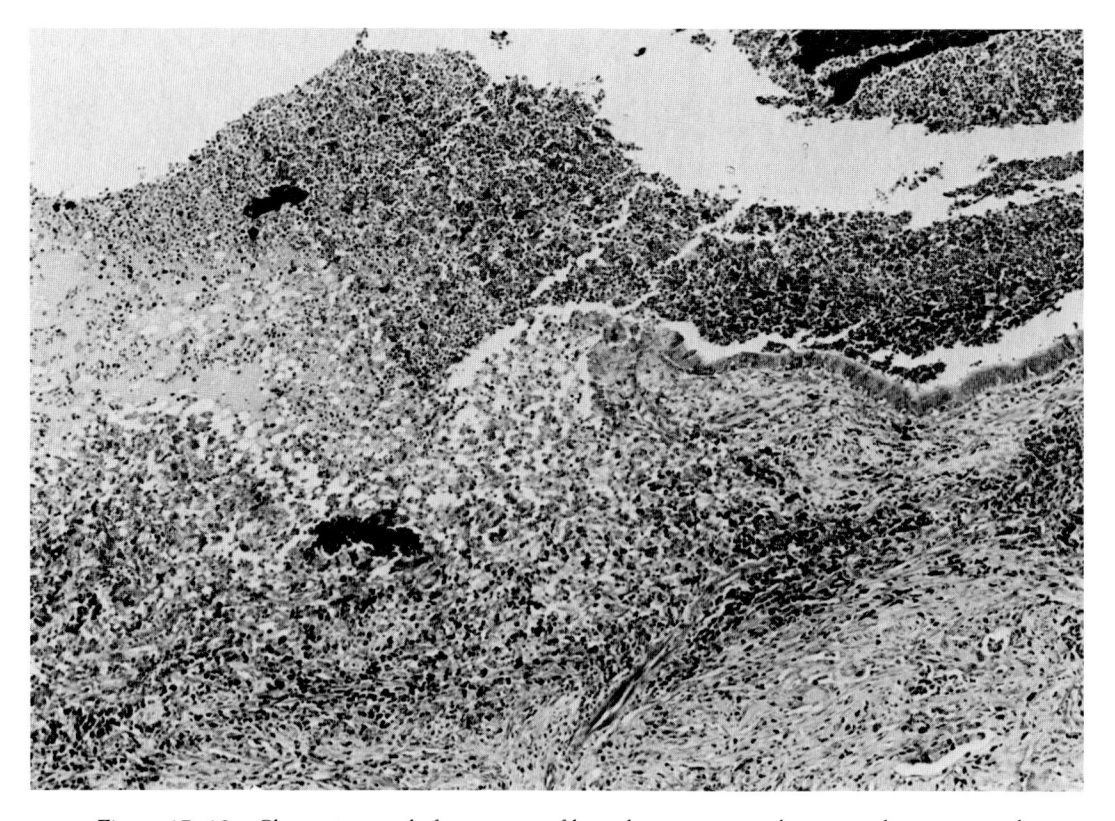

Figure 17–18. Photomicrograph from a case of bronchocentric granulomatosis showing partial replacement (left) of bronchiolar mucosa by epithelioid histiocytes (H&E, ×45).

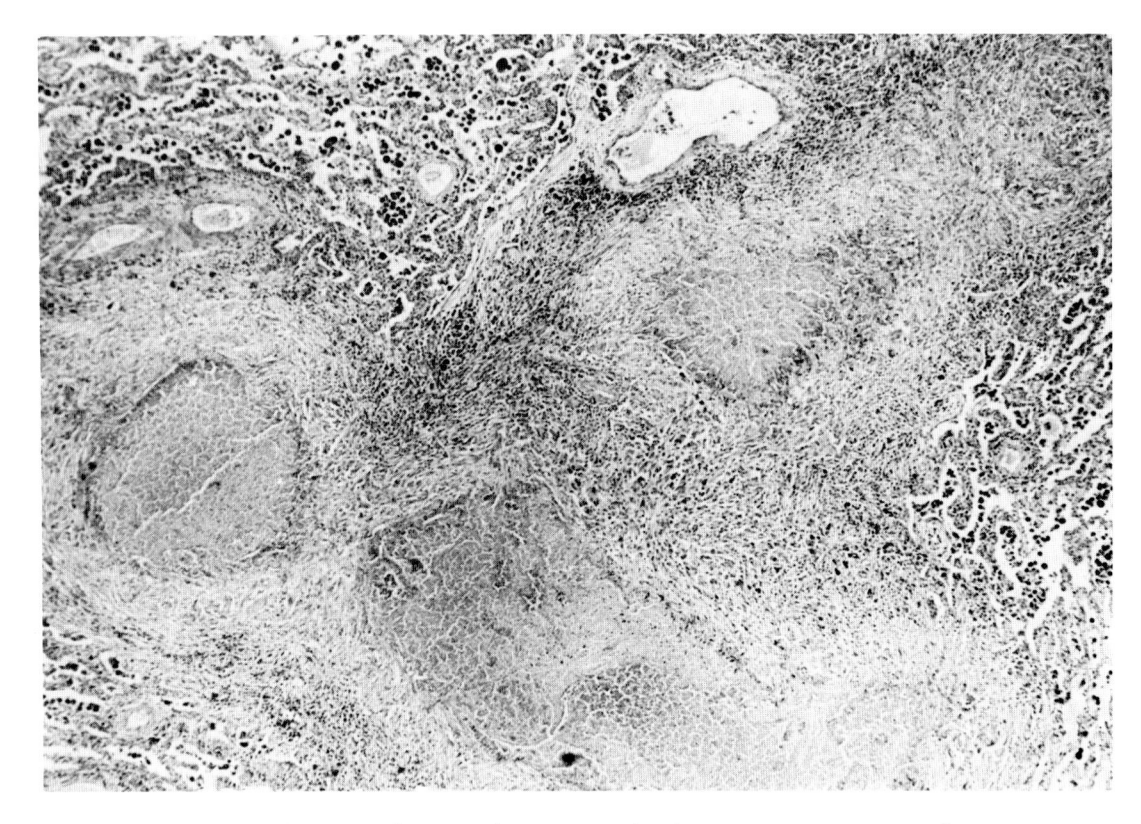

Figure 17–19. Low-magnification photomicrograph showing necrotizing granulomas in bronchocentric granulomatosis. Each granuloma is located next to a pulmonary artery in the position normally occupied by a bronchiole (H&E, ×70).

epithelial and inflammatory cells, numerous eosinophils arranged in clusters and layers, and Charcot-Leyden crystals. The latter structures are hexagonal in cross-section and bipyramidal in longitudinal section. They vary considerably in size and are thought to result from the agglutination of loose eosinophil granules. By means of special stains, scattered fungal hyphae can be identified within the mucus in most asthmatics, but invasion of the bronchial wall is not found. The bronchial wall is compressed and becomes thinned, and there is atrophy of bronchial cartilage. An infiltrate of eosinophils and other chronic inflammatory cells is usually present surrounding the bronchi and there may also be associated fibrosis.

In a few instances, small, well-circumscribed necrotic granulomas can be found in the submucosa of otherwise intact bronchi. A granulomatous reaction has also been noted in rare cases to surround and destroy bronchial cartilage.

Differential Diagnosis

The presence of bronchocentric granulomas per se is not diagnostic of bronchocentric granulomatosis. Such granulomas may be found in fungal and tuberculous infections, nodular rheumatoid disease, in certain other angiitides and granulomatoses.[2, 10, 89] To make the diagnosis of bronchocentric granulomatosis, *all* the granulomas should be centered on bronchioles. The finding of randomly placed granulomas elsewhere in the parenchyma, even if there are not many, should arouse the suspicion of another disease process.

Asthma, evidence of atopy, peripheral blood or tissue eosinophilia, and associated mucoid impaction of bronchi are strong supportive features for the diagnosis of bronchocentric granulomatosis. In their absence the diagnosis should be made only after all other lesions in the differential diagnosis have been carefully excluded. The blood vessels should be examined for evidence of vasculitis to exclude another type of angiitis and granulomatosis. Multiple special stains should be searched for acid-fast bacilli and fungi, and the tissue cultured to rule out an infectious etiology. We have seen several examples of infection where all the granulomas were bronchocentric, and in which the lesions would have been labeled bronchocentric granulomatosis if the special stains had not been performed.

Pathogenesis

It is currently well established that most examples of bronchocentric granulamatosis in asthmatic patients are due to allergic bronchopulmonary aspergillosis (*see* Chapter 14).[92–94] The pathogenesis of the disease in the

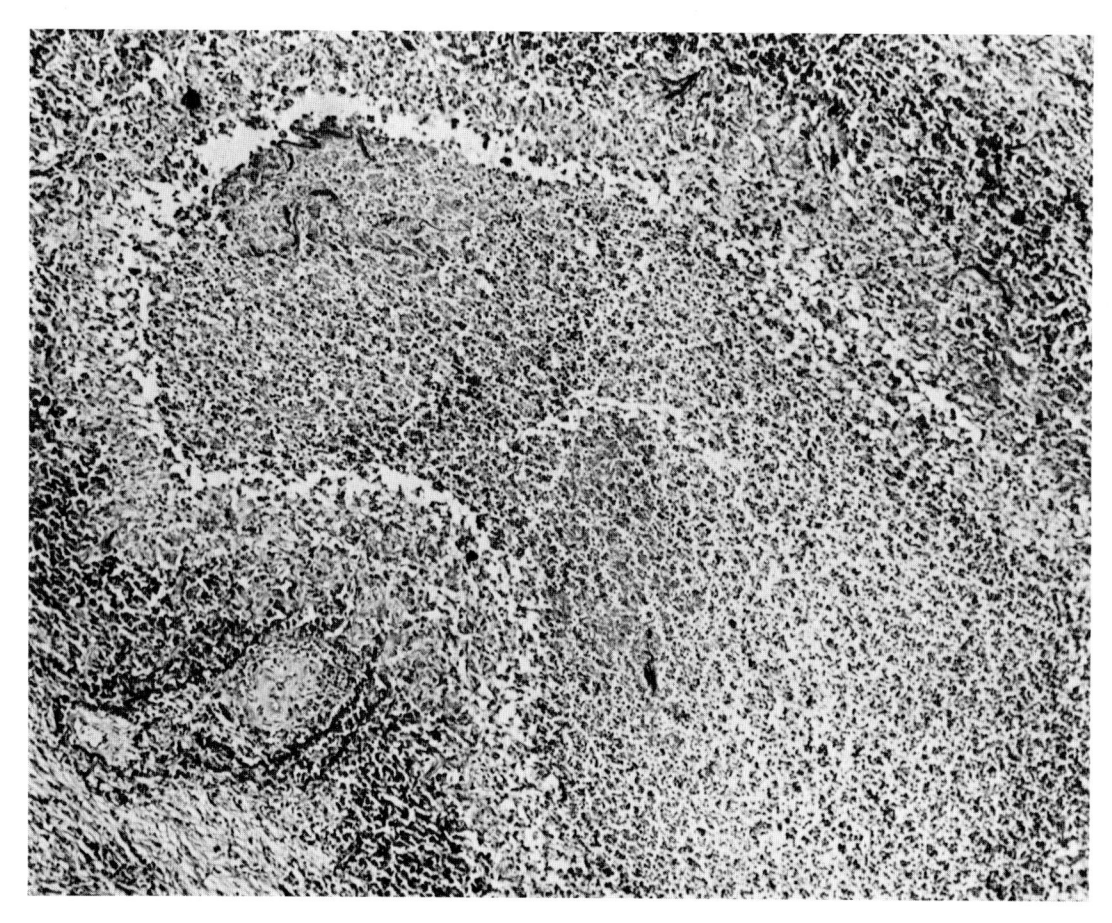

Figure 17–20. Elastic tissue stain showing necrotizing granuloma adjacent to a small pulmonary artery (left). The wall of the artery is secondarily inflamed (Verhoeff van Gieson's stain, ×70).

nonasthmatics has not been elucidated, although it is thought to be a hypersensitivity reaction to an as yet unidentified inhaled antigen. It may represent an uncontrolled reaction to tuberculous or fungal organisms (histoplasma, and so forth) that initially had been present within the airways but are longer identifiable.

References

1. Liebow A: The J. Burns Amberson Lecture: Pulmonary angiitis and granulomatosis. Am Rev Respir Dis 108:1, 1973.

2. Katzenstein A: The histologic spectrum and differential diagnosis of necrotizing granulomatous inflammation in the lung. In Fenoglio CM, Wolff M (eds): *Progress in Surgical Pathology*, vol 2. New York: Masson, 1980, pp 42–70.

3. Katzenstein A: Necrotizing granulomas of the lung. Hum Pathol 11:596, 1980.

4. Fauci A, Haynes B, Katz P: The spectrum of vasculitis. Clinical, pathologic, immunologic, and therapeutic considerations. Ann Intern Med 89:660, 1978.

5. DeRemee R, Wieland L, McDonald T: Respiratory vasculitis. Mayo Clin Proc 55:492, 1980.

6. Herman P, Hillman B, Pinkus G, Harris G: Unusual noninfectious granulomas of the lung. Radiology 121:287, 1976.

7. Israel H, Patchefsky A, Saldana M: Wegener's granulomatosis, lymphomatoid granulomatosis, and benign lymphocytic angiitis and granulomatosis of lung. Recognition and treatment. Ann Intern Med 87:691, 1977.

8. Saldana M, Patchefsky A, Israel H, Atkinson G: Pulmonary angiitis and granulomatosis. The relationship between histological features, organ involvement, and response to treatment. Hum Pathol 8:391, 1977.

9. Alarcon-Segovia D: The necrotizing vasculitides. A new pathogenetic classification. Med Clin North Am 61:241, 1977.

10. Ulbright T, Katzenstein A: Solitary necrotizing granulomas of the lung: Differentiating features and etiology. Am J Surg Pathol 4:13, 1980.

11. Fauci A, Wolff S: Wegener's granulomatosis: Studies in eighteen patients and a review of the literature. Medicine 52:535, 1973.

12. Godman G, Churg J: Wegener's granulomatosis. Pathology and review of the literature. Arch Pathol 58:533, 1954.

13. Landman S, Burgener F: Pulmonary manifestations in Wegener's granulomatosis. AJR 122:750, 1974.

14. Wolff S, Fauci A, Horn R, Dale D: Wegener's granulomatosis. Ann Intern Med 81:513, 1974.

15. Asin H, Wagenaar J, Swierenga J: The mitigated form of Wegener's disease. Scand J Respir Dis 53:367, 1972.

16. Blennerhassett J, Borrie J, Licter I, Taylor A: Localized

pulmonary Wegener's granuloma simulating lung cancer: Report of four cases. Thorax 31:576, 1976.
17. Carrington C, Liebow A: Limited forms of angiitis and granulomatosis of Wegener's type. Am J Med 41:497, 1966.
18. Cassan S, Coles D, Harrison E Jr: The concept of limited forms of Wegener's granulomatosis. Am J Med 49:366, 1970.
19. DeRemee R, McDonald T, Harrison E Jr, Coles D: Wegener's granulomatosis. Anatomic correlates, a proposed classification. Mayo Clin Proc 51:777, 1976.
20. Israel H, Patchefsky A: Wegener's granulomatosis of lung: Diagnosis and treatment. Experience with 12 cases. Ann Intern Med 74:881, 1971.
21. Moorthy A, Chesney R, Segar W, Groshong T: Wegener's granulomatosis in childhood: Prolonged survival following cytotoxic therapy. J Pediatr 91:616, 1977.
22. Roback S, Herdman R, Hoyer J, Good R: Wegener's granulomatosis in a child. Observations on pathogenesis and treatment. Am J Dis Child 118:608, 1969.
23. Maguire R, Fauci A, Doppman J, Wolff S: Unusual radiographic features of Wegener's granulomatosis. AJR 130:233, 1978.
24. Haynes B, Fishman M, Fauci A, Wolff S: The ocular manifestations of Wegener's granulomatosis. Fifteen years experience and review of the literature. Am J Med 63:131, 1977.
24A. Coutu R, Klein M, Lessel S, et al.: Limited form of Wegener's granulomatosis. Eye involvement as a major sign. JAMA 233:868, 1975.
25. Drachman D: Neurological complications of Wegener's granulomatosis. Arch Neurol 8:145, 1963.
26. Sahn E, Sahn S: Wegener's granulomatosis with aphasia. Arch Intern Med 136:87, 1976.
27. Fienberg R: The protracted superficial phenomenon in pathergic (Wegener's) granulomatosis. Hum Pathol 12:458, 1981.
28. Hu C, O'Loughlin S, Winkelmann R: Cutaneous manifestations of Wegener's granulomatosis. Arch Dermatol 113:175, 1977.
29. Pritchard M, Gow P: Wegener's granulomatosis presenting as rheumatoid arthritis (two cases). Proc R Soc Med 69:15, 1976.
30. Kedziora J, Wolff M, Chang J: Limited form of Wegener's granulomatosis in ulcerative colitis. Am J Roentgenol Radium Ther Nucl Med 125:127, 1975.
31. Flye M, Mundinger G, Fauci A: Diagnostic and therapeutic aspects of the surgical approach to Wegener's granulomatosis. J Thorac Cardiovasc Surg 77:331, 1979.
32. Harrison H, Linshaw M, Lindsley C, Cuppage F: Bolus corticosteroids and cyclophosphamide for initial treatment of Wegener's granulomatosis. JAMA 244:1599, 1980.
33. Israel H, Patchefsky A: Treatment of Wegener's granulomatosis. Am J Med 58:671, 1975.
34. Novack S, Pearson C: Cyclophosphamide in Wegener's granulomatosis. Engl J Med 284:938, 1971.
35. Raitt J: Wegener's granulomatosis: Treatment with cytotoxic agents and adrenocorticoids. Ann Intern Med 74:344, 1971.
36. Reza M, Dornfeld L, Goldberg L, et al.: Wegener's granulomatosis. Long-term follow-up of patients treated with cyclophosphamide. Arthritis Rheum 18:501, 1975.
37. Steinman T, Jaffe B, Monaco A, et al.: Recurrence of Wegener's granulomatosis after kidney transplanation. Successful reinduction of remission with cyclophosphamide. Am J Med 68:458, 1980.
38. Donald K, Edwards R, McEvoy J: An ultrastructural study of the pathogenesis of tissue injury in limited Wegener's granulomatosis. Pathology 8:161, 1976.
39. Shasby D, Schwarz M, Forstot J, et al: Pulmonary immune complex deposition in Wegener's granulomatosis. Chest 81:338, 1982.
40. Conn D, Gleich G, DeRemee R, McDonald T: Raised serum immunoglobulin E in Wegener's granulomatosis. Am Rheum Dis 35:377, 1976.
41. Howell S, Epstein W: Circulating immunoglobulin complexes in Wegener's granulomatosis. Am J Med 60:259, 1976.
42. Niinaka T, Okachi T, Watanabe Y, et al.: Chemotactic defect in Wegener's granulomatosis. J Med 8:161, 1977.
43. Shillitoe E, Lerner T, Lessof M, Harrison D: Immunological features of Wegener's granulomatosis. Lancet 1:281, 1974.
44. Rose G, Spencer H: Polyarteritis nodosa. Q J Med 26:43, 1957.
45. Chumbley L, Harrison E Jr, DeRemee R: Allergic granulomatosis and angiitis (Churg-Strauss syndrome). Report and analysis of 30 cases. Mayo Clin Proc 52:477, 1974.
46. Churg J: Allergic granulomatosis and granulomatous-vascular syndromes. Ann Allergy 21:619, 1963.
47. Churg J, Strauss L: Allergic granulomatosis, allergic angiitis, and periarteritis nodosa. Am J Pathol 27:277, 1951.
48. Cooper B, Bacal E, Patterson R: Allergic angiitis and granulomatosis. Prolonged remission induced by combined prednisone-azathioprine therapy. Arch Intern Med 138:367, 1978.
49. Rosenberg T, Medsger T Jr, De Cicco F, Fireman P: Allergic granulomatous angiitis (Churg-Strauss syndrome). J Allergy Clin Immunol 55:56, 1975.
50. Sokolov R, Rachmaninoff H, Kaine H: Allergic granulomatosis. Am J Med 31:131, 1962.
51. Veevaete F, van der Straeten M, de Vos M, Roels H: Allergic granulomatous angiitis. Scand J Respir Dis 59:287, 1978.
52. Koss M, Antonovych T, Hochholzer L: Allergic granulomatosis (Churg-Strauss syndrome). Pulmonary and renal morphologic findings. Am J Surg Pathol 5:21, 1981.
53. Dicken C, Winkelmann R: The Churg-Strauss granuloma. Cutaneous, necrotizing palisading granuloma in vasculitis syndromes. Arch Pathol Lab Med 102:576, 1978.
54. Kelalis P, Harrison E Jr, Greene L: Allergic granulomas of the prostate in asthmatics. JAMA 188:963, 1964.
55. Kelalis P, Harrison E Jr, Utz D: Allergic granulomas of the prostate: Treatment with steroids. J Urol 96:573, 1966.
56. Clausen K, Bronstein H: Granulomatous pulmonary arteritis. A hypereosinophilic syndrome. Am J Clin Pathol 62:82, 1974.
57. Moskowitz R, Baggenstoss A, Slocumb C: Histophahtological classification of periarteritis nodosa: A study of 56 cases confirmed at necropsy. Mayo Clin Proc 38:345, 1963.
58. Churg A, Carrington C, Gupta R: Necrotizing sarcoid granulomatosis. Chest 76:406, 1979.
59. Koss M, Hochholzer L, Feigin D, et al.: Necrotizing sarcoid-like granulomatosis. Clinical, pathologic, and immunopathologic findings. Hum Pathol 11(suppl):510, 1981.
60. Stephen J, Braimbridge M, Corrin B, et al.: Necrotizing "sarcoidal" angiitis and granulomatosis of the lungs. Thorax 31:356, 1976.
61. Beach R, Corrin B, Scopes J, Graham E: Necrotizing sarcoid granulomatosis with neurologic lesions in a child. J Pediatr 97:950, 1980.
62. Rosen Y, Moon S, Huang C, et al.: Granulomatous pulmonary angiitis in sarcoidosis. Arch Pathol Lab Med 101:170, 1977.

63. Liebow A, Carrington C, Friedman P: Lymphomatoid granulomatosis. Hum Pathol 3:457, 1972.
64. Bone R, Vernon M, Sobonya R, Rendon H: Lymphomatoid granulomatosis. Report of a case and review of the literature. Am J Med 65:709, 1978.
65. Katzenstein A, Carrington C, Liebow A: Lymphomatoid granulomatosis. A clinicopathologic study of 152 cases. Cancer 43:360, 1979.
66. Patton W, Lynch J III: Lymphomatoid granulomatosis. Clinicopathologic study of four cases and literature review. Medicine 61:1, 1982.
67. Gibbs A: Lymphomatoid granulomatosis — a condition with affinities to Wegener's granulomatosis and lymphoma. Thorax 32:71, 1977.
68. Lee S, Roth L, Brashear R: Lymphomatoid granulomatosis. A clinicopathologic study of four cases. Cancer 38:846, 1976.
69. Prabhu R, Berger H, Subietas A, Lee M: Lymphomatoid granulomatosis. Report of a patient with severe anemia and clubbing. Chest 78:833, 1980.
70. Schjolseth S, Bloom G: Lymphomatoid granulomatosis of the lung, liver, and spleen. Scand J Haematol 21:104, 1978.
71. Wall C, Goff A, Carrington C, Gaensler E: Lymphomatoid granulomatosis. Case report from the Thoracic Services, Boston University Medical School. Respiration 38:332, 1979.
72. Cohen M, Dawkins R, Henderson D, et al.: Pulmonary lymphomatoid granulomatosis with immunodeficiency terminating as malignant lymphoma. Pathology 11:537, 1979.
73. Hammar S, Gortner D, Sumida S, Bockus D: Lymphomatoid granulomatosis. Association with retroperitoneal fibrosis and evidence of impaired cell mediated immunity. Am Rev Respir Dis 115:1045, 1977.
74. Hammar S, Mennemeyer R: Lymphomatoid granulomatosis in a renal transplant recipient. Hum Pathol 9:111, 1976.
75. Weisbrot I: Lymphomatoid granulomatosis of the lung, associated with a long history of benign lymphoepithelial lesions of the salivary glands and lymphoid interstitial pneumonitis. Report of a case. Am J Clin Pathol 66:792, 1976.
76. James W, Odom R, Katzenstein A: The cutaneous manifestations of lymphomatoid granulomatosis: Report of forty-four patients and a review of the literature. Arch Dermatol 117:196, 1981.
77. Kay S, Fu Y, Minars N, Brady J: Lymphomatoid granulomatosis of the skin: Light microscopic and ultrastructural studies. Cancer 34:1675, 1974.
78. Crissman J: Midline malignant reticulosis and lymphomatoid granulomatosis. Arch Pathol Lab Med 103:561, 1979.
79. DeRemee R, Weiland L, McDonald T: Polymorphic reticulosis, lymphomatoid granulomatosis. Two entities or one? Mayo Clin Proc 53:634, 1978.
80. Stamenkovic I, Toccanier M, Kapanci Y: Polymorphic reticulosis (lethal midline granuloma) and lymphomatoid granulomatosis: Identical or distinct entities? Virchows Arch [A] 390:81.
81. Fauci A, Haynes B, Costa J, et al.: Lymphomatoid granulomatosis. Prospective clinical and therapeutic experience over 10 years. Engl J Med 306:68, 1982.
82. Fuller P, Hafermann D, Byrd R, Jenkins D: Use of irradiation in lymphomatoid granulomatosis. Chest 74:105, 1978.
83. Shank B, Kelley C, Nisce L, Nori D: Radiation therapy in lymphomatoid granulomatosis. Cancer 42:2572, 1978.
84. Pena C: Lymphomatoid granulomatosis with cerebral involvement. Light and electron microscopic study of a case. Acta Neuropathol 37:193, 1977.
85. Bender B, Jaffe R: Immunoglobulin production in lymphomatoid granulomatosis and relation to other benign lymphoproliferative disorders. Am J Clin Pathol 73:41, 1980.
86. Colby T, Carrington C: Pulmonary lymphomas simulating lymphomatoid granulomatosis. Am J Surg Path 6:19, 1982.
87. Nathwani B, Rappaport H, Moran E, et al.: Malignant lymphoma arising in angioimmunoblastic lymphadenopathy. Cancer 41:578, 1978.
88. Reddick R, Fauci A, Valsamis M, Mann R: Immunoblastic sarcoma of the central nervous system in a patient with lymphomatoid granulomatosis. Cancer 42:652, 1978.
89. Katzenstein A, Liebow A, Friedman P: Bronchocentric granulomatosis, mucoid impaction, and hypersensitivity reactions to fungi. Am Rev Respir Dis 111:497, 1975.
90. Koss M, Robinson R, Hochholzer L: Bronchocentric granulomatosis. Hum Pathol 12:632, 1981.
91. Irwin R, Thomas H III: Mucoid impaction of the bronchus. Am Rev Respir Dis 108:955, 1973.
92. Goodman D, Sacca J: Pulmonary cavitation, allergic aspergillosis, and bronchocentric granulomatosis. Chest 72:368, 1977.
93. Hanson G, Flod N, Wells I, et al.: Bronchocentric granulomatosis: A complication of allergic bronchopulmonary aspergillosis. J Allergy Clin Immunol 59:83, 1977.
94. Rosenberg M, Patterson R, Mintzer R, et al.: Clinical and immunologic criteria for the diagnosis of allergic bronchopulmonary aspergillosis. Ann Intern Med 86:405, 1977.

18 Diffuse Pulmonary Hemorrhage

Roberta R. Miller

Hemoptysis is a common presenting complaint of either localized or diffuse pulmonary hemorrhage. While aspiration of blood from a localized source may superficially mimic diffuse pulmonary hemorrhage, the former can be distinguished from the latter by clinical, radiologic, and bronchoscopic findings. It is critical that this distinction be made promptly and accurately since the differential diagnosis and implications of the two are entirely different.

Localized pulmonary hemorrhage is most often due to tumors, bronchiectasis, chronic bronchitis, tuberculosis, or other infections. Treatment is directed towards the underlying cause, and is sometimes a thoracic surgical emergency.

In contrast, diffuse pulmonary hemorrhage (DPH) is a syndrome with several defining features.[1-3] Patients with DPH often present with iron deficiency anemia and usually quite a significant degree of hemoptysis, which may even be life threatening. Chest radiographs show a diffuse fluffy alveolar filling pattern often with rapid worsening and clearing. Bronchoscopy shows blood issuing from all lobes and no endobronchial lesions. The unifying histologic feature is the presence of recent blood and hemosiderin in alveolar spaces.

Considerable advances have been made recently and it is no longer appropriate to think of DPH as being mostly comprised of two diseases, Goodpasture's disease and idiopathic pulmonary hemosiderosis. Rather, one should recognize that there is a syndrome of diffuse pulmonary hemorrhage which is complex and multifactorial. The first step in the differential diagnosis of DPH is to determine the presence and nature of any associated renal disease and/or associated immunologic abnormalities. Table 18-1 illustrates the six basic categories of DPH using this approach.[3] These six categories are antiglomerular basement membrane disease with and without nephropathy, collagen vascular disease with demonstrated immune complexes in some cases with and without nephropathy, and no apparent immunologic abnormality with and without nephropathy. The relative proportions of these six categories varies considerably according to patient selection in any given series. In the most comprehensive series to date,[2] 38% had antiglomerular basement membrane disease and 35% had systemic necrotizing vasculitis (half with nonspecified necrotizing vasculitis, and about one-third with Wegener's granulomatosis). However, it should be noted that no cases of idiopathic pulmonary hemosiderosis or DPH in the immunocompromised host were included in this series.

The various diseases in these categories are discussed in detail below.

Antiglomerular Basement Membrane Disease (Goodpasture's Syndrome)

The triad of antiglomerular basement membrane antibody, diffuse pulmonary hemorrhage, and glomerulonephritis is commonly referred to as Goodpasture's syndrome (and perhaps erroneously since the case included by Goodpasture in his study of deaths due to influenza showed systemic vasculitis).[4] The vast majority of patients are young adult males.[1,5,6] Most patients present with symptoms referrable to DPH rather than renal disease, although laboratory evidence of renal dysfunction is present early on in the majority of patients.[7] It is also of interest that AGBMD presents as DPH particularly in smokers whereas disease activity is more likely to be confined to the kidney in nonsmokers.[2]

The diagnosis of antiglomerular basement membrane disease (AGBMD) requires the demonstration of antiglomerular basement membrane antibody. This antibody can be detected in the serum by radioimmunoassay

Table 18–1. Classification of Diffuse Pulmonary Hemorrhage

Immune Abnormality	Nephropathy	No Nephropathy
Antiglomerular basement membrane	Classic Goodpasture's syndrome	Early or atypical Goodpasture's syndrome
Collagen vascular disease of presumed immune etiology	Systemic necrotizing vasculitis, Wegener's granulomatosis, systemic lupus erythematosis, other	
None	Uremia, Rapidly progressive glomerulonephritis without immune complexes	Idiopathic pulmonary hemosiderosis, Miscellaneous

in over 90% of cases.[2,3] However, some patients will have a false negative serum test, and demonstration of linear deposition of the antibody on the glomerular basement membrane in renal biopsy tissue remains the gold standard for diagnosis.[1,2]

Renal biopsy is a relatively noninvasive method establishing the diagnosis of AGBMD, particularly in cases with negative serology. The usual renal finding by light microscopy is a focal or diffuse, necrotizing, proliferative glomerulonephritis often accompanied by crescent formation.[2,6,8] By immunofluorescence, linear staining for IgG and complement and less commonly for IgM or IgA, is found along glomerular capillary basement membranes. A lung biopsy is most commonly done in those cases in which renal involvement is not prominent. Usually open lung biopsies are performed, but success in diagnosis has been reported with the use of immunofluorescence on small transbronchial lung biopsies.[9,10]

As mentioned above, most patients with AGBMD actually present with chest related complaints rather than overt renal disease. In a few cases, clinically significant renal disease does not occur, and kidney abnormalities are found only by means of a renal biopsy.[11,12] These renal abnormalities may either be microscopic glomerulopathy or simple linear immunoglobulin deposition on the glomerular basement membrane without apparent reaction. Exceptionally, a patient with DPH may have circulating AGBM antibody without actual deposition in the kidney or lung.[13] Some of these patients may progress to overt renal disease in time and some may not. However, it seems reasonable to view such cases as variants of AGBMD as indicated in Table 18–1.

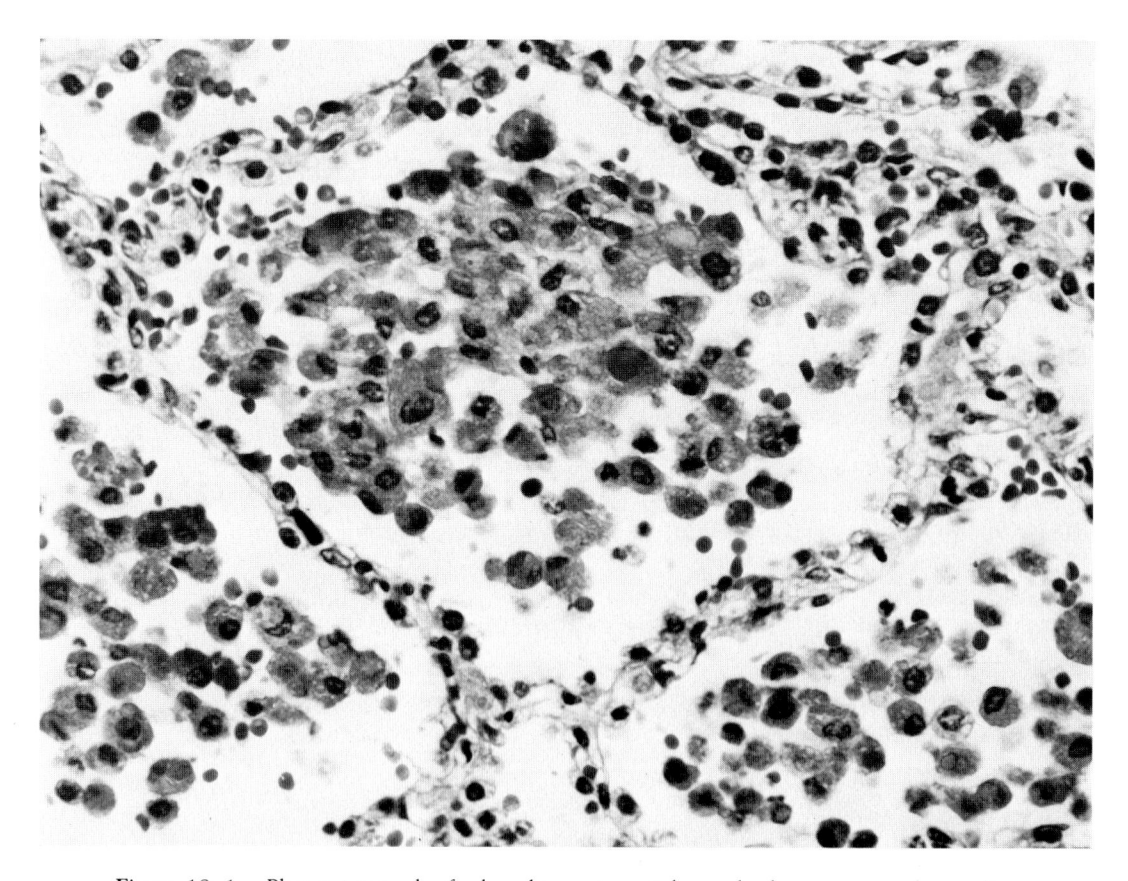

Figure 18–1. Photomicrograph of a lung biopsy in antiglomerular basement membrane disease showing numerous hemosiderin filled macrophages within the alveolar spaces. There is mild thickening of the alveolar septa, and scattered reactive alveolar pneumocytes are seen (H&E ×180). Courtesy of Dr. A-L. A. Katzenstein.

AGBMD was originally associated with a fulminant course and a dismal prognosis, but over the years there has been a gratifying improvement in patient outcome.[1] Those patients with minimal renal abnormalities and mild symptoms at presentation generally have a favorable outcome. There is also some evidence that the combination of immunosuppressive therapy and plasmapheresis (to remove the antigomerular basement membrane antibody) can produce a remission if instituted early in the disease. High doses of corticosteroids appear to stop the pulmonary hemorrhage. The role of bilateral nephrectomy in this disease is controversial, but may no longer be necessary with the use of the above mentioned therapeutic modalities.[1, 14, 15]

Lung Histopathology

The major histologic finding is the presence of blood or blood products within the alveolar spaces (Fig. 18–1). Hemosiderin is prominent if the process has been present for more than a week, and it occurs as clumps either free within alveolar spaces or engulfed by alveolar macrophages. The alveolar septa may be thickened by mild interstitial fibrosis or chronic inflammation combined with alveolar lining cell hyperplasia. This finding is thought to represent a nonspecific reaction to the presence of intraalveolar blood. There is no evidence of vasculitis or other blood vessel abnormalities to explain the bleeding, and significant acute inflammation is not seen. Linear staining for IgG (or occasionally IgA or IgM) and complement within alveolar capillary basement membranes has been described (Fig. 18–2).[6, 9, 10, 16] Nonspecific changes have been noted by electron microscopy within the capillary basement membranes, but electron dense deposits suggestive of immune complex deposition have not been identified.[13, 17, 18]

Diffuse Pulmonary Hemorrhage Associated with Collagen Vascular Diseases

In this group of diseases, diffuse pulmonary hemorrhage has been most clearly established as a complication of systemic lupus erythematosis (SLE)[1, 2, 3, 19–27] but DPH appears to be more frequently associated with systemic necrotizing vasculitis.[2] In most instances, the diagnosis of SLE is well established and the patients have active lupus nephritis as well as other sites of involvement. Rarely, SLE may present as DPH and in such cases the correct diagnosis may be elusive for some time.[19, 24] The mortality rates due to pulmonary hemorrhage in SLE are high,[2, 3] although some patients respond to immunosuppressive therapy, corticosteroids, or plasmapheresis.

Other collagen vascular-like diseases are rarely complicated by DPH.[1, 2, 3] These include systemic vasculidities of various types,[28] cryoglobulinemia,[29] scleroderma, mixed connective tissue disease, idiopathic rapidly progressive glomerulonephritis with immune complex-

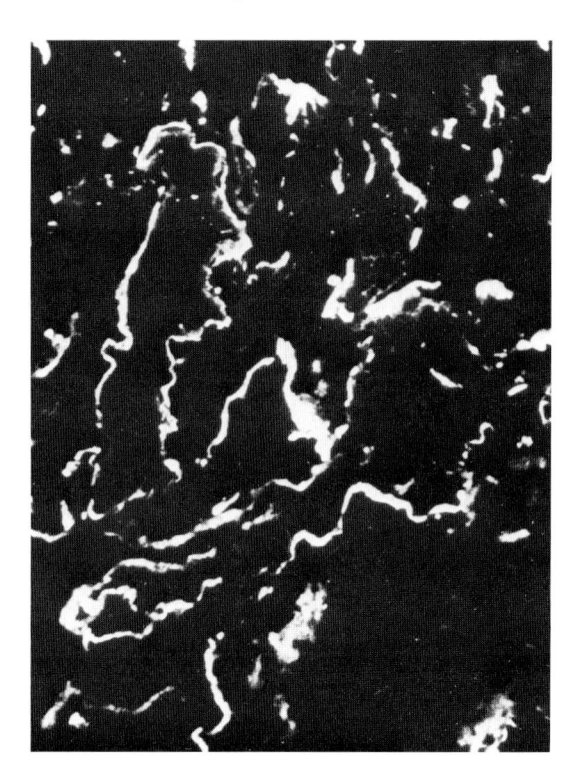

Figure 18–2. Photomicrograph showing immunofluorescence pattern in antiglomerular basement membrane disease. Bright linear staining is seen along the alveolar septa (Anti-IgG, ×180). Courtesy of Dr. A-L. A. Katzenstein.

es,[2, 29a] and proliferative glomerulonephritis with immune complexes.[29b] The latter two conditions can simulate AGBMD very closely clinically, the major difference being that renal biopsy shows granular rather than linear immune deposits. The lung lesion is presumed but not proven to be related to immune complexes as well. Massive lung hemorrhage also occurs in Wegener's granulomatosis, and a lung biopsy may be needed to establish the correct diagnosis.[2, 30] The characteristic features of necrotizing granulomatous inflammation and necrotizing vasculitis serve to distinguish Wegener's granulomatosis from the other entities in the differential diagnosis.

As indicated in Table 18–1, DPH associated with collagen vascular disease is not necessarily accompanied by nephropathy. When present, the nature of the nephropathy becomes important as one is faced with the differential diagnosis of the "pulmonary-renal syndromes."[30] The absence of nephropathy, however, does not alter the likelihood of a lung hemorrhage-collagen vascular disease association.

There is a clinical syndrome that occurs in patients with SLE termed acute lupus pneumonitis. This syndrome is characterized by the sudden onset of dyspnea, hypoxemia and diffuse alveolar infiltrates and is sometimes accompanied by hemoptysis. The pathologic findings in this syndrome vary but in most cases they resemble diffuse alveolar damage rather than DPH.[31, 32]

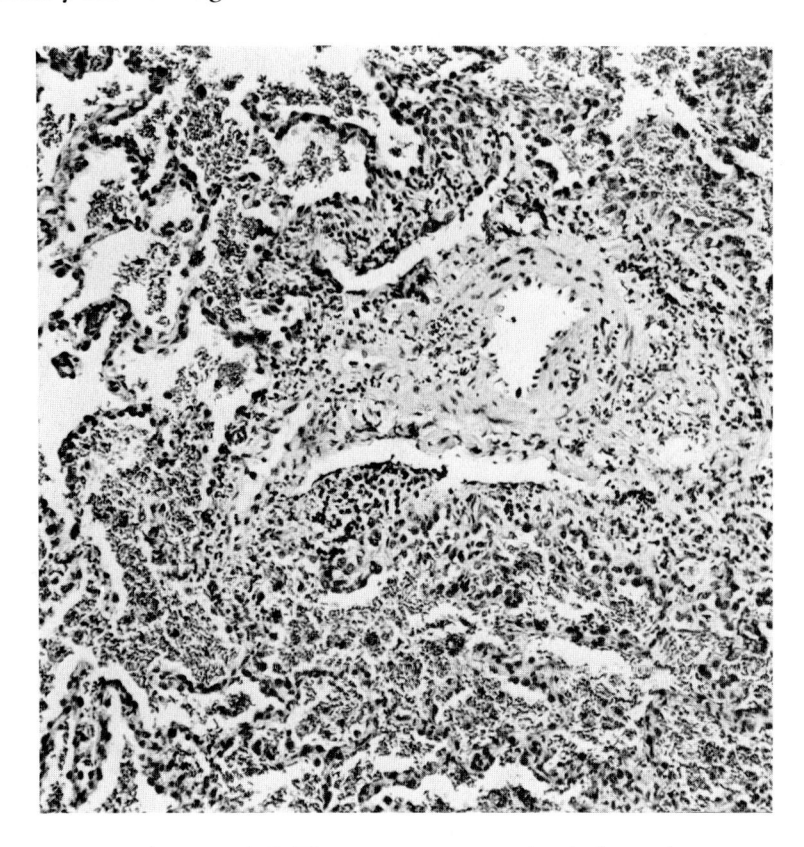

Figure 18–3. Lung changes in SLE. There is extensive intraalveolar hemorrhage associated with interstitial pneumonia. In addition, there is an acute necrotizing vasculitis involving a small pulmonary artery (center) (H&E, ×150). Courtesy of Dr. A-L. A. Katzenstein.

This syndrome is thus in the clinical differential diagnosis of SLE-related DPH, but the correct diagnosis should not be difficult histopathologically.

Lung Histopathology of SLE-Associated Pulmonary Hemorrhage

By light microscopy, diffuse hemorrhage and hemosiderin deposition are seen within alveolar spaces. Hemosiderin filled macrophages are also usually numerous. Several nonspecific findings are common, including chronic interstitial pneumonia, alveolar lining cell hyperplasia and scattered hyaline membranes. Vasculitis involving small arteries and venules as well as alveolar septal capillaries has been found in one case.[20] This vasculitis resembles so-called hypersensitivity angiitis and is characterized by neutrophil infiltration of vessel walls accompanied by abundant nuclear dust (Fig. 18–3). Neutrophils are also seen focally within alveolar septa where they are presumed to have originated around inflamed capillaries.

Immunofluorescence studies in most cases have demonstrated granular staining for IgG (and occasionally IgM and IgA) and complement along alveolar capillary walls.[20, 27] Sometimes granular staining for IgG can be observed within the nuclei of alveolar lining cells or mesothelial cells.[31] This finding is thought to represent a form of in situ antinuclear antibody test. By electron microscopy, dense deposits have been noted within the endothelial basement membranes (Fig. 18–4).[20–22, 24] Some of these deposits possess an internal structure composed of concentric rings that resemble the fingerprint pattern characteristic of the deposits found within glomerular basement membranes in SLE.[20, 22]

Diffuse Pulmonary Hemorrhage and Nephropathy Without Collagen Vascular Disease or Immunologic Abnormality

Diffuse pulmonary hemorrhage may occur in patients with uremia due to a combination of hypervolemia and uremic coagulopathy.[33] In these instances, the uremia antedates any sign of DPH in contrast to the usual course of events in AGBMD.

Rarely, patients with rapidly progressive glomerulonephritis and no demonstrable immune deposits on renal biopsy may develop DPH.[2] These patients are clinically similar to those described above with granular immune

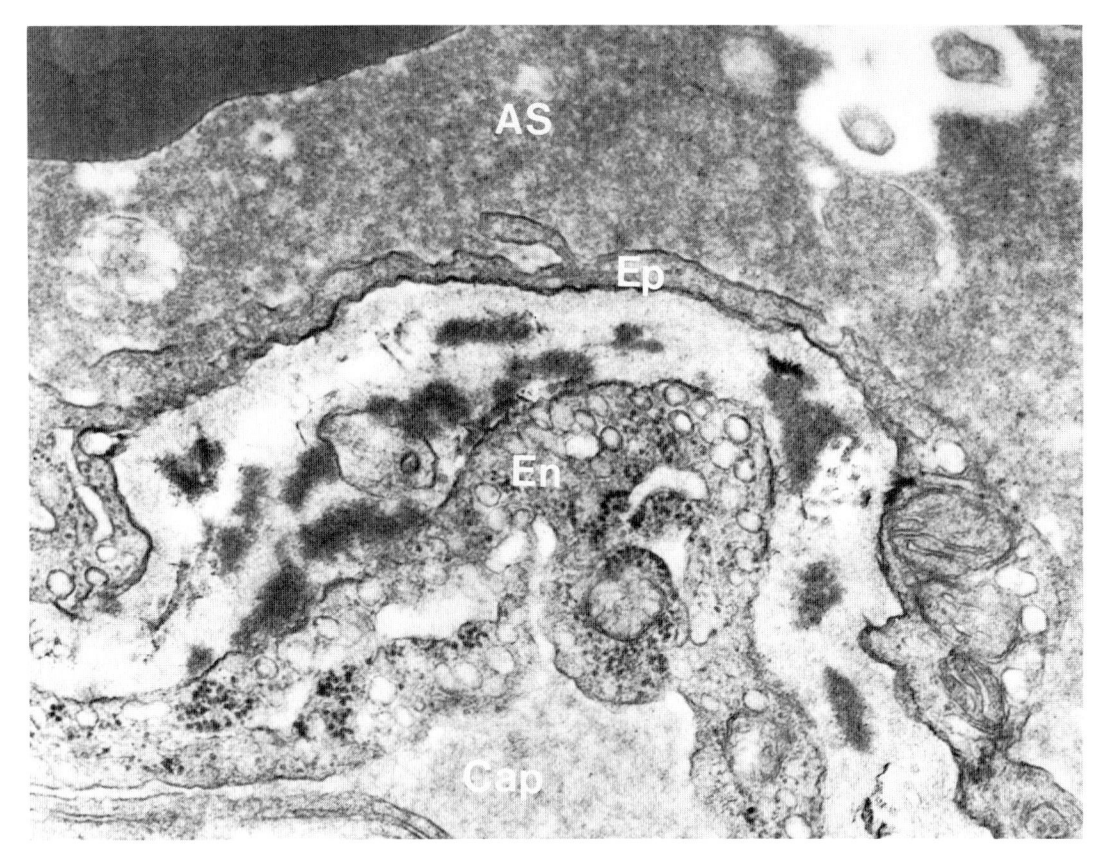

Figure 18-4. Electron micrograph from the patient with SLE whose light microscopic findings are shown in Figure 18-3. Amorphous electron dense deposits are seen in the capillary endothelial basement membrane (AS - alveolar space, Ep - type 1 alveolar pneumocyte, En - endothelial cell, Cap - capillary lumen; ×10,500). Courtesy of A-L. A. Katzenstein.

deposits except for negative renal immunofluorescence. However, they tend to be older with a median age of 53 years, and 50% have a previous history of recent upper respiratory tract infections.[2] Whether this disease is truly nonimmunologic or is too subtle for current detection techniques is an unresolved issue. Again, the distinction between these patients and AGBMD patients lies in the absence of antiglomerular basement membrane antibody.

Diffuse Pulmonary Hemorrhage Without Nephropathy or Immunologic Abnormality

Idiopathic Pulmonary Hemosiderosis

Diffuse pulmonary hemorrhage is the major manifestation of idiopathic pulmonary hemosiderosis (IPH). Antiglomerular basement membrane antibody is not present, and glomerulonephritis is usually not found.[1-3]

IPH occurs predominantly in two age groups: children less than 10 years and young adults in the second to third decades, although older adults can be affected as well.[34,35] Familial cases have been reported.[36,37,38] There is an equal sex incidence in children, while in adults males are affected somewhat more frequently than females. Hemoptysis is the usual presenting complaint, and dyspnea, malaise, and pallor are common associated findings. A hypochromic, microcytic anemia is present in almost all cases. Fluffy, often transient, alveolar infiltrates are found on chest radiographs in the acute stage, while interstitial reticulonodular infiltrates may be seen in the chronic stages. Clinically apparent renal disease is not found, although evidence of IgA nephropathy has been reported in a renal biopsy from one case.[39]

Approximately 50% of patients have elevated serum IgA.[2] Rare examples of celiac disease have been documented in patients with IPH.[40]

The course of IPH is usually chronic, with remissions and recurrences occuring over several years. The long-term prognosis of this disease is poor, with a median survival of three years, although survival rates are somewhat better in the adults.[34,35] In a few cases, death occurs during an episode of acute massive hemorrhage. The results of therapy are difficult to evalute in this disease because of the frequency of spontaneous remission. Corticosteroid and immunosuppressive therapy have been utilized with apparent success in some cases.

Histopathology

By light microscopy, IPH is indistinguishable from antiglomerular basement membrane disease. The alveolar spaces are filled with blood, free hemosiderin, and macrophages containing hemosiderin. Nonspecific alveolar septal thickening and alveolar lining cell hyperplasia are also common. There is no evidence by immunofluorescence of immunoglobulin deposition along alveolar capillary basement membranes. Various nonspecific abnormalities of alveolar capillary and epithelial basement membranes have been noted by some investigators with electron microscopy, including reduplication, smudging, and fragmentation.[41-44] Other studies have failed, however, to confirm the presence of any abnormality of the basement membranes.[18,36-45] Immune complex deposition has not been noted in any cases.

Miscellaneous Causes of Diffuse Pulmonary Hemorrhage

Drug Reactions

Fatal massive pulmonary hemorrhage along with crescentic glomerulonephritis is a rare complication of penicillamine therapy and may represent an unusual hypersensitivity reaction to this drug.[46] The usual pathologic findings reported in these cases are intraalveolar blood and hemosiderin with negative immunofluorescent staining for immunoglobulins and complement. Exposure to large amounts of trimellitic anhydride (TMA), a substance used in the plastics industry, has been reported to cause pulmonary hemorrhage and hemolytic anemia.[47] High titers of circulating antibody to TMA have been found in this disorder. Lymphangiography is rarely complicated by DPH which may be severe or even fatal.[2]

Cardiovascular

Diffuse pulmonary hemorrhage may occur in the setting of severe heart disease of various etiologies[48] although it is generally not massive. Hemoptysis is a particularly common occurrence in mitral stenosis. Intraalveolar hemosiderin deposition may be so prominent in certain cases of pulmonary veno-occlusive disease (Chapter 24)[49] that the biopsy findings may be confused with idiopathic pulmonary hemosiderosis. The two diseases are distinguishable when the venules are examined by means of an elastic tissue stain. In IPH, the venules are normal, while in pulmonary veno-occlusive disease, many are occluded by fibrous tissue. Also, evidence of pulmonary hypertension is usually found in the latter condition. DPH has also been described in amyloidosis involving the pulmonary vasculature.[50]

Blood Dyscrasias

DPH occurs occasionally in leukemic patients, bone marrow transplant patients, and other immunocompromised patients[51,52,53] and should be included in the differential diagnosis of diffuse pulmonary infiltrates in this unfortunate population (Chapter 15). In view of the profound degrees of thrombocytopenia that many of these patients have, DPH is not clinically manifest as often as one might anticipate. It is thought that, at least in most instances, an additional abnormality such as some degree of diffuse alveolar damage must be present also to "tip the patient over the edge" into overt intra-alveolar bleeding.[52] DPH has also been described with anticoagulation therapy.[54]

Acute Lung Injury

Blunt trauma to the chest can result in DPH. Sepsis with or without disseminated intravascular coagulation may result in DPH, presumably due to diffuse endothelial damage. Diffuse alveolar damage of various causes may also be complicated by massive DPH.[52]

Tumors

Primary or, more commonly, metastatic vasoformative tumors may present as DPH[55,56] The diagnosis of malignancy in such cases is by no means always obvious and these patients present tremendous clinical and pathological challenges. As the acquired immune deficiency syndrome becomes more common, primary or metastatic Kaposi's sarcoma in the lung is anticipated to become an important differential diagnostic consideration in the syndrome of diffuse pulmonary hemorrhage.[55]

References

1. Bradley JD: The pulmonary hemorrhage syndromes. Clin Chest Med 3:593–605, 1982.
2. Leatherman JW, Davies SF, Hoidal JR: Alveolar hemorrhage syndromes: Diffuse microvascular lung hemorrhage in immune and idiopathic disorders. Medicine 63:343–61, 1984.
3. Albelda SM, Gefter WB, Epstein DM, Miller WT: Diffuse pulmonary hemorrhage: A review and classification. Radiology 154:289–97, 1984.
4. Goodpasture EW: The significance of certain pulmonary lesions in relation to the etiology of influenza. Am J Med Sci 158:863–70, 1919.
5. Benoit FL, Rulon DB, Theil GB, et al.: Goodpasture's syndrome: A clinicopathologic entity. Am J Med 37:424–44, 1964.
6. Briggs WA, Johnson JP, Teichman S, et al.: Antiglomerular basement membrane antibody-mediated glomerulonephritis and Goodpasture's syndrome. Medicine 58:348–61, 1979.
7. Teague CA, Doak PB, Simpson IJ, Rainer SP, Herdson PB: Goodpasture's syndrome: An analysis of 29 cases. Kidney Int 13:492, 1978.
8. Duncan D, Drummond K, Michael A, Vernier R: Pulmonary hemorrhage and glomerulonephritis. Report of six cases and study of the renal lesion by the fluorescent antibody technique and electron microscopy. Ann Int Med 62:920, 1965.

9. Abboud R, Chase W, Ballon H, et al.: Goodpasture's syndrome: Diagnosis by transbronchial lung biopsy. Ann Int Med 89:635, 1978.
10. Beechler C, Enquist R, Hunt K, et al.: Immunofluorescence of transbronchial biopsies in Goodpasture's syndrome. Am Rev Respir Dis 121:869, 1980.
11. Mathew TH, Hobbs JB, Kalowski S, et al.: Goodpasture's syndrome: Normal renal diagnostic findings. Ann Int Med 82:215–8, 1975.
12. Zimmerman SW, Varanasi UR, Hoff B: Goodpasture's syndrome with normal renal function. Am J Med 66:163–71, 1979.
13. Brambilla C, Brambilla E, Stoebner P, Dechelette E: Idiopathic pulmonary hemmorrhage. Ultrastructural and mineralogic study. Chest 81:120, 1982.
14. Espinosa-Melendez E, Forbes R, Hollomby D, et al.: Goodpasture's syndrome treated with plasmapheresis. Report of a case. Arch Int Med 140:542, 1980.
15. Teichman S, Briggs W, Knieser M, Enquist R: Goodpasture's syndrome: Two cases with contrasting early course and management. Am Rev Respir Dis 13:223, 1976.
16. Border W, Baehler R, Bhathena D, Glassock R: IgA antibasement membrane nephritis with pulmonary hemorrhage. Ann Int Med 91:21, 1979.
17. Botting A, Brown A, Divertie M: The pulmonary lesion in a patient with Goodpasture's syndrome as studied by electron microscopy. Amer J Clin Path 42:387, 1964.
18. Donlan C, Srodes C, Duffy F: Idiopathic pulmonary hemosiderosis. Electron microscopic immunofluorescent and iron kinetic studies. Chest 68:577, 1975.
19. Byrd R, Trunk G: Systemic lupus erythematosus presenting as pulmonary hemosiderosis. Chest 64:128, 1973.
20. Churg A, Franklin W, Chan K, et al.: Pulmonary hemorrhage and immune-complex deposition in the lung. Complications in a patient with systemic lupus erythematosus. Arch Pathol Lab Med 104:388, 1980.
21. Eagen J, Memoli V, Roberts J, et al.: Pulmonary hemorrhage in systemic lupus erythematosus. Medicine 57:545, 1978.
22. Elliott M, Kuhn C: Idiopathic pulmonary hemosiderosis. Ultrastructural abnormalities in the capillary walls. Am Rev Respir Dis 102:895, 1970.
23. Gould D, Soriano R: Acute alveolar hemorrhage in lupus erythematosus. Ann Int Med 83:836, 1975.
24. Kuhn C: Systemic lupus erythematosus in a patient with ultrastructural lesions of the pulmonary capillaries previously reported in the Review as due to idiopathic pulmonary hemosiderosis. Am Rev Respir Dis 106:931, 1972.
25. Marino C, Pertschuk L: Pulmonary hemorrhage in systemic lupus erythematosus. Arch Intern Med 141:201, 1981.
26. Mintz G, Galindo L, Fernandex-Diaz J, et al.: Acute massive pulmonary hemorrhage in systemic lupus erythematosus. J Rheumatol 5:39, 1978.
27. Rogriquez-Iturbe B, Garcia R, Rubio L, Serrano H: Immunohistologic findings in the lung in systemic lupus erythematosus. Arch Pathol Lab Med 101:342, 1977.
28. Thomashow B, Felton C, Navarro C: Diffuse intrapulmonary hemorrhage, renal failure and a systemic vasculitis: A report and review of the literature. Am J Med 68:279, 1980.
29. Martinez J, Kohler P: Variant "Goodpasture's syndrome." The need for immunologic criteria in rapidly progressive glomerulonephritis and hemorrhagic pneumonitis. Ann Intern Med 75:67, 1971.
29a. Loughlin G, Taussig L, Murphy S, et al.: Immune-complex mediated glomerulonephritis and pulmonary hemorrhage simulating Goodpasture's syndrome. J Pediatr 93:181, 1978.
29b. Goldstein J, Weil J, Liel Y: Intrapulmonary hemorrhages and immune complex glomerulonephritis masquerading as Goodpasture's syndrome. Hum Pathol 17:754–7, 1986.
30. Schachter E, Finkelstein F, Bastl C, Smith G: Diagnostic problems in pulmonary renal syndromes. Am Rev Respir Dis 115:155, 1977.
31. Pertschuk L, Moccia L, Rosen Y, Lyons H, Marion C, Rashford A, Wollschlager C: Acute pulmonary complications in systemic lupus erythematosus. Immunofluorescence and light microscopic study. Am J Clin Pathol 68:553, 1977.
32. Matthay R, Schwarz M, Petty T, Stanford R, Gupta R, Sahn S, Steigerwald J: Pulmonary manifestations of systemic lupus erythematosus: Review of twelve cases of acute lupus pneumonitis. Medicine 54:397, 1974.
33. Schwartz E, Teplick J, Oresti G, Schwartz A: Pulmonary hemorrhage in renal disease. Goodpasture's syndrome and other causes. Radiology 122:39, 1977.
34. Morgan P, Turner-Warwick M: Pulmonary haemosiderosis and pulmonary haemorrhage. Br J Dis Chest 75:225, 1981.
35. Soergel K, Sommers S: Idiopathic pulmonary hemosiderosis and related syndromes. Am J Med 32:499, 1962.
36. Beckerman R, Taussig L, Pinnas J: Familial idiopathic pulmonary hemosiderosis. Am J Dis Child 133:609, 1979.
37. Breckenridge R, Ross J: Idiopathic pulmonary hemosiderosis. A report of familial occurrence. Chest 75:636, 1979.
38. Thaell J, Greipp P, Stubbs S, Siegal G: Idiopathic pulmonary hemosiderosis. Two cases in a family. Mayo Clin Proc 53:113, 1978.
39. Yum M, Lamptom L, Bloom P, Edwards J. Asymptomatic IgA nephropathy associated with pulmonary hemosiderosis. Am J Med 64:1056, 1978.
40. Wright P, Menzies I, Pounder R, Keeling P. Adult idiopathic pulmonary haemosiderosis and coeliac disease. Q J Med 197:95, 1981.
41. Donald K, Edwards R, McEvoy J: Alveolar capillary basement membrane lesions in Goodpasture's syndrome and idiopathic pulmonary hemosiderosis. Am J Med 59:642, 1975.
42. Gonzalez-Crussi F, Hull M, Grosfeld J: Idiopathic pulmonary hemosiderosis: Evidence of capillary basement membrane abnormality. Am Rev Respir Dis 114:689, 1976.
43. Hyatt R, Adelstein E, Halazun J, Lukens J: Ultrastructure of the lung in idiopathic pulmonary hemosiderosis. Am J Med 52:822, 1972.
44. Yeager H, Powell D, Weinberg R, et al.: Idiopathic pulmonary hemosiderosis. Ultrastructural studies and response to azathioprine. Arch Int Med 136:1145, 1976.
45. Irwin R, Cottrell T, Hsu K, et al.: Idiopathic pulmonary hemosiderosis: An electron microscopic and immunofluorescent study. Chest 65:41, 1974.
46. Sternlieb I, Bennet B, Scheinberg I: D-penicillamine-induced Goodpasture's syndrome in Wilson's disease. Ann Int Med 82:673, 1975.
47. Ahmad D, Patterson R, Morgan W, et al.: Pulmonary hemorrhage and hemolytic anemia due to trimellitic anhydride. Lancet 2:328, 1979.
48. Buja LM, Freed TA, Berman MA, Morrow AG, Roberts WC: Pulmonary alveolar hemorrhage: A common finding in patients with severe cardiac disease. Am J Cardiol 27:168–72, 1971.
49. Carrington C, Liebow A: Pulmonary veno-occlusive disease. Hum Pathol 1:322, 1970.

50. Road JD, Jacques J, Sparling JR: Diffuse alveolar septal amyloidosis presenting with recurrent hemoptysis and medial dissection of pulmonary arteries. Am Rev Respir Dis 132:1368–70, 1985.

51. Drew W, Finley T, Golde D: Diagnostic lavage and occult pulmonary hemorrhage in thrombocytopenic immunocompromised patients. Am Rev Resp Dis 116:215, 1977.

52. Smith L, Katzenstein A: Pathogenesis of massive pulmonary hemorrhage in acute leukemia. Arch Intern Med 142:2149–52, 1982.

53. Cardonnier C, Bernaudin J-F, Bierling P, Huet Y, Vernant J-P: Pulmonary complications occurring after allogeneic bone marrow transplantation: A study of 130 consecutive transplanted patients. Cancer 58:1047–54, 1986.

54. Finley TN, Aronow A, Cosentino AM, Golde DW: Occult pulmonary hemorrhage in anticoagulated patients. Am Rev Respir Dis 112:23–9, 1975.

55. Nash G, Fligiel S: Kaposi's sarcoma presenting as pulmonary disease in the acquired immunodeficiency syndrome: Diagnosis by lung biopsy. Hum Pathol 15:999–1001, 1984.

56. Yousem SA. Angiosarcoma presenting in the lung. Arch Pathol Lab Med 110:112–5, 1986.

19 Tumors of the Lung

Andrew Churg

Introduction

In this chapter tumors of the lung will be reviewed, particularly new findings derived from ultrastructural and immunohistochemical examinations; some controversial issues that confront pathologists, such as histologic subtyping, will also be discussed. Some areas will receive only short consideration; the sections on epidemiology and on the clinical features of bronchogenic carcinomas, in particular, provide only brief summaries. Interested readers can find extensive reviews in the References section. Excellent coverage of the historical development of modern concepts of pathologic features of lung tumors, especially bronchogenic carcinomas, may be found in Spencer.[1]

I have chosen to use the term "bronchogenic" carcinoma, although this is sometimes criticized as an inaccurate anachronism, since it is quite evident that many so-called tumors are not derived from the bronchial epithelium per se. Nonetheless, I believe that bronchogenic is a useful name for a group of tumors that are clearly related to cigarette smoke and other known inhaled carcinogens and that have a number of histogenetic as well as behavioral characteristics in common. "Lung cancer" and "carcinoma of the lung" are used as synonyms for bronchogenic carcinoma.

Bronchogenic Carcinoma

Epidemiology

Incidence

At the turn of the century, carcinoma of the lung was a rare disease; Adler, cited in Spencer[1] was only able to find 394 cases in a review of the literature in 1912. In 1981 it was estimated that between 130,000 and 140,000 new cases of lung cancer occurred in the United States alone,[2] the largest number of tumors for any single organ. In 1980, bronchogenic cancers accounted for 22 percent of all cancers in men and 8 percent of all cancers in women; bronchogenic cancers also caused 34 percent of all cancer deaths in men and 14 percent of all cancer deaths in women. In men this is the most common cancer (1977 incidence rate of approximately 55 per 100,000 male population)[3]; in women, it is third in frequency (1977 incidence rate of approximately 15 per 100,000 female population)[3] after tumors of the breast and large bowel.

Although the overall number of new cases of lung cancer in women is only about 25 percent of that in men, the incidence rates in women are increasing at a more rapid rate, so that the ratio of men to women developing the disease has dropped from 10:1 in 1962 to 5:1 in 1975.[4] Among young men and women (ages 35 to 44) the ratio dropped from 4.7:1 in 1945 to 1.9:1 in 1970 and 0.9:1 in 1975.[5] This phenomenon presumably reflects increased smoking among younger women in the population.

Epidemiologic Factors: Cigarette Smoke

The association between carcinoma of the lung and cigarette smoking was suspected from case reports in the 1930s and firmly established by numerous large-scale epidemiologic studies in the 1950s and 1960s.[6–8] An exceptional fact about these studies is the large size of the populations involved, the variations of different studies to eliminate possible bias, and the remarkably consistent results: at this point the only viable theory that would deny the causative effect of cigarette smoke on lung cancer is the so-called "constitutional hypothesis"; namely, that some persons are prone because of genetic factors to both smoke cigarettes and develop lung cancer as independent events. By its very nature this theory is

Table 19–1. Lung Cancer Mortality Ratios for Smokers Age 35 to 84[a]

	Nonsmokers	Cigarette Smokers	Cigarette and Other Smokers	Pipe Smokers	Pipe and Cigar Smokers	Cigar Smokers
Men	1.00	10.08	8.25	2.23	1.23	2.15
Women	1.00	2.63	—	—	—	—

[a] Based on the results of Hammond.[10]

Table 19–3. Lung Cancer Mortality by Depth of Inhalation of Cigarette Smoke[a]

			Inhalation		
	Nonsmoker	Noninhaler	Slight	Moderate	Deep
Men	1.00	8.00	8.92	13.08	17.00
Women	1.00	2.00	2.25	3.50	7.13

[a] Based on the results of Hammond.[10]

difficult to disprove; however, indirect evidence against it may be derived from the extremely rapid increases in lung cancer rates over a short period of time, a period in which gene pools could not possibly change, and the constant association of cigarette smoking with other forms of disease, especially coronary heart disease. To deny the association then requires that one postulate a genetic propensity to smoke, and to develop lung cancer, and to develop coronary disease, and so forth, all independent events. A recent study by Friedman and colleagues[9] has tackled this problem. They examined a group of 5200 patients in the Kaiser-Permanente Medical Care Program; mortality for smokers vs. nonsmokers for a variety of diseases was compared for 48 different characteristics. An increased mortality from lung cancer and coronary heart disease was again demonstrated for smokers, and could not be accounted for by any other variable or combination of variables.

Because of the large scale of the studies involved, the effects of smoking have been demonstrated statistically for different situations in great detail. I shall illustrate some of these effects using data from only a few studies; the interested reader is particularly referred to the summary by Hoover[11] for comparison between studies. The most basic and consistent finding has been the association between the fact of smoking cigarettes and the development of lung cancer (Table 19–1); if the standard mortality rate (SMR) from lung cancer is arbitrarily set as 1 for nonsmokers, male cigarette smokers as a whole have been found to have SMRs on the order of 10 to 20. Pipe or cigar smokers, by comparison, have only about a twofold risk over nonsmokers. A similar trend, but of lesser magnitude, holds for women. The risk of death from lung cancer has also been shown to be closely related to the number of cigarettes smoked (Table 19–2);

again the risks increase for both men and women, but are numerically smaller for women. Similarly (Tables 19–3, 19–4) depth of inhalation and age at which smoking was started also correlate well with lung cancer mortality.

These data all suggest that lung cancer develops as a result of inhaling a carcinogen present in the smoke, and that the greater the amount delivered to the lung, either as a result of more years of smoking, more cigarettes smoked, or more smoke inhaled, the greater the carcinogenic risk. The reason for the smaller SMRs in women is not entirely clear but is probably due in part to the fact that smoking became socially acceptable for women later than for men. As noted above, younger women; that is, those whose smoking habits have probably been more like their male counterparts of comparable age, have incidence rates for lung cancer that are much closer to the rates in men.

This idea that lung cancer is produced by carcinogens in cigarette smoke is again supported by the data on the smoking of filter cigarettes, and on the effects of stopping smoking. In one recent study, (Table 19–5) it was shown that persons smoking filter cigarettes had less risk of developing lung cancer compared to those smoking an equal number of nonfilter cigarettes. It has also been demonstrated (Table 19–6) that with cessation of smoking, the risk of death from cancer progressively drops, so that by 10–20 years after cessation this risk probably approximates that of the general population.

One last point is that the effects of smoking outweigh each of the other epidemiologically associated variables by at least an order of magnitude. The one possible exception to this rule is persons in certain high-risk occupations (see Epidemiologic Factors: Geography and Air Pollution, below) where the effects of cigarette smoke and occupational agent appear to be multiplicative; for

Table 19–2. Lung Cancer Mortality by Number of Cigarettes Smoked[a]

	Cigarettes per Day				
	0	1–9	10–19	20–30	40+
Men	1.00	4.62	8.62	14.69	18.77
Women	1.00	1.25	2.38	4.88	7.50

[a] Based on the results of Hammond.[10]

Table 19–4. Lung Cancer Mortality by Age of Beginning to Smoke[a]

	Age Began to Smoke			
	25+	20–24	15–19	<15
Men	4.05	10.08	14.69	16.77
Women	2.25	3.38	5.00	2.50

[a] Based on the results of Hammond.[10]

Table 19-5. Lung Cancer Mortality for Smokers of Filter Vs. Nonfilter Cigarettes[a]

	No. Cigarettes per Day			
	1-10	11-20	21-40	41+
Filter	1.00[b]	1.8	3.0	6.0
Nonfilter	1.20	2.2	4.2	6.8

[a] Based on the results of Wynder and Hoffman.[12]
[b] Standard mortality rate set at 1.00 for one to ten filter cigarettes per day.

Table 19-6. Lung Cancer Mortality in Ex-Cigarette Smokers[a]

	Years Since Stopped Smoking				Non-smokers	Current Smokers
	1	1-4	5-9	10+		
Men who smoked 1-19 cigarettes per day	7.12	3.13	1.25	0.44	1.00	7.5
Men who smoked 20+ cigarettes per day	17.68	10.12	6.50	1.81	1.00	16.9

[a] Based on the results of Hoover.[11]

example, asbestos exposure. Doll and Peto[2] estimate that tobacco usage causes about 30 percent of all cancer deaths in the United States each year, and at least 80 percent (and probably more) of lung cancer deaths.

Epidemiologic Factors: Geography and Air Pollution

Lung cancer rates vary both by country and by location within a country. A listing of rates for various countries is shown in Figure 19-1. The countries with the highest rates are the most part Westernized countries with high per capita cigarette consumption; in this regard the inclusion of the Maori tribe of New Zealand is of interest, since in this tribe both men and women smoke large amounts of tobacco, and the corresponding incidence rates are high for both sexes. Another fact that emerges from Figure 19-1 is that risk relates to both the country of residence and country of origin (for example, see the three entries for Israel); in general, in emigrants risk changes from that of the original country to that of the new country.[7,13]

The most consistent cause of variation of lung cancer rates within countries is probably urban/rural differences. It has been repeatedly shown that lung cancer rates are higher in urban areas than in rural areas, and within rural areas, nonfarm regions have higher rates than farm regions. In a recent report the age-adjusted lung cancer mortality rates for white males in geographic regions of the United States that were more than 75 percent urbanized was 39.9 per 100,000 compared to 31.3 per 100,000 for regions that were less than 25 percent urbanized, and 24.6 per 100,000 for regions that were less than 25 percent urbanized and had more than 25 percent rural farm population.[14] A similar pattern was

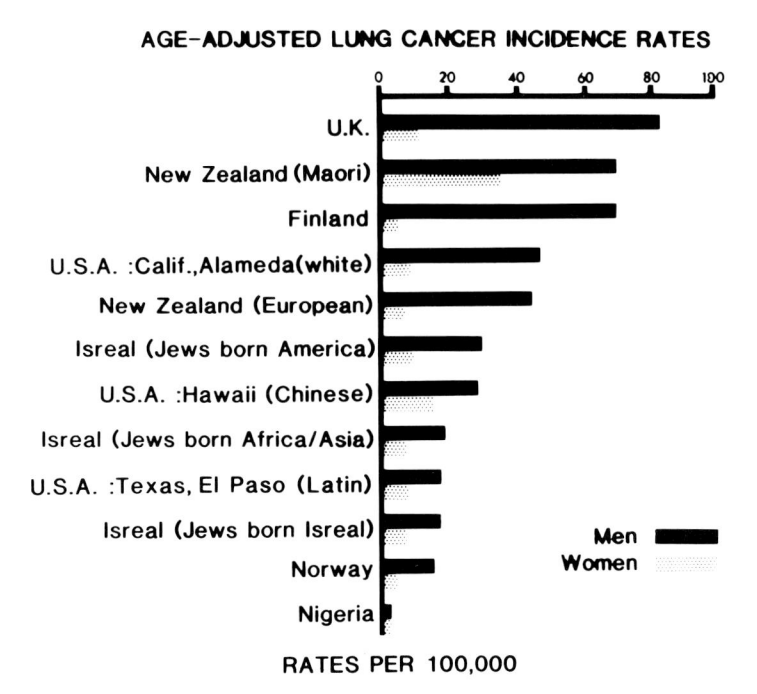

Figure 19-1. Age-adjusted lung cancer incidence rates in various countries. From Burbank and Fraumeni.[28]

found for white women, and also for nonwhites. For the latter group rates were considerably higher than for white males, pointing out the effects of race on lung cancer incidence.[15]

This difference in lung cancer rates has been commonly ascribed to greater air pollution in urban areas, but the hypothesis is controversial. One can divide air pollution into two general categories: known carcinogens, and substances such as sulfur dioxide and soot that are not in themselves carcinogens but may act in some fashion as promoters.[16] For example, there is considerable evidence that substances such as iron oxide particles, a common form of air pollution, increase the yield of benzpyrene-induced lung tumors in experimental animals, even though iron oxide particles are not in themselves carcinogenic.[17] Such findings suggest that much of the particulate and gaseous pollution in cities might augment the effects of specific carcinogens such as cigarette smoke. Actual studies attempting to relate measured air pollution indices and cancer rates have been few; correlations have been found in some instances with smoke levels, or with sulfate levels, but about an equal number of studies have found no correlation.[18-21] Epidemiologic studies have also failed to consistently show that increased duration of residence in urban areas is associated with a high lung cancer rate, and marked urban/rural differences can be found in countries such as Denmark and Norway where there is relatively little pollution.[7] Doll and Peto[2] have pointed out that what urban/rural differences may really reflect are differences in smoking habits of persons living in such locations 50 years ago, a time when smoking was just becoming a widespread habit. At this point the importance of air pollution is unclear.[7,13] Vena[22] concluded that air pollution by itself probably has little effect, but that the combination of heavy smoking and heavy air pollution increased risk by a factor of about 4, compared to a low air pollution exposure. Doll and Peto[2] have suggested that, in large cities, air pollution contributes to about 10 percent of lung cancers, presumably in conjunction with cigarette smoking.

A publication that sheds considerable light on the question of causes of lung cancer is the *Atlas of Cancer Mortality of U.S. Counties: 1950–1969*.[23,24] The maps showing lung cancer rates by county for white males and white females are reproduced in Figure 19–2. It is apparent that there are large differences among different areas in the United States. Many of the "hot spots" are large urban centers such as Chicago, New York, and San Francisco, where the effects of urban/rural differences would be expected. Other high-rate areas such as Miami may be explained on the basis that these are retirement centers in which the population has artificially been shifted to an older age group at high risk for many diseases.

There remain, however, areas such as the Gulf Coast and the southeastern coast where none of the above factors can be applied. The higher rates in many of these counties correlate with the presence of paper, chemical petroleum, and shipbuilding industries.[11,14,25-27] Figure 19–3 shows the lung cancer mortaldity rates for males in counties with petroleum industries separated by percentage of population employed in the specific industry and by urbanization of the county. It is evident that there is a dramatic increase in lung cancer incidence in rural counties in which more than 1 percent of the population is employed in petroleum industries; this effect disappears in urbanized areas. Similar graphs showing the effects of smelters, chemical plants, and paper manufacturing plants are illustrated in Hoover.[11] It is noteworthy that the effects of paper and chemical industries do not disappear with increasing urbanization. In some of these examples the specific carcinogen and the specific group affected can be identified; for example, asbestos used in the shipbuilding industry (*see* Epidemiologic Factors: Occupation, below) appears to affect only those in the industry itself. In other instances, for example, counties with nonferrous metal smelters, it is probable that arsenic released into the air from the smelters affects the entire local population, most of whom are not employed in the industry.[14,25] Such persons might be considered to be exposed to carcinogenic forms of air pollution.

Epidemiologic Factors: Genetic Factors

The role of genetic factors in lung cancer is disputed. There is no doubt that race and sex have some influence.[28-31] For example, lung cancer incidence rates are increasing in the United States more rapidly among blacks than white.[31] Another example is the Chinese in Hong Kong who show a marked predominance of adenocarcinoma; excessive rates are seen among Chinese women in several countries.[11,30] Lung cancer also appears to be more frequent in first-degree relatives of patients with lung cancer. Recent studies suggest, however, that this observation probably reflects either the smoking habits of the subjects themselves or the carcinogenic effects of low levels of someone else's cigarette smoke.[32]

Of particular interest is the possibility of finding a genetic marker that would indicate a predisposition to lung cancer. Kellerman and colleagues[33] suggested that such a marker might be inducibility of aryl hydrocarbon hydroxylase, an enzyme system that metabolizes polycyclic hydrocarbons of the type found in cigarette smoke to more potent carcinogens. In an initial report, lymphocytes from 96 percent of patients with lung cancer as opposed to 55 percent of control subjects showed high levels of inducibility. This report has been criticized on a number of bases including the fact that lymphocytes rather than bronchial epithelial cells were used in the assay, the fact that one-fourth of the patients had adenocarcinoma, a type claimed to show less association with smoking, and a misreading of the genetics of the enzyme, which turns out to have several alleles.[31] Attempts to reproduce the data have not generally been successful.

Epidemiologic Factors: Socioeconomic Status

A higher rate of lung cancer has consistently been found in patients of lower socioeconomic status[31,35]; in large part this probably reflects a remarkably strong correla-

Bronchogenic Carcinoma 315

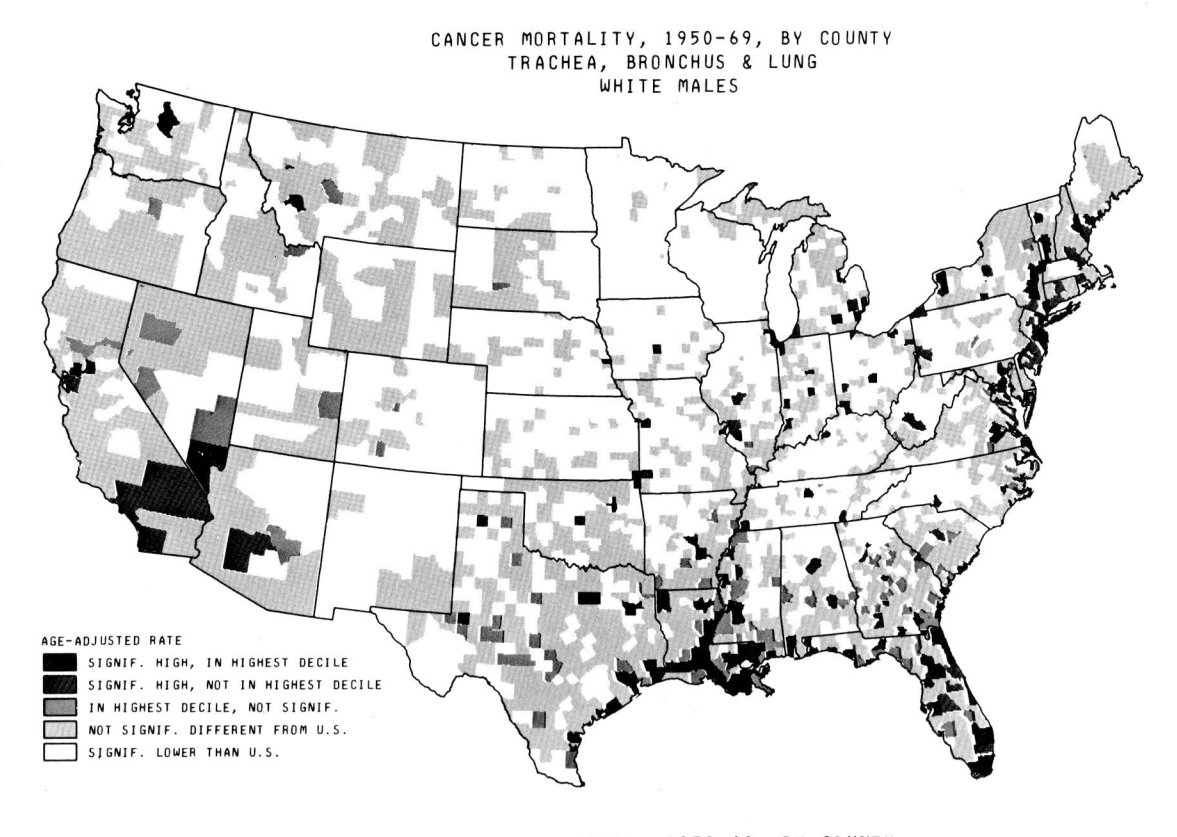

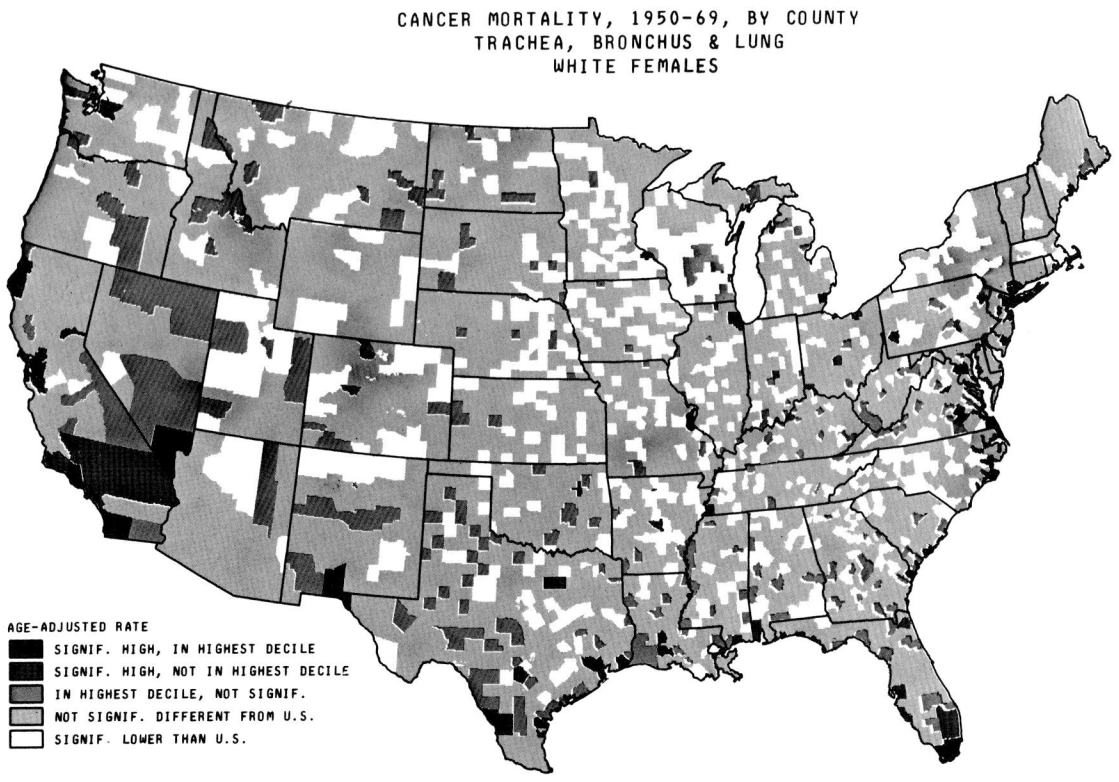

Figure 19–2. Cancer mortality, 1950–1969 by U.S. county for trachea, bronchus, and lung for white males (A) and for white females (B). Reproduced with permission from *Atlas of Cancer Mortality of U.S. Counties 1950–1969.* Courtesy of Dr. T. J. Mason.

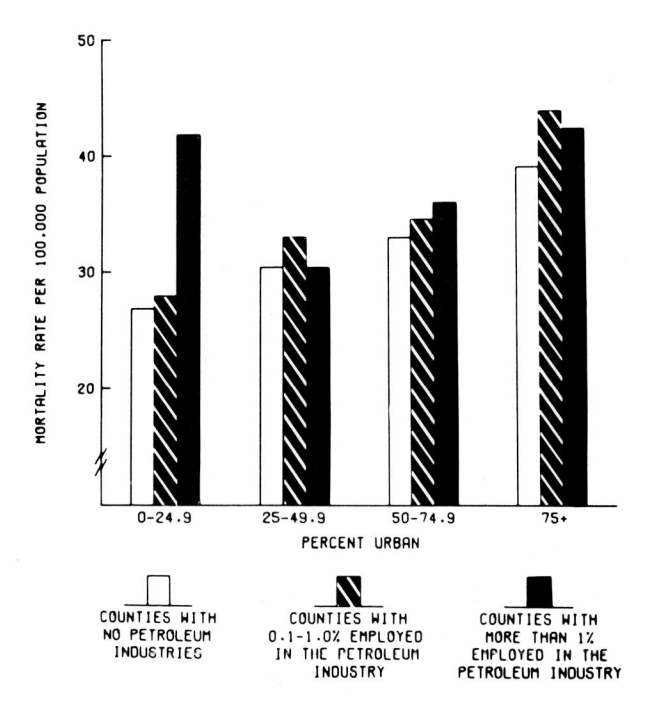

Figure 19–3. Lung cancer mortality as a function of urbanization in the presence of petroleum industries (see Epidemiologic Factors, text). Reproduced with permission from Blot and Fraumeni.[14]

tion between cigarette smoking habits and specific occupations or socioeconomic groups.[36]

Epidemiologic Factors: Occupation

The predominant role of cigarette smoking in causing lung cancer has been discussed. Most of the other factors that have been shown epidemiologically to relate to lung cancer are much less strong; typically the mortality ratios for such factors (for example, urban vs. rural) are less than 2. The major exception to this observation is direct occupational exposure to a number of different pulmonary carcinogens; here the risk factors, either by themselves or in conjunction with cigarette smoking, may range up to almost one hundred times that of the general population. Table 19–7 shows the risks of developing lung cancer for various well-established occupational agents. A variety of other substances, for example, beryllium, chloroprene, isopropyl oil, chloroanilines, and nitrosamines are either known to cause respiratory cancer in animals or are strongly suspected in humans, and there are undoubtedly many more potential respiratory carcinogens used industrially.[37] Many of the agents listed in Table 19–7 are by themselves more potent carcinogens than cigarette smoke; others, particularly radiation and asbestos, appear to act synergistically with cigarette smoke.

Whether occupational carcinogens can be implicated in 25 to 30 percent of lung cancers, as suggested by the National Cancer Institute[38] is questionable; the figure of approximately 15 percent of male lung cancers and 5 percent of female lung cancers arrived at by Doll and Peto[2] seems more reasonable. Even at this lower limit, however, occupational agents could be implicated in at least 15,000 cases per year in the United States alone. In certain specific populations, for instance, asbestos workers and uranium miners, bronchogenic carcinomas clearly account for a large number of deaths; in some high-exposure groups, 20 percent of asbestos workers die of lung cancer.[39,40]

A number of general observations can be made of occupational pulmonary carcinogens. First, a fairly consistent finding is the long latent period between the onset

Table 19–7. Lung Cancer After Exposure to Occupational Agents[a]

Agent	Relative Risk[b]	Tumor	Dose-Response	Occupations at Risk
Tobacco smoke	10	All types (more in upper lobes)	+	Cigarette smokers
Asbestos				
Nonsmokers	5	All types	+	Shipyard, construction workers, asbestos miners,
Smokers	20–50	All types	+	millers, many others
Coke				
Work at side of oven	2		+	Steelworkers, roofers, rubber workers
Work at top of oven	7			
Arsenic	7	All types (more in upper lobe)		Smelter workers
Chromium	9			Chromium ore refiners
Chloromethyl ether	29	Many small cell	+	Chloromethyl ether workers
Mustard gas	37			Mustard gas workers
Nickel	8	Also association with nasal and laryngeal cancer		Nickel refinery workers
Radiation	25[c]	Many small cell	+	Uranium miners

[a] Based on the results of Frank,[37] Hammond et al.,[40] Archer et al.,[41] and Weiss.[42]
[b] Relative to the general population.
[c] For oat cell carcinoma; author's interpretation of the data of Archer et al.[41]

of exposure and the appearance of carcinoma: the average time is in the range of 25 to 30 years, and may range up to 50 years.[37] A long latent period is also, of course, true of the effects of cigarette smoke.

Second, some of these agents are associated with a specific type of carcinoma; for example, it has been shown that exposure to radiation or exposure to chloromethyl ethers produces a very high fraction of oat cell carcinomas.[27,37,41,42] Morton and Treyve have suggested that in most high-risk occupations only one or two histologic types of lung cancer are increased in frequency, and that the observation of such a selected increase should bring an occupational agent to mind.[44] However, some agents, for example, asbestos, appear to produce an increase in all types of lung cancers.

Third, a dose-response relationship is present for many of these carcinogens, as it is for cigarette smoke: arsenic, asbestos, chloremethyl ether, coke oven exposure and, probably, radiation exposure, all follow such a pattern. The dose-response relationship has been customarily measured simply as a matter of time employed in the given industry, but in fact can be considerably refined. For example, for coke oven workers the risk varies by about a factor of 3 depending on whether the worker works above the oven, and hence gets a higher dose, or works at the side of the oven.[42] Enterline[45] showed that for asbestos workers with less than 125 million particles per cubic foot-years (mppcf-year) of exposure, the standard mortality ratio compared to a general population was 1.67; this rose to 5.56 for workers with greater than 750 mppcf-year.

Fourth, the effects of cigarette smoking are quite variable. Chloromethyl ether and nickel appear to act independently of cigarette smoke, and tumors may be found in nonsmokers.[42] Asbestos, on the other hand, is a relatively small danger to nonsmokers (risk factor of about 5 compared to nonsmoking control subjects[40]), but shows a marked multiplicative effect when combined with cigarette smoke (risk factor about 50 compared to nonsmoking control subjects.[40]) Radiation probably is multiplicative as well.[41,46]

Fifth, it is not entirely clear whether these various agents are dangerous only to those directly handling the material, or whether they may also affect nearby workers or even the population at large. Blot and Fraumeni[25] have suggested that increased levels of cancer in counties with smelters probably reflect exposure of the entire population to atmospheric arsenic. Gottlieb and co-workers[48] demonstrated an increased risk for individuals living near petroleum and chemical plants, and equivocal increases associated with proximity to food, grain, canning, and paper industries.[48]

Histogenesis and Development of Bronchogenic Carcinoma

The Origin of Bronchogenic Carcinoma

The normal bronchial epithelium consists of basal cells with no specialized differentiation, and specialized cells that may secrete mucus, bear cilia, or contain neurosecretory granules. Other specialized cells such as Clara cells are found in the distal portion of the bronchial tree. The exact pathway whereby one or more of these various cells give rise to squamous cell, adenocarcinoma, and small-cell carcinomas is disputed (as described below, large-cell carcinomas are poorly differentiated versions of the squamous and adenocarcinomas, and hence do not need a separate category). The traditional theory is that unspecialized cells give rise directly to metaplastic squamous cells or to neoplastic squamous cells (reviewed in McDowell and co-workers[49]), small-cell carcinomas are derived from neurosecretory granule-containing amine precursor uptake and decarboxylation (APUD) cells that have migrated from the neural chest, and adenocarcinomas are presumably derived from cells related to the glands or goblet cells of the bronchus. McDowell and associates,[49] Barrett and colleagues,[50] and Becci and co-workers[51] have raised the alternate possibility, namely, that a differentiated mucus-secreting cell, the small mucus granule cell (SMGC) is the parent of bronchogenic carcinomas. These investigators believe that squamous metaplasia evolves by a sequence of hyperplasia of mucus-secreting cells followed by direct metasplasia of SMGC to squamous cells. Their evidence is based largely on the finding of "mucous granules" in what appears to be metaplastic squamous epithelium of the bronchus. However, my interpretation of their photographs is that the material that stains is really glycocalyx, seen as both an obvious surface layer and in "granules" that are really superficial invaginations of the surface. I would prefer, therefore, to interpret these SMGCs as ordinary metaplastic squamous cells that fall within the range of the traditional theories. These observations do not, in any event, alter the important point made by McDowell and co-workers[52] that the precursor cell can differentiate into combined forms; that is, mucous and neurosecretory granule-containing cells, mucous and squamous cells, and so on, and that all bronchogenic carcinomas are potentially derived from the same cell. Bell and Seetharam[53] have shown that all types of lung carcinomas can express antigens related both to endodermally derived and neural crest–derived cells, regardless of histologic type, a finding in accord with the above hypothesis. This issue is discussed at length by Yesner,[54] and is considered again below and in the sections on small-cell and carcinoid tumors.

Development of Squamous Carcinoma

A variety of hyperplastic, atypical, and dysplastic changes can be found in the epithelium of the trachea and bronchial tree, and in the periphery of the lung, particularly in relation to scars. Most of the lesions found within the epithelium of conducting airways are probably related to smoking, although environmental pollutants such as ozone and sulfur dioxide may also play a role. Auerbach and co-workers[55–57] have extensively (35 to 55 sections per case) studied the tracheobronchial tree from a large group of smokers and matched control subjects, and have shown that a variety of atypical and hyperplastic

Table 19–8. Cigarette Smoking and Changes in Airway Epithelium[a]

	Non-smokers	Smoking Level (%)		
		0–1 pack/day	1–2 packs/day	>2 packs/day
Marked basal hyperplasia				
Persons dying 1955–1960	0	0.1	12.2	66.6
Persons dying 1970–1977	0	0	0.1	0.1
Marked dysplastic lesions				
Persons dying 1950–1955	0	2.6	13.2	22.5
Persons dying 1970–1977	0	0.1	0.8	2.2

[a] Based on the results of Auerbach et al.[55,57]

lesions such as basal cell hyperplasia, loss of cilia, and cytologic dysplasia, occur more frequently and with greater extent and degree in smokers than in nonsmokers; the process can be directly related to the number of cigarettes smoked per day (Table 19–8). They also compared the changes in persons autopsied in 1955–1960, a period in which most cigarettes were nonfilter, and in 1970–1977, when most patients smoked cigarettes that were filtered, and found that such changes were less frequent in the 1970s. Presumably this finding reflects the fact that filters remove part of the irritating/carcinogenic substances found in cigarette smoke.

It should be pointed out that the significance of lesions such as basal cell hyperplasia, squamous metaplasia, and minor degrees of dysplasia is unclear, and in fact it is likely that most such changes are reactive rather than neoplastic. Nonetheless, serial cytologic studies have demonstrated that squamous carcinoma appears to arise from a sequence of increasingly dysplastic metaplastic cells, eventuating first in squamous carcinoma in situ (CIS) and then in invasive carcinoma[58]; this sequence, however, is almost never traceable on resected specimens examined histologically. As a rule if such specimens show carcinoma in situ, lesser degrees of dysplasia are not present.[59] Details of the cytologic and dysplastic changes and their time sequence are presented in Chapter 27.

Histologically, the only clearly defined in situ carcinoma of the tracheobronchial tree is squamous CIS.[59,60] The lesion consists of cytologically malignant squamous cells that replace the whole thickness of the epithelium (Figure 19–4B). Although these cells may keratinize, they do not show the usual sequence of maturation seen in simple metaplastic squamous epithelium. The nuclei are of quite varied and often bizarre sizes and shapes, and mitoses may be numerous. An important point from the view of treatment is that the process extends into the underlying glands; thus stripping the epithelium, as might be done for dysplastic lesions of the vocal cords, will leave residual neoplasm behind in the bronchus. Such glands are often the earliest site of invasion of tumor into the bronchial wall.[59,61,62]

Squamous cell carcinoma in situ (CIS) may be apparent grossly (Figure 19–4A). The earliest and most subtle lesion is loss of bronchial ridges, followed by thickening of the mucosa. This progresses to heaping up of the mucosa and often eventual obstruction of the lumen. However, studies in which many areas or all of the tracheobronchial tree are sectioned[59] indicate that CIS may not be apparent grossly, and that the lesions are commonly multifocal and most frequently involve segmental bronchi. Thus careful selection of biopsy sites via the bronchoscope is necessary to define the extent of needed resection, and careful examination by the pathologist, particularly careful examination of resected margins, is necessary to determine if resection is incomplete.

Carcinoma in situ is identified in a clinical setting in two different ways. One is by examination of multiple sequential sputum cytology samples from asymptomatic patients who are at risk of developing lung cancer. These studies are discussed further in Chapter 27. The other setting is the symptomatic individual who may present with cough or hemoptysis, and who often shows radiographic evidence of obstruction, but no clear mass lesion. Cytologic examination of the sputum indicates that a malignancy is present, but even with this knowledge, visualization of the lesion may be extremely difficult; Pearson and colleagues[63] were able to find the neoplasm in only 21 of 41 such patients. Cortese and colleagues[64] have suggested that lesions may be visualized by fluorescence of hematoporphyrin which is preferentially localized in tumor tissue.

Cytologic studies indicate that severe dysplasia and CIS are relatively slowly progressive lesions; Saccomanno and co-workers[58] found that the average time from the appearance of severe dysplasia or CIS to the appearance of invasive carcinoma was 4 to 5 years. Thus patients in whom only CIS is present should, in theory, have an excellent prognosis if the lesion is detected and resected. The actual prognosis for symptomatic patients who have radiographically occult lesions resected in uncertain; results from several of the larger studies are shown in Table 19–9. In probably more than half these patients, early invasive carcinoma was present along with the in situ lesions, and a small number also had metastases to regional lymph nodes. Even in this situation, resection may be curative; Martini and colleagues[65] report two patients alive and well 6 years after resection of lesions that had metastasized to hilar nodes. An unknown fraction of these patients also develop a second invasive primary; in some series[59,65] this phenomenon was observed in as many as 25 percent of patients. This finding is not surprising, given the tendency for CIS to be a multifocal lesion. Nonetheless, the data presented in Table 19–9 indicate that the prognosis for those patients with "early" lesions is clearly far superior to that expected for patients with the usual radiographically visible tumor. An additional important conclusion to be drawn from these studies is that the usual symptomatic, radiographically visible lung cancer is first seen by the physician in a late stage of the disease.[59,61,62]

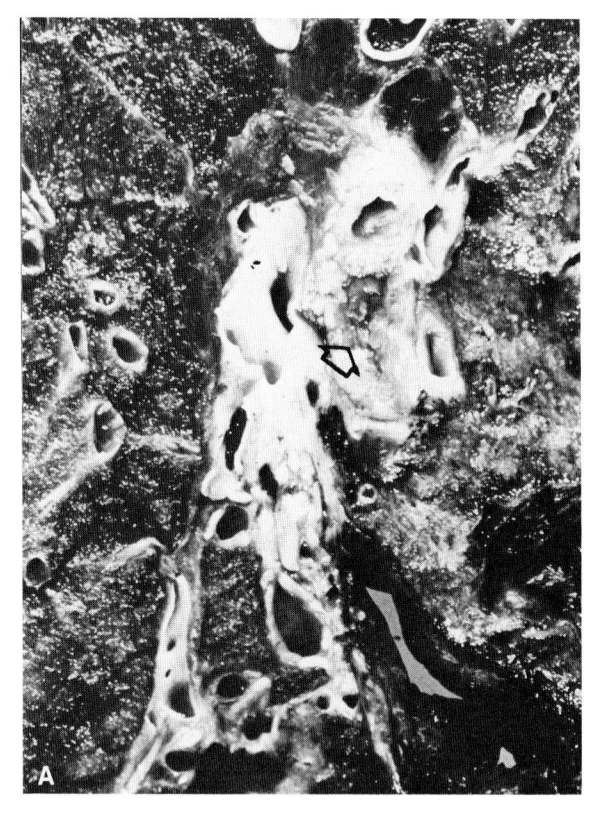

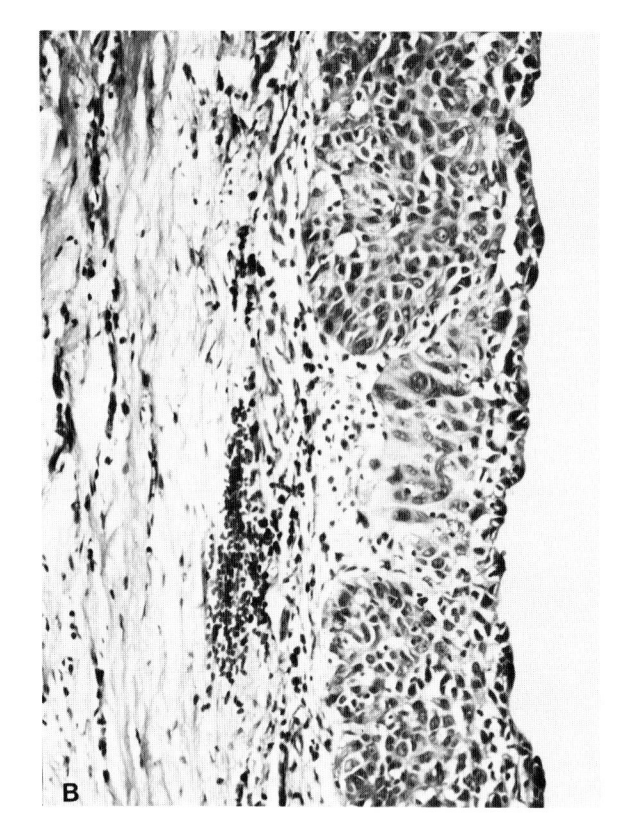

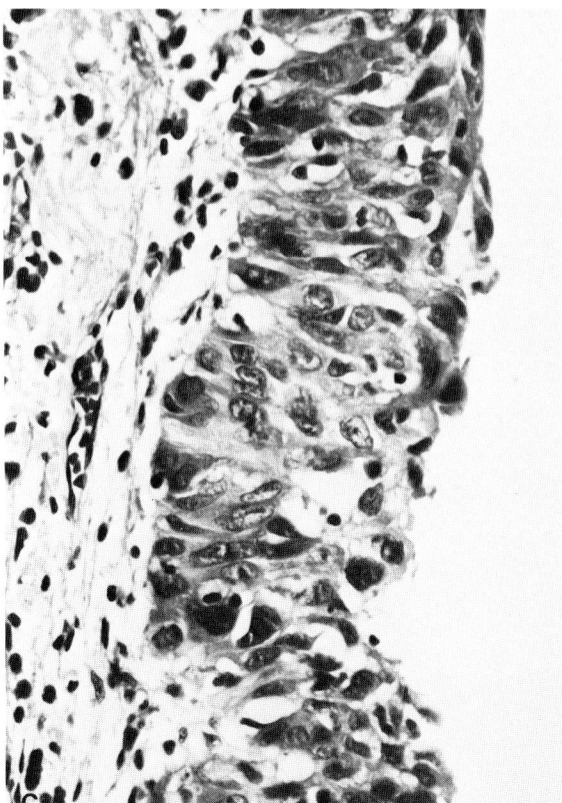

Figure 19–4. Carcinoma in situ. A. Gross appearance of lesion showing thickened bronchial mucosa (arrow); B and C. microscopic appearance of carcinoma in situ. Note the replacement of the epithelium by cytologically malignant cells which extend from the basement membrane through the surface. A possible focus of early invasion is present in B. (B ×160, C ×400).

Table 19–9. In Situ and Early Squamous Carcinomas

Author	No. Patients	Symptomatic	Abnormal Chest X-Ray Film	Resected	Dead	Second Primary	Survival	Invasive Cancer
Pearson et al.[63]	41	25		19				14 of 21
Woolner et al.[66]	28	12 of 13	8 of 28	28	3 of 28		Mean 6 years	14 of 28
Martini et al.[65]	26		4 of 26	?18	6 of 18	7	Mean 5 years	
Carter et al.[59]	20			19	3 of 20	4 or 5		12 of 20

Development of Adenocarcinomas and Small-Cell Carcinomas

The precursor lesion for other histologic types of carcinoma arising in bronchi is clinically and histologically poorly defined. Occasionally one finds evidence of widespread proliferation of neurosecretory granule-containing cells, the presumed precursor cells of small-cell carcinoma, in lungs resected for such tumors. Ranchod[67] reported a case in which multiple tumorlets (minute carcinoids) were present along with an oat cell carcinoma. However, the carcinoid tumors, although malignant, are much lower-grade lesions than the carcinoma, and are probably not an in situ form of oat cell carcinoma. It is also possible that small-cell anaplastic carcinomas (and by analogy, adenocarcinomas) arise from lesions which histologically appear to be squamous cell CIS. Some circumstantial evidence for this idea comes from the studies by Saccomanno and colleagues[46,56] in uranium miners. This group has a much higher incidence of small-cell carcinomas than the usual group of nonmining smokers; however, cytologic and histologic studies in such persons show dysplastic squamous cells and lesions which appear to be squamous carcinoma in situ. The frequency of the squamous carcinoma in situ lesions is in fact about the same in the miners and nonminers, and the lesion is present even in those who do develop small-cell carcinoma. It is also possible that a definite histologic small-cell in situ lesion is present briefly, as opposed to the relatively long time course for dysplastic squamous lesions, but is destroyed by the rapidly growing tumor.

The precursor lesion for tumors arising in the periphery of the lung, which are most frequently adenocarcinomas, is uncertain, but is commonly thought to be related to scarring. The scarring may be of any cause including bronchiectasis,[68,69] infarcts,[70] old tuberculous scars,[71] and even trauma, as in the tumor arising in an old bullet wound reported by Raeburn and Spencer.[72]

The details of this histologic process have been studied by Meyer and Liebow.[73] In areas of scarring the normal epithelium is replaced by a variety of different cell types: these may resemble the cells of terminal bronchiolar epithelium, type II cells, or squamous epithelium. Assembling series of cases, it is possible to find instances of progressively greater cytologic atypia in these cells, in particular in the squamous metaplastic cells, until obvious carcinoma is present. Sometimes a similar process can be observed in mucus-secreting cells with the formation of obvious adenocarcinoma, but this is relatively unusual. More common is the problem of finding a scar lined by atypical but not clearly malignant cells of the type which may be seen in bronchioloalveolar carcinoma. Discrimination between some of the cytologic atypias and carcinoma can be extremely difficult.

The definition of a tumor as a scar carcinoma is also somewhat arbitrary; such a tumor should either arise in an area of old honeycombing, or in a solitary scar. Such scars are usually hyalinized and frequently contain large amounts of pigment. Because tumors tend to evoke a desmoplastic response, it is sometimes difficult to determine whether a scar was preexisting or produced by tumor.

Meyer and Liebow[73] found that of 153 surgical patients who had carcinoma of the lung, scarring in the form of honeycombing was present in 32 (21 percent), whereas only 19 (4.7 percent) of 384 control autopsy lungs showed honeycombing. Of these latter 19 patients, lung cancer was present in 4. A history of pneumonia 5 years before was twice as common in persons with carcinoma and honeycombing as with only carcinoma. In the surgical series, 10 of 32 tumors were adenocarcinomas, and all of the tumors occurred in men. Bennett and colleagues[74] examined one hundred adenocarcinomas of the lung in men, a figure at that time accounting for only 9 percent of lung tumors in their local male population. Sixty-five percent of the tumors were peripheral and half appeared to be associated with preformed scars.

More recently, Auerbach and colleagues[75] reviewed Veterans Administration material and found 82 scar carcinomas constituting 7 percent of autopsied lung tumors over 21 years. Whereas in the period 1955–1959 only 2 percent of tumors were considered to be associated with scars, this figure increased to 16 percent in 1970–1973. Three-fourths of the tumors were adenocarcinomas, with the remainder large-cell and squamous cell carcinomas. They believed that the scar cancers were not related to smoking, but were largely related to infarcts.

The notion that peripheral carcinomas associated with collagen and pigment have arisen in preexisting scars has recently been challenged by Shimosato and colleagues[76]. They examined 50 peripheral tumors less than 3 cm in diameter; 38 of these tumors were adenocarcinomas, 2 large-cell carcinomas, and 8 squamous carcinomas. In the adenocarcinomas, greater amounts of collagen and the presence of hyalinized collagen correlated directly with tumor size; the bigger the tumor, the bigger the "scar." The larger tumors also had a higher incidence of nodal metastases and pleural invasion. Shimosato and colleagues also reviewed the relevant chest radiographs and found that arteries and bronchi tend to converge (that is, collapse) around a "scar" after the appearance of a tumor, and not before. These authors concluded that most "scars" in scar adenocarcinomas are actually desmoplastic responses to the neoplasm, and that so-called markers for scars, for example, pigment, merely reflect collapse of a large amount of parenchyma into a small area. Interestingly, these correlations were not found for squamous carcinomas.

There is a definite association between scarring from some chronic interstitial lung diseases and carcinoma of the lung. Turner-Warwick and associates[77] found 20 lung cancers in 205 cases of cryptogenic fibrosing alveolitis, a prevalance rate of 9.8 percent. Contrary to previous reports[78,79] all histologic types of tumors were present, and their relative frequency was about the same as seen in ordinary bronchogenic carcinomas. Comparison with expected incidence values for smokers and nonsmokers who do not have interstitial fibrosis suggested that diffuse scarring increased the risk of developing lung cancer by about a factor of 8.[77] Other causes of diffuse scarring or honeycombing also give rise to an increased incidence of lung cancer. These causes include: asbestosis (which some authors[80] believe is associated primarily with adenocarcinomas, a fact denied by others[81]), sarcoid,[82] rheumatoid lung,[83] and scleroderma.[78,79] Tumorlets (minute carcinoids) are frequently found in scars of all varieties[84,85]; they should not be mistaken for oat cell carcinomas.

Pathological Features of Bronchogenic Carcinomas

Classification of the Common Types of Lung Cancer

The common carcinomas of the lung may be subdivided into squamous or epidermoid, small-cell anaplastic, adenocarcinomas, and large-cell undifferentiated carcinomas.[86] The World Health Organization (WHO) classification scheme[86] is shown in Table 19–10 along with the modification suggested by the Working Party for Therapy of Lung Cancer (WPL).[87] A revised version of the WHO classification has just been published[88] and is very similar to that of the WPL. The latter system has the advantage of including well, moderately, and poorly differentiated subcategories for adenocarcinomas and squamous cell carcinomas, a feature lacking in the original WHO system. Carcinomas with clear-cut combinations of adenocarcinoma and squamous carcinoma features also occur but are relatively rare (about 0.2 percent of cases according to Yesner[89]).

The value of such classification schemes in the realm of patient therapy and also in comparing results from institution to institution is clear.[90] However, most pathologists are equally familiar with the fact that lung cancers tend to be histologically heterogeneous, so that the degree of differentiation may vary considerably from area to area, and, in the case of poorly differentiated tumors, the direction of differentiation may not be obvious. Feinstein and colleagues[91] reported the classifications assigned to 50 different tumors which were read by five experienced pathologists. The well-differentiated adenocarcinomas and squamous carcinomas were almost universally agreed on. However, the rate of disagreement rose to approximately 25 percent of readings for small-cell anaplastic and large-cell undifferentiated carcinomas, and to approximately 40 percent each for the tumors called by the majority poorly differentiated squamous and poorly differentiated adenocarcinomas. Similarly Yesner[92] found that only 43 percent of poorly differentiated adenocarcinomas and 47 percent of poorly differentiated squamous carcinomas, 34 percent of polygonal small-cell carcinomas, and 10 percent of large-cell carcinomas were unanimously classified by a panel of pathologists.

These facts should especially be kept in mind when attempting to classify lung cancers on the basis of endobronchial or transbronchial biopsies. In addition to the pleomorphism of the usual lung cancer, such biopsies frequently are scanty or show marked artifactual distortions. A number of authors have compared the results obtained by such biopsies with the diagnosis

Table 19–10. Classification of Lung Cancers

WHO[a]	WPL[b]	Revised WHO[c]
Epidermoid Carcinoma	Epidermoid Carcinoma 　Well differentiated 　Moderately differentiated 　Poorly differentiated	Squamous Carcinoma 　Well differentiated 　Moderately differentiated 　Poorly differentiated
Small-Cell Anaplastic 　Fusiform 　Polygonal 　Lymphocyte-like	Small-Cell Anaplastic 　Lymphocyte-like 　　(oat) 　Intermediate cell	Small-Cell Carcinoma 　Oat cell type 　Intermediate cell type 　Combined oat cell types
Adenocarcinoma 　Bronchogenic 　　Acinar 　　Papillary 　Bronchioloalveolar	Adenocarcinoma 　Well differentiated 　Moderately differentiated 　Poorly differentiated	Adenocarcinoma 　Acinar type 　Papillary type 　Bronchioloalveolar 　Solid carcinoma with mucus production
Large-Cell Carcinoma 　Solid with mucin 　Solid without mucin 　Giant cell 　Clear cell	Large-Cell Carcinoma 　With mucin production 　With stratification 　Giant cell 　Clear cell	Large-Cell Carcinoma 　Giant cell carcinoma 　Clear cell carcinoma
Adenosquamous Carcinoma	Adenosquamous Carcinoma	Adenosquamous Carcinoma

Abbreviations: WHO, World Health Organization; WPL, Working Party for Therapy of Lung Cancer.
[a] Based on the results of Kreyberg et al.[86]
[b] Based on the results of Matthews.[87]
[c] Based on the results of the World Health Organization.[88]

Table 19–11. Results of Histologic Typing: Biopsy Vs. Resected Tumor

	Squamous Cell Carcinoma			Small-Cell Carcinoma			Adenocarcinoma			Large-Cell Cancer		
Series	#C	#I	%I	#C	#I	%I	#C	#I	%I	#C	#I	%I
Rilke et al.[93]	33	2	6%	3	1	25%	2	2	50	3	2	40%
Hinson et al.[94]	143	10	7%	40	6	13%	3	0	0	0	5	100%

Abbreviations: #C, no. patients correctly diagnosed on biopsy; #I = no. patients incorrectly diagnosed; %I = percentage of patients incorrectly diagnosed.

Table 9–13. Histologic Subtypes in Surgical and Autopsy Specimens from the Same Series of Patients[a]

	Surgical Cases	Autopsy Cases
Squamous cell carcinoma	47.8	34.5
Small-cell carcinoma	19.1	23.2
Adenocarcinoma	16.0	25.6
Large-cell carcinoma	16.0	14.7

[a] Based on the results of Yesner.[92]

based on a resection specimen (Table 19–11). As shown in Table 19–11, the diagnosis of squamous carcinoma is generally accurate, and the diagnosis of small-cell carcinoma less so. Confusion between squamous and small-cell carcinomas appeared to be the most common error in these two series. It should be noted that in both of these reports there were relatively few adenocarcinomas and large-cell carcinomas, hence the accuracy of conclusions for these two tumor types is uncertain.

In my experience, which has been accumulated in institutions where the proportion of adenocarcinomas, and in particular of large-cell carcinomas is much higher than that just cited, it is not uncommon that one is able only to distinguish small-cell from non-small-cell carcinomas in small biopsy specimens. Since at present this distinction is the major one in terms of clinical therapy, there seems to be little gain in arbitrarily subclassifying the non-small-cell tumors on inadequate samples. Examination of cytologic specimens may be of use in this circumstance.

Frequency of Different Histologic Types of Lung Cancer

Despite the difficulties cited above, there is remarkable agreement concerning frequencies of the major different histologic types in most large series. Overall most such series show squamous carcinomas accounting for 30 to 40 percent of all cases, small-cell carcinomas for 29 to 35 percent, adenocarcinomas for 20 to 30 percent, and large-cell tumors for 10 to 15 percent. True mixed adenocarcinoma and squamous carcinomas make up less than 1 percent of the total.[94–97] A summary of several different reports is shown in Table 19–12.

The incidence of the various types of carcinoma of the lung are different when surgical and autopsy series are compared, and as noted above, when biopsies are compared to resection specimens. The series listed in Table 19–11 from Hinson and co-workers[94] is a surgical series, a fact which may in part account for the peculiar distribution of cases they report. Because small-cell carcinomas are not commonly resected, surgical series will show considerably fewer of these tumors than autopsy series. Similarly, because many adenocarcinomas are peripheral, surgical biopsy series tend to show a lower frequency of adenocarcinoma than surgical resection or autopsy series. Yesner's[92] data (Table 19–13) for 617 cases for which both surgical and autopsy material were available illustrate the differences. This series spans a considerable time and probably includes more small-cell carcinomas than would currently be resected. More recent data from the Veterans Administration study cited by Matthews[98] show only 3 percent small-cell carcinomas out of 244 surgical specimens.

Another factor that may account for the differences between autopsy and surgical series is the effect of therapy on the histologic appearances of lung tumors. Radiation, for example, regularly induces the formation of giant cells, sometimes to the point where the original histologic picture is unrecognizable (*see* p. 328). Several recent reports have considered the differences between the appearance of small-cell carcinoma in cytology/biopsy specimens and the finding of tumor with squamous or adenocarcinoma features at autopsy. In part this phenomenon may reflect poor sampling of the original tumor, but it may also be a manifestation of therapy-induced histologic alterations (see p. 337 and references 99–101).

Table 19–12. Frequency of Bronchogenic Carcinomas by Histologic Subtype[a]

	Series			
	Auerbach et al.[95]	Vincent[b] et al.[97]	Cox and Yesner[96]	Hinson et al.[94]
Squamous cell carcinoma	35.2	38.0	33.0	70.9
Small-cell carcinoma	24.6	19.2	22.1	11.6
Adenocarcinoma	25.2	26.5	28.2	8.6
Large-cell carcinoma	14.2	9.3	16.6	7.2
No. patients	656	1682	1017	740
Time period	1955–1972	1962–1975	1958–1977	?

[a] All values as percent of total.
[b] 6.9% mixed and unclassified tumors not included.

Histologic Types and Secular Trends

Although most series of reports encompassing the last 15 to 25 years show a preponderance of squamous carcino-

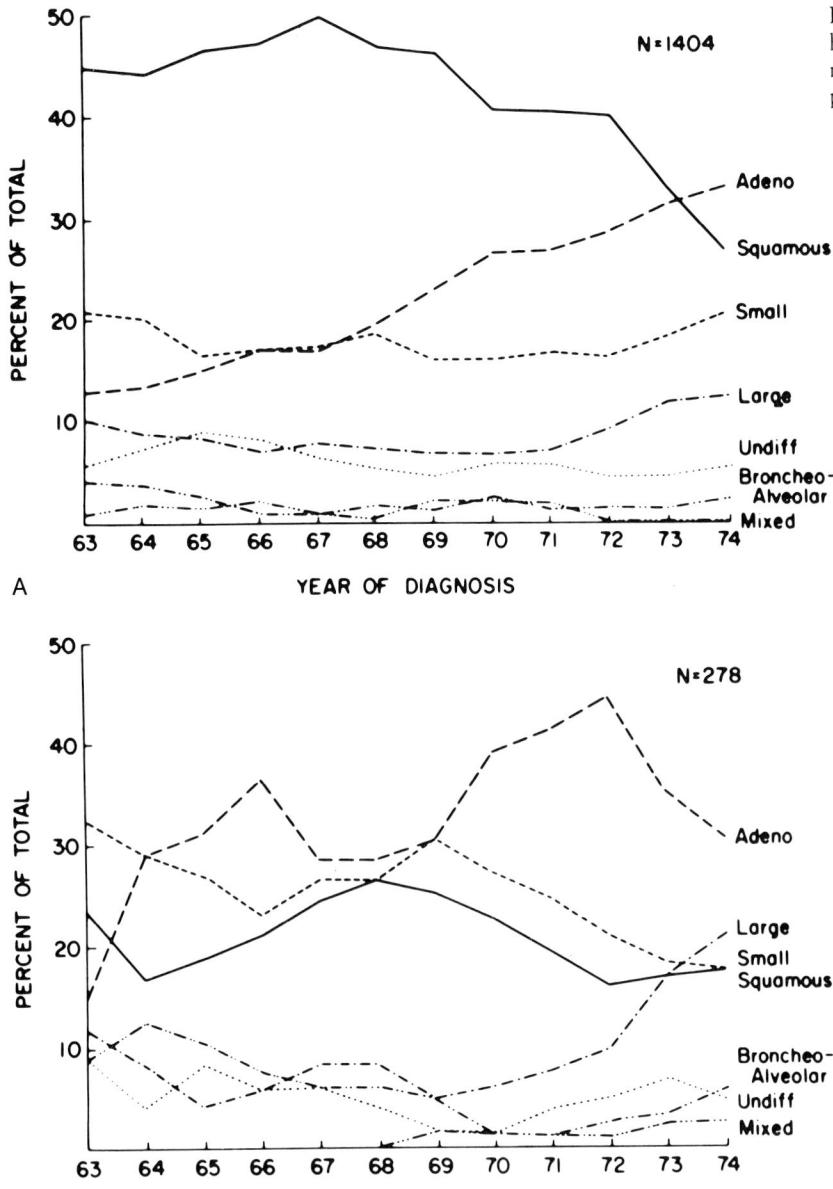

Figure 19–5. Changing incidence of different histologic types of bronchogenic carcinoma in males (A) and females (B). Reproduced with permission from Vincent et al.[97]

mas (see Table 19–12), when some of these series are broken down by date of accession, a distinct decrease in the number of squamous carcinomas and an increase in the number of adenocarcinomas is observed.[96,97] Cox and Yesner[96] compared 617 patients autopsied between 1958 and 1967 to 400 patients autopsied from 1968 to 1977; the percentage of squamous carcinomas dropped from 34.5 to 30.8, while the adenocarcinomas rose from 25.6 to 32.3. Similarly, in a series of patients from the Roswell Park Memorial Institute, squamous carcinomas constituted 48.6 percent of the total in 1962 but only 25.5 percent in 1975, while adenocarcinomas rose from 17.6 to 29.8 percent over that period[97] (Figure 19–5).

It is apparent that adenocarcinoma is becoming the most frequent histologic type. Possible reasons for this trend have been considered by Vincent and co-workers[97]. They were unable to find consistent errors in histologic diagnosis that would artifactually produce such a change. The data could neither be accounted for by the increased numbers of women with lung cancer, as shown in Figure 19–5; nor apparently by smoking. The data suggest that occupational factors may be involved, however, as shown in Table 19–7, adenocarcinoma is not specifically increased with any of the usual occupational carcinogens. The possibility that such changes reflect use of filter cigarettes should be considered, since, as discussed below in Incidence by Sex and Smoking, there seems to be some association between amount of cigarette smoking and the development of squamous and small-cell carcinomas.

Incidence by Sex and Smoking

The frequencies of the various histologic subtypes of lung cancer are related both to sex and to smoking. Although all histologic types may be found in women, there is a definite predominance of adenocarcinomas both in smokers and nonsmokers and this predominance has not changed with time[97] (see Figure 19–5). In women who do not smoke, adenocarcinomas usually account for more than 75 percent of tumors, whereas they account for 30 to 40 percent in those who do smoke.[97,102] In male nonsmokers there is also a preponderance of adenocarcinomas, although not to the degree found in women.

Although the overall association of smoking with lung cancer is not disputed, there is some disagreement about the association with specific cell types. Kreyberg[103] originally proposed that squamous and small-cell tumors were related to smoking, while adenocarcinomas were not. Such a theory is hard to reconcile with the obvious increasing incidence of adenocarcinoma in smokers and the relatively small absolute number of adenocarcinomas seen in nonsmokers. Whether there is a dose-response relationship between number of cigarettes smoked and type of carcinoma is unclear. Weiss and colleagues[104], in a study of 6136 men, showed a distinct dose-relationship type of response for squamous carcinoma, and equivocal results for small-cell carcinoma and adenocarcinomas. Auerbach and associates[95] claimed that small-cell carcinomas increased with cigarette consumption, but that the other types did not. Both these studies agree that adenocarcinomas are definitely associated with cigarette smoking. At present, it appears safe to say that all of the common histologic types of lung cancer are related to cigarette smoking, although there may be variations in the strength of the relationship.

Pathologic Features of Specific Tumor Types

Squamous or Epidermoid Carcinomas

Strictly speaking, the term "squamous" carcinoma should refer to any tumor composed of flattened cells.[49,105] The proper term for the type of tumor described here is "epidermoid," indicating that it mimics the differentiation of epidermis. However, the use of squamous carcinoma is so widespread that there seems little point in attempting to change terminology.

The WHO[86] histologic requirements for the diagnosis of squamous carcinoma include: (1) formation of keratin and/or (2) formation of intercellular bridges (prickles). Squamous carcinomas are commonly divided into subgroups of well, moderately, and poorly differentiated. The separation points for these subcategories are nebulous: in general, tumors that form large amounts of keratin or have many cells with intercellular bridges are called well or moderately differentiated, but some authors include in the poorly differentiated group tumors that do not form keratin or bridges, but merely show some stratification.[98] Nonetheless, the subtype breakdown for resection specimens from several different series is quite similar, as shown in Table 19–14. This type of separation is useful clinically, since it correlates well with prognosis (see p. 358).

Table 9–14. Breakdown of Squamous Carcinomas into Well, Moderately, and Poorly Differentiated Types in Various Reported Series

	Hinson et al.[94]	Rilke et al.[93]	Reinila and Dammert[106]	Matthews and Gordon[98]
Total no. patients	525	109	95	244
Well differentiated	19.4%	30.3%	71.6%	14%
Mod. differentiated	44.8%	36.6%	Included above	53%
Poorly differentiated	35.8%	33.0%	28.4%	33%

The majority of squamous cell carcinomas arise in the central portions of the lung, commonly in association with the main, segmental, or subsegmental bronchi[107,108] (Figure 19–6A to C). However, about one-third of squamous cell carcinomas arise in the periphery of the lung,[1] commonly in association with focal scars or with more diffuse honeycombing. Like the other forms of bronchogenic carcinoma, squamous carcinoma is more common in the upper than the lower lobes. Squamous carcinomas have been reported arising in walls of bronchiectatic cavities and in sequestra. These tumors may be variably necrotic or cystic; this is particularly true of so-called Pancoast's tumors arising in the apex of the lung (Figure 19–7).[109]

Within the bronchi, squamous carcinomas appear as heaped-up intraluminal growths. In most resection specimens obvious invasion out of the bronchial wall is present. Compared to adenocarcinomas, squamous cell carcinomas feel either smooth or gritty, rather than mucoid. Squamous carcinomas appear to grow along the bronchial tree in a proximal direction, often reaching hilar lymph nodes by direct extension.

The well-differentiated squamous carcinomas resemble those seen elsewhere: the tumor cells are generally arranged in nests which are composed of cells stratified into epithelium-like structures, with evidence of maturation to an eosinophilic keratin-producing cell (see Figure 19–6D). Masses of acellular keratotic debris may form necrotic-appearing centers of the nests or of larger cavitary lesions. The moderately and poorly differentiated tumors generally show no or very focal keratin production, the latter sometimes in the form of squamous pearls. Poorly differentiated tumors tend to be quite anaplastic and often lose the nesting arrangement, forming instead large sheets of cells (Figure 19–6F,G). Such tumors are frequently quite difficult to separate from large cell carcinomas, and many slides may have to be searched to find an acceptable area of squamous differentiation. The process is sometimes made easier by use of plastic-embedded 1-μM-thick sections; either because of superior resolution, differences in refractive index, or

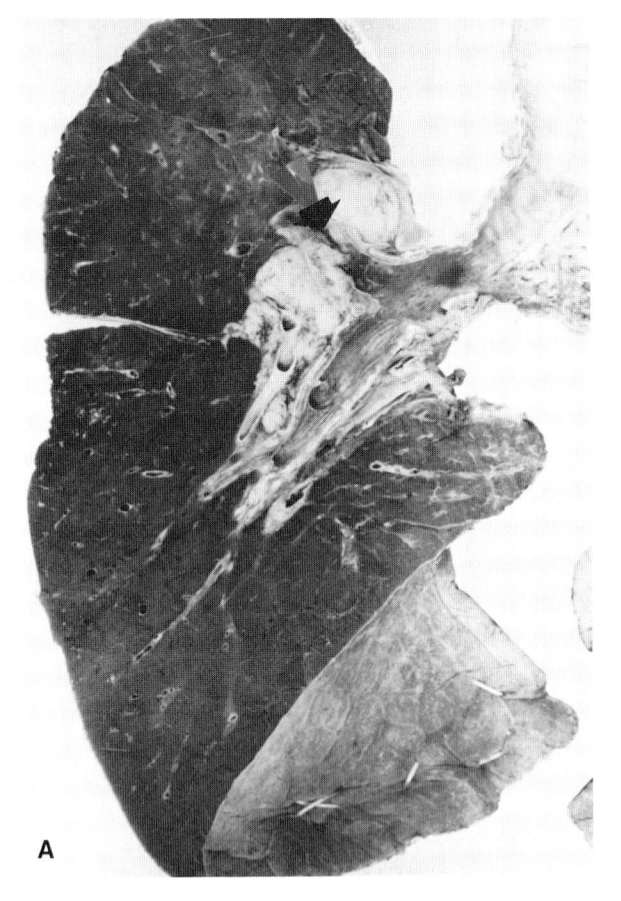

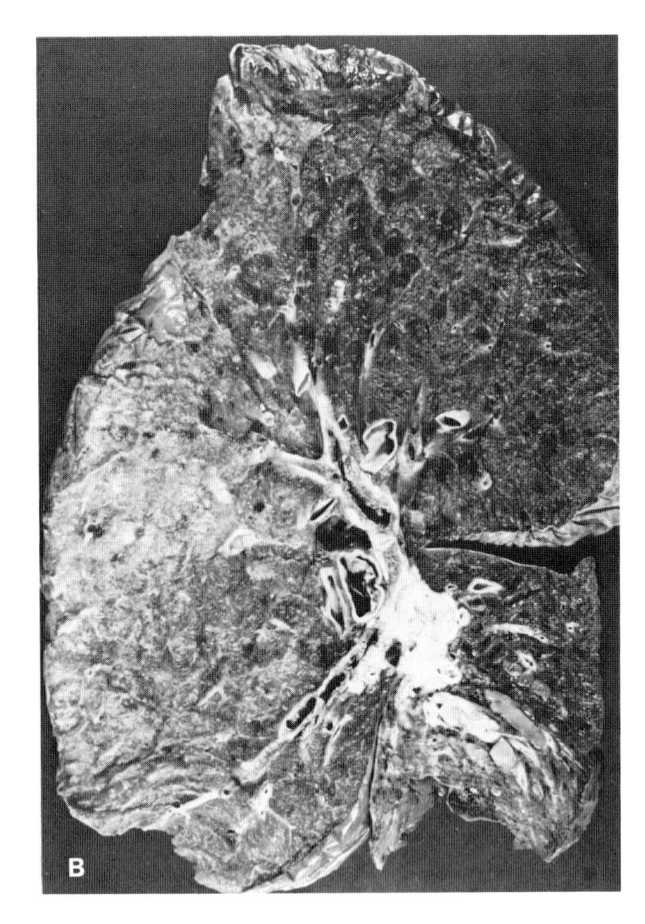

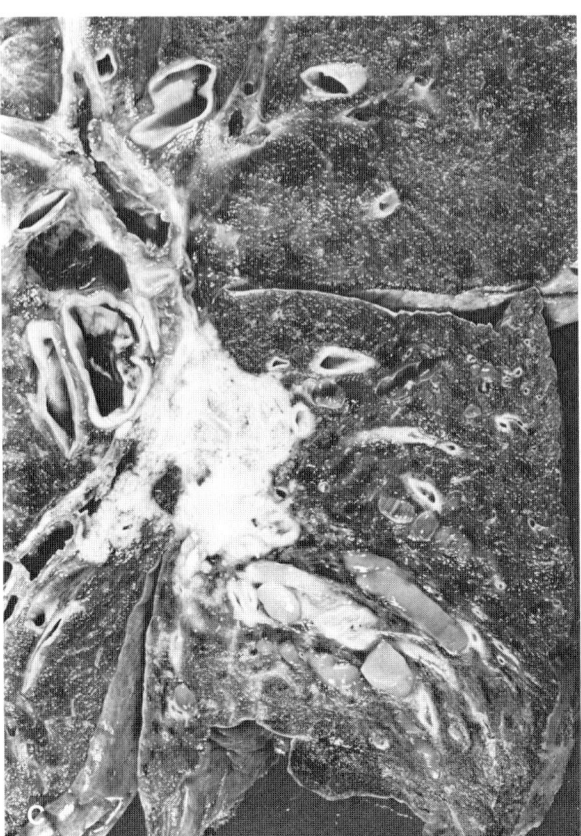

Figure 19–6A–C. Squamous carcinoma. A. Gross appearance of a central tumor arising in the main upper lobe bronchus (arrow). The tumor has already spread to hilar lymph nodes. B and C. Squamous carcinoma arising in the lower lobe bronchus. The lower lobe is partially collapsed and purulent bronchiectasis is present behind the tumor.

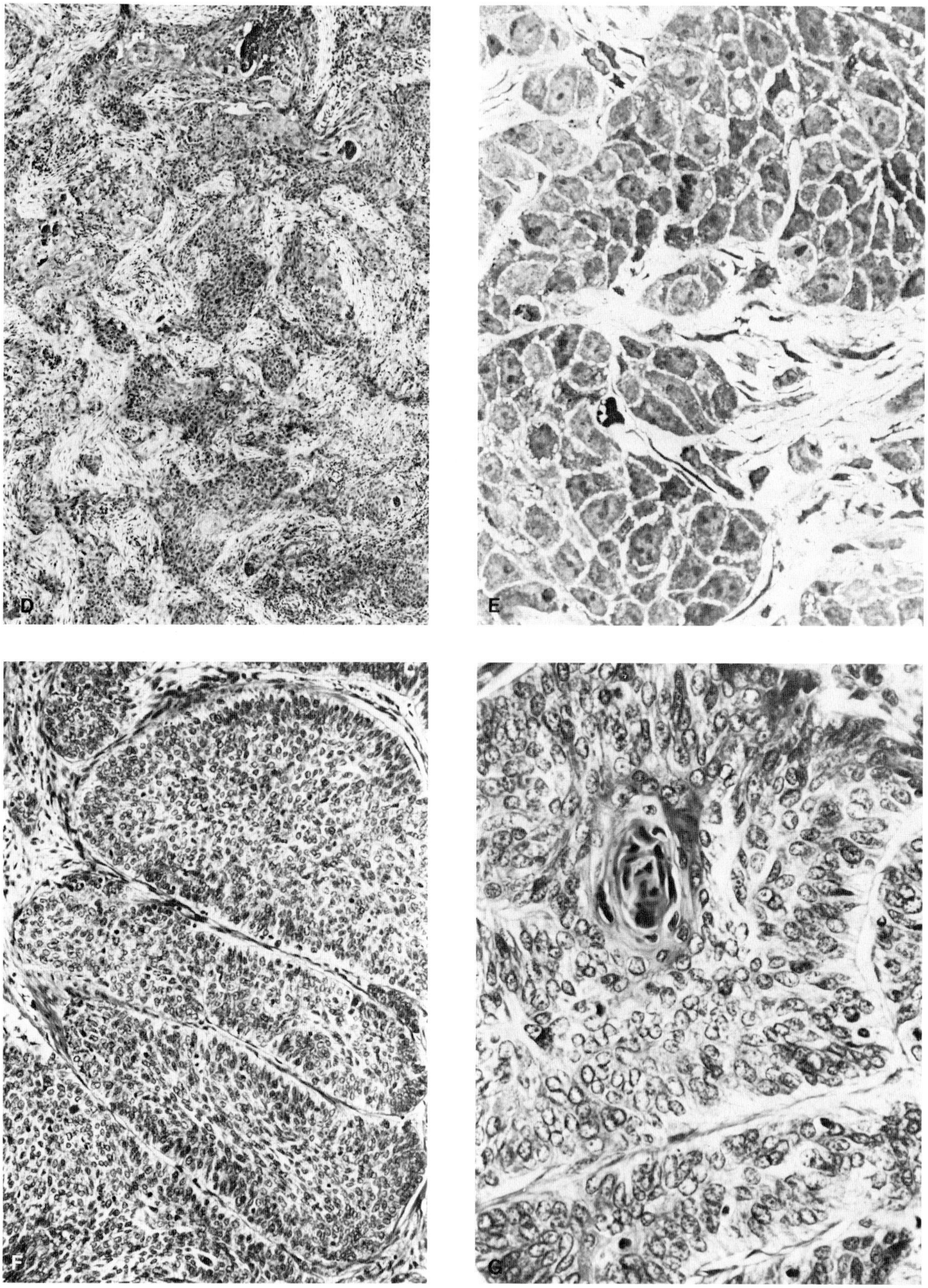
D
E
F
G

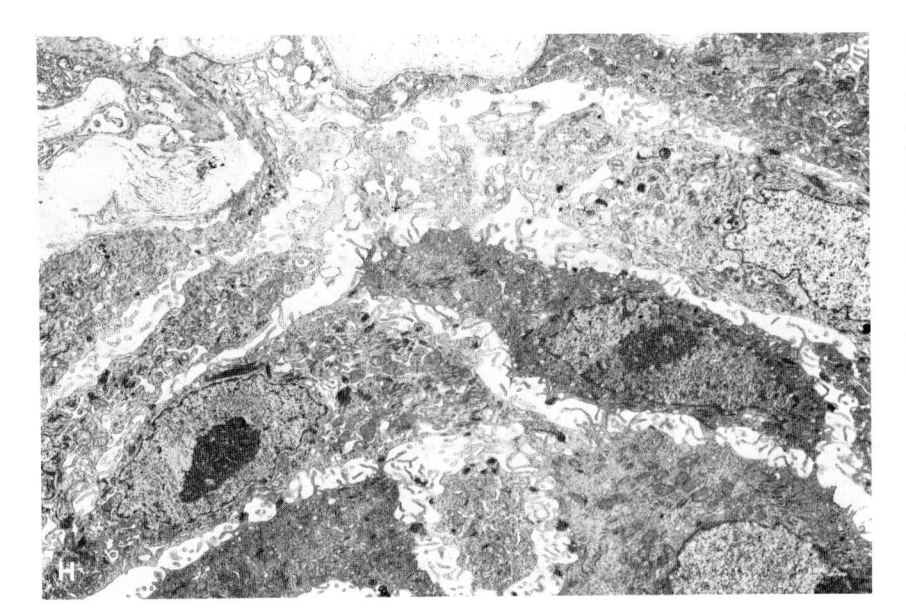

Figure 19–6H,I. Electron micrographs of squamous carcinoma. H. A well-differentiated squamous carcinoma at low power. I. A poorly differentiated squamous carcinoma at low power. Note that despite the light microscopic differences, both tumors show the defining ultrastructural features of numerous well-formed desmosomes and intercellular bridges (long arrows), as well as the formation of so-called interfacial canals (short arrows), spaces that mimic lumina. These spaces are not, however, bounded by tight junctions but by well-formed desmosomes.

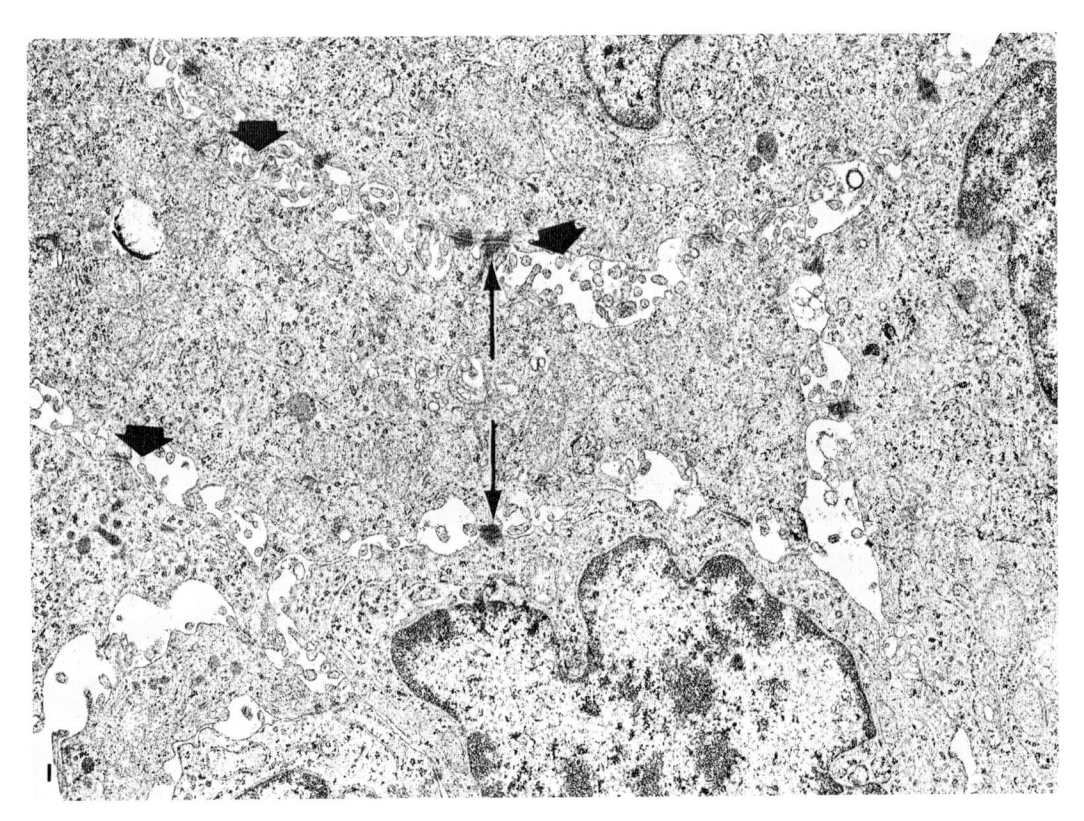

Figure 19–6D–G. D and E. Moderately well-differentiated squamous carcinoma showing the diagnostic features of keratinization and formation of intercellular bridges or prickles (D ×64, E ×400). F and G, Poorly differentiated squamous carcinoma. The bulk of the tumor appears similar to F, but rare foci of keratinization are present (G). Although some pathologists would classify this as a squamous carcinoma simply on the appearances in Field F, strictly speaking one needs to find either intercellular bridges or evidence of keratinization such as is shown in G (F ×160, G ×400).

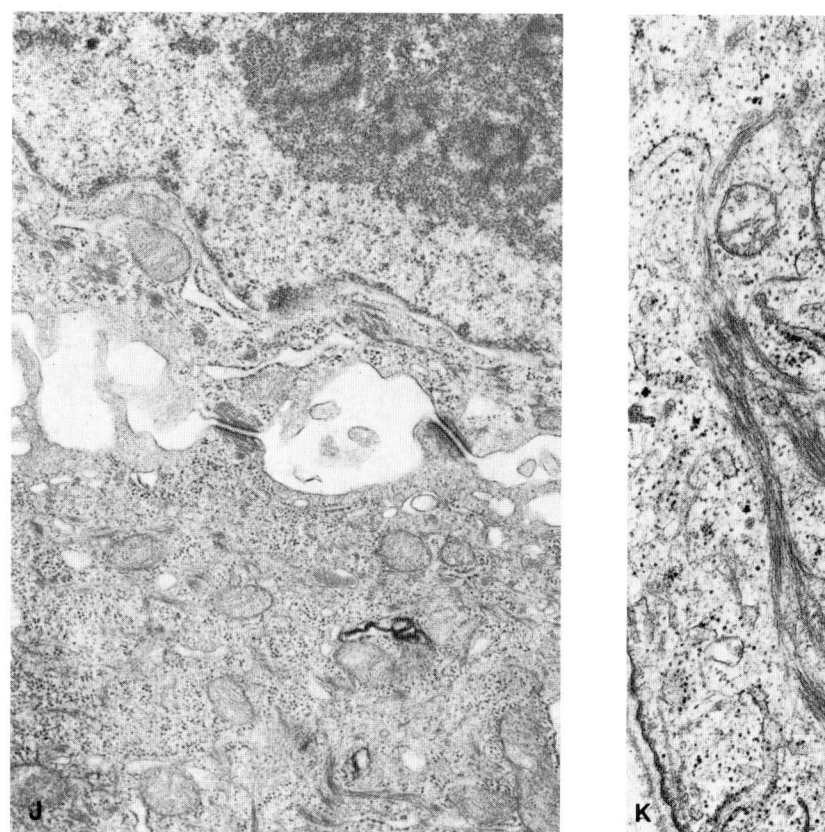

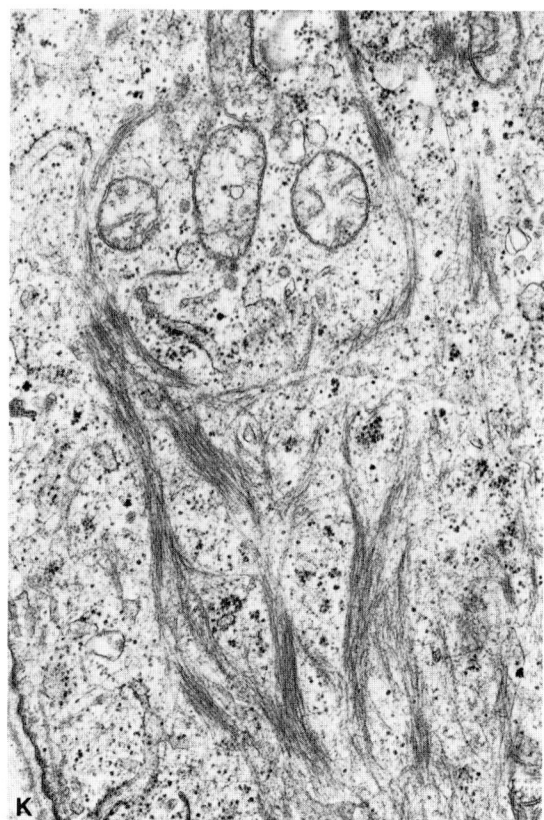

Figure 19–6J,K. The outpouchings of cytoplasm connected by desmosomes as shown in J constitute the intercellular bridges. K. Numerous tonofilament bundles, another characteristic ultrastructural feature of squamous carcinoma (H ×2000, I ×10,000). Reproduced with permission from Churg.[111]

differences in tissue shrinkage, intercellular bridges may be quite obvious in such preparations when they are completely inapparent in 5-μM-thick paraffin sections (Figure 19–6E).

A number of unusual variants of squamous cell carcinoma have been defined. Papillary forms are usually classified under the heading "papillary tumors of the surface epithelium"; WHO class VIII.[86] These tumors are probably smoking associated, but have a considerably different prognosis. They are therefore considered separately on p. 360. The so-called transitional cell type of squamous tumor forms stratified nests resembling the pattern of transitional cell carcinoma of the bladder.[86] These tumors may show no or only very scattered areas of squamous differentiation. Their behavior appears to be similar to other poorly differentiated squamous carcinomas. The same is true of "basal-celled carcinoma" of the bronchus.[1] These tumors resemble keratotic basal cell carcinomas of the skin, but behave with the agressiveness of the usual squamous carcinoma of the lung. Lastly, mention must be made of giant cell change in squamous carcinomas that have been irradiated. This phenomenon is commonly encountered in Pancoast's tumors that are radiated and then resected.[1,109] (Figure 19–7D). A similar change occurs in adenocarcinomas. In my experience, it is usually possible to find areas without giant cell change in these tumors; except for their location, they are in no way different from ordinary squamous carcinomas (or adenocarcinomas) of the lung and should not be called "giant cell" carcinomas.

Special stains are generally of little help in squamous carcinomas. Although some authors[86,110] employ histochemical stains for keratin, I have found these unreliable and difficult to interpret. Immunohistochemical stains for keratin should, in theory, stain all epithelial tumors, and are at present of little use in this context. Stains for mucin should be negative in squamous carcinoma; however, if one stains many (10 to 20) sections of an otherwise ordinary squamous carcinoma, rare droplets of mucin may occasionally be observed within the cytoplasm of tumor cells. Whether these droplets represent phagocytized material or true focal differentiation toward mucin production is unclear. I prefer not to use the term adenosquamous carcinomas for such tumors, reserving it for tumors in which biphasic differentiation is unequivocal in hematoxylin and eosin (H&E)–stained slides (*see*

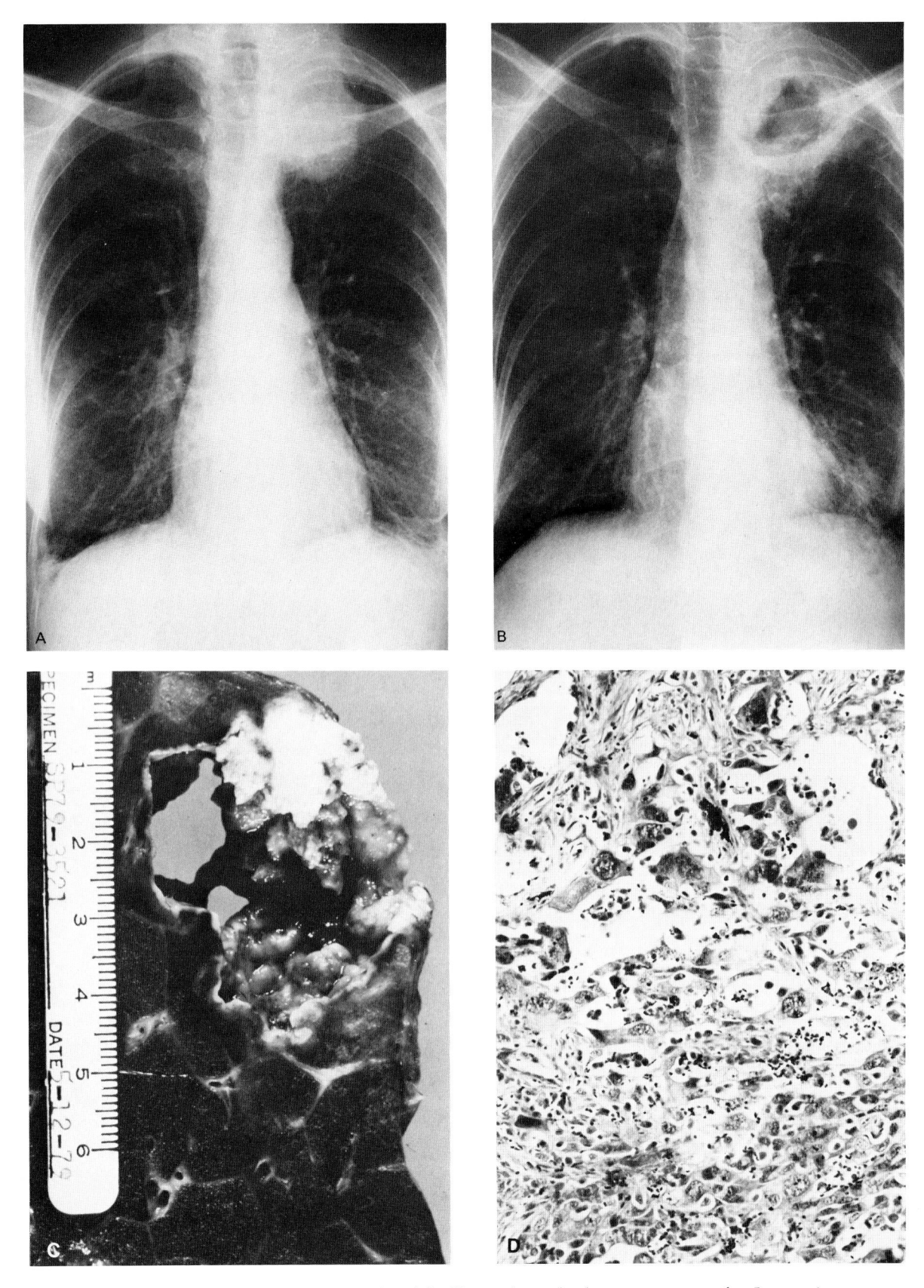

Figure 19–7. Pancoast's tumor. A and B. Chest radiographs showing a patient wih a Pancoast's tumor before and after radiation. C. Gross appearance of the same tumor. The center of the tumor mass has become completely necrotic and has liquified and disappeared. D. Radiation change in the same tumor. The peculiar giant cells produced by radiation mimic the appearance of so-called giant cell tumor of the lung but are a common finding in any radiated adenocarcinoma or squamous carcinoma ($\times 400$).

McDowell and colleagues[49] and p. 331 for discussion of this point). The ordinary adenocarcinoma, by contrast, contains easily demonstrable mucin.

The ultrastructure of squamous carcinoma of the lung resembles that of squamous carcinoma in other organs.[105,111–114] Well-differentiated tumors show abundant intracellular keratin. Most tumors, however, demonstrate only the presence of numerous desmosomes and intracytoplasmic tonofilament bundles (see Figure 19–6H to K). The intercellular bridge, an outpouching of cytoplasm from two adjacent cells connected by a well-formed desmosome, is commonly found in even poorly differentiated squamous carcinomas, and is a helpful diagnostic feature. The separation of squamous from adenocarcinoma by the presence of desmosomes is not absolute, since these structures are seen in both types[114]; however, in squamous carcinomas they are larger and more numerous. Care should be taken not to overdiagnose intercellular lumina by electron microscopy. True lumens must be bounded by tight junctions; the mere presence of microvilli between cells is not diagnostic of either tumor type, and in fact circular structures lined by microvilli (so-called interfacial canals) are commonly found between squamous cells of both normal and neoplastic epithelium (see Table 19–17 and Figure 19–6).

Small-Cell Squamous Carcinoma

Most squamous carcinomas are composed of relatively large cells; such tumors merge, at the poorly differentiated end of the scale, into large-cell undifferentiated carcinomas. There is, however, a group of squamous tumors composed of relatively small cells; it appears that such tumors are always very poorly differentiated, and can be difficult to distinguish from small-cell anaplastic carcinomas[86] (Figure 19–8A to C). A series of such tumors has been described by Churg and co-workers[101] and I have since observed several additional cases (Churg, unpublished data). Out of the five cases originally described, two were believed to be small-cell anaplastic carcinomas on the basis of cytology and five on the basis of light microscopy. However, electron microscopy demonstrated that four tumors had no cells containing neurosecretory granules but many cells connected by well-formed desmosomes, and sometimes containing tonofilament bundles, all features of squamous carcinoma (Figure 19–8D, E). A fifth tumor was composed of a mixture of squamous cells and cells containing neurosecretory granules. The importance of these tumors lies in the fact that they probably behave more like squamous than small-cell carcinomas.[101]

Immunohistochemical Findings. When this chapter was first compiled in late 1980, immunohistochemical staining of paraffin-embedded material was, so to speak, in its infancy. At the time of writing (early 1984), the infant has reached the adolescent stage and is getting larger every day, but is also experiencing a variety of growing pains. Different reports of immunohistochemical staining for the same antigen have used different antisera with (apparently) different staining properties, and in many cases these antisera are home-grown and available to only a few investigators. Additionally, variations in fixation, processing, and staining techniques can give drastically different results, even using the same antisera. Many of the published observations are undoubtedly scientifically valid, but their diagnostic applicability at this point is often problematic. In the area of diagnosis, the comments below and in other parts of this chapter must be interpreted with great caution.

Keratin is the intermediate filament considered to be the archetype of epithelial cells. Nonetheless, the demonstration of keratin in human lung cancers has been inconsistent, and depends on the antibody used and whether tissue is embedded or frozen. Said and colleagues[114A] claim that only squamous carcinomas stain with antibody to stratum corneum keratin; however, their antibody appears to have a peculiar specificity and others have found that most types of bronchogenic carcinoma, including small-cell carcinoma, do stain for keratin.[114B–114D] Use of antibodies to Mallory body–type keratin increases the number of tumors that stain, and is potentially valuable for poorly differentiated lesions.[114E] It has been suggested that squamous and adenocarcinomas may produce keratins of different molecular weight: Said and co-workers[114F] suggest that only squamous carcinomas produce 63-kilodalton keratin, whereas Banks-Schlegel and colleagues[114G] have found a 44-kilodalton keratin which appears to be confined to squamous carcinomas. At this point the most general use for keratin immunostaining is probably to determine that a poorly differentiated malignant neoplasm is indeed a carcinoma, rather than a lymphoma or mesenchymal tumor[114B,114E]; an example is the separation of a spindled lung carcinoma from a sarcoma. However, it should be borne in mind that nonepithelial neoplasms such as mesotheliomas and synovial sarcomas also stain for keratin.

It has been suggested that keratin staining (positive in mesotheliomas, negative in adenocarcinomas) may be useful in separating these two types of tumor[114H]; however, subsequent investigations[114I,114J] have failed to confirm this idea.

Carcinoembryonic antigen (CEA) is the other antigen that has been repeatedly examined in lung carcinomas. Carcinoembryonic antigen appears to be present in many bronchogenic carcinomas; its major use is probably in separating mesotheliomas, which are weakly reactive or nonreactive for this antigen, from carcinomas[114H–114J] (see Holden and Churg[114I] for a tabulation of other studies).

Small-Cell Carcinomas

Histogenesis. The cell of origin and exact site of origin of small-cell carcinoma has been and remains controversial. It was initially believed that small-cell carcinomas were actually sarcomas arising in the mediastinum until Barnard[115] pointed out their epithelial origin from lung. Despite recognition of their distinctive behavioral pattern, these tumors were frequently regarded as variants of adenocarcinoma because of their tendency to form rosettes and similar structures (reviewed in detail in

Azzopardi[116]). The work of Azzopardi[116] in particular helped to establish oat cell carcinoma as a separate histologic subclass and they were formally incorporated into the WHO scheme as small-cell carcinomas; the suggested subtypes are shown in Table 19–10 and discussed below.

Bensch and colleagues[117] and Hattori and co-workers[118] were the first to report the presence of neurosecretory granules in small carcinomas; this finding followed the discovery by Bensch and colleagues[117] of the presence of such granules in carcinoids and certain cells, which they referred to as Kultschitzky (K) cells, of the bronchial and bronchiolar epithelium (reviewed in Bonikos and Bensch[119]). These authors believed that a continuous spectrum existed from the K cells to the carcinoid of variable malignancy to the oat cell carcinoma. Pearse[120] included the oat cell tumors as the most malignant type of what he termed the APUD system, a series of cells distributed throughout the body (previously described by Feyter[121] as the Hellenzellen or clear-cell system) and characterized by common biochemical properties, particularly the abilities to produce catecholamines and peptide hormones, as well as a supposed origin from the neural crest.

The evidence for the neural crest origin of many of the cells involved in the APUD system has been seriously questioned (see reports by Tischler[122] Sidhu,[123] and Gould and associates[123A,123B]. For example, formalin-induced fluorescence of catecholamines was suggested by Pearce[120] to be a feature of cells migrating from the neural crest, but recent observations indicate that in fact such fluorescence activity does not begin until the migrating cell has reached its destination, so that differentiation in situ rather than migration cannot be ruled out. More recently LeDourain and Teillet[124] grafted neural anlage from Japanese quails onto chick embryos; the quail cells are distinctive in chick tissue. Using this system, it appears that, although many of the supposed APUD cells including ganglia, adrenal medulla, thyroid C cells, and carotid body cells do indeed migrate from the neural crest, cells of the pancreas and gut, including cells of the bronchial mucosa, differentiate in situ. Tischler[122] suggests that such cells be regarded as "neuroendocrine programmed"; that is, although they do not originate in neural crest, in their fully differentiated form they share many biochemical and some structural features with true neural crest cells in other locations. This concept is supported by the finding of neurofilaments in small-cell carcinomas, but not in the other types,[125] as well as by the demonstration of neuron-specific enolase,[123A,123B,125A,126] bombesin,[127] serotonin,[123A,123B] and a variety of other "neuroendocrine" peptide hormones[123A] in small-cell carcinomas. However, small-cell carcinomas also express surface antigens associated with endodermally derived tumors, as noted previously,[53] and both neuroendocrine peptide hormones and occasionally even neurosecretory granules and catecholamines are produced by non-small-cell tumors.[54,114,123A,123B,128] It appears that the exact direction of differentiation of any given bronchogenic carcinoma is variable, and that mixtures of neuroendocrine and endodermal features may be present.

The types and numbers of granule-containing cells in normal lung and lung tumors have been matters of considerable dispute (see Gould and colleagues[123A,123B] for a review). It is clear that these cells exist in the airway epithelium in two forms: as solitary cells with clear cytoplasm, often referred to as K cells, and as clusters of similar cells; the latter have been named "neuroepithelial bodies" by Lauweryns and co-workers[131]. The neuroepithelial bodies have been shown to discharge their granule contents in response to hypoxia or hypercapnea, and are presumed to act as chemoreceptors[131]; the role of the K cells is less certain but they may be important in local functional modulation in the airway. Immunochemical examination shows that both the K cells and the neuroepithelial bodies can produce bombesin, serotonin, calcitonin, and neuron-specific enolase,[123A,123B,130] while the K cells also produce leu-enkephalin.

Ultrastructurally, Bensch and colleagues[117,119] claim that only one morphological type of neurosecretory granule is seen in these cells in the adult lung, but Hage[129] has reported finding at least three different types of granule-containing cells in the bronchial epithelium of human fetuses. Whether there are specific morphologic features that define the different hormone-producing cells is a problem that requires ultrastructural immunohistochemical examination. McDowell and associates[49] found bronchial epithelial cells containing dense core granules as well as mucin. This is an important observation, since it lends additional evidence to the notion that granule-containing cells differentiate in situ from the basal cells of the bronchial epithelium; sometimes such cells differentiate toward combined forms, and sometimes tumors composed of combined types (for example, small cell and squamous cell) are produced.

As mentioned above, the precursor lesion of small-cell carcinoma is unknown, and some small-cell carcinomas arise in a setting of squamous dysplasia. Gould and co-workers,[123A,123B] using immunohistochemical markers, have suggested that lungs containing both carcinoids and small-cell carcinomas show increased numbers of stainable K cells and neuroepithelial bodies, as well as what they called cytologically dysplastic foci of proliferating K cells. The latter can produce adrenocorticotropic hormone (ACTH), a substance Gould and associates regard as "ectopic" (that is, to the lung), and that may prove to be a marker of malignancy (see Carcinoid and Related Tumors, below).

Relation to Carcinoid Tumors. The relation of carcinoids and small-cell carcinomas, although occasionally disputed, has generally been accepted, largely because both tumors have the ability to produce neurosecretory granules, and both may produce peptide hormones and biogenic amines.[49,117,122,123A,123B,132] Histologically, both may also form rosettes and trabeculae, and, as described in Carcinoids and Related Tumors, below, a continuous spectrum of cytologically malignant forms from carcinoid to oat cell carcinoma can be found. There are differences between the two types of tumor: the granules in oat cell carcinoma are much smaller and sparser than in

Figure 19-8A-C. Small-cell squamous carcinoma. A. Chest radiograph showing a right lower lobe coin lesion found incidentally in an asymptomatic male smoker. B and C. Microscopic appearance of the lesion shown in A. By light microscopy this appears to be an ordinary small-cell carcinoma (B ×160, C ×400).

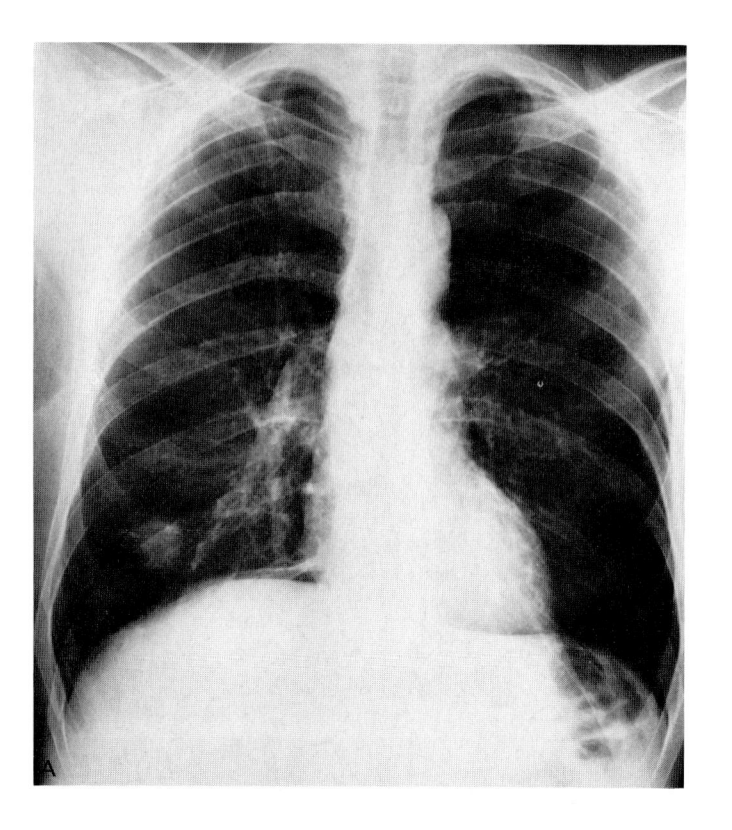

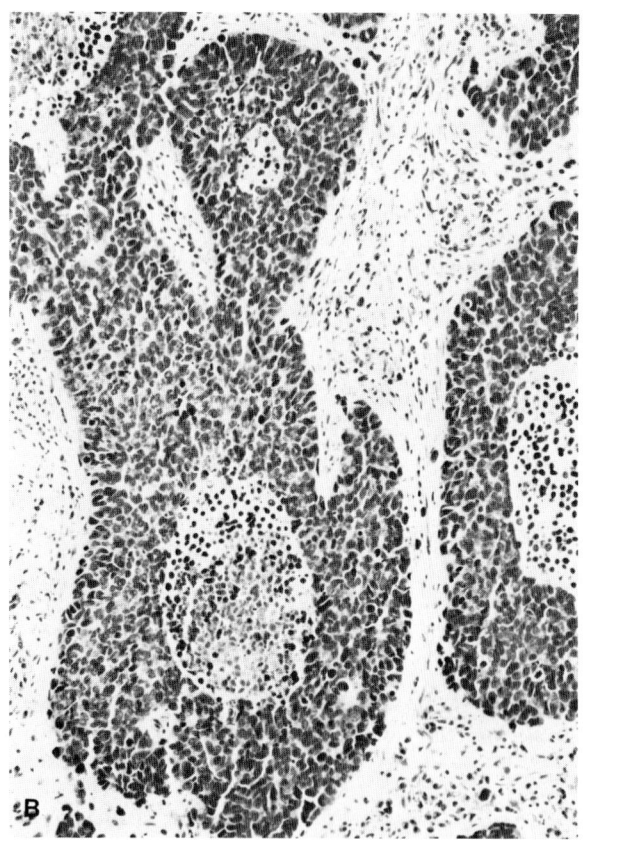

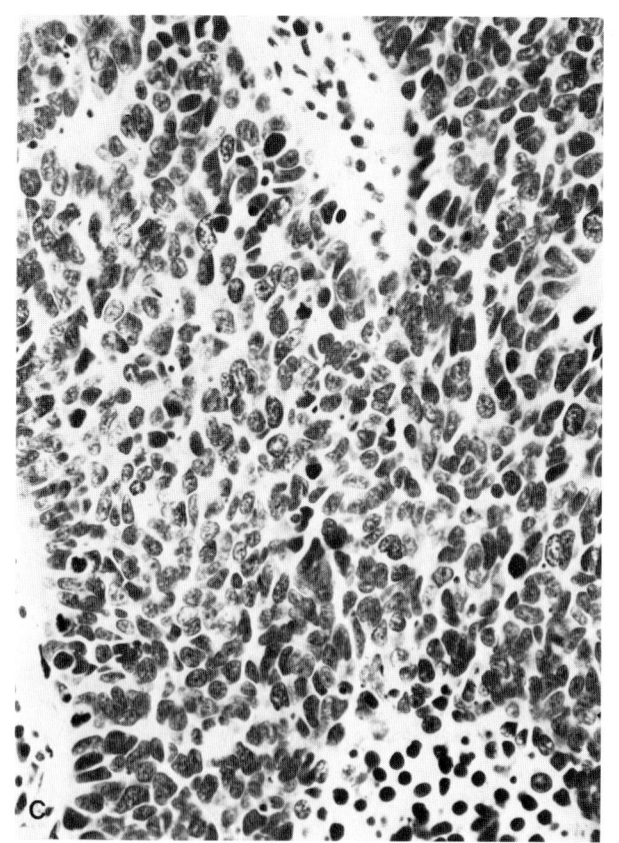

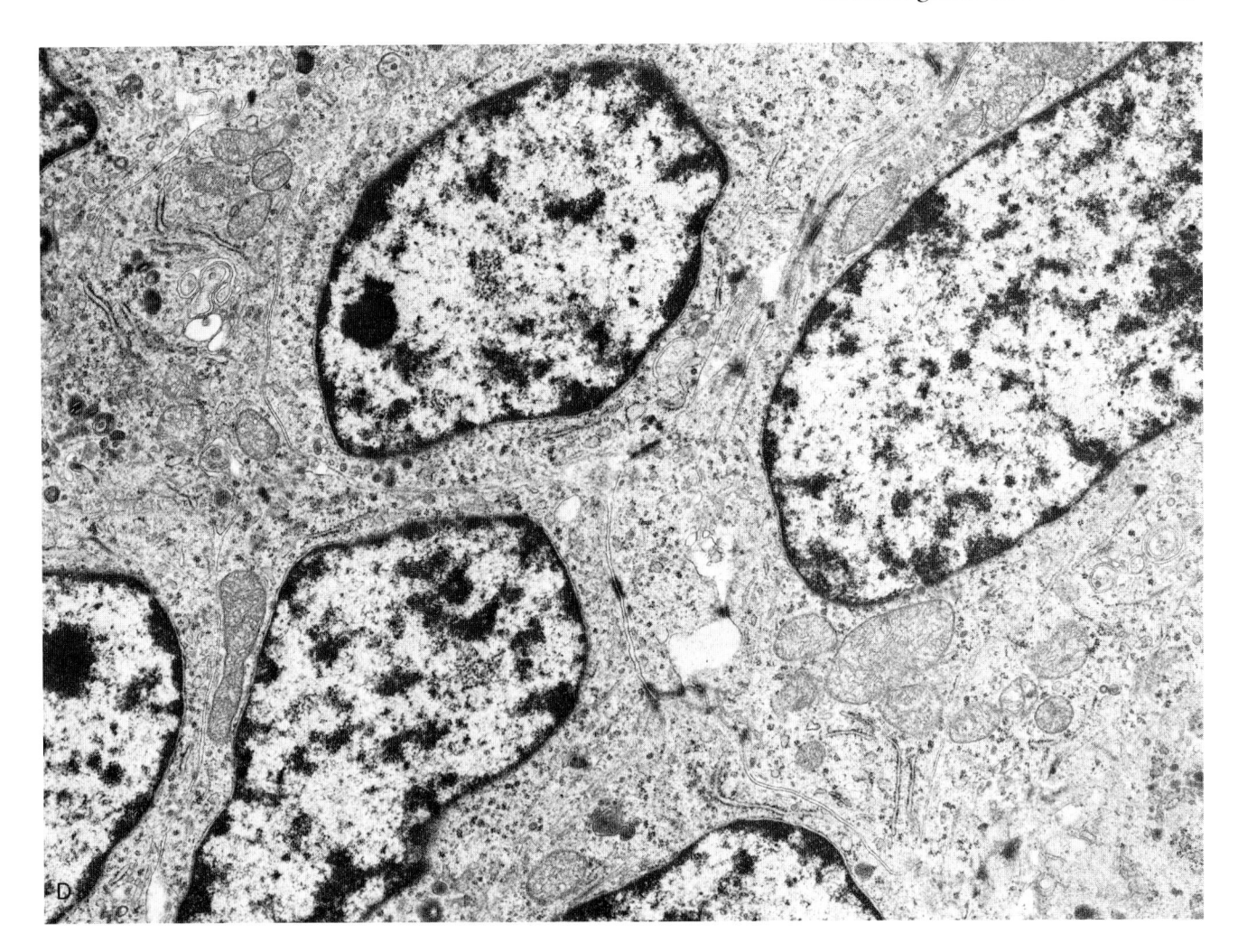

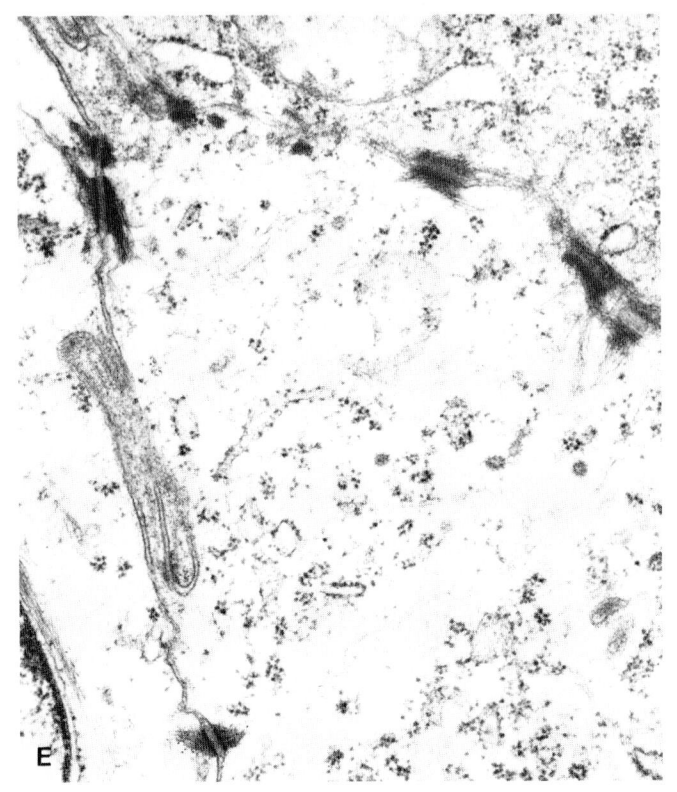

Figure 19–8D,E. Electron micrographs of the same tumor showing cells connected by numerous well-formed desmosomes but no neurosecretory granules. A diagnosis of small-cell squamous carcinoma was made. The patient survived for 2½ years with no further therapy before recurrence of the tumor at the resection margin (D ×6000, E ×16000. D and E from Churg et al.[101]).

334 Tumors of the Lung

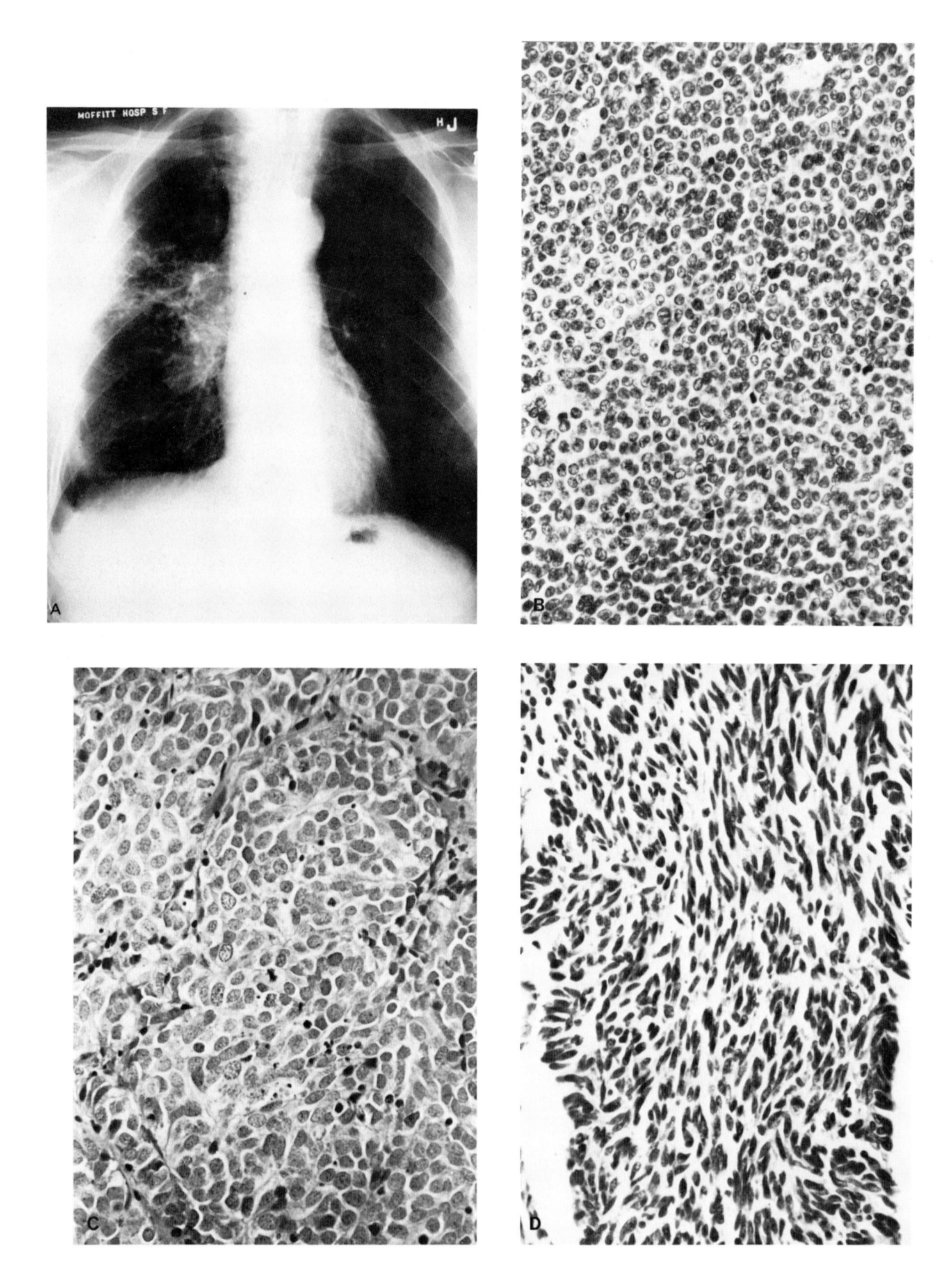

carcinoids; in my experience granule number decreases in direct proportion to increasing anaplasia of the tumor cells, and Gould and colleagues[123A,123B] have reached a similar conclusion. It is noteworthy that small-cell carcinoma is clearly related to smoking and occupational carcinogens, but carcinoids are not related to known carcinogens.[133]

However, this relationship is one of direction of differentiation, not one of direct lineage; that is, small-cell carcinomas do not arise from carcinoids, and it is likely that both types of tumor arise from undifferentiated cells of the bronchial epithelium, rather than from the granule-containing cells, since the latter appear to be differentiated nondividing cells.[123A,123B]

Pathologic Features. The vast majority of small-cell carcinomas are central tumors (Figure 19–9A) but peripheral lesions are occasionally observed.[134] Although they may form large intrabronchial masses, this event is infrequent and is usually only seen with very large bulky tumors at autopsy. More commonly the mucosa at the time of bronchoscopic exploration is smooth or only slightly elevated. Small-cell tumors typically grow around the bronchus of origin and thence to surrounding structures. Bronchoscopic biopsy may nonetheless be positive even in the face of an apparently normal mucosa; Kato and colleagues[135], obtained positive bronchial biopsies in 22 of 41 cases in which no gross lesion was visible.

Small-cell carcinomas show a variety of light microscopic cell types (Table 19–10). The most typical is the so-called "oat cell" or "lymphocyte-like" (Figure 19–9B) and the term oat cell carcinoma is frequently, albeit incorrectly, used for the entire group of tumors. The oat cell is typically about twice the size of a lymphocyte. The cytoplasm is scanty, and the nuclei hyperchromatic. In well-fixed preparations the chromatin is finely granular; poorly fixed or autopsy specimens may show intensely hyperchromatic nuclei without chromatin detail. Nuclear molding is common. The other forms of small-cell tumor are identified as fusiform or polygonal in the old WHO classification,[86] and intermediate cell type in the WPL[87] and new WHO[88] classification (Figure 19–9C, D). The fusiform cells tend to be spindled and the polygonal cells have somewhat larger nuclei and distinctly more cytoplasm than the oat cells. Giant cells may occasionally be formed.[136] The chromatin pattern of the individual cells is similar to that of well-fixed oat cell tumors; I believe that the finding of finely stippled chromatin (*see* Figure 19–9C) is a helpful feature in separating small-cell carcinomas from other carcinomas, all of which tend to have vesicular chromatin.

Transitions between the various histologic subtypes are not unusual and exact subclassification may be difficult. Table 19–15 illustrates the proportions of the various types found in several different series; it is evident that there is considerable variation from series to series. Hirsch and co-workers[137] showed that, while three experienced observers arrived at a unanimous diagnosis of small-cell carcinoma in 94 percent of a series of test cases, unanimity in regard to subclassification was achieved in only 38 percent of cases using the old WHO classification, and 54 percent of cases using the new classification. Vollmer[138] pointed out that, if one measures cell size, there is a continuous distribution from "small-cell" to "large-cell" carcinomas, and that the apparent cell size depends somewhat on the type of biopsy, suggesting that these rather fragile cells are subject to considerable handling artifact. I believe that if a firm diagnosis of small-cell carcinoma can be made, there is little to be gained from subclassification, but some authors claim there are prognostic differences associated with different histologic subtypes (*see* p. 358).

The histologic patterns of small-cell carcinoma are described in detail by Azzopardi[116] and are common to all the histologic subtypes. The tumor cells tend to form ribbons and rosettes (Figure 19–9E). Sometimes the latter resemble acini and occasionally contain mucus. The tumor cells themselves are fragile and smudge easily; however, care should be exercised in interpreting this phenomenon as specific since lymphocytes and other types of lung tumors may also show smudge artifact. Matthews and Gordon[98] require that well-preserved tumor cells be identified before a diagnosis of small-cell carcinoma is made. Mitoses are usually numerous, and extensive necrosis of tumor is the rule. A characteristic feature is the presence of a hematoxophylic staining of blood vessel walls; this is particularly common in areas of tumor necrosis (Figure 19–9F). Azzopardi[116] has shown that the hematoxophylic material is DNA which is apparently released in massive amounts from tumor cells. This phenomenon, although typical of small-cell carcinoma of the lung, should not be regarded as diagnostic, since it occasionally occurs in other rapidly proliferating and necrosing tumors.

The ultrastructural features of small cell carcinoma are also common to all the histologic subtypes (McDowell and colleagues[49], Mackay and associates[112]). The tumor cells are polygonal to elongated and generally contain relatively few organelles, primarily mitochondria and polyribosomes (Figure 19–9G). Frequently the cells possess thin cytoplasmic processes which extend for long distances and can be seen in thin sections interdigitating between tumor cells. The characteristic feature of small-

Figure 19–9A–D. Small-cell carcinoma. A. Chest radiograph of a patient with small-cell carcinoma showing enlargement of the right hilus and hilar lymph nodes and obstructive pneumonia in the right lung. B. Oat cell type of small-cell carcinoma. In this surgical specimen the chromatin does not have the hyperchromatic appearance frequently found in autopsy material (×400). C. Polygonal (intermediate) cell type of small-cell carcinoma. Note the more extensive cytoplasm than seen in the oat cell form and the finely stippled chromatin (×400). D. Fusiform (intermediate) cell type of small-cell carcinoma. In this autopsy specimen the chromatin is hyperchromatic (×400).

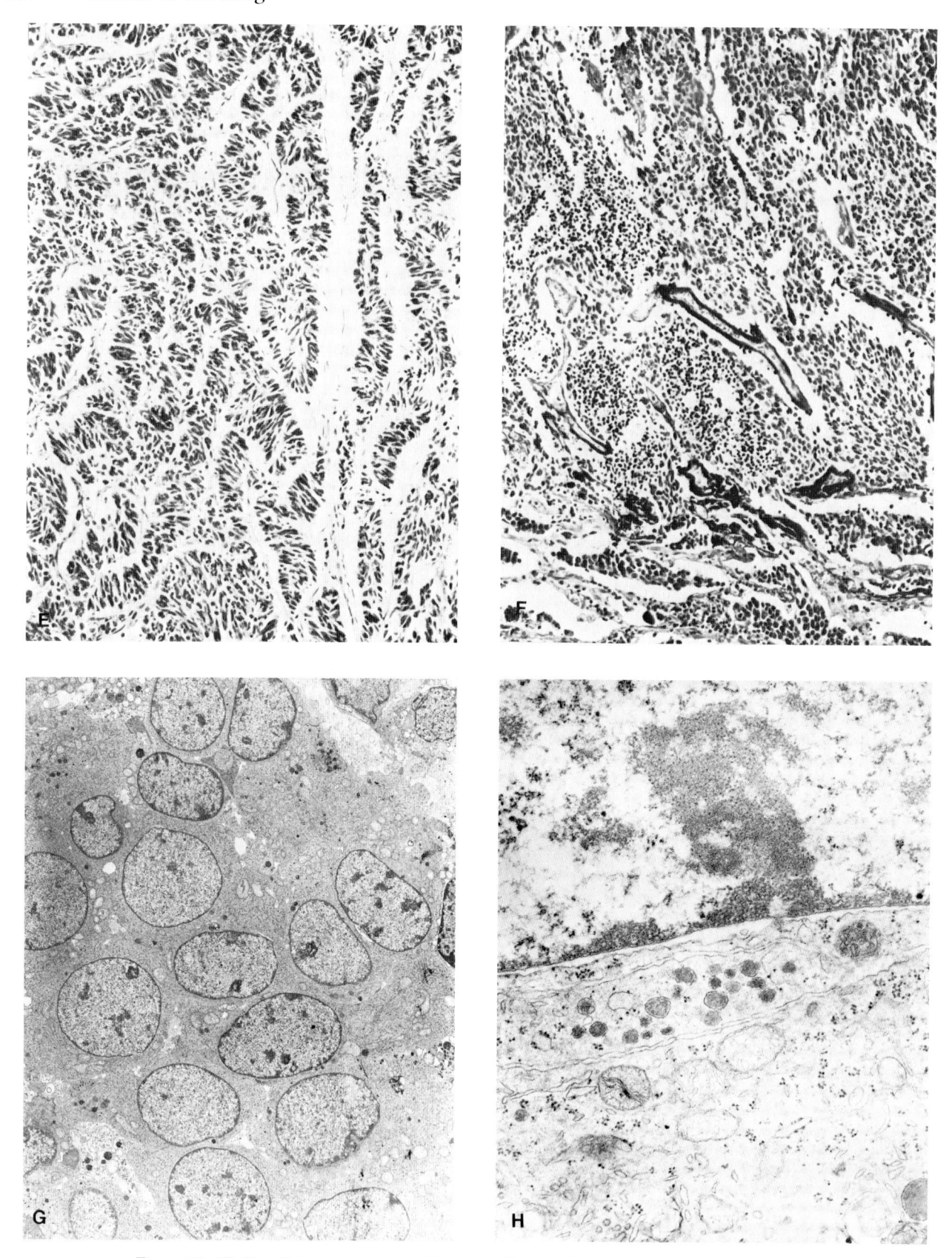

Figure 19–9E–H. E. Low-power view of the tumor illustrated in D, showing formation of ribbons and rosettes, a characteristic finding of small-cell carcinoma (×100). F. Low-power view of another field of the same tumor showing DNA staining of vessels (×64). G and H. Electron micrographs of small-cell carcinoma. G shows a low-power view of the polygonal tumor cells; H demonstrates characteristic neurosecretory granules in a longitudinal cell process (G ×2000, H ×22,000).

Table 9–15. Proportions of Subtypes of Small-Cell Carcinoma in Various Series

	Hinson et al.[94]	Carney et al.[139]	Davis et al.[140]	Burdon et al.[141]	Hirsch et al.[141]
Oat cell	16.2%	54%	73.1%	52.1%	53%
Fusiform cell[a]	45.3%	41%[a]	26.9%[a]	17.3%	47%[a]
Polygonal cells[a]	38.3%			30.4%	
Total cases	86	103	626	46	200

[a] These series use the new World Health Organization classification which combines the fusiform and polygonal cell types into the intermediate cell type.

cell carcinoma is the presence of neurosecretory granules (Figure 19–9H). As originally described by Bensch and colleagues[117] in 22 of 22 tumors and Hattori and colleagues[118] in 22 of 24 tumors, the granules vary from about 800 to 2000 A in diameter and when well preserved have a dense core and surrounding halo under the limiting membrane. Recent work by Hage and colleagues suggests that, like the K cells themselves and like carcinoid tumors, small-cell carcinomas may contain different types of granules, presumably producing different substances. The granules may be found in the main body of the cell, but tend to be particularly concentrated in the elongate processes, and cross-sections of such processes are valuable areas to examine to establish the diagnosis. Care should be taken not to overdiagnose neurosecretory granules, since primary lysosomes are frequently ultrastructurally very similar. I insist on finding clusters of granules within the cytoplasm; a solitary granule-like structure must be interpreted with great caution.

The cells of small-cell carcinomas are generally connected by scanty and poorly formed junctions; occasionally there are true desmosomes with clearly demarcated tonofilament bundles, but more commonly macula adherens or close junctions are observed. The presence of numerous well-formed desmosomes should lead to the suspicion that one is actually dealing with a small-cell squamous carcinoma, as described on p. 330. It should also be appreciated that granules are never numerous in small-cell carcinoma and in fact can be exceedingly difficult to identify[54,114]; Sidhu[114] was able to find granules in only 30 percent of tumors. My rule of thumb is that a tumor that appears to be a small-cell carcinoma but apparently contains neither granules nor well-formed junctions (or any other differentiating feature) is classified as a small-cell carcinoma.

The ability of small-cell carcinomas to produce immunochemically demonstrable neuron-specific enolase may prove to be of diagnostic value but all of the caveats previously raised concerning the state of the art of immunostaining need to be kept in mind here also. The few published reports on the topic suggest that a variable proportion of small-cell carcinomas will stain for neuron-specific enolase[123A,123B,125A,126]; in the series of Sheppard and colleagues,[125A] 18 of 31 small-cell carcinomas stained positively. Whether the negative tumors are really negative or are only poorly preserved is unclear, but the method of fixation definitely influences the frequency of positive results.[123A,123B] It is also unclear whether neuron-specific enolase is only found in small-cell carcinomas; Sheppard and colleagues[125A] were unable to demonstrate it in any of 30 squamous carcinomas, adenocarcinomas, and large-cell carcinomas, but Dhillon and colleagues[141B] did find staining in some non-small-cell tumors. This critical issue needs to be further examined before the specificity of this type of staining can be accepted, and it is also critical to whether the presence or absence of such staining can be related to clinical outcome.

Mixed Types of Small-Cell Carcinoma. In recent years the notion of small-cell carcinomas as a histogenetically separate group of tumors has been challenged by the light microscopic and ultrastructural findings of tumors of combined histologic type or of transition from one type to another (some examples are illustrated in Figure 19–10). Brereton and colleagues[100] reported 5 of 21 biopsy-proven small-cell carcinomas which at autopsy were mixtures of small-cell and squamous carcinoma. Matthews[142] found mixtures of histologic types at autopsy in 23 of 91 patients. In 18 patients there was a combination of small-cell carcinoma and another histologic type, and in 5 patients only a non-small-cell carcinoma was present. Abeloff and colleagues[99] reviewed 40 cases for which biopsy and autopsy material was available. In five patients, a completely different type of tumor was found at autopsy (squamous carcinoma, adenocarcinoma, or large-cell carcinoma) and in six cases a mixture of small-cell and other cell types was present (Table 19–16).

The presence of combined forms (small-cell carcinoma and squamous carcinoma) has been confirmed ultrastructurally by Mackay and co-workers,[112] Saba and associates,[143] and Sidhu.[114] Hashimoto and associates[144] report a case in which squamous carcinoma, adenocarcinoma, and small-cell carcinoma were all present. Additional cases in which the light microscopic appearance was homogeneous but different elements were present by electron microscopy have been reported by Churg and co-workers,[101] Saba and colleagues,[143] and Leong and Canny.[145]

It has been suggested that mixed types of tumors may in some instances arise consequent to chemotherapy and radiation therapy.[99,100,142] However, there is no doubt that some cases (for instance, case 5 of Churg and associates,[101] the case of Hashimoto and colleagues,[144] case 2 of Saba and colleagues,[143] and the case of Mackay and co-workers[112]) are mixed before any therapy is administered. As noted above, one conclusion that may be drawn from the existence of such mixed tumors is that small-cell

Figure 19–10A,B. Mixed types of small-cell carcinoma. A. Light micrograph of a mixed small-cell and squamous carcinoma (×160). B and C. Electron micrographs of a tumor that by light microscopy appeared to be an intermediate type of small-cell carcinoma. B shows a cell containing tonofilament bundles and joined to its neighbors by numerous desmosomes; this is consistent with squamous differentiation. (B ×8000).

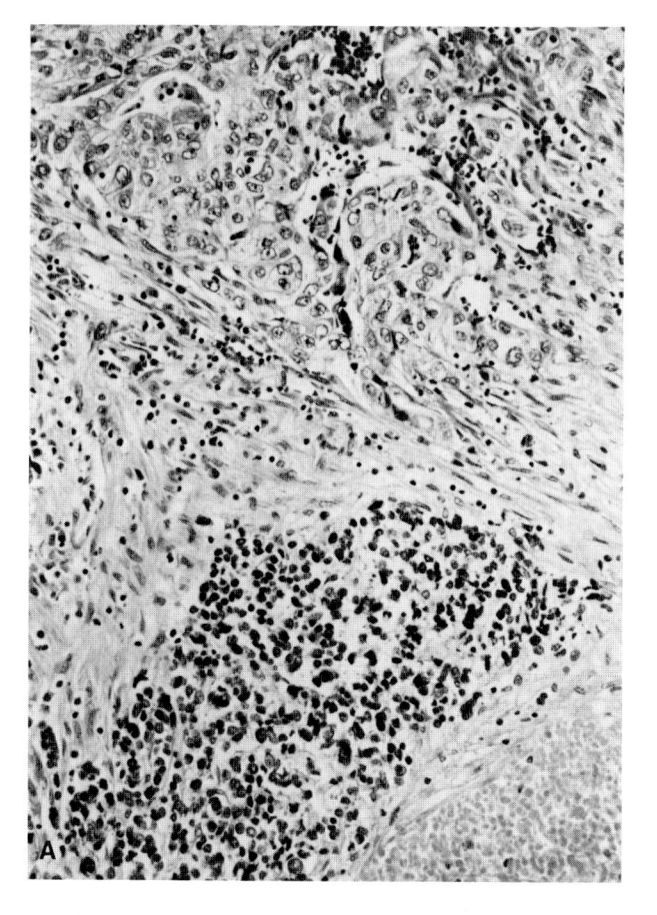

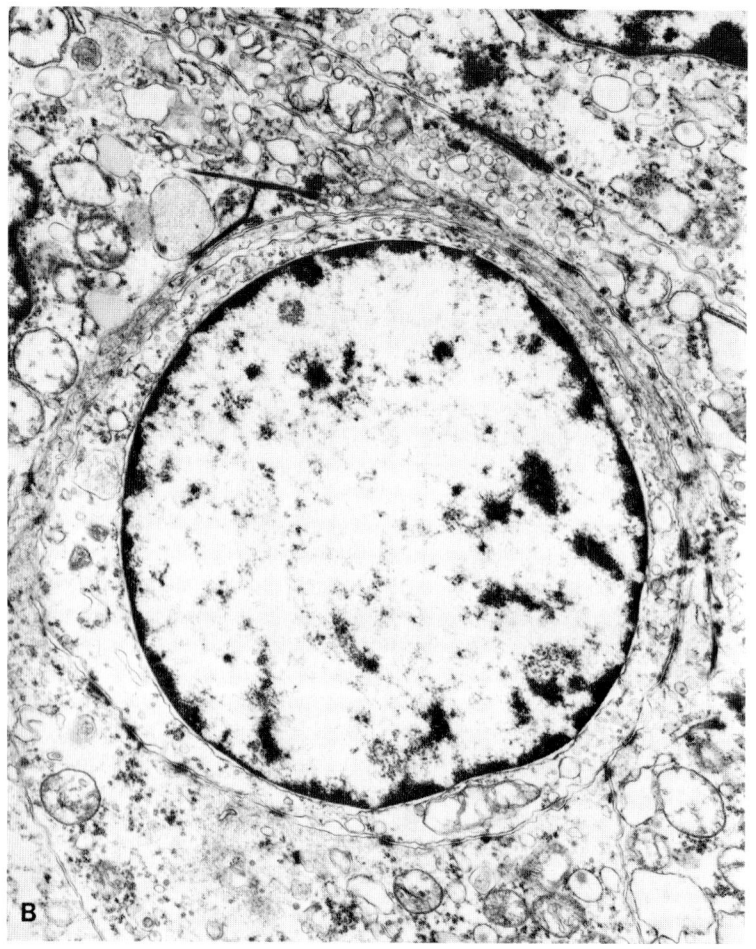

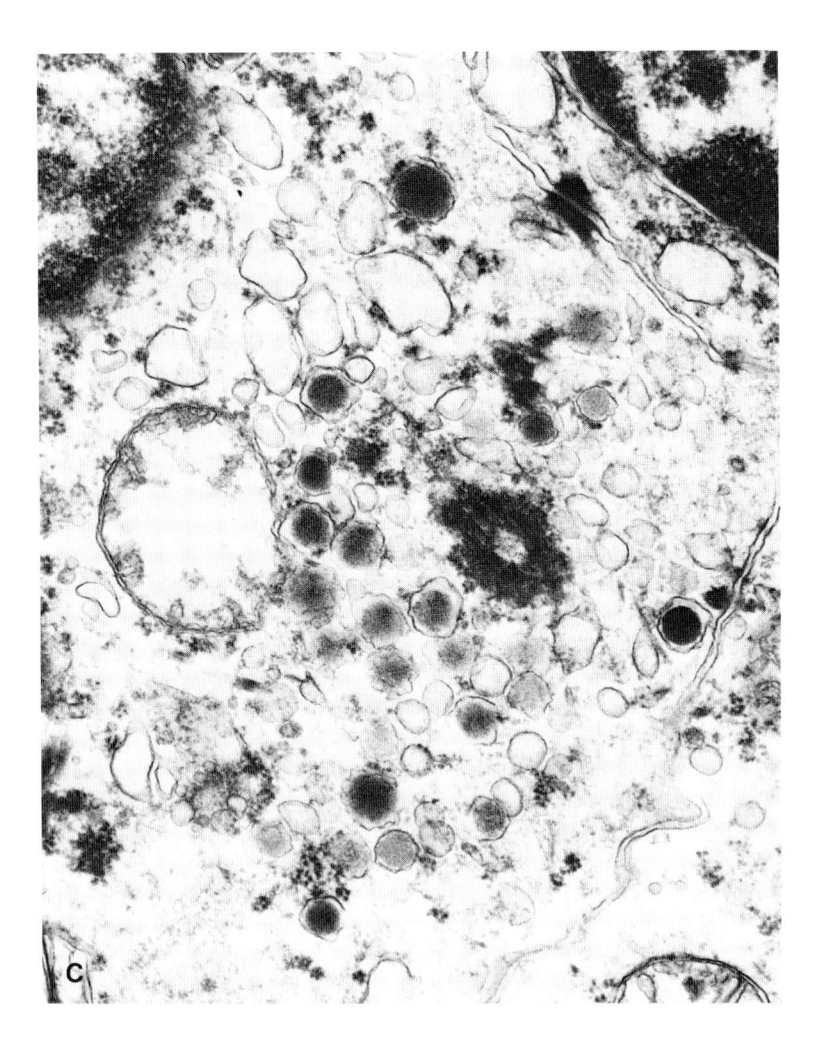

Figure 19–10C. Numerous neurosecretory granules in a nearby cell, an appearance consistent with small-cell carcinoma (C ×16,000). Reproduced by permission from Churg et al.[101]

carcinomas arise from bronchial cells which may differentiate toward any type of tumor, rather than from "neuroendocrine-committed" cells of the neural crest. There is also the suggestion[99] that tumors that are initially of mixed type may have a somewhat better prognosis than pure small-cell forms; however, Radice and coworkers[146] found that the mixed types of tumors had lower response rates to chemotherapy and shorter survivals.

Adenocarcinomas

Although some adenocarcinomas arise as central lesions that occlude bronchi, three-fourths are said to occur in the periphery of the lung[1] (Figure 19–11A). Whether this phenomenon will continue to be true with the increase in frequency of adenocarcinomas is unclear. Grossly, adenocarcinomas may range from less than 1 cm to many centimeters and are usually fairly firm, but they may be soft mucoid lesions. Necrosis is common, but cavitary lesions are relatively infrequent. The peripheral lesions often have central pigmented scars, and usually do not show any clearly defined bronchus of origin. Scar carcinomas are discussed on p. 320.

Adenocarcinomas arising in the proximal bronchi obstruct the lumen and spread toward the hilum much in the manner of squamous cell carcinoma. Tumors arising in the periphery show more tendency to grow toward the pleura, and sometimes onto the pleura. Harwood and co-workers[147] and Babolini[148] describe so-called pseudomesotheliomatous carcinoma of the lung (Figure 19–11B). These tumors grow out over the pleura and surround the lung; occasionally a small nodule is visible

Table 19–16. Reports of Combined Small-Cell Carcinomas with Other Histologic Types[a]

Series	No. Patients	Mixed Small-Cell Carcinoma and Another Type Present at Autopsy	Only Another Histologic Type Present at Autopsy
Abeloff et al.[99]	40	6	5
Matthews[142]	91	18	5
Brereton et al.[100]	21	5	—

[a] Light microscopic series.

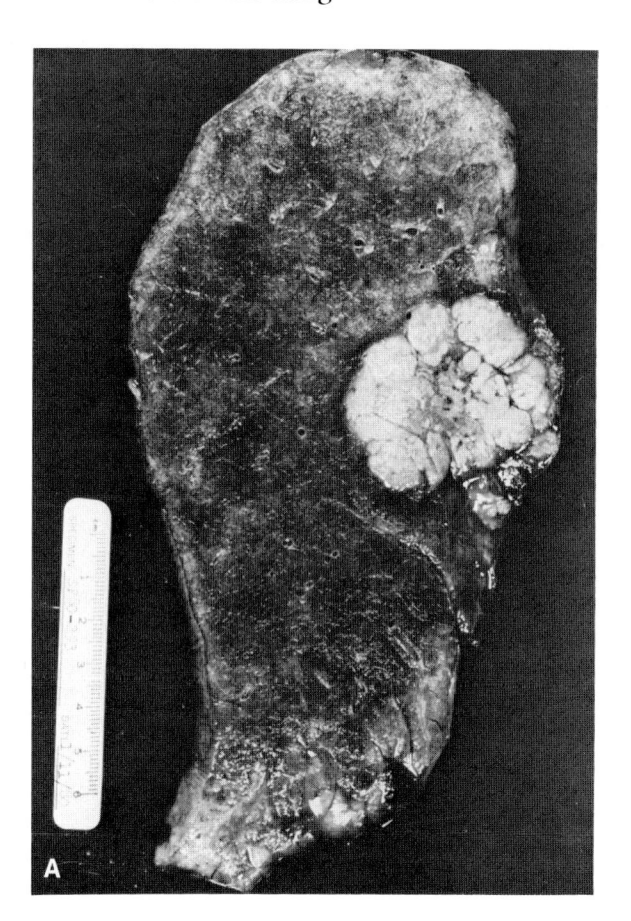

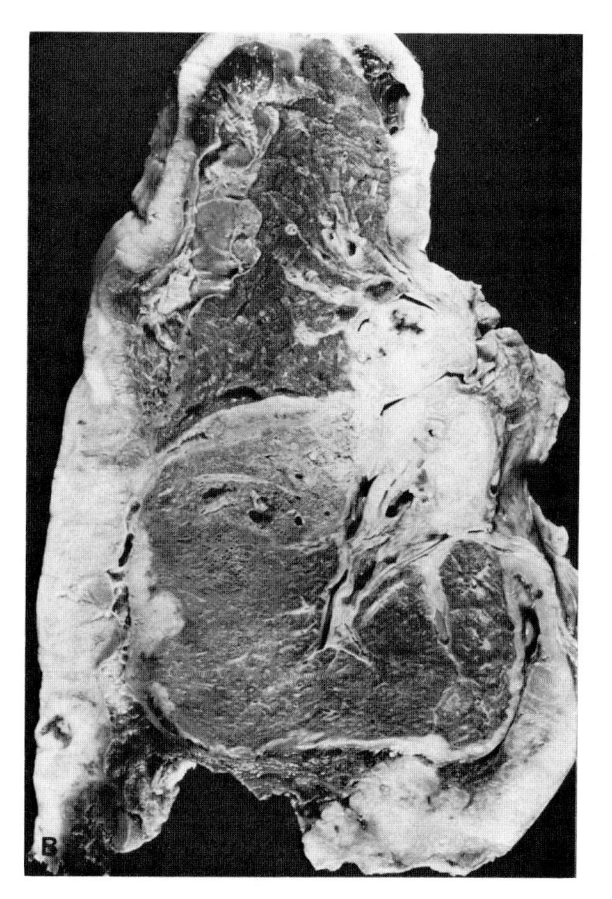

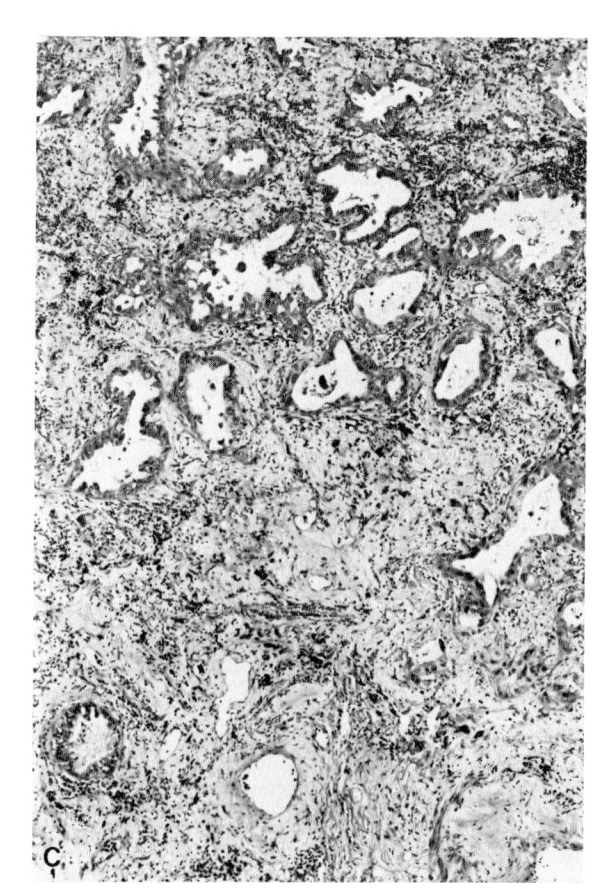

Figure 19–11A–C. Adenocarcinoma. A. Peripheral adenocarcinoma. This is the usual gross appearance of this type of tumor. B. So-called pseudomesotheliomatous form of adenocarcinoma. The tumor has spread around the periphery of the lung in a fashion mimicking malignant mesothelioma. C. Moderately well-differentiated adenocarcinoma showing gland formation. The tumor does not respect preexisting pulmonary architecture (×64).

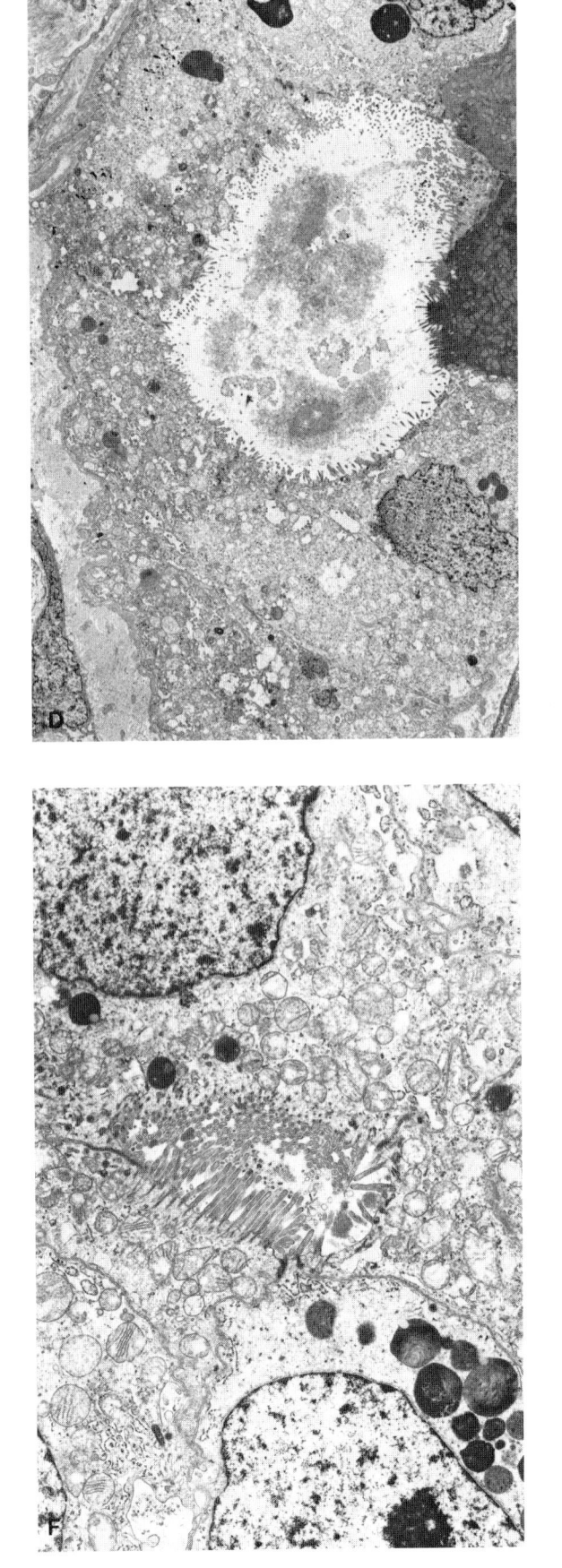

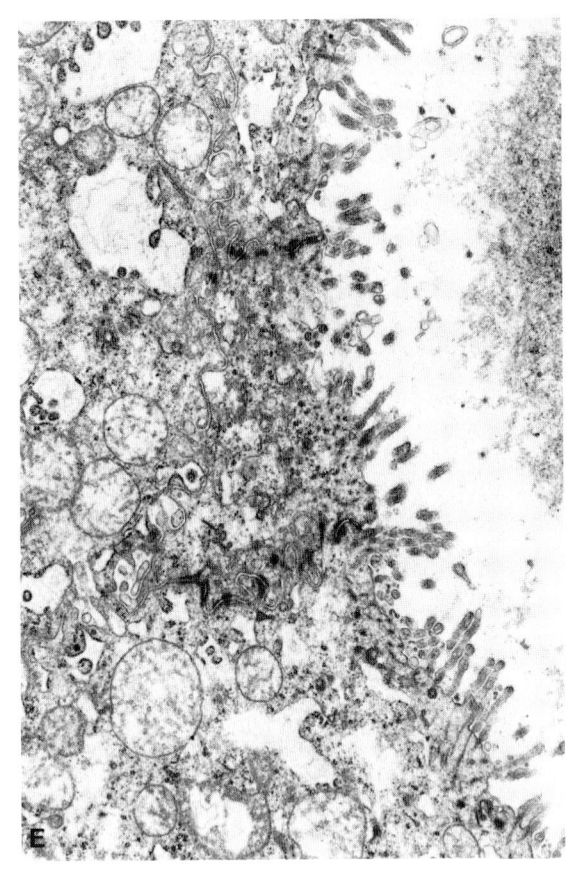

Figure 19–11D–F. D and E. Electron micrograph showing a formation of an intercellular lumen. This structure, which is bounded by junctional complexes (shown at higher power in E), is the ultrastructural prerequisite for the definition of a tumor as an adenocarcinoma (D ×2000, E ×10,000). F. Electron micrograph of another poorly differentiated adenocarcinoma of the lung showing formation of an intercellular lumen. Note the long microvilli. Compare this figure to Figure 26–9. This morphologic appearance casts doubt on the theory that mesotheliomas have longer and thinner microvilli than adenocarcinomas of the lung (*see* Chapter 26).

Table 19–17. Ultrastructural Features of Bronchogenic Carcinomas

Type	Desmosomes/ Tonofilament Bundles	Micro- villi	Tight Junctions	Lumina	Secre- tory RER	Neuro- secretory Granules
Squamous carcinoma	Many, well formed	+	–	–	–	–
Small-cell carcinoma	Small, poorly formed	Rare	–	–	–	+
Adenocar- cinoma	Many, small well formed	+	+	+	+	–

Abbreviations: RER, rough endoplasmic reticulum.

in the parenchyma on the radiograph or on gross examination. Histologically, five of six cases reported by Harwood and colleagues[147] were bronchioloalveolar carcinoma; the carcinomatous nature of the tumor was proved by periodic acid-Schiff (PAS) staining. Harwood and associates suggest that this form of tumor spreads through the subpleural lymphatics to encase the lung.

The histologic appearances of adenocarcinomas of the lung are quite variable, and there may be differences either in histologic appearance or in diagnostic criteria between Europe and the United States.[94,98] I use the WPL classification scheme (see p. 321) which groups the tumors into well, moderately, and poorly differentiated, and includes bronchioloalveolar and papillary forms as a separate group.

The basic criterion for the diagnosis of adenocarcinoma is the formation of glands or acini (Figure 19–11C); most adenocarcinomas in lung also secrete mucin.[95] In the new WHO classification,[88] any tumor that secretes mucin is classified as an adenocarcinoma, even if it does not form glands. A variety of patterns are seen, ranging from tumors that form extremely well-differentiated glands with little tissue disruption, to forms resembling large-cell carcinomas except for the presence of a few clearly defined glandular elements. The distinction between well and moderately, and between moderately and poorly differentiated forms is arbitrary, and probably tumor stage is of considerably greater importance in determining survival. Auerbach and associates[95] classified 118 of 167 adenocarcinomas as well differentiated and an additional 47 as moderately differentiated. Such subtyping probably depends on whether tumors are central or peripheral; in my experience, the central tumors are usually poorly differentiated.

Histologically the cells of pulmonary adenocarcinomas are quite heterogeneous. Occasionally the central tumors are formed of cells resembling bronchial glands; more commonly the cells are large, polygonal, and possessed of variably clear to eosinophilic cytoplasm which frequently contains mucin droplets. In most instances clear cytoplasm is the result of glycogen accumulation; this phenomenon is particularly common in poorly differentiated tumors and has no prognostic significance.[149] Nuclear characteristics are again variable; the poorly differentiated tumors tend to have vesicular nuclei with large nucleoli.

As a rule, the growth pattern of adenocarcinoma is such as to disrupt the pulmonary architecture to a greater or lesser extent; the majority of tumors, even well-differentiated ones, show little regard for preexisting architecture (see Figure 19–11C). However, such tumors may in part grow in lepidic fashion along the alveolar walls; this does not qualify them for the term bronchioloalveolar carcinoma. In particular, I regard carcinomas that invade scars and form multiple back-to-back nests as adenocarcinomas, even if the remainder of the tumor is lepidic. Primary adenocarcinomas of the lung may be papillary and may have psammoma bodies,[150] although these features are much more typical of bronchioloalveolar tumors. It should also be pointed out that histologically there is no absolute method of separating most primary adenocarcinomas of the lung from metastases, although the finding of epithelial dysplasia within surrounding bronchial epithelium[106] or the presence of tumor in a pigmented scar are at least suggestive of a primary origin. Lepidic growth in itself is not a definitive sign of a primary tumor. Foster[151] has found differences in the types of mucins secreted by primary lung cancers and metastatic mimics, and this approach is worthy of further exploration.

Mucin stains are invaluable for the diagnosis both of adenocarcinoma and for excluding malignant mesothelioma. Both digested PAS and mucicarmine are suitable for tumors arising in lung; Kreyberg[110] claims, however, that mucin staining may fade with time in paraffin-embedded material.

Ultrastructurally adenocarcinomas show the features of secretory cells to a greater or lesser extent, depending on degree and type of differentiation.[49,111,112] (Table 19–17). In general, such cells are bounded by well-formed, usually small, desmosomes with well-formed short tonofilament bundles. The cytoplasm frequently contains strands of rough endoplasmic reticulum, and occasionally this is stacked in the fashion of some exocrine secretory cells. Secretory product is often present. Kimula[152] has attempted to separate lung adenocarcinomas by histochemistry and ultrastructure of the secretory product; he believes that the typical flocculent 0.5-μM secretory granules which by light microscopy stain with PAS-Alcian blue indicate origin from goblet cells whereas the tumors with numerous low-density granules and microvilli are derived from mucous cells of the bronchial glands. Kimula has also suggested that some adenocarcinomas are made up of cells with whorled lipid inclusions similar to those seen in type II cells, but the majority (21 of 25) of Kimula's adenocarcinomas were composed of cells with long microvilli and electron-opaque granules measuring 0.4 to 1 μm in diameter, which he regards as derived from Clara cells. Bolen and Thorning[153] also found tumors with Clara type granules, and type II cell granules, as well as the more common flocculent granules. Churg[111] examined a series of poorly differentiated adenocarcinomas and found that secretory product, when present, was of the flocculent type; Mackay and colleagues[112] point out that the appearance of secre-

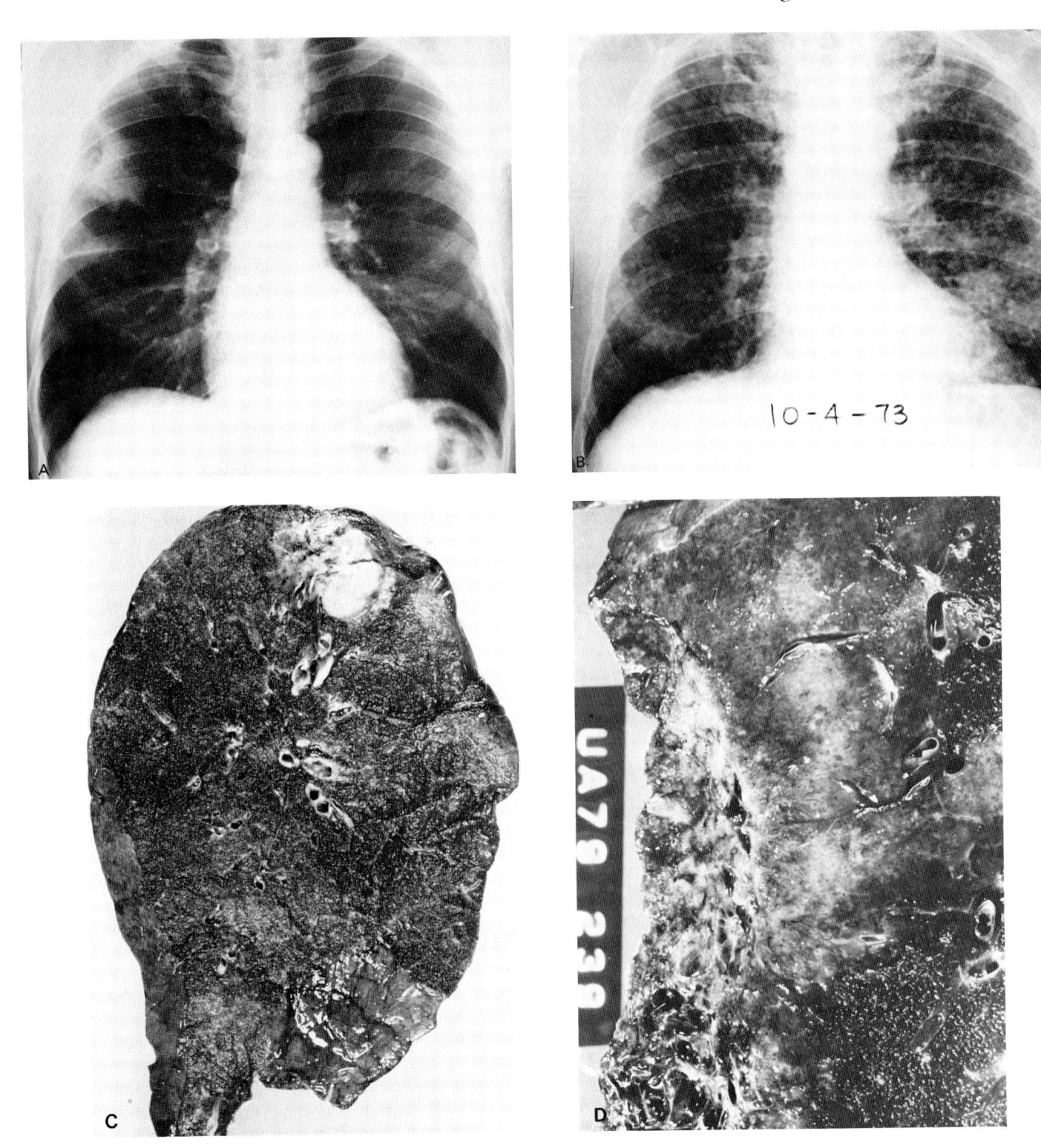

Figure 19–12A–D. Bronchioloalveolar carcinoma. A. Chest radiograph of a patient with bronchioloalveolar carcinoma presenting as a localized mass infiltrate. Note the extension of the tumor torward the pleura. B. Chest radiograph of a patient with bronchioloalveolar tumor presenting as multiple bilateral nodules. C and D. Gross appearance of bronchioloalveolar carcinoma presenting as a solitary nodule. In D the association with a pre-existing area of honeycomb scarring is apparent. In this figure the tumor appears as a diffuse poorly defined infiltrate.

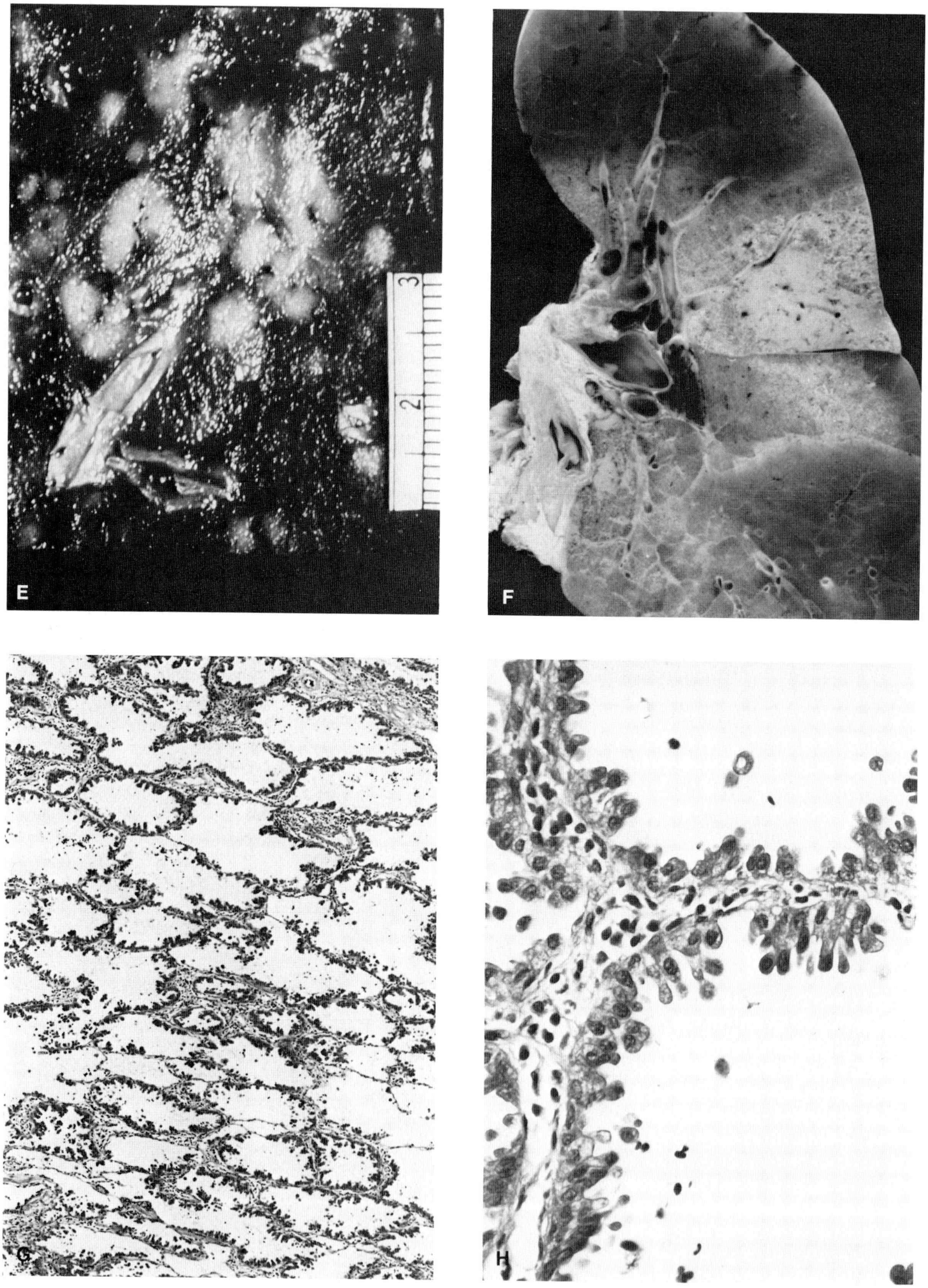
E
F
G
H

tory product reflects very much the manner of fixation and is not reliably identified in most adenocarcinomas.

The conclusion that some adenocarcinomas are derived from cells with type II cell differentiation is supported by studies using immunohistochemical staining for surfactant apoprotein; Espinoza and co-workers[154] found staining in 4 of 14 primary adenocarcinomas of the lung. Similar staining has been reported in bronchioloalveolar tumors (see Bronchioalveolar Carcinoma, below). However, I am loathe to accept the specificity of the cells thought to be Clara cells. At present, their identification depends entirely on the finding of a secretory granule that by definition greatly resembles a secondary lysosome,[155] and such structures are common in malignant cells of many types. Indeed, Sidhu[114] describes granules with "overlapping" features of type II cell and Clara cell granules, and these are almost certainly secondary lysosomes. Definitive classification of the origin of such tumors will require a better means of identifying Clara cells.

More useful at the ultrastructural level, and more basic to the definition of adenocarcinoma, is the presence of true lumens.[49,111,112] These are defined as inter- or intracellular spaces, usually having a rim of microvilli, and bounded by tight junctions (see Fig. 19–11D to F). The latter is a critical feature since, as discussed in the section on squamous carcinomas, microvillous-lined spaces may be seen in squamous carcinomas. In my experience, the number of lumens that may be observed is a direct reflection of the degree of differentiation of the tumor. It also becomes apparent from comparison of light microscopic and electron microscopic material that many structures which appear to be lumens by light microscopy are merely spaces from which necrotic cells have disappeared, but generally the number of lumens appears to parallel the number of mucin droplets visible by light microscopy.

Bronchioloalveolar Carcinoma

Bronchioloalveolar cell tumor (BAT) is generally classified as a subcategory of adenocarcinoma, and can itself be subdivided into the pure and papillary forms, although in practice the two histologic patterns often overlap.[156] In most cases, BAT is both clinically and pathologically similar to other forms of bronchogenic carcinoma, but a number of distinctive variations are found. Thus, although the mean age for the appearance of this tumor is similar to that for smokers in general, the age range is extraordinarily wide, ranging from the second to the ninth decades. The majority of such tumors are associated with smoking,[102] but there is a substantial proportion, especially in women, arising in nonsmokers. The half-dozen tumors reported in teenagers also appear to be unrelated to smoking.[157,158]

An interesting ultrastructural finding reported by Hammar and co-workers[159] is the presence of Langerhans cells in 7 of 37 bronchioloalveolar tumors examined by electron microscopy. Five of the seven patients also had precipitating antibodies against aspergillus species. Hammar and co-workers[159] conclude that the tumors in these instances are originating in scars that represent the residua of allergic reactions, perhaps eosinophilic granuloma. This idea is intriguing, although eosinophilic granuloma commonly produces multiple scars rather than solitary scars, and is not associated with antibodies to aspergillus.

Bronchioloalveolar carcinoma shows three different growth patterns. (1) Growth as a solitary peripheral nodule (Figure 19–12C, D), two-thirds of which occur in the upper lobes. Radiographically, these lesions appear as nodules, often associated with puckering of the overlying pleura (Figure 19–12A). About half of such tumors appear to be associated with a preexisting scar.[160,161] Depending on their association with a preexisting scar, BAT may be firm or instead soft and even gelatinous. (2) Multiple nodules of similar appearance, apparent both on chest radiograph and on gross examination (Figure 19–12B, E). These are frequently bilateral. Because the tumor evokes no or little desmoplastic response, such tumors are usually soft, slightly raised yellowish nodules which may be nearly confluent in areas. (3) So-called "pneumonic pattern" (Figure 19–12F). In this form of growth there is filling of the alveolar spaces by mucus producing a pneumonic consolidation on x-ray examination and a firm gelatinous mass in the pulmonary parenchyma.

The defining microscopic feature of bronchioloalveolar tumor is lepidic growth; that is, growth along preexisting structures of the lung without destroying the underlying framework (see, Figure 19–12G). In its simplest form, this phenomenon is seen as tumor cells growing along alveolar walls replacing the normal lining cells without altering the interstitial tissues. Sometimes a desmoplastic response is observed in the underlying alveolar walls and in other instances a lymphocytic response; however, the underlying architecture is still preserved in these tumors. In areas of preexisting scar, the growth pattern may become somewhat more irregu-

Figure 19–12E–H. E. Gross appearance of bronchioloalveolar carcinoma presenting as multiple tumor nodules, corresponding to the chest radiograph shown in B. F. Gross appearance of bronchioloalveolar carcinoma presenting in its so-called pneumonic form. No distinct tumor mass is seen but the involved area of lung appears lighter and homogeneous. G and H. Light micrograph showing growth of bronchioloalveolar carcinoma in typical lepidic fashion along alveolar walls. The higher-power view shows the peg-like cells often found in this tumor (G ×64, H ×400).

lar; however, tumors that form solid masses of back to back glands are probably best classified as well-differentiated adenocarcinomas, even if the majority of the tumor grows in a lepidic fashion.

The cells of bronchioloalveolar tumor are quite variable in appearance. Typically that are tall cells with mucus-filled apices and small, remarkably bland-appearing nuclei. In other instances the cells are cuboidal or peg-like (see Figure 19–12G, H). Mitoses are usually difficult to find, but the nuclei may be fairly anaplastic and mitoses relatively plentiful. In some instances the cells are goblet type (Figure 19–12I). Giant cells are occasionally seen. The nuclei may contain inclusions (see below).

The papillary forms of bronchioloalveolar carcinoma are composed of similar cells which are heaped up on an intact underlying stroma; sometimes the tumors appear to form by budding papillary projections off the alveolar walls (Figure 19–12J).

Mucus secretion is present in about 80 percent of bronchioloalveolar tumors and may be extensive enough to produce the mucoid pneumonia described above (Figure 19–12K, L). In such tumors the numbers of cells may be remarkably scanty. Psammona bodies may also be present; their frequency has been estimated at 15 to 50 percent of tumors.[98,150]

An attempt to grade BAT using cytologic characteristics have been made by Dunn and colleagues.[162] They found that patients with high-grade tumors had the shortest survival; however, these investigators' illustration of a high-grade tumor appears to me to be that of an ordinary adenocarcinoma. Tao and associates[163] also claim a poorer prognosis when the lesion is histologically higher grade, but their results probably reflect the fact that most of their patients had multiple nodules (that is, disseminated disease). As with other forms of adenocarcinoma, prognosis likely depends more on stage than on cytologic grade.

Some authors[1] describe a lesion known as "benign pulmonary adenomatosis." This lesion appears structurally and cytologically identical to the usual BAT, although usually much smaller in size. I know of no evidence to suggest that such lesions are benign, and I prefer to regard them as small BATs. Bronchioloalveolar cell tumors of this type must be separated from reactive bronchiolar and type II cell epithelial proliferations that occur in any focus of scarring, but which are not cytologically atypical.

The histogenesis of bronchioloalveolar carcinoma, indeed its very existence, has been a source of controversy, with some authors claiming that neither pathologic nor behavioral features separate BAT from ordinary adenocarcinoma.[156,160,161,164,165] Part of the evidence for the existence of this tumor comes from similar-appearing diseases of animals. In the mouse, for example, adenomas are found that reproduce the histologic patterns of BATs, including the papillary forms.[166,167] Ultrastructurally the animal tumors appear to be derived either from Clara cells in which case the neoplasm is usually papillary in nature, or from type II cells, in which instances they show an alveolar pattern.[166] A closer counterpart is the virus-induced disease of sheep, Jaagsiekte.[168] This lesion appears to be derived from type II cells and occasionally metastasizes. It was initially believed that the peculiar inclusions found in the nuclei of some bronchioloalveolar carcinomas represented viral particles,[169–171] but Singh and co-workers[172] suggest that they are actually nuclear inclusions of surfactant apoprotein and that their presence indicates a tumor with type II cell differentiation.

The cell of origin of the human tumors is less obvious (the cells found by various authors are summarized in Table 19–18 and illustrated in Figure 19–12M to O). By ultrastructural examination, the most common cell is tall and contains apical mucous granules, as well as occasional microvilli or cilia on the surface. This cell appears to be derived from the goblet cells of the bronchial epithelium. Cells of this type have been observed in almost all the BATs examined (see Table 19–18), as well as in ordinary adenocarcinomas.[49,111,152] Indeed, Bedrossian and colleagues[173] concluded that, ultrastructurally, they were not able to distinguish their eight BATs from more centrally occurring adenocarcinomas. A second cell type which is less constantly observed has surface microvilli and the dense osmiophilic granules of Clara cells. Kuhn[170] concluded that some tumors had cells in this category, and most of the subsequent reports describe such cells (see Table 19–18). Of interest is the study of Kimula,[152] who believed that not only the majority of BATs but the majority of ordinary adenocarcinomas he examined were composed of Clara cells; only two of Kimula's nine BATs appeared to be derived from mucous cells. The nonspecificity of this type of ultrastructural identification has been discussed in the section on adenocarcinomas (see p. 345).

The question of whether human BATs ever contain neoplastic type II cells has also been a source of great controversy, but one that is now resolved. Early reports[165,174] concluded that the human tumors were indeed derived from type II cells, but these findings were challenged by Kuhn[170] and by Bedrossian[173]; as Mackay and co-workers[112] illustrate, it is easy to chance upon reactive type II cells at the edges of a tumor and conclude

Figure 19–12I–L. I, Bronchioloalveolar tumor composed of goblet-type cells (×64). J, Papillary form of bronchioloalveolar carcinoma (×64). K and L, Pneumonic form of bronchioloalveolar carcinoma. Note filling of alveolar spaces by mucus and relatively scanty tumor cells seen best in L (K ×64, L ×160).

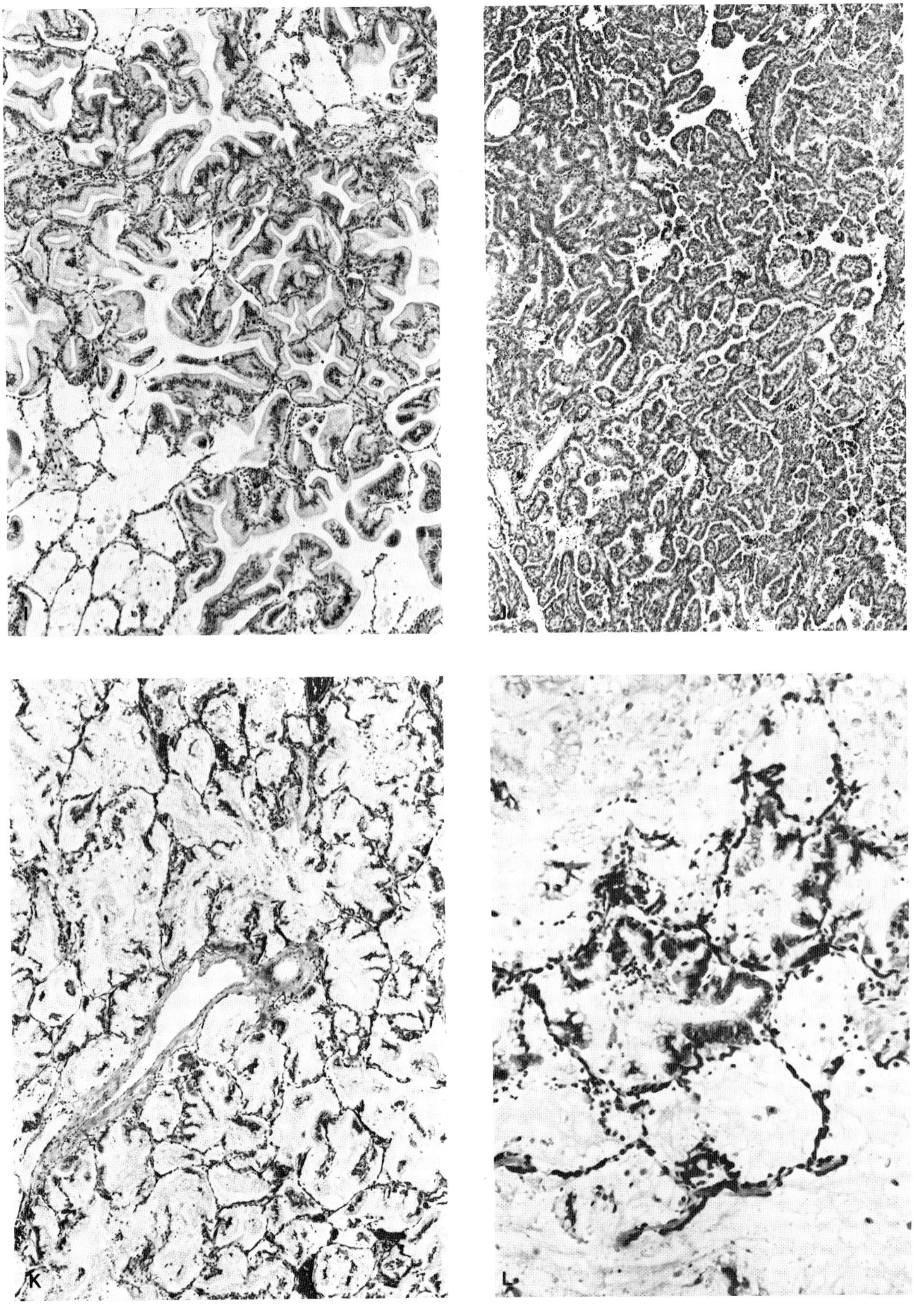
I
J
K
L

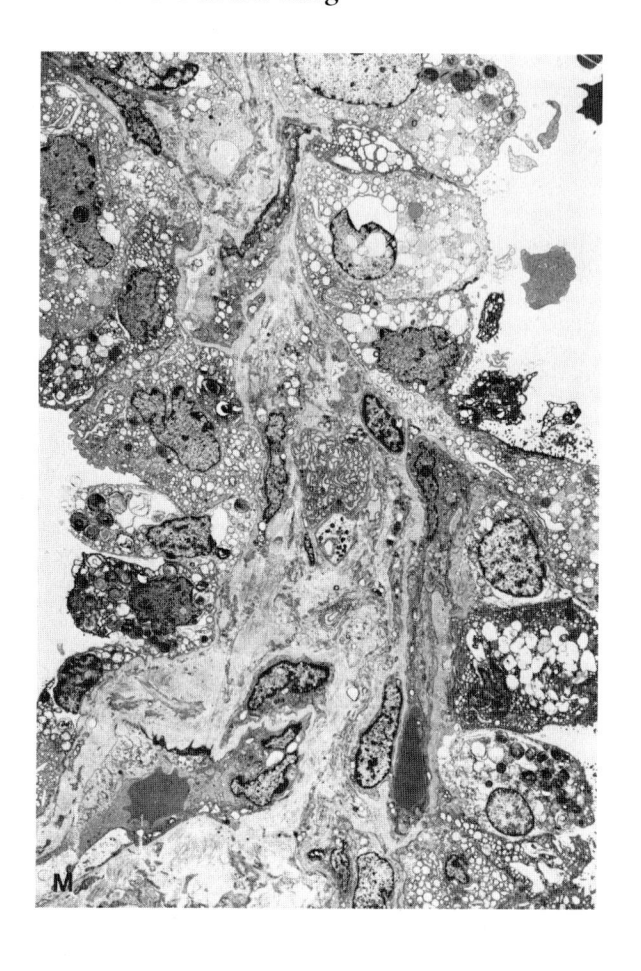

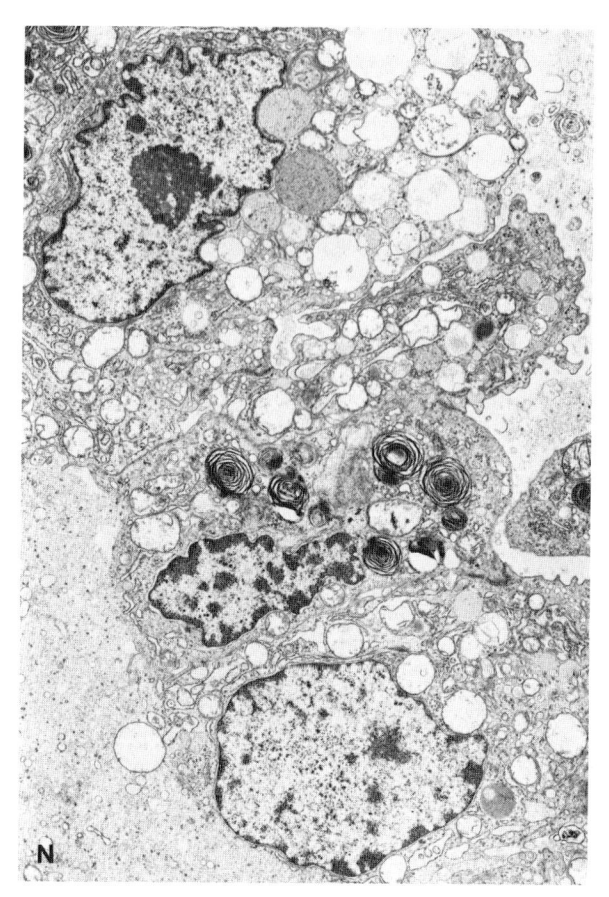

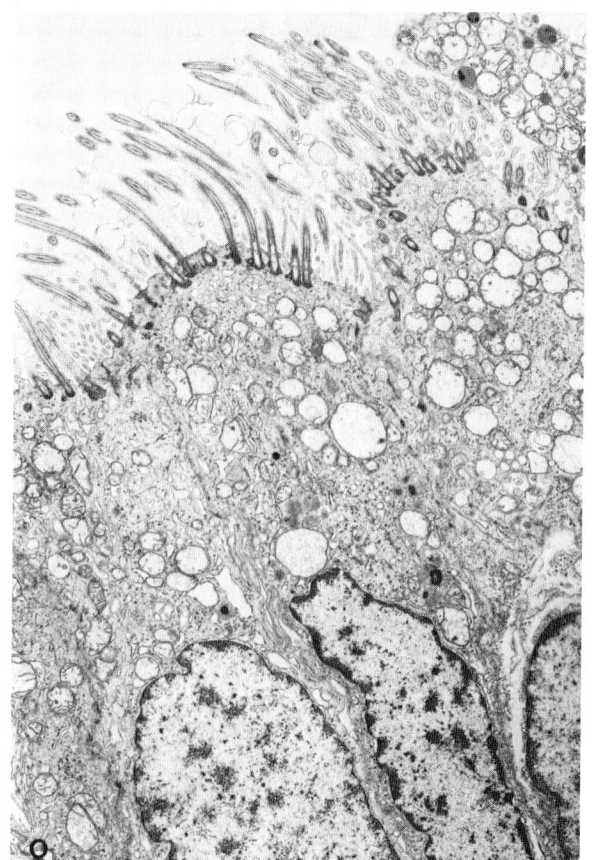

Figure 19–12M–O. Electron micrographs of bronchioloalveolar tumor. Low-power view (M) shows numerous tumor cells lining alveolar wall. A mixture of cell types can be seen. Higher-power view (N) shows type II cells containing lamellated inclusions intermixed with mucus-secreting cells. O. Another area of the same tumor in which the cells bear cilia (M ×2000, N ×8000, O ×8000).

they are part of the neoplasm. It is also easy to find occasional myelin whorls in many types of neoplastic cells[170]; these are probably an artifact of fixation and should not be considered evidence of the formation of lamellar bodies. Nonetheless, recent evidence indicates that malignant human tumors containing cells with the features of type II cells do occur. Bonikos and associates[175] reported a case in which the tumor cells were clearly of type II cell origin and maintained formation of lamellar bodies for several months in tissue culture. Morningstar and Hassan[176] presented a case in which type II cells were found in metastases in a lymph node, a finding that obviates arguments against accidental inclusion of reactive type II cells in tissue samples. Singh and Katyal,[177] using immunohistochemical staining for surfactant apoprotein, found staining in 26 percent of 45 tumors. Both the nuclear inclusions and the cytoplasm stained, and staining correlated with the presence of type II cell lamellated inclusions. I have examined the tumor illustrated in Figure 19–12J and M to O. The sample was taken from deep within a papillary type of bronchioloalveolar tumor, but mucus-secreting cells, Clara-like cells, type II cells, and ciliated cells were all present, mixed in a somewhat jumbled disarray.

In summary, it appears that the majority of bronchioloalveolar tumors show differentiation toward cells that resemble those of other mucus-secreting adenocarcinomas, and less frequently toward type II cells, ciliated cells, and cells resembling Clara cells. Rarely, one of these nonmucous secreting types is the only cell present. Thus one may conclude that, morphologically, bronchioloalveolar tumor does indeed exist, albeit with considerable overlap into the sphere of ordinary adenocarcinoma.

Large-Cell Carcinomas

Large-cell carcinomas in both the WHO and WPL classifications (see Table 19–10) are tumors that do not show the intercellular bridges or keratin formation of squamous carcinoma, nor the gland formation of adenocarcinoma. They are further broken down as tumors with or without mucin production, clear-cell tumors, and giant cell tumors. As Yesner[92] has pointed out, this essentially negative definition permits large-cell carcinoma to become an umbrella term for any tumor that has not been conveniently classified. An additional problem arises in biopsy material where only poorly or undifferentiated elements of a tumor may be present, yet a resection specimen shows definable foci, indeed, one may need to sample many blocks to find subclassifiable tumor in such a situation. As noted above, in the new WHO classification,[88] tumors that produce mucin but do not form glands are classified as adenocarcinomas.

Large-cell carcinomas are frequently large and peripherally located,[98] but central tumors, in my experience, are not uncommon. Necrosis is common. The central tumors may be associated with large bronchi.

Microscopically, the usual large-cell carcinoma is composed of sheets of variably anaplastic cells which may be spindled or oval but tend to be polygonal (Figure

Table 19–18. Cell Types Found in Bronchioloalveolar Carcinomas

Report	Ciliated	Mucus Secreting	Clara	Type II
Adamson et al.[174]				+
Bedrossian et al.[173]	+	+		
Bolen and Thorning[153]			+	
Bonikos et al.[175]				+[a]
Greenberg et al.[178]	+	+	+	
Jacques and Currie[179]				+
Kimula.[152]		+	+	
Kuhn[170]		+	+	
Mackay et al.[112]	+	+	+	
Montes et al.[180]		+		
Morningstar and Hassan[176]				+ (metastatic tumor)
Nash et al.[165]				+
Sidhu and Forrester[181]		+	+	
Singh and Katyal[177]				+

[a] Both in original tumor and in tissue culture.

19–13A, B). In many instances the tumor is remarkably uniform, despite the atypical features of the nuclei. Sometimes the tumor cells are arranged in stratified sheets, and are called by some pathologists poorly differentiated squamous carcinomas, despite the lack of other defining features. Mucin droplets are easily demonstrable in about half the cases. According to the new WHO classification[88] these tumors would now be called adenocarcinoma.

Large-cell carcinomas may be partly or entirely composed of clear cells (see Figure 19–13A, B), although, as Katzenstein and colleagues[149] point out, areas of clear-cell change are even more common in ordinary adenocarcinoma and squamous cell carcinoma. They studied 15 tumors composed of more than 50 percent clear cells and found that such tumors behaved identically to tumors of similar histologic type but with fewer than 50 percent clear cells. As a rule, the clear-cell change reflects cytoplasmic glycogen.[111] Probably the most important aspect of clear cell tumors is the resemblance to metastatic renal cell carcinoma, a lesion which must be ruled out when the overall pattern is adenocarcinoma or undifferentiated carcinoma. Rarely malignant primary lung tumors are encountered which are composed of clear cells which do not contain glycogen.

The ultrastructure of large-cell carcinomas has been studied by Churg,[111] Horie and Ohta,[182] and Sidhu.[114] Churg examined eight large-cell carcinomas and found that the majority of cells were undifferentiated polygonal cells which often contained large amounts of cytoplasmic glycogen but no specific features. However, scattered cells did show more differentiation; either formation of true lumens (Figure 19–13C) (four of eight cases) or presence of intercellular bridges and numerous desmosomes (four cases) (Figure 19–13D to E). No overlapping cases were observed. The major ultrastructural difference between the differentiated (by light mi-

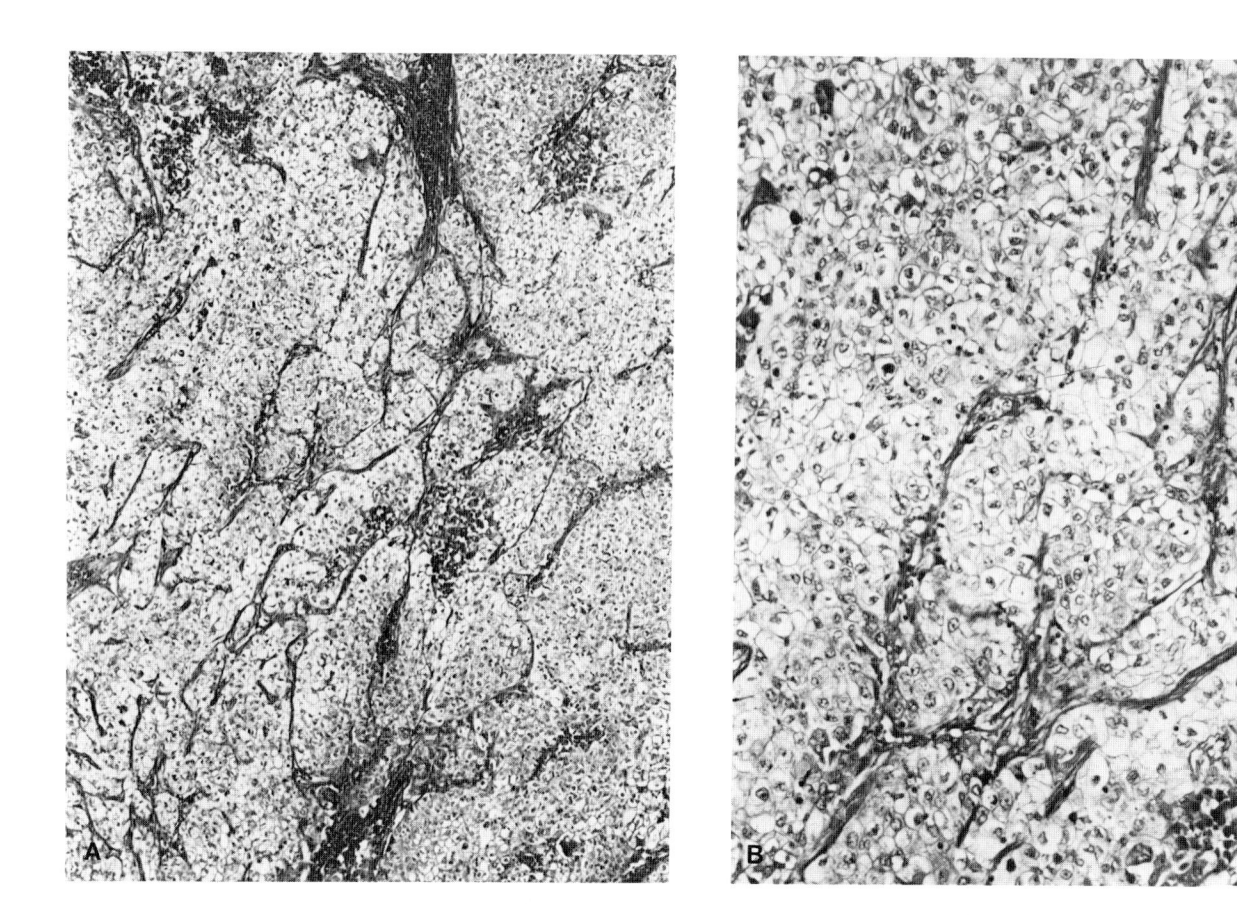

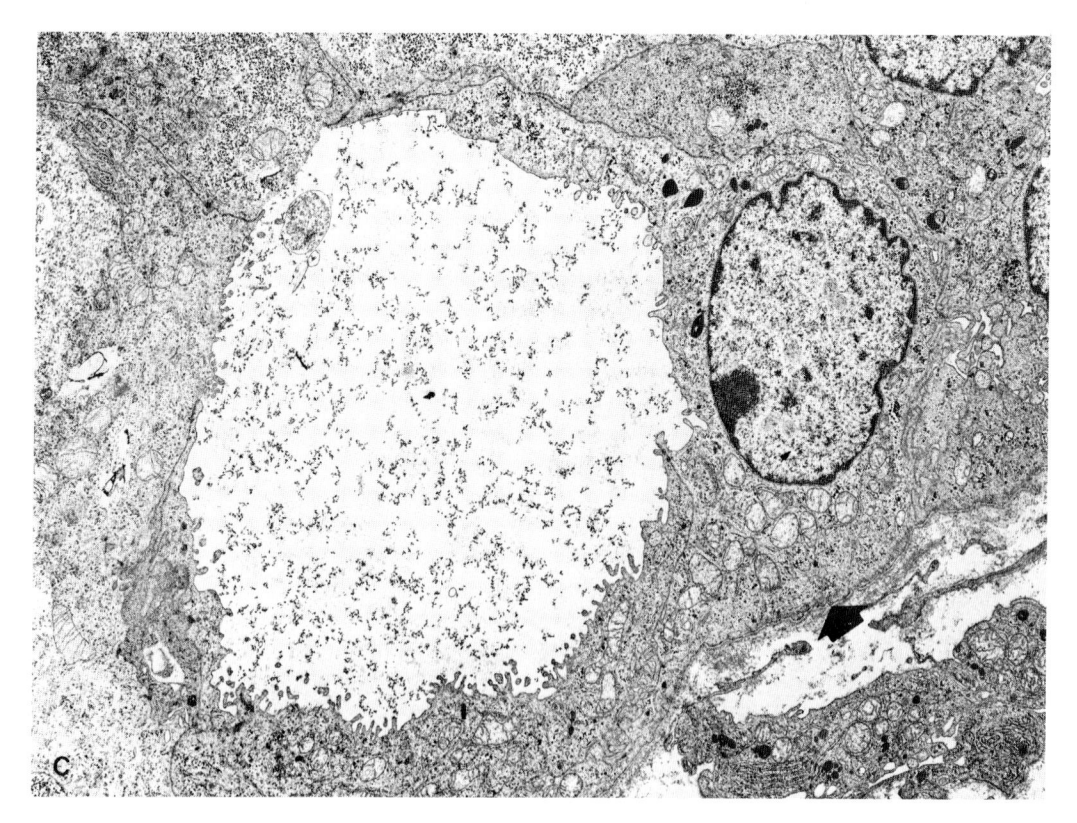

Figure 19–13A–C. Large-cell undifferentiated carcinoma. Light micrographs of typical large-cell carcinoma of the lung. Note polygonal cells without any evidence of differentiation that would entitle the tumor to be classified as squamous or adenocarcinoma. This particular example is composed of clear cells; ultrastructurally they contain large amounts of glycogen which produces the clear appearance (A ×40, B ×160). Ultrastructural appearance of different large-cell carcinomas of the lung. C shows a tumor similar to that in A which forms an intercellular lumen thus classifying it as an adenocarcinoma.

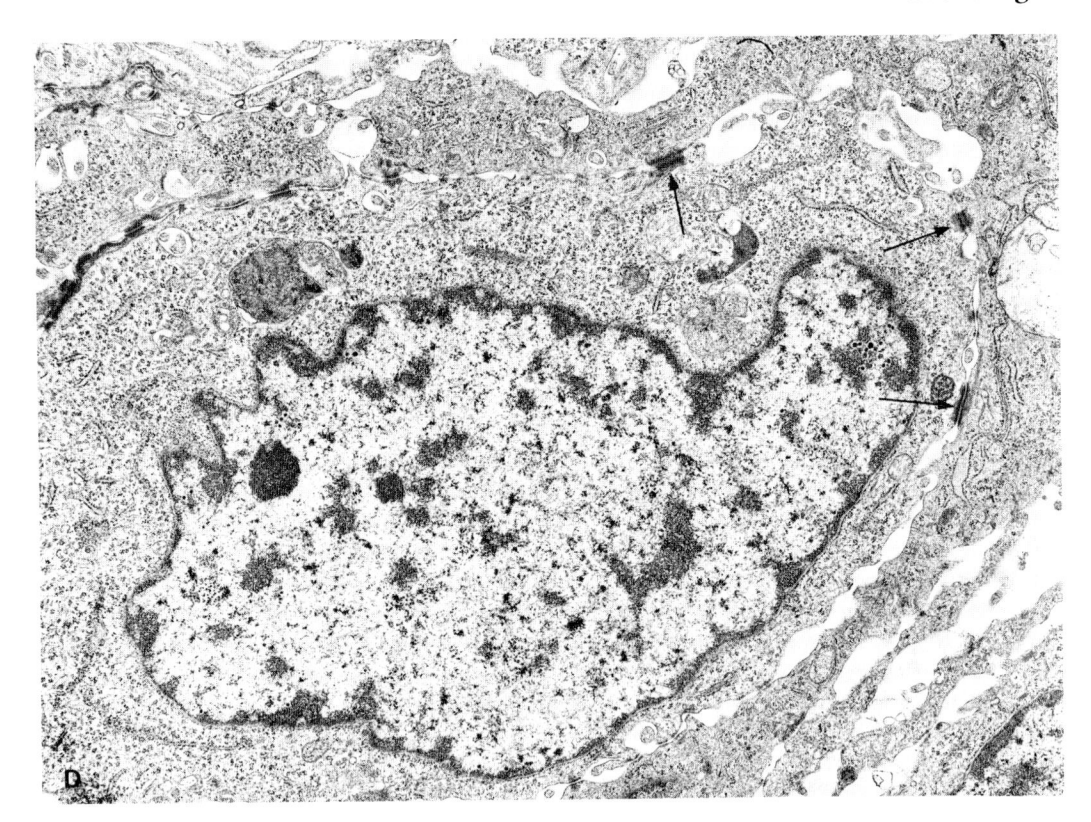

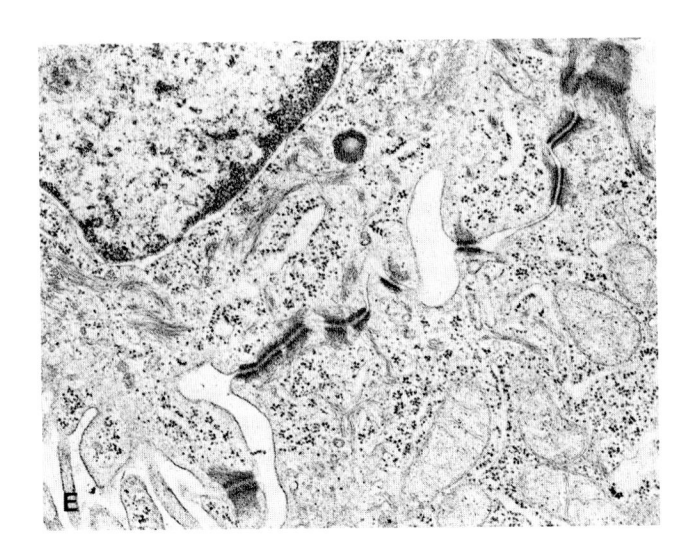

Figure 19–13D–E. Ultrastructural appearance of different large-cell carcinomas of the lung. D and E show a tumor that was also similar to that in A but which ultrastructurally forms numerous desomsomes and intercellular bridges (arrows), thus classifying it as a squamous carcinoma (C ×1600, D ×1600, E ×12000). Reproduced with permission from Churg.[111]

croscopy) and the large-cell tumors was the greater frequency of differentiated cells at the ultrastructural level in the definable tumors. Horie and Ohta[182] examined 24 cases; they concluded that 5 showed features of squamous carcinoma, 9 features of adenocarcinoma, and 10 were mixed tumors. Both these articles conclude that large-cell carcinomas are poorly differentiated versions of the ordinary adenocarcinomas and squamous cell carcinomas. However, McKay and co-workers[112] believe that they are all poorly differentiated adenocarcinomas. Sidhu[114] was unable to find any differentiating structures in some large cell carcinomas, and in one case he observed neurosecretory type granules. These structural differences may reflect behavioral differences (see Prognosis of Bronchogenic Carcinoma, below).

Giant cell carcinoma was initially described as a separate type of tumor by Nash and Stout,[183] but is currently classified with the large-cell carcinomas. Hathaway and colleagues[184] reviewed 139 cases in the literature and found that the age and sex ratios were in general similar to those for other types of bronchogenic carcinoma. Giant cell carcinoma is composed partly or entirely of pleomorphic giant cells, often of extremely bizarre shape (Figure 19–14). Phagocytosis of red cells and white cells is common. In some instances the tumor cells are heavily infiltrated with polymorphonuclear leukocytes, and other inflammatory cells, a pattern that resembles inflammatory fibrous histiocytoma. Transitions to clearcut adenocarcinoma are sometimes seen; Razzuk and colleagues[185] found foci of adenocarcinoma in four of nine cases and an area resembling bronchioloalveolar carcinoma in one additional case. In some tumors the giant cells contain mucin droplets.

Razzuk and colleagues[185] and Wang and associates[186] studied the ultrastructure of giant cell carcinoma. By electron microscopy, the cells had numerous profiles of rough endoplasmic reticulum and an extensive Golgi system, and were considered to represent poorly differentiated cells of epithelial origin. Horie and Ohta[182] concluded that one of two tumors examined had the ultrastructural features of squamous carcinoma. It seems likely that giant cell carcinoma is a morphologic variant of ordinary adenocarcinoma and squamous carcinoma; its major importance lies in its aggressive behavior; Hathaway and colleagues[184] found a median survival of about 5.5 months for the 139 cases they tabulated; Razzuk and associates[185] were unable to find significant differences in survival between supportive treatment, and surgery or radiation therapy. Giant cell carcinomas must be distinguished from squamous carcinomas or adenocarcinomas (usually Pancoast's tumors) which have been irradiated and undergone giant cell transformation, since the latter have a relatively favorable prognosis.[109]

Mixed Adenocarcinoma and Squamous Carcinoma

Mixed tumors with unequivocal histologic features of adenocarcinoma and squamous cell carcinoma are relatively rare: they accounted for 5 of 740 cases in the series of Hinson and colleagues[94] and 200 of 10,000 cases in the series reported by Yesner and associates.[187] As noted above, Horie and Ohta[182] claim that half of the large-cell carcinomas they studied by electron microscopy had mixed features. McDowell and colleagues[49] contend that 46 percent of the lung cancers they examined were of mixed type, and they propose various ultrastructural subdivisions (well-differentiated squamous component with poorly differentiated adenocarcinoma component, and so on). I believe that the structural basis for this sort of breakdown is nebulous and may represent a misreading of some rather nondescript ultrastructural features; unless such divisions can be shown to be of prognostic or therapeutic significance, they only serve to confuse the classification of lung cancers. At present the behavioral characteristics of mixed tumors are not known. An example of adenosquamous carcinoma is illustrated in Figure 19–15.

Clinical Manifestations of Bronchogenic Carcinoma

Radiographic Abnormalities

Any detailed discussion of radiographic abnormalities is beyond the scope of this chapter; the present material is based on the short review by Miller.[188]

Lung cancers in general produce different radiographic signs depending on peripheral or central location. The earliest peripheral lesions are ill-defined nodules; in practice about the smallest tumor that is readily detectable is at least 1 cm in diameter. In general, the outlines of such a tumor are ragged, but a smooth contour, although suggesting a granuloma or other benign lesion, is no guarantee against malignancy. Early central tumors may be very difficult to detect on plain films, the earliest sign sometimes being a small mass that obliterates the space between the mediastinum and the pulmonary artery.

Large but still operable tumors may appear as tumors themselves, or through their obstructive effects. Tumor in a mainstem bronchus or metastatic to a hilar node will frequently appear as increased size or density of the hilus. Such findings are seen with 40 percent of squamous cell carcinomas, 78 percent of small-cell carcinomas, 32 present of large-cell carcinomas, and 17 percent of adenocarcinomas.[189] Peripheral nodules are more likely to be adenocarcinomas or large-cell carcinomas. Tomography is helpful in the exact delineation of the tumor, as well the detection of cavitation, a frequent finding in squamous carcinomas, or of subtle soft tissue extension, particularly with Pancoast's tumors. Evidence of obstruction in the form of atelectasis or nonresolving pneumonic infiltrates are also common signs of central tumors that obstruct bronchi.

Bronchioloalveolar carcinoma presents an unusually wide spectrum of radiographic appearances.[190] In its simplest form it appears as a sharply defined or irregular nodule. Frequently the nodule is subpleural and a linear density extends to the pleura, the so called "rabbit ear" sign. The tumor may also appear as multiple nodules that are usually bilateral, but may be unilateral; when growing close together these may coalesce into large masses. Such masses may at first appear "pneumonic," but careful examination usually reveals that the edge of the infiltrate is actually still nodular. Cavitation may occur in such large lesions. In other instances a true pneumonic picture is present when the tumor produces large amounts of mucus that fill the air spaces. Less frequently BAT will grow along bronchi in the fashion of other types of lung cancer, producing obvious rigidity of the bronchi on inspiration as well as bronchial obliteration.

Mass screening radiographic studies have been performed by several groups[191–193] with generally disappointing results. In the studies of Nash and co-workers[192] and Brett,[191] 4-year survival rates were 18 and 15 percent, respectively. The Philadelphia project[193] screened 6136 men and found 94 cases of lung cancer. Only 37 percent

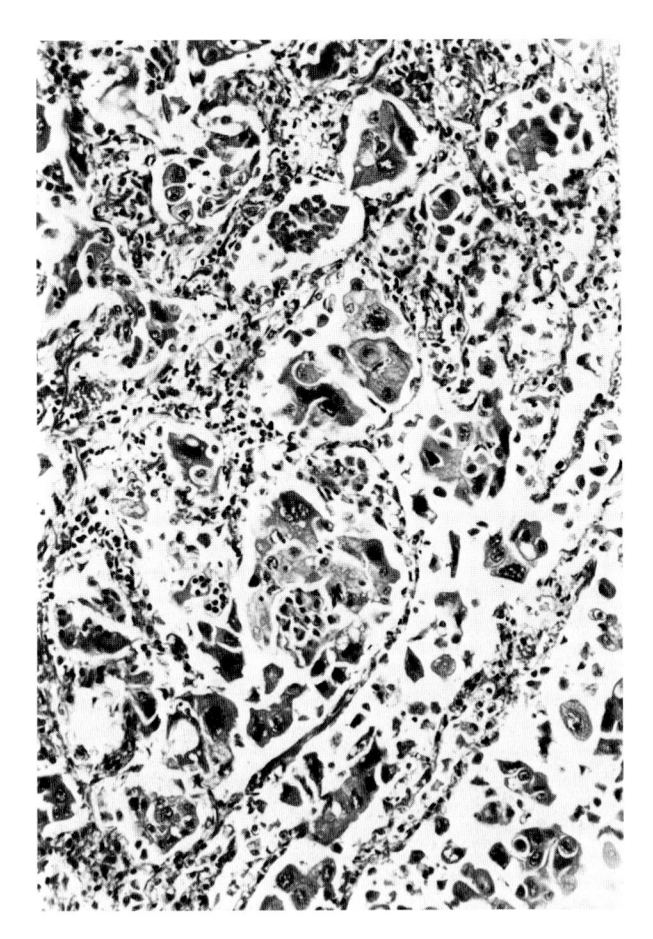

Figure 19–14. Giant cell carcinoma of the lung. Note the bizarre giant cells and the numerous phagocytized red and white cells, a finding typical of this tumor (×160).

were resectable at the time of discovery and the overall survival was only 6 percent.

Manifestations of the Local Spread of Lung Cancers

A summary of some of the common signs and symptoms produced by intrapulmonary growth and direct extrapulmonary extension of bronchogenic carcinoma, and the correlation of these signs and symptoms with pathologic features, is shown in Table 19–19. Details may be found in Cohen.[194,195] Any of the signs, symptoms, or syndromes listed may be found as a presenting complaint, or may be seen late in the course of the disease.

Intrapulmonary Effects. Tumors of the lung may produce a variety of effects secondary to intrapulmonary growth. These include cough, probably related to irritation of bronchial irritant receptors, hemoptysis from erosion of pulmonary or tumor vessels, wheezing related to obstruction of bronchi, and dyspnea, probably secondary to loss of lung volume. Pain is a frequent manifestation, although its origin in the instance of purely intrapulmonary tumors is not entirely clear. All the above features are typical of central lesions, whereas peripheral carcinomas are more likely to present with pain as a result of transpleural spread.

Because the central tumors tend to obstruct bronchi, either by direct filling of a bronchus, or by enlargement of lymph nodes with bronchial compression,[196] infectious lesions are common. These include unremitting pneumonia, bronchiectasis, and sometimes abscess formation.

Effects Related to Direct Spread from the Lung. Growth of a tumor in the apical portion of the lung, so-called Pancoast's tumor, may lead to Pancoast's syndrome. This involves extension into the brachial plexus to produce pain in the shoulder and arm, extension into the sympathetic ganglia to produce Horner's syndrome, and rib destruction.[197]

Extension of tumor into the pleura commonly causes a pleural effusion to form; after cardiac failure and infection, malignant neoplasm is probably the most common cause of pleural effusion, and a large portion of such neoplasms originate in the lung (see Chapter 26). Spread within the mediastinum may cause hoarseness secondary to involvement of the recurrent laryngeal nerve, particularly on the left. The diaphragm can be paralyzed if the phrenic nerve is involved. Compression or invasion of the superior vena cava produces superior vena caval syndrome; this syndrome is particularly common with small-cell carcinoma.[198] Extension into the esophagus may present as dysphagia; occasionally tumors are extensive enough that determination of an esophageal vs. lung primary is difficult.

Effects Not Mediated by Direct Spread of Tumor: Paraneoplastic Syndromes

A variety of effects not mediated by physical invasion of tumor are common with lung cancers (Table 19–20). Most of these are presumably mediated through production of specific substances by tumor cells, although the exact nature of the substances involved has been clearly defined only for the various endocrine and neuroendocrine syndromes discussed below, and for the mucins produced by some adenocarcinomas. In other paraneoplastic syndromes (particularly the neurologic syndromes) no mediator has yet been identified but resection of the tumor may alleviate the symptoms, supporting the idea of circulating tumor-produced effectors.[89,199,200]

Nonendocrine Syndromes. Coagulation disorders may take the appearance of migratory thrombophlebitis and/or nonbacterial thrombotic endocarditis. These types of thrombosis are most common with mucin-producing adenocarcinomas, both of lung and other organs. Disseminated intravascular coagulation of a chronic low-grade variety may also be encountered.[201–203]

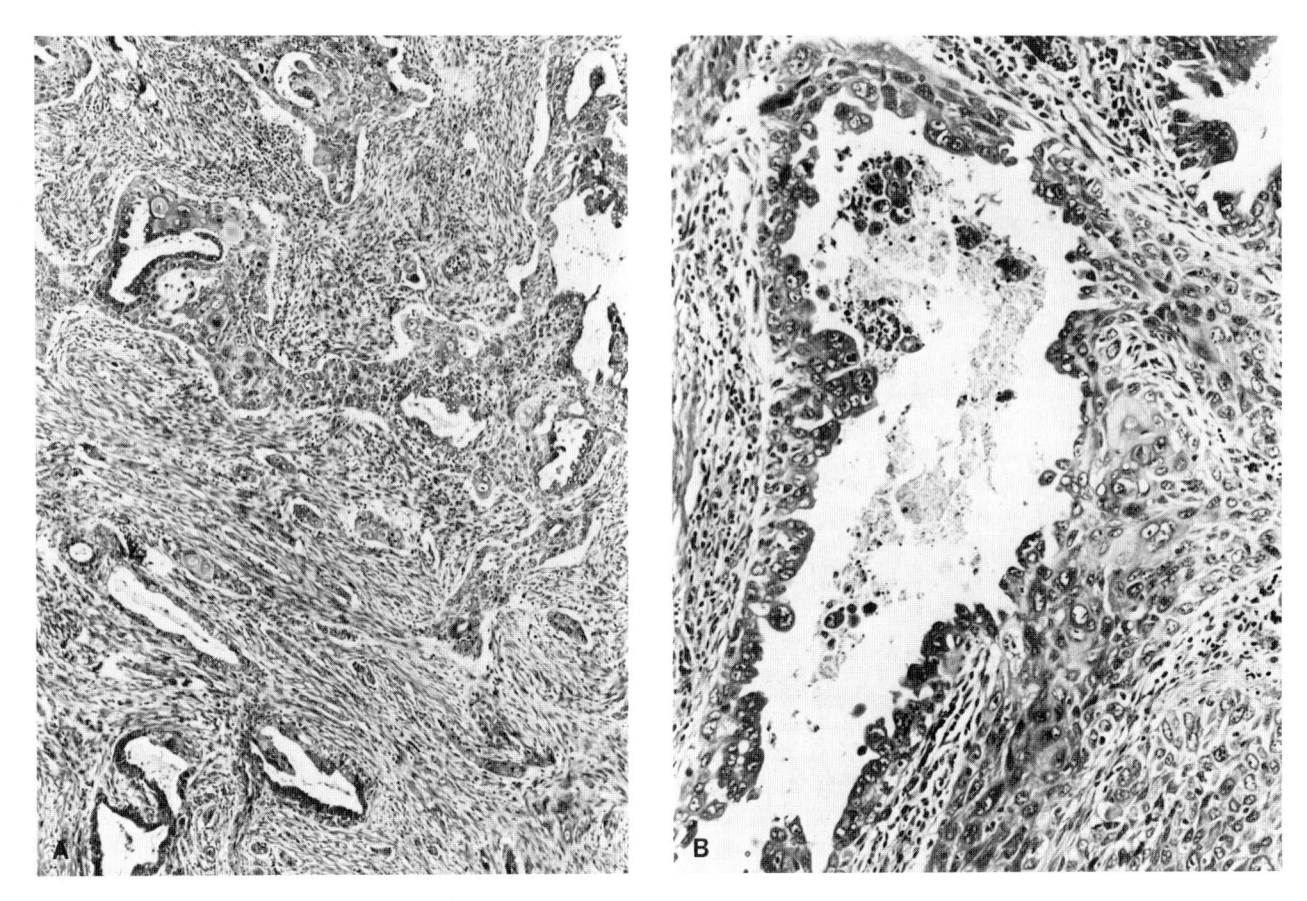

Figure 19–15. Adenosquamous carcinoma. Long high-power views of a tumor that demonstrates a clear glandular configuration as well as defnite areas of keratinization. Mucin staining was positive in the glandular areas (A ×64, B ×160).

Hypertrophic pulmonary osteoarthropathy consists of periostitis of the long bones and clubbing of the fingers, sometimes associated with polyarthritis.[204] It is said to be more frequent with adenocarcinoma but is seen with other tumors and non-neoplastic conditions.[205–208] The mediator is unknown, but manifestations may disappear with removal of the tumor. It should be noted that hypertrophic pulmonary osteoarthropaphy is encountered with benign conditions.

Acanthosis nigricans,[209,210] scleroderma, and tylosis[211] are associated with squamous cell carcinoma. Dermatomyositis is associated with a variety of visceral malignancies including bronchogenic carcinoma.

Neurologic manifestations include encephalopathy, cerebellar degeneration apparently secondary to loss of Purkinje cells, and a variety of peripheral neuropathies and myopathies.[212–214] All types of tumors may produce these syndromes, but they are most common with small-cell carcinomas.[215] Remission of cerebellar dysfunction may occur after treatment of the tumor[216,217]; similarly, Croft and Wilkinson[218] have reported remission of peripheral neuropathies.

Endocrine and Neuroendocrine Syndromes. A wide variety of peptide and steroid hormones and related substances are produced by lung cancers (Table 19–21; *see also* Yesner[89] and Primack and co-workers[200]). As assays become more sensitive, it becomes apparent that production of such substances can be demonstrated in a large fraction of tumors, although actual clinical manifestation are considerably less common. Gropp and colleagues[219] analyzed 110 patients and found that an elevated level of at least one of seven substances was present in 65 percent of all patients and 78 percent of patients with oat cell carcinoma. Morphologically, reports of secretory granules in tumors other than small-cell carcinoma are rare, and the exact mode of secretion of these substances is unknown. Attempts to use some of these hormones as markers of tumor presence or activity are reviewed in Yesner[89] and Richardson and colleagues.[220] Many have been promoted as specific markers of the presence of tumors or of specific histologic types, but none as yet has actually proved to be diagnostically reliable. Lokich[221] notes that the presence of ectopic hormone syndromes in small-cell carcinoma is associated with a worse survival, compared to those without the syndromes.

Adrencorticotropic Hormone and Big Adrenocorticotropic Hormone. Cushing's syndrome is probably the most common of the paraneoplastic syndromes, accounting for up to 2 percent of patients in large series.[222] Big

Table 19–19. Signs and Symptoms of Bronchogenic Carcinoma: Pathologic Correlation

Sign/Symptom/Syndrome	Pathologic Feature
Features Related to Intrapulmonary Disease	
Cough	? Invasion of bronchial walls
Dyspnea	Volume loss secondary to obstruction
Chest pain	Nerve involvement in lung
Hemoptysis	Invasion of pulmonary or bronchial vessels
Wheeze or stridor	Airway obstruction by tumor
Pneumonia	Airway obstruction by tumor
Bronchiectasis or abscess	Airway obstruction by tumor
Lobar collapse	Usually airway obstruction by tumor; sometimes RML syndrome secondary to hilar node metastases
Features Related to Direct Extension from Lung	
Pleural effusion	Pleural spread
Hoarseness	Invasion of recurrent laryngeal nerve
Diaphragmatic paralysis	Invasion of phrenic nerve
Superior vena caval syndrome	Invasion or compression of SVC
Dysphagia	Invasion of esophagus
Chest pain	Invasion of chest wall
Cardiac tamponade	Invasion of pericardium
Pain or weakness of arm or shoulder[a]	Invasion of brachial plexus
Rib destruction[a]	Invasion of chest wall
Horner's syndrome[a]	Invasion of sympathetic ganglia

Abbreviations: RML, right middle lobe; SVC, superior vena cava.
[a] This combination of features comprises Pancoast's syndrome.

Table 19–20. Paraneoplastic Syndromes Produced by Lung Cancers[a]

General
  Anorexia
  Weight loss
  Fever
Vascular
  Disseminated intravascular coagulation
  Migratory thrombophlebitis
  Marantic endocarditis
Cutaneous
  Acanthosis nigricans
  Dermatomyositis
  Tylosis
Osseous
  Hypertrophic osteoarthopathy
  Clubbing
Neurologic
  Cerebellar degeneration
  Peripheral neuropathies
  Encephalopathy
  Myositis
  Myasthenia gravis–like syndromes
Endocrine/Neuroendocrine
  Cushing's syndrome
  Inappropriate secretion of ADH
  Hypercalcemia
  Gynecomastia
  Others (numerous hormones produced; only a fiew yield clinical disease)

Abbreviations: ADH, antidiuretic hormone.
[a] Based on the results of Cohen.[194]

or pro-adrenocorticotropic hormone (pro-ACTH), the precursor of the active ACTH molecule, can be found in 75 percent of tumors in some reports.[222–224] When levels of ACTH are measured in different types of tumor, the greatest amounts are always found in the small-cell carcinomas and clinically, Cushing's syndrome is almost always seen in patients with oat cell tumors or carcinoids,[222,225] and rarely with other types of tumor. Gropp and colleagues[219] found elevated levels of serum ACTH in 30 percent of patients with oat cell carcinoma.

Chorionic Gonadotrophin. About 5 percent of patients with lung cancer develop gynecomastia.[200] Any type of lung tumor may produce this hormone, but it is said to be seen especially with variants of giant cell or large-cell carcinoma[226]; the possibility that some of the latter are actually germ cell neoplasms arising in the lung should be considered (see p. 408). Gropp and colleagues[219] found elevated levels of chorionic gonadotrophin in 33 percent of patients with oat cell carcinoma, 26 percent of patients the large-cell carcinoma, and 19 percent of patients with squamous carcinoma.

Calcitonin. Silva and co-workers[227] report elevated levels of serum calcitonin in 62 percent of 26 men with lung cancer. Elevated levels were found largely with the small-cell and adenocarcinomas, and in some patients the calcitonin level varied directly with progression and regression of the tumor.

Parathyroid Hormone. Hypercalcemia is common in patients with lung cancer, even in the absence of bone involvement. It appears to be commonly mediated via production of parathormone or parathormone-like materials, and it more common with squamous and small-cell carcinomas. Gropp and colleagues[219] found that 32 percent of patients with squamous carcinoma and 27 percent of patients with oat cell carcinoma had elevated serum levels. Other substances, including prostaglandin E_2, also appear to be responsible in some instances for hypercalcemia.[228]

Antidiuretic Hormone. The vast majority of tumors producing the syndrome of inappropriate secretion of ADH are small-cell carcinomas.[89] George and colleagues[229] claim to illustrate an adenocarcinoma with what appear to be secretory granules in a patient with inappropriate ADH secretion; however, to me this tumor appears to be a carcinoid.

Histaminase and L-Dopa Decarboxylase. These enzymes are increased in small-cell carcinoma of the lung[230] and in medullary carcinoma of the thyroid, emphasizing the biochemical similarities if the not embryologic origin of the so-called APUD tumors. Of particular interest is the report of Abeloff and colleagues[231]

Table 19–21. Endocrine and Neuroendocrine Substances Produced by Lung Cancers

ACTH
MSH
Calcitonin
ADH
Chorionic gonadotropin
Growth hormone
Estradiol
Insulin
Glucagon
Renin
Gastrin
Erythropoietin
Histaminase
Dopa-decarboxylase
Alphafetoprotein
Carcinoembryonic antigen
Bombesin
Neuron-specific enolase

Abbreviations: ACTH, adrenocorticotropic hormone; ADH, antidiuretic hormone; MSH, melanocyte stimulating hormone.

comparing small-cell carcinomas that maintain their morphology with tumors that become either mixed or purely non-small-cell at autopsy; in these latter tumors the histaminase and dopadecarboxylase activities drop almost to zero.

Catecholamines. 5-hydroxytrophytophan, 5-hydroxytryptamine, and their metabolites have been reported in tissue and serum of small-cell carcinomas.[89,200] Gould and Chejfec[128] found 5-hydroxy 3-indolacetic acid, vanillylmandelic acid, and catecholamine activity in a series of "undifferentiated" lung tumors (*see* p. 331). All showed amine activity, despite the fact that no neurosecretory granules could be found in two of the small-cell tumors. They suggest that failure to observe granules may indicate insufficient sampling, inability of the tumor cells to properly store secretory product, or a cyclic mode of catecholamine production. Carcinoid syndrome, commonly ascribed to secretion of serotonin but more likely due to secretion of kinins, has occasionally been described in patients with small-cell carcinoma.[232]

Neuron-Specific Enolase and Bombesin. These substances have been described in small cell carcinomas[126,127] and may prove to be of use in the diagnosis of this type of tumor.

Miscellaneous Hormones. Estradiol, renin, insulin, glucagon, erythropoietin, and gastrin have all been described in lung cancers, but are exceedingly unusual.[200]

Fetoproteins. Alphafetoprotein is occasionally found in lung cancer,[200] but CEA is much more common. Initially thought to be specific for carcinoma of the colon, CEA has been shown to be elevated in all types of lung cancer. In the series of Vincent and colleagues,[233] 60 percent of patients with lung cancer did not have an elevated CEA, hence it is not useful as a screening marker. However, it was found that very high levels of CEA in the presence of a suspicious lesion were a good predictor of the presence of lung cancer, and levels as high as 15 ng/ml implied a very poor prognosis.

Patterns of Metastatic Spread

Details of the pattern of lymphatic spread are discussed by Spencer.[1] As a rule, the initial nodal metastases of bronchogenic carcinomas are to the hilar and mediastinal chains, but spread to nodes of the abdomen and cervical region is common. The direction and extent of spread is a function of location of the tumor and of histologic type. Ochsner and DeBakey[234] reviewed lymphatic spread in 1298 tumors and found that the tracheobronchial nodes were involved in 70 percent, the abdominal nodes in 20 percent, the cervical nodes in 17 percent, the auxillary nodes in 6 percent, and the supraclavicular nodes in 4 percent.

The routes of spread to hilar and mediastinal nodes are analyzed by Borrie[235] and are shown diagrammatically in Figure 19–16. In general, tumors spread initially to the ipsilateral hilar lymph nodes, and thence to the corresponding paratracheal lymph nodes. However, tumors from the left lung not infrequently cross the mediastinum to involve the right-sided lymph nodes. Lower lobe tumors may also spread to paraesophageal and paraphrenic lymph nodes.

Lung tumors may also spread outside the chest by direct lymphatic extension. Tumors in the apices that extend to the chest wall can penetrate supraclavicular and axillary node groups. Meyer[236] showed that direct pathways connect the lower lobes of the lung with the celiac and para-aortic lymph nodes.

In addition to almost universal lymphatic metastases, early widespread hematogenous dissemination of lung cancer is the rule. Careful examination of resection specimens reveals invasion of the pulmonary veins in the vast majority of cases[237]; once tumor has entered the veins it may spread to almost any organ in the body; presentation at distant locations, such as the tip of a digit, is not rare.

Patterns of Spread as a Function of Histologic Type of Tumor

As shown in Tables 19–22 and 19–23, the pattern of disease spread varies with histologic type of lung tumor. The data of Auerbach and co-workers[95] in Table 19–22 are derived from a large autopsy series and reflect the end stage of the disease. Overall in this series, metastatic disease was found in 96.3 percent of patients, with figures of 94 percent for squamous carcinoma, 99.4 percent for small-cell carcinoma, 96.4 percent for adenocarcinoma, and 96.8 percent for large-cell carcinoma. The data in Table 19–22 have been grouped into sites of regional and distant spread, and, except for a slightly higher value of pleural spread in adenocarcinomas (reflecting their initial peripheral location), the values for local spread are much the same for all types of tumor. Greater differences are seen in the metastases to distant sites: here the small-cell carcinomas clearly metastasize most fre-

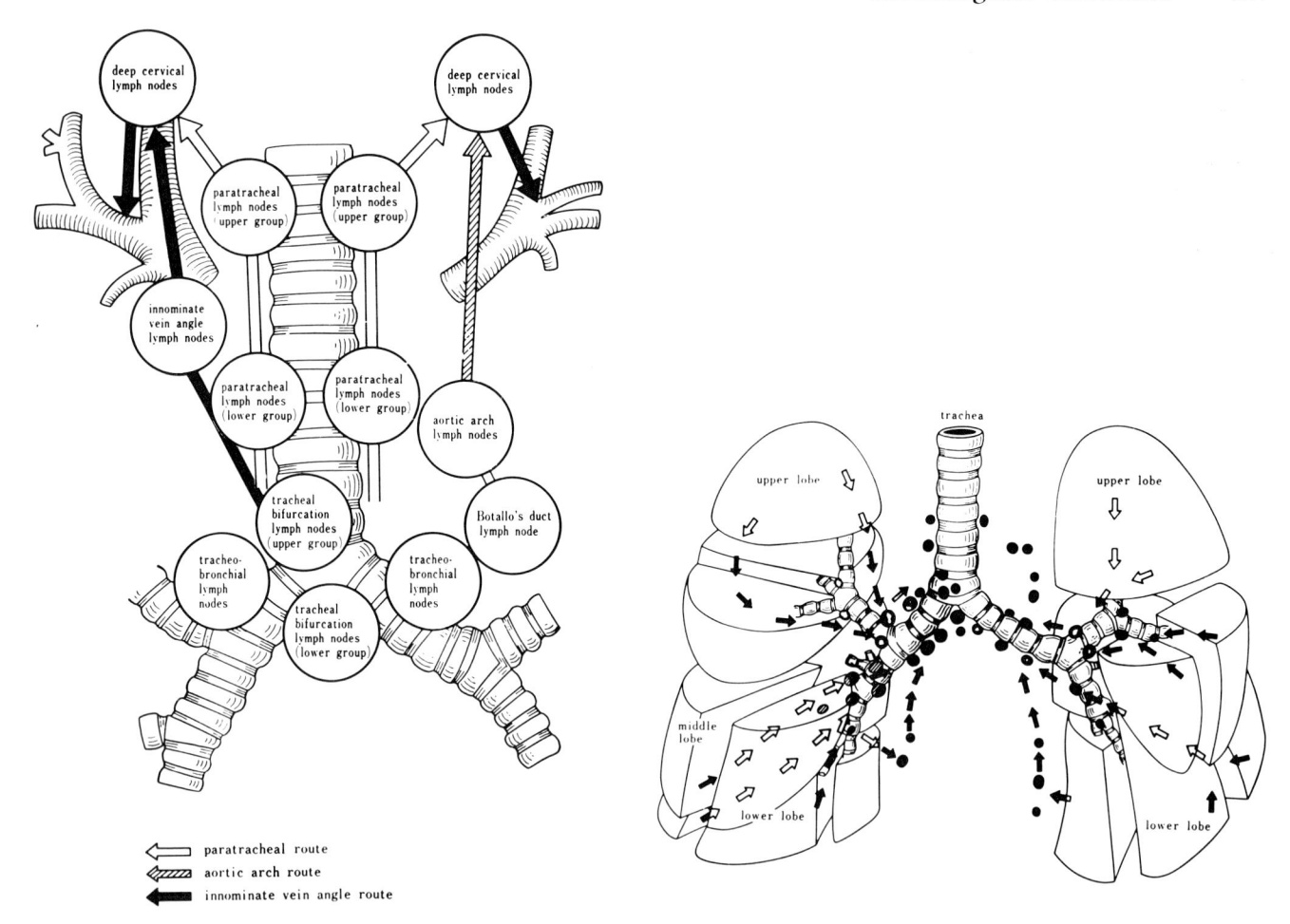

Figure 19–16. Lymphatic flow in the lung. Left. The various lymph node groups. Right. A schematic representation of the direction of lymph flow. Reproduced with permission from Nagaishi C: *Functional Anatomy and Histology of the Lung.* Tokyo: Igaku-Shoin.

quently, followed by the adenocarcinomas and large-cell carcinomas.

These differences are seen more clearly in the data of Matthews and colleagues[238] derived from a study of 202 patients dying within 1 month of a "curative" resection. Ignoring the values for large-cell carcinoma, which are based on few patients, it becomes apparent that at the very least one-third of patients (32.6 percent of those with squamous carcinoma, 68.4 percent of those with small-cell carcinoma, and 43.3 percent of those with adenocarcinoma) have residual disease after such a resection. In the patients with squamous carcinoma, about half have disease localized to the chest, whereas the vast majority of patients with adenocarcinoma and small-cell carcinoma who have residual disease already have metastases.

Matthews[136] has also examined patterns of spread as a function of histologic subtype. Matthews found that while about half of well-differentiated squamous carcinomas tended to remain in the chest, poorly differentiated tumors spread widely. Similarly, poorly differentiated adenocarcinomas behaved more aggressively than the well-differentiated forms, although the differences were

Table 19–22. Patterns of Lymphatic and Hematogenous Spread of Lung Cancer (Autopsy Series of 662 Patients)[a]

		Cell Type (% in Each Category)			
Site	Total	Squamous Carcinoma	Small-Cell Carcinoma	Adeno- carcinoma	Large-Cell Carcinoma
Regional nodes	89.1	83.3	95.7	91.0	89.4
Pleura	24.3	23.6	22.7	29.9	18.1
Chest wall	15.6	15.9	12.3	18.0	13.8
Pericardium	17.5	15.0	20.3	18.6	17.0
Esophagus	13.1	13.7	17.8	10.2	8.5
Distant nodes	44.6	29.2	62.0	47.9	44.7
Brain	44.7	35.9	50.0	46.8	49.2
Liver	44.1	37.1	61.7	42.4	33.3
Adrenal	33.7	20.0	44.4	41.2	35.5
Bone	29.5	25.6	35.0	43.7	24.5
Kidney	23.6	23.0	24.7	25.5	19.4

[a] Based on the results of Auerbach and co-workers.[95]

358 Tumors of the Lung

not as striking as for squamous cancers. Values for survival as a function of subtype are given in Prognosis of Bronchogenic Carcinoma, below.

Prognosis of Bronchogenic Carcinoma: Stage, Histologic Type, and Survival

As a general rule, survival with bronchogenic carcinoma is a function both of tumor stage and of the specific type of tumor. Staging of lung cancer is based on the system devised by the American Joint Committee for Cancer Staging and End Results Reporting[239]; a summary is shown in Table 19–24. The staging system is based on a T value which reflects size and direct extension of tumor, and N and M values which reflect the presence of nodal or distant metastases, respectively. As a rule, only stage I and II non-small-cell tumors are resected. Small-cell tumors are treated with radiation and chemotherapy (see Small-Cell Carcinomas, below), as are stage III non-small-cell tumors. For brief reviews of the results of radio and chemotherapy in non-small-cell tumors, see Muggia and Rozencweig.[240]

Hyde and colleagues[241] have reviewed the natural course of inoperable lung cancer treated only with supportive therapy. In a group of 1068 patients, the median survival rate was best related to cell type: small- and large-cell tumors had median survivals of approximately 7 weeks, squamous cell tumors of 10 weeks, and adenocarcinomas of 14 weeks.

The breakdown of patients presenting in each of the clinical stages is shown in data from the American Joint Committee for Cancer Staging and End Results Reporting[239] (Table 19–25). Overall, in this series of almost 2000 patients, 64 percent presented in stage III, 29.4 percent in stage I, and 6.6 percent in stage II. The preponderance of patients in stage III was found for all cell types, although it was greatest for small-cell carcinoma (83.9 percent) and least for squamous and large-cell cancers (56.9 percent and 57.0 percent, respectively). Since stage III cancers are generally not resected, only about one-third of all patients presenting with lung cancer can be considered as candidates for a potentially curative procedure.

The overall 5-year survivals for a slightly larger group of patients from the same study are listed in Table 19–26 and the actual survival curves are illustrated in Figure 19–17. For all clinical stages squamous carcinomas fare somewhat better than adenocarcinoma or large-cell carcinomas; small-cell carcinomas do very poorly, although recent chemotherapeutic regimes have improved survival (see below). However, as described above, the majority of patients present in stage III, and the overall survival for bronchogenic carcinoma in most series is less than 10 percent. Except for small-cell carcinomas, few changes in survival appeared to have occurred in the last 30 years. Wilkins and colleagues[242] reviewed the experience at the Massachusetts General Hospital and came to the disappointing conclusion that between 1941 and 1970 no improvement had occurred in the survival of resectable cases. Between 1964 and 1970, thoracotomy for cure was attempted in 29 percent of 1126 patients, and resection in 22 percent. The 5-year survival for those resected was 30 percent, producing an overall 5-year survival of about 7 percent. Glenn and colleagues[243] tabulated the results of seven different reports published between 1963 and 1971. Of 5754 patients, 47 percent were submitted to exploratory thoracotomy, and of those explored 62 percent had some sort of resection (that is, 29 percent of the original 5754 patients). The overall survival was again about 7 percent.

Detailed data on the effects of subtype are relatively scanty. Table 19–27 shows the 5-year survivals for subclasses of squamous carcinoma and adenocarcinoma from two different series. These data indicate that the well-differentiated squamous tumors tend to fare better than the poorly differentiated varieties. Overall it appears that, ignoring stage, poorly differentiated squamous carcinomas, most adenocarcinomas, and probably large-cell carcinomas have about the same behavior patterns and prognosis, and, therefore, histologic separation of these entities is not critical. The value, if any, of subtyping large-cell carcinomas is uncertain: Horie and Ohta[182] suggest that large-cell carcinomas that are squamous tumors by electron microscopy have a more favorable prognosis than those which turn out to be either adenocarcinomas or mixtures. However, their data are based on a small number of cases in which the majority of adenocarcinomas and mixed tumors were in stage III, whereas half the squamous tumors were stage I.

Small-Cell Carcinomas. Initially, small-cell carcinoma was treated by surgical resection with poor results. A report by the Medical Research Council[246] demonstrated that equal results could be obtained by radiation therapy (4 percent 5-year survival with mean survival of 284 days for patients treated with radiation, and 1 percent 5-year survival with mean survival of 199 days for patients treated surgically). Since that time surgery has generally been considered contraindicated,[247] although surgery is once again being suggested for the few patients who present with limited-stage disease.[248] For most cases, a variety of multidrug chemotherapeutic regimes along with local radiation are now used for these tumors. Overall, 3-year survival is now reported in 15 to 20 percent of those with limited-stage disease, but few or no patients with extensive-stage disease.[248] Reviews of current results may be found in Hande and Des Prez,[248] Lichter and Bunn,[249] Greco and Oldham,[250] and Cohen and Matthews.[251]

The importance of light microscopic subtyping of small-cell carcinomas is disputed. As shown in Table 19–28, this question has been addressed in five different series, three of which[139,141,141a] found essentially no differences in survival for patients treated with radiotherapy and chemotherapy. However, Nixon and colleagues[252] found that the oat cell and fusiform types of tumors had a longer median survival than the polygonal cell tumors, which they believed behaved more like non-small-cell carcinomas. Davis and associates[140] indicated that the oat cell type had longer survivals than the intermediate type. It should be noted that Carney and co-workers[139] examined the concordance between the histologic appearance

Table 19-23. Patterns of Spread of Lung Cancer in a Series of 202 Patients Dying Within 1 Month of a "Curative" Resection[a]

Site	Cell Type (% in Each Category)			
	Squamous Carcinoma	Small-Cell Carcinoma	Adeno-carcinoma	Large-Cell Carcinoma
Nodes	3.4	31.5	13.3	4.5
Adrenal	3.8	21.0	23.3	9.0
Liver	1.5	36.8	6.7	9.0
Brain	1.5	10.5	16.7	0
Kidney	1.7	10.5	3.3	13.6
Contralateral lung	1.7	5.2	0	9.0
Vertebra	0	5.2	10.0	4.5
Total with residual disease	32.6	68.4	43.3	13.7
Local disease only	16.8	5.2	3.3	0
Metastatic disease	16.8	63.2	40.0	13.7

[a] Based on the results of Matthews et al.[238]

Table 19-24. Staging of Lung Cancer[a]

T_x Categories (Tumor Size and Extent)
  T_x: Tumor proven by cytologic examination of bronchial secretions, but not visualized bronchoscopically or radiographically
  T_1: Tumor less than 3.0 cm in diamter
  T_2: Tumor larger than 3.0 cm in diamter
  T_3: Tumor of any size with direct extension out of lung or endobronchially within 2 cm of the carina, or associated with pleural effusion
N Categories (Regional Nodal Metastases)
  N_0: No metastases to regional or distant nodes
  N_1: Metastases to ipsilateral hilar lymph nodes
  N_2: Metastases to mediastinal nodes
M Categories (Distant Metastases)
  M_0: No distant metastases
  M_1: Distant metastases
Clinical Stages Based on TNM Categories
  Occult carcinoma: $T_xN_0M_0$
  Stage I
    $T_1N_1M_0$
    $T_1N_1M_0$
    $T_2N_0M_0$
  Stage II
    $T_2N_1M_0$
  Stage III
    T_3 with any N or M
    N_2 with any T or M
    M_1 with any T or N

[a] Based on the results of the American Joint Committee for Cancer Staging and End Results Reporting.[239]

of the primary tumor and of metastases, and found that in 26 percent of patients an additional or different subtype was present in the metastases. Hirsch and associates[141a] suggested that when large cells were also present (14 percent of their cases), survival was somewhat poorer, but they could not find differences between the oat cell and intermediate forms. One possible reason for these discrepancies is that the pure oat cell tumors may be the ones that respond well to chemotherapy, and that the subset of patients that consistently fail to respond[98] may be those who have a polygonal cell tumor which is actually a small-cell squamous carcinoma (see p. 330) or a mixed small-cell–squamous cell tumor. The problems of histologic subclassification are discussed on p. 335.

Bronchioloalveolar Carcinomas. Whether the behavior of these tumors is different from that of well-differentiated adenocarcinomas is difficult to determine, in large part because of uncertainties in the standards used by various authors for histologic classification, and because many authors fail to separate the disseminated tumors (which in some series, for example, that of Liebow,[156] account for almost 50 percent of cases) from the localized forms. Recent reports of 5-year survival for tumors that presented as solitary nodules, range from 23 percent[245] to 47 percent[253] and 100 percent.[254] The disseminated tumors are rapidly fatal.

Pancoast's Tumors. Paulson[197,255] has reported a 34 percent 5-year survival, Miller and colleagues[256] a 31 percent 5-year survival rate, and Attar and co-workers[257] a 23 percent 3-year rate for these tumors. The squamous

Table 19-25. Proportion of Patients Presenting with Various Stages of Lung Cancer[a]

Cell Type	No. Patients	Stage I (%)	Stage II (%)	Stage III (%)
Squamous	921	35.9	7.2	56.9
Small cell	360	10.5	5.6	83.9
Adenocarcinoma	513	9.4	5.5	65.1
Large cell	181	33.7	9.3	57.0
Total in stage I: 581 patients (29.4%)				
Total in stage II: 131 patients (6.6%)				
Total in stage III: 1263 patients (64.0%)				

[a] Based on the results of the American Joint Committee for Cancer Staging and End Results Reporting.[239]

Table 19–26. 5-Year Survivals for 2155 Patients with Lung Cancer by Stage and Cell Type[a]

Group	Squamous Carcinoma (%)	Adenocarcinoma (%)	Large-Cell Carcinoma (%)
All patients (N = 2155)	25	12	13
Surgically resected patients (N = 835)	37	27	27
Stage I patients	40	31	30
Stage II patients	17	7	6
Stage III patients	9	3	5
Resected stage I patients	54	51	
Resected stage II patients	35	18	
Resected stage III patients	19	10	

[a] Based on the results of the American Joint Committee for Cancer Staging and End Results Reporting[239] and Mountain.[244]
[b] Combined adenocarcinoma and large-cell carcinoma.

Table 19–27. Survival by Histologic Subtype for Squamous Carcinoma and Adenocarcinoma

	Katlic and Carter[245] %	Feinstein et al.[90] %
Squamous carcinoma (all)	18	16
Well differentiated	39	20[a]
Moderately differentiated	20	
Poorly differentiated	7	13
Adenocarcinoma	23	7
Well/moderately differentiated	24	10
Poorly differentiated	26	2

[a] Includes both well and moderately differentiated.

Table 19–28. Survival in Small-Cell Tumors by Histologic Subtype

Series	No. Cases	Outcome
Nixon et al.[252]	61	Oat cell and fusiform cell survived longer than polygonal cell
Burdon et al.[141]	46	No differences in survival
Carney et al.[139]	103	No differences in survival
Davis et al.[140]	626	When extensive disease present, survival longer for oat cell than intermediate cell group. No difference for limited disease.
Hirsch et al.[141a]	200	No differences, except those with admixed large cells (14%) had shorter survival

tumors apparently survive longer than the adenocarcinomas and large-cell carcinomas[197,255]. The occasional small-cell carcinoma presenting as a Pancoast's tumor appears to behave much as do central small-cell carcinomas.[258]

Uncommon Tumors of the Lung

Papillary Tumors of the Surface Epithelium

A variety of papillary tumors arise from the bronchial epithelium. Some have myxoid or inflammatory cores and a single bland-appearing layer of epithelial cells and are obviously benign.[259] More worrisome are the forms with multilayered epithelia, and determination of the malignancy of those neoplasms is difficult (Figure 19–18). In approximately 2 percent of patients with laryngotracheal papillomatosis, spread occurs to the bronchial tree,[260] and on rare occasions "papillomas" in this setting turn out to be malignant.[261–264] Spencer and co-workers[264] have recently reviewed the topic of papillary tumors of the bronchus and has presented 19 new cases of tumors that were noninvasive. These occurred in adults, with one exception, and were clinically characterized by cough, sputum production, and recurrent pneumonias. Several were incidental findings at autopsy or routine chest radiography. Histologically, most of the tumors were covered by squamous epithelium, or by a combination of squamous and mucus-secreting epithelia (so-called mucoepidermoid papillary tumors). The majority appeared cytologically benign, but dysplastic epithelium was not uncommon, and several cases demonstrated CIS.

Papillary endobronchial tumors of undoubted malignancy have been described by Sniffen and colleagues,[265] Sherwin and associates,[266] and Smith and Dexter.[267] Sherwin and associates[266] reported a frequency of nine papillary tumors among 85 bronchogenic carcinomas, but the ratio of 7 in 714 noted by Smith and Dexter[267] is a more realistic estimate of their frequency. These lesions largely occurred in middle-aged smokers; the presentation and radiographic appearance were similar to those described above. Grossly, several of the tumors were noted to extend for many centimeters along the bronchus, and usually obviously invaded the bronchial wall as well. Histologically the tumors were either squamous or mucoepidermoid; in some instances they appeared deceptively bland despite microscopic invasion of the bronchial wall; other examples were clearly cytologically malignant. The patients in these series were treated by resection; only 1 of 18 appears to have died of their initial tumor, although 2 developed subsequent tumors in the contralateral lung. These tumors are also extremely radiosensitive (C. B. Carrington, personal communication).

Because they may be histologically deceptive, papillary tumors of the bronchus in adults should always be

Uncommon Tumors of the Lung   361

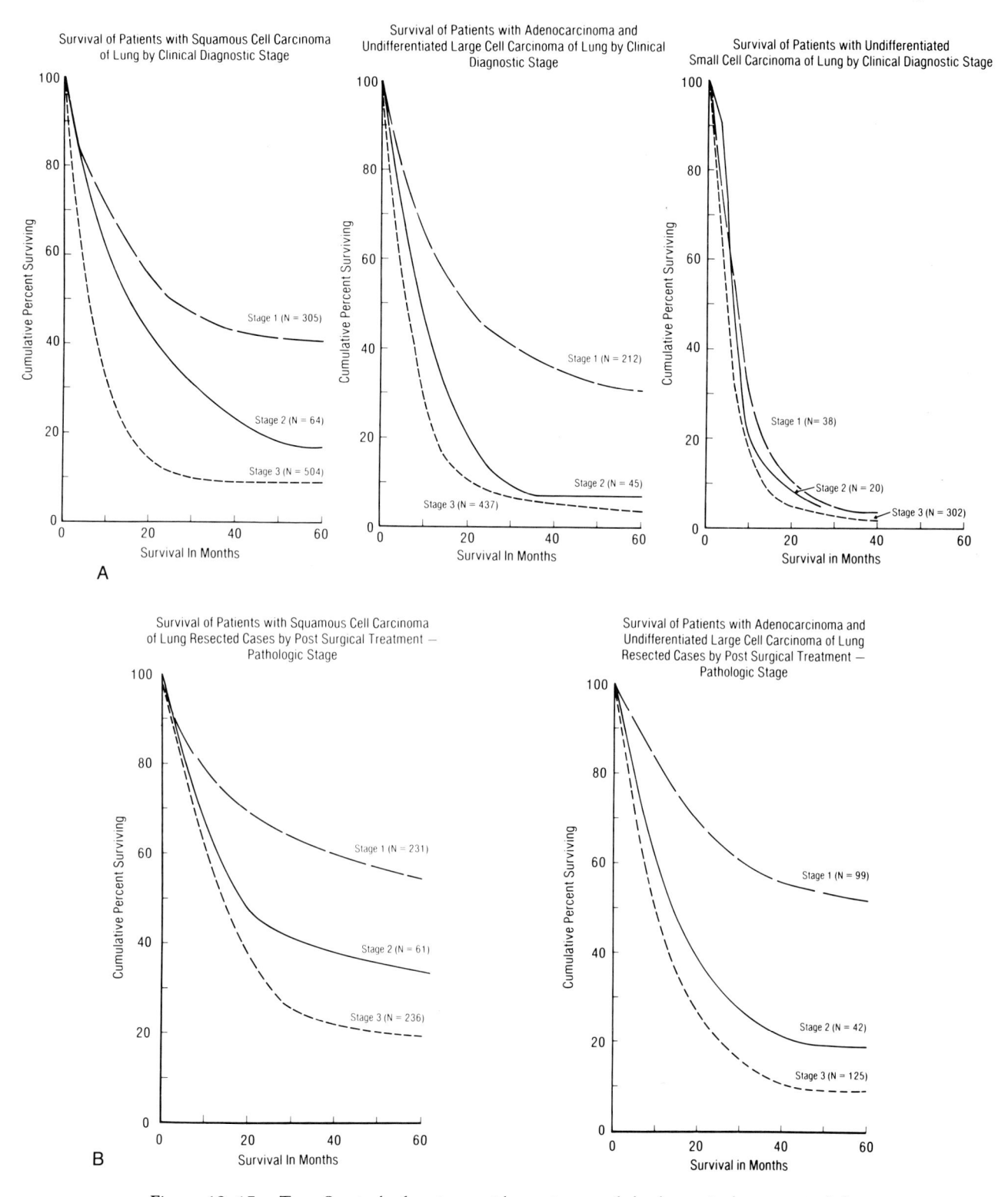

Figure 19–17. Top. Survival of patients with carcinoma of the lung. A shows survival for different histologic types of tumor by clinical stage. Bottom. Survival by postsurgical pathologic stage. Note that for any type of staging and any given stage squamous carcinomas tend to fare better than adenocarcinomas or large-cell carcinomas, all of which fare better than small-cell carcinomas. Reproduced with permission from American Joint Committee for Cancer Staging and End Results Reporting: *Straging of Lung Cancer 1979*.

viewed with suspicion and the diagnosis of benignancy made with great caution.

Carcinoid and Related Tumors

Carcinoids are the major subset of the group of tumors that previously were labeled "bronchial adenoma." Since none of these tumors (carcinoids, mucoepidermoid carcinomas, or adenoid cystic carcinomas) are benign, the term adenoma should not be used for the group. True bronchial adenomas do exist and are discussed on p. 379.

Of the unusual tumors of the lung, carcinoids as a whole are probably among the most frequent, accounting for 1 percent of all lung tumors.[268] Carcinoids may conveniently be divided into several groups: so-called tumorlets, peripheral carcinoids, central carcinoids, and atypical or high-grade carcinoids (Table 19–29). All share common morphologic and biochemical features.

Subclassification of the Carcinoids: Histogenesis and Ultrastructure. Carcinoids, like small-cell carcinomas, are generally considered to be related to the granule-containing K cells and neuroepithelial bodies of the bronchial epithelium[269–274] (also see Small-Cell Carcinomas, above). Experimental evidence (see p. 331) favors the notion that the immediate precursor cell of bronchial carcinoids, like that of small-cell carcinoma, differentiates from indifferent bronchial epithelial cells[123A,123B,275] rather than from so-called APUD cells that have migrated from the neural crest.[120]

Within the last few years, it has become apparent from a variety of morphologic, histochemical, and immunohistochemical evidence that "carcinoids" of the lung are not a homogeneous group of tumors.[276] Not all carcinoids of the lung and other organs possess the same structure, either at the light microscopic or submicroscopic level. Attempts have been made to subclassify the tumors in ways that will predict staining properties and eventually functional properties. Soga and Tazawa[277] evaluated 62 carcinoids from bronchus and gut and separated them into tumors with nodular solid nests (A type), tumors with trabecular or ribbon pattern (B type), tumors with tubular, acinar, and rosette-like structures (C type), and tumors of other structures (D type). Almost all of their bronchial carcinoids were B or D type. Correlations with staining showed that A-type carcinoids, which were the predominant forms in the midgut, were argentaffin positive and were considered to store serotonin, while the remaining types were argyophil positive and were considered to store 5-hydroxytryptophan, the precursor of serotonin. These findings were challenged by Jones and Dawson[278] who found that most bronchial carcinoids fell into Soga and Tazawa's[277] A or B groups. Nonetheless, argentaffin staining and formalin-induced fluorescence for the demonstration of 5-hydroxytryptamine were found only in the midgut tumors, regardless of pattern. It appears that, at least for bronchial carcinoids, serotonin production is not easily related to light microscopic pattern and that this type of pattern analysis is much less useful than immunohistochemical staining; for example, Warren and colleagues[277] found serotonin in 21 of 25 carcinoids by staining. Nonetheless, the light microscopic pattern may prove to have clearly defined functional (immunochemical) correlations with other substances.

The morphologic heterogeneity suggested by the observations just described has also become apparent in recent reports of the ultrastructure of bronchial carcinoids. The ultrastructure of bronchial carcinoids was first examined by Bensch and colleagues[296] and Gmelich and associates[280] who showed that the tumor cells were characterized in general by long cellular processes, small but well-formed desmosomes, and the presence of numerous neurosecretory granules. More recent studies have made it apparent that several different types of cells containing several different morphologic types of granules are found in these tumors[129,270,281–283] although the terminology used by various authors for these different granules is confusing and somewhat contradictory and it is difficult to be certain how many different granule types actually exist. Detailed illustrations of the different types of granules can be found in Hage and co-workers[281] and Capella and associates.[282]

Not only are there different types of granules in different carcinoid tumors, but there are differences in cell organization at the ultrastructural level as well.[281,282] At least two different forms have been described[281,282] so-called trabecular, and so-called paragangloid. The trabecular forms were composed of polygonal cells that formed microacini in the traditional carcinoid pattern, whereas the two tumors of the "paragangloid" type were composed of cells with long processes, often containing empty vesicles as well as dense core granules. Granules and vesicles were grouped near focal thickenings of the membranes and fusions of the membranes of adjacent cells were observed. This structure is claimed to resemble that of true paragangliomas and suggests that some tumors that appear to be bronchial carcinoids are actually paragangliomas.[281,282] The criteria by which one might make such a distinction are not entirely clear; presumably true pulmonary paragangliomas, by analogy with other true APUD tumors, would be composed of cells that had indeed migrated from the neural crest, and presumably these cells would be producing epinephrine or norepinephrine. Occasional tumors producing these substances have been described in the lung (see p. 373).

Substances Produced by Carcinoids

As noted in the section on Small-Cell Carcinomas, above, differences in granule type presumably correspond to secretion of different peptides, and it is clear from immunochemical studies that carcinoids can produce a wide variety of peptide products. Cutz and co-workers[284] showed that the small carcinoids commonly called tumorlets contained bombesin, calcitonin, and serotonin when examined by immunohistochemical staining, but these investigators were only able to demonstrate serotonin in larger tumors. Presumably this result is a fixation or methodologic problem, since Warren and associates[279] found a variety of substances including serotonin, neuron—specific enolase, bombesin, vasoactive intestinal polypeptide (VIP), gastrin, leu-enkephalin, MSH, so-

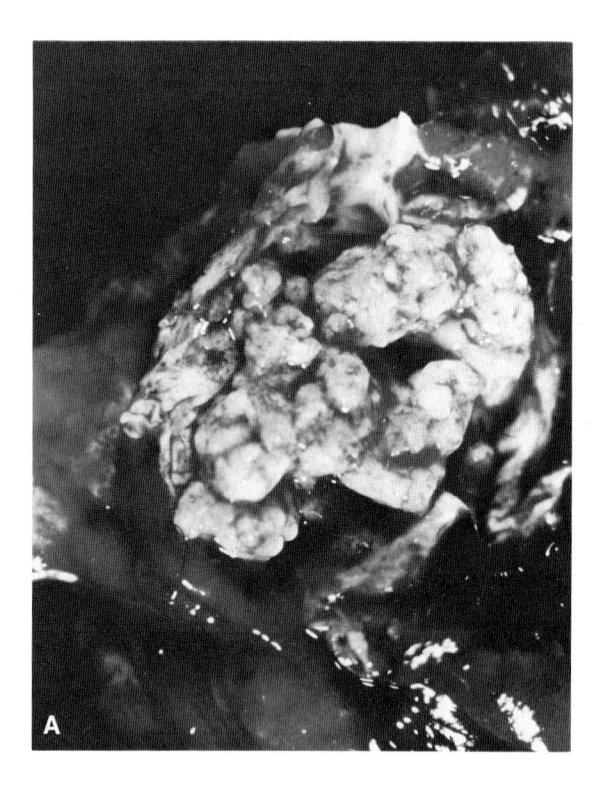

Figure 19–18A–C. Papillary tumors of the surface epithelium. A. Gross appearance of a large multilobulated tumor that distends the bronchus. B and C. A papillary intrabronchial tumor of obvious cytologic malignancy. Note the presence of carcinoma in situ as well as obvious cytologic atypia in C (B ×40, C ×160).

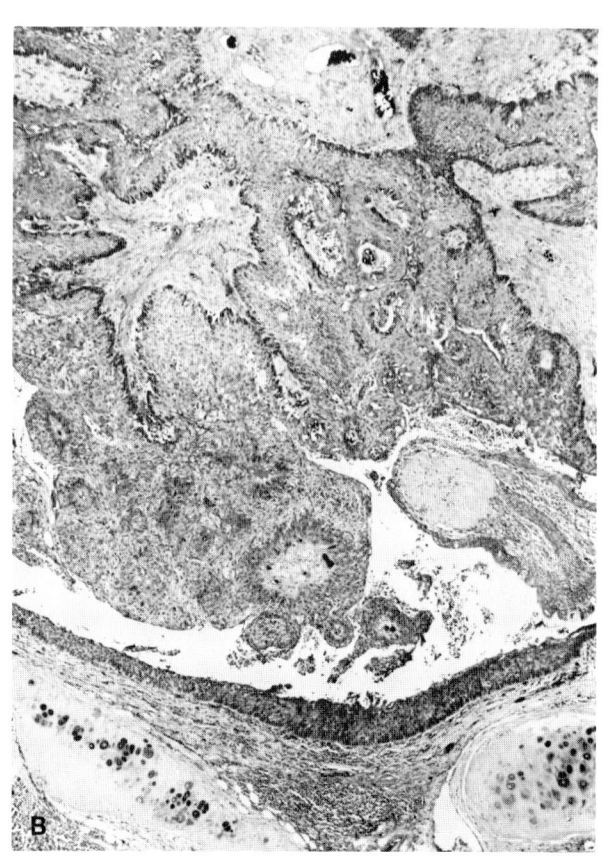

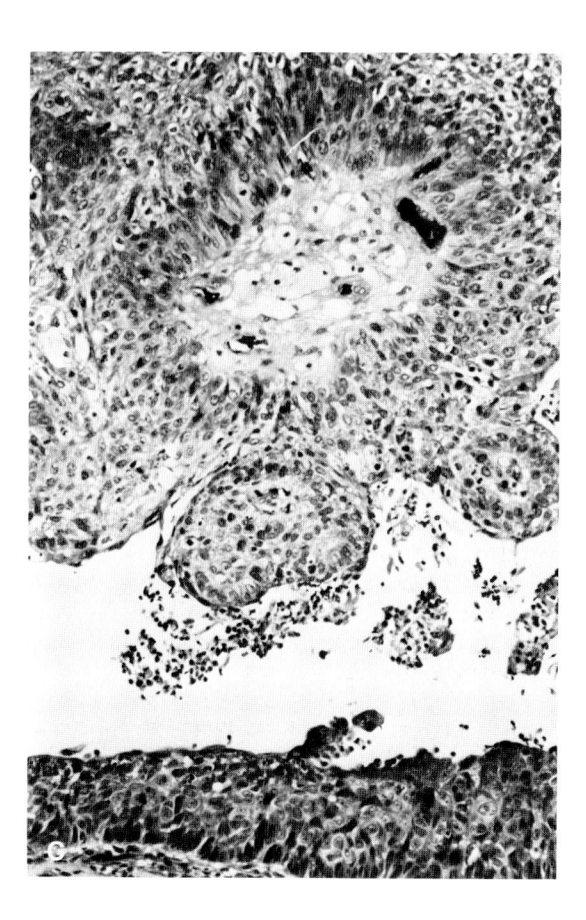

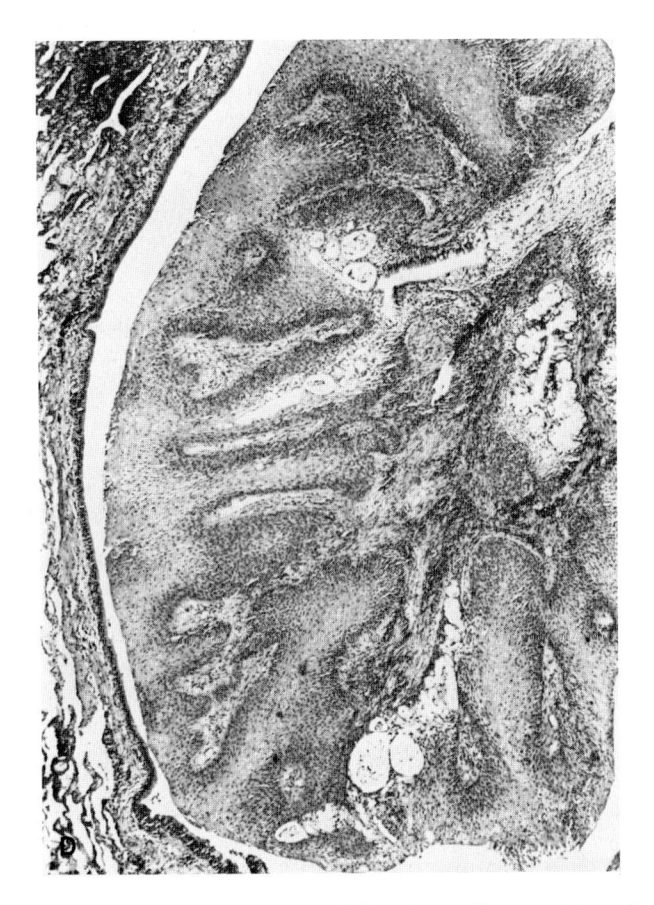

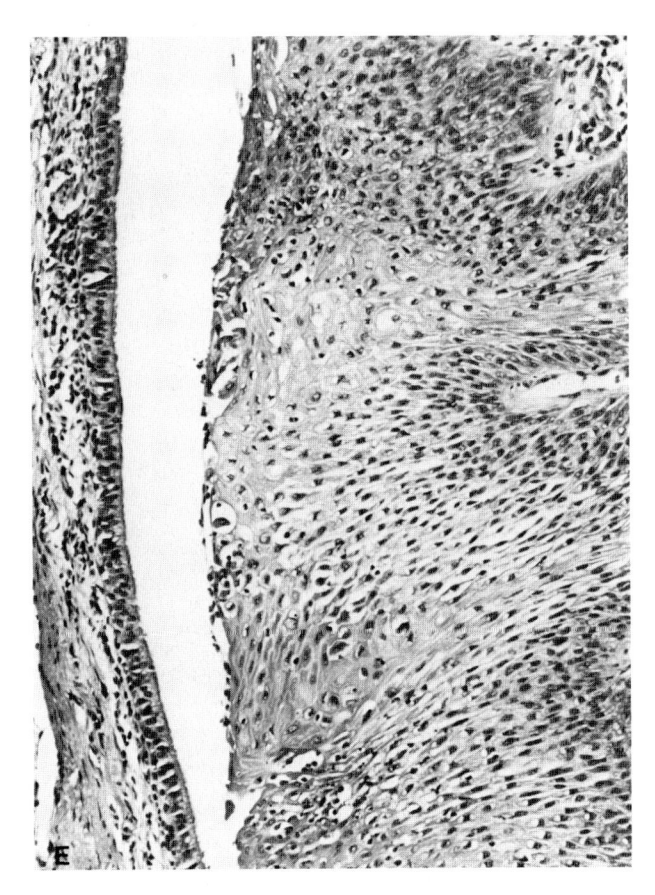

Figure 19–18D,E. A papillary endobronchial tumor of deceivingly bland appearance. A low-power view is shown in D and a higher-power view in E. Although this tumor appears to be histologically innocuous it had invaded out of the bronchus of origin (D ×40, E ×160).

matostatin, substance P, and calcitonin in a series of ordinary low-grade carcinoids; in 24 of 25 cases at least two hormones were produced, and in some cases up to eight different hormones were found. Neuron-specific enolase is probably the best current marker for these tumors: Sheppard and colleagues[125A] found it in 16 of 18 cases and Warren and associates[279] in 24 of 25 cases. Adrenocorticotropic hormone was not found in any of the tumors studied by Warren and associates,[279] and Gould and associates[123A,123B] suggest that the appearance of "ectopic" hormones, particularly ACTH, signifies a tumor of high grade, a suggestion of practical diagnostic importance. However, Tsutsumi and co-workers[284A] claim that low-grade carcinoids also produce ACTH.

Correlations of ultrastructural granule type with substances produced have thus far been based on biochemical or functional rather than immunohistochemical studies. The P_1 (type I) granules apparently store catecholamines[271,272,283] (see Hage[281] and Capella and co-workers[282,283] for definitions of granule types). Some carcinoids with large granules also probably store catecholamines.[129,285] The carcinoids and oat cell carcinomas that have been studied and that have produced ACTH, MSH, growth hormone, vasopressin, and corticotropin-releasing factor have all had P_a-type granules.[229,286–289]

Intestinal carcinoids classically produce the carcinoid syndrome, a combination of diarrhea, intestinal obstruction, and fibrous proliferation on the endocardium and valves of the heart, all thought to be mediated by serotonin production,[290] and flushing, especially of the face, believed to be mediated by catecholamine activation of kallikrein.[291,292] Normally the lung inactivates seroto-

Table 19–29. Types of Carcinoid Tumors Found in the Lung

Tumorlet
Peripheral carcinoid
Central carcinoid
High-grade carcinoid
Oncocyte carcinoid
Carcinoid resembling medullary carcinoma of thyroid

nin and cardiac fibrosis is not usually seen with bronchial carcinoids; rarely endocardial fibrosis on the left side is seen with primary pulmonary tumors.[293] As opposed to intestinal carcinoids, carcinoid syndrome is relatively rare with bronchial tumors (2 to 7 percent of cases,[294–296] and is usually found only when extensive liver metastases are present (62 of 64 cases summarized by Ricci and co-workers.[294]) Most bronchial carcinoids secrete relatively little serotonin (although, as noted above, many produce it) and contain relatively large amounts of its inactive precursor, 5-hydroxytryptophan, instead. In addition to serotonin, at least some symptoms of carcinoid syndrome appear to be mediated by kinin release,[297] and some serotonin-negative tumors may produce effects via these mediators.

Cushing's syndrome is the next most frequent of the ectopic hormone syndromes produced by bronchial carcinoids. Mason and co-workers[298] record 28 cases. In Mason's series, only 10 of 26 tumors were seen radiographically during the first 6 months after the diagnosis of hypercorticism, hence the diagnosis may be difficult. It is my impression from observation of clinical cases that ACTH producing carcinoids are likely to be of relative high-grade malignancy, a theory in accord with the ideas of Gould and colleagues[123A,123B] mentioned above. Carcinoids may also produce corticotropin-releasing factors.[289]

Other substances are sometimes secreted by carcinoid tumors in amounts sufficient to cause clinical symptoms; Warren and associates[279] suggest that these syndromes are, like Cushing's syndrome, markers of high-grade rather than low-grade tumors. Sonksen and co-workers[286] discuss acromegaly produced by bronchial carcinoids. This may be caused either by the production of growth hormone or growth hormone–like substances by the tumor, or by the production of a growth hormone releasing factor. Melanocyte stimulating hormone can be found in many carcinoids that produce ACTH.[289] George and co-workers[229] report production of antidiuretic hormone from a tumor which, from the illustration, appears to be a carcinoid, probably of high grade.

A variety of other substances have been described in bronchial carcinoids, largely as individual case reports: these include prolactin, parathormone, calcitonin, insulin, glucagon, and VIP.[282,283]

Occasionally bronchial carcinoids are found in the multiple endocrine adenomatosis syndromes, and even more rarely produce a carcinoid syndrome in this situation.[299–302]

Central Carcinoids

The common carcinoids are central carcinoids. These comprised 168 of 203 morphologically typical carcinoids reported by Okike and colleagues,[303] a figure that is probably representative of the relative distribution of carcinoids in the lung. Salyer and Salyer[304] found 22 central and 6 peripheral carcinoids in another series. Most series show a roughly equal male/female distribution. The age range is wide, varying from childhood[305] to the seventh, eighth, and ninth decades; the median age is around 50 (58 in Okike's series), a figure not unlike that for lung cancer, despite the absence of any relationship between carcinoids and smoking.

The majority of patients with central carcinoids are symptomatic, presenting variably with cough, hemoptysis, pneumonia secondary to obstruction, and fever. Frequently symptoms have been present for many months to years before the tumor is discovered. X-ray examination demonstrates a mass lesion in one-third to half the cases (Fig. 19–19A to C), but it is not uncommon for the tumor to be radiographically invisible. Such cases may show no lesion or evidence of obstruction or bronchiectasis.

Carcinoids are soft fleshy tumors which may be yellow, pink, or grey on cut section. Traditionally the tumor is seen by the bronchoscopist as a mass lesion covered by smooth-surfaced bronchial epithelium which may be partially ulcerated (see Fig. 19–17F, G). Sometimes the tumor is pedunculated and entirely intraluminal (3 of 16 of the cases of Salyer and colleagues,[304] 50 of 168 of Okike's[303] cases) but this appearance is deceptive and attempts at resection by scraping through a rigid bronchoscope are almost certain to leave residual neoplasm. More commonly the tumor is a sessile mass broadly attached to the bronchial wall, and frequently extending through it (Fig. 19–19D, E). The tumor may also take the form of an iceberg, with the majority lying extraluminally, a situation not unlike that of oat cell carcinoma to which it is probably related. Tumor sizes range from 0.5 to 6 to 8 cm. There is a predilection for the segmental bronchi of the lower lobes, but central carcinoids may also occur in mainstem bronchi.

Microscopically the typical central carcinoid is composed of polygonal cells with pale or eosinophilic cytoplasm (Fig. 19–19H). The nuclei have stippled to vesicular chromatin. The cells are commonly arranged in nests, ribbons, trabeculae, and sometimes in acini which secrete mucin.[306] Electron microscopic examination reveals numerous neurosecretory granules (Fig. 19–19I), as described above. Staining with argyrophilic stains demonstrates the cytoplasmic granules with comparative ease; argentaffin stains are occasionally positive as well. Hosoda and co-workers,[285] have suggested that this phenomenon indicates those tumors that actually produce serotonin, as opposed to the majority of bronchial carcinoids in which amine metabolism proceeds only as far as the production of 5-hydroxytryptophan. The stroma of bronchial carcinoids of the central type is most commonly composed of a fine network of capillary channels, rendering the tumor quite vascular. In other instances, the stroma may be composed of fibrous or fibroelastic tissue and occasionally is ossified, calcified, or hyalinized.[307] Rarely amyloid may be present. It has been argued that ossification merely reflects previous necrosis and calcification, but it is also likely that some tumors secrete substances that cause osteoblastic reactions, a phenomenon seen with metastases to bone as well.[307]

Figure 19–19A,B. Central carcinoid tumor. A. Carcinoid tumor presenting with a radiographically visible mass in the right lower lobe. B. Carcinoid tumor presenting with evidence of obstruction on the left side.

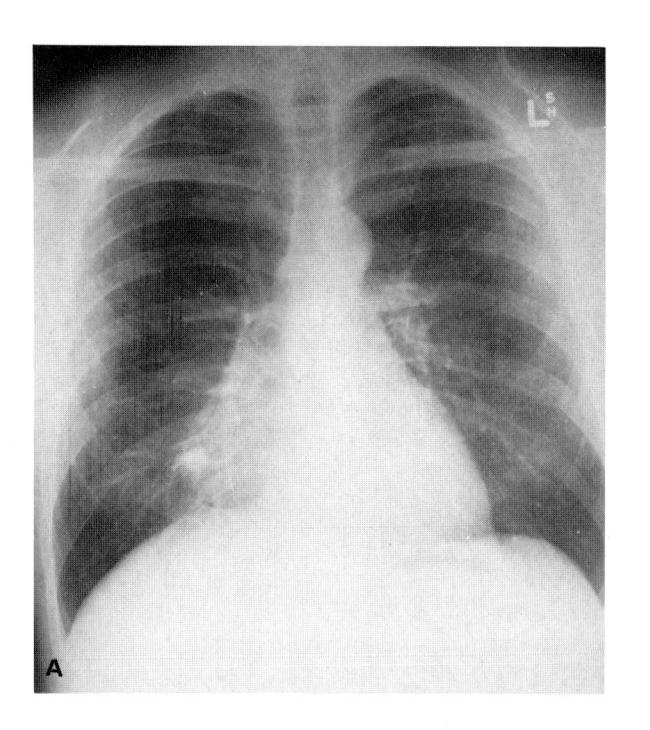

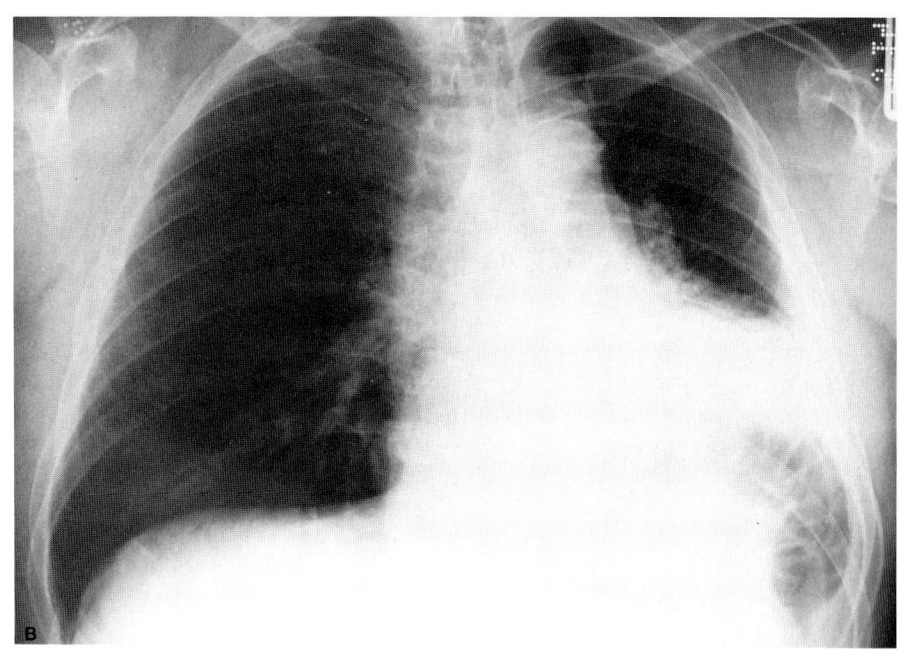

Peripheral Carcinoids

If one defines peripheral carcinoids as tumors located beyond the segmental bronchi, then probably one-fourth of macroscopic carcinoids occur in this location. Peripheral carcinoids show a remarkable microscopic heterogeneity, and should always be considered in the differential diagnosis of peripheral lung tumors.

The smallest of the peripheral carcinoids are the so-called tumorlets, also referred to originally by Liebow[308] as "carcinoid atypical proliferation." In general, tumorlets are incidental findings in lungs resected for other reasons; they are almost invariably multiple. They are not uncommonly associated with other larger peripheral carcinoids, and occasionally have been associated with Cushing's syndrome.[309] Tumorlets may occur both in scars and otherwise normal lung (Fig. 19–20A, B).

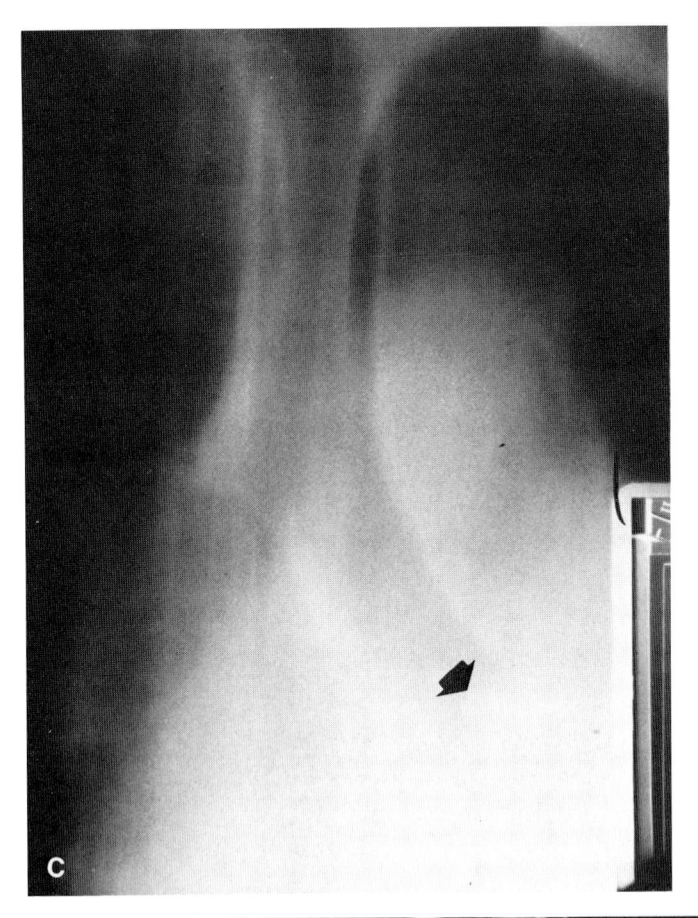

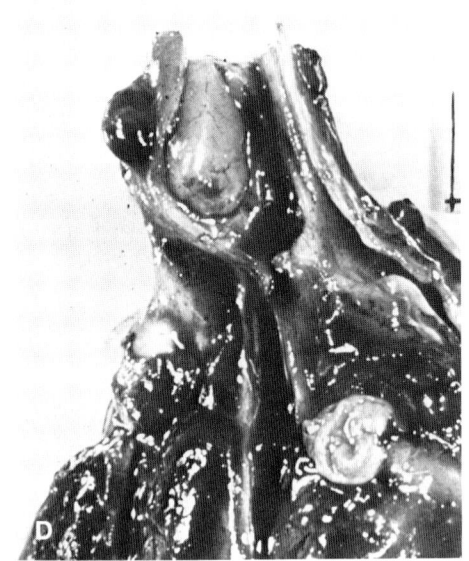

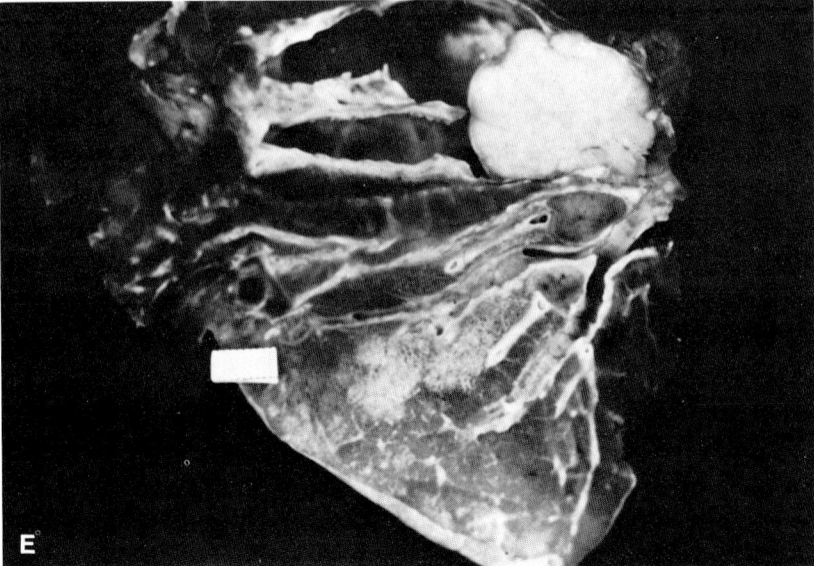

Figure 19–19C–E. Tomogram (C) shows a round mass completely occluding the lumen of the bronchus. D. Gross appearance of carcinoid tumor in a resection specimen; note the smooth surface appearance. E. Carcinoid tumor producing bronchiectasis as a result of obstruction. Obstructive pneumonia is also visible as a lighter area in the parenchyma.

Rare instances of tumorlet nests in hilar nodes have been noted; these have no clinical significance.

Tumorlets were initially regarded as forms of early invasive or in situ oat cell carcinoma, but it was soon realized that such patients never showed other evidence of oat cell carcinoma. Various other names such as peripheral adenoma and atypical proliferation of bronchiolar epithelium were also applied until Whitwell[77] coined the term "tumorlet" which has remained in the literature. Morphologically the usual tumorlet consists of nests of small spindled cells arranged in arrays. The nuclei are elongate and the chromatin stippled and fairly hyperchromatic. Mitoses are almost never observed. The cytoplasm is scanty and eosinophilic (Fig. 19–20C).

The nature of tumorlets has been debated, but recent studies have made clear their relationship to larger carcinoids and to granule-containing cells of the bron-

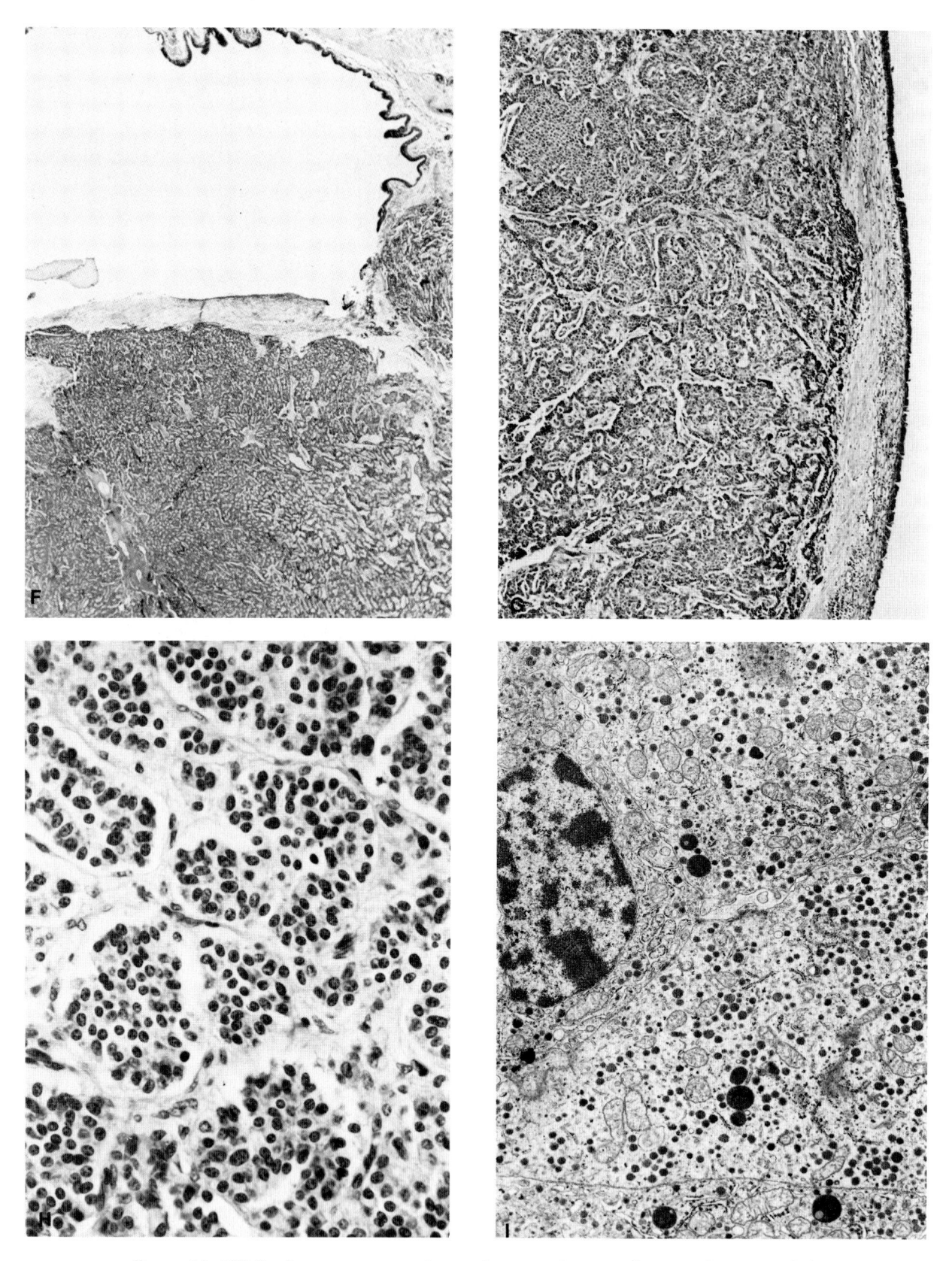

Figure 19–19F–I. Low-power view of central carcinoid tumor showing ulceration of the bronchial mucosa over the tumor mass (×20). G. Central carcinoid tumor underlying intact bronchial epithelium. When the bronchial epithelium is intact the tumor appears to have a smooth grey surface, such as that shown in D (×64). H. Histologic appearance of typical central carcinoid showing regular cells arranged in nests (×400). I. Electron micrograph of central carcinoid tumor showing numerous neurosecretory granules (×4000).

chial tree. Churg and Warnock[84] examined 20 cases and showed that although one-third occurred in association with bronchiectatic scarring or other inflammatory processes, in fact the majority were found in unscarred lungs, contrary to previously held notions. Three cases were examined by electron microscopy and neurosecretory granules were found; these averaged about 900 A in diameter in material reprocessed from paraffin. Argyrophilic granules were demonstrated in the remaining cases. These authors concluded that tumorlets were indeed forms of peripheral carcinoid. A similar conclusion was reached by Bonikos and associates[310] who also found small granules in the tumor cells. Ranchod[67] presented an unusual case which demonstrates the origin of the tumorlet. In a patient with an oat cell carcinoma, multiple tumorlets were observed. In addition, he showed that one could find proliferation of granule-containing cells in varying numbers in many bronchioles; these proliferations ranged from linear groups to small aggregates, the latter representing the earliest "tumorlet." The proliferation of the tumorlet cells was accompanied by formation of elastic tissue and scarring in the underlying bronchiolar wall; the lumen was soon obliterated. Finally the cells nests spread into the immediately surrounding lung and into the bronchial scar, producing the typical tumorlet pattern.

As described above, there are differences in the secretory products demonstrable in tumorlets and larger carcinoids by immunohistochemical staining. Cutz and co-workers[284] suggest that the pattern of staining in tumorlets is more like that of normal bronchial epithelium, and hence that tumorlets are actually hyperplastic rather than neoplastic. Although this hypothesis fits the facts, so does the theory that tumorlets are merely better "differentiated" than large carcinoids.

Macroscopic peripheral carcinoid tumors blend into tumorlets and the dividing line is arbitrary. I generally call any carcinoid tumor larger than 3 or 4 mm a carcinoid and use tumorlet for the smaller sizes. Radiographically they are usually coin lesions (Fig. 19-20H). Peripheral carcinoids may range up to 6 cm in size and macroscopically are similar to central carcinoids (Fig. 19-20D). Careful observation frequently discloses a small bronchiole to one side of the tumor; if this is not visible grossly it can usually be found microscopically. Peripheral carcinoids are characterized microscopically by a wide variety of patterns (Fig. 19-20E, F, I, J). The most easily identified are those that resemble central tumors and are composed of similar nests of polygonal cells. More frequently, however, other patterns are found. Spindle carcinoids are one of the most common; the cells resemble those of tumorlets. More interesting are the forms in which the cells are considerably larger and appear more like smooth muscle or nerve cells; often the cytoplasm of such tumors is copious and eosinophilic[311-313] (Fig. 19-20E, F). Other forms that have been described resemble vascular tumors, either with cells arranged around vascular cores, a pattern similar to that of sclerosing hemangioma, or arranged in a fashion that mimics hemangiopericytoma[314] (Fig. 19-20I, J). The cells of such tumors vary from spindled to cuboidal and the granules are usually in the order of 1100 to 1400 A in diameter (Fig. 19-20G). Electron microscopically a variety of patterns are seen, varying from cuboidal cells with microvilli and no processes to cells demonstrating elaborate interdigitations.

Both peripheral and central carcinoids are commonly surrounded by a capsule of fibrous and elastic tissue and invasion of this capsule is almost universal; however, there is no prognostic significance to this finding.

Prognosis of Carcinoids and High-Grade Forms

The prognosis for carcinoids is related to histologic features to a large extent. However, like other endocrine tumors, they are also somewhat unpredictable in behavior. Okike and colleagues[303] cite a 94 percent 5-year survival for 160 patients with typical bronchial carcinoids; the survival rate for the central tumors was 96 percent at 5 years and for the peripheral tumors 87 percent at 5 years. A partial breakdown of the figures of Okike and colleagues[303] is shown in Table 19-30.

Godwin[268] found in a series of more than 200 tumors a 96 percent 5-year survival for those tumors confined to lung, and a 71 percent 5-year survival for those with metastases to regional nodes. In Okike's[303] series of morphologically typical tumors, 5.4 percent had nodal metastases at the time of resection. These figures are in contrast to some in the literature in which survival rates as low as 59 percent[315] are cited for carcinoids. The descriptions in these instances suggest that at least some were high-grade tumors, either carcinoids or ordinary carcinomas.

By contrast, a group of carcinoid tumors exists that exhibit histologically malignant features (Fig. 19-21) and behave aggressively. These tumors are commonly referred to as "atypical" carcinoids; since this term is also used for some of the low-grade but histologically unusual peripheral forms, I prefer to label the clearly malignant forms: "High-grade carcinoid." Gould and colleagues[123A,123B] suggest that they be called "well-differentiated neuroendocrine carcinomas," a term that emphasizes both their histogenesis and behavior. In some instances high-grade carcinoids are difficult to distinguish from small-cell carcinomas.

Most of these tumors have been reported as individual cases, but Arrigoni and colleagues[316] investigated 23 such patients from the larger group reported by Okike and associates,[303] and Mills and colleagues[317] have recently added 17 more cases. It is of interest that 16 of 17 of the

Table 19-30. Survival for Patients with Central Carcinoid Tumors[a]

	5 Years	10 Years	20 Years	25 Years
Peripheral	87	83	70	60
Central	96	88	77	67

[a] Based on the results of Okike et al.[303]

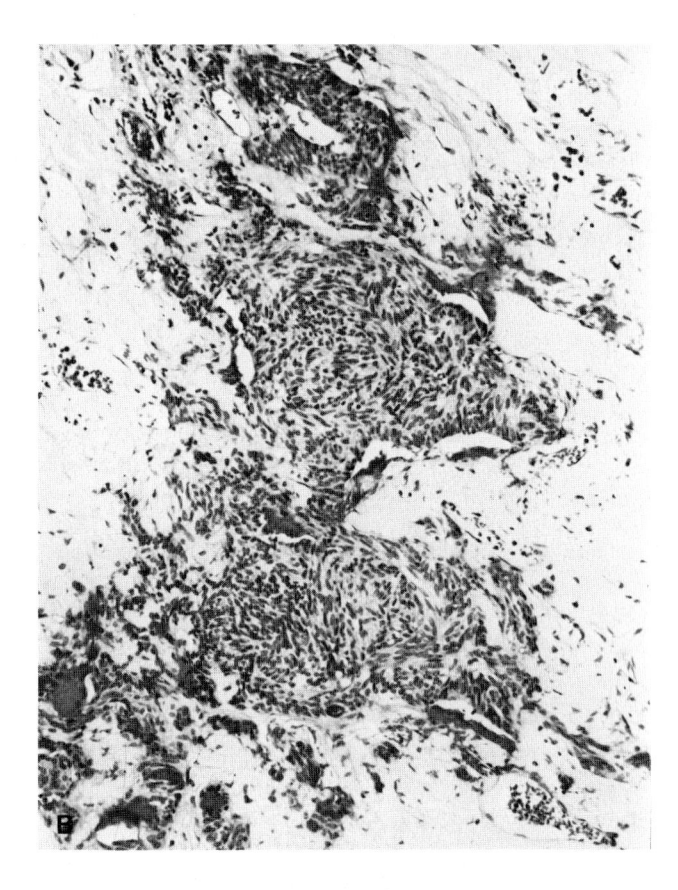

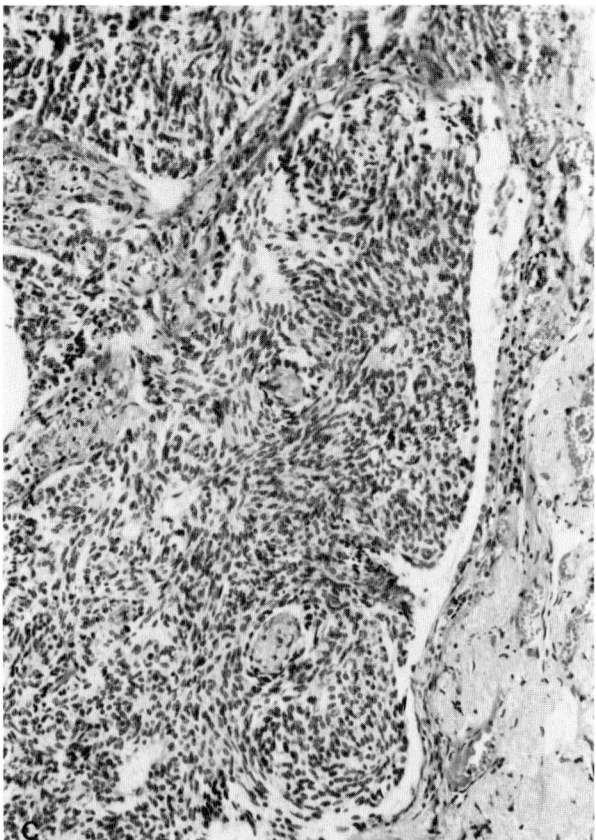

Figure 19–20A–C. Peripheral carcinoid tumors. A and B, So-called tumorlet type of carcinoid, occurring in otherwise normal lung (A) and in a scar (B). The tumor consists of nests of spindled cells. The appearance of invasion of lymphatics is common in these lesions but is probably of no clinical significance (A ×40, B ×64). C. Higher-power view of typical tumorlet cells. These are spindled, uniform, and bland (×160).

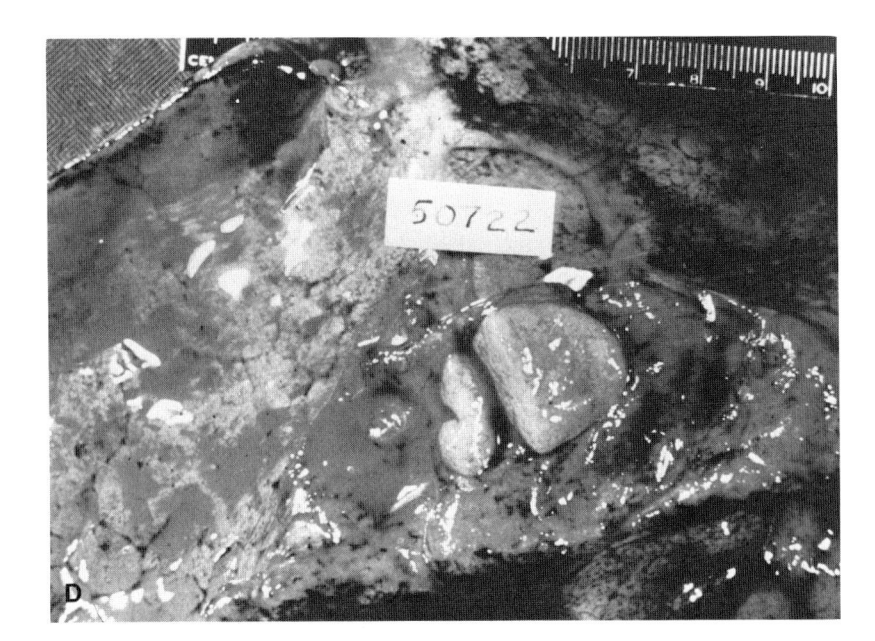

Figure 19–20D–F. D. Gross appearance of a peripheral carcinoid arising in a young woman. E and F. Microscopic appearance of the tumor shown in D, note the resemblance to smooth muscle or neural tissue (E ×40, F ×400).

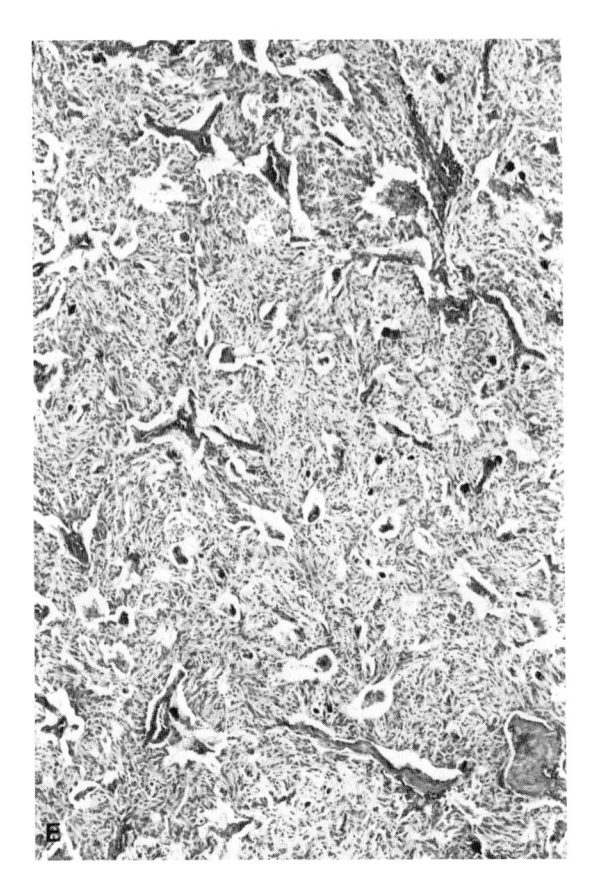

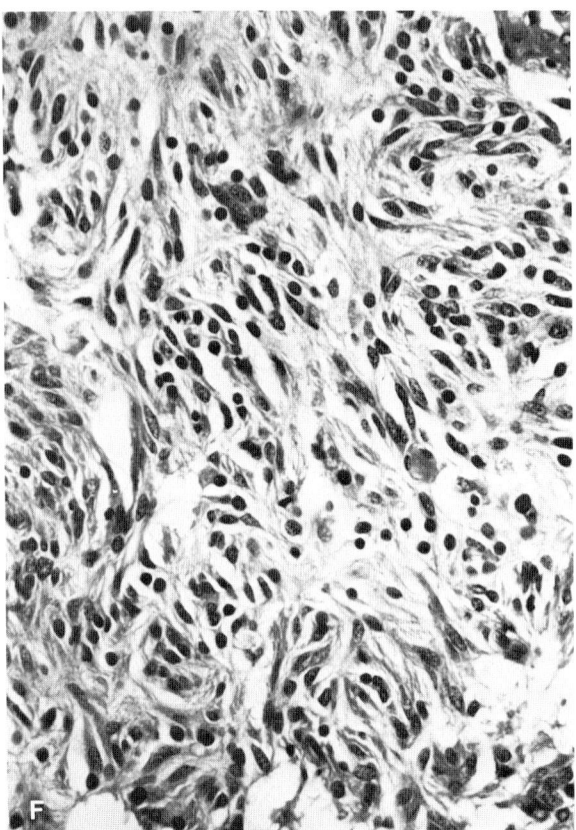

patients reported by Mills and colleagues[317] smoked cigarettes, since low-grade carcinoids are not associated with cigarette smoking.

Grossly, some of the tumors showed necrosis, but were not otherwise different from the low-grade forms; they averaged 4 to 5 cm in size, comparable to that of the typical tumors. Half the tumors in the series of Arrigoni and co-workers [316] were central. Histologically the distinctive features were cytologic evidence of malignancy, and included increased mitotic rate, nuclear abnormalities, and high cellularity. In some instances a spindled or oat cell pattern highly resembling that of small-cell carcinoma was present.

Peripheral carcinoids composed of spindled cells have

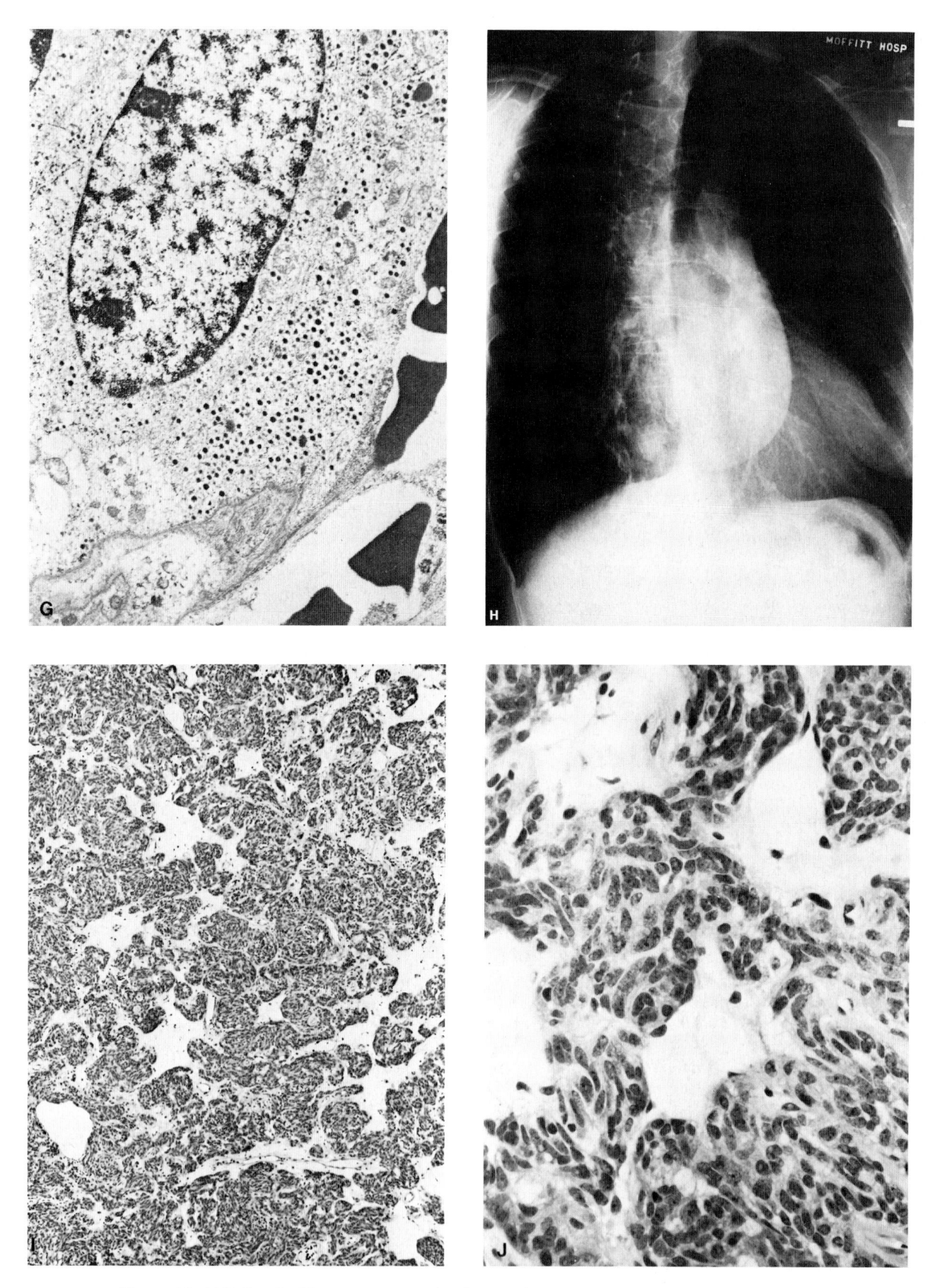

Figure 19–20G–J. G. Electron micrograph of tissue from the same tumor reprocessed from paraffin. Numerous neurosecretory granules are obvious even in this quality of preparation (×3000). H. Chest radiograph showing a lesion found behind the heart in a patient presenting with cough. I and J. Microscopic appearance of tumor shown in H. Histologically this resembles a hemangiopericytoma, but electron microscopy revealed numerous neurosecretory granules (I ×40, J ×400).

been labeled "atypical," with the implication of aggressive behavior. Spindled shape probably does not imply high-grade malignancy. Ranchod and Levine[313] examined 35 spindled peripheral carcinoid tumors and found 3 with metastases (2 to regional nodes, 1 to bone), but none of these patients appears to have died of his or her tumor. However, Gillespie and co-workers[318] found three metastases in 13 spindled peripheral tumors.

By contrast, metastases developed in 16 of 23 of the patients described by Arrigoni and co-workers,[316] a 70 percent rate, and 30 percent of the patients were dead at follow-up with an average survival of only 27 months. In the series of Mills and colleagues,[317] 8 of 17 patients died of metastatic tumor.

Unusual Variants of Carcinoids

Oncocytic carcinoids are tumors composed of large eosinophilic oncocytes variably mixed with more typical cells of central carcinoids (Fig. 19–22). These tumors tend to occur in the same distribution as carcinoid tumors. Ultrastructural studies have not always confirmed the diagnosis: Fechner and Bentinck[319] and Santos-Bris and associates[320] failed to find neurosecretory granules in purely oncocytic tumors, but Black[321] and Sajjad and colleagues[322] did demonstrate granules in such tumors. Walter and associates[323] and Sklar and colleagues[324] were able to find granules in the carcinoid cells and none in the oncocytic cells, with variable numbers in intermediate-appearing cells. Gordon[325] has reported a tumor that appeared identical to medullary carcinoma of the thyroid. The stroma contained extensive amyloid and the cells contained secretory granules.

Chemodectomas, Real and Imagined

Physiologic studies indicate that chemoreceptor organs exist within the lung. The corresponding cellular structures are unclear, although some may be paraganglia found within the parenchyma near branchpoints of the pulmonary arteries. Blessing and Hora[326] described 68 such "glomera" in the lungs of a fetus; however, they did not examine these structures with electron microscopy or silver stains, so that such identification is tentative. It also appears that at least some of the individual K-type cells of the bronchial epithelium as well as the neuroepithelial bodies of Lauweryns and Goddeeris[272] and Gould and Linnoila[327] serve a chemoreceptor function. Thus great interest was evoked by the report of Korn and colleagues[328] of a neoplasm of the chemoreceptor organ which they labeled "minute pulmonary chemodectoma." Zak and Chabes[329] and Ichinose[330] added additional series of cases. Barroso-Moguel and Costero[331] claimed that the tumors possessed neural connections and argentaffin granules, but Kuhn and Askin[332] and Churg and Warnock[333] have refuted this notion.

The so-called minute pulmonary chemodectoma consists of nests of spindled cells with copious pale-staining cytoplasm and regular nuclei containing finely vesicular chromatin (Fig. 19–23A, B). The nests are embedded in and appear to spread through the interstitium of the lung; the cells in the nests are arranged in what have been termed *Zellballen*, a counterpart to the structure seen in paragangliomas. It was on this basis that the name chemodectoma was applied.[328]

Churg and Warnock[333] and Kuhn and Askin[332] examined a further series of such cases and described their ultrastructure. Churg and Warnock found a female preponderance (22 female to 1 male) and a rate of 1/360 autopsies. About half the cases had multiple tumors. Electron microscopically, the results are quite surprising. No neurosecretory granules were observed. Instead the tumor was found to consist of a jigsaw-puzzle-like arrangement of large cells with long complicated interdigitating processes (Fig. 19–23C, D). The cells were filled with 60-A filaments and were bordered by pinocytotic vesicles. The lack of secretory granules, as well as the lack of any organization resembling the cells of the true paragangliomas at the fine structure level ruled out the possibility of a chemoreceptor tumor. Instead, both sets of authors agreed that the ultrastructural pattern was indistinguishable from that of meningioma.

Two large primary tumors with the light and ultrastructural features of meningioma have been reported by Chumas and Lorelle[334] and by Kemnitz and co-workers.[335] Why meningeal cells should be found in this location, and what their proliferation might indicate remains obscure. Mirra and Miles[336] report an intracranial meningioma with meningotheleal and hemangiopericytic differentiation, and discuss the close relationship of these two tumors. This observation raises the possibility that both the microscopic and macroscopic intrapulmonary tumors are actually variants of hemangiopericytoma.

Possible True Paragangliomas. A variety of other solitary macroscopic tumors have been reported as paragangliomas. Singh and co-workers reviewed nine cases.[337] Their own tumor arose from a pulmonary artery, but several of the other lesions so labeled appeared to arise from small bronchioles. All of the tumors were composed of epithelioid cells forming Zellballen. In the case of Singh and co-workers,[337] electron microscopy revealed neurosecretory granules. Of particular interest is the case reported by Blessing and associates[338] in which both granules and norepinephrine were demonstrated within the tumor.

In general, however, it is difficult to be certain whether such tumors should be classified as paragangliomas or carcinoids; their identification as paragangliomas is based almost entirely on the presence of a Zellballen pattern by light microscopy. As noted in the section on Carcinoids and Related Tumors, above, the ultrastructural and biochemical distinction between these two types of tumor is not entirely clear. It is also necessary to be wary of metastatic paragangliomas, especially from carotid body.[339]

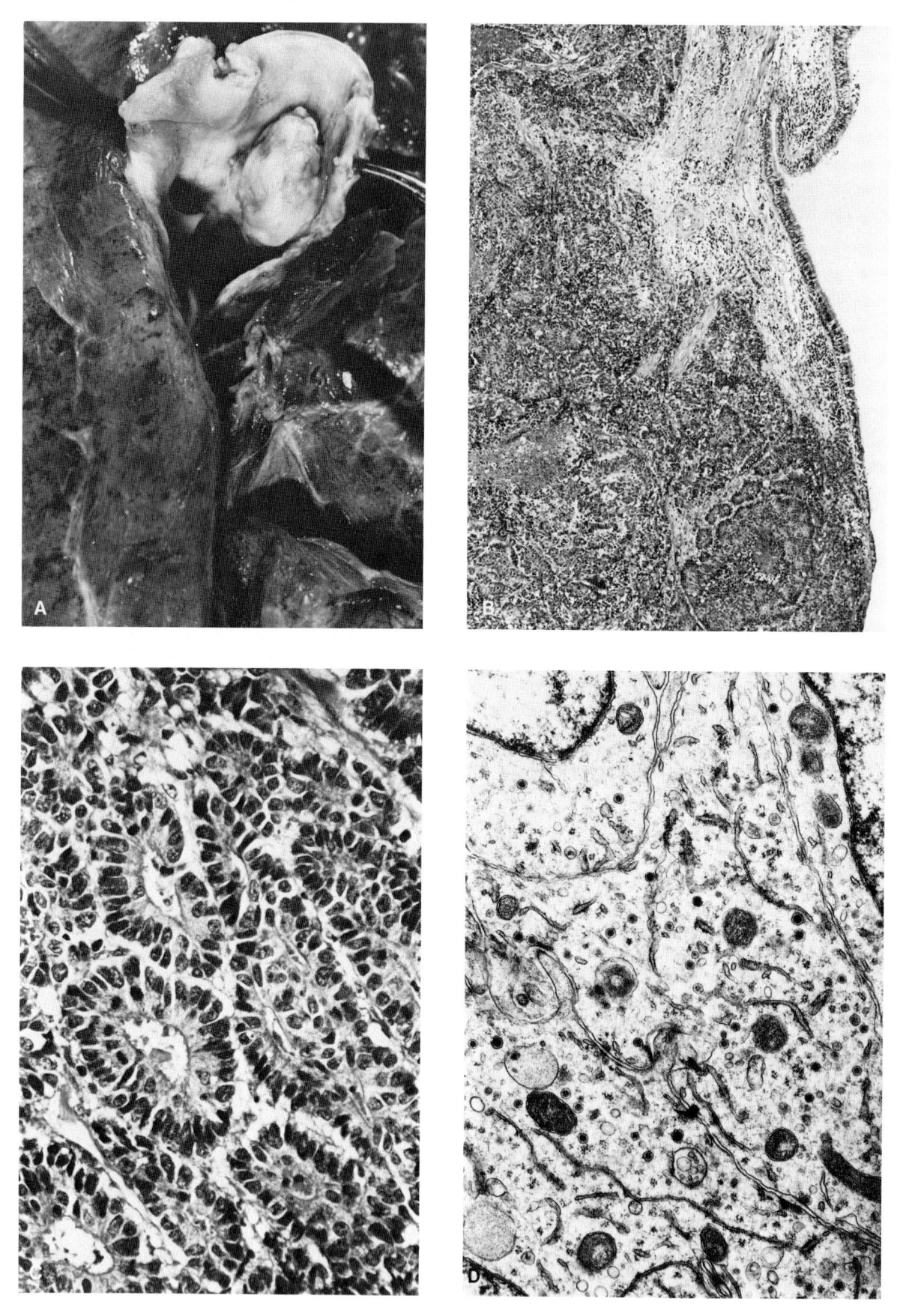

Figure 19–21A–D. High-grade carcinoid. A. Gross appearance of a high-grade carcinoid presenting as a polypoid, partially endobronchial mass. B and C. Microscopic appearance of a high-grade carcinoid showing subepithelial tumor. Note the evident areas of necrosis at low power in B. The high-power view (C) shows typical carcinoid type of tubules, but with mitotically active and cytologically atypical cells (B ×40, C ×400). D. Electron micrograph of the same tumor shown in B, demonstrating small neurosecretory granules (×12,000).

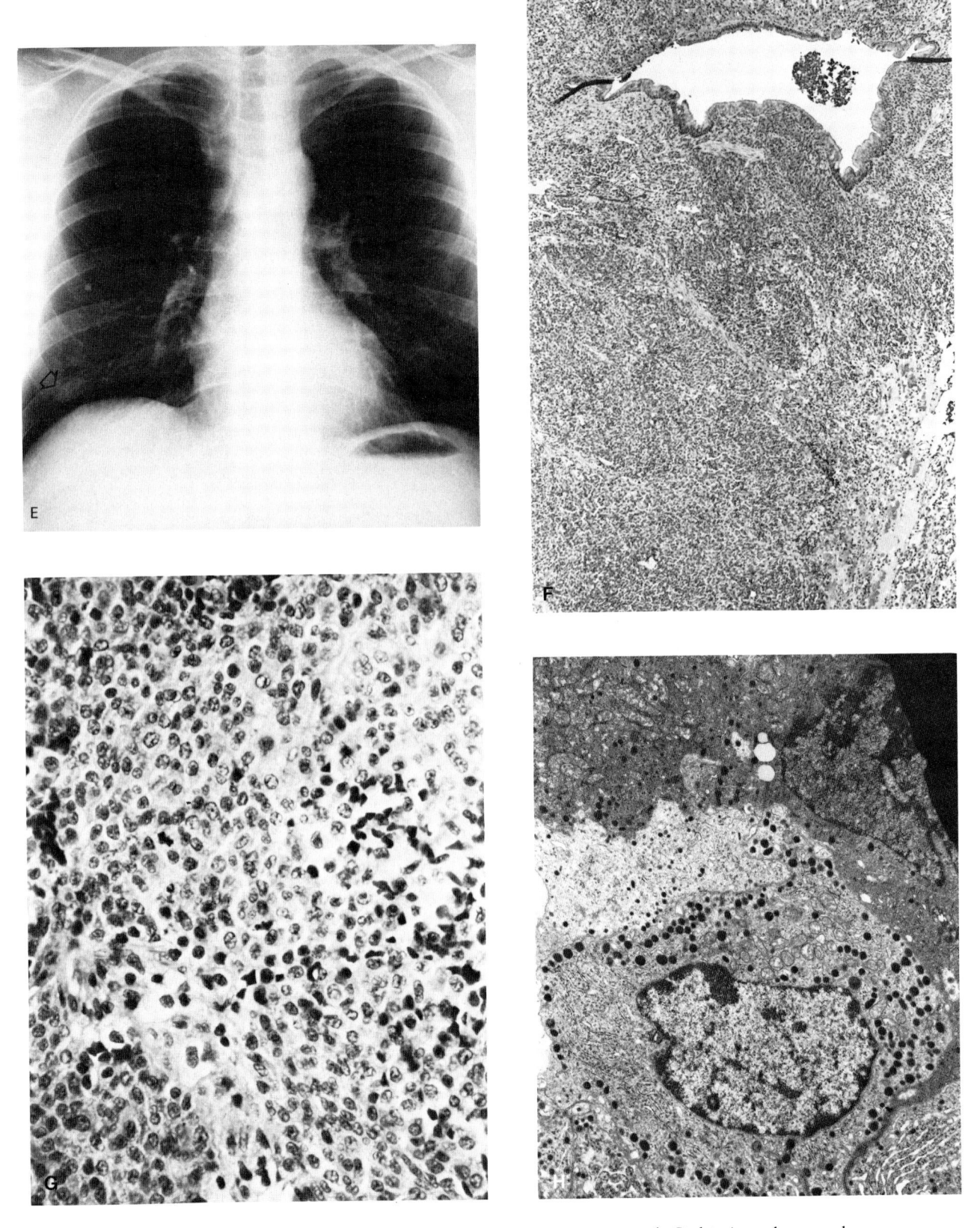

Figure 19–21E–H. E. Chest radiograph of a patient presenting with Cushing's syndrome and found to have a vaguely defined right lower lobe nodule (arrow). F and G. Histologic appearance of the tumor shown in E. Note the mitotic figures in the high-power view (F ×40, G ×400). H. Electron micrograph of the same tumor showing various types of neurosecretory granules. Immunohistochemical staining at a light microscopic level indicated that at least some of these granules contained adrenocorticotropic hormone (×6000).

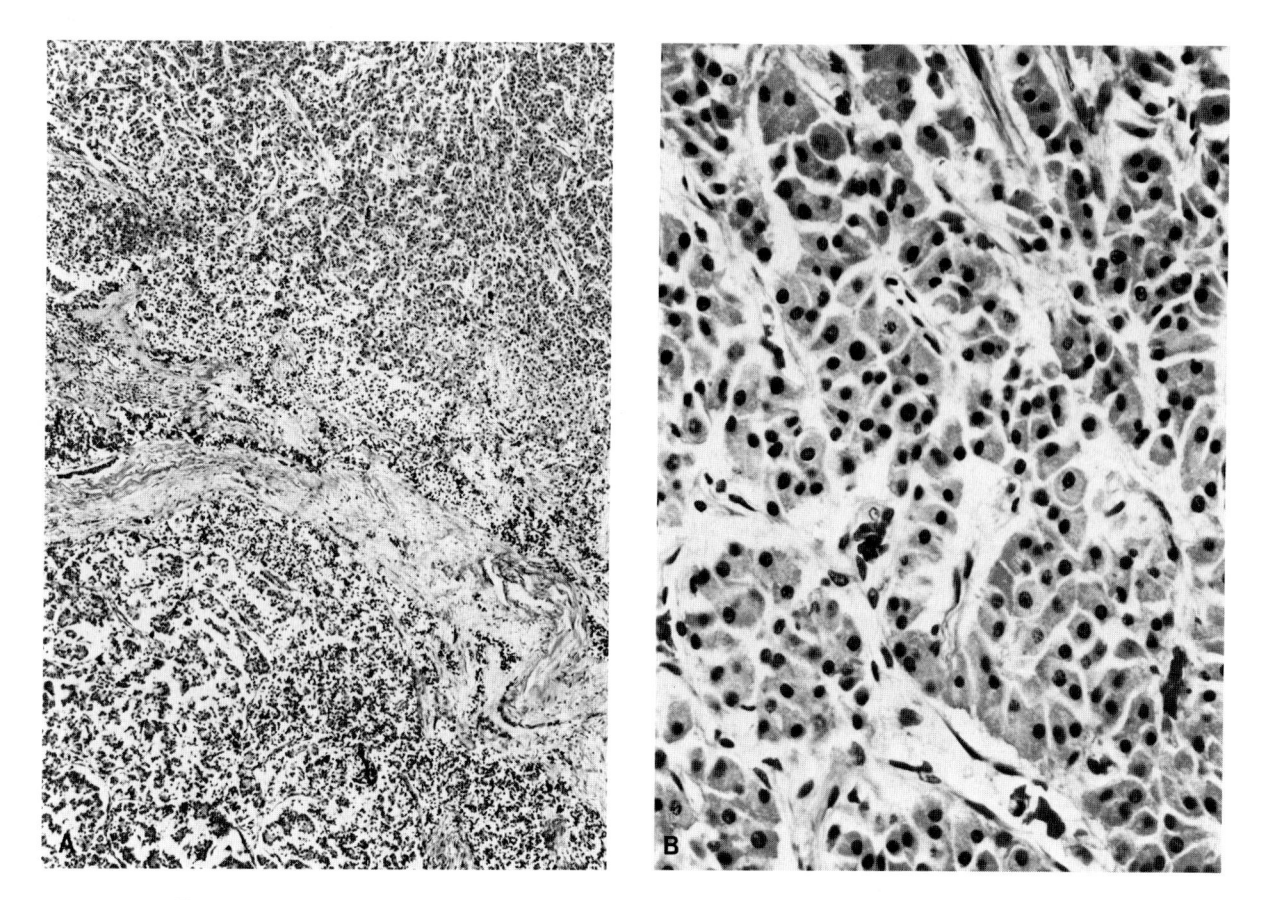

Figure 19–22. Oncocytic carcinoid tumor. Microscopic appearance of a peripheral coin lesion discovered incidently at autopsy. The lower-power view (A) shows two histologic patterns. The one in the lower portion o the field resembles cytologically the spindle cells of the tumorlet illustrated in Figure 18–20C. The cells in the upper portion of the field are shown at high power in B and appear to be oncocytes. Electron microscopy demonstrated that the spindled cells, but not the oncocytic cells, contained neurosecretory granules (A ×40, B ×400).

Tumors of Salivary Gland Type

A variety of tumors that are histologically and functionally identical to those of salivary gland are found in the lung; presumably all arise from the bronchial glands. Traditionally, the mucoepidermoid and adenoid cystic carcinomas have been included with carcinoids in the misnamed group of bronchial "adenomas." Since both of these entities are malignant, the term adenoma should not be used.

Mucoepidermoid Carcinomas. Mucoepidermoid carcinoma was first described in lung by Liebow[340] and Smetana.[341] Fewer than 100 cases have been reported: Leonardi and co-workers were able to find seven new cases among 4250 primary carcinomas; Conlan and associates[343] found only 12 examples during a 50-year period at the Mayo Clinic. The topic has recently been reviewed by Klacsmann and colleagues.[344]

The age range is wide, ranging from childhood to the sixth and seventh decade. The majority of patients present with respiratory symptoms such as cough or hemoptysis; evidence of systemic disease is unusual. Radiographically, the tumors are sometimes seen as ill-defined masses but more often the chest film shows only atelectasis or pneumonic infiltrate.

Grossly, the tumors are varied in appearance: many are smooth-surfaced pedunculated masses, while others are ragged and invasive. A smooth-surfaced gross appearance apparently does not predict a low-grade lesion, but the ragged lesions are always high grade (Fig. 19–24A).

Histologically, the tumors can be classified much as those in the salivary gland into low, moderate, and high grade. The low-grade tumors are characterized by a high proportion of mucus-secreting cells, and relatively few squamous type cells (Fig. 19–24B, C). The high-grade tumors show the reverse pattern. In some high-grade tumors the distinction between mucoepidermoid and adenosquamous carcinoma may be difficult, as in the series of Axelsson and colleagues.[345] This problem has been considered by Klacsmann and co-workers.[344] Since the high-grade mucoepidermoid tumors are highly ag-

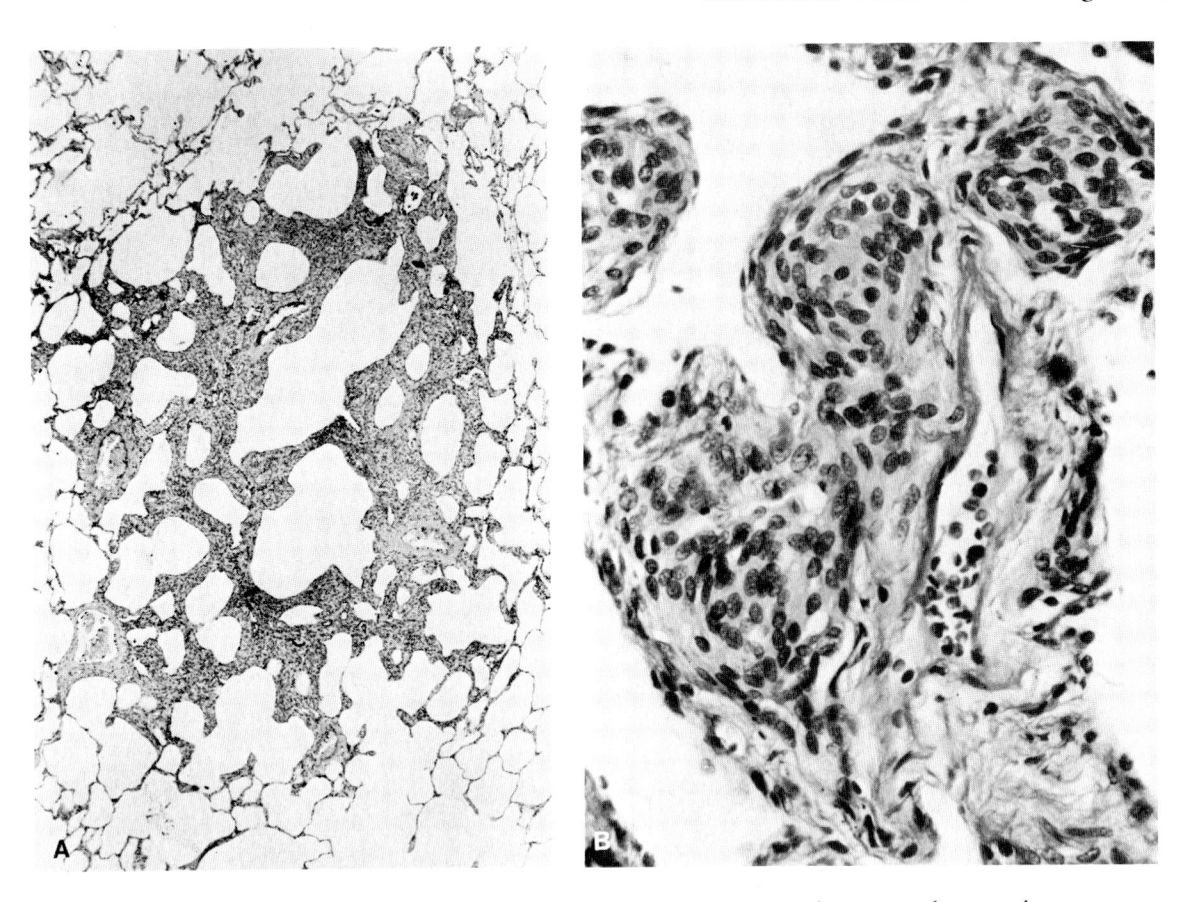

Figure 19–23A,B. Minute pulmonary chemodectoma. Light micrographic views of a typical so-called minute pulmonary chemodectoma. The tumor cells proliferate in the interstitium where they appear as nests or *Zellballen* (A ×25, B ×400).

gressive, this separation is probably not of great practical importance.

Survival appears to depend on tumor grade and also on the age of the patient. Mullins and Barnes[346] reviewed seven cases in children under 16: all were histologically low grade and all had benign clinical courses. In adults, the results are closely related to the grade of tumor. Conlan and colleagues[343] report patients with grade 1 neoplasms alive up to 28 years postoperatively, while those with grade 2 and 3 tumors tend to be dead within a few months to years. Their overall survival was 8 of 12 patients. Similarly, Leonardi and associates[342] found that their one patient with a high-grade tumor was dead within 28 months, while those with low-grade tumors, including a tracheal tumor, were alive 5 to 23 years after resection. Reichle and Rosemond[347] reviewed the older literature and found 13 of 18 evaluable patients alive from 1½ to 16½ years after resection. Wilkins and co-workers[348] reported five of five survivors.

Mucoepidermoid tumors occasionally occur in the trachea.[349]

Adenoid Cystic Carcinoma (Cylindroma). Judging from the Mayo Clinic experience,[343] adenoid cystic carcinomas make up fewer than 10 percent of the so-called bronchial "adenomas."

Patients with adenoid cystic carcinomas may present with cough and sputum production or evidence of pneumonia, but systemic complaints including malaise and weight loss are not unusual.[315,343] Radiographically, mass lesions are probably less common than changes of obstruction.

There is controversy in the literature about the gross appearance of these tumors, perhaps because of their relative rarity. Conlon and colleagues[343] found polyploid broad-based necrotic tumors that mimicked ordinary bronchogenic carcinomas. Spencer[350] describes growths that are infiltrative rather than occlusive. Examination of a small number of cases suggests to me that the tumor is always extensively invasive, even if it appears as a smooth surfaced polypoid lesion. Extension into the mediastinum is not uncommon.

Microscopically the tumors are essentially identical to those found in the salivary gland and are composed of sheets or nests of darkly staining cells which form small lumina (Fig. 19–25A, B). Like the tumor in the salivarygland, the adenoid cystic carcinoma of the bronchus tends to be infiltrative and particularly tends to surround and invade nerves.

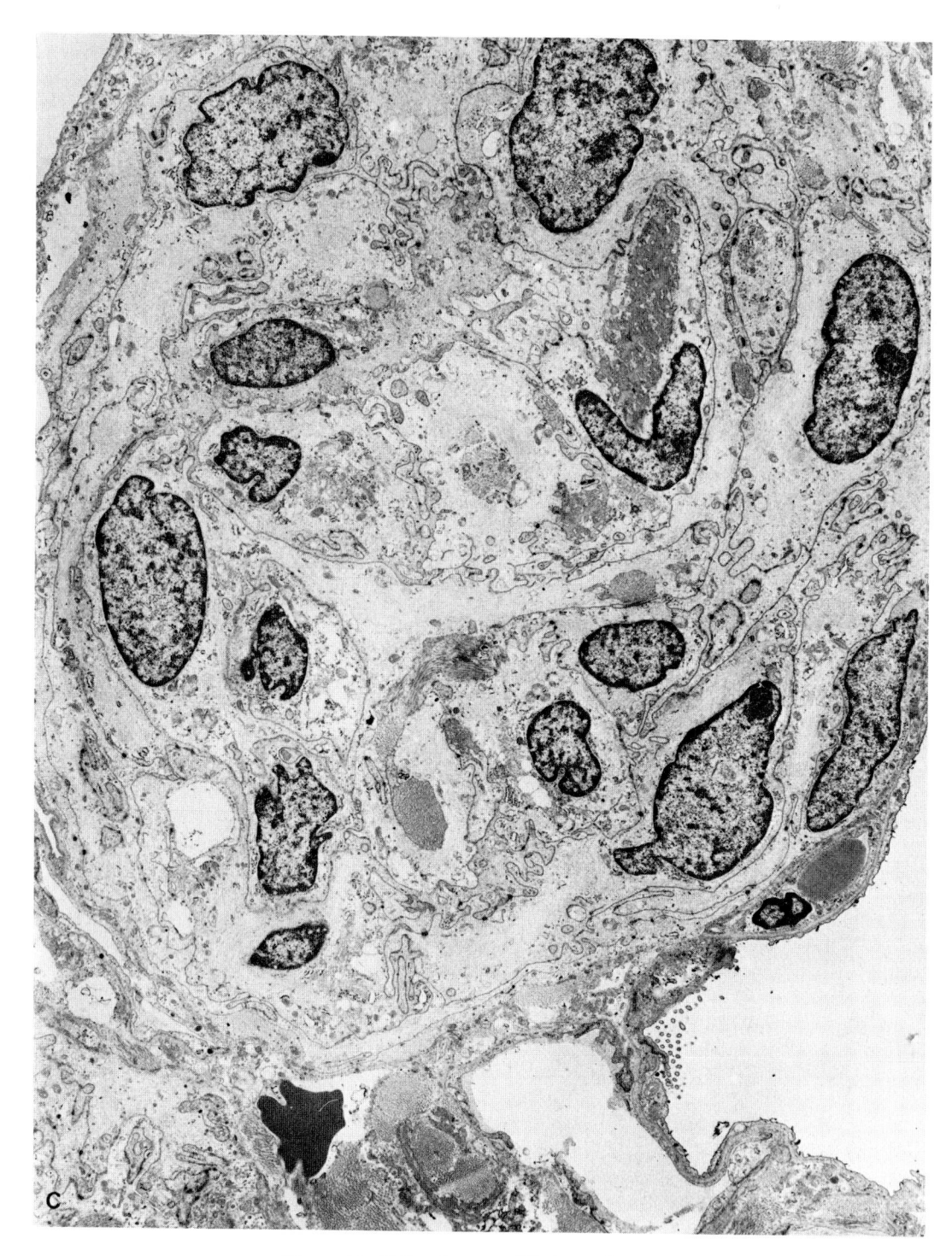

Figure 19–23C. See page 379 for explanation.

Survival data are scanty (Table 19–31), but as in salivary gland, adenoid cystic carcinoma of the tracheobronchial tree is slowly but relentlessly progressive. All of Conlon and colleagues'[343] patients died of tumor eventually, although some survived as long as 16 years. More recent results form Gaillard,[351] who assembled 69 such tumors from the trachea and bronchi, suggest that curative surgery will salvage about one-third of patients, and even those who are inoperable may survive as long as 10 years with radiotherapy.

Adenoid cystic carcinoma is secondary only to squamous carcinoma in frequency as a primary tracheal tumor.[243]

Other Neoplasms Arising from Bronchial Glands and Analogous to Salivary Gland Tumors. Fechner and colleagues[354]

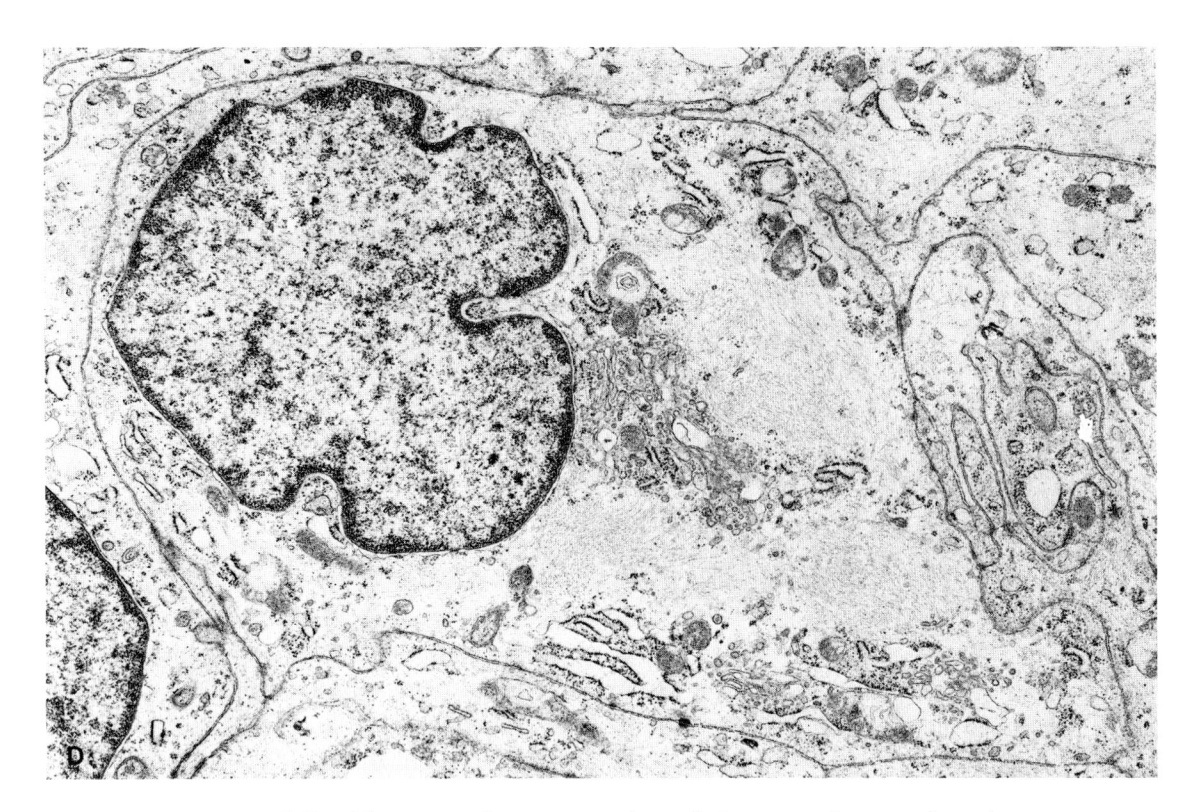

Figure 19–23C,D. Ultrastructural appearance of so-called minute pulmonary chemodectoma. Note the numerous irregular cells which fit together like a jigsaw puzzle. At high power the cells are filled with fine filaments and are connected by small well-formed junctions. This ultrastructural appears is identical to that of meningioma (C ×4400, D ×9700). Reproduced with permission from Churg and Warnock.[333]

and Katz and Buris[355] have described acinic cell tumors characterized by cells with large (800-nm) PAS-positive granules; these tumors are morphologically similar to some forms of salivary gland acinic cell tumor. Mixed tumors, again identical to those in salivary gland, have been described by Spencer,[350] Payne and co-workers,[356] and Verska and colleagues.[357] Spencer[350] illustrates an oxyphil adenoma of the bronchus, a tumor difficult to distinguish by light microscopy from an oncocytic carcinoid, and also includes the true bronchial adenoma in this group of tumors.

True Mucous Gland Adenoma. I am following the convention of Spencer[350] and including this tumor under the general heading of tumors of salivary gland type, although no analogous tumor actually exists in salivary gland. This is one of the few true bronchial adenomas, as opposed to the misuse of the term for carcinoids, mucoepidermoid, and adenoid cystic carcinomas. Kroe summarizes 11 cases in the literature.[358] They appear as smooth-surfaced rounded masses which are entirely endobronchial in location. They may cause cough, wheezing, hemoptysis, and sometimes protracted pneumonia. In reported cases symptoms have been present for months to up to 10 years. Flap-like motion of the tumor on its pedicle may produce a check-valve effect such that progressive hyperinflammation of a lung of lobe ensues.

The microscopic pattern is invariably a collection of small, mucus-filled cysts with a lining of cuboidal to columnar cells. Many of the lining cells are goblet type (Fig. 19–26). These lesions are benign, and are almost never diagnosed prior to surgical removal.

Table 19–31. Survival in Adenoid Cystic Carcinoma of Bronchus

	Cases	5 Years (%)	10 Years (%)	15 Years (%)	20 Years (%)
Gaillard et al.[351]	69	67			
Conlan et al.[342]	20	30	30		25
Wilkins et al.[348]	5		60		
O'Grady et al.[352]	4	0			
Goodner et al.[353]	5	40			
Turnbull et al.[315]	12	25			

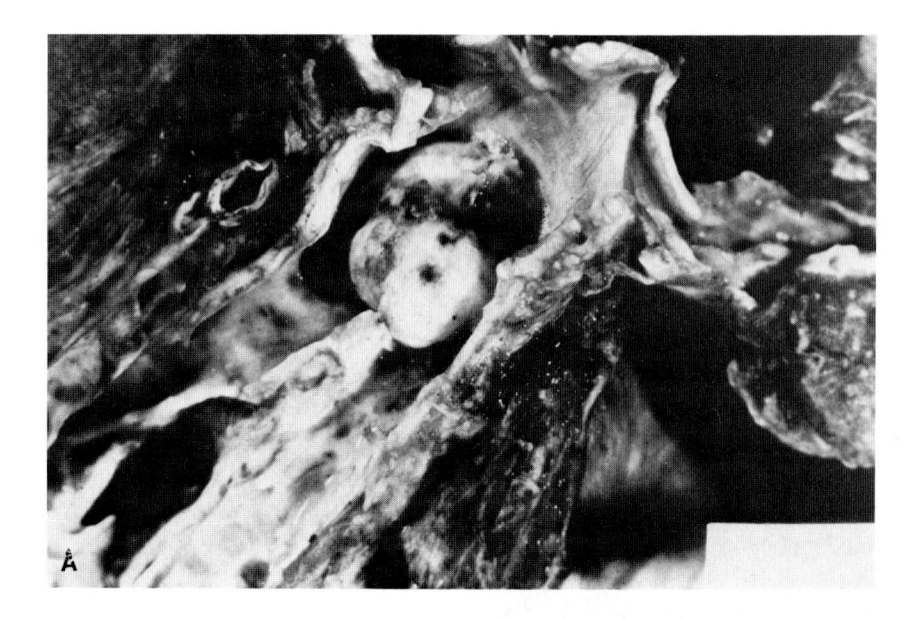

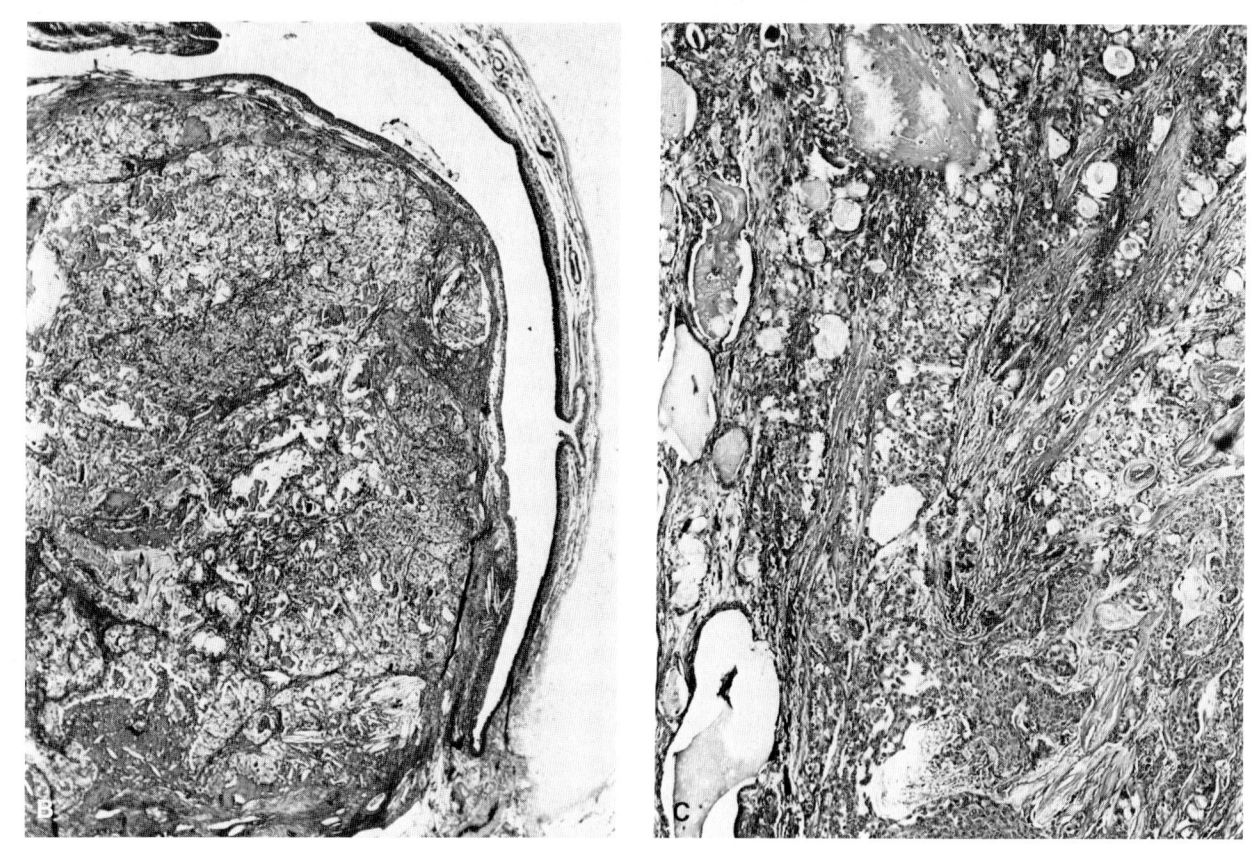

Figure 19–24. Mucoepidermoid tumor of the bronchus. A. Gross appearance of a mucoepidermoid tumor. B and C. Microscopic appearance of the same tumor. Note how the mucosa is stretched over the tumor; the gross appearance of a smooth surfaced endobronchial mass is no guarantee that a tumor is a carcinoid. Higher-power view (C) shows a typical appearance of a low-grade mucoepidermoid tumor (B ×20, C ×64).

Benign Mesenchymal Tumors

Lipomas

The literature on pulmonary lipomas has been recently reviewed by Politis and colleagues.[359] Endobronchial lipomas are uncommon; approximately 50 have been reported in the literature and only 3 were found in 3000 surgical lung specimens by Horanyi and co-workers.[360] Clinically the majority of patients present with cough, chest pain, or dyspnea. Pulmonary lipomas are found in

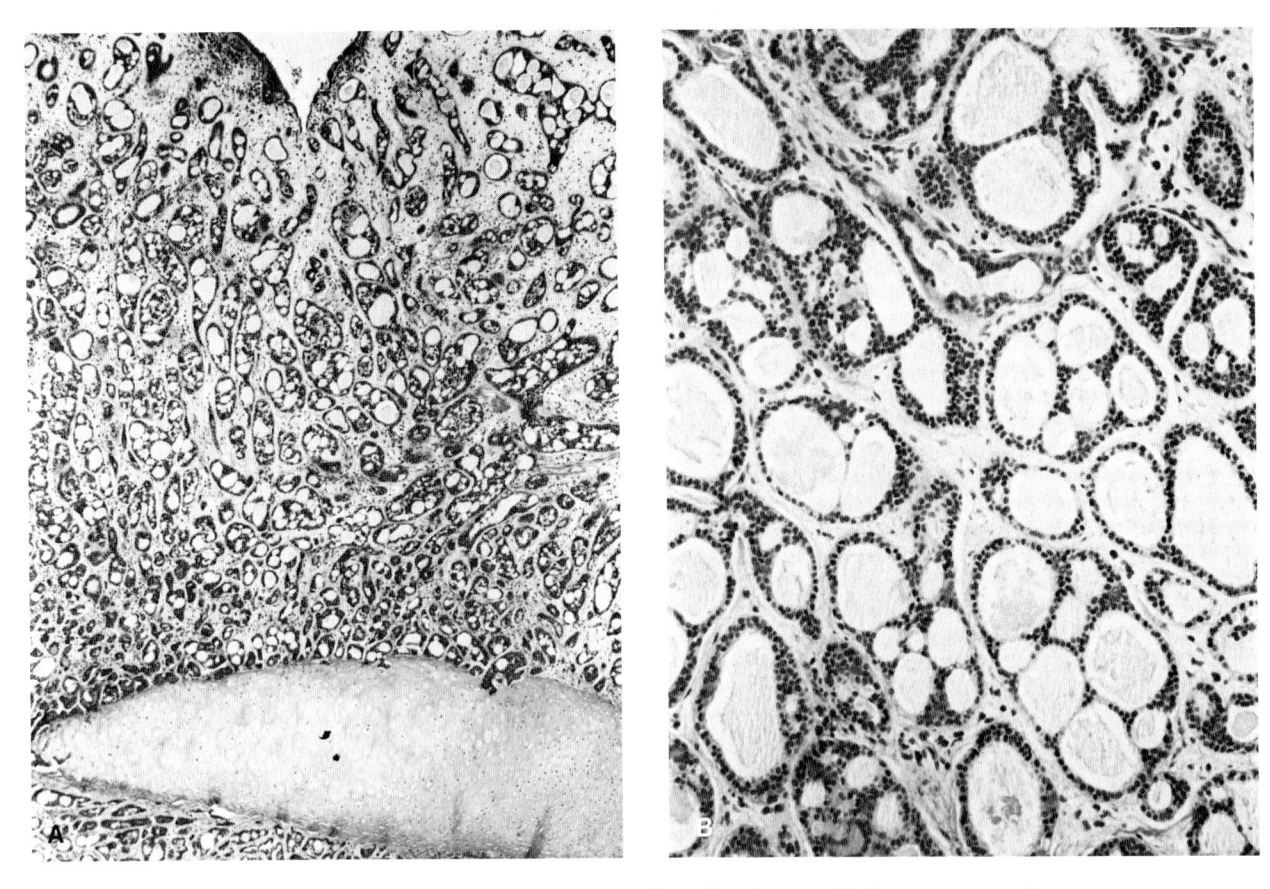

Figure 19–25. Adenoid cystic carcinoma of the bronchus. Low- and high-power views of a tumor that is histologically identical to the adenoid cytic carcinoma of salivary gland (A ×40, B ×160).

adults, and approximately 90 percent have occurred in men. In several instances symptoms have been present for up to 20 years. Destruction of the parenchyma secondary to infection and even absence of perfusion have been reported with these tumors.[361]

At bronchoscopy or gross examination, endobronchial lipomas are usually pedunculated tumors covered with bronchial epithelium. Histologically they are composed of mature fat (Fig. 19–27). Three cases have been found in which peribronchial extension occurred,[362–364] but all appeared to behave as benign lesions.

Lipomas of the pleura and parenchyma are even more uncommon.[359,365,366] These tumors are almost always diagnosed postoperatively.

Solitary Leiomyomas

Fifty-one cases of solitary leiomyomas were summarized by Orlowski and colleagues.[367] The age range was very wide, with tumors reported from childhood to the seventh decade. There was a 2:1 female/male predominance. About half of the lesions were endobronchial, causing cough, sputum production, and symptoms of obstruction. Virtually all the parenchymal tumors were asymptomatic. Whether in fact these tumors are actually examples, at least in women, of so-called benign metastasizing leiomyoma is unclear. Forty percent of the women in these series had a history of uterine leiomyomas; however, none of these cases were accepted by Wolff and co-workers[368] in their extensive review.

Neural Tumors

Bartley and Arean[369] have summarized the literature regarding these tumors. They found 24 neurofibromas, of which they believed 8 were actually neurilemmomas and 7 were actually malignant neoplasms.

Clinically, about one-third of neurofibromas are asymptomatic, while the rest present with a variety of pulmonary symptoms. The majority of the neurilemmomas present with cough, fever, and sputum production. The age range for both types of tumor is wide but there appears to be a predilection for young adults. Radiographically, most of the patients have had round or

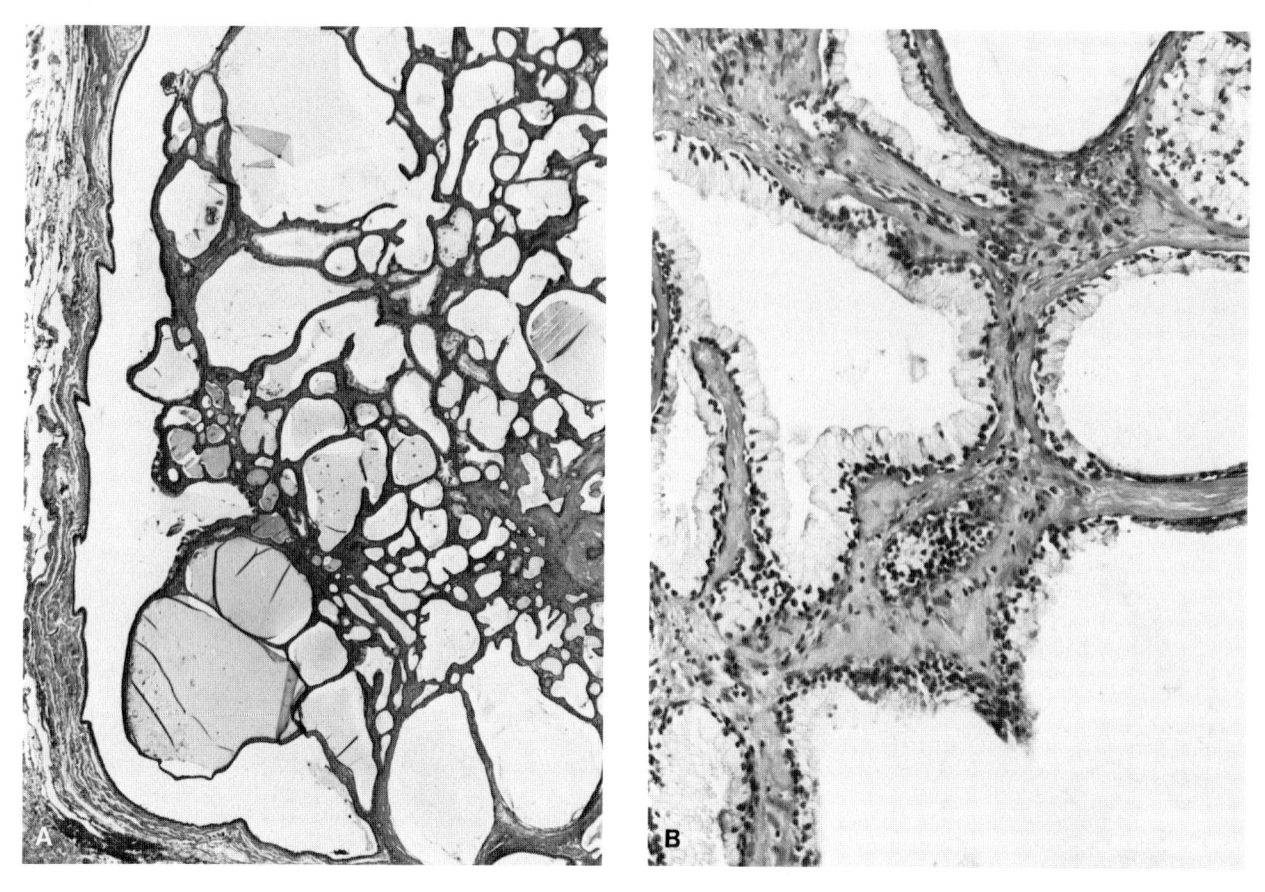

Figure 19–26. True bronchial mucous gland adenoma. The tumor is composed of cystic spaces lined by bland-appearing mucus-secreting cells (A ×20, B ×160).

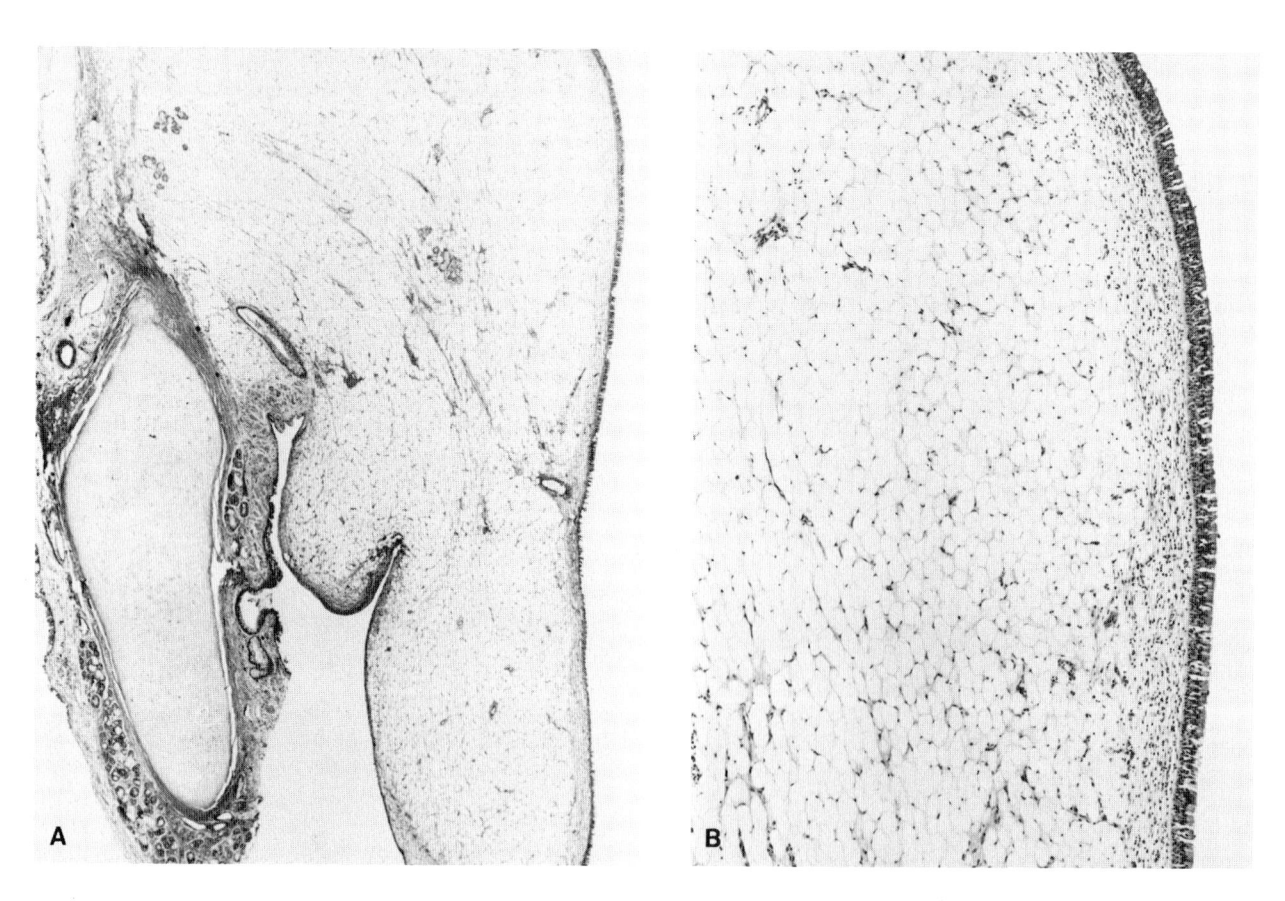

Figure 19–27. Intrabronchial lipoma. Low- and high-power views of a polypoid intrabronchial mass. Note again that the tumor is covered by bronchial epithelium (A ×20, B ×64).

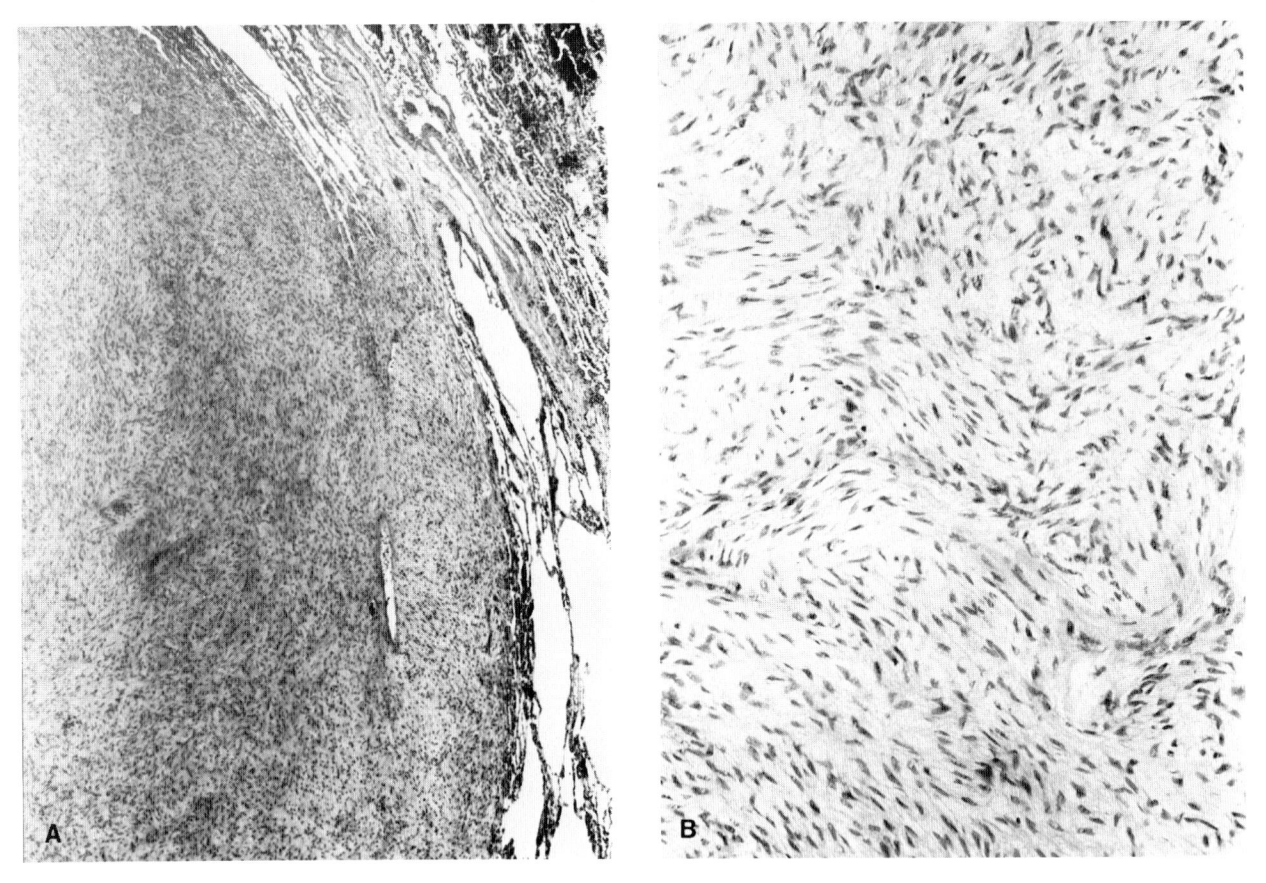

Figure 19–28. Intrapulmonary neurolemmoma. Low- and high-power views of a circumscribed intrapulmonary tumor in a patient with neurofibromatosis (A ×40, B ×160).

oval masses measuring up to 13 cm. They tend to be associated with the bronchial tree and may bulge into the lumen; the neurilemmomas sometimes penetrate the bronchial wall to produce a dumbbell shape. Most cases appear to have no association with generalized neurofibromatosis.

Histologically, the appearances are typical of those seen in either solitary neurofibroma, or in neurilemmoma, the latter usually showing Antoni A- and B-type tissue (Fig. 19–28). Older neurilemmomas may show areas of hemorrhage and cystic change, along with hyalinization of the vessels. Silverman and colleagues[370] examined a neurilemmoma ultrastructurally and confirmed its identity.

Clinically, the benign tumors do not recur. The nature of the malignant tumors described as malignant schwannomas is unclear and they would probably be classified differently today.

Cooney[371] has described a ganglioneuroma derived from a neuroblastoma primary in lung.

Intrapulmonary Fibromas

Spencer[1] discusses and illustrates this entry; however, it is unclear just what type of tumor is implied. Most likely these tumors should be classified as either plasma cell granulomas or fibrous histiocytomas.[372,373] Some may also be neurofibromas.

Malignant Mesenchymal Tumors

Primary Sarcomas of the Lung

Sarcomas of the lung are uncommon tumors, with estimates of frequency ranging from 1 per 500 lung cancers[374] to 1 in 8000 cases.[375] Interpretation of data regarding incidence and behavior of specific varieties of sarcoma must be interpreted with extreme caution. For most specifically defined types, only small numbers of cases have been reported. Classification of sarcomas has also changed greatly over the past 25 years and new entities such as malignant fibrous histiocytoma, which is probably the most frequent sarcoma of the soft tissues, have been described. It has also been recognized that some of the older literature identified small-cell carcinomas as sarcomas. As a result, relatively little data are actually available to indicate prognosis for specific types of tumor.

Clinical Features. The clinical and radiographic features of most pulmonary sarcomas are similar. The age range is very wide, with cases reported from infancy to old age. The majority of tumors appear to occur in middle age; there is no evidence that they are related to smoking. Cough, chest pain, and hemoptysis are common, and expectoration of tumor fragments is not an unusual event, since many of these tumors are endobronchial or may be so large as to erode into a bronchus. However, even huge tumors may be asymptomatic; in the series of Meade and colleagues,[376] 10 of 24 hemangiopericytomas were incidental findings. There does not appear to be any clear-cut sex predominance.

Radiographically, the parenchymal tumors tend to be rather sharply defined lobulated or smooth contoured masses which may occupy most of a hemithorax (Figs. 19–29, 19–30). Cavitation occasionally occurs. The intrabronchial tumors frequently produce obstruction with atelectasis or pneumonic infiltrates.

Hemangiopericytoma. This tumor was first described by Stout and Murray[377] as a neoplasm of the soft tissues. It is believed, largely on the basis of histologic pattern, to arise from the pericyte. Grossly, the pulmonary tumors are white and firm; the size ranges from 2 to 15 cm (*see* Fig. 19–29). Most hemangiopericytomas arise in the parenchyma, and endobronchial primaries appear to be rare. Large tumors frequently involve the pleura. Micrscopically, the tumor in the lung is similar to that in soft tissues (*see* Fig. 19–29). It is composed of sheets of polygonal to spindled cells which tend to whorl around small blood vessels. Reticulum stain demonstrates that the tumor cells always are situated outside the endothelial basement membrane, and that there is a separate, probably non-neoplastic endothelial cell. A distinctive feature of hemangiopericytoma is the vascular pattern that is classically described as branching or glove-like, and is a helpful diagnostic finding.

The prognosis for hemangiopericytoma of the soft tissue depends to a large extent on the measurable features of size, cellular atypica, mitotic frequency, and necrosis[378]; this is presumably true of hemangiopericytoma in the lung as well, but no studies have examined the problem. In the collected series of Meade and co-wokers,[376] 11 of 24 patients died of their disease from 3 months to 13 years after diagnosis.

Fibrosarcoma and Leiomyosarcoma. Guccion and Rosen,[374] Cameron,[379] Dowell,[380] and Nascimento and colleagues[381] have reviewed pulmonary fibrosarcomas and leiomyosarcomas. These tumors may be endobronchial or parenchymal. Roughly one hundred cases have been reported, and the two types of tumor appear to occur with about equal frequency. Among the fibrosarcomas, approximately one-third occur as endobronchial lesions, but only one-sixth of leiomyosarcomas do so. Of interest is the fact the vast majority of endobronchial fibrosarcomas have occurred in young adults, whereas the intrapulmonary fibro- and leiomyosarcomas are lesions of middle-aged to elderly individuals.

Grossly, the endobronchial tumors are polypoid lesions, usually not larger than 2.5 cm. Ulceration and hemorrhage are common. Some of these tumors grossly invade the bronchial wall. They are more common on the right side. The intrapulmonary lesions are usually round to oval, rather sharply circumscribed masses which are not encapsulated. They range up to 24 cm in diameter. Hemorrhage and necrosis are frequent in the larger tumors. Large tumors may extend into the chest wall. The histologic features are identical to fibrosarcomas and leiomyosarcomas of the soft tissues.

The behavior of these tumors has been studied by Cameron,[379] Guccion and Rosen,[374] and Nascimento and colleagues.[381] Cameron[379] found a 45 percent 5-year survival for fibrosarcoma and a 64 percent 5-year survival for leiomyosarcoma. Seven of nine patients with fibrosarcoma in the series of Nascimento and co-workers died of their tumor, generally within 1 to 2 years, but one patient survived 19 years. Guccion and Rosen[374] examined numbers of mitotic figures and found this to be a useful criterion. The endobronchial lesions generally had fewer than three mitoses per 10 high-power fields (hpf) and most appeared to behave in a benign fashion, but metastases may occur.

The intrapulmonary leiomyosarcomas are much more aggressive lesions in adults, and even small tumors may metastasize. The large intrapulmonary leiomyosarcomas are usually inoperable and tend to metastasize rapidly. These authors found that tumors with fewer than eight mitoses/10 hpf grew slowly. In their series the 5-year survival rate was about 50 percent for adults, but in children the tumors were generally of low-grade malignancy.

Intrapulmonary fibrosarcomas are also more malignant lesions than the endobronchial forms; the majority metastasize, but oddly enough the larger tumors metastasize less frequently and tend to kill by local extension. Again, a level of about eight mitoses per 10 hpf signifies the point at which the tumors become aggressive.

Malignant Fibrous Histiocytoma. This is a recently described neoplasm[382,383] and only a few cases have been reported in the lung.[384,385] The cases reported thus far have been highly aggressive parenchymal tumors, but it seems likely from previously published descriptions that endobronchial varieties also occur, and also that many of the tumors with giant cells that were called fibrosarcoma in the past are actually malignant fibrous histiocytoma. Prognosis of this tumor in the soft tissues does not correlate well with mitotic index, but with tumor size and location.[383] Criteria for behavior in the lung have yet to be developed. An example is illustrated in Fig. 19–30.

Chondrosarcoma. Chondrosarcomas of the lung are rare: Daniels and co-workers[386] found 14 cases in the literature and added a case arising at the carina. The intrapulmonary tumors are highly malignant: 10 of 12 traceable patients were dead within 1 year. The one endobronchial lesion had not recurred after 3 years.

Sarcomas of the Pulmonary Trunk. These are unusual tumors; approximately 60 are reported in the literature.[387–389] The clinical history is typically that of progressive unexplained heart failure; the diagnosis is usually not made until autopsy. Grossly the tumors are polypoid lesions which may be multifocal and usually involve the bifurcation of the pulmonary artery; these lesions may grow down through the pulmonary valve as well as distally into the small branches of the pulmonary artery. Histologically, a variety of forms are seen, including leiomyosarcomas, rhabdomyosarcomas, chondrosarcomas, and mixed sarcomas (malignant mesenchymomas). Bleisch and Kraus[387] suggest that these tumors originate from the bulbus cordis and should be termed "myenchymomas."

Rhabdomyosarcomas. Many cases reported as rhabdomyosarcoma have been either pulmonary blastomas or malignant fibrous histiocytomas. The scanty literature is reviewed by Drennan and McCormack.[390] The tumors have been invariably large and most have been intraparenchymal. The diagnostic feature is the presence of tumor cells with muscle-type cross-striations.

Sclerosing Vascular Sarcoma (Intravascular and Sclerosing Bronchioloalveolar Tumor). First described by Dail and Liebow[391] and Farinacci and colleagues,[392] these peculiar tumors are actually unrelated to bronchioloalveolar carcinomas. Dail and colleagues[393] have reported a series of 20 cases.

Clinically, most of the patients have been female and more than half were under 40 at the time of presentation. Although some patients present with systemic disease, many cases are detected because of incidental observation of nodules on chest radiographs. The tumors are almost invariably multifocal at the time of presentation.

Grossly, the tumor nodules are firm, translucent, and have somewhat the appearance of cartilage. Microscopically, the tumor nodules have a distinct organization: at the periphery are cellular areas in which large polygonal eosinophilic cells fill the alveoli (*see* Fig. 19–30). Careful observation indicates that similar cells may be found within the interstitium; this is best seen in 1-μm plastic sections. The cellular areas secrete a mucin-like product which stains with PAS. Toward the center of the nodule, the secreted material becomes progressively hyalinized but leaves the alveolar walls intact. In the very center of the nodules, few tumor cells are present, and these are often stellate. Some tumor cells appear to contain vacuoles, but mucin stains of such cells are negative. The tumor nodules are, microscopically, always multiple. In addition, invasion of arteries, veins, and lymphatics, often at large distances from tumor nodules, is always present (Fig. 19–31).

Electron microscopic studies[394–396] indicate that the initial proliferative processes appears to take place within the interstitium. The proliferating cells are polygonal to jigsaw-puzzle-shaped, and are connected by small junctions (*see* Fig. 19–31). Some are surrounded by basement membrane. The cytoplasm is filled with fine filaments and pinocytotic vesicles line the cell membranes. In some areas the tumor cells form sheets or linear arrays; in other areas the same cells wrap around each other and form lumen-like spaces (*see* Fig. 19–31). The product secreted by the cells appears as finely granular low-density material which traverses the basement membrane of the pulmonary alveolar walls, entrapping the type II and type I cells.

Immunohistochemical staining for factor VIII–related antigen has been positive in a number of cases.[393]

The ultrastructural features and immunohistochemical reactions just described seem to fit best with a vascular tumor of the interstitium which spreads out into the alveolar spaces as well as into vessels.[394–396] The fine structure of the tumor cells and the attempts at lumen formation suggest that the cell of origin is endothelial or pericytic. The nature of the secretory material is not clear, but the morphology of the cells is analogous to that seen in mixed tumors of salivary gland. I believe that a much more appropriate name for this tumor is "sclerosing vascular sarcoma of lung."

Because it is a widespread tumor at presentation, sclerosing vascular sarcoma is not amenable to surgical therapy. However, it is often slow-growing and some patients live many years with disease; in the series of Dail and co-workers,[393] 8 of 17 patients lived for 5 years and 2 of 17 for 10 years after initial diagnosis. Clinically significant metastases are uncommon, and death results from local tumor spread.

Other Vascular Sarcomas. Wagenvoort and co-workers[397] have reported a case that they labeled as "capillary hemangiomatosis" of the lungs. This lesion consisted of multiple proliferating capillary-type vessels which involved and destroyed vascular parenchyma. The exact relationship of this process to angiomatosis of the soft tissues is unclear, since the latter tends to present more like a hamartoma than a true neoplasm. The topic is reviewed by Enzinger and Weiss.[398]

Pulmonary Blastoma and Carcinosarcoma. Carcinosarcomas are defined as malignant tumors in which both adult-type epithelial and stromal elements are malignant and have the potential to metastasize either together or independently. The occurrence of such tumors has been taken to imply the simultaneous occurrence of malignant change in cells derived from two different germ layers.[399,400] Pulmonary blastoma, which was first described as "embryoma" by Barnard[401] and later called "blastoma" by Spencer[402] is a neoplasm in which a mature or immature adenocarcinoma-like epithelium is mixed with a primitive-appearing stroma (*see* Fig. 19–33). The classical appearance of blastoma resembles that of fetal lung, and the tumor was initially thought to be derived from pluripotential mesenchyme (that is, a blastema or a single germ layer) in accordance with the experiments of Waddell.[403] However, electron microscope examination of the growing lung has made it clear that the pulmonary alveolar cells as well as the proximal bronchial epithelium are derived from endoderm, whereas the interstitial cells originate in mesoderm.[404–406] Thus the blastoma is in fact a carcinosarcoma, albeit of a histologically distinct type.

Carcinosarcomas are reviewed by Stackhouse and associates,[399] Chaudhuri,[402] Chaudhuri and associates,[408] Kakos, Davis and colleagues,[410] Razzuk and co-workers,[411] and Roth and Elguezabel.[412] About 30 cases have been reported to date. The patients are in general

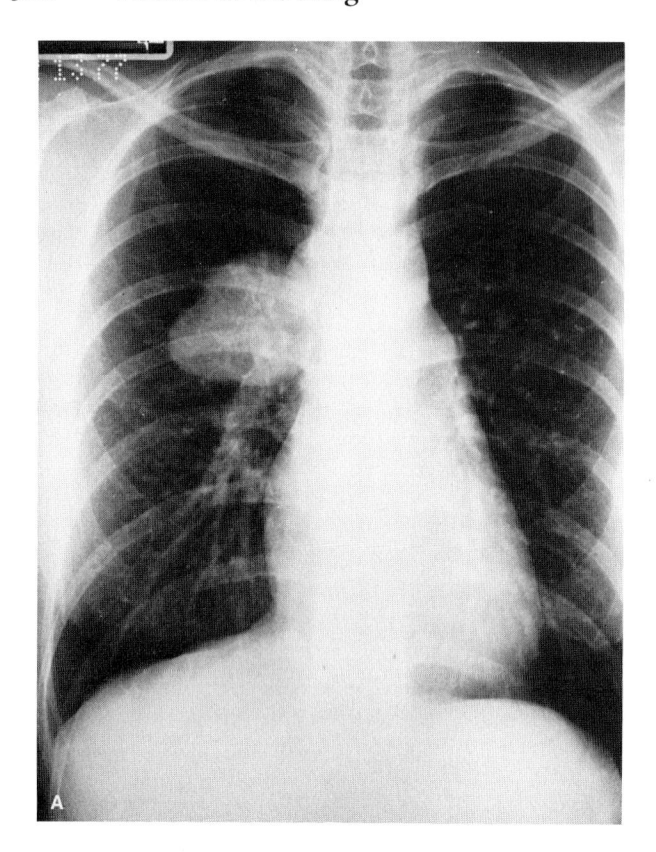

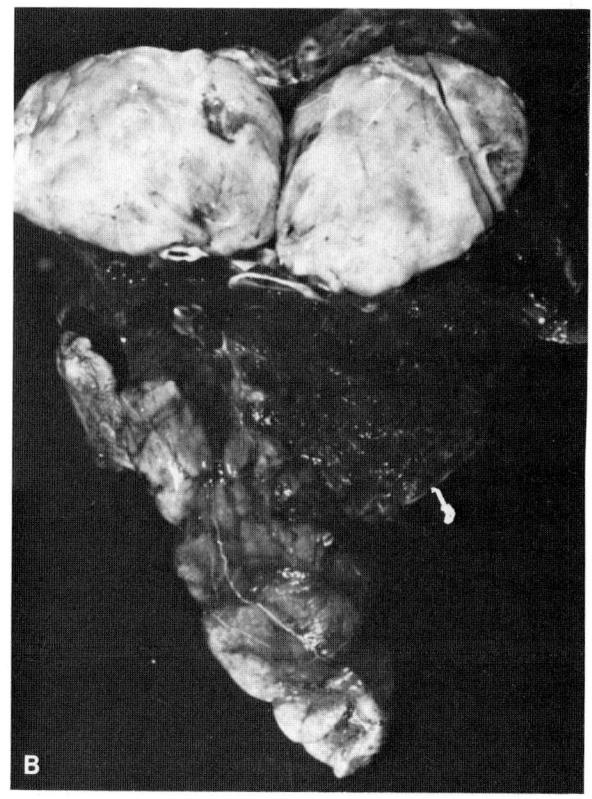

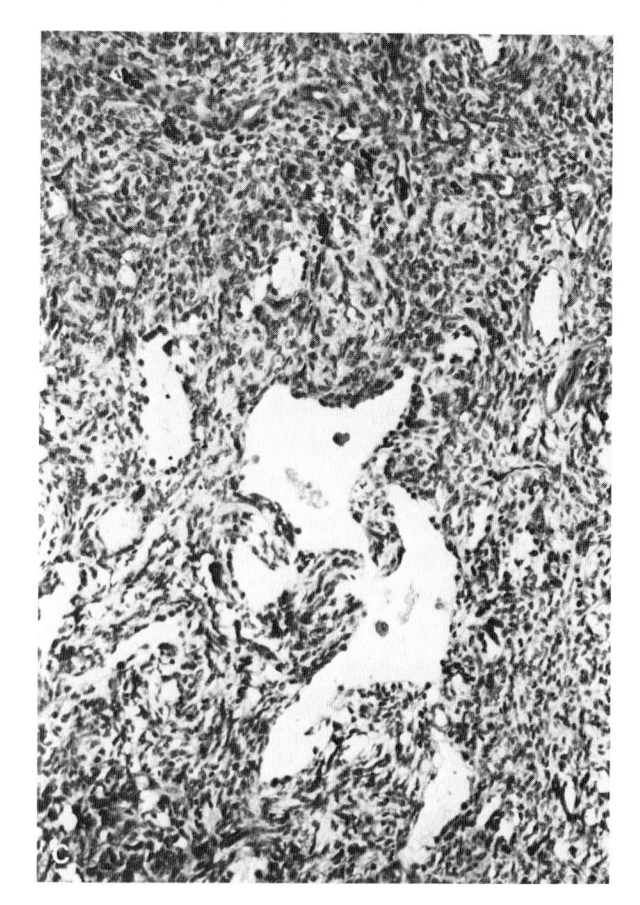

Figure 19–29. Primary hemangiopericytoma of lung. A. Chest radiograph showing a sharply circumscribed tumor mass arising in a young woman. She presented with expectoration of a tumor fragment. B. Gross appearance of resected specimen showing a distinct circumscription of the tumor mass. C. Microscopic appearance demonstrating vessels and spindle cells, typical of hemangiopericytoma (×160).

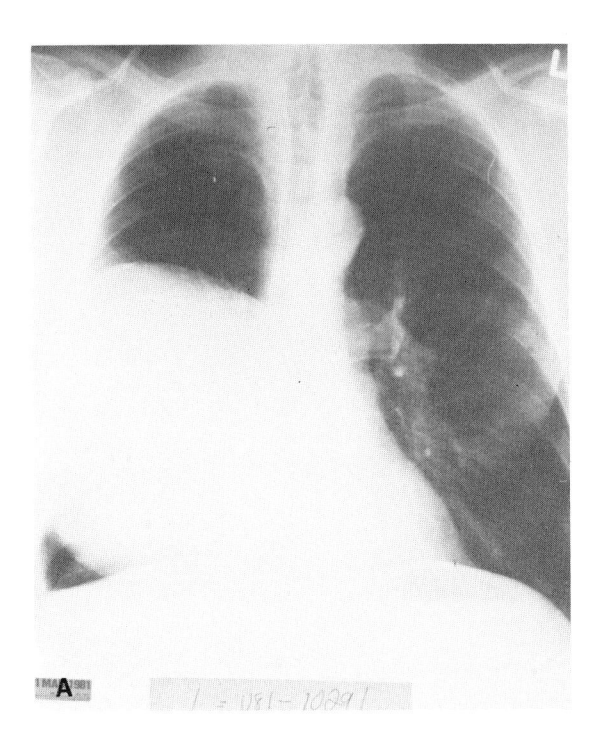

Figure 19–30. Primary malignant fibrous histiocytoma of lung. A. Radiograph of huge right-sided tumor found in an elderly man who presented with weight loss. B and C. Microscopic appearance of the same tumor shown in A. This particular tumor has formed a capsule, visible on the low-power view. The high-power micrograph demonstrates combination of spindle and giant cells, typical of malignant fibrous histiocytoma (B ×40, C ×160).

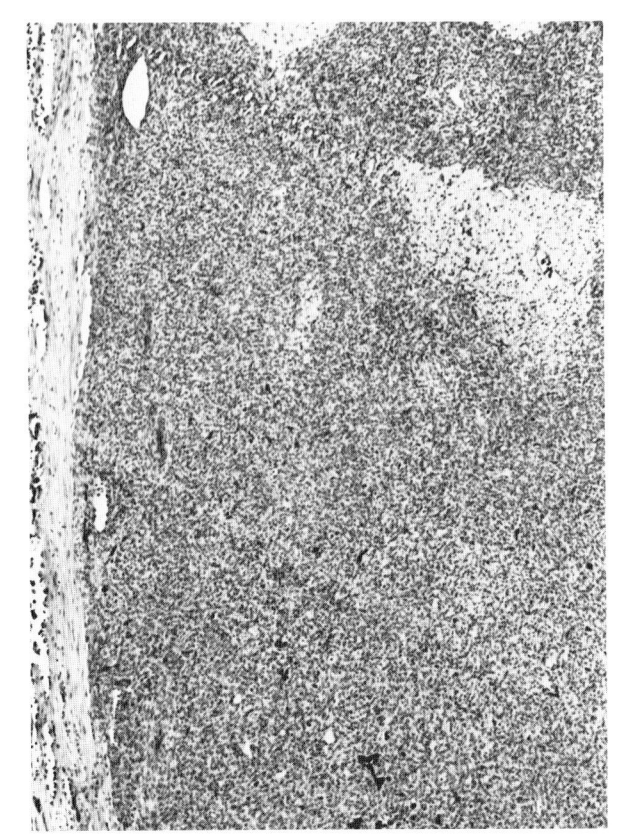

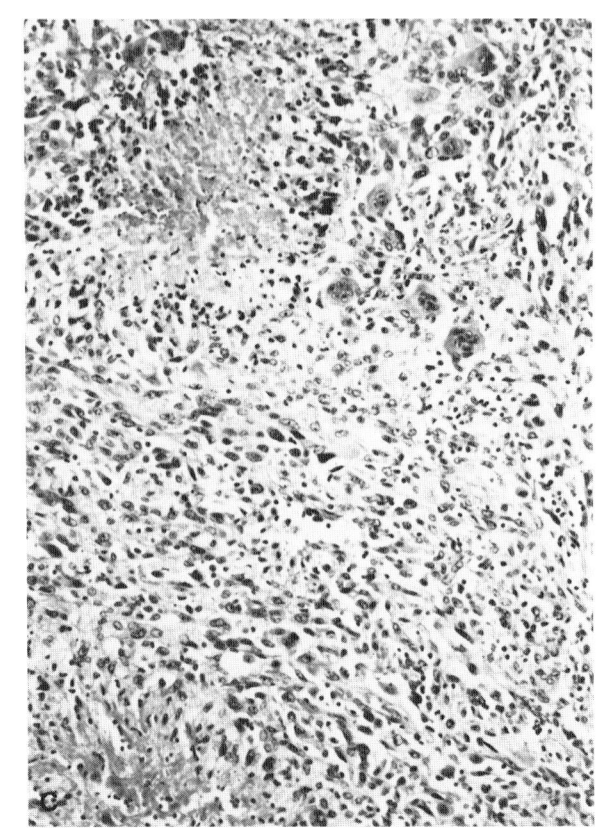

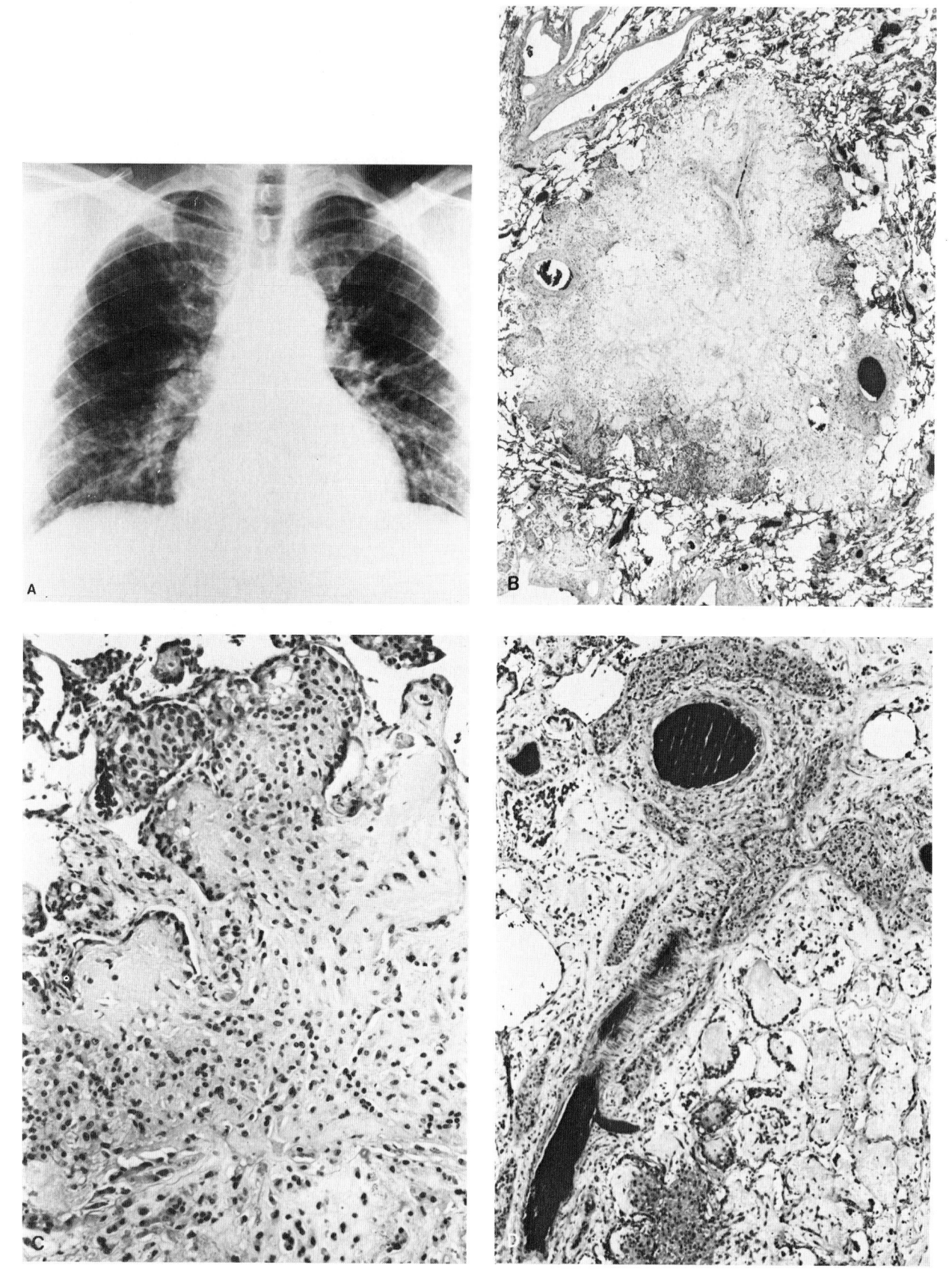

Figure 19–31A–D. Sclerosing vascular sarcoma (intravascular and sclerosing bronchioloalveolar tumor). A. Chest radiograph showing sclerosing vascular sarcoma presenting as multiple small intrapulmonary nodules. B and C. Low- and high-power views of a typical nodule. At the periphery the tumor is composed of polygonal cells, while the central portion of the nodule is composed of a hyaline matrix (B ×20, C ×160). D. Another area from the same slide showing lymphangitic spread of tumor. This focus is far distant from any obvious tumor nodule (×40).

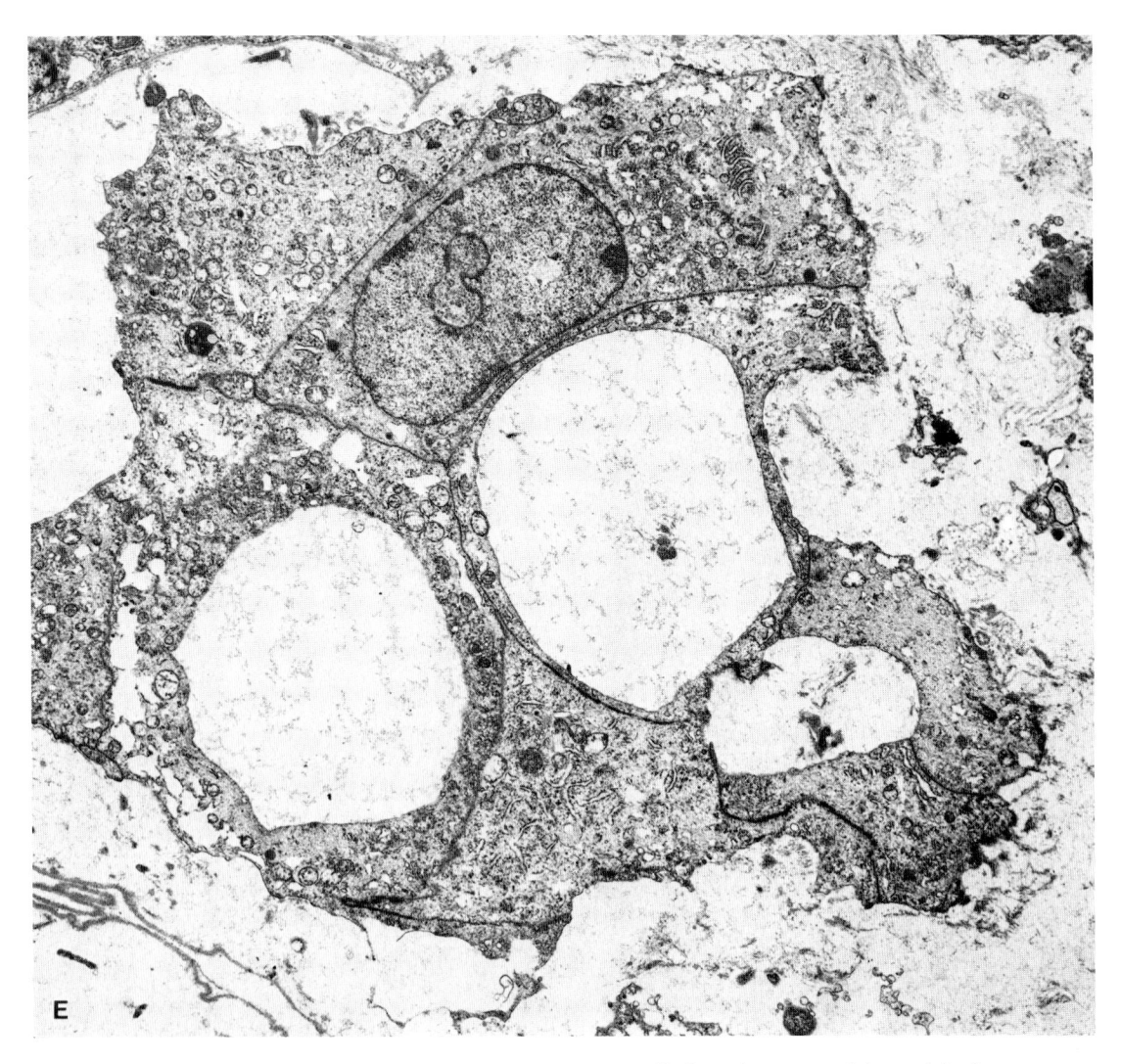

Figure 19–31E. Ultrastructural appearance of tumor cells from the center of the nodule shown in B. Note the formation of lumen-like structures indicating the vascular origin of this tumor (×4500p). Reproduced by permission from Azumi and Churg.[394]

middle-aged to elderly. Those with endobronchial tumors tend to present with symptoms of obstruction, whereas those with parenchymal lesions may present with pulmonary symptoms such as shortness of breath, hemoptysis, chest pain, or with signs of systemic disease. Radiographically the endobronchial lesions generally show evidence of obstruction, whereas the parenchymal lesions appear as large, usually sharply circumscribed masses.

Reported tumors measure up to 14 cm and are usually white to yellow with areas of hemorrhage and necrosis. Microscopically, the vast majority are a combination of squamous carcinoma with a stroma resembling fibrosarcoma, although elements of cartilage and bone may be present as well (Fig. 19–32). In some instances the epithelial component resembles adenocarcinoma or undifferentiated carcinoma.[407,408]

The distinction between a carcinosarcoma and an ordinary bronchogenic carcinoma of the lung with a spindled component may be difficult, particularly when the neoplasm in question appears to be either a squamous carcinoma with spindled elements or a carcinosarcoma with squamous carcinoma and fibrosarcoma. Most of the literature on this topic concerns tumors of the head and neck, and esophagus rather than lung, but presumably the same conclusions apply. The histologic distinctions which have been proposed; for example, whether the two components are totally separate or intermingle, do not appear to indicate tumors with different behavior in the esophagus.[413] Ultrastructural reports are contradictory: Lichtiger and colleagues[414] examined 13 tumors and found features of squamous cells in the spindled component, whereas Leifer and associates[415] were only able to demonstrate

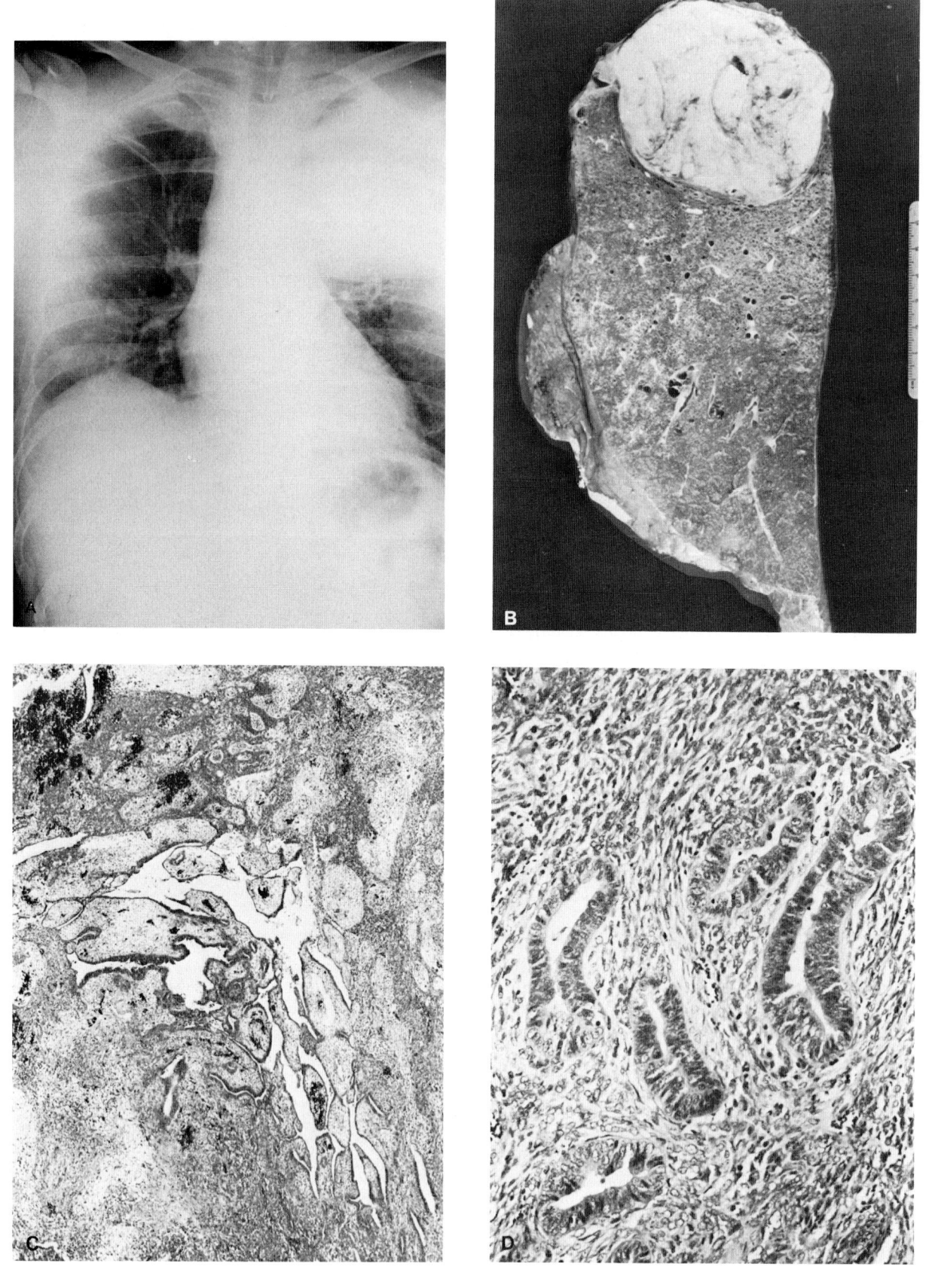

Figure 19–32. Pulmonary blastoma. A. Chest radiograph of a blastoma presenting as a left upper lobe mass in a middle-aged smoker. Note the sharp circumscription of the tumor. B. Gross appearance of the tumor shown in A. C and D. Microscopic appearance of blastoma. A low-power view shows a complicated pattern of stroma and overlying epithelium. The high-power view demonstrates the classic pattern of primitive-appearing glands in an immature stroma (C ×20, D ×160).

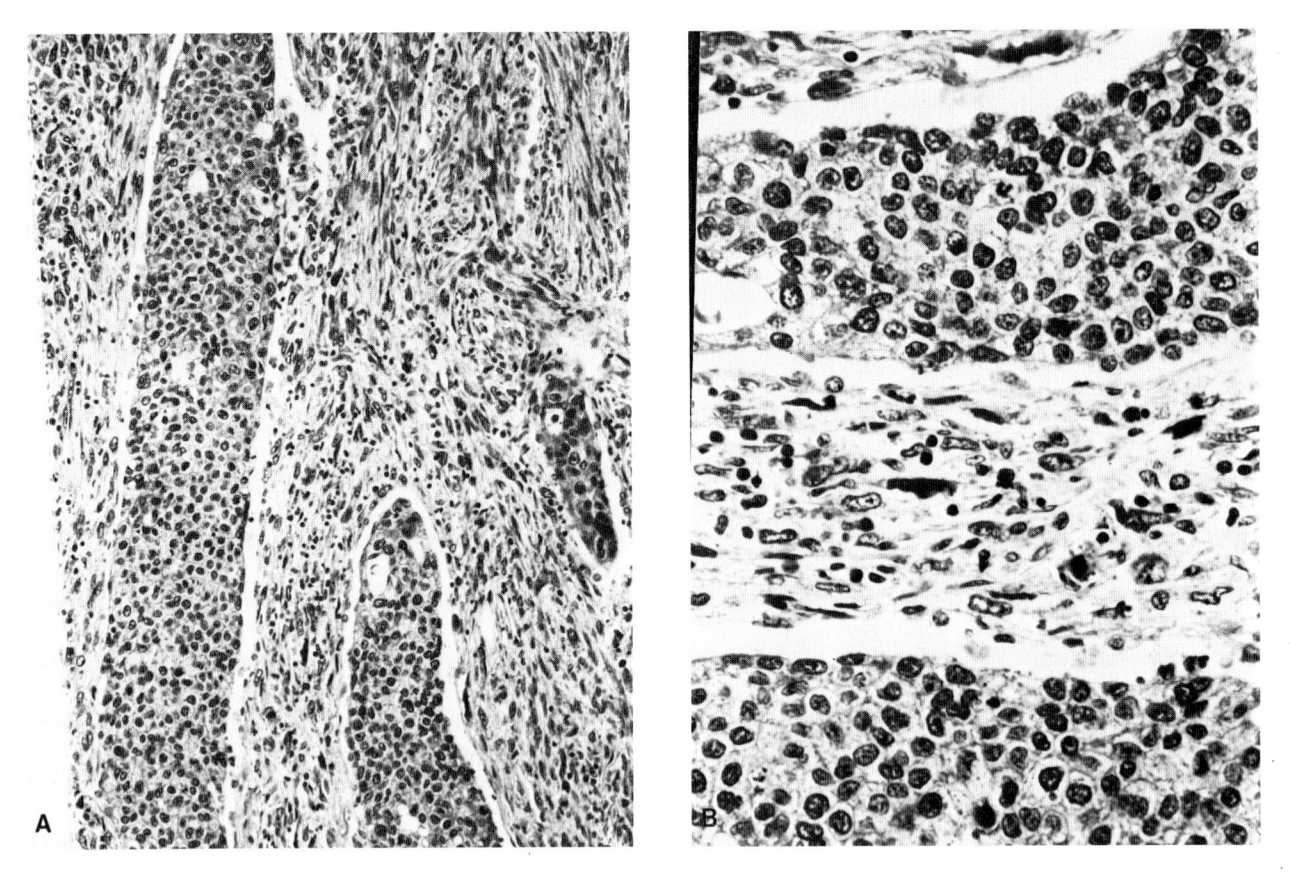

Figure 19–33. Carcinosarcoma. The light micrographs show a tumor composed of a distinctly epithelial as well as a distinctly sarcomatous component (A ×160, B ×400).

fibroblast-like cells in the spindle cell metastases from two similar tumors. Battifora[416] suggested that the spindled component was composed of fibroblasts, squamous cells, and forms transitional between the two. Unless mucin stain reveals mucin, or immunohistochemical staining for keratin is positive in the spindled component, currently there does not seem to be any clear-cut method of separating these neoplasms.

Blastomas typically present over a much wider age range: they have been found in children of 2 months and patients as old as 77 years.[412,417,418] There is a marked male predominance. About 50 cases are now in the literature. Blastomas typically present with a variety of pulmonary complaints including fever, chills, and chest pain. However, a number have been asymptomatic findings, and in rare instances have been present as radiographic lesions for many years. They are almost invariably peripheral lesions which appear well circumscribed radiographically, and may be so large as to occupy almost an entire lobe (Fig. 19–33). Occasionally multiple nodules are present.[419,420] Rare endobronchial forms have been described.[402,421]

McCann and colleagues[422] examined a case of blastoma ultrastructurally and found that two distinct cell types, epithelial and mesenchymal, were present. The epithelial component appeared to differentiate toward ciliated cells, thus imitating the bronchial epithelium, and was separated by a basement membrane from primitive-appearing stromal cells. The stromal cells appeared to be differentiating toward cartilage. Fung and associates[423] concluded that the ultrastructural features were those of fetal lung prior to the fourth gestational month. Tamai and associates[424] transplanted a quite typical-appearing blastoma into nude mice and found that after several passages the stromal cells disappeared and the epithelial component differentiated into squamous cells, mucus-secreting cells, and cells containing neurosecretory granules. They concluded that blastoma is actually a neoplasm of the bronchial epithelium. Marcus and associates[425] found somewhat similar features in a human tumor and concluded that the neoplasm shows intestinal epithelial differentiation.

The notion that blastoma is basically an epithelial tumor has been taken one step further by Kradin and colleagues[426] who reported a purely epithelial neoplasm containing granulated and mucus-secreting cells. Although this tumor may indeed be a blastoma, I believe the histologic features are equally compatible with a diagnosis of peripheral carcinoid, and that the term should in general not be used for monophasic purely epithelial tumors.

In some instances the distinction between blastoma and carcinosarcoma has been difficult: Roth and Elguezabel,[412] Davis and co-workers,[410] and Edwards and associates[427] have reported cases in which the lining epithelium was mature, usually squamous carcinoma, and the stroma was primitive, or in which the reverse occurred. Cartilaginous foci are not uncommon in otherwise typical blastomas. These findings support the notion that blastoma is merely a special variety of carcinosarcoma.

Prediction of clinical course in these tumors is difficult. Roth and Elguezabel[412] have summarized the literature. One case of a patient known to have a blastoma for 24 years has been reported[428] and other patients are living more than 10 years postoperatively. Survival appears better for those with smaller tumors. The overall survival is around 50 percent at 5 years.

The survival for carcinosarcoma appears to be worse than that of blastoma. Of 33 patients summarized by Carter and Eggleston,[429] 27 died of tumor and the longest period of survival was 6 years. All seven patients reported by Bull and Grimes[430] died of tumor with a mean survival of 7 months. Ludwigsen[431] found that four of six patients with endobronchial tumors died within 1 year of diagnosis. This prognosis is not dissimilar to that of carcinoma of the lung, hence there is probably little reason to attempt separation of carcinosarcoma and carcinoma with spindled component if this is not readily obvious.

Malignant Small-Cell Tumor of the Thoracopulmonary Region. Askin and colleagues[432] described 20 examples of a small-cell tumor arising in the thorax in children and adolescents. Only two of the tumors appeared to originate in the lung; the rest were most likely pleural or soft tissue primaries. The ultrastructural features were most consistent with a neuroepithelial origin. The median survival was 8 months.

Secondary Sarcomas in the Lung

The lung is the most common site of metastasis of most sarcomas of the soft tissue and bone; histologic distinction between primary and secondary tumors for the forms which are also primary in lung is not usually feasible, but it should be remembered that metastases outnumber primary tumors by a considerable margin.

Metastasizing Leiomyoma/Multiple Leiomyomatous Hamartomas. These terms have been used to refer to single or multiple cytologically bland-appearing tumors composed of smooth muscle.[368,433] Clinically, these are most commonly seen in the lungs of women of reproductive age or older, but Wolff and colleagues[368] have now reported the same phenomenon in three males. Patients may have a variety of symptoms including cough, dyspnea, and cyanosis; some are asymptomatic. Radiographically the most common finding is the presence of one or more sharply circumscribed nodules; roughly half the cases have multiple nodules. Occasional cases show a fine reticulonodular pattern instead.[434]

The critical features are the pathologic ones. The tumors are, when grossly visible, firm yellow-white, and whorled. They range in size from microscopic to 10 cm. Microscopically they consist of clearly recognizable smooth muscle cells arranged in intersecting bundles (Fig. 19–34). Most reports in the literature claim that mitotic activity is lacking or mimimal, but Wolff and colleagues[368] specifically counted mitotic figures and found that they varied from 0.25 to 12.5 per 10 hpf and were present in every case.

Another typical feature is the presence of slit-like spaces within the masses of smooth muscle. The spaces tend to be more frequent near the periphery of the nodules. They are lined by low cuboidal cells which appear similar to those seen in many reactive conditions, and which may be derived from terminal bonchiolar epithelium or sometimes from reactive alveolar type II cells.

Electron microscopic studies have shown that the cells making up the neoplasm are smooth muscle cells of varying degrees of maturity, often interspersed with a variable amount of fibrous tissue.[435] The entrapped epithelium ultrastructurally resembles cells (Clara cells) of terminal bronchiole; but a few cells with clearly defined lamellar inclusions indicative of type II cells are illustrated by Wolff and colleagues.[368]

The nature of these lesions is controversial; the major issue is whether they represent leiomyomatous hamartomas or metastases. The argument for a hamartomatous nature has largely centered around the absent or low mitotic rate and the presence of glandular elements within the tumor, a finding claimed by some to indicate a pulmonary origin. Piccaluga and Capelli[436] demonstrated by careful study the origin of the glandular structures: the expanding tumor mass causes a reactive proliferation of cellular elements and then entraps these elements by growing within the interstitium around the former air space or bronchiole. The presence of carbon-filled macrophages in these spaces indicates communication with if not origin from the lung.

The argument for a malignant nature has come from the fact that many lesions are multiple and increase in size and number, as is the case with other types of hematogenous metastases. On close inspection the lung lesions always turn out to have at least one and often an appreciable number of mitoses.

Clinically, patients reported with both labels appear to be similar in regard to age, sex, and symptoms; the major differences are that the tumor nodules are present in considerably greater number in patients having recognized metastatic disease.[368,433] Such patients also tend to have a much greater frequency of bilateral disease. Of the documentable cases labeled as hamartoma or a similar lesion, two-thirds had a history of surgery for removal of uterine leiomyomas or purported leiomyomas. Of 20 patients in this category, 8 showed an increase in the size of the lesions remaining after removal of some of the lesions. Among 30 reported cases of benign-appearing smooth muscle tumors that were interpreted as metastases, all the patients had had uterine surgery or were found to have multiple uterine tumors at autopsy. Half

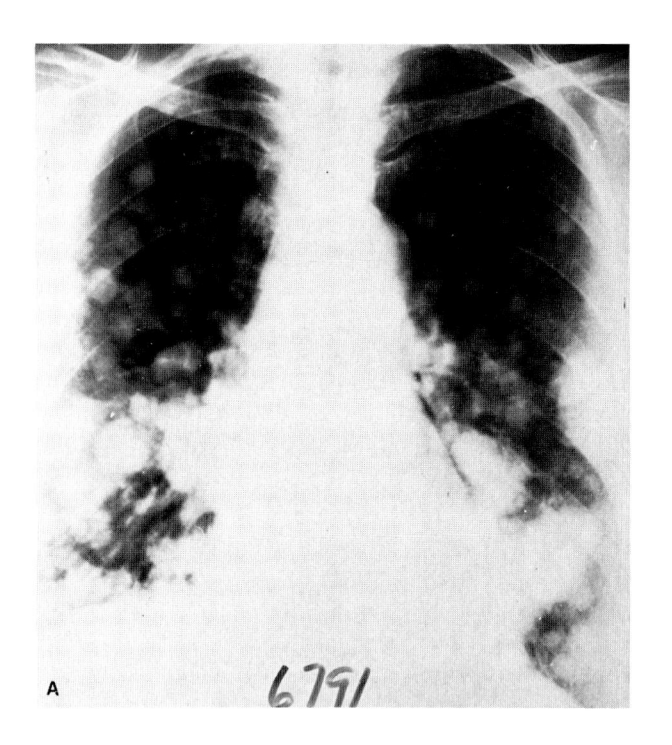

Figure 19–34. Benign metastasizing leiomyoma. A. Chest radiograph of a patient with benign metastasizing leiomyoma which appears radiographically as multiple large intrapulmonary nodules. B and C. Light micrographs from a case of benign metastasizing leiomyoma in which most of the nodules are microscopic to a few millimeters in size. Note the occasional entrapped glands visible in B and atypical spindle cells in C. Electron microscopy confirmed that the cells were smooth muscle (B ×20, C ×160).

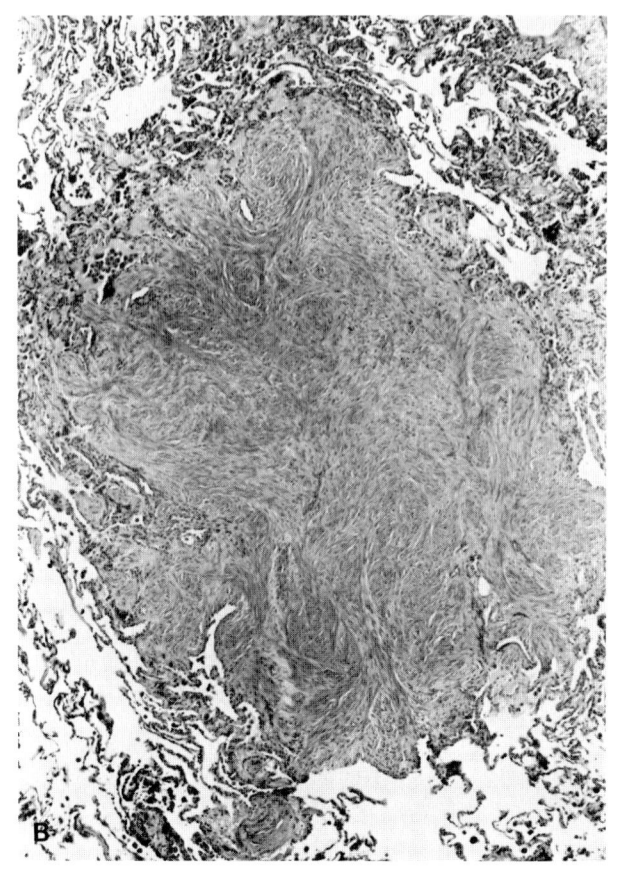

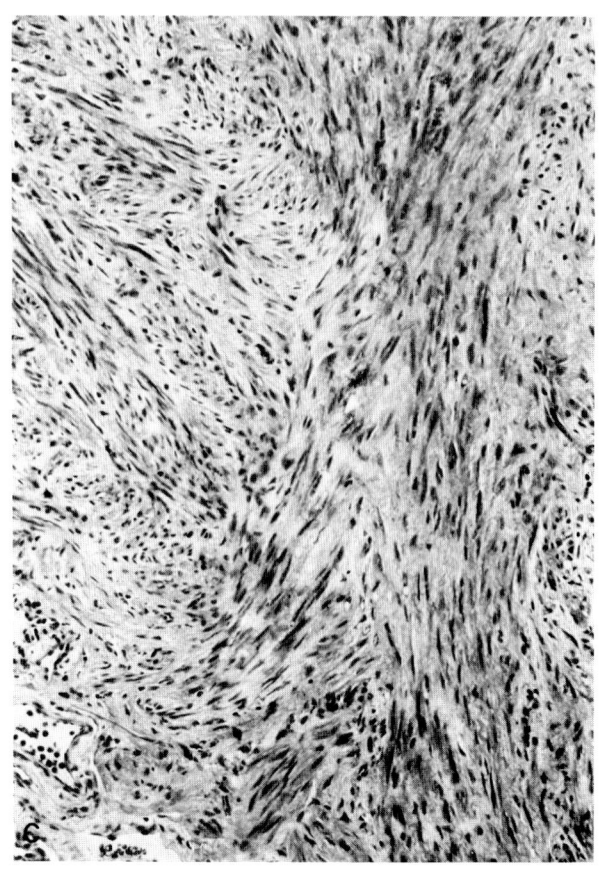

these patients died of their disease. Horstmann and colleagues[433] point out that age has an effect on prognosis: the disease process in the postmenopausal group tends to remain stationary or may be only slowly progressive, while in the premenopausal group pulmonary insufficiency or death is considerably more likely. Of particular interest is the case reported by Horstmann and colleagues.[433] Multiple nodules were found on radiography in a 30-year-old pregnant woman; during pregnancy they regressed spontaneously and became even smaller during postpartum breast feeding. Horstmann and co-workers[433] suggest that these lesions, like those in the uterus, are under hormonal influence. Cramer and associates[437] measured the estrogen receptor content of a very bland-appearing tumor and found that it was near the upper level for a series of uterine leiomyomas. The incorporation of thymidine was much lower than that seen in a leiomyosarcoma, thus confirming the hormonal sensitivity and low growth rate of these neoplasms.

The majority opinion at the present time is that the lesions are in fact all metastases. This finding is supported by Wolff's[368] data on three males with "metastasizing leiomyoma"; all had documented soft tissue primaries. Histologically the pulmonary lesions in the males appeared bland, but the primary tumors (gluteal region, saphenous vein, diaphragm) were clearly malignant. Benign-appearing metastases in women have been seen concomitantly in areas outside the lungs, including the retroperitoneum, lymph nodes, thoracic vessels, and pelvic viscera.[438]

When the nodules of metastasizing leiomyoma are microscopic, the process may be confused with lymphangioleiomyomatosis.[434]

Kaposi's Sarcoma. In the general population, Kaposi's sarcoma metastatic to lung is extremely rare; however, it is seen frequently in patients with acquired immunodeficiency syndrome (AIDS) and is often associated in this condition with pulmonary infections. The tumor itself may prove fatal. References to and illustrations of this process are provided in Chapter 15.

Lymphoproliferative Processes

Intrapulmonary Lymph Nodes

Lymph nodes in humans are normally found in the mediastinum and around the main bronchi at the hilum of the lung. Occasionally, true lymph nodes with capsule and sinusoids may be found deep in the pulmonary parenchyma. Trapnell[439] has examined a series of postmortem lungs by angiography and found that intrapulmonary nodes could be demonstrated in 6 of 92 cases, an incidence of 7 percent. In one of these cases the node could be seen as a lesion on routine chest film. Their clinical importance stems from the fact that they may appear as coin lesions.[440] Angiofollicular lymph node hyperplasia of Castleman may also occasionally be found within the lung; the histologic appearance is similar to that of angiofollicular hyperplasia in other sites.[441]

Lymphomas and Pseudolymphomas

All types of lymphoid and hematopoietic malignancies may involve the lung, but only a few are primary lesions. Freeman and colleagues[442] found that primary pulmonary lymphomas accounted for only 3.6 percent of a series of 1467 extranodal lymphomas. In general, primary lymphomas in the lung take the form of well-differentiated lymphocytic or lymphoplasmacytic lymphomas[443-445] or histiocytic lymphomas[443,444]; occasionally one also finds cases of primary Hodgkin's disease. Poorly differentiated lymphocytic lymphomas, although common as nodal primaries, are uncommon as primary lymphomas in the lung. The diagnosis of Hodgkin's disease and of histiocytic lymphoma is usually obvious; the major difficulty in the lung consists of separating well-differentiated lymphocytic lymphomas from pseudolymphomas.

Pseudolymphoma and Well-Differentiated Lymphocytic Lymphoma. Pseudolymphomas, by definition, are lesions that simulate the histologic appearance of lymphomas. The concept of pseudolymphomas as mimics of lymphomas derives from the work of Saltzstein,[446,447] but Colby and Carrington[448] have questioned whether any such tumors exist. This problem is partially a matter of definition: at one end of the spectrum are tumors composed of a mixture of inflammatory cells, fibrous tissue, and sometimes giant cells, which shade off into obvious inflammatory pseudotumors and plasma cell granulomas. When there is a major lymphoid component, some would refer to such tumors as pseudolymphomas. Difficulties arise when the tumors are composed entirely or nearly entirely of lymphoid cells. Saltzstein[446,447] suggested that the presence of a mixed inflammatory infiltrate along with germinal centers indicated the benign nature of the lesion. A highly polymorphous cell population still appears to be a reliable indicator of pseudolymphoma, and the presence of numerous germinal centers scattered through the lesion also favors a benign diagnosis if the intervening cell population is polymorphous (Table 19–32). However, there is no doubt that germinal centers, arising either as a reaction to tumor or from some other process (such as obstruction) in the lung, may be seen in or around true lymphomas. When associated with lymphomas, they are usually present only in small numbers. Other features of pseudolymphomas are sparing of the pleura (at least to the extent that plaques of tumor cells are not formed), lack of lymphangitic spread within the lung, and minor degrees of vascular infiltration. The latter feature may be seen with any lymphoid infiltrate in the lung, and is not specific. In some instances pseudolymphomas contain large areas of scarring (Table 19–32). Individual fields of pseudolymphomas may be identical in appearance to lymphoid interstitial pneumonia, but the former process is localized and the latter diffuse.[449]

Well-differentiated lymphocytic lymphoma (WDL) or lymphoplasmacytic lymphoma grossly appears as single or multiple yellow to grey masses. Microscopically, these neoplasms are characterized by a monomorphous proliferation of well-differentiated mature lymphocytes (*see* Fig. 19–36). In the nodules the underlying pulmonary architecture is effaced; at the periphery, tumor cells spread through the interstitium, expanding it at the expense of air spaces. Vascular involvement is common but neither spectacular nor specific. Involvement of the pleura by large numbers of tumor cells with the formation of plaques on the visceral pleura is a finding

Table 19–32. Separation of Pseudolymphoma from Well-Differentiated Lymphocytic Lymphoma

Well-Differentiated Lymphocytic Lymphomas	Pseudolymphoma
Monomorphous proliferation of mature lymphocytes	Polymorphous mixture of lymphocytes, plasma cells, histiocytes
Germinal centers few or absent	Germinal centers often present in large numbers
Large areas of scarring may be present	Scarring not usually seen
May form pleural tumor plaques	Tumor plaques not present
Monoclonal cell population by marker studies	Polyclonal cell population
Minor degrees of vasculitis may be present	Minor degrees of vasculitis may be present
Tumor cells spread lymphangitically	Lymphangitic spread not present

indicative of true lymphoma (Table 19–32). Another feature strongly suggesting lymphoma is tracking of lymphoid cells along lymphatic routes[445,448,450,451] (that is, the bronchovascular bundles and the lobular septa); this phenomenon should be looked for away from tumor nodules, since any sort of lymphoid nodule in lung can expand interstitially immediately around its periphery.

One further feature that, when present, aids in the separation of pseudolymphomas from true lymphomas, is involvement of the regional lymph nodes. A finding of lymphoma in a regional node is clear indication of the nature of the process in the lung; however, most WDL presenting in the lung do not have nodal involvement[448] and a negative finding should not be interpreted as indicating that the pulmonary process is benign.

Attempts have been made to separate true and pseudolymphoma using immunohistochemical techniques to demonstrate monoclonal or polyclonal cell lines: by analogy with nodal lesions, pseudolymphomas should be polyclonal proliferations and true lymphomas monoclonal proliferations. The results suggest that the methods are bedeviled by technical problems (particularly attempting to examine cell surface markers in formalin-fixed, paraffin-embedded tissue), but also that the criteria for separating pseudolymphoma and lymphoma need revision. Faguet and co-workers[452] describe what they believe is a benign lymphoid proliferation which nonetheless exhibited monoclonal markers in a patient wth Sjögren's syndrome. Twenty-two months later the patient developed an overt lymphoma. Similarly, Julsrud and colleagues[453] using immunoperoxidase staining on paraffin-embedded tissue, found that three of six lesions believed to be pseudolymphomas exhibited monoclonal staining. One of these patients eventually developed lymphoma. However, Herbert and co-workers[454] found monoclonal staining in four of four tumors examined. I believe that one of the problems in the diagnosis of lymphoid malignancies in the lung is the presence of benign lymphoid reactions that hide tumor cells, and that, not surprisingly, exhibit polyclonal staining. Engulfment of tumor cells by benign-reacting cells would also account for the appearance of some cases of so-called lymphomatoid granulomatosis, a lesion that appears to be a form of malignant lymphoma (*see* below).

Radiographically, pseudolymphomas are localized lesions which appear as nodules or irregular infiltrates[443–455] (Fig. 19–35). Most patients present with pulmonary symptoms including cough, sputum production, and fever, but some lesions are incidental findings. Sometimes pseudolymphomas appear radiographically at the site of a previous episode of pneumonia.

Well-differentiated lymphocytic lymphomas are characterized radiographically by localized infiltrates which may be well circumscribed and sometimes nodular (Fig. 19–36); the average size in the series of Julsrud and colleagues[453] was 6.2 cm. Multiple nodules were visible in one-fourth of 36 patients reviewed by Colby and Carrington.[456] Hilar adenopathy is apparently rare. Clinically, collected series of patients with pulmonary WDL indicate that most occur in middle-aged patients.[443–445] The presenting complaints are nonspecific and include cough, chest pain, and recurrent bouts of pneumonia. Some patients are asymptomatic and the tumors are incidental findings on chest x-ray examination.

Recent studies indicate that the prognosis of these lesions is usually excellent, with 80 percent 10-year and up survivals in some series (Table 19–33). To a certain extent, this finding may lessen the importance of separating these types of low-grade lymphomas from pseudolymphomas.

Histiocytic Lymphoma. Less data is available concerning histiocytic lymphoma primary in the lung. Freeman[442] reported that these lesions constituted 15% of primary pulmonary lymphomas. L'Hoste and colleagues[444] found 12 cases in a series of 36 lymphomas, but Koss and associates[443] only identified 8 in a series of 120 lymphoid malignancies. Colby and Carrington[450] reported 20 patients with a male/female ratio of 2:1. The average age was 53 years. Three-fourths of the patients were symptomatic, and most symptoms related to the thorax. Single or multiple nodules were found on chest films in 14 patients and diffuse infiltrates in the other 6 (Fig. 19–37).

Microscopically, the usual histiocytic lymphoma of lung resembles that of other organs (*see* Fig. 19–37). In contrast to the well-differentiated lymphocytic lymphomas, the histiocytic tumors are considerably more destructive; they are not confined to the interstitium but instead obliterate the architecture completely. Necrosis is common (13 of 20 cases of Colby and Carrington), and a destructive vasculitis caused by tumor cells is also a frequent finding (*see* Fig. 19–37). Lymphatic tracking of the sort seen in WDL is also found with histiocytic lymphoma. In the series of Colby and Carrington,[450] tumor was seen in hilar nodes in one of seven cases. Nine of 20 patients died of their disease, almost all within 1 year, and the prognosis in other recent series appears equally poor.[443,444]

Many cases of histiocytic lymphoma or immunoblastic

Figure 19–35. Pseudolymphoma. A. Chest radiograph showing a vaguely defined right upper lobe infiltrate (circled) which had been present for 6 months. The patient had recently had a bout of pneumonia which radiographically appeared to be in the same location. B and C. Microscopic appearance of pseudolymphoma showing numerous germinal centers, as well as cholesterol clefts and included gland-like spaces derived from pulmonary epithelium (B ×40, C ×160).

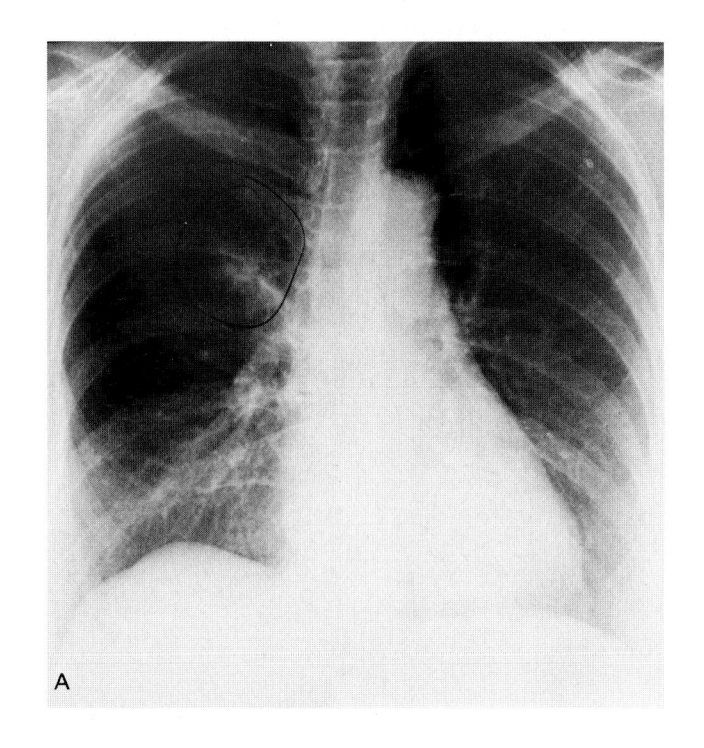

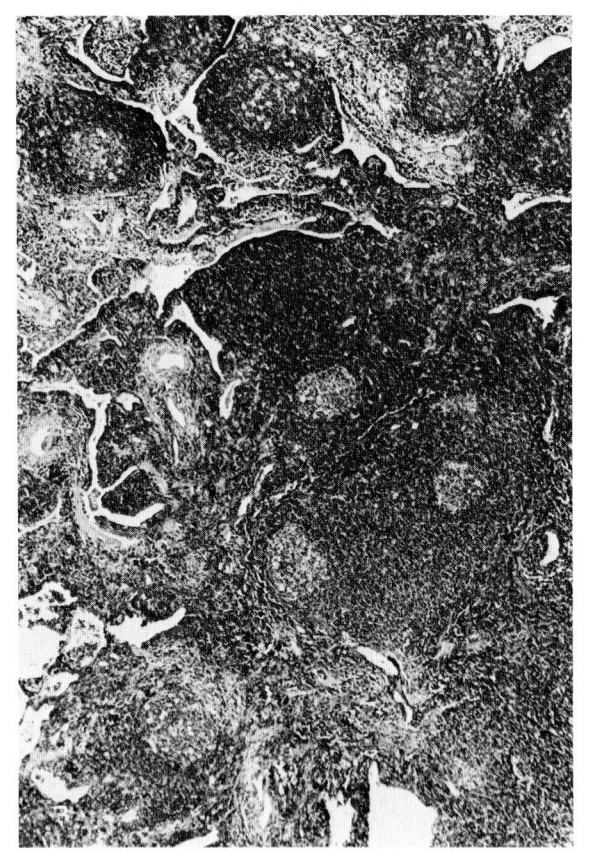

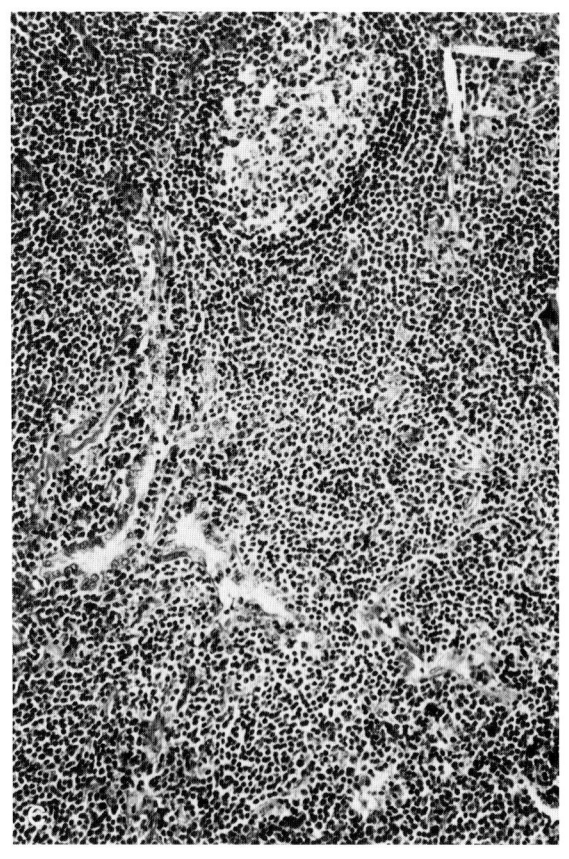

'sarcoma in the lung show the features (vasculitis, necrosis, and atypical cells) of so-called lymphomatoid granulomatosis (LYG). However, recent studies suggest that most examples of LYG turn out to be lymphoma or lymphoproliferative processes such as angioimmunoblastic lymphadenopathy when carefully examined, and it is doubtful that LYG actually represents a separate disease.[448,450,456,457] Lymphatoid granulomatosis is described in Chapter 17; the issue of its existence is considered at length by Churg.[457] My rule of thumb is that

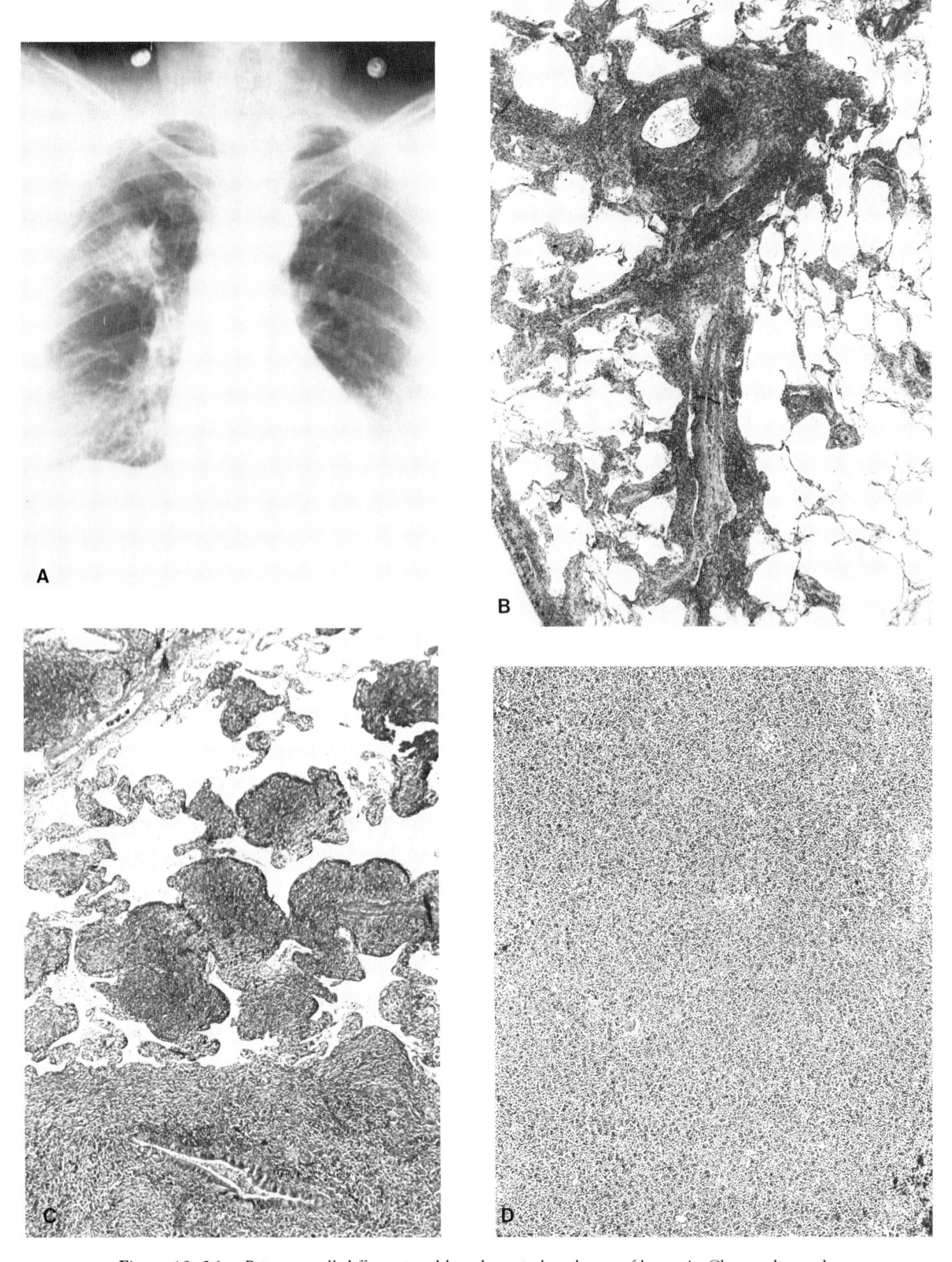

Figure 19–36. Primary well-differentiated lymphocytic lymphoma of lung. A. Chest radiograph showing well-differentiated lymphocytic lymphoma presenting as a localized right upper lobe lesion. B. Low-power appearance of the same tumor away from the mass lesion, demonstrating lymphangitic spread of tumor along the bronchovascular bundles. This histologic appearance is strongly suggestive of malignant lymphoma, either primary or secondary. C through E. Another case of well-differentiated lymphocytic lymphoma. C shows the tendency of tumor to spread in the interstitium away from the large nodular masses. In the center of the large masses (D and E) the tumor forms monotonous sheets of well-differentiated lymphocytes. The presence of a monomorphous cell population is also strongly indicative of malignant lymphoma (B ×20, C ×40, D ×64, E ×400).

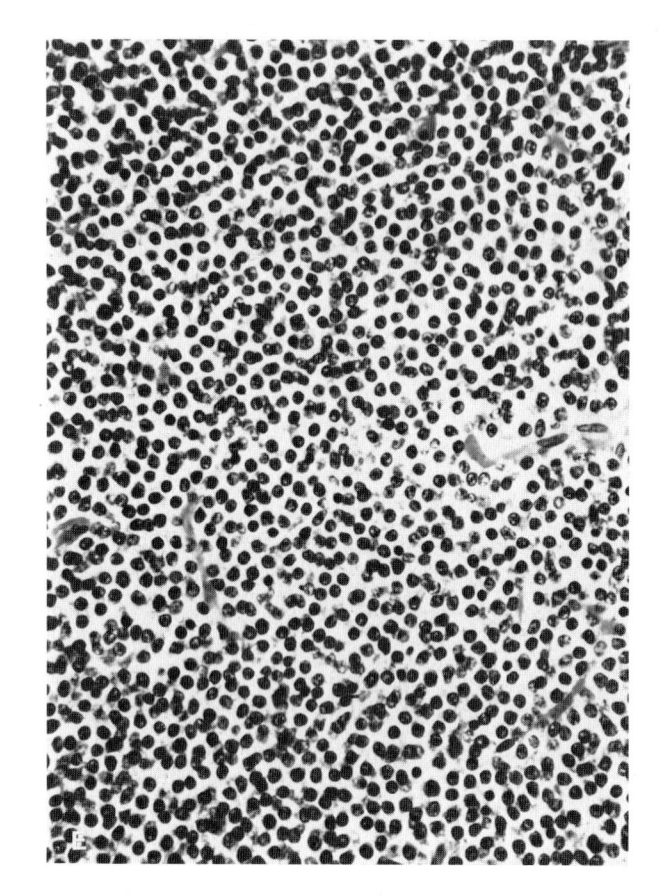

Figure 19–36E. See page 397 for explanation.

Table 19–33. Survival in Primary Well-Differentiated Lymphocytic or Lymphoplasmacytic Lymphomas

Report	Outcome
Koss et al.[443]	80% survival at 11 years
Turner et al.[445]	1 of 33 dead of disease
L'Hoste et al.[444]	88% alive at 5 years
Colby and Carrington[456]	3 of 34 dead of disease

mass lesions showing vasculitis, necrosis, and atypical lymphoid cells should be diagnosed and treated as high-grade lymphomas, since most seem to behave as such.

Hodgkin's Disease. Primary pulmonary Hodgkin's disease is rare.[458–460] Wood and Coltman[461] reported 28 cases with 6 five year survivors. Histologically, most of these lesions appear to be of nodular sclerosis type. The diagnostic criteria are similar to those of nodal Hodgkin's disease. As is true of other lung lymphomas, there is a distinct tendency for the tumors to spread in a lymphangitic fashion.

Plasmacytoma. Primary solitary plasmacytomas of the lung are rare. Romanoff and Milwidsky[462] reviewed 14 cases and added 1 of their own; however, their case, as well as a number of others in their listing appear to be plasma cell granulomas or manifestations of systemic multiple myeloma. A recent primary case has been reported by Wile and colleagues.[463] The number of correctly identified cases appears too small to permit assessment of their behavior.

Lung: Secondary Involvement by Lymphomas

Secondary involvement of the lung by lymphomas of all types is common, and, more important, is histologically indistinguishable from primary tumor. As a practical matter, secondary involvement should be one's first thought when encountering a hematopoietic neoplasm in the lung. Secondry involvement has been reported not only in the usual types of lymphocytic lymphoma and Hodgkin's disease (in almost half of primary nodal cases),[458] but in mycosis fungoides (Fig. 19–38), malignant histiocytosis,[448] and angioimmunoblastic lymphadenopathy.[464] Colby and associates[448] point out that lymphatic tracking (lymphangitic spread) by tumor is an extremely useful diagnostic feature, since this phenomenon is apparently not seen in benign conditions, and may occasionally be the only clue to the diagnosis (see Fig. 19–38). Leukemias may also produce clinical pulmonary disease, usually of a restrictive type; histologically this type of involvement is characterized by extensive interstitial infiltration with formation of tumor aggregates along lymphatic routes.

Miscellaneous Tumors and Tumor-Like Lesions of the Lung

Tumor-Like Lesions that May be Reactive or Neoplastic

Plasma Cell Granuloma. This lesion is known by a variety of terms including inflammatory pseudotumor, histiocytoma, vascular endothelioma, and fibroxanthoma. The name plasma cell granuloma was coined by Bahadori and Liebow,[465] and is probably worth preserving, since pseudolymphomas, amyloid nodules, and a variety of other inflammatory processes (see below) have been labeled as "inflammatory pseudotumors." Occasionally the term plasmacytoma has been used, but this should be reserved for the true hematopoietic neoplasm of that nature.

Bahadori and Liebow[465] presented 40 cases; the sex ratio showed a slight female predominance. Although the age range runs from infancy to the seventh decade, one-third of their patients were less than 20 years of age and 11 were 10 years old or younger. Patients presented with cough, hemoptysis, and shortness of breath, the latter sometimes resulting from obstructing intrabronchial lesions. Chest pain, cyanosis and clubbing were also noted; clubbing was seen in only one patient and disappeared after removal of the lesion. Rarely a history of infection precedes the appearance of the tumor.

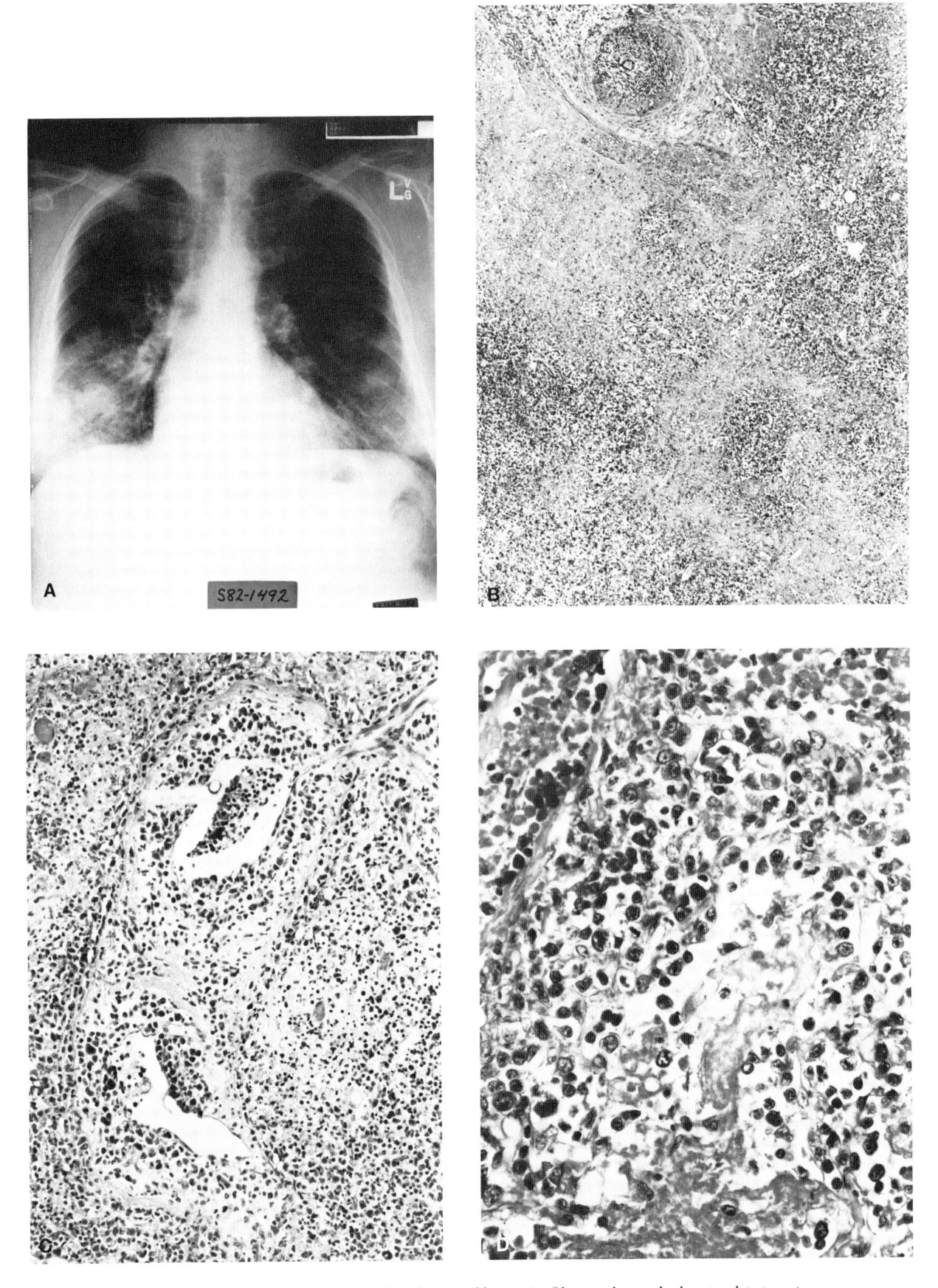

Figure 19–37. Primary histiocytic lymphoma of lung. A. Chest radiograph showing histiocytic lymphoma presenting as multiple bilateral nodules. B through D. Microscopic appearance of primary histiocytic lymphoma of lung. Note extensive necrosis (B) and vasculitis (C and D). The cells are obviously cytologically malignant. Except for the question of cytologic malignancy, the histologic appearance is identical to lymphomatoid granulomatosis which this author believes to be a form of malignant lymphoma (B ×40, C ×160, D ×400).

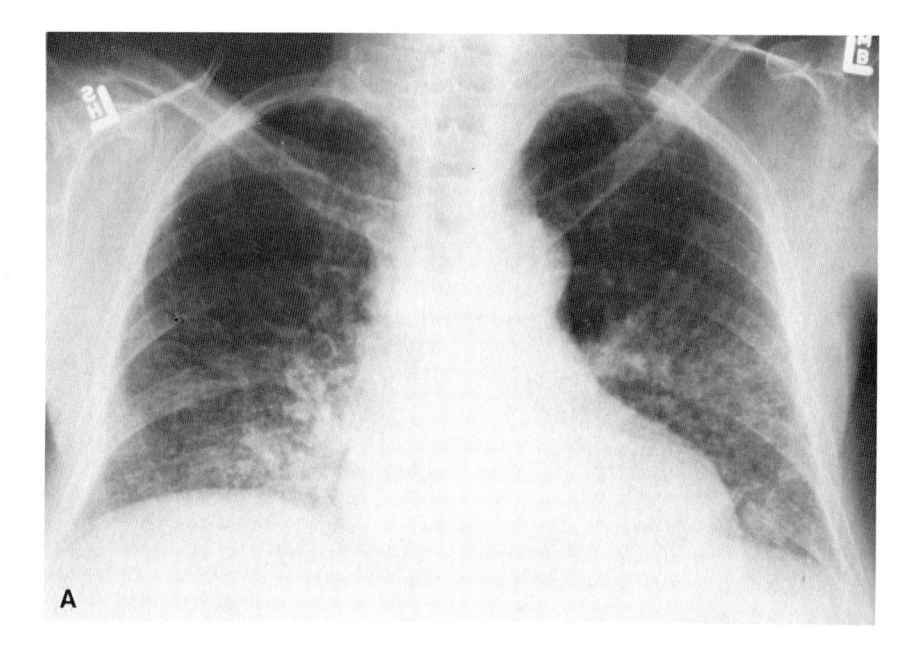

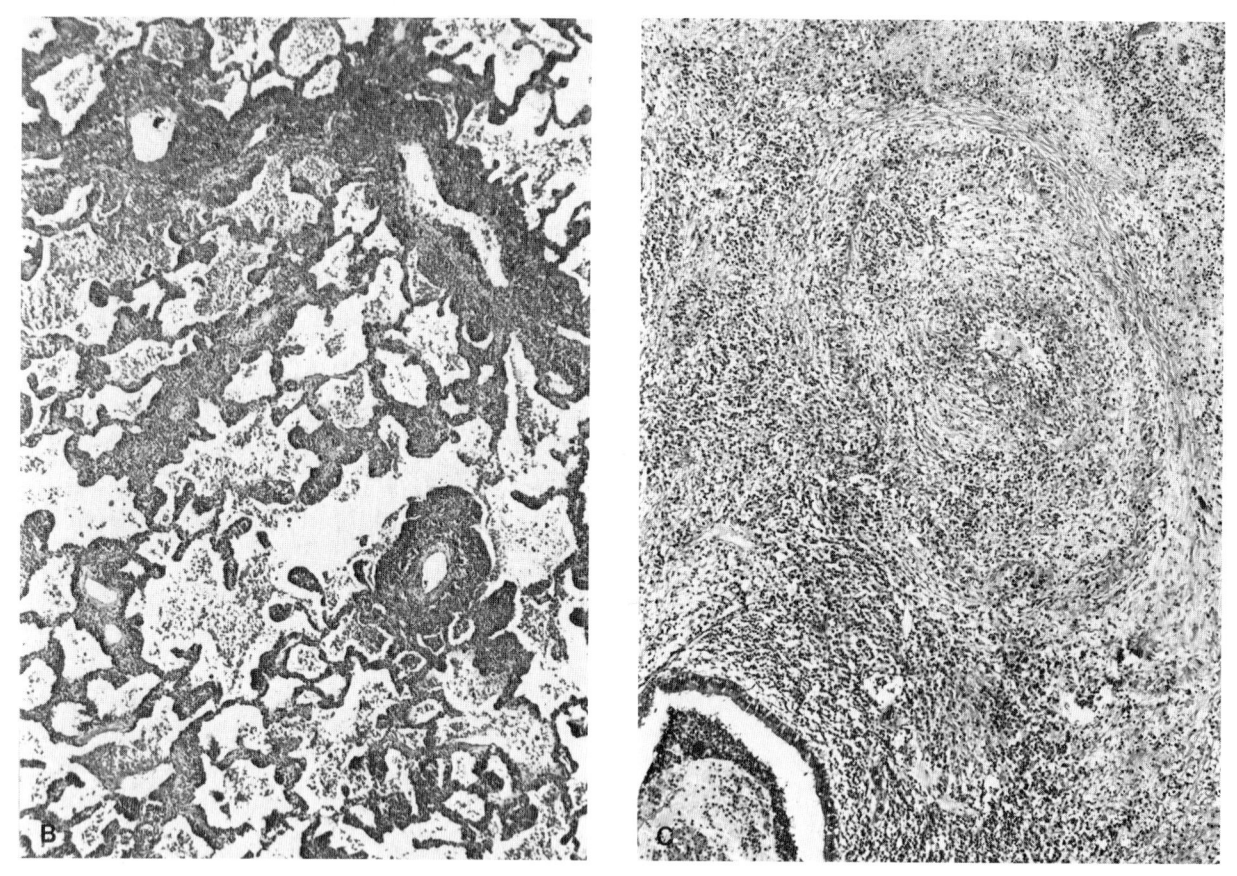

Figure 19–38A–C. Secondary lymphoma in the lung. A. Chest radiograph showing a pattern of lymphangitic spread of tumor in a patient with extensive mycosis fungoides. B through D. Microscopic appearance of the tumor shown in A. Note the pattern of lymphangitic spread (B) and the destructive vasculitis (C) (B ×40, C ×64). See Figure 19–38D on page 401.

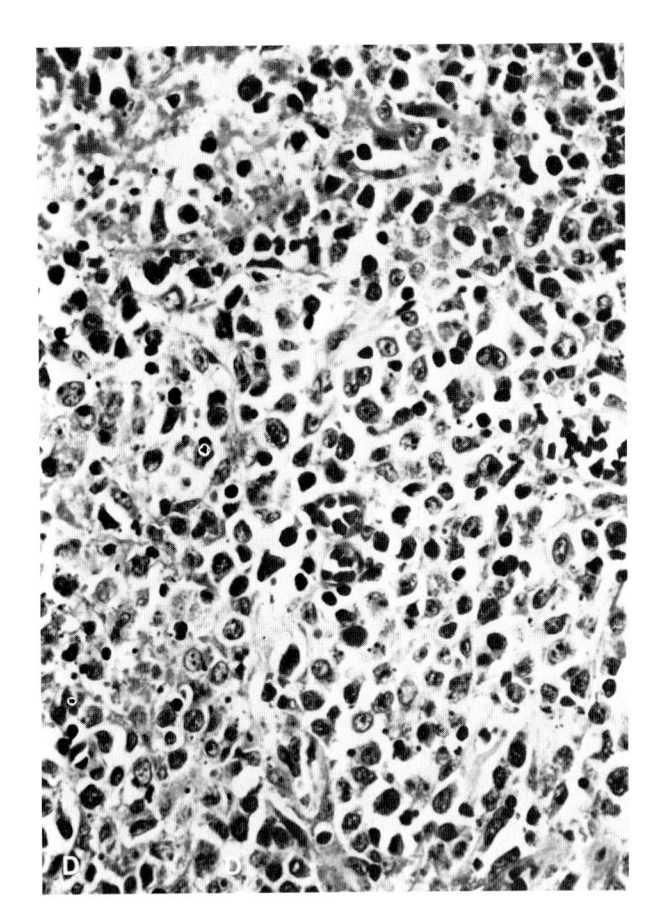

Figure 19–38D. Vasculitis as well as necrosis may be seen in secondary lymphomas involving the lung and is not a specific finding (D ×400).

Radiographically, the majority of lesions are coin lesions or discrete solitary masses (Fig. 19–39); several were followed for up to 2 years and the lesions increased slowly in size. Occasionally the tumors are so large as to occupy an entire lung field; they may also be calcified. Cavitation is occasionally observed.[465–467]

Plasma cell granulomas macroscopically appear as well-circumscribed masses and are somewhat more frequent in the lower lobes. They may grow through the pleura or into the mediastinum, and may also obstruct a bronchus or even the trachea or esophagus.[468] Obliteration of bronchi within the masses is common. The color is variable but commonly white-yellow; evidence of old and recent hemorrhage may be present, as well as foci of necrosis and calcification. Microscopically, the tumor is not as sharply defined as it appears grossly in most instances and usually does not possess a capsule (see Fig. 19–39). The striking features are a combination of fibrous tissue which may be exceedingly dense and calcified, interspersed to a variable degree with inflammatory cells and almost always with large numbers of plasma cells (see Fig. 19–39). Amyloid may be present. In other instances the stromal component is composed of very loose connective tissue. The lymphoid cells are occasionally dense and arranged in the form of germinal centers. Histiocytes and foamy macrophages may be seen. The distinction between plasma cell granuloma and benign fibrous histiocytoma can be extremely difficult; the latter presumably have a minimal inflammatory component and a prominent fibrous stroma.

These lesions are benign; recurrence is unusual, but I have seen this phenomenon in one patient. Radiation has been used to shrink the tumor in some instances.[469]

The etiology of plasma cell granulomas is unknown; some are clearly postinflammatory. Recently Buell and co-workers[470] examined a plasma cell granuloma ultrastructurally and found what they believed to be possible viral particles on some of the cells, a finding that suggests that the original process could be a viral infection.

It is possible that old plasma cell granulomas eventually become hyalinized and are included in the rather nonspecific groups of pseudotumors called "hyalinizing granuloma."[471] The latter are nodules of hyaline connective tissue with variable amounts of inflammatory cells; most likely they represent an end stage of many different pulmonary processes. As noted above, the term inflammatory pseudotumor is also used for a variety of other conditions, ranging from pseudolymphoma,[472] to pulmonary infarction,[473] to amyloid nodule.[474] Also in this category are lesions that histologically resemble an organizing pneumonia, but that present as vaguely defined nodular masses radiographically.[467] These tumors are probably foci of resolving or persisting pneumonia (Fig. 19–40).

Sclerosing Hemangioma. This lesion was first named by Liebow and Hubbell[475] who described seven cases. Further cases were collected by Arean and Wheat[476] and by Katzenstein and colleagues.[477] These tumors have also been called xanthomas and histiocytomas.

The recorded cases indicate that sclerosing hemangioma is most likely to occur in women (about two-thirds of cases). The age range is wide, varying from young children to the fifth and sixth decades, but the majority occur around 30 to 40 years of age. Often the history suggests that the neoplasm has been present for many years before diagnosis.

A variety of presenting complaints are found; of these hemoptysis, which may be severe, is the most common. A few patients have symptoms such as fever, anorexia, night sweats, chest pain, and pneumonia. Radiographically the process usually appears as a sharply demarcated lesion, most frequently seen in the lower right lobe. On occasion, a diffuse lesion is seen, most likely as a result of bronchial compression. In several cases, extremely slow radiographic progression has been noted over a period of several years.

Grossly, the sclerosing hemangioma is a sharply demarcated lesion, usually surrounded by a fibrous capsule which is probably derived from organization of old and recent hemorrhage. The bulk of the tumor may be hemorrhagic or yellow to grey or pink. Not infrequently the tumor bulges into the pleural cavity and occasionally

Figure 19–39. Plasma cell granuloma. A. Chest radiograph showing plasma cell granuloma seen as a sharply circumscribed mass (the typical radiographic appearance) in a young man who presented with cough. B and C. Microscopic appearance of the tumor shown in A. This particular example is predominantly fibrous with a scattering of plasma cells between the collagen bundles. However, other examples of plasma cell granuloma may be predominantly cellular with little fibrous tissue (B ×40, C ×160).

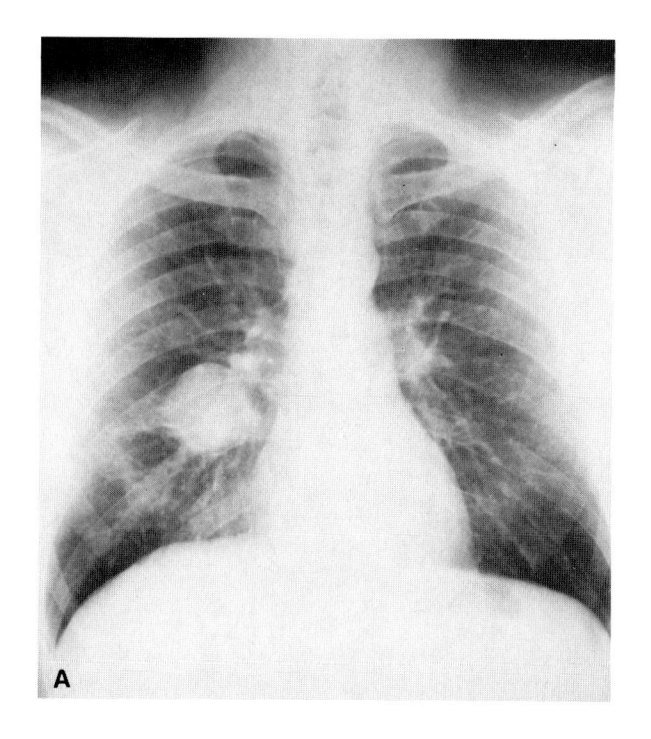

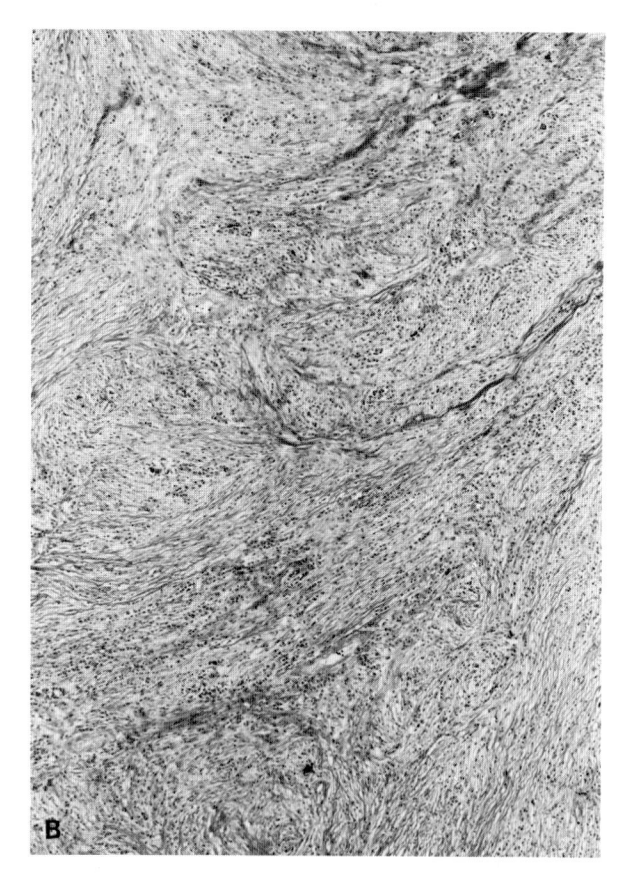

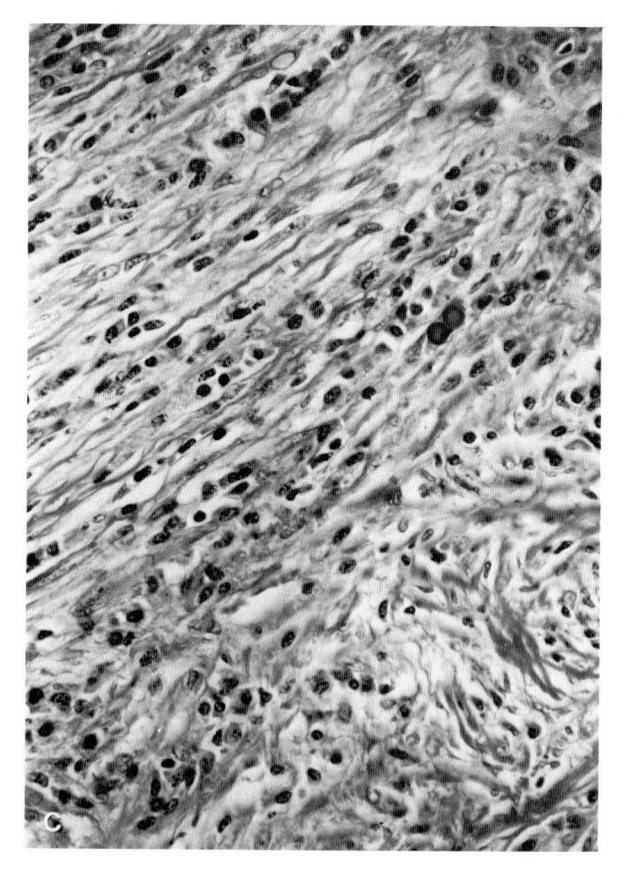

into the mediastinum. A few cases with multiple apparently separate lesions have been reported.[476,478]

Microscopically, the sclerosing hamangioma consists of a combination of elements, sometimes organized from the periphery of the tumor (Fig. 19–41). At low power the lesions have the overall appearance of a vascular tumor with numerous blood-filled channels. The proliferating cells appear as monotonous sheets of polygonal cells with eosinophilic cytoplasm which some authors describe as pale-staining; sheets are best seen at the periph-

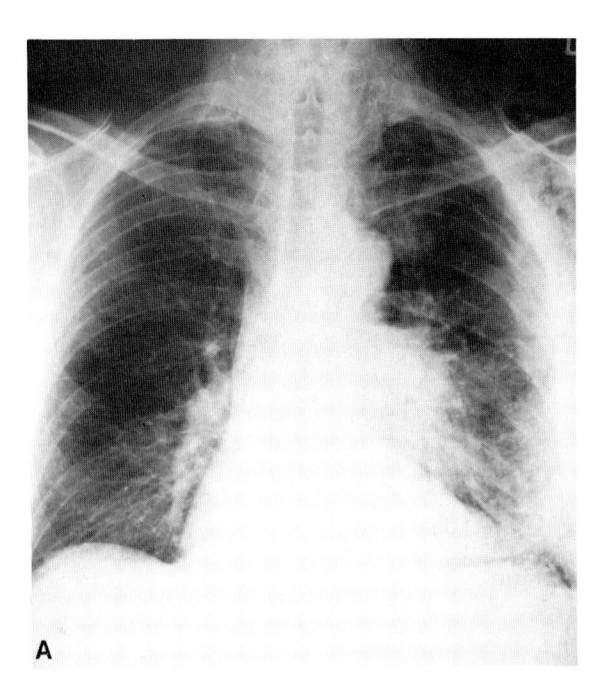

Figure 19–40. Inflammatory pseudotumor. A. Chest radiograph of a middle-aged smoker who presented with a left lower lobe pneumonia. The initial pneumonia resolved but 3 months later the patient's chest radiograph appeared as is shown in this radiograph. B. Microscopic appearance of the lesion shown in A. This appears to be a combination of bronchiolitis obliterans and interstitial pneumonia, a nonspecific pattern of reaction (×64).

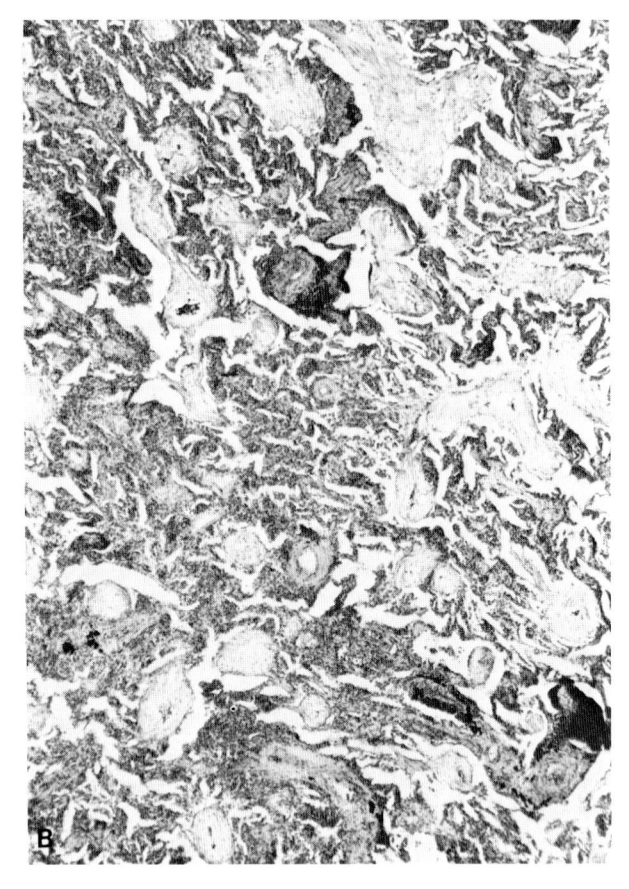

ery of the lesions. Within the masses of polygonal cells are areas of hemorrhage and numerous lipid-laden macrophages, undoubtedly reflecting present or past hemorrhage, as well as hemosiderin-laden macrophages. In areas, papillary formations appear, composed initially of cuboidal cells lining a fibrous and cellular core; the core cells are similar to the sheets. With time the core becomes progressively fibrotic. Eventually it appears that, if clinical symptoms or massive hemorrhage do not ensue, the whole lesion becomes sclerotic; it is possible that some persist and end up under the general category of hyalinizing granuloma.

The nature of the proliferating epithelial element has been a matter of dispute. Hill and Eggleston[479] found two cellular elements, described by them as dark and light cells; the former appeared to possess the ultrastructural features of type II cells, whereas the nature of the light cells was uncertain. The authors concluded that the tumor was a proliferation of primitive epithelial cells of the alveoli, some of which might differentiate into type II cells. Palacios and colleagues[480] found similar type II cells in an additional patient, as did Kennedy[481] in two separate patients. Haas and colleagues[482] and Kay and associates[483] found cells similar to the light cells and, in the case reported by Kay and co-workers, supposed Weibel-Palade rodlets were found. These authors concluded that the tumor is a proliferation of endothelial cells. As Palacios and associates[480] pointed out, the differences in description between those who favor an endothelial tumor and those who favor an epithelial tumor are minor and accurate identification is difficult. The type II cells are probably included in the tumor by accident, as was discussed in Bronchioloalveolar Carcinoma, above.

Recently Katzenstein and associates[484] concluded that sclerosing hemangioma is of mesothelial origin. Their conclusions are based in large part on the use of a glycosaminoglycan extraction and analysis technique which is questionable, and on ultrastructural findings which they admit are also consistent with an epithelial derivation. At present the cell of origin and even the neoplastic versus reactive nature of this lesion is unsettled.

Hamartomas

Spencer states that "A hamartoma is the result of unbalanced co-ordinated expansile but non-invasive growth confined to a limited anatomical field. The component tissues follow the general plan of development and may reach varying degrees of maturity and functional ability. Further growth of a hamartoma may continue after similar normal tissues have reached maturity."[1] The common pulmonary hamartoma is a mixture of cartilaginous core and a covering epithelium. A variety of synonyms are used for these tumors including adenochondroma, chondromatous hamartoma, fibroade-

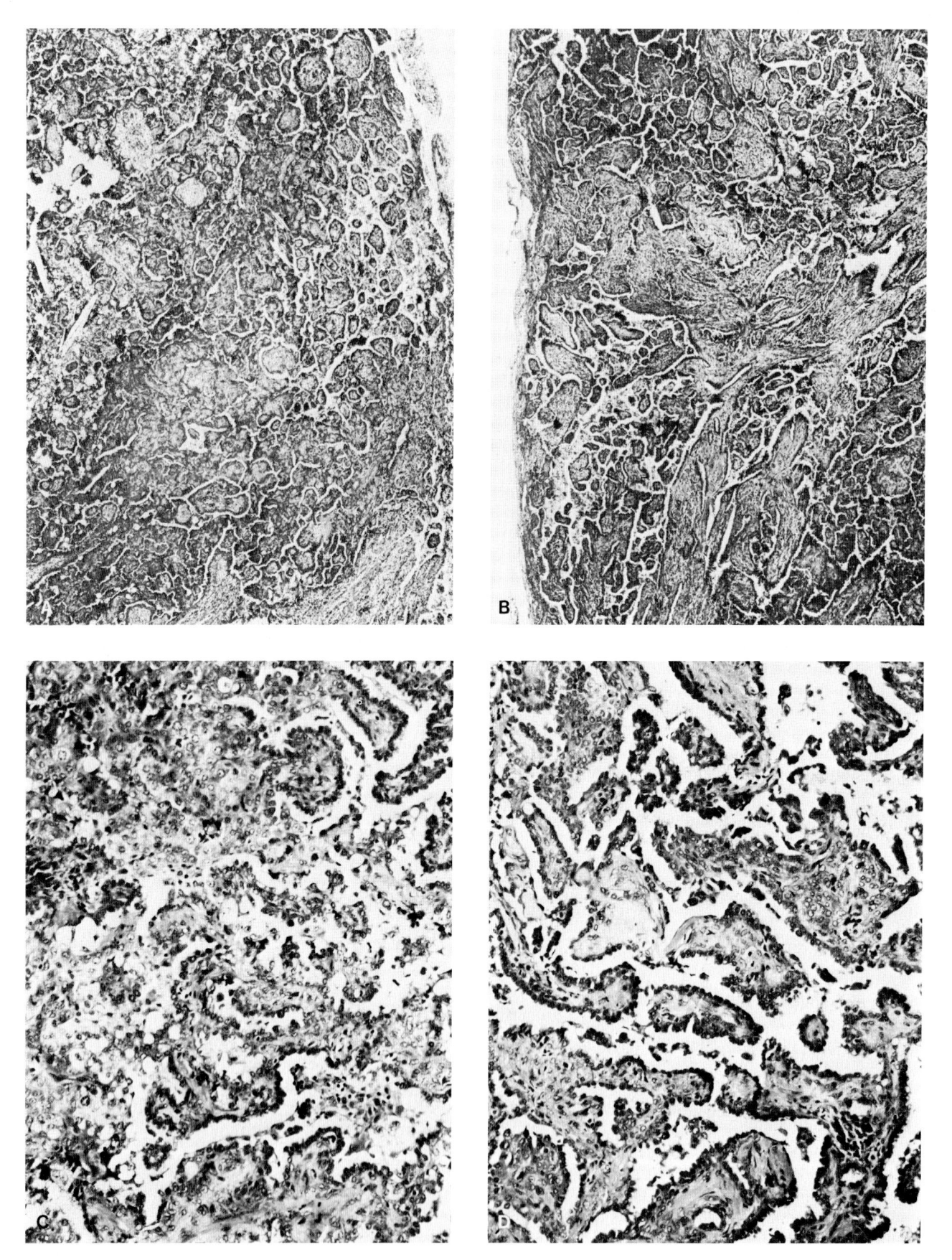

Figure 19–41. Sclerosing hemangioma of lung. The low-power appearance of numerous papillary projections interspersed with what appear to be blood-filled channels and foamy macrophages are shown in A and C and the eventual sclerotic appearance of the papillary structures in B and D. The actual tumor cells are polygonal forms (C and D) which appear to fill the papillary structures (A ×40, B ×40, C ×160, D ×160).

noma of the lung, lipochondroadenoma, and mixed pulmonary tumor. These tumors may be found in as many of 0.25 percent of autopsies, most commonly in middle-aged to elderly adults.[485] The tumors are usually single, and are more commonly found near the pleura; however, essentially identical lesions labeled enchondromas occur within the bronchial tree. Radiographically, the peripheral hamartomas appear as coin or lobulated lesions which are frequently calcified. Minasian[486] has recently reported a patient with both endobronchial and parenchymal hamartomas. Most tumors are 1 to 3 cm in size but occasionally are much larger. Grossly they are cartilaginous lobulated tumors which shell out easily from the surrounding parenchyma (Fig. 19–42).

Microscopically, the usual hamaratoma has a cartilaginous core (see Fig. 19–42). Calcium, bone, fat, muscle, lymphocytes, and cleft-like spaces may also be present. Surrounding the core is a layer of loose mesenchymal tissue covered by an epithelium which dips down into clefts within the core. Rarely, the core is entirely composed of some noncartilaginous element such as fat (see Fig. 19–42). By light microscopy the epithelium is composed of cuboidal cells, some of which contain mucin and some of which are ciliated.

Whether these lesions are neoplasms or hamartomas, and, if neoplasms, whether they are tumors of cartilage which "pick up" a non-neoplastic component from the surrounding lung, tumors of epithelial origin that induce mesenchyme, or true mixed tumors has been a matter of dispute, as has the question of whether the bronchial and parenchymal lesions are the same.

The few studies that have examined these questions in detail imply that hamartomas of this type are indeed neoplasms. Bateson[487,488] has studied the formation of hamartomas and attempted to explain the complex arrangement of clefts and connective tissue. Bateson suggested that the tumors form by proliferation of mesenchymal, usually cartilaginous, components of the bronchial wall, which evaginate the overlying epithelium. As the connective tissue mass proliferates and twists on itself, the epithelium becomes trapped within the cartilage. In this scheme the basic proliferating component is an undifferentiated mesenchymal tissue which may then take any of the forms detailed above. Butler and Kleinerman[489] also concluded that the neoplasm was of mesenchymal origin and noted that the cartilage showed signs of immaturity, evidence consistent with a neoplastic rather than a developmental origin. They concluded that there was no difference between the endobronchial and peripheral types of tumor from a morphologic point of view, a notion that accords with Bateson's theories of the formation of these lesions. Tomashefski[490] agreed that all of the variants were derived from bronchi of different sizes.

The ultrastructure of a peripheral hamartoma was examined by Stone and Churg[491] who concluded that the epithelium was a mixture of elements that line the distal bronchiole and alveoli, including immature epithelial cells, secretory cells, ciliated cells, Clara cells, and some type II cells (see Fig. 19–42). The underlying stroma showed primitive-appearing mesenchymal cells which could be observed to transform into typical chondroid cells with a chondroid matrix. Stone and Churg noted that many of the lining epithelial cells were more like those encountered in fetal or developing lung, and suggested that the tumor might indeed be a mixed neoplasm arising from epithelial and mesenchymal elements.

Benign Clear-Cell Tumor of the Lung

These tumors were first described by Liebow and Castleman[492] who reviewed 12 cases. The age range is wide, but the tumor is one of adults. The sex distribution is roughly equal. Except for the patient of Ozdemir and associates,[493] who presented with cough and hemoptysis, none of the patients reported have had symptoms related to the tumor. Most of the tumors have been in the lower lobes. Chest films show, as a rule, coin-type lesions or lobulated lesions; all shell out easily at surgery. Tumors measure up to 6.5 cm. Gross examination usually fails to reveal a capsule. The cut surfaces vary from pink to red, grey, or brown, but are never the yellow color of metastatic renal cell carcinoma. Necrosis has been seen in the cases of Zolliker and associates[494] and of Sale and Kurlander.[495]

The microscopic appearance of benign clear-cell tumor is distinctive (Fig. 19–43). The cells are arranged as large masses with very scanty stroma. The cell shape is quite variable, ranging from polygonal to elongated to spindle shaped. Multinucleated giant cells resembling Touton giant cells are common. The cytoplasm of the cells making up the tumor is distinctive; at low power it appears pale to clear, but at higher power is sometimes made up of fine eosinophilic granules. Sometimes the granules radiate from the nucleus in so-called "spider cells." Occasionally cells resembling neurons are also encountered. The nuclei may be quite variable in appearance, but only one mitosis was found in the original set of 12 tumors described by Liebow and Castleman,[492] and one in the report of Zolliker and co-workers.[494] Frequently the nuclei contain eosinophilic inclusions of cytoplasm or intranuclear glycogen masses.

Benign clear-cell tumors contain tremendous amounts of glycogen, hence the nickname "sugar tumors." One of Liebow and Castleman's original cases was analyzed and found to contain almost 11,000 μmol of glycogen per 100 g wet tissue or roughly 500 times that of normal lung tissue.

An important distinguishing feature separating benign clear-cell tumors from metastatic renal carcinomas, an obvious choice of differential, is the peculiar vascular supply. This consists of dilated thin-walled sinusoidal channels with the tumor cells separated from the lumen by an endothelial cell and a very small amount of connective tissue (see Fig. 19–43). This feature is not seen in metastatic renal cell carcinoma, which, in addition, is frequently yellow in gross appearance, and usually, but not always, has clear cells, necrosis, cytologic features of malignancy, and intracellular lipid. Reticulum is said to surround every cell of the benign clear-cell tumor but surrounds groups of cells of metastatic renal cell carcinoma.[492]

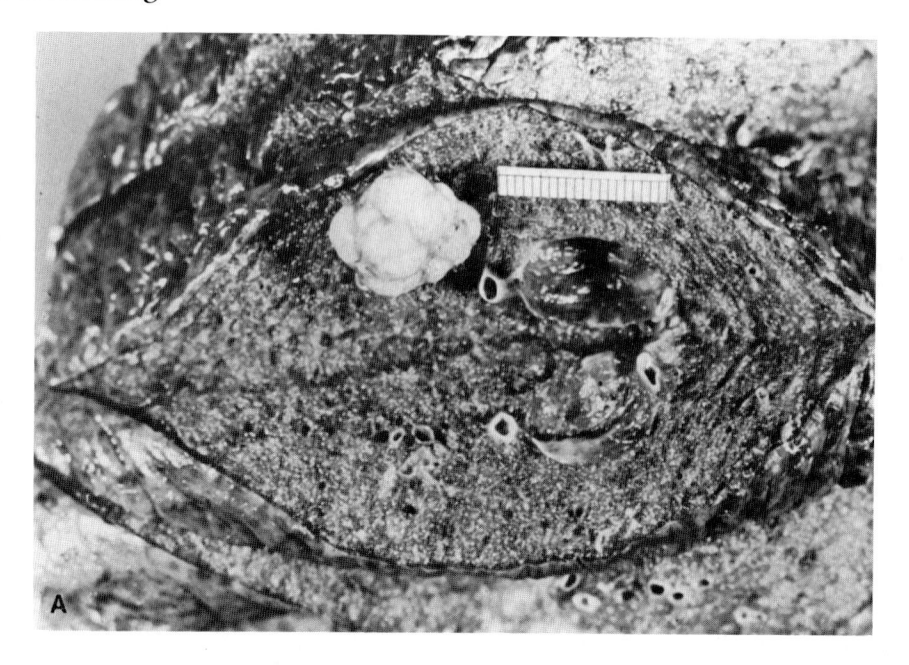

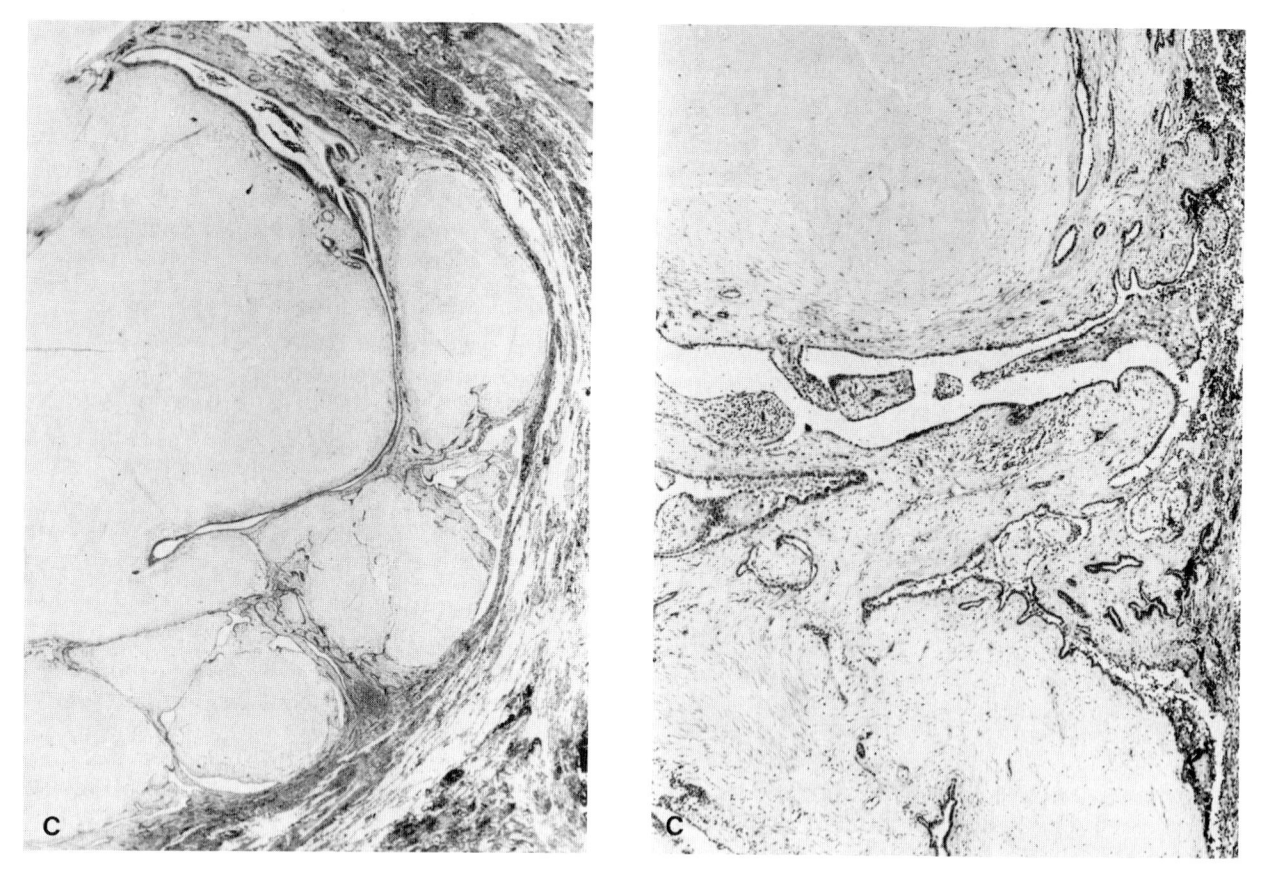

Figure 19–42A–C. Hamartoma. A. Gross appearance of typical cartilaginous hamartoma showing lobulated structure. This tumor has popped out of the lung as is commonly the case. B and C. Low-power appearance of usual chondromatous hamartoma showing cartilaginous or myxoid cores with overlying epithelium (B ×20, C ×64).

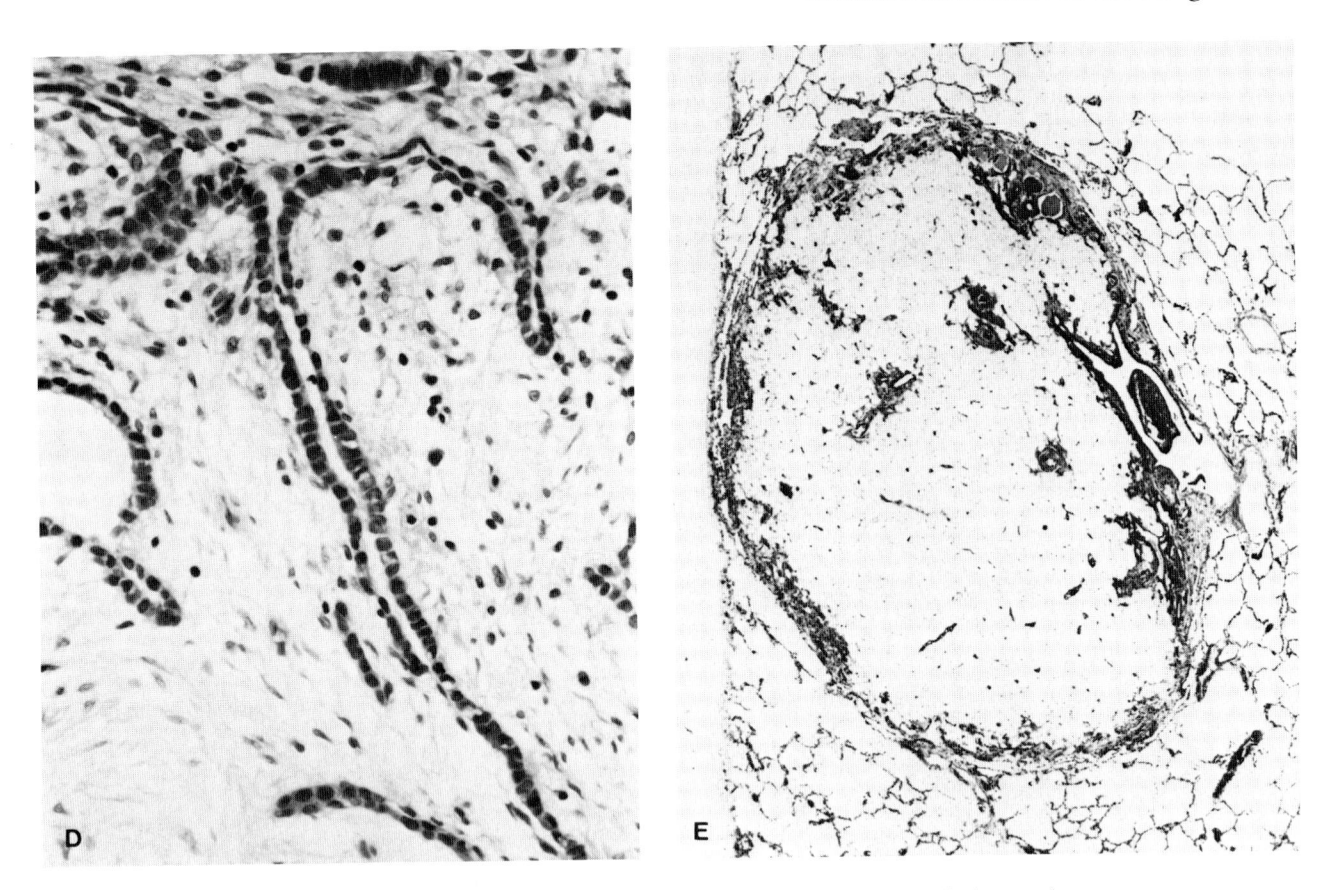

Figure 19–42D,E. D. High-power view of epithelium showing cuboidal cells dipping down into clefts within the tumor (×160). E. Hamartoma composed entirely of adipose tissue. The tumor had an epithelial covering which dips into clefts within the tumor in the same fashion as is seen with the cartilaginous types (×20).

Ultrastructural examination of a few lesions has produced interesting results. Becker and colleagues[496] found that the glycogen was both free and membrane bound, the latter a peculiar phenomenon seen otherwise only in type II glycogen storage disease (Pompe's disease). Becker and co-workers[496] believe that their tumor also contained neurosecretory granules, and suggested that the tumor was really a variant of carcinoid; however, it is unclear from their published photographs whether the neurosecretory granules might in fact be lysosomes. Zolliker and co-workers[494] failed to find membrane-bound glycogen. Hoch and co-workers[497] found not only membrane-bound glycogen, but individual tumor cells surrounded by basement membrane material, and containing filaments and dense bodies resembling those of smooth muscle, as well as pinocytotic vesicles. Hoch and associates concluded that the tumor was an aberrant form of smooth muscle tumor. At this point the histogenesis of the tumor is obscure.

The important distinction of benign clear-cell tumors from metastatic renal cell carcinoma has been discussed above. The other major differential diagnosis is an ordinary lung cancer with clear cells. Such tumors may be distinguished by their obvious cytologic malignancy, as well as the absence of the distinctive sinusoidal vascular pattern.

Granular Cell Tumors

Also called granular cell myoblastomas, fewer than 40 reports describing bronchial tumors have been published. The patients have been adults. The usual clinical presentation has been that of bronchial obstruction or pneumonia.

Grossly the tumors are usually polypoid masses arising from the bronchial wall. The histologic appearance is similar to that of granular cell tumors of other organs, and in common with granular cell tumors of other sites, for example, skin and oral cavity, the overlying epithelium may be hyperplastic and occasionally mimics a carcinoma.

Granular cell tumors are most commonly found in the skin, tongue, and subcutaneous tissue. Multiple tumors are fairly frequent; Moscovic and Azar[498] estimated their incidence at between 7 and 16 percent. A few cases have been reported in which a granular cell tumor of the

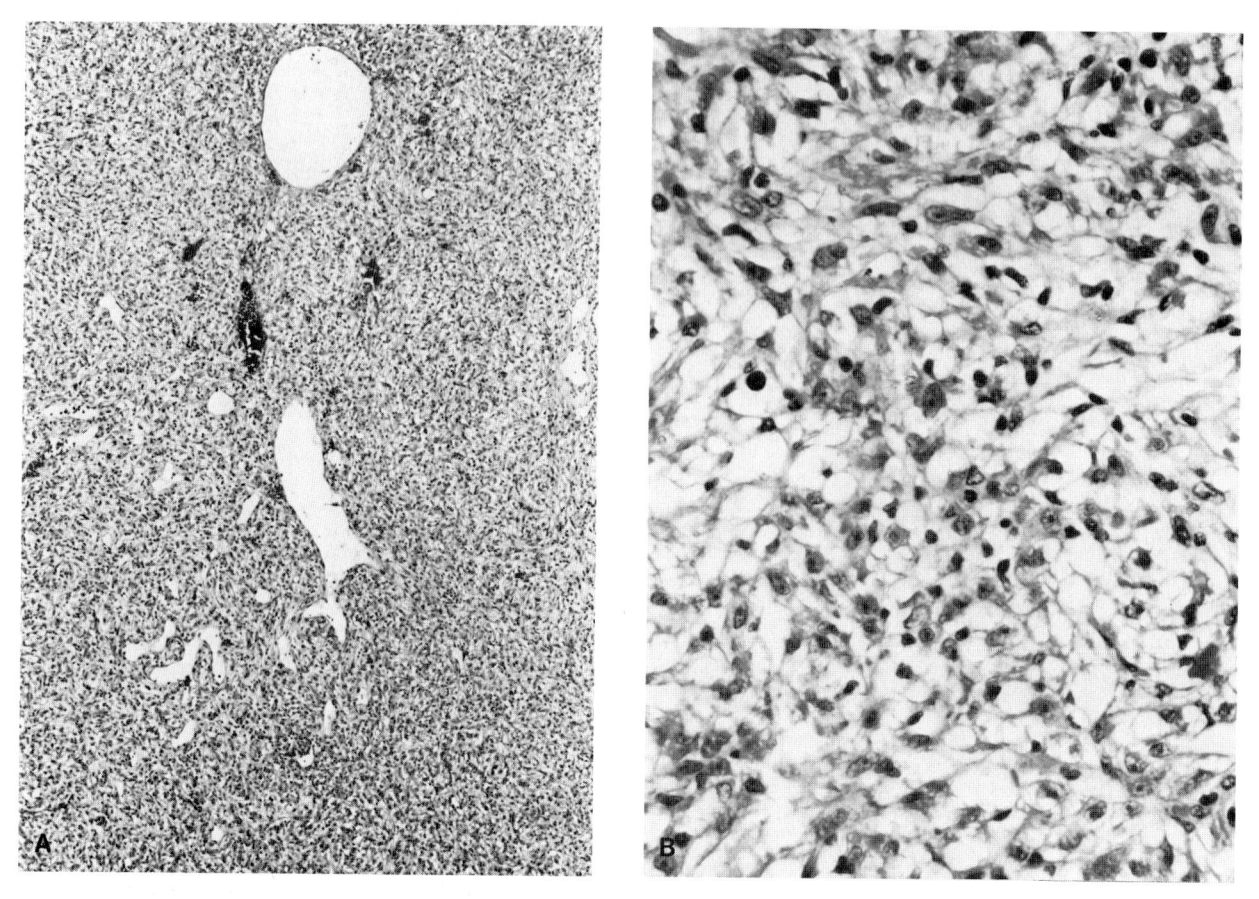

Figure 19–43. Benign clear cell tumor of lung. Low- and high-power views showing the distinctive sinusoidal vascular supply and the clear cells that make up this tumor (A ×40, B ×400).

bronchus was found in addition to tumors elsewhere in the body. Bush and Plain[499] report a case of three such tumors within the bronchial tree and note several reports of multiple pulmonary tumors. O'Connell and colleagues[500] report a case in which multiple tumors were found in the bronchi and the gastrointestinal tract.

These tumors are benign.

Malignant Melanoma

Taboada and associates[501] reviewed 11 cases of supposed primary malignant melanoma of the lung. Because of the frequency of metastasis of melanoma, particularly metastasis from an occult primary, such cases must be accepted with extreme caution. Taboada and colleagues concluded that most likely only 4 of the 11 cases were true primary tumors. Two of the cases are alive 10 and 11 years after resection.

Intrapulmonary Teratoma

These are extremely rare tumors; fewer than ten examples have been reported. The benign lesions constitute about half the total and typically include skin and skin appendages; similar to teratomas of the ovary or mediastinum, they may be filled with sebaceous material. Pancreatic and bronchial tissue may also be present. These tumors may be endobronchial.[502] The cases reported by Day and Taylor[503] and Holt and co-workers[504] were of interest because of the identification of thymic tissue; this finding suggests that midline germ cells were carried along with thymic tissue into the lung during embryogenesis. Although other germ cell tumors are not generally thought to arise in lung, Fox and associates[505] suggest that some large-cell carcinomas which secrete human chorionic gonadotropin and alphafetoprotein actually fall into this category.

Tumors of the Trachea

A variety of tumors occur in the trachea; about 45 percent are squamous carcinoma and about 35 percent are adenoid cystic carcinomas. Rarely, carcinoids, mucoepidermoid carcinomas, mixed tumors, and a variety of other tumors possibly related to bronchial glands are found.[243,506–509] Benign tumors also occur: these include papillomas, benign mesenchymal tumors such as lipomas

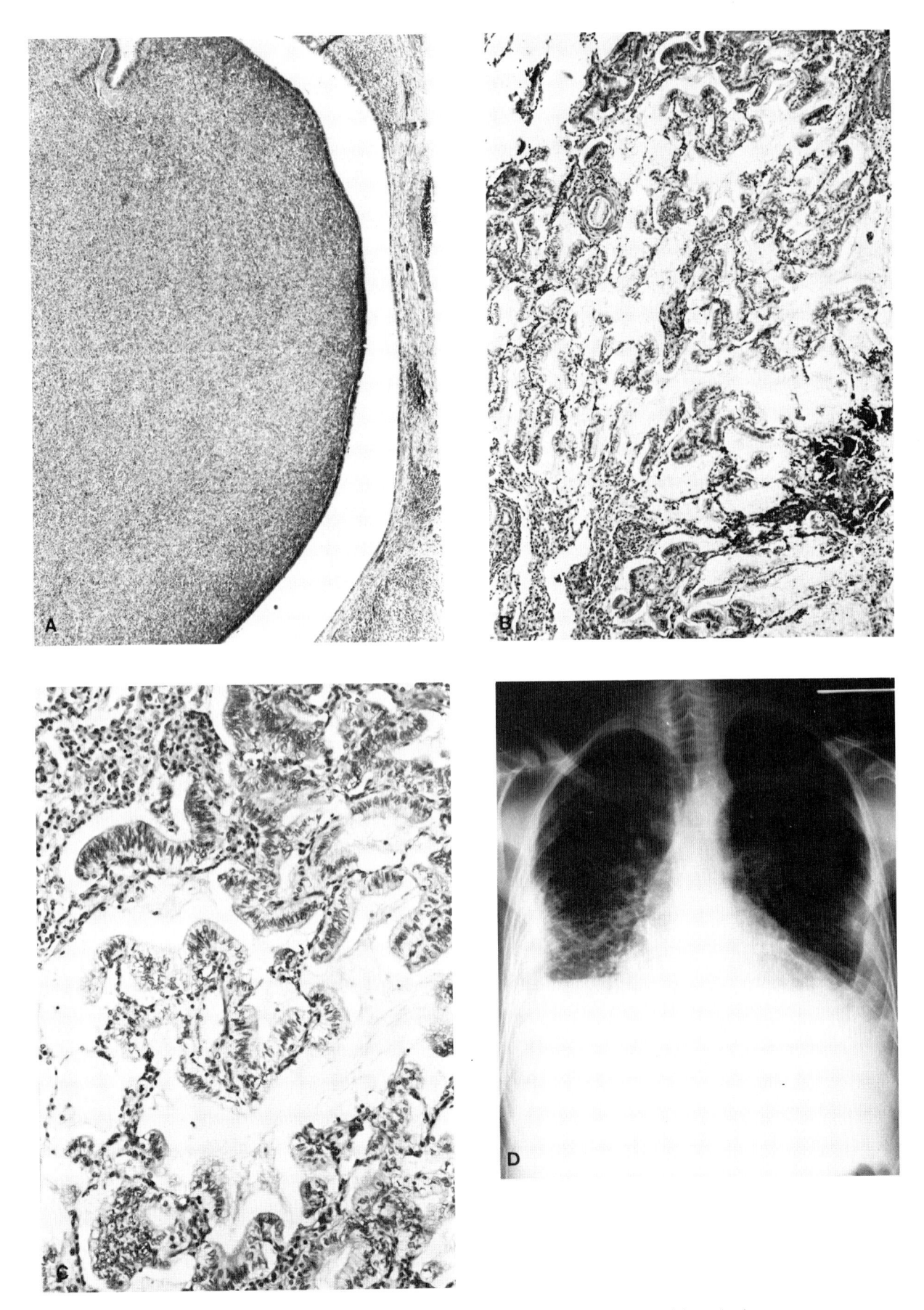

Figure 19–44A–D. Secondary tumors in the lung. A. An example of endobronchial metastases from an extrapulmonary tumor, in this case a malignant melanoma (×20). B and C. Metastatic adenocarcinoma mimicking bronchioloalveolar tumor. The patient presented with a pulmonary mass which is illustrated in this figure. After biopsy, workup revealed it to be a metastasis from a pancreatic primary. Compare this figure to Figure 19–12G,H on p. 34 (B ×64, C ×160). D. Chest radiograph showing lymphangitic spread of a carcinoma of the bladder in an elderly male.

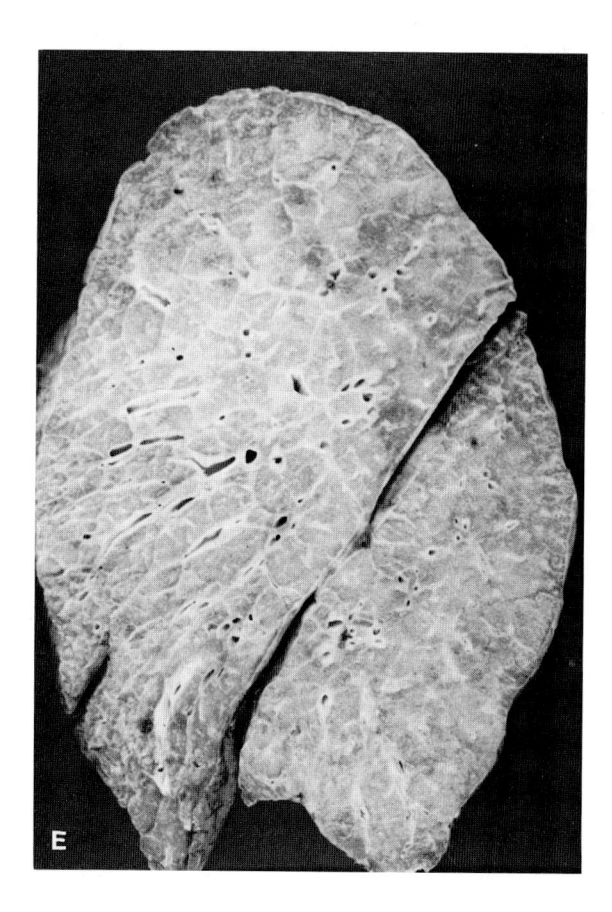

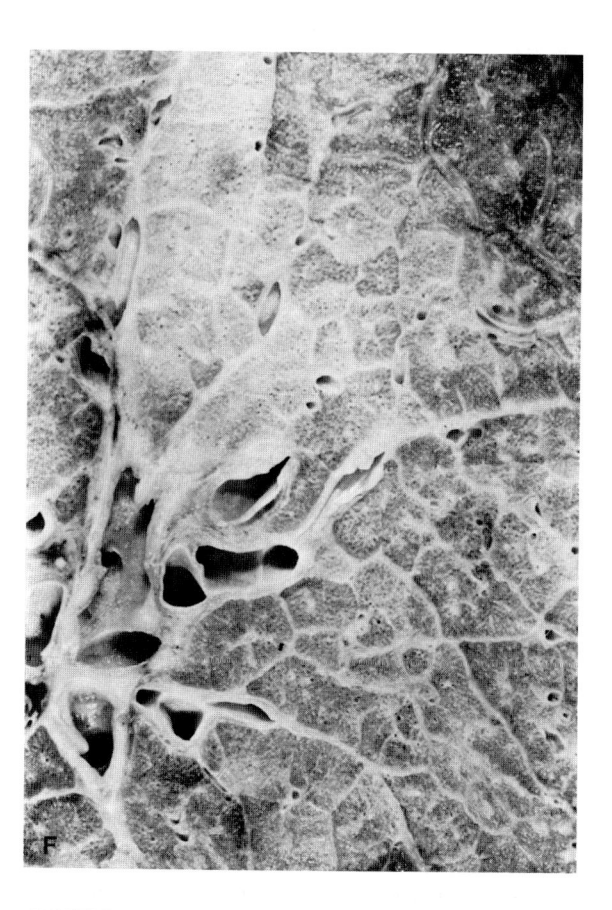

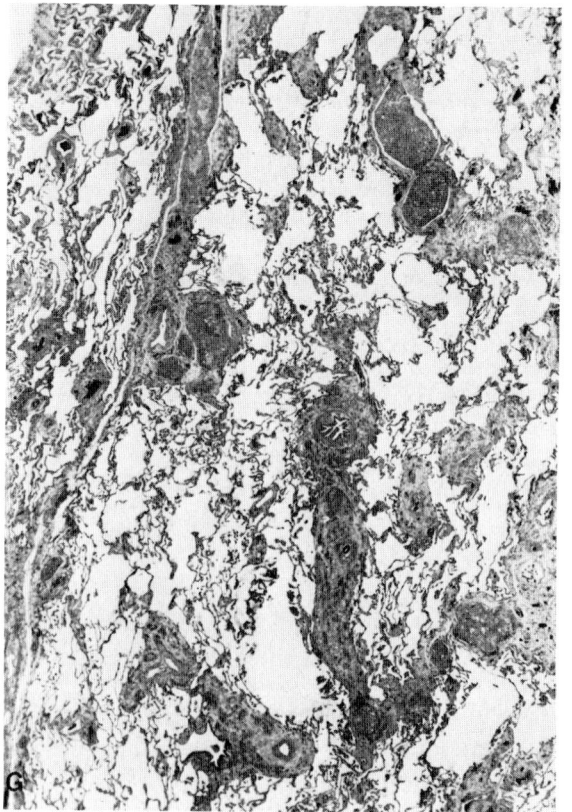

Figure 19–44E–G. E and F. Gross appearance of the tumor shown in D. Note the outlining of the septal lymphatics. G. Microscopic appearance of the tumor shown in D. Note tumor filling septal and peribronchial perivascular lymphatics (×20).

and leiomyomas, and a variety of inflammatory tumors such as hemangiomas and inflammatory pseudopolyps. The latter are usually encountered after a tracheostomy tube has been in place.[243,507]

Secondary Tumors

Tumors may reach the lung from other sites either through the lymphatics or blood vessels, or, relatively infrequently, through direct spread from a neighboring organ. The topic of lymphatic spread and its possible routes is reviewed in detail by Spencer,[1] who notes that, on occasion, lymphatic tumors from other organs may reach the bronchial submucosal lymphatics, producing a fraction of these tumors.[511] Cassiere and associates[512] reported that 3.4 percent of 294 patients with pancreatic carcinomas presented with radiographic and clinical features of a lung primary, particularly mediastinal widening and hilar adenopathy. As mentioned above, histologic separation of primary and secondary adenocarcinomas in the lung is frequently impossible; an example is shown in Fig. 19–44.

Lymphangitic carcinoma has a typical appearance, with outlining of the peribronchial, septal, and pleural lymphatics by a trail of tumor tissue; the lung is frequently quite firm if the permeation is extensive (see Fig. 19–44). Most instances of lymphangitic carcinoma apparently result from blood-borne emboli with extensive invasion and retrograde filling of lymphatics.[1] Occasional tumors also spread through the coeliac lymph nodes, through the diaphragm, and thence to the mediastinal and hilar nodes, again producing retrograde filling of lymphatics. Lymphangitic tumor is particularly common with carcinomas of the stomach, breast, lung, prostate, pancreas, and ovary. Secondary involvement by lymphoma should also be considered a form of lymphangitic tumor, since it tends to follow exactly the same routes. Lymphangitic tumor may present as an occult cause of restrictive lung disease; in such patients the chest radiograph may show a reticulonodular pattern (see Fig. 19–44), although eventual formation of large nodules is probably common.

Hematogenous metastases are also commonly seen with tumors of the breast, ovary, colon, kidney, testis, and sarcomas of all varieties.[243] Spencer[1] notes that about 20 percent of patients with malignant neoplasms of all sorts will show metastases at autopsy. Occult hematogenous metastases with extensive obstruction of small pulmonary vessels may occasionally present as pulmonary hypertension of unknown origin.[513,514]

A number of reports have discussed resection of pulmonary metastases. Gall and co-workers[515] removed 120 metastases from 67 patients compared to a control group in which metastases were not removed. The 5-year survival for the test group was 58 percent for those patients undergoing lobular resection and 25 percent for those undergoing wedge resection. Katzenstein and colleagues[516] showed that patients with a solitary metastasis from a renal cell carcinoma had a 39-month mean survival after resection. Mountain and associates[517] found a 29 percent 5-year survival rate for patients undergoing resection of a metastatic carcinoma and a 16 percent survival rate for those undergoing resection of a metastatic sarcoma. Similarly, McCormack and co-workers[518] found a 27 percent 5-year survival rate for patients undergoing resection of metastatic osteosarcoma. Morrow and colleagues[519] pointed out that survival rate depends particularly on tumor type; sarcomas, testicular, and renal cell carcinomas have relatively favorable prognoses, while melanomas, and carcinomas of the colon, rectum, and cervix have relatively poor prognoses.

References

1. Spencer H: *Pathology of the Lung*, 3rd ed. London: Pergamon Press, 1977.

2. Doll R, Peto R: The causes of cancer: Quantitative estimates of avoidable risks of cancer in the United States today. J Natl Cancer Inst USA 66:1192, 1981.

3. Cancer Statistics, 1979. CA 29:6, 1979.

4. Vincent RG, Pickren JW, Lane WW, et al.: The changing histopathology of lung cancer. A review of 1962 cases. Cancer 39:1647, 1977.

5. Meigs JW: Epidemic lung cancer in women (editorial). JAMA 238:1055, 1977.

6. Doll R, Hill AB: Mortality in relation to smoking: Ten years' observations of British doctors. Br Med J 1:1399, 1964.

7. Higgins ITT: *Epidemiological Evidence on the Carcinogenic Risk of Air Pollution*. INSERM Symposia Series, vol 52. Lyon: International Agency for Research on Cancer, 1976, p 41.

8. Hammond EC, Horn D: Smoking and death rates—report on forty four months of follow-up of 187,783 men. JAMA 166:1159, 1958.

9. Fiedman GD, Dales LG, Ury H: Mortality in middle-aged smokers and nonsmokers. N Engl J Med 300:213, 1979.

10. Hammond E: Smoking habits and air pollution in relation to lung cancer. In Lee DHK (ed): *Environmental Factors in Respiratory Disease*. New York: Academic Press, 1972, p 177.

11. Hoover R: Tobacco and geographic pathology. In Harris CC (ed): *Pathogenesis and Therapy of Lung Cancer*. New York: Marcel Dekker, 1978, p 3.

12. Wynder EL, Hoffman D: Tobacco and tobacco smoke. Semin Oncol 3:5, 1976.

13. Higginson J, Jensen OM: Epidemiological review of lung cancer in man. In Mohn U (ed): *Air Pollution and Cancer in Man*. Lyon: International Agency for Research on Cancer, 1971, p 169.

14. Blot WJ, Fraumeni JF: Geographic patterns of lung cancer: Industrial correlations, Am J Epidemiol 103:539, 1976.

15. Schneiderman MA, Levin DL: Trends in lung cancer—mortality, incidence, diagnosis, treatment, smoking and urbanization. Cancer 30:1320, 1972.

16. Chahinian AP, Chretien J: Present incidence of lung cancer: epidemiologic data and etiologic factors. In Israel L, Chahinian AP (eds): *Lung Cancer—Natural History, Prognosis and Therapy*. New York: Academic Press, 1976, p 1.

17. Nettesheim P, Creasia D, Mitchell T: Studies on the carcinogenic and co-carcinogenic effects of inhaled synthetic smog and ferric oxide particles. J Natl Cancer Inst 55:159, 1975.

18. Hitogusi M: Epidemiological study of lung cancer with special reference to the effect of air pollution and smoking habit. Inst Public Health Bull (Jpn) 17:237, 1968.

19. Menck HR, Casagrande JT, Henderson BD: Industrial air pollution: Possible effect on lung cancer. Science 183:210, 1974.

20. Winkelstein W, Kantor S, Davis EW, et al.: The relationship of air pollution and economic status to total mortality and selected respiratory system mortality in men. I. Suspended particulates. Arch Environ Health 14:162, 1967.

21. Zeidberg LD, Horton RJM, Landau V: The Nashville air pollution study. V. Mortality from disease of the repsiratory tract in relation to air pollution. Arch Environ Health 15:214, 1967.

22. Vena JE: Air pollution as a risk factor in lung cancer. Am J Epidemiol 116:42, 1982.

23. Mason TJ, McKay FW, Hoover R, et al.: *Atlas of Cancer Mortality of U.S. Counties: 1950—1969*, DHEW Publications No. (NIH) 75. Washington DC, U.S. Government Printing Office, 1975.

24. Mason TJ, McKay FW, Hoover R, et al.: *Atlas of Cancer Mortality Among U.S. Nonwhites: 1950—1969*, DHEW Publication No. (NIH) 76. Washington DC, U.S. Government Printing Office, 1976.

25. Blot WJ, Fraumeni JF: Arsenical air pollution and lung cancer. Lancet 2:142, 1975.

26. Blot WJ, Harrington JM, Toledo A, et al.: Lung cancer after employment in shipyards during WWII. N Engl J Med 229:620, 1978.

27. Hoover R, Fraumeni JF: Cancer mortality in U.S. counties with chemical industries. Environ Res 9:196, 1975.

28. Burbank F, Fraumeni JF Jr: U.S. cancer mortality: Nonwhite predominance. J Natl Cancer Inst 49:649, 1972.

29. Creagan ET, Fraumeni JF Jr.: Cancer mortality among American Indians, 1950–1967. J Natl Cancer Inst 49:959, 1972.

30. Fraumeni JF Jr, Mason TJ: Cancer mortality among Chinese Americans, 1950–1969. J Natl Cancer Inst 52:659, 1974.

31. Mulvihill JJ: Host factors. In Harris CC (ed): *Pathogenesis and Therapy of Lung Cancer*. New York: Marcel Dekker, 1978, p 53.

32. Hammond EC, Selikoff IJ: Passive smoking and lung cancer with comments on two new papers. Environ Res 24:444, 1981.

33. Kellerman GH, Shaw CR, Luytein-Kellerman M: Aryl hydrocarbon hydroxylase inducibility and bronchogenic carcinoma. N Engl J Med 289:934, 1973.

34. Paigen B, Gurtoo HL, Monowada J, et al.: Questionable relation of aryl hydrocarbon hyroxylase to lung-cancer risk. N Engl J Med 297:344, 1977.

35. Brown SM, Selvin S, Winkelstein W Jr: The association of economic status with the occurrence of lung cancer. Cancer 36:1903, 1975.

36. Fox AJ, Adelstein AM: Occupational mortality: Work or way of life? J Epidemiol Community Health 32:73, 1978.

37. Frank AL: Occupational lung cancer. In Harris CC (ed): *Pathogenesis and Therapy of Lung Cancer*. New York: Marcel Dekker, 1978. p 25.

38. Bridbord K, Decoufle P, Fraumeni JF, et al.: *Estimates of the Fraction of Cancer in the United States Related to Occupational Factors*. Bethesda, MD, National Cancer Institute, 1978.

39. Becklake ML: Asbestos-related diseases of the lung and other organs: Their epidemiology and implication for clinical practice. Am Rev Respir Dis 114:187, 1976.

40. Hammond EC, Selikoff IJ, Seidman H: Asbestos exposure, cigarette smoking and death rates. Ann NY Acad Sci 330:473, 1979.

41. Archer VE, Saccomanno G, Jones JH: Frequency of different histologic types of bronchgenic carcinoma as related to radiation exposure. Cancer 34:2056, 1974.

42. Weiss W: Lung cancer due to chemicals. Comp Therapy 5:18, 1979.

43. Selikoff IJ, Hammond EC: Asbestos-associated disease in United States shipyards. CA 28:87, 1978.

44. Morton WE, Treyve EL: Histologic differences in occupational risks of lung cancer incidence. Am J Indust Med 3:441, 1982.

45. Enterline P: Respiratory cancer in relation to occupation among retired asbestos workers. Br J Indust Med 30:162, 1973.

46. Saccomanno G, Archer VE, Auerbach O, et al.: Histologic types of lung cancer among uranium miners. Cancer 27:515, 1971.

47. Deleted during publication.

48. Gottlieb MS, Shear CL, Seale DB: Lung cancer mortality and residential proximity to industry. Environ Health Perspect 45:157, 1982.

49. McDowell EM, Becci PJ, Barrett LA, Trump BF: Morphogenesis and classification of lung cancer. In Harris CC (ed): *Pathogenesis and Therapy of Lung Cancer*. New York: Marcel Dekker, 1978, p 445.

50. Barrett LA, Becci PJ, Glavin F, et al.: The respiratory epithelium. III. Histogenesis of epidermoid metasplasia and carcinoma in situ in the human. J Natl Cancer Inst 61:563, 1978.

51. Becci PJ, McDowell EM, Trump BF: The respiratory epithelium. IV. Histogenesis of epidermoid metasplasia and carcinoma in situ in the hamster. J Natl Cancer Inst 61:577, 1978.

52. McDowell EM, Sorokin SP, Hoyt RF, Trump BF: An unusual bronchial carcinoid tumor: Light and electron microscopy. Hum Pathol 4:338, 1981.

53. Bell CE, Seetharam S: Expression of endodermally derived and neural crest-derived differentiation antigens by human lung and colon tumors. Cancer 44:13, 1979.

54. Yesner R: The dynamic histopathologic spectrum of lung cancer. Yale J Biol Med 54:447, 1981.

55. Auerbach O, Hammond EC, Garfinkel L: Changes in bronchial epithelium in relation to cigarette smoking. 1955–1960 vs. 1970–1977. N Engl J Med 300:381, 1979.

56. Auerbach O, Saccomanno G, Kuschner M, et al.: Histologic findings in the tracheobronchial tree of uranium miners and non-miners with lung cancer. Cancer 42:483, 1978.

57. Auerbach O, Stout AP, Hammond EC, Garfinkel L: Changes in bronchial epithelium in relation to cigarette smoking and in relation to lung cancer. N Engl J Med 265:253, 1961.

58. Saccomanno G, Archer VE, Auerbach O, et al.: Development of carcinoma of the lung as reflected in exfoliated cells. Cancer 33:257, 1974.

59. Carter D: Pathology of early squamous cell carcinoma of the lung. Pathol Annu 13:131, 1978.

60. Mason MK, Jordan JW: Carcinoma in situ and early invasive carcinoma of the bronchus. Thorax 24:461, 1969.

61. Carter D, Marsh BR, Baker RR, et al.: Relationships of morphology to clinical presentation in ten cases of early squamous cell carcinoma of the lung. Cancer 37:1389, 1976.

62. Marsh BR, Frost JK, Erozan YS, Carter D: New horizons in lung cancer diagnosis. Cancer 37:437, 1976.

63. Pearson FG, Thompson DW, Delarue NC: Experience with the cytologic detection, localization and treatment of radiographically undemonstrable bronchial carcinoma. J Thorac Cardiovasc Surg 54:371, 1967.

64. Cortese DA, Kinsey JH, Woolner LB, et al.: Clinical application of a new endoscopic technique for detection of in situ bronchial carcinoma. Mayo Clin Proc 54:635, 1979.

65. Martini N, Beattie EJ, Cliffton EE, Melamed MR: Radiologically occult lung cancer—report of 26 cases. Surg Clin N Am 54:811, 1974.

66. Woolner LB, David E, Fontana RS, et al.: In situ and early invasive bronchogenic carcinoma—report of 28 cases with postoperative survival data. J Thoracic Cardiovasc Surg 60:275, 1970.

67. Ranchod M: The histogenesis and development of pulmonary tumorlets. Cancer 39:1135, 1977.

68. Berkheiser SW: Bronchiolar proliferation and metaplasia associated with bronchiectasis, pulmonary infarcts and anthracosis. Cancer 12:449, 1959.

69. Berkheiser SW: The significance of bronchiolar atypia and lung cancer. Cancer 18:516, 1965.

70. Balo J, Juhasz E, Temes J: Pulmonary infarcts and pulmonary carcinoma. Cancer 9:918, 1956.

71. Kreus KE, Hakama M, Saxen E: Association of pulmonary tuberculosis and carcinoma of the lung. Scand J Respir Dis 51:276, 1970.

72. Raeburn C, Spencer H: Study of origin and development of lung cancer. Thorax 8:1, 1953.

73. Meyer EC, Liebow AA: Relationship of interstitial pneumonia honey-combing and atypical epithelial proliferation to cancer of the lung. Cancer 18:322, 1965.

74. Bennett DE, Sasser WF, Ferguson TB: Adenocarcinoma of the lung in men. A clinicopathologic study of 100 cases. Cancer 23:431, 1969.

75. Auerbach O, Garfinkel L, Parks VR: Scar cancer of the lung. Increase over a 21 year period. Cancer 43:636, 1979.

76. Shimosato Y, Hashimoto T, Kodama T, et al.: Prognostic implications of fibrotic focus (scar) in small peripheral lung cancers. Am J Surg Pathol 4:365, 1980.

77. Turner-Warwick M, Lebowitz M, Burrows B, Johnson A: Cryptogenic fibrosing alveolitis and lung cancer. Thorax 35:496, 1980.

78. Batsakis JG, Johnson HA: Generalized scleroderma involving lungs and liver with pulmonary adenocarcinoma. Arch Pathol 69:633, 1960.

79. Siegel A: Scleroderma. Med Clin North Am 61:283, 1977.

80. Whitwell F, Newhouse M, Bennett DR: A study of the histological types of lung cancer in workers suffering from asbestosis in the United Kingdom. Br J Indust Med 31:298, 1974.

81. Kannerstein M, Churg J: Pathology of carcinoma of the lung associated with asbestos exposure. Cancer 30:14, 1972.

82. Brincker H, Wilbek E: The incidence of malignant tumors in patients with respiratory sarcoidosis. Br J Cancer 29:247, 1974.

83. Moolten SE: Scar cancer of lung complicating rheumatoid lung disease. Mt Sinai J Med 40:736, 1973.

84. Churg A, Warnock ML. Pulmonary tumorlet. A form of carcinoid tumor. Cancer 37:1469, 1976.

85. Whitwell F: Tumorlets of the lung. J Pathol Bacteriol 70:529, 1955.

86. Kreyberg L, Liebow AA, Uehlinger EA: *Histological Typing of Lung Tumours*. Geneva: World Health Organization, 1967.

87. Matthews MJ: Morphologic classifcation of bronchogenic carcinoma. Cancer Chemother Rep 4:299, 1973.

88. World Health Organization: The World Health Organization Histological Typing of tumours. Am J Clin Pathol 77:123, 1982.

89. Yesner R: Spectrum of lung cancer and ectopic hormones. Pathol Annu 13:217, 1978.

90. Feinstein AR, Gilfman NA, Yesner R: The diverse effects of histopathology on manifestations and outcome of lung cancer. Chest 66:225, 1974.

91. Feinstein AR, Gelfman NA, Yesner R, et al.: Observer variability in diagnosis of lung cancer. Rev Respir Dis 101:671, 1970.

92. Yesner R: Observer variability and reliability in lung cancer diagnosis. Cancer Chemother Rep 4(part 3):55, 1973.

93. Rilke F, Carbone A, Clemente C, Pilotti S: Surgical pathology of resectable lung cancer. In Muggia F, Rozencweig M (eds): *Lung Cancer, Progress in Therapeutic Research*. New York: Raven Press, 1979, p 129.

94. Hinson KFW, Miller AB, Tall R: An assessment of the World Health Organization classification of the histologic typing of lung tumors applied to biopsy of diagnosis and resected material. Cancer 35:399, 1975.

95. Auerbach O, Garfinkel L, Parks UR: Histologic type of lung cancer in relation to smoking habits, year of diagnosis and sites of metastases. Chest 67:382, 1975.

96. Cox JD, Yesner RA: Adenocarcinoma of the lung: Recent results from the Veterans Administration Lung Group. Am Rev Respir Dis 120:1125, 1979.

97. Vincent RG, Pickren JW, Lane WW, et al.: The changing histopathology of lung cancer. A review of 1682 cases. Cancer 39:1647, 1977.

98. Matthews MJ, Gordon PR: Morphology of pulmonary and pleural malignancies. In Straus MJ (ed): *Lung Cancer. Clinical Diagnosis and Treatment*. New York: Grune & Stratton, 1977, pp 49–69.

99. Abeloff MD, Eggleston JC, Mendelsohn G, et al.: Changes in morphologic and biochemical characteristics of small cell carcinoma of the lung. A clinicopathologic study. Am J Med 66:757, 1979.

100. Brereton HD, Mathews MM, Costa J, et al.: Mixed anaplastic small-cell and squamous-cell carcinoma of the lung. Ann Intern Med 88:805, 1978.

101. Churg A, Johnston WH, Stulbarg M: Small cell squamous and mixed small cell squamous—small cell anaplastic carcinomas of the lung. Am J Surg Pathol 4:255, 1980.

102. Rosenow III EC, Carr DT: Bronchogenic carcinoma. CA 29:233, 1979.

103. Kreyberg L: Relationship of different histological lung tumor groups to tobacco smoking. Br J Cancer 15:51, 1961.

104. Weiss W, Altan S, Rosenzweig M, Weiss WA: Lung cancer in relation to cigarette dosage. Cancer 39:2568, 1977.

105. Ham AW, Cormack DH: *Histology*, 8th ed., Philadelphia, JB Lippincott, 1979.

106. Reinila A, Dammert K: An attempt to use the WHO typing in the histological classification of lung carcinomas. Acta Path Microbiol Scand, Sect A 82:783, 1974.

107. Walter JB, Pryce DM: The site of origin of lung cancer and its relation to histological type. Thorax 10:117, 1955.

108. Walter JB, Pryce DM: The histology of lung cancer. Thorax 10:107, 1955.

109. Paulson DL: Carcinomas of the superior pulmonary sulcus. J Thorac Cardiovasc Surg 70:1095, 1975.

110. Kreyberg L: Comments on the histochemical typing of lung tumors. Acta Path Microbiol Scand, Sect A 79:409, 1971.

111. Churg A: The fine structure of large cell undifferentiated carcinoma of the lung. Evidence for its relation to squamous cell carcinomas and adenocarcinomas. Hum Pathol 9:143, 1978.

112. MacKay B, Osbourne BM, Wilson RA: Ultrastructure of lung neoplasms. In Straus MJ (ed): *Lung Cancer. Clinical Diagnosis and Treatment.* New York: Grune & Stratton, 1977, p 71.

113. Sasaki M, Hayashi N, Yamori T: Electron microscopic studies on human pulmonary carcinoma. Gann 55:109, 1964.

114. Sidhu GS: The ultrastructure of malignant epithelial neoplasms of the lung. Pathol Annu 17:229, 1982.

114A. Said JW, Nash G, Tepper G, Banks-Schlegel S: Keratin proteins and carcinoembryonic antigen in lung carcinoma. Hum Pathol 14:70, 1983.

114B. Nagle RB, McDaniel KM, Clark VA, Payne CM: The use of antikeratin antibodies in the diagnosis of human neoplasms. Am J Clin Pathol 79:458, 1983.

114C. Espinoza CG, Azar HA: Immunohistochemical localization of keratin-type proteins epithelial neoplasms. Am J Clin Pathol 78:500, 1982.

114D. Saba SR, Espinoza GC, Richman AV, Azar HA: Carcinomas of the lung: An Ultrastructural and immunocytochemical study. Am J Clin Pathol 80:6, 1983.

114E. Kahn JH, Huang S-N, Hanna WM, et al.: Immunohistochemical localization of epidermal and Mallory body cytokeratin in undifferentiated epithelial tumors.

114F. Said JW, Nash G, Banks-Schlegel S, et al.: Keratin in human lung tumors: Patterns of localization of different-molecular-weight keratin proteins. Am J Pathol 113:27, 1983.

114G. Banks-Schlegel SP, McDowell EM, Wilson TS, et al.: proteins in human lung carcinomas. Am J Pathol 1114:273, 1984.

114H. Corsun JM, Pinkus GS: Mesothelioma: Profile of keratin proteins and carcinoembryonic antigen. Am J Pathol 108:80, 1982.

114I. Holden J, Churg A: Immunohistochemical staining for keratin and carcinoembryonic antigen in the diagnosis of malignant mesothelioma. Am J Surg Pathol 8:277, 1984.

114J. Battifora H, Kopinski MI: Distinction of mesothelioma and reactive mesothelial cells from adenocarcinoma: An immunohistochemical study. Lab Invest 50:4a, 1984.

115. Barnard WG: Nature of oat-celled sarcoma of mediastinum. J Pathol 29:241, 1926.

116. Azzopardi JG: Oat-cell carcinoma of the bronchus. J Pathol Bacteriol 78:513, 1960.

117. Bensch KG, Corrin B, Pariente R, Spencer H: Oat-cell carcinoma of the lung. Its origin and relationship to bronchial carcinoid. Cancer 22:1163, 1968.

118. Hattori S, Minoru M, Tateishi R, et al.: Oat cell carcinoma of the lung. Clinical and morphological studies in relation to its histogenesis. Cancer 30:1014, 1972.

119. Bonikos DS, Bensch KG: Endocrine cells of bronchial and bronchiolar epithelium. Am J Med 63:765, 1977.

120. Pearce AGE: The cytochemistry and ultrastructure of polypeptide hormone-producing cells of the APUD series and the embryologic, physiologic, and pathologic implications of the concept. J Histochem Cytochem 17:303, 1969.

121. Feyter F: *Uber die peripheren endocrinen (Parakrinen) Drusen des Menschen.* Vienna: W Maudrich, 1954.

122. Tischler AS: Small cell carcinoma of the lung. Cellular origin and relationship to other neoplasms. Semin Oncol 5:244, 1978.

123. Sidhu GS: The endodermal origin of digestive and respiratory tract APUD cells—Histopathologic evidence and a review of the literature. Am J Pathol 96:5, 1979.

123A. Gould VE, Linnoila RI, Memoli VA, Warren WH: Neuroendocrine components of the bronchopulmonary tract: Hyperplasias, dysplasia, and neoplasms. Lab Invest 49:519, 1983.

123B. Gould VE, Linnoila RI, Memoli VA, Warren WH: Neuroendocrine cells and neuroendocrine neoplasms of the lung. Pathol Annu 18(part I):287, 1983.

124. LeDourain N, Teillet MA: The migration of neural crest cells to the disgestive tract in avian embryo. J Embryol Exp Morphol 30:31, 1973.

125. Lehto VP, Stenman S, Miettinen M, et al.: Expression of a neural type of intermediate filament as a distinguishing feature between oat cell carcinoma and other lung cancer. Am J Pathol 110:113, 1983.

125A. Sheppard MN, Corrin B, Bennett MH, et al.: Immunocytochemical localization of neuron specific enolase in small cell carcinomas and carcinoid tumors of the lung. Histopathology 8:171, 1984.

126. Wick MR, Scheithauer BW: Neuron-specific enolase in neuroendocrine tumors of the thymus, bronchus, and skin. Lab Invest 48:93A, 1983.

127. Moody TW, Pert CB, Gazdar AF, et al.: High levels of intracellular bombesin characterize human small-cell lung carcinoma. Science 214:1246, 1981.

128. Gould VE, Chejfec G: Ultrastructural and biochemical analysis of "undifferentiated" pulmonary carcinomas. Hum Pathol 9:377, 1978.

129. Hage E, Hansen M, Hirsch FR: Electron microscopic sub-classification of small cell carcinoma of the lung. Acta Pathol Jpn 33:671, 1983.

130. Cutz E, Chan W, Track NS: Bombesin, calcitonin, and leu-enkephalin in endocrine cells of human lung. Experimentia 37:765, 1981.

131. Lauweryns JM, Goddeeris P: Neuroepithelial bodies in the human child and adult lung. Am Rev Respir Dis 111:469, 1975.

132. Fisher ER, Palekar A, Paulson JD: Comparative histopathologic, histochemical, electron microscopic, and tissue culture studies of Bronchial carcinoids and oat cell carcinomas of lung. Amer J Clin Pathol 69:165, 1978.

133. Godwin JD, Brown CC: Comparative epidemiology of carcinoid and oat-cell tumors of the lung. Cancer 40:1671, 1977.

134. Higgins GA, Shields TW, Keehn RJ: The solitary pulmonary nodule. Ten-year follow-up of Veterans Administration–Armed Forces Comparative Study. Arch Surg 110:570, 1975.

135. Kato Y, Ferguson TB, Bennett DE, Burford TH: Oat cell carcinoma of the lung—review of 138 cases. Cancer 23:517, 1969.

136. Matthews MJ: Morphology of lung cancer. Semin Oncol 1:175, 1974.

137. Hirsch FR, Matthews J, Yesner R: Histopathologic classification of small cell carcinoma of the lung. Cancer 50:1360, 1982.

138. Vollmer RT: The effect of cell size on the pathologic diagnosis of small and large cell carcinomas of the lung. Cancer 50:1380, 1982.

139. Carney DN, Matthews MJ, Ihde DC, et al.: Influence of histologic subtype of small cell carcinoma of the lung on clinical presentation, response to therapy, and survival. J Natl Cancer Inst 65:1225, 1980.

140. Davis S, Stanley KE, Yeser R, et al.: Small cell carcinoma of

the lung. Survival according to histologic subtype. Cancer 47:1863, 1981.

141. Burdon JGW, Sinclair RA, Henderson MM: Small cell carcinoma of the lung—prognosis in relation to histologic subtype. Chest 76:302, 1979.

141A.Hirsch FR, Osterlind K, Hansen HH: The prognostic significance of histopathologic subtyping of small cell carcinoma of the lung according to the classification of the World Health Organization. Cancer 52:2144, 1983.

141B.Dhillon AP, Rode J, Dhillon DP, Moss E, Thompson RJ: Neural markers in carcinoma of the lung. Br J Cancer 51:645, 1985.

142. Matthews MJ: Effects of therapy on the morphology and behavior of small cell carcinoma of the lung—a clinicopathologic study. In Muggia F, Rozencweig M (eds): *Lung Cancer: Progress in Therapeutic Research.* New York; Raven Press, 1979, p 155.

143. Saba SR, Azar HA, Richman AV, et al.: Dual differentiation in small cell carcinoma (oat cell carcinoma) of the lung. Ultrastruct Pathol 2:131, 1981.

144. Hashimoto T, Fukuoka M, Nagasawa S, et al.: Small cell carcinoma of the lung and its histological origin. Am J Surg Pathol 3:343, 1979.

145. Leong ASY, Canney AR: Small cell anaplastic carcinoma of the lung with glandular and squamous differentiation. Am J Surg Pathol 5:307, 1981.

146. Radice PA, Matthews MJ, Ihde DC, et al.: The clinical behavior of "mixed" small cell/large cell bronchogenic carcinoma compare to "pure" small cell subtypes. Cancer 50:2894, 1982.

147. Harwood, TR, Gracey DR, Yokoo H: Pseudomesotheliomatous carcinoma of the lung. A variant of peripheral lung cancer. Am J Clin Pathol 65:159, 1976.

148. Babolini G: The pleural form of primary cancer of the lung. Dis Chest 29:314, 1956.

149. Katzenstien ALA, Prioleau PG, Askin FB: The histologic spectrum and significance of clear cell change in lung carcinoma. Cancer 45:943, 1980.

150. Untermann DH, Reingold IM: The occurrence of psammoma bodies in papillary adenocarcinoma of the lung. Am J Clin Pathol 57:297, 1972.

151. Foster CS: Mucus-secreting 'alveolar-cell' tumor of the lung: A histochemical comparison of tumours arising within and outside the lung. Histopathology 4:567, 1980.

152. Kimula Y: A histochemical and ultrastructural study of adenocarcinoma of the lung. Am J Surg Pathol 2:253, 1978.

153. Bolen JW, Throning D: Histogenetic classification of pulmonary carcinomas: Peripheral adenocarcinomas studied by light microscopy, histochemistry, and electron microscopy. Pathol Annu 17:77, 1982.

154. Espinoza CG, Saba SR, Shelley SA, et al.: Antibodies to surfactant apoprotein as a diagnostic tool for identifying carcinomas of the lung with alveolar cell differentiation. Lab Invest 46:21A, 1983.

155. Cutz E, Conen PE: Ultrastructure and cytochemistry of Clara cells. Am J Pathol 62:127, 1971.

156. Liebow AA: Bronchiolo-alveolar carcinoma. Adv Intern Med 10:329, 1960.

157. Case Records of the Massachusetts General Hospital. N Engl J Med 294:210, 1976.

158. Donaldson JC, Stoop DR, Kaminsky DB: Bronchiolar carcinoma in a 20-year-old man. Chest 71:111, 1977.

159. Hammar SP, Bockus D, Remington F, et al.: Langerhans cells and serum precipitating antibodies against fungal antigens in bronchioloalveolar cell carcinoma: Possible association with pulmonary eosinophilic granuloma. Ultrastruct Pathol 1:19, 1980.

160. Bennett DE, Sasser WF: Bronchiolar carcinoma: A valid clinicopathologic entity? A study of 30 cases. Cancer 24:876, 1969.

161. Delarue NC, Anderson W, Sander D, Starr J: Bronchioloalveolar carcinoma. A reappraisal after 24 years. Cancer 29:90, 1972.

162. Dunn D, Hertel B, Norwood W, Nicoloff DM: Bronchioalveolar cell carcinoma of the lung: A clinicopathological study. Ann Thorac Surg 26:241, 1978.

163. Tao LC, Delarue NC, Sanders D, Weisbrod G: Bronchioloalveolar carcinoma. A correlative clinical and cytologic study. Cancer 42:2759, 1978.

164. Donaldson JC, Kaminsky B, Elliott RC: Bronchiolar carcinoma. Cancer 41:250, 1978.

165. Nash G, Langlinais PC, Greenawald KA: Alveolar cell carcinoma. Does it exist? Cancer 29:322, 1972.

166. Kauffman SL, Alexander L, Sass L: Histologic and ultrastructural features of the Clara cell adenoma of the mouse lung. Lab Invest 40:708, 1979.

167. Kennedy AR, McGandy RB, Little JB: Histochemical, light and electron microscopic study of plonium-210 induced peripheral tumors in hamster lungs: Evidence implicating the Clara cell as the cell of origin. Eur J Cancer 13:1325, 1977.

168. Hod I, Herz A, Zimber A: Pulmonary carcinoma (Jaagsiekte) of sheep. Ultrastructural study of early and advanced tumor lesions. Am J Pathol 86:545, 1977.

169. Coalson RE, Nordquist RE, Coalson JJ, et al.: Alveolar cell carcinoma. An *in vitro* study. Lab Invest 28:38, 1973.

170. Kuhn C: Fine structure of bronchiolo-alveolar carcinoma. Cancer 30:1107, 1972.

171. Torikata C, Ishiwata K: Intranuclear tubular structures observed in the cells of an alveolar cell carcinoma of the lung. Cancer 40:1194, 1977.

172. Singh G, Katyal SL, Torikata C: Carcinoma of type II pneumocytes. Am J Pathol 102:195, 1981.

173. Bedrossian CWM, Weilbaecher DG, Bentinck DC, Greenbery SD: Ultrastructure of human bronchiolo-alveolar cell carcinoma. Cancer 36:1399, 1975.

174. Adamson JS, Senior RM, Merrill T: Alveolar cell carcinoma—an electron microscopic study. Am Rev Respir Dis 100:550, 1969.

175. Bonikos DS, Hendrickson M, Bensch KG: Pulmonary alveolar cell carcinoma. Fine structural and in vitro study of a case and critical review of this entity. Am J Surg Pathol 1:93, 1977.

176. Morningstar WM, Hassan MO: Bronchiolo-alveolar carcinoma with nodal metastases. An ultrastructural study. Am J Surg Pathol 3:273, 1979.

177. Singh G, Katyal SL: Surfactant apoprotein in alveolar proteinosis and pulmonary tumors. Lab Invest 48:79A, 1983.

178. Greenberg SD, Smith MN, Spjut HJ: Bronchiolo-alveolar carcinoma—cell of origin. Am J Clin Pathol 63:153, 1975.

179. Jacques J, Currie W: Bronchiolo-alveolar carcinoma: A Clara cell tumor? Cancer 40-2171, 1977.

180. Montes M, Binette JP, Chaudry AP, et al.: Clara cell adenocarcinoma. Am J Surg Pathol 245:76, 1977.

181. Sidhu GS, Forrester EM: Glycogen-rich clara cell-type bronchiolo-alveolar carcinoma. Cancer 40:2209, 1977.

182. Horie A, Ohta M: Ultrastructural features of large cell

carcinoma of the lung with reference to the prognosis of patients. Hum Pathol 12:423, 1981.

183. Nash AD, Stout AP: Giant cell carcinoma of the lung. Report of 5 cases. Cancer 11:369, 1958.

184. Hathaway BM, Copeland K, Gurley J: Giant cell adenocarcinoma of the lung—Report of 21 and analysis of 139 cases. Arch Surg 98:24, 1969.

185. Razzuk MA, Lyon JA, Kingsley WB, et al.: Giant cell carcinoma of the lung. J Thorac Cardiovasc Surg 59:574, 1970.

186. Wang N-S, Seemayer TA, Ahmed MN, Knaack J: Giant cell carcinoma of the lung. Hum Pathol 7:3, 1976.

187. Yesner R, Gerstl B, Auerbach O: Application of the World Health Organization classification of lung carcinoma to biopsy material. Ann Thorac Surg 1:33, 1965.

188. Miller WE: Roentgenographic manifestations of lung cancer. In Straus MJ (ed): *Lung Cancer—Clinical Diagnosis and Treatment.* New York: Grune & Stratton, 1977, p 129.

189. Byrd RB, Carr DR, Miller WE, et al.: Radiographic abnormalities in carcinoma of the lung as related to histological cell type. Thorax 24:573, 1969.

190. Berkmen YM: The many faces of bronchiolo-alveolar carcinoma. Semin Roentgenol 12:207, 1977.

191. Brett GZ: Earlier diagnosis and survival in lung cancer. Br Med J 4:260, 1969.

192. Nash FA, Morgan JM, Tomkins JG: South London lung cancer study. Br Med J 2:715, 1968.

193. Weiss W, Boucot K: The Philadelphia pulmonary neoplasm research project: Early roentgenographic appearance of bronchogenic carcinoma. Arch Intern Med 134:306, 1974.

194. Cohen MH: Signs and symptoms of bronchogenic carcinoma. In Straus MJ (ed): *Lung Cancer—Clinical Diagnosis and Treatment.* New York: Grune & Stratton, 1977, p 85.

195. Cohen MH: Diagnosis, staging and therapy. In Harris CC (ed): *Pathogenesis and Therapy of Lung Cancer.* New York: Marcel Dekker, 1978, p 653.

196. Bartelsen S, Struve-Christensen E, Annet A, Jorgen S. Isolated middle lobe atelectasis: Aetiology, pathogenesis, and treatment of the so-called middle lobe syndrome. Thorax 35:449, 1980.

197. Paulson DL: Carcinomas in the superior pulmonary sulcus. J Thorac Cardiovasc Surg 70:1095, 1975.

198. Polackwich RJ, Straus MJ: Superior vena caval syndrome. In Straus MJ (ed): *Lung Cancer—Clinical Diagnosis and Treatment.* New York: Grune & Stratton, 1977, p 249.

199. Morgan WKC, Andrews CE: Extrapulmonary syndromes associated with tumors of the lung. In Baum GL (ed): *Textbook of Pulmonary Diseases,* 2nd ed. Boston: Little, Brown, 1974, p 819.

200. Primack A, Broder LE, Diasio RB: Production of markers by bronchogenic carcinoma. A review. In Straus MJ (ed): *Lung Cancer—Clinical Diagnosis and Treatment,* New York: Grune & Stratton, 1977, p 33.

201. Goodnight SH: Bleeding in intravascular clotting in malignancy—a review. Ann NY Acad Sci 230:271, 1974.

202. Holyoke ED, Frank AL, Weiss L: Tumor thromboplastin activity in vitro. Int J Cancer 9:959, 1972.

203. Mersky C: Pathogenesis and treatment of altered blood coagulability in patients with malignant tumors. Ann NY Acad Sci 230:271, 1974.

204. Greenfield GB, Schorsch HA, Shkolnik A: The various roentgen appearances of pulmonary hypertrophic osteoarthropathy. Am J Radiol 101:927, 1967.

205. Carroll KB, Doyle L: A common factor in hypertrophic osteoarthropathy. Thorax 29:262, 1974.

206. Ennis GC, Cameron DP, Burger HG: On the aetiology of hypertrophic pulmonary osteoarthropathy in bronchogenic carcinoma—lack of relationship to elevated growth hormone levels. Aust NZ J Med 3:157, 1973.

207. Jao JY, Barlow JJ, Krant MJ: Pulmonary hypertrophic osteoarthropathy, spider angiomata and estrogen hypersecretion in neoplasms. Ann Intern Med 70:581, 1969.

208. Yacoub MH: Relation between the histology of bronchial carcinoma and hypertrophic pulmonary osteoarthropathy. Thorax 20:537, 1965.

209. Brown J, Winkelman RK: Acanthosis nigricans—a study of 90 cases. Medicine 47:33, 1968.

210. Ellenbogen BK: Acanthosis nigricans associated with bronchial carcinoma. Report of two cases. Br J Dermatol 61:251, 1949.

211. Schwindt WD, Bernhardt LC, Johnson SAM. Tylosis and intrathoracic neoplasms. Chest 57:590, 1970.

212. Morton DL, Itabashi HH, Grimes OF: Nonmetastatic neurological complications of bronchogenic carcinoma. The carcinomatous myopathies. J Thorac Cardiovasc Surg 51:14, 1966.

213. Overholt BF, Green RA: Bronchogenic carcinoma and peripheral neuromyopathies. Postgrad Med 40:13, 1966.

214. Tyler HR: Paraneoplastic syndromes of nerve, muscle and neuromuscular junction. Ann NY Acad Sci 230:348, 1974.

215. Dayan AD, Croft PB, Wilkinson M: Association of carcinomatous neuromyopathy with different histological types of carcinoma of the lung. Brain 88:435, 1965.

216. Jenkyn LR, Brooks PL, Forcier J, et al.: Remission of the Lambert-Eaton syndrome and small cell anaplastic carcinoma of the lung induced by chemotherapy and radiotherapy. Cancer 46:1123, 1980.

217. Paone JF, Jeyasingham K: Remission of cerebellar dysfunction after pneumonectomy for bronchogenic carcinoma. N Engl J Med 302:156, 1980.

218. Croft PB, Wilkinson M: Carcinomatous neuromyopathy: Its incidence in patients with carcinoma of the lung and breast. Lancet 1:184, 1965.

219. Gropp C, Havemann K, Scheuer A: Ectopic hormones in lung cancer patients at diagnosis and during therpay. Cancer 46:347, 1980.

220. Richardson RL, Greco FA, Oldham RK, Liddle GW: Tumor products and potential markers in small cell carcinoma. Semin Oncol 5:253, 1978.

221. Lokich JJ: The frequency and clinical biopsy of the ectopic hormone syndromes of small cell carcinoma. Cancer 50:2111, 1982.

222. Wolfson AR, Odell WD: ProACTH: Use for early detection of lung cancer. Am J Med 66:765, 1979.

223. Ayvazian LF, Schneider B, Gewirtz G, Yalow RS: Ectopic production of big ACTH in carcinoma of the lung—its clinical usefulness as a biologic marker. Am Rev Respir Dis 111:279, 1975.

224. Yalow RS, Eastridge CE, Higgins G Jr, Wolf J: Plasma and tumor ACTH in carcinoma of the lung. Cancer 44:1789, 1979.

225. Hauger-Klevene JH: Asymptomatic production of ACTH—radio immunoassay in squamous cell, oat cell and adenocarcinoma of the lung. Cancer 22:1262, 1968.

226. Cottrell JC, Becker KL, Matthews MJ, Moore C: Histology of

gonadotropin-secreting bronchogenic carcinoma. Am J Clin Pathol 52:720, 1969.

227. Silva OL, Becker KL, Primack A, et al.: Increased serum calcitonin levels in bronchogenic cancer. Chest 69:495, 1976.

228. Seyberth HW, Segre GV, Morgan JL, et al.: Prostaglandins as mediators of hypercalcemia associated with certain types of cancer. N Engl J Med 293:1278, 1975.

229. George JM, Capen C, Phillips AS: Biosynthesis of vasopressin in vitro and ultrastructure of a bronchogenic carcinoma. J Clin Invest 51:141, 1972.

230. Baylin SB, Abeloff MD, Wieman KC, et al.: Elevated histaminase (diamine oxidase) activity in samll-cell carcinoma of the lung. N Engl J Med 293:1286, 1975.

231. Abeloff MD, Eggleston JC, Mendelsohn G, et al.: Changes in morphologic and biochemical characteristics of small cell carcinoma of the lung. A clinicopathologic study. Am J Med 66:757, 1979.

232. Salyer DC, Eggleston JC: Oat cell carcinoma of the bronchus and the carcinoid syndorme. Arch Pathol 99:513, 1975.

233. Vincent RG, Chu TM, Lane WW: The value of carcinoembryonic antigen in patients with carcinoma of the lung. Cancer 44:685, 1979.

234. Ochsner A, DeBakey M: Significance of metastases in primary carcinoma of the lung. J Thorac Surg 11:357, 1941–1942.

235. Borrie J: Primary carcinoma of the bronchus. Prognosis following surgical resection. Ann R Coll Surg Engl 10:165, 1952.

236. Meyer KK: Direct lymphatic connections from lower lobe of lung to abdomen. J Thorac Sug 35:726, 1958.

237. Ballantyne AJ, Clagett OT, McDonald JR: Vascular invasion in bronchogenic carcinoma. Thorax 12:294, 1957.

238. Matthews MJ, Kanhouwa S, Pickren J, Robinette D: Frequency of residual and metastatic tumor in patients undergoing curative surgical resection for lung cancer. Cancer Chemother Rep 4:63, 1973.

239. American Joint Committee for Cancer Staging and End Results Reporting: *Classification and Staging of Lung Cancer of Site*. Chicago: American Joint Committee for Cancer Staging and End Results Reporting, 1976.

240. Muggia F, Rozencweig M: *Lung Cancer, Progress in Therapeutic Research*. New York: Raven Press, 1979.

241. Hyde L, Wolf J, McCracken S, Yesner R. Natural course of inoperable lung cancer. Chest 64:309, 1973.

242. Wilkins EW, Scannell JG, Craver JG: Four decades of experience with resections for bronchogenic carcinoma at the Massachusetts General Hospital. J Thorac Cardiovasc Surg 76:364, 1978.

243. Glenn WWL, Liebow AA, Linskog GF: *Thoracic and Cardiovascular Surgery with Related Pathology*, 3rd ed. New York: Appleton-Century-Crofts, 1975.

244. Mountain CF: Surgical therapy. In Fishman AP (ed): *Pulmonary Disease and Disorders*. New York: McGraw-Hill, 1980, p 1422.

245. Katlic M, Carter D. Prognostic implications of histology, size, and location of primary tumors. In Muggia F, Rozencweig M (eds): *Lung Cancer, Progress in Therapeutic Research*. New York: Raven Press, 1979, p 143.

246. Miller AB, Fox W, Tall R: Five-year follow-up of the medical research council comparative trial of surgery and radiotherapy for the primary treatment of small-celled or oat-celled carcinoma of the bronchus. Lancet 1:501, 1969.

247. Weiss RB: Small-cell carcinoma of the lung: Therapeutic management. Ann Intern Med 88:522, 1978.

248. Hande KR, Des Prez RM: Current perspectives in small cell lung cancer. Chest 85:669, 1984.

249. Lichter AS, Bunn PA: The management of small-cell carcinoma of the lung. In: Fishman AP (ed): *Update: Pulmonary Diseases and Disorders*. New York: McGraw-Hill, 1982, p 300.

250. Greco FA, Oldham RK: Current concepts in cancer—small cell lung cancer. N Engl J Med 301:355, 1979.

251. Cohen MH, Matthews M: Small cell bronchogenic carcinoma: A distinct clinicopathologic entity. Semin Oncol 5:234, 1978.

252. Nixon DW, Murphy GF, Sewell CW, et al.: Relationship between survival and histologic type in small cell anaplastic carcinoma of the lung. Cancer 44:1045, 1979.

253. Carter D, Eggleston JC: *Tumors of the Lower Respiratory Tract*. Washington, DC, Armed Forces Institute of Pathology, 1979.

254. Munnell ER, Dilling E, Grantham RN, et al.: Reappraisal of solitary bronchiolar (alveolar cell) carcinoma of the lung. Ann Thorac Surg 25:287, 1978.

255. Paulson DL: Carcinoma in the superior pulmonary sulcus. Ann Thorac Surg 28:3, 1979.

256. Miller JL, Mansour KA, Hatcher CR: Carcinoma of the superior pulmonary sulcus. Ann Thorac Surg 28:44, 1979.

257. Attar S, Miller JE, Satterfield J, et al.: Pancoast's tumor: Irradiation or surgery? Ann Thorac Surg 28:578, 1979.

258. Johnson DH, Hainsworth JD, Greco FA: Pancoast's syndrome and small cell lung cancer. Chest 82:602, 1982.

259. Ashley DJB, Danino EA, Davies HD: Bronchial polyps. Thorax 18:45, 1963.

260. Singer DB, Greenberg SD, Harrison GM: Papillomatosis of the lung Am Rev Respir Dis 94:777, 1966.

261. Al-Saleem T, Peale AR, Norris CM: Multiple papillomatosis of the lower respiratory tract. Clinical and pathologic study of 11 cases. Cancer 22:1173, 1968.

262. DiMarco AF, Montenegro H, Payne CB Jr, Kwon KH: Papillomas of the tracheobronchial tree with malignant degeneration. Chest 74:464, 1978.

263. Kaufman G, Klopstock R: Papillomatosis of the respiratory tract. Am Rev Respir Dis 88:839, 1963.

264. Spencer H, Dail DH, Arneaud J: Non-invasive bronchial epithelial papillary tumors. Cancer 45:1486, 1980.

265. Sniffen RC, Soutter L, Robbins LL: Muco-epidermoid tumors of the bronchus arising from the surface epithelium. Am J Pathol 34:671, 1958.

266. Sherwin RP, Laforet EG, Strieder JW: Exophytic endobronchial carcinoma. J Thorac Cardiovasc Surg 43:716, 1962.

267. Smith JF, Dexter D: Papillary neoplasms of the bronchus of low grade malignancy. Thorax 18:340, 1963.

268. Godwin JD: Carcinoid tumors—an analysis of 2837 cases. Cancer 36:560, 1975.

269. Bensch KG, Gordon GB, Miller LR: Electron microscopic and biochemical studies on the bronchial carcinoid tumor. Cancer 18:592, 1965.

270. Hage E, Hage J, Juel G: Endocrine-like cells of the pulmonary epithelium of the human adult lung. Cell Tissue Res 178:39, 1977.

271. Lauweryns JM, Cokelaere M, Theunynck P: Serotonin producing neuro-epithelial bodies in rabbit respiratory mucosa. Science 180:410, 1973.

272. Lauweryns JM, Goddeeris P: Neuroepithelial bodies in the human child and adult lung. Am Rev Respir Dis 111:469, 1975.

273. McDowell EM, Barrett LA, Trump BF: Observations on small granule cells in adult human bronchial epithelium and in carcinoid and oat cell tumors. Lab Invest 34:202, 1976.

274. Terzakis JA, Sommers SC, Anderson B: Neurosecretory appearing cells of human segmental bronchi. Lab Invest 26:127, 1972.

275. McDowell EM, Sorokin SP, Hoyt RF, Trump BF: An unusual bronchial carcinoid tumor: Light and electron microscopy. Hum Pathol 4:338, 1981.

276. Bensch KG: The problem of classifying peripheral endocrine tumors. Hum Pathol 14:383, 1983.

277. Soga J, Tazawa K: Pathologic analysis of carcinoids. Cancer 28:990, 1971.

278. Jones RA, Dawson IMP: Morphology and staining patterns of endocrine cell tumors in the gut, pancreas and bronchus and their possible significance. Histopathology 1:137, 1977.

279. Warren WH, Memoli VA, Gould VE: Immunohistochemical and ultrastructural analysis of bronchopulmonary neuroendocrine neoplasms. I. Carcinoids. Ultrastructural Pathol 6:15, 1984.

280. Gmelich JT, Bensch KG, Liebow AA: Cells of Kultschitzky type in bronchioles and their relation to the origin of peripheral carcinoid tumor. Lab Invest 17:88, 1967.

281. Hage E: Histochemistry and fine structure of bronchial carcinoid tumors. Virchows Arch [A] 361:121, 1973.

282. Capella C, Gabrielli M, Polak JM, et al.: Ultrastructure and histological study of 11 bronchial carcinoids. Evidence for different types. Virchows Arch [A] 381:313, 1979.

283. Capella C, Hage E, Solcia E, Usellini L: Ultrastructural similarity of endocrine-like cells of the human lung and some related cells of the gut. Cell Tissue Res 186:25, 1978.

284. Cutz E, Chan W, Kay JM, Chamberlain DW: Immunoperoxidase staining for serotonin, bombesin, calcitonin, and leuenkephalin in pulmonary tumorlets, bronchial carcinoids, and oat cell carcinomas. Lab Invest 46:16A, 1983.

284A. Tsutsumi Y, Osamura RY, Watanbe K, Yanaihara N: Immunohistochemical studies on gastrin releasing peptide and adreno-corticotropic hormone-containing cells in the human lung. Lab Invest 48:623, 1983.

285. Hosoda S, Nakamura W, Suzuki H, et al.: A bronchial carcinoid having low serotonin concentration. Arch Pathol 90:320, 1970.

286. Sonksen PH, Ayres AB, Braimbridge M, et al.: Acromegaly caused by pulmonary carcinoid tumors. Clin Endocrinol 5:503, 1976.

287. Ratcliffe JG, Scott AP, Bennett HPJ, et al.: Production of a corticotrophin-like intermediate lobe peptide and of corticotrophin by a bronchial carcinoid tumor. Clin Endocrinol 2:51, 1973.

288. Gewirtz G, Yalow RS: Ectopic ACTH production in carcinoma of the lung. J Clin Invest 53:1022, 1974.

289. Imura H, Matsukura S, Yamamoto H, et al.: Studies on ectopic ACTH-producing tumors. II. Clinical and biochemical features of 30 cases. Cancer 35:1430, 1975.

290. Tilson MD: Carcinoid syndrome. Surg Clin North Am 54:409, 1974.

291. Said SI: Endocrine role of the lung in disease. Am J Med 57:453, 1974.

292. Oates JA, Melmon K, Sjoerdsma A, Mason DT: Release of a kinin peptide in the carcinoid syndrome. Lancet 1:514, 1964.

293. Bernheimer H, Ehringer H, Heistracher P, et al.: Biologish asktives, nicht metastasierendes Bronchuscarcinoid mit Linksherzsyndrom. Wien Klin Wochenschr 72:867, 1960.

294. Ricci C, Patrassi N, Massa R, et al.: Carcinoid syndrome in bronchial adenoma. Am J Surg 126:671, 1973.

295. Stanford WR, Davis JE, Gunter JU, Hobart SG Jr: Bronchial adenoma (carcinoid type) with solitary metastasis and associated functioning carcinoid syndrome. South Med J 51:449, 1958.

296. Pichel Warner RR, Kirschner PA, Warner GM: Serotonin production by bronchial adenomas without the carcinoid syndrome. JAMA 178:1175, 1961.

297. Sherry S. The kallikrein system: A basic defense mechanism. Hosp Pract June:75–85, 1970.

298. Mason AMS, Ratcliffe JG, Buckle RM, Mason AS: ACTH secretion by bronchial carcinoid tumors. Clin Endocrinol 1:3, 1972.

299. Hansen OP, Hansen M, Hansen HH, Rose B: Multiple endocrine adenomatosis of mixed type. Acta Med Scand 200:327, 1976.

300. Kaneko HM, Hojo H, Ishikawa S, Kikuchi M: Bronchial carcinoid accompanied by thyroid adenomas and adrenal adenomas. Acta Pathol Jpn 27:375, 1977.

301. Southern AL: Functioning metastatic bronchial carcinoid with elevated levels of serum and cerebronspinal fluid serotonin and pituitary adenoma. J Clin Endocrinol 20:298, 1960.

302. Williams ED, Celestin LR: The association of bronchial carcinoid and pluriglandular adenomatosis. Thorax 17:120, 1962.

303. Okike N, Bernatz PE, Woolner LB: Carcinoid tumors of the lung. Ann Thorac Surg 22:270, 1976.

304. Salyer DC, Salyer WR, Eggleston JC: Bronchial carcinoid tumors. Cancer 36:1522, 1975.

305. Lack EE, Harris GBC, Erkalis AJ, Vawter GF: Primary bronchial tumors in childhood. Cancer 51:492, 1983.

306. Whitehead R, Cosgrove C: Mucins and carcinoid tumours. Pathology 11, 473, 1979.

307. Thomas CP, Morgan AD: Ossifying bronchial adenoma. Thorax 13:286, 1958.

308. Liebow AA: *Tumors of the Lower Respiratory Tract. Fascicle 17, Atlas of Tumor Pathology.* Washington, DC Armed Forces Institute of Pathology, 1952.

309. Rodgers-Sullivan RF, Weiland LH, Palumbo PJ, Hepper GG: Pulmonary tumorlets associated with Cushing's syndrome. Am Rev Respir Dis 117:799, 1978.

310. Bonikos DS, Archibald R, Bensch KG: On the origin of the so-called tumorlets of the lung. Hum Pathol 7:461, 1967.

311. Churg A: Large spindle cell variant of peripheral bronchial carcinoid tumor. Arch Pathol 101:216, 1977.

312. Dube VE: Peripheral bronchial carcinoid with a spindle-cell pattern. Report of a case. Arch Pathol 89:374, 1970.

313. Ranchod M, Levine GD: Spindle-cell carcinoid tumors of the lung. A clinicopathologic study of 35 cases. Am J Surg Pathol 4:315, 1980.

314. Bonikos DS, Bensch KG, Jamplis RW: Peripheral pulmonary carcinoid tumors. Cancer 37:1977, 1976.

315. Turnbull AD, Huvos AG, Goodner JT, Beattie EJ Jr: The malignant potential of bronchial adenoma. Ann Thorac Surg 14:453, 1972.

316. Arrigoni MG, Woolner LB, Bernatz PE: Atypical carcinoid tumors of the lung. J Thorac Cardiovasc Surg 64:413, 1972.

317. Mills SE, Cooper PH, Walker AN, Kron IL: Atypical carcinoid tumor of the lung. Am J Surg Pathol 6:643, 1982.

318. Gillespie JJ, Luger AM, Gallaway LA: Peripheral spindled carcinoid tumor: A review of its ultrastructure, differential diagnosis, and biologic behavior. Hum Pathol 10:601, 1979.

319. Fechner RE, Bentinck BR: Ultrastructure of bronchial oncocytoma. Cancer 31:1451, 1973.

320. Santos-Briz A, Terron J, Sastre R, et al.: Oncocytoma of the lung. Cancer 40:1330, 1977.

321. Black III WC: Pulmonary oncocytoma. Cancer 29:1347, 1969.

322. Sajjad SM, Mackay B, Lukeman JM: Oncocytic carcinoid tumor of the lung. Ultrastruct Pathol 1:171, 1980.

323. Walter P, Warter A, Morand G: Carcinoide oncocytaire bronchique. Virchows Arch [A] 379:85, 1978.

324. Sklar JL, Churg A, Bensch KG: Oncocytic carcinoid tumor of the lung. Am J Surg Pathol 4:287, 1980.

325. Gordon HW, Miller R Jr, Mittman C: Medullary carcinoma of the lung with amyloid stroma: A counterpart of medullary carcinoma of the thyroid. Hum Pathol 4:431, 1973.

326. Blessing MH, Hora BI: Gomera in der lunge des menschen. Z Zellforsch 87:526, 1968.

327. Gould VE, Linnoila RI: Pulmonary neuroepithelial bodies, neuroendocrine cells, and pulmonary tumors. Hum Pathol 13:1064, 1982.

328. Korn D, Bensch K, Liebow AA, Castleman B: Multiple minute pulmonary tumors resembling chemodectomas. Am J Pathol 37:641, 1960.

329. Zak FG, Chabes A: Pulmonary chemodectomatosis. JAMA 183:887, 1963.

330. Ichinose H, Hewitt RL, Drapanas T: Minute pulmonary chemodectomas. Cancer 28:692, 1971.

331. Barroso-Moguel R, Costero I: Quimiorreceptores y otras estructuras intra- pulmonares argentafines relacionadas con la regulacion de la circulacion pulmonar. Arch Inst Cardiol 38:337, 1968.

332. Kuhn C III, Askin FB: The fine structure of minute pulmonary chemodectomas. Hum Pathol 6:681, 1975.

333. Churg A, Warnock ML: So-called "minute pulmonary chemodectomas." Cancer 37:1759, 1976.

334. Chumas JC, Lorelle CA: Pulmonary meningioma. Am J Surg Pathol 6:795, 1982.

335. Kemnitz P, Spormann H, Heinrich P: Meningioma of lung: First report with light and electron microscopic findings. Ultrastruct Pathol 3:359, 1982.

336. Mirra SS, Miles ML: Unusual pericytic proliferation in a meningotherliomatous meningioma. Am J Surg Pathol 6:573, 1982.

337. Singh G, Lee RE, Brooks DH: Primary pulmonary paraganglioma. Report of a case and review of the literature. Cancer 40:2286, 1977.

338. Blessing MH, Borchard F, Lenz W: Glomustumor (sog. Chemodektom) der lunge. Pathologisch-anatomische und biochemische befunde. Virchows Arch [A] 359:315, 1973.

339. Tu H, Bottomley RH: Malignant chemodectoma presenting as a miliary pulmonary infiltrate. Cancer 33:244, 1974.

340. Liebow AA: *Tumors of the Lower Respiratory Tract. Fascicle 17, Atlas of Tumor Pathology.* Washington, DC Armed Forces Institue of Pathology, 1952.

341. Smetana HF, Iverson L, Swan LL: Bronchogenic carcinoma—analysis of 100 autopsy cases. Milit Surg 111:335, 1952.

342. Leonardi HK, Jung-Legg Y, Legg MA, Neptune WB: Tracheobronchial mucoepidermoid carcinoma. J Thorac Cardiovasc Surg 78:431, 1978.

343. Conlan AA, Payne WS, Woolner LB, Sanderson DR: Adenoid cystic carcinoma (cylindroma) and mucoepidermoid carcinoma of the bronchus. Factors affecting survival. J Thorac Cardiovasc Surg 76:369, 1978.

344. Klacsmann PG, Olson JL, Eggleston JC: Mucoepidermoid carcinoma of the bronchus. Cancer 43:1720, 1979.

345. Axelsson C, Burcharth F, Johansen AA: Mucoepidermoid lung tumors. J Thorac Cardiovasc Surg 65:902, 1973.

346. Mullins JD, Barnes RP: Childhood bronchial mucoepidermoid tumors. Cancer 44:315, 1979.

347. Reichle FA, Rosemond GP: Mucoepidermoid tumors of the bronchus. J Thorac Cardiovasc Surg 51:443, 1966.

348. Wilkins EW, Darling RC, Souter L, Sniffen RC: A continuing clinical survey of adenomas of the trachea and bronchus in a general hospital. J Thorac Cardiovasc Surg 46:279, 1963.

349. Trentini GP, Palmeri B: Mucoepidermoid tumor of the trachea. Chest 62:336, 1972.

350. Spencer H: Bronchial mucous gland tumors. Virchows Arch [A] 383:101, 1979.

351. Gaillard J, Levasseur P: Treatment of adenocystic carcinomas (cylindromas) of the trachea and bronchi. Bronchopneumologie 28:430, 1978.

352. O'Grady WP, McDivitt RW, Homan CW, Moore SW: Bronchial adenomas. Arch Surg 101:558, 1970.

353. Goodner JT, Berg JW, Watson WL: The nonbenign nature of bronchial carcinoids and cylindromas. Cancer 14:539, 1961.

354. Fechner RE, Bentinck BR, Askew JB Jr: Acinic cell tumor of the lung. A histologic and ultrastructural study. Cancer 29:501, 1972.

355. Katz DR, Buris JJ: Acinic cell tumor of the bronchus. Cancer 38:830, 1976.

356. Payne WS, Schier J, Woolner LB: Mixed tumors of the bronchus (salivary gland type). J Thorac Cardiovasc Surg 49:663, 1965.

357. Verska JJ, Connolly JE: Bronchial adenomas in children. J Thorac Cardiovasc Surg 55:411, 1968.

358. Kroe DJ, Pitcock JA: Benign mucous gland adenoma of the bronchus. Arch Pathol 84:539, 1967.

359. Politis J, Funahashi A, Gehlsen JA, et al.: Intrathoracic lipomas. Report of 3 cases and review of the literature with emphasis on endobronchial lipoma. J Thorac Cardiovasc Surg 77:550, 1979.

360. Horanyi J, Horlay B, Molnar J: Endobronchial lipoma. Thoraxchirurgie 8:573, 1961.

361. Guidice JC, Gordon R, Komansky HJ: Endobronchial lipoma causing unilateral absence of pulmonary perfusion. Chest 77:104, 1980.

362. Bellin HJ, Libshitz HI, Patchefsky AS: Bronchial lipoma—report of two cases showing chondroitic metaplasia. Arch Pathol 92:20, 1971.

363. Crutcher RR, Waltuch TL, Ghosh AK: Bronchial lipoma—report of a case and literature review. J Thorac Cardiovasc Surg 55:422, 1968.

364. MacArthur CGC, Cheung DLC, Spiro SG: Endobronchial lipoma. A review with four cases. Br J Dis Chest 71:93, 1977.

365. Plachta A, Hershey H: Lipoma of the lung—review of the literature and report of a case. Am Rev Respir Dis 86:912, 1962.

366. Shapiro R, Carter MG: Peripheral lipoma of the lung—rerpot of a case. Am Rev Respir Dis 69:1042, 1954.

367. Orlowski T, Stasiak K, Kolodziej J: Leiomyoma of the lung. J Thorac Cardiovasc Surg 76:257, 1978.

368. Wolff M, Kaye G, Silva F: Pulmonary metastases (with

admixed epithelial elements) from smooth muscle neoplasms. Report of nine cases, including three males. Am J Surg Pathol 3:325, 1979.

369. Bartley TD, Arean VM: Intrapulmonary neurogenic tumors. J Thorac Cardiovasc Surg 50:114, 1965.

370. Silverman JF, Leffers BR, Kay S: Primary pulmonary neurilemona—report of a case with ultrastructural examination. Arch Pathol Lab Med 100:644, 1976.

371. Cooney TP: Primary pulmonary ganglioneuroblastoma in an adult: Maturation, involution, and the immune response. Histopathology 5:451, 1981.

372. Viguera JL, Pujol JL, Reboiras SD, et al.: Fibrous histiocytomas of the lung. Thorax 31:475, 1976.

373. Grossman RE, Bemis EL, Pemberton AH, Narodick BG: Fibrous histiocytoma or xanthoma of the lung with bronchial involvement. J Thorac Cardiovasc Surg 65:653, 1973.

374. Guccion JG, Rosen SH: Bronchopulmonary leiomyosarcoma and fibrosarcoma. A study of 32 cases and review of the literature. Cancer 30:836, 1972.

375. Carswell J, Kraeft NH: Fibrosarcoma of the bronchus. J Thorac Surg 19:117, 1950.

376. Meade JB, Whitwell F, Bickford BJ, Waddington JKB: Primary haemangiopericytoma of lung. Thorax 29:1, 1974.

377. Stout AP, Murray MR: Hemangiopericytoma. A vascular tumor featuring Zimmermann's pericytes. Ann Surg 116:26, 1942.

378. Enzinger FM, Smith BH: Hemangiopericytoma. An analysis of 106 cases. Hum Pathol 7:61, 1976.

379. Cameron EWJ: Primary sarcoma of the lung. Thorax 30:516, 1975.

380. Dowell AR: Primary pulmonary leiomyosarcoma. Ann Thorac Surg 17:384, 1974.

381. Nascimento AG, Unni KK, Bernatz PE: Sarcomas of the lung. Mayo Clin Proc 57:335, 1982.

382. Kempson RL, Kyriakos M: Fibroxanthosarcoma of the soft tissues. A type of malignant fibrous histiocytoma. Cancer 29:961, 1972.

383. Weiss SC, Enzinger F: Malignant fibrous histiocytoma. Analysis of 200 cases. Cancer 41:2250, 1978.

384. Bedrossian CWM, Verani R, Unger KM, Salman J: Pulmonary malignant fibrous histiocytoma—light and electron microscopic studies of one case. Chest 75:186, 1979.

385. Kern WH, Hughes RK, Meyer BW, Harley DP: Malignant fibrous histiocytoma of the lung. Cancer 44:1793, 1979.

386. Daniels AC, Conner GH, Straus FH: Primary chondrosarcoma of the tracheobronchial tree. Arch Pathol 84:615, 1967.

387. Bleisch VR, Kraus FT: Polypoid sarcoma of the pulmonary trunk. Analysis of the literature and report of a case with leptomeric organelles and ultrastructural features of rhabdomyosarcoma. Cancer 46:314, 1980.

388. Shmookler BM, Marsh HB, Roberts WC: Primary sarcoma of the pulmonary trunk and/or right or left main pulmonary artery—a rare cause of obstruction to right ventricular outflow. Report on 2 patients and analysis of 35 previously described patients. Am J Med 63:263, 1977.

389. Wackers FJT, VanDerSchoot JB, Hampf JF: Sarcoma of the pulmonary trunk associated with hemorrhagic tendency. Cancer 23:339, 1969.

390. Drennan JM, McCormack RJM: Primary rhabdomyosarcoma of the lung. J Pathol Bacteriol 79:147, 1960.

391. Dail D, Liebow A: Intravascular bronchioloalveolar tumor. Am J Pathol 78:6a(abstr), 1975.

392. Farinacci DJ, Blauw AS, Jennings EM: Multifocal pulmonary lesions of possible decidual origin (so-called pulmonary deciduosis). Am J Clin Pathol 59:508, 1973.

393. Dail DH, Liebow AA, Gmelich JT, et al.: Intravascular, bronchiolar, and alveolar tumor of the lung (IVBAT). Cancer 51:452, 1983.

394. Azumi N, Churg A: Intravascular and sclerosing bronchioloalveolar tumor. A pulmonary sarcoma of probable vascular origin. Am J Surg Pathol 5:587, 1981.

395. Corrin B, Manner B, Millard M, Weaver L: Histogenesis of the so-called "intravascular bronchioloalveolar tumor." J Pathol 128:163, 1979.

396. Weldon-Linne CM, Victor TA, Christ ML, Fry WA: Angiogenic nature of the 'intravascular bronchioloalveolar tumor' of the lung. Arch Pathol Lab Med 105:174, 1981.

397. Wagenvoort CA, Beetstra A, Spijker J: Capillary haemangiomatosis of the lungs. Histopathology 2:401, 1978.

398. Enzinger FE, Weiss SW: *Soft Tissue Tumors.* New York: CV Mosby, 1983.

399. Stackhouse EM, Harrison EG Jr, Ellis FH Jr: Primary mixed malignancies of lung: Carcinosarcoma and blastoma. J Thorac Cardiovasc Surg 57:385, 1969.

400. Willis RA: *Pathology of Tumors*, 4th ed. London: Butterworths, 1967.

401. Barnard WG: Embryoma of the lung. Thorax 7:299, 1952.

402. Spencer H: Pulmonary blastoma. J Pathol Bacteriol 82:161, 1961.

403. Waddell WR: Organoid differentiation of the fetal lung—a histologic study of the differentiation of mammalian fetal lung in utero and in transplants. Arch Pathol 27:227, 1949.

404. Campiche M, Gautier A, Hernandez EI, Reymond A: An electron microscopic study of the fetal development of human lung. Pediatrics 32:976, 1963.

405. Leeson JS, Leeson CR: A light and electron microscopic study of developing respiratory tissue in the rat. J Anat 98:183, 1964.

406. O'Hare KH, Sheridan MN: Electron microscopic observations on the morphogenesis of the albino rat lung: With special reference to epithelial cells. Am J Anat 127:181, 1970.

407. Chaudhuri MR: Bronchial carcinosarcoma. J Thorac Cardiovasc Surg 61:319, 1971.

408. Chaudhuri MR, Eastham WN, Frediksz PA: Pulmonary blastoma with diverse mesenchymal proliferation. Thorax 27:487, 1972.

409. Kakos GS, Williams TE, Assor D, Vasko JS: Pulmonary carcinosarcoma—etiologic, therapeutic and prognostic considerations. J Thorac Cardiovasc Surg 61:777, 1971.

410. Davis PW, Briggs JC, Seal RME, Storring FK: Benign and malignant mixed tumors of the lung. Thorax 27:657, 1972.

411. Razzuk MA, Urschel HC, Race GJ, et al.: Carcinosarcoma of the lung—report of two cases and review of the literature. J Thorac Cardiovasc Surg 61:541, 1971.

412. Roth JA, Elguezabel A: Pulmonary blastoma evolving into carcinosarcoma—a case study. Am J Surg Pathol 2:407, 1978.

413. Matsusaka T, Watanabe H, Enjoji M: Pseudosarcoma and carcinosarcoma of the esophagus. Cancer 37:1546, 1976.

414. Lichtiger B, MacKay B, Tessmer CF: Spindle-cell variant to squamous carcinoma—a light and electron micrscopic study of 13 cases. Cancer 26:1311, 1970.

415. Leifer C, Miller AS, Putong PB, Min BH: Spindle cell

carcinoma of the oral mucosa. A light and electron microscopic study of apparent sarcomatous metastasis to cervical lymph nodes. Cancer 34:597, 1974.

416. Battifora H: Spindle cell carcinoma—ultrastructural evidence of squamous origin and collagen production by the tumor cells. Cancer 37:2275, 1976.

417. Iverson RE, Straehley CJ: Pulmonary blastoma: Longterm survival of juvenile patient. Chest 63:436, 1973.

418. Valderrama E, Saluja G, Shende A, et al.: Pulmonary blastoma. Report of two cases in children. Am J Surg Pathol 2:415, 1978.

419. Karcioglu ZA, Someren AO: Pulmonary blastoma—a case report and review of the literature. Am J Clin Pathol 61:287, 1974.

420. Kern WH, Stiles QR: Pulmonary blastoma. J Thorac Cardiovasc Surg 72:801, 1976.

421. Kennedy A, Prior AL: Pulmonary blastoma—a report of two cases and a review of the literature. Thorax 31:776, 1976.

422. McCann MP, Fu YS, Kay S: Pulmonary blastoma. A light and electron microscopic study. Cancer 38:789, 1976.

423. Fung CH, Lo JW, Yonan TN, et al.: Pulmonary blastoma. An ultrastructural study with a brief review of literature and a discussion of pathogenesis. Cancer 39:153, 1977.

424. Tamai S, Kameya T, Shimosato Y, et al.: Pulmonary blastoma—an ultrastructural study of a case and its transplanted tumor in athymic nude mice. Cancer 46:1396, 1980.

425. Marcus PB, Dieb TM, Martin JH: Pulmonary blastoma: An ultrastructural study emphasizing intestinal differentiation in lung tumors. Cancer 49:1829, 1982.

426. Kradin RL, Young RH, Dickersin GR, et al.: Pulmonary blastoma with argyrophil cells and lacking sarcomatous features (pulmonary endodermal tumor resembling fetal lung). Am J Surg Pathol 6:163, 1982.

427. Edwards CW, Saunders AM, Collins F: Mixed malignant tumor of the lung. Thorax 34:629, 1979.

428. Bauermeister DE, Jennings ER, Beland AH, Judson HA: Pulmonary blastoma, a form of carcinoma. Am J Clin Pathol 46:322, 1976.

429. Carter D, Eggleston J: *Tumors of the Lower Respiratory Tract*. Washington, DC, Armed Forces Institute of Pathology, 1980.

430. Bull JC, Grimes OF: Pulmonary carcinosarcoma. Chest 65:9, 1974.

431. Ludwigsen E: Endobronchial carcinosarcoma. Virchows Arch [A] 373:293, 1977.

432. Askin FB, Rosai J, Sibley RK, et al.: Malignant small cell tumor of the thoracopulmonary region in childhood. Cancer 43:2438, 1979.

433. Horstmann JP, Pietra GG, Harman JA, et al.: Spontaneous regression of pulmonary leiomyomas during pregnancy. Cancer 39:314, 1977.

434. Banner A, Carrington CB, Emory WB, et al.: Efficacy of oophorectomy in lymphangioleiomyomatosis and benign metastasizing leiomyoma. N Engl J Med 305:204, 1981.

435. Silverman JF, Kay S: Multiple pulmonary leiomyomatous hamartomas. Cancer 38:1199, 1976.

436. Piccaluga A, Capelli A: Fibroleiomiomatosi metastatizzante dell'utero. Arch Ital Anat Istolog Patol 41:99, 1967.

437. Cramer SF, Meyer JS, Kraner JF, et al.: Metastasizing leiomyoma of the uterus. S-phase fraction, estrogen receptor, and ultrastructure. Cancer 45:932, 1980.

438. Bachman D, Wolff M: Pulmonary metastases from benign smooth muscle tumors of the uterus. AJR 127:441, 1976.

439. Trapnell DH: Recognition and incidence of intrapulmonary lymph nodes. Thorax 19:44, 1964.

440. Greenberg HB: Benign subpleural lymph node appearing as a pulmonary 'coin' lesion. Radiology 77:97, 1961.

441. Anagnostou D, Harrison CV: Angiofollicular lymph node hyperplasia (Castleman). J Clin Pathol 25:306, 1972.

442. Freeman C, Berg JW, Cutler SJ: Occurrence and prognosis of extranodal lymphomas. Cancer 29:252, 1972.

443. Koss MN, Hochholzter L, Nichols PW, et al.: Primary non-Hodgkin's lymphoma and pseudolymphoma of lung. Hum Pathol 14:1024, 1983.

444. L'Hoste RJ, Filippa DA, Lieberman PH, Bretsky S: Primary pulmonary lymphomas. Cancer 54:1397, 1984.

445. Turner RR, Colby TV, Doggett RS: Well-differentiated lymphocytic lymphoma. A study of 47 persons with primary manifestation in the lung. Cancer 54:2088, 1984.

446. Saltzstein SL: Extranodal malignant lymphomas and pseudolymphomas. Pathol Annu 4:159, 1969.

447. Saltzstein SL: Pulmonary malignant lymphomas and pseudolymphomas: Classification, therapy and prognosis. Cancer 16:928, 1963.

448. Colby TV, Carrington CB: Pulmonary lymphomas: Current concepts. Hum Pathol 14:884, 1983.

449. Liebow AA, Carrington CB: Diffuse pulmonary lymphoreticular infiltrates associated with dysproteinemia. Med Clin North Am 57:809, 1973.

450. Colby TV, Carrington CB: Pulmonary lymphomas simulating lymphomatoid granulomatosis. Am J Surg Pathol 6:19, 1982.

451. Colby TV, Carrington CB, Mark GJ: Pulmonary involvement in malignant histiocytosis. Am J Surg Pathol 5:61, 1981.

452. Faguet GB, Webb H, Agee JF, et al.: Immunologically diagnosed malignancy in Sjögren's pseudolymphoma. Am J Med 65:424, 1978.

453. Julsrud PR, Brown LR, Li Chin-Yang, et al.: Pulmonary processes of mature-appearing lymphocytes: Pseudolymphoma, well-differentiated lymphocytic lymphoma, and lymphocytic interstitial pneumonitis. Radiology 127:289, 1978.

454. Herbert A, Wright DH, Isaacson PG, Smith JL: Primary malignant lymphoma of lung. Hum Pathol 15:415, 1984.

455. Hutchinson WB, Friedenberg MJ, Saltzstein S: Primary pulmonary pseudolymphoma. Radiology 82:48, 1964.

456. Colby TV, Carrington CB: Lymphoreticular tumors and infiltrates of the lung. Pathol Annu 18(PTE):87, 1983.

457. Churg A: Pulmonary angiitis and granulomatosis revisited. Hum Pathol 14:868, 1983.

458. MacDonald JB: Lung involvement in Hodgkin's disease. Thorax 32:664, 1977.

459. Monahan DT: Hodgkin's disease of the lung. J Thorac Cardiovasc Surg 49:173, 1964.

460. Whitcomb ME, Schwarz MI, Keller AR, et al.: Hodgkin's disease of the lung. Am Rev Respir Dis 106:79, 1972.

461. Wood NL, Coltman CA: Localized primary extranodal Hodgkin's disease. Ann Intern Med 78:113, 1973.

462. Romanoff H, Milwidsky H: Primary plasmocytoma of the lung. Bri J Dis Chest 56:139, 1962.

463. Wile A, Olinger G, Peter JB, Dornfeld L: Solitary intrapanrenchymal pulmonary plasmacytoma associated with production of an M-protein. Cancer 37:2338, 1976.

464. Frizzera G, Moran EM, Rappaport H: Angio-immunoblastic lymphadenopathy. Am J Med 59:803, 1975.

465. Behadori M, Liebow AA: Plasma cell granulomas of the lung. Cancer 31:191, 1973.

466. McCall IW, Woo-ming M: The radiological appearances of plasma cell granuloma of the lung. Clin Radiol 29:145, 1978.

467. Pearl M: Postinflammatory pseudotumor of the lung in children. Pediatr Radiol 105:391, 1972.

468. Hutchins GM, Eggleston JC: Unusual presentation of pulmonary inflammatory pseudotumor (plasma cell granuloma) as esophageal obstruction. Am J Gastroenterol 71:501, 1979.

469. Hoover SV, Granston AS, Koch DF, Hudson TR: Plasma cell granuloma of the lung, response to radiation therapy. Cancer 39:123, 1977.

470. Buell R, Wang NS, Seemayer TA, Ahmed MN: Endobronchial plasma cell granuloma (xanthomatous pseudotumor). Hum Pathol 17:411, 1976.

471. Engleman P, Liebow AA, Gmelich J, Friedman PJ: Pulmonary hyalinizing granuloma. Am Rev Respir Dis 115:997, 1977.

472. Cox IL, Chang CHJ, Mantz F: Pseudotumor of the lung. Chest 67:6, 1975.

473. Erdman S, Vidne B, Levy MJ: Lung pseudotumor caused by pulmonary infarction. Geriatrics 30:103, 1975.

474. Rabin IJ, Hilfer CL, Scheinman HZ, McKenna PJ: Amyloid pseudotumor of the lung. Mt Sinai J Med 43:168, 1976.

475. Liebow AA, Hubbell DS: Sclerosing hemangioma (histiocytoma xanthoma) of the lung. Cancer 9:53, 1956.

476. Arean VM, Wheat MW: Sclerosing hemangioma of the lung. Am Rev Respir Dis 85:261, 1962.

477. Katzenstein ALK, Gmelich JT, Carrington CB: Sclerosing hemangioma of the lung. Am J Surg Pathol 4:343, 1980.

478. Joshi K, Shankar SK, Gopinath N, Kumar R, Chopra P: Multiple sclerosing hemangiomas of the lung. Postgrad Med J 56:50, 1980.

479. Hill GS, Eggleston JC: Electron microscopic study of so-called "pulmonary sclerosing hemangioma." Report of a case suggesting epithelial origin. Cancer 30:1092, 1972.

480. Palacios JJN, Escribano PM, Toledo J, et al.: Sclerosing hemangioma of the lung. Cancer 44:949, 1979.

481. Kennedy A: "Sclerosing haemangioma" of the lung. An alternative view of its development. J Clin Pathol 26:792, 1973.

482. Haas JE, Yunis EJ, Totten RS: Ultrastructure of a sclerosing hemangioma of the lung. Cancer 30:512, 1972.

483. Kay S, Still WJS, Borochovitz D: Sclerosing hemangioma of the lung: An endothelial or epithelial neoplasm? Hum Pathol 8:468, 1977.

484. Katzenstein ALA, Weise DL, Fulling K, Battifora H: So-called sclerosing hemangioma of the lung. Evidence for its mesothelial origin. Am J Surg Pathol 7:3, 1983.

485. McDonald JR, Harrington SW, Clagett OT: Hamartoma (often called chondroma) of the lung. J Thorac Surg 14:128, 1945.

486. Minasian H: Uncommon pulmonary hamartomas. Thorax 32:360, 1977.

487. Bateson EM: Histogenesis of intrapulmonary and endobronchial hamartomas and chondromas (cartilage-containing tumors): A hypothesis. J Pathol 101:77, 1970.

488. Bateson EM: Relationship between intrapulmonary and endobronchial cartilage-containing tumors (so-called hamartomata). Thorax 20:447, 1965.

489. Butler C, Kleinerman J: Pulmonary hamartoma. Arch Pathol 88:584, 1969.

490. Tomashefski JF: Benign endobronchial mesenchymal tumors. Their relationship to parenchymal pulmonary hamartomas. Am J Surg Pathol 6:531, 1982.

491. Stone F, Churg A: The ultrastructure of pulmonary hamartoma. Cancer 39:1064, 1977.

492. Liebow AA, Castleman B: Benign clear cell ("sugar") tumors of the lung. Yale J Biol Med 43:213, 1971.

493. Ozdemir IA, Zaman NU, Rullis I, Webb WR: Benign clear cell tumor of lung. J Thorac Cardiovasc Surg 68:131, 1974.

494. Zolliker A, Jacques J, Goldstein AS: Benign clear cell tumor of the lung. Arch Pathol Lab Med 103:526, 1979.

495. Sale GE, Kulander BG: Benign clear cell tumor of lung with necrosis. Cancer 37:2355, 1976.

496. Becker NH, Soifer I: Benign clear cell tumor ("sugar tumor") of the lung. Cancer 27:712, 1971.

497. Hoch WS, Patchefsky AS, Takeda M, Gordon G: Benign clear cell tumor of the lung. Cancer 33:1328, 1974.

498. Moscovic EA, Azar HA: Multiple granular cell tumors ("myoblastomas"). Case report with electron microscopic observations and review of the literature. Cancer 20:2032, 1967.

499. Bush RW, Plain GL: Granular cell tumors (myoblastomas) involving the bronchus and skin—report of a case. Am J Clin Pathol 50:563, 1968.

500. O'Connell DJ, MacMahon H, DeMeester TR: Multicentric tracheobronchial and oesophageal granular cell myoblastoma. Thorax 33:596, 1978.

501. Taboada CF, McMurray JD, Jordan RA, Seybold WD: Primary melanoma of the lung. Chest 62:629, 1972.

502. Jamieson MPG, McGowan AR: Endobronchial teratoma. Thorax 37:157, 1982.

503. Day DW, Taylor SA: An intrapulmonary teratoma associated with thymic tissue. Thorax 30:532, 1975.

504. Holt S, Deverall PB, Boddy JE: A teratoma of the lung containing thymic tissue. J Pathol 126:85, 1978.

505. Fox RM, Woods RL, Tattersall MNH, McGovern VJ: Undifferentiated carcinoma in young men: The atypical teratoma syndrome. Lancet 1:1316, 1979.

506. Briselli M, Mark GJ, Grillo HC: Tracheal carcinoids. Cancer 42:2870, 1978.

507. Houston HE, Payne WS, Harrison EG: Primary tumors of the trachea. Arch Surg 99:132, 1969.

508. Ma CK, Lewis J, Lee MW: Benign mixed tumor of the trachea. Cancer 44:2260, 1979.

509. Heard BE, Dewar A, Firmin RK, Lennox SC: One very rare and one new tracheal tumour found by electron microscopy: Glomus tumor and acinic cell tumour resembling carcinoid tumours by light microscopy. Thorax 37:97, 1982.

510. King N, Castleman B: Bronchial involvement in metastatic pulmonary malignancy. J Thorac Surg 12:305, 1943.

511. Albertini RE, Ekberg NT: Endobronchial metastases in breast cancer. Thorax 35:435, 1980.

512. Cassiere SG, McLain DA, Emory WB, Hurst HB: Metastatic carcinoma of the pancreas simulating primary bronchogenic carcinoma. Cancer 46:2319, 1980.

513. Case Records of the Massachusetts General Hospital. New Engl J Med 303:1049, 1980.

514. Kane RD, Hawkins HK, Miller JA, Noce PS: Microscopic pulmonary tumor emboli associated with dyspnea. Cancer 36:1473, 1975.

515. Gall FP, Muhe E, Angermann B: Surgical treatment for lung metastases. Dtsch Med Wochenschr 104:835, 1979.

516. Katzenstein AL, Purvis R, Gmelich J, Askin F: Pulmonary resection for metastatic renal adenocarcinoma. Pathologic findings and therapeutic value. Cancer 41:712, 1978.

517. Mountain CF, Khalil KG, Hermes KE, Frazier OH: The contribution of surgery to the management of carcinomatous pulmonary metastases. Cancer 41:833, 1978.

518. McCormack PM, Bains MS, Beattie EJ, Martini N: Pulmonary resection in metastatic carcinoma. Chest 73:163, 1978.

519. Morrow CE, Vassilopoulos PP, Grage TB: Surgical resection for metastatic neoplasms of the lung. Cancer 45:2981, 1980.

20 Infiltrative Lung Disease

Thomas V. Colby
Charles B. Carrington

Introduction

General Definitions and Terms

Diffuse infiltrative lung disease is a generic term for a large group (Table 20–1) of lung diseases with several clinical features in common.[1] Some of these diseases, including the adult respiratory distress syndrome (ARDS) and a few others, are acute in terms of a relatively sudden onset and a course measured in days or weeks. Far more of them are chronic in nature. With a few exceptions, this chapter is concerned primarily with chronic lesions.

Clinically, dyspnea is the predominant symptom, and on examination, frequently the only finding is "dry rales." Radiographs generally show a diffuse "infiltration" by irregular lines, small nodules, or "ground glass" shadows. Physiologically, the abnormalities primarily affect oxygen exchange and result in hypoxemia, whereas the mechanics of breathing are little impaired. None of the names used to designate this group is entirely accurate. Diffuse lung disease does not exclude the much more common obstructive disorders which are also diffuse yet specifically excluded here. The term interstitial is misleading because most of these disorders also have intra-alveolar abnormalities, and in some these abnormalities predominate. Finally, alveolar-capillary block does not correspond to recent interpretation of the pathophysiologic process involved. The term diffuse infiltrative is the most appropriate, although sometimes the disease is more or less localized. Both interstitial lung disease and restrictive lung disease are terms well embedded in general usage which are hard for many to abandon despite their inaccuracy. The overall prevalence of these diseases is difficult to estimate, but even together they are much less common than diseases associated with chronic airflow obstruction. The number of cases and also the breakdown into subcategories seen in any one practice or clinic are considerably influenced by the local patient population and by a particular clinician's known special interests. Thus, a hospital or ward that sees many cases of acute trauma encounters many related examples of ARDS. In Gaensler's laboratory at Boston University, about 20 percent of all referrals seen over a 25-year period concerned chronic infiltrative lung disease, an experience that is clearly weighted by the special interests of that laboratory's director.[1]

Acute Vs. Chronic

Diffuse infiltrative lung disease may be acute or chronic. This is a first and major fork in classification of disease in any given patient, because it strongly influences the likelihood of particular diagnoses and etiologies. In several previous analyses of chronic cases, the authors used a duration of 6 months (by any evidence such as symptoms, radiographs, and so on) as the dividing point between acute and chronic. This works reasonably well, but rare cases are difficult to classify so.

Although morphologists tend to use the terms acute and chronic, the morphologist obviously must infer duration. This is less accurate than clinical measurement of the time course, and it is useful for the clinician and pathologist to confer on this point. For example, both usual interstitial pneumonia (UIP) and bronchiolitis obliterans with organizing pneumonia have organization leading to scars; however, patients with UIP rarely come to biopsy until the disease has been present for many months or years, whereas those with the latter are often seen after an illness of only a few weeks' or months' duration. Awareness of the natural history of such diseases and comparison with the clinical duration in a

Table 20–1. Diffuse Infiltrative Lung Disease[a]

	Percent	Total No. Patients	With Biopsy
Infections	3.2		
Military tuberculosis		15	5
Fungal and amebic		10	2
Viral?		14	2
"Allergic" reactions	3.1		
Chronic eosinophilic pneumonia		30	21
Asthma with infiltration and drug reactions		8	1
Malignant neoplasms	2.4		
Leukemia and lymphoma		9	3
Bronchoalveolar carcinoma		4	4
Carcinomatosis, metastatic		16	7
Environmental diseases	24.8		
Allergic alveolitis		15	5
Silicosis, coal, and graphite		65	21
Asbestosis (excluding survey cases)		115	58
Other silicates		17	4
Berylliosis		63	16
Toxic gases (NO_2, SO_2, Br, Cl) and smoke		31	2
Connective tissue disorders	7.9		
Progressive systemic sclerosis		43	10
Systemic lupus erythematosus		26	2
Rheumatoid disease		22	4
Other combined		7	2
Sarcoidosis	20.8	257	65
Interstitial pneumonias	12.8		
Acute		7	6
Usual (UIP)		76	61
Usual, due to radiation (radiation fibrosis)		24	6
Desquamative (DIP)		47	45
Lymphocytic (LIP)		4	4
Unusual specific disorders	3.8		
Wegener's granulomatosis		6	5
Idiopathic hemosiderosis		3	3
Goodpasture's syndrome		5	5
Pulmonary alveolar proteinosis		13	13
Pulmonary alveolar microlithiasis		1	1
Eosinophilic granuloma		15	15
Tuberous sclerosis		1	1
Lymphangioleiomyomatosis (LAM)		3	3
Pulmonary vascular diseases	6.4		
Arteriolitis		3	2
Veno-occlusive		3	3
Multiple emboli and idiopathic hypertension		73	12
Chronic passive congestion	1.9	23	7
Nonspecific reactions	5.8		
Honeycombing, etiology unknown		18	16
Focal fibrosis		22	20
Primarily small-airway disease		12	12
Cystic fibrosis		10	2
Primarily emphysema		3	3
Aspiration (oil, blood, food)		4	4
Normal lung		2	2
No diagnosis	7.2	89	5
		1234	490

[a] Based on the results of Carrington and Gaensler.[1]

specific patient is one more step that helps to achieve the correct diagnosis.

Causes and Classification of Diffuse Infiltrative Lung Disease

The spectrum of disorders included in this category is very large and constantly growing. How this vast list should be subdivided to provide some sort of order is in part a logistical problem: there are between 150 and 200 separate diseases, and some can be subcategorized in several different ways. It is also a philosophical problem: many of the individual reactions (for example, bronchiolitis obliterans) have multiple causes, known and unknown, but often inapparent to the histologist, whereas many individual agents (for example, bleomycin) can produce a variety of reactions, each of which can also be due to other agents.

Is it better to classify by reaction or by cause? This question is especially difficult since many causes can be determined only at the clinical level (the lesions look alike), but only if someone asks the right questions or make's the right associations. Many causes are convincing in epidemiologic studies but unprovable in specific cases; some "causes" are of uncertain relationship to the lesion even when an association is clear. The best approach to classification of this unwieldy group is to adapt the scheme to the purpose at hand. No scheme is best for every purpose. For some years, the authors followed an etiologic grouping suggested by Buechner.[2] With clarification of certain etiologies, description of new histologic patterns, characterization of allergic and immunologically mediated disorders, and growth of the list of environmental lung diseases, the authors have recently used a classification based on their own experience (Table 20–1). This is something of a hybrid scheme, but it provides a useful framework for getting a grasp on the overall problem.

There are a few diagnoses in Table 20–1 that are irrelevant to the clinical picture of diffuse interstitial lung disease, but which, in the authors' series, were the only abnormality seen on some lung biopsies. Thus, emphysema is a perfectly sound diagnosis in the right circumstances, but in the context of the reasons for biopsy in these patients, it did not explain the symptoms, dysfunctions, or radiographs.

Irrespective of the way diseases are grouped, the labels selected for specific cases are often helped by adding a phrase or so: bronchiolitis due to adenovirus; allergic alveolitis due to bleomycin; bleomycin toxicity — diffuse alveolar damage type; bronchiolitis obliterans in a patient with rheumatoid disease; rheumatoid lung — UIP type. These may sound cumbersome, but they convey considerable information. In contrast, the diagnoses bronchiolitis, allergic alveolitis, or rheumatoid lung may provide incomplete or misleading information.

Some disorders in Table 20–1 are not discussed here since they are included in other chapters.

Clinical Manifestations of Chronic Diffuse Interstitial Lung Disease and the Clinical Approach to Diagnosis*

In most instances, disease is discovered by chest roentgenogram obtained because of respiratory symptoms. Discovery was incidental during routine examination or because of symptoms suggestive of a systemic disorder in about 20 percent of cases in one series.[3] The chief complaint in more than half of the cases in Gaensler's laboratory was dyspnea, sometimes with cough, expectoration, and weight loss, and less frequently with fever, night sweats, or other evidence of toxicity. Joint pains, with or without swelling and redness, were the only other relatively common chief complaint, occurring in about 6 percent prominently in sarcoidosis and quite often in the interstitial pneumonias.[4]

The history is the most productive part of the examination and, in earlier experience, has led to a diagnosis in 32 percent of all cases.[3] Apart from the conventional present, past, and family histories, the most important aspect concerns environmental and occupational review. This should include all materials handled, tools, and any intermediary compound used, such as cutting oils, graphite, or talc.[5-7] Similar symptoms in other workers, the use of masks, and frequency of state inspections are important clues to potentially dangerous exposure. A review of recreational activities, hobbies, and geographic locations must be included here. Historical information is as important to the pathologist as it is to the clinician, since there are many ways in which the lung can be injured, but only a few stereotyped ways in which it can react. A few of these tissue reactions, such as the dust macule with or without fibrosis, are diagnostic of an environmental insult, especially when they contain abundant dust. Virtually all other lung reactions may or may not be related to the environment. For example, the sarcoid reaction may be idiopathic or it may result from exposure to beryllium; UIP may be cryptogenic or it may be caused by exposure to fibrous silicates; and bronchiolitis obliterans may be the consequence of a viral pneumonia or may result from acute or chronic exposure to oxides of nitrogen. If the pathologist is more familiar with the causes of occupational lung injury than the clinician, direct questions or those implied by the tentative diagnoses may help focus the investigation and stimulate renewed efforts when the original history is inadequate. Such questions are especially important when the original history is inadequate. Such questions are especially important when there is only a litle dust in the lung tissue or when the histologic pattern is compatible with an environmental insult and there is no pathognomonic dust. In such cases, the correct diagnosis can be made only with the aid of epidemiologic data.

The chest roentgenogram may be normal even when there is severe interstitial lung disease. This was true in 7.7 percent of 508 patients who had lung biopsy in Gaensler's series,[8] including patients with UIP, desquamative interstitial pneumonia (DIP), sarcoidosis, bronchiolitis obliterans, allergic alveolitis, asbestosis, and lymphangioleiomyomatosis (LAM). As a corollary, the severity of radiographic infiltration correlates poorly both with physiologic abnormalities and pathologic estimates of severity.[4,9,10]

Radiographic opacities may consist of the linear or irregular markings[11] that are most often seen in interstitial pneumonias. Alternatively, they may be rounded, as in silicosis,[12] or reticulonodular — perhaps a combination of linear and rounded opacities — as seen most often in granulomatous disorders.[13] Additionally, and most importantly, the entire lungs or parts thereof may have a ground glass appearance.[10] Such opacities have been referred to as alveolar pattern or airlessness and may indeed result from displacement of alveolar gas by cellular or amorphous debris, as in pulmonary edema, or from patchy or diffuse atelectasis. However, a similar ground glass pattern also may be seen when the alveoli are smaller than normal, as in full expiration, and when alveolar walls are diffusely thickened by cells or scars. Finally, a honeycomb pattern is well recognized both radiologically[14] and morphologically.[15,16]

These radiographic patterns, together with their predominant location, can be related statistically to certain pathologic entities, but in individual cases, they are rarely diagnostic. A few exceptions include pulmonary alveolar microlithiasis, recognized by the sand-like appearance of the roentgenogram, or a ground glass pattern involving the lung periphery, which is diagnostic for chronic eosinophilic pneumonia.[17] Other radiographic patterns may be diagnostic when supported by minimal clinical information[18]; for example, a reticulonodular pattern with bilateral hilar adenopathy in young black persons represents a combination of findings diagnostic of sarcoidosis.

A review of previous radiographs often is the most revealing diagnostic procedure in the study of pulmonary disease. The pathologist should share in this information or ask for older films for an indication of the natural history of the disease. Most persons have had such roentgenograms during previous unrelated admissions, for insurance examinations or in connection with pre-employment screening. The time and expense involved in correspondence and travel to obtain such films is paltry compared with the alternatives of lengthy hospitalization, extensive laboratory investigations, or discharge and later readmission with the hope of establishing the natural history prospectively. Recent films frequently enable differentiation of acute from chronic disease; films spanning many years often document the onset of diffuse lung disease many years before the appearance of symptoms.

Physical examination does not often aid in diagnosis. Dry rales with a "close-to-the-ear" sound or "cellophane rales" may be heard early during the course of interstitial disease but are nonspecific. Digital clubbing, exercise cyanosis, and signs of cor pulmonale merely are indicative of advanced disease. More specific findings, such as

---

* This section, in part written by Gaensler, is used with permission of the author and the International Academy of Pathology.[1]

hepatosplenomegaly, enlarged lymph nodes, and especially signs suggesting connective tissue disorders, are important leads to further examination. Cardiac examination may reveal the diffuse lung disease to be consequence of heart disease, most often mitral stenosis.

Urinalysis or anemia may provide diagnostic leads. Polycythemia generally is secondary and nonspecific as is a reversed albumin/globulin ratio or an elevated sedimentation rate. Eosinophila suggests an allergic disorder or the presence of parasites. However, allergic reactions such as chronic eosinophilic pneumonia may be seen without eosinophilia,[17] although this finding is common in infections such as tuberculosis or coccidioidomycosis. Additionally, screening tests for connective tissue disorders and biologic dust antigens are useful in selected cases.

There are other routine examinations that can be done quickly, inexpensively, and painlessly. They include skin testing for anergy, tuberculosis, and fungal infections, repeated examination of the sputum by aerobic and anaerobic culture for bacteria and fungi, and multiple cytologic examinations.

Physiologic examination, particularly of respiratory gas exchange, is useful in detecting diffuse infiltrative lung disease, especially if the chest roentgenogram is normal. Furthermore, such studies characterize the severity of the disease much more accurately than either clinical examination or the chest roentgenogram. Therefore, pulmonary functions tests are useful for monitoring the natural course of disease and for evaluating the results of therapy. They are, however, not helpful for specific diagnosis because the type of physiologic derangement observed is common to all of the disorders shown in Table 20–1. The pathophysiology has been well described.[19–21] Generally there is no overt obstruction, and restriction of lung volumes is variable and usually is seen only in advanced disease. The characteristic abnormalities consist of diminution or diffusing capacity and increased alveolar-arterial oxygen pressure difference (P[A-a]O_2) resulting in hypoxemia. This is accompanied by alveolar hyperventilation and a compensated respiratory alkalosis stimulated perhaps by chronic hypoxemia or excessive reflexes from the lung or other sites. The principal abnormality, hypoxemia, was attributed for years to a decrease of the diffusing capacity from thickening of the alveolar-capillary membrane.[19–21] More recently this theory has fallen into disrepute because:

1. The diffusing capacity of the lung membrane is so large that normally complete equilibration of oxygen partial pressure between alveolar gas and capillary blood occurs in one-fourth the time available for gas exchange. Therefore, a marked reduction of diffusing capacity, say to half of normal, would not result in alveolar-end capillary PO_2 "gradient"; yet such patients commonly have an elevated P(A-a)O_2. From this it has been reasoned that the P(A-a)O_2 must be due to postcapillary venous admixture rather than to impaired diffusing capacity.[22]
2. At least half of the total resistance to diffusion is caused by the slowness of the reaction rate of oxygen with hemoglobin,[23] and this is not altered by lung disease.
3. If impaired diffusion were the sole cause of an elevated P(A-a)O_2, this would always increase with exercise, which causes an accelerated flow rate of blood through capillaries.[19,20] Actually, in about one-third of studied patients,[4] (P(A-a)O_2 decreased with exercise.
4. The histologic picture evoked by the term alveolar-capillary block — a uniform thickening of the blood-gas barrier — is rarely seen. Occasionally alveolar walls are uniformly lined by epithelial cells, and sometimes there are selected fields in which the walls are diffusely thickened by cellular infiltration or amyloid. Most often there are focal solid lesions and much normal intervening lung tissue, as in sarcoidosis and silicosis; sometimes the alveoli appear to be completely filled by granular debris or macrophages, as in proteinosis. Even in interstitial pneumonia, cellular thickening and fibrosis generally are quite uneven. Sometimes the alveolar walls are thick, but the capillaries are seen to spiral around the periphery of the fibrous tissue, which then does not contribute to an increased diffusion distance. Thus, edema and cellular infiltration may not alter the thickness of the blood-air barrier, a possibility confirmed by electron microscopic studies.[24]

For these reasons, it is now assumed that hypoxemia in this group of disorders is largely the result of ventilation/perfusion discrepancies.[22,25] Such mismatching of gas and blood is easily explained on histologic grounds considering the very uneven involvement in most cases and the predilection of some lesions for the bronchovascular bundles.[26] These ventilation-perfusion discrepancies undoubtedly fully explain hypoxemia at rest. During exercise, however, the contact time between alveolar gas and capillary blood is greatly reduced, especially in patients with a compromised pulmonary capillary bed. Then impaired diffusing capacity may contribute to hypoxemia in some cases.

Bronchoalveolar lavage and gallium-67 scanning of the lung have been used in the evaluation of patients with interstitial lung disease.[26a] (These methods are further discussed with specific diseases.) Cells retrieved by bronchoalveolar lavage are thought to reflect the inflammatory cell population of the lung at the alveolar level and therefore are representative of the effector cells of parenchymal inflammation (alveolitis).[26a,26b] In gallium scanning, the nucleide is thought to localize selectively to sites of inflammation, both acute and chronic, whereas there is little if any localization in the normal lung.[26a]

Morphologic Approach to Diffuse Infiltrative Lung Disease

Some examples of infiltrative lung disease have specific structures, such as dust macules, or nearly specific structures, such as granulomas in sarcoid; these enable diagnosis on small transbronchial biopsies. In other examples of diffuse infiltrative lung disease, however, one must rely on a constellation of histologic features. Together, these display a bewildering array of characteristic pictures whose recognition requires examination of tissue pieces of the size obtainable only from open biopsy techniques.

The lung has a limited number of responses to injury, although these may be combined to form numerous composite pictures. The following discussion concentrates on these fundamental components, despite the fact that any one rarely occurs alone. The combination that characterize each disease will be discussed later in the chapter.

Gross Pathology

With some notable exceptions (proteinosis, lymphangioleiomyomatosis, sarcoidosis, miliary tuberculosis, microlithiasis, silicosis), the gross findings in infiltrative lung disease are of little help in differential diagnosis even in whole lungs. In small surgical biopsies, gross lesions may not even by discernible.

Histologic Features

General Evaluation

The process of histologic diagnosis is simplified by first assessing the broad categories and questions listed in Table 20–2. In many cases, one can quickly decide wether a lesion is acute or chronic, interstitial or alveolar or both, granulomatous or not, exudative or organizing. Thus, a lesion dominated by hyaline membranes and proteinaceous debris is more likely to be an acute reaction. The presence of tumor, dust, or infectious agents is also easily decided in most cases, although a few simple aids such as special stains may be needed and cultures should always be done. The authors scan sections under polarized light; birefringent crystals are readily missed without high-intensity illumination. (Special studies that may aid in analyzing dusts are discussed in Chapter 23.)

Table 20–2. Broad Categories and Questions

Acute or chronic?
Alveolar filling only?
Interstitial only?
Both?
Granulomatous or not?
Exudative or organizing?
Diffuse or focal?
Random or site specific?
Infectious agents?
Dust?
Tumor?

Distribution of Lesions

The distribution of lesions (Table 20–3) and structures affected (Fig. 20–1) are evaluated. Few lesions are exclusively localized at certain sites; others tend to center along particular structures, although less exclusively; many affect a variety of structures, apparently unselectively. For example, some pneumoconioses, sarcoidosis, lymphoreticular infiltrates, and lymphangitic carcinoma are the only diseases in which the lesions commonly tend to concentrate along the lymphatic pathways. It is important to note lesions of blood vessels and conducting airways (in most biopsies this means bronchioles). It must then be decided whether these are the dominant lesions or simply components of a more diffuse reaction. Bronchiolitis obliterans, for example, may result from infection, toxic injury, or allergy; the resolution of this differential depends more on the associated parenchymal changes than on the morphology of the bronchioles.

Most of the categories in Table 20–3 are self-explanatory, but the question of interstitial as opposed to alveolar filling merits special explanation. Most infiltrative lung diseases have both interstitial and alveolar components. In bacterial infections, the lesions are essentially alveolar. In UIP the intersititium appears to be the main site of fibroblast proliferation and scar formation; however, some of the air spaces are filled with fluid and serum proteins, macrophages, regenerating epithelium, and fibroblasts. Thus, the reaction is by no means purely interstitial, and the alveolar components contribute importantly to the radiographic and clinical findings as well as to the anatomic pathogenesis of the ultimate scars.

Individual Histologic Features

After noting the distribution of lesions, the specific features listed in Table 20–4 should be investigated.

The significance of some features in Table 20–4 may be difficult to assess from the biopsy alone. The presence of widespread alveolar hemorrhage may be the only apparent lesion in an early stage of pulmonary hemosiderosis, but more often it is an irrelevant result of the trauma of the biopsy. Radiographic and hematologic data clarify this situation. Epidemiologic data are needed to interpret the significance of a few dust particles.

Cellular Infiltrates and Epithelial Proliferation. A single cell type strongly dominates the infiltrating cell population in

Table 20–3. Distribution of Lesions

1. Even or uneven throughout the available tissue
2. Random or targeted on specific normal structures
3. Airways: large, intermediate, or small
4. Pulmonary arteries: large, intermediate, or small
5. Pulmonary veins: large, intermediate, or small
6. Lymphatics or along lymphatic routes
7. Alveolar wall and general interstitium
8. Intra-alveolar and other small air spaces

Figure 20–1. Normal lung. Important landmarks for evaluation in infiltrative lung disease including the pleura, septa, bronchovascular bundles, pulmonary vein, alveolar ducts, alveoli, and alveolar walls (neonatal lung, H & E, ×30).

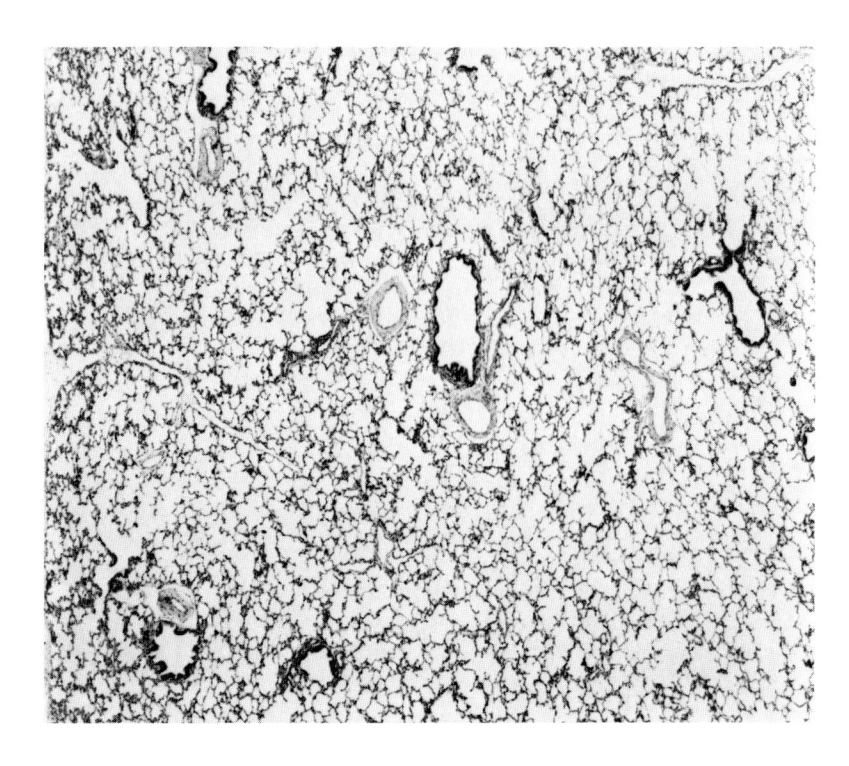

only a few instances, such as chronic eosinophilic pneumonia (interstitial and alveolar eosinophils). In the majority of lesions, cellular infiltrates are seen in mixtures that vary from one microscopic field to another. The precise composition of the cell population is useful less often in differential diagnosis than knowing the overall pattern of the infiltrate and the other components of the lesion.

Interstitial cells and alveolar epithelium are on opposite sides of the epithelial basement membrane, but they are sometimes difficult to distinguish by light microscopy; they may jointly account for the cellularity of individual alveolar walls. Mild interstitial cellular infiltrates can be difficult to detect. Two steps are useful. The first is to inspect the small interlobular septae and the perivascular zones (Fig. 20–2) around the small blood vessels. These regions represent unequivocal interstitium that are close to alveoli but are normally sparsely populated by cells. Slight infiltrates are more easily recognized in these locations, and they usually correlate with changes in the alveolar walls. The second step in uncertain cases is to count nuclei in 20 to 30 well-sectioned, discrete, representative alveolar walls. Most alveolar walls contain six to 10 nuclei exclusive of intracapillary leukocytes. If more than 10 percent of the counted walls have more than ten nuclei, the alveolar walls are hypercellular.

Despite the presence of marked interstitial infiltrates, there may be only a small change in the air to tissue ratio. The normal tissue volume is so small that a several-fold increase still leaves a high air/tissue ratio, assuming no change in the intracapillary blood volume and no significant alveolar filling. In practical terms, this is reflected by the difficulty of demonstrating interstitial lesions radiographically unless they are extremely severe or are accompanied by appreciable air space exudates, congestion and edema, or loss in air volume.

Epithelial Necrosis and Proliferation. Necrosis of type I pneomonocytes and reparative proliferation of type II pneumonocytes are best seen in acute reactions, particularly in cases of diffuse alveolar damage. Acute epithelial necrosis is rarely observed in chronic diffuse infiltrative lung disease, but the various stages of repair are so commonly observed that one assumes that the necrosis, too, is fairly common. In the repair process, type II cells divide to repopulate alveolar surfaces, and the regenerated type II cells gradually transform into normal type I cells. In the interim, however, the alveolar wall is lined by an increased number of plump type II cells. While regenerating, the cells often have large, blast-like nuclei that sometimes appear quite bizarre or atypical. Such an appearance is especially marked when the injury is produced by ionizing radiation or chemotherapeutic agents. Other types, including bronchiolar and squamous epithelium, may line air spaces during repair. For simplicity, the general inclusive term is metaplastic alveolar epithelium.

Normal or regenerating type II cells or metaplastic epithelial cells may become detached from the alveolar walls and be mistaken for alveolar macrophages. A useful clue to their epithelial nature is that they are often still connected to one another in long chains (*see* Fig. 20–12). Nonetheless, in any given case, the majority of intraalveolar cells are macrophages.

Capillary and Endothelium Pericytes. These cells account for a substantial part of the cellularity of the normal

Table 20-4. Histologic Features Assessed in Diffuse Infiltrative Lung Disease

> Alveoli, small air spaces
> > Hyaline membranes
> > Proteinaceous exudates
> > Stasis of secretions
> > Epithelial regeneration (type II pneumonocytes)
> > Hemorrhage
> > Hemosiderosis (macrophages)
> > Alveolar cell population (kind and number)
> > Organisms, inclusion bodies
> > Dust
>
> Interstitium
> > Edema
> > Diffuse cell population
> > Localized lymphoid follicles
> > Dust
> > Granulomas, with or without necrosis
> > Destruction
> > Organization, fibrosis, honeycombing
>
> Conducting airways
> > Narrowing by mural or external lesions
> > Intralumenal granulation tissue
> > Intralumenal mucus
> > Cellular infiltrates
> > Granulomas
> > Loss
>
> Vessels
> > Diffuse hypertrophy, intimal proliferation
> > Thrombi, emboli
> > Fibrous obliteration
> > Angiitis
>
> Tumor

alveolar wall and individually are hard to distinguish from interstitial infiltrates.

Air Space Exudates. Cells in the small air spaces are more easily identified and enumerated than those infiltrated in the interstitium. The majority are alveolar macrophages. They may contain phagocytosed debris, hemosiderin, or exogenous dust. When macrophages are actively phagocytizing, they usually develop a vacuolated cytoplasm because of the numerous phagosomes. A few fatty (foamy) macrophages are thus commonly seen in many different lung reactions. Large numbers of them are associated with proximal airways obstruction. In most instances, when alveoli contain moderate or large numbers of macrophages, a few appear as multinucleated giant cells. The presence of a few giant cells in the company of numerous alveolar macrophages is neither unusual nor specific.

Granulomas. The presence of granulomas is an important diagnostic clue, and the presence or absence of necrosis is a major factor in further differential diagnosis. Non-necrotizing or sarcoid-type granulomas are the main feature of sarcoidosis, but they are also seen in many other disorders. Necrotizing granulomas (with necrosis or neutrophils) are usually caused by infectious agents such as mycobacteria or fungi, but they may also be due to such idiopathic syndromes as Wegener's granulomatosis or necrotizing sarcoidal granulomatosis. The distribution of granulomas relative to other structures is also important in differential diagnosis.

The sarcoid-type or noncaseating granuloma (which is by no means restricted to sarcoidosis) consists of a nodule of mononuclear cells of the macrophage-histiocyte type, sometimes resembling epithelium (epithelioid cells). They are associated with small amounts of reticulum or collagen in such a way that the nodule has a structured arrangement. Usually there are also moderate numbers of lymphocytes, plasma cells, multinucleated giant cells, and fibroblasts in the granuloma; these may be diffusely scattered or concentrated in a peripheral cuff. The giant cells may be Langerhans type with peripherally arranged nuclei, foreign body type with randomly scattered nuclei, Touton type with xanthomatous cytoplasm and wreath of nuclei, or a mixture. Often the giant cells contain a few birefringent crystals. Mineralized structures rich in calcium and occasionally iron are also fairly common (*see* p. 504). Cholesterol clefts may also be present in giant cells.

Judging from the clinical recovery of many patients and from the occasional chance opportunity to study their lung tissue years later, some granulomatous lesions can apparently resolve without leaving any residue. Others heal leaving barely visible stellate scars or more extensive destruction and honeycombing.

Necrosis. Visible necrosis of either the cellular infiltrates or the parenchyma is uncommon in chronic, nongranulomatous infiltrative lung disease. Its presence is of great significance, however, and narrows the differential diagnosis. Most chronic necrotizing infections are granulomtous, but the granulomatous component is occasionally inapparent because of chance sampling or is markedly altered by treatment, as with steroids. Miliary lesions with necrosis are especially suspect for infection irrespective of their precise cell composition, demarcation, or location. Both the infiltrate and the parenchyma undergo necrosis in Wegener's granulomatosis and related diseases, although the granulomatous nature is occasionally obscured on a biopsy sample. Necrosis of exudate (but not alveolar walls) is a prominent feature of some cases of eosinophilic pneumonia; occasionally it also affects the cells in pooled secretions in honeycombing, probably because of superimposed infection.

Organization and Scarring. The appearance of fibroblasts, myxomatous fibrous tissue, fibrillar collagen, and dense old scars is usually seen in the lung only when there has been parenchymal necrosis or when there is an interstitial cellular infiltrate. The appearance of organization and collagen deposition connotes severe injury and often results in permanent scarring or honeycombing. These changes may be focal or widespread and may or may not be progressive depending on the underlying cause. Thus, the mere presence of organization in one region does not assure severe or irreversible dysfunction at the clinical level.

Organization of alveolar exudates also occurs. Since

Figure 20–2. Assessing the presence of an interstitial infiltrate in two cases of diffuse alveolar damage. A. The alveolar wall has too many nuclei, but they are in endothelial cells and pneumonocytes since no interstitial infiltrate is seen around the small vein to left of center (H&E, ×400). B. Although nuclei of endothelial cells and alveolar lining cells are prominent, the presence of an interstitial infiltrate is confirmed by the interstitial cells around the small vein to left of center (H&E, ×400).

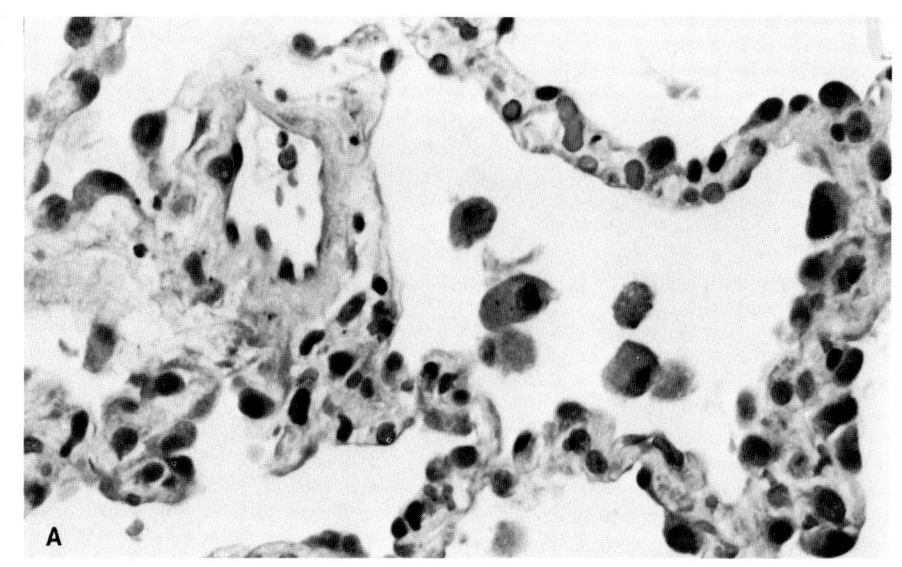

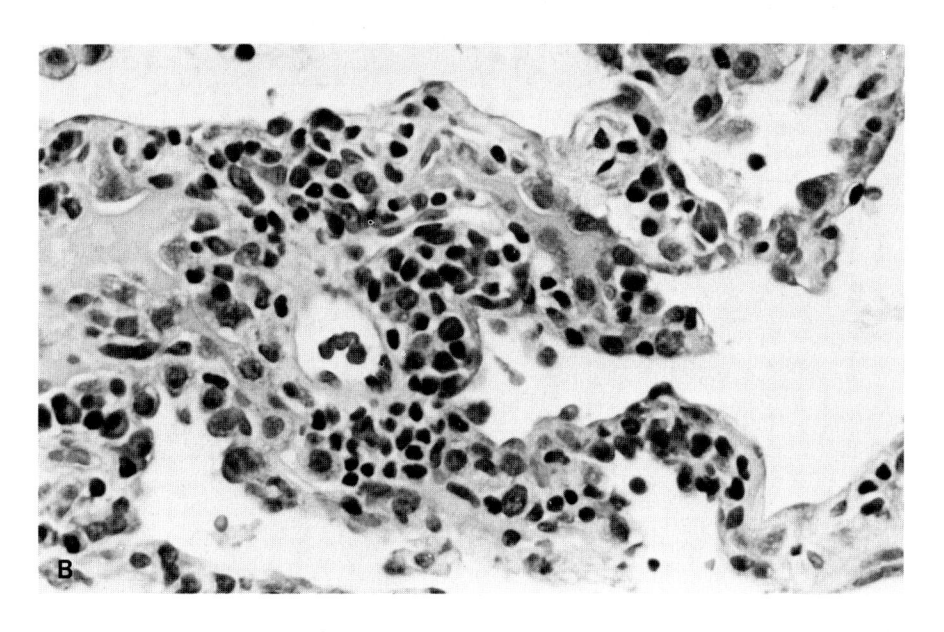

many chronic infiltrative lung diseases have both alveolar exudates and interstitial lesions, organization of the two often occurs simultaneously. Fibroblasts become recognizable in the air spaces, intermixed with scattered macrophages and lymphocytes within the clumped masses of proteinaceous debris. As this debris is lysed and phagocytized, the exudate becomes edematous and myxomatous in appearance. In time collagen fibrils can be identified. The regenerating alveolar epithelium proliferates over these clumps of organizing exudates, and the exudates are thus gradually incorporated into the interstitium. The exudate gradually contracts into a smaller, dense, and relatively acellular interstitial scar. When there is organization of abundant exudates filling several adjacent air spaces, it is possible that the several structures are fused into one contracted scar and that this is how some reduction in the number of alveolar walls occurs.

Honeycombing. Honeycombing is the end result of destruction, obliteration, organization, regeneration, repair, and revision of the architecture of the lung (Fig. 20–3).[15] The gas-exchanging part of the lung (the acinus) is transformed into an interconnecting labyrinth of variably sized spaces lined by scarred walls. There is considerable variation in the size of the holes and in the density of the scar tissue in the walls from lung to lung and from one focus to another in the same lung. Three-dimensional reconstructions suggest that many of the holes are due to bronchiolectasis;[27] however, this could be a secondary change following the destruction and reorganization of the surrounding parenchyma. In any case, lung architecture is permanently destroyed and the tissue is function-

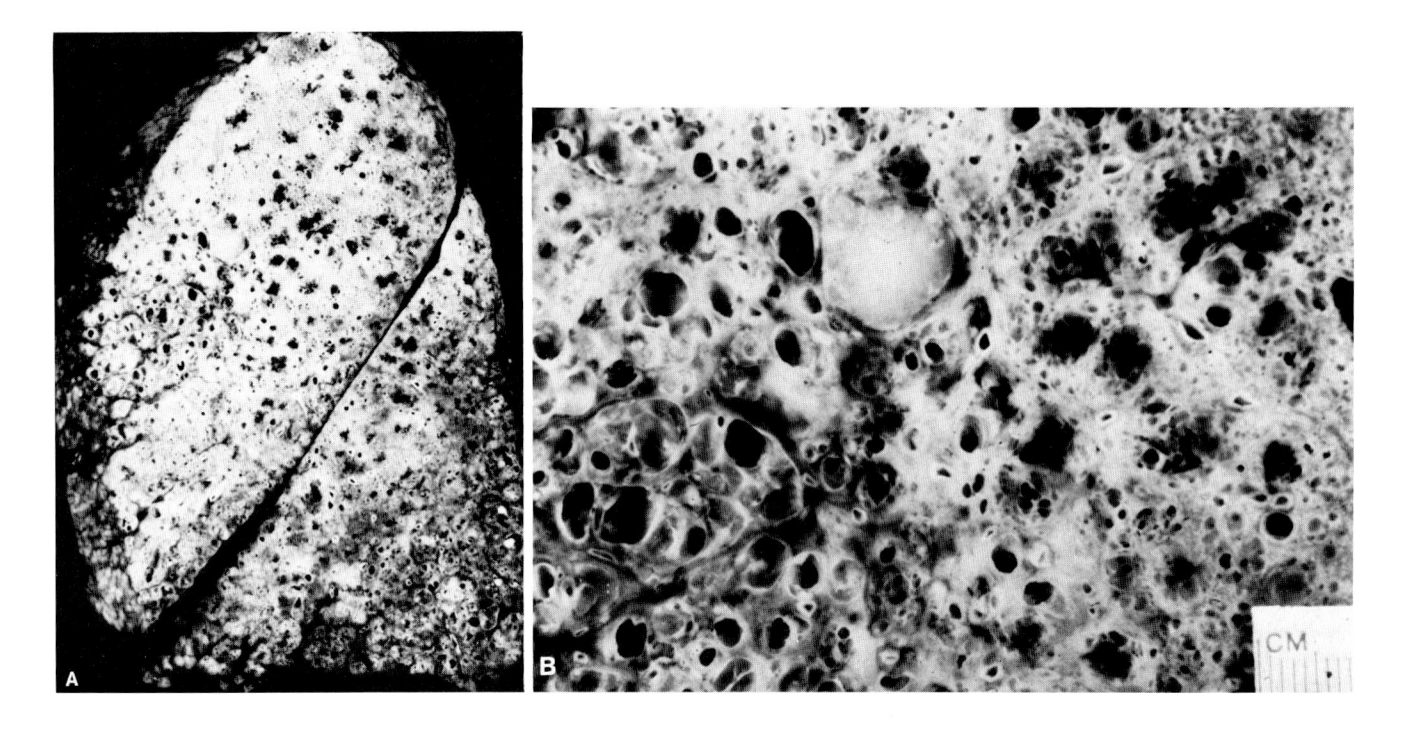

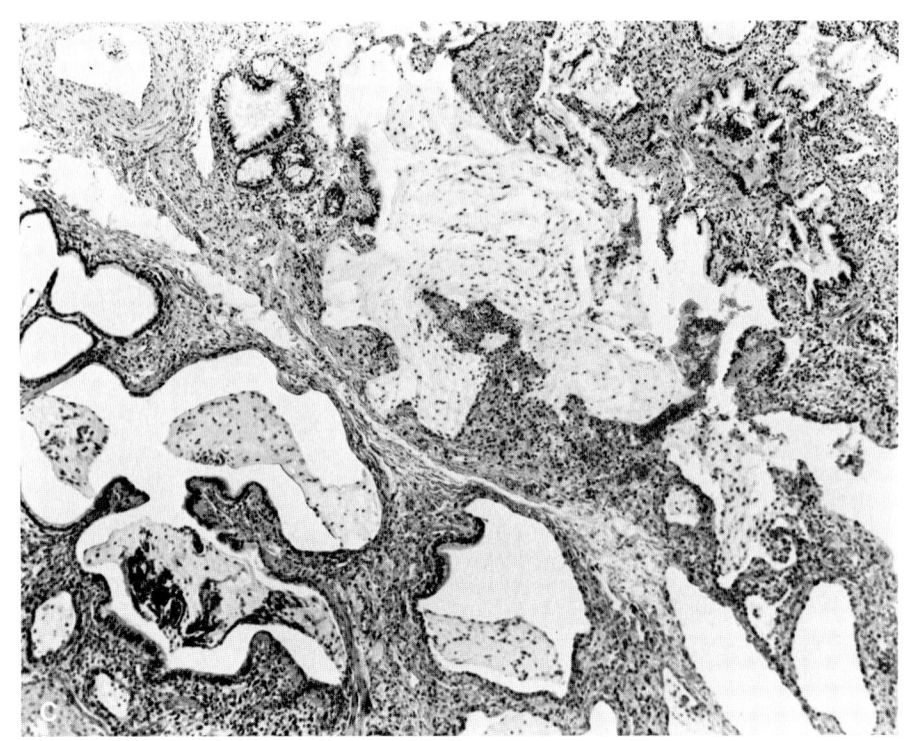

Figure 20-3. Honeycombing. Note the knobby pleural surface caused by the septal retraction. The honeycombing is patchy and varies in severity. Histologically (C) there is scarring, inflammation, and abnormal air spaces with mucus statis and partial lining by metaplastic epithelium (H&E, ×50).

ally useless. The features of honeycombing include metaplastic epithelium of the spaces, stasis of secretions, interstitial proliferation of muscle and elastic tissue, and changes in the vessels, somewhat analogous to endarteritis obliterans. A problem which sometimes arises is to separate metaplastic epithelium from neoplasia, especially bronchiolar alveolar cell tumors. The epithelial cell population in tumors is usually relatively homogenous compared with the population of cells in metaplasia, which is usually variegated: thus the greater the variety, the more likely is the lesion to be benign. The striking architectural changes in honeycombing undoubtedly interfere with normal clearance mechanisms, leading to pooling of secretions in the abnormal spaces. The lining of such spaces by secretory epithelium obviously compounds the problem.

Pulmonary scars contain an admixture of smooth muscle and elastic fibers. Sometimes the smooth muscle is extremely prominent, and even grossly apparent as red-brown, resilient tissue (muscular cirrhosis of the lung). The origin of this smooth muscle is uncertain but may originate from myofibroblasts, since such cells are prominent in the interstitium in chronic fibrotic lung disorders.[28]

Pulmonary vessels in zones of honeycombing often have markedly narrowed lumens. This is usually due in large part to intimal thickening. In some kinds of lung injury, the vessels are involved and subsequently scarred. Liebow[29] suggested that most of the intimal thickening seen in honeycombing represented an endarteritis type of response due to the loss of the distal capillary bed normally supplied by such arteries.

Miscellaneous Structures. Several curious endogenous structures may be encountered in air spaces. These included corpora amylacea and blue bodies, which are discussed in Pulmonary Calcification and Ossification, this chapter.

Acicular crystals of cholestrol esters are sometimes admixed in alveolar exudates. They are sometimes surrounded by foreign body giant cells. Such deposits and fat-laden macrophages are nonspecific and should not be confused with the aspirated lipids of exogenous lipid pneumonia (*see* Chapter 24).

Special Stains in Interstitial Lung Disease

Even the experienced morphologist derives information from special stains in diffuse infiltrative lung disease. Elastic tissue stains are useful in delimiting the location and extent of scarring and assessing the state of vessels. Ferruginous bodies are much easier to identify on iron stains, and in any patient who is immunocompromised, a full battery of special stains for microorganisms should be performed.

lesions are actually patchy in distribution with large amounts of normal intervening parenchyma. Loss of all functioning air spaces would not be compatible with life. Sometimes the etiology of the honeycombing can be suspected on the basis of gross pattern, as in the cases of asbestosis with subpleural honeycoming and lower lobe involvement (*see* Chapter 23), sarcoidosis with upper lobe involvement, and eosinophilic granuloma with sparing of the costophrenic angles (*see* Sarcoidosis, and Eosinophilic Granuloma (Histiocytosis X) Involving the Lung, below).

The causes of honeycombing are shown in Table 20–5. A number of other lesions that grossly resemble honeycombing are excluded: extensive congenital cystic disease of the lung, cystic adenomatoid malformations, lymphangiectasis, interstitial emphysema, and the diffuse multicystic lesions seen in LAM and tuberous sclerosis.

In some cases of honeycombing, attention to morphologic detail may be sufficient for diagnosis. In the majority of cases, however, morphologic clues must be correlated with clinical (and occupational) and radiologic data to make a specific diagnosis. Structurally preserved parenchyma showing features of UIP or DIP suggests they are the cause of the honeycombing. Honeycombing due to drugs or collagen vascular disease may show prominent plasma cells and, in the case of rheumatoid arthritis, numerous germinal centers (*see* subsection Rheumatoid Arthritis, in section on Pulmonary Involvement in Collagen Vascular Disease, below).

Bizarre metaplastic alveolar lining cells are characteristic of honeycombing due to chemotherapeutics or radiation. Numerous asbestos bodies (best appreciated with an iron stain) are seen in the honeycombing of asbestosis. Sarcoidosis and berylliosis are morphologically indistinguishable, and honeycombing associated with them may or may not have residual granulomas; a lymphatic distribution of granulomas or hyaline scars along lymphatic routes raises the possibility. A rare granuloma in honeycombing is nonspecific. In the ab-

Honeycomb Lung (End-Stage Lung Disease)

The term honeycomb lung is usually reserved for lungs with extensive bilateral honeycombing. Focal pulmonary parenchymal scarring grossly resembling honeycombing (focal honeycombing) is sometimes an incidental finding at autopsy which has no discernible clinical correlate. Subpleural scars (subpleural blebs) associated with pneumothorax in otherwise healthy young adults are an exception in which focal honeycombing does have a clinical correlate. It is somewhat arbitrary at what point the term focal honeycombing is more appropriate than focal scarring. Extensive bilateral honeycombing is rarely asymptomatic (*see* Fig. 20–3). Affected patients have infiltrative lung disease that varies in severity with the extent of the anatomic lesion. Radiologically such cases represent diffuse bilateral disease; however, the gross

Table 20–5. Causes of Honeycomb Lung[a]

Usual or desquamative interstitial pneumonia
Interstitial pneumonias associated with
   Collagen-vascular disease
   Drugs
Asbestosis
Sarcoidosis
Berylliosis
Chronic granulomatous infections
Chronic allergic alveolitis
Eosinophilic granuloma
Lymphocytic interstitial pneumonia
Lymphocytic lymphomas
Diffuse alveolar damage (toxic, infectious, radiation induced)
Chronic interstitial pulmonary edema
Recurrent aspiration of gastric acid
Idiopathic

[a] Based on the results of Katzenstein and Askin and personal observations.[30]

sence of granulomas, Schaumann bodies and fragments thereof in the scar tissue may be the only hint of previous granulomatous disease. Honeycombing caused by chronic allergic alveolitis may be nondescript or show active foci with all the histologic features of allergic alveolitis. Honeycombing caused by eosinophilic granuloma may or may not have active lesions. Honeycombing in lymphocytic interstitial pneumonia (LIP) usually still has abundant lymphoplasmacytic infiltrates. Some examples of honeycombing have massive monomorphic infiltrates of lymphocytes and may represent examples of honeycombing caused by lymphocytic lymphoma (personal observations), a situation which may be analogous to cirrhosis of the liver associated with infiltrates of chronic lymphocytic leukemia.[31] Severe diffuse alveolar damage can cause extensive honeycombing as it organizes. Rapid development of honeycombing from diffuse alveolar damage is characteristic of paraquat poisoning. Honeycombing has also been attributed to chronic interstitial pulmonary edema and recurrent bouts of aspiration. In a sizable proportion of cases, the cause for honeycombing is not identified. It remains to be shown whether such cases of idiopathic honeycombing represent a distinct clinicopathologic entity.

Table 20–6. Chronic Interstitial Pneumonias[a]

Usual interstitial pneumonia
Desquamative interstitial pneumonia
Lymphocytic interstitial pneumonia
Giant cell interstitial pneumonia
Bronchiolitis with interstitial pneumonia

[a] Based on the results of Liebow et al.[33]

Table 20–7. Synonymns of Usual Interstitial Penumonia[a]

Cryptogenic fibrosing alveolitis[b]
Idiopathic pulmonary fibrosis[b]
Hamman-Rich syndrome
Organizing interstitial pneumonia
Chronic interstitial penumonitis
Acute diffuse interstitial fibrosis of the lungs
Bronchiolar emphysema
Muscular cirrhosis of the lung

[a] Based on the results of Gaensler et al.[34]
[b] Currently in use by some investigators.

Usual Interstitial Pneumonia and Desquamative Interstitial Pneumonia

Background

The original description of Hamman and Rich[32] focused attention on a mysterious diffuse lung disorder which led to extensive scarring. It became gradually apparent that there was a certain inhomogeneity among cases regarded as examples of Hamman-Rich disease. The first significant refinement in classification came with the gradual recognition of the syndrome now called adult hyaline membrane disease or ARDS. The next major attempt at subdivision was presented over a period of years by Liebow[33] who established five subcategories (Table 20–6) for those cases with more chronic course than that seen with ARDS.

Usual interstitial pneumonia derives its name from the observation that it is the most common or usual type of chronic interstitial pneumonia that the pathologist encounters. Some of the terms previously used synonymously with UIP are shown in Table 20–7.[34]

Although Liebow's classification represents a tidy grouping of lesions, the interrelationship between the lesions is not so clear-cut. The separation of UIP and DIP, which is followed by many North American physicians, remains controversial and is little used in the United Kingdom where they are grouped together under such names as chronic diffuse (cryptogenic) fibrosing alveolitis and various synonyms. For reasons to be described below, the authors believe the separation of UIP and DIP is still useful and employ it in practice.

However named, most cases of chronic interstitial pneumonia fall into the UIP and DIP categories. Lymphocytic interstitial pneumonia is considerably less common; although the patients with LIP have the usual features of infiltrative lung disease, a significant number also have autoimmune disease, especially Sjögren's syndrome. Many cases once classified as LIP are now known to represent lymphomas or other lymphoproliferative disorders diffusely involving the lungs. Those still called LIP are described separately below. Giant cell interstitial pneumonia represents a histologic curiosity which is very rare. The lesion originally called bronchiolitis obliterans with inerstitial pneumonia is much more familar now due to the accumulation of many biopsies taken early in this disease's relatively brief course. With these new data, the descriptive name of bronchiolitis (with or without obliterans) with patchy organizing pneumonia has been adopted as more appropriate (see Bronchiolitis Obliterans and Organizing Interstitial Pneumonia, below). This lesion is no longer considered strictly as an interstitial pneumonia, although it is obviously a diffuse infiltrative disease. Nevertheless, because bronchiolitis with patchy organizing pneumonia is often mistaken for UIP histologically, it is discussed below.

Clinical Features of Usual Interstitial Pneumonia and Desquamative Interstitial Pneumonia

Several series of patients with UIP and DIP have been published, and a characteristic clinicopathologic syndrome has emerged.[4,34–39]

Most patients are older than age 40. However, onset in teenage years is well known. The average age at diagnosis of DIP is younger than that for UIP (42 years versus 51 years). Men are affected roughly twice as often as women. Familial cases are well described in both adults and children.[39a,39b]

The signs and symptoms are nonspecific and reflect the presence of diffuse infiltrative lung disease. Early in the course, there is an insidious onset of dyspnea and progressive shortness of breath with exertion and a dry cough. Hyperpnea is usually present. These symptoms progress slowly over months or years, and in the late stages, clubbing, cyanosis, and signs and symptoms of cor pulmonale develop. The characteristic findings on auscultation are crackles close to the ear and increased breath sounds. Other nonspecific symptoms include fatigue, exhaustion, weight loss, and occasionally pleuritic chest pain. These symptoms can be so subtle in onset and slow in progression as to go unnoticed by the patient or are ascribed simply to aging until the disease is quite advanced. In some patients, the presentation and course are punctuated by episodes of pneumonia, and these may be the presenting complaint.

Chest radiographs show bilateral, widespread reticular or reticulonodular infiltrates that are usually accentuated at the lung bases (Fig. 20-4; see Fig. 20-6A). A diffuse or patchy ground glass pattern is recognized in occasional cases. Rarely the chest radiograph is normal (especially in DIP); however, signs, symptoms and pulmonary functions in such patients belie the presence of diffuse infiltrative lung disease. In late stages, the lung volumes are decreased. Honeycombing is evident radiologically at the time of diagnosis in 20 percent of patients with DIP and 57 percent of patients with UIP.[4] Usual interstitial pneumonia and DIP cannot be distinguished radiographically.

Pulmonary functions reflect diffuse infiltrative lung disease. There is abnormal gas exchange with decreased diffusing capacity. Lung volumes are characteristically decreased in UIP but may be normal initially in DIP. In addition to restriction, obstructive changes may also be present, especially in smokers with UIP.[4]

Laboratory changes are nonspecific. Over 90 percent of patients have an elevated erythrocyte sedimentation rate. Positive tests for antinuclear antibody (7 percent), rheumatoid factor (14 percent), cryoglobulinemia (41 percent), and Lupus erythematosus cells may be seen even in patients who lack any other findings of collagen vascular disease.[38] Overall, 20 percent of patients with UIP have overt manifestations of collagen vascular disease. The percentage for DIP is much less. Serum protein electrophoresis is frequently abnormal with a nonspecific elevation of one or several fractions.

Gallium scanning is used to detect sites of inflammation,[26a,37-39] and the absence of pulmonary disease, there is no localization in the lungs. Positive gallium scans may be seen in many infiltrative lung disease including UIP and DIP.[37-39]

Differential cell counts on bronchopulmonary lavage fluid in patients with UIP and DIP show increased cellularity with relative increase in neutrophils and occasionally eosinophils and lymphocytes.[26a,37-42] The value of these observations is still limited by the sparse data correlating lavage with long-term clinical course, but some interesting observations have been assembled. In a prospective study of 21 patients, Haslam and colleagues[40] showed that differential cell counts on lavage fluid did not correlate with quantitative cell counts in the alveolar spaces or interstitium, but nevertheless steriod responsiveness correlated with the percentage of lymphocytes in the lavage fluid and a complementary fall in the percentage of macrophages. In a separate report of 120 patients, Rudd and associates[41] showed that response to steriods was associated with an increase in proportions of lymphocytes in the lavage fluid, and failure to respond to steriods was associated with an increase in eosinophils or neutrophils without a lymphocytosis.

At present, lavage is best considered as a research tool for which the clinical role remains to be established. Therapeutic decisions based on lavage data represent clincial research today, not established practice, and they should be made within sound protocols and the usual safeguards for patient research. The reasons for continuing such research are simple. Serial open lung biopsies are not practical. Even transbronchial biopsies have limited practicality in terms of multiple repetitions. Serial studies by lavage are practical, hence their enormous appeal. Furthermore, lavage instead of biopsy would clearly be preferable if it provided information of equal or greater value for treatment and for establishing prognosis, even if it did not provide diagnosis in the classic sense. If lavage works as a reliable guide to treatment and or prognosis, it will be very useful.

Pathogenesis

Usual interstitial pneumonia and DIP are idiopathic. In both there is a progressive, gradually destructive process that permanently alters pulmonary parenchyma and smolders for many years. Their histologic patterns represent manifestations of tissue injury and repair.

Research into the causes of UIP and DIP has centered on "alveolitis."[26a] Considerable evidence suggests that immunologic factors are involved, but no specific conclusions can yet be drawn. It is also unknown whether the hypothesized immune reactions are primary or are initiated by some other and possibly transient events. Humoral immune mechanisms are implicated by the relative frequency of a positive rheumatoid factor and antinuclear antibody, clinical evidence of collagen vascular disease in many cases, granular deposition of immunoglobulin-like material ultrastructurally in the alveolar walls in some cases, and the presence of circulating immune complexes and/or serum cryoglobulins.[26a,37,39] Macrophages release chemotactic factors for other inflammatory cells and also may be involved in direct cytotoxic injury to parenchymal lung cells.[26a] Neutrophils also may be involved in injury to parenchymal cells, and

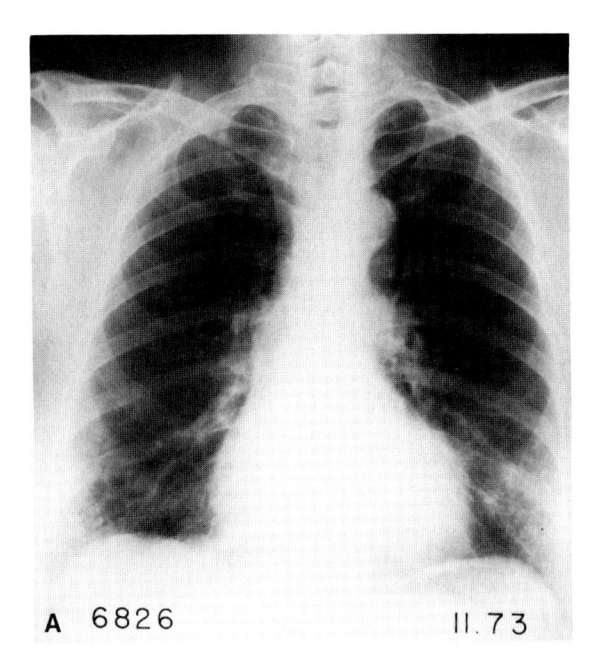

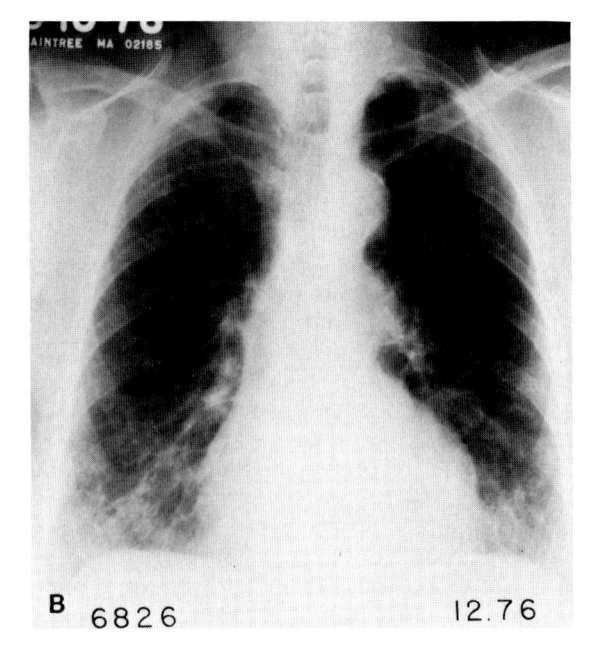

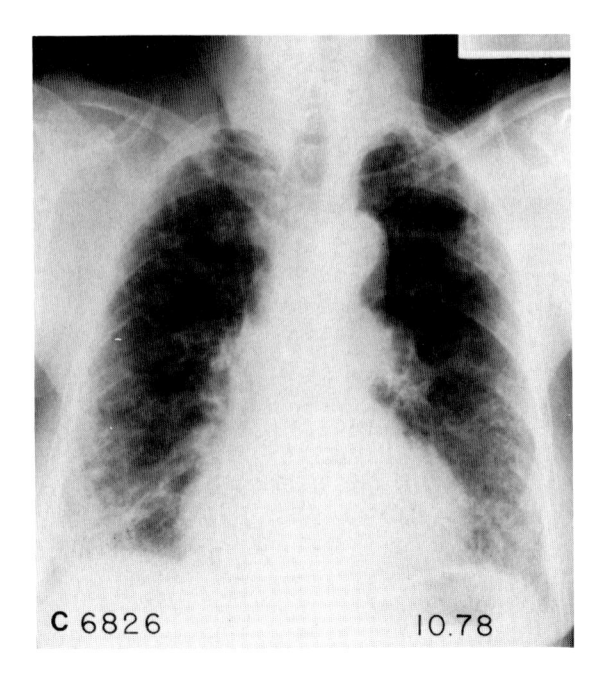

Figure 20–4. Radiographic progression of usual interstitial pneumonia (UIP) over 5 years. The difference between consecutive radiographs is relatively subtle, although the difference between the 1973 and 1978 films is much more apparent. Courtesy of Drs. Gaensler and Epler, Boston.

their numbers are increased in bronchoalveolar lavage fluid from patients with UIP.[26a] None of these observations is yet fully established in terms of relevance to the nature of the basic injury or to perpetuation of the lung's reaction. There is no evidence that the scarring process is abnormal when compared with other scarring diseases in the lung, such as chronic tuberculosis.

Gross Morphology

The gross pathologic features of UIP and DIP are entirely nonspecific and reflect the degree of involvement and stage of the lesion. In early cases, the gross appearance may be nearly normal, whereas late cases are associated with extensive honeycombing. Characteristically at autopsy one finds large zones of honeycombing alternating with less involved and even normal pulmonary parenchyma. Gross abnormalities parallel the radiographs and are usually worse in the lower lobes. The lungs are firm, rubbery, and contracted and have a nodular pleural surface resembling the surface of cirrhotic liver.

Figure 20–5A,B. Histology of UIP. A. The patchy and random location of the scarring is apparent. Several microscopic foci of complete architectural destruction (honeycombing) are present. The scarring is irregular and poorly demarcated and merges with normal parenchyma. (H&E, ×5). B. Focus of honeycombing (H&E, ×160)

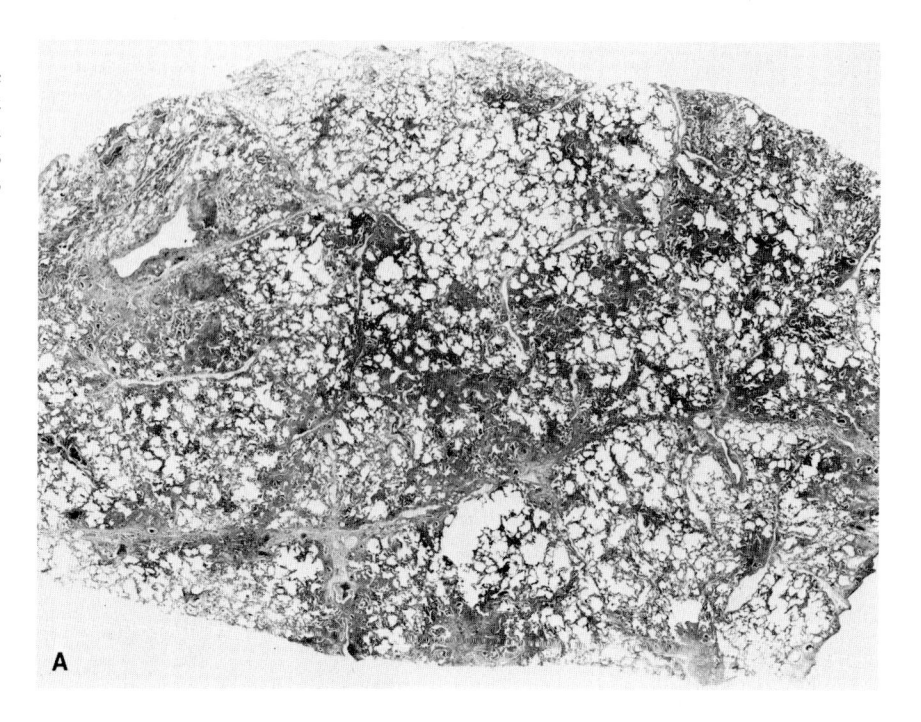

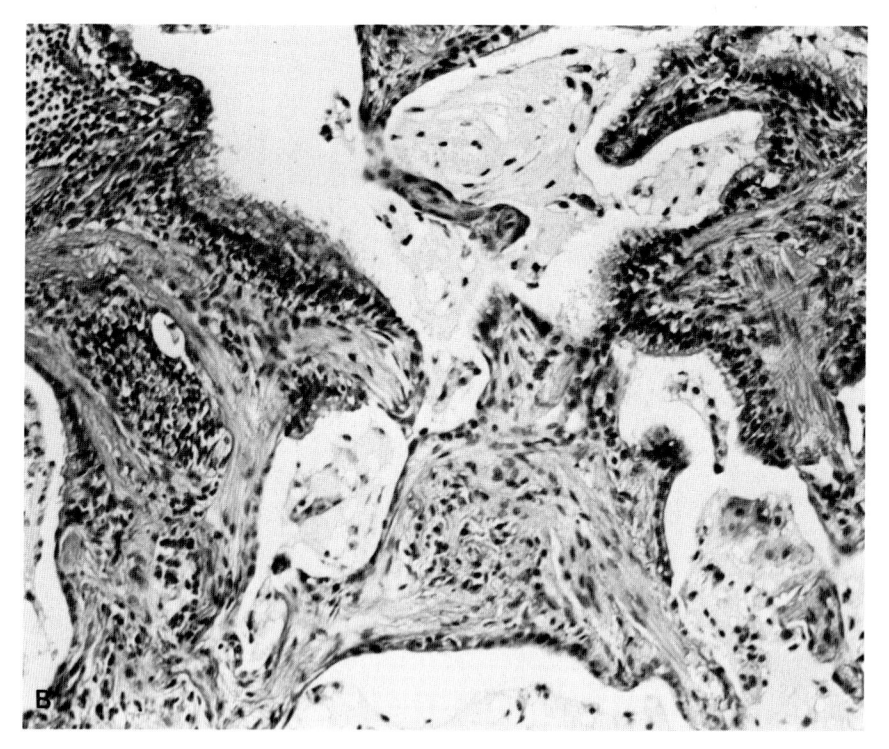

Histology of Usual Interstitial Pneumonitis (Fig. 20–5)

The site of lung injury in UIP is presumed to be alveolar wall, but the nature of the injury, the specific cellular or acellular target, and the way in which the injury spreads to more alveoli with time are all unknown. Consider first a single focus of injury. The mildest, and presumably earliest, histologic change that is apparent is an increase in cellularity of alveolar walls, due to both interstitial and epithelial changes. The interstitial infiltrate is composed of a mixture of lymphocytes, monocytes, and occasionally plasma cells and eosinophils. Neutrophils are not prominent in the interstitial infiltrate. Initially the interstitial infiltrate is subtle, but it becomes increasingly dense. Then fibroblasts are seen and gradually fibrillar collagen as the scarring progresses. The last stage is a dense, nearly acellular, interstitial scar with no more than an occasional nodule or scattering of lymphocytes. Honey-

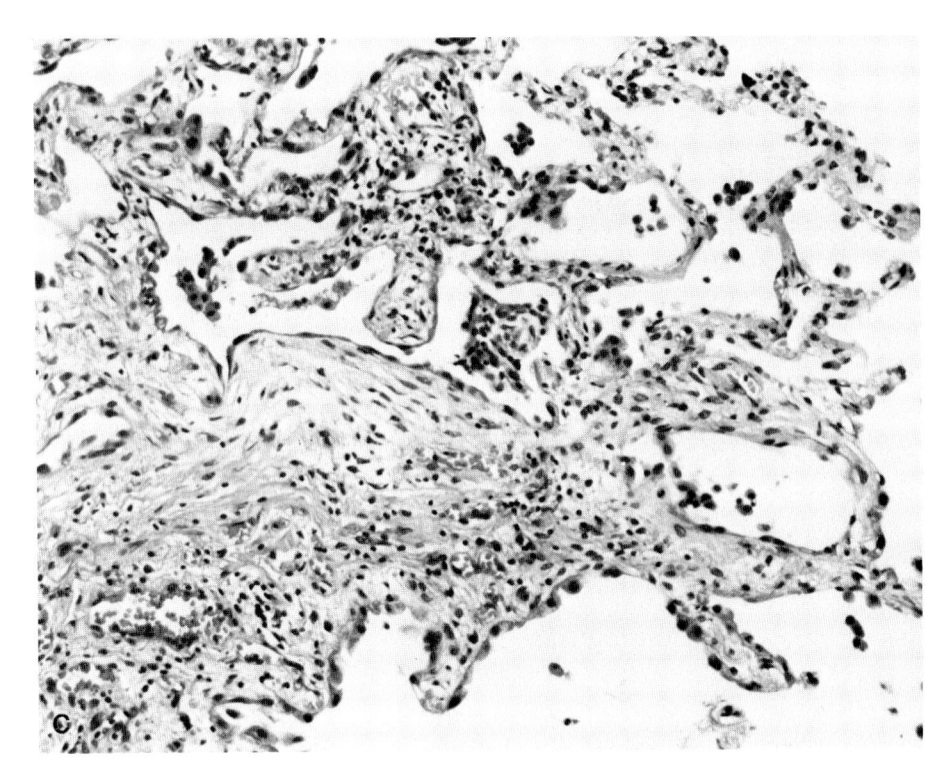

Figure 20–5C,D. C. Focus of active interstitial pneumonia with young cellular connective tissue and inflammatory cells in the interstitium, prominent type II alveolar lining cells, and a nonspecific increase in alveolar macrophages (H&E, ×160). D. Adjacent normal parenchyma (H&E, ×160).

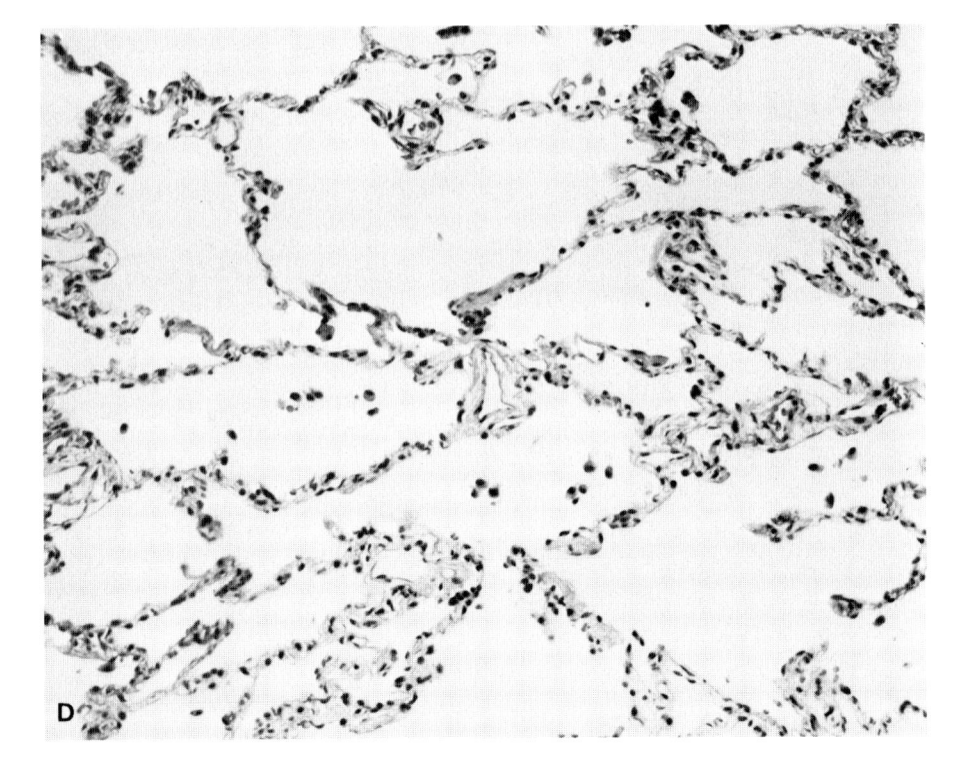

combing is the end result of interstitial pneumonitis. Neutrophils may be numerous in foci of honeycombing and mucus statis, but in the authors' experience, they are not a prominent feature of the interstitial infiltrate except in occasional cases in which they appear to represent an acute reaction to the trauma of the biopsy.

Although the interstitial and epithelial changes are the most dramatic, there is also an air space lesion that progresses simultaneously. The initial feature here is a patchy exudate of proteinaceous debris with only a few monocytes and very rarely other cells. This protein-rich exudate implies that endothelium also is a target of injury in UIP. Where adherent to the alveolar walls, this air space exudate tends to be overgrown by the regenerating alveolar epithelium and thereby is incorporated into the interstitium. Here it too is infiltrated by fibroblasts and gradually changed to scar. Granulation tissue within airways and alveoli, typical of bronchiolitis obliterans with patchy organizing pneumonia (discussed below) is a focal and generally inconspicuous feature in UIP. The final interstitial scars thus have a dual genesis, the end result looking the same whatever their origin(s).

Although there is not a good experimental model of UIP, current approximations and models of various other forms of lung injury suggest that these changes from initial infiltrate to honeycombing can probably be completed in a matter of weeks. The clinical course of slow progression over many years appears to result from a random recruitment into the process of additional groups of alveoli day after day, year after year: progression is cumulative. The anatomic sign of this is the random distribution and the mixture of ages of lesions that can be seen at any one time. *This marked variegation or lack of uniformity is one of the most important features of UIP* both for diagnosis, which cannot be made without this feature, and for understanding the nature of the progressive disease. Once established, this UIP type of reaction usually continues until the patient dies of the lung disease or some unrelated disorder. (When death is related to the lung disease, such added factors as cor pulmonale, bacterial pneumonia, pulmonary emboli, and lung carcinoma may be important.) The rate at which UIP progresses varies considerably from patient to patient, although a total course of 1 year or less is extremely rare.[4] The speed of progression correlates to some extent with the activity seen microscopically in biopsies. Mixed-cell interstitial infiltrates, fibroblastic proliferation, and epithelial regeneration and reliable indicators of activity. Residual lymphoid follicles and the secondary features noted below are not useful in judging activity.

Pulmonary hypertension and cor pulmonale often develop after the honeycombing is so extensive that over half of the capillary bed is gone. As pulmonary hypertension appears, the characteristic vascular lesions of that process are superimposed as well.

Usual interstitial pneumonia has a distinctive overall histologic pattern despite the fact that no one component is specific. This pattern must be recognized in order to make the diagnosis microscopically: nondescript chronic inflammation, scarring, or honeycombing alone is not sufficient. In the terminal part of the course, foci with active components of UIP may be difficult to find. In that instance, only honeycombing can be recognized, and the nature of the process cannot be determined unless an earlier biopsy or additional tissue provides evidence of the essential variegated and active components as well as the scar. Since an established progression to scarring is part of the requirement for diagnosis, an absence of scarring early in the course or in an ill-chosen biopsy with only a early focus also may preclude accurate diagnosis, although this problem is uncommon. (For further discussion, see the section on cellular interstitial pneumonia below.)

Histology of DIP (Fig. 20-6)

Desquamative interstitial pneumonia microscopically has a relative uniformity from field to field. The most striking change is the presence of large numbers of macrophages within the small air spaces. Most of the macrophages within alveoli have eosinophilic to slightly pigmented cytoplasm. These cells may have small amounts of iron or tan-brown residual bodies and are periodic acid-Schiff (PAS) positive. Occasional giant cells may be seen. Foamy histiocytes are not prominent, nor usually is proteinaceous exudate. The alveoli are lined by prominent type II alveolar pneumocytes; the name DIP came from the early idea that a massive desquamation of this epithelium produced the cells in the air spaces. Ultrastructural studies set this concept to rest by showing that most of the air space cells have the features of macrophages.[43,44] Although the name DIP persists and evokes a familiar mental picture of the lesion, it is nevertheless a misnomer.

The second essential part of DIP is the interstitial infiltration, although this is less striking than the air space exudate. As in UIP, this infiltrate is a mixture of various round cells with occasional eosinophils, but both plasma cells and eosinophils tend to be more prominent than in UIP; here is an essential feature for diagnosis. In biopsies, interstitial fibrosis is often mild, and honeycombing is usually less extensive than in UIP. In advanced cases, usually seen after many years of progression, the scarring and honeycombing are more extensive and may eventually dominate the histologic picture. In diagnosis, the hallmark of DIP is air space filling by macrophages in a monotonous fashion in which there is a cellular infiltrate in the interstitium *but fibrosis and honeycombing are absent or slight*. The filling of air spaces by macrophages in zones of honeycombing is nonspecific. Abundant granulation within airways is not a feature of DIP.

UIP and DIP Vs. Cryptogenic Fibrosing Alveolitis

The British concept of fibrosing alveolitis states that DIP is an early phase of UIP.[45,46] In contrast, in reference to the descriptions just given, both UIP and DIP are distinguishable lesions early but both can progress to honeycombing. In so doing, they become less and less easily separated, and finally neither can be reliably identified. Until a better understanding of the essential components of these reactions is achieved, these different views cannot be reconciled. Regardless of whether UIP and DIP are part of a continous spectrum or two separate lesions, however, patients whose biopsies have the pattern of DIP are significantly more steroid-responsive than those who have the pattern of UIP (*see* below). Thus, recognition of these two patterns has practical application.

Histologic Diagnosis of UIP and DIP

Usual interstitial pneumonia and DIP are associated with distinctive clinical, functional, and radiologic findings, and a diagnosis should not be made without knowledge of these features. A slide alone can be misleading. Although most cases are idopathic, DIP and particulary UIP also represent patterns of pulmonary reaction with a number of different causes or associations which should be considered. Desquamative interstitial pneumonia generally has less scarring than UIP. Although classically DIP has large fields with the alveoli uniformly stuffed with macrophages, some cases have a patchy alveolar filling by macrophages.

Differential Diagnosis of UIP

Although most cases of UIP are idiopathic, certain causes and associations have been made for some cases. There is no histologic clue to separate most of these cases from those that are in every sense idiopathic. Thus, the connection between a UIP reaction and drug or other chemical exposure, collagen-vascular disease, metal fume inhalation, or the presence of other familial cases must be found by a careful history. The chronic pneumonia induced by ionizing radiation may have a few tell-tale marks such as bizarre fibroblasts, degenerative changes in bronchial glands, or excessive vascular injury, but in the majority, the histologic changes mimic UIP exactly. The distinction can be made by history and by distribution of the lesion: in the authors' experience, radiation pneumonia is confined to the radiation fields.

When a UIP type of reaction is known to be due to dust exposure, it is traditionally given a specific pneumoconiosis name. Although a few cases of silicosis have extensive, diffuse, interstitial changes as well as the characteristic silicotic nodules, the only common pneumoconiosis that often presents with a UIP is asbestosis. Whether such cases of asbestosis are called asbestosis or UIP due to asbestos is a semantic argument. The histologic identification is based on the finding of asbestos bodies. These may be numerous and obvious, but at times they are found only after careful examination of slides stained with iron, and it is the authors' policy to do such stains on every case of UIP.

Many of the lesions that should be considered in the differential diagnosis of UIP are shown in Table 20–5. The differential diagnosis of UIP from bronchiolitis obliterans with organizing pneumonia is discussed in Bronchiolitis Obliterans and Organizing Interstitial Pneumonia, below. Allergic alveolitis is characterized by a histologic triad of bronchiolitis, interstitial infiltrates, and randomly scattered granulomas. The interstitial infiltrate in allergic alveolitis is usually greater both in number of cells and proportion of plasma cells than in UIP. Typically allergic alveolitis is much more uniform in its distribution and (in early cases) lacks interstitial fibrosis and architectural destruction. Eosinophilic granuloma produces focal discrete scars which contain clusters of Langerhans cells and eosinophils. Usual interstitial pneumonia produces a much more irregular scarring without the discrete nodules of eosinophilic granuloma and lacks clusters of Langerhans cells.

Some of the original cases reported by Hamman and Rich[32] appear in retrospect to have been cases of diffuse alveoli damage, that is, adult hyaline membrane disease or ARDS. Although widespread injury may be present in both, time has failed to provide evidence of a significant relationship between ARDS and UIP. Observation of thousands of patients with ARDS has shown that organization of that lesion can indeed produce scarring, even honeycombing, but there is no evidence that these cases transform into progressive lesions like UIP. Rather, the ARDS patients tend to die quickly or survive with stable or gradually improving function. Hyaline membranes can be seen in UIP, but they are sparse and confined to a few cases. When ARDS does organize, the resulting lesion tends to be homogenous in age: the scars look very much alike and the same is true of the infiltrate. Bronchioles are often injured in ARDS also, so that scarring is often partially within the small airways which are spared in UIP. Typically the history of an acute, explosive onset in ARDS is different from the insidious slow appearance of the symptoms in UIP. This is especially useful information in cases in which the biopsy is equivocal, which occasionally is true. Because of infection, oxygen therapy, or other factors, ARDS sometimes complicates the terminal course of UIP; then the picture is mixed. Such cases are especially difficult to interpret without a detailed history and even then may defy solution.

Localized lesions, most of which are probably due to infection or aspiration, can progress to localized honeycombing when necrosis is sufficient. Occasionally such lesions in biopsy are microscopically similar to UIP, but their course is to end as a stable local scar. Such localized lesions affect function only in these rare instances when they are very extensive. Even then, the course is characterized by rapid stabilization without subsequent progression. Thus, the history, radiographic distribution, and serial studies of function help greatly in such cases.

Late stages of sarcoidosis may be associated with interstitial fibrosis as well as nonspecific honeycombing. The presence of even a few granulomas, the tendency of the fibrosis to follow lymphatic routes, and the identification of Schaumann (conchoidal) bodies embedded in the fibrous tissue favor a diagnosis of sarcoidosis, as does a predominantly upper lobe distribution.

The interstitial infiltrate of LIP is much more extensive and uniform than that seen in UIP.

The term cellular interstitial pneumonia characterizes lesions in which there is an interstitial infiltrate lacking specific features and that have not resulted in appreciable scarring or destruction of parenchyma. The outcome of cases of cellular interstitial pneumonia cannot be predicted on the basis of histology. Some may represent a slowly healing viral pneumonia; several have been shown to be allergic or drug reactions which were largely reversible. Still others have become typical examples of UIP in time. Whether in the latter cases there actually was no scarring at the time of biopsy or it was missed in the sample is unknown.

Pulmonary veno-occlusive disease occasionally presents a pattern suggesting an interstitial penumonia. The interstitium is thickened, and there is a scant inflammatory infiltrate and prominent type II alveolar lining cells.

Figure 20–6A,B. DIP. A. Nonspecific bilateral reticulonodular infiltrates, worse in lower lobes. B. Uniform involvement of lung parenchyma by an interstitial and alveolar-filling process (H&E, ×32).

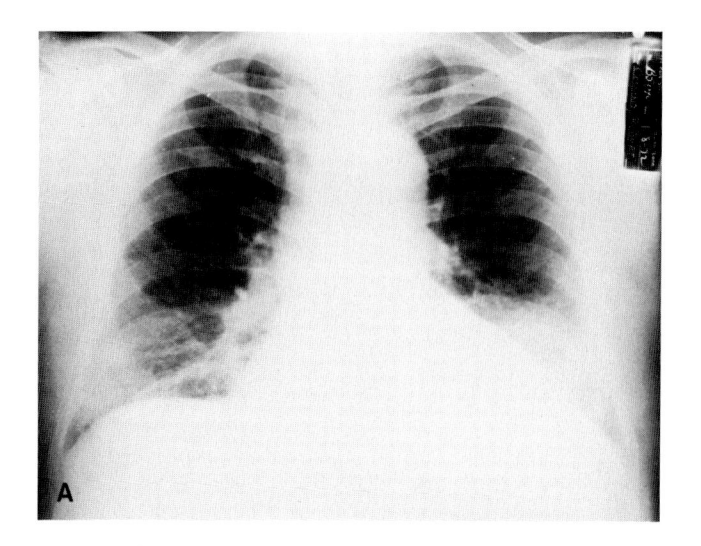

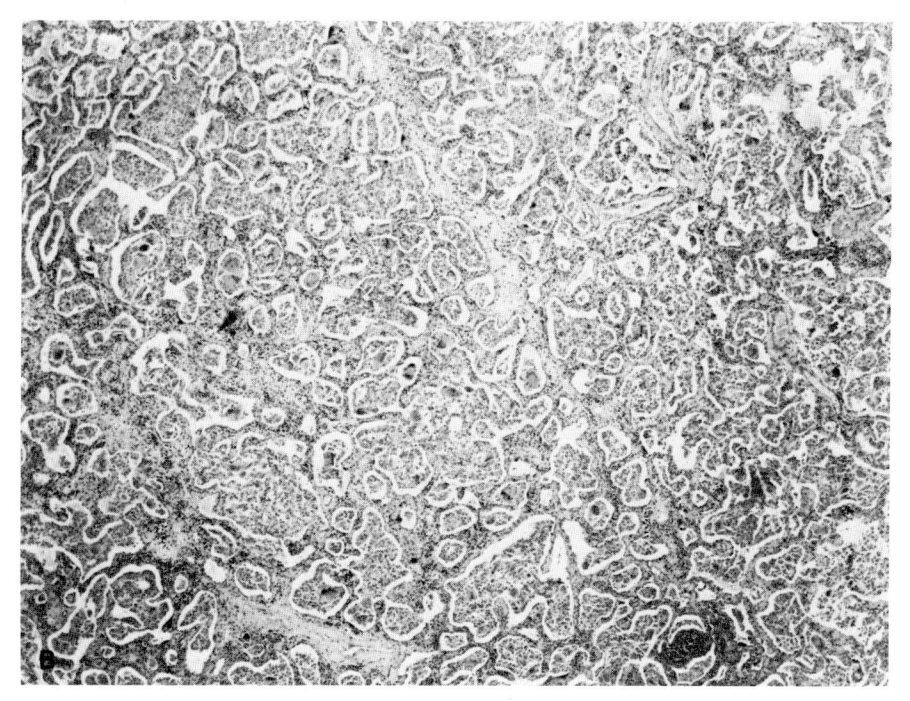

Careful attention to the preservation of pulmonary architecture, clusters of hemosiderin-filled macrophages, and the fact that much of the apparent interstitial prominence is due to abnormal vessels, edema, and metaplastic epithelium should lead to a suspicion of pulmonary veno-occlusive disease. Elastic tissue stains facilitate recognition of the true nature of the process.

Differential Diagnosis of DIP

Foci resembling DIP may be seen around mass lesions as focal nonspecific reaction, and an erroneous diagnosis of DIP can be made. Such a pseudo-DIP reaction may be seen around rheumatoid nodules, the nodules of eosinophilic granuloma (Fig. 20–7), and adjacent to intrapulmonary lymph nodes or a cartilagenous hamartoma.[47] It has also been seen next to primary and metastatic tumors, abscesses, and sarcoid granulomas. A focal DIP-like reaction is of no diagnostic significance, and one should not be misled by its presence, particularly in small specimens such as transbronchial biopsies. In addition, increased alveolar macrophages and nonspecific changes in the alveolar walls are frequent in many diffuse lung diseases, especially in foci of scarring and honeycombing, again reflecting the histologic nonspecificity of this reaction. Such an appearance focally in UIP is common. Asbestosis rarely takes the form of DIP reaction,[48] so including iron stains may be advisable. In a single patient with asbestosis studied in Gaensler's laboratory, steroid therapy failed to produce any slowing in the patient's course, which was similar to that of other

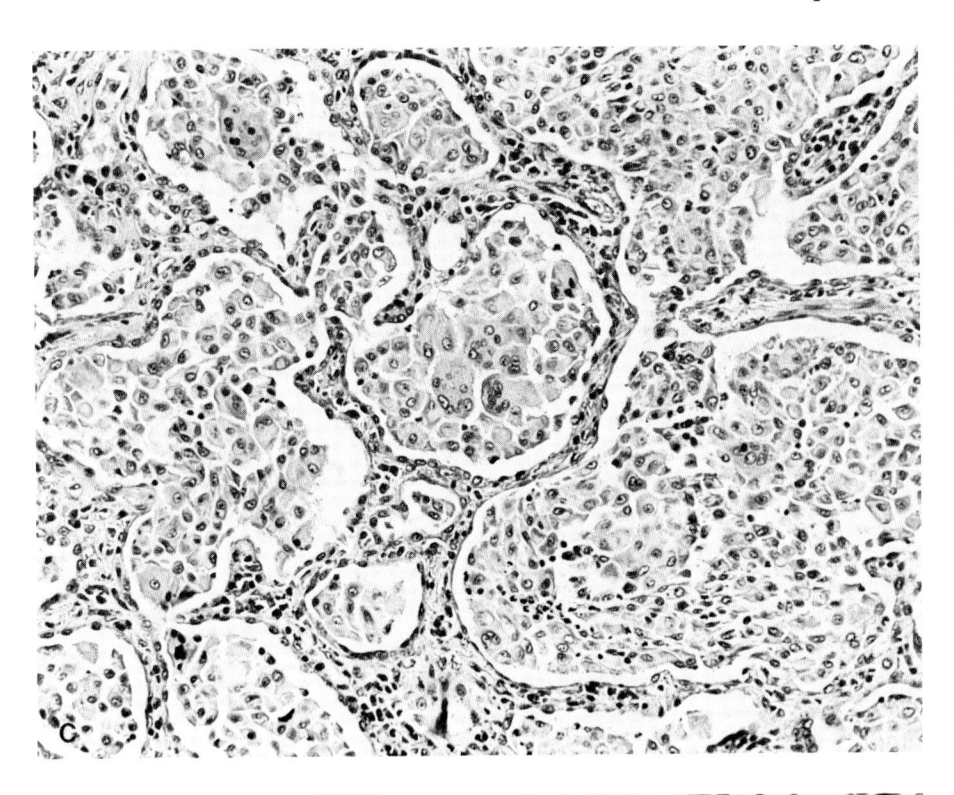

Figure 20–6C,D. C. Multinucleation of some of the alveolar macrophages can be seen (H&E, ×160). D. Detail shows prominence of type II cells and interstitial thickening with an infiltrate composed predominantly of mononuclear cells (H&E, ×400).

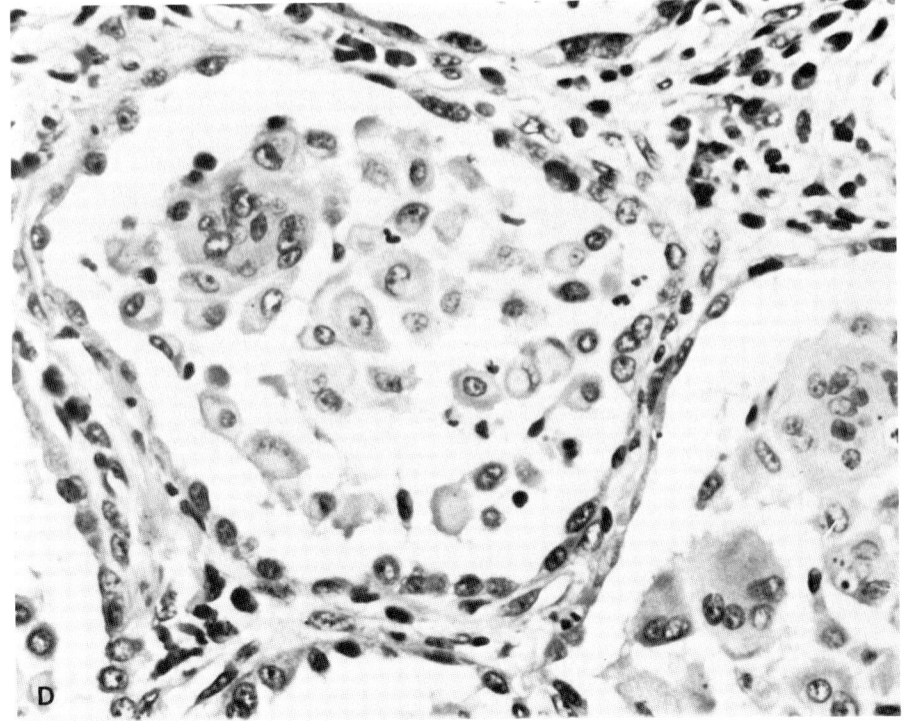

patients with asbestosis. Occasionally in cases of DIP, other dusts have been seen in excessive amounts, including hard metals, silica, talc, and aluminum.[49] Rarely DIP has been mistaken for idiopathic hemosiderosis because of the numerous macrophages with faintly brown pigment. An iron stain usually clarifies this since the amount of blue staining in DIP is usually far less than in hemosiderosis. Clinically patients with hemosiderosis are usually anemic children; patients with DIP have normal hematocrits or polycythemia from chronic hypoxemia.

Treatment of UIP and DIP

Steroids are of considerable benefit in DIP and often result in cure of the disease.[4,44,45] Nevertheless, some patients with DIP will ultimately progress to respiratory failure.[4] Steroids are of little benefit in UIP, although cases caused by drugs or associated with collagen vascular disease represent groups in which response may rarely occur.[4] This pessimistic view toward therapy in UIP is not shared by all, but it is derived from a large number of cases.[4] There are other series that have claimed some steroid-responsiveness in UIP,[37,38,40,41,46,50] and some prognostic factors have been identified. In the study by Rudd and associates,[41] response to steroids was correlated with more abnormal initial forced vital capacity, a more recent onset of disease, and relative lymphocytosis in bronchoalveolar lavage fluid. The prognosis of DIP is significantly better than that associated with UIP, as illustrated in Table 20–8. These data reflect the slow but relentless progression of the lesions and the fact that many smolder for as long as 15 years yet ultimately prove fatal. The usual cause of death is different, in that most patients with UIP die directly or indirectly of the disease, whereas deaths of patients with DIP are caused by unrelated, intercurrent diseases in more than half the cases.[44] An excess in mortality from lung cancer has been noted in patients with UIP compared with a control population, and this may reflect propensity for lungs with scarring to develop carcinoma.[51]

Bronchiolitis Obliterans and Organizing Interstitial Pneumonia

Introduction

This section discusses a lesion in which bronchiolitis obliterans is associated with a variable degree of organizing pneumonia in a patchy but often widespread distribution. Since the bronchiolitis obliterans component is so important to this lesion, it is necessary first to give some consideration to bronchiolitis obliterans in general. Diffuse panbronchiolitis, recently described from Japan,[52] represents a completely different lesion with mononuclear infiltrates around the bronchioles without bronchiolitis obliterans. The topic of bronchiolitis obliterans as an airway lesion associated with chronic airflow obstruction is discussed on p. 151.

Bronchiolitis Obliterans

Bronchiolitis obliterans is a lesion that results when injury to small conducting airways is repaired by proliferation of granulation tissue, which at one stage often produces spectacular, polypoid masses protruding into and filling the airways' lumens. Bronchiolar necrosis has probably occurred, but at the stage of repair, this may be apparent only from defects in the musculoelastic structure of the wall. The regularity with which this luxurious proliferation of granulation tissue can be produced after fume-induced injury spontaneously (as in silo filler's disease) or experimentally suggests that this is the usual and appropriate reaction to this injury at this site rather than an inappropriate reaction seen only in special hosts.

Like granulation tissue generally, bronchiolitis obliterans is a rapidly changing dynamic lesion; the edematous, intraluminal polyp is but one transient stage. The first stage has necrosis and, at least in some reactions, a more or less ordinary acute inflammatory exudate. Seen alone, this would be called acute bronchiolitis or acute necrotizing bronchiolitis. This stage is followed by repair in which the familiar granulation tissue polyps appear, often accompanied by epithelial regeneration or metaplasia. The early granulation tissue is richly cellular and edematous and may be interspersed with residual exudate. Later this tissue markedly shrinks and contracts leaving variable amounts of scarring.

In those instances on which the necrosis is very mild and focal and the polyp is attached to the wall only by a narrow stalk, the end scar can be trivial in size and damage. With more extensive injury and ulceration, the granulation tissue can attach widely and lead to permanent obliteration of the entire lumen. Every degree of bronchiolar narrowing can occur, and a wide variety is commonly seen in any one case. When small airways obliterated by old, fibrous scars are widespread in the lung, there is often clinical evidence of airflow obstruction.[54-58] However, it is exceedingly difficult to predict the extent of scarring and narrowing that will eventually occur from observations made at the stage of polypoid masses of granulation tissue. This is further hampered by the fact that the functional outcome depends on how many bronchioles are impaired as well as the extent of the injury in each. Even with generous open biopsies, only a few bronchioles are included, so the sample is always small. The lesion can be localized and involve bronchioles in one region but not in another. Finally, even in widespread disease, the lesion in one bronchiole may affect so short a segment as to be detected only with the use of serial sections.[53] In this instance, the sparsity of microscopic lesions is in fact misleading in terms of functional effect.

Although the name bronchiolitis obliterans clearly implies bronchiolar location, the site ranges from small (more or less terminal) bronchioles to alveolar ducts. In the former, recognition of the bronchiolar wall, or remnants thereof, and the adjacent pulmonary arterioles facilitates identification of the lesion, especially on slides stained for elastic tissue. Identification of lesions in alveolar ducts depends on recognition of the characteristic branching shapes. Alveoli surrounding the conducting airways are frequently involved also. By convention, when involvement of the distal air spaces is most pronounced, the term organizing pneumonia is used; when the reaction in the bronchioles is most pronounced, bronchiolitis obliterans is the favored term. In fact, the changes are part of a continuum.

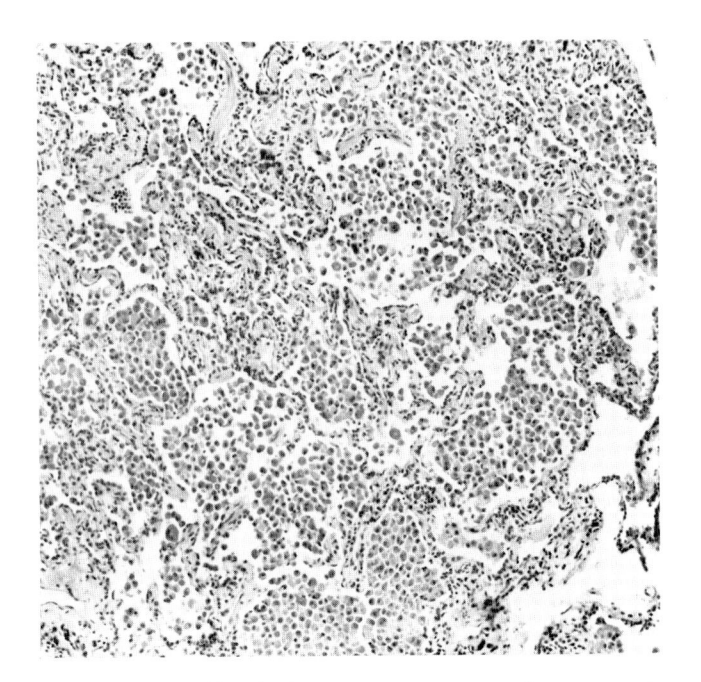

Figure 20-7. Pseudo-desquamative interstitial pneumonia (DIP) in pulmonary eosinophilic granuloma. Pulmonary parenchyma adjacent to a nodule of eosinophilic granuloma shows an interstitial infiltrate and increase in alveolar macrophages reminiscent of DIP (H&E, ×80).

Etiology of Bronchiolitis Obliterans

Bronchiolitis obliterans, with or without organizing penumonia, may be a focal lesion in the lung or may involve the pulmonary parenchyma as a diffuse bilateral process. The reaction is common and monospecific; it is seen in organizing infections (bacterial, fungal, viral, mycoplasma), aspiration of gastric contents, toxic fume inhalation, allergic reactions (eosinophilic pneumonia, extrinsic allergic alveolitis), organizing diffuse alveolar damage, drug reactions, and collagen vascular diseases. It is also seen distal to bronchiectasis or large airway obstruction, probably due to smoldering low-grade infection, and finally as a focal reaction adjacent to other lesions such as abscesses or tumors. Occasionally the histology of the bronchiolitis obliterans is suggestive of the cause. The best example is probably toxic fume exposure, which leads to a relatively pure bronchiolitis obliterans of terminal and first-generation respiratory bronchioles and their immediately surrounding alveoli with practically no involvement of distal parenchyma. Such cases appear as scattered inflammatory nodules centering on small airways on biopsy, which correspond to the miliary small nodules that may be seen radiologically.

In most instances of bronchiolitis obliterans, the underlying diagnosis is determined by the associated components of the overall reaction, history, and other laboratory data rather than by morphology of the orga-nizing bronchiolitis. For example, in allergic alveolitis, the bronchiolitis obliterans is accompanied by a diffuse interstitial infiltrate, prominent plasma cells, randomly scattered small granulomas, and, with sufficient probing, a telltale history. Cultures or serial serologic studies can help to pinpoint infectious causes, and clinical evidence of specific collagen vascular disease can help establish that assocation despite poor understanding of the exact relationship. When there are neither anatomic nor historic data to support a more specific diagnosis, bronchiolitis obliterans, with or without an associated organizing pneumonia, remains as a descriptive diagnosis by exclusion.

When bronchiolitis and organizing penumonia present as a radiologically localized lesion, the term focal organizing pneumonia has traditionally been applied. This lesion is well known to pathologists and clinicians alike, and it may be seen following a clinically recognized episode of pneumonia or as an incidental finding. When the lesion has suggested a neoplasm on radiographs, the term inflammatory pseudotumor is sometimes applied by the pathologist.

Bronchiolitis Obliterans and Patchy Organizing Pneumonia

Although bronchiolitis obliterans is an appropriate descriptive diagnosis for situations in which an etiology (such as a specific infection) or an associated cause (such as rheumatoid arthritis) can be identified, it is preferable to add the modifying phrase "due to . . . ." Bronchiolitis obliterans and patchy organizing pneumonia may also be widespread in the lung when no etiology is found, even following extensive clinical evaluation. Labels for such cases are many and have included bronchiolitis obliterans with interstitial pneumonia or diffuse alveolar damage,[33] bronchiolitis obliterans,[54,57,58–62] idiopathic pulmonary fibrosis or interstitial fibrosis,[63] organizing pneumonia,[64,65] and cryptogenic organizing pneu-

Table 20-8. Usual Interstitial Pneumonia Vs. Desquamative Interstitial Penumonia Survival and Response to Steroids[a]

	UIP	DIP
No. patients	53	40
No. deaths	48 (94%)	14 (39%)
Mean years to death	6.2	16.8
Follow-up (years)	8–12	7–28
Response to steroids[b]		
Mean years of therapy	2.1 (±2.3)	3.1 (±2.8)
Long-term improvement	8%	68%

[a] Based on a 1982 update of patients reported in Gaensler et al.[34]
[b] Based on 26 patients with UIP and 26 patients with DIP who received adequate therapy

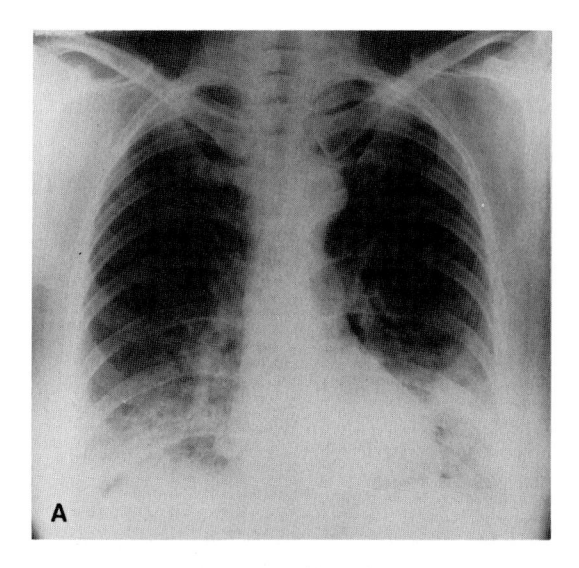

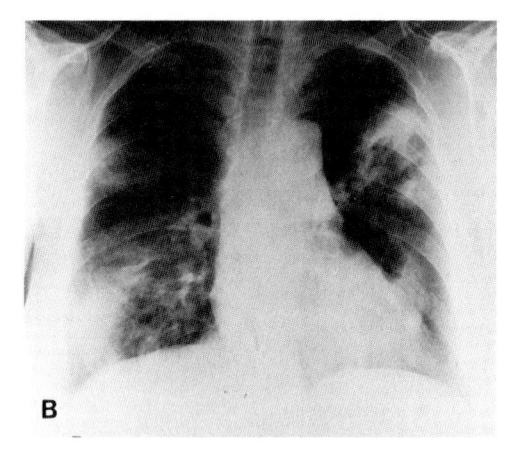

Figure 20–8. Two cases of bronchiolitis obliterans with patchy organizing pneumonia: radiographic findings. A. Bilateral lower lobe infiltrates (left) that cleared after steroid therapy (right). B. Patchy bilateral infiltrates. Courtesy of Dr. Epler, Boston.

monitis[65a]. The label bronchiolitis obliterans with patchy organizing pneumonia, however, is descriptive and less likely to be confused with other forms of infiltrative lung disease. Recognition of these cases is important, since their etiology, course, treatment, and prognosis can be very different from some of the chronic interstitial pneumonias, notably UIP, with which they are often confused. The following discussion is based on the authors' experience with a large series of cases[66] and other reported cases.[54,56–60,65]

Patients with bronchiolitis obliterans and organizing pneumonia may be asymptomatic and may have incidental radiologic abnormalities. However, the majority have significant respiratory complaints, including cough, fever, shortness of breath, and rarely hemoptysis. Often these symptoms have followed what seemed to be an upper respiratory tract infection. In other instances, a clinical diagnosis of pneumonia had been made, and the lesion failed to resolve in the usual fashion. By the time a biopsy was performed, symptoms had usually been present for weeks or months. Laboratory findings were nonspecific. However, occasional cases have eosinophilia or immunoglobulin deficiencies.

Radiologically alveolar or reticular infiltrates are seen in patchy distribution often either involving multiple lobes or as a diffuse bilateral process (Fig. 20–8). Waxing and waning may be seen, and infiltrates sometimes appear at one site while they are regressing in others. The radiologist's impression is often one of an atypical or unresolving pneumonia.

Despite the prominence of bronchiolitis obliterans histologically, those patients who have functional deficits usually show restrictive disease with decreased diffusing capacity rather than airflow obstruction. Airflow obstruction is seen acutely in a small number of patients; in a few cases, chronic airflow obstruction is a lasting sequel of bronchiolitis obliterans and organizing pneumonia.[57,63]

The gross appearance of biopsies is nonspecific. The involved tissue is firm and grey on cut surface. The foci of consolidation by young connective tissue may impart a mucoid appearance. The striking feature histologically is the presence of numerous uniform, edematous plugs of granulation tissue filling bronchioles and alveolar ducts in a patchy distribution (Figs. 20–9 through 20–12). Despite the abundance of active lumenal fibrosis, elastic tissue stains usually show relative preservation of the pulmonary parenchyma. When present, interstitial fibrosis is concentrated in the peribronchiolar regions. Terminal bronchioles commonly have a mural cellular infiltrate composed predominantly of mononuclear cells, sometimes with neutrophils in the lumen. Acute inflammation and fibrinous exudate may be present in some of the alveoli (see Fig. 20–10) as may histolgic changes of obstructive pneumonia. An alveolar interstitial infiltrate of lymphocytes and plasma cells is also frequent (see Fig. 20–11). In cases in which this feature is mild, it appears related to the obstruction and resembles that seen in ordinary obstructive pneumonia. In other cases, it is so severe (compared with that seen in simple obstruction), that it suggests a true interstitial pneumonia: a primary alveolar interstitial response to the injury. Eosinophils characterize some cases, whereas plasma cells and lymphocytes predominate in most. Scattered granulomas may be present. Extensive necrosis is unusual and should stimulate a careful search for an active infection.

Although some cases of bronchiolitis obliterans and organizing pneumonia have a history spanning several months, the histologic features do not often appear that old. Late lesions of bronchiolitis obliterans and organizing pneumonia presumably look like simple scars, but there have been few opportunities to see such lesions after having seen the typical early lesion in the same patient. Judging from the clinical course in the majority of patients, the process can heal with little if any resultant functional abnormality. A few cases appear to progress to chronic obstructive pulmonary disease.[57,63]

Etiology of Idiopathic Bronchiolitis Obliterans and Organizing Pneumonia

Even when no direct evidence of an infectious cause is found clinically, an occasional case responds favorably to an intensified and prolonged (2 weeks) course of antibiotics. This suggests that a few of the "idiopathic" cases are actually due to infection. The majority of favorable responses are induced by steroids rather than antibiotics, which suggests that many of the cases are somehow immunologically mediated. Especially instructive are the two cases reported by Grinblat and colleagues[65] in which cessation of steroid therapy resulted in relapses which again underwent remissions when steroid therapy was resumed.

Differential Diagnosis

One frequent error in the diagnosis of bronchiolitis obliterans with organizing pneumonia is to call it UIP. The clinical, radiologic, and histologic differences of UIP and bronchiolitis obliterans with patchy organizing pneumonia are summarized in Table 20–9.

The most important histologic feature in separating bronchiolitis obliterans and organizing pneumonia from UIP is the temporal uniformity of the former with its distinctive, evenly spaced plugs of young connective tissue within airways (see Fig. 20–12). Air space organization occurs in UIP as a focal inconspicuous finding relative to the foci of honeycombing and interstitial scarring. Foci of honeycombing are unusual in bronchiolitis obliterans and organizing pneumonia. In the few cases in which differentiation is difficult, review of the clinical and radiographic findings may solve the problem.

Two important clinical features that differentiate UIP from bronchiolitis obliterans and organizing pneumonia are the prognosis and response to therapy. Whereas more than 75 percent of patients with bronchiolitis obliterans and organizing pneumonia do well, usually with steroid therapy, the vast majority of patients with UIP show no such response and have a uniformly bad prognosis if followed for a long enough period of time (see Table 20–8).

A few patients with bronchiolitis obliterans and organizing pneumonia (less than 10 percent) develop progressive respiratory failure and die despite all attempts at therapy, including the use of immunosuppressive drugs. Most deaths occur with a few months of the onset of symptoms. Such fatal cases comprise the old reports of bronchiolitis obliterans by Blumgart and MacMahen,[58] Liebow,[33] and probably some of those reported by Hamman and Rich.[32] The increased use of lung biopsy, especially early in the course of undiagnosed disease, has dramatically increased the number of cases recognized in living patients.

Bronchiolitis obliterans is common in ARDS, and organizing diffuse alveolar damage may be identical to bronchiolitis obliterans and organizing pneumonia field for field. The greater uniformity of diffuse alveolar damage and the characteristic clinical history usually allow separation, but in a few instances, these disorders are truly inseparable. Some examples of allergic alveolitis or eosinophilic pneumonia show bronchiolitis obliterans and organizing pneumonia in addition to their other characteristic features. Focal bronchiolitis obliterans and organization may be seen in close proximity to mass lesions such as infectious granulomas, Wegener's granulomatosis, or tumor. Correlation of clinical, radiologic, and histologic information is often helpful in avoiding these pitfalls.

Bronchiolitis obliterans and organizing pneumonia is currently a frequent finding in open lung biopsies, but it is by no means a new entity; many cases have been previously reported but under a number of different titles.

Table 20–9. Bronchiolitis Obliterans with Patchy Organizing Pneumonia Versus Usual Interstitial Penumonia

	BOOP	UIP
Symptoms and signs	Develop over weeks or few months; may follow or simulate respiratory tract infection	Insidious dyspnea over months or years
Pulmonary function tests	Variable; may be normal, restrictive, or rarely obstructive	Progressive restrictive lung disease
Chest radiograph	Variable; patchy, wandering, or bilateral and diffuse alveolar and/or reticular infiltrates	Bilateral reticular infiltrates progressing to honeycombing
Histology	Uniform age; always involves small conducting airways	Lesions of varying age; conducting airways rarely involved except with secondary infections
Therapy	Steroids; rarely antibiotics	No good therapy
Prognosis	Much better on average. Less than 10% die of disease; most deaths occur within a few months	Very poor; almost all die of the disease or its complications; most deaths occur after many years.

Abbreviations: BOOP, bronchiolitis obliterans with patchy organizing pneumonia; UIP, usual insterstitial pneumonia.

[a] Based on the results of Epler et al.[66]

448 Infiltrative Lung Disease

Figure 20–9A,B. Bronchiolitis obliterans with patchy organizing pneumonia. A. Plugs of young connective extend from a respiratory bronchiole into an alveolar duct (H&E, ×40). B. Adjacent alveolar ducts are involved (H&E, ×40).

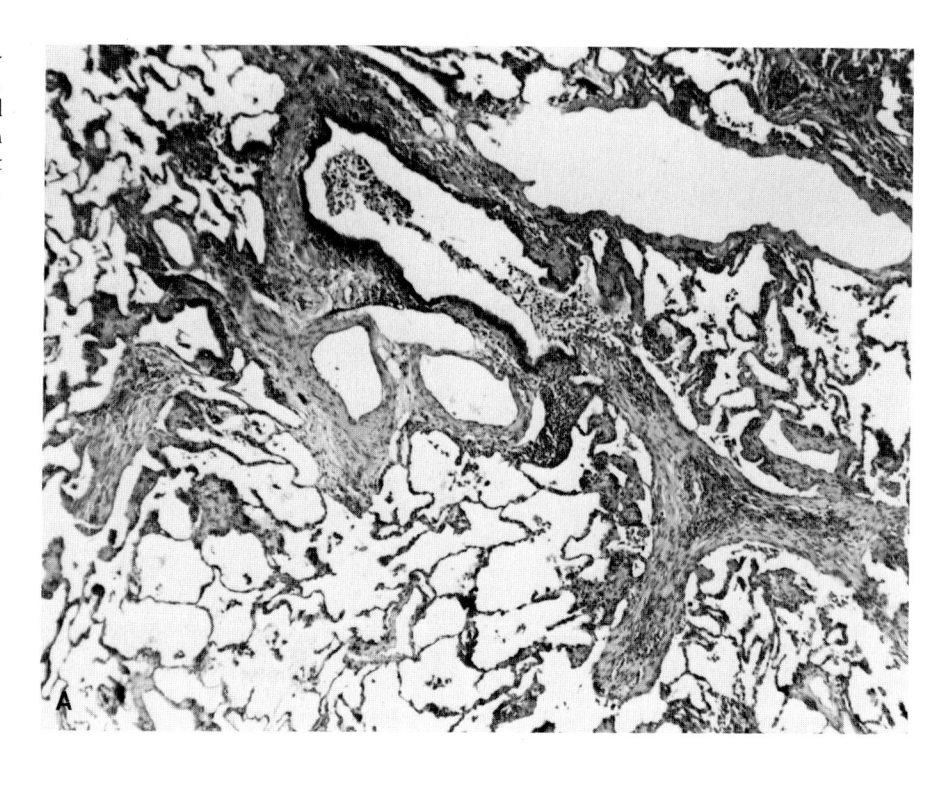

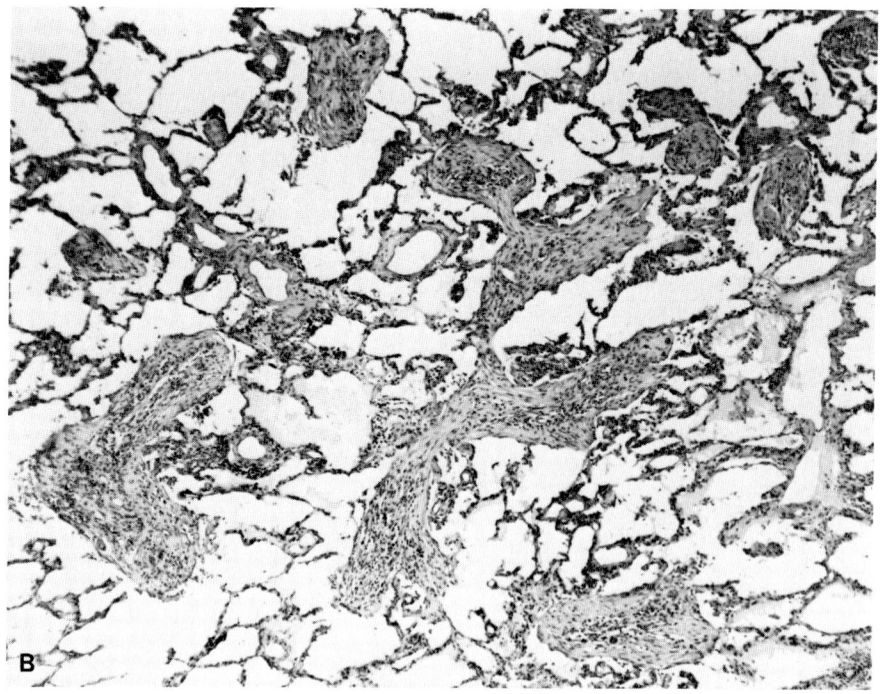

Giant Cell Interstitial Pneumonia

Giant cell interstitial pneumonia is a very uncommon pattern and probably a histologic curiosity, as illustrated by the fact that Liebow[33] mentioned having seen only two cases by 1968. It produces infiltrative lung disease that is distinguished by its histologic appearance. The interstitium and alveolar walls are thickened and infiltrated by mononuclear cells. The diagnostic feature is the presence of large numbers of giant cells filling the air spaces (Fig. 20–13). Some of the giant cells appear cannibalistic and have other cells, including lymphocytes and macrophages, within their cytoplasm.

Figure 20–9C. Detail of intra-airway connective tissue proliferation shows fibroblasts, lymphocytes, and plasma cells (H&E, ×400).

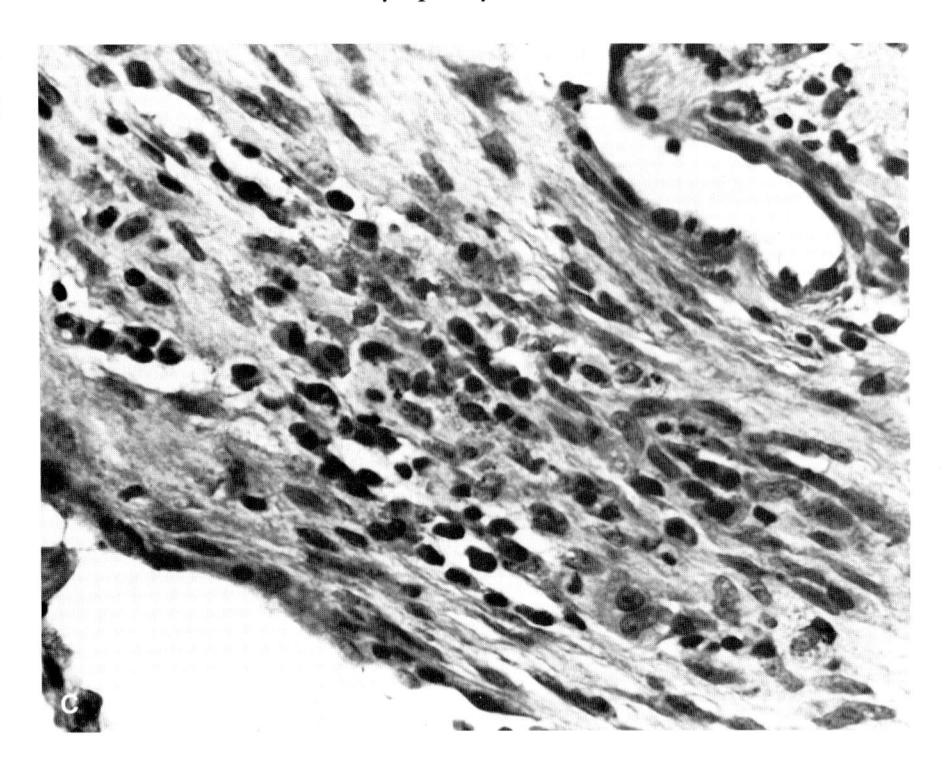

Recent studies[67,67a,67b] suggest that giant cell interstitial pneumonia may be associated with exposure to inorganic particulates, especially hard metals (*see* Chapter 23).

Lymphocytic Interstitial Pneumonia

Lymphocytic interstitial pneumonia (LIP) is a chronic, scarring, interstitial pneumonia characterized by bilateral massive interstitial infiltrates of heterogenous composition.[16,33,68–80] Lymphocytic interstitial pneumonia likely includes cases of diverse etiology but nonetheless comprises a relatively homogenous group histologically with distinct clinical features.

Lymphocytic interstitial pneumonia is more common in women than men and has been described in patients as young as 14 months and as old as 77 years.[16,69,70,75] Familial cases have been reported.[79] Symptoms include cough, dyspnea, weight loss, and progressive shortnesses of breath.[16,70,75] Fever, chest pain, and hemoptysis are unusual. Symptoms have usually been present for more than a year and often several years before the diagnosis is made.

Chest radiographs are variable.[16,70,75,77] Coarse bibasilar reticulonodular infiltrates with nodules less than 1 cm in diameter characterize some cases, whereas others have soft, fluffy infiltrates that become confluent.[77] Ultimately honeycombing develops. Air bronchograms are unusual in LIP, being more common in lymphomas.[77]

Pulmonary function studies are typical of diffuse infiltrative lung disease: restriction with abnormal gas exchange.

Dysproteinemia is frequent in LIP, usually as serum protein elevation but occasionally as hypogammaglobulinemia.[70,75,80] A selective serum immunoglobulin, such as IgA, may be depressed. Lymphocytic interstitial pneumonia is a concomitant finding in some patients with abnormal immunologic states.[72,81] Eosinophilia was seen in two patients reported by Liebow.[70]

The cause of LIP is unknown, but the frequent association of autoimmune disease suggests that immunologic factors are important. Sjögren's syndrome is present in up to one-third of cases.[70] Nodular lymphoid hyperplasia of the intestine, amyloidosis, Hashimoto's thryoiditis, myasthenia gravis, pernicious anemia, autoerythrocyte sensitivity syndrome, chronic active hepatitis, agammaglobulinemia, systemic lupus erythematosus, and salivary gland enlargement are other reported concomitants.[70,72,75,76]

The course and response to therapy are inconsistent. Although some studies showed little long-term response to steroid therapy,[70] others found steroids produced long-term remissions in some patients.[75] Strimlan and colleagues[75] found a better prognosis in younger patients in their study. A few patients have been placed on immunosuppressives with variable results. Some patients do have progressive disease and ultimately die of respi-

Figure 20–10. Bronchiolitis obliterans with patchy organizing pneumonia. Fibrinous alveolar exudate is undergoing organization into fibrous connective tissue in the center of the alveolar duct (H&E, ×160).

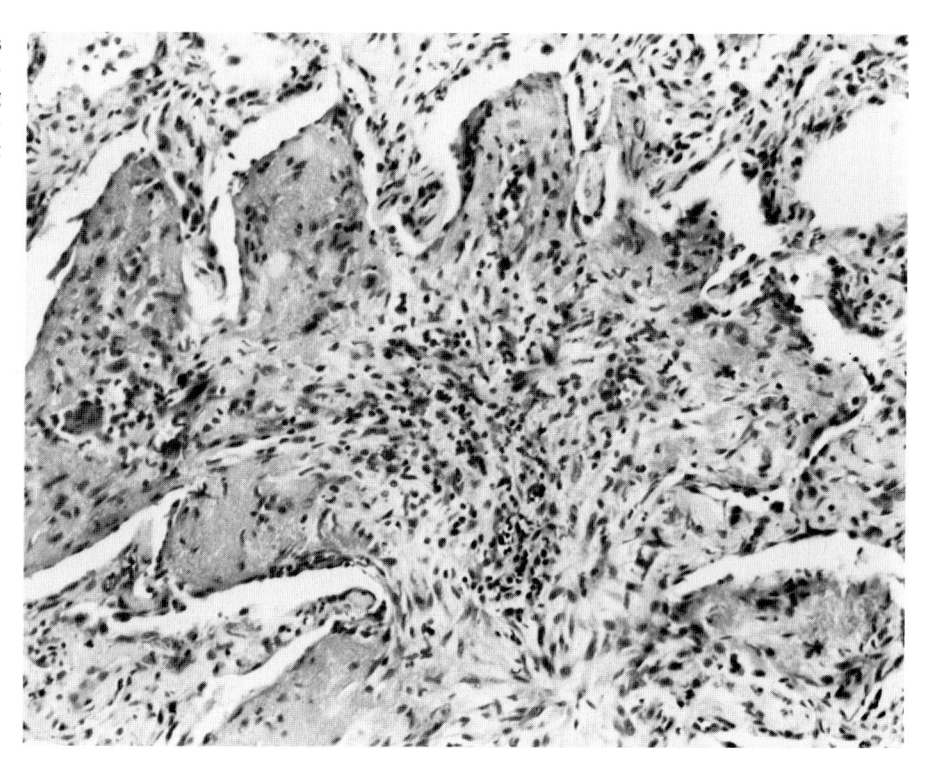

ratory failure; however, a review of Liebow's material by Hecht[77] showed that the majority of patients did not die of lung disease. O'Brodovich and associates[79] described LIP in two brothers, one of whom died after 10 years of disease, while the other was still alive with few symptoms 11 years after diagnosis.

Since the first description of LIP, its exact relationship to lymphocytic and lymphoplasmactic lymphomas (well-differentiated lymphocytic lymphomas) has been unclear. Much of this uncertainty derived from unreliable histologic criteria which resulted in mislabeling a number of cases of lymphoma as LIP.

Most cases of LIP and malignant lymphoma can now be distinguished by reproducible histologic techniques; the available immunologic marker studies supported this approach.[82] Many lymphomas show monoclonal surface markers on the lymphocytes, whereas LIP is polyclonal.[73,74,78] Some lymphomas do not stain at all, limiting the usefulness of marker studies. Despite the fact that lymphomas are considered malignant and LIP is deemed benign, Julsrud and co-workers[74] found that the ultimate prognosis with LIP was worse than that associated with well-differentiated lymphocytic lymphomas presenting in the lung.

Even when lymphomas are separated from real cases of LIP, there appears to be real progression to malignant lymphoma in a small percentage of LIP cases. This is not surprising since LIP is often associated with autoimmune conditions such as Sjögren's syndrome in which an increased incidence of lymphoma is well known. Nevertheless, there is always the possibility of misdiagnosis over, and discussion of, such progression.

Grossly lungs of patients with LIP show varying amounts of nonspecific honeycombing and ill-defined yellow-tan or grey foci of consolidation. The distinctive histologic features of the lymphoid infiltrate in LIP are the degree, the polymorphous composition, and the fact that the entire interstitium is involved (Fig. 20–14). The amount of infiltrate in LIP is much greater than in other interstitial pneumonias. The infiltrate is polymorphous and has a mixture of lymphocytes, plasma cells, and histiocytes in variable numbers, and occasionally granulomas and giant cells. Lymphoid follicles with germinal centers may be scattered throughout the interstitum. In some cases plasma cells predominate.[68] Amyloid or amyloid-like material (para-amyloid) may be found. The infiltrate involves the interstitium diffusely and does not show a predilection to follow the lymphatic routes as is seen in lymphocytic lymphomas. Secondary obstructive pneumonia, bronchiolitis, or bronchiolitis obliterans is uncommon.

The differential diagnosis of LIP includes lymphocytic lymphomas, allergic alveolitis, follicular bronchiolitis, and angioimmunoblastic lymphadenopathy. Lymphocytic lymphomas are monomorphous and show a tendency to follow the lymphatics. They do not often show the uniform diffuse involvement of LIP. The interstitial infiltrate in allergic alveolitis is generally less dense than that associated with LIP, and the bronchiolitis with bronchiolitis obliterans is more prominent. Granulomas may be seen in both conditions. The histologic appearance of allergic alveolitis is occasionally identical to LIP, and differentiation is impossible without clinical correlation. Follicular bronchiolitis is often misinterpreted as LIP. In follicular bronchiolitis, there are prominent germinal centers that follow the airways. The intervening

Figure 20–11. Bronchiolitis obliterans with patchy organizing pneumonia. The alveolar walls are hypercellular with an interstitial infiltrate surrounding an alveolar duct containing a plug of granulation tissue (H&E, ×160).

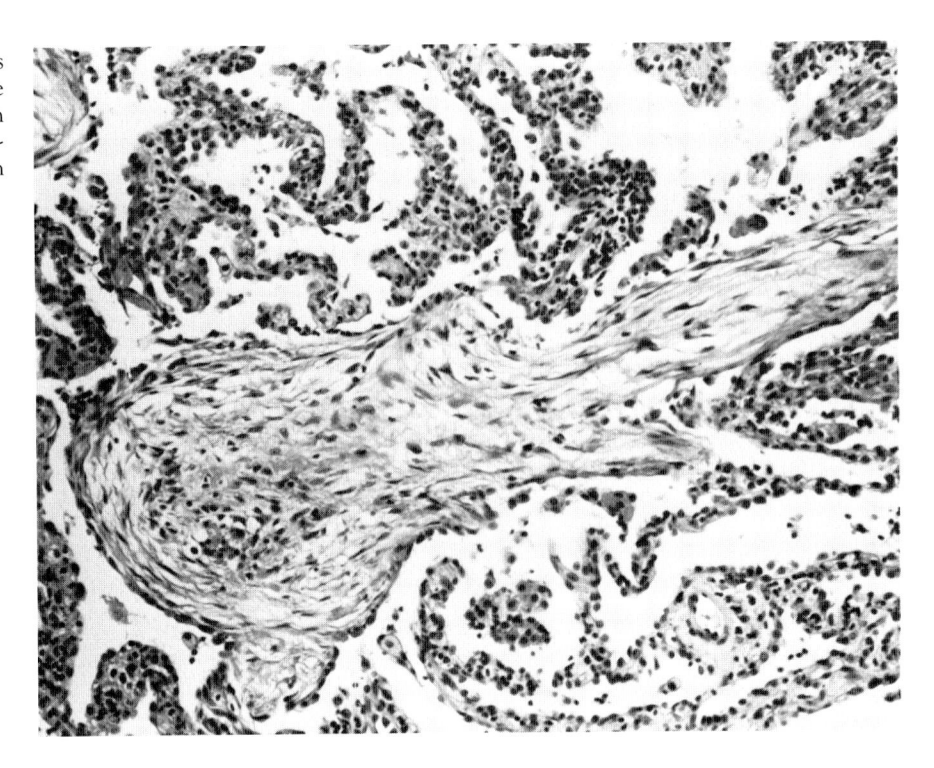

parenchyma is generally uninvolved, but it may be so atelectatic and compressed that it creates an impression of a "diffuse" lymphoid infiltrate with prominent germinal centers. Like LIP, follicular bronchiolitis may be associated with hypogammaglobulinemia. The polymorphous immunoblastic infiltrate of angioimmunoblastic lymphadenopathy and lymphomas with a similar appearance may involve the lung and bear a superficial resemblance to LIP. Like lymphocytic lymphomas, the infiltrates in these lesions tend to follow the lymphatic routes.

Pulmonary Involvement in Collagen Vascular Disease

Collagen vascular disease represents a diverse group of chronic inflammatory conditions, many of which are thought to be immunologically mediated.[83] They are associated with both localized and diffuse pulmonary lesions, and the latter accounts for a significant part of the diffuse infiltrative lung disease spectrum (see Table 20–1).

The pulmonary changes associated with rheumatoid arthritis and systemic lupus erythematosus are the most widely recognized. However, pleuropulmonary involvement is also found in most collagen vascular disease.[83,84]

The morphologic changes are summarized in Table 20–10.

Rheumatoid Arthritis

Pleuropulmonary Involvement in Adult Rheumatoid Arthritis

The incidence of pleuropulmonary disease in rheumatoid arthritis varies with the method of assessment: clinical episodes, abnormal pulmonary functions, abnormal chest radiographs, or abnormal histology.[83,136a] Although 40 percent of patients have abnormal pulmonary function tests[107,109,110,124,125] and nearly that many demonstrate some clinical evidence of pleural involvement,[83,126] no more than 5 percent of adults with rheumatoid arthritis have clinically significant parenchymal pulmonary disease.[83,93,100,102,110,126] Despite the general female predominance, both the absolute and relative frequencies of pleuropulmonary involvement appear to be greater in men.[83,93,98,101,120,126]

Of the pulmonary lesions seen in rheumatoid arthritis, only rheumatoid nodules have specific histologic features. The other pulmonary lesions associated with rheumatoid arthritis are nonspecific in the sense that they are encountered in nonrheumatoid patients. Proving an association of such lesions with a disease as common as rheumatoid arthritis has been difficult, since large numbers of cases are required to exclude a chance association. The generally accepted pulmonary lesions associated with rheumatoid arthritis are shown in Table 20–11. Table 20–12 outlines the entire spectrum of histologic lesions that have been reported and gives their presumed clinical correlates. Since the morphology of most of the lesions is described elsewhere, the discus-

Figure 20–12. Bronchiolitis obliterans with patchy organizing pneumonia. A. connective tissue plugs in alveolar ducts are cut transversely in field (left) and longitudinally (right). In the atelectatic lung (left), the alveolar duct granulation tissue proliferations are recognized by their edematous, pale appearance and even spacing at low power (H&E ×32). B. Detail of bronchiolitis obliterans from the field depicted on the left in A (H&E, ×160).

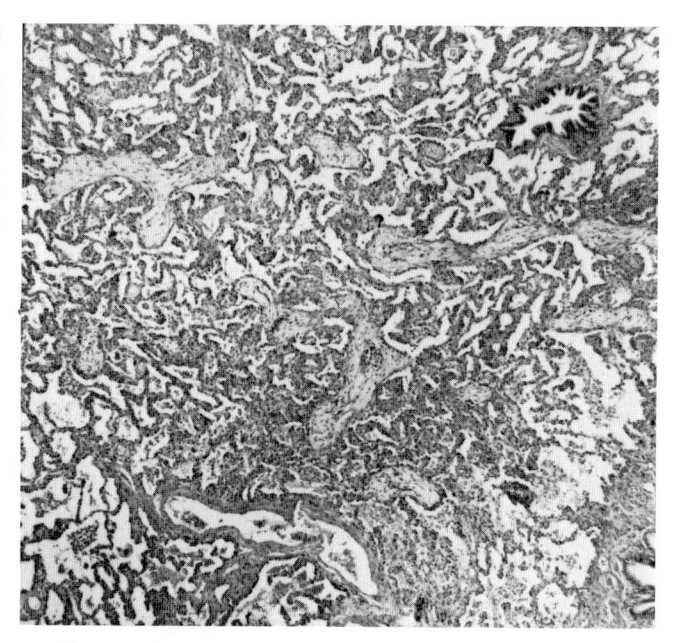

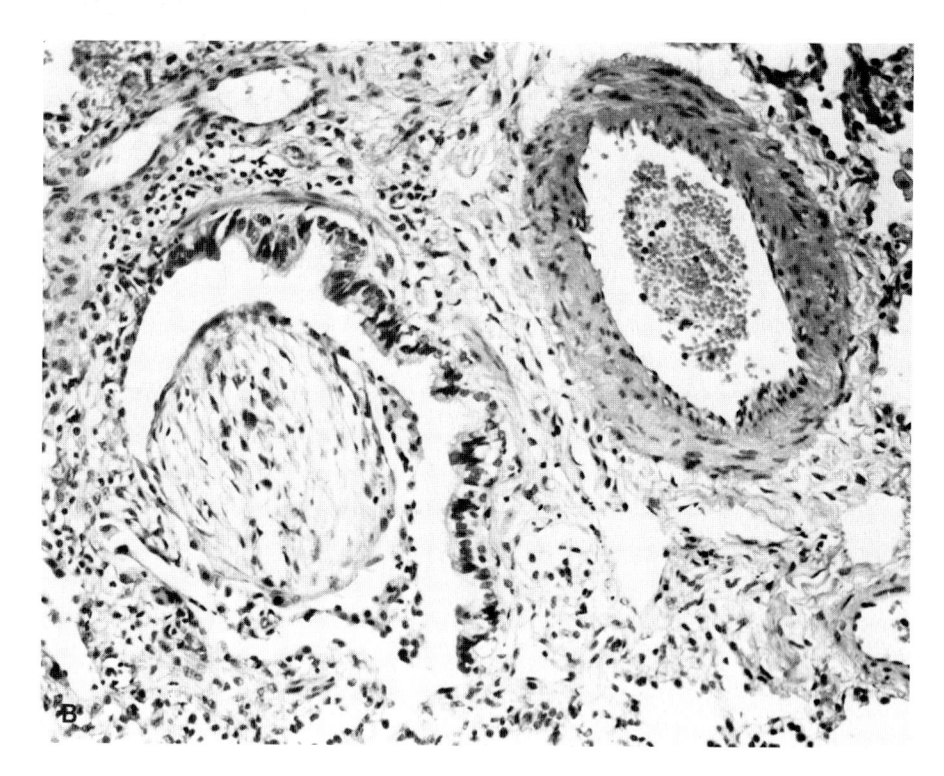

sion here concerns primarily the association with rheumatoid arthritis.

Pleurisy and/or pleural effusions are the most common form of pleuropulmonary disease in rheumatoid arthritis.[83] Histologically there is a fibrinous pleuritis that may be acute, organizing, or fibrotic. Twenty-one percent of rheumatoid arthritis patients relate a history of pleurisy; 40 percent of patients with rheumatoid arthritis who are autopsied have fibrous pleural adhesions.[126] Pleural effusions in rheumatoid arthritis characteristically show low glucose and complement levels.[126]

The clinical significance of airway lesions in rheumatoid arthritis has only recently been emphasized.[121] Nonspecific cell infiltrates in and around airways are common, and when germinal centers are prominent, the terms follicular bronchitis and follicular bronchiolitis are appropriate. Bronchitic episodes are relatively common in rheumatoid arthritis, as is evidence of mild obstructive disease on pulmonary function tests. Collins and colleagues[112] have shown a synergistic effect of smoking in producing the airway obstruction. They also found an increased frequency of the PiMS alpha-1-antitrypsin phenotype in rheumatic patients with obstructive pulmonary functions. The most serious airway lesion in rheumatoid arthritis is progressive bronchiolitis obliterans which cause the death of five of six patients reported by Geddes and co-workers.[53] Three of the six had been on penicillamine.

Interstitial lung disease usually develops during active arthritis. Only rarely does the interstital process precede the articular manifestations.[91,98] Histologic classification is difficult in some cases as the histology may vary from field to field.[53] Many cases are inseparable from idiopathic examples of UIP. A preponderance of honeycombing prevents further classification. Plasma cells and germinal centers[106] are often prominent. Germinal centers may be along airways (follicular bronchitis/bronchiolitis), scattered through the parenchyma, or in the septa (Fig. 20–15).[136a,136b]

Bronchiolitis obliterans with organizing pneumonia in rheumatoid arthritis has received little attention since it has usually been included as the generic diffuse interstitial fibrosis; however, it is a relatively common reaction pattern in rheumatoid arthritic patients with pulmonary disease.[136a] Bronchiolitis obliterans with organizing pneumonia may cause an acute and occasionally progressive process in rheumatic patients, either de novo or superimposed on another lesion, such as UIP. The three cases of Beck and Hoffbrand[94] and one of Petty and Wilkins[95] probably had bronchiolitis obliterans with organizing pneumonia which was steroid responsive. Not all patients respond to steroids, and a few die of a rapidly progressive process. Brannan and associates[91] described fluffy infiltrates as an early finding in the interstitial pneumonia of rheumatoid arthritis. The infiltrates either progressed or cleared spontaneously, and although histology is lacking, the histology may have been bronchiolitis obliterans with organizing pneumonia. Although labeled bronchiolitis obliterans, the patient of Herzog and colleagues[61] had a restrictive deficit, and a histologic description is more consistent with bronchiolitis obliterans with organizing pneumonia.

Eosinophilia of the peripheral blood is uncommon in rheumatoid arthritis, and when present is associated with an increased incidence of extra-articular manifestations.[96,136] Three cases of eosinophilic pneumonia with prominent bronchiolitis obliterans in patients with rheumatoid arthritis were reported by Cooney.[129]

Primary vascular lesions, particularly when limited to the lung, are rare in rheumatoid arthritis. Arteritis in most cases is probably the result of pulmonary hypertension. Cor pulmonale and pulmonary hypertension also occur as a nonspecific consequence of advanced interstitial disease.[117] Scarring and thickening of pulmonary blood vessels has been seen,[86] but such findings in scarred lungs are so frequent and nonspecific that their significance is questionable.

Bronchogenic carcinoma occurs in rheumatoid lung disease,[98,103,126] and in such cases probably represents an example of "scar carcinoma," analogous to that seen in patients with scleroderma and UIP.

Several immunofluorescent studies of pulmonary tissue in patients with rheumatoid arthritis have shown granular deposits of IgM or IgG and complement. Linear IgG in alveolar walls in a single case was reported by Herzog and colleagues.[61] Cervantes-Perez and associates[128] reported positive immunofluorescence findings in two patients who lacked clinical, radiographic, and functional evidence of pulmonary disease, and also described patients with no immunofluorescent findings despite infiltrative lung disease. Circulating immune complexes in rheumatoid arthritis are associated with an increased incidence of pulmonary disease,[83,84] but their role in its pathogenesis is not established. Rheumatoid factor is also markedly elevated in patients with pulmonary disease.[84]

Any discussion of pulmonary involvement in rheumatoid arthritis must include consideration of the lesions associated with gold and penicillamine therapy.[53,61,115,123,130–132,135] Pulmonary lesions in rheumatics given gold therapy have usually been associated with evidence of a systemic hypersensitivity reaction.[132] Bilateral interstitial infiltrates and restrictive pulmonary functions are usually present.[132] In the 20 patients reviewed by Scott and co-workers,[132] only one died and most showed improvement or resolution when the gold was stopped. Morphologic descriptions are scant and incomplete. An interstitial infiltrate of lymphocytes and plasma cells associated with interstitial fibrosis was described by Winterbauer and associates[115] in two patients, only one of whom had an open lung biopsy. The demonstration of gold in the lung tissue of such patients is of unknown significance, since there has been little study of the gold content in the lungs of similarly treated patients who do not develop pulmonary disease.

Reactions to penicillamine have been more varied and serious. Both obstructive and restrictive syndromes have been observed.[53,130–132] Histologically bronchiolitis obliterans is seen in those with obstructive disease.[122,136,138] Two of three patients on penicillamine reported by Geddes and colleagues died.[53] Radiographically diffuse interstitial infiltrates were present; Scott and co-workers[132] speculated that the histologic features were those of an acute interstitial pneumonia, subsequently confirmed in a report by Camus and associates.[135] Three of the four patients reported by Scott and co-workers[132] showed improvement or resolution of their pulmonary process.

Many of the histologic lesions in Tables 20–10 and 20–12 may be found together. In most cases, it is possible to identify the clinically significant process, but in some even this is difficult. The lack of histologic specificity of the lesions and a history of gold or penicillamine therapy are compounding factors. The term rheumatoid lung is vague since it could be applied to all of the syndromes in Tables 20–12. Unmodified, it fails to convey anything meaningful. A recent histologic study identified five prognostically significant categories of pathology in rheumatoid lung disease; rheumatoid nodules, UIP, bronchiolitis obliterans with patchy organizing pneumonia, lymphoid (follicular) hyperplasia, and nonspecific cellular interstitial infiltrates.[136a] Patients with rheumatoid nodules, lymphoid hyperplasia, and cellular interstitial infiltrates had a relatively favorable prognosis; those with UIP had a poor prognosis; and those who had bronchiolitis obliterans with patchy organizing pneumonia had an intermediate prognosis.[136a]

Figure 20–13. Giant cell interstitial pneumonia. There is interstitial thickening and cell infiltrates, prominence of type II pneumonocytes (some of which have artifactually sloughed in chains), and preponderance of giant cells, some cannibalistic (H&E: A ×160, B ×160).

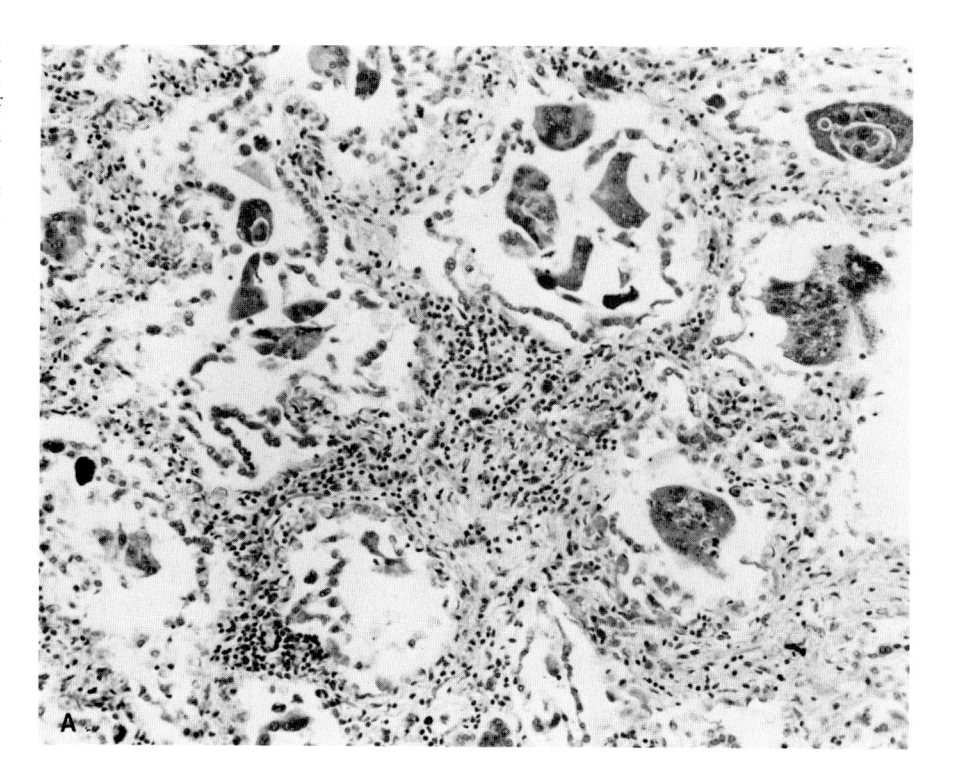

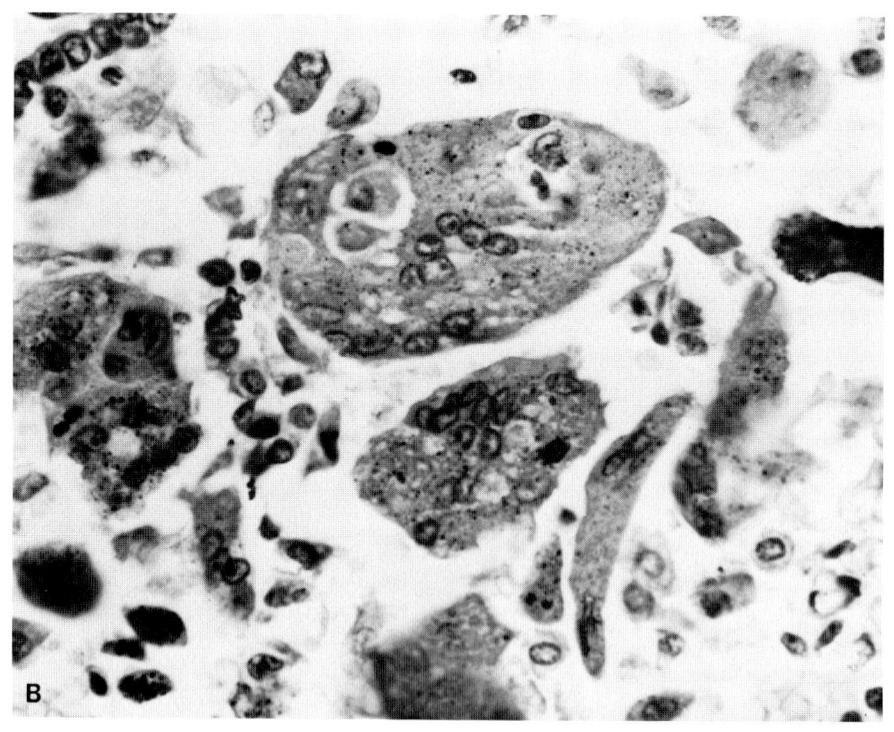

Juvenile Rheumatoid Arthritis

The sparsity of reports[98, 100, 120, 137–140] of pulmonary involvement in juvenile rheumatoid arthritis is reflected by the fact that Athreya and colleagues[139] could collect only 16 cases, of which was tissue examined histologically in only 6. Eight of the 16 cases were from their own clinic population of 191 patients with juvenile rheumatoid arthritis for an incidence of 4 percent, although a figure as high as 8 percent was suggested in one study.[139] The patients varied in age from 11 months to 19 years, with all but two under the age of 12 years. In most, pulmonary involvement occurred during active joint disease. Martel

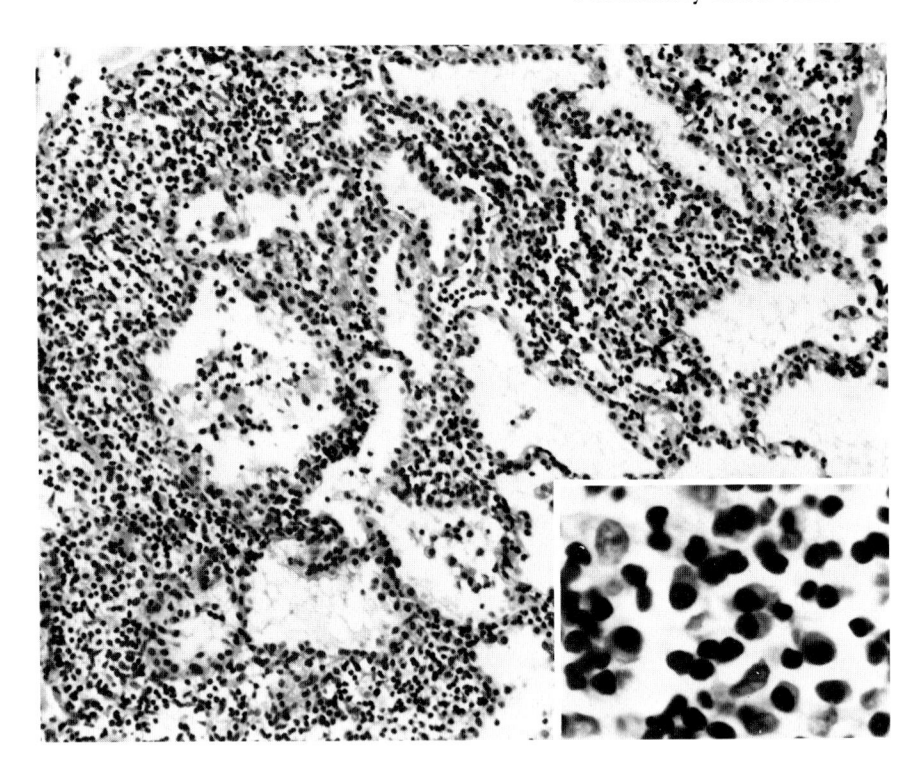

Figure 20–14. Lymphocytic interstitial pneumonia. There is a massive diffuse interstitial infiltrate that is polymorphous in composition (H&E, ×160; Inset ×640).

and colleagues,[98] however, reported a patient in whom lung disease preceded joint disease by 7 years. Clinical and pathologic features of the pulmonary lesions in juvenile rheumatoid arthritis are summarized in Table 20–13.

The presence of abnormal pulmonary functions in more than 50 percent of patients with juvenile rheumatoid arthritis[140] suggests histologic abnormalities may be more prevalent than the few cases reported would suggest. Parenchymal nodules, pulmonary hypertension with arthritis, and idiopathic pulmonary hemosiderosis are present in isolated reports, and no association with juvenile rheumatoid arthritis has been clearly established.

Pulmonary Involvement in Systemic Lupus Erythematosis

Although pleuropulmonary disease is said to be more common in systemic lupus erythematosus (SLE) than any of the other collagen diseases, involving 50 to 70 percent of patients, the number of patients with significant parenchymal lesions is probably less.[83,84,106,141–164] Pleural disease is very common.[141,149] Hematoxylin bodies are pathognomonic of systemic lupus erythematosus but they are so uncommon in the lungs (1 of 120 cases in one study[161]) that for practical purposes with ordinary light microscopy, there are no pathognomonic histologic features of pulmonary involvement.[144,164] Morphologic lesions and their clinical correlates are outlined in Table 20–14. Secondary lesions such as pulmonary edema, infection, and pulmonary emboli, although common in patients with systemic lupus erythematosus[141,161] are not included. Generally infections are the most frequent cause of pulmonary infiltrates in patients with systemic lupus erythematosis[161] and, along with pulmonary emboli, may also be associated with cavitation.[163]

The clinical syndrome of acute lupus pneumonitis has been used to encompass a number of histopathologic lesions (see Table 20–14), some of which may or may not be related to systemic lupus erythematosus; as a rule, radiographic infiltrates in systemic lupus erythematosus are usually not directly related to lupus.[161] The term lupus pneumonitis should be modified by the specific morphologic lesion. Other than infections, lesions that may cause an acute process in systemic lupus erythematosus include diffuse alveolar damage (hyaline membrane disease, ARDS), pulmonary hemorrhage, nonspecific interstitial infiltrates, pulmonary vasculitis, and bronchiolitis with patchy organizing pneumonia.

Lesions resembling idiopathic UIP are uncommon in systemic lupus erythematosus, 1 to 6 percent on review.[84] Although the incidence of patchy nonspecific interstitial inflammation and fibrosis is said by some to be almost universal in autopsy material,[83,106,141] the authors' experience has not demonstrated an increase in such lesions when compared with the general population as seen in adult autopsies. Abnormal pulmonary function with decreased diffusing capacity is relatively common in patients with systemic lupus erythematosus; 31 of 43 patients (72 percent) in one study had abnormal diffusion.[160] The abnormal pulmonary functions are probably multifactorial, and pulmonary vascular disease and diaphragmatic dysfunction are contributing factors.[152]

Pulmonary hypertension is seen in patients with systemic lupus erythematosus, 4 of 43 patients followed by Perez and associates[162] developed this complication.

Table 20–10. Pleuropulmonary Histologic Lesions in the Collagen Vascular Diseases[a]

Pulmonary Lesions	Rheumatoid Arthritis	Juvenile Rheumatoid Arthritis	Systemic Lupus Erythematosus	Scleroderma	Dermatomyositis/ Polymyositis	Mixed Connective Tissue Disease	Sjögren's Syndrome	Behçet's Syndrome	Ankylosing Spondylitis
Pleural									
Pleuritis, effusions	X	X	X	X					
Airway									
Inflammation; lymphoid hyperplasia	X	X	X	X			X		
Bronchiolitis obliterans	X				X				
Alveolar/Parenchymal									
Diffuse alveolar damage			X						
Hemorrhage		X	X	X					
Chronic interstitial pneumonia (UIP, DIP, LIP, cellular insertitial pneumonia)	X	X	X	X	X	X	X		X
Bronchiolitis obliterans with organizing pneumonia	X		X	X	X		X		
Eosinophilic infiltration (eosinophilic pneumonia)	X								
Vascular (hypertension, vasculitis)	X	X	X	X		X	X	X	
Miscellaneous									
Parenchymal nodules	X	X							
Apical fibroibullous disease	X								X
Lymphoid proliferations							X		

Abbreviations: DIP, desquamative interstitial pneumonia; LIP, lymphocytic interstitial pneumonia; UIP, usual interstitial pneumonia.
[a] See text for definitions.

Histologically the lesions are identical to those in other examples of pulmonary hypertension. In some cases, pulmonary hypertension is associated with clinical evidence of interstitial disease, whereas in others it may be the only pulmonary finding. Fayemi[151] assessed vascular lesions in 20 autopsies; abnormal vasculature was identified in eight cases including necrotizing vasculitis in four. In only one of the 20 cases had there been respiratory complaints that could have been attributed to the vascular disease. Fayemi[151] suggests that hypertension may develop from these vascular lesions, but the patients may already have had subclinical pulmonary hypertension.

Immune complexes are thought to play a significant role in the tissue injury in patients with lupus.[155] Pulmonary deposits have been identified both ultrastructurally and by immunofluorescence in vessel walls, alveolar walls, alveolar lining cells, and mesothelial cells.[148–150,153,157–159] Deposits are mainly in the alveolar interstitium.[84] Most studies[83,153,159] have shown granular deposition of IgG, IgM, IgA, and C3. IgE was also seen in cases of bronchiolitis in systemic lupus erythematosus.[153] A role for immune complexes in the pathogenesis of pulmonary hemorrhage in lupus seems likely,[159] but their role in other forms of pulmonary disease seen in lupus is less clear. Tuboloreticular inclusions have been seen ultrastructurally in a number of tissues in patients with systemic lupus erythematosus, and they may occasionally be seen in the lung.[164a]

Pulmonary Involvement in Scleroderma (Progressive Systemic Sclerosis, CREST Syndrome)

Clinical evidence of pulmonary disease in scleroderma is common, and autopsy findings in the lung are almost universal.[83,84,106,165–179a] Clinical pulmonary involvement is a major cause of morbidity and imports a poor prognosis.[178] Lung involvement is more frequent and more severe in patients with systemic forms of the disease than in those with more localized scleroder-

Table 20–11. Pulmonary Lesions Associated with Rheumatoid Arthritis[53,83,89,100,120]

Pleural reactions
Pulmonary rheumatoid nodules
Caplan's syndrome
Diffuse interstitial disease
Bronchiolitis obliterans
Arteritis

Table 20–12. Pulmonary Lesions in Rheumatoid Arthritis[a]

Histologic Lesions	Clinical Correlates

Pleural Lesions
  Fibrinous pleuritis, acute or organized
  Fibrous pleural adhesions and thickening[126]
	Pleurisy, pleural effusions, healed pleurisy
	Empyema[110]

Parenchymal Nodules (see chapters 13 and 16)
  Rheumatoid nodules,[101,119,126] usually septal or pleural
    Occasionally minute and peribronchial[87]
    Occasionally associated with sarcoid-like granulomas
 	
  Caplan's syndrome[106,107,126]
	Radiographic coin lesion(s) in majority[97,126] with or without cavitation
	
	Normal chest radiograph or interstitial markings only in some patients[97]
	Effusion, empyema (pyo)pneumothorax[97,99,110]
	Rheumatoid arthritis complicating pneumoconiosis[85,108,126]
	Cavitation and calcification on x-ray film

Airway Lesions
  Chronic cellular bronchitis, peribronchitis, bronchiolitis, peribronchiolitis[86,126]
  Follicular bronchitis/bronchiolitis[106,131,136b]
  Bronchiolitis obliterans[53,55,86,106,129,133]
  Peribronchial fibrosis and muscular hyperplasia[128]
  Bronchiectasis[100]
	Increased frequency of bronchitis and pneumonia in patients with rheumatoid arthritis[92,100,120,133,134]
	Increased frequency of functional obstruction and small-airways disease in rheumatoid arthritis[53,112,125,133]
	Asthmatic episodes[124]
	Fatal obstructive airways disease[53]
	Cryptogenic bronchiolitis obliterans[55]

Alveolar/Parenchymal Lesions[83–85,87,95,104,106,114,121]
  Honeycomb lung
  UIP (some foci resembling DIP), LIP, and combinations thereof
  Cellular interstitial pneumonia (see text)
  Characteristic features
    Numerous plasma cells
    Prominent germinal centers[87,93,106,136a,163b]
	Clinically and radiographically progressive interstitial disease indistinguishable from idiopathic UIP.[90,100,102,126] Rare cases appear to be more responsive to steroids than idiopathic UIP[90,100,102,116]
	Increased frequency of subclinical restrictive disease in rheumatoid arthritis[109]
	"Shrinking lung" in rheumatoid arthritis[120]
	?Associated with pneumothorax[98]
	Bilateral upper lobe infiltrates[120]

Miscellaneous
  Nonspecific parenchymal or subpleural scarring[86,92,97]
  Metaplastic ossification[86]
  Bronchiolitis obliterans with patchy organizing pneumonia[95,106,136a]
    (overlap with airway lesions—see text)
 	
  Eosinophilic infiltrations[129]
  Septal infiltration
  Eosinophilic pneumonia
  Pulmonary arteritis/venulitis (± infarction)[96,100,113,122]
  Pulmonary hypertension[100,117,118]
  Arterial intimal and/or adventitial fibrosis[86]
  No histology
  Bronchopulmonary amyloidosis
  Bronchogenic carcinoma[98,103,126]
	History of increased frequency of bronchitis, pneumonia, pleurisy in patients with rheumatoid arthritis[92,100,120]
	Acute, occasionally progressive and fatal pulmonary disease in rheumatoid arthritis presenting as localized, patchy, or diffuse infiltrates. Some cases steroid responsive.[94,95]
	Peripheral eosinophilia pneumonia radiographically and clinically[96,129,136]
	Increased frequency of pleuropulmonary involvement in rheumatoid patients with hypereosinophilia[96]
	Clinical findings of pulmonary hypertension or rapidly progressive respiratory failure[122]
	
	Apical fibrobullous disease[84,89,127]
	See pp. 491.
	See Chapter 19.

[a] Based on the results of Cruickshank,[88] Gardner,[105] personal observations, and references as shown.

ma.[179a] The majority of patients are women, and most give a history of well-established extrapulmonary manifestations of scleroderma prior to the development of significant pulmonary disease.[168] Most patients are older than age 50 years, but pulmonary involvement under the age of 10 has been well documented.[177] The most common symptoms are dyspnea, orthopnea, cough, and, less commonly, recurrent pneumonias. In patients with severe pulmonary vascular disease, signs and symptoms of cor pulmonale develop. Spontaneous pneumothorax may occur.

Chest x-ray films are abnormal in up to 80 percent of patients with scleroderma.[170] Typical radiographic changes include bilateral, lower lobe, reticulonodular infiltrates, sometimes with subpleural honeycombing or pleural thickening. Right ventricular hypertrophy from pulmonary hypertension may be superimposed.

Abnormal pulmonary function tests usually precede the clinical and radiographic abnormalities.[83] Restrictive disease with decrease diffusing capacity is seen[84,179a]; abnormal diffusion may be the only finding in some cases.[84,167] Evidence of airflow obstruction may be seen in the later stages of scleroderma.[84,172]

The two major lesions in pulmonary scleroderma are vascular disease with pulmonary hypertension and interstitial fibrosis.[83,167,168,174,175,179] The latter is indistinguishable from UIP and is the more common of the two. Some degree of interstitial fibrosis was present in all 28 autopsy cases studied by Weaver and colleagues,[168] and this was associated with subpleural honeycombing in 26 patients,

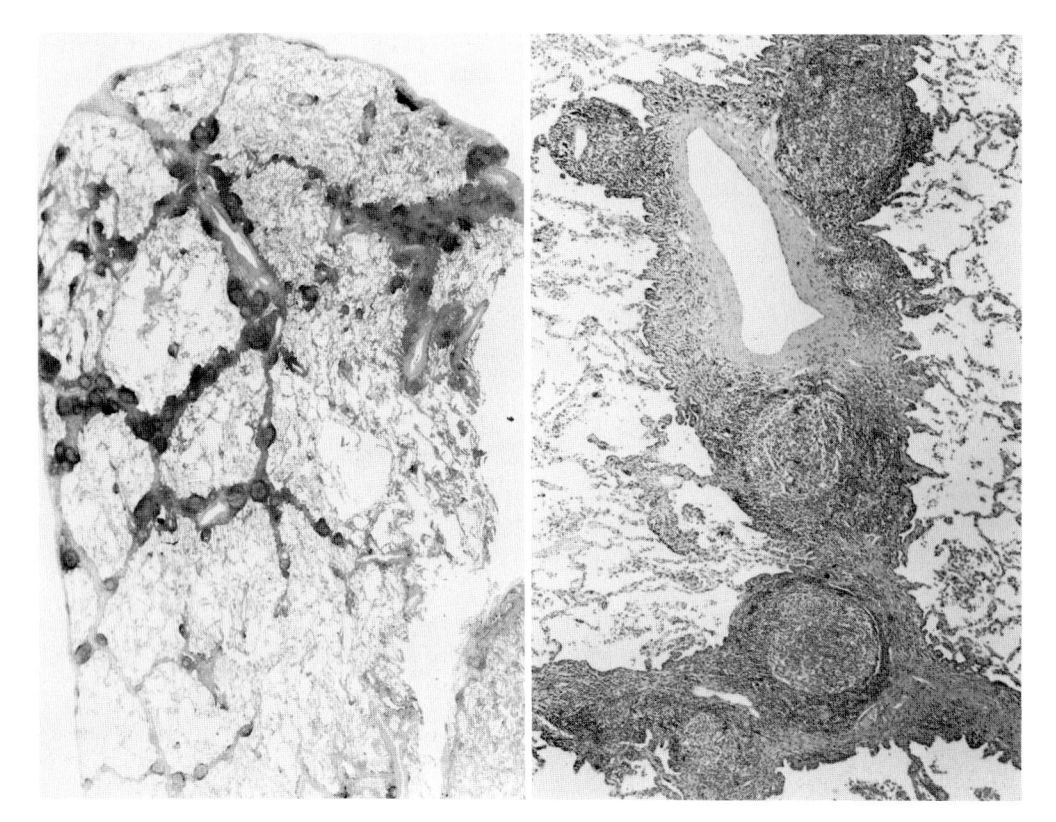

Figure 20-15. Lymphoid hyperplasia in rheumatoid arthritis. Marked reactive follicular hyperplasia follows a lymphangitic distribution. An interstitial infiltrate of eosinophils (not illustrated) was also present (H&E: left ×5, right ×32).

although these features were rarely a direct cause of death. Subpleural honeycombing is characteristic of scleroderma and is thought to predispose to spontaneous pneumothorax.[165] Interstitial fibrosis in scleroderma appears from some studies[83,170] to be more indolent and more slowly progressive than UIP. Conversely some cases may be recognized earlier because lung disease is specifically sought. Rapidly progressing interstitial pneumonia has also been reported.[176]

Although less common than interstitial disease, pulmonary vascular lesions in scleroderma are more often the cause of symptoms.[175] Minor changes in vessels are found in nearly all patients with scleroderma at autopsy.[166,168] However, severe morphologic changes are seen in less than half and clinically significant lesions in still fewer. These findings correlate with clinical studies[166] that show increased pulmonary vascular resistance in about half the patients, most of whom also have some degree of right ventricular hypertrophy. Somewhat less than 10 percent of patients with scleroderma develop severe and fulminant pulmonary hypertension with vascular lesions similar to those in the kidneys in malignant hypertension, although there is no correlation between the two.[175] Salerni and co-workers[174] described ten patients with pulmonary hypertension in scleroderma and maintained that clinically significant pulmonary hypertension is usually associated with the CREST (calcinosis, Raynaud's Phenomenon esophageal dysfunction, sclerodactyly, and telangiectasia) variant of scleroderma. In one case, pulmonary hypertension developed in a patient who had had the syndrome for 40 years. Pulmonary venoocclusive disease has also been described in scleroderma.[179]

The morphologic changes in the pulmonary vessels are characteristic and almost pathognomonic.[166,168,175] There is some medial thickening, but the most distinctive change is onion-skin proliferation of the intima with depostion of PAS-positive and Alcian blue–positive material between the cells.[166] Intimal proliferation may entirely occlude the lumen of the vessel. Fibrinoid necrosis and plexiform lesions, both of which are seen in idiopathic primary pulmonary hypertension and pulmonary hypertension associated with systemic lupus erythematosus, are not seen in scleroderma.[175] Interstitial fibrosis and pulmonary vascular disease in scleroderma are commonly found in the same lung, but they do not appear to be causally related[163,175] except in the cases of secondary pulmonary hypertension due to widespread interstitial fibrosis.

A number of other pleuropulmonary changes have been described in scleroderma.[168] Fibrous pleural thickening is common and was seen at autopsy in 24 of the 28 cases reported by Weaver and associates,[168] but the incidence of pleural effusion is much lower than in other

Table 20-13. Pulmonary Lesions in Juvenile Rheumatoid Arthritis[a]

Pathologic Lesions	Clinical Correlates

Pleural Lesions
  Fibrinous pleuritis (± organization)
  Adhesions[137]
	Pleurisy, effusions

No Histology	Multiple bilateral cavitary nodules on chest x-ray films
Airway Lesions Follicular bronchiolitis (lymphoid bronchiolitis)	Bilateral reticulonodular infiltrates Patchy infiltrates

Alveolar/Parenchymal Lesions
  Cellular interstitial infiltrates
  Interstitial fibrosis
  Lymphocytic interstitial pneumonia
	More than 50% of patients with juvenile rheumatoid arthritis have abnormal functions: abnormal ventilation to perfusion flow rates, or low diffusing capacity[140]
	Progressive (and fatal) interstitial disease

No histology	Patchy infiltrates clearing spontaneously or on steroids; syndrome of pleuritis, pericarditis, migratory pneumonitis[138]

Miscellaneous Lesions
  Vascular lesions
  Arteritis and pulmonary hypertension[100]
	Chest pain, dyspnea, sudden death

Pulmonary hemosiderosis (diagnosis confirmed only by presence of hemosiderin-filled macrophages in sputum) Amyloidosis[120,137]	Clinical features of idiopathic pulmonary hemosiderosis

[a] Based on the results of Athreya et al.[139] and references as shown.

Table 20-14. Pulmonary Involvement in Systemic Lupus Erythematosus

Histologic Lesion	Clinical Correlate
Pleura Fibrinous pleuritis ± organization, adhesions, chronic inflammatory cells	Polyserositis Pleural effusions
Parenchymal Nodules No histologic correlate	Radiologic atelectasis—especially peripheral basal segments[143,149]

Airway Lesions
  Follicular bronchiolitis[153]
  Peribronchiolitis[153]
	Acute cough, dyspnea[153]

Alveolar/Parenchymal Lesions
  Diffuse alveolar damage ± organization[106]
  Bronchiolitis obliterans with organizing pneumonia[164]
	Unilateral or bilateral infiltrates, fever, hypoxia

Pulmonary edema[145,162]	Pulmonary edema

Alveolar hemorrhage[150,154,158,160]
(see chapter 18)
  Acute
  Recurrent resembling idiopathic pulmonary hemosiderosis[146]
	"Acute lupus pneumonitis"
	Bilateral infiltrates
	Acute and fulminant or chronic with waxing and waning

Cellular interstitial pneumonia[157]	"Lupus pneumonitis"
Patchy nonspecific interstitial[144] inflammation	—
UIP[84,142,147,153,162] LIP[148,159] DIP[153]	Clinical, radiologic, and functional features of chronic interstitial pneumonia[84,142,143,147,161,163]

Miscellaneous lesions
  Vascular thickening medial and intimal[144,151,163]
  Acute vasculitis[144]
	Pulmonary hypertension[163]
	"Acute lupus pneumonitis"[144]

No histologic correlate	Diaphragm dysfunction with elevation and loss of volume[143,152]

Abbreviations: As in Table 20-10.
[a] After Hunninghake,[83] personal observations, and references as noted.

collagen vascular diseases. Weaver and associates also noted evidence at autopsy of acute bronchitis, chronic bronchitis, and bronchiolectasis in more than half of their 28 patients. Peribronchial fibrosis was present in four. Bronchiolitis obliterans and granulation tissue in alveolar ducts was noted by Nozawa.[106] Some of these lesions may represent the morphologic correlate of airway obstruction described in 42 percent of patients by Guttadauria and colleagues.[172] Kallenbach and co-workers[173] reported a patient with scleroderma and recurrent hemoptysis that remitted with steroid therapy.

There have been a number of reports of bronchogenic carcinoma in patients with scleroderma.[83,171] The majority of these have been bronchoalveolar carcinomas, and they are thought to arise from the atypical metaplastic epithelium associated with pulmonary fibrosis.[171] Patients who develop carcinoma typically show an abrupt deterioration in pulmonary status.

Abnormal esophageal motility is characteristic of scleroderma. This predisposes to recurrent bouts of aspiration pneumonia which may lead to recurrent patchy infiltrates and complicate any of the lesions already described.

Pulmonary Involvement in Eosinophilic Fascitis

Eosinophilic fascitis is a syndrome related to scleroderma. Intrinsic pulmonary disease has not been described in eosinophilic fascitis; however, Epler and associates[123] described a patient with eosinophilic fascitis who developed bronchiolitis obliterans while on penicillamine therapy.

460   Infiltrative Lung Disease

Table 20–15. Pulmonary Lesions in Sjögren's Syndrome[a]

Tracheobronchitis, submucosal gland atrophy[83]
Asthma[187]
Peribronchiolitis with airway narrowing[133,185]
Bronchiolitis obliterans[133]
Bronchiolitis obliterans with patchy organizing pneumonia[b]
Recurrent infections
  Bronchitis
  Bronchiectasis
  Pneumonia
Discoid atelectasis
UIP (diffuse interstitial fibrosis)
LIP
Granulomas[187]
Pseudolymphoma
Malignant lymphoma
Amyloidosis[186]
Vasculitis
Pleural effusions

Abbreviations: As in Table 20–10.
[a] Based on the results of Strimlan et al.[184] and as noted.
[b] Personal observations.

Pulmonary Involvement in Mixed Connective Tissue Disease

Mixed connective tissue disease shares some features with other collagen vascular disease but is distinguished from them by the serologic finding of antibody to extractable nuclear antigen.[180] Only a few cases of pulmonary disease in mixed connective tissue disease have been reported, but the incidence of pulmonary involvement appears to be significant.[83,181–183] In one series, 84 percent of patients had either abnormal chest radiographs, abnormal pulmonary function tests, or both.[181] Pulmonary function studies[181] have shown decreased diffusing capacity and restriction, and chest radiographs show diffuse infiltrates with or without evidence of effusion. In one study,[182] steroid-responsive segmental consolidation was described. Although Harmon[181] reported an excellent response to steroids in 12 of 14 patients with resolution of all abnormalities in 6 patients, Wiener-Kronish and co-workers[183] reported five cases with severe rapidly progressive lung disease that was not steroid responsive. Three of the patients in this latter series had only severe pulmonary hypertension.

Morphologic descriptions of the lungs in mixed connective disease are incomplete. Histologic changes appear to be those of UIP and pulmonary hypertension.[83,182,183] The vascular changes described are similar to those seen in the pulmonary hypertension associated with systemic lupus erythematosus. Unlike in lupus, immune complexes have not been found in the cases of interstitial disease.[183]

Pulmonary Involvement in Sjögren's Syndrome

Defining pulmonary involvement in Sjögren's syndrome is difficult because Sjögren's syndrome is commonly associated with other collagen vascular diseases.[83,184–189] About half of patients with Sjögren's syndrome have evidence of rheumatoid arthritis.[83,187] Pulmonary function abnormalities in patients with primary biliary cirrhosis have been attributed to coexisting Sjögren's syndrome.[188]

The majority of patients with Sjögren's syndrome are women with known collagen vascular disease who have insidiously developed the syndrome.[83] Pulmonary disease is frequent, with pleurisy or interstitial lung disease seen in up to 15 percent of patients.[83,184] Most lesions are similar, if not identical, to those associated with rheumatoid arthritis; however, atrophy of tracheobronchial submucosal glands and lymphocytic interstitial pneumonia are characteristic of Sjögren's syndrome (Table 20–15).[83]

As in the salivary gland, there is a diffuse lymphocytic infiltrate of the bronchial submucosal glands. This is associated with atrophy of the glands and stasis in the small airways with atelectasis, secondary infection, and ultimately peribronchial scarring.[83,185] The patients have cough, problems expectorating, and recurrent bouts of bronchitis. Pulmonary function tests show peripheral airflow obstruction.[83,185,187] A restrictive ventilatory defect has been found in up to 60 percent of patients.[187] The symptoms may be steriod responsive.[83] Hyperinflation is a radiographic finding in some.[189]

The largest reported series of pulmonary involvement in Sjögren's syndrome is that a Strimlan and colleagues[184] who studied 343 patients with a history of Sjögren's syndrome from one month to 23 years. Thirty-one (9 percent) had evidence of pulmonary disease (including those with lesions of tracheobronchial submucosal glands). Their symptoms were cough, dyspnea, recurrent pneumonia, and pleurisy. Radiographically diffuse interstitial infiltrates were seen in 16, diffuse alveolar infiltrates in 4, and pleural effusions in 5. Eighteen patients showed evidence of restriction or decreased diffusing capacity. Histologic findings were available in 13 patients, lymphocytic interstitial pneumonia in 3, amyloidosis in 2, pseudolymphoma in 1, malignant lymphoma in 3, UIP in 2, and bronchopneumonia in 4. Fairfax and associates[187] noted pulmonary parenchymal granulomas in 2 of 15 patients with Sjögren's syndrome; both had positive antimitochondrial antibody titers, and 1 had proven primary biliary cirrhosis.

Pulmonary Involvement in Polymyositis/Dermatomyositis

Overall pleuropulmonary involvement in polymyositis/dermatomyositis (PM/DM) is considerably less frequent than in other collagen vascular diseases.[64,83,190–197]

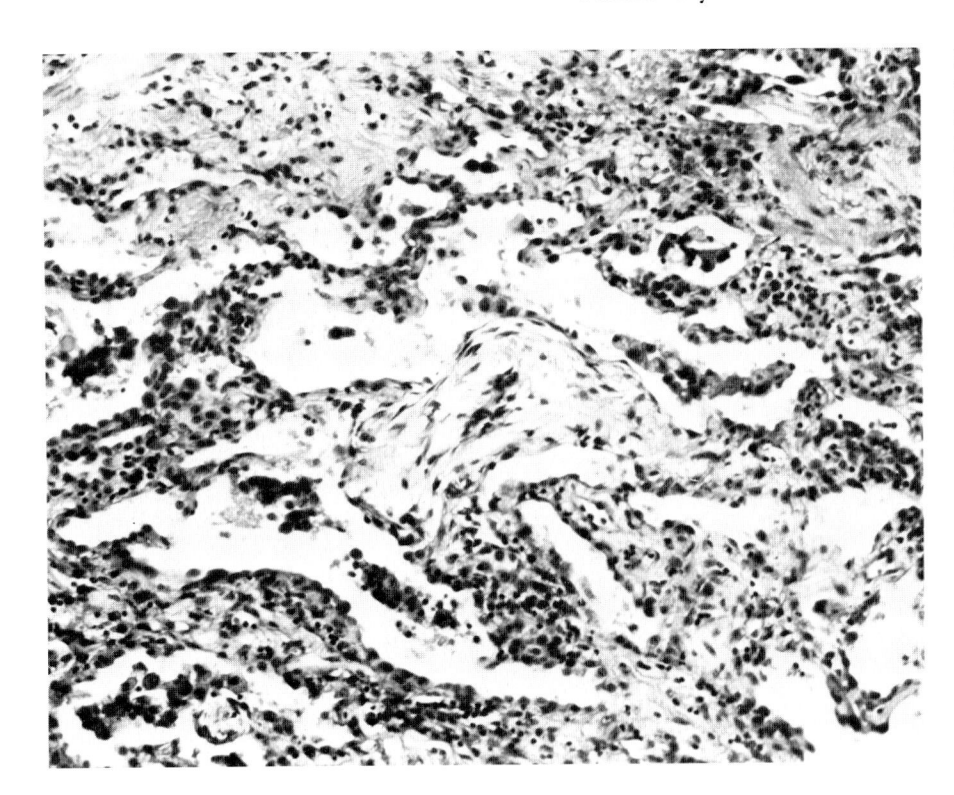

Figure 20–16. Bronchiolitis obliterans with patchy organizing pneumonia in polymyositis. Young connective tissue partially fills an alveolar duct. The adjacent alveolar walls have an interstitial infiltrate and prominent type II alveolar lining cells. This lesion was steroid-responsive (H&E, ×160).

Although the percentage of patients with infiltrative lung disease may be roughly the same (5 percent), a figure of 9 percent was found in one series.[208] Not included among these are cases of aspiration (which are common) and hypoventilation secondary to muscle disease.[83,100,197a] In 1976 Schwarz and colleagues[64] cited 500 cases of PM/DM that did not have associated pulmonary disease, but they were able to find another 37 cases, including 6 of their own, in which pulmonary involvement was present. The patients ranged from 5 to 76 years of age. In nearly 40 percent, the pulmonary symptoms preceded evidence of skin or muscle disease by as much as 3 years. In 20 percent of the patients, lung and skin or muscle involvement developed concurrently. About twice as many women as men were affected. Presenting symptoms included progressive dyspnea and cough. Chest radiographs showed bilateral lower lobe reticulonodular infiltrates without effusions. Alveolar infiltrates, which were often steroid responsive, were also described. Pulmonary function tests showed restriction with decreased diffusing capacity. Pulmonary involvement in PM/DM does not appear to correlate with severity of muscle disease.[83]

The histology in most cases of PM/DM has been described as UIP; however, there is probably more than one lesion. A cellular inflammatory lesion termed organizing pneumonia has also been described.[64,106,193] By description and illustration, this appears to be bronchiolitis obliterans with patchy organizing pneumonia (Fig. 20–16). Three of the six patients reported by Schwarz and colleagues[64] had this pattern in addition to interstitial fibrosis. The presence of this lesion was correlated with a better response to steroid therapy. Approximately 50 percent of patients with interstitial lung disease in PM/DM respond to steroids.[83] Schwarz and colleagues[64] and Duncan and colleagues[193] postulate that the responders have the more acute process (bronchiolitis obliterans with organizing penumonia) in which there is significantly less fibrosis. Some have referred to this as acute fibrile pneumonitis.[192] The second lesion in PM/DM is interstitial fibrosis associated with relatively little inflammation, essentially UIP. Whether the former develops into the latter or whether they are two separate processes is not clear. Schwarz and associates[64] speculated that they were related and the acute lesion was the early stage of the UIP, using this as an argument for early steroid therapy in interstitial lung disease in PM.

In most patients the evolution of the interstitial lung disease in PM is relatively slow; few patients die of their pulmonary disease,[64,197] although fulminant fatal cases have been reported.[194] Electron microscopy in two cases showed no evidence of immune complexes.[197] Pleural fibrosis at autopsy is common, and acute pleuritis may be seen on biopsies.[197] Other forms of pulmonary involvement in PM/DM are unusual. Bunch and co-workers[196] reported a woman with PM with fulminant pulmonary hypertension.

Pulmonary Involvement in Ankylosing Spondylitis

Two broad categories of pulmonary abnormality in ankylosing spondylitis are recognized: chest wall restriction leading to chronic hypoventilation and parenchymal pulmonary disease, primarily upper lobe fibrobullus change.[83,198–206] The latter is characteristic of ankylosing spondylitis. Although some studies[205] have reported an incidence of pulmonary disease as high as 30 percent, the largest study, that of Rosenow and associates,[205] which included 2080 cases, gave a figure of 1.3 percent. Twenty-eight cases were identified: 26 with apical fibrobullous disease, 3 with transient pleural effusions, and 1 with severe pleural fibrosis leading to respiratory failure. Two patients gave a history of pneumothorax.[205] Cromptom and co-workers[201] reported two cases with extensive pleural fibrosis.[201]

Patients with ankylosing spondylitis and upper lobe fibrobullous disease are usually men and all are adults; reported cases show an age range from 38 to 83 years. Average age at recognition of pulmonary disease is 60 years.[205] In most patients, bony involvement has been present for many years, up to 58 years in one study,[201] and the majority of patients with apical fibrobullous disease have complete ankylosis of the spine and inactive arthritis.[203,205] Apical fibrobullous disease is usually asymptomatic;[83,205] shortness of breath from chest wall restriction may be present. The apical fibrobullous disease is usually identified radiologically.[205] Patients with complications such as pneumothorax or fungus ball may have fever, cough, or hemoptysis.[200]

The lesion usually begins in one upper lobe and eventually becomes bilateral; however, a significant number of patients have only one upper lobe involved at the time of recognition. There is initially an increase in interstitial markings associated with pleural thickening. Cysts, cavities, and ultimately bullae develop.[205] Occasionally the process involves the midlung fields.[200] Severe scarring may result in elevation of the hilar.[83] The radiologic rate of progression of the changes is variable, and the lesions often remain static for many years.[205]

Pulmonary function tests show decrease in vital capacity and increase in residual volume.[198,205] The proportion of such changes that are related to fixation of the chest wall is not always clear.[83]

The morphologic features of the changes in the upper lobe are nonspecific.[198–200,202,204] Grossly the lungs show honeycombing and bullae. Histologically there is interstitial fibrosis, stasis of secretion, organization, metaplastic epithelium, and bullae. Bronchiectasis has been described.[202]

Few patients die directly of pulmonary parenchymal disease. Complications of fibrobullous disease and ankylosing spondylitis include pneumothorax with an occasional presenting symptom and secondary infection which is a significant cause of morbidity and mortality.[198,200,201,204–206] Of the 26 patients with apical changes described by Rosenow and associates, 5 had aspergillomas.[205] In addition to *Aspergillus fumigatus*, *Aspergillus terreus*, *Metshnikowia pulcherrima*, and *Allescheria boydii*, various species of mycobacteria may be secondary pathogens.[83,206] An unfortunate problem with surgery in these patients is that up to 50 percent develop postoperative chronic empyema or bronchopleural fistula.[83] The relatively high incidence of cavitary tuberculosis reported in the past in patients with ankylosing spondylitis was probably due to the misinterpretation of apical fibrobullous disease for the changes of tuberculosis.[212,216]

Pulmonary Involvement in Behcet's Syndrome

Descriptions of pulmonary involvement in Behcet's syndrome are few and incomplete.[83] Transient infiltrates, reticulonodular opacities, and rounded densities associated with exacerbation of the extrapulmonary disease have been described.[83,208] Pleurisy, pleural effusions, and hemoptysis may be present, and hemoptysis may be severe.[83,208] These findings have been attributed to pulmonary vasculitis.[208] Slavin and de Groot[207] reported the histologic findings in the lung in one patient with Behçet's syndrome who had a localized infiltrate and severe hemorrhage requiring lobectomy. Histologic study showed a necrotizing lymphocytic or neutrophilic vasculitis involving arteries, veins, and capillaries. Early and healed vasculitis was seen, attesting to the episodic nature of the lesion. The authors compiled the following list of complications of Behcet's syndrome in the lung: aneurysms of the elastic arteries, venous and arterial thromboses, infarcts, and erosion of airways by aneurysms.[207] Steroids may suppress some of the inflammatory changes but do not appear to alter the ultimate course of the disease.[208]

Pulmonary Involvement in Essential Mixed Cryoglobulinemia

Essential mixed cryoglobulinemia is associated with purpura, arthralgias, weakness, serum cryoglobulins, and rheumatoid factor activity.[209] In a report of 23 patients with essential mixed cryoglobulinemia by Bombardieri and associates,[209] significant pulmonary complaints were present in 9 patients, including cough, dyspnea, and, less commonly, asthma, pleurisy, or hemoptysis. Some degree of interstitial lung disease on chest radiograph was present in 18 patients. Pulmonary function tests showed evidence of peripheral airflow obstruction. Histologic studies were not obtained in any of these patients. Circulating cryoglobulins are found in a significant number of patients with UIP.[38]

Sarcoidosis

Classic Pulmonary Sarcoidosis

Sarcoidosis is a systemic granulomatous disease with protean clinical manifestations and frequent pulmonary manifestations.[210-245] Sarcoidosis has been histologically defined by Mitchell and Scadding[211] as "a disease characterized by the presence in all of several affected organs and tissue of noncaseating epithelioid cell granulomas, proceeding either to resolution or to conversion into hyaline connective tissue." A more encompassing definition, in reality a description, was adopted in 1975 at the Seventh International Conference on Sarcoidosis[241]:

> Sardoidosis is a multisystem granulomatous disorder of unknown etiology, most commonly affecting young adults and presenting most frequently with bilateral hilar lymphadenopathy, pulmonary infiltration, skin or eye lesions. The diagnosis is established most securely when clinical and radiographic findings are supported by histologic evidence of widespread, non-caseating epitheloid cell granulomas in more than one organ, or positive Kveim-Siltzbach skin test. Immunologic features are depression of delayed type hypersensitivities suggesting impaired cell mediated immunity, and raised or abnormal immunoglobulins. There may also be hypercalcuria with or without hypercalcemia. The prognosis may correlate with the mode of onset: an acute onset with erythema nodosum heralds a self limiting course and spontaneous resolution, whereas an insidious onset may be followed by relentless, progressive fibrosis. Corticosteroids relieve symptoms and suppress inflammation and granuloma formation.

Sarcoidosis is capable of resolving spontaneously without a recognizable residual lesion. There are also a number of individuals whose sarcoidosis is asymptomatic or at least subclinical. It is not known how often these events occur together, but the frequency of accidental discovery of sarcoidosis suggests that there is a substantial number of affected individuals who are never detected. The following descriptions are based on detected cases, but the prevalence of the disease is understated and the frequency of one manifestation or another correspondingly overstated.

The following description is based on three large clinical reviews.[211,222,239] In the United States, blacks are affected more frequently than whites, and among blacks, female patients predominate. In Europe sarcoidosis is more common in northern countries. Ninety percent of cases occur between the ages of 20 and 40 years. Onset before age 10 or after 60 is unusual,[243] although 1 percent are older than age 70 at the time of diagnosis.[216] Approximately 40 cases per 100,000 population are seen in the United States.

Of recognized cases, slightly less than 10 percent are asymptomatic and are discovered during evaluation for other conditions. Some patients have a fulminant course with high fever and arthralgias, but in the majority, the onset is insidious with symptoms varying depending on the organs most severely affected. In one study[245c] the frequency of symptoms was greater in older women than in other groups. Respiratory symptoms include shortness of breath, cough, chest pain, and, less commonly,

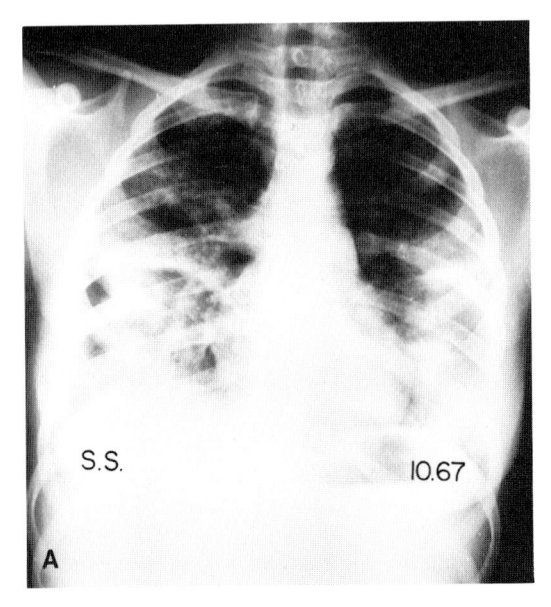

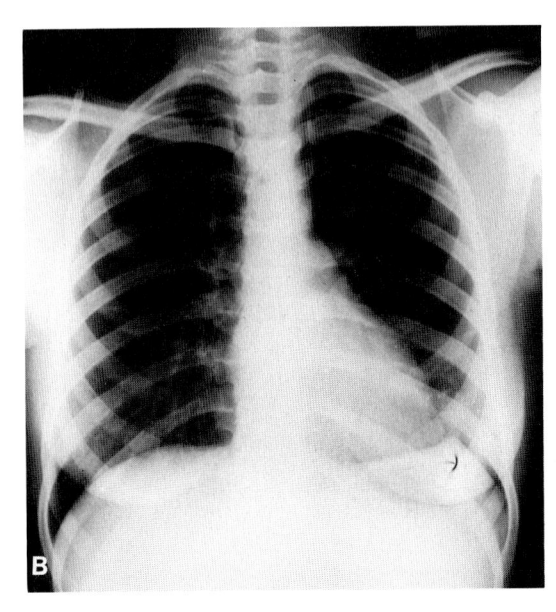

Figure 20–17. Sarcoidosis. A. An extensive bilateral reticular and fluffy infiltrate was seen on the chest radiograph at presentation. B. This patient's chest radiograph was normal 2½ years later. A, reproduced with permission of Lippincott, Harper & Row.

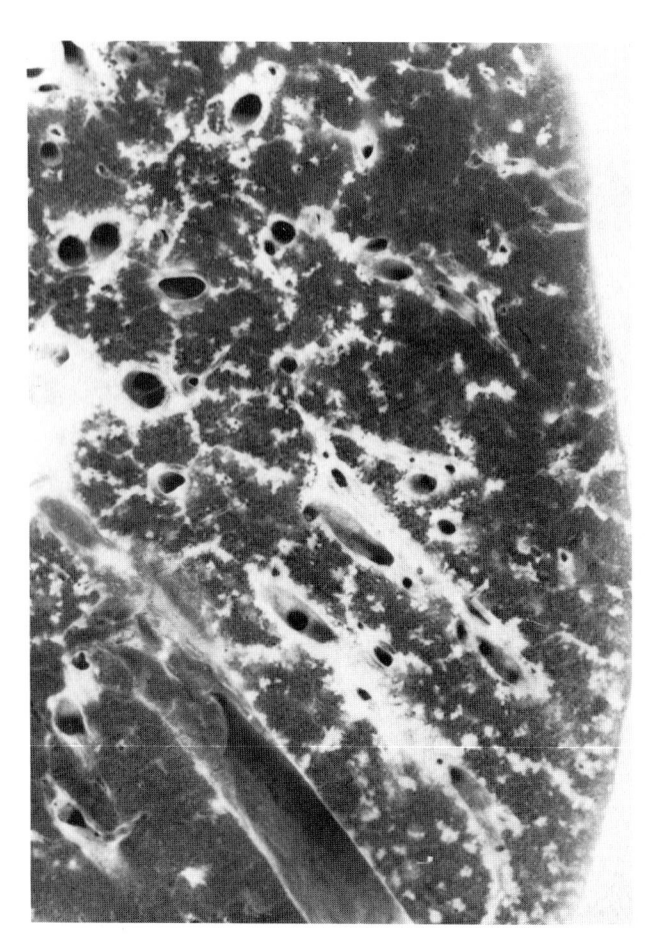

Figure 20–18. Sarcoidosis. A delicate lacework of granulomas follows the lymphatic routes in the pleura and septa and along veins and bronchovascular rays. Courtesy of Dr. Bensch, Stanford, CA.

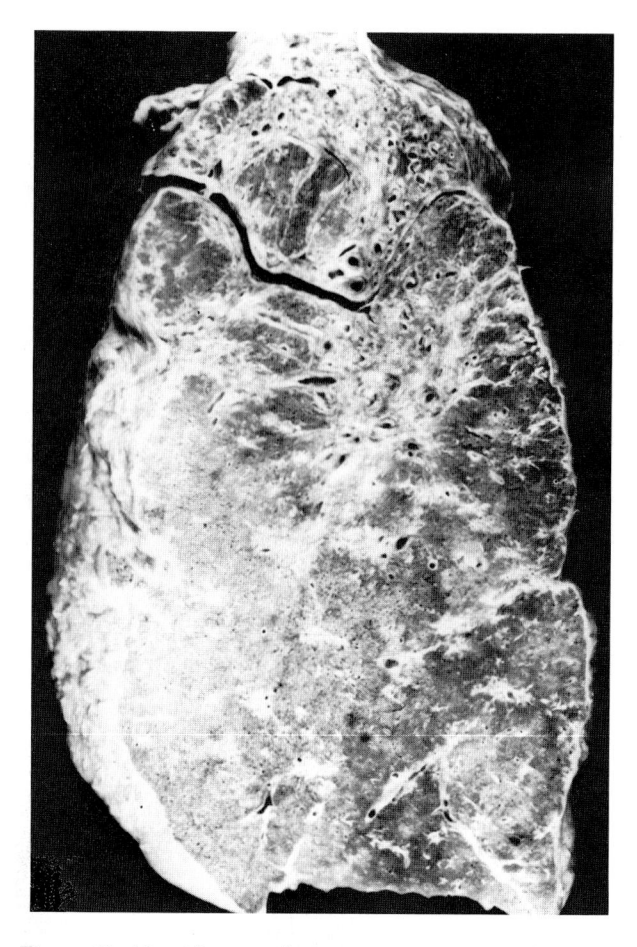

Figure 20–19. Honeycombing at autopsy in sarcoidosis. More severe disease is shown in the upper lobe. A tracery of scarring and granuloma remains around the vessels (lymphatic routes) in the lower lobe.

hemoptysis which can be massive.[245d] Whites are more frequently asymptomatic than blacks.

The chest radiographic findings vary enormously: 5 to 10 percent of patients have normal chest radiographs despite the fact that granulomas in the lungs are identified histologically. One-third of all patients (40 percent of black patients) have both pulmonary infiltrates and bilateral hilar lymph node enlargement. Another one-third have hilar or mediastinal lymph node enlargement alone, which is unilateral in 5 percent. Pulmonary infiltrates may be reticular, reticulonodular, alveolar (Fig. 20–17), or show a ground glass appearance,[26] and are not necessarily bilteral.[238] Peripheral pulmonary infiltrates were recently described in eight patients with sarcoidosis.[245b] Nodules larger than 1 cm are seen in 2 to 4 percent of cases, and cavitation has occasionally been noted. Honeycombing, apical fibrocystic disease, bullae, and giant bullous emphysema (vanishing lung) may be seen in progressive disease.[234] Pleural effusions are seen in slightly less than 10 percent of patients.

Nearly half the patients have abnormal liver function tests, 70 percent have hypergammaglobulinemia, 25 percent have positive antinuclear antibodies, and 20 percent show either hypercalcemia, hypercalcuria, or both. Cutaneous anergy is present in 40 percent. A majority of patients with active sarcoidosis have elevation of the serum angiotension converting enzyme (ACE).[229,240,242] Since ACE elevation serum may be seen in conditions other than sarcoid, its use as a diagnostic tool is limited and histologic confirmation is still recommended.[229,242] Serum ACE may be useful in following disease activity in individual patients. ACE has been identified immunohistologically in sarcoid granulomas.[245] Immunologic abnormalities in sarcoidosis have been recognized for many years since many patients have erythema nodosum, cutaneous anergy, or hypergammaglobulinemia.[221,222,237,239] Recent studies[230–232,244,245a] suggest that the number of helper T-cells is increased at sites of active disease and that such cells release lymphokines that recruit monocytes and macrophages which ultimately form the granulomas.

Pulmonary function tests are abnormal in 60 percent of patients (75 percent of blacks), although significant abnormalities are present in less than one-third. Pulmonary

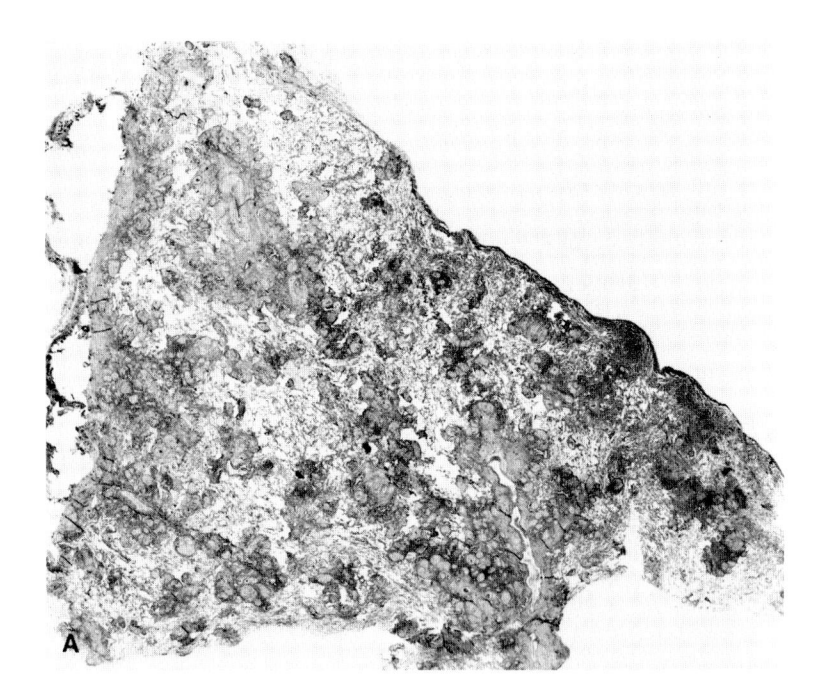

Figure 20–20. Sarcoidosis. Confluent aggregate of well-formed granulomas follows the lymphatic routes. Note the perivascular tracking in B (H&E A ×6, B ×32).

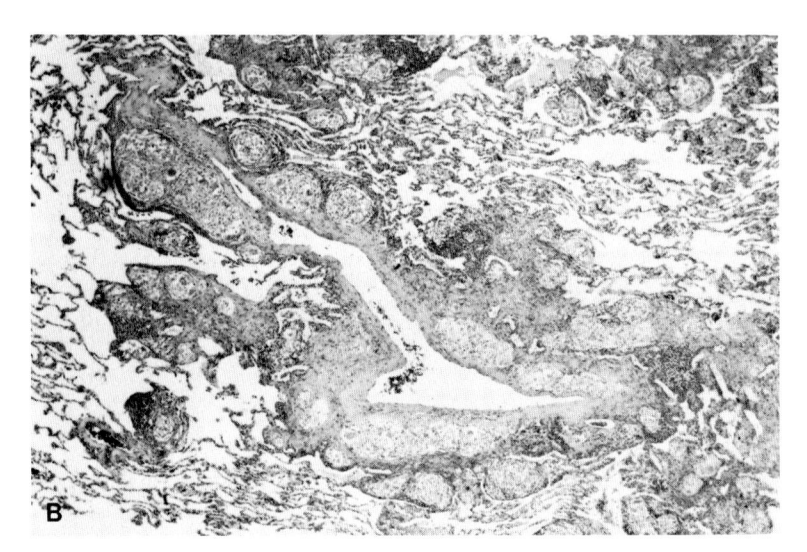

function abnormalities include progressive decrease in lung capacity, abnormal gas exchange, airflow obstruction, and increased compliance.[215] Airflow obstruction may even be seen in patients with normal chest radiographs who have endobronchial lesions.[212]

Gross findings (Figs. 20–18, 20–19) parallel the radiologic findings. In minimally affected cases, the gross apperance may be almost normal or reveal only tiny white nodules corresponding to granulomas. In other cases, masses of granulomas as large as several centimeters may be seen, as may secondary changes of honeycombing, which is commonly in the upper lobes (see Fig. 20–19) and occasionally unilateral. In cases with grossly recognizable granulomas, a lymphangitic distribution reminiscent of lymphangitic carcinoma is characteristic (see Fig. 20–18).

Granulomas in sarcoid are tight, well formed, and often lack significant surrounding inflammation. The granulomas are distributed along the pulmonary lymphatics (Fig. 20–20) in the pleura, septa, and along pulmonary arteries, veins, and bronchi.[26] This distribution along lymphatic routes is one of the most helpful features in recognizing sarcoidosis and distinguishing it from other forms of granulomatous pulmonary disease. Small foci of fibrinoid necrosis may be seen in the granulomas. Giant cells in the granulomas frequently contain inclusions (see 20–51) which may or may not be birefringent. Many of the inclusions are irregular basophilic Schaumann bodies (see below), whereas lucent birefringent calcium oxalate crystals and other calcium salts may also be present. Esthetically appealing, although nonspecific, is the star-shaped asteroid body,

Figure 20–21. Vascular involvement in sarcoidosis. A. The media of a medium-sized pulmonary artery is extensively replaced by granulomas (H&E, ×160). B. Disruption of the elastica by granulomas in a pulmonary vein (elastic van Geson [EVG], ×160).

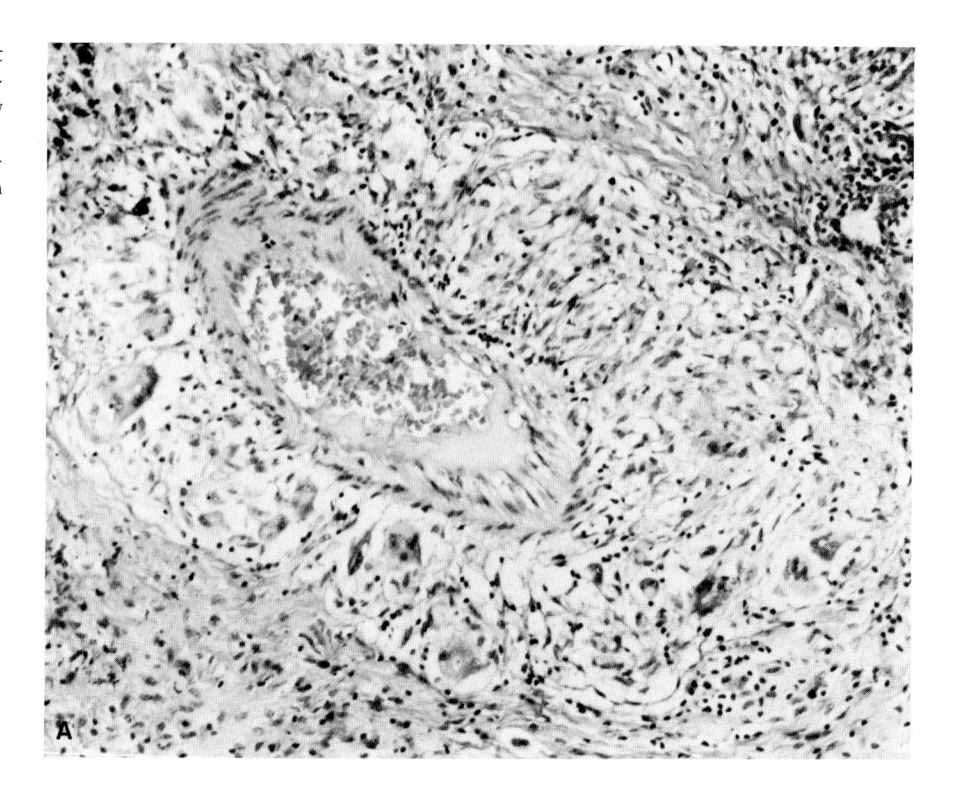

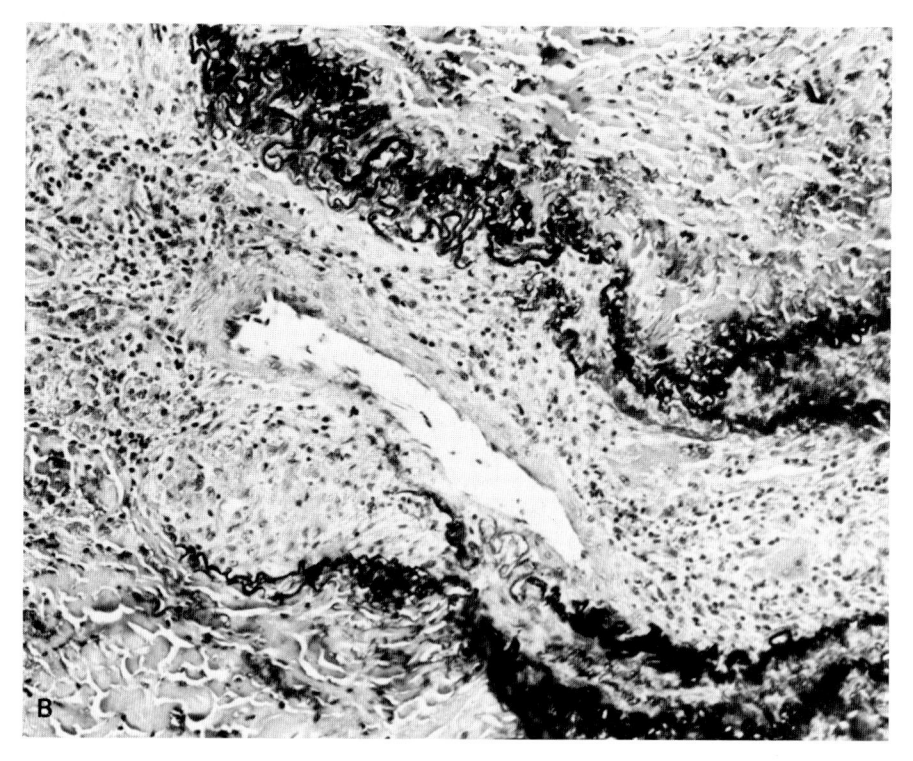

which also may be seen in the giant cells of sarcoid. Granulomas identified histologically often correlate with the chest radiograph changes but not necessarily with pulmonary function tests.[26] Lung sections from patients with sarcoid proven at an extrapulmonary site and normal chest radiographs usually have scattered granulomas, either single or as small confluent masses along lymphatic routes.

The presence of granulomas along the lymphatic routes probably explains why the frequency of vascular involvement is so common (Fig. 20–21). More than half the cases of pulmonary sarcoidosis show involvement of pulmonary arteries or veins, usually the latter (*see* Fig. 20–21).[26,219] Pulmonary hypertension caused by extensive vascular involvement in sarcoidosis is extremely rare.[210,212,237,245] More commonly pulmonary hypertension is related to massive lung fibrosis and honeycombing with loss of more than half of the capillary bed. Airways are also frequently involved by granulomas, and measurable airflow obstruction occurs in a small percentage of cases.[221]

A mild interstitial infiltrate of lymphocytes and plasma cells is frequent in cases of sarcoidosis, especially around the granulomas.[223] The extent of this infiltrate appears to show better correlation with pulmonary function tests than does the extent of the granulomas.[26] Patients with a more extensive interstitial infiltrate may also be the ones who are more likely to develop extensive fibrosis but, as a generalization, the histologic findings are a poor predictor of the patients who will progress to extensive honeycombing.

The granulomas either resolve and disappear completely or leave behind a hyaline scar. Scattered Schaumann bodies may be the only clue to the previous presence of granulomas. Granulomas may or may not be found in cases that have progressed to honeycombing.[236]

The presence of granulomas in the pleura in patients with sarcoidosis is common, although clinical evidence of pleural disease is unusual.[211,222,239] Less than 10 percent of patients have evidence of pleural effusion, which may be small, asymptomatic, and transient or massive and associated with significant symptomatology.[213] In three cases described by Nicholls and associates,[228] pleural effusions in two responded to steroids and one resolved spontaneously. Kanada and colleagues[227] described a case of sarcoidosis in which there was massive pleural thickening by granulomas and severe respiratory compromise.

Although the clinical and radiologic features often are so typical that a presumptive diagnosis of sarcoidosis can be made without it, histologic confirmation should be obtained prior to institution of steroid therapy.[222,239] About one-third of patients with sarcoidosis are diagnosed by examination of lung tissue, usually by transbronchial biopsy[239]; however, the proportion diagnosed by lung biopsy varies. Transbronchial biopsies will show features compatible with or diagnostic of sarcoidosis in 65 to 80 percent of cases, with the highest positive rate being found in patients with both hilar lymphadenopathy and pulmonary infiltrates.[239] One study[226] found that four or more transbronchial biopsies yielded a diagnostic rate of 90 percent. Transbronchial biopsy may be positive even in patients with normal chest radiographs. *In the correct clinical setting*, a transbronchial biopsy is diagnostic of sarcoidosis if the characteristic well-formed confluent masses of granulomas are seen in a lymphangitic distribution. If only one or a few granulomas are present, the tissue is consistent with sarcoidosis. In the absence of the right clinical circumstances, a diagnosis of sarcoidosis based solely on transbronchial biopsy is risky, particularly if poorly formed or only a few granulomas are present. In some hands, the Kveim reaction is a good diagnostic test for sarcoidosis; however, only two-thirds of patients with active sarcoid will show a positive reaction.[239] The antigen is also difficult to obtain.

Despite the low frequency of positive results, in every case of sarcoidosis, cultures should be taken and followed for a full eight weeks to rule out tuberculosis.[222] Special stains are justified when there is necrosis or other atypical features. Although sarcoidosis is usually different from granulomatous infections in the lung, there is sufficient histologic overlap in a small percentage of cases such that differentiation is impossible. Allergic alveolitis is associated with pulmonary parenchymal granulomas. Unlike sarcoidosis the granulomas are random in distribution (do not follow lymphatics), are usually small and poorly formed, and do not show a tendency to coalesce. Allergic alveolitis has a more prominent interstitial infiltrate and significant bronchiolitis, often with bronchiolitis obliterans, and evidence of obstructive pneumonia. A few cases of allergic alveolitis have large numbers of granulomas which may show some coalescence, and differentiation from sarcoidosis on histologic grounds alone may be extremely difficult if not impossible.[214,217,233] Drug reactions may cause granulomas, but the pattern is usually more reminiscent of allergic alveolitis than sarcoidosis. Chronic berylliosis is histologically indistinguishable from sarcoidosis, and differentiation rests on clinical grounds.[26] Aspiration of foreign material may result in a granulomatous reaction centered on airways. The foreign material may or may not be identified in the granulomas. Occasional granulomas of the sarcoid type may be seen in bronchocentric granulomatosis and also in numerous other allergic lung reactions, however. They may also be associated with tumors or without apparent explanation. Caution is therefore required in basing a diagnosis exclusively on the occasional finding of such granulomas.

Paradoxically, severe acute cases of sarcoidosis often resolve completely (*see* Fig. 20–17) whereas patients who develop chronic lung disease often have had an insidious and slowly progressive course.[222,239] The majority of patients have a favorable prognosis, although hilar lymph nodes may remain enlarged for decades, and pulmonary infiltrates may wax and wane in severity. Once the pulmonary infiltrates clear completely, they generally do not return. In the past several decades, there has been a reported marked decrease in both morbidity and mortality in sarcoidosis. A recent report of 775 cases of sarcoidosis in Japan found that half the patients were clear of signs and symptoms after 1 year, and two-thirds were free of disease after 4 to 6 years.[220] Long-term follow-up showed that 86 percent of patients ultimately became asymptomatic, although identifiable lesions remained in a few; 11 percent had continuing symptoms, 3 percent had died, less one-third of these as a direct result of sarcoidosis.[220] A particularly good prognostic sign in that series was the clearance of hilar adenopathy within 6 months,[220] although complete resolution may take several years in some cases.[245c] In another study of 1090 patients, 2.8 percent died as a result of sarcoidosis during the period of follow to up (0 to 17 years).[236] The average course in those who died was 10 years. Causes of death included cor pulmonale, pneumonia, hemorrhage associated with a mycetoma, or cardiac complications.[222,225,236] Although patients with sarcoid have impaired immunity, this does not appear to be a major factor contributing to mortality.[222]

Although generally used as a mainstay of therapy in sarcoidosis, steroids remain controversial and unproven in rigorously controlled studies.[239]

Variants of Pulmonary Sarcoidosis

Nodular Pulmonary Sarcoidosis

Small nodules on chest x-ray films are extremely common in sarcoidosis. In 2 to 4 percent of cases, large nodules are seen.[241,246-248] They are usually bilateral and multiple but may be unilateral and solitary.[246-248] They may measure 4 to 5 cm in diameter and are well circumscribed. Hilar lymph nodes may also be enlarged. Most patients with nodular sarcoid are 20 to 40 years old, and in the United States, the majority are black. The radiologic appearance may resemble metastatic disease. Patients may be entirely asymptomatic or have all the symptoms seen in other patients with sarcoid. The nodules may either resolve spontaneously or during steroid therapy. Histologically the nodules are composed in varying proportions of masses of granulomas and hyalinized connective tissue (Fig. 20–22).

Necrotizing Sarcoid Granulomatosis (Sarcoidal Wegener's Granulomatosis)

Necrotizing sarcoid granulomatosis (NSG) is an unusual pulmonary lesion originally described by Liebow as sarcoidal Wegener's granulamatosis and thought to be a variant of Wegener's granulomatosis.[249-258a] Several reports have appeared since, one speculating that it is a variant of sarcoidosis,[253] another that it is a form of hypersensitivity pneumonitis.[256] It is defined histopathologically as a mass of confluent granulomas associated with necrosis and vascular involvement, usually granulomatous vasculitis.[249] (Fig. 20–23). (NSG is also discussed in Chapter 17.)

In the three largest series[252,253,256] the age at presentation varied from 21 to 75 years; the mean age in all series was between 48 to 50. Males predominated 2:1. The proportion of patients who were asymptomatic at presentation varied from 2 of 13 in Koss and colleagues' series[256] to two-thirds of the 24 patients in Saldana's series.[252] Symptoms were cough, dyspnea, fever, chest pain, and occasionally other constitutional symptoms. Signs and symptoms of upper respiratory disease or renal involvement were uniformly lacking. Two children (ages 11 and 12), described in individual case reports, are the youngest patients described to date.[254,258]

Radiographically, most patients have multiple pulmonary nodules which are either unilateral or bilateral.[252,253,256] Single nodules or diffuse nodular infiltrates are uncommon. Hilar lymph node enlargement, pleural effusions, and cavitation may be present.

A few of the patients described have had evidence of extrapulmonary disease such as enlarged hilar lymph nodes, uveitis, and spinal cord or hypothalamic lesions. The two patients with spinal cord lesions were children.[254,258]

Grossly, the lung lesions of necrotizing sarcoid granulomatosis are firm, grey-white, well-circumscribed masses which may be quite large and show evidence of necrosis. They are composed of sheets of granulomas associated with necrosis (see Fig. 20–23) which is far more extensive than the occasional foci of fibrinoid necrosis seen in typical sarcoidosis.[253,256] The necrosis may appear suppurative.[258a] The necrosis may be caseous, infarct-like or fibrinoid, and may be surrounded by palisaded histiocytes. Vascular involvement is seen in three forms: compression of blood vessels by granulomas; a true granulomatous angiitis in which granulomas involve the wall, and may obliterate the lumen of vessels; and a lymphoplasmocytic angiitis, in which the vessels are infiltrated by mononuclear cells with or without granulomas.[253] Giant cells may rim the vascular adventitia. Noncaseating granulomas in a lymphatic distribution are commonly found away from the mass lesions, a feature taken as support for a relationship between necrotizing sarcoid granulomatosis and sarcoid.[253] The granulomatous process may extend through the pleura.[253]

All series have stressed the relatively favorable prognosis of necrotizing sarcoid granulomatosis, particularly in relation to Wegener's granulomatosis,[252,253,256] and in patients with single lesions surgery seems to be adequate treatment. In those with multiple lesions, resolution may occur spontaneously or with steroid therapy.

Necrotizing sarcoid granulomatosis is a diagnosis of exclusion: special stains *and* cultures are negative. Necrotizing sarcoid granulomatosis must also be separated from Wegener's granulomatosis. Wegener's granulomatosis does not have the well-formed granulomas seen in NSG, is associated with more extensive necrosis of vessel walls, and in the foci of necrosis is marked by prominent granular basophilic material rimmed by palisaded histiocytes. In bronchocentric granulomatosis careful examination shows the bronchocentricity of the process. Rheumatoid nodules only rarely have sarcoid-like granulomas, they are usually septal or subpleural and there is usually a long history of rheumatoid arthritis. Innes and co-workers recently described necrotizing sarcoid granulomatosis-like pulmonary lesions in a patient with osteosarcoma on methotrexate and Adriamycin therapy.[255] Despite the aforementioned "rules" some necrotizing granulomas defy accurate classification when first encountered and are clarified only as the patient is followed clinically.

The etiology of necrotizing sarcoid granulomatosis is unknown. Since cavitation is known to occur in nodular sarcoid,[251,257] necrotizing sarcoid granulomatosis may

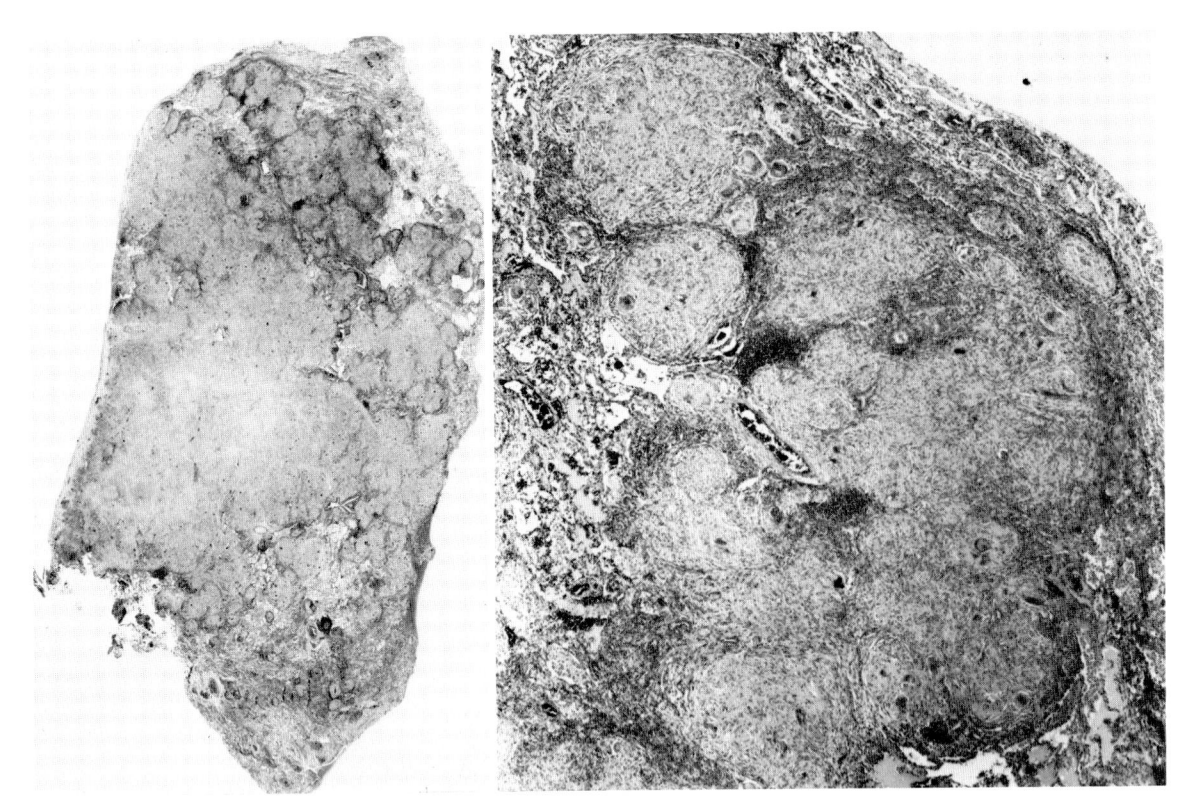

Figure 20–22. Nodular sarcoid. A large (radiographically visible) nodule with hyalinized center (left) is composed of confluent masses of granulomas which surround a vessel (right) (H&E: left ×5, right ×32).

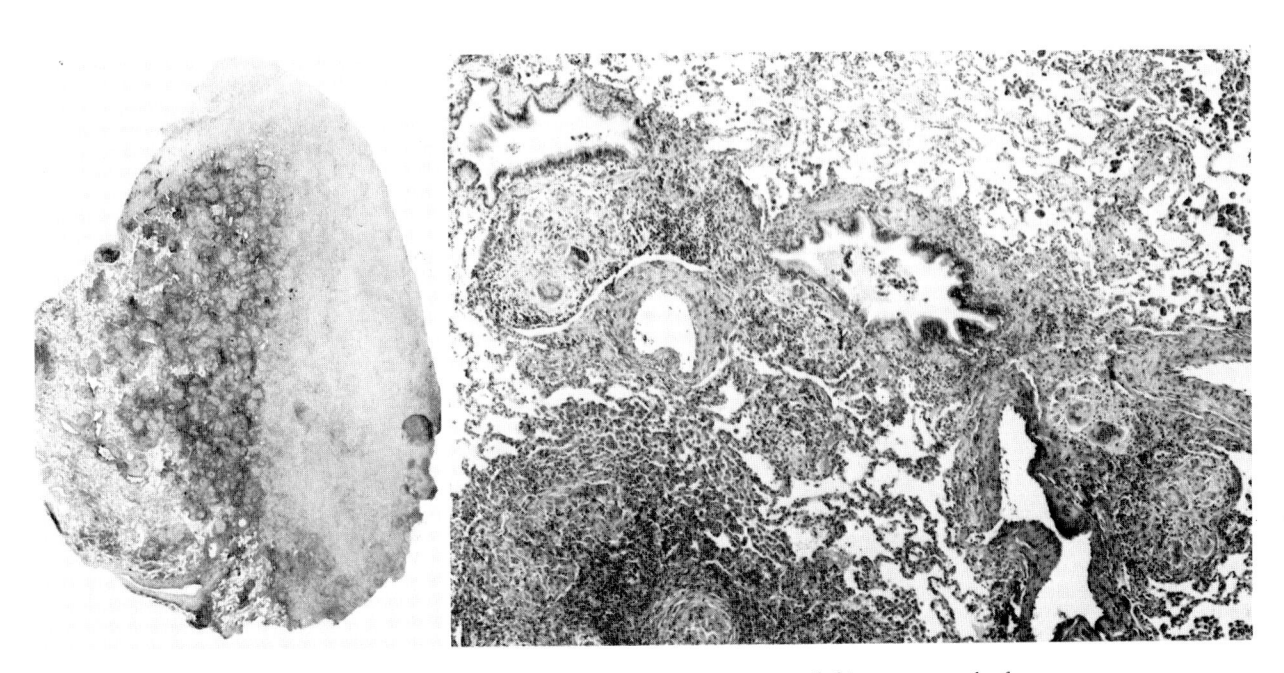

Figure 20–23. NSG. A large nodule with a necrotic center (left) is composed of numerous confluent granulomas which, at the edge, follow lymphatic routes along bronchovascular bundles (H&E: left ×6, right ×48).

merely represent nodular sarcoid with necrosis. While this may be true in a portion of the cases, there are some differences between the two groups. Most patients with nodular sarcoid are 20 to 40 years old and black; those with NSG are older, and in only one of the three series was race given: 4 of 13 patients in Koss's series were black.[256]

In the absence of an appreciable eosinophilic pneumonia, the main problem in differential diagnosis is with periarteritis nodosa. The latter affects arteries only and has a prominent infiltrate of polymorphonuclear leukocytes (PMNs) at the height of the necrosis. Although a neutrophilic capillaritis may be seen in Wegener's granulomatosis, in larger vessels neutrophils are usually associated with the necrotic granulomatous foci in the vessel wall. The necrosis is often eccentric, involving only part of the vessel, which itself is surrounded by a predominantly mononuclear cell infiltrate, occasionally containing eosinophils. The necrosis in Wegener's granulomatosis is more a coagulative than a fibrinoid necrosis and may start as punctuate foci of granular basophilic necrosis surrounded by histiocytes, but it tends to become more extensive to the point of forming large grossly evident infarct-like masses with geographic necrosis rather than merely microscopic foci.

Eosinophilic Granuloma (Histiocytosis X) Involving the Lung

The term histiocytosis X (Hx) was coined by Lichtenstein to encompass a group of clinical entities including localized eosinophilic granuloma, Hand-Schüller-Christian disease, and Letterer-Siwe disease.[259] Pulmonary involvement in Hx is seen either as the sole site of disease or as part of multisystemic syndromes, but in the majority of cases, Hx is limited to the lung.[260-264] A characteristic histiocyte (Hx cell) is seen in infiltrates of Hx along with other inflammatory cells, most frequently eosinophils.[260-263,265] The exact histogenesis of Hx and its cause are unknown, but Hx cells are similar if not identical to Langerhans cells of the skin,[265] and the cellular proliferation may represent the manifestation of abnormal responses in the monocyte-phagocyte system.[245a]

The majority of patients with pulmonary Hx are adults with nonspecific respiratory complaints: dyspnea, cough, chest pain, and increased sputum production.[260-263,265,266] A minority present with wheezing or hemoptysis; up to 20 percent with pneumothorax.[266] Nonspecific systemic complaints including weight loss, malaise, and fever are present in one-third of patients. Clubbing is a rare but occasional finding at presentation.[266] As many as one-fifth of patients are asymptomatic and have abnormal chest radiograph on routine examination.[262,263]

All patients with symptomatic pulmonary Hx have abnormal chest radiographs[261-264] (Fig. 20–24), with one known exception.[8] The infiltrates are bilateral and symmetric, often spare the costophrenic angles, and are reticular or reticulonodular with nodules up to 1.5 cm in diameter. The majority of nodules are smaller than 0.5 cm in diameter and typically stellate in configuration.[262] Cysts and honeycombing on chest radiographs are superimposed in 1 to 15 percent of cases.[263]

Pulmonary function tests in patients with pulmonary Hx may be normal or show changes of restrictive or obstructive disease.[261,263,267] The most common abnormality is decreased diffusing capacity.

Gross findings in pulmonary Hx are nonspecific; small palpable nodules with either normal or fibrotic intervening pulmonary parenchyma may be found. The histologic diagnosis of pulmonary Hx can often be made at scanning power (Figs. 20–25, 20–26), but it is confirmed by identification of the Hx cells at high power.[260-263] One of the most useful diagnostic features is the low-power assessment of the nodules which are roughly symmetric, discrete, and usually have a fibrotic center with cellular peripheral interstitial tentacles. The earliest lesions are interstitial accumulations of Hx cells with varying numbers of eosinophils, often adjacent to a small airway. The lesions show a histologic evolution with peripheral extension of the infiltrate and central scarring; the infiltrate eventually disappears, and a nonspecific focal scar is left behind. Pigmented macrophages are often caught up in the fibrosis. The characteristic Hx cells (Figs. 20–27, 20–28) are most easily found in the cellular periphery of lesions, and considerable search may be required to find small pockets of them in extensively fibrotic lesions. In cellular lesions, mitotic figures may be numerous. The number of eosinophils varies among patients and among lesions in the same patient. True eosinophilic abscesses are seen occasionally, but giant cells are uncommon. Other inflammatory cells which may be present include lymphocytes, plasma cells, and neutrophils. Necrosis is rarely seen in pulmonary Hx. Vascular infiltration (angiitis) by mononuclear inflammatory cells is sometimes present.

A typical histologic feature of pulmonary Hx is the accumulation of intra-alveolar macrophages at the periphery of the lesions (see Figs. 20–7, 20–26). Sometimes this reaction may be so extensive that it stimulates DIP and the term pseudo-DIP reaction is appropriate.[48] Another characteristic feature of pulmonary Hx is the presence of active cellular lesions adjacent to burned-out lesions (see Fig. 20–25). A biopsy may show only nonspecific scars, and a definite diagnosis of Hx is impossible; examination of all the tissue sampled and step sections may show diagnostic foci of Hx cells.

One finding in pulmonary Hx, which is yet to be adequately explained, is the presence of cysts or cavities arising within the lesions[268] (see Fig. 20–26). Whether they represent the residue of distorted airways or constitute a new phenomenon is not known. In early lesions, the cavity may be entirely rimmed by Hx cells, whereas older lesions have a fibrotic wall.

The pulmonary lesions in the limited multisystem variants of Hx, such as Hand-Schüller-Christian disease, are identical to those just described. Lesions in Letterer-Siwe disease tend to be more cellular and less fibrotic and have relatively fewer eosinophils.[269] Histiocytosis X

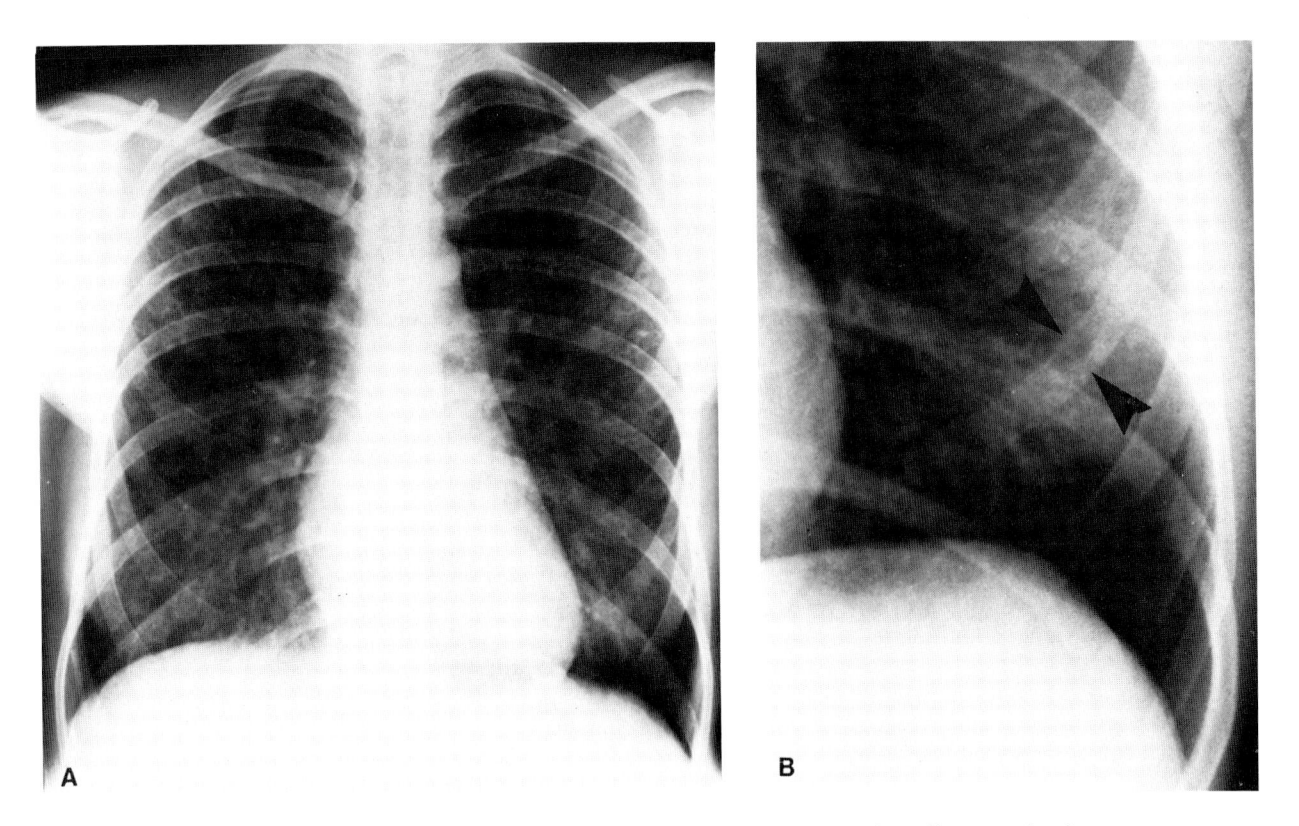

Figure 20–24. Pulmonary eosinophilic granuloma. A. Bilateral reticular infiltrates with relative sparing of the costophrenic angles are seen on the chest radiograph. B. In another case, an incidental bony lesion of eosinophilic granuloma was seen in a rib (arrow). Reticular infiltrates and sparing of the costophrenic angles are also apparent.

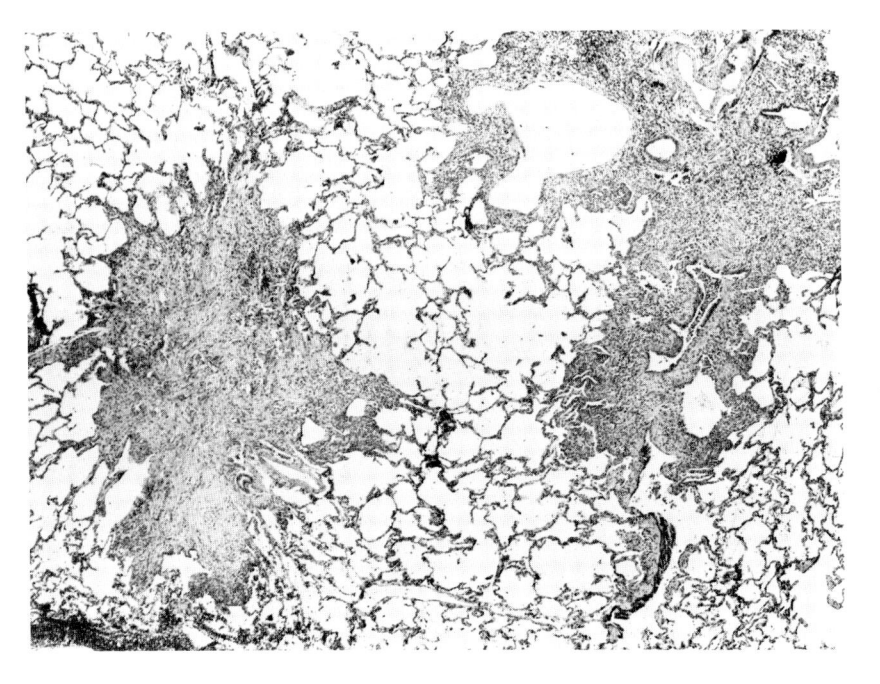

Figure 20–25. Pulmonary eosinophilic granuloma. Two lesions are present; the left one shows the classic discrete stellate scar. Langerhans cells are present only focally at the periphery in the interstitium. The other lesion is early, with little scarring and a cell population rich in eosinophils, and Langerhans cells infiltrating along a small airway. A small cavity has developed at upper right center (H&E, ×32).

cells in Letterer-Siwe disease still maintain the characteristic cytologic features, but they show somewhat more pleomorphism. Clincial and cytologic features should allow separation of Letterer-Siwe disease from childhood lymphomas and malignant histiocytosis, which have sometimes been confused with it.

The Hx cell has distinctive cytologic features [260–263,268] (see Figs. 20–27, 20–28). The nucleus has a delicate nuclear membrane, which is often elongated and folded with single or sometimes multiple small nucleoli. The cytoplasm is abundant and faintly eosinophilic with a poorly demarcated cell membrane. Histiocytosis X cells do not show significant phagocytosis, and the cytoplasm is much paler than that of alveolar macrophages. The nuclei of pulmonary macrophages also tend to be more rounded or oval, with slightly more prominent nucleoli and without the delicate folding. With suboptimal fixation, the nuclei of Hx cells may be ballooned and have more prominent nucleoli. The interstitial location, indistinct cell borders, lack of phagocytosis, and tendency of Hx cells to cluster allow differentiation from alveolar macrophages.

The histologic differential diagnosis of pulmonary Hx includes DIP, UIP, eosinophilic pneumonia, eosinophilic pleuritis,[270] bronchiolitis obliterans, and nonspecific subpleural scarring.[263] The pseudo-DIP reaction in pulmonary Hx[47] may be so extensive that the lesions of Hx are missed without careful searching. The fibrosis in UIP is less discrete and less symmetric than in Hx, and Hx cells are lacking. Eosinophilic pneumonia is an intraalveolar exudative process. Eosinophilic pleuritis is a pleural reaction that frequently follows pneumothorax.[270] There is a proliferation of mesothelial cells and infiltration of eosinophils and histiocytes. The cytologic featues, location, and clinical history usually allow separation. Nonspecific airway-centered scars from burned-out Hx may be indistinguishable from other old inflammatory processes such as bronchiolitis obliterans. The most common histologic lesion in young adults with idiopathic pneumothorax is focal nonspecific subpleural scarring. Histiocytosis X may also produce similar subpleural scarring, but deeper intraparenchymal and active lesions can usually be found.

The Hx cell has a characteristic ultrastructural appearance due to the presence of Langerhans cell or Birbeck's granules[260,261,263] (Fig. 20–29). Confirmation of a diagnosis of pulmonary Hx is possible with the electron microscope, but the light microscopic features are so characteristic as to preclude the need for it. Ultrastructural evaluation is complicated by the fact that Hx cells are occasionally seen in non-Hx fibrotic lung disease.[260,271]

Pulmonary Hx is analogous to sarcoidosis, since patients may be asymptomatic throughout the course and spontaneous clearing often occurs. Number of patients have radiologic abnormalities, yet the infiltrates clear and therapy is never required. Patients with symptoms are usually treated with steroids that appear to be beneficial, although no controlled study has proven their efficacy. The prognosis of patients with Hx limited to the lungs is good; as many as 90 percent have complete resolution or stabilization of signs, symptoms, functions, and radiographic findings without severe deficits.[262,263] A small proportion develop progressive pulmonary disease resulting in end-stage honeycombing and its consequences. Such cases may show active lesions or nonspecific honeycombing at autopsy. A peculiarity of pulmonary Hx is that the various parameters may change independently of one another, such as radiographic clearing despite persistence of symptoms and vice versa.[267] The prognosis for patients who have pulmonary Hx as part of multisystemic disease depends on the extent and severity of extrapulmonary disease; in general it is worst in children with Letterer-Siwe disease.[272,273]

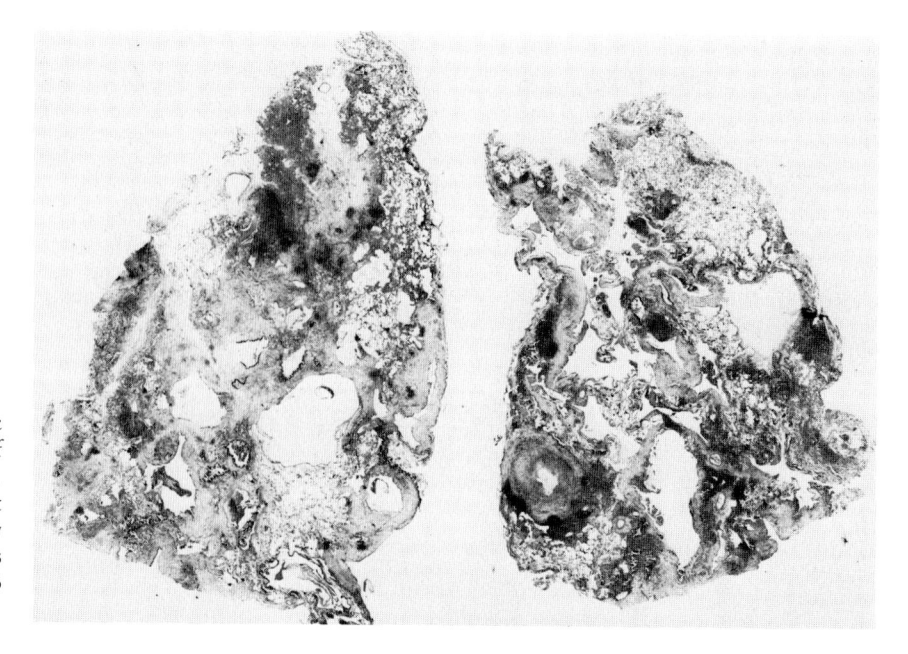

Figure 20–26. Pulmonary eosinophilic granuloma. Several large cavities and foci of honeycombing have developed in this case. Some of the lesions have coalesced and lost their discrete character. Most are still richly cellular with large numbers of Langerhans cells (H&E, ×4). With permission of WB Saunders).

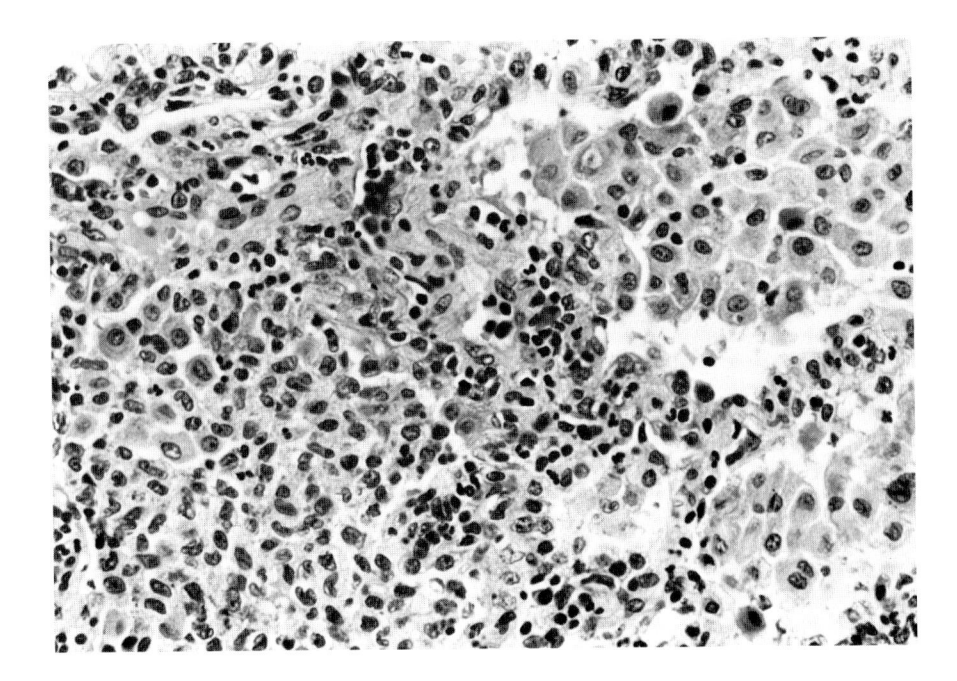

Figure 20–27. Pulmonary eosinophilic granuloma. Cytologic features of Langerhans cells (left) and alveolar macrophages (right) are contrasted. The nuclei of the Langerhans cells are delicately folded and more irregular in shape and the cytoplasmic borders less distinct. A few scattered alveolar macrophages are discernible among the Langerhans cells (H&E, ×320).

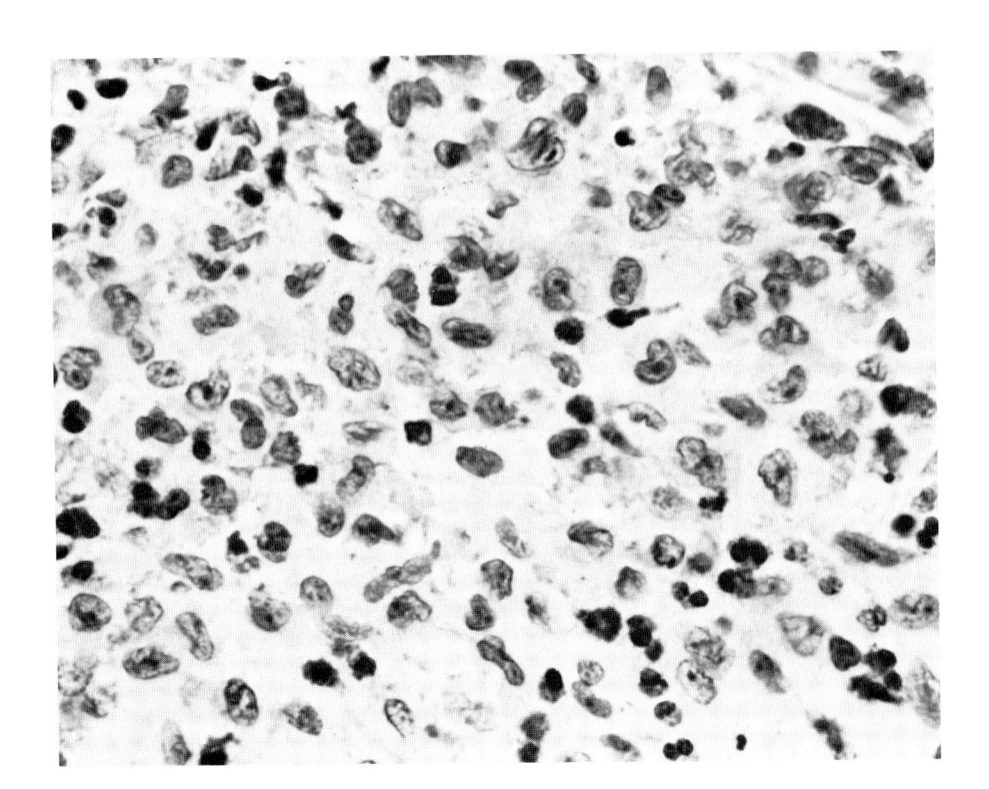

Figure 20–28. Pulmonary eosinophilic granuloma. Cytologic detail of the the Langerhans cells. A few cells have relatively prominent nucleoli. The darker cells are eosinophils; a bilobed nucleus is discernible in some (H&E, ×640).

Figure 20–29. Pulmonary eosinophilic granuloma: ultrastructure. Three Langerhans cells with characteristic nuclear features are present in the upper half of the illustration (×6400). Inset, characteristic cytoplasmic Langerhans cell granule (×69,000). Courtesy of Dr. Hammar, Seattle.

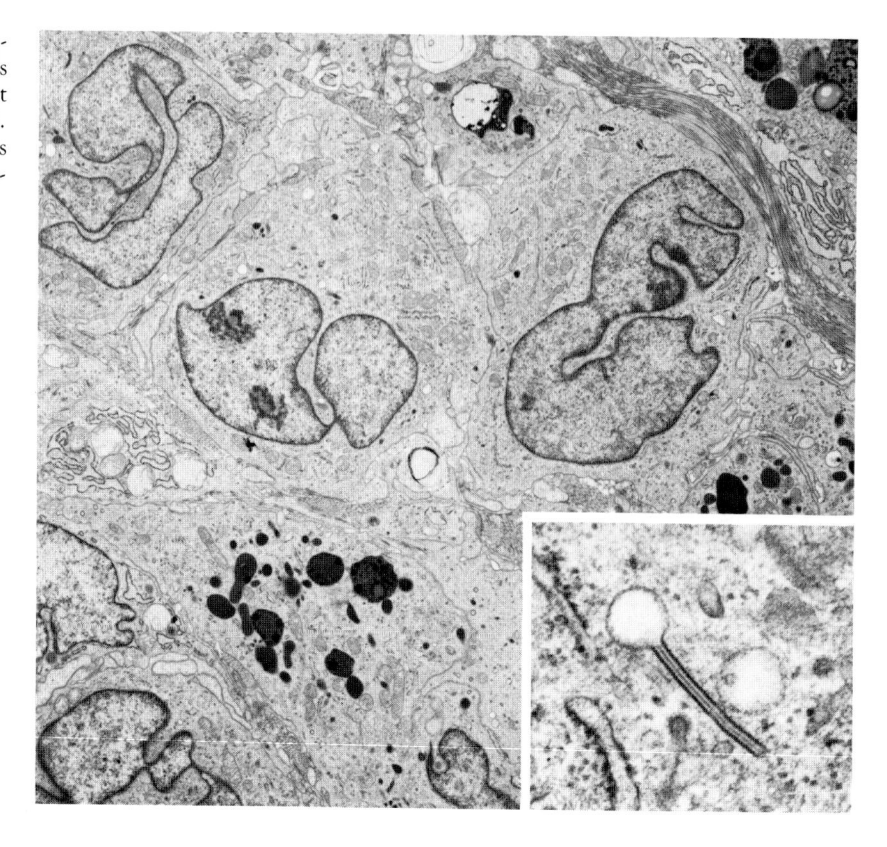

Eosinophilic Pneumonia

This term here designates pulmonary parenchymal infiltrations that contain an appreciable number of eosinophils (at least at some stage). Eosinophilic pneumonia is often associated with an increased number of eosinophils in the circulating blood; however, there are cases in which all blood white cell and differential counts are normal.[273,275] In terms of basic immunology and mechanisms of cell biology, the nature of the eosinophilic pneumonias is not yet clear. An excellent review of the eosinophil is provided by Schatz and colleagues.[276] Results of searches for IgE, other immunoglobulins, complement, and immune complexes in eosinophilic pneumonias and in the angiitis seen with some of them have given mixed results.[227–281]

Several relatively distinct syndromes are recognized in association with eosinophilic pneumonia (Table 20–16). A few other cases, including some of the first cases with histology reported by Harkavy,[282] have other features and do not readily fit in any of the classification schemes.

Löffler's Syndrome

Löffler's syndrome is defined in terms of its brevity and mild manifestations. Crofton and colleagues[283] included a detailed review of this syndrome in their report on pulmonary eosinophilia. Symptoms are mild or absent. Shadows are always seen on the radiograph vary from small to massive, and may shift from one location to another. The blood eosinophil count is always elevated. All manifestations are transient and vanish without treatment within 1 month. Admittedly, their cut-off point is arbitrary, but in the authors' experience, it has been consistently useful. Most cases of pulmonary eosinophilia either fall into the brief duration of Löffler's syndrome or are clearly much more chronic. Hence when a patient is still afflicted after 1 month, the problem will probably be something other than Löffler's syndrome.

Circumstantial and objective evidence indicates that Löffler's syndrome is frequently related to infestation by *Ascaris lumbricoides*.[283] These worms mature and deposit ova in the stool several weeks after the time of pulmonary migration, which is apparently the time that Löffler's syndrome usually occurs. The diagnosis of ascariasis by demonstration of such ova cannot be accomplished until the lung disease is gone; in turn, the absence of ova during the lung infiltration is meaningless. The variety of other causes include other worms, pollen, bacteria, and drugs (sulfonamides).[283] One case

Table 20–16. Syndromes Associated with Eosinophilic Pneumonia

Löffler's syndrome
Chronic eosinophilic pneumonia
Churg-Strauss' allergic angiitis and granulomatosis
Tropical eosinophilia
Hypereosinophilic syndrome
Periarteritis nodosa and polyarteritis

was due to a reaction of an ingested nickle-containing coin.[284]

There have been few opportunities to study the lung tissue directly in Löffler's syndrome because of the mild and transient disease. Von Meyenburg's report[285] probably was an example, but there were no clinical data in those cases. The case described by Bedrossian and associates[286] clearly qualifies with spontaneous and complete remission in 4 weeks from onset of symptoms. These sparse data suggest that the lesions in Löffler's syndrome are identical, except perhaps for extent and severity, to those in chronic eosinophilic pneumonia.

Chronic Eosinophilic Pneumonia

Patients in whom eosinophilic pneumonia persists for longer periods were divided into prolonged pulmonary eosinophilia and pulmonary eosinophilia with asthma in Crofton's series.[283] The authors[274,275,287] have not found the separation of those with and without wheezing to be useful and have placed all of these cases in the category of chronic eosinophilic pneumonia, although the distinction of those with asthma has been continued by Pearson and Rosenow.[288] Patients with chronic eosinophilic pneumonia have a disease of not only greater duration but usually also of much greater severity than patients with Löffler's syndrome. They usually present with dyspnea, cough with mucoid sputum, and severe weight loss.[287] Fever is universal and frequently high, and many patients have drenching sweats. Some patients have mild hemoptysis, and tuberculosis is often suspected at the inital clinical examination. Even within this group, there is some diversity. Occasionally the illness is relatively mild and lasts only 6 to 8 weeks, but more often it is severe and disabling, lasting 3 months or longer. Some patients have spontaneous remissions and recurrences over many years. Others have a severe, relentless progressive disease with high fever, prostration, extreme dyspnea, and even respiratory failure.[287,289]

A characteristic radiographic picture with peripheral, nonsegmental, ground glass–like opacifications (Fig. 20–30), often most apparent toward the apices and axillae (like a photographic negative of pulmonary edema), is pathognomonic of chronic eosinophilic pneumonia and is seen in about two-thirds of cases.[287] Its recognition has greatly diminished the need for lung biopsy in these cases. Radiographic abnormalities, always present, are less characteristic in the remaining cases and provide little help in diagnosis. The response to steroids in patients with chronic eosinophilic pneumonia is so prompt and dramatic as to constitute both another feature of this syndrome and a diagnostic test. The majority of patients are middle-aged women, but typical cases have also been desribed in men and at every age from infancy to the late 70s.

The cause of chronic eosinophilic pneumonia is rarely discovered. Cases have been associated with chronic use of drugs, infection (atypical mycobateria,[290] Coccidioides, Corynebacterium[278]), parasitic infestations, and collagen vascular disease, but the vast majority are idiopathic. A

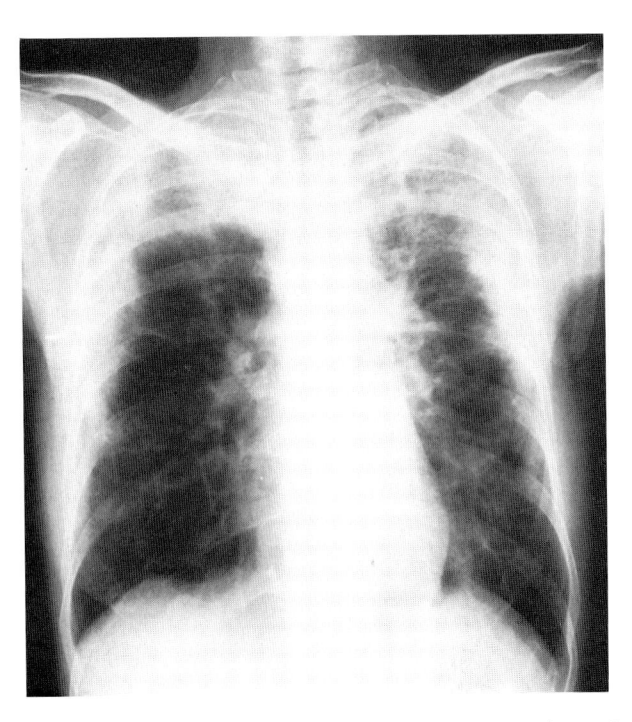

Figure 20–30. Eosinophilic pneumonia. Chest radiograph shows peripheral fluffy infiltrates.

relationship to other allergic manifestations in the same patient is often difficult to interpret. Thus, chronic eosinophilic pneumonia sometimes occurs in patients who have long-standing asthma or rheumatoid arthritis. Approximately 10 percent of cases[291] have occurred during desensitization therapy for hay fever. Although this seems to be an inordinately large proportion, the meaning of the association remains obscure. A few examples of chronic eosinophilic pneumonia appear to be due to Aspergillus allergy and are then sometimes included in the syndrome of bronchopulmonary aspergillosis. That syndrome is usually dominated by bronchial symptoms and lesions, but a few foci of eosinophilic pneumonia nearby are not rare. This problem of overlapping syndromes and lesions is discussed by Katzenstein and associates.[292]

The histology of chronic eosinophilic pneumonia has been described (Figs. 20–31, 20–32).[274,275,277,279,291] The typical lesion include infiltrates in both small air spaces and in interstitium. The most striking feature under low magnification is a massive filling of air spaces with a mixture of eosinophils and macrophages, a pneumonic consolidation which accounts for most of the radiographic shadow. In a few cases, there are proteinaceous debris and even fibrin admixed with the cells, but usually these are insignificant. A few randomly scattered, small, multinucleated giant cells are often present, especially when the marcrophages are numerous, but these are not organized into any structured arrangement. A small number of lymphocytes and plasma cells are also seen. Necrosis is usually confined to small foci in the exudate,

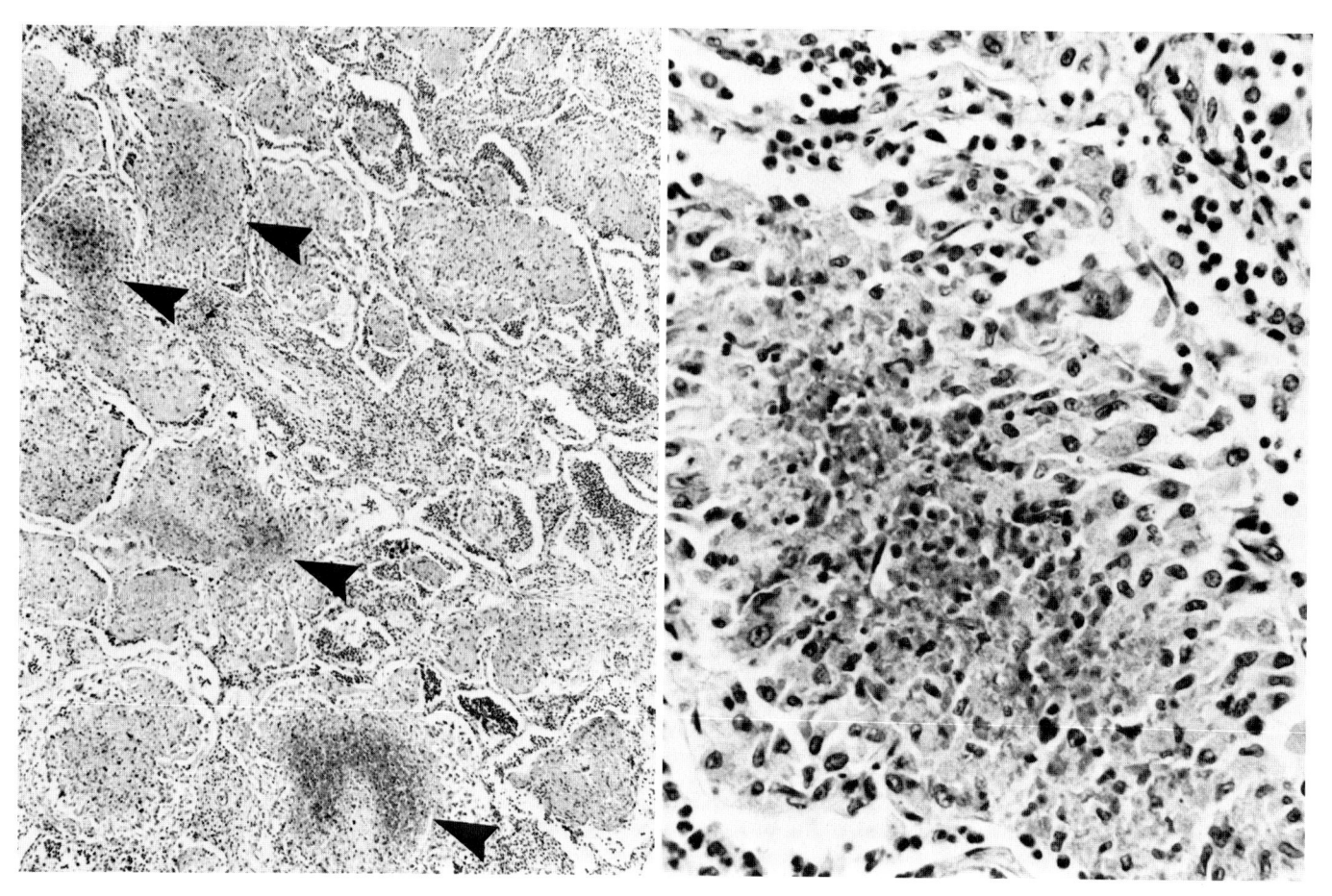

Figure 20–31. Eosinophilic pneumonia. There is an extensive alveolar exudate with foci of necrosis (arrows) associated with a scant but definite interstitial infiltrate in intact alveolar walls. The alveolar exudate is composed predominantly of eosinophils; where necrosis of the exudate has occurred, there is a palisaded histiocytic (granulomatous) response to the eosinophil debris (right) (H&E: left ×48, right ×320).

consisting of eosinophilic debris and disintegrating eosinophils. The necrotic material is surrounded by macrophages, sometimes with the appearance of epithelioid cells and sometimes in a palisaded arrangement. Broadly these are granulomas, but they lack the structured appearance of sarcoid-like granulomas. Another name that more accurately describes these foci is eosinophilic microabscess.

Cavitation has been described radiographically in a few cases, implying that true tissue necrosis can occur, but the authors have never seen this in a specimen. An interesting phenomenon is the accumulation within macrophages of eosinophilic granules and debris.[274,275] Whether this results simply from phagocytosis of material from eosinophils which have disintegrated or whether the granules are "passed" between intact cells has not been established. In any event, the macrophages process this material to form small Charcot-Leyden crystals.[279] These are sometimes best seen if the microscope condenser is racked down. An interstitial infiltrate is a constant but less impressive feature. It too is composed predominantly of eosinophils and macrophages, but plasma cells and lymphocytes account for a somewhat greater proportion than they do in the air space exudate. Sparse organization by proliferation of fibroblastic tissue is common, but notable amounts are more likely to occur after recurrent or very prolonged episodes. The authors have seen functionally significant, severe, permanent damage with scarring in only two or three consultation cases and never in their own series.

Additional features which are inconstant and rarely prominent include bronchiolitis obliterans and non-necrotizing sarcoid-like granulomata. A microangiitis, usually of venules and consisting of a perivascular cuff of lymphocytes and eosinphils with only a few cells actually infiltrated into the media, can be found by careful searching in two-thirds of cases. Angiitis more severe than this is rare. A similar microangiitis affecting venules and arterioles is occasionally found in nonpulmonary tissues, but anything more extensive than that should immediately raise the question of Churg-Strauss's angiitis and granulomatosis or periarteritis nodosa.

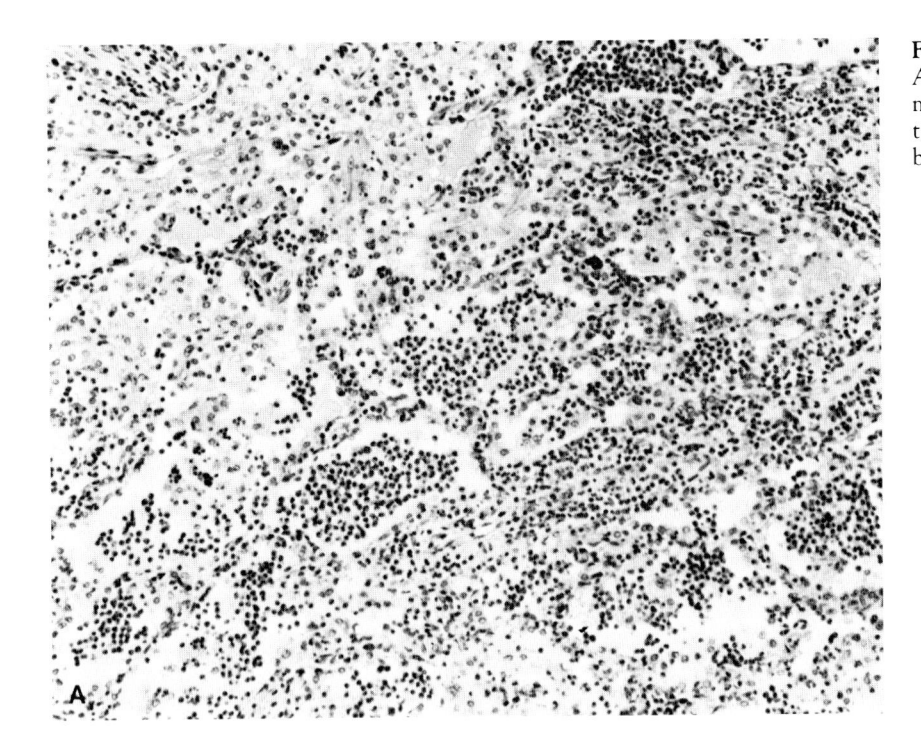

Figure 20–32. Eosinophilic pneumonia. A. Air spaces are flooded by eosinophils and macrophages (H&E, ×100). B. An interstitial infiltrate is present, but it is overshadowed by the alveolar filling (H&E, ×320).

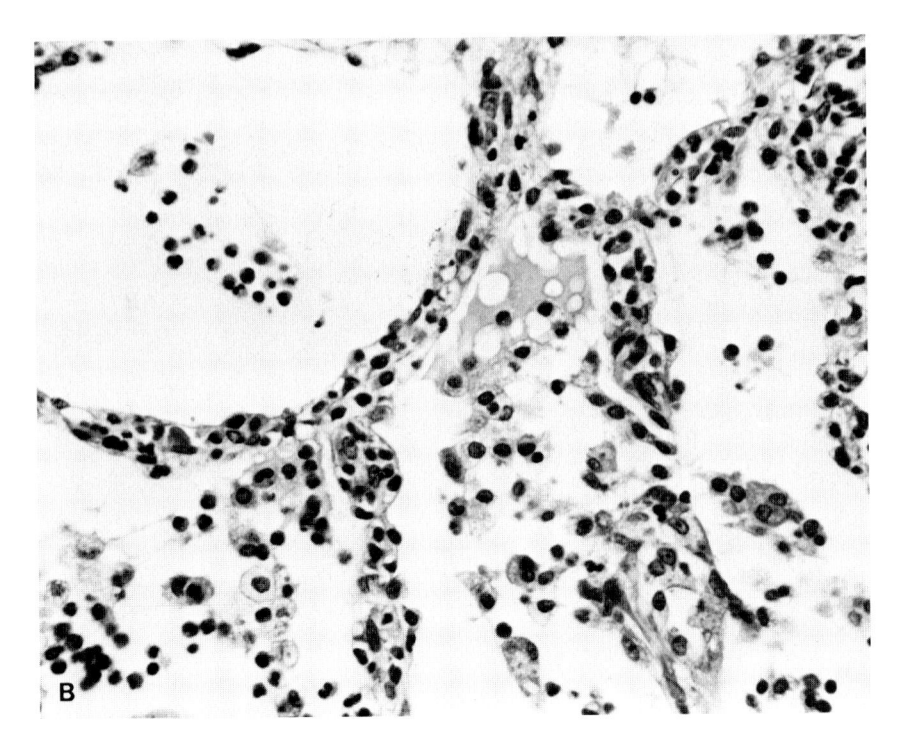

Differential Diagnosis of Chronic Eosinophilic Pneumonia

The separation of Löffler's syndrome and chronic eosinophilic pneumonia must be made clinically. This is probably true also of tropical eosinophilia, although the lesions in that condition are more likely to have a miliary, nodular pattern. Normally the eosinophils far outnumber the monocytes in eosinophilic pneumonia, but when the lesions fade spontaneously or during steroid therapy, the eosinophils depart more rapidly than do the macrophages. The result is that the lesion can transiently resemble DIP. Occasionally some parts of a single biopsy resemble DIP, whereas others are more typical of eosinophilic pneumonia.

An eosinophilic pneumonia-like picture may complicate granulomatous infections. The infectious granuloma and the so-called granuloma or eosinophilic abscess of eosinophilic pneumonia can usually be separated easily. The infectious granuloma is more structured (but not so much as the sarcoid granuloma), typically has several giant cells within its margin of epithelioid cells, and destroys parenchyma (a necrotizing granuloma) and alveolar exudate. In some instances, special stains will demonstrate organisms, but not always. If the infectious focus is not in the biopsy, there is little the histologist can do.[290]

Bronchiolitis obliterans is usually a minor part of the lesion of eosinophilic pneumonia, but once in a while it is more dramatic. Since both bronchiolitis and eosinophilic pneumonia have been observed in rheumatoid arthritis[53,123,293] Cooney[129] speculated on possible interrelationships of these problems.

Eosinophilic granuloma is another lesion in which both large mononuclear cells and eosinophils are prominent. Recognition of the focal and destructive nature of the lesions and the characteristic Hx cell which is interstitial makes this a realtively easy separation.

Biopsy is less often employed in patients with chronic eosinophilic pneumonia now that the clinical syndrome and radiographic picture are better recognized.[294] When necessary, a transbronchial biopsy can sometimes suffice, but successful differentiation of eosinophilic pneumonia from Churg-Strauss's allergic angiitis and granulomatosis, a reaction associated with periarteritis nodosa and one associated with infection, is not likely with such a small biopsy.

Churg-Strauss's Allergic Angiitis and Granulomatosis

Since Churg and Strauss[295] reported their finding of angiitis and granulomatosis in a series of asthmatic patients, there has been a steady but sparse stream of case reports and small series of more or less similar cases with discussion of how such cases should be classified. A key feature is the presence of a widespread, systemic, necrotizing angiitis; the classification debates concern the relationship to periarteritis nodosa, polyarteritis, and Wegener's granulomatosis. Fienberg[296,297] resolved at least part of the problem by proposing pathergic granulomatosis as an overall classification to bracket a spectrum of manifestations, but most authors continue to separate the various syndromes. As generally defined, allergic angiitis and granulomatosis are restricted to patients with bronchial asthma and are characterized by eosinophilia in the blood and several tissues, necrotizing angiitis, and extravascular granulomas. A few cases are classified as periarteritis nodosa and polyarteritis by some authors and as allergic angiitis and granulomatosis by others. It is clear from reviewing reported cases, including the large series from the Mayo Clinic,[281,295,298–303] that this is a systemic disorder with protean manifestations (see Chapter 16).

The lung lesion consists of angiitis, granulomatosis, and eosinophilic pneumonia in various combinations. The necrotizing angiitis affects small and medium-sized vessels, some considerably larger than those described in chronic eosinophilic pneumonia, and usually veins as well as arteries. The cell infiltrate in these vessels is mixed but includes prominent eosinophils, epithelioid monocytes, and usually giant cells as in giant cell arteritis. The granulomas can be anywhere, but some must be extravascular. The necrotic centers of these contain many eosinophils and are surrounded by epithelioid and various other cells. They may be inseparable from the eosinophilic microabscesses in chronic eosinophilic pneumonia. The tissue eosinophilia can vary from trivial to an extensive pneumonic consolidation as described in chronic eosinophilic pneumonia. Hence angiitis is of paramount importance in differential diagnosis. It is possible to miss this in a lung biopsy because of sampling, especially in a transbronchial biopsy. It is also possible that not all cases include pulmonary angiitis. For these reasons, striking extrapulmonary visceral or skin manifestations or a course atypical for chronic eosinophilic pneumonia should bring this diagnosis to mind even if a lung biopsy does not. However, a microangiitis without appreciable tissue eosinophilia or granulomas is occasionally seen in skin, pleura, or synovium of patients with otherwise ordinary chronic eosinophilic pneumonia.

Tropical Eosinophilia

Since the initial description of tropical eosinophilia, it has become apparent that this is usually a manifestation of filariasis, and some evidence of such infestation is usually required for the diagnosis. The syndrome was reviewed in detail by Udwadia[304] and more recently by Neva and Ottesen.[305] Patients usually have wheezing and cough with little sputum and often some systemic symptoms such as weight loss, low-grade fever, fatigue, and lymph node enlargement. Laboratory studies are notable for extremely high blood eosinophil counts (more than 3000 per milliliter), high titers of antifilarial antibodies, and high IgE levels (at least 1000 U/ml). Microfilaria usually cannot be demonstrated in the blood, however. Less specific findings, such as an elevated erythrocyte sedimentation rate, are also common. Chest radiographs may be normal, or may have increased bronchovascular markings, diffuse 1 to 3 mm miliary nodulations, or mottled opacities. In terms of function, less than a third of cases have airflow obstruction, most have restricted lung volumes, and patients with long-standing disease have abnormal gas exchange. Eighty percent of patients are men, usually in their 20s or 30s. A favorable response to diethylcarbamazine, usually within days, is the final proof of diagnosis, although this may also occur with other round worm infestations whose antigens also can cross-react with those of Filaria. Cases of tropical eosinophilia encountered in North America are acquired elsewhere, usually in India, Indonesia, Sri Lanka, Pakistan, and southeast Asia. Neva and Ottesen[305] emphasize that exposure to an endemic area must be for months rather than days or weeks, because filarial infections are not efficiently transmitted. Untreated, the disease continues for weeks or months but may remit and recur months or years later. Histologically these cases are described as having interstitial and air space histiocytic infiltrates in the first few weeks, then an eosinophilic bronchopneumonia with eosinophilic abscesses. After several months, a mixed-cell exudate organized in nodular patterns evolves to predominantly histiocytic granulomatous response with increasing fibrosis.[304] It is doubtful that the bronchopneumonia stage can be separated from chronic eosinophilic pneumonia unless there is a miliary, nodular pattern. The other stages do not sound specific. The yield of finding Filaria in biopsies is low.[304,305] For these reasons, lung biopsies appear to have little use in the diagnosis of tropical eosinophilia.

Hypereosinophilic Syndrome

The hypereosinophilic syndrome is less well characterized than the aforementioned entities. According to Chusid and associates,[306] it is characterized by persistent marked or "hyper" eosinophilia of the blood associated with diffuse organ infiltration of eosinophils. It is associated with prominent cardiac and hematologic problems and has significant morbidity and mortality. Only 40 percent of the patients reviewed[306] actually had pulmonary disease, and half of those had pleural effusions. Only 10 or 15 percent of cases had pulmonary infiltrates on radiographs, usually associated with cough. Some patients had pulmonary emboli. Thirty-nine cases in this series had autopsies, and 40 percent of these had lung involvement, usually an interstitial eosinophilic infiltrate. More rarely, there were necrotic areas in the parenchyma which they attributed to microemboli.

Periarteritis Nodosa and Polyarteritis

Although polyarteritis nodosa is sometimes linked with pulmonary eosinophilia, the lesions do not often fit well with other cases of eosinophilic pneumonia. Alternatively there are examples in the literature[283,307] in which eosinophilic pneumonia was the presenting problem or a serious complication in the course of periarteritis nodosa. Apparently in some such cases, the pulmonary lesions are indistinguishable from the usual form of chronic eosinophilic pneumonia, although the systemic vascular lesions and their manifestations reveal the true nature of the disease. However, there are instances of eosinophilic pneumonias that have a few small inflamed vessels, usually venules, resembling those called sensitivity angiitis by Zeek[308] as described in chronic eosinophilic pneumonia, but this hardly represents periarteritis nodosa as described by Kussmaul and Maier.[309] Furthermore, these cases appear to behave identically to other examples of chronic eosinophilic pneumonia. In the authors' experience, patients with true periarteritis nodosa are rare, even more rarely have lung lesions, and then have mainly an acute arteritis with numerous neutrophils with little if any pneumonitis.

Both clinically and anatomically, they are seldom a problem in differential diagnosis. Some patients with vascular lesions and pneumonia and others with eosinophil infiltrates in the lung without vascular lesions still defy classification as outlined in Table 20–1. These include some of the cases described by Harkavy,[282] Bergstrand,[310] Rose and Spencer,[311] and the case discussed in a clinical pathologic conference at the Massachusetts General Hospital.[312]

Treatment of Eosinophilic Pneumonia

Proper managment of these patients depends critically on the syndrome in Table 20–1 in which they best fit. In Löffler's syndrome, the pneumonia itself does not require treatment, but an effort should be made to identify the cause. In chronic eosinophilic pneumonia, the cause should also be sought, but success is not likely. The pneumonia in this syndrome responds marvelously to steroid therapy, but even there, treatment is not always necessary, as noted by Dines[294] who also suggested a detailed regimen. Since severe fibrosis is an uncommon and late event in this syndrome, the authors agree there is no need for rushing to treat these cases. Progression to respiratory failure obviously must be prevented, however. Whenever response to treatment is slower or less complete than anticipated, the search for an underlying or complicating factor or an alternate diagnosis such as allergic angiitis and granulomatosis should be reconsidered.

Pulmonary Alveolar Proteinosis

Pulmonary alveolar proteinosis[313–341] is associated with progressive shortness of breath, bilateral radiographic infiltrates resembling pulmonary edema, and histologic filling of alveoli by dense, granular, eosinophilic, PAS-positive, glycoproteinaceous material.[313]

Pulmonary alveolar proteinosis was described by Rosen and colleagues[313] in 1958 in 127 patients, which is still one of the largest series reported. Most patients present between the ages of 20 and 50; however, newborns and patients as old as 65 have been described.[335,338] Clinical findings are minimal.[313] The majority of patients have insidious dyspnea that progresses slowly over months and sometimes years. There is often cough productive of thick sputum. Fatigue, chest pain, weight loss, mild fever, clubbing, and cyanosis may develop eventually. Approximately half of the patients relate an episode of pneumonia prior to the development of symptoms. A minority have a fulminant illness which progresses rapidly to respiratory failure.[322,333] Patients may be asymptomatic despite extensive radiologic findings.[313] Most cases are sporadic; however, several familial cases, particularly in children, have been reported.[317,336,338] The condition may mimic neonatal respiratory distress syndrome.[331]

Chest radiographs show a "fine, diffuse, perihilar,

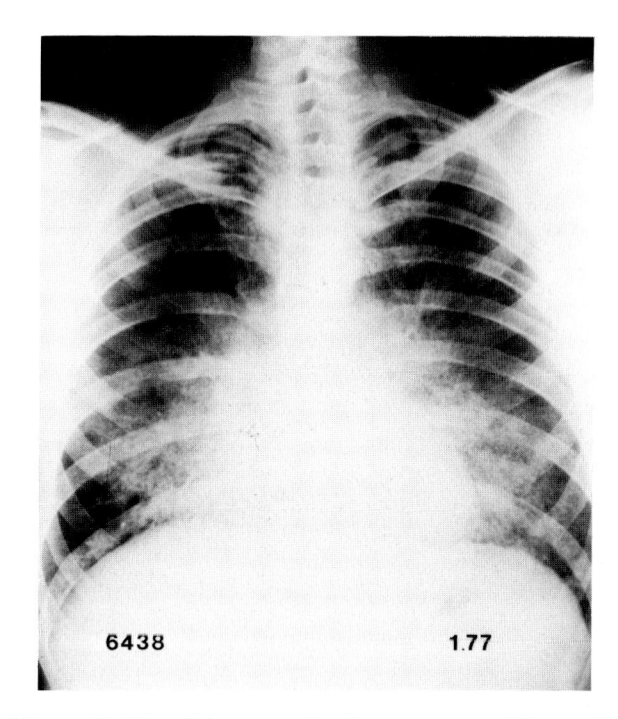

Figure 20–33. Pulmonary alveolar proteinosis. Chest radiograph shows a fluffy perihilar infiltrate. Courtesy Dr. Gaensler, Boston.

radiating, feathery or vaguely nodular, soft density, resembling in its 'butterfly' distribution the patterns seen in severe pulmonary edema" (Fig. 20–33).[313] Reticular infiltrates may be present at the edge of the main shadows.[333] Most cases are bilateral and symmetric; asymmetry in the radiologic findings is unusual.[333] An interstitial infiltrate may be the only finding in some cases.[337] Radiographic changes may clear spontaneously, remain stable, or progress. Clearing usually begins peripherally.

Pulmonary functions in PAP reflect alveolar filling with impaired gas exchange, decreased total lung capacity, and normal flow rates. Diffusing capacity is severely depressed. Ventilation/perfusion mismatching is marked, and low PO_2 levels are characteristic. Functional abnormalities improve as the disease clears spontaneously or following bronchopulmonary lavage, the treatment of choice.[326]

Prior to the development of bronchopulmonary lavage, approximately one-third of patients with PAP died.[313] Various forms of therapy have been tried,[335] but only bronchopulmonary lavage, first described in 1963, offers promise for the majority of patients.[335] Some patients with few or no symptoms clear without receiving therapy.[326] Fatal cases are due to progressive respiratory failure or superimposed infection.[313] Pulmonary alveolar proteinosis in children has a significantly worse prognosis than in adults, since children show poor response to lavage.[317]

Pulmonary alveolar proteinosis is characterized grossly by yellow-grey zones of consolidation with thick fluid that may be misinterpreted as purulent. In biopsies the zones are nodular and rarely over 2 cm in diameter, whereas at autopsy there is extensive consolidation, unless PAP is not the cause of death. Microscopically the alveoli are stuffed with dense eosinophilic granular material (Fig. 20–34) that is PAS-positive and diastase resistant[313,318] and stains positively with fat stains.[327] Frozen sections stained with hematoxyin and eosin (H&E) may occasionally show basophilic staining of this material.[341c] Mucicarmine and alcian stains are negative. Within the granular material are larger lamellated eosinophilic bodies. Cholesterol clefts, macrophages, and degenerating cells are also present. The alveolar walls are normal or show only a slight mononuclear cell infiltrate. Interstitial fibrosis is a rare sequel (Fig. 20–35)[319,338] and has also been reported early in the course of the disease.[341a] Giant cells with cholesterol clefts are frequently associated with

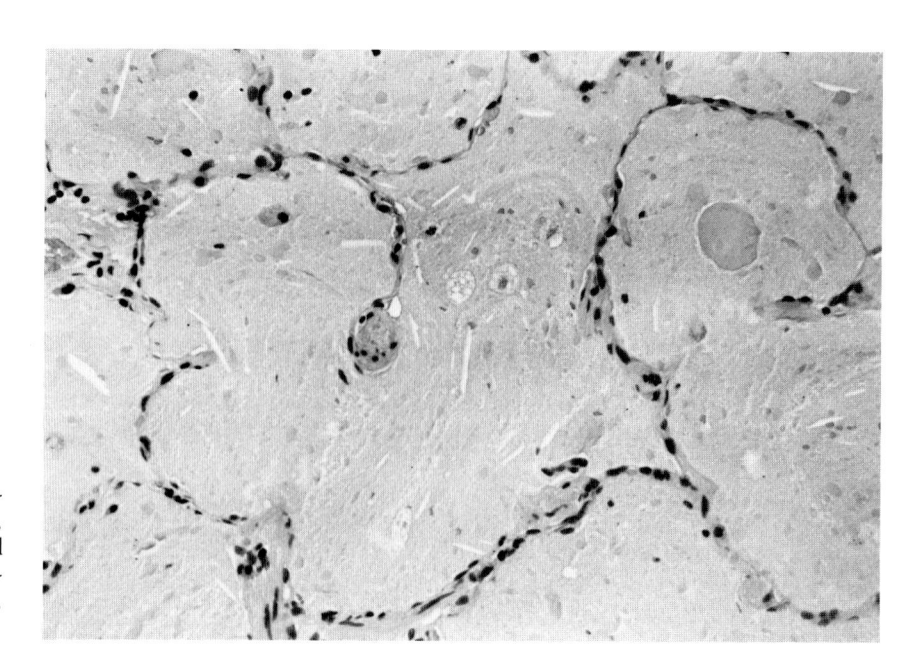

Figure 20–34. Pulmonary alveolar proteinosis. Dense material fills the alveoli: cells, eosinophilic bodies, cellular debris, and acicular clefts also characterize it. The interstitium has a slight increase in nuclei (H&E, ×200).

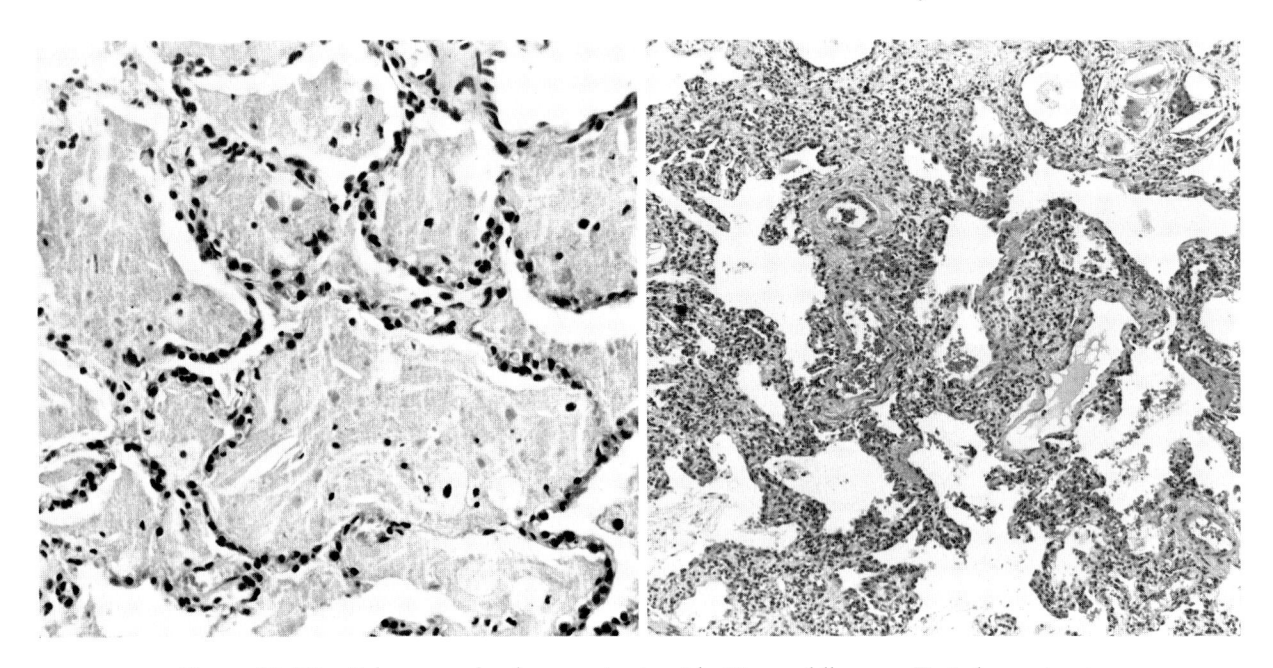

Figure 20–35. Pulmonary alveolar proteinosis with 12-year follow-up. Typical proteinosis, clinically and histologically (left) was seen at presentation. The initial biopsy shows classic proteinosis with a prominent alveolar lining cells. The follow-up biopsy done at the time of cardiac surgery shows interstitial inflammation and fibrosis. A cholesterol granuloma is present at upper right (H&E: left ×200, right ×80). Courtesy of Dr. Emory, New Orleans.

interstitial fibrosis that is seen in PAP. Histologic examination of sputum and lavage fluid from patients shows the intra-alveolar material and, in the right clinical setting, may confirm a diagnosis.[332]

In its full blown state, PAP does not have a histologic differential diagnosis. Other intra-alveolar eosinophilic substances include edema, fluid, hyaline membranes, and mucus. Edema fluid is only slightly PAS-positive, mucus is positive with alcian or mucicarmine stains, and hyaline membranes rarely fill alveoli and are usually associated with interstitial changes. Microscopic foci identical to PAP, rarely occupying more than a few air spaces, may be an occasional incidental finding in biopsies or autopsies, especially in foci of interstitial fibrosis, and they are apparently of no significance.

Electron microscopy shows widespread cellular degeneration and an electron-dense granular background with numerous lamellar bodies up to 5 μm in diameter[314,320,323,324,327] (Fig. 20–36). The lamellar bodies resemble those found in granular pneumonocytes. Cells free within the alveolar material include degenerating granular pneumonocytes and macrophages.

The intra-alveolar material in PAP has been extensively analyzed owing to its accessibility by lavage. It is a phospholipid, largely phosphatidylcholine with abundant lecithin rich in palmitic acid and cholesterol. It is not simply a transudate of plasma proteins nor a hypersecretion of normal products found within the air spaces, but is similar to surfactant[314,315,318,323–325,334,339] and has been found to stain positively for surfactant apoprotein.[334,339]

Pulmonary alveolar proteinosis in experimental animals can be caused by a variety of mineral and metal dusts, certain drugs, and oxygen.[316,323,329,333,341,341d] Although the cause in humans remains unknown, interest in its pathogenesis has centered on the alveolar macrophages, since they show impaired intracellular killing of bacteria and increased amounts of fat as well as morphologic abnormalities in the lysosomes.[321,327] The macrophage defects are thought to be acquired in the pulmonary environment and to result in impaired clearing of intra-alveolar consitituents that leads to progressive accumulation. Immunologic phenomena have been implicated as contributing factors since IgG is elevated in the lavage fluid, and this is associated with a decreased serum IgG.[324,328] Up to 30 percent of children with PAP have thymic alymphoplasia or other immune deficiency[322,336]; it is also associated with lymphoreticular malignancy and the immunosuppressed state.[330] In one study,[341] several different inorganic particulates were associated with PAP. Such an diversity of associations suggest that PAP is a nonspecific reaction pattern to a variety of different injuries that may be acquired or are inborn errors. This possibility was raised in the initial description of the condition.[313]

Pulmonary alveolar proteinosis is sometimes associated with hematolymphoid malignancies and opportunistic infections,[322,330] and has recently been reported with virus-associated adult T-cell lymphoma/leukemia.[341b] Of the 260 reported cases reviewed by Bedrossian and associates in 1981,[330] 22 (8 percent) were associated with

Figure 20-36. Pulmonary alveolar proteinosis. The heterogenous composition of the intra-alveolar material is apparent at the ultrastructural level. A type II pneumonocyte can be seen discharging vacuoles (arrow) into the alveolar space (×3500). Courtesy of Dr. Bausch Stanford, Calif.

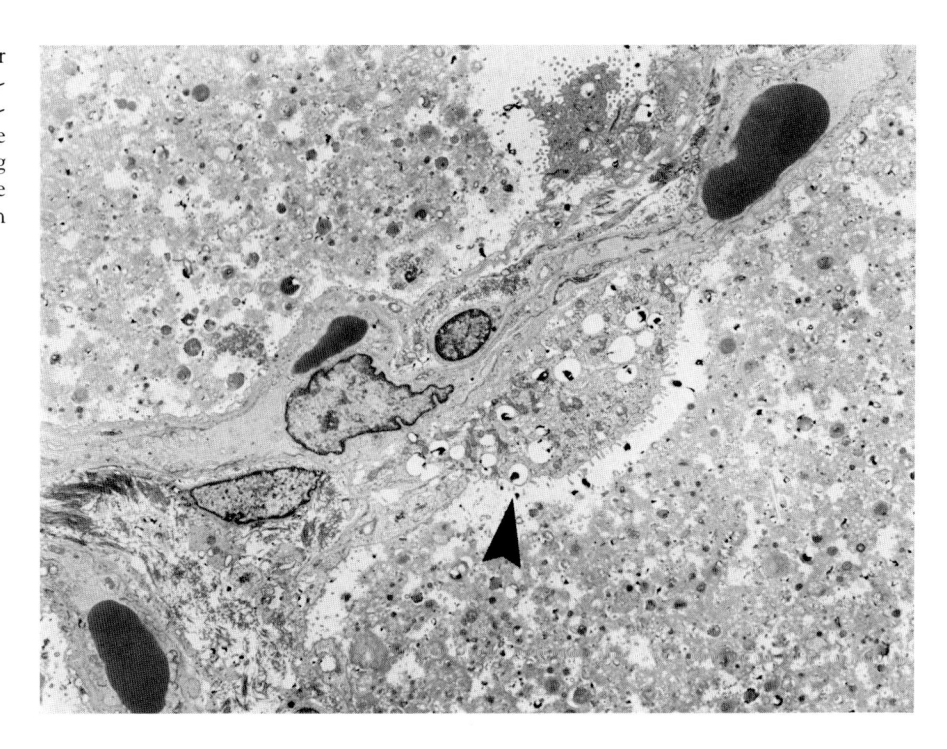

leukemia or lymphoma. Since such cases are more likely to be reported, this may represent an exaggeration of actual incidence. A recent study suggests that the lesion in these patients is different since staining for surfactant-specific apoprotein is only focal in contrast to the uniform staining seen in primary PAP.[339] This finding raises questions about the specificity of the morphologic features of PAP.[340] PAP is also associated with primary immunoglobulin deficiencies, and it has been suggested that patients and their relatives should be evaluated for immunodeficiency.[336] Bedrossian's group[330] also found 40 cases associated with opportunistic infections. These included cryptococcosis, tuberculosis, candidiasis, mucormycosis, nocardiosis, histoplasmosis, aspergillosis, pneumocystosis, atypical mycobacterial infections, streptomyces infections, cytomegalovirus, and Herpes.[330] The authors' experience with PAP in immunosuppressed patients shows minor morphologic differences from normal hosts. In the former, there is considerably more edematous widening of alveolar walls and increased numbers of nuclei, predominantly of reactive type II pneumonocytes. The appearance of PAP on a lung biopsy from a compromised host should prompt a vigorous search for infection, and step sections may be necessary to locate a small focus of organisms that are overshadowed by an extensive PAP reaction.

Lymphangioleiomyomatosis and Tuberous Sclerosis

Lymphangioleiomyomatosis is rare and limited to women in the reproductive years.[342-355] Spindle cells resembling immature smooth muscle proliferate in the lung and along axial lymphatics in the thorax and abdomen.[345,349]

The clinical features are uniform.[344,345,349] All patients reported have been women, nearly all between the ages of 17 and 47 at the time of diagnosis. Rare cases present after age 50.[344] There is no familial association. Progressive shortness of breath, cough, and repeated pneumothoraces are characteristic. Less common presenting features include chyloptysis and hemoptysis. Symptoms may be present even in the absence of chest radiograph abnormalities.[352] Pleural effusions are common during the course of the disease, presenting in 27 of 34 patients reviewed by Corrin and colleagues,[345] among which the effusion was chylous in 8. Lymphedematous swelling of the lower extremities was reported in two patients.[352]

Most patients have chest radiographic abnormalities at presentation: these include fine reticular or linear and nodular densities, greater at the bases, without sparing of the costophrenic angles[345,349] (Fig. 20-37). The changes are progressive, and the later stages show cyst-like spaces and a pattern resembling honeycombing. The radiologic abnormality usually correlates with the clinical symptoms, although pneumothorax may occur in patients with an otherwise normal chest radiograph.[352] Progressive lung enlargement with an increasing reticulonodular infiltrate is characteristic.[349] (Fig. 20-38). Abnormal lymphatics and lymph nodes in the chest and abdomen are seen on lymphangiogram.[345]

Pulmonary functions are distinctive.[345,349,352] Lung volumes are normal or only slightly increased when measured by spirometry but are abnormally large by chest radiograph and plethysmography, indicating air trapping. Flow rates are decreased and lung compliance in-

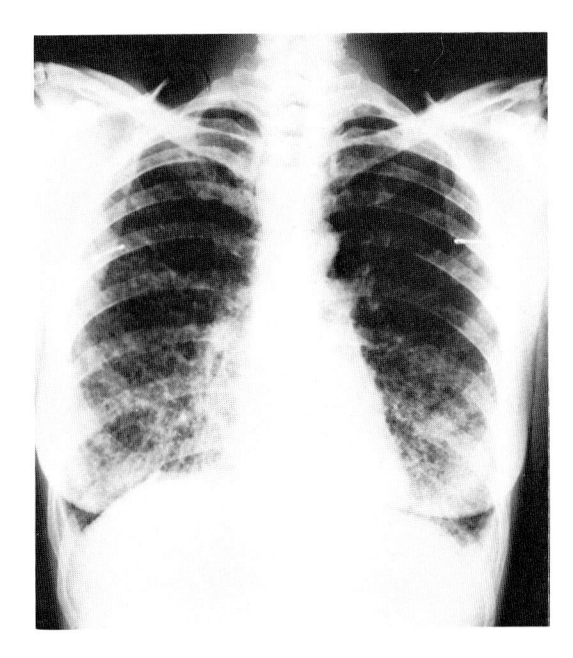

Figure 20–37. Lymphangioleiomyomatosis (LAM). Typical chest radiograph showing diffuse, bilateral reticular infiltrates with roughly normal lung volume.

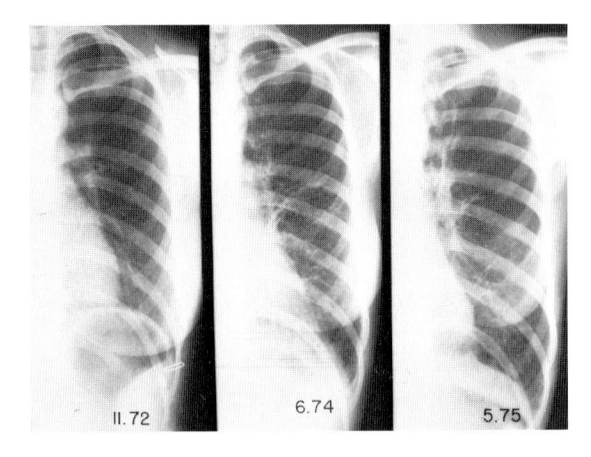

Figure 20–38. Radiographic progression of LAM. Note increasing lung volume and infiltrates. Courtesy Dr. Gaensler, Boston.

creased.[352] There is a disproportionately low diffusion capacity relative to total lung capacity, in contrast to most chronic interstitial pneumonias in which the decrease in diffusion generally correlates with the decrease in volume.[349]

Most patients with LAM die within 10 years of diagnosis; however, survival for longer than 15 years occurs, and one patient remained asymptomatic for 9 years following the diagnosis.[345,349] Most deaths are ascribed to progressive respiratory insufficiency associated with mild pulmonary hypertension and right ventricular hypertrophy.[345] In one patient, retroperitoneal hemorrhage was a significant factor.[349]

No therapeutic promise has been shown by radiation, steroids, androgens, immunosuppressives, or palliative surgery.[345,349] Since the lesion is limited to women, the possibility of hormonal influence has been recognized.[344,345,349,351] Several recent reports[353–355d] have suggested that estrogen suppression and particularly oophorectomy may have a significant role in arresting the disease.

The lungs grossly resemble honeycombing in LAM, being firm and having numerous abnormal air spaces linked by thick walls. Careful observations reveals tan smooth muscle rather than grey-white fibrous tissue, and the lungs are much larger than those with honeycombing. Honeycombing is also more patchy and irregular in extent. Nodular masses of smooth muscle are found along the axial lymphatics in the chest and abdomen, and the lymphatics are cord-like and exude milky lymphatic fluid.[345]

The histologic findings in LAM are unique[343,345,349] (Figs. 20–39 through 20–42). The lesion begins as a focal cellular proliferation along the lymphatic routes in the pleura, septa, and bronchovascular rays. Eventually discrete micronodular proliferations involve the parenchyma extensively, and their distribution is difficult to discern. The cells are cytologically distinctive and do not resemble normal smooth muscle cells (see Fig. 20–40). They are shorter, plumper, and have a higher nucleus/cytoplasm ratio than normal smooth muscle; in every cellular myoblastic foci the cells are polygonal. Endothelial-lined clefts are found among the spindle cells (see Figs. 20–39A and C, 20–40). These spaces lack erythrocytes and have been interpreted as newly formed lymphatic spaces. Airway obstruction produces foci of emphysema and subpleural blebs (see Fig. 20–39A). Irregular emphysematous cavities partially surrounded by uniform fascicles of plump spindle cells are so characteristic at scanning power magnification as to be diagnostic (see Fig. 20–39A). Small vein obstruction causes microhemorrhages and hemosiderin accumulation, a common feature of LAM.[349] The amount of smooth muscle progressively increases and results in thick bands between the irregular emphysematous spaces, giving a superficial resemblance to honeycombing (see Fig. 20–42).

When the diagnosis of LAM is suspected preoperatively or at frozen section, tissue should be saved for estrogen and progesterone receptor analysis, although negative receptor analysis may not preclude a response to hormonal manipulation.[355b] Although the unique features of LAM allow for recognition on transbronchial biopsy, most cases are diagnosed by open biopsy, sometimes undertaken at the time of evaluation and therapy for recurrent pneumothoraces. The differential diagnosis of LAM includes fibrosis, smooth muscle metaplasia, and benign metastasizing leiomyoma. The cellular proliferation in LAM is different from smooth muscle metaplasia in

Figure 20–39A,B. Lymphangioleiomatosis (LAM) at biopsy. A. Emphysematous spaces partially surrounded by bundles of smooth muscle and partially by normal alveolar walls (arrows). Slit-like lymphatic spaces are present in many of the bundles (H&E, ×32). B. The smooth muscle proliferation partially involves a septal lymphatic (H&E, ×60).

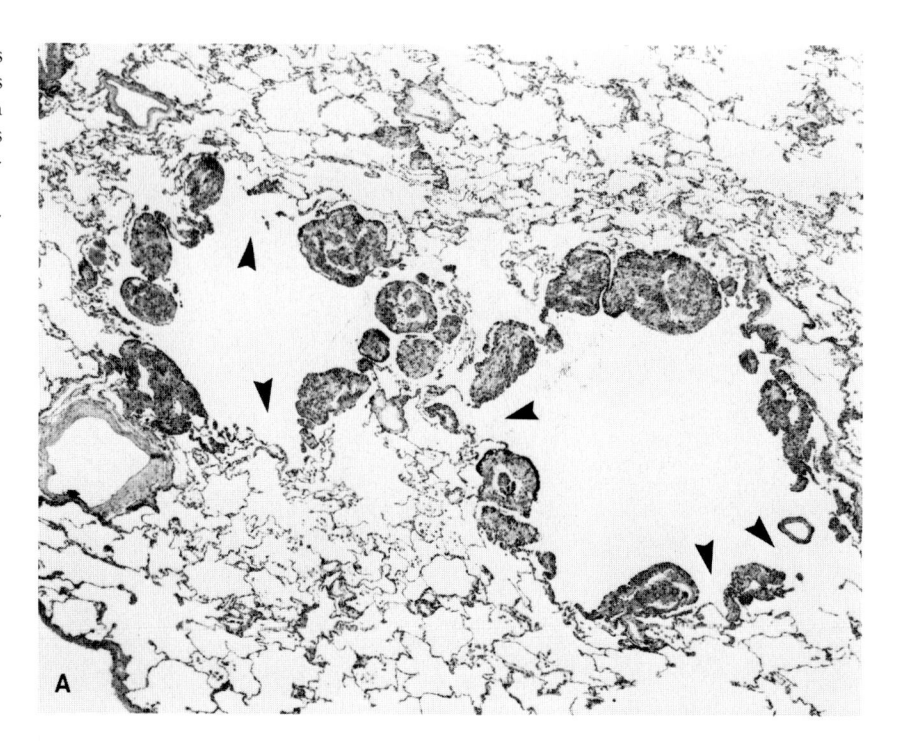

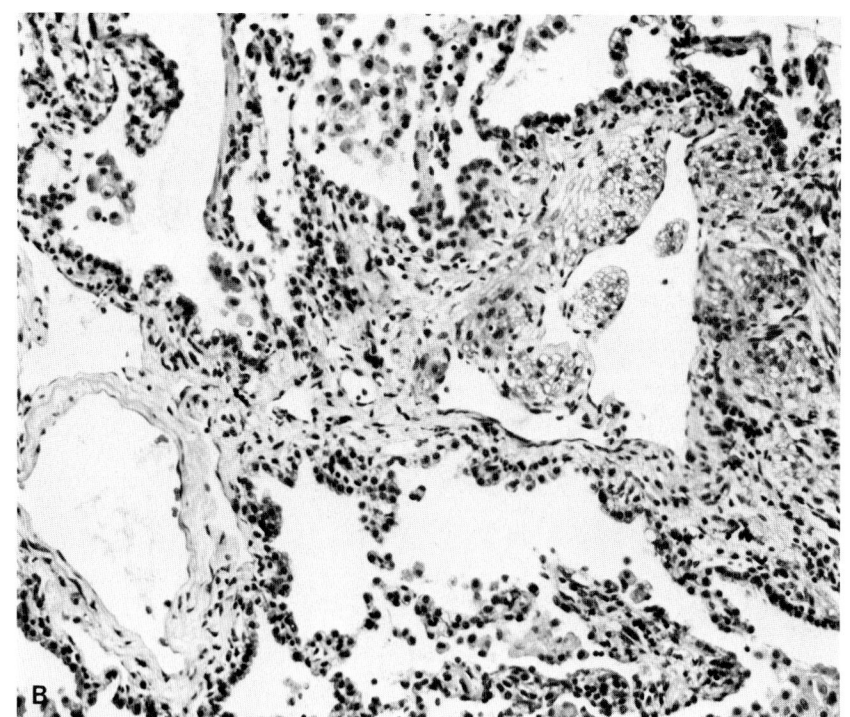

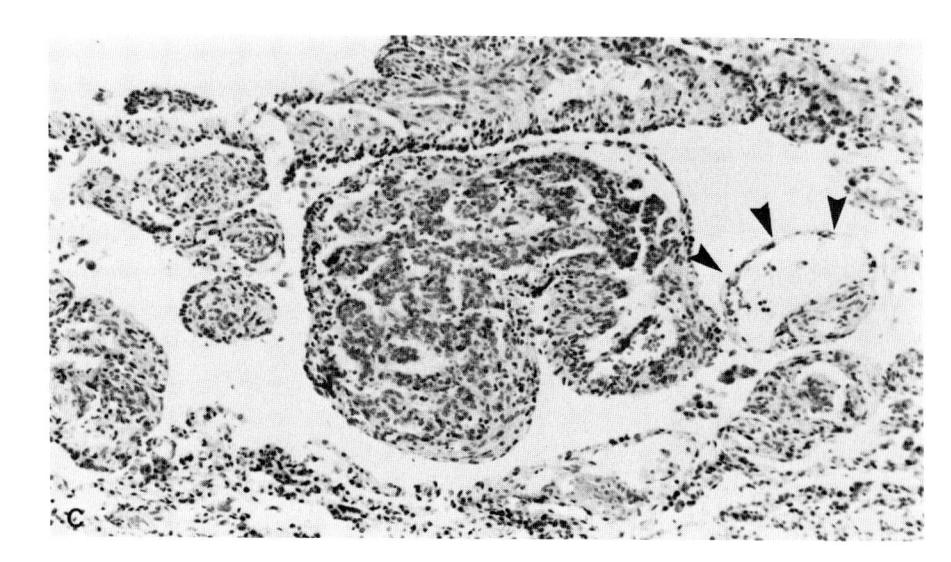

Figure 20–39C. In addition to the more spindled cells around it, a nodule of more polygonal cells (myoblastic focus) is seen. A slit-like space distened with lymph node is seen at the right (arrows) (H&E, ×120).

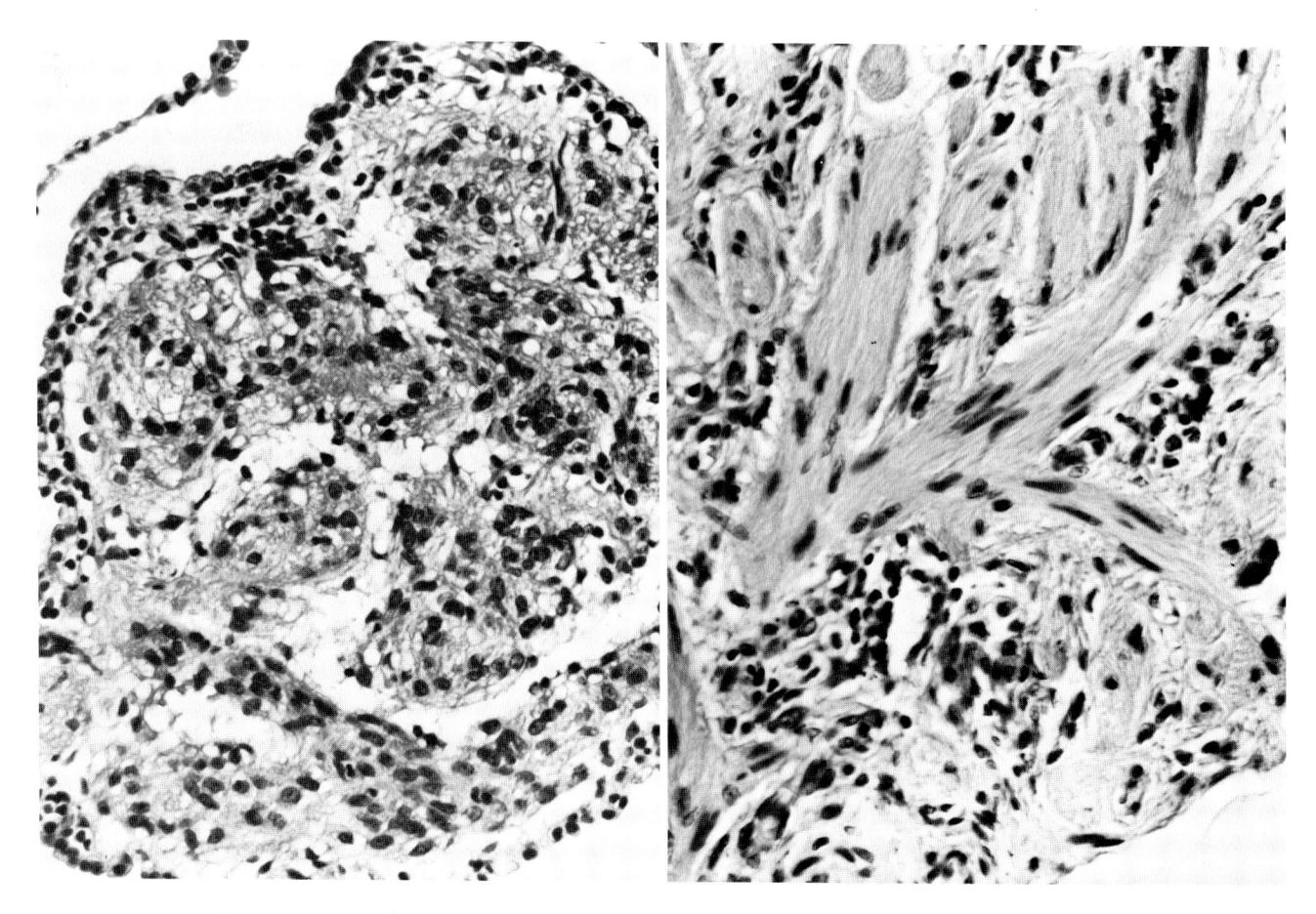

Figure 20–40. The spindle cell proliferation of LAM (left is compared with metaplastic smooth muscle in the lung in a case of UIP (right) (both H&E, ×300).

Figure 20–41. Lymph node involvement in LAM. Only rare islands of lymphocytes remain (arrows) (H&E, ×32).

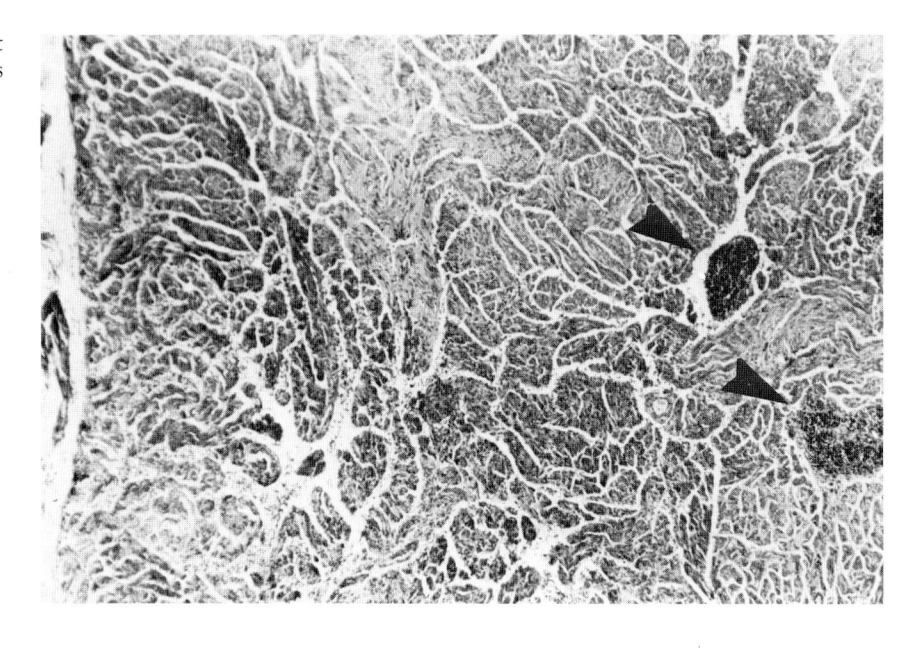

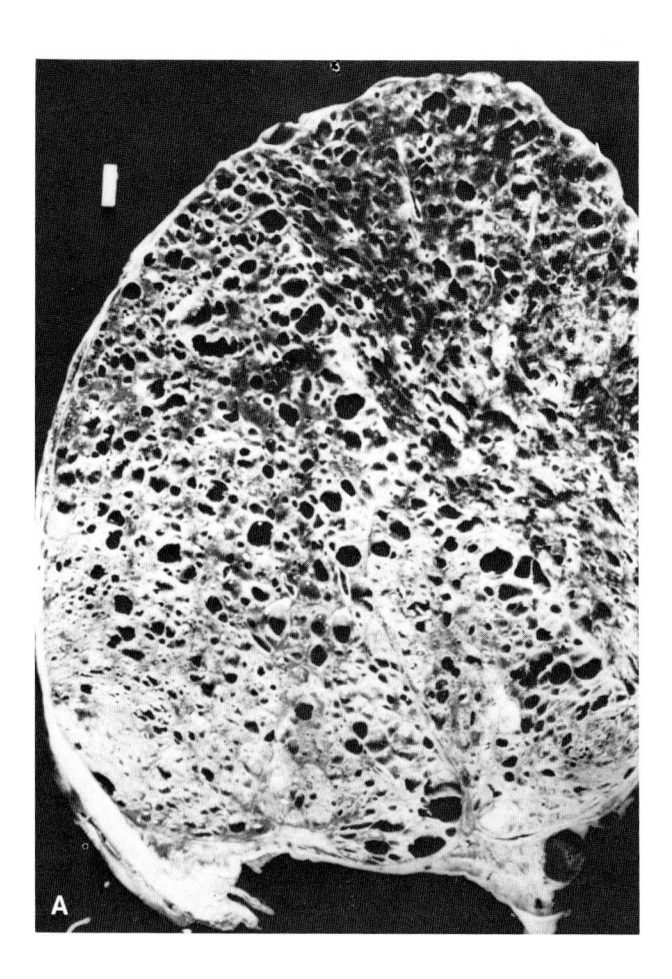

Figure 20–42A. Lymphangioleiomyomatosis at autopsy. A. Gross section of lung showing uniform involvement with superficial resemblance to honeycombing.

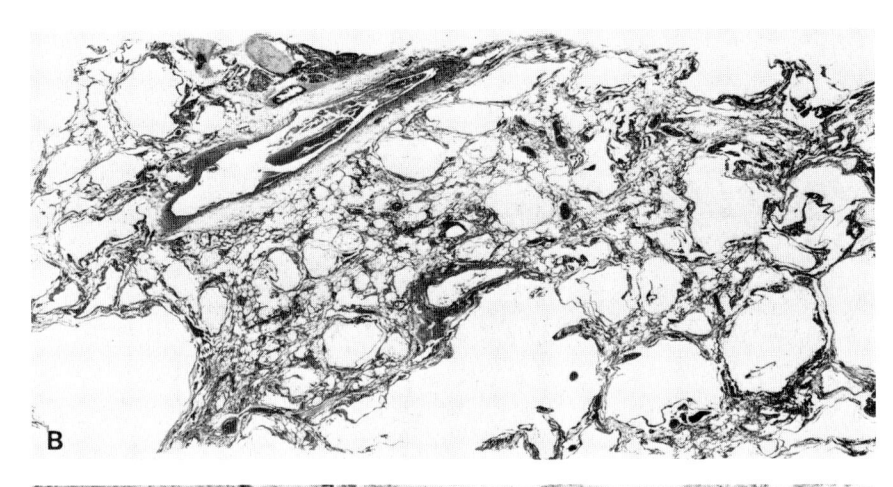

Figure 20–42B,C. B. Section of inflated lung showing that many of the cavities are lined by relatively normal parenchyma (emphysema), whereas others have thickened walls due to the smooth muscle proliferation. C. Another case showing more extensive muscle proliferation, involving much of the parenchyma at autopsy. Collections of hemosiderin-filled macrophages are present (arrows) (H&E, ×32).

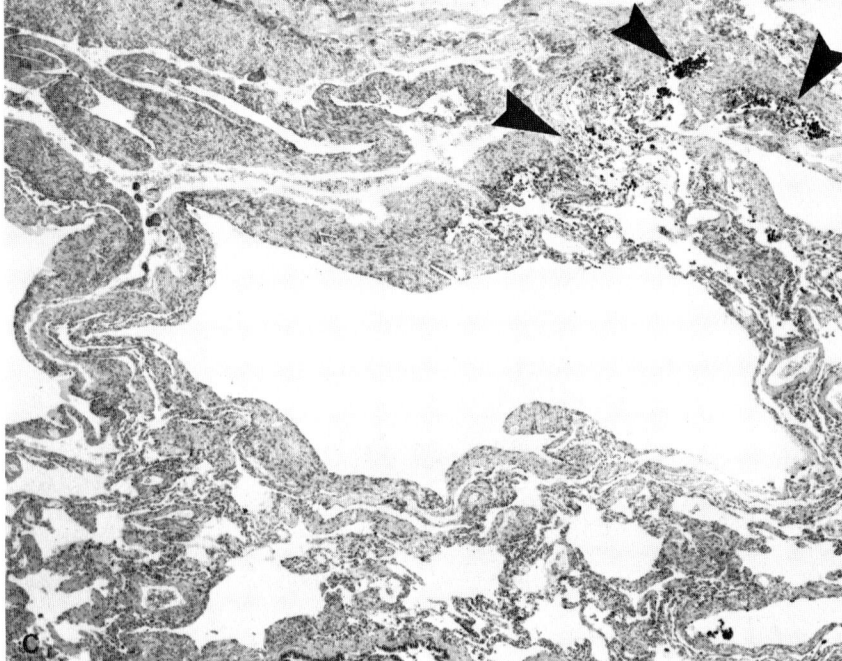

fibrotic lungs, although it does show the special staining characteristics of smooth muscle. Metaplastic smooth muscle resembles normal smooth muscle with elongated cells, abundant pink cytoplasm, and cigar-shaped nuclei. Benign metastasizing leiomyoma produces randomly scattered nodules, usually 1 cm or larger, that are separated by normal parenchyma, whereas LAM rarely produces more than microscopic nodular proliferations, tends to involve the parenchyma much more diffusely, and is oriented along lymphatics. The distinction between LAM and benign metastasizing leiomyoma is usually not difficult, although in rare cases it is almost impossible both histologically and clinically.[355]

Thoracic and abdominal lymphangiomyomas, composed of masses of smooth muscle surrounding irregular lymphatic spaces and lymph node involvement, also occur in patients with LAM[352] (see Fig. 20–41). Metaplastic alveolar epithelium, so-called adenomatous proliferation, is also seen.[345] Lymphangiomeiomatosis has also been associated wtih ureteral involvement and chyluria, hyperparathyroidism, and angiomyolipomas of the kidney.[345,346,352]

The histologic findings in LAM explain the clinical, radiologic, and functional changes (Table 20–17).[349]

Ultrastructural studies have confirmed smooth muscle differentiation in LAM.[347,348,350] Some cells contain features of myofibroblasts. One study claimed that the pulmonary interstitial stromal cell rather than smooth muscle cells from vascular walls was the progenitor cell in LAM.[350]

The relationship between LAM and tuberous sclerosis has been debated. Since the pulmonary lesions in tuberous sclerosis are similar to those in LAM,[356–360] LAM may be a forme fruste of tuberous sclerosis.[344–347] Typically

Table 20-17. Clinical, Physiologic, and Radiographic Consequences of Lymphangioleiomyomatosis[a]

Histologic Features	Clinical	Physiologic	Radiographic
Hyperplasia of smooth muscle along lymphatic routes with:			Reticulonodular pattern
Lympatic obstruction	Rupture of lympatics with chylous effusion, ascites, chyloptysis, abdominal masses, dyspnea	Decreased lung volume from effusion	Abnormal lymphangiogram, pleural effusions, coarse reticulation
Venous obstruction with focal hemorrhage and hemosiderosis	Hemoptysis, dyspnea	Uneven perfusion, ventilation/perfusion mismatch	Reversible coarse, infiltration
		Hypoxemia and decreased diffusing capacity of the lung	
Bronchiolar obstruction, distal alveolar lesions, emphysema	Emphysema, recurrent pneumothorax, dyspnea	Increased TLC and RV, airflow obstruction, uneven ventilation, and ventilation/perfusion mismatch	Enlarged lung volume, "microcysts," pneumothorax

Abbreviations: RV, residual volume; TLC, total lung capacity.
[a] Based on the results of Carrington et al.[349]

tuberous sclerosis is associated with epilepsy, mental retardation, and sebaceous adenomas of the skin.[359] Tuberous sclerosis affects both men and women, and familial cases show autosomal dominant inheritance, although sporadically occurring cases outnumber those with family histories.[359] Pulmonary involvement in tuberous sclerosis is rare and probably affects less than 1 percent of patients.[356] Interestingly, affected patients are usually women in the reproductive years in whom central nervous system lesions and mental retardation are less frequent.[360] Although there are minor differences, the clinical signs and symptoms, chest radiographic findings, pulmonary functions, and clinical course are similar in the two conditions.[342,356-360] According to some authors, the histologic changes in the lung are identical in the two conditions, whereas others have found differences.[358] Stovin and coworkers[358] claim that vascular smooth muscular proliferates in tuberous sclerosis and that the perilymphatic cells are involved in LAM; both axial and peripheral structures are involved in tuberous sclerosis, whereas only axial structures are involved in LAM; and localized nodular proliferations of smooth muscle occur in tuberous sclerosis, as opposed to the more diffuse proliferation in LAM. Adenomatous foci of metaplastic epithelium, similar to those seen in LAM, have also been described in tuberous sclerosis.[359]

Valensi[357] has summarized the similarities and differences between tuberous sclerosis with pulmonary involvement and with LAM. The similarities noted included sex and age distribution, histologic features, the presence of renal angiomyolipomas, and the involvement of lymphatics and lymph nodes; the differences included absence of brain lesions, retardation, seizures, adenoma sebaceum, and family history in LAM. As Corrin and associates[345] and Lie and associates[359] indicated, the relationship between tuberous sclerosis and LAM is yet to be resolved.

Pulmonary Involvement in Neurofibromatosis

Clinical, radiographic, functional, and morphologic features of UIP were first described in neurofibromatosis in 1965 in a woman and her son.[361] Several other reports have documented the occurrence of lung disease in neurofibromatosis.[362-366] In the study of Massaro and Katz, 20 of 88 patients with neurofibromatosis had either radiologic or histologic abnormalities.[362] All but one of the patients were men, and the most frequent radiographic abnormality was apical bullous disease which was associated with an interstitial infiltrate in 11 cases. The histologic findings were "alveolitis and fibrosis," but these terms were used descriptively, and the histologic findings in most of the cases were focal and nonspecific. Simarily, in the study of 70 patients by Webb and Goodman,[365] 7 showed radiologic interstitial infiltrates; chronic interstitial pneumonia (UIP) was apparently present in 4; and 5 had apical bullae combined with interstitial infiltrates. Of the six cases reported by Sagel and colleagues,[364] only two appear to represent a progressive chronic interstitial pneumonia (UIP), whereas three had only mild pulmonary disease, and in one the pulmonary symptoms were clearly related to bullae alone. The youngest patient with neurofibromatosis and UIP was a 28-year-old woman reported by Patchefsky and coworkers.[363]

Two separate patterns of pulmonary involvement occur in neurofibromatosis, interstitial disease, and apical bullae, and they may occur together or independently. Most cases have the pattern of UPI, but a few resemble DIP.[380] The actual incidence is probably less than 10 percent. Apical bullous change is often unilateral and may be extensive enough to be associated with significant airflow obstruction. Patients who have evidence of both bullae and interstitial pneumonia may show a peculiar combination of obstructive and restrictive disease.[364]

Pulmonary Amyloidosis

Amyloid is a chemically diverse glycoprotein that is deposited extracellulary.[367-369] Deposits may be focal and localized to a single organ or part of a widespread systemic disease.[368] Amyloidosis may be idiopathic or associated with chronic inflammatory disease or lymphoproliferative disorders. Familial cases occur. Structurally amyloid is a beta-pleated sheet of fibrils; the term beta fibrilloses has been proposed to encompass all examples of amyloidosis.[368,369] The beta-pleated configuration gives amyloid its light microscopic staining properties as well as its characteristic ultrastructure of 75 to 100 Å diameter woven fibrils.[370,371] In histologic sections, amyloid stains red with the Congo red stain which gives an apple-green color with birefringence.

Pulmonary amyloidosis occurs as a localized process restricted to the lung (primary pulmonary amyloidosis) or part of systemic infiltration.[371-374] Isolated pulmonary anyloidosis may be divided into the following groups: tracheobronchial, nodular parenchymal, diffuse alveolar septal, and senile. The first three constitute relatively well-defined, clinicopathologic entities with little overlap among them. Their clinical features are outlined in Table 20–18.

Primary Pulmonary Amyloidosis

Tracheobronchial Amyloid

Tracheobronchial amyloid (Fig. 20–43) is the most common form of amyloid limited to the respiratory tract.[372,375-380] Most patients have symptoms of airway obstruction, and some relate having had symptoms for 35 to 40 years. Laryngeal involvement is frequently a concomitant finding and accounts for the high frequency (33 percent) of hoarseness and stridor.[372] Characteristically there is diffuse involvement of the tracheobronchial tree, although localized lesions are occasionally seen. In the latter group, the distinction between localized tracheobronchial amyloid and nodular parenchymal amyloid secondarily occluding an airway is somewhat arbitrary.

Chest radiographs usually show nonspecific changes secondary to airway obstruction but are normal in up to one-quarter of patients. Bronchograms demonstrate radiographically nonspecific focal obstruction(s). Pulmonary function studies show airflow obstruction.[378] Abnormal serum proteins are not found.[376]

The gross features of tracheobronchial amyloidosis are distinctive.[376] There are discrete, occasionally pedunculated, irregular nodules and plaques with intact overlying mucosa. The largest deposits are found in the immediate subglottic region. Large lesions may distort and erode cartilage, and in severe cases, extensive stenoses involve many airways.

Histologically the amyloid is deposited in the submucosa in and around vessels, bronchial glands, and connective tissue adjacent to the cartilage. There may also be deposition in the walls of pulmonary arteries. Secondary calcification and ossification occur, and metaplasia in the overlying epithelium is common. In late lesions, bone and calcification may be so prominent that amyloid is difficult to find, and differential diagnosis from tracheopathia osteoplastica may be nearly impossible. On small biopsies, amyloid may be easily overlooked unless specifically considered and sought.

Patients will diffuse tracheobronchial amyloidosis have a slow but relentless course. Palliative surgery to relieve local obstruction may be long-lasting in a few cases, but it is not curative and recurrences are frequent. Of the reported cases, approximately one-third of patients have died as a direct result of the disease or its therapy[372]; although rare, spontaneous regressions have been reported.[380] Patients do not develop systemic amyloidosis.[379]

Nodular Parenchymal Amyloid

Nodular parenchymal amyloid (Fig. 20–44) presents as single or multiple discrete nodules in one or both lungs.[372,375,381-388] Most cases represent incidental radio-

Table 20–18. Primary Pulmonary Amyloidosis[a]

Type	No. Cases	Male/Female Ratio	Mean Age (Range)	Dyspnea	Percent of Patients Presenting with:	
					Couch	Hemoptysis
Tracheobronchial	41	2:1	53 (16–76)	60	74	51
Nodular parenchymal	31	1.3:1	65 (38–95)	12	30	4
Diffuse alveolar septal	4	1:1	55 (39–67)	100	100	0

[a] Based on the results of Rubinow et al.[372].

Figure 20–43. Tracheobronchial amyloidosis. A. A mucosally covered plaque is present near a bronchial bifurcation. B. The bronchial lumen (top) is filled with inspissated mucus and inflammatory cells. Under the intact mucosa are nodular deposits of amyloid (lower left) some of which are calcified (arrows) (H&E, ×32).

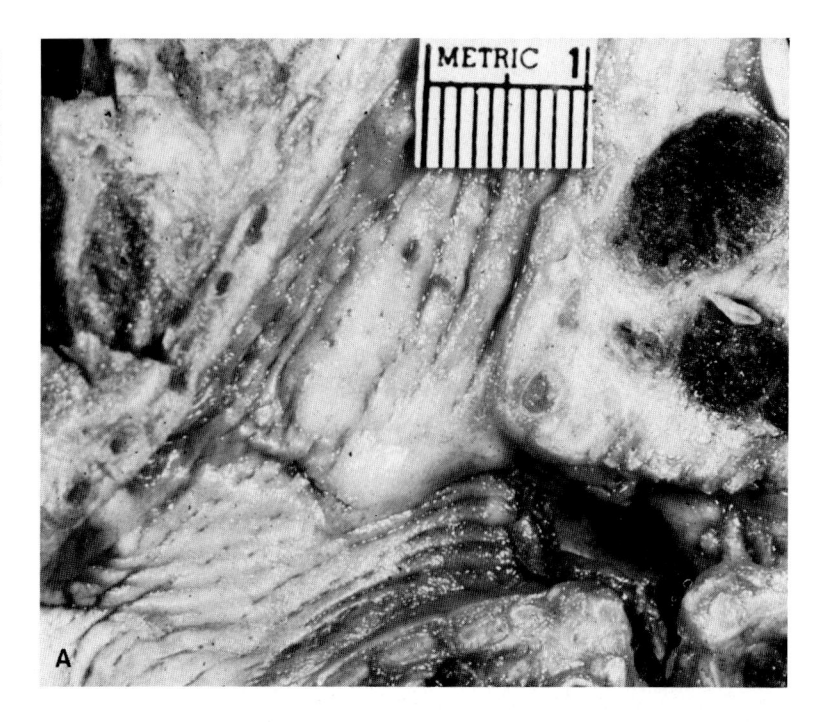

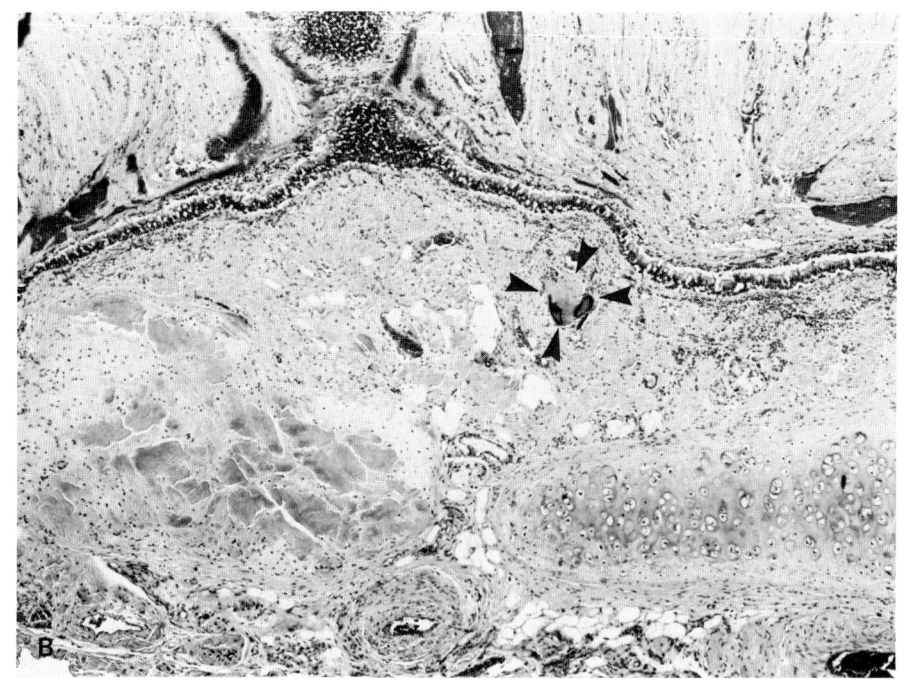

graphic findings, although a small percentage are symptomatic (see Table 20–18) and respiratory insufficiency has been reported.[388a] Biopsy or resection is performed to exclude a neoplasm.

Radiographically any lobe may be involved. The nodules generally are only a few centimeters in diameter. Approximately one-quarter show calcification on chest radiograph; cavitation is rare.

Laboratory studies usually show no serum protein abnormalities, but some patients have a benign monoclonal gammopathy, macroglobulinemia, or hypergammaglobulinemic purpura.[387] Pulmonary function tests have been normal in the few patients in whom they were evaluated.[386]

Grossly the nodules are wedge-shaped or rounded with grey-yellow translucence on cut section.[375,381] Some have opaque calcified zones. Histologically irregular, amorphous, and predominantly acellular masses of amyloid replace the pulmonary parenchyma.[375,385–386] Most lesions are sharply demarcated, although interstitial

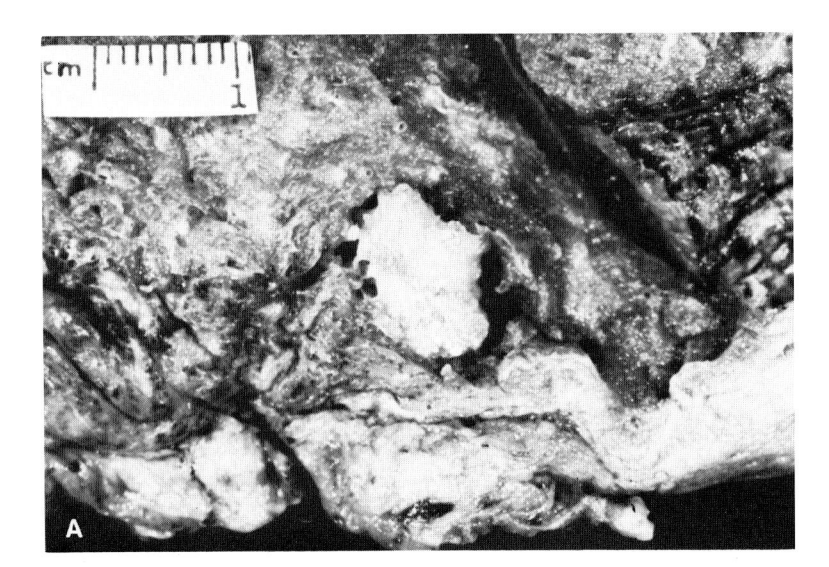

Figure 20–44. Nodular parenchymal amyloidosis. A. A grey-white subpleural nodule is sharply demarcated from the adjacent parenchyma (courtesy of Dr. Gmelich, Pasadena, CA). B. Metaplastic bone with marrow (right center) has developed in the nodule of amyloid (H&E, ×32). C. Amyloid (upper left) merges with metaplastic bone (lower left). The cell infiltrate is predominantly mononuclear but includes a giant cell reaction (arrow) to the amyloid (H&E, ×200).

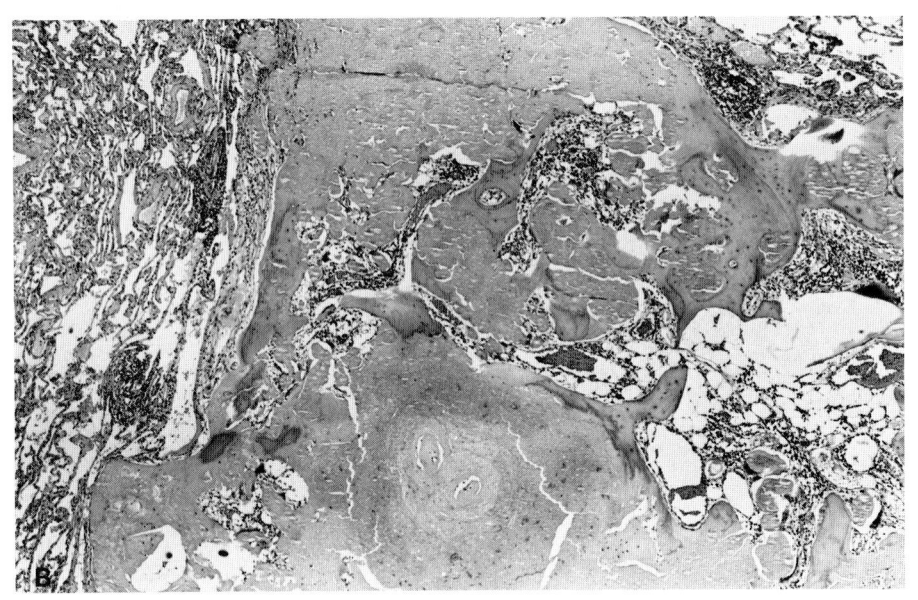

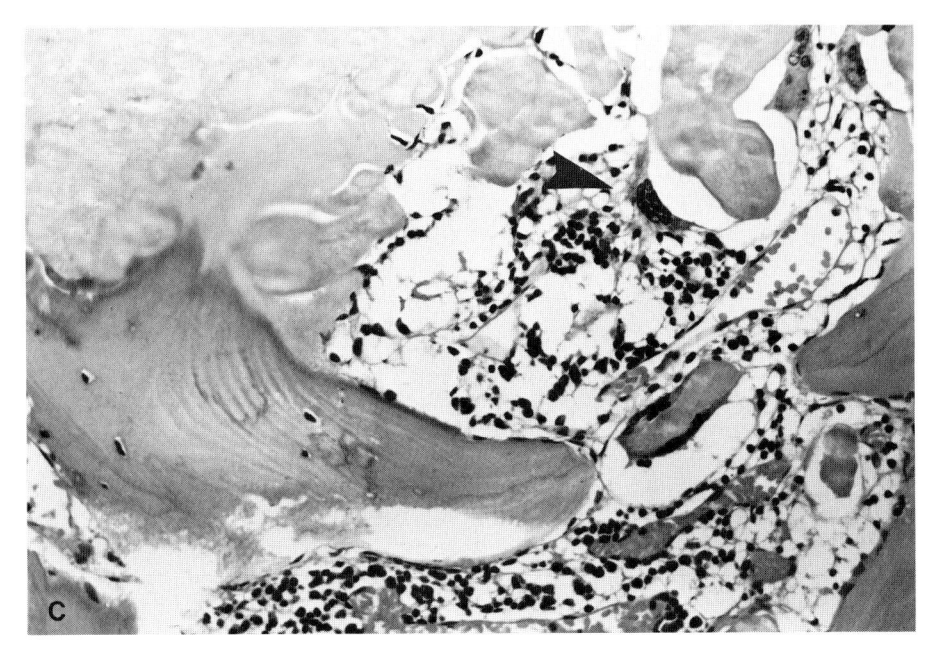

accumulations of amyloid may be seen at the edges of some, suggesting an interstitial origin of the nodules. Amyloid is frequently present in vessel walls within the nodule. Fibrosis, calcification, ossification, and chondroid metaplasia may occur and are more frequent than radiographic changes might suggest.[381] Giant cell reaction to the amyloid is frequent as are scattered infiltrates of plasma cells, lymphocytes, and histiocytes. Electron microscopy shows the characteristic fibrillary structure of amyloid.[388]

The differential diagnosis includes all eosinophilic nodular lesions: hyalinized scars and old healed granulomas, plasma cell granulomas, and pulmonary hyalinizing granulomas, a few of which were reported to have amyloid and may actually represent a nodular amyloidosis.[389] The differential diagnosis also includes unrelated lesions that are associated with amyloid deposition, such as LIP and lymphocytic lymphomas; amyloid is not the most prominent histologic finding in these conditions.

The prognosis for nodular parenchymal amyloid is excellent. A few of the reported patients have died but from other causes. The lesions may recur[385]; although they do not recur following lobectomy,[385] such surgical therapy may be excessive. Patients with nodular parenchymal amyloid do not develop systemic amyloidosis, multiple myeloma, or serum protein abnormalities (if these were not evident at presentation), but data are few and most of the reported follow-up is short.

Diffuse Alveolar Septal Amyloid

Diffuse alveolar septal amyloid (Fig. 20–45) is the least common form of isolated pulmonary amyloidosis, and only a few cases have been reported.[372,390–395] Patients have signs, symptoms, pulmonary function findings, and radiologic features of interstitial lung disease. The few patients reported have all been symptomatic (see Table 20–18). Radiologically they have reticular or reticulonodular infiltrates of varying severity. Pleural effusions may be present and occasionally dominate the clinical course.[393]

Serum protein abnormalities may or may not be present. Pulmonary function studies have shown impaired gas transfer.

The gross findings are identical to those seen in diffuse alveolar septal amyloid associated with systemic amyloidosis.[371,394,395] The lungs are firm and distended and have a "uniform rubbery sponge-like appearance.[394]

Histologically there is diffuse deposition of amyloid in the alveolar walls, interstitium, and tracheobronchial tree.[391] The amount of deposition may vary, and small nodules may be found.[392] Giant cell reaction and infiltrate of plasma cells, lymphocytes, and histiocytes are sometimes present. Nodules may become calcified or ossified. Massive pleural involvement occurs in some cases.[393] Electron microscopy has shown the typical fibrillary structure of amyloidosis.[391] The few reported patients with primary diffuse alveolar septal amyloidosis have died of progressive respiratory insufficiency in less than a year.

Senile Amyloid Deposition

Focal deposition of amyloid seen in elderly patients, so-called senile amyloidosis, is an incidental finding at autopsy in several organs including the lung.[367,369,374,396,396a] The incidence of this form of amyloid increases with age and is seen in at least one site in approximately 50 percent of autopsies of individuals aged 90 or more.[396] In patients older than age 70, 36 percent show focal amyloid deposition. Incidental identification of amyloid in the lungs at autopsy is most

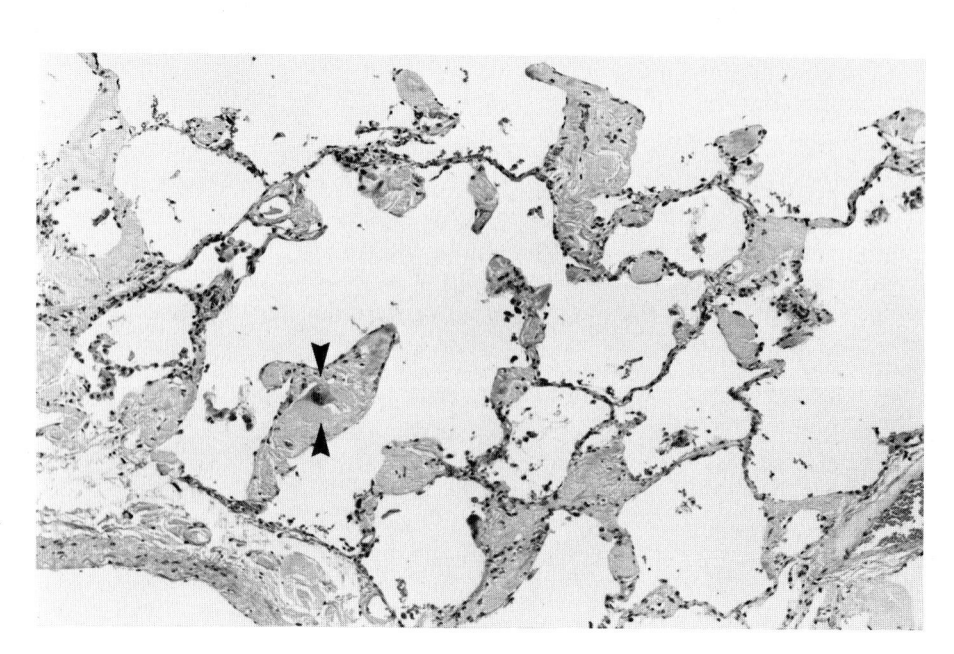

Figure 20–45. Diffuse alveolar septal amyloidosis. Micronodular massas of amyloid distend alveolar wall. An occasional giant cell is present (arrows) (H&E, ×80).

frequently associated with similar deposits in the heart.[374] In a study[396] in which the cardiac and pulmonary amyloid deposits (in the absence of systemic amyloidosis) were specifically evaluated, 20 percent of autopsies on patients older than age 80 demonstrated cardiac or pulmonary lesions or both, with involvement of the heart alone being slightly more frequent than only the lung. An immunohistochemical study showed that senile amyloidosis may be more widespread than previously appreciated, and the term senile systemic amyloidosis may be more appropriate.[396a]

Pulmonary Amyloidosis Occurring as Part of Multisystemic or Systemic Amyloidosis

The lung is frequently involved in systemic amyloidosis,[367,369–371,373,374,397,398,398a] estimates being from 30 percent to more than 90 percent of cases. The higher figure is probably more accurate. The sex incidence is roughly equal. Most patients are older than age 50, but one report[373] describes a 16-year-old patient with systemic amyloidosis who died of progressive alveolar septal deposition. In only a few patients do the effects of pulmonary infiltration dominate the clinical picture, and in most there are few if any symptoms related to it. Pulmonary symptoms are more frequent in patients with associated lymphoproliferative disorders compared with chronic inflammatory processes. Cough and dyspnea are the most frequent complaints. Radiographic findings generally correlate with the clinical symptoms, and radiography of patients with symptoms invariably shows pulmonary infiltrates that are described as interstitial reticular or reticulonodular. The chest radiographs may suggest UIP. Other effects of systemic amyloidosis such as pulmonary edema due to left-side heart failure may produce superimposed radiographic findings and make a significant contribution to the symptomatology. Asymptomatic patients may have a normal chest radiograph or may show a mild interstitial infiltrate.

Pulmonary function tests reflect the severity of involvement and manifest as impaired gas transfer.[397,398]

The pathologic features are those of diffuse alveolar septal amyloidosis. Patients with amyloid secondary to underlying chronic inflammatory conditions tend to have less severe histologic changes.[373] There is involvement of alveolar walls, tracheobronchial tree, and pulmonary vasculature, although the degree of involvement of these sites varies among cases. Small nodules with secondary calcification and metaplastic bone may be found. Electron microscopic examination has shown that early deposits in the alveolar wall are associated with focal widening of the basal membrane.[398a]

Monoclonal gammopathy is usually seen in patients with idiopathic amyloidosis and in amyloidosis associated with lymphoproliferative disorders, but is uncommon in amyloidosis associated with chronic inflammatory conditions.[373]

Amyloidosis Involving the Hilar Lymph Nodes

Amyloidosis of the hilar nodes is rarely seen in patients with systemic amyloidosis and pulmonary infiltrates.[399] Hilar lymph nodes are also a rare site of a localized amyloid deposition.[400]

Pulmonary Involvement in Inborn Errors of Metabolism

Extrapulmonary manifestations usually account for signs and symptoms in most inborn errors of metabolism, although clinically inapparent involvement of the lung is common. When signs and symptoms of respiratory involvement are present, they most frequently manifest as diffuse interstitial lung disease.

Gaucher's Disease

Abnormal amounts of sphingolipid are deposited in lysosomes of the reticuloendothelial system in Gaucher's disease, which is familial and transmitted as an autosomal recessive trait.[401–408] Clinically significant pulmonary disease is more common in infantile forms of Gaucher's, and a miliary or interstitial infiltrate is seen on chest radiograph.[403] Pulmonary involvement in adult forms of the disease is much rarer,[406] although patients with pulmonary manifestations have presented after 50 years of age.[404] The major symptom is increasing shortness of breath.[406] Chest radiographs show diffuse reticular, nodular, or reticulonodular infiltrates more extensive at the bases.[402,404,406,407] Pulmonary function tests show decreased vital capacity and lowered PO_2.[406,408] Cyanosis and clubbing have been reported in the late stages of severe cases. Involvement of lungs only, heart and lungs, and nervous system and lungs may be seen in adults with pulmonary Gaucher's disease.

Grossly the lungs are firm and pale. Gaucher's cells stuff the alveoli and infiltrate the alveolar septa, airways, and pleura.[402,405–407] Some of the cells stain positively for iron. Interstitial fibrosis occasionally develops.[402] The characteristic morphology of the Gaucher cell allows for cytologic diagnosis by needle aspiration.[408]

Gaucher's disease is occasionally associated with pulmonary hypertension, supposedly caused by Gaucher cells occluding the pulmonary capillary network.[401,407]

Niemann-Pick Disease

Sphingomyelin accumulates in reticuloendothelial cells throughout the body in Niemann-Pick disease.[402,409–412] The disease is autosomal recessive in inheritance, and several infantile and adult forms have been described.[410]

Pulmonary disease in infantile forms of Niemann-Pick disease is common.[411] Among 28 cases of Niemann-Pick disease collected by Lachman and associates,[411] 18 had pulmonary disease described as diffuse nodular infiltrates, sometimes with honeycombing and linear stranding. All 18 patients presented in infancy and died before age 8. None of the cases in later childhood or adolescent had pulmonary involvement. Long and colleagues[412] described three cases of adult Niemann-Pick disease with interstitial infiltrates and honeycombing on chest radiographs and decreased diffusing capacity.

The lungs are pale and heavy and infiltrated by masses of foamy Niemann-Pick cells.[409] Alveoli are stuffed, and there is infiltration of alveolar septa, air spaces, and pleura (Fig. 20–46). Fibrosis may be a late finding. Electron microscopy has shown the characteristic features of Niemann-Pick disease.[410]

Fabry's Disease (Angiokeratoma Corporis Diffusum Universale)

Fabry's disease is an X-linked, recessive disorder of glycolipid metabolism with deposition of sphingolipid in endothelial, smooth muscle, and vascular-supporting cells.[413–416] The existence of pulmonary involvement in Fabry's disease has been controversial. Bartimmo and associates[464] do not believe that pulmonary symptoms in most patients are directly related to Fabry's disease, but Kariman and colleagues[415] and Rosenberg and colleagues[416] claim that airway obstruction is a significant part of the disease and that it is more severe than would be expected when environmental factors, such as smoking, are taken into account. Rosenberg and associates[416] have shown Fabry's-like inclusions in epithelial cells from the airways, but they do not relate this finding to clinical symptomatology.

Hermansky-Pudlak Syndrome

Hermansky-Pudlak syndrome is an autosomal recessive disorder that includes oculocutaneous (tyrosine-positive) albinism, a defect in the second stage of platelet aggregation and accumulation of ceroid-filled histiocytes in body tissues.[417–420] Some patients have a lesion which clinically and histologically resembles idiopathic UIP.[417–419] Granulomatous colitis has also been associated with the syndrome.[420] The exact incidence of pulmonary involvement is hard to ascertain; two of six patients reported by Davies and Tuddenham[417] had a UIP-like clinical picture. Some patients who lack albinism but have the defect in the second stage of platelet aggregation have also been found to have a chronic interstitial pneumonia.[417] Clinical signs, symptoms, and functional findings are indistinguishable from idiopathic UIP.[417–419] According to Garay and associates,[418] most patients in the United States are Puerto Rican; in western Europe, the majority are from southern Holland.

The histology is said to be similar to UIP except that increased numbers of ceroid-filled histiocytes may be present in the air spaces and interstitium.[418,419] The relationship between the ceroid deposition and the interstitial fibrosis is not known, and from the descriptions, it is not clear if the histology is sufficiently distinctive to be recognized as different from UIP. In any case, the diagnosis of Hermansky-Pudlak syndrome requires knowledge of the clinical and family history.

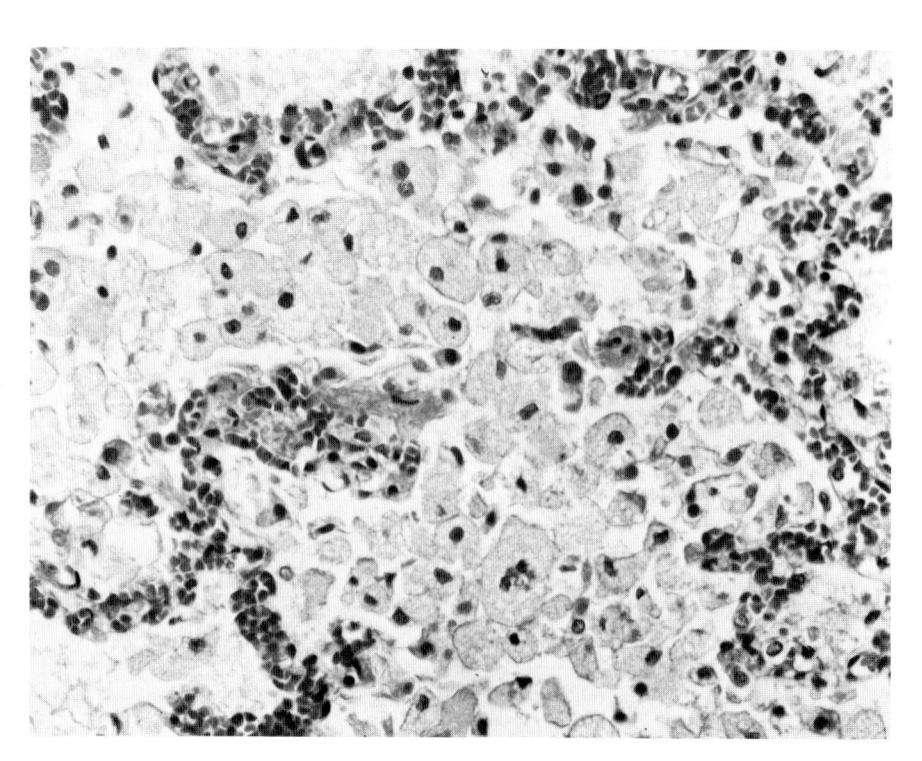

Figure 20–46. Pulmonary Niemann-Pick disease. The alveoli are stuffed with foamy macrophages (H&E, ×300).

Infantile GM₁-Gangliosidosis

Matsumoto and colleagues[421] described a 14-month-old infant with GM_1 gangliosidosis who died of progressive respiratory insufficiency. Autopsy showed massive accumulations of foamy cells in the alveoli with fewer in the interstitum.

Chronic Diffuse Infiltrative Lung Disease and Renal Tubular Acidosis

Thirteen patients with at least partial renal tubular acidosis were studied by Mason and colleagues.[422] Abnormal pulmonary function tests were present in eight, and patients who were severely affected had a clinical illness similar to idiopathic UIP. All eight patients also had associated autoimmune disease, including Sjögren's syndrome, primary biliary cirrhosis, and Hashimoto's disease among others. Zalin and co-workers[423] reported a patient in whom renal tubular acidosis developed after the chronic infiltrative lung disease had already been recognized.

Krabbe's Disease

Clark and co-workers[424] reported a case of Krabbe's disease (globoid leukocystrophy) with progressive respiratory insufficiency and found a similar case in the literature. The air spaces were filled with macrophages with dense eosinophilic cytoplasm and amber-brown inclusions which were PAS- and Sudan black–positive. Although typical globoid cells were not seen in the lung, the lesion was interpreted as pulmonary Krabbe's disease.

Pompe's Disease (Type II Glycogenosis, Acid Maltase Deficiency)

Lightman and Schooley[425] reported an adult with Pompe's disease who had dyspnea, a restrictive pulmonary function defect, and diaphragmatic paralysis. No histologic description was given, and it is not clear if there was intrinsic lung disease unrelated to the muscle disease. Spencer[426] described accumulation of glycogen in the alveolar macrophages in Pompe's disease.

Farber's Disease (Disseminated Lipogranulomatosis)

Farber's disease is a rare storage disease associated with granulomatous infiltrates throughout tissues of the body.[427] Lung involvement is unusual although occasionally noted.[402,408] Rutsaert and associates[428] described a patient who died of severe respiratory distress at 21 months of age. The lung contained multiple lesions. The granulomatous infiltrate is composed of sheets of histi-

Table 20–19. Pulmonary Calcification and Ossification

Lesion	Histologic Features (on H&E-Stained Sections)
Calcification	
Dystrophic calcification	Deposition of basophilic granular calcium phosphate in sites of tissue injury, scars, etc. (see Fig. 20–47)
Metastatic calcification	Diffuse alveolar septal, perivascular, and intimal calcification (see Fig. 20–48)
Pulmonary alveolar microlithiasis	Laminated, intra-alveolar, basophilic, calcified concretions, 0.1–0.3 mm in diameter, involving 25–80% of the alveoli (see Fig. 19–49)
Blue bodies (intra-alveolar conchoidal bodies)	Pale blue to blue-grey, intra-alveolar concretions, 15–40 μm, occurring singly and in clusters in foci of interstitial scarring; associated with histiocytes and giant cells (see Fig. 19–50)
Schauman (conchoidal) bodies	Deeply basophilic, irregular, amorphous, and laminated masses found in giant cells in granulomas; may be birefringent; may persist in interstitium after disappearance of the granuloma (see Fig. 20–51)
Calcium oxalate	Lucent, birefringent crystals in giant cells in granulomas
Ossification	
Dystrophic ossification (heterotopic or metaplastic bone formation)	Ossification in sites of old injury or hemorrhage commonly associated with dystrophic calcification (see Fig. 20–52, 19–53)
Clinicopathologic entities Nodular parenchymal ossification	Intra-alveolar bony nodules occurring in air spaces, often bilaterally; most cases associated with chronic passive congestion (see Fig. 20–54)
Dendriform pulmonary ossification	Irregular branching, coral-like ossification usually occurring in association with interstitial fibrosis; may be bilateral and extensive in chronic interstitial pneumonias
Tracheobronchial ossification Submucosal ossification (tracheopathia osteoplastica)	Diffuse submucosal metaplastic bone formation (see Chapter 21)
Ossification of tracheobronchial cartilages	Ossification of tracheobronchial cartilages occurring as an aging change
Corpora Amylacea	Eosinophilic, intra-alveolar, laminated spheroidal and ellipsoidal bodies, 30–200 μm, may calcify (see Fig. 20–55)

ocytes with a background of lymphocytes and plasma cells. With progression, the histiocytes enlarge, become foamy, then degenerate leaving a fibrous scar.[427]

Pulmonary Calcification and Ossification

Calcification and ossification occur in the lung in a variety of forms (Table 20-19).

Pulmonary Calcification

Calcification on H&E stained sections of the lung is similar to that in other organs. Affected tissues show granular, lamellar, or plate-like basophilic material. Most tissue calcification is composed at least partially of calcium and phosphate and is therefore positive with the von Kossa stain, which stains the phosphate. The alizarin red stain is more specific for calcium.

Dystrophic Calcification

Dystrophic Calcification (Fig. 20-47) is a common occurrence at sites of injury throughout the body. It may be seen in acute necrosis, organizing exudate, and old scars. A particularly common site is in old healed granulomas accounting for the radiologic identification of healed granulomatous disease. The residual necrotic center and the fibrous wall are the sites of calcification. Calcification has been observed in the hilar lymph nodes of a significant number of patients with a previous history of sarcoid involving lung and hilar nodes.[429] Dystrophic calcification may follow pneumonias as multiple discrete calcified nodules. Dystrophic calcification is also seen in parasitic infections, silicosis, and berylliosis and is a consequence of many other inflammatory reactions. Other than serving as a marker for tissue injury, dystrophic calcification is usually of little clinical significance.

Metastatic Calcification

Metastatic calcification (Fig. 20-48), however, may be a significant clinical problem.[430-456a] Calcium salts are deposited in previously normal tissues as a result of abnormal serum levels of calcium, phosphate, and possibly magnesium. Local tissue alkalinity is thought to predispose to metastatic calcification, explaining why the stomach, kidney, and lung are the sites most frequently involved.[436] Metastatic calcification is usually associated with an identifiable disease which affects calcium and phosphate metabolism.[430,431,436] Examples include chronic bone disease, particularly extensive bone involvement by tumors; chronic renal disease, particularly with chronic renal failure or after renal transplantation; and primary or tertiary hyperparathyroidism. Other causes of metastatic calcification include hypervitaminosis D, steroid and phosphate therapy in patients with known hypercalcemia, sarcoidosis, milk-alkali syndrome, and prolonged immobilization. In a small number of patients, no cause is found. The key factor in the development of metastatic calcification is the saturation point of calcium and phosphate, which depends on the product

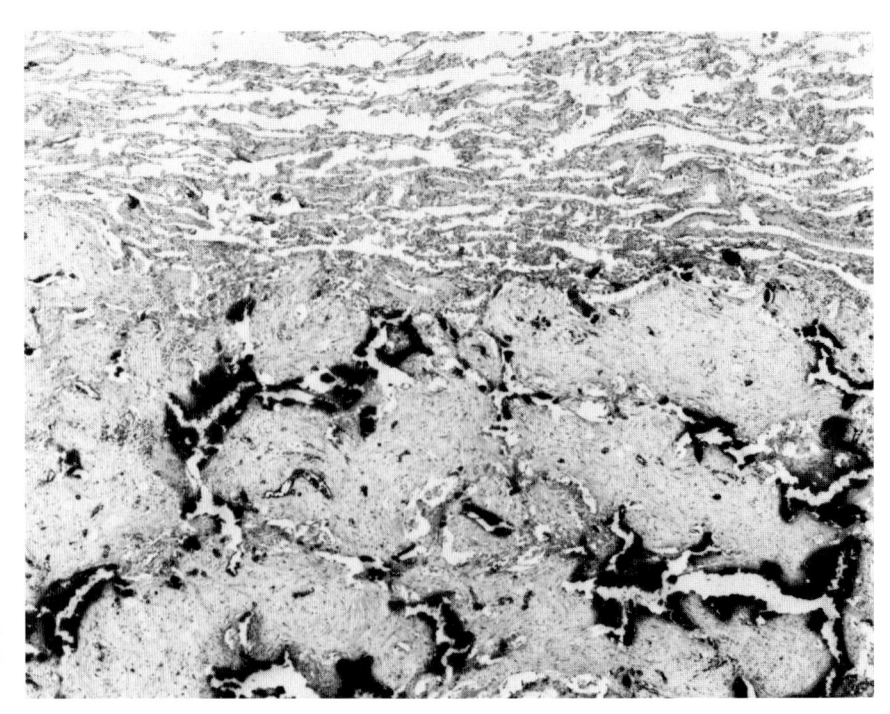

Figure 20-47. Dystrophic calcification occurring in a focus of organizing pneumonia (H&E, ×32).

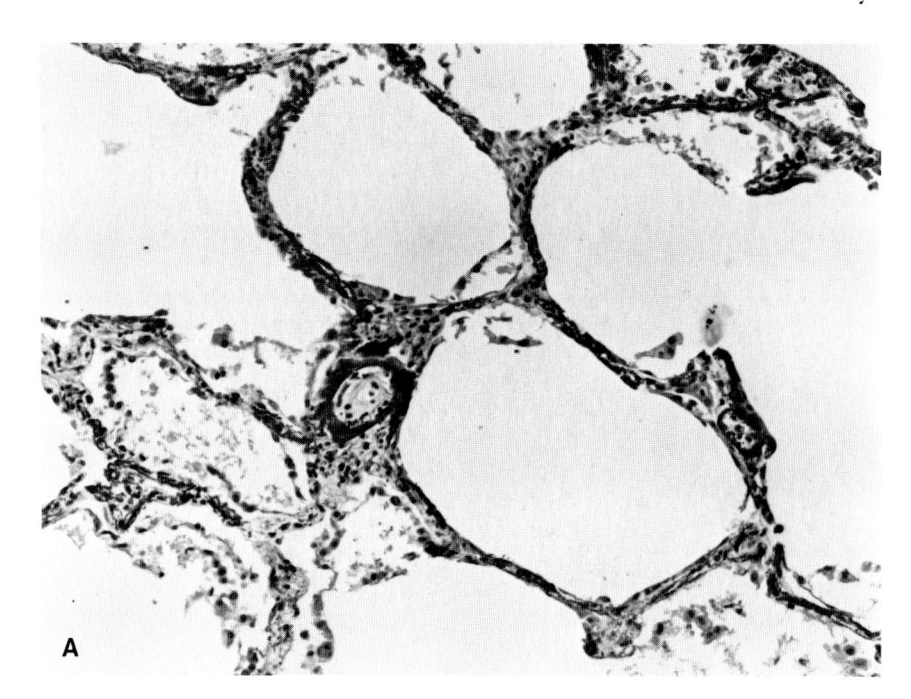

Figure 20–48. Metastatic calcification diffusely involves alveolar and vessel walls (A, H&E, ×120; B, Von Kossa, ×75).

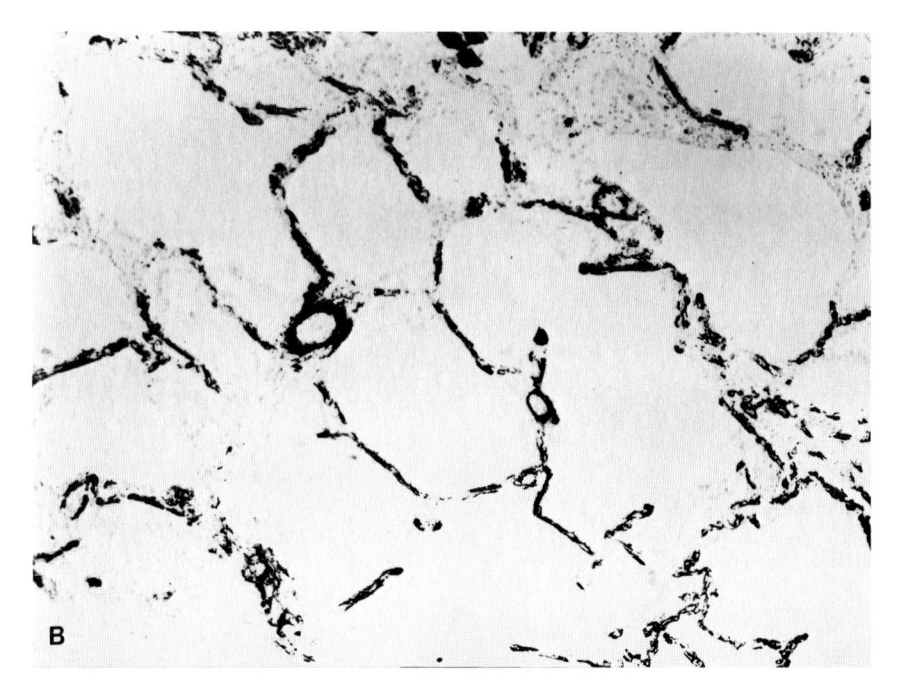

of both serum calcium and phosphate. Thus, metastatic calcification may be seen in patients with normal or low serum calcium levels when the serum phosphate level is markedly elevated.[436] Justrabo and associates[438] claim that nonvisceral metastatic calcificaiton tends to be hydroxyapatite, whereas visceral metastatic calcification is often associated with elevated serum magnesium, and the deposits are in the form of Whitlockite $(CaMg)_3(PO_4)_2$.

Metastatic calcification of the lung is a significant problem in patients on chronic hemodialysis.[434,436,438,456b] Affected patients usually have secondary hyperparathyroidism and the metabolic derangements caused by dialysis. Most of those who develop metastatic calcification of the lung will have no related clinical signs or symptoms. Fifteen of 31 patients on chronic dialysis studied by Conger and associates[434] died; 9 of them showed metastatic pulmonary calcification at autopsy. This incidence far exceeded the clinical suspicion as radiograph abnormalities were present in only one patient. The serum calcium was only slightly greater in those patients found at autopsy to have metastatic calcification than in those without calcification at autopsy. Patients on chronic dialysis who develop clinical evidence of metastatic calcification had significant morbidity: 7 of the 13 patients reviewed by Justrabous group[438] died of pulmonary insufficiency.

Metastatic calcification of the lung is uncommon, although the lung is involved in 75 percent of cases with metastatic calcification[430] and is its most frequent site.[433] Kaltreider and colleagues[431] found only 13 cases among 7221 autopsies; however, the incidence in any given series will depend heavily on selection factors and the population studied. Most cases are incidental autopsy findings, and none of the 13 cases was identified by chest radiograph. A few patients develop significant signs and symptoms, usually progressive dyspnea.[431] These patients may have either localized or diffuse infiltrates; the former may simulate a pneumonia and the latter may mimic pulmonary edema.[436] The characteristic feature is the unchanging nature of the infiltrates. Rarely are the pulmonary infiltrates nodular or wedge-shaped.[436] Calcification is usually not recognized as such on radiographs.[436]

Functional changes in pulmonary metastatic calcification include decreased diffusing capacity and restriction; these precede symptoms.[434] Many patients show a sudden clinical deterioration, as if a threshold point were reached beyond which the course is rapid.[431,435] A few cases have an abrupt and fulminant course.[432,435,456a] Arrhythmias caused by metastatic calcification in the heart may contribute to morbidity.[436]

Severely affected lungs are rigid and gritty with calcific granules and plates on cut section.[431,437] Less severely involved lungs may appear grossly normal.[431] Microscopically the deposition of calcium may be focal and patchy or extensive and widespread.[430,431,433,434,438,456b] Calcification occurs in alveolar and vessel walls, more extensively in the former. The calcification appears in linear bands or granular humps. The elastica of vessels may be encrusted. Calcification is occasionally found in airways. If an intraalveolar exudate is present, it may also become calcified. Giant cells are seen occasionally. Septal thickening and fibrosis with mild inflammatory infiltrates have sometimes been attributed to chronic metastatic calcification.[434] Ossification is seldom seen. Electron microscopy has shown rough edges (suggesting active growth) in small foci of calcification, whereas large foci are polycyclic and have a smooth edge, suggesting that growth decreases as the foci of calcification become larger.[437,456b] Early deposits may occur among elastic fibers.[456b] Nodular masses larger than 100 μm are unusual.

Neff and associates[433] reported an unusual case of metastatic pulmonary calcification in a patient with normal serum calcium and phosphorus. The calcified material was von Kossa-negative, alizarin red-positive, and chemically composed of calcium carbonate. No explanation was offered for this unusual case.

Pulmonary Alveolar Microlithiasis

Pulmonary alveolar microlithiasis derives its name from the unique histologic finding of innumerable laminated calcific bodies filling up to 80 percent of alveoli.[439–454] A few more than 100 case have been documented, and there has been a definite familial association.[440–444] The rarity of the disease is reflected in the fact that only eight cases were seen at the Mayo Clinic in a 46-year period.[454] Sex incidence is roughly equal except in familial cases, which show a 2:1 female predominance.[444,449] Age has ranged from premature infants[444] to 80 years.[448] Familial cases generally present at a younger age than nonfamilial cases[446] and are usually restricted to siblings.[454] The cause is unknown; however, one report described pulmonary alveolar microlithiasis in users of a particular snuff in Thailand.[441] Serum calcium levels are normal in the disease.

Less than half of patients are symptomatic at the time of diagnosis.[440–454] The majority present with an abnormal chest radiograph. The most common presenting symptom is cough. As the disease progresses, the patients develop dyspnea and occasionally hemoptysis; some may have repeated bouts of pneumonia or pleurisy.[451] Pneumothorax may occur. Terminally, patients have symptoms of end-stage interstitial pneumonia with cyanosis, clubbing, and congestive heart failure with cor pulmonale.[440,444]

The radiologic findings have been considered diagnostic.[440,451] They show a "sandstorm" throughout the lung, worse at the bases. The fine granular densities have the same radiodensity as calcium and show no tendency to coalesce.

Pulmonary function tests parallel the clinical severity and may be nearly normal at presentation.[448,449] Abnormal function precede symptoms.[446] As the disease progresses, the patients develop restrictive lung disease with decreased vital capacity, abnormal diffusion, and features of uneven ventilation.[443,445,446,448,449] Airflow obstruction has been an unusual finding.[453] The course is slow but progressive[440,449,451]; some cases may show very slow progression or apparent arrest of the disease for an extended period of time.[452] The longest course on record is 25 years.[440,442] A variety of therapeutic modalities has been tried, but nothing has been found to be beneficial other than palliative treatment of complications.[449,451]

Grossly the lungs may show pleural adhesions and subpleural blebs.[449,451] They are extremely difficult to cut, and a saw is occasionally required.[449,451] Cut surfaces are hard and gritty with innumerable 0.2- to 0.3-mm yellow-brown, sand-like grains. The cut surface has been compared to sandpaper.[440] Histologically 25 to 80 percent of the alveoli are filled with the characteristic laminated calcospherites[439,440,448,452] (Fig. 20–49). The calcospherites often contain a PAS-positive central core, which is presumed to be polysaccharide, whereas the surrounding laminations are von Kossa-positive and PAS-negative. Most microliths are 50 to 200 μm, rarely as large as 3 mm. They are composed of tricalcium phosphate with small amounts of magnesium and aluminum.[449,453,454] There may be a mild chronic inflammatory infiltrate and an increase in interstitial fibrous tissue. The calcospherites are birefringent, giving a Maltese cross pattern. The spherites are occasionally seen in the bronchial wall. In only one case have they been described outside the lung:

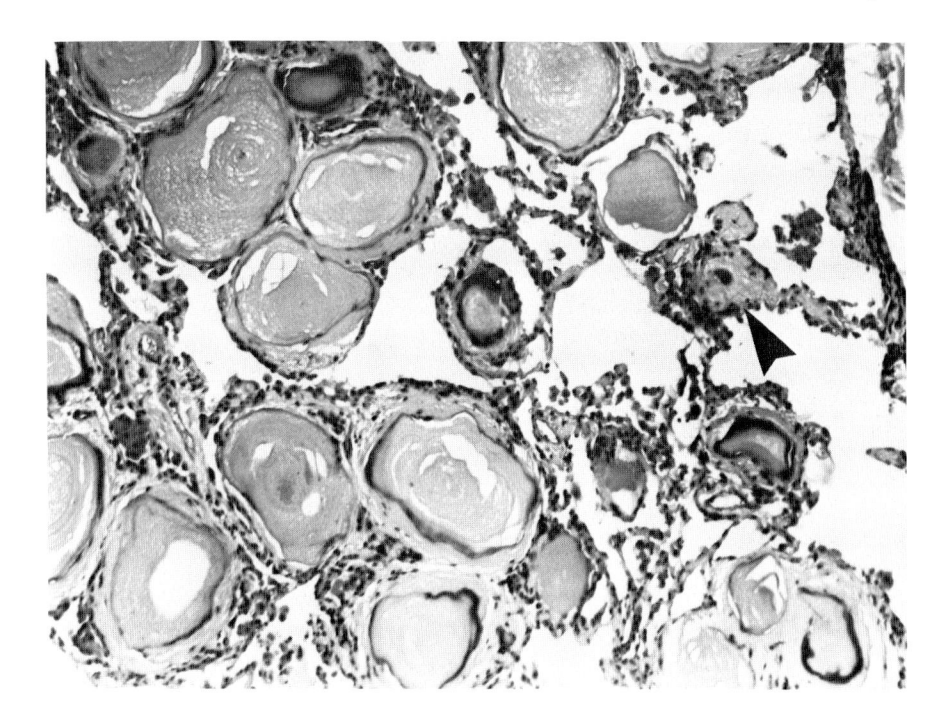

Figure 20–49. Pulmonary alveolar microlithiasis. Large, laminated, partially calcified concretions are found in many alveoli. A small (? early) concretion is seen within the interstitium (arrow) (H&E, ×120).

in lumbar sympathetic ganglion and testes.[447] The microliths are occasionally associated with macrophages and giant cells, and metaplastic bone formation has been described in confluent clusters.[439] The microliths should be distinguished from blue bodies and corpora amylacea.

Intra-Alveolar Blue Bodies

These are intra-alveolar, pale blue to blue-grey calcific concretions occurring singly or in clusters[455,456] (Fig. 20–50). Their size varies from 15 to 40 μm. A positive

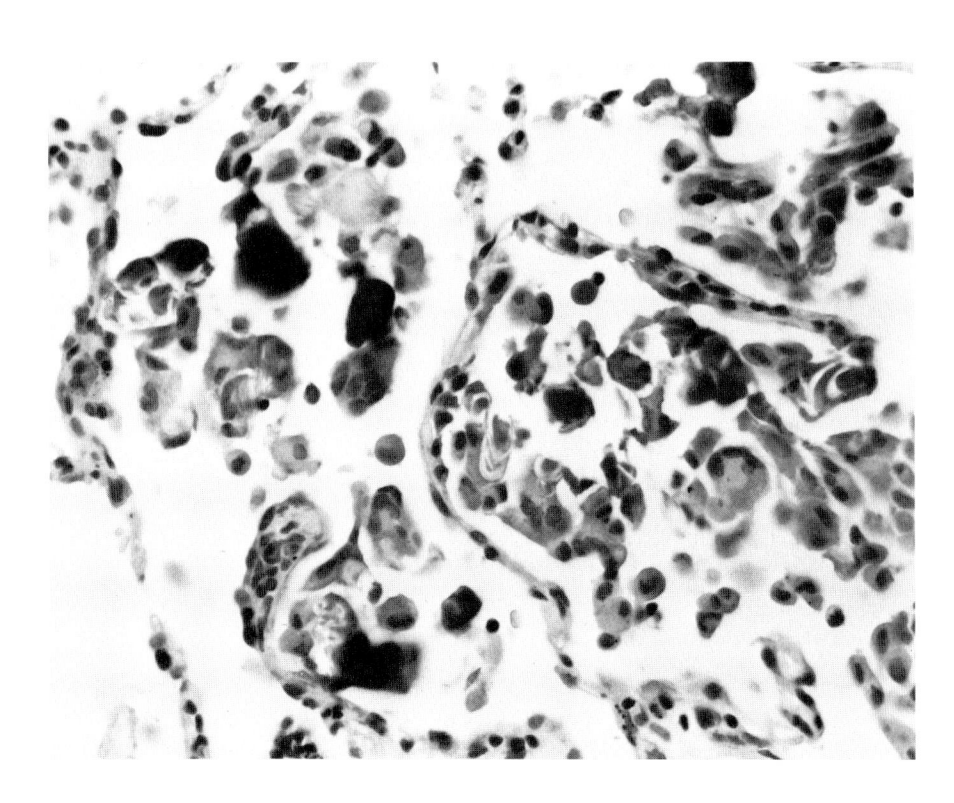

Figure 20–50. Blue bodies. Intra-alveolar calcified laminated bodies are associated with giant cells and numerous alveolar macrophages (H&E, ×320).

stain for iron may be seen in the outer rim. Blue bodies are always contained in histiocytes and occasionally giant cells. They are birefringent in unstained sections, acid-soluble, and have a mucopolysaccharide matrix. They are PAS- and Alcian-blue positive confirming the presence of mucopolysaccharide in the matrix. Koss and associates[456] have reviewed the ultrastructure of blue bodies. Their cause if unknown, but it is suspected that they are related to the inflammatory process, possibly histiocyte catabolism[456] and they may represent a residue of prior granulomas as they are common in cases of allergic alveolitis. There is no diagnostic significance of blue bodies; they have been seen in cases of DIP (most commonly), UIP, extrinsic allergic alveolitis, and other conditions.[456]

Schaumann Bodies

Schaumann (conchoidal) bodies are irregular, amorphous, and partially laminated calcospherites occurring in giant cells in granulomatous inflammation[456] (Fig. 20–51). Some show birefringence, and they give a positive reaction to alizarin, von Kossa, and iron stains. When granulomas have vanished, interstitial Schaumann bodies may be the only residual markers of the previous granulomatous inflammation. In some cases of honeycomb lung, this may be the only clue to the diagnosis of inactive sarcoid or healed tuberculosis. More importantly, Schaumann bodies should not be interpreted as exogenous in origin (i.e. a pneumoconiosis).

Calcium Oxalate

Calcium oxalate crystals are another inclusion that may be seen in giant cells in granulomas. The crystals are shiny and lucent and give a bright birefringence.[456] They lack calsopheric lamination and do not stain with alizaren red.[456] Giant cells containing calcium oxalate crystals have irregular holes in their cytoplasms up to 40 or 50 μm in diameter which on careful examination have lucent, irregular, plate-like crystals which are better appreciated with birefringence.

Pulmonary Ossification

Dystrophic Ossification

Like dystrophic calcification, dystrophic calcification may be seen at sites of previous injury. Well-formed bone with marrow is frequently seen and may be intra-alveolar or interstitial. Focal ossification (metaplastic bone) is a frequent insignificant and incidental finding at autopsy at many sites, including the lung (Figs. 20–52, 20–53). The degree of metaplastic bone may be extensive, and two clinicopathologic lesions, which themselves show some overlap, are recognized.[457]

Dendriform Pulmonary Ossification.[457–459] Cases of extensive interstitial fibrosis, either unilateral or bilateral, may occasionally be associated with extensive branching ossification, which may give a coral tree or dichotomous branched appearance to the bone. Various theories have been put forth in an effort to explain this form of ossification. The process is now generally thought to be dystrophic ossification occurring in foci of fibrosis. Unfortunately this does not explain cases that show no significant scarring. Some cases occur in chronic passive congestion that is associated with interstitial thickening and fibrosis in the lower lobes.

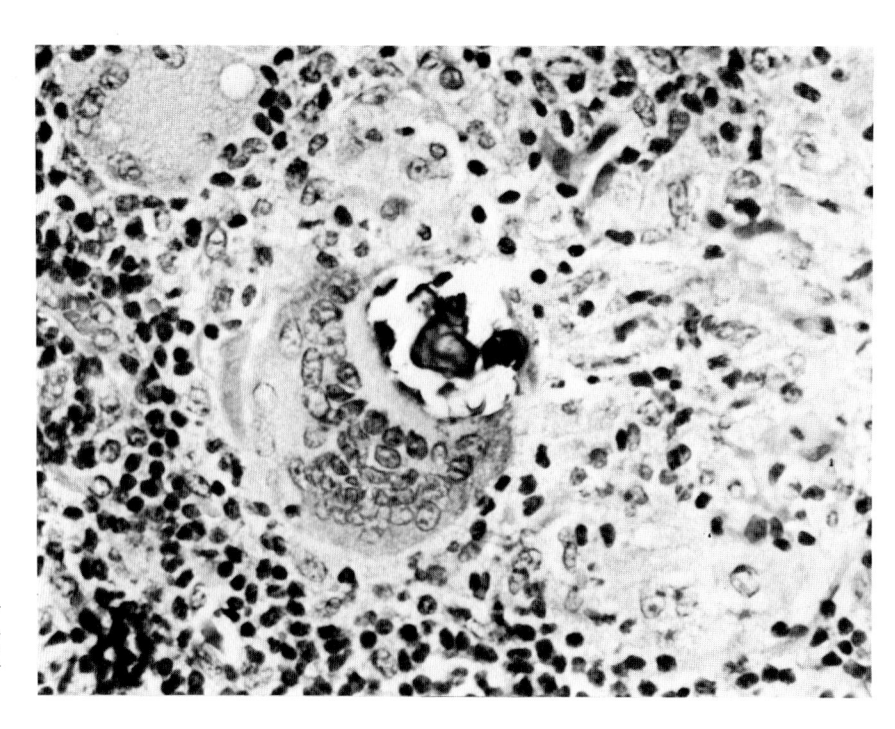

Figure 20–51. Schaumann body (conchoidal body). An irregular, partially laminated calcified body is present in a giant cell from a case of sarcoidosis (H&E, ×400).

Pulmonary Calcification and Ossification

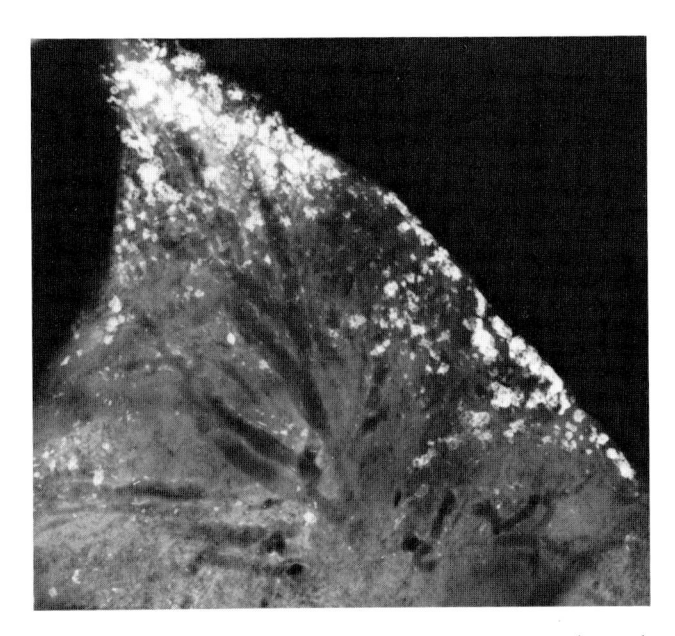

Figure 20–52. Ossifying pneumonia. A specimen radiograph shows extensive ossification which histologically was found to be occurring at sites of organizing pneumonia (slightly reduced from actual size).

Disseminated Nodular Pulmonary Ossification. Disseminated intra-alveolar nodules of well-formed bone are the usual forms of metaplastic ossification associated with chronic passive congestion[457,460–463] (Fig. 20–54). In the past, chronic mitral stenosis caused the majority of cases. The typical patient presents with a chest radiograph showing disseminated calcific densities, most prominent in the lower lobes, and a history of mitral stenosis. Most are men (4:1) with an average age of 35 years. The calcifications vary from a fine stippling to diffuse nodularity, and the radiograph may resemble healed granulomatous disease.

In one autopsy study,[457] 50 percent of patients with mitral valve disease were found to have some degree of diffuse ossification. Grossly changes of chronic passive congestion are combined with numerous tiny bony nodules up to 2 to 3 mm in size. Histologically intra-alveolar woven bone is identified. The nodules may involve one or several alveoli or an alveolar duct. Unusually the nodules may reach 1 cm or more in diameter. Patchy fibrosis may be present in the pulmonary parenchyma, but it generally does not appear to be related to the bony nodules. Occasionally inflammatory changes in the small vessels and vascular proliferation around bony nodules have been described. A peculiar feature is the consistent lack of cartilage. The pathogenesis of the metaplastic bone has been assumed to be dystrophic ossification occurring in organized intra-alveolar exudate or related to the hemosiderosis of chronic passive congestion.

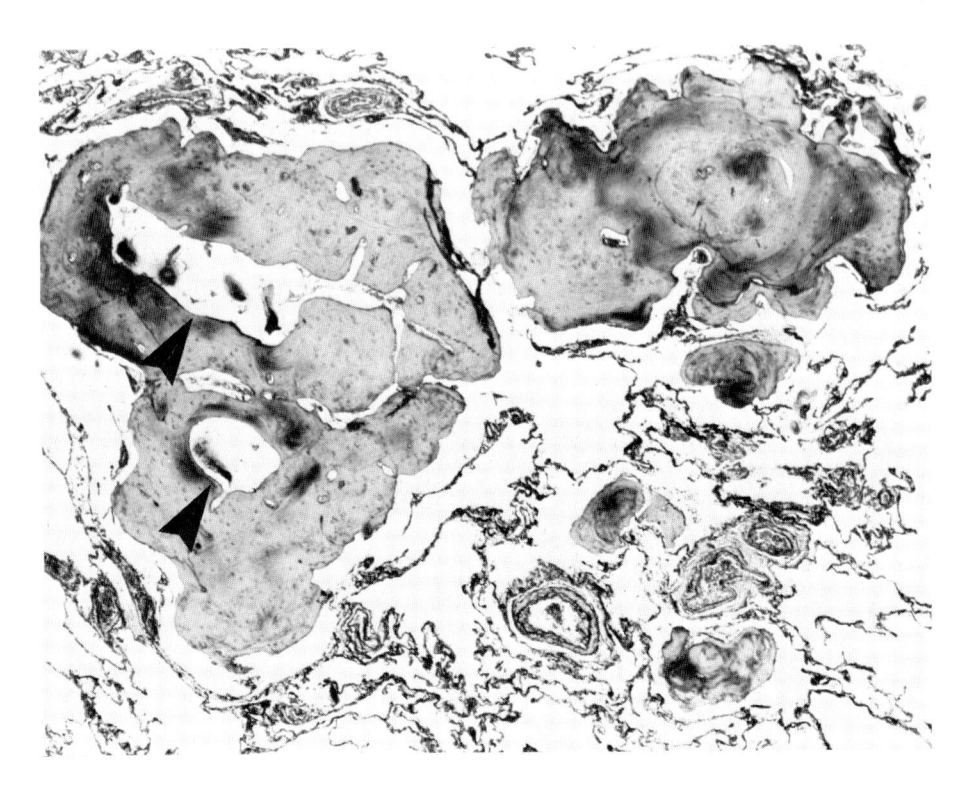

Figure 20–53. Dystrophic ossification (heterotopic bone). Large irregular nodules of well-formed occupy air spaces. Marrow (arrows) has developed in the nodule of the left. The stimulus for the development of the bone is no longer apparent (EVG ×32).

502 Infiltrative Lung Disease

Disseminated nodular pulmonary ossification may also be associated with chronic pulmonary fibrosis, left-atrial myxoma, constrictive pericarditis, systemic hypertension, coronary artery disease, aortic regurgitation, idiopathic hypertrophic subaortic stenosis, or a sequela of ARDS.[462] This form of pulmonary ossification is sometimes seen in patients without any predisposing condition, and such cases may be idiopathic or the result of some healed previous inflammatory process.[463]

Tracheobronchial Ossification

Bronchial Submucosal Bony Metaplasia[464](*Tracheopathic Osteoplastica*). This lesion, which should be distinguished from ossification in cases of tracheobronchial amyloidosis, is discussed in Chapter 21.

Ossification of Tracheobronchial Cartilages. This is a frequent aging change occasionally seen on chest radiograph which is of little clinical significance.

Corpora Amylacea

Corpora amylacea[465-467] were named for their staining similarity to starch. They are intra-alveolar laminated spherical and ellipsoidal bodies varying from 30 to 200 μm (Fig. 20-55). They may be found within the alveolar wall. They are PAS positive and only rarely stain for calcium salts. Corpora are usually surrounded by a ring of histiocytes. A central particle 15 to 20 μm is frequently present. They are birefringent, giving a Maltese cross pattern with polarization. Faint light and dark rings may be seen in some. Their number varies from one to two per section to one or two per high-power field. They may occur in sputum cytology specimens.

Corpora amylacea represent an incidental finding in adult lungs. Their cause is unknown, although aspirated spores of *Lycopodium clavatum*, a common ingredient in dusting powders, were implicated in one study.[467] Others believe corpora are a product of macrophages.[466] Their incidence varied from 0.6 percent in the 6000 autopsies studied by Hollander and Hutchins[467] to 3.8 percent in the 1070 autopsies studied by Michaels and Levene.[466] The youngest patient in these two studies was 21, although the authors have seen them in younger patients.

Drug Reactions in the Lung

Many drugs, both therapeutic and illicit, have been found to produce an array of morphologic reactions in the lung.[468-477] Their effects may be primary or secondary. Secondary effects (opportunistic infections in patients on chemotherapy, aspiration, and ventilatory problems associated with the central nervous system and drug-related thromboembolic phenomena) are not included here. Lung lesions in the immunocompromised host are considered as a separate entity in Chapter 14. Pulmonary drug reactions can be approached from several points of view such as by pharmacologic class of drug, the clinical or clinicopathologic syndromes that are produced, or the histologic changes alone. Most reviews include only the clinical or clinicopathologic syndromes of drug-related pulmonary disease.

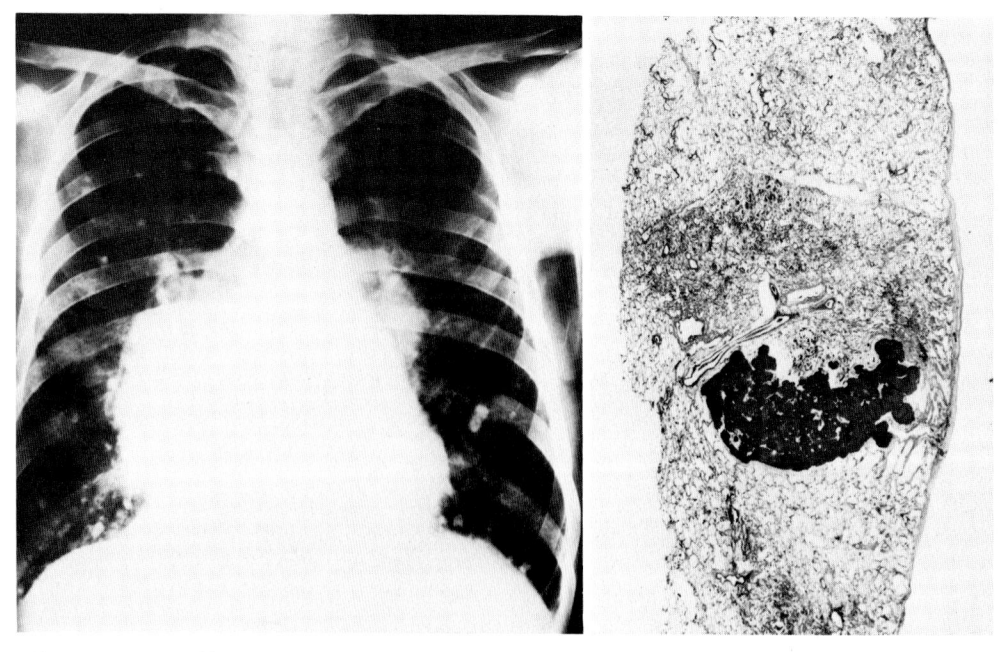

Figure 20-54. Chronic passive congestion (from mitral stenosis) with multiple ossified nodules. The bony lesion at the right represents the same one seen in the left mid-lung field (right, H&E, ×3).

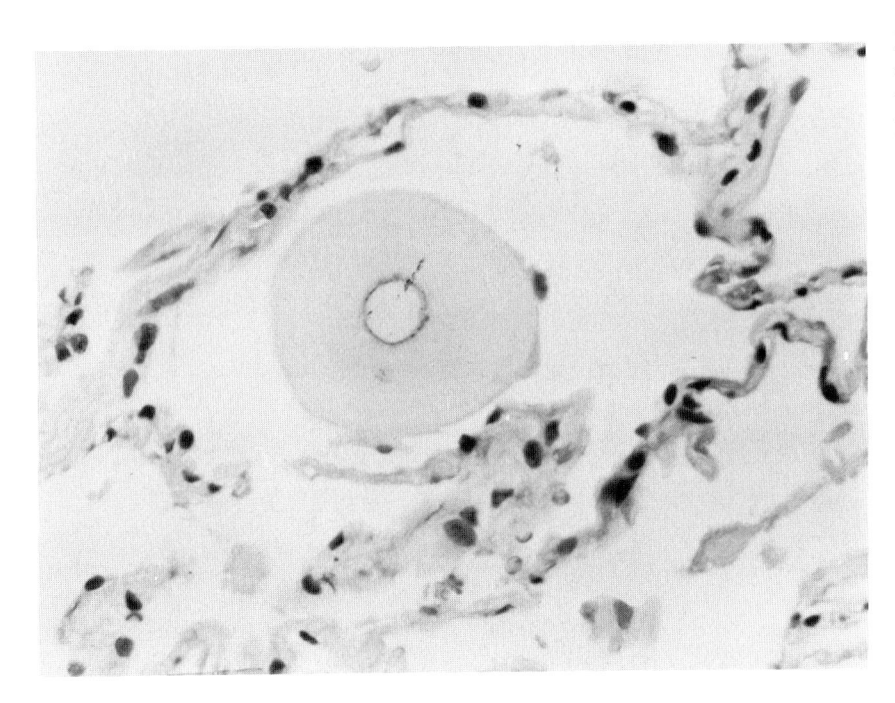

Figure 20–55. Corpora amylacea. There is a laminated eosinophilic intra-alveolar body with central basophilic granule. A macrophage (nucleus at right) tries to engulf it (H&E, ×300).

The lung's response patterns to injury are limited, and none of the lesions associated with drugs is unique. Identification of a drug reaction requires knowledge of the clinical course of events and does not rest on identification of any specific morphologic features. Proving a drug reaction is difficult and requires a rigorous approach that is rarely available. Two principles apply to drug reactions. The first is that drugs can probably cause a wide variety of pulmonary lesions and no morphologic appearance completely excludes a drug reaction. The second is that the lack of published reports of a reaction to a specific drug should not absolutely exclude the drug as the offending agent.

Histologic patterns that may be associated with drug reactions are shown in Table 20–20, and two are illustrated in Fig. 20–56. This list is far from complete since combinations of the patterns shown occur, and new patterns are sure to be described. Drug-induced diffuse alveolar damage is considered in more detail in Chapter 16.

The clinical-pathologic syndromes associated with drug reactions are shown in Table 20–21. This list is derived from several recent reviews, and information about the specific drugs can be found in the references. There is some overlap between Tables 20–20 and 20–21 since some of the clinical-pathologic syndromes are, of necessity, defined morphologically. Unfortunately, in most cases, the morphology is not known, and many of the drugs in Table 20–21 are there only by virtue of the clinical syndrome. Probably more than one of the morphologic patterns in Table 20–20 are represented in the given clinical pathologic syndrome in Table 20–21. Diffuse alveolar damage and pulmonary fibrosis (UIP) are grouped together for convenience, as many of the cases of pulmonary fibrosis are the result of organized diffuse alveolar damage. As used in Table 20–21, hypersensitivity pneumonitis is defined loosely in a clinical sense, and it probably overlaps with diffuse alveolar damage and airway disease. The drug-induced systemic lupus erythematosus syndrome is included in Table 20–21 since pulmonary findings in such cases are said to be more impressive than in idiopathic systemic lupus erythematosus.

Table 20–20. Pulmonary Pathology Associated with Drugs[a]

Edema
Hemorrhage
Metastatic calcification
Asthmatic changes
Bronchiolitis obliterans
Bronchiolitis obliterans with patchy organizing pneumonia
Diffuse alveolar damage: acute, organizing, or organized
Usual interstitial pneumonia
Cellular interstitial pneumonia
Allergic alveolitis
Eosinophilic pneumonia
Parenchymal necrosis
Parenchymal granulomas (microgranulomatosis)
Foreign body granulomas (talcosis)
Pulmonary hypertension (± vasculitis)
Small- or large-vessel angiitis
Pleuritis, pleural fibrosis

[a] Based on the results of Gillett and Ford[470] Demeter et al.,[471–473] Kilburn,[474] Whimster and de Poitiers,[476] and Pollak and Saomi,[4776] and personal observations

Diffuse alveolar damage caused by chemotherapeutic agents is the best known and most common drug reaction encountered in lung biopsies, as indicated in several recent reviews.[469,472,473,475] If the injury is severe enough or if the drug is continued, fatal pulmonary fibrosis may ensue. Bizarre regenerative alveolar lining cells are characteristic of this form of chemotherapy-induced diffuse alveolar damage but are nonspecific. Another reaction that is relatively common in patients on chemotherapy is bronchiolitis obliterans with patchy organizing pneumonia, and its distinction from organizing diffuse alveolar damage is arbitrary in some cases. Less commonly, hypersensitivity reactions are due to chemotherapeutic agents. The patterns of eosinophilic pneumonia and allergic alveolitis may be produced.

In most drug reactions, pulmonary injury ceases when the offending drug is removed; however, scarring may remain as a permanent residue. Occasionally, especially with chemotherapeutic agents, putative drug-induced injury may progress even after the drug is discontinued.

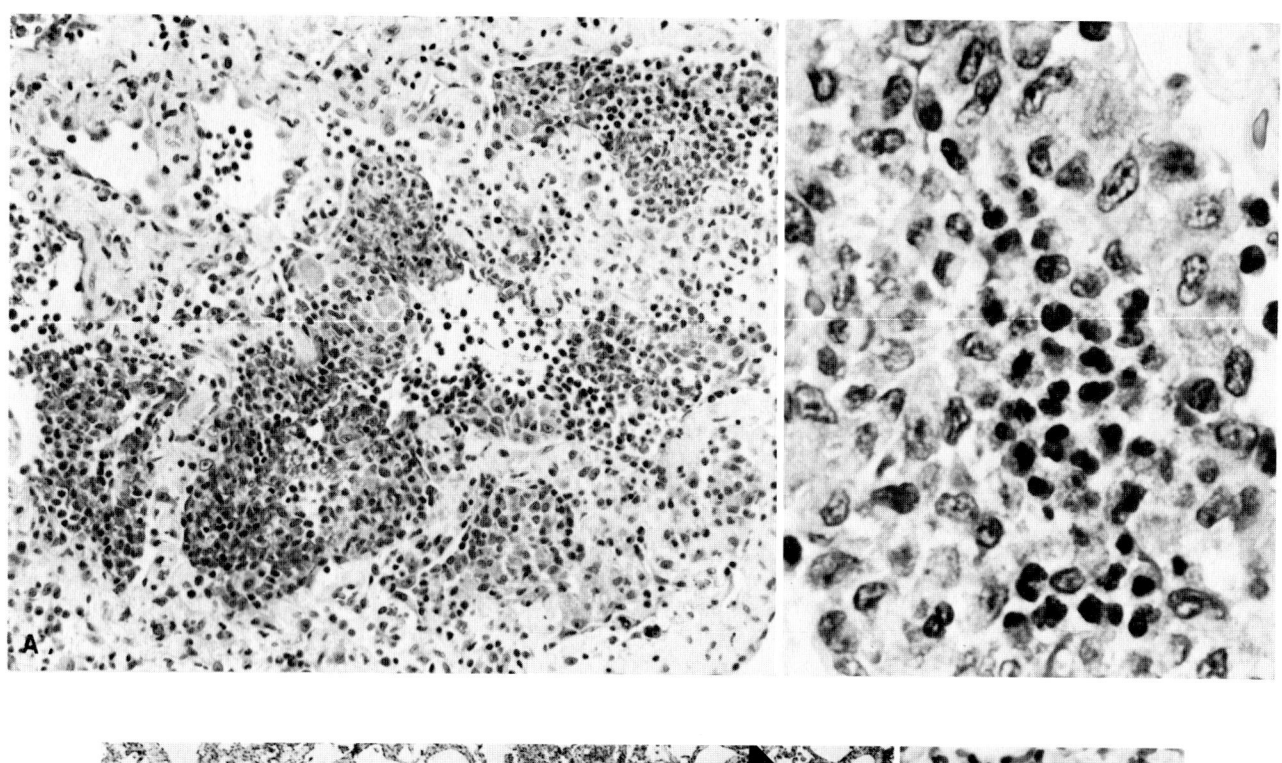

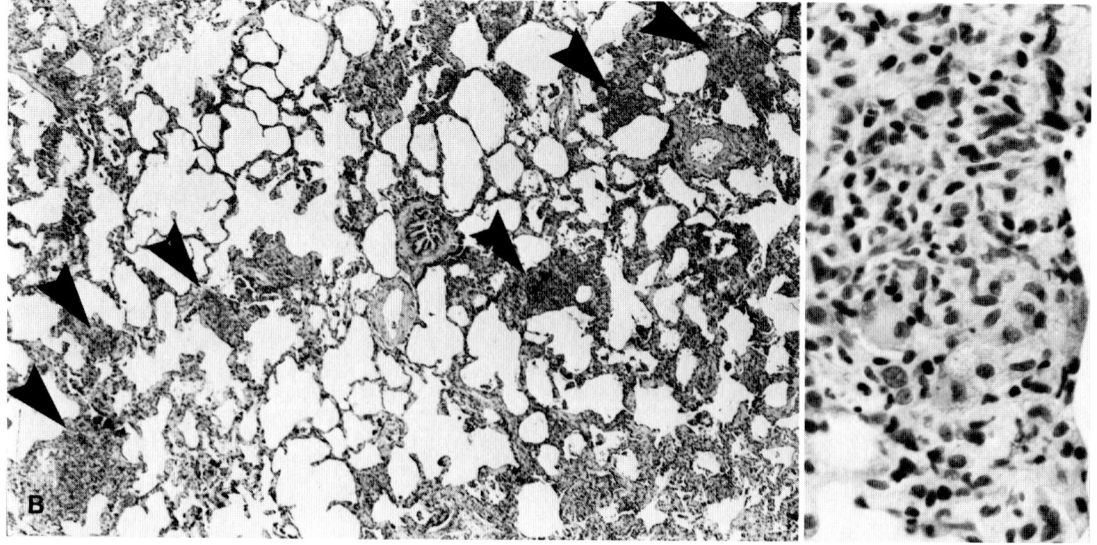

Figure 20–56. Pulmonary drug reaction. A. Eosinophilic pneumonia associated with bleomycin therapy (H&E: left ×160, right ×640). B. Disseminated microgranulomas (arrows) associated with cyclophosphamide therapy (H&E: left ×32, right ×320).

Table 20–21. Pulmonary Drug Reactions: Clinicopathologic Syndromes[a]

Syndrome	Implicated Drugs
Noncardiogenic pulmonary edema	Amitriptyline
	Bromocarbamide
	Chlordiazepoxide
	Colchicine
	Dextran
	Epinephrine
	Ethchlorvynol
	Fluorescein
	Halothane
	Heroin/morphine
	Hydrochlorothiazide
	Iodinized oils (Lipiodol)
	Metaraminol
	Methadone
	Nitrofurantoin
	Nitrogen mustard
	Oxygen
	Pentazocine
	Phenylbutazone
	Propoxur
	Propoxyphene
	Salicylates
	Saline (hypertonic intrathecal)
	Sodium diatrizoate (Hypaque)
	Tranylcypromine (+ cheese)
Hemorrhage	Anticoagulants
	Lymphangiographic dyes
	Mineral oil
	Oxygen
	Penicillamine (Goodpasture's-like syndrome)
Metastatic calcification	Antacids
	Calcium salts
	Phosphorus
	Vitamin D
	Milk-alkali syndrome
Asthma/wheezing	Acetoaminophen
	Althesin
	Ampicillin
	Chlorine thiazole
	Diazepam
	Ethyl ether
	Formalin
	Halothane
	Indomethacin
	Isoproteronol
	Methacholine
	Mefenamic acid
	Neostigmine
	Pancreatin
	Penicillin
	Pentazocine
	Phenylbutazone
	Piperazine
	Pituitary snuff
	Propoxyphene
	Propranolol
	Prostaglandin F3a
	Salicylates
	Serum
	Succinylcholine

Table 20–21. (Continued)

Syndrome	Implicated Drugs
	Tartrazine
	Trypsin
	Tween
Bronchiolitis obliterans	Penicillamine[468]
Diffuse alveolar damage (ARDS), pulmonary fibrosis (acute and/or chronic interstitial pneumonia)	Alpha-adrenergic nasal sprays
	Amiodarone[477–477b]
	Amitriptyline
	Azathioprine
	BCNU
	Bleomycin
	Busulfan
	Carbamazepine
	Chlorambucil
	Cromoglycate
	Cyclophosphamide
	Diphenylhydantoin
	Gold
	Hexamethonium
	Intravenous drugs
	Iodine (radioactive)
	Mecamylamine
	Melphalan
	6-Mercaptopurine
	Methotrexate
	Methysergide
	Mineral oil
	Mitomycin
	Nitrofurantoin
	Oxygen
	Paraquat
	Pencillamine
	Pentolinium
	Pindolol
	Pituitary snuff
	Practolol
	Procarbazine
	Sulfasalazine
Hypersensitivity pneumonitis[b] With eosinophilia	
	Aminosalicylic acid
	Ampicillin
	Antitetanus serum
	Bleomycin
	Carbamazepine
	Chlorpropamide
	Cromolyn
	Diphenylhydantoin
	Disodium chromoglycate
	Gold
	Hydralazine
	Imipramine
	Isoniazid
	Mecamylamine
	Mephenesin
	Niridazole
	Nitrofurantoin
	Para aminosalicyclic acid
	Penicillin
	Pituitary snuff
	Procarbazine
	Salicylazosulfapyridine

Infiltrative Lung Disease

Table 20–21. (Continued)

Syndrome	Implicated Drugs
	Sulfadimethoxine
	Sulfanilamide
	Sulfasalazine
	Sulfonamides
	Tetracycline
Without eosinophilia	Azathioprine
	BCG therapy
	Bulsulfan
	Colchicine
	Gold
	Ibuprofen
	Methotrexate
	Nitrogen mustard
	Penicillamine
	Procarbazine
Infiltrates with (lipo)granulomas	Cromolyn
	Lipids/oils
	Methotrexate
	Nitrofurantoin
	Phenylbutazone
	Pituitary snuff
	Quinicrine talc
	Talc
	Visciodol
Systemic lupus erythematosus-like syndrome: pleurisy, pleural effusions, cough, dyspnea, fever, alveolar atelectasis	
	Aminosalicylic acid
	Chlorpromiazine
	Chlorthalidone
	Digitalis
	Diphenylhydantoin
	Ethosuximide
	Gold
	Griseofulvin
	Guanoxan
	Hydralazine
	Hydrochlorothiazide
	Isoguanazepan
	Isoniazid
	Levodopa
	Mephenytoin
	Methyldopa
	Methysergide
	Methylthiouracil
	Nitrofurantoin
	Oral contraceptives
	Oxphenisatin
	Para-aminosalicylic acid
	Pencillin
	Phenylbutzone
	Practolol
	Primidone
	Procainamide
	Propylthiouracil
	Quinidine
	Reserpine
	Streptomycin
	Sulfonamides
	Tetracycline
	Tolazamide

Table 20–21. (Continued)

Syndrome	Implicated Drugs
	Trimethadione
Pulmonary hypertension	
	Alpha-adrenergic nasal sprays
	Aminorex
	Estrogens (embolic hypertension)
	Talc (IV drug addicts) (secondary to drug-induced diffuse pulmonary fibrosis)
Pulmonary angiitis	Busulfan
	Chlorophentermine
	Cromoglycate
	Intravenous illicit drugs
	Sulfonamides
Pleural: pleuritis, effusions	
	Drug-induced SLE-like syndrome (*see above*)
	Anticoagulants (hemorrhagic)
	Bleomycin
	Ibuprofen
	Methotrexate
	Methysergide (pleural fibrosis)
	Mitomycin
	Nitrofurantoin
	Oxyprenolol (fibrosis)
	Procarbazine
	Practolol (fibrosis)

Abbreviations: ARDS, adult respiratory distress syndrome; BCG, bacillus Calmette-Guérin; BCNU.

[a] Based on the results of Gillett and Ford,[470] Demeter et al.,[471–473] Kilburn,[474] Whimster and dePoitiers,[476] and other references as shown.

[b] See text.

References

1. Carrington CB, Gaensler EA: Clinical-pathologic approach to diffuse infiltrative lung disease. In Thurlbeck WM, Abell MR (eds): *The Lung: Structure, Function, and Disease.* Baltimore: Williams & Wilkins, 1978, pp 58–87.

2. Buechner HA: The differential diagnosis of miliary disease of the lung. Med Clin North Am 43:89–112, 1959.

3. Gaensler EA: Diagnostic techniques in diffuse or miliary lung diseases. Experience with 381 patients. In Banyai AL, Gordon BL (eds): *Advances in Cardiopulmonary Disease*, vol III. Chicago: Year Book, 1966, pp 81–122.

4. Carrington CB, Gaensler EA, Coutu RE, et al: Natural history and treated course of usual and desquamative interstitial pneumonia. N Engl J Med 298:801–810, 1978.

5. FitzGerald MX, Carrington CB, Gaensler EA: Environmental lung disease. Med Clin North Am 57:593–622, 1973.

6. Morgan WKC, Seaton A: *Occupational Lung Diseases.* Philadelphia: WB Saunders, 1975.

7. Parkes WR: *Occupational Lung Disorders.* London: Butterworth, 1974.

8. Epler GR, McLoud TC, Gaensler EA, et al: Normal chest roentgenograms in chronic diffuse infiltrative lung disease. N Engl J Med 298:934–939, 1978.

9. Gaensler EA, Carrington CB, Coutu RE, FitzGerald MX: Radiographic-physiologic-pathologic correlations in interstitial pneumonias. Prog Respir Res 8:223–241, 1975.

10. Gaensler EA, Carrington CG, Coutu RE, et al: Pathological, physiological and radiological correlations in the pneumoconioses. Ann NY Acad Sci 200:574–607, 1972.

11. Andersen HA, Fontana RS: Transbronchioscopic lung biopsy for diffuse pulmonary disease: Technique and results in 450 cases. Chest 62:125–128, 1972.

12. Jacobson G, Lainhart WS (eds): ILO U/C 1971 international classification of radiographs of the pneumoconioses. Med Radiogr Photogr 48:65–76, 1972.

13. Jefferson FR III, Lawton BR, Myers WO, et al.; Open pulmonary biopsy: 19-year experience with 416 consecutive operations. Chest 69:43–47, 1976.

14. Genereux GP: The end-stage lung: Pathogenesis, pathology and radiology. Radiology 116:279–289, 1975.

15. Heppleston AG: The pathology of honeycomb lung. Thorax 11:77–93, 1956.

16. Liebow AA, Carrington CB: The interstitial pneumonias. In Simon M, Potchen EJ, LeMay M (eds): *Frontiers of Pulmonary Radiology*. New York: Grune & Stratton, 1969, pp 102–141.

17. Gaensler EA, Carrington CB: Peripheral opacities in chronic eosinophilic pneumonia: The photographic negative of pulmonary edema. AJR 128:1–13, 1977.

18. McLoud TC, Carrington CB, Gaensler EA: Diffuse infiltrative lung disease: A new scheme for description. Radiology 149:353–363, 1983.

19. Austrian R, McClement JH, Renzetti AD Jr, et al.: Clinical and physiologic features of some types of pulmonary diseases with impairment of alveolar-capillary diffusion. The syndrome of "alveolar-capillary block." Am J Med 11:667–685, 1951.

20. Marks A, Cugell DW, Cardigan JB, Gaensler EA: Clinical determination of the diffusion capacity of the lungs. Comparison of methods in normal subjects and patients with "alveolar-capillary block" syndrome. Am J Med 22:5–73, 1957.

21. Comroe JH, Forster RE, DuBois AB, et al.: *The Lung: Clinical Physiology and Pulmonary Function Tests*. Chicago: Year Book, 1962, pp 111–139.

22. Finley TN, Swenson EW, Comroe JH Jr: The cause of arterial hypoxemia at rest in patients with "alveolar-capillary syndrome." J Clin Invest 41:618–622, 1962.

23. Roughton FJW, Forster RE: Relative importance of diffusion and chemical reaction rates in determining rate of exchange of gases in the human lung, with special reference to true diffusing capacity of pulmonary membrane and volume of blood in the lung capillaries. J Appl Physiol 11:290–302, 1957.

24. Kuhn C: Ultrastructure and cellular function in the distal lung. In Thurlbeck WM, Abell WR (eds): *The Lung: Structure, Function, and Disease*. Baltimore: Williams & Wilkins, 1978, pp 1–20.

25. Wagner PD, Dantzker DR, Dueck R, et al.: Distribution of ventilation-perfusion ratios in patients with interstitial lung disease. Chest 69:256–257, 1976.

26. Carrington CB, Gaensler EA, Mikus JP, et al.: Structure and function in sarcoidosis. Ann NY Acad Sci 278:265–283, 1976.

26a. Crystal RG, Bitterman PB, Rennard SI, et al.: Interstitial lung diseases of unknown cause, Part I. N Engl J Med 310:154–166, 1984.

26b. Martin WJ, Williams DE, Dines DE, Sanderson DR: Interstitial lung disease: Assessment by broncho-alveolar lavage. Mayo Clin Proc 58:751–757, 1983.

27. Pimentel JC: Tridimensional photographic reconstruction in a study of the pathogenesis of honeycomb lung. Thorax 22:444–452, 1967.

28. Adler KB, Craighead JE, Vallyathan NV: Actin-containing cells in human pulmonary fibrosis. Am J Pathol 102:427–437, 1981.

29. Liebow AA. Arteriosclerosis of the pulmonary circulation. In Blumenthal HT (ed): *Cowdry's Arteriosclerosis*. Springield, IL: Charles C Thomas, 1966, pp 248–328.

30. Katzenstein ALA, Askin FB: *Surgical Pathology of Nonneoplastic Lung Disease*. Philadelphia: WB Saunders, 1982.

31. Schwartz JB, Shamsuddin AM: The effects of leukemic infiltrates in various organs in chronic lymphocytic leukemia. Hum Pathol 12:432–440, 1981.

32. Hamman L, Rich AR: Acute diffuse interstitial fibrosis of the lungs. Bull Johns Hopkins Hosp 74:177–212, 1944.

33. Liebow AA: New concepts and entities in pulmonary disease. In Liebow AA (ed): *The Lung*. Baltimore: Williams & Wilkins, 1968, pp 332–365.

34. Gaensler EA, Carrington CB, Coutu RE: Chronic interstitial pneumonias. Clinical notes on respiratory disease. Am Thorac Soc, Spring, 1972.

35. Livingstone JL, Lewis JG, Reid L, Jefferson KE: Diffuse interstitial pulmonary fibrosis. Q J Med 33:71–103, 1964.

36. Liebow AA, Steer A, Billingsley JG: Desquamative interstitial pneumonia. Am J Pathol 39:369–404, 1965.

37. Jackson LK: Idiopathic pulmonary fibrosis. Clin Chest Med 3:579–592, 1982.

38. Crystal RG, Fulmer JD, Roberts WC, et al.: Idiopathic pulmonary fibrosis—Clinical, histologic, radiographic, physiologic, scintigraphic, cytologic, and biochemical aspects. Ann Intern Med 85:769–788, 1976.

39. Crystal RG, Gadek JE, Ferrans VJ, et al: Interstitial lung disease: Current concepts of pathogenesis, staging and therapy. Am J Med 70:542–568, 1981.

39a. Solliday NH, Williams JA, Gaensler EA, et al.: Familial chronic interstitial pneumonia. Am Rev Respir Dis 108:193–204, 1973.

39b. Tal A, Maor E, Bar-Ziv J, Gorodischer R: Fatal desquamative interstitial pneumonia in three infant siblings. J Pediatr 104:873–876, 1984.

40. Haslam PL, Turton CWG, Heard B, et al.: Bronchoalveolar lavage in pulmonary fibrosis: Comparison of cells obtained with lung biopsy and clinical features. Thorax 35:9–18, 1980.

41. Rudd RM, Haslam PL. Turner-Warwick M: Cryptogenic fibrosing alveolitis—Relationships of pulmonary physiology and bronchoalveolar lavage to response to treatment and prognosis. Am Rev Respir Dis 124:1–8, 1981.

42. Fulmer JD: Bronchoalveolar lavage. Am Rev Respir Dis 126:961–963, 1982.

43. Farr GH, Harley RA, Henningar GR: Desquamative interstitial pneumonia. Am J Pathol 60:347–358, 1970.

44. Tubbs RR, Benjamin SP, Reich, NE, et al.: Desquamative interstitial pneumonitis—Cellular phase of fibrosing alveolitis. Chest 72:159–165, 1977.

45. Scadding JG, Hinson KFW: Diffuse fibrosing alveolitis (diffuse interstitial fibrosis of the lungs). Thorax 22:291–304, 1967.

46. Turner-Warwick M, Burrows B, Johnson A: Cryptogenic fibrosing alveolitis: Response to corticosteroid treatment and its effect on survival. Thorax 35:593–599, 1980.

47. Bedrossian CWM, Kuhn C, Luna MA, et al.: Desquamative interstitial pneumonia-like reaction accompanying pulmonary lesions. Chest 101:166–169, 1977.

48. Corrin B, Price AB: Electron microscopic studies in desquamative interstitial pneumonia associated with asbestos. Thorax 27:324–331, 1972.

49. Abraham JL, Hertzberg MA: Inorganic particles associated with desquamative interstitial pneumonia. Chest 80(Suppl):67S–70S, 1981.

50. Lillington GA, Siefkin AM: Fibrosing alveolitis—Causes, characteristics, and consequences. Postgrad Med 71:128–137, 1982.

51. Turner-Warwick M, Lebowitz M, Burrows B, Johnson A: Cryptogenic fibrosing alveolitis and lung cancer. Thorax 35:496–499, 1980.

52. Homma H, Yamanaka A, Tanimoto, et al.: Diffuse panbronchiolitis. Chest 83:63–69, 1983.

53. Geddes DM, Corrin B, Brewerton DA, et al.: Progressive airway obliteration in adults and its association with rheumatoid disease. J Med 46:427–444, 1977.

54. Gosink BB, Friedman PJ, Liebow AA: Bronchiolitis obliterans roentgenologic-pathologic correlation. AJR 117:816–832, 1973.

55. Turton CW, Williams G, Green M: Cryptogenic obliterative bronchiolitis in aduls. Thorax 36:805–810, 1981.

56. Green M, Turton CW: Bronchiolitis and its manifestations. Eur J Respir Dis 63(Suppl):36–42, 1982.

57. Seggev JS, Mason UG, Worthen S, et al.: Bronchiolitis obliterans: Report of three cases with detailed physiologic studies. Chest 83:169–174, 1983.

58. Blumgart HL, MacMahon HE: Bronchiolitis fibrosa obliterans: A clinical and pathologic study. Med Clin North Am 13:197–214, 1929.

59. Dale RC, Auchincloss JH, Gilbert R, Markarian B: Bronchiolitis literans: Longterm follow-up. NY State J Med 14:85–88, 1977.

60. Hawley PC, Whitcomb ME: Bronchiolitis fibrosa obliterans in adults. Arch Intern Med 141:1324–1337, 1981.

61. Herzog CA, Miller RR, Hoidal JR: Case reports—bronchiolitis and rheumatoid arthritis. Am Rev Respir Dis 124:636–639, 1981.

62. Tukianen P, Poppius H, Taskinen E: Slowly progressive bronchiolitis obliterans: A case report with detailed pulmonary function studies. Eur J Respir Dis 61:77–83, 1980.

63. McCarthy DS, Ostrow DN, Hershfield ES: Chronic obstructive pulmonary disease following idiopathic pulmonary fibrosis. Chest 77:473–477, 1980.

64. Schwarz MI, Matthay RA, Sahn SA, et al.: Interstitial lung disease in polymyositis and dermatomyositis: Analysis of six cases and review of the literature. Medicine 55:89–104, 1976.

65. Grinblat J, Mechlis S, Lewitus Z: Organizing pneumonia-like process: An unusual observation in steroid responsive cases with features of chronic interstitial pneumonia. Chest 80:259–263, 1981.

65a. Davison AG, Heard BE, McAllister WAC, Turner-Warwick MEH. Cryptogenic organizing pneumonitis. QJ Med 52:382–394, 1983.

66. Epler GR, Colby TV, McLoud TC, et al.: Idiopathic bronchiolitis obliterans with organizing pneumonia. N Engl J Med 312:152–159, 1985.

67. Abraham JL, Spragg RG: Documentation of environmental exposure using open lung biopsy, transbronchial biopsy and bronchopneumonary lavage in giant cell interstitial pneumonia (GIP). Am Rev Respir Dis 119(Abstr):197, 1979.

67a. Davison AG, Haslam PL, Corrin B, et al.: Interstitial lung disease and asthma in hard-metal workers: Broncho-alveolar lavage, ultrastructural and analytical findings and results of bronchial provocation tests. Thorax 38:119–128, 1983.

67b. Demedts M, Gheyseus B, Nagels J, et al.: Cobalt lung in diamond polishers. Am Rev Respir Dis 130:130–135, 1984.

68. Moran TJ, Totten RS: Lymphoid interstitial pneumonia with dysproteinemia: Report of two cases with plasma cell predominance. Am J Clin Pathol 54:747–756, 1970.

69. Greenberg SD, Haley MD, Jenkins DE, Fischer SP: Lymphoplasmacytic pneumonia with accompanying dysproteinemia. Arch Pathol 96:73–80, 1973.

70. Leibow AA, Carrington CB: Diffuse pulmonary lymphoreticular infiltration associated with dysproteinema. Med Clin North Am 57:809–843, 1973.

71. Binette JP, Montes M: Lymphoid interstitial pneumonia. J Can Med Assoc 114:810–812, 1976.

72. Dukes RJ, Rosenow EC, Hermans PE: Pulmonary manifestations of hypogammaglobulinemia. Thorax 33:603–607, 1978.

73. Faguet GB, Webb HH, Agee JF, et al.: Immunologically diagnosed malignancy in Sjögren's pseudolymphoma. Am J Med 65:424–429, 1978.

74. Julsrud PR, Brown LR, Li C-Y, et al.: Pulmonary processes of mature-appearing lymphocytes: Pseudolymphoma, well differentiated lymphocytic lymphoma, and lymphocytic interstitial pneumonitis. Radiology 127:289–296, 1978.

75. Strimlan CV, Rosenow EC, Weiland LH, Brown LR: Lymphocytic interstitial pneumonitis. Ann Intern Med 88:616–621, 1978.

76. Benisch B, Peison B: The association of lymphocytic interstitial pneumonia and systemic lupus erythematosus. Mt Sinai J Med (NY), 46:398–401, 1979.

77. Hecht S: Lymphoid interstitial pneumonia: A clincial-radiologic-pathologic correlation. Medical student thesis in cooperation with PJ Friedman MD. University of California, La Jolla Medical School, 1980.

78. Nichols PW, Koss MN, Taylor CR, Hochholzer L: Immunoperoxidase studies in the diagnosis of 51 primary pulmonary lymphoid lesions. Lab Invest 44(Abstr):48, 1980.

79. O'Brodovich HM, Moser MM, Lu L: Familial lymphoid interstitial pneumonia: A longterm follow-up. Pediatrics 65:523–528, 1980.

80. Church JA, Isaacs H, Saxon A, et al.: Lymphoid interstitial pneumonitis and hypogammaglobulinemia in children. Am Rev Respir Dis 124:491–496, 1981.

81. Kohler PF, Cook RD, Brown WR, Manguso RL: Common variable hypogammaglobulinemia with T-cell nodular lymphoid interstitial pneumonitis and B-cell nodular lymphoid hyperplasia: Different lymphocyte populations with a similar response to prednisone therapy. J Allergy Clin Immunol 70:299–305, 1982.

82. Turner R, Colby TV, Doggett RS: Well differentiated lymphocytic lymphoma of the lung. Cancer 54:2088–2096, 1984.

83. Hunninghake GW, Fauci AS: State of the art — Pulmonary involvement in the collagen vascular disease. Am Rev Respir Dis 119:471–503, 1979.

84. Eisenberg H: The interstitial lung disease associated with the collagen-vascular disorders. Clin Chest Med 3:565–578, 1982.

85. Caplan A: Certain unusual radiological appearances in the chest of coal-miners suffering from rheumatoid arthritis. Thorax 8:29–37, 1953.

86. Price TML, Skelton MO: Rheumatoid arthritis with lung lesions. Thorax 11:234–240, 1956.

87. Brinkman GL, Chaikof L: Case reports: Rheumatoid lung disease. Am Rev Respir Dis 80:732–737, 1959.

88. Cruickshank B: Interstitial pneumonia and its consequences in rheumatoid disease. Br J Dis Chest 53:226–236, 1959.

89. Editorial. Lancet 1:812, 1960.

90. Doctor L, Snider GL: Diffuse interstitial pulmonary fibrosis associated with arthritis. Am Rev Respir Dis 85:413–422, 1962.

91. Brannan HM, Good CA, Divertie MB, Baggenstoss AH: Pulmonary disease associated wtih rheumatoid arthritis. JAMA 189:914–918, 1964.

92. Talbott JA, Calkins E: Pulmonary involvement in rheumatoid arthritis. JAMA 189:911–913, 1964.

93. Patterson CD, Harville WE, Pierce JA: Rheumatoid lung disease. Ann Intern Med 62:685–697, 1965.

94. Beck ER, Hoffbrand BI: Acute lung changes in rheumatoid arthritis. Ann Rheum Dis 25:459–462, 1966.

95. Petty TL, Wilkins M: The five manifestations of rheumatoid lung. Dis Chest 49:75–82, 1966.

96. Portner MM, Gracie WA Jr: Rheumatoid lung disease with cavitary nodules, pneumothorax and eosinophilia. N Engl J Med 275:697–700, 1966.

97. Rubin EH, Gordon M, Thelmo WL: Nodular pleuropulmonary rheumatoid disease. Am J Med 42:567–581, 1967.

98. Martel W, Abell MR, Mikkelsen WM, Whitehouse WM: Pulmonary and pleural lesions in rheumatoid disease. Radiology 90:641–653, 1968.

99. Panettiere F, Chandler BF, Libcke JH: Pulmonary cavitation in rheumatoid disease. Am Rev Respir Dis 97:89–95, 1968.

100. Walker WC, Wright V: Pulmonary lesions and rheumatoid arthritis. Medicine 47:501–519, 1968.

101. Scadding JG: The lungs in rheumatoid arthritis. Proc Soc Med 62:227–238, 1969.

102. Walker WC, Wright V: Diffuse interstitial pulmonary fibrosis and rheumatoid arthritis. Ann Rheum Dis 28:252–259, 1969.

103. Winchester RJ, Litwin SD, Koffler D, Kunkel HG: Observations on the eosinophilia of certain patients with rheumatoid arthritis. Arthritis Rheum 14:650–655, 1971.

104. DeHoratius RJ, Abruzzo JL, Williams RC: Immunofluorescent and immunologic studies of rheumatoid lung. Arch Intern Med 129:441–446, 1972.

105. Gardner DL: *The Pathology of Rheumatoid Arthritis*. Baltimore: Williams & Wilkins, 1972, pp 137–143.

106. Nozawa Y: Histopathological findings of the lung in collagen disease—Especially on their differential diagnosis. Acta Pathol Jpn 22:843–858, 1972.

107. Popper MS, Bogdonoff ML, Hughes RI: Interstitial rheumatoid lung disease. Chest 62:243–249, 1972.

108. Benedek TG: Rheumatoid pneumoconiosis. Am J Med 55:515–524, 1973.

109. Frank ST, Weg JG, Harkelroad LE, Fitch RF: Pulmonary dysfunction in rheumatoid disease. Chest 63:27–34, 1973.

110. Laitinen O, Nissila M, Salorinne Y, Aalto P: Pulmonary involvement in patients with rheumatoid arthritis. Scand J Respir Dis 56:297–304, 1975.

111. Dieppe PA. Empyema in rheumatoid arthritis. Ann Rheum Dis 34:181–185, 1975.

112. Collins RL, Turner RA, Johnson AM, et al.: Obstructive pulmonary disease in rheumatoid arthritis. Arthritis Rheum 19:623–628, 1976.

113. Glass D, Soter NA, Schur PH: Rheumatoid vasculitis. Arthritis Rheum 19:950–952, 1976.

114. Wang SC: Pseudolymphomatous pulmonary infiltrates in rheumatoid arthritis. Mt Sinai J Med (NY) 43:157–162, 1976.

115. Winterbauer RH, Wilske KR, Wheelis RF: Diffuse pulmonary injury associated with gold treatment. N Engl J Med 294:919–921, 1976.

116. Cohen JM, Miller A, Spiera H: Interstitial pneumonitis complicating rheumatoid arthritis. Chest 72:521–524, 1977.

117. Kay JM, Banik S: Unexplained pulmonary hypertension with pulmonary arteritis in rheumatoid disease. Br J Dis Chest 71:53–59, 1977.

118. Wagenvoort CA, Wagenvoort N: *Pathology of Pulmonary Hypertension*. New York: John Wiley & Sons, 1977.

119. Eraut D, Evans J, Caplin M: Pulmonary necrobiotic nodules without rheumatoid arthritis. Br J Dis Chest 72:301–306, 1978.

120. Macfarlane JD, Dieppe PA, Rigden BG, Clark TJH: Pulmonary and pleural lesions in rheumatoid disease. Br J Dis Chest 72:288–300, 1978.

121. Editorial: Airways in Rheumatoid Disease. Lancet II:192–193, July 22, 1978.

122. Baydur A, Mongan ES, Slager UT: Acute respiratory failure and pulmonary arteritis without parenchymal involvement. Chest 75:518–520, 1979.

123. Epler GR, Snider GL, Gaensler EA, et al.: Bronchiolitis and bronchitis in connective tissue disease. JAMA 242:528–532, 1979.

124. Geddes DM, Webley M, Emerson PA: Airways obstruction in rheumatoid arthritis. Ann Rheum Dis 38:222–225, 1979.

125. Hills EA, Davies S, Geary M: Frequency dependence of dynamic compliance in patients with rheumatoid arthritis. Thorax 34:755–761, 1979.

126. Hurd ER: Extra-articular manifestations of rheumatoid arthritis. Semin Arthritis Rheum 8:151–176, 1979.

127. Strohl KP, Feldman NT, Ingram RH Jr: Apical fibrobullous disease with rheumatoid arthritis. Chest 75:739–741, 1979.

128. Cervantes-Perez P, Toro-Perez AH, Rodriquez-Jurado MP: Pulmonary involvement in rheumatoid arthritis. JAMA 243:1715–1719, 1980.

129. Cooney TP: Interrelationship of chronic eosinophilic pneumonia, bronchiolitis obliterans, and rheumatoid disease: A hypothesis. J Clin Pathol 34:129–137, 1981.

130. Stein HB, Patterson C, Offer RC, et al.: Adverse effects of d-penicillamine in rheumatoid arthritis. Ann Intern Med 92:24–29, 1980.

131. Murphy KC, Atkins CJ, Offer RC, et al.: Obliterative bronchiolitis in two rheumatoid arthritis patients treated with penicillamine. Arthritis Rheum 24:557–560, 1981.

132. Scott DL, Bradby GVH, Aitman TJ, et al.: Relationship of gold and pencillamine therapy to diffuse interstitial lung disease. Ann Rheum Dis 40:136–141, 1981.

133. Begin R, Masse S, Cantin A, et al.: Airway disease in a subset of nonsmoking rheumatoid patients—Characterization of the disease and evidence of an autoimmune pathogenesis. Am J Med 72:743–750, 1982.

134. Case records of the Massachusetts General Hospital: Case 3-1982. N Engl J Med 306:157–165, 1982.

135. Camus P, Degat R, Justrabo E, Jeannin L: D-Penicillamine-induced severe pneumonitis. Chest 81:376–378, 1982.

136. Crisp AJ, Armstrong RD, Grahame R, Dussek JE: Rheumatoid lung disease, pneumothorax, and eosinophila. Ann Rheum Dis 41:137–140, 1982.

136a. Yousem SA, Colby TV, Carrington CB: Lung biopsy in rheumatoid arthritis. Am Rev Respir Dis 131:770–777, 1985.

136b. Yousem SA, Colby TV, Carrington CB: Follicular bronchitis/bronchiolitis. Hum Pathol 16:700–706, 1985.

137. Romicka A, Maldyk E: Pulmonary lesions in the course of rheumatoid arthritis in children. Pol Med History Bull 18:263–268, 1975.

138. Yousefzadeh DK, Fishman PA: The triad of pneumonitis, pleuritis, and pericarditis in juvenile rheumatoid arthritis. Pediatr Radiol 8:147–150, 1979.

139. Athreya BH, Doughty RA, Bookspan M, et al.: Pulmonary manifestations of juvenile rheumatoid arthritis. Clin Chest Med 1:361–374, 1980.

140. Wagener JS, Taussig LM, DeBenedetti C, et al.: Pulmonary function in juvenile rheumatoid arthritis. J Pediatr 99:108–110, 1981.

141. Purnell DC, Baggenstoss AH, Olsen AM: Pulmonary lesions in disseminated lupus erythematosus. Ann Intern Med 42:619–628, 1955.

142. Newcomer AD, Miller RD, Hepper NGG, Carter ET: Pulmonary dysfunction in rheumatoid arthritis and systemic lupus erythematosus. Dis Chest 46:562–570, 1964.

143. Hoffbrand BI, Beck ER: "Unexplained" dyspnoea and shrinking lungs in systemic lupus erythematosus. Br Med J 1:1273–1277, 1965.

144. Gross M, Esterly JR, Earle RH: Pulmonary alterations in systemic lupus erythematosus. Am Rev Respir Dis 105:572–577, 1972.

145. Olsen EGJ, Lever JV: Pulmonary changes in systemic lupus erythematosus. Br J Dis Chest 66:71–77, 1972.

146. Byrd RB, Trunk G: Systemic lupus erythematosus presenting as pulmonary hemosiderosis. Chest 64:128–129, 1973.

147. Eisenberg H, Dubois EL, Sherwin RP, Balchum OJ: Diffuse interstitial lung disease in systemic lupus erythematosus. Ann Intern Med 79:37–45, 1973.

148. Matthay RA, Schwarz MI, Petty TL, et al.: Pulmonary manifestations of systemic lupus erythematosus: Review of twelve cases of acute lupus pneumonitis. Medicine 54:397–409, 1974.

149. Turner-Warwick M: Immunological aspects of systemic diseases of the lungs. Proc Soc Med 67:541–547, 1974.

150. Gould DB, Soriano RZ: Acute alveolar hemorrhage in lupus erythematosus. Ann Intern Med 83:836–837, 1975.

151. Fayemi AO: Pulmonary vascular disease in systemic lupus erythematosus. Am J Clin Pathol 65:284–290, 1976.

152. Gibson GJ, Edmonds JP, Hughes GRV: Diaphragm function and lung involvement in systemic lupus erythematosus. Am J Med 63:926–932, 1977.

153. Pertschuk LP, Moccia LF, Rosen Y, et al.: Acute pulmonary complications in systemic lupus erythematosus: Immunofluorescence and light microscopic study. Am J Clin Pathol 68:553–557, 1977.

154. Rodriquez-Iturbe B, Garcia R, Rubio L, Serrano H: Immunohistologic findings in the lung in systemic lupus erythematosus. Arch Pathol Lab Med 101:342–344, 1977.

155. Eagen JW, Roberts JL, Schartz MM, Lewis EJ: The composition of pulmonary immune deposits in systemic lupus erythematosus. Clin Immunol Immunopathol 12:204–219, 1979.

156. Eagen JW, Memoli VA, Roberts JL, et al.: Pulmonary hemorrhage in systemic lupus erythematosus. Medicine 57:545–560, 1978.

157. Inoue T, Kanayama Y, Ohe A, et al.: Immunopathologic studies of pneumonitis in systemic lupus erythematosus. Ann Intern Med 91:30–34, 1979.

158. Mintz G, Galindo LF, Fernandez-Diaz J, et al.: Acute massive pulmonary hermorrhage in systemic lupus erythematosus. J Rheumatol 5:39–50, 1978.

159. Churg AC, Franklin W, Chan KW, et al.: Pulmonary hemorrhage and immune-complex deposition in the lung. Arch Pathol Lab Med 104:388–391, 1980.

160. Silberstein SL, Barland P, Grayzel AI, Koerner SK: Pulmonary dysfunction in systemic lupus erythematosus: Prevalence, classification and correlation with other organ involvement. J Rheumatol 7:187–195, 1980.

161. Haupt HM, Moore GW, Hutchins GM: The lung in systemic lupus erythematosus. Am J Med 71:791–798, 1981.

162. Perez HD, Kramer N: Pulmonary hypertension in systemic lupus erythematosus: Report of four cases and review of the literature. Semin Arthritis Rheum 11:177–181, 1981.

163. Webb WR, Gamsu G: Cavitory pulmonary nodules with systemic lupus erythematosus. AJR 136:27–31, 1981.

164. Kinney WW, Angelillo VA: Bronchiolitis in systemic lupus erythematosus. Chest 82:646–649, 1982.

164a. Lyon MG, Bewtra C, Kenik JG, Hurley JA: Tubuloreticular inclusions in systemic lupus erythematosus. Arch Pathol Lab Med 108:599–600, 1984.

165. Getzowa S: Cystic and compact pulmonary sclerosis in progressive scleroderma. Arch Pathol 40:99–106, 1945.

166. Naeye RL: Pulmonary vascular lesions in systemic scleroderma. Dis Chest 44:374–380, 1963.

167. Wilson RJ, Rodnan GP, Robin ED: An early pulmonary physiologic abnormality in progressive systemic sclerosis (diffuse scleroderma). Am J Med 36:361–369, 1964.

168. Weaver AL, Divertie MB, Titus JL: Pulmonary scleroderma. Dis Chest 54:4–12, 1968.

169. D'Angelo WA, Fries JF, Masi AT, Shulman LE: Pathologic observations in systemic sclerosis (scleroderma): A study of fifty-eight autopsy cases and fifty-eight matched controls. Am J Med 46:428–440, 1969.

170. Colp CR, Riker J, Williams MH: Serial changes in scleroderma and idiopathic interstitial lung disease. Arch Intern Med 132:506–515, 1973.

171. Bookman AAM, Urowitz MB, Mitchell RI: Alveolar cell carcinoma in progressive systemic sclerosis. J Rheumatol 1:466–472, 1974.

172. Guttadauria M, Ellman H, Emmanuel G, et al.: Pulmonary function in scleroderma. Arthritis Rheum 20:1071–1079, 1977.

173. Kallenbach J, Prinsloo I, Zwi S: Progressive systemic sclerosis complicated by diffuse pulmonary haemorrhage. Thorax 32:767–770, 1977.

174. Salerni R, Rodnan GP, Leon DF, Shaver JA: Pulmonary hypertension in the CREST syndrome variant of progressive systemic sclerosis (scleroderma). Ann Intern Med 86:394–399, 1977.

175. Young RH, Mark GJ: Pulmonary vascular changes in scleroderma. Am J Med 64:998–1004, 1978.

176. Bettmann MA, Kantrowitz F: Selected reports: Rapid onset of lung involvement in progressive systemic sclerosis. Chest 75:509–510, 1979.

177. Case records of the Massachusetts General Hospital: Case 43-1979. N Engl J Med 301:929–936, 1979.

178. Schneider PD, Wise RA, Hochberg MC, Wigley FM: Serial pulmonary function in systemic sclerosis. Am J Med 73:385–394, 1982.

179. Case records of the Massachusetts General Hospital: Case 14-1983. N Engl J Med 308:823–834, 1983.

179a. Konig G, Luderschmidt C, Hammer C, et al.: Lung involvement in scleroderma. Chest 85:318–324, 1984.

180. Sharp GC, Irvin WS, Tan EM, et al.: Mixed connective tissue disease—An apparently distinct rheumatic disease syndrome associated with a specific antibody to an extractable nuclear antigen (ENA). Am J Med 52:148–159, 1972.

181. Harmon C: Pulmonary involvement in mixed connective tissue disease. Arthritis Rheum 19:801, 1976.

182. O'Connell DJ, Bennett RM: Mixed connective tissue disease—Clinical and radiological aspects of 20 cases. Br J Radiol 50:620-625, 1977.

183. Wiener-Kronish JP, Solinger AM, Warnock ML, et al.: Severe pulmonary involvement in mixed connective tissue disease. Am Rev Respir Dis 124:499–503, 1981.

184. Strimlan CV, Rosenow EC, Divertie MB, Harrison EG: Pulmonary manifestations of Sjögren's syndrome. Chest 70:354–361, 1976.

185. Newball HH, Brahim SA: Chronic obstructive airway disease in patients with Sjögren's syndrome. Am Rev Respir Dis 115:295–304, 1977.

186. Polansky SM, Ravin CE: Nodular pulmonary infiltrate in patients with Sjögren's syndrome. Chest 77:411–412, 1980.

187. Fairfax AJ, Haslam PL, Pavia D, et al.: Pulmonary disorders associated with Sjögren's syndrome. QJ Med 50:279–295, 1981.

188. Rodriquez-Roisin R, Pares A, Bruguera M, et al.: Pulmonary involvement in primary biliary cirrhosis. Thorax 36:208–212, 1981.

189. Segal I, Fink G, Machtey I, et al.: Pulmonary function abnormalities in Sjögren's syndrome and the sicca complex. Thorax 36:286–289, 1981.

190. Hepper NGG, Ferguson RH, Howard FM Jr.: Three types of pulmonary involvement in polymyositis. Med Clin North Am 48:1031–1042, 1964.

191. Olsen GN, Swenson EW: Polymyositis and interstitial lung disease. Am Rev Respir Dis 105:611–617, 1972.

192. Frazier AR, Miller RD: Interstitial pneumonitis in association with polymyositis and dermatomyositis. Chest 65:403–407, 1974.

193. Duncan PE, Griffin JP, Garcia A, Kaplan SB: Fibrosing alveolitis in polymyositis: A review of histologically confirmed cases. Am J Med 57:621–626, 1974.

194. Park S, Nyhan WL: Fatal pulmonary involvement in dermatomyositis. Am J Dis Child 129:723–726, 1975.

195. Songcharoen S, Raju SF, Pennebaker JB: Interstitial lung disease in polymyositis and dermatomyositis. J Rheumatol 7:353–360, 1980.

196. Bunch TW, Tancredi RG, Lie JT: Pulmonary hypertension in polymyositis. Chest 79:105–107, 1981.

197. Salmeron G, Greenberg SD, Lidsky MD: Polymyositis and diffuse interstitial lung disease: A review of the pulmonary histopathologic findings. Arch Intern Med 141:1005–1010, 1981.

197a. Dickey BF, Myers AR: Pulmonary disease in polymyositis/dermatomyositis. Semin Arthritis Rheum 14:60–76, 1984.

198. Lauritzen H, Medina J, Loken MD, MacDonald FM: Pulmonary disease in patients with ankylosing spondylitis. Am Rev Respir Dis 98:126, 1968.

199. Cohen AA, Natelson EA, Fechner RE: Fibrosing interstitial pneumonitis in ankylosing spondylitis. Chest 59:369–371, 1971.

200. Davies D: Ankylosing spondylitis and lung fibrosis. J Med 41:395–417, 1972.

201. Crompton GK, Cameron SJ, Langlands AO: Pulmonary fibrosis, pulmonary tuberculosis and ankylosing spondylitis. Br J Dis Chest 68:51–56, 1974.

202. Appelrouth D, Gottlieb NL: Pulmonary manifestations of ankylosing spondylitis. J Rheumatol 2:446–453, 1975.

203. Chakera TMH, Howarth FH, Kendall MJ, et al.: The chest radiograph in ankylosing spondylitis. Clin Radiol 26:455–460, 1975.

204. Wolson AH, Rohwedder JJ: Upper lobe fibrosis in ankylosing spondylitis. Am J Roentgenol 124:466–471, 1975.

205. Rosenow EC, Strimlan CV, Muhm JR, Ferguson RH: Pleuropulmonary manifestations of ankylosing spondylitis. Mayo Clin Proc 52:641–649, 1977.

206. Libshitz HI, Atkinson GW: Pulmonary cystic disease in ankylosing spondylitis: Two cases with unusual superinfection. J Can Radiol Assoc 29:266–268, 1978.

207. Slavin RE, de Groot WJ: Pathology of the lung in Behçet's disease. Am J Surg Pathol 5:779–788, 1981.

208. Dreisen RB: Pulmonary vasculitis. Clin Chest Med 3:607–618, 1982.

209. Bombardieri S, Paoletti P, Ferri C, et al.: Lung involvement in essential mixed cryoglobulinemia. Am J Med 66:748–756, 1979.

210. Levine BW, Saldana M, Hutter AM: Pulmonary hypertension in sarcoidosis — a case report of a rare but potentially treatable cause. Am Rev Respir Dis 103:413–417, 1971.

211. Mitchell DN, Scadding JG: Sarcoidosis. Am Rev Respir Dis 110:774–802, 1974.

212. Schachter EN, Smith GJW, Cohen GS, et al.: Pulmonary granulomas in a patient with pulmonary veno-occlusive disease. Chest 67:487–489, 1975.

213. Beekman JF, Zimmet SM, Chun BK, et al.: Spectrum of pleural involvement in sarcoidosis. Arch Intern Med 136:323–330, 1976.

214. Burke GW, Gaensler EA, Carrington CB, et al.: Hypersensitivity pneumonitis or sarcoidosis? Chest 70:421, 1976.

215. Levinson RS, Metzger LF, Stanley NN, et al.: Airway function in sarcoidosis. Am J Med 62:51–59, 1977.

216. Case Records of the Massachusetts General Hospital: Case 4-1977. N Engl J Med 296:215–221, 1977.

217. Cohen SH, Fink JN, Garancis JC, et al.: Sarcoidosis in hypersensitivity pneumonitis. Chest 72:588–592, 1977.

218. Mitchell DN, Scadding JG, Heard BE, Hinson KFW: Sarcoidosis: Histopathological definition and clinical diagnosis. J Clin Pathol 30:395–408, 1977.

219. Rosen Y, Moon S, Huang CT, et al.: Granulomatous pulmonary angitis in sarcoidosis. Arch Pathol Lab Med 101:170–174, 1977.

220. Yamamoto Y, Kosuda T, Yanagawa H, et al.: Longterm follow-up in sarcoidosis in Japan. Z Erkr Atmungsorgane 149:191–196, 1977.

221. Dines DE, Stubbs SE, McDougall JC: Obstructive disease of the airways associated with stage 1 sarcoidosis. Mayo Clin Proc 53:788–791, 1978.

222. Israel HL, Atkinson GW: Sarcoidosis. Am Lung Assoc, Basics Respir Dis 7:1–6, 1978.

223. Rosen Y, Athanassiades TJ, Moon S, Lyons HA: Nongranulomatous interstitial pneumonitis in sarcoidosis. Chest 74:122–125, 1978.

224. Huang CT, Heurich AE, Rosen Y, et al.: Pulmonary sarcoidosis. Respiration 37:337–345, 1979.

225. Kaplan J, Johns CJ: Mycetomas in pulmonary sarcoidosis: Non-surgical management. John Hopkins Med J 145:157–161, 1979.

226. Gilman MJ, Wang KP: Transbronchial lung biopsy in sarcoidosis. Am Rev Respir Dis 122:721–724, 1980.
227. Kanada DJ, Scott D, Sharma OP: Unusual presentations of pleural sarcoidosis. Br J Dis Chest 74:203–205, 1980.
228. Nicholls AJ, Friend JAR, Legge JS: Sarcoid pleural effusion: Three cases and review of the literature. Thorax 35:277–281, 1980.
229. Rohatgi PK: Significance of serum angiotensin converting enzyme and gallium scan in noninvasive diagnosis of sarcoidosis. Eur J Repir Dis 62:223–230, 1980.
230. Crystal RG, Roberts WC, Hunninghake GW, et al.: Pulmonary sarcoidosis: A disease characterized and perpetuated by activated lung T-lymphocytes. Ann Intern Med 94:73–94, 1981.
231. Godard P, Clot J, Jonquet O, et al.: Lymphocyte subpopulations in bronchoalveolar lavages of patients with sarcoidosis and hypersensitivity pneumonitis. Chest 80:447–452, 1981.
232. Hunninghake GW, Crystal RG: Pulmonary sarcoidosis. A disorder mediated by excess helper T-lymphocyte activity at sites of disease activity. N Engl J Med 305:429–434, 1981.
233. Konig G, Baur X, Fruhmann G: Sarcoidosis or extrinsic allergic alveolitis? Respiration 42:150–154, 1981.
234. Miller A: The vanishing lung syndrome associated with pulmonary sarcoidosis. Br J Dis Chest 75:209–214, 1981.
235. Pertschuk LP, Silverstein E, Friedland J: Immunohistologic diagnosis of sarcoidosis. Am J Clin Pathol 75:350–353, 1981.
236. Huang CT, Heurich AE, Sutton AL, Lyons HA: Mortality in sarcoidosis. Eur J Respir Dis 62:231–238, 1981.
237. Davies J, Nellen M, Goodwin JF: Reversible pulmonary hypertension in sarcoidosis. Postgrad Med J 58:282–285, 1982.
238. Demicco WA, Fanburg BL. Sarcoidosis presenting as a lobar or unilateral lung infiltrate. Clin Radiol 33:663–669, 1982.
239. Harkleroad LE, Young RL, Savage PJ, et al.: Pulmonary sarcoidosis: Long-term follow-up of the effects of steroid therapy. Chest 82:84–87, 1982.
240. James DG, Williams WJ: Immunology of sarcoidosis. Am J Med 72:5–8, 1982.
241. Kataria YP, Shaw RA, Campbell PB: Sarcoidosis: An overview II. Clin Notes Respir Dis 20:3–15, 1982.
242. Rohrback MS, DeRemee RA: Pulmonary sarcoidosis and serum angiotensin-converting enzyme (Editorial). Mayo Clin Proc. 57:64–66, 1982.
243. Margolis ML, Israel HL: Sarcoidosis in older patients—Clinical characteristic and course. Geriatrics 38:121–128, 1983.
244. Pinkston P, Bitterman PB, Crystal RG: Spontaneous release of interleukin-2 by lung T-lymphocytes in active pulmonary sarcoidosis. N Engl J Med 308:793–800, 1983.
245. Smith LJ, Lawrence JB, Katzenstein ALA: Vascular sarcoidosis: A rare cause of pulmonary hypertension. Am J Med Sci 285:38–44, 1983.
245a. Crystal RG, Bitterman PB, Rennard SI, et al.: Interstitial lung diseases of unknown cause, Part II. N Engl J Med 310:235–244, 1984.
245b. Glazer HS, Levitt RG, Shackelford GD: Peripheral pulmonary infiltrates in sarcoidosis. Chest 86:741–744, 1984.
245c. Hillerdal G, Nou E, Osterman K, Schmekel B: Sarcoidosis: Epidemiology and prognosis. Am Rev Respir Dis 130:29–32, 1984.
245d. McLeod DT, Hilton Am, Large DM: Pulmonary sarcoidosis presenting with large haemoptysis. Br J Dis Chest 78:292–294, 1984.
246. Sharma OP, Hewlett R, Gordonson J: Nodular sarcoidosis: An unusual radiographic appearance. Chest 64:189–192, 1973.
247. Onal E, Lopata M, Lourenco RV: Nodular pulmonary sarcoidosis: Clinical roentgenographic, and physiologic course in five patients. Chest 72:296–300, 1977.
248. Romer FK: Sarcoidosis with large nodular lesions simulating pulmonary metastases. Scand J Respir Dis 58:11–16, 1977.
249. Liebow AA: Pulmonary angitis and granulomatosis. Am Rev Respir Dis 108:1–18, 1973.
250. Stephen JG, Braimbridge MV, Corrin B, et al.: Necrotizing "sarcoidal" angitis and granulomatosis of the lung. Thorax 31:356–360, 1976.
251. Tellis CJ, Putnam JS: Cavitation in large multinodular pulmonary disease. Chest 71:792–793, 1977.
252. Saldana MJ: Necrotizing sarcoid granulomatosis: Clinicopathologic observations in 24 patients. Lab Invest 38(Abst):364, 1978.
253. Churg A, Carrington CB, Gupta R: Necrotizing sarcoid granulomatosis. Chest 76:406–413, 1979.
254. Beach RC, Corrin B, Scopes JW, Graham E: Necrotizing sarcoid granulomatosis with neurologic lesions in a child. J Pediatr 97:950–953, 1980.
255. Innes DJ Jr, Feldman PS, Sabio H: Nodular sarcoid-like pulmonary lesions associated with chemotherapy. Am J Clin Pathol 74:501, 1980.
256. Koss MN, Hochholzer L, Feigin DS, et al.: Necrotizing sarcoid-like granulomatosis: Clinical, pathologic, and immunopathologic findings. Hum Pathol 11:510–519, 1980.
257. Rohatgi, PK, Schwab LE: Primary acute pulmonary cavitation in sarcoidosis. AJR 134:1199–1203, 1980.
258. Singh N, Cole S, Krause PJ, et al.: Necrotizing sarcoid granulomtosis with extrapulmonary involvement. Am Rev Respir Dis 124:189–192, 1981.
258a. Rolfes DB, Weiss MA, Sanders MA: Necrotizing sarcoidosis with suppurative features. Am J Clin Pathol 82:602–607, 1984.
259. Lichtenstein L: Histiocytosis X. Arch Pathol 56:84–102, 1953.
260. Corrin B, Basset F: A review of histiocytosis X with particular reference to eosinophilic granuloma of the lung. Invest Cell Pathol 2:137–146, 1979.
261. Basset F, Corrin B, Spencer H, et al.: Pulmonary histiocytosis X. Am Rev Respir Dis 118:811–820, 1978.
262. Friedman PJ, Liebow AA, Sokoloff J: Eosinophilic granuloma of the lung. Medicine 60:385–396, 1981.
263. Colby TV, Lombard C: Histiocytosis X presenting in the lung. Hum Pathol 14:847–856, 1983.
264. Lacronique J, Roth C, Battesti J-P, et al.: Chest radiological features of pulmonary histiocytosis X: A report based on 50 adult cases. Thorax 37:104–109, 1982.
265. Nezelof C: Histiocytosis X: A histologic and histogenetic study. In Rosenberg HS, Bolade RP (eds): *Perspectives in Pediatric Pathology*, vol 5. New York: Masson, 1979, pp 153–178.
266. Lewis JG: Eosinophilic granuloma and its variants with special reference to lung involvement. Q J Med 33:337–359, 1964.
267. Hoffman L, Cohn JE, Gaensler EA: Respiratory abnormalities in eosinophilic granuloma of the lung. N Engl J Med 267:577–588, 1962.
268. Brody AR, Kanich RE, Graham WG, Craighead JE: Cyst wall formation in pulmonary eosinophilic granuloma. Chest 66:576–578, 1974.
269. Enriques P, Dahlin DC, Hayles AB, Henderson ED: Histiocytosis X: A clinical study, Mayo Clin Proc 42:88–99, 1967.

270. Askin FB, McCann BG, Kuhn C: Reactive eosinophilic pleuritis. Arch Pathol Lab Med 101:187–191, 1977.

271. Kawanami O, Basset F, Ferrans VJ et al.: Pulmonary Langerhans cells in patients with fibrotic lung disorders. Lab Invest 44:227–233, 1981.

272. Lahey ME: Prognostic factors in histiocytosis X. Am J Pediatr Hematol Oncol 3:57–60, 1981.

273. Greenberger JS, Crocker AC, Vawter G, et al.: Results of treatment of 127 patients with systemic histiocytosis (Letterer-Siwe Syndrome, Schüller-Christian syndrome and multifocal eosinophilic granuloma). Medicine 60:311–338, 1981.

274. Liewbow AA, Carrington CB: The eosinophilic pneumonias. Medicine 48:251–285, 1969.

275. Carrington CB, Addington WW, Goff Am, et al.: Chronic eosinophilic pneumonia. N Engl J Med 280:786–798, 1969.

276. Schatz M, Wasserman S, Patterson R: The eosinophil and the lung. Arch Intern Med 142:1515–1519, 1982.

277. Fox B, Seed WA: Chronic eosinophilic pneumonia. Thorax 35:570–580, 1980.

278. Keslin MH, McCoy EL, McCusker JJ, Lutch JS: Corynebacterium pseudotuberculosis — A new cause of infections and eosinophilic pneumonia. Am J Med 67:228–231, 1979.

279. Kanner RE, Hammar SP: Chronic eosinophilic pneumonia — Ultrastructural evidence of marked immunoglobulin production plus macrophagic ingestion of eosinophils and eosinophilic lysosomes leading to intracytoplasmic Charcot-Leyden crystals. Chest 71:95–98, 1977.

280. Conn DY, McDuffie FC, Holley KE, Schroeter Al: Immunologic mechanisms in systemic vasculitis. Mayo Clin Proc 51:511–581, 1976.

281. Koss MN, Antonovych T, Hochholzer L: Allergic granulomatosis (Churg-Strauss syndrome). Am J Surg Pathol 5:21–28, 1981.

282. Harkavy J: Vascular allergy. III. J Allergy 14:507–537, 1943.

283. Crofton JW, Livingstone JL, Oswald NC, Roberts ATM: Pulmonary eosinophilia. Thorax 7:1–35, 1952.

284. Gray J: Brief reports: Löffler's syndrome following ingestion of a coin. Can Med Assoc J 127:999–1000, 1982.

285. Von Meyenburg V: Das H. Eosinophile Lungeninfiltrat: Pathologische anatomie und pathogenese. Schweiz Med Wochenschr 23:809–811, 1942.

286. Bedrossian CWM, Greenberg SD, Williams LJ: Ultrastructure of the lung in Loeffler's pneumonia. Am J Med 58:438–443, 1975.

287. Gaensler EA, Carrington CB: Peripheral opacities in chronic eosinophilic pneumonia: The photographic negative of pulmonary edema. AJR 128:1–13, 1977.

288. Pearson DJ, Rosenow EC: Chronic eosinophilic pneumonia (Carrington's) — A follow-up study. Mayo Clin Proc 53:73–78, 1978.

289. Libby DM, Murphy TF, Edwards A, et al.: Chronic eosinophilic pneumonia: An unusual cause of acute respiratory failure. Am Rev Respir Dis 122:497–500, 1980.

290. Wright JL, Pare PD, Hammond M, Donevan RE: Eosinophilic pneumonia and atypical myobacterial infection. Am Rev Respir Dis 127:497–499, 1983.

291. Rogers RM, Christiansen JR, Coalson JJ, Patterson CD: Eosinophilic pneumonia — Physiologic response to steroid therapy and observation on light and electron microscopic findings. Chest 68:665–671, 1975.

292. Katzenstein AL, Liebow A, Friedman PJ: Bronchocentric granulomatosis, mucoid impaction, and hypersensitivity reactions to fungi. Am Rev Respir Dis 111:497, 1975.

293. Payne CR, Connellan SJ: Chronic eosinophilic pneumonia complicating longstanding rheumatoid arthritis. Postgrad Med 56:519–520, 1980.

294. Dines DE: Chronic eosinophilic pneumonia: A roentgenographic diagnosis. Mayo Clin Proc 53:129–130, 1978.

295. Churg J, Strauss L: Allergic granulomatosis, allergic angitis, and periarteritis nodosa. Am J Pathol 32:277–301, 1950.

296. Fienberg R: Pathergic granulomatosis. Am J Med 19:829–831, 1955.

297. McCluskey RT, Fienberg R: Vasculitis in primary vasculitides, granulomatoses, and connective tissue diseases. Hum Pathol 14:305–315, 1983.

298. Chumbley LC, Harrisson EG, DeRemee RA: Allergic granulomatosis and angitis (Churg-Strauss syndrome). Report and analysis of 30 cases. Mayo Clin Proc 52:477–484, 1977.

299. Clausen K, Bronstein H: Granulomatous pulmonary arteritis—A hypereosinophilic syndrome. Am J Clin Pathol 62:82–87, 1974.

300. Veevaete F, Van Der Straeten M, De Vox, Roels H: Allergic granulomatous angitis. Scand J Resp Dis 59:297–296, 1978.

301. Olsen KD, Neel HB, DeRemee RA, Weiland LH: Nasal manifestations of allergic granulomatosis and angitis (Churg-Strauss syndrome). Otolaryngol Head Neck Surg 88:85–89, 1980.

302. Sale S, Patterson R: Recurrent Churg-Strauss vasculitis with exopthalmos, hearing loss, nasal obstruction, amyloid deposits, hyperimmunoglobulinemia E, and circulating immune complexes. Arch Intern Med 141:1363–1364, 1981.

303. Wishnick MM, Valensi Q, Doyle EF, et al.: Churg-Strauss syndrome — Development of cardioymopathy during corticosteroid treatment. J Dis Child 136:339–344, 1982.

304. Udwadia FE: Pulmonary eosinophila. Prog Respir Res 7: Basel, Munchen, Paris, London, New York, Sidney. S. Karger 1975. 286 pp.

305. Neva FA, Ottesen EA: Current concepts in parasitology — Tropical (filarial) eosinophilia. N Engl J Med 298:1129–1131, 1978.

306. Chusid MJ, Dale DC, West BC, Wolff SM: The hypereosinophilic syndrome: Analysis of fourteen cases with review of the literature. Medicine 54:1–27, 1975.

307. Hennell H, Sussman ML: Roentgen features of eosinophilic infiltrations in the lungs. Radiology 44:328–334, 1945.

308. Zeek PM: Periarteritis nodosa. A critical review. Am J Clin Pathol 22:777, 1952.

309. Kussmaul A, Maier R: Uber eine bisher nicht beschriebene eigentumliche Arterienerkrankung (Periarteritis nodosa) die mit Morbus Brightu und rapid fortschreitender allgemeinder Muskellahmung einhergeht. Dtsch Arch Klin Med 1:484–517, 1866.

310. Bergstrand H: Morphological equivalents in polyarteritis rheumatica, periarteritis nodosa, transient eosinophilic infiltration of the lung and other allergic syndromes. J Pathol Bacteriol 58:399–409, 1946.

311. Rose GA, Spencer H: Polyarteritis nodosa. J Med 26:43–81, 1957.

312. Scully RE, Galdabini JJ, McNeely BU: Case records of the Massachusetts General Hospital. N Engl J Med 303:1218–1225, 1980.

313. Rosen SH, Castleman B, Liebow AA: Pulmonary alveolar proteinosis. N Engl J Med 258:1123–1142, 1958.

314. Kuhn C, Gyorkey F, Levine R, Ramirez-Rivera J: Pulmonary alveolar proteinosis. A study using enzyme histochemistry,

electron microscopy, and surface tension measurement. Lab Invest 15:492–509, 1966.

315. Ramirez RJ, Harlan WR Jr: Pulmonary alveolar proteinosis. Nature and origin of alveolar lipid. Am J Med 45:502–512, 1968.

316. Corrin B, King E: Pathogenesis of experimental pulmonary alveolar proteinosis. Thorax 25:230–236, 1970.

317. Colon AR Jr, Lawrence RD, Mills SD, O'Connell EJ: Childhood pulmonary alveolar proteinosis (PAP): Report of a case and review of the literature. Am J Dis Child 121:481–485, 1971.

318. Case records of the Massachusetts General Hospital. Weekly clinicopathological exercises. N Engl J Med 291:464–469, 1974.

319. Hudson AR, Halprin GM, Miller JA, Kilburn KH: Pulmonary interstitial fibrosis following alveolar proteinosis. Chest 65:700–702, 1974.

320. Costello JF, Moriarty DC, Branthwaite MA, et al.: Diagnosis and management of alveolar proteinosis: The role of electron microscopy. Thorax 30:121–132, 1975.

321. Golde DW, Territo M, Finley TN, Cline MJ: Defective lung macrophage in pulmonary alveolar proteinosis. Ann Intern Med 85:304–309, 1976.

322. Carnovale R, Zornoza J, Goldman AM, Luna M: Pulmonary alveolar proteinosis: Its association with hematologic malignancy and lymphoma. Diagn Radiol 122:303–306, 1977.

323. Jacobovitz-Derks D, Corrin B: Degenerative processes in the pathogenesis of pulmonary alveolar lipoproteinosis. Virchows Arch [A] 376:165–174, 1977.

324. Hook GER, Bell DY, Gilmore LB, et al.: Composition of bronchoalveolar lavage effluents from patients with pulmonary alveolar proteinosis. Lab Invest 39:342–357, 1978.

325. Ito M, Takeuchi N, Ogura T, et al.: Pulmonary alveolar proteinosis: Analysis of pulmonary washings. Br J Dis Chest 72:313–320, 1978.

326. Rogers RM, Levin DC, Gray BA, Moseley LW Jr: Physiologic effects of broncho-pulmonary lavage in alveolar proteinosis. Am Rev Respir Dis 118:255–264, 1978.

327. Hocking WG, Golde DW: Medical Progress. II. The pulmonary-alveolar macrophage. N Engl J Med 301:639–645, 1979.

328. Bell DY, Hook GER: Pulmonary alveolar proteinosis: Analysis of airway and alveolar proteins. Am Rev Respir Dis 119:979–990, 1979.

329. Ranchod M, Bissell M: Pulmonary alveolar proteinosis and cytomegalovirus infection. Arch Pathol Lab Med 103:139–142, 1979.

330. Bedrossian CWM, Luna MA, Conklin RH, Miller WC: Alveolar proteinosis as a consequence of immunosuppression. A hypothesis based on clinical pathologic observations. Hum Pathol 11:527–535, 1980.

331. Coleman M, Dehner LP, Sibley RK, et al.: Case Reports. Pulmonary alveolar proteinosis: An uncommon cause of chronic neonatal respiratory distress. Am Rev Respir Dis 121:583–586, 1980.

332. Martin RJ, Coalson JJ, Rogers RM, et al.: Pulmonary alveolar proteinosis: The diagnosis by segmental lavage. Am Rev Respir Dis 121:819–825, 1980.

333. Rubin E, Weisbrod GL, Sanders DE: Pulmonary alveolar proteinosis. Relationship to silicosis and pulmonary infection. Radiology 135:35–41, 1980.

334. Singh G, Katyal SL: Surfactant apoprotein in nonmalignant pulmonary disorders. Am J Pathol 101:51–61, 1980.

335. Smith LJ, Ankin MG, Katzenstein AL, Shapiro BA: Clinical conference in pulmonary disease. Management of pulmonary alveolar proteinosis. Chest 78:765–770, 1980.

336. Webster JR, Battifora H, Furey C, et al.: Pulmonary alveolar proteinosis in two siblings with decreased immunologlobulin A. Am J Med 69:786–789, 1980.

337. Miller PA, Ravin CE, Smith GJW, Osborne DRS: Pulmonary alveolar proteinosis with interstitial involvement. AJR 137:1069–1071, 1981.

338. Teja K, Cooper PH, Squires JE, Schnatterly PT: Medical intelligence. Pulmonary alveolar proteinosis in four siblings. N Engl J Med 305:1390–1392, 1981.

339. Singh G, Katyal SL, Bedrossian CWM, Rogers RM: Pulmonary alveolar proteinosis: Staining for surfactant apoprotein in alveolar proteinosis and in conditions simulating it. Chest 83:82–86, 1983.

340. Harris JO: Pulmonary alveolar proteinosis: Specific or nonspecific response? (Editorial) Chest 84:1–2, 1983.

341. Abraham JL, McEuen DD: Inorganic particulates associated with pulmonary alveolar proteinosis. Am Rev Respir Dis 119:196, 1979.

341a. Clague HW, Wallace AC, Morgan WKC: Pulmonary fibrosis associated with alveolar proteinosis. Thorax 38:865–866, 1983.

341b. Case records of the Massachusetts General Hospital. Case 14. N Engl J Med 310:906–916, 1984.

341c. Corsello BF, Choi H: Basophilic staining in pulmonary alveolar proteinosis. Arch Pathol Lab Med 108:68–70, 1984.

341d. Miller RR, Churg AC, Hutcheon M, Lam S: Pulmonary alveolar proteinosis and aluminin dust exposure. Am Rev Respir Dis 130:312–315, 1984.

342. Malik SK, Neely P, Martin CJ: Involvement of the lungs in tuberous sclerosis. Chest 58:538–540, 1970.

343. Wolff M: Lymphangiomyoma: Clinicopathologic study and ultrastructural confirmation of its histogenesis. Cancer 31:988–1007, 1973.

344. Silverstein EF, Ellis K, Wolff M, Jaretzki A III. Pulmonary lymphangiomyomatosis. Am J Roentgenol Radium Ther Nucl Med 120:832–850, 1974.

345. Corrin B, Liebow AA, Friedman PJ: Pulmonary lymphangiomyomatosis. A review. Am J Pathol 79:348–367, 1975.

346. Gray SR, Carrington CB, Cornog JL Jr: Lymphangiomyomatosis: Report of a case with ureteral involvement and chyluria. Cancer 35:490–498, 1975.

347. Basset F, Soler P, Marsac J, Corrin B: Pulmonary lymphangiomyomatosis: Three new cases studied with electron microscopy. Cancer 38:2357–2365, 1976.

348. Vazquez JJ, Fernandez-Cuervo L, Fidalgo G: Lymphangiomyomatosis: Morphogenetic study and ultrastructural confirmation of the histogenesis of the lung lesion. Cancer 37:2321–2327, 1976.

349. Carrington CB, Cugell DW, Gaensler EA, et al.: Lymphangioleiomyomatosis: Physiologic-pathologic-radiologic correlations. Am Rev Respir Dis 116:977–995, 1977.

350. Kane PB, Lane BP, Cordice JWV, Greenberg GM: Ultrastructure of the proliferating cells in pulmonary lymphangiomyomatosis. Arch Pathol Lab Med 102:618–622, 1978.

351. Shuman RL, Engleman R, Kittle CF: Pulmonary lymphangiomyomatosis. Ann Thorac Surg 27:70–75, 1979.

352. Bradley SL, Dines DE, Soule EH, Muhm JR: Pulmonary lymphangiomyomatosis. Lung 158:69–80, 1980.

353. Kitzsteiner KA, Mallen RG: Pulmonary lymphangiomyomatosis: Treatment with castration. Cancer 46:2248–2249, 1980.

354. McCarty KS, Mossler JA, McLelland R, Sieker HO: Pulmo-

nary lymphangiomyomatosis responsive to progesterone. N Engl J Med 303:1461–1465, 1980.

355. Banner AS, Carrington CB, Emory WB, et al.: Efficacy of oopherectomy in lymphangioleiomyomatosis and benign metastasizing leiomyoma. N Engl J Med 305:204–209, 1981.

355a. Brentani MM, Carvalho RR, Saldiva PH, et al.: Steroid receptors in pulmonary lymphangiomyomatosis. Chest 85:96–99, 1984.

355b. Dishner W, Cordasco EM, Blackburn J, et al.: Pulmonary lymphangiomyomatosis. Chest 85:796–799, 1984.

355c. Graham ML, Spelsberg TC, Dines DE, et al.: Pulmonary lymphangiomyomatosis: With particular reference to steroid-receptor assay studies and pathologic correlation. Mayo Clin Proc 59:3–11, 1984.

355d. Svendsen TL, Viskym K, Hansborg N, et al.: Pulmonary lymphangioleiomyomatosis: A case of progesterone receptor positive lymphangioleiomyomatosis treated with medroxyprogesterone, oophorectomy and tamoxifen. Br J Dis Chest 78:264–271, 1984.

356. Dwyer JM, Hickie JB, Garvan J: Pulmonary tuberous sclerosis. Q J Med 40:115–125, 1971.

357. Valensi QJ: Pulmonary lymphangiomyoma, a probable form fruste of tuberous sclerosis. Am Rev Respir Dis 180:1411–1415, 1973.

358. Stovin PGI, Lum LC, Flower CDR, et al.: The lungs in lymphangiomyomatosis and in tuberous sclerosis. Thorax 30:497–509, 1975.

359. Lie JT, Miller RD, Williams DE: Cystic disease of the lungs in tuberous sclerosis clinicopathologic correlation, including body plethysmographic lung function tests. Mayo Clin Proc 55:547–553, 1980.

360. Rudolph RI: Pulmonary manifestations of tuberous sclerosis. Cutis 27:82–84, 1981.

361. Israel-Asselain J, Chebat J, Sors C, et al.: Diffuse interstitial pulmonary fibrosis in a mother and son and von Recklinghausen's disease. Thorax 20:153–157, 1965.

362. Massaro D, Katz, S: Fibrosing alveolitis: Its occurrence, roentgenographic and pathologic features in von Recklinghausen's neurofibromatosis. Am Rev Respir Dis 93:934–942, 1966.

363. Patchefsky AS, Atkinson WG, Hoch WS, et al.: Interstitial pulmonary fibrosis and von Recklinghausen's disease. An ultrastructural and immunofluorescent study. Chest 64:459–464, 1973.

364. Sagel SS, Forrest JV, Askin FB: Interstitial lung disease in neurofibromatosis. South Med J 68:647–649, 1975.

365. Webb WR, Goodman PC: Fibrosing alveolitis in patients with neurofibromatosis. Radiology 122:289–293, 1977.

366. Davis SA, Kaplan RL: Neurofibromatosis and interstitial lung disease. Arch Dermatol 114:1368–1369, 1978.

367. Kyle RA, Bayrd ED: Amyloidosis: Review of 236 cases. Medicine (Baltimore) 54:271–299, 1975.

368. Glenner GG: Amyloid deposits and amyloidosis (Part 1). N Engl J Med 302:1283–1292, 1980.

369. Glenner GG: Amyloid Deposits and amyloidosis (part II). N Engl J Med 302:1333–1344, 1980.

370. Rajan VT, Kikkawa Y: Alveolar septal amyloidosis in primary amyloidosis. Arch Pathol Lab Med 89:521–525, 1970.

371. Toriumi J: The lung in generalized amyloidosis. Acta Pathol Jpn 22:141–153, 1972.

372. Rubinow A, Celli BR, Cohen AS, et al.: Localized amyloidosis of the lower respiratory tract. Am Rev Respir Dis 118:603–611, 1978.

373. Celli Br, Rubinow A, Cohen AS, Brody JS: Patterns of pulmonary involvement in systemic amyloidosis. Chest 74:543–547, 1978.

374. Smith RRL, Hutchins GM, Moore GW, Humphrey RL: Type and distribution of pulmonary parenchymal and vascular amyloid: Correlation with cardiac amyloidosis. Am J Med 66:96–104, 1979.

375. Whitwell F: Localized amyloid infiltrations of the lower respiratory tract. Thorax 8:309–315, 1953.

376. Prowse CB: Amyloidosis of the lower respiratory tract. Thorax 13:308–320, 1958.

377. Antunes ML, Vieira Da Luz JM: Primary diffuse tracheobronchial amyloidosis. Thorax 24:307–311, 1969.

378. Gottlieb LS: Gold WM: Primary tracheobronchial amyloidosis. Am Rev Respir Dis 105:425–429, 1972.

379. Attwood HD, Price CG, Riddell RJ: Primary diffuse tracheobronchial amyloidosis. Thorax 27:620–624, 1972.

380. Hof DG, Rasp FL: Spontaneous regression of diffuse tracheobronchial amyloidosis. Chest 76:237–239, 1979.

381. Weiss L: Isolated multiple nodular pulmonary amyloidosis. Am J Clin Pathol 33:318–329, 1960.

382. Cotton RE, Jackson JW: Localized amyloid "tumours" of the lung simulating malignant neoplasms. Thorax 19:97–103, 1964.

383. Hayes WT, Bernhardt H: Solitary amyloid mass of the lung. Cancer 24:820–825, 1969.

384. Saab SB, Burke J, Hopeman A, Almond C: Primary pulmonary amyloidosis: Report of two cases. J Thorac Cardiovasc Surg 67:301–307, 1974.

385. Dyke PC, Demaray MJ, Delavan JW, Rasmussen RA: Pulmonary amyloidoma. Am J Clin Pathol 64:301–305, 1974.

386. Lee SC, Johnson HA: Multiple nodular pulmonary amyloidosis: A case report and comparison with diffuse alveolar-septal pulmonary amyloidosis. Thorax 30:178–185, 1975.

387. Bignold LP, Martyn M, Basten A: Nodular pulmonary amyloidosis associated with benign hypergammaglobulinemic purpura. Chest 2:334–336, 1978.

388. Schoen FJ, Alexander RW, Hood CI, Dunn LJ: Nodular pulmonary amyloidosis: Description of a case with ultrastructure. Arch Pathol Lab Med 104:66–69, 1980.

388a. Laden SA, Cohen ML, Harley RA: Nodular pulmonary amyloidosis with extrapulmonary involvement. Hum Pathol 15:594–597, 1984.

389. Engleman P, Liebow AA, Gmelich J, Friedman PJ: Pulmonary hyalinizing granuloma. Am Rev Respir Dis 115:997–1008, 1977.

390. Zundel WE, Prior AP: An amyloid lung. Thorax 26:357–363, 1971.

391. Eshun-Wilson K, Frandsen NE, Christensen HE: Pulmonary alveolar septal amyloidosis: A scanning and transmission electron microscopy study. Virchows Arch 371:89–99, 1976.

392. Lewinsohn G, Bruderman I, Bohadana A: Primary diffuse pulmonary amyloidosis with monoclonal gammopathy. Chest 69:682–685, 1976.

393. Case records of the Massachusetts General Hospital. Case 48. N Engl J Med 297:1221–1228, 1977.

394. Gonzalez-Cueto DM, Rigoli M, Gioseffi LM, et al.: Diffuse pulmonary amyloidosis. Am J Med 48:668–670, 1970.

395. Poh SC, Tjia TS, Seah HC: Primary diffuse alveolar septal amyloidosis. Thorax 3:186–191, 1975.

396. Kunze WP: Senile pulmonary amyloidosis. Pathol Res Pract 164:413–422, 1979.

396a. Ptikanen P, Westermark P, Cornwell GG: Senile systemic amyloidosis. Am J Pathol 117:391–399, 1984.

397. Crosbie WA, Lewis ML, Ramsay ID, Doyle D: Pulmonary amyloidosis with impaired gas transfer. Thorax 27:625–630, 1972.

398. Kanada DJ, Sharma OP: Long-term survival with diffuse interstitial pulmonary amyloidosis. Am J Med 67:879–882, 1979.

398a. Monreal FA: Pulmonary amyloidosis: Ultrastructural study of early alveolar septal deposits. Hum Pathol 15:388–390, 1984.

399. Wilson SR, Sanders DE, Delarue NC: Intrathoracic manifestations of amyloid disease. Radiology 120:283–289, 1976.

400. Desai RA, Mahajan VK, Benjamin S, et al.: Pulmonary amyloidoma and hilar adenopathy. Chest 76:170–173, 1979.

401. Roberts WC, Frederickson DS: Gaucher's disease of the lung causing severe pulmonary hypertension with associated acute recurrent pericarditis. Circulation 35:783–789, 1967.

402. Genereux GP: Lipids in the lungs: Radiologic-pathologic correlation. J Can Assoc Radiol 21:1–15, 1970.

403. Kirkpatrick JA, Capitanio MA: Pulmonary manifestations of systemic disease in infants. Semin Roentgenol 7:149–172, 1972.

404. Wolson AH: Pulmonary findings in Gaucher's disease. AJR 123:712–715, 1975.

405. Lee RE, Peters SP, Glew RH: Gaucher's disease: Clinical, morphologic, and pathogenetic considerations. Pathol Annu 12:309–339, 1977.

406. Schneider EL, Epstein CJ, Kaback MJ, Brandes D: Severe pulmonary involvement in adult Gaucher's disease. Am J Med 63:475–480, 1977.

407. Smith RL, Hutchins GM, Sack GH, Ridolfi RL: Unusual cardiac, renal and pulmonary involvement in Gaucher's disease. Am J Med 65:352–360, 1978.

408. Rahal F, McWilliams NB: Pulmonary Gaucher's disease diagnosed ante mortem. Va Med 108:186–187, 1981.

409. Crocker AC, Farber S: Niemann-Pick disease: A review of eighteen patients. Medicine 37:1–95, 1958.

410. Skikne MI, Prinsloo I, Webster I: Electron microscopy of lung in Niemann-Pick disease. J Pathol 106:119–122, 1972.

411. Lachman R, Crocker A, Schulman J, Strand R: Radiological findings in Niemann-Pick disease. Radiology 108:659–664, 1973.

412. Long RG, Lake BD, Pettit JE, et al.: Adult Niemann-Pick disease: Its relationship to the syndrome of the sea-blue histiocyte. Am J Med 62:627, 1977.

413. Bagdade JD, Parker F, Ways PO, et al.: Fabry's disease—A correlative clinical, morphologic, and biochemical study. Lab Invest 18:681–688, 1968.

414. Bartimmo EE, Guisan M, Moser EM: Pulmonary involvement in Fabry's disease: A reappraisal. Am J Med 53:755–764, 1972.

415. Kariman K, Singletary WV, Sieker HO: Pulmonary involvement in Fabry's disease. Am J Med 64(lett):911–912, 1978.

416. Rosenberg DM, Ferrans VJ, Fulmer JD, et al.: Chronic airflow obstruction in Fabry's disease. Am J Med 68:898–905, 1980.

417. Davies BH, Tuddenham EGD: Familial pulmonary fibrosis associated with oculocutaneous albinism and platelet function defect. J Med 45:219–232, 1976.

418. Garay SM, Gardella JE, Fazzini EP, Goldring RM: Hermansky-Pudlak syndrome. Am J Med 66:737–747, 1979.

419. Hoste P, Willems J, Devriendt J, et al.: Familial diffuse interstitial pulmonary fibrosis associated with oculocutaneous albinism. Scand J Respir Dis 60:128–134, 1979.

420. Schinella RA, Greco MA, Cobert BL, et al.: Hermansky-Pudlack syndrome with granulomatous colitis. Ann Intern Med 92:20–23, 1980.

421. Matsumoto T, Matsumori H, Taki T, et al.: Infantile GM_1-gangliosidosis with marked manifestation of lungs. Acta Pathol Jpn 29:269–276, 1979.

422. Mason AMS, McIllmurray MB, Golding PL, Hughes DTD: Fibrosing alveolitis with renal tubular acidosis. Br Med J 4:596–599, 1970.

423. Zalin AM, Weeple J, Gumpel M: Fibrosing alveolitis and renal tubular acidosis. Br Med J 4(lett):804, 1970.

424. Clarke JTR, Ozere RL, Krause VW: Early infantile variant of Krabbe globoid cell leucodystrophy with lung involvement. Arch Dis Child 56:640–642, 1981.

425. Lightman NI, Schooley RT: Adult-onset acid maltase deficiency. Chest 72:250, 1977.

426. Spencer H: *Pathology of the Lung.* Oxford: Pergamon Press, 1977.

427. Abul-Haj SK, Martz DG, Douglas WF, Geppert LJ: Farber's disease. J Pediatr 61:221–232, 1962.

428. Rutsaert J, Tondeur M, Vamos-Hurwitz E, Dustin P: The cellular lesions of Farber's disease and their experimental reproduction in tissue culture. Lab Invest 36:474–480, 1977.

429. Israel HL, Lenchner G, Stiner RM: Late development of mediastinal calcification in sarcoidosis. Am Rev Respir Dis 124:302–305, 1981.

430. Mulligan RM: General reviews: Metastatic calcification. Arch Pathol 43:177–230, 1947.

431. Kaltreider HB, Baum GL, Bogaty G, et al.: So-called "metastatic" calcification of the lung. Am J Med 46:188–196, 1969.

432. Mootz JR, Sagel SS, Roberts TH: Roentgenographic manifestations of pulmonary calcifications. Radiology 107:55–60, 1973.

433. Neff M, Yalcin S, Gupta S, Berger H: Extensive metastatic calcification of the lung in an azotemic patient. Am J Med 56:103–109, 1974.

434. Conger JD, Hammond WS, Alfrey AC, et al.: Pulmonary calcification in chronic dialysis patients. Ann Intern Med 83:330–336, 1975.

435. Cohen AM, Maxon HR, Goldsmith RE, et al.: Metastatic pulmonary calcification in primary hyperparathyroidism. Arch Intern Med 137:520–522, 1977.

436. Firooznia H, Pudlowski R, Golimbu C, et al.: Diffuse interstitial calcification of the lungs in chronic renal failure mimicking pulmonary edema. AJR 129:1103–1105, 1977.

437. Heath D, Robertson AJ: Pulmonary calcinosis. Thorax 32:606–611, 1977.

438. Justrabo E, Genin R, Rifle G: Pulmonary metastatic calcification with respiratory insufficiency in patients on maintenance haemodialysis. Thorax 34:384–388, 1979.

439. Sharp ME, Danino EA: An unusual form of pulmonary calcification: "Microlithiasis alveolaris pulmonum." J Pathol Bacteriol 65:389–399, 1953.

440. Sosman MC, Dodd GD, Jones WD, Pillmore GU: The familial occurrence of pulmonary alveolar microlithiasis. Am J Roentgenol Rad Ther Nuc Med 77:947–1012, 1957.

441. Chinachoti N, Tangchai P: Case report section: Pulmonary alveolar microlithiasis associated with the inhalation of snuff in Thailand. Dis Chest 32:687–689, 1957.

442. Thomson WB: Pulmonary alveolar microlithiasis. Thorax 14:76–81, 1959.

443. Lebacq E, Lauweryns J, Billiet L: Pulmonary alveolar microlithiasis case report with lung function studies. Br J Dis Chest 58:31–35, 1964.

444. Caffrey PR, Altman RS: Pulmonary alveolar microlithiasis occurring in premature twins. J Pediatr 66:758–763, 1965.

445. O'Neill RP, Cohn JE, Pellegrino ED: Pulmonary alveolar microlithiasis — A family study. Ann Intern Med 67:957–967, 1967.

446. Fuleihan FJD, Abboud RT, Balikian JP, Nucho CKN: Pulmonary alveolar microlithiasis: Lung function in five cases. Thorax 24:84–90, 1969.

447. Coetzee T: Pulmonary alveolar microlithiasis with involvement of the sympathetic nervous system and gonads. Thorax 25:637–642, 1970.

448. Sears MR, Chang AR, Taylor AJ: Pulmonary alveolar microlithiasis. Thorax 26:704–711, 1971.

449. Ghavamian M: Pulmonary alveolar microlithiasis: A report of two cases. Nebr Med J 259–264, 1972.

450. Kino T, Kohara Y, Tsuji S: Pulmonary alveolar microlithiasis: A report of two young sisters. Am Rev Respir Dis 105:105–110, 1972.

451. Hossein E: Pulmonary alveolar microlithiasis. Mich Med 72:691–694, 1973.

452. Thind GS, Bhatia JL: Pulmonary alveolar microlithias. Br J Dis Chest 72:151–154, 1978.

453. Saputo W, Zocchi M, Mancosu M, et al.: Pulmonary alveolar microlithiasis: A case report with a discussion of differential diagnosis. Helv Pediatr Acta 34:245–255, 1979.

454. Prakash UBS, Barham SS, Rosenow EC, et al.: Pulmonary alveolar microlithiasis. Mayo Clin Proc 58:290–300, 1983.

455. Gardiner IT, Uff JS: "Blue bodies" in a case of cryptogenic fibrosing alveolitis (desquamative type)—An ultra-structural study. Thorax 33:806–813, 1978.

456. Koss MN, Johnson FB, Hochholzer L: Pulmonary blue bodies. Hum Pathol 12:258–266, 1981.

456a. Margolin RJ, Addison TE: Hypercalcemia and rapidly progressive respiratory failure. Chest 86:767–769, 1984.

456b. Bestetti-Bosisio M, Cotelli F, Schiaffino E, et al.: Lung calcification in long-term dialysed patients: A light and electron microscopic study. Histopathology 8:69–79, 1984.

457. Popelka CG, Kleinerman J: Diffuse pulmonary ossification. Arch Intern Med 137:523–525, 1977.

458. Jacobs AN, Neitzschman HR, Nice CM: Metaplastic bone formation in the lung. AJR 118:344–347, 1973.

459. Muller KM, Friemann J, Stichnoth E: Dendriform pulmonary ossification. Pathol Res Pract 168:163–172, 1980.

460. Elkeles A, Glynn LE: Disseminated parenchymatous ossification in the lungs in association with mitral stenosis. J Pathol 58:517–522, 1946.

461. Daugavietis HE, Mautner LS: Disseminated nodular pulmonary ossification with mitral stenosis. Arch Pathol 63:7–12, 1975.

462. Buja LM, Roberts WC: Pulmonary parenchymal ossific nodules in idiopathic hypertrophic subaortic stenosis. Am J Cardiol 25:710–715, 1970.

463. Green JD, Harle TS, Greenberg D, et al.: Disseminated pulmonary ossification: A case report with demonstration of electron-microscopic features. Am Rev Respir Dis 101:293–298, 1970.

464. Ashley DJB: Bony metaplasia in trachea and bronchi. J Pathol 102:186–188, 1970.

465. Baar HS, Ferguson EF: Microlithiasis alveolaris pulmonum. Arch Pathol 76:81–88, 1963.

466. Michaels L, Levene C: Pulmonary corpora amylacea. J Pathol Bacteriol 74:49–58, 1957.

467. Hollander DH, Hutchins GM: Central spherules in pulmonary corpora amylacea. Arch Pathol Lab Med 102:629–630, 1978.

468. Siegel H: Human pulmonary pathology associated with narcotic and other addictive drugs. Hum Pathol 3:55–66, 1972.

469. Lippmann M: Pulmonary reactions to drugs. Med Clin North Am 61:1353–1367, 1977.

470. Gillett DG, Ford GT: Drug-induced lung disease. In Thurlbeck WM, Abell MR (eds): *The Lung—Structure, Function and Disease.* Baltimore: Williams & Wilkins, 1978.

471. Demeter SL, Ahmad M, Tomashefski JF: Drug-induced pulmonary disease part I: Patterns of response. Cleve Clin Q 46:89–99, 1979.

472. Demeter SL, Ahmad M, Tomashefski JF: Drug-induced pulmonary disease part II, Categories of drugs. Cleve Clin Q 46:101–112, 1979.

473. Demeter SL, Ahmad M, Tomashefski JF: Drug-induced pulmonary disease part III: Agents used to treat neoplasms or alter the immune system including a brief review of radiation therapy. Cleve Clin Q 46:113–124, 1979.

474. Kilburn KH: Pulmonary disease induced by drugs. In Fishman AP (ed): *Pulmonary Diseases and Disorders.* New York: McGraw-Hill, 707–724, 1980.

475. Weiss RB, Muggia FM: Cytotoxic drug-induced pulmonary disease: Update 1980. Am J Med 68:259–266, 1980.

476. Whimster WF, dePointers W: The lung. In Riddell RH (ed): *Pathology of Drug-Induced and Toxic Diseases.* New York: Churchill Livingstone, 1982, pp 167–200.

477. Sobol SM, Rakita L: Pneumonitis and pulmonary fibrosis associated with amiodarone treatment: A possible complication of a new anti-arrhythmic drug. Circulation 65:819–824, 1982.

477a. Darmanata JI, van Zandwijk N, Dureu DR, et al.: Amiodarone pneumonitis: Three further cases with a review of published reports. Thorax 39:57–64, 1984.

477b. Pollak PT, Sami M: Acute necrotizing pneumonitis and hyperglycemia after amiodarone therapy. Am J Med 76:935–939, 1984.

21 Chronic Airflow Obstruction

William M. Thurlbeck

Introduction

A number of terms have been used to encompass those diseases and lesions associated with chronic airflow obstruction; often included are chronic obstructive pulmonary disease, chronic obstructive lung disease, chronic airways disease, chronic nonspecific lung disease, and chronic airflow limitation. These terms recognize the fact that one is dealing with a functional abnormality; a diminished ability to expire air. In the 1950s, British physicians used the term chronic bronchitis to describe the same condition that U.S. physicians referred to as emphysema. In 1958 a number of prominent physicians met to address the problem. They proposed definitions of chronic bronchitis, emphysema, and asthma and used the term chronic nonspecific lung disease to encompass conditions that were often associated with chronic airflow obstruction.[1] Except in the Netherlands, where the term CARA (the acronym for the Dutch translation of chronic nonspecific lung disease) is used, chronic nonspecific lung disease is no longer in vogue, although there is much to recommend it, as not all patients with chronic bronchitis, emphysema, or asthma have chronic airflow obstruction.

Chronic airflow obstruction, the term that will be used here, is characterized by persistent abnormalities of tests of expiratory flow; the conditions associated with these abnormalities are the subject of this chapter. In addition to the classic causes of chronic airflow obstruction, the chapter will also deal with other and rarer conditions that may be associated with obstruction to airflow. Chronic airflow obstruction is a functional syndrome, not a specific condition, and it should be approached in the same way as anemia, jaundice, or fever. The differential diagnosis is complicated by the fact that many lesions may be associated with chronic airflow obstruction. They occur together in various combinations, often with differing severity, so that it is usually not possible to define precisely the role of each particular lesion in a given patient. Furthermore, since therapy for the lesions is not particularly effective, many question the reasons for trying to identify the responsible lesions. The main justification for the exercise is precision in the practice of medicine; if the effectiveness of therapeutic intervention was used as a criterion of practice, there would be little justification for a considerable part of medicine.

Flow is determined by two factors—the force applied to the system and the resistance to flow, which mainly depends on the caliber of the conduits through which flow occurs. In the lung, pulmonary elastic recoil determines the force,[2] and the dimensions of the airways determine the resistance to flow. Dimensions of the airways should be regarded as dynamic rather than fixed; thus, airflow resistance may be increased by lesions which affect the dynamic properties of the airways.

The anatomy of the airways and lung parenchyma are shown diagrammatically in Figure 21–1, and airway anatomy is discussed in further detail in Chapters 2 and 4. As discussed in Chapter 2, there are three categories of airways. The major or large airways are bronchi, characterized by having cartilage and mucous glands in their walls. They are succeeded by (membranous) bronchioles which lack cartilage, mucous glands, and gas-exchanging structures (alveoli). The final category of airways has, to a greater or lesser extent, alveoli in the walls and constitutes the acinus or the gas-exchanging structure of the lung (*see* Fig. 2–1, p. 12). Because of the complexity of the lung, the precise arrangement and dimensions of the various structures are not known. The total cross-sectional areas of the airways that are predicted by the simplest model of regular dichotomy[3] are shown in Figure 3–3 (p. 53), which indicates a rapid increase in the total cross-sectional area of the airways as the periphery is approached. This increase occurs because the number of airways increases much more than the diameter of the

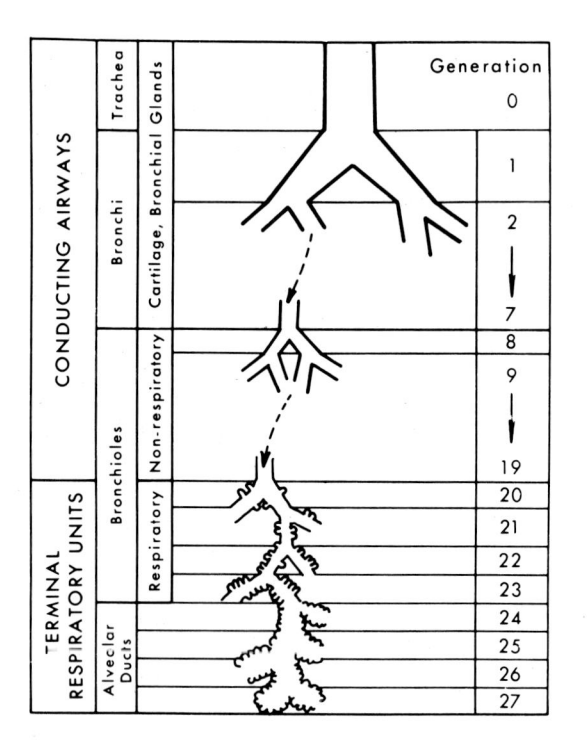

Figure 21–1. A diagrammatic representation of the airways is shown, using a pattern of regular dichotomy. Airflow obstruction may result from lesions in the bronchi, nonrespiratory bronchioles, or within the acinus (beyond generation 19 in this model). From Murray.[359]

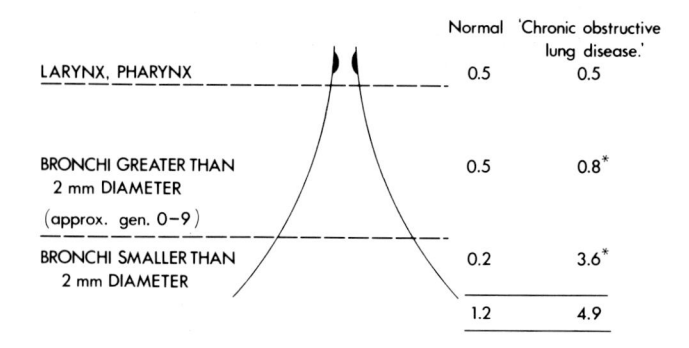

*Average of 7 lungs studied by Hogg, Macklem, and Thurlbeck (1968).

Figure 21–2. Partitioning of airway resistance in normal subjects and those with chronic obstructive lung disease (chronic airflow obstruction). In normal lungs, there is relatively little resistance of flow in airways less than 2 to 3 mm in diameter (small bronchi and bronchioles). In patients with chronic obstructive lung disease, obstruction is mainly peripheral (see text). Data derived from Hogg et al.[7]

	Normal	'Chronic obstructive lung disease.'
LARYNX, PHARYNX	0.5	0.5
BRONCHI GREATER THAN 2 mm DIAMETER (approx. gen. 0–9)	0.5	0.8*
BRONCHI SMALLER THAN 2 mm DIAMETER	0.2	3.6*
	1.2	4.9

individual airways decreases. The functional consequence is that resistance to flow should diminish markedly in the peripheral airways.

Airways, however, do not branch dichotomously, nor are the pathways the same length to the periphery of the lung. In axial pathways[4] that proceed in a fairly straight line from the lobar bronchus to the most distant lung periphery (such as to the posterior basal segment of the lung), there may be as many as 28 orders of conducting airways from the first respiratory bronchiole to tracheal carina. In lateral or spiral pathways, such as to the medial aspect of the lung, there may be as few as ten orders. Horsfield and Cumming[5] studied a bronchial cast of the lung of one subject and showed the wide variations in numbers of branches and distances of airways. (Their data are discussed in Chapter 3). These variations indicate a considerably smaller total cross-sectional area of the peripheral airways than the Weibel model. Thus, the Horsfield-Cumming model predicts a larger peripheral resistance.

Macklem and Mead,[6] in their classic 1967 study, were able to partition airway resistance in the dog by wedging a pressure-sensing catheter in peripheral airways in excised lungs. They found, as would be predicted by the Weibel model, that resistance to flow in the wedged catheter was only a small proportion of total airflow resistance. Hogg and co-workers[7] performed similar experiments in normal excised human lungs and found that resistance to flow was only 10 to 15 percent of total flow resistance (Fig. 21–2). They also showed that, in patients with chronic airflow obstruction, the major increase in flow resistance occurred in the airways peripheral to the wedged catheter.

Their report introduced two important concepts. The catheter wedged in airways 2 to 3 mm in diameter so that the airways peripheral to the catheter were the smallest bronchi and bronchioles. A wide variety of lesions was present in the peripheral airways in patients with chronic airflow obstruction, including inflammation, fibrosis, narrowing, and plugging by mucus and exudates. They coined the term small airways disease to describe the changes since both bronchi and bronchioles were involved and inflammation (bronchiolitis) was an inadequate term. The second concept was that, since peripheral airways constituted so small a proportion of airway resistance, considerable disease could be present in these airways without there being a measurable increase in resistance to flow. It also followed that classic tests of expiratory flow, such as the forced expiratory volume in 1 second (FEV_1), could be normal although the peripheral airways might be structurally and functionally abnormal. This finding led to the development of tests that assessed the function of peripheral airways. These tests include analysis of the expiratory concentration of an inhaled bolus of ^{133}Xe, re-emphasis of the Fowler single breath nitrogen test, analysis of expiratory flow rates at low lung volumes, and analysis of expiratory flow rates breathing air compared with breathing helium-oxygen mixtures.

The validity of the observation concerning the low values of peripheral airway resistance and the value of tests of small airway function are now being questioned.[8-11] FEV_1 may also be abnormal with relatively mild lesions in the peripheral airways.[12] However, there is compelling evidence, as reviewed below, that lesions in peripheral airways are associated with abnormalities of tests of small airway function.

Bronchiolitis

The mildest (and presumably earliest) lesions associated with chronic airflow obstruction are in bronchioles, and the major site of severe chronic airflow obstruction lies in the peripheral airways. Discussion of lesions producing chronic airflow obstruction should therefore start with bronchioles. Lesions in these airways are less well and more recently studied than chronic bronchitis and emphysema, the classic associations of chronic airflow obstruction. Emphysema, however, is the most important association of moderately severe and severe chronic airflow obstruction.[13–15] Besides occurring in typical patients with chronic airflow obstruction, bronchiolitis has certain particular associations, such as with rheumatoid arthritis, diffuse panbronchiolitis, and bronchiolitis obliterans. These conditions are associated with chronic airflow obstruction as well, but the clinical associations are different, and the conditions have specific clinical and morphologic features.

Lesions in Peripheral Airways in Usual Chronic Airflow Obstruction (Small Airways Disease)

A variety of lesions have been described in the peripheral airways of patients with chronic airflow obstruction (Tables 21–1 and 21–2). Relating these lesions to specific functional abnormalities is a difficult task and not directly relevant here. The structure-functional correlations have been reviewed in detail elsewhere.[14]

Bronchiolitis and Its Sequelae

Inflammation of the bronchioles has been a consistent finding in patients with both mild and severe chronic airflow obstruction (see Tables 21–1 and 21–2). Few precise data are available, perhaps reflecting the difficulty of study. Terminal infection in autopsy lungs is frequent, making analyses hard to interpret; surgically derived lungs nearly all come from subjects with lung cancer who are smokers, so control material is not easy to find. The degree of inflammation is usually slight but may become severe (Fig. 21–3 through 21–5). Since lymphocytes and some plasma cells are normally present in bronchioles, it took a long time for the abnormality to be documented adequately because a quantitative rather than qualitative phenomenon was involved.

However, airway inflammation per se is associated with airflow obstruction. This was first properly documented by Cosio and colleagues,[12] who showed that the major difference between their patients with a low score for bronchiolar lesions and normal tests of small airway function (group I) and patients with evidence of mild bronchiolar lesions and abnormal tests of small airway function (group II) was the presence of inflammation. Berend and associates[26] found that bronchiolitis was the single best correlate of abnormal tests of small airway function. It is still uncertain how inflammation per se causes airflow obstruction. Bronchioles behave as though they are lined by surface active material rendering them relatively resistant to closure,[58] and osmiophilic material resembling surfactant has been observed lining bronchioles.[59] Inflammation may result in displacement of this material rendering the airways functionally unstable.[60] Inflammation may also result in release of mediators that may act directly on bronchiolar smooth muscle leading to constriction or may induce a reflexly mediated bronchiolar constriction.[26]

A variety of consequences of bronchiolar inflammation leads to further airflow obstruction. Cosio and co-workers[12] found that the major difference between patients with mild (group II) and moderate (group III) severity of peripheral airway lesions was the presence of fibrosis and squamous metaplasia of the bronchioles, suggesting that these were temporal sequelae. Similarly when Cosio and colleagues[25] compared peripheral airway lesions in older smokers with younger ones,[19] they found increased fibrosis in the airways of older smokers.

A predictable consequence of airway fibrosis is narrowing. This may be an important cause of increased airflow resistance, because according to Poiseuille's law, narrowing will increase resistance to the fourth power of the reduction in radius. Thus, reducing airway lumen by one-half will increase airway resistance 16 times, whereas obliteration of half the airways will only double flow resistance. Reduction in mean airway bronchiolar diameter is hard to demonstrate even in patients with severe chronic airflow obstruction.[53] However, a reduction in the volume proportion of bronchiolar lumen (the proportion of bronchiolar lumen to the volume of the lung) has been shown in patients with chronic bronchitis and little clinical evidence of airflow obstruction,[18] in patients with severe emphysema and severe chronic airflow obstruction,[53,56] and in patients with cor pulmonale due to chronic airflow obstruction.[55,56] Narrowing of airways results in a disproportionate number of the smallest airways (Fig. 21–6 and 21–7); several authors have expressed airway narrowing as the proportion of airways that are less than 350 μm or 400 μm in diameter.[25,45] When narrowing is expressed in this way, an increased proportion of airways smaller than 400 μm in diameter has been found in older smokers[25] and in patients with cor pulmonale.[45] Fibrosis of the bronchial wall may be responsible for thickening of bronchioles noted in some patients with panacinar emphysema,[57] and Linhartova and Anderson have produced a model that would account for closure of airways at relatively high lung volumes.

Florey and colleagues[61] pointed out that the inflammatory response of mucous membranes to irritation included hypersecretion of mucus.[61] The morphologic counterpart of increased secretion of mucus into bronchioles is an increase in the number of goblet cells within their surface epithelium. Normally only 1 percent

Table 21-1. Lesions in Peripheral Airways in Patients Thought or Known to Have Mild Chronic Airflow Obstruction

Year	Authors	Clinical or Functional Abnormalities	Morphologic Abnormalities in Peripheral Airways
1955	Reid[16]	Chronic bronchitis	Excess intralumenal mucus, narrowing and obliteration
1970	Martin et al.[17]	Shortness of breath, RV/TLC increase	Narrowing of airways 0.2–0.4 mm
1973	Matsuba and Thurlbeck[18]	Chronic productive cough, no emphysema, no clinical airflow obstruction	Narrowing, excess intralumenal mucus
1974	Niewoehner et al.[19]	Male smokers under age 40 dying suddenly	Inflammation, respiratory bronchiolitis
1974	Niewoehner and Kleinerman[8]	Conductance	Mean bronchiolar diameter
1975	Thurlbeck et al.[20]	Chronic bronchitis and no emphysema	No goblet cell metaplasia
1975	Ebert and Terracio[21]	Smokers	Loss of Clara cells, increase in goblet cells
1978	Cosio et al.[12]	Volume at isoflow, slope of phase III, closing capacity	Inflammation, fibrosis, squamous metaplasia, goblet cell metaplasia, ulceration, increased muscle, pigmentation
1979	Berend et al.[22]	CV % VC, FEF_{25-75}	Narrowing
1980	Hale et al.[23]	Increased intimal and medial area, increased number of vessels <200 μm	In smokers, vascular lesions related to severity of peripheral airway disease and to emphysema
1980	Petty et al.[24]	Closing capacity, slope of phase III of SBNT	Inflammation, increased muscle
		Slope of phase III	Intralumenal mucus
1980	Cosio et al.[25]	Smokers	Inflammation, increase in goblet cells, increase in proportion of airways of less than 400 μm in diameter, increased muscle
1981	Berend et al.[26]	FEV_1, FEF_{25-75}, CV % VC, slope of phase III of SBNT	Inflammation
1982	Salmon et al.[27]	Slope of phase III, $V_2{}^*$	Peripheral airway diameter
1982	Petty et al.[28]	Increased closing capacity	Increase in proportion of airways 400 μm in diameter
		Closing capacity ($r = -0.38$), FEV_1 ($r = 0.59$), FEF_{25-75} ($r = 0.53$)	Bronchiolar diameter
1982	Berend and Thurlbeck[29]	Max. flow at P_L5	Inflammation, fibrosis (not muscle or airway dimensions)
1983	Wright et al.[30]	Smokers	Goblet cell metaplasia, respiratory bronchiolitis, no increased inflammation of bronchioles
1983	Wright et al.[31]	Smokers; increased intima, media, and adventitia of pulmonary arteries	Bronchiolitis
1984	Wright et al.[32]	Decrease of FEV_1	Inflammation of respiratory and membranous bronchioles, goblet cell metaplasia, decreased muscle in respiratory bronchioles
		FEV_1 80% of that predicted Two tests of small airway function abnormal	Inflammation of walls of respiratory bronchioles
		Three tests abnormal	Increase in bronchiolar and respiratory bronchiolar inflammatory cells
1984	Lumsden et al.[33]	Smokers	Goblet cell metaplasia; decreased Clara cells in bronchioles and respiratory bronchioles

Abbreviations: CV% VC, Closing volume as a percentage of vital capacity; FEF_{25-75}, flow rate between 75% and 25% of a forced vital capacity (FVC); FEV_1, volume of air expired in the first second of FVC; P_L5, lung distending pressure of 5 cm H_2O, RV/TLC, ratio of residual volume to total lung capacity; SBNT, single-breath nitrogen test, $V_2{}^*$ approximately the equivalent of closing volume.

or less of the cells of the surface epithelium of bronchioles are formed by goblet cells. Karpick and associates[46] were the first to report the significance of an increased number of goblet cells in the peripheral airways. They compared the lungs of patients dying in an intensive care unit with control patients and found that the most significant difference between the two groups was an increase in the number of goblet cells. Most of the former were patients with chronic airflow obstruction dying of respiratory failure. They referred to this change

Table 21-2. Abnormalities of Small Airways in Patients with Severe Chronic Airflow Obstruction

Year	Authors	Disease Investigated	Abnormalities Found
1835	Laennec[34]	Emphysema	Air-trapping due to obstruction in peripheral airways
1953	Spain and Kaufman[35]	Emphysema	Mural inflammation and fibrosis of bronchioles
1954	Reid[36]	Chronic bronchitis	Bronchiolitis, bronchiolar obliteration, and mucous plugging
1957	Leopold and Gough[37]	Centrilobular emphysema	Inflammation, fibrosis with narrowing of 60% of bronchioles supplying centrilobular space
1958	McLean[38]	Emphysema	Inflammation of proximal respiratory bronchioles, mucous plugging, and loss of bronchioles.
1961, 1965	Pratt et al.[39,40]	Centrilobular emphysema	Loss or distortion because of loss of radial support of bronchioles
1962	Anderson and Foraker[41]	Emphysema	Narrowing of smallest bronchioles associated with loss of alveolar attachments
1967	Anderson and Foraker[42]	Emphysema	Loss of bronchioles in patients under age 70
1968	Hogg et al.[7]	Chronic airflow obstruction	Inflammation and fibrosis of bronchi and bronchioles and mucous plugging
1968	Mitchell et al.[43]	Chronic airflow obstruction	Inflammation, atrophy, goblet cell metaplasia, squamous metaplasia, and mucus plugs in bronchioles
1969, 1970	Bignon et al.[44,45]	Cor pulmonale and centrilobular emphysema	Inflammatory narrowing and fibrosis, loss of bronchioles, and mucous plugging
1970	Karpick et al.[46]	Respiratory failure	Goblet cell metaplasia
1971	Linhartova et al.[47]	Emphysema	Plugging of bronchioles with inflammatory cells and mucus
1971, 1973, 1974, 1977, 1982	Linhartova et al.[48-52]	Emphysema	Distortion, tortuosity and irregular narrowing of bronchioles, loss of alveolar wall attachments
1972	Matsuba and Thurlbeck[53]	Severe emphysema and chronic airflow obstruction	Loss of lumen of airways less than 2 mm in diameter diameter due primarily to narrowing and mucous plugs
1972	Depierre et al.[54]	Emphysema	Increase in proportion of airways less than 350 μm in diameter
		Centrilobular and panlobular emphysema	Decrease in number of airways
1975	Thurlbeck et al.[20]	Chronic bronchitis and emphysema	Increased goblet cells especially in symptomatic subjects
1975	Scott and Steiner[55]	Cor pulmonale	Lack of bronchographic filling of bronchioles of less than 1 mm
1976	Scott[56]	Chronic airflow obstruction	Loss of airway lumen
1976	Mitchell et al.[13]	Chronic airflow obstruction	Chronic inflammation ($r = 0.48$), narrowing ($r = 0.29$), fibrosis ($r = 0.27$), goblet cell metaplasia ($r = 0.24$), and decreased number of small airways ($r = -0.18$)
1983	Linhartova and Anderson[57]	Panlobular emphysema	Thickening of bronchiolar walls and chronic inflammation

in brochiolar epithelium as goblet cell metaplasia. Thurlbeck and co-workers[20] noted an increase in goblet cells in patients with chronic bronchitis and emphysema and even more in patients with severe chronic airflow obstruction. An increase in goblet cells has also been observed in smokers.[30,33]

Obstruction of airflow from goblet cell metaplasia may result from one or both of two mechanisms. Increased intralumenal mucus has been observed in patients with chronic bronchitis and no emphysema,[18] patients with chronic bronchitis and emphysema, and patients with emphysema and no bronchitis[53]; the likely source of this mucus is goblet cells, perhaps compounded by poor peripheral airway clearance. In addition, mucus may

Figure 21–3. Grade I inflammation of a membranous bronchiole. From Wright et al.[360]

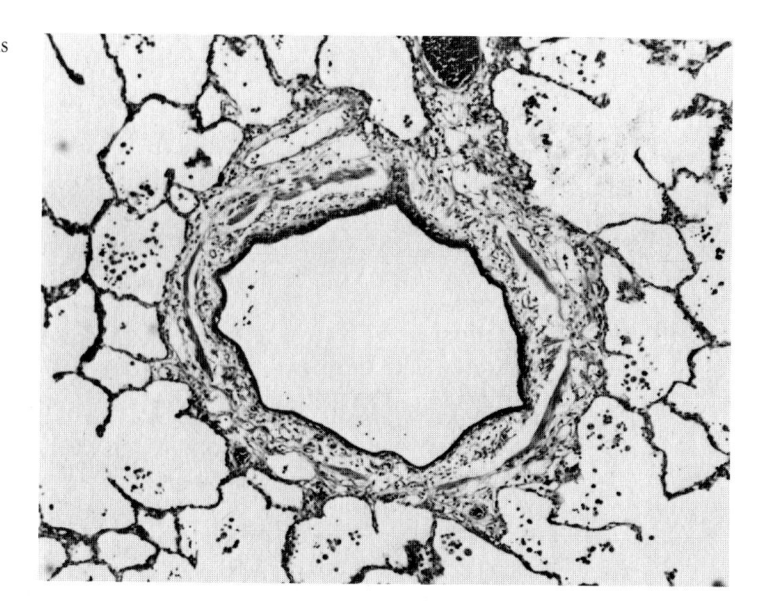

displace the surfactant layer of bronchioles and alter the mechanical properties of the airways.

Increased muscle has also been associated with mild chronic airflow obstruction.[24] It is less clear that increased muscle is a result of inflammation, but it appears to be one of the components of a complex pattern of changes in the airways of patients with chronic airflow obstruction. Liebow and colleagues[62] described an increase in bronchiolar muscle in some patients with emphysema.

Bronchiolar obliteration has been described, mainly in emphysematous lungs.[36,38,53] Since the airways disappear, obliteration can only be demonstrated by dissection or counting the number of airways. By correlating bronchograms with serial reconstructions, Reid[36] showed that a bronchographic-filling defect characterized by a tapering appearance was associated with bronchiolar obliteration and noted this change in patients with chronic bronchitis and emphysema. Counting bronchioles has serious theoretic and practical problems, but a small and inconstant loss of airways has been described in severely emphysematous lungs.[53] Extensive lack of filling of peripheral airways in postmortem bronchograms has been observed in patients with chronic airflow obstruction, related in particular to cor pulmonale.[55] Most lack of filling is due to intralumenal mucus and inflammatory exudate.

Respiratory bronchiolitis involves the proximal part of

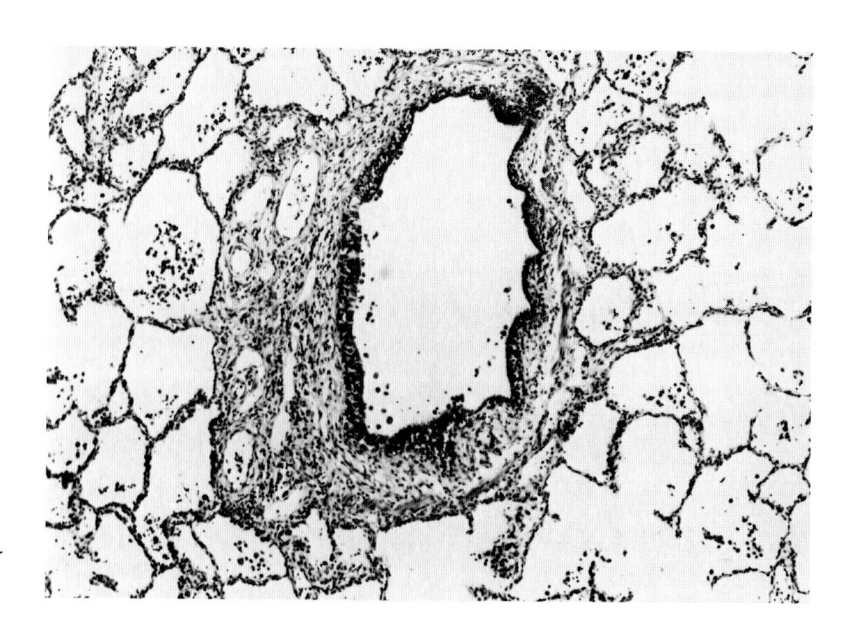

Figure 21–4. Grade II inflammation of a membranous bronchiole. From Wright et al.[360]

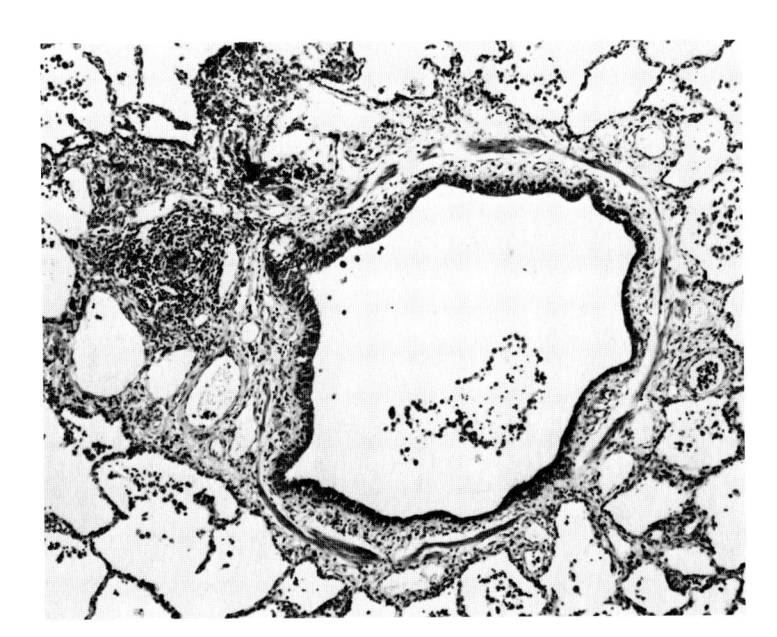

Figure 21–5. Grade III inflammation of a membranous bronchiole. Courtesy of Dr. J. L. Wright.

the acinus (*see* Fig. 2–1, p. 12) and thus is not strictly speaking a lesion of the conducting airways, but it is conveniently discussed at this point. It was first described by Niewoehner and co-workers[19] in the lungs of smokers younger than age 40 years who died suddenly by violence. It consists of mild inflammation and the accumulation of pigmented macrophages in the lumen and walls of respiratory bronchioles and in adjacent air spaces (Figs. 21–8, 21–9). The lesion has profound implications concerning the pathogenesis of emphysema and will be discussed further below. Despite the fact that the total cross-sectional area at the respiratory bronchiolar level is large and the narrowing of respiratory bronchioles has not been observed in association with respirtory bronchiolitis, there is recent evidence[32] that respiratory bronchiolitis may be responsible for abnormalities of tests of small airway function, particularly when the FEV_1 is more than 80 percent of predicted.

Numerous studies have correlated abnormal tests of pulmonary function with lesions in the bronchioles. There is evidence that inflammation per se may produce mild chronic airflow obstruction, although a recent report[32] has not shown a difference in bronchiolar inflammation between smokers and nonsmokers, although the smokers had evidence of airflow obstruction. In most patients, flow obstruction is probably due to a combination of the sequelae of inflammation occurring in varying degrees of severity. Fibrosis, narrowing, and goblet cell

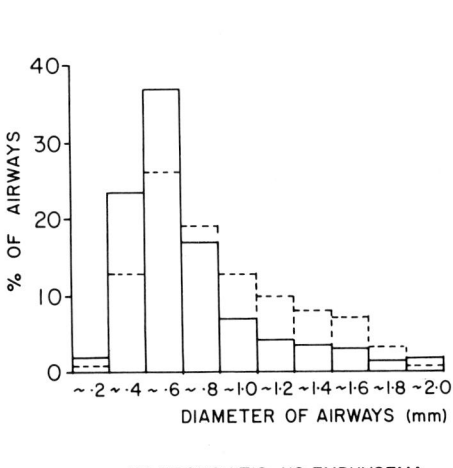

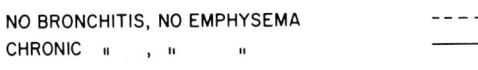

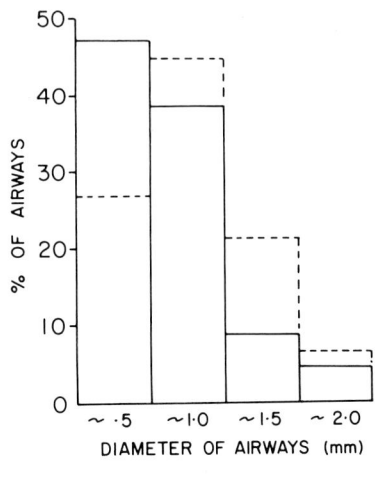

Figure 21–6. The size distribution of airways less than 2 mm in internal diameter is shown in patients with chronic bronchitis but no emphysema and is compared with normal subjects (no bronchitis and no emphysema). There is an excessive proportion of airways less than 0.5 mm in diameter and between 0.2 and 0.6 mm in internal diameter. From Matsuba and Thurlbeck.[18]

Figure 21-7. The size distribution of airways less than 2 mm in internal diameter is shown in patients with chronic bronchitis and emphysema and is compared with normal subjects (no bronchitis and no emphysema). There is an excessive proportion of airways less than 0.5 mm in internal diameter due to an excess proportion of airways less than 0.4 mm in internal diameter. From Matsuba and Thurlbeck.[53]

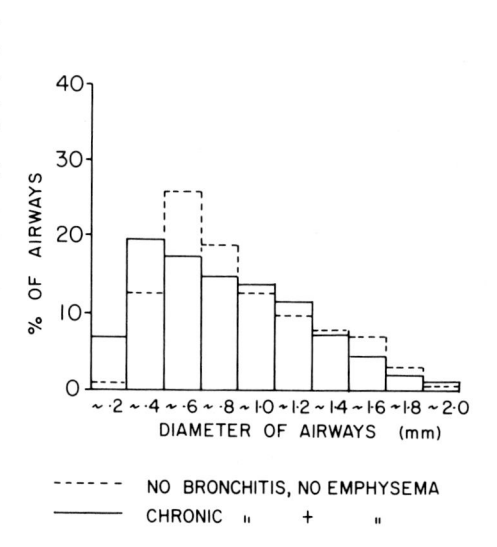

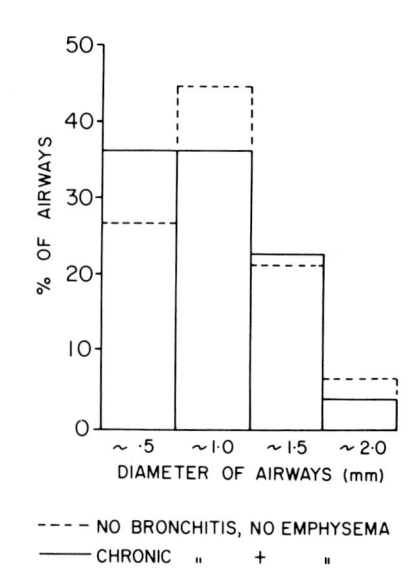

metaplasia play a more important role in patients with severe chronic airflow obstruction.

By far the most important cause of bronchiolitis and its consequences is tobacco smoke. Bronchiolar lesions, notably bronchiolitis, have generally been found to be increased in frequency and severity in smokers.[19,25,30] However, bronchiolitis can occur in nonsmokers, so other factors may be involved.[25] The pathogenesis of bronchiolitis is less clear, but it is probably a direct effect of one or more constituents of tobacco smoke. There is little evidence that it is due to infection predisposed to by tobacco smoke.[63]

Bronchiolar Lesions in Emphysema

The mechanical properties of bronchioles are largely determined by their interconnection with the elastic framework of the lung. Dayman[64] was the first to implicate the peripheral airways as the major cause of physiologically determined airflow obstruction in patients with emphysema; Pratt and colleagues[39] and Anderson and Foraker[41] were the first to suggest that peripheral airway patency might be compromised by loss of alveolar walls in emphysema. A specific effect of emphysema interfered with the normal radial traction exerted by the elastic framework of the lung.[41] In nonemphysematous lungs and lungs with mild and moderate emphysema, the distance between alveolar attachments to bronchiolar walls averaged 0.146 mm; in moderately severe and severe emphysema, this distance increased to 0.173 mm and 0.209 mm, respectively.[52] In normal lungs, the alveolar attachments formed a regular polyhedral net as seen on serial section reconstructions,[52] whereas in severe emphysema, the attachments formed irregularly shaped patterns of variable size (Fig. 21-10). A direct correlation between loss of alveolar attachments and airway narrowing has been demonstrated.[48]

A related lesion is tortuosity and irregularity of the lumens of bronchioles in emphysema[49-51] which may be a reflection of irregularity of alveolar wall attachments.

The significance of these lesions is still not certain. The irregular narrowing of the airways will result in an underestimation of their functional effects; since measurements reflect the average diameter of airways, whereas the minimal diameter is a significant dimension in causing airflow obstruction. It has been speculated that lack of alveolar support causes collapse of the unsupported airways on expiration with resultant air trapping. Some corroboration has come from the observation that maximum flow is diminished at given elastic recoil pressures in emphysematous lungs.[22,29] This suggests that some particular feature of emphysema results in increased flow resistance. Also postmortem bronchographic studies have shown undue narrowing of the stenotic regions of the airways.[65] Expert physiologic opinion does not favor the air-trapping hypothesis, and expiratory and inspiratory resistance was the same in the peripheral airways of excised lungs from patients with chronic airflow obstruction.[7]

Special Forms of Bronchiolitis

Rheumatoid Bronchiolitis

Geddes and colleagues[66] described six patients, five of whom had rheumatoid arthritis and the other a positive rheumatoid factor, who developed chronic airflow obstruction and rapidly progressive dyspnea. These patients died of respiratory failure five to 18 months after the onset of symptoms. Similar cases have been reported,[67] and it has been observed that chronic airflow obstruction is more frequent in patients with rheumatoid arthritis than in control populations.[68] The first reported cases thus appear to be an extreme example of a more common condition.

The lesions described in the original patients were inflammation of airways 1 to 6 mm in diameter with occlusion of the lumens by loose fibrous tissue. The

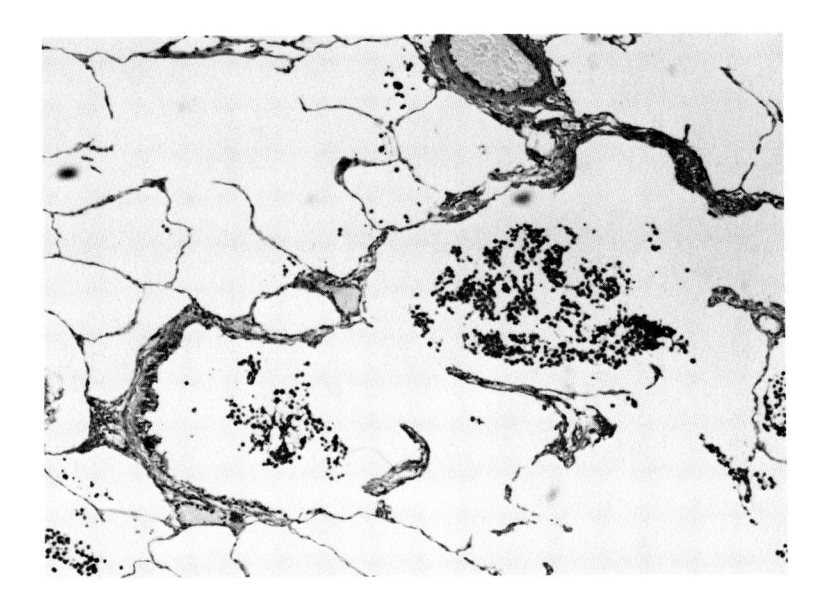

Figure 21-8. Respiratory bronchiolitis. Pigmented macrophages are present in the lumen of respiratory bronchioles and adjacent air spaces. From Wright et al.[360]

lesions are patchy and may easily be missed on random histologic sections, and they are best demonstrated by a systematic dissection of the bronchi. The etiology of the lesions is controversial. They may be a complication of D-penicillamine therapy,[67,69] as similar lesions have been seen in patients treated with D-penicillamine for conditions other than rheumatoid arthritis.[69] However, fatal rheumatoid bronchiolitis can occur in patients not treated with D-penicillamine.[66] The patients reported by Geddes and colleagues[66] had severe airflow obstruction, especially at low lung volumes, and their chest radiographs showed grossly overinflated lungs without alteration of the peripheral pulmonary vasculature. Lung elastic recoil and diffusing capacity were normal.

Cryptogenic Obliterative Bronchiolitis

Isolated chronic bronchiolitis may also occur from causes other than rheumatoid bronchiolitis. Turton and co-workers[70] studied 2094 patients who had chronic airflow obstruction as defined by an FEV_1 of less than 60 percent predicted. They excluded all patients with known causes of chronic airflow obstruction such as emphysema, bronchitis, bronchiectasis, asthma, other lung disease, and cigarette smoking. Ten patients remained, five with rheumatoid arthritis and five with chronic airflow obstruction presumably due to bronchiolitis caused by other agents. They applied the term cryptogenic obliterative bronchiolitis to this latter group. The observed functional abnormalities suggested obstruction to flow in

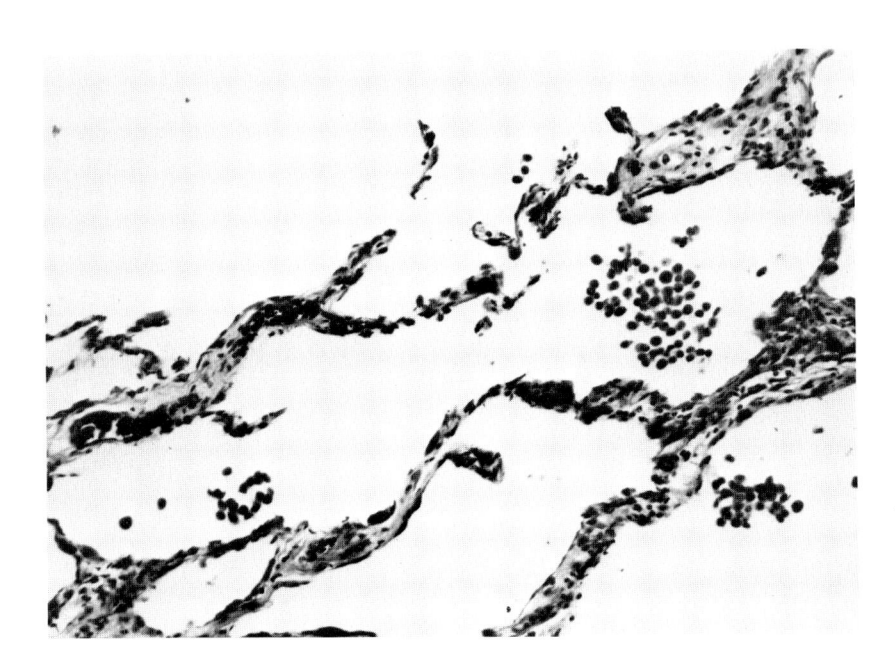

Figure 21-9. Respiratory bronchiolitis. Pigmented macrophages are apparent in the walls of bronchioles as well as in air spaces. Note the mild thickening and fibrosis of bronchiolar walls. Courtesy of Dr. J. L. Wright.

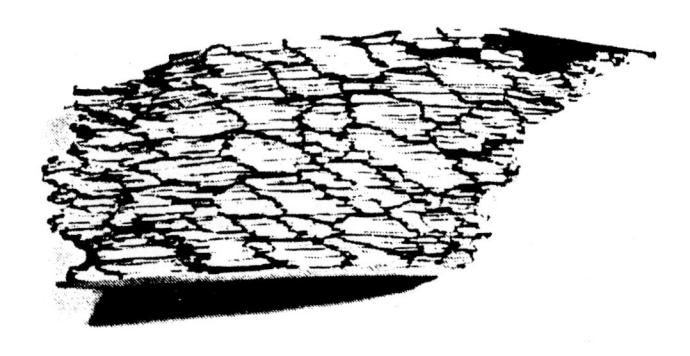

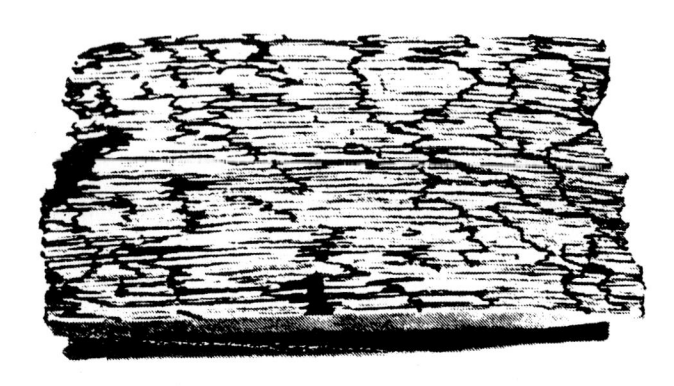

Figure 21–10. The pattern of alveolar attachments to the wall of membranous bronchioles in a nonemphysematous lung (top) is compared with an emphysematous lung (bottom). Note the loss of regularity of alveolar wall attachments and their sparsity. From Linhartova et al.[52]

the peripheral airways. Their cases differed from those of Geddes and colleagues[66] in that the obstruction was less severe and the course of the disease more benign.

Diffuse Panbronchiolitis

Between 1978 and 1980, 1238 probable cases, 82 with histologic confirmation, of diffuse panbronchiolitis were collected in Japan.[71] The lesions of the lung consisted of severe chronic inflammation of the proximal respiratory bronchioles, which was thought to extend subsequently to involve more proximal bronchioles. There was thickening and fibrosis of the walls of the airways and an infiltrate of lymphocytes, plasma cells, and histiocytes. With further progression of the disease, narrowing of the respiratory bronchioles and dilation of the more proximal airways occurred. The lesions were diffusely disseminated through the lung, but they were more common in the lower lobes. The condition occurred about twice as frequently in men as in women most often between 20 and 60 years of age. Chronic cough, sputum, and dyspnea were the chief symptoms, and three-quarters of their patients had chronic sinusitis. Chest radiographs characteristically showed nodular densities less than 2 mm in diameter, together with varying degrees of overinflation. There was marked airflow obstruction, hypoxemia, and, in the later stages, hypercapnia.

Homma and colleagues[71] pointed out that, in North America, four of the cases reported by Macklem and associates[72] and two reported by Gosink and associates[73] closely resembled their cases. Two of the four patients of Macklem and co-workers[72] had bronchiectasis at autopsy, and a third subsequently died and was found to have extensive bronchiectasis. Thus, there may be an overlap between cases diagnosed as panbronchiolitis in Japan and those diagnosed as bronchiectasis in North America. This is to be expected since diffuse panbronchiolitis and bronchiectasis[74] are both associated with distal bronchiolitis and proximal airway dilation. Bronchiectasis differs in that both the dilation and bronchiolitis are more proximal and symptoms of bronchiectasis usually date to childhood. Physicians from the United States who have visited Japan have been impressed by the frequency of diffuse panbronchiolitis and the paucity of similar cases in their own experience.

Bronchiolitis Obliterans

The term bronchiolitis obliterans (Table 21–3) has been used to describe both the presence of granulation tissue plugs in small bronchi and bronchioles, extending to alveolar ducts at times, as well as complete destruction of bronchi or bronchioles leaving only a scar. Initially bronchiolitis obliterans was used to describe an idiopathic case, then lesions associated with oxides of nitrogen, subsequently as a variant of interstitial pneumonia, and finally as a condition including a heterogeneous group of cases.[73] The last two developments provide a starting point for discussion about this confusing term. (The association between bronchiolitis obliterans and infiltrative lung disease is discussed in Chapter 20.).

Liebow and Carrington[75] used the term bronchiolitis obliterans interstitial pneumonia (BIP) to describe cases of bronchiolitis obliterans with a prominent component of interstitial pneumonia. Although such cases exist, they are probably uncommon. Granulation tissue in alveolar spaces is a described part of fibrosing alveolitis or usual interstitial pneumonia (UIP) (*see* Chapter 20) but is seldom a dominant feature; when this is the case, BIP may be the appropriate diagnostic term. Functionally BIP cases are examples of restrictive rather than obstructive lung disease. The majority of cases reported by Gosink and associates[73] had accumulation of granulation tissue in alveolar ducts and sacs, and many observers would refer to these as organizing pneumonia. Epler and Colby[76] have suggested that such cases should be referred to as examples of bronchiolitis with organizing pneumonia. These patients often have a previous history of pulmonary infection, and airflow obstruction is usually not an important part of their disease. The distinction between bronchiolitis with organizing pneumonia and

Table 21–3. Spectrum of Bronchiolitis Obliterans

Fibrosis of the lumen or total obliteration of bronchioles
Emphysema
Bronchiectasis
Toxic gases, especially oxides of nitrogen, ammonia, and sulfur dioxide
Infections, especially adenovirus, measles, mycoplasma
Allergic alveolitis
Esoinophilic pneumonia
Esoinophilic fasciitis
Sjögren's syndrome
Graft versus host disease
Heart-lung transplantation
Connective tissue diseases, especially rheumatoid arthritis
Penicillamine
Cryptogenic bronchiolitis
Diffuse panbronchiolitis
Bronchiolitis obliterans and organizing pneumonia

BIP or UIP is an important one since the former has a better prognosis and may respond to steroids.[77]

In contrast to BIP and bronchiolitis obliterans with organizing pneumonia, bronchiolitis obliterans, primarily involving the airways, is often due to known agents. These include inhalation of toxic gases such as oxides of nitrogen,[78-80] sulfur dioxide,[81] and ammonia.[82] Viral infections, especially adenovirus infections[83] and measles, and mycoplasma infections[84] may also lead to extensive bronchiolitis obliterans with subsequent chronic airflow obstruction. Bronchiolitis obliterans is an integral part of bronchiectasis, notably in saccular and varicose bronchiectasis.[74] The obliterative lesions, rather than the ectatic bronchi and their contents, are primarily responsible for the associated airflow obstruction. Similarly the Swyer-James syndrome (see p. 545) is associated with bronchiolar obliteration. Bronchiolitis obliterans is often present in extrinsic allergic alveolitis and may be a prominent feature of eosinophilic pneumonia,[85] eosinophilic fasciitis,[86] or Sjögren's syndrome[87] and is responsible for the component of chronic airflow obstruction in these conditions.

Bronchiolitis obliterans is now recognized as a complication of graft versus host disease following bone marrow transplantation.[88-93] It is an uncommon complication compared with the occurrence of interstitial pneumonia due to cytomegalovirus, Herpes, and pneumocystis infections. The reported patients have developed dyspnea some months after bone marrow transplantation without radiographic evidence of interstitial lung disease; they also have developed rapidly progressive airflow obstruction. A lymphocytic infiltrate in and around bronchioles together with epithelial necrosis has been described[91]; intralumenal proliferation of fibrous tissue, fibrin, lymphocytes, plasma cells, and the occasional polymorph were also seen.

Most recently bronchiolitis obliterans has been described in patients receiving heart-lung transplants.[94] This occurred (or was presumed to occur) in 5 of 14 patients surviving the postoperative period. These patients had recurrent bronchopulmonary infections with subsequent development of dyspnea; airflow obstruction appeared 6 months to more than 2 years following transplantation. Chest radiographs have shown peribronchial and interstitial infiltrates. Total lung capacity was decreased in all cases. The morphologic details have not been specifically described, but bronchiolitis obliterans was widespread. In two cases, extensive bronchiectasis was found. The etiology is unknown, and the features are quite different from lung transplant rejection.

In a proportion of cases of bronchiolitis obliterans, no etiologic agent is apparent, and the course generally slows and may be associated with scattered small nodular opacities on the chest radiograph.[95,96] In many respects, these cases resemble examples of diffuse panbronchiolitis and may be the same entity.

Chronic Bronchitis (Chronic Hypersecretion of Mucus)

There is little reason to use the term chronic bronchitis. The term is ambiguous and it designates a symptom to be a disease. The ambiguity arises from the fact that chronic bronchitis was used by the British in the past synonymously with chronic airflow obstruction, and this habit still lingers. A suggested subclassification into simple chronic bronchitis, chronic or recurrent mucopurulent bronchitis, and chronic obstructive bronchitis[97] suggested that there might be different syndromes and perhaps implied chronic bronchitis was a cause of chronic airflow obstruction.

The accepted definition of chronic bronchitis is chronic or recurrent excess secretion of mucus into the bronchial tree.[1] No method is available of measuring the amount of mucus secreted, so a clinical definition of increased sputum production has been adopted. Arbitrarily, the production of any sputum, whether expectorated or swallowed, is regarded as abnormal and is usually associated with cough. Chronic has been defined as occurring on most days for 3 months in the year for at least 2 successive years. Chronic sputum production should not be the result of other known disease such as tuberculosis or bronchiectasis. Considerable clarification would occur if these two terms—chronic sputum production and chronic productive cough—were used rather than chronic bronchitis, but ingrained habits are such that this is unlikely to be changed.

Enlargement of Tracheobronchial Mucous Glands

Intrabronchial mucus is secreted by both tracheobronchial mucous glands and surface goblet cells. The former constitute about 98 percent of the volume of mucus-secreting cells and thus are thought to be more important as a source of mucus.[98] It is thus logical to anticipate an increase in size of mucous glands in patients with chronic hypersecretion of mucus. Reid[98] was the first to quanti-

Figure 21–11. The appearance of a bronchial wall of a nonbronchitic subject (A,C) is compared with that of a chronic bronchitic (B,D). A. The mucous glands form only a small proportion of the thickness of the bronchial wall ($\times$ 80). C. The mucous and serous tubules are shown more clearly, and scattered lymphocytes are apparent ($\times$ 150). B. and D. The glands form a much higher proportion of the wall. The bronchial submucosa is increased by approximately the increase in thickness of the gland. Note the increased number of inflammatory cells (B $\times$ 80, C $\times$ 120). From Angus.[361]

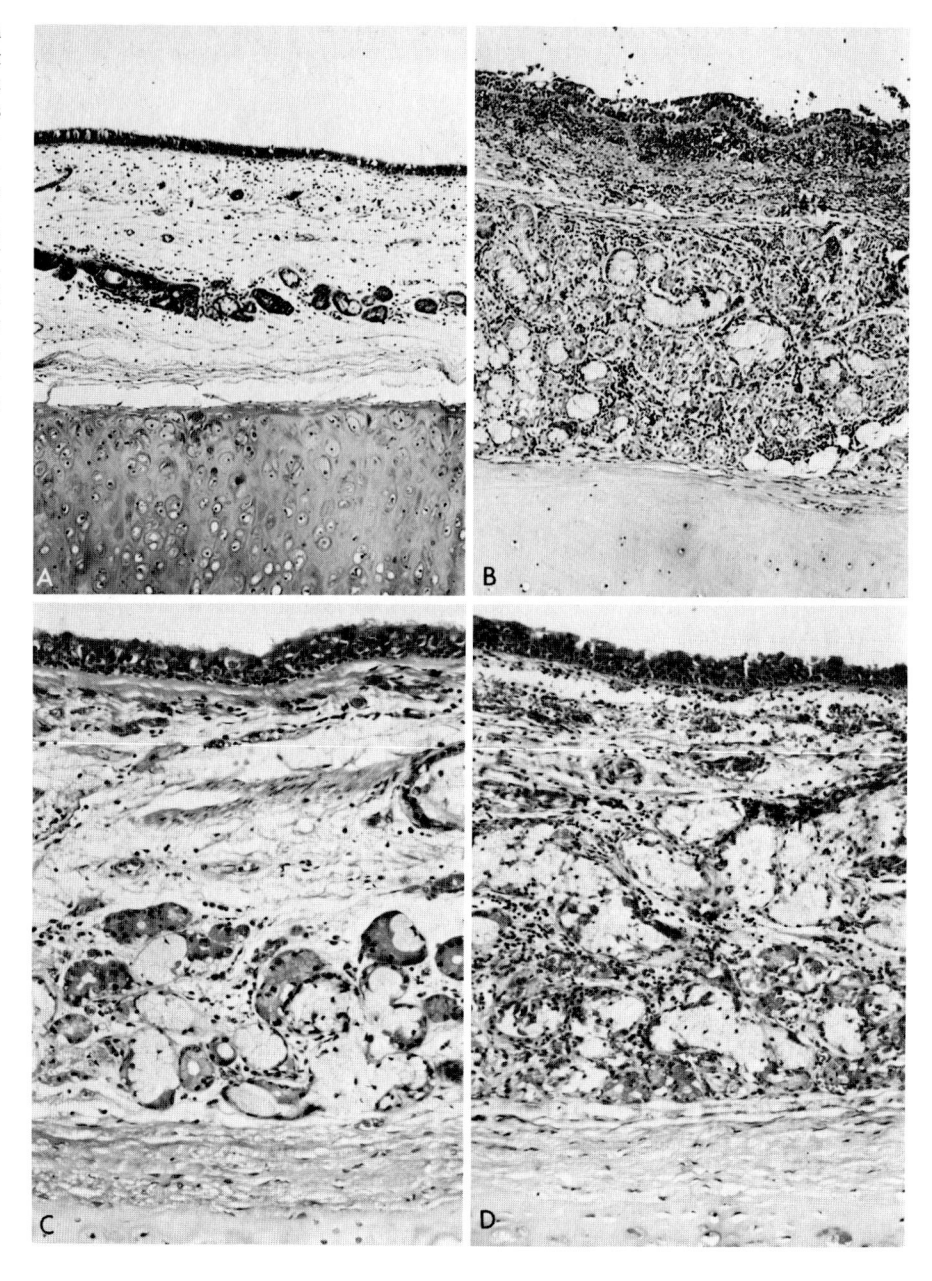

tate the increase in gland size. The enlargement of mucous glands is primarily due to hyperplasia of cells rather than hypertrophy.[99] Some enlargement of cells occurs, so it is best to speak of mucous gland hypertrophy or mucous gland hyperplasia. The changes that occur in chronic bronchitis are illustrated in Figure 21–11. There is obvious enlargement of the mucous glands, an increase in the diameter of the individual "acini" (in reality branched tubules) of the glands, and an increased proportion of mucous cells compared with serous cells. The ducts of the mucous glands may be dilated and plugged with mucus.

Reid Index

Reid[98] quantitated the change in gland size by calculating the ratio of the thickness of the bronchial mucous glands to the thickness of the bronchial wall as seen on histologic sections. The bronchial wall was defined as the distance from the inner perichondrium to the basement membrane of the bronchial epithelium, and the ratio is generally referred to as the Reid index. As glands enlarge, their thickness (a cube root function of volume) increases, and since this is the numerator of the Reid index,

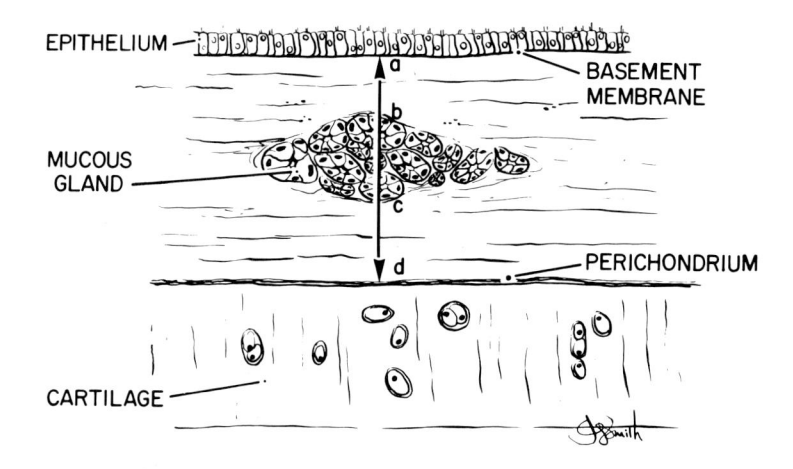

Figure 21–12. The Reid index is calculated by measuring the maximum thickness of a bronchial mucous gland internal to the cartilage (b to c) and by dividing this by the bronchial wall thickness (a to d). From Thurlbeck.[207]

the Index increases. Reid found that the mean ratio in nonbronchitics was 0.26, with a range of 0.14 to 0.36. There was no overlap with the value in chronic bronchitis, who had a mean of 0.59 and a range of 0.41 to 0.79. Subsequent work has extended the original observations, and a reasonable consensus has emerged concerning the meaning of the Reid index.

The exact way in which the Reid index has been measured has generally not been described. Individual glands vary considerably in thickness in a single section of a bronchus, and they often are located other than between the cartilage and basement membrane. In addition, terminal inflammation and hemorrhage may occur, and often there is artifactual separation of lamina propria from the cartilage. Because of these problems, others[13,100] have suggested that a simple subjective assessment of gland size might be as effective as measurement of the Reid index. Thurlbeck and colleagues[101] found that it was essential to adopt a rigid method of measurement if intra- and interobserver variations are to be kept at a minimum and to distinguish bronchitics from nonbronchitics. Acutely inflamed and hemorrhagic bronchi were discarded as were bronchi with separation of lamina propria from cartilage. Glands were measured in which epithelium and cartilage were approximately parallel. The maximum thickness of every gland was measured, and the wall thickness was measured at exactly the same line (Fig. 21–12).

Results are shown in Table 21–4. The increase in Reid index in chronic bronchitis has not been as dramatic in the subsequent series as it was in Reid's original one, and in two the differences between bronchitics and nonbronchitics has been small. More importantly, the Reid index shows a unimodal distribution curve[102] (Fig. 21–13), which has been confirmed by others.[103–108] This is perhaps to be expected. The division of the population into two sharply defined categories, bronchitics and nonbronchitics, is artifical and represents the arbitrary definition of bronchitis as sputum production. It seems more likely that if intrabronchial secretion of mucus could be measured directly, it would show a unimodal distribution curve as well.

The concept that there is a gradual transition between normal (no sputum production) and disease (sputum production) is an important one. It indicates that there may be subclinical chronic bronchitis. The frequency distribution of the Reid index in chronic bronchitics and nonbronchitics in a random population is shown in Figure 21–14; both categories have a unimodal distribution curve, but when the Reid Index is less than 0.36, only 6 percent of patients have chronic bronchitis, and when it is over 0.55, 70 percent are chronic bronchitis. Similar results have been found by others: Scott[106] found that 18 percent of patients with a Reid index of less than 0.36 had chronic bronchitis, and 64 percent of patients with a Reid index of more than 0.49 had chronic bronchitis. Burton

Table 21–4. Reported Reid Index Values

Authors	Bronchi Used for Measurement	Nonbronchitics	Bronchitics	Nonminers	Miners
Reid[98]	Main, lobar, segmental	0.26	0.59		
Thurlbeck and Angus[102]	Main, lobar	0.44	0.52		
McKenzie et al.[103]	Intrapulmonary	0.29	0.43		
Hayes[104]	Main			0.31	
Ryder et al.[105]	Main			0.42	0.44
Scott[106]	Right main	0.40	0.49		

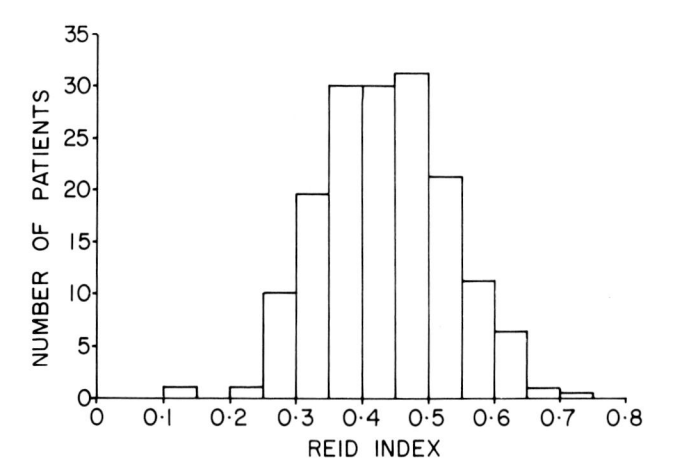

Figure 21–13. The frequency distribution of the Reid index and random cases is unimodal. From Angus.[361]

and Dixon[107] found that 15 percent of patients with a Reid Index of less than 0.45 had chronic bronchitis, whereas the incidence was 73 percent in patients with a Reid Index greater than this value. Mitchell and colleagues[109] found that 74 percent of patients with a Reid index of greater than 0.6 in one bronchus or greater than 0.5 in two bronchi had chronic bronchitis. Figure 21–14 also indicates the predictability of chronic bronchitis from the Reid index. Predictability is good at high and low levels, but in the range of 0.36 to 0.55, in which the bulk of patients are found (see Fig. 21–13), prediction is about random.

The Reid index is usually the same in different bronchi of the same patient, but variations may occasionally occur.[107,110–113] Niewoehner and colleagues[112] suggested that this "regional chronic bronchitis" might result in severe abnormalities of ventilation/perfusion ratios with resultant cor pulmonale, which was a feature of their patients.

Other Measurements of Gland Size

Rather than express gland thickness as a ratio, absolute values can be used. The theoretic advantage of this approach is that the Reid index is affected by the denominator: bronchial wall thickness. An increase in wall thickness because of edema might obscure increases in gland thickness, or atrophy of the bronchial wall might produce an apparently abnormally high Reid index. A theoretic disadvantage is that absolute gland thickness should be normalized for the size of the bronchus in individuals and among individuals, and this is accomplished by the Reid index. In practice, the Reid index discriminates better between bronchitics and nonbronchitics than does gland thickness.[110]

The other most commonly used measurement of gland size is the volume proportion of glands in which the areas of mucous glands are measured on histologic sections and compared with the total bronchial wall area. The relative area of glands can be assessed by point counting,[106,112,114,115] tracing images of the glands or bronchi onto paper or cardboard and weighing their cutouts, and planimetry,[100] which is now greatly expedited by computer-assisted digitizers. Measurement of area has many apparent advantages over the Reid index. All glands can be counted; it is not necessary to make arbitrary decisions where to measure glands; and the artifactual space separating lamina propria from cartilage is no longer a problem since this area can be measured and then omitted from total bronchial wall. Theoretically area measurements also have the advantage over thickness measurements in that they involve two dimensions. Thus, a gland that increases in volume eight times would quadruple in cross-sectional area and double in linear dimension. Measurement of area has the advantage that other components of the bronchial wall, such as cartilage and muscle, can be measured and expressed as a proportion of bronchial wall.

Table 21–5 shows available reports and indicates the wide variation reported by different observers in bronchitics and nonbronchitics, which is generally greater than the Reid index. The increase in chronic

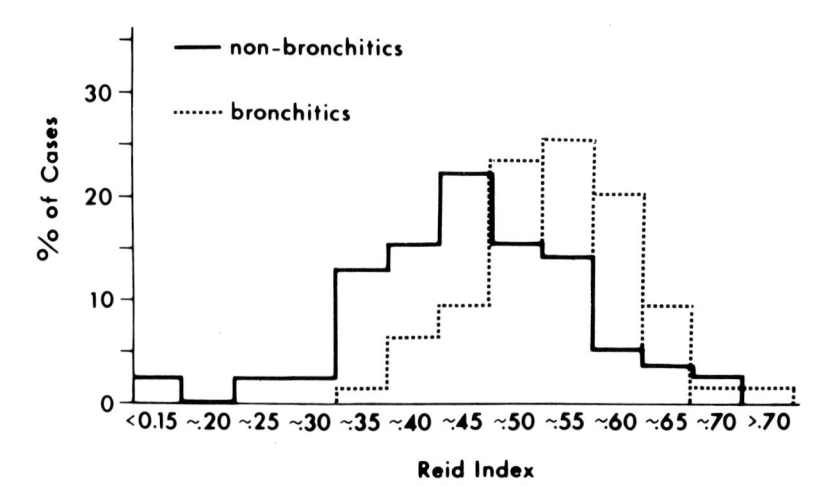

Figure 21–14. The Reid index in chronic bronchitics is compared with nonbronchitics. Note that the Reid index is shifted to the right in the chronic bronchitics. Below a Reid index of 0.35, patients are seldom bronchitic and above 0.55 patients are usually chronic bronchitics. However, in the intervening range, where most values are found, the Reid index is poorly predictive of the presence of chronic bronchitis. From Thurlbeck.[362]

Table 21-5. The Mucous Gland Proportion of Bronchi[a]

Authors	Bronchi Examined	Non-bronchitics	Chronic Bronchitics	All Cases
Hale et al.[113]	Segmental	6.5		
Dunnill et al.[114]	Segmental	12.7	27.8	
Takizawa and Thurlbeck[115]	Main, lobar	8.8	16.9	
Niewoehner et al.[112]	Lobar, segmental	9.8	25.5	
Sobonya and Kleinerman[116]	Lobar, segmental			10.4
Scott[106]	Right main	12.9	16.0	
Ryder et al.[117]	Main, lobar			17.0
Restrepo and Heard[118,141]	Bronchus to basal segments,	13.4	25.8	
	inferior lingular	11.2	23.4	

[a]The proportion quoted from Hale et al.[113] is from their Figure 6; from Restrepo and Heard is calculated from two separate papers[118,141]; from Sobonya and Kleinerman[116] from their Figure 3.

bronchitis is also generally greater than that noted using the Reid index. The Reid index and mucous gland proportion have found to be statistically correlated,[45,106,115] although a more recent study[119] has found a different result. The Reid index is quicker, although computer-assisted digitizers have speeded up the process of area measurement and perform the calculations. The relative value of the measurements depends on the clinical association with chronic sputum production. Recently a stronger correlation was found between the volume proportion of glands and the amount of sputum produced than between the Reid index and amount of sputum.[119] The volume proportion of mucous glands has generally been found to be the same in main, lobar, and segmental bronchi, but a recent report[120] found that the mucous gland proportion may be smaller in the lower lobe segmental bronchi in nonbronchitic lungs and larger in main and upper lobe bronchi in bronchitic lungs.

Absolute area may be a better measurement than volume proportion because of alterations in the denominator of the latter which might produce abnormal results. However, the disadvantage is similar to that of thickness because absolute measurements of area are not normalized for bronchial wall size or size of individuals. Different ways of measuring absolute area are significantly related to each other.[100] They are also related to gland proportion, but not to the Reid index.[100]

The tubules (acini) that form the mucous glands increase in diameter in chronic bronchitis and the number of tubules per unit area decreases.[98] These measurements discriminate less well between bronchitic and nonbronchitic lungs than the Reid index does.[98,101]

Mucous glands are formed by mucus and serous cells, the latter also secreting mucosubstances. Subjective descriptions indicate an increase in the relative proportion of mucous cells. Takizawa and Thurlbeck[115] quantitated the relative proportions of mucous cells and found an increase from 39 percent in nonbronchitics to 48 percent in chronic bronchitics. Because of the wide range of values in both bronchitics and nonbronchitics, the difference was not significant. An increased proportion of cells secreting acid mucosubstances has been reported.[121]

Mucous Gland Enlargement and Airflow Obstruction

Clinically chronic bronchitis may be associated with all degrees of airflow obstruction from none to severe, and airflow obstruction gets worse as the amount of sputum increases.[41] The reason for the varying severity of obstruction in chronic bronchitis is mostly related to associated emphysema and, to a lesser extent, to peripheral airway lesions.[13-15] However, mucous gland enlargement probably should cause airflow obstruction by narrowing airways at the major site of flow resistance in the lung. Several studies have compared the severity of airflow obstruction and mucous gland enlargement; about two-thirds have shown a statistically significant (although rather poor) relationship, and the remainder have not.[14] Loss of the volume proportion of bronchial lumen has been described in chronic bronchitis together with an increased proportion of bronchial wall tissue.[121a] Both were related to increased airways resistance and diminished FEV_1. These results suggest that encroachment on the bronchial lumen by increased size of mucous glands and perhaps inflammatory thickening results in obstruction to airflow. At one stage, it was thought that there was a close, perhaps causative, association between mucous gland enlargement and cor pulmonale. This is no longer the case. Mucus within the major airways clearly cannot be beneficial, but intralumenal mucus is difficult or impossible to quantitate, so no information is available. Intralumenal mucus, often infected, is a common finding in bronchi and bronchioles in patients dying of chronic airflow obstruction, representing the terminal episode.

Other Airway Changes

Changes in Goblet Cells

Goblet cell metaplasia of bronchioles has been described earlier. It might be anticipated that the increase in goblet cells would occur in the surface epithelium of bronchi in chronic bronchitis. One narrative comment[36] suggested that goblet cells were increased, but this has not been the case in other narrative comments.[98,108,111] No quantitative data are available.

Airway Inflammation

Chronic Inflammation. Inflammation of the peripheral airways is well related to airflow obstruction, and one might anticipate that the same might be true for central airways. The occurrence of inflammatory cells in patients with chronic bronchitis and/or in cigarette smokers is not well documented. Reid[98] stated that inflammation was not obvious in the bronchi of patients with chronic bronchitis. No consistent relationship existed between the estimates of mucous gland size and the extent of inflammation in earlier studies.[111,122] A heavy infiltrate of lymphocytes and occasional eosinophils and neutrophils was noted by Salvato[123] in chronic bronchitis; however, a heavy infiltrate of lymphocytes was also seen by him in normal lungs. Martin and colleagues[124] found a positive correlation between inflammation of the bronchi and a subjective assessment of bronchial gland enlargement, but not with the Reid index. Similar results were found by Mitchell and associates[13] who noted a significant relationship between a subjective assessment of mucous gland enlargement and large airway inflammation; no association was found between inflammation and the Reid index. More recently Linhartova and colleagues[125] found intense infiltration with chronic inflammatory cells and thickening of bronchi primarily in association with severe panacinar emphysema. No increased inflammation was found in the bronchi of lungs with severe centrilobular emphysema, but some bronchial wall thickening was recorded. (This did not reach conventional levels of significance.) Because of the association of chronic bronchitis and mucous gland enlargement with emphysema, these changes could be interpreted as being an association between inflammation and bronchitis. This suggestion is, however, very tenuous and Linhartova and colleagues[125] suggested that the inflammation may have pathogenetic implications in panacinar emphysema.

Only one group[13] has assessed the association between central airway inflammation and clinically assessed chronic airflow obstruction; no relationship was found.

Eosinophilia. The presence of large numbers of eosinophils in the airways is indicative of asthma,[123,126] and a heavy bronchial infiltrate of eosinophils is a characteristic feature of status asthmaticus.[123,126–132] This diagnosis should not be entertained in the absence of bronchial eosinophilia. Eosinophils may be seen in the airways of patients with chronic bronchitis[123,133]; thus, the change is a quantitative one rather than a qualitative one. Salvato[123] suggested the diagnosis of asthma is "definitely indicated" when eosinophils constitute more than 3 percent of the bronchial wall infiltrate. Leopold[126] found that eosinophils formed 4.5 to 44 percent of the cellular infiltrate in patients dying of status asthmaticus and that they constituted less than 2.6 percent of cells in chronic bronchitics. In absolute terms, he found that the eosinophil count was 10.3 to 441.6 per square millimeter in bronchi in patients with status asthmaticus and less than 3.2 in patients with chronic bronchitis. A larger overlap among eosinophil count in the bronchial walls in asthmatics without status, normal subjects, and chronic bronchitics has been reported.[134]

Increase in Muscle

The status and significance of increased smooth muscle in chronic bronchitis is still not certain. Dunnill and co-workers[114] found no increase in the mean value of smooth muscle in chronic bronchitis, but one of their patients had about a threefold increase in muscle, in the range that was found in their patients with status asthmaticus. Heard and colleagues[135,136] measured absolute area of smooth muscle and found that the mean value of the amount of muscle was approximately doubled in lobar and segmental bronchi in their patients with chronic bronchitis but there was no increase in tracheal smooth muscle. Takizawa and Thurlbeck[137] found increased smooth muscle in one of five chronic bronchitic patients and in three of four chronic bronchitic patients with episodes of wheezing. More recently Carlile and Edwards[120] found that the average proportion of muscle in main, lobar, and segmental bronchi was approximately doubled in patients with chronic bronchitis and airflow obstruction. There thus appears to be little doubt that there is increased muscle in some patients with chronic bronchitis, but the precise incidence is still in doubt. Interestingly, the increase in muscle is due to hyperplasia of muscle cells rather than hypertrophy.[136]

Since there is evidence of airway hyperreactivity in patients with chronic bronchitis, the increased muscle may be the morphologic counterpart. This hypothesis has never been adequately tested. In one study, increased bronchial muscle was associated with a decreased FEV_1 and an increased residual volume.[121a]

Cartilage Atrophy

As is the case of muscle, the status of cartilage atrophy in chronic bronchitis is unclear, and the subject has to be discussed in the context of emphysema. Wright[138] described obvious airway atrophy, including atrophy of cartilage, in patients with chronic airflow obstruction all of whom had severe emphysema. The changes were particularly apparent in subsegmental bronchi. Presumably most of the patients also had chronic bronchitis. Subsequently, with Stuart[139] he described cartilage atrophy in patients with chronic bronchitis, but the majority of patients had severe emphysema, although in 8 of 37 it was minimal. Tandon and Campbell[140] dissected bronchi and stained the cartilage from chronic bronchitic and nonbronchitic lungs. They found diminished cartilage in the subsegmental bronchi in chronic bronchitis and a highly significant negative correlation (-0.85) between the Reid index and the distance circumferentially placed cartilage extended peripherally in the airways. Other observers[111,114,115,141] who assessed the proportion or absolute amounts of cartilage from histologic sections of bronchi have found no diminution of cartilage in patients who had chronic bronchitis, most of whom also had emphysema. Because of the difficulty in interpreting the relative role of emphysema and chronic bronchitis in cartilage atrophy, Thurlbeck and associates[147] studied a group of random cases, several of whom had no emphysema or chronic bronchitis; none had severe emphysema. They found no difference in the amount of cartilage between bronchitics and nonbronchitics or between patients with high and low Reid index scores, even when bronchi were dissected open and the cartilage stained. In contrast, changes were obvious in emphysema, although the emphysema was not severe. There was consistently less cartilage in the bronchi in emphysematous lungs, and this reached significant levels in the segmental and subsegmental bronchi to the lower lobe. Present physiologic evidence ascribes no functional abnormality in association with cartilage atrophy.

Pits in the Bronchial Wall

The openings of the tracheobronchial glands into the bronchial epithelium can be seen using a hand lens or a dissecting microscope. In chronic bronchitis, the ducts may be distended with mucus that may protrude into the lumen and be visible grossly. Wang and Ying[143,144] have suggested a sequence of events that begins with dilation of gland ducts, depressions in the epithelium, and finally herniation of the bronchial epithelium through the muscularis. The duct lumens may be increased in diameter and become visible with the naked eye. These herniations form pits up to 1 mm in diameter that can be demonstrated radiographically as diverticulum-like outpouchings which are characteristically seen along with the inferior margins of the major bronchi. The ducts of several mucous glands enter into them. The precise significance of these pits has never been documented, but both small pits (dilated ducts) and large pits are commonly seen in chronic bronchitis and also in bronchiectasis. Wang and Ying[143,144] pointed out that these abnormalities could be seen in patients without chronic bronchitis. They also indicated that the glands opened into depressions that lay between mucosal bulges that consisted of transverse bundles of smooth muscle.

Peripheral Airway Lesions

Airway narrowing is easy to demonstrate in patients with chronic bronchitis but no emphysema, even in the absence of clinically apparent chronic airflow obstruction. Excess mucus within the peripheral airways is also found.[18]

Emphysema and Chronic Bronchitis

The concept of the relationship between bronchitis and emphysema has changed over the years. Since patients with chronic airflow obstruction characteristically develop chronic productive cough in the third or fourth decade and clinical evidence of emphysema in the sixth and seventh decade, it was logical to think that bronchitis led to emphysema, probably because of the development of airway infection. This is no longer widely believed. Patients with chronic productive cough may never develop emphysema, and severe emphysema may occur without bronchitis. There is no evidence that patients with chronic or recurrent mucopurulent bronchitis are particularly prone to develop chronic airflow obstruction or emphysema.[63] Bronchiolitis and respiratory bronchiolitis also occur in nonbronchitics.[25,30] These conditions are primarily associated with tobacco smoking.

The most likely connection among chronic bronchitis, emphysema, and bronchiolitis is tobacco smoking. Irritant(s) within tobacco smoke produce inflammation in various parts of the lung. In the bronchi, this results in hypersecretion of mucus from bronchial mucous glands, inflammation and narrowing in the peripheral airways, and emphysema in the parenchyma. Under these circumstances, emphysema and chronic bronchitis are fairly closely linked. Figure 21–15 contrasts the frequency of emphysema in patients with chronic bronchitis to those without bronchitis. The frequency of emphysema is more than doubled in patients with chronic productive cough. The figure indicates that the association between bronchitis and emphysema is stronger in older male smokers and that panlobular emphysema appears randomly associated, irrespective of the frequency of bronchitis. The association between emphysema and chronic bronchitis is more apparent when milder grades of emphysema are excluded (Fig. 21–16). This figure shows that the frequency of emphysema of more than 25 percent severity, using their grading system, is only 12 percent in nonbronchitics but increases six times to 72 percent in chronic bronchitics.[109]

Another way to express the relationship is to compare the incidence of chronic bronchitis as the severity of emphysema gets worse (Fig. 21–17). As emphysema gets worse, the incidence of chronic bronchitis increases, but only to a certain point. There is no increase in the last categories in which the frequency of chronic bronchitis is approximately 80 percent. Since the frequency of chronic bronchitis was determined by retrospective survey of patient's charts, this may be an underestimation.

The relationship between mucous gland enlargement and emphysema is less certain, but the majority of series (Table 21–6) have shown an increase in mucous gland size in patients with emphysema, but the change is small. Any relationship between mucous gland enlargement and emphysema is not direct, as there is no increase in gland size with patients with severe emphysema com-

Table 21–6. Mucous Gland Enlargement in Emphysema

Authors	Measurement	Nonemphysematous Lungs (%)	Emphysematous Lungs (%)
Thurlbeck and Angus[144a]	Reid index	0.43	0.48
Greenberg et al.[111]	Reid index	0.38	0.47
Hernandez et al.[145]	Reid index	0.41	0.40
Ryder et al.[117]	Mucous gland volume	14.80	18.30

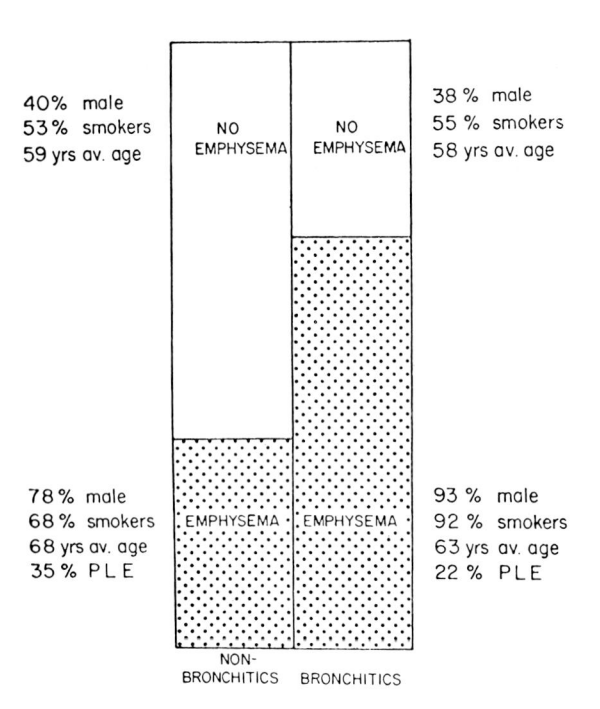

Figure 21-15. Emphysema is about twice as frequent in subjects with chronic bronchitis (chronic productive cough) compared with nonbronchitics (those without). Chronic bronchitics with emphysema are more frequently men and smokers compared with those without emphysema. Nonbronchitics with emphysema are older than bronchitics with emphysema and are less frequently smokers and have a higher frequency of panacinar emphysema. From Thurlbeck.[363]

Figure 21-16. The frequency of emphysema of mild degree or more is increased 12 times in chronic bronchitics. From Thurlbeck.[159]

pared with moderate emphysema.[111] Indeed, there may even be atrophy of bronchial glands in most severe degrees of emphysema.

The association among chronic bronchitis, peripheral airway disease, and emphysema makes it hard to determine the role of chronic bronchitis in producing chronic airflow obstruction.

Epidemiologic Relationships of Mucous Gland Enlargement

Although tobacco smoke is overwhelmingly important in the production of chronic bronchitis, increase in mucous gland size has not been found consistently in cigarette smokers (Table 21-7). There is a general trend for smokers to have mucous gland enlargement which has often been significant, but usually the enlargement has been modest. Only two series compared mucous gland size in heavy smokers with light smokers. One found a difference between the two groups[102], but the other found no significant enlargement in the heavy smokers.[98]

Both the Reid index and mucous gland proportion are higher in children than in adults,[148,149] and the volume proportion of mucous glands in children with bronchiolitis and fibrocystic disease was more than 20 percent[149] a level seldom found in adults with chronic

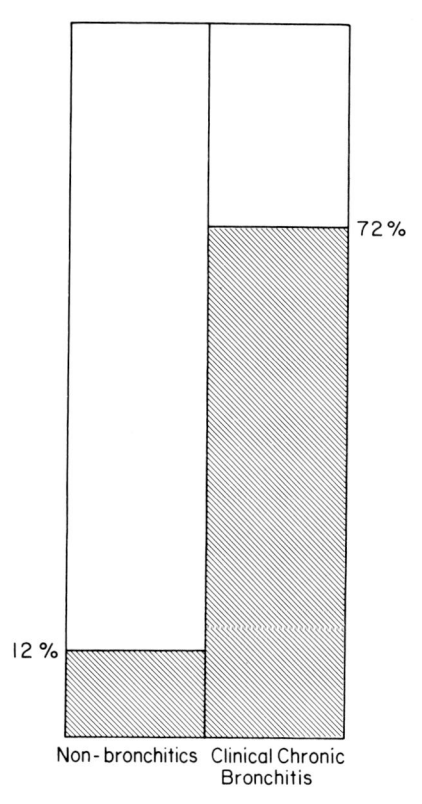

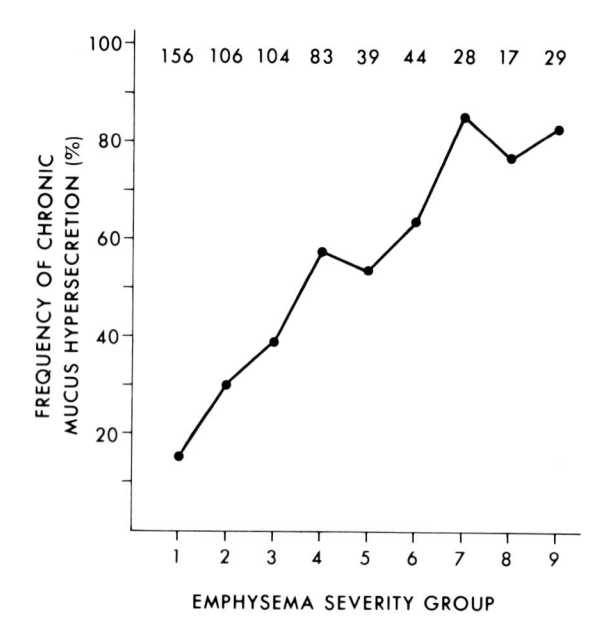

Figure 21-17. The frequency of chronic bronchitis increases from about 15 percent in patients with no emphysema (group 1) to about 80 percent in the patient with the worst emphysema (groups 7 to 9). From Thurlbeck.[362]

Table 21-7. Mucous Gland Enlargement in Smokers and Nonsmokers

Assessment	Authors	Nonsmokers	Smokers	Light and Moderate Smokers	Heavy Smokers
Reid index	Reid[98]			0.46	0.43
	Thurlbeck et al.[101]	0.43	0.50	0.45	0.53
	Thurlbeck and Angus[102]	0.44	0.49		
	Bath and Yates[108]	0.45	0.49		
	Hayes[104]	0.32	0.33		
	Scott[106]	0.41	0.46		
Mucous gland proportion	Ryder et al.[117]				
(Men)		14.5%	17.8%		
(Women)		14.5%	17.1%		
	Sobonya and Kleinerman[116]	11.2%	10.7%		
	Scott[106]	14.1%	14.4%		
Frequency of cases expressed as a percentage of cases in the group	Field et al.[122]				
(Men)		12%	37%		
(Women)		18%	26%		
Megahed et al.[146]		14%	61%		
Petty et al.[147]		8.8%	37%		

bronchitis. The Reid Index is increased in children with atelectasis, suggesting that mucous plugging may be a cause of atelectasis.[148] The frequency of mucous gland enlargement, as assessed by the Reid index of more than 0.40, was 42 percent in patients with bronchopneumonia, 54 percent in patients with pneumoconiosis, and 66 percent in patients with lung cancer.[122] (It was 15 percent in patients without lung disease and 72 percent in patients with chronic bronchitis.) The increase in the Reid index in coal miners was small and not significant in one study,[150] but a more recent study[151] has shown that mucous gland enlargement correlated with dust exposure. The Reid index has also been found to be increased in proximal bronchi in patients with bronchiectasis.[98,152] The increase in the frequency of mucous gland enlargement in patients with bronchopneumonia may represent a predisposition to pulmonary infection in chronic bronchitics but may also represent acute enlargement of glands. Helgason and associates[153] showed that the mean Reid index increased from 0.44 to 0.49 in 24 patients who died following pneumonectomy or lobectomy. There was also more evidence of airway inflammation at autopsy. The increased Reid index in patients with lung cancer is attributable to smoking since the frequency of chronic bronchitis is about doubled in patients with lung cancer.[154] Mucous gland enlargement in bronchiectasis is likely due to proximal spread of inflammation. The enlargement of mucous glands in coal miners substantiates the increased frequency of chronic bronchitis in miners and other workers in dusty occupations.[155-158]

Epidemiology of Chronic Bronchitis

Extensive surveys have been made of the incidence of chronic bronchitis using a standard questionnaire. Although there are difficulties with the questionnaire and there may be subjective interpretations made by both patient and observer, a fairly reasonable consensus has evolved.[159] Chronic bronchitis is a common condition affecting between 10 and 25 percent of adults. It is more common in men than in women and more frequent in those older than 40 years than younger. Tobacco smoking is by far the most important association of chronic bronchitis, but up to 10 percent of patients with chronic bronchitis may be nonsmokers. Even allowing for smoking, chronic bronchitis is more common in the United Kingdom than in the United States, and more common in urban than rural areas. Only one report[122] has examined mucous gland size in relation to the environment and found no difference between urban and rural dwellers. A low average Reid index was recorded in a Jamaican autopsy series,[104] but it is not clear whether this represented low environmental pollution, racial differences, or observer variation.

Long-term follow-up of patients with chronic bronchitis has shown remarkable variations in changes in expiratory flow rate.[63] In the best known study,[63] deterioration was primarily determined by smoking and by the severity of the initial airflow obstruction. In general, the worse the initial airflow obstruction, the more severe the decline. Chronic bronchitis by itself was not related to the development of airflow obstruction. This has lead to the concept of the obstructive component of chronic bronchitis as opposed to the hypersecretory component. This concept should not obscure the fact that bronchial wall lesions and intralumenal mucus may be responsible for at least some airflow obstruction.

Etiology and Pathogenesis

Knowledge of the etiology of chronic bronchitis is derived from epidemiologic studies. Typical studies[157,158,160] showed a frequency of chronic bronchitis of about 5 percent in nonsmokers, rising to about 20 percent in light (1 to 14 cigarettes a day), and 30 percent in smokers of 15 or more cigarettes daily. In the same series, the frequency of chronic bronchitis was increased by 50 to 100 percent in industrial workers. Tobacco smoke presumably induces an inflammatory response, but the mechanism by which hypersecretion of mucus by glands and multiplication of their cells occur is not known. Secretion of mucus is under control of the autonomic nervous system, but it is not clear whether hypersecretion is mediated by this system or whether the action is a more direct local one.

Emphysema

Definition and Recognition

In contrast to chronic bronchitis, which is defined functionally, emphysema is defined strictly in anatomic terms. It thus becomes important to consider abnormal structure as the variable to which other variables—clinical, functional, radiologic, etiologic—must be related. Since emphysema is an abnormality of anatomy, the normal anatomy of the structures involved must be known.

The conducting airways are divided into two categories: bronchi and bronchioles (see Fig. 20-1). The last purely conducting structure is the terminal bronchiole, and the structures distal to the terminal bronchiole constitute the acinus, the terminal gas-exchanging structure of the lung (see Fig. 2-1, p. 12). Emphysema is defined in terms of the acinus as permanent, abnormal enlargement of any part or all of the acinus accompanied by destruction of respiratory tissue.[1,161] This definition has four component parts. The first is enlargement and this should be permanent. Thus enlargement of the acinus that accompanies an asthma attack and may reverse would not constitute emphysema. Enlargement in emphysema should be abnormal; since enlargement of air spaces occurs, perhaps inevitably, with age, this should not be considered emphysema.

Perhaps the most important part of the definition is the concept of destruction. The initial definition of emphysema by the Ciba Symposium[1] included enlargement by dilation alone as well as destruction, but this definition has fallen into disuse, largely because of clinical concepts. The acinus may become abnormally, permanently enlarged in the contralateral lung following pneumonectomy or in the rest of the lung in atelectasis. The clinical and functional abnormalities in such lung tissue have little resemblance to those found when there is enlargement of the acinus accompanied by destruction. A recent workshop sponsored by the National Heart Lung and Blood Institute (NHLBI) redefined emphysema as well as destruction (see below). This is not a published document, but if its recommendations are considered acceptable by the pulmonary community, it will make some difference in concepts and classifications. This chapter will follow the traditional view, and the new definitions and their consequences will be discussed on page 557.

There are problems in the precise use of this definition, and this has been discussed in detail elsewhere.[162] Fortunately, it probably matters little. Although it may be difficult to draw the line precisely between nonemphysematous lungs and lungs with the mildest grade of emphysema, the latter has little clinical significance. (However, the argument will be made later that loss of recoil may be associated with subtle morphologic changes rather than the lesions of emphysema, and some might like to define these changes as emphysema for functional reasons.) The precise definition of destruction is important, however, for epidemiologic and pathogenetic reasons. Very discrepant assessments of the incidence of emphysema have been provided in various populations. This doubtlessly reflects true differences, but perhaps in greater part represents differences in observer assessment of the presence of emphysema.[163,164]

Destruction has never been defined precisely (see commentary on the NHLBI workshop). It is often obvious because emphysema is characteristically localized and there is a contrast between the emphysema and adjacent normal lung tissue (Fig. 21-18, 21-19). However, it is not clear whether the apparently nonemphysematous tissue is normal or less abnormal than the adjacent emphysematous tissue. The first approach at the recognition and definition of destruction was made by Boren[165] who suggested that fenestrae, holes in the alveolar wall more than 20 μm in largest diameter, constituted evidence of emphysema. Smaller holes were considered normal structures, the pores of Kohn. Pump[166] extended these observations and described various stages of fenestrae, all of which he regarded as abnormal. Grade I fenestrae were rounded or oval with smooth margins that were formed by capillaries. If two stage I fenestrae were adjacent, the intervening capillary was thin and bloodless. With enlargement of the fenestrae, the margins became more irregular, and often degenerated elastic fibers could be seen at the margins. The largest fenestrae involved the entire wall of an alveolus. He measured the summed surface area of pores and plotted this against age and found a steady increase with age; he concluded that emphysema was a normal accompaniment of age. In patients with clinical symptoms attributed to emphysema, the summed surface area of pores was even greater.

The reason for choosing an arbitrary size of alveolar wall defect as abnormal is unclear. There are two distinct approaches to the definition of disease or abnormality. One is a qualitative one—a person is either sick or well—as with infectious diseases. The other is a quantitative one, as in hypertension or mucous gland enlargement, in which there is a gradual transition between normal and abnormal. Choosing an arbitrary size of pore as the upper limit of normal represents the first approach;

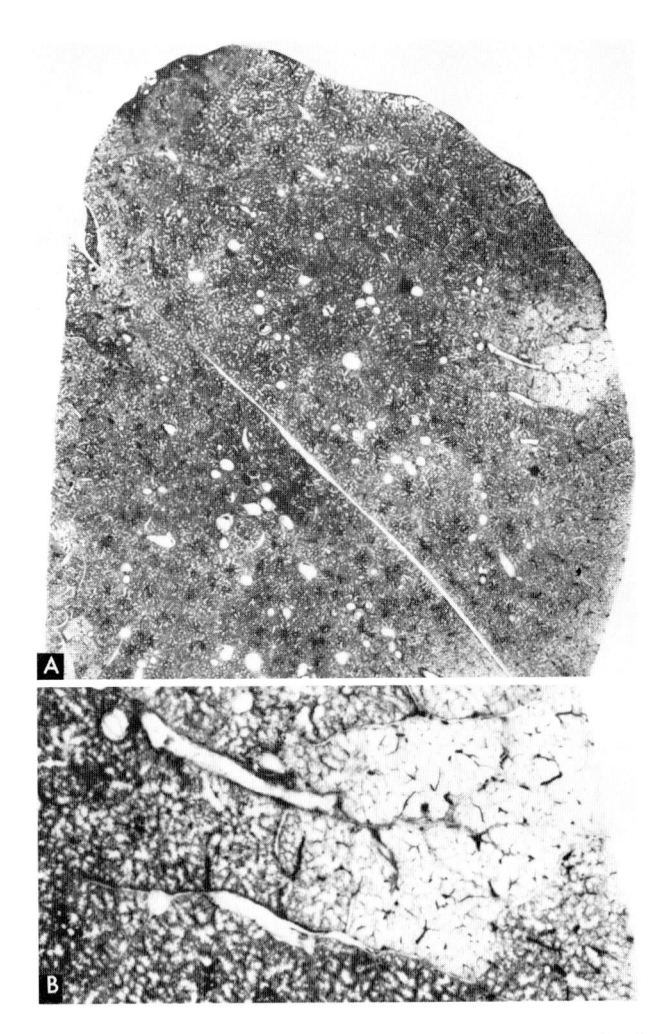

Figure 21–18. A. Localized panacinar emphysema is seen distal to an obliterative small bronchiole in the anterior segment of the upper lobe. B. The lesion is seen better in which the obliterated airways can be recognized in the area of emphysema. Emphysema is readily recognized in contrast to the normal adjacent parenchyma. From Thurlbeck.[159]

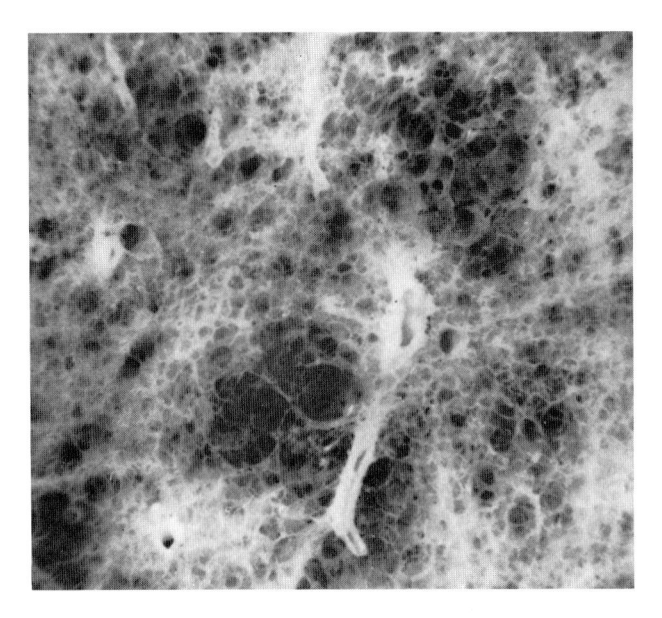

Figure 21–19. Several mild centrilobular emphysematous spaces are apparent. Minimal fibrosis is present and the lesions are readily recognized in contrast to the normal adjacent parenchyma. From Thurlbeck.[159]

developing a normal range in pore size or summed size of alveolar pores represents the latter.

In both instances, the definition of normal subjects is imperative. Presumably they should be nonsmokers without respiratory symptoms, with normal serum protease inhibitor, and perhaps living in a nonpolluted environment. Two results may be found: it may be that no pores greater than 20 μm in diameter will be found in the study group so that a qualitative definition could be used. Alternatively there may be a variation in pore size, perhaps age or sex related; under these circumstances, a distribution curve of pore size would have to be constructed. The definition of emphysema could then either be size of pores outside the normal range, or some arbitrary upper limit could be set, such as 1.74 standard deviations above normal. In the latter circumstance, 5 percent of the normal subjects, as defined, would thus become abnormal. Dimensions need to be studied to determine abnormal enlargement of air spaces in the definition of emphysema. The same problems arise as in the case of pores. Animal studies suggest an early increase in pore size and number in normals, but little or no increase after the age of onset of sexual maturity. (Changes in dimensions with age are discussed on p. 555.)

Although the definition of emphysema is clear, its application may be difficult, and more normative data are needed. These data would be extremely hard to obtain. Despite the lack of totally acceptable data, it is possible to approach emphysema on a more pragmatic basis. Emphysema, both enlargement and destruction, is recognized by comparison with (relatively) normal lung.

Classification of Emphysema

Emphysema is classified by the way the acinus is involved and four patterns are recognized:

1. In proximal acinar emphysema, respiratory bronchioles forming the "stem" or proximal part of the acinus are abnormally enlarged and destroyed (Fig. 21–20).
2. In panacinar emphysema, the process of enlargement and destruction in the acinus involves the acinus more or less uniformly (Fig. 21–21).

3. In distal acinar emphysema, alveolar ducts are dominantly affected (Fig. 21–22).
4. In irregular emphysema, there is irregular enlargement and destruction of the acinus (Fig. 21–23).

Different clinical associations may occur with each type of emphysema, and similar clinical associations may be found with different types of emphysema.

Other Definitions and Conditions that are not Emphysema

Changes associated with age or pneumonectomy should not be regarded as emphysema but should be referred to as aging lung and (compensatory) overinflation, respectively. A bleb is a collection of air within the layers of the pleura; a cyst is a closed cavity lined by bronchiolar epithelium or fibrous tissue. Interstitial emphysema is characterized by collections of air in the interstitium of the lung. It is similar to a bleb in concept; therefore it is appropriate to redefine bleb as collections of air within the connective tissue of the lung. Then one could refer more specifically to pleural blebs and multiple interstitial blebs; the latter would be the definition of interstitial emphysema.

A *bulla* has been defined as an emphysematous space with a diameter of more than 1 cm in the distended state. (This topic will be discussed further in Bullae and Blebs, below.)

Proximal Acinar Emphysema

Two forms of proximal acinar emphysema are recognized—centrilobular (nonindustrial) emphysema and simple coal workers' pneumoconiosis, best described as proximal acinar emphysema, due to dust.

Figure 21–20. In proximal acinar (centrilobular) emphysema, respiratory bronchioles are dominantly involved. RB = respiratory bronchiole (subscript indicates order); TB = terminal bronchioles. From Thurlbeck.[207]

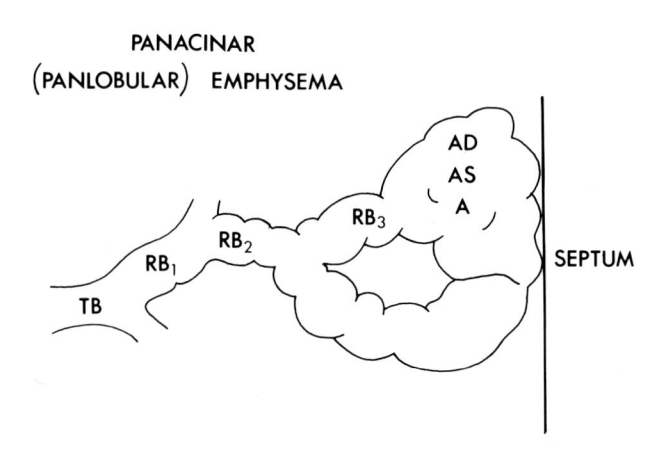

Figure 21–21. In panacinar (panlobular) emphysema, enlargement and destruction of the air spaces involve the acinus more or less uniformly. Abbreviations as in Fig. 21–20, except A = alveoli, AD = alveolar duct A. From Thurlbeck.[207]

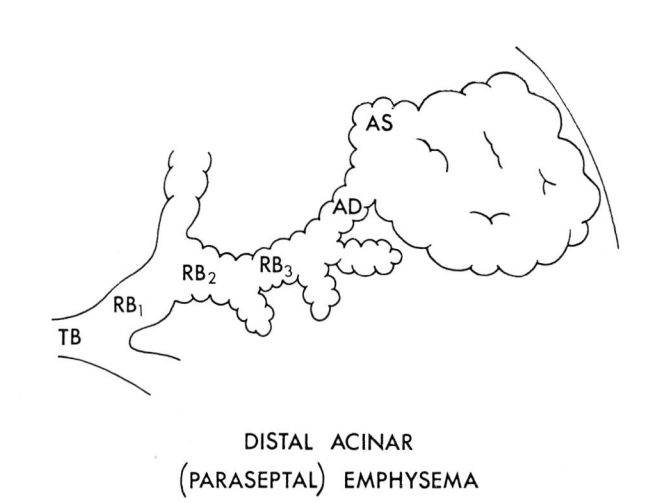

Figure 21–22. In distal acinar (paraseptal) emphysema, the peripheral part of the acinue is dominantly involved. From Thurlbeck.[159]

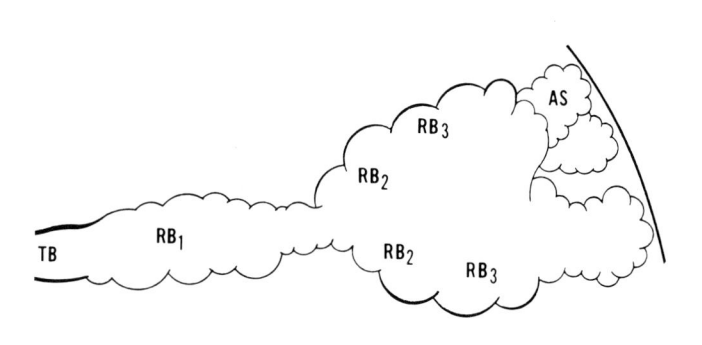

Figure 21–23. In irregular emphysema, the components of the acinus are randomly destroyed and enlarged. Fibrosis is a usual accompaniment of this lesion. From Thurlbeck.[159]

Centrilobular Emphysema

Morphology. Centrilobular emphysema was described briefly in 1952 by Gough[167] and amplified by Leopold and Gough in 1957.[37] In Australia, McLean[168] provided a detailed description of centrilobular emphysema using the term focal emphysema. It is surprising that this distinctive lesion was not recognized previously. Its recognition was primarily due to examination of fixed, inflated lungs, either grossly or using the whole lung, paper-mounted technique of Gough and wentworth.[169] The characteristic lesion results from enlargement and destruction of respiratory bronchioles leading to emphysematous spaces that become confluent in series and in parallel (Fig. 21–24 through 21–27). The primary change is one of destruction of the respiratory tissue as opposed to the primary dilation that occurs in proximal acinar emphysema due to dust (*see* p. 607).

In classic examples, the emphysematous spaces lie near (but not precisely at) the center of the secondary lobules. Thus the term centrilobular emphysema is, strictly speaking, a misnomer, but it is traditional and widely accepted. The term centriacinar emphysema has also been proposed,[170] but it is really the proximal part of the acinus that is involved.

The lung tissue distal to the emphysematous spaces is often apparently normal; thus, the spaces are separated from each other, from the septa of the secondary lobules, and from the margins of the acini along vessels and airways by apparently normal-looking lung tissue. Although the distal parenchyma may look normal, Leopold and Gough[37] pointed out that generalized (panacinar) emphysema was usually present in the intervening tissue, and there is greater loss of alveolar surface area than can be accounted for by the centrilobular emphysematous spaces.[171] Second- and third-order respiratory bronchioles are more severely affected than the first order respiratory bronchiole. Characteristically there is a striking variation in the severity of emphysema among lobules and even within the same lobule.[37] The lesions are more frequent and become more severe in the upper zones of the lungs than in the lower zones.[172] The lesions in the superior segment of the lower lobe resemble the upper lobe rather than the lower lobe, and the posterior and superior segment of the upper lobe are affected most frequently and most severely. Varying degrees of pigmentation may be present in the walls of the spaces, but this is usually only modest compared with proximal acinar emphysema due to dust.

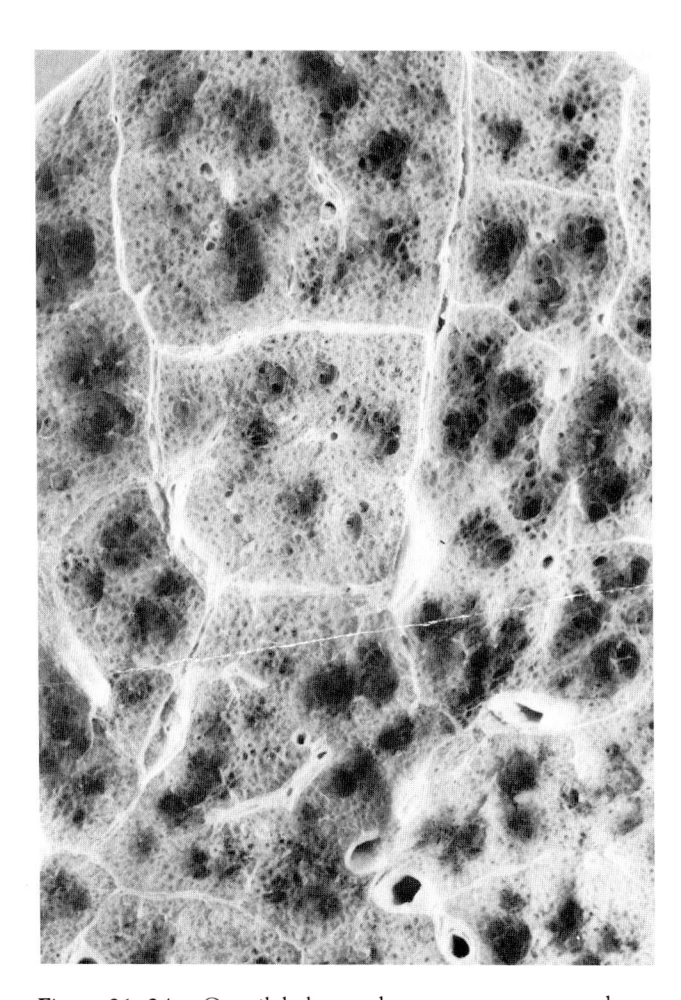

Figure 21–24. Centrilobular emphysematous spaces are shown in a lung with well-demarcated lobular septa. Note that the spaces lie midway between the center of the lobules and the periphery of the lobules. Normal-appearing respiratory tissue lies between the spaces and between them and the periphery of the lobule. Note that from time to time there is encroachment and destruction of alveolar ducts and sacs (×2.5 approximately). From Thurlbeck.[159]

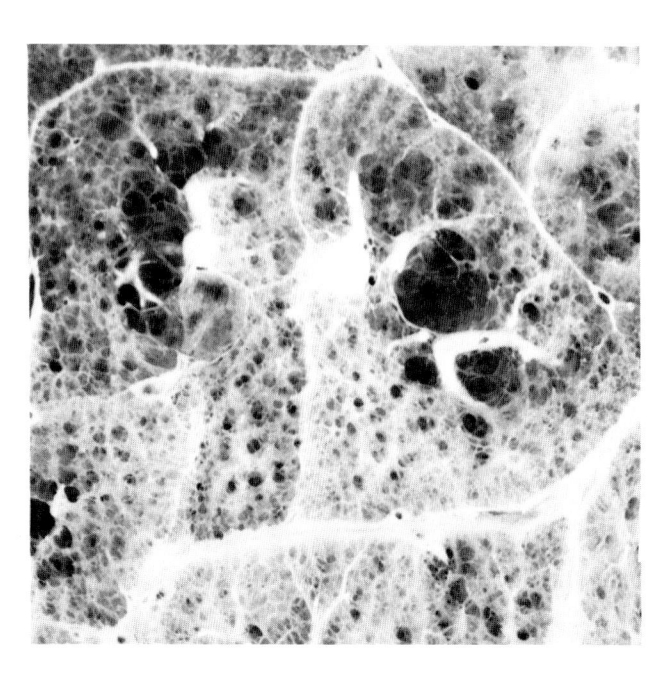

Figure 21–25. In this specimen, the pulmonary arterial system has been filled with contrast medium. Note the obvious destructive nature of centrilobular emphysema. The acinar periphery appears normal (to the right), whereas at top left there appears to be enlargement and destruction of the acinar periphery (×5 approximately).

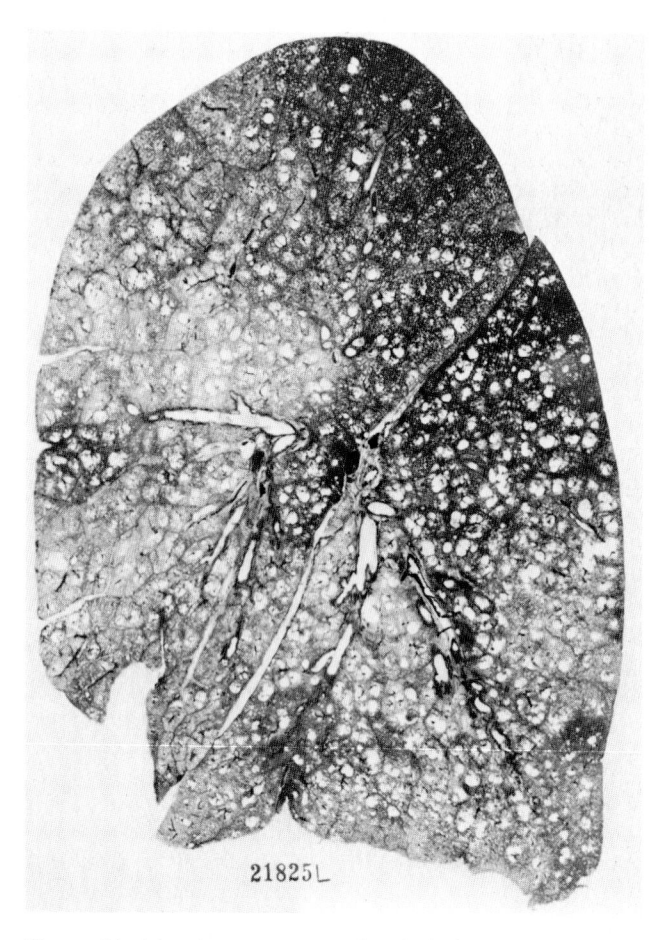

Figure 21–26. A paper-mounted, whole lung section shows widespread centrilobular emphysema more or less uniformly distributed through the lung (×5 approximately). From Thurlbeck.[171]

Atypical examples of centrilobular emphysema predominate over classic ones, and this has led to differing classification of emphysema in the same lungs by expert observers.[163,173] Although the peripheral part of the acinus is maintained intact in classic examples of centrilobular emphysema, more often there is variable encroachment on the alveolar ducts and sacs that form the acinar periphery. Even in lesions that all observers would consider examples of centrilobular emphysema, the margins of the emphysematous spaces may lie close to the lobular septa and structures limiting the border of the acinus. Clearly alveolar ducts have been destroyed, but the lesions still involve the proximal part of the acinus dominantly. As emphysematous spaces get larger, the spaces tend to become confluent, but usually a rim of acinar tissue can be seen between the spaces. A further problem is that in many lungs, both centrilobular and panacinar emphysema may coexist, and apparent (or real) transitions may be seen between the two lesions (see p. 545).

Leopold and Gough[37] stressed that inflammation was usually present in the airways supplying the emphysematous spaces and that inflammation also occurred in the major airways. Evidence of chronic inflammation and fibrosis of the walls of the emphysematous spaces can nearly always be found if sought. In 60 percent of cases, Leopold and Gough found that the supplying bronchiole was narrowed, but in the remainder, these airways were normal or even dilated.

Associations of Centrilobular Emphysema. There is general consensus that centrilobular emphysema is the most common form of emphysema associated with symptomatic and fatal chronic airflow obstruction,[37,40,44,152,174–183] although this is occasionally denied by some authors.[170,185] There is also a general consensus that centrilobular emphysema is more common than panacinar emphysema.[159,186] Centrilobular emphysema is rarely encountered in nonsmokers.[187] In the author's experience, it is frequently associated with chronic productive cough. It also occurs more commonly in men,[37,188–190] probably reflecting past smoking habits. An interrelationship among smoking, age, sex, and bronchitis is shown in Fig. 21–15.

Proximal Acinar Emphysema due to Dust

This condition is fully described on pp. 609 to 614 as is the distinction between it and centrilobular emphysema. The terms simple pneumoconiosis of coal workers and focal emphysema have also been applied to this lesion. The former can be ambiguous because it has been used to describe the apperance of pneumoconiosis on chest radiographs in coal workers; the latter has no precise interpretation.

Panacinar Emphysema

Various terms have been used to describe a form of emphysema that involves the acinus more or less uniformly, and these include panlobular emphysema, diffuse emphysema, generalized emphysema, vesicular emphysema, and alveolar emphysema. Panacinar emphysema is the best term since it describes the lesion in terms of the acinus as is done in other forms of emphysema. Panacinar emphysema occasions the most difficulty in recognition since the precise distinction (if there is one) between normal and the mildest grade of emphysema is very difficult. This in part accounts for the wide discrepancy in the reported incidence of panacinar emphysema.[186] Most animal models of emphysema result in panacinar emphysema, and in animals it is not always clear whether destruction of respiratory tissue is present.

Morphology

It has been suggested that the earliest stage of panacinar emphysema primarily involves alveolar ducts and sacs[172,191] and that subsequently other parts of the acinus are involved. Mild panacinar emphysema is best recog-

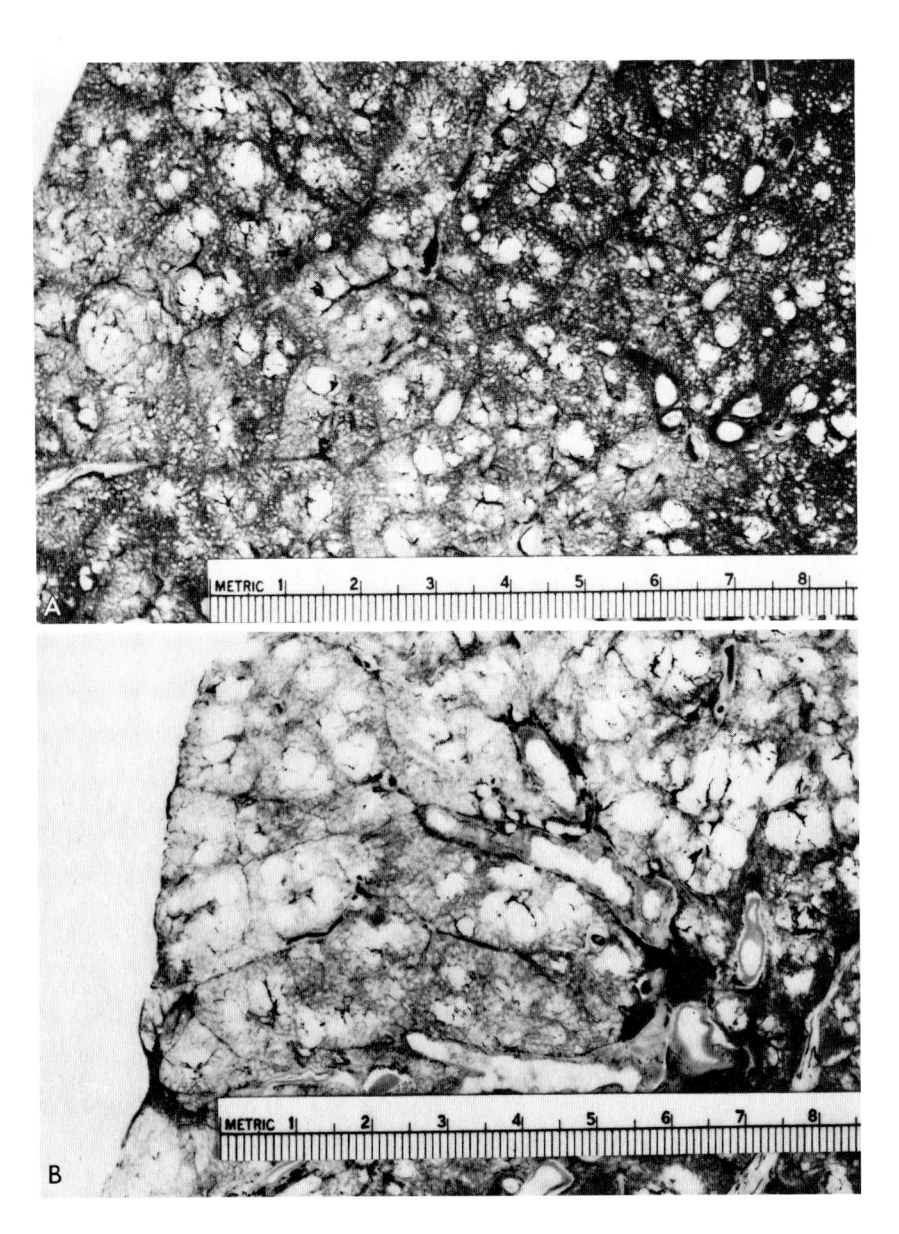

Figure 21–27. A. A close up of Fig. 20–26 shows the lesions more clearly. B. Larger centrilobular emphysematous spaces are shown. In some instances, the acinar periphery appears normal, whereas in others the lesions extend almost to the lobular septums. From Thurlbeck et al.[215]

nized by examining a barium sulfate-impregnated slice of lung immersed in water.[192] A normal lung examined in this way has a characteristic appearance. Alveoli are recognized as the smallest air spaces and are multifaceted structures. They are dispersed among larger air spaces that are transversely sectioned alveolar ducts and respiratory bronchioles. In examples of the mildest, clearly recognizable panacinar emphysema, alveoli are enlarged and flattened, and the sharp distinction between alveolar ducts and alveoli is lost (Fig. 21–28). With progression, all air spaces enlarge, and destruction of lung parenchyma becomes evident (Fig. 21–29).

Even lesions as apparently severe as those in Fig. 21–29F may not be recognizable by naked eye examination of fixed distended lung slices. When the slices are not immersed in water, panacinar emphysema can be suspected because the lung parenchyma falls away from supporting structures such as the airways, vessels, and lobular septa so that they protrude slightly above the cut surface. The precise division between normal and abnormal may be difficult. One of the best criteria is the contrast between the abnormal lung and normal lung since the mildest grade of emphysema is usually not uniformly dispersed through the lung.

Most observers[4,189,190,192,193] have stated that panacinar emphysema is more common in the lower zones and anterior margins of the lungs. In the author's experience,[172] panacinar emphysema tended to be more frequent in the lower zones of the lungs in random cases, but this was not statistically significant (Fig. 21–30). However, panacinar emphysema was clearly more frequent in the lower zones of the lungs of patients with severe emphysema, and panacinar emphysema characteristically was more severe in the same zones.

Panacinar emphysema occurs in very different clinical situations although the anatomic lesions may be identical. Not all of the associations are agreed on, as will be discussed below.

Figure 21–28. A normal lung (A ×13, B ×26 approximately) is compared with an example of mild panacinar emphysema (C ×13 approximately, D ×26 approximately). Note the effacement of normal lung structure; the sharp distinction among alveoli (the smallest polygonal structures) and alveolar ducts and respiratory bronchioles (the large spaces) is lost in mild panacinar emphysema. B from Thurlbeck.[364]

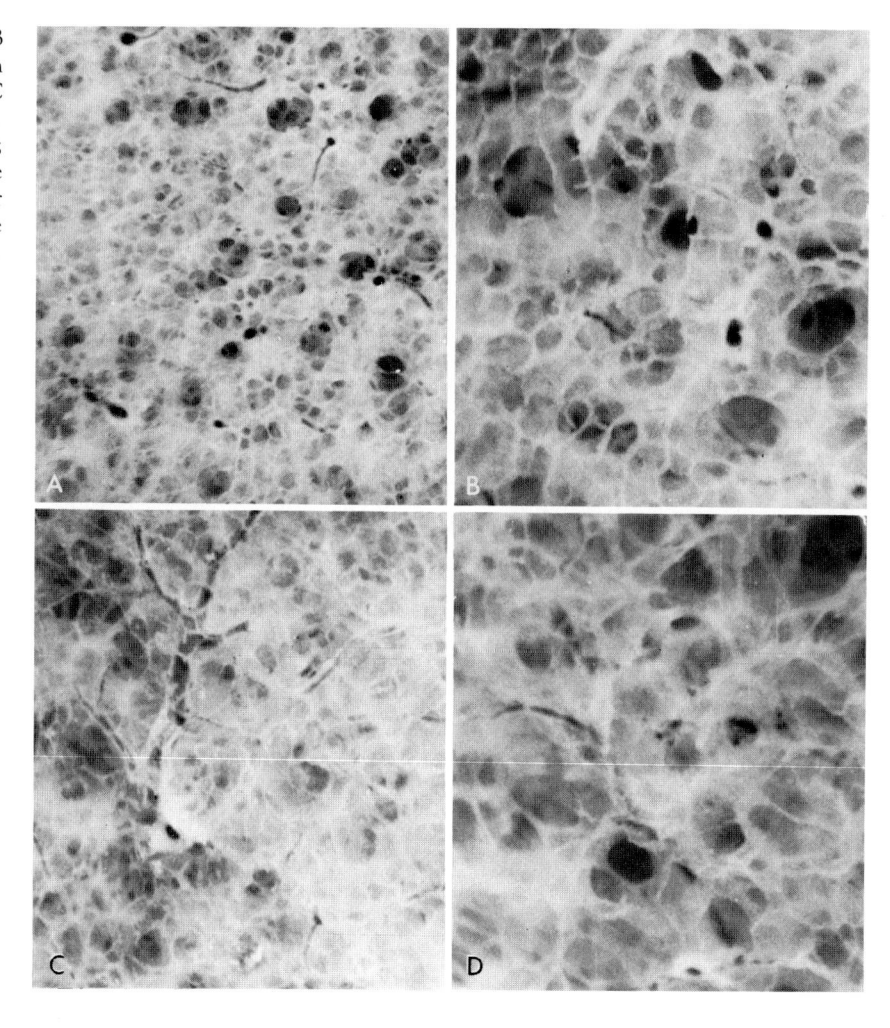

Associations

Familial Emphysema Associated with Alpha-1-Antitrypsin Abnormalities. One of the major breakthroughs in the understanding of the pathogenesis of emphysema was the discovery, on routine survey of sera using electrophoresis, that some subjects had diminished levels of alpha-1 macroglobulin.[194] Subsequent analysis of the subject disclosed that the defect as familial, associated with diminished antitrypsin activity in the serum and a high frequency of chronic airflow obstruction. The other important observation, made at about the same time and equally serendipidous, was that intratracheal installation of papain, instead of ameliorating experimental silicosis, resulted in emphysema.[195] These two observations led to the now widely held protease-antiprotease theory of the pathogenesis of emphysema (*see* p. 555).

The amount and type of alpha-1-antitrypsin in the blood is determined by a pair of codominant alleles. The abbreviation Pi, for proteinase inhibitor, is usually given to the alleles which are then further described by a superscript. The Pi^M allele is the most common with a gene frequency of about 0.95, and the common phenotype is a Pi^{MM}. More correctly the term Pi^M is used since the phenotype may be the expression of Pi^{MM} or Pi^{MO}. The phenotypes are detected by crossed immunoelectropheresis, and thus far 30 alleles have been detected.[196] The most important allele is Pi^Z which in the homozygous condition is associated with extremely low levels of alpha-1-antitryptic activity in the blood. In the heterozygous state of Pi^{MZ}, there is an intermediate level between Pi^Z and Pi^M. Pi^Z has a varying geographic gene frequency, with a result that the frequency of Pi^{MZ} is about 3 percent in adults in the United Kingdom,[197] 4.7 percent in Sweden,[198] and 5 to 9 percent in U.S. residents of North European extraction. Pi^{MZ} is extremely uncommon in blacks, Jews, Indians, and those of Italian descent.[199,200] Similarly Pi^Z is most common in North Europe where it has been found in about 1 in 1000 to 5000 births. It is correspondingly less common in the previously mentioned populations and unknown in Japan and African blacks.[201] Pi^S is the most common allelic variant in Spain and Portugal with a gene frequency of 0.1124 and 0.1410, respectively, compared with 0.023 in Norway.[202]

Pi^Z is associated with cirrhosis of the liver in infancy and a high frequency of emphysema in adult life. Not all

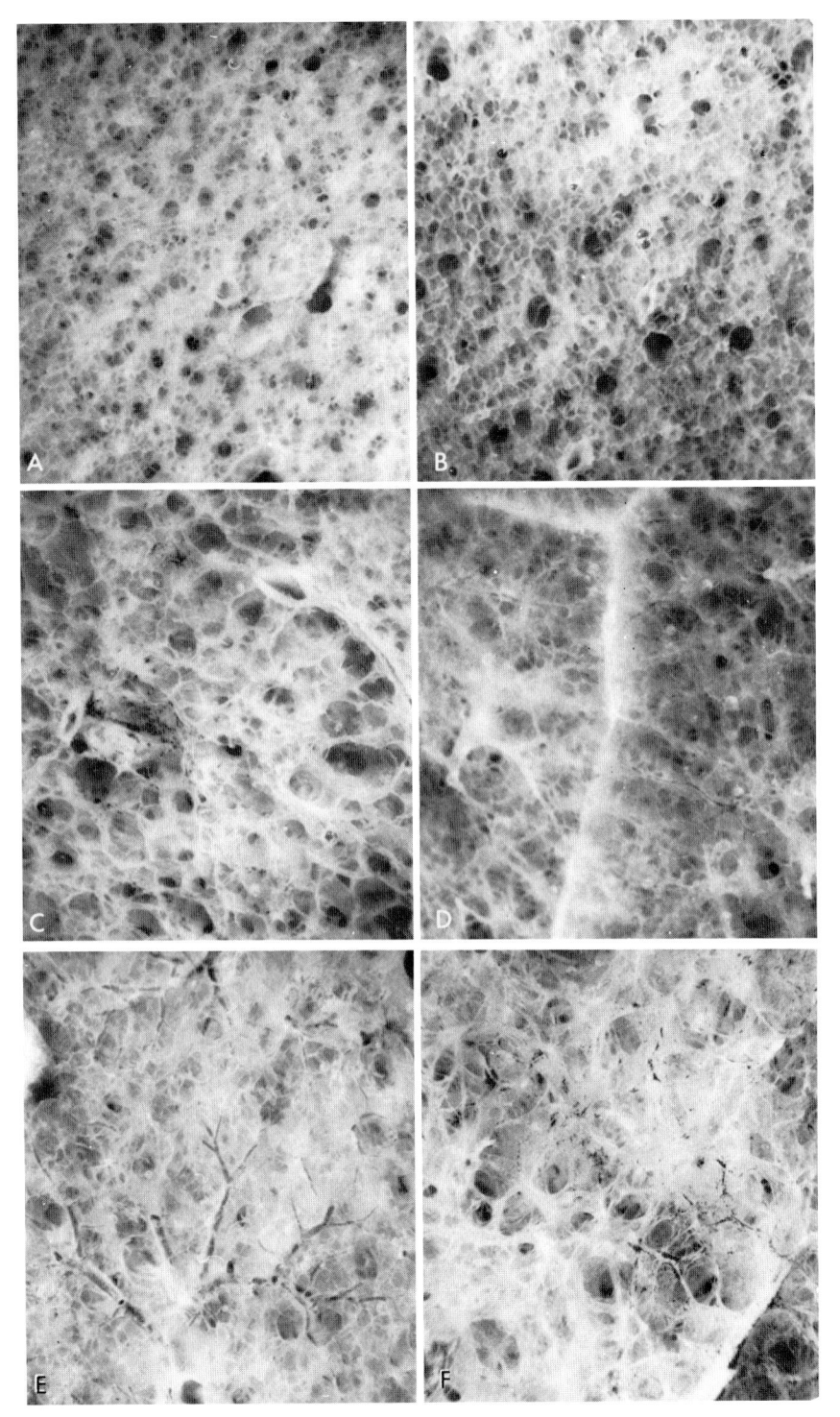

Figure 21–29. Normal lungs are shown in A (55-year-old woman) and B (75-year-old woman). Alveolar ducts and respiratory bronchioles appear enlarged (compare Fig. 20–28). C to F show varying grades of mild panacinar emphysema. Dilation appears to be the predominant phenomenon in C, whereas destruction of alveolar tissue is clearly apparent in D to F. From Thurlbeck.[159]

patients develop clinical emphysema, and the frequency is increased in smokers. The pattern of chronic airflow obstruction is characteristic: the onset of dyspnea starts in or before the fourth decade, usually preceding the onset of chronic productive cough, and the average age of presentation to a physician is 45 years compared with 57 years in the average patient with chronic airflow obstruction.[200,203] Patients with Pi^Z form the minority of patients with chronic airflow obstruction, but those younger than age 40 may comprise as much as 40 to 50 percent of patients with severe chronic airflow obstruction.[204] The chest roentgenograms may be characteristic with greatly enlarged lung volumes and radiologic emphysema which is symmetric and worse at the bases. The latter appear-

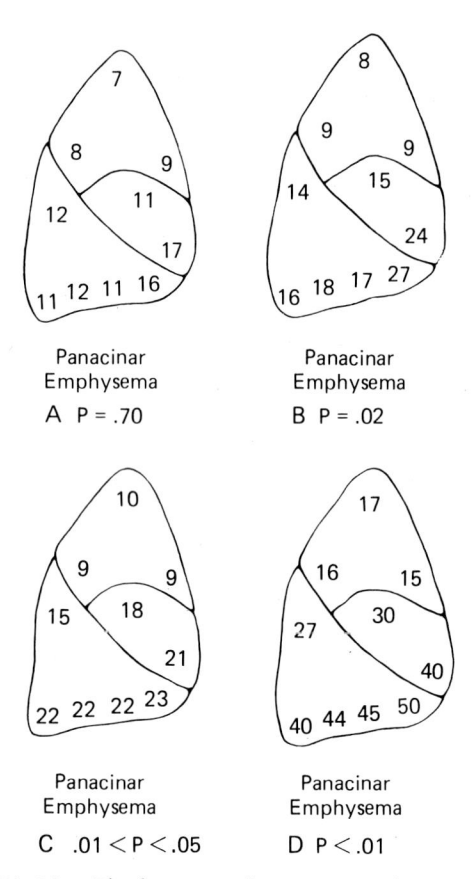

Figure 21–30. The frequency of panacinar emphysema is shown in 138 random cases (A) and in 30 cases with severe emphysema (B). In the random cases, the panacinar emphysema tends to be more common in the lower zones of the lung, but not significantly so. In severe emphysema, panacinar emphysema is more common in the lower zones of the lung. When severity of emphysema is assessed, panacinar emphysema becomes more severe in the lower zones of the lung in both random cases and patients with severe emphysema (C and D). From Thurlbeck.[1]

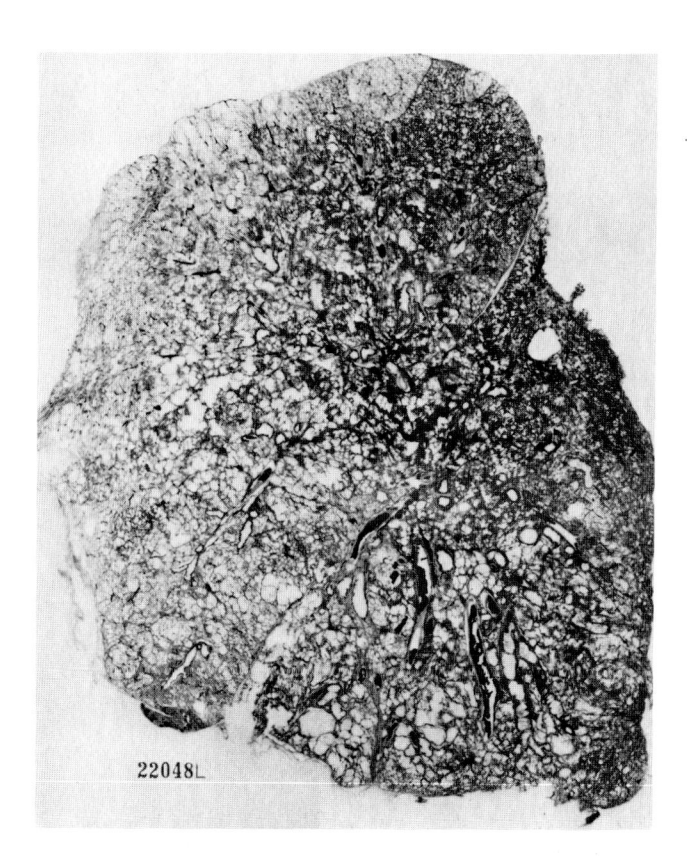

Figure 21–31. A patient with alpha-1-antitrypsin deficiency has widespread panacinar emphysema which is worse in the lower zones of the lung. From Thurlbeck.[171]

ance may be accentuated by redistribution of blood to the upper zones of the lung.

Patients with Pi^{SZ} hve low levels of alpha-1-antitrypsin activity and have a predisposition to emphysema, which has similar characteristics although this is not as well documented. The Pi^S phenotype is also associated with an increased frequency of chronic airflow obstruction. The major interest, however, has centered on Pi^{MZ} because of the frequency of this phenotype. More than 20 surveys have been conducted assessing the frequency of chronic airflow obstruction in this phenotype with conflicting results. Proper epidemiologic surveys performed on random populations show no increased frequency of chronic airflow obstruction in these subjects,[196] although surveys derived in whole or part from known subjects with Pi^Z have shown an increased frequency of chronic airflow obstruction. The latter phenomenom results from socioeconomic, environmental, and smoking factors.

With one exception,[183] the type of emphysema that occurs in Pi^Z (and probably Pi^{SZ} and Pi^S) is panacinar. In patients with severe chronic airflow obstruction, it is characteristically widespread through the lung and is worse in the lower zones (Fig. 21–31). Since cigarette smoking aggravates emphysema in alpha-1-antitrypsin deficiency and smoking is also associated with centrilobular emphysema, centrilobular emphysema is also found in some instances, as in the case reported by Schleusener and colleagues.[205] Severe pure panacinar emphysema without evidence of centrilobular emphysema is uncommon, and this finding should raise the suspicion of alpha-1-antitrypsin deficiency.

Severe Panacinar Emphysema in Young Subjects. Martelli and colleagues[206] have described the occurrence of severe panacinar emphysema in three young subjects with a clinical presentation similar to alpha-1-antitrypsin deficiency but with normal alpha-1-antitrypsin activity. There was no obvious familial association, but the data were incomplete in this study.

Other Forms of Familial Emphysema. Clinical familial emphysema unassociated with alpha-1-antitrypsin deficiency is well recognized. The morphologic correlates are unknown.

Incidental Panacinar Emphysema. If careful examination is made of lungs, focal areas of mild panacinar emphysema may be found in 5 to 10 percent of random autopsies.[207] In the seventh and eighth decades, the incidence increases to about 20 percent when it approximates the frequency of centrilobular emphysema. Under these circumstances, panacinar emphysema is most common at the bases and anterior margins of the lungs. It is not associated with symptoms nor particularly related to chronic bronchitis or smoking. It is best regarded is a variant of the aging lung, perhaps an exaggeration of the normal aging process that affects a small proportion of the population (*see* p. 556).

Panacinar Emphysema Associated with Centrilobular Emphysema and Chronic Airflow Obstruction. There is evidence that the parenchyma distal to centrilobular emphysematous spaces frequently displays a mild grade of panacinar emphysema which is hard to recognize and is overshadowed by the more obvious lesion of centrilobular emphysema. In addition, however, a characteristic finding in patients with chronic airflow obstruction is the presence of centrilobular emphysema in the upper zones of the lung and panacinar emphysema in the lower zones (Fig. 21-32). Such patients have the typical associations of chronic bronchitis and cigarette smoking, as in centrilobular emphysema. This combination of lesions has led to considerable difficulties. Apparent transition zones can be found when both types of emphysema are present, and many areas are found in which it is difficult to categorize the lesions. It is logical to suppose that one is observing a transition from centrilobular emphysema to panacinar emphysema, and some refer to such lungs as examples of centrilobular emphysema.[183]

However, since the acinus is more or less uniformly involved, it seems more appropriate to refer to this lesion as panacinar emphysema and question whether it indeed represents a progression from centrilobular emphysema. An additional difficulty is that it may be hard to classify such lungs, and they may be regarded as examples of centrilobular emphysema, panacinar emphysema, dominantly centrilobular emphysema, dominantly panacinar emphysema, or equally mixed depending on the perception of the observer.

Emphysema Associated with Bronchial and/or Bronchiolar Atresia. Occasional localized areas of emphysema may be found in the lung distal of obliterated bronchi and bronchioles (*see* Fig. 21-18). These represent an incidental autopsy finding, but widespread bronchial and bronchiolar obliteration may occur resulting in the Swyer-James[208] or MacLeod[209] syndrome. Patients with this syndrome are usually asymptomatic and present with an abnormal chest radiograph. The affected lung is hyperlucent, and blood flow is redistributed to the opposite lung which, because of the increased radiologic opacity, may be regarded as the abnormal one. Similarly the remarkable shunt of blood from the affected side may delay or prevent angiographic filling, so these cases may be incorrectly regarded as examples of pulmonary artery atresia. The most characteristic feature occurs on expiration when the affected lung traps air so that the mediastinum shifts toward the normal side and the difference in vascularity between the two sides becomes even more marked.

The syndrome results from extensive bronchial and bronchiolar obliteration, usually as a consequence of severe airway inflammation in childhood. The nature of the airway obliteration is such that most of the lung parenchyma remains distended with air via collateral channels. Postinfective or idiopathic bronchiectasis (*see* p. 558) has a similar etiology, but airway obliteration is such that collapse of the parenchyma ensues. In the Swyer-Jones syndrome, the bronchi are abnormally dilated, and some have referred to this condition as bronchiectasis without atelectasis. The functional abnormalities are due to bronchial and bronchiolar obliteration.

Since surgical resection is not indicated, descriptions of the anatomic pathology are few. In the one example seen by the author, there was limited panacinar emphysema at the base of the lung. Since emphysema may not be an invariable accompaniment of the airway obliterative lesions, a preferable term is unilateral pulmonary transradiancy which describes the condition most precisely. The airway lesions are not strictly unilateral, although they are dominantly so: that is, both lungs may be affected, one more than the other. The lung clinically apparently affected is not affected uniformly throughout. The pathogenesis of emphysema has not been established in this condition. Since air-trapping—continued overexpansion on expiration—occurs, increased intra-alveolar pressure may be responsible. It may be that intra-alveolar pressure exceeds pulmonary artery pressure, resulting in stoppage of blood flow and ischemic atrophy of the lung parenchyma. This facile explanation does not account for filling of the air spaces since airway pressure must exceed alveolar pressure of the air spaces to fill.

Congenital Bronchial Atresia. This is a well-recognized condition, usually involving the apicoposterior segmental bronchus of the left upper lobe. Other lobes may also be involved. Figure 21-33 illustrates involvement of the lateral segment of the right lower lobe. Distal to the atretic bronchus, there characteristically is mucous impaction and bronchial dilation. The bronchial mucous plug may be seen radiologically as a mass. The lung parenchyma distal to the atretic bronchus is overinflated and, over the course of years, may develop panacinar emphysema. Alveolar multiplication may be abnormal so that the complement of alveoli present at birth overexpand and become disrupted.

Distal Acinar Emphysema

A variety of terms have been used to describe distal acinar emphysema, and they reflect the way that the lesions affect the acinus and where the peripheral part of

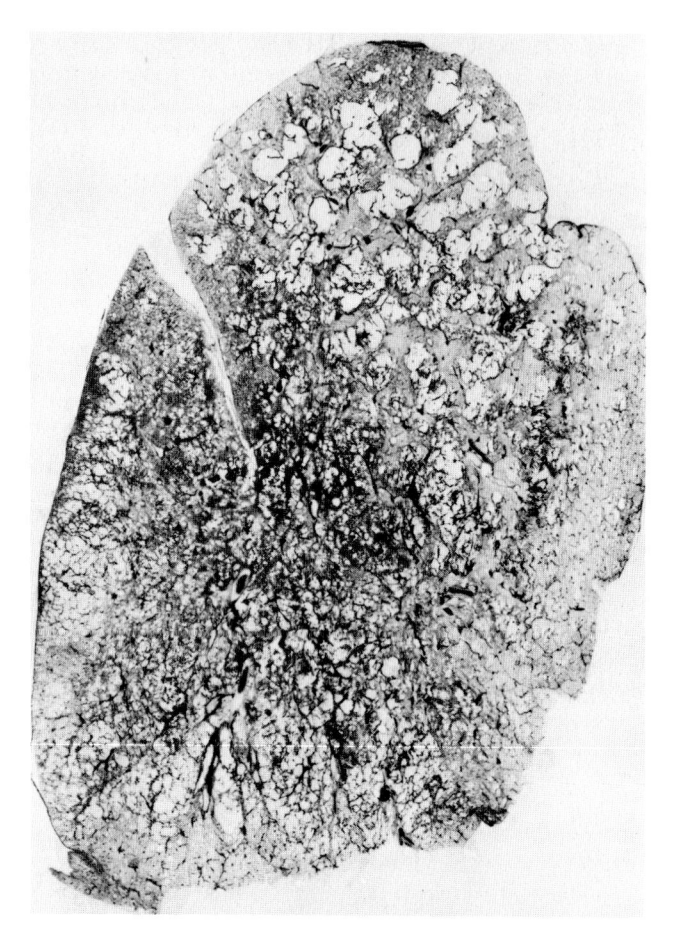

Figure 21–32. Severe centrilobular emphysema is seen in the upper zones of the lung, whereas the emphysema in the lower zones of the lung is panacinar in type. From Thurlbeck.[207]

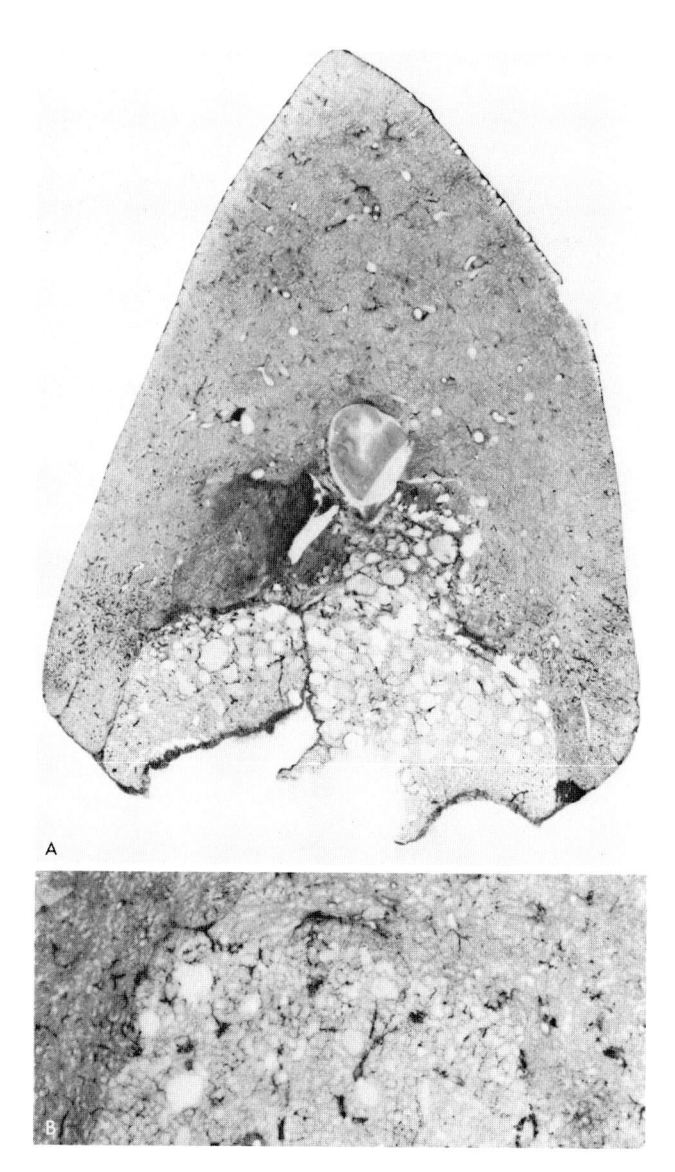

Figure 21–33. Congenital atresia of the lateral segmental bronchus of the right lower lobe has produced a dilated proximal bronchus with mucoid impaction (center of A). Emphysema is readily apparent in the affected segmented and is best seen (B) in contrast with the adjacent normal lung (left). From Thurlbeck.[159]

the acinus lies. It has been referred to as superficial or mantel emphysema, reflecting its subpleural location; as paraseptal or linear emphysema, indicating its involvement of the acinar periphery along lobular septums, airways, and vessels; and also as periacinar emphysema, involving the periphery of the acinus. It is the least common form of emphysema and the least well described. It may occur alone or in association with panacinar or centrilobular emphysema.

Alone, distal acinar emphysema is usually limited in extent, occurs most commonly along the posterior or anterior margins of the upper part of the lung, and is often associated with fibrosis. Because of this, some might like to refer to this form of emphysema as scar or paracicatrical emphysema. However, if the distal part of the acinus is dominantly involved, it appears more appropriate to refer to this lesion as distal acinar emphysema (Fig. 21–34). Its characteristic association is with spontaneous pneumothorax of young adults.[210] The upper zonal location exposes the lesions to more negative intrapleural pressure, and its subpleural location predisposes it to rupture into the pleura (forming blebs, see p. 549) and subsequent rupture into the pleural space. The classic association of spontaneous pneumothorax with exercise in tall young men emphasizes the importance of large negative intrapleural pressures, since these are greater in tall subjects and at large lung volumes. In addition, the more diffuse form of distal acinar emphysema is probably the type of emphysema associated with bullous disease of the lung, as described by Laurenzi and colleagues.[211] This term applied to young adults with multiple bullae visualized radiologically and only mild chronic airflow obstruction.

Distal acinar emphysema may be associated with panacinar emphysema, centrilobular emphysema, and

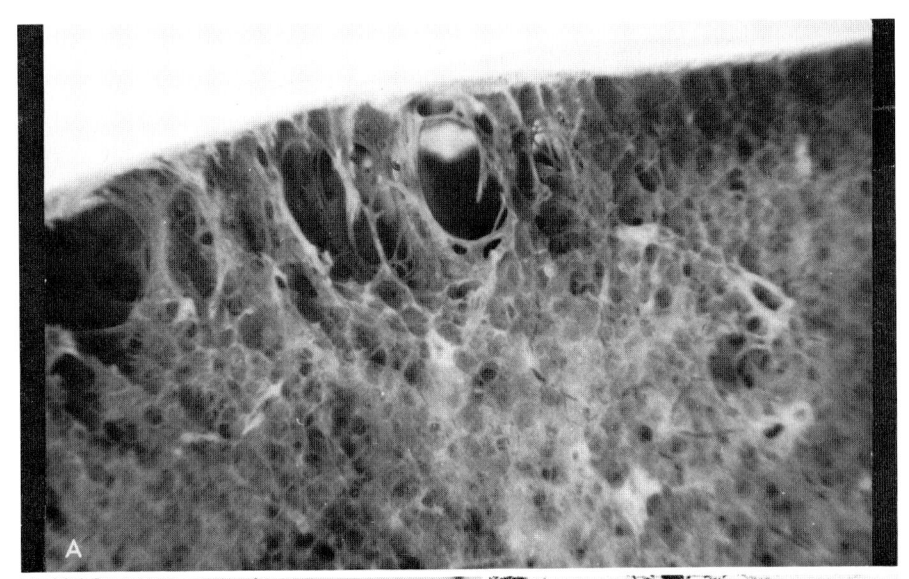

Figure 21–34. A. Distal acinar emphysema involves the acinus adjacent to the pleura (×7 approximately). Histologic sections (B ×12 approximately, C ×25 approximately) illustrate the involvement of the distal part of the acinus. Fine fibrosis is readily apparent. From Thurlbeck.[159]

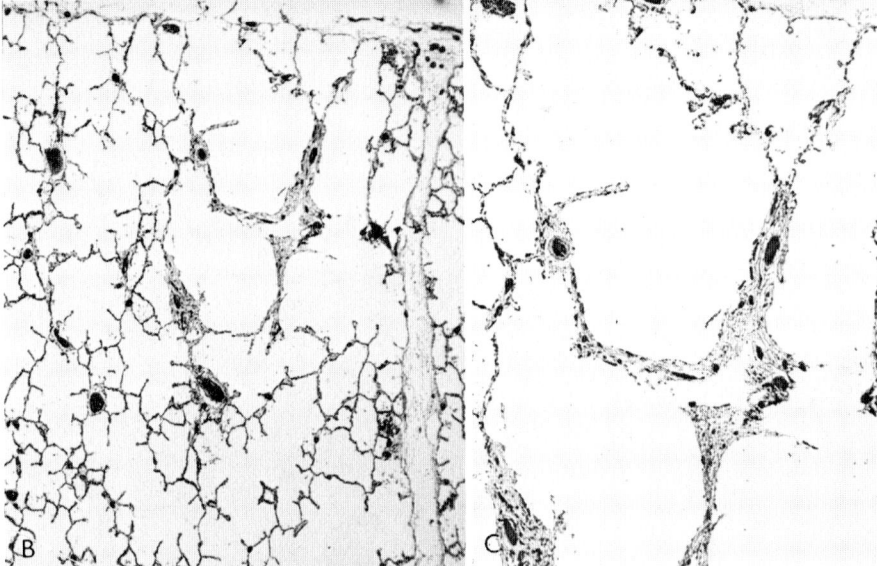

hence chronic airflow obstruction. Occasionally distal acinar emphysema may occur alone and be associated with chronic bronchitis and severe chronic airflow obstruction (Fig. 21–35) The illustrated case is of historical interest in that it may be the first structure-functional correlation in chronic airflow obstruction. (The patient's pulmonary function was studied at St. Bartholomew's Hospital in London; Dr. David Bates sent the lung to Dr. Jethro Gough in Cardiff.)

Irregular Emphysema

Irregular emphysema is always associated with scarring and is the most common form of emphysema, since scars with associated irregular enlargement of the acinus are usually found in the lung at autopsy if a careful examination is made (Fig. 21–36). Most of these lesions are not associated with symptoms. Occasionally there may be widespread scarring within the lung and extensive irregular emphysema leading to symptomatic airflow obstruction. This is found in granulomas of the lung such as tuberculosis, histoplasmosis, or pneumoconiosis. Some examples of eosinophilic granuloma[159] or sarcoidosis may also present in this way.

Although irregular emphysema is invariably associated with scarring, the reverse is not true; scarring may be associated with specific involvement of the acinus such as proximal acinar emphysema in pneumoconiosis,[212] panacinar emphysema, or paraseptal emphysema.

Bullae and Blebs

Although bullae and blebs are terms that are frequently used clinically and radiologically, they are uncommonly

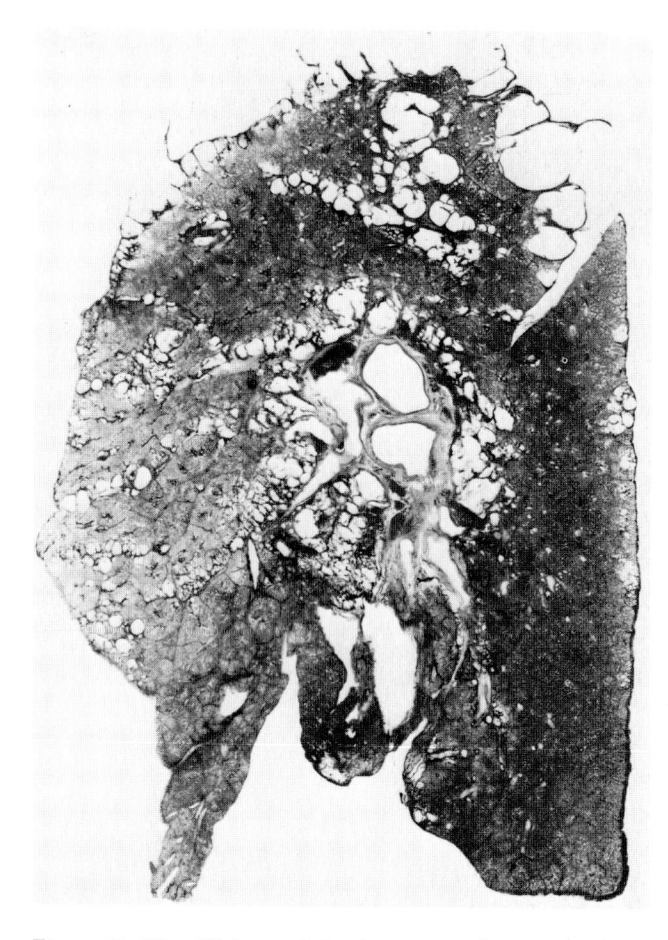

Figure 21–35. Widespread distal acinar can be recognized and is situated deep to the pleura, along lobular septa, and around vessels and airways. This patient had chronic bronchitis and died of chronic airflow obstruction.

encountered pathologically. A bulla has been defined as an emphysematous space more than 1 cm in diameter in the distended state. However, most bullae recognized radiologically are not bullae as assessed morphologically. Those seen radiologically in the lower zone of the lung represent severe panacinar emphysema, but the radiologic margins represent lobular septa, and there is attenuated respiratory tissue within the "bullae." Radiologically determined upper zonal bullae usually represent centrilobular emphysematous spaces,[213] but even then there is often respiratory tissue within the space.

Bullae may occur as isolated lesions in otherwise normal lungs, but this is uncommon. Usually they are associated with varying degrees of emphysema and represent the radiologic appearance of a more severe area of a usual form of emphysema. Since surgery may be curative in the case of isolated bullae, it is important to recognize these patients compared with those whose radiologic bullae are part of a generalized process. The two extremes are generally easy: in one, airflow obstruction is absent or mild (such a patient may even have a restrictive pulmonary function defect), and isolated large bullae are present; in the other, there is evidence of severe chronic airflow obstruction with several scattered radiologic bullae. Between these two extremes, all degrees of combination are found.

Reid[170] has classified bullae into three types. Type I bullae occur independently of widespread emphysema. They are subpleural and occur more commonly in the upper lobes and along the medial surface of the lung. Characteristically they have a narrow neck at the junction of the normal lung, and the diameter of the neck is narrower than the diameter of the bulla. They contain little respiratory tissue, their margins are formed by fibrous tissue and lobular septa and probably represent greatly expanded emphysematous lobules. In excised specimens, they form a large mushroom-like projection on the surface of the lungs, but in vivo they are inverted into the lung parenchyma and, if large enough, compress adjacent lung. Type II and III bullae represent local exaggerations of widespread emphysema; type II bullae are subpleural, whereas type III bullae occur elsewhere in the lung parenchyma.

Blebs, collections of air in the pleura (*see* p. 540), are usually described by surgeons in patients with spontaneous pneumothorax. However, these may not be found on examination of resected specimens[170] and may be erroneous descriptions of distal acinar (subpleural) emphysema. Interstitial emphysema (first distinguished from emphysema proper by Laennec) is air in the interstitial tissue of the lung, in lobular septa, and in the bronchovascular bundle. If one extends the definition of blebs to include air within interstitial tissue, interstitial emphysema can be conveniently described as multiple blebs. (Interstitial emphysema is discussed further in Chapter 10.)

Prevalence of Emphysema

The prevalence of emphysema in 30 autopsy series has been reviewed,[159] and since then two further surveys have been reported.[186] The reported prevalence of emphysema and the relative frequency of various types of emphysema has been discrepant. The former is due to the care and the methods used to examine the lung and the latter to different interpretations of the types of emphysema present. If careful search of the lungs is made of barium-impregnated inflated slices of lungs using a dissecting microscope and localized irregular emphysema is included, nearly all lungs from adults will have emphysema.[172] If irregular emphysema and equivocal emphysema are omitted, roughly half of lungs in adult autopsy populations will have emphysema. About two-thirds of men and 15 percent of women will have emphysema. Centrilobular emphysema has usually been found to be more common than panacinar emphysema. Emphysema increases in frequency with age, and it is found most frequently in patients in the seventh decade (Fig. 21–37).

Another way of examining the incidence of emphysema is to express it as average severity[214] using the panel grading method that subjectively assesses emphysema from 0 to 100.[215] Under these circumstances, the average

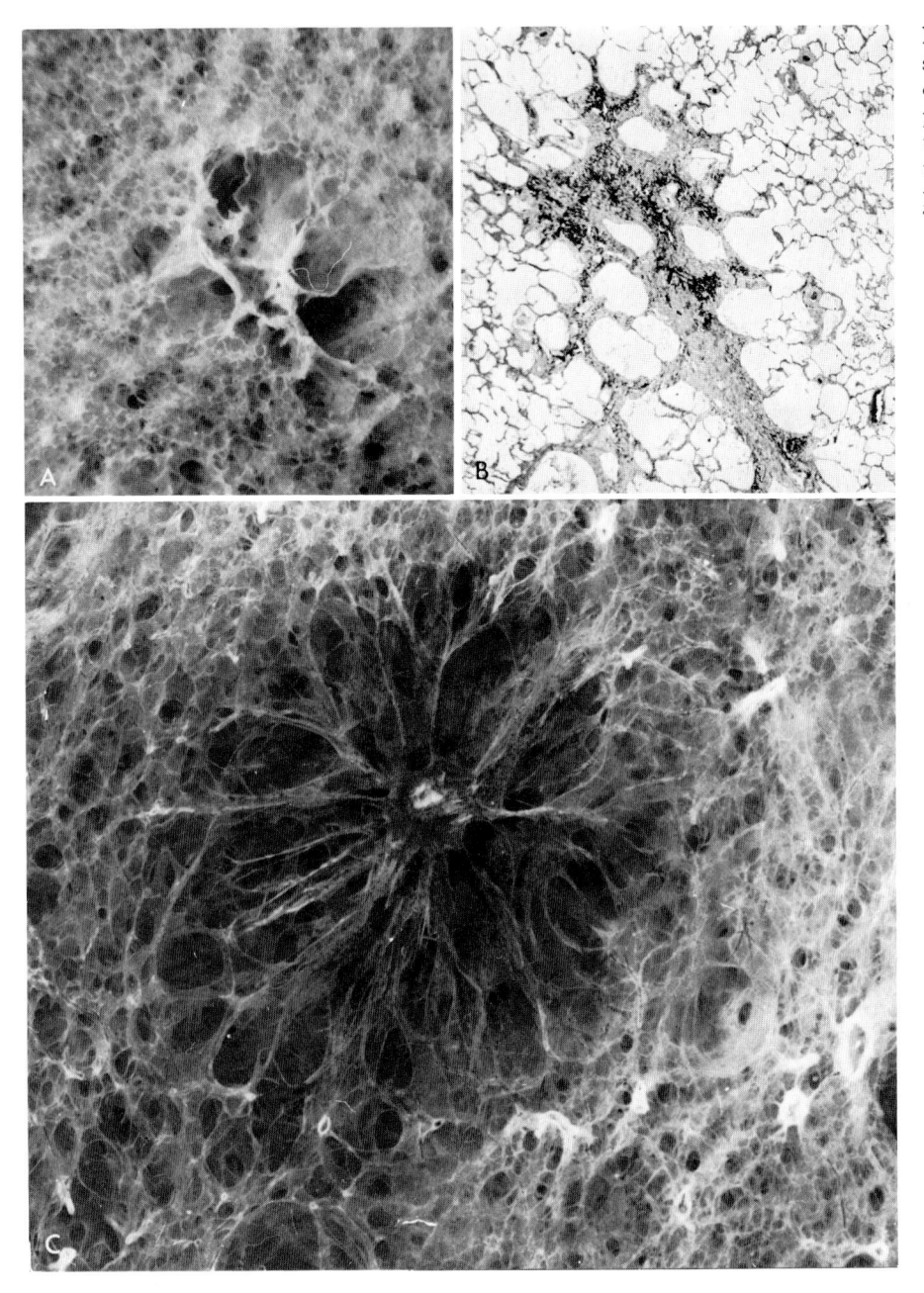

Figure 21–36. A. An isolated scar is seen in the lung with associated irregular emphysema (×7 approximately). B. A photomicrograph of the lesion illustrates the scarring ×10). C. A granuloma in the lung is associated with adjacent emphysema (×7 approximately). From Thurlbeck.[159]

emphysema score is substantial in men and higher than in women (Fig. 21–38). Emphysema is more severe and more common in smokers (Fig. 21–39), and emphysema of anything more than a mild degree is nearly always associated with tobacco smoking.

Differences in the incidence of emphysema have been reported in different parts of the world, but these are hard to interpret because of interobserver variation. (For example, the incidence of emphysema was found to vary from 42.5 to 85 percent in the same set of lungs examined by different observers.[163]) Certain geographic variations may exist. For example, the same observers compared lungs from two cities and found a much higher frequency of emphysema in lungs from St. Louis, Missouri, with high environmental pollution, compared with Winnipeg, Manitoba, which has clean air.[216] The incidence of emphysema is extremely low in Nigeria[217] and Uganda.[218] The differences between these two populations and studies in industrial cities are so large that geographic variations are probably real. The highest frequency and severity of emphysema has been noted in Cardiff, Wales.[214]

Clinicopathologic Correlations

An extensive literature exists which has related clinical, radiologic, and pulmonary function findings to the

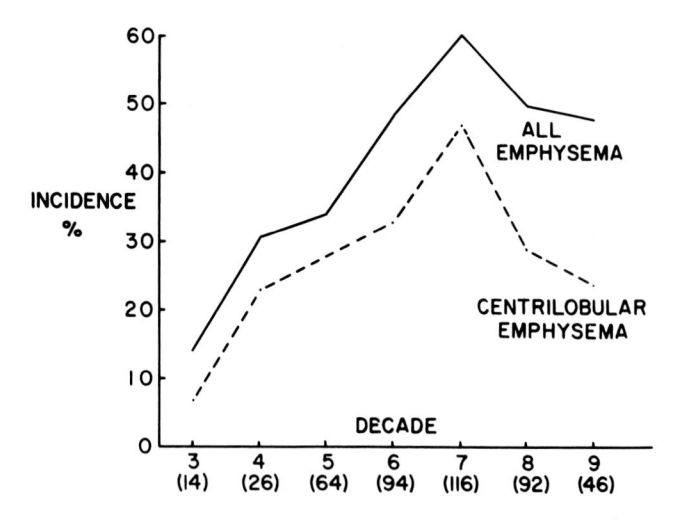

Figure 21-37. When the incidence of panacinar and centrilobular emphysema (all emphysema) is plotted against age, there is an increase to about 60 percent in the seventh decade. Following this there is a decrease in the incidence of centrilobular emphysema. The incidence of panacinar emphysema (the difference between the two lines) increase with increasing age. From Thurlbeck.[207]

amount and type of emphysema. This literature has been reviewed in detail,[14,159] and only a broad outline will be dealt with here.

Lesions of the bronchi, bronchiolitis, and emphysema occur together more often than chance will allow. Each of the three components has several different lesions, so that in any one patient, there are numerous variables, each of varying severity.

Emphysema is the major determinant of clinically recognized, severe chronic airflow obstruction.[13,15] It is relatively uncommon to find severe chronic airflow obstruction in patients with little or no emphysema; severe emphysema is usually accompanied by clinical evidence of chronic airflow obstruction. Exceptions, however, must continually be expected. Figure 21-40 indicates that one-third of patients with the most severe grade of emphysema were not recognized as having severe chronic airflow obstruction from a retrospective survey of the patients' charts. How truly asymptomatic these patients were is uncertain. By the nature of the study, they had other severe diseases that may have obscured the diagnosis of chronic airflow obstruction. The frequency of mild chronic airflow obstruction did not increase as emphysema became more severe, suggesting that mild chronic airflow obstruction and therefore also severe chronic airflow obstruction were substantially underdiagnosed.

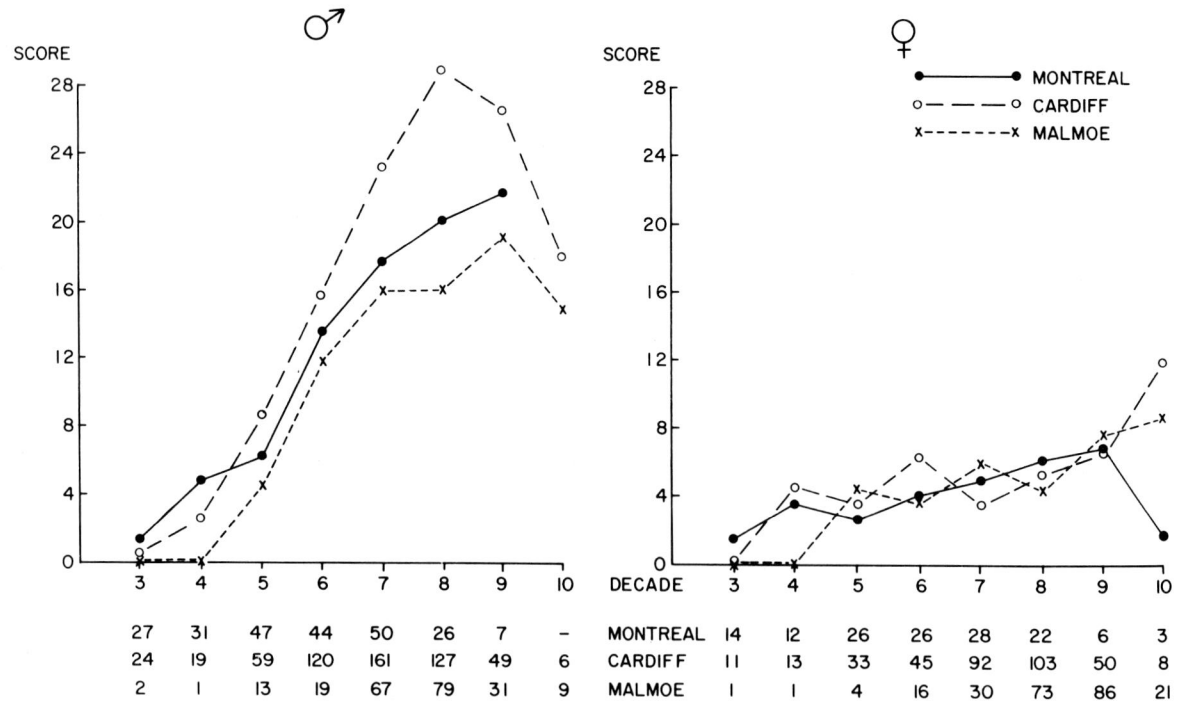

Figure 21-38. The average severity of emphysema (score) is compared in men and women in three different cities. The average emphysema score was determined from the panel grading method.[145] The numbers under the figure indicate the number of subjects in each decade. The average emphysema score in men in the eighth decade varied from about 16 to 28. Note the much lower average emphysema score in women. From Thurlbeck et al.[214]

Emphysema 553

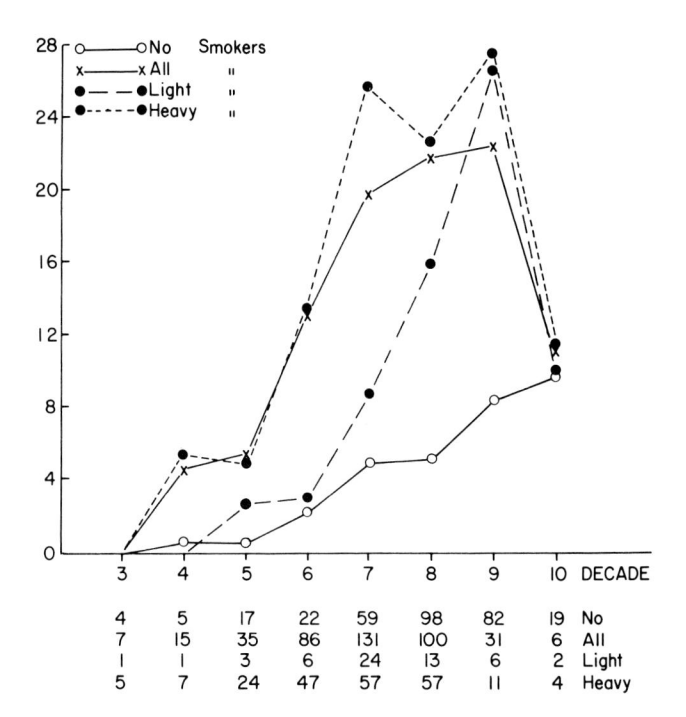

Figure 21-39. The average emphysema score for men and women in the three cities illustrated in Fig 20-38 is shown in various categories of smokers. Note the striking effect of smoking and that average emphysema severity increases with age even in nonsmokers. The effect is greater in men than in women.[140] From Thurlbeck et al.[214]

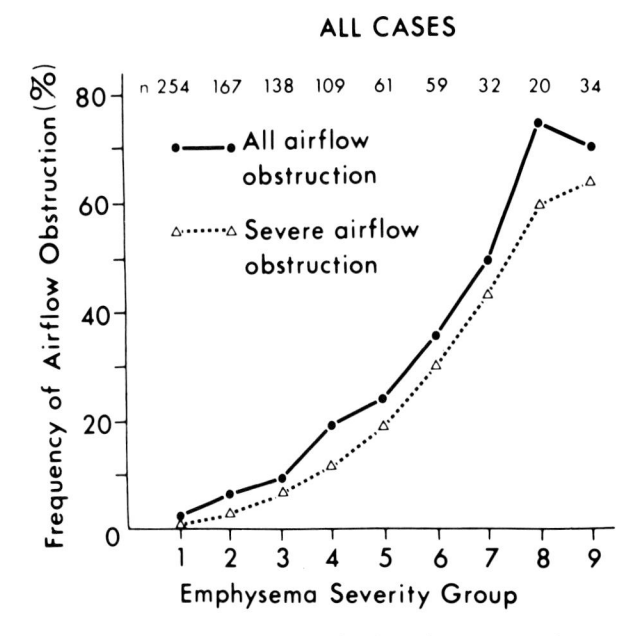

Figure 21-40. The frequency of airflow obstruction is shown in patients with increasing severity of emphysema. Emphysema severity group 1 are patients without emphysema and group 9 have the worst emphysema. The numbers of patients in each group are shown at the top. Severe airflow obstruction increases as emphysema increases, but lesser grades of airflow obstruction (difference between all airflow obstruction and severe airflow obstruction) do not. From Thurlbeck.[362]

The relationship between cor pulmonale and emphysema has undergone radical revision in the past two decades. Cor pulmonale, when defined as right ventricular hypertrophy, is more common in patients with emphysema than those without and is more common with increasing severity of emphysema.[159,219] This is in contrast to the old view that emphysema was not related to cor pulmonale; indeed, one study suggested a negative correlation.[220]

The relationship between emphysema and cor pulmonale is probably an indirect one. As emphysema gets worse, so does the frequency and severity of chronic airflow obstruction. Cor pulmonale is related to the severity of chronic airflow obstruction as it is found only in patients with moderate and severe chronic airflow obstruction. The reasons why some patients with comparable degrees of chronic airflow obstruction develop cor pulmonale whereas others do not are uncertain, but evidence suggests that this is related to the severity of bronchiolar narrowing.

Hypoxemia is intimately related to the development of cor pulmonale and is presumably primarily related to ventilation/perfusion mismatch due to the bronchiolar lesions. Recent data have suggested that radiologic evidence of emphysema was related to pulmonary arterial pressure irrespective of hypoxemia, again raising the old hypothesis of reduction of a capillary bed as being part of the cause of cor pulmonale in emphysema.[221]

Part of the problem in assessing the cardiac complications of emphysema is the confusion between cor pulmonale (increase right-ventricular weight) and the "blue bloater" syndrome. Patients with equally severe chronic airflow obstruction could present, as extremes, in one of two ways. In one case, patients have relatively well-maintained blood gases, are often thin, with increased minute ventilation; these patients were colloquially referred as "pink puffers." In the other case, patients may have severe hypoxemia, often hypercarbia, polychythemia, and right-ventricular failure; these are referred to as "blue bloaters." The latter instance was at one time thought to be associated with mucous gland enlargement, but this association has been abandoned even by some of the original proponents.[13,43,109,219]

The problem is that syndromes have not been properly defined. A rigorous approach divided patients with severe chronic airflow obstruction into type A (resembling the pink puffers) and type B (resembling blue bloaters).[222] The type A subjects had severe emphysema substantially more frequently than those with the type B syndrome, which was thought to be due to airway lesions.[222] Only one other study[159] has used these precise criteria, and the difference of emphysema severity between the groups was much less. A similar, but not identical, classification of the clinical syndrome showed that a substantial proportion of patients with the blue bloater syndrome had severe emphysema[223] The nature of the bronchiolar lesion has never been examined in detail in the two syndromes.

The precision of the radiologic diagnosis of emphysema has also undergone revision. Although different criteria were used (overinflation in some instances, attenuation of the peripheral vasculature in others), the diagnosis was initially thought to be very precise.[159] Overinflation, especially as assessed by diaphragmatic flattening, appears to recognize a high proportion of patients with severe emphysema but may produce false-positives, particularly in patients with asthma. Peripheral arterial deficiency when present is highly suggestive of severe emphysema,[213] but a substantial portion of patients with severe emphysema will not show this sign.

The correct recognition of peripheral arterial deficiency probably requires a high degree of reader proficiency, and interobserver variation is large[159,224]; the same is true of irregular lucencies (bullae). Increased total lung capacity is an early event in emphysema[39,40,225] and well recognized by chest radiography.[225] These observations suggest that the chest radiograph should be highly useful in the diagnosis of emphysema. The latest evidence is that the chest radiograph achieves about 80 percent sensitivity, specificity, and accuracy when two of five criteria for the recognition of emphysema are used.[226] The same was true of a subjective diagnosis of emphysema. This is in contrast to a study which indicated a 100 percent specificity and sensitivity in distinguishing grades 0, I, and II emphysema from grades III and IV using mainly peripheral arterial deficiency.[227] Arterial deficiency achieved a sensitivity of 45 percent and specificity of 81 percent in another study.[224] A problem is that it is not clear what is meant by the diagnosis of emphysema. Using the criterion of the presence of emphysema as assessed by arterial deficiency, data[213] show that the diagnosis is highly specific but very insensitive. Correlation coefficient between emphysema severity and radiologic diagnosis have been modest ($r = +0.69$ for depression of the diaphragm; $r = +0.46$ for arterial deficiency).[228] The chest radiograph has to be regarded as an integral part of the diagnosis of emphysema and to be used in conjunction with the clinical and functional data.

The best way of recognizing emphysema is by pulmonary function testing.[14] Diminution of expiratory flow rates is primarily used to assess the severity of chronic airflow obstruction but is also related to the severity of emphysema. Subdivisions of lung volume, notably total lung capacity and functional residual capacity, are good indicators of emphysema. Residual volume is increased in mild emphysema but may be increased in peripheral airway disease; however, it is seldom greatly increased except in emphysema. In most clinical studies, total lung capacity has only been increased in severe emphysema. However, these studies have utilized the helium dilution method of measuring total lung capacity. Total lung capacity is consistently increased in mild emphysema, and an increase determined plethysmographically or radiologically should be regarded as good evidence of emphysema, especially in the absence of asthma. Increase in functional residual capacity is a relatively sensitive method of recognizing emphysema and is, like residual volume, seldom greatly increased except in emphysematous lungs.

Recent evidence has shown a good correlation among functional residual capacity static lung mechanics, total lung capacity at maximum inflation, and diffusing capacity.[229] Consistently the best relationship to the severity of emphysema has been to the diffusing capacity (transfer factor) for carbon monoxide, measured in a variety of ways. Relationships between emphysema and loss of elastic recoil have generally not been good, but there was initial enthusiasm for a close relationship between the shape of the volume-pressure curve as expressed by fitting an exponential[230] or an empirical equation.[231] Subsequent investigators[232,233] have not confirmed this early promise.

The clinical assessment of the severity of anatomic emphysema depends on an integrated approach. Cigarette smoking, age, and chronic bronchitis are important in the patient's history. The absence of cigarette smoking, chronic bronchitis, or a young age make the diagnosis of emphysema suspect. Physical examination is of limited value, but a grossly overdistended, hyperresonant chest with distant heart sounds and diminished diaphragmatic excursion are important positive findings. Radiologic appearance may be useful, and function residual capacity, total lung capacity, and the diffusing capacity for carbon monoxide are good indicators. In many instances, these factors may enable one to make the diagnosis of severe emphysema with considerable certainty. As each of the individual variables become less characteristic, so the diagnosis of emphysema becomes less certain.

Etiology and Pathogenesis[234]

Epidemiologic and postmortem studies[159] have established beyond doubt the role of tobacco smoking as the major cause of emphysema. It appears that cigarette smoking is particularly important. Inhalation of coal dust and inflammatory fibrosis may result in emphysema, but these are relatively infrequent causes of anything other than relatively mild emphysema.

If tobacco were introduced as a new product at the present time, it might receive acceptance by the U.S. Food and Drug Administration since there is no convincing evidence of experimental emphysema (or cancer) resulting from tobacco smoke. The only present issue is how tobacco smoke produces emphysema. The general view is that some component(s) in tobacco smoke produce inflammation in lung parenchyma, and the best known example is respiratory bronchiolitis. The observed inflammatory response consists mainly of macrophages, which are greatly increased in numbers in smokers and are biochemically more active with increased proteolytic activity. As the cells die, they release their proteolytic enzymes digesting the lung parenchyma. In addition, cigarette smokers have been shown to have decreased activity of alpha-1-antitrypsin activity in their bronchoalveolar lavage fluid due to oxidation of methionine in alpha-1-antitrypsin. This in turn maximizes the damage due to the release of enzymes. This hypothesis, however, ignores the fact that polymorphonuclear, leukocyte-derived elastase is the most effective elastolytic agent and that an increase in polymorphonuclear leukocyte has not been consistently shown in the alveolar walls of smokers or in emphysema.

The proteolysis-antiproteolysis hypothesis of the pathogenesis of emphysema stemmed from two serendipidous observations made almost simultaneously and referred to previously (see p. 543). Gross and co-workers[195] instilled papain into animals with experimental silicosis hoping to ameliorate the lesions. Instead, emphysema resulted. Laurel and Eriksson[194] found that patients with alpha-1-antitrypsin deficiency had a marked predisposition to develop emphysema. It transpired that papain acted mainly on elastin and that elastase was a potent cause of experimental emphysema. Alpha-1-antitrypsin has a potent antielastase activity and, if administered simultaneously with elastase, obviates the development of emphysema.

Why tobacco smoke should produce centrilobular emphysema in the upper zones of the lung and panacinar emphysema in the lower zones of the lung is less clear. Stresses are greater in the upper zones of the lung and thus may produce rupture in the weakened alveolar walls in patients with respiratory bronchiolitis.[235] The reason for the development of panacinar emphysema is less clear. There may be diffuse subtle alveolar wall inflammation, or some component of tobacco smoke may act directly on the interstitial tissue of the alveolar walls.

The role of bronchial inflammation and narrowing in the pathogensis of emphysema has now been markedly de-emphasized. Although bronchiolar narrowing is easy to document in patients with emphysema (see p. 526), this may represent a separate effect of tobacco smoke on the airways resulting in inflammation and subsequent narrowing. Irregularity in shape of airways may be the result of emphysema rather than its cause.

Emphysema-Like Conditions

The Aging Lung

With age, the lung undergoes a predictable set of morphologic and functional changes. Since these change occur in the great majority of subjects, they are thought to be normal. Thus, the enlargement of air spaces that occurs with old age is usually not referred to as emphysema since the definition of emphysema requires abnormal enlargement (see p. 537). It has never been shown, however, that these changes are indeed normal. For example, skin wrinkling and degeneration of elastic tissue are seen in areas consistently exposed to the sun, such as the face, and in areas with intermediate exposure, such as the arms; changes are slight or absent in unexposed areas, such as the buttocks. It may be that the changes in the lung with age are due to environmental pollutants rather than to aging alone. Aging mice brought up in an environment free of pollution and infection did not show the classic changes of aging.[236] No study has compared lung structure in aging humans in a polluted and a clean environment. An alternate approach is to refer to the changes that occur with age as panacinar emphysema.[170]

Changes that Occur in the Lung

Change in Shape. With increasing age, the lung "rounds out."[237] These authors observed an increase in the anteroposterior diameter, perimeter, area, and height until age 59 years in whole lung, paper-mounted sections. Beyond this age, anteroposterior diameter increased more than height; thus, the lung appeared more rounded.

Increase in Alveolar Duct Air. A characteristic change occurs with age in the lung as seen on whole lung, paper-mounted sections. These sections are about 0.25 to 0.5 mm in thickness. Alveoli, being smaller than this, form the solid background of parenchyma in which small air spaces can be seen. These represent respiratory bronchioles, alveolar ducts, and alveolar sacs. As lungs age, these spaces increase in size. This change has been referred to as "ductectasia,"[238] has been documented morphometrically,[3] and is accompanied by a relative decrease in the volume proportion of alveolar air (Fig. 21–41).

Decrease in Complexity of the Alveolar Surface. A consistent finding in humans and animals has been an increase in the mean linear intercept or the average distance between alveolar walls.[159] This distance is reciprocally related to the surface/volume ratio of alveoli. There is also a decrease in alveolar surface area with age (Fig. 21–42) which begins in the third decade. The change in surface/volume ratio also reflects the change in abnormal geometry of the lung.

Loss of Alveolar Wall Tissue. The proportion that alveolar walls form of the lung decreases steadily from about 11 percent at age 20 years to about 8 percent at age 80 years.[159] The precise reason for this loss of tissue is unknown. It may represent the loss of capillary bed which occurs in other organs with age. The proportion of the alveolar wall formed by interalveolar communications (pores of Kohn or fenestrae, see p. 538) has been found by one observer to increase with age in the human,[166] and this may contribute to alveolar wall loss. The author has, in an unpublished study, found that the number of alveoli per unit volume decreased with age. This was initially attributed to increse in lung volume with age, but this is now known not to occur.[225] Thus several causes of loss of alveolar wall tissue exist.

Loss of Elastic Tissue. A decreased amount of elastic tissue fibers in alveoli with age has been described.[239] However, this has not been substantiated biochemically, but there appears to be an increase in elastic tissue in blood vessels, bronchi, and pleura as assessed biochemically. Alveolar wall elastin is unchanged.[159]

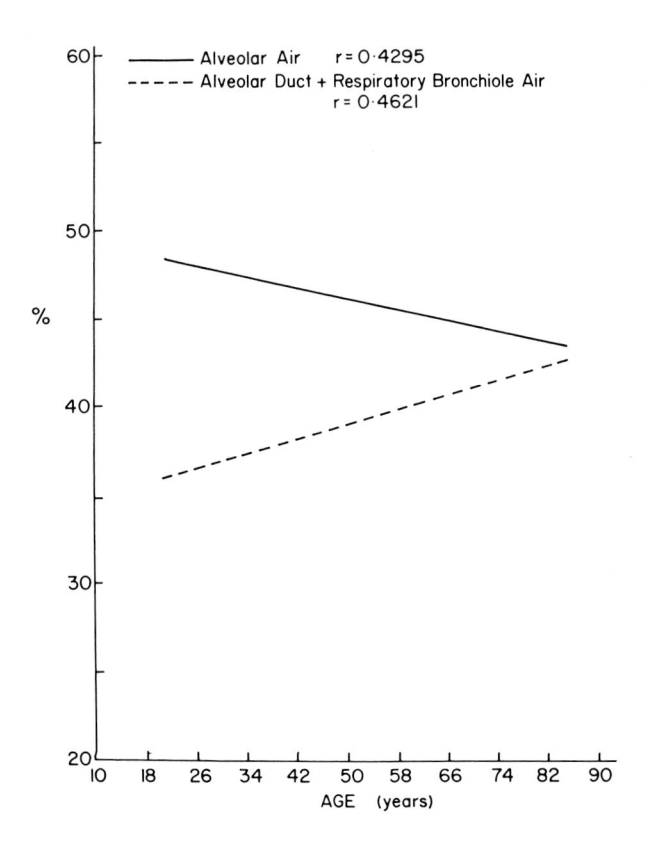

Figure 21–41. When the proportion of the lung that alveolar air and alveolar duct plus respiratory bronchiolar air are expressed as proportion of the lung, alveolar air decreases with age and alveolar duct air increases. From Thurlbeck.[159]

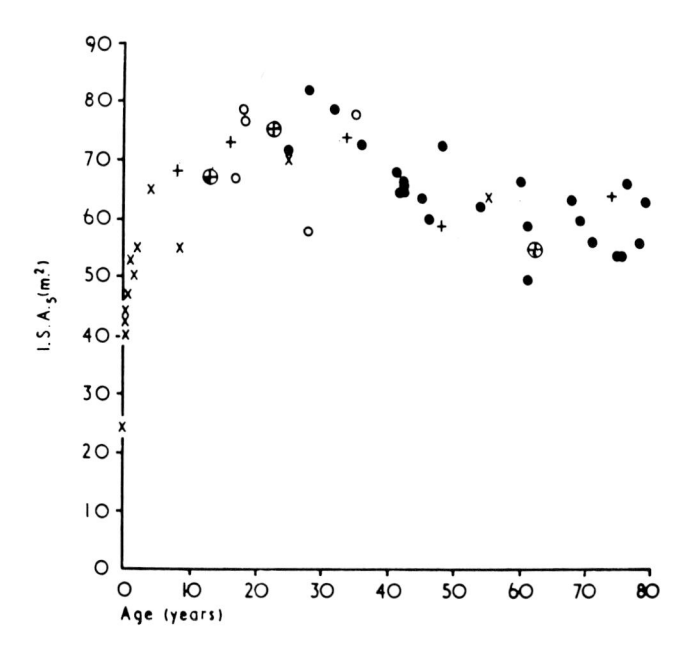

Figure 21–42. When alveolar surface area is expressed at a standard lung volume of 5 L (ISA$_5$) there is a steady decline with age starting at about age 20 years. The symbols represent data from different observers. From Thurlbeck.[171]

Increased Frequency of Emphysema. As shown in Figure 21–43 and discussed on p. 544, with increasing age there is an increase in frequency of emphysema in nonsmokers, mostly panacinar in type. This is perhaps one of the best reasons for referring to the changes that occur in the lung with age in most subjects as the aging lung. Panacinar emphysema is clearly distinguishable from the changes that occur with age, and panacinar emphysema involves only a minority of subjects.

Overinflation of the Lung

Overinflation of the lung may occur in a number of different circumstances, and the acinus may thus be abnormally enlarged. These conditions are not usually referred to as emphysema, however, since there is no destruction of alveolar walls. Also the change may not be detectable. Linear changes are one dimensional and thus will change with the cube root of the changes in volume. Doubling of lung volume, for example, will result in only a 25 percent increase in linear dimensions. Since linear dimensions are variable among individuals, changes due to overinflation will be hard to recognize. Overinflation of the lung occurs in a number of different clinical conditions.

Congenital Lobar Overinflation

This condition, also referred to as congenital lobar emphysema, usually presents as a dramatic clinical syndrome. Shortly after birth, a lobe rapidly overinflates, compressing the remaining lung tissue producing severe respiratory distress. Less commonly, lobar overinflation occurs later in infancy or childhood. The left upper lobe is the most commonly affected one, followed by the right upper lobe.

The lower lobes are rarely affected. Usually only one lobe is involved, but in 10 percent of cases, more than one lobe is affected and the condition may be bilateral.[240] It is much more common in males, and there are associated congenital cardiac anomalies in about 50 percent of patients.

There are several causes of congenital lobar overinflation. In a small number of cases, an obvious cause of obstruction, such as a flap value in the bronchus or vascular compression, may be apparent. The majority of cases may be due to defects in bronchial cartilage.[241,242] The morphologic findings in the affected lobe are not well described. Interstitial fibrosis has been described by some authors[243]; others[244] have described an increase in alveolar size and an increase in number of alveolar above normal—polyalveolar lobe.

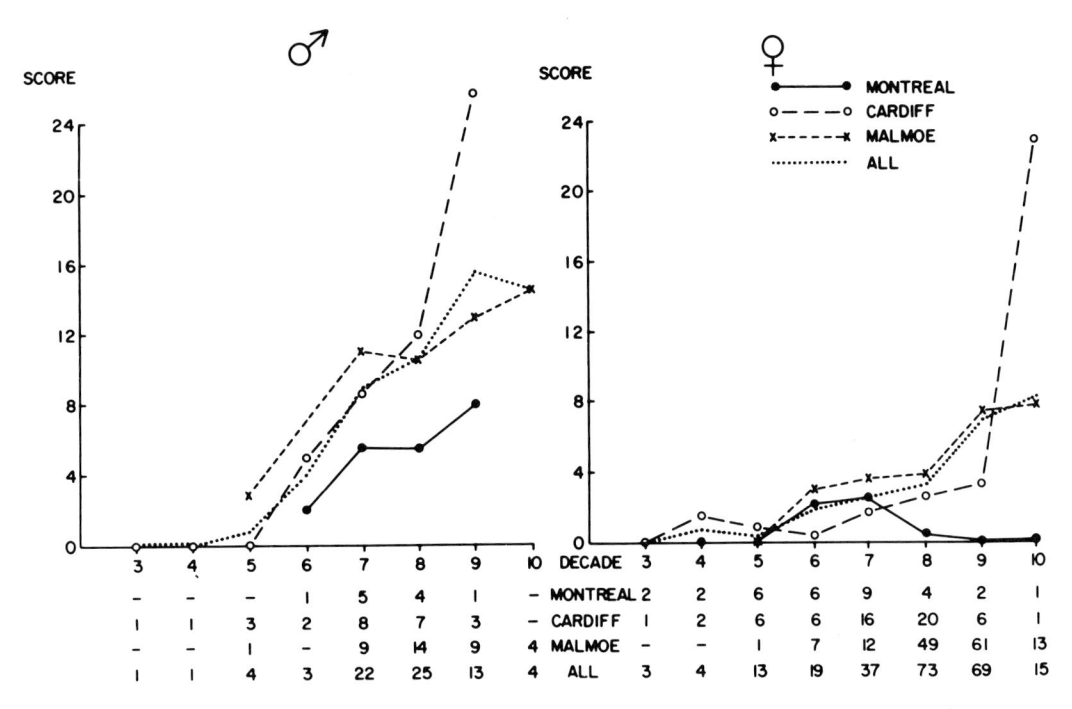

Figure 21–43. The average severity of emphysema by decade in men and women nonsmokers is shown (see Fig. 21–37). ("All" is the average of the three cities). At all ages, the average emphysema score is greater in men than in women and reaches an average score of approximately 15 in males and 6 in women. From Thurlbeck et al.[214]

Acquired Obstructive Overinflation

Overinflation of the lung may result from acquired bronchial obstruction, such as a tumor or inhaled foreign body. Bronchial and bronchiolar obliteration may also produce panacinar emphysema (see page 545). The differences probably reflect the length of time between insult and examination of the specimen. Acute obstruction results in overinflation. If the condition persists, emphysema may intervene.

Compensatory Overinflation

If a lobe collapses or a lung is removed, the remaining lung increases in volume. The increase in volume of the contralateral lung is modest (16 to 40 percent) in humans following pneumonectomy,[245–247] although in animals the lung may expand to equal the volume of both lungs. The changes in the lung have not been described completely in humans. In animals, the appearance of the lung may be confused by compensatory alveolar multiplication.[248] Since pneumonectomy is usually performed in humans after aveolar multiplication has ceased, alveolar enlargement probably occurs, but the changes in linear dimension are likely to be small.

The NHLBI Workshop on the Definition of Emphysema

This workshop, the proceedings of which are unpublished at the present time, may have significant impact on current concepts of emphysema. The definition of emphysema was largely unchanged, but the workshop indicated that the airspace enlargement should not be associated with "obvious" fibrosis. The main reason for introducing this notion was that there appeared to be confusion in the minds of clinicians between honeycomb lung (see Chapter 20) and emphysema. The term air space enlargement with fibrosis was used to describe abnormally enlarged air spaces when there was fibrosis, whether they were lined by alveolar epithelium or not. To pathologists, the confusion between emphysema and honeycomb lung seems a trivial and unlikely event, but this definition has other consequences. More importantly, it raised the question about the amount of fibrosis that may be found in emphysema. Focal areas of fibrosis have been described in centrilobular emphysema, panlobular emphysema, distal emphysema, and even coalworkers' pneumoconiosis; it now becomes imperative to develop an accurate assessment of the amount of fibrosis usually present in emphysema.

The other important concept was the definition of destruction in emphysema. The participants recognized the problems addressed previously in this chapter and thought that the appropriate definition was "loss of the orderly architecture of the acinus of the lung." This implied the distinction between mild emphysema and normal lung by comparison between the two. It also implied that overinflation of the lung or changes in alveolar duct or alveolar dimensions with age were normal since the orderly architecture remains intact.

The impact of this workshop thus remains small. The recognition of emphysema still remains empirical and subjective on the basis of comprison with normal lung tissue, and irregular emphysema becomes irregular air space enlargement with fibrosis.

Bronchiectasis

Once a relatively common condition, bronchiectasis is seldom a clinical problem in the industrialized world. As is the case of emphysema, bronchiectasis is defined as an abnormality of anatomy, has several different associations, and may also be categorized under other disease designations. Bronchiectasis is defined as permanent, abnormal, dilation of bronchi (airways with cartilage and usually bronchial mucous glands in their walls). The qualification permanent is important since bronchial dilation may occur as a consequence of bacterial or viral pneumonia.[249-251] Bronchographically the airways may resemble the usual forms of bronchiectasis but revert to normal within weeks.[252] This is important to recognize. Since bronchiectasis predisposes to infection and pneumonia, surgical resection may be indicated; however, surgery is not required in temporary bronchial dilation following pneumonia.

Bronchial dilation accompanies a variety of other lesions, although the primary cause rather than bronchiectasis may be applied to the condition. For example, bronchial obstruction by tumors or foreign bodies may produce bronchial dilation. Varying degrees of atelectasis may complicate such lesions, and bronchial dilation is usually part of atelectasis but the latter term is usually applied to them. Bronchial dilation occurs in the syndrome of unilateral pulmonary transradiancy (MacLeod's syndrome, Swyer-James syndrome), but these terms are usually used rather than bronchiectasis (see p. 545.). The same is true for intralobar sequestration of the lung (see Chapter 10). Scarring of the lung, as with healed tuberculosis or fibrosing alveolitis (UIP), may have associated bronchial dilation, although the term bronchiectasis is usually not used. In cystic fibrosis (see Chapter 10), widespread bronchiectasis is a common finding but will often not be diagnosed. In cystic fibrosis, the pathogenesis and cause of airflow obstruction—obliteration of peripheral bronchi and bronchioles—are similar to the forms of bronchiectasis discussed below. The same is true of bronchiectasis associated with the immotile cilia syndrome (see p. 564). In both chronic airflow obstruction may be an important feature of the disease. The association of bronchiectasis is shown in Table 21–8.

These examples represent only a minority of examples of bronchiectasis. The remainder occur in patients under consideration, but no satisfactory, more specific terms have been widely adopted. A commonly used term is postinfective bronchiectasis, but a substantial number of patients do not date their symptoms from an infectious episode. Surgical bronchiectasis has also been used, but surgery is seldom performed today. The term idiopathic bronchiectasis will be used, although this has the defect that in many cases the etiology is known or suspected.

Etiology and Pathogenesis of Bronchiectasis

Bronchiectasis occurs in a number of situations in which the term bronchiectasis is not used, and in these an etiologic factor often is apparent. In the remaining cases, infection plays an important role. A history of severe bronchopulmonary infection in childhood has been documented in up to 70 percent of cases, and many of these patients date their symptoms from this episode.[253-256] Whooping cough and measles were common antecedent infections, but with the development of vaccines, these two causes have become much less frequent, and this probably accounts for the diminution in the frequency of bronchiectasis. Adenovirus infection is now an important cause of bronchiectasis, but the most frequent antecedent infection is a nonspecific bronchopneumonia. In the immotile cilia syndrome, the attendant bronchiectasis is similar to the postinfectious form of bronchiectasis described later[257] and its development is greatly modified by treatment.[257,258] Thus, it is probably a consequence of repeated pulmonary infection. Similarly, bronchiectasis in intralobar sequestration is probably due to superimposed infection.

The inflammatory episode may severely affect major bronchi and weaken them, but the major event is obliteration of distal bronchi and bronchioles. This produces varying degrees of atelectasis and results in bronchial dilation. It is the obliterative lesions rather than dilated bronchi that result in obstruction to airflow. Mucus accumulates in the ectatic bronchi for several reasons. Cough is relatively ineffective since the obliterated airways obviate high airflow. Ciliary damage impairs mucus transport, and the distorted shape of airways probably contributes to clearance difficulty. The pools of mucus are susceptible to bacterial colonization, and a vicious cycle is set up with infection further weakening bronchial walls, obliterating further airways, and increasing secretion of mucus.

Classification of Idiopathic Bronchiectasis

A variety of classifications of bronchiectasis have been proposed, but the best is that Reid[74] since it is relatively simple and is clinically relevant. She divided bronchiectasis into three categories (Table 21–9). This classification, which is not widely used, is different from the more usual one of cylindrical and saccular bronchiectasis. The latter

Table 21–8. Classification of Bronchiectasis

1.	Postinfective	Measles
		Pertussis
		Adenovirus
		Tuberculosis
2.	Bronchial obstruction[a]	Foreign bodies
		Tumors
		Mucous plugs
3.	Irritants[a]	Ammonia
4.	Aspiration, especially in heroin addicts	
5.	Hereditary abnormalities[a]	
		Cystic fibrosis
		Immotile cilia syndrome
6.	Cogenital abnormalities	
		Intralobar sequestration[a]
		Congenital bronchiectasis
7.	Immunologic abnormalities	
		Hypogammaglobulinemia
		Neutrophil and macrophage abnormalities
8.	Swyer-James or MacLeod syndrome[a]	
9.	Idiopathic bronchiectasis	

[a] Often not included under bronchiectasis.

becomes uncommon and the most common form is varicose bronchiectasis using the Reid classification.

Saccular Bronchiectasis

The degree of bronchial dilation increases progressively as one proceeds distally. Three to four generations (with the segmental bronchus being generation one) are involved, and the bronchial tree ends in blind sacs. Further airways are seldom found on microscopic examination, so there is extensive bronchial and bronchiolar obliteration.

Varicose Bronchiectasis

In this category, the bronchi are irregularly dilated, and there are sites of relative constriction, and the bronchographic pattern resembles varicose veins. The ectatic bronchi terminate with bulbous ends. About four generations of bronchi can be visualized bronchographically, but further generations can be identified on gross examination; 3 to 12 generations have been found with a mean of 6.5. Histologic sections may show a few more generations.

Cylindrical Bronchiectasis

In this form of bronchiectasis, the bronchi are enlarged and are cylindrical in shape, but they do not diminish in size in a regular fashion as they proceed distally. Bronchographically, the distal airways end abruptly with square ends which are due to obstruction by mucous plugs. The distal bronchi and bronchioles do not fill with contrast material. Substantially more generations of bronchi are visualized bronchographically (6 to 10 generations), grossly (8 to 15), and grossly plus microscopically (15 to 18) compared with other forms of bronchiectasis. The distinction between cylindrical bronchiectasis and broncial dilation in emphysema is not clear, and this question has never been rigorously examined. In full inflation, bronchi are often increased in dimension as visualized bronchographically in subjects with emphysema, but may be unduly narrowed on expiration.[259] Airway occlusion from mucous plugging because of associated bronchitis is common in emphysema. Many cases of cylindrical bronciectasis should probably be considered as emphysema with incidentally associated enlarged airways on inspiration. From 18 to 27 percent of patients with severe emphysema and chronic airflow obstruction will have localized saccular or varicose bronchiectasis.[132,152] In these patients, the bronchiectasis should be regarded as a relatively minor complication of their major disease. This is separate from the observation that bronchiectasis may be primarily responsible for 12 to 14 percent of such patients with severe chronic airflow obstruction.[152,222] These series were from patients who died in the early 1960s, and the frequency of bronchiectasis as a cause of severe chronic airflow obstruction is probably substantially less today.

Gross Lesions

In bronchiectasis the lower lobes are more commonly involved, and the left lower lobe is involved approximately twice as often as the right.[253,260,261] Bronchiectasis is bilateral in 18 to 41 percent of cases.[260–262] More than one lobe on the same side is involved in 20 to 25 percent of cases.[260] The posterior basal segment is particularly involved and in one series, it was involved in more than 90 percent of left lungs.[253] Varying degrees of severity and patterns of bronchial dilation may be observed in the different forms of bronchiectasis. The surfaces of the bronchi are obviously abnormal, and there is usually obvious transverse ridging of the bronchi (Fig. 21–44). In normal bronchi, longitudinal striations are present due to elastic fiber bundles, and these are destroyed in bronchiectasis. Numerous pits in the mucosa are apparent representing a common opening of several dilated ducts of mucous glands (see p. 535). The bronchial epithelium may be reddened due to inflammation and congestion, and secretions are present in the dilated bronchi. This may be mucus, but often in saccular and varicose bronchiectasis, it may be obviously purulent.

Microscopic Lesions

Varying degrees of inflammation are present with bronchiectasis, usually chronic inflammation is obvious, although occasionally inflammation may be minimal. Lymphoid follicles are frequently present in the bronchial walls. Extensive destruction of the bronchial wall is present; muscle, cartilage, and bronchial glands may disappear, and the walls then are formed by fibrous

Table 21–9. Relative Incidence of Types of Bronchiectasis and Extent of Airway Lesions in Each[a]

Type of Bronchiectasis	n	Average No. (Range) of Airway Generations		
		Bronchogram	Gross Examination	Plus Microscopic
Cylindrical	12	7.5 (6–10)	11 (8–13)	16 (15–18)
Varicose	28	4 (2–8)	6.5 (3–12)	8 (3–11)
Saccular	5	3.5 (3–4)	4 (3–4)	4 (3–5)

[a] From Reid.[74]

Bronchiectasis tissue. These changes are most marked in saccular bronchiectasis and mildest in cylindrical bronchiectasis.[263] Bronchial wall atrophy has been noted in severe emphysema; the changes in cylindrical bronchiectasis are similar, further emphasizing the association between emphysema and cylindrical bronchiectasis. Varying degrees of acute inflammation together with ulceration and squamous metaplasia are present, and these changes are more prominent in saccular bronchiectasis.

Lesions in Other Airways

Inflammatory lesions may be present in bronchi that appear normal on bronchography.[264] These lesions may be responsible for the sometimes progressive course of bronchiectasis following resection of bronchiectasis segments or lobes. Airways peripheral to the dilated ones are always abnormal. Extensive obliteration of bronchi and bronchioles is the rule, and this is particularly severe in saccular bronchiectasis.[74,253,258,265] These lesions are pathogenetically important and are responsible for airflow obstruction in bronchiectasis. The airflow obstruction is compounded by secretions in the airways. Peribronchiolar fibrosis and lymphoid follicles are often present in the peripheral airways, and the diagnosis of proximal bronchiectasis can frequently be made when these findings are present in a lung biopsy.

Other abnormalities in the airways include mucous gland enlargement in airways central to the dilated ones[98,152,266] and reflect airway inflammation and may be responsible for the hypersecretion of mucus. It is inappropriate to refer to these changes as chronic bronchitis since mucus hypersecretion in these patients has a specific cause (see p. 529).

Tumorlets are common findings in bronchiectasis.[267] There are proliferation of K (Kulchitsky or argentaffin) cells that result in clusters of spindle, oat, or round cells that resemble carcinoids or oat cells carcinomas. They are usually found in distal bronchioles or respiratory bronchioles, associated with scarring. Clusters of similar cells may be found in lymphatics. It used to be thought that these lesions represented an early stage of oat cell carcinoma, but the frequent finding of tumorlets in young subjects with bronchiectasis make this unlikely.

Parenchymal Lesions

Lesions in the lung parenchyma are the rule in bronchiectasis, but they vary widely in severity and type. At one extreme, there may be almost complete loss of alveolated tissue which is replaced by fibrous tissue. At the other extreme, the lung parenchyma may be overinflated or even emphysematous. Unilateral pulmonary transradiancy (Swyer-James or MacLeod syndrome) is a form of bronchiectasis in which distal bronchiolar obliteration but not parenchymal collapse ensues (see p. 545).

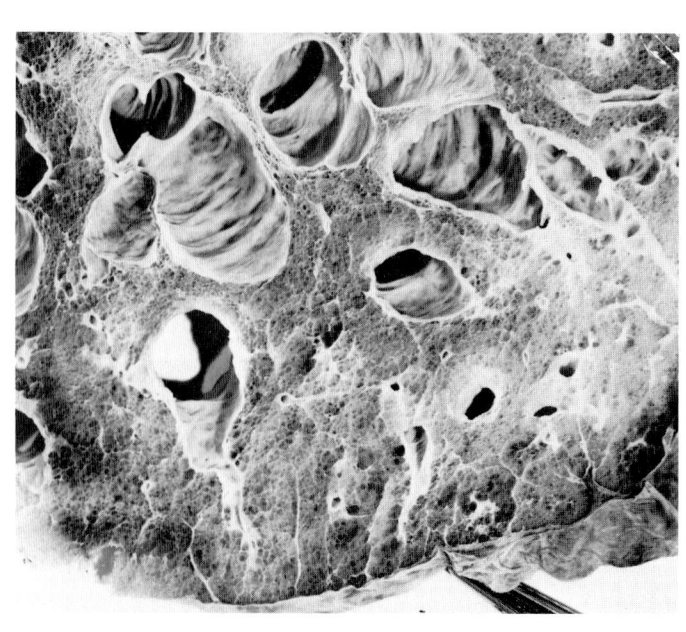

Figure 21–44. An example of varicose bronchiectasis illustrates the irregular dilation of proximal bronchi, with transverse ridging together with pits in their walls. Note narrowed and obliterated distal bronchi and bronchioles (below). From Thurlbeck.[159]

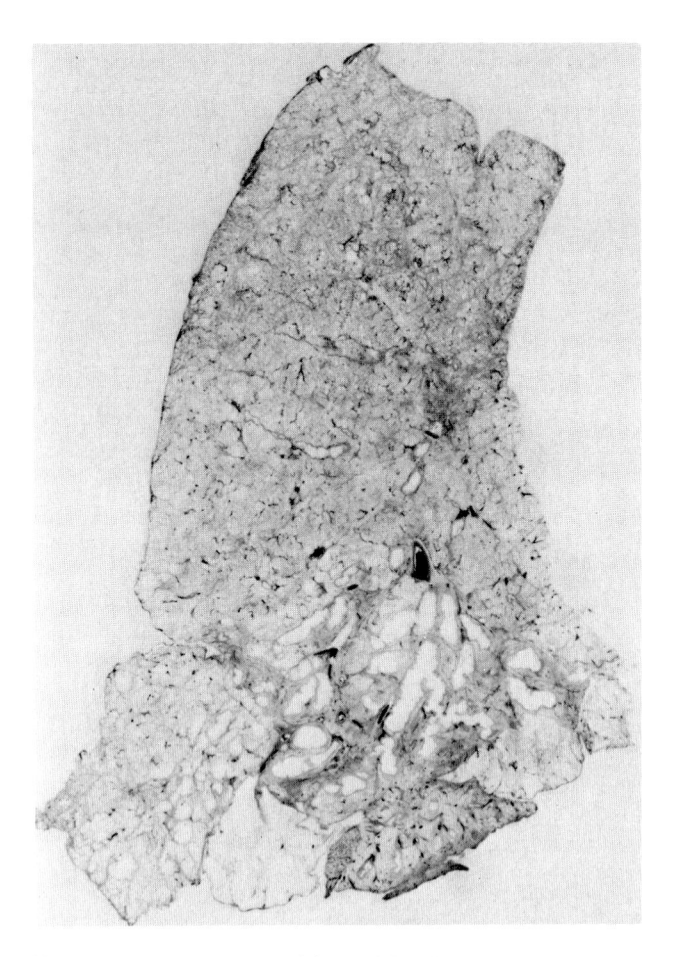

Figure 21–45. A resected lower lobe shows bronchiectasis in the basal segments associated with obvious emphysema. From Thurlbeck.[159]

In the usual case, collapse and fibrosis of parenchyma are dominant, but varying degrees of emphysema may be present (Fig. 21–45).

There is a distinct overlap between patients whose primary abnormality is emphysema and those whose primary abnormality is bronchiectasis. Localized bronchiectasis is commonly found in emphysema, and emphysema is a complication of bronchiectasis. The distinction is usually easy since in the former, emphysema is widespread and bronchiectasis is localized, and in the latter, emphysema is localized to the bronchiectatic regions. In some instances, it may be impossible to decide which is the primary lesion and what is mainly responsible for the patients pulmonary dysfunction.[152] Cylindrical bronchiectasis and widespread bronchial dilation in severe emphysema may be the same condition.

Bronchial Arteries in Bronchiectasis

Characteristically there is considerable enlargement of the bronchial arteries in bronchiectasis,[268] representing the response to continued inflammation, blood supply to granulation tissue, and the development of fibrous tissue (bronchial arteries supply new tissue, even tumors, that arises in the lung). There is an appropriate increase in the size of bronchial veins, and this may lead to an increased left to right shunt. In addition extensive anastomoses develop between pulmonary arteries and bronchial arteries, and these may occasionally be so extensive that there may be retrograde flow of blood in the pulmonary artery.

Clinical Features

Bronchiectasis may be regarded as an incidental feature in a patient characterized as having another disease such as fibrocystic disease, right middle lobe syndrome, or Swyer-James syndrome, among others. In the usual case, the symptoms date from childhood or infancy, often to an episode of bronchopulmonary infection. The key symptom is chronic productive cough. Sputum production may be profuse and is often purulent. Hemoptysis may occur. Intermittent pulmonary infections are frequent. Clubbing is a feature of extensive, long-standing bronchiectasis. In most instances, the overall effect on function is slight but when bronchiectasis is widespread, a significant impairment may result with concomitant dyspnea and cyanosis. Radiologically abnormalities are present in more than 90 percent of instances on the plain roentgenogram. These consist of increased bronchial markings, overcrowding of bronchi, and loss of lung volume locally. Cystically dilated bronchi may be visualized. The changes are well visualized bronchographically. Surprisingly, computed tomography has not been useful.[269] Pulmonary function effects are variable. Some loss of total lung capacity is usual, and other changes depend on the degree of airflow obstruction. In some instances, the defect appears to be entirely restrictive; rarely it may be almost entirely obstructive. In most instances, varying combinations are found. (Some other aspects of bronchiectasis, notably pathogenesis and treatment, are included in Chapter 25.)

Congenital Bronchiectasis

The existence of congenital bronchiectasis has been challenged,[270] although a congenital basis for bronchiectasis dates to 1880.[271] The reason for the doubt includes a lack of symptoms or findings of bronchiectasis in the newborn period and lack of familial cases.[270] Many cases claiming to be congenital bronchiectasis have several of the features of idiopathic bronchiectasis. However, Williams and Campbell[272] described bronchiectasis associated with cartilage deficiency, and further cases have been reported by Williams and colleagues[273] and Wayne and Taussig[274]; the latter described two clinical cases in siblings who dated their symptoms from infancy.

The cases described by Williams and Campbell[272] and Williams and colleagues[273] had many of the usual features of idiopathic bronchiectasis, including persistent productive cough, rales, and crowding of bronchi radiographically. Unusual features included the onset of symptoms usually in the first year of life and airway dilation and collapse of the third to eighth generation bronchi during tidal breathing. The bronchographic abnormalities were disproportionately abnormal compared with the duration of infections. The findings were bilateral, and the lungs appeared overinflated radiographically. Morphologic examination has only been performed in two cases,[272,275] and these showed a uniform lack of cartilage in the bronchi but persistence of cartilage at bronchial bifurcations, lack of destruction of other components of the bronchial wall, and extension to involve the first and second segmental orders in which dilation was not found. The evidence indicates that this syndrome (Williams-Campbell syndrome) exists and that it is congenital in nature.

Congenital bronchiectasis may be recognized grossly. Usually an entire lobe or lung is involved. The lung is pink and inflates and deflates readily.[276] In contrast, in acquired bronchiectasis, the lesions are segmental or sublobar, the lung is firm and dull slate blue, and it fails to inflate.[276]

Asthma

Asthma is covered elsewhere (see Chapter 22), but reference to it should be made here. Asthma is distinguished from other diseases associated with chronic airflow obstruction by the reversibility of the airflow obstruction. In asthma, airflow obstruction varies in severity, whereas the other diseases discussed in this chapter have fixed airflow obstruction. Patients with typical asthma usually do not develop emphysema or fixed airflow obstruction. Important overlaps do exist, however. Although asthmatic attacks are usually readily reversible, there is often evidence of some expiratory flow obstruction between attacks although the patient may appear well. Similarly about 15 percent of patients with typical chronic airflow obstruction due to bronchitis, bronchiolitis, or emphysema will have a significant reversible component to their chronic airflow obstruction with bronchodilators. Patients with asthma have an increase in size of mucous glands as do bronchitics, and some patients with bronchitis have the increased bronchial muscle so characteristic of patients with asthma. From 15 to 20 percent of patients with asthma have saccular bronchiectasis and subpleural fibrosis most commonly in the upper lobe, an uncommon site for bronchiectasis.[126,132,277] The pathogenesis is uncertain. Dunnill[132] ascribed it to bronchial obstruction and atelectasis because of mucous plugs, but Leopold[126] attributed it to organization of eosinophilic pneumonia. Recently it has been suggested that patients with long-standing history of asthma but dying of other causes may have lesions in their peripheral airways.[278] Although asthma and diseases associated with chronic airflow obstruction may have different etiologies, lesions, and clinical features, there is a small group of patients that is difficult to define clinically, and asthma should always be regarded as integral part of chronic airflow obstruction.

Alterations in Other Organs in Chronic Airflow Obstruction

At this stage, it is appropriate to describe changes in other organs that are found in chronic airflow obstruction. Generally these have not been identified with specific conditions associated with chronic airflow obstruction, but when possible the correlations will be made.

The Cardiovascular System

The clinicopathologic correlations of cardiac disease in chronic airflow obstruction have been dealt with in part previously (see page 552). Other aspects will be dealt with here.

Cor Pulmonale

The term cor pulmonale is an ambiguous one and is often applied to right ventricular hypertrophy as assessed morphologically, electrocardiographically, or radiologically, but it is also applied to apparent heart failure as judged by raised jugular venous pressure, hepatomegaly, or peripheral edema in patients with chronic airflow obstruction. Because of the confusion, two expert committees have defined cor pulmonale.[279,280] A functional definition was thought inappropriate since features such as pulmonary hypertension and increased pulmonary vascular resistance were extremely variable from time to time and because of the difficulty of their measurement. The committee thus chose an anatomic basis, and cor pulmonale was defined as "hypertrophy of the right ventricle resulting from disease affecting the function and/or structure of the lung, except where the pulmonary alterations are the result of diseases that primarily affect the left side of the heart or of congenital heart disease."

Right ventricular hypertrophy is traditionally measured by thickness of the right ventricle at autopsy. This assessment has serious defects since it is a one-dimensional measurement of a three-dimensional change and depends on the obliquity of section of the right ventricle and where the measurement is made. Right ventricular thickness will also be diminished if there is dilation of the ventricle. In 1952 Fulton and associates[281] dissected off the right ventricle and compared it with the weight of the left ventricle and septum. The heart is divided at the atrioventricular ring. The right ventricle is cut flush with the septum, and the trabeculae are included in its weight. Fulton and associates also separated the left ventricle from the septum. This is not necessary for routine purposes. They also dissected off the fat and superficial vessels, but this step is usually omitted. They suggested that the upper limit of the weight of the right ventricle was 65 g, the left ventricle 125 g, and the septum 60 g. They found that right ventricular hypertrophy so defined occurred in 94 percent of patients with left ventricular failure and suggested that a ratio of left ventricle plus septal weight was the best way of assessing right ventricular hypertrophy. They suggested that the normal range was 2.3 to 3.3, and a ratio below this indicated right ventricular hypertrophy and above this, left ventricular hypertrophy.

Pulmonary Arterial System

Cor pulmonale in chronic airflow obstruction is primarily a consequence of hypoxemia[159] which in turn leads to pulmonary arterial muscle contraction and pulmonary hypertension. The role of hypercarbia and acidosis is less clear.[159] Other factors involved include increased blood volume,[282] polycythemia, and an increase in frequency of thromboemboli with an incidence between 13 and 62 percent being reported.[43,44,46,152,182] Restriction of the vascular bed due to destruction in emphysema cannot be excluded.[221]

Despite the frequent occurrence of right ventricular hypertrophy, morphologic changes in the pulmonary arterial system are generally slight in chronic airflow obstruction compared with other causes of pulmonary hypertension. This is also true of pulmonary hypertension due to hypoxemia of other causes such as high altitude and kyphoscoliosis.[283] An increase in muscle was found in the smallest pulmonary arteries (less than 100 μm in diameter) in which muscle is usually scanty or absent. Authors[283] pointed out that these vessels may be directly exposed to alveolar air and may respond directly to alveolar hypoxia. An increase in muscle in the small muscular pulmonary arteries (100 to 300 μm in diameter), so characteristic of other forms of pulmonary hypertension, was not reported by them. They attributed the relatively minor changes in the pulmonary arteries to the mild and episodic nature of pulmonary hypertension in chronic airflow obstruction.

Wagenvoort and Wagenvoort found an increase in medial thickness of 60 percent of patients with chronic airflow obstruction and hypoxemia and an increase in number of arteries less than 70 μm in diameter.[284] In patients with emphysema, abnormal longitudinal muscle appeared in the intima of arteries up to 800μ in diameter,[285] and sometimes longitudinal muscle was found external to the outer elastic lamina. With progression of the lesion, there was fibrosis in and around the intimal longitudinal muscle, together with splitting of the internal elastic lamina and fibrosis. These changes occurred in emphysema whether or not it was associated with right ventricular hypertrophy, and Hicken and his colleagues attributed these changes to stretching of the vessels in emphysematous lungs.[285]

Hale and co-workers[23] found an increase in arterial media and intima and proportion of vessels less than 200 μm in diameter in smokers; this was related to both local lesions in peripheral airways and emphysema. Similar abnormalities were noted by Wright and associates[31] in smokers, and these were also related to peripheral airway lesions. In another study (Russell L, Cooney TP, Thurlbeck WM, unpublished data), the major change in patients with chronic airflow obstruction and hypoxemia in the National Institutes of Health Intermittent Positive Pressure Breathing Trial was an increase in arterial intimal area and an increase in proportion of vessels less than 100 μm in diameter. Changes in the pulmonary arterial system in emphysema, high altitude, and hypoxia are also discussed elsewhere (*see* Chapter 24).

Pulmonary Veins

Changes in pulmonary veins have also been described in about half of patients with chronic airflow obstruction and right ventricular hypertrophy.[286] These changes consisted of medial hypertrophy and arterialization (a distinct internal and external elastic lamina at least on part of the circumference) of pulmonary veins less than 150 μm in diameter. Similar changes were seen in high-altitude residents and a patient with a Pickwickian syndrome. This finding suggests that either hypoxemia induces vasoconstriction or left ventricular failure (*see* later).

Bronchial Arteries and Veins

Bronchial arteries have been found to be increased in patients with chronic airflow obstruction by most observers,[287–289] but decreased in emphysema in one study.[290] The most likely explanation for this is bronchial inflammation associated with chronic bronchitis. Bronchial veins have also been found to be enlarged in chronic airflow obstruction[287,289,291]; this may result in a significant right to left shunt, aggravating preexisting hypoxemia.[291]

Left Ventricular Hypertrophy

Left ventricular hypertrophy has been encountered consistently in patients dying of chronic airflow obstruction, and an incidence of 15 to 30 percent has generally been reported.[159] Similarly clinical evidence of left ventricular dysfunction and raised pulmonary wedge pressure has been reported, although the issue is controversial.[159] In many instances, these changes are due to coincidental cardiac disease, but in a small proportion of cases, the left ventricular hypertrophy appears to be due to chronic airflow obstruction.[159] Left ventricular hypertrophy usually occurs in those patients with severe hypoxemia and massive right ventricular hypertrophy. Under these circumstances, the left ventricle plus septum/right ventricular weight ratio may be misleading.

Cardiac Atrophy

One study has shown diminished left ventricular size in patients with severe emphysema, although the right ventricle was enlarged[292]; this has been attributed to lowered systemic blood pressure in patients with severe emphysema.[293] As will be indicated later, loss of body weight occurs in patients with chronic airflow obstruction, especially with emphysema, and this may be the cause of, or contribute to, cardiac atrophy.

Loss of Body Weight

As emphysema increases in severity as assessed at necropsy, body weight decreases, and this is apparent even in relatively mild grades of emphysema.[294] Diminished body weight is a feature of patients with chronic airflow obstruction, especially those with clinically apparent severe emphysema[159,295–297] and is related to diminution of FEV_1, FEV_1/FVC ratio and diffusing capacity.[295–297] About 27 percent of patients with chronic obstructive lung disease have loss of weight, and there is loss of muscle as well as fat; evidence of anergy was present in about a quarter.[295,297,298] Several reasons have been suggested. Smoking and consequent reduction of appetite may play a role, but the loss of weight in smokers was found only in those with airflow obstruction.[296] Increased oxygen consumption was related to loss of body weight,[297] and nutritional intake appeared normal[298]; thus, increased work of breathing may be the main factor. The observation that starvation produces emphysema-like changes in rats[299] suggests that undernutrition may aggravate emphysema in humans.

Diaphragm

The earlier literature was conflicting, with some observers finding hypertrophy or thickening of the diaphragm in patients with emphysema or chronic airflow obstruction[300,301] and others finding the diaphragm was smaller and weighed less.[302,303] Recent data have indicated that diaphragm area and mass are reduced in emphysema[294,304,305] and that diaphragm muscle mass, area, thickness, and length were reduced in some patients with chronic airflow obstruction.[305] Diaphragm weight has been found to be closely related to loss of body weight and body muscle mass,[294,305] although there may be further diminished diaphragm weight in patients with severe emphysema.[294] Diaphragm fiber diameter has been found to be significantly decreased in patients with chronic airflow obstruction.[306] These changes are significant ones because of the central role of the diaphragm in respiration, and nutritional depletion has been shown to be associated with respiratory muscle weakness.[307]

Peptic Ulceration

Numerous studies have shown an increased frequency of peptic ulceration in patients with chronic airflow obstruction, and prevalences between 15.4 and 42.9 percent have been recorded.[159] These ulcers have been described in the stomach and duodenum with about the same distribution as in patients without chronic airflow obstruction. Ulceration tends to be particularly severe and was the primary cause of death in 12 percent of patients with chronic airflow obstruction in one series.[308] High carbon dioxide content of the blood has been shown to increase secretion of gastric acid[309] and may account for the particularly high frequency of peptic ulcer, often acute, in patients with cor pulmonale and hypercapnea.[310,311] An alternate link is through cigarette smoking[312] which produces gastric hypersecretion or because of a personality type liable to both cigarette smoking and ulcer.

Kidney and Glomerular Enlargement

Kidney enlargement was noted in 22 percent of an autopsy series of patients with chronic airflow obstruction.[313] Glomerular enlargement was noted, and this was confirmed by Ishikawa and coworkers[314] who, however, did not find renal enlargement in patients with severe emphysema and cor pulmonale. Glomerular enlargement, increased glomerular cellularity and lobulation, and mesangial widening were reported in another series without renal enlargement.[315] Increased glomerular size was described recently in patients with hypoxic cor pulmonale, but no increase in kidney size was found.[316] The proportion of glomeruli with an identifiable juxtaglomerular apparatus was increased with increasing glomerular size. Arterial oxygen tension was closely related to glomerular size. These authors suggested glomerular changes reflected changes in renal salt and water metabolism. Patients treated with long-term domicilliary oxygen had slightly smaller glomeruli (although not significantly) than those not so treated, and the authors suggested that the glomerular lesions were potentially reversible with oxygen therapy. Since glomeruli form a small proportion of the kidney, it seems unlikely that the consistently observed changes would result in enlargement of the kidneys.

Tracheobronchopathica Osteoplastica

As a symptomatic condition, tracheobronchopathica osteoplastica is extremely rare; however, it was an incidental finding in about 1 of 200 autopsies.[317] It is more common in men and is usually found in subjects older than 50 years, but it has been described in children. Numerous irregularly shaped masses of cartilage and bone are found in the submucosa of trachea and bronchi. They are in continuity with the cartilage rings and plates of the trachea and bronchus which may in turn may be ossified. On gross examination, the affected airways are stiffened, and there are numerous protrusions visible below the surface of the airway epithelium (Fig. 21–46). They are hard, 2 to 3 mm in diameter, and may follow tracheal rings or lie between them. The lower two-thirds of the trachea are mainly involved, but the process may extend into the major bronchi, and the larynx and true vocal cords may also be involved. The overlying surface epithelium is usually intact.

Microscopically the nodules consist of mature bone and cartilage, and in the former, bone marrow is present. The epithelium over the nodules may be thinned to a single layer of cuboidal epithelium,[318] show basal cell hyperplasia or squamous metaplasia,[319] or be ulcerated.[320] Amyloid may be seen in the airway, and it has been suggested that tracheobronchopathica osteoplastica and bronchial amyloidosis are the same conditions.[321–322a] More recent evidence indicates that they are separate.[318,322b] The evidence cited included the lack of amyloid in at least some, and possibly most, cases,

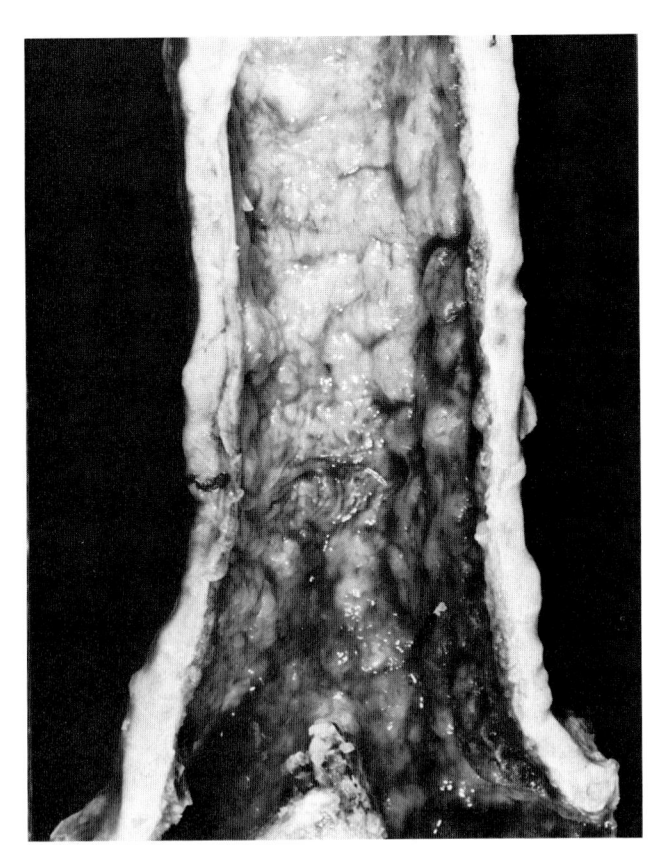

Figure 21-46. Tracheobronchopathica osteoplastica. Numerous nodules of ossified cartilage can be seen deep to the epithelium. The lesion extends into proximal bronchi (below). Courtesy Dr. A Churg.

especially early ones; the nodules in amyloidosis represent stromal metaplasia, whereas in tracheopathica osteoplastica they are ecchondroses; the disappearance of amyloid has not been noted, so it seems unlikely that tracheal amyloid could evolve to tracheopathica osteoplastica without a trace of amyloid. The nature and etiology of tracheobronchopathica osteoplastica are unknown. Symptoms when present are nonspecific and include cough, sputum, wheezing, and dyspnea[319]; hemoptysis has been described. In some subjects, there may be extensive involvement of the airways, and airflow obstruction results.[322c]

Bronchial Amyloidosis

Amyloid may be found in airways as well as in lung parenchyma (see Chapter 20). In the latter situation, it may be nodular or diffuse. The nodular form may present clinically as multiple nodules in the lung mimicking mestastases; the diffuse form, which is extremely rare, is usually associated with diffuse amyloidosis and cardiac amyloid. Bronchial amyloid may be localized and produce localized obstruction. Diffuse bronchial deposits are more common and have a gross appearance similar to tracheobronchopathica osteoplastica, and there may be ossification of the amyloid.

Tracheobronchomegaly (Mournier-Kuhn Syndrome)

Tracheobronchomegaly is a rare condition; 57 cases had been reported by 1973.[323] As its name denotes, it is characterized by marked dilation of trachea, bronchi, and even the larynx. Other terms used to describe this condition include megatrachea, tracheobronchiectasis, and tracheomalacia. It can be regarded as a form of cylindrical bronchiectasis, but it is distinguished by the fact that the trachea is also greatly dilated and by the absence of peripheral airway lesions. Although it is a disease affecting mostly men, the majority whom are in the third and fourth decade,[324,328] it is thought to be a congenital disorder and a familial occurrence has been noted.[325] The trachea and major bronchi are involved, and histologically there is atrophy of all components of the bronchial wall. Clinically there is marked collapsability of the airways on expiration, patients suffer from repeated bronchopulmonary infections, and there may be associated chronic airflow obstruction.

Tracheal Stenosis

Tracheal stenosis is a common complication of prolonged intubation and assisted ventilation, and stridor is noted in 5 percent of patients after intratracheal intubation.[329] It occurs both in infants with the infantile distress syndrome and adults with the adult respiratory distress syndrome who require prolonged ventilation.

Tracheal stenosis may occur at the level of the tracheostomy site, at the level of the inflated cuff, or where the tip of the tracheostomy tube rubs against the tracheal mucosa. About two-thirds occur at the tracheostomy site and nearly all of the remainder at the level of the cuff.[330] Only rarely does the stenosis occur at the site of the tip of the tube. Stenosis at the tracheostomy site is a consequence of direct injury which results in fibrosis. The pressure within the cuffed balloon may exceed capillary pressure with resultant ischemic necrosis of the mucosa, and this may extend to involve tracheal cartilage.[331] Narrowing may result from fibrous stenosis, granulation tissue, or expiratory collapse due to tracheomalacia.[332] Usually no symptoms are present when the tracheostomy tube is removed, but shortly afterward dyspnea, stridor, and difficulty raising secretions may be noted. Upper airway obstruction may not be noted for several weeks, and resection may be required.[333]

Relapsing Perichondritis

This is an inflammatory disease that affects cartilage of the tracheobronchial tree, ribs, ear lobes, nose, and joints. Its etiology is unknown, but the association of vasculitis, iritis, and aortitis suggests that it may be related to the collagen vascular diseases.[334] Involvement of the trachea and bronchi may result in severe airflow obstruction, and airway involvement is responsible for death and disability in this condition. Histologically there is a round cell infiltrate in and around the cartilage, destruction of cartilage, and fibrosis.[335]

Immotile Cilia Syndrome*

The Basic Defect

In the immotile cilia syndrome, heritable structural abnormalities of the axoneme lead to ineffective or absent beating of respiratory cilia. The predictable results are failure of mucociliary clearance and recurrent upper and lower respiratory tract infections. Half the affected subjects have complete situs inversus or dextrocardia and thus fulfill Kartagener's triad. Men with this syndrome are usually sterile. In fact, the syndrome was originally discovered during the investigation of sterility in men who proved to have normal spermatoza except that they exhibited no flagellar movement.[336,337] Electron microscopy showed absence of dynein arms on the flagellar axoneme. Most of these patients had situs inversus and repeated sinobronchial infections.[336,338]

A number of different structural abnormalities of the axoneme are now known to give rise to the immotile cilia syndrome. The most common is absence of both dynein arms (Fig. 21–47). Alternatively there may be selective absence of either inner or outer dynein arms.[339] The entire radial spokes may be missing[340] or the spoke heads selectively.[339] Several complex abnormalities have been described including combined absence of the inner dynein arm and spoke head,[341] absence of the entire axoneme,[342,343] and a lesion known as microtubular transposition[344] in which the two central singlet microtubules were absent and one of the peripheral doublets crossed to the center in the lower third of the axoneme to occupy the position of the central pair. In addition to the missing structures, it is common to observe secondary ultrastructural abnormalities in the cilia in affected patients. In normal subjects, it is usual for the plane of the central pair of singlet tubules of the individual cilia to be parallel and for the basal feet to project from the basal bodies all in the same direction. In the immotile cilia syndrome, these orderly orientations are lost.[345] In some patients, many of the cilia have supernumerary microtubules (Fig. 21–48). When the primary defect involves the radial spokes, there is loss of the regular spacing of the peripheral doublets equidistant from the central pair complex.[345]

The arguments for considering the abnormalities hereditary have been summarized by Afzelius.[346] Genetic abnormalities of the axoneme are well documented in lower species, notably the flagellate alga *Clamydomonas reinhardi*. The clinical abnormalities in humans appear early in life. The condition is familial and is particularly common at least in Sweden, in regions where inbreeding is prevalent. The ultrastructural abnormalities of the axoneme are consistent within a given family.[347]

If living ciliated cells obtained from patients with the syndrome are examined microscopically in wet mounts maintained at 37°C, several patterns of ciliary activity can be seen. In some patients, none of the cells beat, but in others a variable fraction of cells (from 1 to 40 percent in various reports) will display abnormal movements. The cilia beat at a diminished frequency, without consistent direction or metachronal coordination.[348–351] Cilia with each type of ultrastructural defect have a different pattern of oscillation or vibration.[351] Because the beat is so often abnormal and ineffective rather than absent, there is

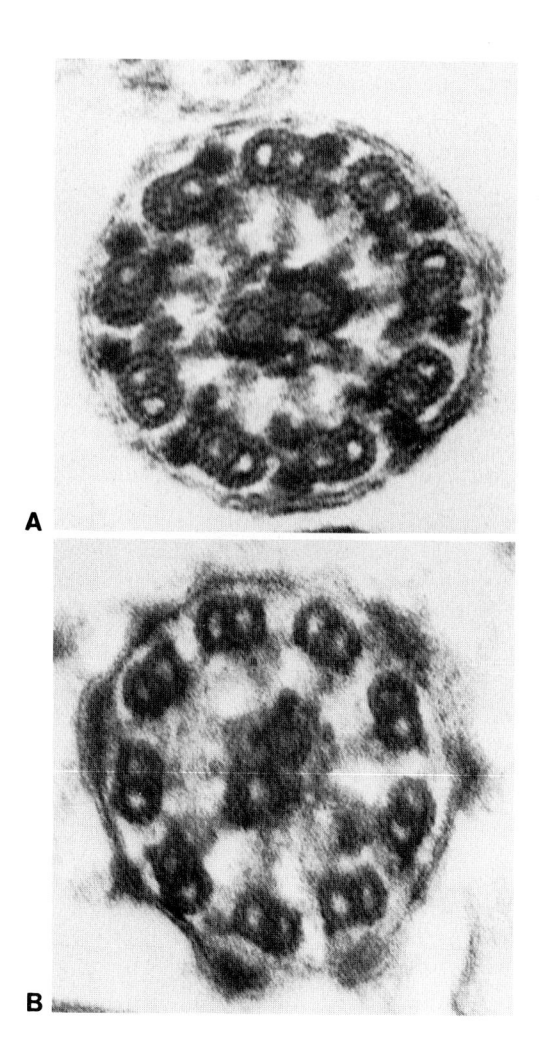

Figure 21–47. A. Cross-section of a normal cilium with two dynein arms projecting in a clockwise rotation from each of the nine peripheral doublet microtubules. B. Immotile cilia syndrome lacking both inner and outer dynein arms. Both electron micrographs after fixation with tannic acid and glutaraldehyde ($\times 250{,}000$).

---

*The section on *Immotile Cilia Syndrome* was written by Charles Kuhn III.

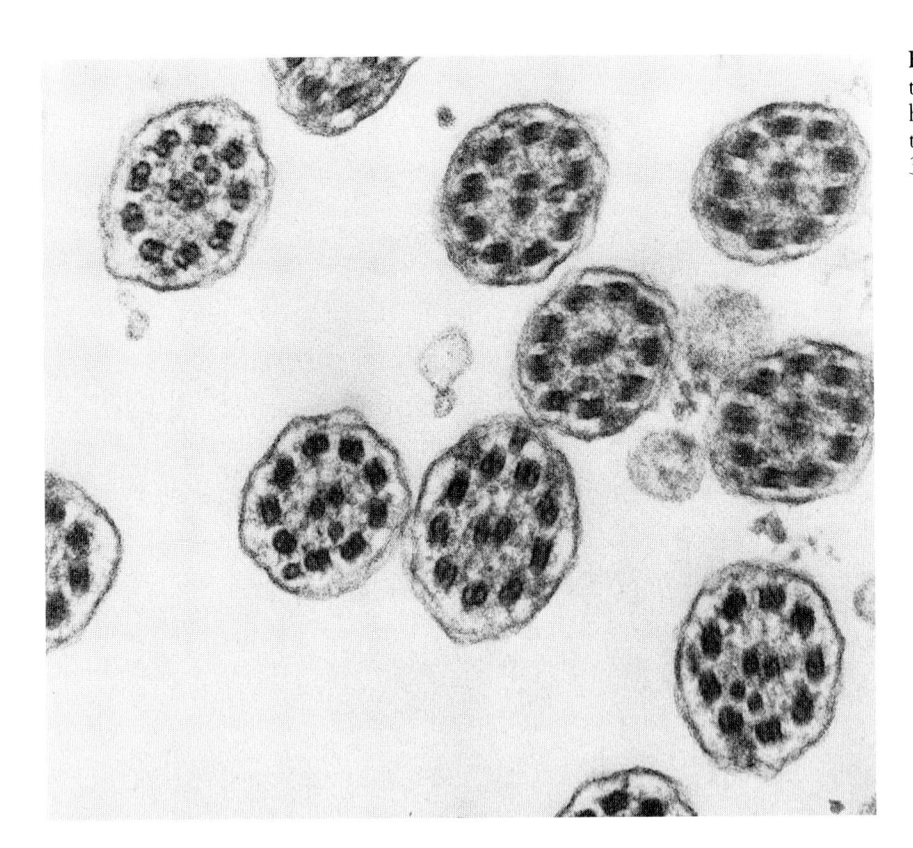

Figure 21-48. Immotile cilia syndrome due to dynein arm deficiency. Note that most cilia have an extra singlet microtubules giving them a 9 + 3, 9 + 4, 1 + 9 + 2, or 1 + 9 + 3 structure (×110,000).

current enthusiasm for replacing the term immotile cilia syndrome with ciliary dyskinesia.

Clinical Features[352-354]

In the immotile cilia syndrome, symptoms begin early in life, often in infancy. Patients suffer from repeated bouts of otitis media, sinusitis, chest infections, and pneumonia; 50 percent have situs inversus or dextrocardia. Nasal polyps are common. Chronic cough is invariably present. Permanent bronchial damage develops after a variable period of time, beginning as cylindrical bronchiectasis which later becomes varicose or saccular. Typically the bronchiectasis is localized and affects the lower lobes, thus resembling the common postinfectious bronchiectasis rather than the diffuse bronchiectasis seen with cystic fibrosis. A minority of patients have clubbing of the digits. Pulmonary function testing shows an obstructive ventilatory pattern with air trapping. Resting hypoxemia is the rule. The abnormalities show little tendency to progress over time, and long-term survival appears to be possible despite chronic symptoms.[352,354]

Diagnosis

The diagnosis of immotile cilia syndrome should be considered in any patient in whom recurrent sinobronchial infections begin early in life, especially when there is situs inversus or a family history and the sweat test is normal. Screening can be carried out by demonstrating impaired mucociliary clearance or by light microscopic examination of the motility of living ciliated epithelial cells. Nasal biopsy frequently fails to provide ciliated epithelium, but an adequate sample for light microscopy can be obtained from the inferior turbinate with a curette or a bronchial brush,[355] and often this tiny sample can be retrieved for electron microscopy.

The addition of 0.1 percent tannic acid to the aldehyde fixative used for electron microscopy improves the visualization of the structure of the axoneme. It is important to study an adequate number of properly oriented cilia to be certain that a consistent abnormality is present in all, or at least the great majority. Some abnormal cilia can be found in normal subjects[356,357] and are more common in those with bronchial disease.[358] Compound cilia, abnormalities of microtubules, especially of the central pair, and minor degrees of dynein arm loss commonly affect a few cilia in those without the immotile cilia syndrome.

References

1. Ciba Guest Symposium Report: Terminology, definitions and classification of chronic pulmonary emphysema and related conditions. Thorax 14:286–299, 1959.

2. Macklem PT: Airway obstruction and collateral ventilation. Physiol Rev 51:368–436, 1971.

3. Weibel ER: *Morphometry of the Human Lung.* New York: Academic Press, 1963.

4. Hayward J, Reid L: Observations on anatomy of intrasegmental bronchial tree. Thorax 7:89–97, 1952.

5. Horsfield K, Cumming G: Morphology of the bronchial tree in man. J Appl Physiol 24:373–383, 1968.

6. Macklem PT, Mead J: Resistance of central and peripheral airways measured by retrograde catheter. J Appl Physiol 22:395–401, 1967.

7. Hogg JC, Macklem PT, Thurlbeck WM: The site and nature of airway obstruction in chronic obstructive lung disease. N Engl J Med 278:1355–1360, 1968.

8. Niewoehner DE, Kleinerman J: Morphologic basis of pulmonary resistance in the human lung and the effects of aging. J Appl Physiol 36:412–418, 1974.

9. Hoppin FG Jr, Green M, Morgan MS: The relationship of central and peripheral airway resistance to lung volume in dogs. J Appl Physiol 44:728–737, 1978.

10. Kappos AD, Rodarte JR, Lai-Fook SJ: Frequency dependence and partitioning of respiratory impedence in dogs. J Appl Physiol 61:621–629, 1981.

11. Van Brabandt H, Cauberghs M, Verbeken E, et al.: Partitioning of pulmonary impedence in excised human and canine lungs. Funcitonal-structural relationships. J Appl Physiol 55:1733–1742, 1983.

12. Cosio MG, Ghezzo H, Hogg JC, et al.: The relations between structural changes in small airways and pulmonary function tests. N Engl J Med 298:1277–1281, 1978.

13. Mitchell RS, Stanford RE, Johnson JM, et al.: The morphologic features of the bronchi, bronchioles and alveoli in chronic airway obstruction. Am Rev Dis 114:137–145, 1976.

14. Thurlbeck WM: In Petty TL (ed): *Chronic Obstructive Pulmonary Disease*, 2nd ed. New York: Marcel Dekker, 1985.

15. Hale KA, Ewing SL, Gosnell BA, Niewoehner DE: Lung disease in long-term cigarette smokers with and without chronic air-flow obstruction. Am Rev Respir Dis 130:716–721, 1984.

16. Reid LM: Correlation of certain bronchographic abnormalities seen in chronic bronchitis with the pathological changes. Thorax 10:199–204, 1955.

17. Martin CJ, Katsura S, Cochran TH: The relationship of chronic bronchitis to the diffuse obstructive pulmonary syndrome. Am Rev Respir Dis 102:362–369, 1970.

18. Matsuba K, Thurlbeck WM: Disease of the small airways in chronic bronchitis. Am Rev Respir Dis 107:552–558, 1973.

19. Niewoehner DE, Kleinerman J, Rice DP: Pathologic changes in the peripheral airways of young cigarette smokers. N Engl J Med 219:755–758, 1974.

20. Thurlbeck WM, Malaka D, Murphy K: Goblet cells in the peripheral airways in chronic bronchitis. Am Rev Respir Dis 112:65–69, 1975.

21. Ebert RV, Terracio MJ: The bronchiolar epithelium in cigarette smokers. Am Rev Respir Dis 111:4–11, 1975.

22. Berend N, Woolcock AJ, Marlin GE: Correlation between the function and structure of the lung in smokers. Am Rev Respir Dis 119:695–705, 1979.

23. Hale KA, Niewoehner DE, Cosio MG: Morphologic changes in the muscular pulmonary arteries: Relationship to cigarette smoking, airways disease and emphysema. Am Rev Respir Dis 122:273–278, 1980.

24. Petty TL, Silvers GW, Stanford RE, et al.: Small airway pathology is related to increased closing capacity and abnormal slope of phase III in excised human lungs. Am Rev Respir Dis 121:449–456, 1980.

25. Cosio MG, Hale, KA, Niewoehner DE: Morphologic and morphometric effects of prolonged cigarette smoking on the small airways. Am Rev Respir Dis 122:265–271, 1980.

26. Berend N, Wright JL, Thurlbeck WM, et al: Small airways disease: Reproducibility of measurement and correlation with lung function. Chest 79:263–268, 1981.

27. Salmon RB, Saidel GM, Inkley SR, Niewoehner DE: Relationship of ventilation inhomogeneity to morphologic variables in excised human lungs. Am Rev Respir Dis 126:686–690, 1982

28. Petty TL, Silvers GW, Stanford RE: Small airway dimension and size distribution in human lungs with an increased closing capacity. Am Rev Respir Dis 125:535–539, 1982.

29. Berend N, Thurlbeck WM: Correlation of maximum expiratory flow with small airway dimensions and pathology. J Appl Physiol 52:346–351, 1982.

30. Wright JL, Lawson LM, Pare PD, et al.: Morphology of peripheral airways in current smokers and ex-smokers. Am Rev Respir Dis 127:474–477, 1983.

31. Wright JL, Lawson L, Pare PD, et al.: The structure and function of the pulmonary vasculature in mild chronic obstructive pulmonary disease. The effect of oxygen and exercise. Am Rev Respir Dis 128:702–707, 1983.

32. Wright JL, Lawson LM, Pare PD, et al.: The detection of small airways disease. Am Rev Respir Dis 129:989–994, 1984.

33. Lumsden AB, McLean A, Lamb D: Goblet and Clara cells of human distal airways: Evidence for smoking induced changes in their numbers. Thorax 39:844–849, 1984.

34. Laennec RTH: *A Treatise on the Diseases of the Chest and on Mediate Auscultation*, 4th ed. New York: Wood, 1835.

35. Spain DM, Kaufman G: The basic lesion in chronic pulmonary emphysema. Am Rev Tuberc 68:24–30, 1953.

36. Reid LMcA: Pathology of chronic bronchitis. Lancet 1:275–278, 1954.

37. Leopold JG, Gough J: The centrilobular form of hypertrophic emphysema and its relation to chronic bronchitis. Thorax 12:219–235, 1957.

38. McLean KH: The pathogenesis of pulmonary emphysema. Am J Med 25:62–74, 1958.

39. Pratt PC, Haque A, Klugh GA: Correlation of postmortem function and structure in normal and emphysematous lungs. Am Rev Respir Dis 83:856–865, 1961.

40. Pratt PC, Jutabha O, Klugh GA: Quantitative relationship between structural extent of centrilobular emphysema and postmortem volume and flow characteristics of lungs. Med Thorac 22:197–209, 1965.

41. Anderson AE, Foraker AG: Relative dimensions of bronchioles and parenchymal spaces in lungs from normal subjects and emphysematous patients. Am J Med 32:218–226, 1962.

42. Anderson AE Jr, Foraker AG: Populations of nonrespiratory bronchioles in pulmonary emphysema. Arch Pathol Lab Med 83:286–292, 1967

43. Mitchell RS, Silvers GW, Dart GA, et al.: Clinical and morphologic correlations in chronic airway obstruction. AC Rev Respir Dis 97:54–62, 1968.

44. Bignon J, Khoury F, Even P, et al.: Morphometric study in chronic obstructive bronchopulmonary disease. Am Rev Respir Dis 99:669–695, 1969.

45. Bignon J, Andre-Bougaran J, Brouet G: Parenchymal, bronchiolar and bronchial measurements in centrilobular emphysema. Relation to weight of right ventricle. Thorax 25:556–567, 1970.

46. Karpick RJ, Pratt PC, Asmundsson T, Kilburn KH: Pathological findings in respiratory failure. Ann Intern Med 72:189–197, 1970.

47. Linhartova A, Anderson AE Jr, Foraker AG: Intraluminal

exudates of non-respiratory bronchioles in pulmonary emphysema. Hum Pathol 2:333–336, 1971.

48. Linhartova A, Anderson AE Jr, Foraker AG: Radial traction and bronchiolar obstruction in pulmonary emphysema. Arch Pathol 92:384–391, 1971.

49. Linhartova A, Anderson AE, Foraker AG: Non-respiratory bronchiolar deformities. Graphic assessment in normal and emphysematous lungs. Arch Pathol Lab Med 95:45–47, 1973.

50. Linhartova A, Anderson AE Jr, Foraker AG: Topology of non-respiratory bronchioles of normal and emphysematous lungs. Hum Pathol 5:729–735, 1974.

51. Linhartova A, Anderson AE Jr, Foraker AG: Further observations on luminal deformity and stenosis of non-respiratory bronchioles in pulmonary emphysema. Thorax 32:53–59, 1977.

52. Linhartova A, Anderson AE Jr, Foraker AG: Affixment arrangements of peribronchiolar alveoli in normal and emphysematous lungs. Arch Pathol Lab Med 106:499–502, 1982.

53. Matsuba K, Thurlbeck WM. The number and dimensions of small airways in emphysematous lungs. Am J Pathol 67:265–275, 1972.

54. Depierre A, Bignon J, Lebeau A, Brouet G: Quantitative study of parenchyma and small conductive airways in chronic nonspecific lung disease. Use of histologic stereology and bronchial casts. Chest 62:699–708, 1972.

55. Scott KWM, Steiner GM: Post mortem assessment of chronic airways obstruction by tantalum bronchography. Thorax 30:405–414, 1975.

56. Scott KWM: A pathological study of the lungs and heart in fatal and non-fatal chronic airway obstruction. Thorax 31:70–79, 1976.

57. Linhartova A, Anderson AE Jr: Small airways in panlobular emphysema: Mural thickening and premature closure. Am Rev Respir Dis 127:42–45, 1983.

58. Macklem PT, Proctor DF, Hogg JC: The stability of peripheral airways. Respir Physiol 8:191–203, 1970.

59. Gil J, Weibel ER: Extracellular lining of bronchioles after perfusion-fixation of rat lungs for electron microscopy. Anat Rec 169:185–199, 1971.

60. Hogg JC, Cosio M: The pathophysiology of small airways. In Sadoul P, Milic-Emili J, Simonsson BG, Clark TJH (eds): *Small Airways Disease in Health and Disease.* Excerpta Medica, 1979.

61. Florey H, Carleton HM, Wells AQ: Mucus secretion in the trachea. Br J Exp Pathol 13:269–284, 1932.

62. Liebow AA, Loring WE, Felton WL II: The musculature of the lungs in chronic pulmonary disease. Am J Pathol 29:885–912, 1953.

63. Fletcher C, Peto R, Tinker C, Speizer FE: *The Natural History of Chronic Bronchitis and Emphysema.* New York: Oxford University Press, 1976.

64. Dayman H: Mechanics of airflow in health and in emphysema. J Clin Invest 30:1175–1190, 1951.

65. Wilson AG, Massarella GR, Pride NB: Elastic properties of airways in human lungs post mortem. Am Rev Respir Dis 110:716–729, 1974.

66. Geddes DM, Corrin B, Brewerton DA, et al.: Progressive airway obliteration in adults and its association with rheumatoid disease. Q J Med 184:427–444, 1977.

67. Epler GR, Snider GL, Gaensler EA, et al.: Bronchiolitis and bronchitis in connective tissue disease. A possible relationship to the use of penicillamine. JAMA 242:528–532, 1979.

68. Geddes DM, Webley M, Emerson PA: Airways obstruction in rheumatoid arthritis. Ann Rheum Dis 38:222–225, 1979.

69. Brewerton D: D-penicillamine. Br Med J 2:1507, 1976.

70. Turton CW, Williams G, Green M: Cryptogenic obliterative bronchiolitis in adults. Thorax 36:805–810, 1981.

71. Homma H, Yamanaka A, Tanimota S, et al.: Diffuse panbronchiolitis. A disease of the transitional zone of the lung. Chest 83:63–69, 1983.

72. Macklem PT, Thurlbeck WM, Fraser RG: Chronic obstructive disease of small airways. Ann Intern Med 74:167–177, 1971.

73. Gosink BB, Friedman PJ, Liebow AA: Bronchiolitis obliterans. Roentgenologic-pathologic correlation. AJR 117:816–832, 1973.

74. Reid LMcA: Reduction in bronchial subdivision in bronchiectasis. Thorax 5:233–247, 1950.

75. Liebow AA, Carrington CB: The interstitial pneumonias. In Simon K, Potchen EJ, LeMay M (eds): *Frontiers of Pulmonary Radiology.* New York: Grune & Stratton, 1969, pp. 102–141.

76. Epler GR, Colby TV: The spectrum of bronchiolitis obliterans. Chest 83:161–162, 1983.

77. Epler GR, Colby TV, McLoud TC, et al.: Bronchiolitis obliterans organizing pneumonia. N Engl J Med 312:152–158, 1985.

78. McAdams AJ Jr: Bronchiolitis obliterans. Am J Med 19:314–322, 1955.

79. Darke CS, Warrack AJN: Bronchiolitis from nitrous fumes. Thorax 13:327–333, 1958.

80. Horvath EP, doPico GA, Barbee RA, Dickie HA: Nitrogen dioxide-induced pulmonary disease. J Occup Med 20:103–110, 1978.

81. Woodford DM, Coutu RE, Gaensler EA: Obstructive lung disease from acute sulfur dioxide exposure. Respiration 38:238–245, 1979.

82. Close LG, Catlin FI, Cohn AM: Acute and chronic effects of ammonia burns of the respiratory tract. Arch Otolaryngol 106:151–158, 1980.

83. Becroft DMO: Bronchiolitis obliterans, bronchiectasis and other sequelae of adenovirus type 21 infection in young children. J Clin Pathol 24:72–82, 1971.

84. Edwards C, Penny M, Newman J: Mycoplasma pneumonia, Stevens-Johnson syndrome, and chronic obliterative bronchitis. Thorax 38:867–869, 1983.

85. Cooney TP: Interrelationship of chronic eosinophilic pneumonia, bronchiolitis obliterans, and rheumatoid disease: A hypothesis. J Clin Pathol 34:129–137, 1981.

86. Epler GR, Snider GL, Gaensler EA, et al.: Bronchiolitis and bronchitis in connetive tissue diseases. JAMA 242:528–532, 1979.

87. Newball HH, Brahim SA: Chronic airway disease in patients with Sjögren's syndrome. Am Rev Respir Dis 115:295–304, 1977.

88. Bradstock KF, Cotes R, Despas P, et al.: Fatal obstructive airways disease after bone marrow transplantation. Transplant Proc 16:1034–1036, 1984.

89. Roca J, Granena A, Rodrigues-Roison R, et al.: Fatal airway disease in an adult with graft-versus-host disease. Thorax 37:77–78, 1982.

90. Ralph DD, Spingmeyer SC, Sullivan KM, et al.: Rapidly progressive airflow obstruction in marrow transplant patients. Am Rev Respir Dis 129:641–644, 1984.

91. Johnson FL, Stokes DC, Ruggiero M, et al.: Chronic obstructive airways disease after bone marrow transplantation. J Pediatr 105:370–376, 1984.

92. Atkinson K, Bryant D, Biggs J, et al.: Obstructive airways disease: A rare but serious manifestation of graft-versus-host disease after allogenic marrow transplantation in humans. Transplant Proc 16:1030–1033, 1984.

93. Wyatt SE, Nunn P, Hows JM, et al.: Airways obstruction

associated with graft versus host disease after bone marrow transplantation. Thorax 39:887–894, 1984.

94. Burke CM, Theodore J, Dawkins KD: Post transplant obliterative bronchiolitis and other late lung sequelae in human heart-lung transplantation. Chest 86:824–829, 1984.

95. Baar HS, Calindo J: Bronchiolitis fibrosa obliterans. Thorax 21:209–214, 1966.

96. Tukiainen P, Poppius H, Taskinen E: Slowly progressive bronchiolitis obliterans. A case report with detailed pulmonary function studies. Eur J Respir Dis 61:77–83, 1980.

97. Definition and classification of chronic bronchitis for clinical and epidemiologic purposes. A report to the Medical Research Council by their committee on the aetiology of chronic bronchitis. Lancet 1:775–779, 1965.

98. Reid L: Measurement of bronchial mucous gland layer: A diagnostic yardstick in chronic bronchitis. Thorax 15:132–141, 1960.

99. Douglas AN: Quantitative study of bronchial mucus gland enlargement. Thorax 35:198–201, 1980.

100. Bedrossian CWM, Anderson AE Jr, Foraker AG: Comparison of method for quantitating bronchial morphology. Thorax 26:406–408, 1971.

101. Thurlbeck WM, Angus GE, Pare JAP: Mucous gland hypertrophy in chronic bronchitis, and its occurrence in smokers. Br J Dis Chest 57:73–78, 1963.

102. Thurlbeck WM, Angus GE: A distribution curve for chronic bronchitis. Thorax 19:436–442, 1964.

103. McKenzie HI, Glick M, Outhred KG: Chronic bronchitis in coal miners: Ante-mortem/post-mortem comparisons. Thorax 24:527–535, 1969.

104. Hayes JA: Distribution of bronchial gland measurements in a Jamaican population. Thorax 24:619–622, 1969.

105. Ryder RC, Lyons JP, Campbell M, Gough J: Bronchial mucous gland status in coal workers' pneumoconiosis. Ann NY Acad Sci 200:370–380, 1972.

106. Scott KWM: An autopsy study of bronchial mucous gland hypertrophy in Glasgow. Am Rev Respir Dis 107:239–245.

107. Burton PA, Dixon MF: A comparison of changes in the mucous glands and goblet cells of nasal, sinus and bronchial mucosa. Thorax 24:180–185, 1969.

108. Bath JCJL, Yates PA: Clinical and pathologic correlations in chronic airways obstruction observations on patients with pulmonary resection. Ninth Aspen Conference. US Public Health Service Publication 1717:293–308, 1968.

109. Mitchell RS, Ryan SF, Petty TL, Filley GF: The significance of morphologic, chronic hyperplastic bronchitis. Am Rev Respir Dis 93:720–729, 1966.

110. Thurlbeck WM, Angus GE: The variation of Reid Index measurements within the major bronchial tree. Am Rev Respir Dis 95:551–55, 1967.

111. Greenberg SD, Boushy SF, Jenkins DE: Chronic bronchitis and emphysema. Correlation of pathologic findings. Am Rev Respir Dis 96:918–928, 1967.

112. Niewoehner DE, Kleinerman J, Knoke JD: Regional chronic bronchitis. Am Rev Respir Dis 105:586–593, 1972.

113. Hale FC, Olsen CR, Mickey MR Jr: The measurement of bronchial wall components. Am Rev Respir Dis 98:978–987, 1968.

114. Dunnill MS, Massarella GR, Anderson JA: A comparison of the quantitative anatomy of the bronchi in normal subjects, in status asthmaticus, in chronic bronchitis, and in emphysema. Thorax 24:176–179, 1969.

115. Takizawa T, Thurlbeck WM: A comparative study of four methods of assessing the morphologic changes in chronic bronchitis. Am Rev Respir Dis 103:774–783, 1971.

116. Sobonya RE, Kleinerman J: Morphometric studies of bronchi in young smokers. Am Rev Respir Dis 105:768–775, 1972.

117. Ryder RC, Dunnill MS, Anderson JA: A quantitative study of the bronchial mucous gland volume, emphysema and smoking in a necropsy population. J Pathol 104:59–71, 1971.

118. Restrepo GL, Heard BE: The size of bronchial glands in chronic bronchitis. J Pathol Bacteriol 85:305–310, 1963.

119. Jamal K, Cooney TP, Fleetham JA, Thurlbeck WM: Chronic bronchitis: Correlation of morphological findings in sputum production and flow rates. Am Rev Respir Dis 129:719–722, 1984.

120. Carlile A, Edwards C: Structural variations in the named bronchi of the left lung. A morphometric study. Br J Dis Chest 77:344–348, 1983.

121. De Haller R, Reid L: Adult chronic bronchitis. Morphology, histochemistry and vascularisation of the bronchial mucous glands. Med Thorac 22:549–567, 1965.

121a. Oberholzer M, Dalquen P, Rohr HP: Morphologic findings in central bronchi correlated to lung function data in obstructive airways disease. Pathol Res Pract 164:58–67, 1979.

122. Field WEH, Davey EN, Reid L, Roe FJC: Bronchial mucous gland hypertrophy: Its relation to symptoms and environment. Br J Dis Chest 60:66–80, 1966.

123. Salvato G: Some histological changes in chronic bronchitis and asthma. Thorax 23:168–172, 1968.

124. Martin CJ, Katsura S, Cochran TH: The relationship of chronic bronchitis to the diffuse obstructive pulmonary syndrome. Am Rev Respir Dis 102:362–369, 1970.

125. Linhartova A, Anderson AE Jr, Foraker AE: Site predilection of airway inflammation by emphysema type. Arch Pathol Lab Med 108:662–665, 1984.

126. Leopold JG: A contrast of bronchitis and asthma. In: *Symposium on the Nature of Asthma*. Midhurst, Sussex, England: King Edward VII Hospital 1964, pp 30–38.

127. Huber HL, Koessler KK: The pathology of bronchial asthma. Arch Intern Med 30:689–760, 1922.

128. Houston JC, de Nevasquez S, Trounce JR: Clinical and pathological study of fatal cases of status asthmaticus. Thorax 8:207–213, 1953.

129. Earle BV: Fatal bronchial asthma: Series of 15 cases with review of literature. Thorax 8:195–206, 1953.

130. Cardell BS: Pathological findings in death from asthma. Int Arch Allergy 9:189–199, 1956.

131. Williams DA, Leopold JG: Death from bronchial asthma. Acta Allergol 14:83–86, 1959.

132. Dunnill MS: The pathology of asthma, with special reference to changes in the bronchial mucosa. J Clin Pathol 13:27–33, 1960.

133. Glynn AA, Michaels L: Bronchial biopsy in chronic bronchitis and asthma. Thorax 15:142–153, 1960.

134. Callerame ML, Condemi JJ, Ishizaka K, et al.: Immunoglobulins in bronchial tissues from patients with asthma, with special reference to immunoglobulin E. J Allergy 47:187–197, 1971.

135. MacLeod LJ, Heard BE: Area of muscle in tracheal sections in chronic bronchitis, measured by point counting. J Pathol 97:157–161, 1969.

136. Hossain S, Heard BE: Hyperplasia of bronchial muscle in chronic bronchitis. J Pathol 101:171–184, 1970.

137. Takizawa T, Thurlbeck WM: Muscle and mucous gland size

in the major bronchi of patients with chronic bronchitis, asthma and asthmatic bronchitis. Am Rev Respir Dis 104:331–336, 1971.

138. Wright RR: Bronchial atrophy and collapse in chronic obstructive pulmonary emphysema. Am J Pathol 37:63–77, 1960.

139. Wright RR, Stuart CM: Chronic bronchitis with emphysema: A pathological study of the bronchi. Med Thorac 22:210–219, 1965.

140. Tandon MK, Campbell AH: Bronchial cartilage in chronic bronchitis. Thorax 24:607–612, 1969.

141. Restrepo GL. Heard BE: Air-trapping in chronic bronchitis and emphysema: Measurement of the bronchial cartilage. Am Rev Respir Dis 90:395–400, 1964.

142. Thurlbeck WM, Pun R, Toth J, Fraser RG: Bronchial cartilage in chronic obstructive lung disease. Am Rev Respir Dis 109:73–80, 1974.

143. Wang NS, Ying WL: Morphogenesis of human bronchial diverticulum. A scanning electron microscopic study. Chest 69:201–204, 1976.

144. Wang NS, Ying WL: The pattern of goblet cell hyperplasia in human airways. Hum Pathol 8:301–311, 1977.

144a. Thurlbeck WM, Angus GE: The relationship between chronic bronchitis and emphysema as assessed morphologically. Am Rev Respir Dis 87:815–819, 1963.

145. Hernandez JA, Anderson AE Jr, Foraker AG: Bronchial characteristics in pulmonary emphysema. Arch Pathol 77:82–92, 1964.

146. Megahed GE, Senna GA, Eissa MH, et al. Smoking versus infection as the aetiology of bronchial mucous gland hypertrophy in chronic bronchitis. Thorax 22:271–278, 1967.

147. Petty TL, Ryan SF, Mitchell RS: Cigarette smoking and the lungs. Relation of post-mortem evidence of emphysema, chronic bronchitis, and black lung pigmentation. Arch Environ Health 14:172–177, 1967.

148. Field WEH: Mucous gland hypertrophy in babies and children aged 15 years or less. Br J Dis Chest 62:11–18, 1968.

149. Matsuba K, Thurlbeck WM: A morphometric study of bronchial and bronchiolar walls in children. Am Rev Respir Dis 105:908–913, 1972.

150. Ryder R, Lyons JP, Campbell H, Gough J: Bronchial mucous gland status in coal workers' pneumoconiosis. Ann NY Acad Sci 200:370–380, 1972.

151. Douglas AN, Lamb D, Ruckley VA: Bronchial gland dimensions in coal miners: Influence of smoking and dust exposure. Thorax 37:760–764, 1982.

152. Thurlbeck WM, Henderson JA, Fraser RG, Bates DV: Chronic obstructive lung disease. A comparison between clinical, roentgenologic, functional and morphologic criteria in chronic bronchitis, emphysema, asthma and bronchiectasis. Medicine 49:81–145, 1970.

153. Helgason AH, Boushy SF, Billing DM, Gyorky F: Changes with time in morphologic chronic bronchitis: comparison of surgically resected lungs and the remaining lung obtained after death. Geriatrics 25:101–106, 1970.

154. Rimington J: Smoking, chronic bronchitis and lung cancer. Br Med J 2:373–375, 1971.

155. Pemberton J: Chronic bronchitis, emphysema and bronchial spasm in bituminous coal workers; Epidemiologic study. Arch Ind Health 13:529–544, 1956.

156. Fletcher CM: Disability and mortality from chronic bronchitis in relation to dust exposure. Arch Ind Health 18:368–373, 1958.

157. Higgins ITT, Cochrane AL, Gilson JC, Wood CH: Population studies of chronic respiratory disease. A comparison of miners, foundryworkers and others in Staveley, Derbyshire. Br J Ind Med 16:255–268, 1958.

158. Higgins ITT, Cochrane AL: Chronic respiratory disease in a random sample of men and women in the Rhondda Fach in 1958. Br J Ind Med 18:93–102, 1961.

159. Thurlbeck WM: *Chronic Airflow Obstruction in Lung Disease.* Philadelphia: WB Saunders, 1976.

160. Higgins ITT: Respiratory symptoms, bronchitis and disability in a random sample of an agricultural population. Br Med J 2:1198–1203, 1957.

161. American Thoracic Society: Chronic bronchitis, asthma and pulmonary emphysema. A statement by the committee on diagnostic standards for nontuberculous respiratory diseases. Am Rev Respir Dis 85:762–768, 1962.

162. Thurlbeck WM: Overview of the pathology of pulmonary emphysema in the human. Clin Chest Med 4:337–350, 1983.

163. Thurlbeck WM, Anderson AE, Janis M, et al.: A co-operative study of certain measurements of emphysema. Am Rev Respir Dis 98:217–228, 1968.

164. Thurlbeck WM, Horowitz I, Siemiatycki J, et al.: Intra- and inter-observer variations in the assessment of emphysema. Arch Environ Health 18:646–659, 1969.

165. Boren HG: Alveolar fenestrae. Relationship to the pathology and pathogenesis of pulmonary emphysema. Am Rev Respir Dis 85:328–344, 1962.

166. Pump KK: Emphysema and its relation to age. Am Rev Respir Dis 114:5–13, 1976.

167. Gough J: Discussion on the diagnosis of pulmonary emphysema. The pathological diagnosis of emphysema. Proc Soc Med 45:576–577, 1952.

168. McLean KH: Macroscopic anatomy of pulmonary emphysema. Aust Ann Med 5:73–88, 1956.

169. Gough H, Wentworth JE: Thin sections of entire organs mounted on paper. Harvey Lect (1957–58) 53:182–185, 1958.

170. Reid L: *The Pathology of Emphysema.* London: Lloyd-Luke, 1967.

171. Thurlbeck WM: Internal surface area and other measurements in emphysema. Thorax 22:483–96, 1967.

172. Thurlbeck WM: The incidence of pulmonary emphysema. With observations on the relative incidence and spatial distribution of various types of emphysema. Am Rev Respir Dis 87:206–215, 1963.

173. Mitchell RS, Silvers GW, Goodman N, et al.: Are centrilobular emphysema and panlobular emphysema two different diseases? Hum Pathol 1:433–441, 1970.

174. Dunnill MS: An assessment of the anatomical factor in cor pulmonale in emphysema. J Clin Pathol 14:246–258, 1961.

175. Sweet HC, Wyatt JP, Kinsella PW: Correlation of lung macrosections with pulmonary function in emphysema. Am J Med 29:277–281, 1960.

176. Jenkins DE, Greenberg SD, Boushy SF, et al.: Correlation of morphologic emphysema with pulmonary function parameters. Trans Assoc Am Phy 78:218–230, 1965.

177. Nash ES, Briscoe WA, Cournand A: The relationship between clinical and physiologic findings in chronic obstructive disease of the lungs. Med Thorac 22:305–327, 1965.

178. Watanabe S, Mitchell M, Renzetti AD Jr: Correlation of structure and function in chronic pulmonary disease. Am Rev Respir Dis 92:221–227, 1965.

179. Burrows B, Fletcher CM, Heard BE, et al.: The emphysematous and bronchial types of chronic airways obstruction. A clinico-pathological study of patients in London and Chicago. Lancet 1:830–835, 1966.

180. Hicken P, Heath D, Brewer D: The relation between the weight of the right ventricle and the percentage of abnormal air space in the lung in emphysema. J Pathol Bacteriol 92:519–528, 1966.
181. Martin CJ, Cochran TH, Katsura S: Tuberculosis, emphysema and bronchitis. Am Rev Respir Dis 97:1089–1094, 1968.
182. Cullen JH, Kaemmerlen JT, Daoud A, Katz HL: A prospective clinical-pathologic study of the lungs and heart in chronic obstructive lung disease. Am Rev Respir Dis 102:190–204, 1970.
183. Pratt PC, Kilburn KH: A modern concept of the emphysemas based on correlations of structure and function. Hum Pathol 1:443–453, 1970.
184. Hasleton PS: Right ventricular hypertrophy in emphysema. J Pathol 110:27–36, 1973.
185. Lamb D: The location of bronchial pathology in obstructive lung disease. In Orie NG, Van Der Lender R (eds): *Bronchitis Three*. Assen: Royal Vangorcum, 1970, pp 149–59.
186. Sobonya RE, Burrows B: The epidemiology of emphysema. Clin Chest Med 4:351–358, 1983.
187. Anderson AE Jr, Hernandez JA, Holmes WL, Foraker AG: Pulmonary emphysema. Prevalence, severity and anatomical patterns in macrosections, with respect to smoking habits. Arch Environ Health 12:569–577, 1966.
188. Wyatt JP, Fischer VW, Sweet HC: Centrilobular emphysema. Lab Invest 10:159–177, 1961.
189. Snider GL, Brody JS, Doctor L: Subclinical pulmonary emphysema. Am Rev Respir Dis 85:666–683, 1962.
190. Hernandez JA, Anderson AE Jr, Holmes WL, Foraker AG: Macroscopic relations in emphysematous and aging lungs. Geriatrics 21:155–166, 1966.
191. Heppleston AG, Leopold JG: Chronic pulmonary emphysema: Anatomy and pathogenesis. Am J Med 31:279–291, 1961.
192. Heard BE: A pathological study of emphysema of the lungs with chronic bronchitis. Thorax 13:136–149, 1958.
193. Wyatt JP, Fischer VW, Sweet HC: Panlobular emphysema: Anatomy and pathodynamics. Dis Chest 41:239–259, 1962.
194. Laurell CB, Eriksson S: The electrophoretic alpha$_1$-globulin pattern of serum in alpha$_1$-antitrypsin deficiency. Scand J Clin Lab Invest 15:132–140, 1963.
195. Gross P, Babyak MA, Tolker E, Kashak M: Enzymatically produced pulmonary emphysema: a preliminary report. J Occup Med 6:481–484, 1964.
196. Idell S, Cohen AB: Alpha-1-antitrypsin deficiency. Clin Chest Med 4:359–375, 1983.
197. Cook PJL: Genetic aspects of alpha-1-antitrypsin. Thorax 26:488, 1971.
198. Eriksson S: Studies in alpha$_1$ antitrypsin deficiency. Acta Med Scand 177(suppl 432):1–85, 1965.
199. Fagerhol MK, Laurell CB: The Pi system-inherited variants of serum alpha$_1$-antitrypsin. Prog Med Genet 7:96–111, 1970.
200. Lieberman J: Alpha$_1$-antitrypsin deficiency. Med Clin North Am 57:691–706, 1973.
201. Kueppers F: Alpha-1-antitrypsin. In Litwin SD (ed): *Genetic Determinants of Pulmonary Disease*. New York: Marcel Dekker, 1978.
202. Fagerhol MK, Tenfjord OW: Serum Pi types in some European, American, Asian and African populations. Acta Pathol Microbiol Scand 72:601–608, 1968.
203. Jones MC, Thomas GO: Alpha antitrypsin deficiency and pulmonary emphysema. Thorax 26:652–662, 1971.
204. Lieberman J: Heterozygous and homozygous alpha$_1$-antitrypsin deficiency in patients with pulmonary emphysema. N Engl J Med 281:279–284, 1969.

205. Schleusener A, Talamo RC, Pare JAP, Thurlbeck WM: Familial emphysema. Am Rev Respir Dis 98:692–696, 1968.
206. Martelli NA, Goldman E, Roncoroni AJ: Lower zone emphysema in young patients without alpha-1-antitrypsin deficiency. Thorax 29:237–244, 1974.
207. Thurlbeck WM: Chronic obstructive lung disease. In Sommers SC (ed) *Pathology Annual*. New York: Appleton-Century-Crofts, 1968, pp 367–398.
208. Swyer PR, James GCW: A case of unilateral pulmonary emphysema. Thorax 8:133–136, 1953.
209. MacLeod WM: Abnormal transradiancy of one lung. Thorax 9:147–153, 1954.
210. Edge J, Simon G, Reid L: Periacinar (paraseptal) emphysema: Its clinical, radiological and physiological features. Br J Dis Chest 60:10–18, 1966.
211. Laurenzi GA, Turino GM, Fishman AP: Bullous disease of the lung. Am J Med 361–378, 1962.
212. Duguid JB, Lambert MW: The pathogenesis of coal miner's pneumoconiosis. J Pathol Bacteriol 88:389–403, 1964.
213. Thurlbeck WM, Simon G: Radiographic appearance of the chest in emphysema. Am J Roentgenol 130:429–440, 1978.
214. Thurlbeck WM, Ryder RC, Sternby N: A comparative study of the severity of emphysema in necropsy populations in three different countries. Am Rev Respir Dis 109:239–248, 1974.
215. Thurlbeck WM, Dunnill MS, Hartung W, et al.: A comparison of three methods of measuring emphysema. Hum Pathol 1:215–226, 1970.
216. Ishikawa S, Bowden DH, Fisher V, Wyatt JP: The "emphysema profile" in two midwestern cities in North America. Arch Environ Health 18:660–666, 1969.
217. Alli AF: Emphysema in Nigeria and in the English Midlands: A comparative incidence study. J Pathol 110:vi, 1973.
218. Jones AW, Madda PJ: Necropsy incidence of emphysema in Uganda. Thorax 29:195–198, 1974.
219. Mitchell RS, Stanford RE, Silvers GW, Dart G: The right ventricle in chronic airway obstruction: A clinico-pathologic study. Am Rev Respir Dis 114:147–154, 1976.
220. Millard J, Reid L: Right ventricular hypertrophy and its relationship to chronic bronchitis and emphysema. Br J Dis Chest 68:103–110, 1974.
221. Williams IP, Boyd MJ, Humberstone AM, et al.: Pulmonary arterial and hypertension. Br J Dis Chest 78:211–216, 1984.
222. Burrows B, Fletcher CM, Heard BE, et al.: The emphysematous and bronchial types of chronic airways obstruction. A clinico-pathological study of patients in London and Chicago. Lancet 1:830–835, 1966.
223. Mitchell RS, Petty TL, Filley GF, et al.: Clinical, physiologic and morphologic correlations in chronic airways obstruction. In Orie NG, Van Der Lende R (ed): *Bronchitis Three*. Assen: Royal Vangorcum, 1970, pp. 164–174.
224. Nicklaus TM, Stowell DW, Christiansen WR, Renzetti AD Jr: The accuracy of the roentgenologic diagnosis of chronic pulmonary emphysema. Am Rev Respir Dis 93:889–899, 1966.
225. Thurlbeck WM: Postmortem lung volumes. Thorax 34:735–739, 1979.
226. Lohela P, Sutinen S, et al.: Diagnosis of emphysema on chest radiographs. Fortschr Rentgenstr 141:395–402, 1984.
227. Reid L, Millard FJC: Correlation between radiological diagnosis and structural lung changes in emphysema. Clin Radiol 15:307–311, 1964.
228. Katsura S, Martin CJ: The roentgenologic diagnosis of anatomic emphysema. Am Rev Respir Dis 96:700–706, 1967.
229. Yip CK, Epstein H, Goldring RM: Relationship of functional

residual capacity to static pulmonary mechanics in chronic obstructive pulmonary disease. Am J Med Sci 287:3–6, 1984.

230. Greaves IA, Colebatch HJH: Elastic behaviour and structure of normal and emphysematous lungs post-mortem. Am Rev Respir Dis 121:127–136, 1980.

231. Niewoehner DE, Kleinerman J, Liotta L: Elastic behaviour of postmortem human lungs: Effects of aging and mild emphysema. J Appl Physiol 36:943–949, 1975.

232. Berend N, Thurlbeck WM: Exponential analysis of pressure-volume relationship in excised human lungs. J Appl Physiol 52:838–844, 1982.

233. Pare PD, Brooks LA, Bates J, et al.: Exponential analysis of the lung pressure-volume curve as a predictor of pulmonary emphysema. Am Rev Respir Dis 126:54–61, 1982.

234. Stone PJ: The elastase-antielastase hypothesis of the pathogenesis of emphysema. Clin Chest Med 4:405–412, 1983.

235. West JB: Distribution of mechanical stress in the lung. A possible factor in localisation of pulmonary disease. Lancet 1:839–841, 1971.

236. Kawakami M, Paul JL, Thurlbeck WM: The effect of age on lung structure in male BALB/cNNia inbred mice. Am J Anat 170:1–21, 1984.

237. Anderson WF, Anderson AE Jr, Hernandez JA, Foraker AG: Topography of aging and emphysematous lungs. Am Rev Respir Dis 90:411–423, 1964.

238. Ryan SF, Vincent TN, Mitchell RS, et al.: Ductectasia: An asymptomatic pulmonary change related to age. Med Thorac 22:181–187, 1965.

239. Wright RR: Elastic tissue of normal and emphysematous lungs. A tridimensional histologic study. Am J Pathol 39:355–367, 1961.

240. Lincoln JCR, Stark J, Subramanian S, et al.: Congenital lobar emphysema. Ann Surg 173:55–62, 1971.

241. Raynor AC, Capp MC, Sealy WC: Lobar emphysema of infancy. Diagnosis, treatment and etiological aspects. Ann Thorac Surg 4:374–385, 1967.

242. Stovin PG: Congenital lobar emphysema. Thorax 14:254–262, 1959.

243. Bolande RB, Schneider AF, Boggs JD: Infantile lobar emphysema. Etiological concept. Arch Pathol 61:289–294, 1956.

244. Hislop A, Reid L: New pathological findings in emphysema of childhood: I. Polyalveolar lobe with emphysema. Thorax 25:682–690, 1970.

245. Friend J: Respiratory insufficiency after pneumonectomy Lancet 2:260–262, 1954.

246. Cournand A, Berry FB: The effect of pneumonectomy upon cardipulmonary function in adult patients. Ann Surg 116:532–552, 1942.

247. Ogilvie C, Harris LH, Meecham J, Ryder G: Ten years after pneumonectomy for carcinoma. Br Med J 1:1111–1115, 1963.

248. Thurlbeck WM: Postpneumonectomy compensatory lung growth. Am Rev Respir Dis 128:965–967, 1983.

249. Pontius JR, Jacobs LG: The reversal of advanced bronchiectasis. Radiology 68:204–208, 1957.

250. Nelson SW, Christoforidis A: Reversible bronchiectasis. Radiology 72:375–382, 1958.

251. Opie EL: The pathologic anatomy of influenza. Based chiefly on American and British sources. Arch Pathol 5:285–303, 1928.

252. Blades B, Dugan JD: Pseudobrochiectasis. J Thorac Surg 13:40–48, 1944.

253. Whitwell F: Study of pathology and pathogenesis of bronchiectasis. Thorax 7:213–239, 1952.

254. Glauser EM, Cook CD, Harris GBC: Bronchiectasis: A review of 187 cases. Acta Pediatr Scand (suppl) 165:1–15, 1966.

255. Fernald GW: Bronchiectasis in childhood. A 10 year survey of cases treated at North Carolina Memorial Hospital. NC Med J 39:368–372, 1978.

256. Lewiston NJ: Bronchiectasis in childhood. Pediatr Clin North Am 31:865–878, 1984.

257. Holmes LB, Blennerhassett JB, Austen KF: A reappraisal of Kartagener's syndrome. Am J Med Sci 255:13–28, 1968.

258. Churchill ED: The segmental and lobular physiology and pathology of the lung. J Thorac Surg 18:279–293, 1949.

259. Fraser RG: Measurements of the calibre of human bronchi in three phases of respiration by cinebronchography. J Can Assoc Radiol 12:102–112, 1961.

260. Ogilvie AG: The nataural history of bronchiectasis. A clinical, roentgenologic and pathologic study. Arch Intern Med 68:395–465, 1941.

261. Perry KMA, King DS: Bronchiectasis: A study of prognosis based on a follow-up of 400 cases. Am Rev Tuberc 41:531–548, 1940.

262. Diamond S, Van Loon EL: Bronchiectasis in childhood. JAMA 118:771–778, 1942.

263. Hayward J, Reid LMcA: The cartilage of the intrapulmonary bronchi in normal lungs, in bronchiectasis and in massive collapse. Thorax 7:98–110, 1952.

264. Moore JR, Kobernick SD, Wiglesworth FW: Bronchiectasis; Study of segmental distribution of pathologic lesions. Surg Gynecol Obstet 89:145–153, 1949.

265. Culiner MM: Obliterative bronchitis and bronchiolitis in bronchiectasis. Dis Chest 44:351–361, 1963.

266. Kourilsky R: Histologie de la muqueuse bronchique au cours des inflammations chroniques non tuberculeuses des bronches (étude sur prelevements biopsiques). Bronches 10:76–116, 1960.

267. Whitwell F: Tumourlets of lung. J Pathol Bacteriol 70:529–541, 1955.

268. Liebow AA, Hales MR, Lindskog GE: Enlargement of the bronchial arteries and their anastomoses with the pulmonary arteries in bronchiectasis. Am J Pathol 25:211–231, 1949.

269. Müller NL, Bergin CJ, Ostrow DN, Nichols DM: Role of computed tomography in the recognition of bronchiectasis. AJR 143:971–976, 1984.

270. Capitanio MA: Commentary. J Pediatr 87:233–234, 1975.

271. Grawitz P: Uber angeborene bronchiektasia. Virchows Arch [A] 82:217–246, 1880.

272. Williams M, Campbell P: Generalized bronchiectasis associated with deficiency of cartilage in the bronchial tree. Arch Dis Child 35:182–191, 1960.

273. Williams HE, Landau LI, Phelan PD: Generalized bronchiectasis due to extensive deficiency of bronchial cartilage. Arch Dis Child 47:423–428, 1972.

274. Wayne KS, Tausig LM: Probable familial congenital bronchiectasis due to cartilage deficiency (Williams-Campbell syndrome). Am Rev Respir Dis 114:15–22, 1976.

275. Mitchell RE, Bury RG: Congenital bronchiectasis due to deficiency of bronchial cartilage (Williams-Campbell syndrome). J Pediatr 87:230–233, 1975.

276. Hentel W, Longfield AN, Gordon J: A re-evaluation of bronchiectasis using fume fixation. 1. The broncho-alveolar structures: A preliminary study. Dis Chest 41:41–45, 1962.

277. Messer JW, Peters GA, Bennett WA: Causes of death and pathologic findings in 304 cases of bronchial asthma. Dis Chest 38:616–624, 1960.

278. Sobonya RE: Concise clinical study. Quantitative structural alterations in long-standing allergic asthma. Am Rev Respir Dis 130:289–292, 1984.
279. World Health Organization: Chronic cor pulmonale: Report of an expert committee. Circulation 27:594–615, 1963.
280. Behnke RH, Blount SG, Bristow JD, et al.: Primary prevention of pulmonary heart disease. Pulmonary heart disease study group. Circulation 41A:17–23, 1970.
281. Fulton RM, Hutchinson EC, Jones AM: Ventricular weight in cardiac hypertrophy. Br Heart J 14:413–420, 1952.
282. Segal N, Bishop JM: The circulation in patients with chronic bronchitis and emphysema at rest and during exercise, with special reference to the influence of changes in blood viscosity and blood volume on the pulmonary circulation. J Clin Invest 45:1555–1568, 1966.
283. Hasleton PS, Health D, Brewer DB: Hypertensive pulmonary vascular disease in states of chronic hypoxia. J Pathol Bacteriol 95:431–440, 1968.
284. Wagenvoort CA, Watgenvoort N: Hypoxic pulmonary vascular lesions in man at high altitude and in patients with chronic respiratory disease. Pathol Microbiol 29:276–282, 1973.
285. Hicken P, Heath D, Brewer DB, Whitaker W: The small pulmonary arteries in emphysema. J Pathol 90:107–114, 1965.
286. Wagenvoort CA, Wagenvoort N: Pulmonary venous changes in chronic hypoxia. Virchows Arch [A] 372:51–56, 1976.
287. Liebow AA: Pulmonary emphysema with special reference to vascular change. Am Rev Respir Dis 80(suppl):67–93, 1959.
288. Turner-Warwick M: Systemic arterial patterns in the lung and clubbing of the fingers. Thorax 18:238–250, 1963.
289. Marchand P, Gilroy JC, Wilson VH: Anatomical study of bronchial vascular system and its variations in disease. Thorax 5:207–221, 1950.
290. Cudkowitz L, Armstrong JB: Bronchial arteries in pulmonary emphysema. Thorax 8:46–58, 1953.
291. Liebow AA: Bronchopulmonary venous collateral circulation with special reference to emphysema. Am J Pathol 29:251–289, 1953.
292. Foraker AG, Bedrossian CWM, Anderson AE Jr: Myocardial dimensions and properties in pulmonary emphysema. Arch Pathol 90:344–347, 1970.
293. Anderson AE Jr, Bedrossian CWM, Foraker AG: Systemic blood pressure in subjects with and without emphysema. Am Rev Respir Dis 103:576–578, 1971.
294. Thurlbeck WM: Diaphragm and body weight in emphysema. Thorax 33:483–487, 1978.
295. Openbrier DR, Irwin MM, Rogers RM, et al: Nutritional status and lung function in patients with emphysema and chronic bronchitis. Chest 83:17–22, 1983.
296. Nemery B, Maovero NE, Brasseur L, Stanescu DC: Smoking, lung function and body weight. Br Med J 286:249–251, 1983.
297. Braun SR, Keim NL, Dixon RM, et al: The prevalence and determinants of nutritional changes in chronic obstructive pulmonary disease. Chest 86:558–563, 1984.
298. Hunter AMB, Carey MA, Larsh HW: The nutritional status of patients with chronic obstructive pulmonary disease. Am Rev Respir Dis 124:376–381, 1981.
299. Sahebjami H, Vassalo CL: Effects of starvation and refeeding on lung mechanics and morphometry. Am Rev Respir Dis 119:443–451, 1979.
300. Wyatt JP, Fischer VW, Sweet HC: The pathomorphology of the emphysema complex. Am Rev Respir Dis 89:533–560, 721–735, 1964.
301. Ishikawa S, Hayes JA: Functional morphometry of the diaphragm in patients with chronic obstructive lung disease. Am Rev Respir Dis 108:135–138, 1973.
302. Steele RH, Heard BE: The size of the diaphragm in chronic bronchitis. Thorax 28:55–60, 1973.
303. Fromme H: Systematische Untersuchungen uber die Gewichsverhaltnisse des Zwerchfells. Virchows Arch [Pathol Anat] 221:117–155, 1916.
304. Butler C: Diaphragmatic changes in emphysema. Am Rev Respir Dis 114:155–159, 1976.
305. Arora NS, Rochester DF: Effect of body weight and muscularity on human diaphragm muscle mass, thickness and area. J Appl Physiol 52:64–70, 1982.
306. Sanchez J, Derenne JP, Bebesse B, et al.: Typology of the respiratory muscles in normal man and in patients with moderate chronic respiratory disease. Bull Europ Physiopathol Respir 18:901–914, 1982.
307. Arora NS, Rochester DF: Respiratory muscle strength and maximal voluntary ventilation in undernourished patients. Am Rev Respir Dis 126:5–8, 1982.
308. Mitchell RS, Filley GF: Chronic obstructive bronchopulmonary disease. I. Clinical features. Am Rev Respir Dis 89:360–371, 1964.
309. Browne JSL, Vineburg AM: The interdependence of gastric secretion and the CO_2 content of the blood. J Physiol (Lond) 75:345–365, 1932.
310. Flint FJ, Warrack AJ: Acute peptic ulceration in chronic emphysema. Lancet 2:178–179, 1958.
311. Fulton RM: The heart in chronic pulmonary disease. Q J Med 22:43–58, 1953.
312. Lowell FC, Franklin W, Michelson AL, Schiller IW: A note on the association of emphysema, peptic ulcer and smoking. N Engl J Med 245:123–124, 1956.
313. Ellis PA: Renal enlargement in chronic cor pulmonale. J Clin Pathol 14:552–556, 1961.
314. Ishikawa S, Bowden DH, Wyatt JP: The glomerular capillary bed in chronic pulmonary emphysema. A pathophysiologic study. Am Rev Respir Dis 100:95–98, 1969.
315. Rosenmann E, Dwarka L, Boss JH: Proliferative glomerulopathy in rheumatic heart disease and chronic lung disease. Am J Med Sci 264:213–223, 1972.
316. Campbell JL, Calverly PMA, Lamb D, Flenley DC: The renal glomerulus in hypoxic cor pulmonale Thorax 37:607–611, 1982.
317. Ashley DJB: Bony metaplasia in trachea and bronchi. J Pathol 102:186–188, 1970.
318. Pounder DJ, Pieterse AS: Tracheopathia osteoplastica: Report of four cases. Pathology 14:429–433, 1982.
319. Young RS, Sandstrom RJ, Mark GJ: Tracheopathia osteoplastica. Clinical, radiological and pathological correlations. J Thorac Cardiovasc Surg 79:537–541, 1980.
320. Eimind K: Tracheopathia osteoplastica. Nord Med 72:1029–1031, 1964.
321. Sakula A: Tracheobronchopathia osteoplastica: Its relationship to primary tracheobronchial amyloidosis. Thorax 23:105–110, 1968.
322. Shuttleworth JS, Self CL, Pershing H: Tracheopathia osteoplastica. Ann Intern Med 52:234–242, 1960.
322a. Alroy GG, Lichtig C, Kaftori JK: Tracheobronchopathia osteoplastica: End stage of primary lung amyloidosis? Chest 61:465–468, 1972.
322b. Pounder DJ, Pieterse AS: Tracheopathia osteoplastica: A study of the minimal lesion. J Pathol 138:235–239, 1982.
322c. Secrest PG, Kendig TA, Beland AJ: Tracheobronchopathia osteochondroplastica. Am J Med 36:815–818, 1964.

323. Bateson EM, Woo-Ming M: Tracheobronchomegaly. Clin Radiol 24:354–358, 1973.

324. Himalstein MR, Gallagher JC: Tracheobronchiomegaly. Ann Otol Rhinol Laryngol 82:223–227, 1973.

325. Johnston RF, Green RA: Tracheobronchiomegaly. Report of five cases and demonstration of familial occurrence. Am Rev Respir Dis 91:35–50, 1965.

326. Guest JL, Anderson JN: Tracheobronchomegaly (Mounier-Kuhn syndrome). JAMA 238:1754–1755, 1977.

327. Katz L, Le Vine M, Herman P: Tracheobronchiomegaly. The Mounier-Kuhn syndrome. 88:1084–1094, 1962.

328. Al-Mallah Z, Quantock OP: Tracheobronchomegaly. Thorax 23:320–324, 1968.

329. Dixon TC, Sando KJW, Bolton JM, Gilligan JE: A report of 342 cases of prolonged intubation. Med J Aust 2:529–533, 1968.

330. Pearson FG, Goldberg M, daSilva AJ: Tracheal stenosis complicating tracheostomy with cuffed tubes. Clinical experience and observations from a prospective study. Arch Surg 97:380–394, 1968.

331. James AE Jr, MacMillan AS Jr, Eaton SB, Grillo HC: Roentgenology of tracheal stenosis resulting from cuffed tracheostomy tubes. Am J Roentgenol 109:455–466, 1970.

332. MacMillan AS Jr, James AE Jr, Stitik FP, Grillo HC: Radiological evaluation of post-tracheostomy lesions. Thorax 26:696–670, 1971.

333. Grillo HC: The management of tracheal stenosis following assisted respiration. J Thorac Cardiovasc Surg 57:52–71, 1969.

334. Gibson GJ, David P: Respiratory complications of relapsing polychondritis. Thorax 29:726–731, 1974.

335. Dolan DL, Lemmon GB Jr, Teitelbaum SL: Relapsing polychondritis. Analytical literature review and studies on pathogenesis. Am J Med 41:285–299, 1966.

336. Pedersen H, Rebbe H: Absence of arms in the axoneme of immobile human spermatozoa. Biol Reprod 12:541–544, 1975.

337. Afzelius B, Eliasson R, Johnsen O, Lindholmer C: Lack of dynein arms in immotile human spermatozoa. J Cell Biol 66:225–232, 1975.

338. Eliasson R, Mossberg B, Camner P, Afzelius B: The immotile cilia syndrome. A congenital ciliary abnormality as an etiologic factor in chronic airway infections and male sterility. N Engl J Med 297:1–6, 1977.

339. Afzelius BA, Eliasson R: Flagellar mutants in man. On the heterogeneity of the immotile-cilia syndrome. J Ultrastruct Res 69:43–52, 1979.

340. Sturgess JM, Chao J, Wong J, et al.: Cilia with defective radial spokes, a cause of human respiratory disease. N Engl J Med 300:53–56, 1979.

341. Schneeberger EE, McCormack J, Issenberg HJ, et al.: Heterogeneity of ciliary morphology in the immotile-cilia syndrome in man. J Ultrastruct Res 73:34–43, 1980.

342. Buccetti B, Burrini AG, Pallini V: Spermatozoa and cilia lacking axoneme in an infertile man. Andrologia 12:525–532, 1980.

343. Fonzi L, Lungarella G, Palatresi R: Lack of kinocilia in the nasal mucosa in the immotile cilia syndrome. Eur J Respir Dis 63:158–163, 1982.

344. Sturgess JM, Chao J, Turner JAP: Transposition of ciliary microtubules. Another cause of impaired ciliary motility. N Engl J Med 303:318–322, 1980.

345. Veerman AJP, Van Delden L, Feenstra L, Leene W: The immotile cilia syndrome, phase contract light microscopy, scanning and transmission electron microscopy. Pediatrics 65:698–702, 1980.

346. Afzelius BA: "Immotile cilia" syndrome and ciliary abnormalities induced by infection and injury. Am Rev Respir Dis 127:107–109, 1981.

347. Chao J, Turner JAP, Sturgess JM: Genetic heterogeneity of dynein deficiency in cilia of patients with respiratory disease. Am Rev Respir Dis 12:302–305, 1982.

348. Rossman CM, Forrest JB, Lee RMKW, Newhouse MT: The dyskinetic cilia syndrome, ciliary motility in immotile cilia syndrome. Chest 78:580–582, 1980.

349. Pedersen J, Mygind N: Ciliary motility in the immotile cilia syndrome. First results of microphoto-oscillographic studies. Br J Dis Chest 74:239, 1980.

350. Rutland J, Cole P: Ciliary dyskinesia. Lancet 2:859, 1980.

351. Rossman CM, Lee RMKW, Forrest JB, Newhouse MT: Nasal ciliary ultrastructure and function in patients with primary ciliary dyskinesia compared with that in normal subjects and in subjects with various respiratory diseases. Am Rev Respir Dis 129:161–167, 1984.

352. Turner JAP, Corkey CWB, Lee JYV, et al.: Clinical expression of immotile cilia syndrome. Pediatrics 67:805–810, 1981.

353. Corkey CWB, Levison H, Turner JAP: The immotile cilia syndrome, a longitudinal survey. Am Rev Respir Dis 124:554–548, 1981.

354. Mossberg B, Afzelius BA, Eliasson R, Camner P: On the pathogenesis of obstructive lung disease. A study on the immotile cilia syndrome. Scand J Respir Dis 59:55–65, 1978.

355. Rutland J, Cole PJ: Non-invasive sampling of nasal cilia for measurement of beat frequency and study of ultrastructure. Lancet 2:564–565, 1980.

356. Fox B, Bull TB, Makey AR, Rawbone R: The significance of ultrastructural abnormalities of human cilia. Chest 80:7965–7995, 1981.

357. Wisseman CL, Simel DL, Spock A, Shelburne JD: The prevalence of abnormal cilia in normal pediatric lungs. Arch Pathol Lab Med 105:552–55, 1981.

358. Howell JT, Schochet SS, Goldman AS: Ultrastructural defects of respiratory tract cilia associated with chronic infections. Arch Pathol Lab Med 104:52–55, 1980.

359. Murray JF: *The Normal Lung: the Basis for Diagnosis and Treatment of Pulmonary Disease.* Philadelphia: WB Saunders, 1976.

360. Wright JL, Cosio M, Wiggs B, Hogg JC: A morphologic grading system for membranous and respiratory bronchioles. Arch Pathol Lab Med 109:163–165, 1985.

361. Angus GE: Morphologic studies of chronic bronchitis. Thesis, McGill University, 1966.

362. Thurlbeck WM: Aspects of chronic airflow obstruction. Chest 72:341–349, 1977.

363. Thurlbeck WM: The anatomy and histology of chronic bronchitis and all forms of emphysema. In deTreville R (ed): *Emphysema in Industry.* Mellon Foundation, 1966, pp 1–20.

364. Thurlbeck WM: Pulmonary emphysema. Am J Med Sci 246:332–353, 1963.

22 Extrinsic Immunologic Lung Disease

James C. Hogg

Although this chapter is entitled "Immunologic Lung Disease," the discussion will focus on the problems of extrinsic allergic alveolitis and asthma. Other diseases that have either a real or putative immunologic basis will be discussed in separate chapters. In particular, immunologic mechanisms may be involved in noninfectious angiitis and granulomatosis (see Chapter 17) and sarcoidosis (see Chapter 20). In considering hypersensitivity reaction of the conducting airways and gas-exchanging surface, it is useful to have some understanding of the deposition of particles in the lung and their subsequent clearance. These matters are dealt with in Chapters 4 and 23. It follows from that discussion that large particles such as ragweed pollen will deposit primarily above the larynx and in the larger airways of the lower respiratory tract. It requires allergenic particles less than 6 μm in diameter to penetrate to the peripheral portions of the lung to produce hypersensitivity pneumonitis.[1] Clearly a mixture of different-sized particles can be expected to produce both asthma and extrinsic allergic alveolitis.

Asthma

Asthma has been difficult to define,[2] but it is usually thought of in terms of reversible airways obstruction. Those who have the propensity to develop asthmatic attacks have hyperresponsive airways, and they can be identified by challenge tests. These tests consist of the administration of increasing doses of either histamine or methacholine as an aerosol for the patient to breathe for a standard period.[3] The forced expiratory volume in 1 second (FEV_1) is measured after the administration of each dose; patients with hyperresponsive airways show a 20 percent fall in their FEV_1 at lower doses of agonist than normal subjects. Patients that have hyperresponsive airways are also known to bronchoconstrict to other stimuli such as exercise[4] or breathing cold air[5] in which heat or water loss are thought to be the factors that precipitate the bronchoconstriction.

Relatively few subjects have a clearly established allergic mechanism for their asthma. The majority seem to acquire hyperreactivity and asthma in a nonspecific fashion. In cases in which an immune mechanism can be demonstrated, it occurs as a result of specific immunoglobulin (Ig) E binding to mast cells. When antigen interacts with this antibody, the mast cells release both preformed mediators such as histamine and also generate a wide variety of other mediators including the leukotrienes. (The subject of mediator release has been well reviewed elsewhere[6-8] and will not be further discussed here.) In recent years, it has become apparent that airways hyperreact when an inflammatory reaction becomes established in them.[9,10] This inflammatory reaction can be induced by either antigen reacting with IgE on mast cells or after the airways have been exposed to nonspecific irritants such as cigarette smoke,[10] viral infections,[11] NO_2,[12] or ozone.[13]

Florey[14] showed that inflammatory reactions in mucous membranes have some features that are similar to inflammatory reactions occurring elsewhere and some that are specific for mucous membranes. The general features are those of edema and cellular infiltration, whereas goblet cell discharge of mucus and shedding of epithelial cells are specific for mucous membranes such as the airways. These features can readily be identified in the airways of patients that die of asthma.

Pathology of Asthma

The pathology of asthma can be discussed under the headings of muscle spasm, airways inflammation with edema, and mucous hypersecretion. Although all three are relatively constant features of asthma, their proportionate contribution in any particular case varies considerably. For example, smooth muscle spasm is undoubtedly the feature of the disease that is rapidly reversible with treatment, whereas inflammatory edema and mucous plugging of the airways appear likely to account for the more slowly reversible or irreversible forms of the disorder.

Smooth Muscle Spasm

In models of asthma such as allergic bronchoconstriction in the guinea pig, the smooth muscle contraction is not associated with airways edema or mucous plugging of the airways, so this reaction can be assumed to be due solely to smooth muscle constriction.[15] This contrasts sharply with human asthmatic deaths, which are nearly always associated with edema of the airway walls and mucous plugging of the airways lumen[16,17] (Fig. 22–1). This suggests that airways smooth muscle contraction may play an important role in cases of asthma when the airways obstruction is easily and rapidly reversible by bronchodilator therapy, whereas inflammation of the wall and mucous plugging of the lumen may be the important anatomic features of asthma as it becomes more severe.

The dominant control of the smooth muscle is provided by the cholinergic system which constricts smooth muscle[18] and the beta-adrenergic system which relaxes it.[19] Alpha-adrenergic receptors are sparse in the airways muscle of most species and probably relate to the bronchial vasculature or mucus-secreting apparatus more than to the smooth muscle. A third system of nerves, the so-called nonadrenergic inhibitory system,[18] has been described more recently; as its name suggests, this system is thought to relax the airways smooth muscle by an unidentified mediator. Several theories of asthma have developed that relate to one or other aspect of the control of airways smooth muscle. One theory[19] has stressed the possibility of a partial beta blockade, another hyperreactive cholinergic pathway,[20] and a third theory[21] has suggested a basic abnormality is a suppression of the nonadrenergic inhibitory system. Finally, it has also been suggested that asthmatic airways may be associated with smooth muscle that functions as a single unit so that the whole network contracts when part of it is stimulated.[18]

Airways Inflammation

Analysis of the protein in the bronchial mucous plugs from asthmatic patients[22] shows large amounts of albumin and large numbers of inflammatory cells which strongly suggests that an inflammatory exudate enters the airways lumen. As this reaction is difficult to study in humans, we must rely on animal studies.

Animal studies have provided several important insights into the development of acquired airways hyperresponsiveness. A single exposure to cigarette smoke in the guinea pig can produce an inflammatory reaction in the airways that has both an exudative and proliferative phase.[23] The exudative phase is associated with an increased wet weight/dry weight ratio of the airway wall due to the inflammatory edema and an immigration of inflammatory cells into the interstitial space and through the epithelium to lie on the mucosal surface. This inflammatory reaction is associated with an increased mucosal permeability which is maximum 30 minutes after the smoke exposure and returns to normal by 24 hours. This change in permeability can be readily measured by the tracer horseradish peroxidase (HRP), and this method has shown that the increase in permeability is associated with increased exposure of the irritant receptors. The hypothesis that the hyperresponsiveness is due to exposure of these nerve endings is attractive, but the evidence is inconclusive to date.[10]

Several workers in Nadel's laboratory have shown that the lower airways can become hyperreactive to nonspecific stimuli such as histamine during an acute upper respiratory tract infection. Empey and associates[11] have shown that the hyperreactivity to histamine seen with respiratory virus infections can be blocked by atropine, and they speculated that the inflammatory reaction caused by virus sensitized the afferent receptors and exaggerated the reflex component of the histamine response. Nitrogen dioxide,[12] ozone,[13] and cigarette smoke[10] have also been shown to enhance bronchial reactivity. Empey and colleagues[11] attributed the acquired hyperreactivity to mucosal damage and speculated that this unspecified damage might be due to inflammation of the mucosa. It seems likely that the common feature of the damage produced by viral infection, NO_2, and ozone inhalation is the inflammatory reaction and that this in some way causes the hyperreactivity. Just what aspect of the inflammation reaction is responsible for the increased hyperresponsiveness is under investigation at the present time.[9,10]

The hyperreactive response can involve more than one mechanism, so inflammation of the airways may induce an abnormal response at more than one site. For example, histamine is capable of stimulating both the irritant receptors to produce reflex bronchoconstriction and of stimulating the airway smooth muscle directly. Methacholine, on the other hand, only stimulates the smooth muscle and is not usually associated with irritant receptor stimulation. This fact has been demonstrated by Vidruk and co-workers[24] who recorded from single nerve fibers and can be clearly seen from the data of Michoud and colleagues[25] on intact animals. They compared antigen, methacholine, and histamine challenge to Ascaris-sensitive monkeys and showed that, while the antigen and histamine caused an increase in airways resistance and rapid, shallow breathing, methacholine only caused increased airways resistant without rapid, shallow breathing. This fact is further brought out by the study of Holtzman and associates[26] who showed that the ganglionic blocker hexmethonium could block the histamine but not the methacholine response.

Mast Cells

As allergic asthmatic attacks are initiated by the interaction of antigen with IgE on mast cells,[6] the relationship of

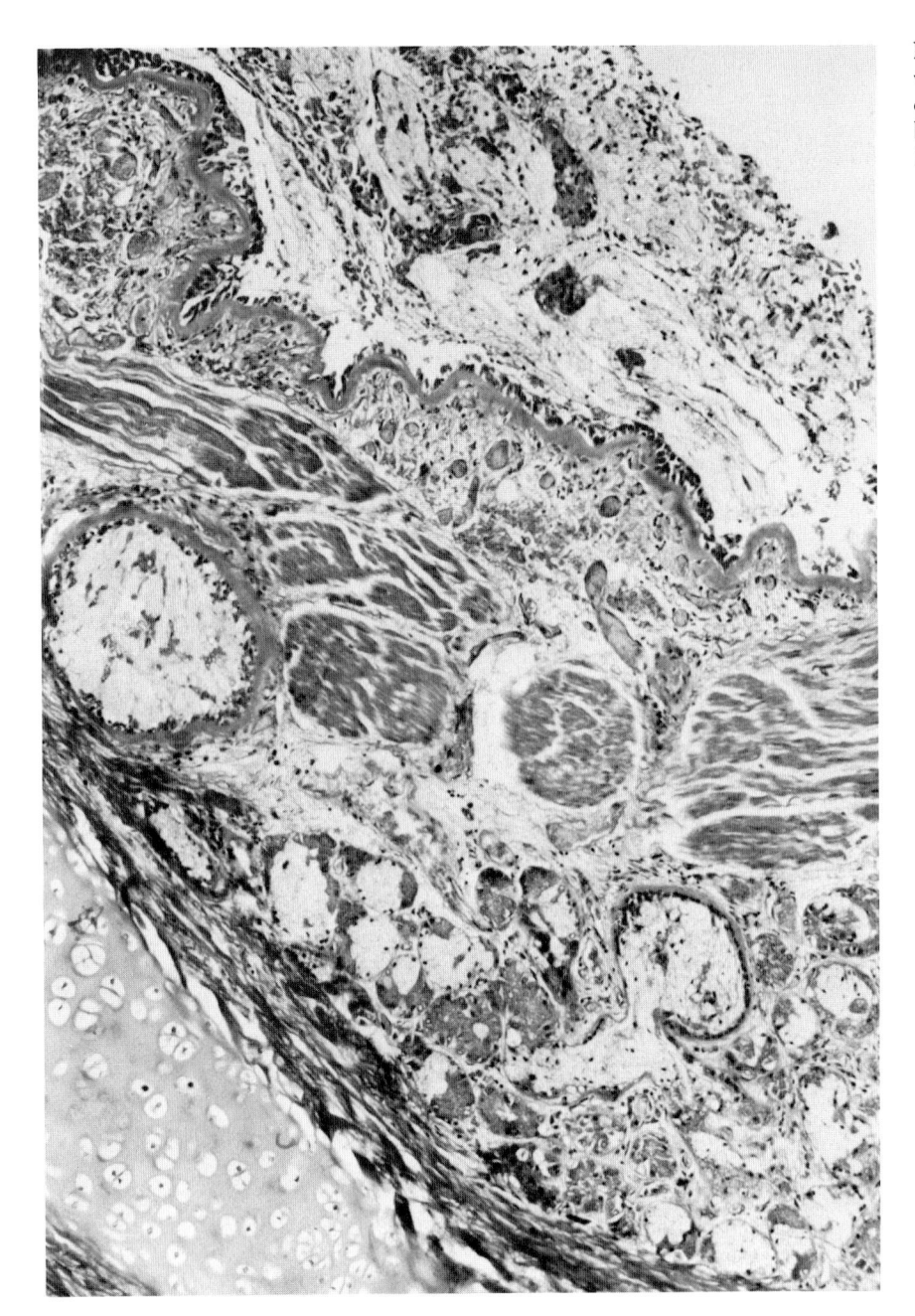

Figure 22–1. A bronchus from a patient who died of asthma showing inflammatory exudate in the lumen, thick basement membrane, and hypertrophic smooth muscle (H&E, ×25).

the mast cell to the airway lumen is of critical importance in the initiation of these attacks. Studies on mast cell distribution are not easy because their fixation requires alcohol-based rather than water-based fixatives, and these are seldom in routine use. Salvato[27,28] has demonstrated that mast cells are depleted in asthma and those that remain are markedly degranulated. Guerzon and associates[29] have shown that there are relatively few mast cells in the mucosa compared with the large concentration of mast cells in the submucosa of the airways. Although there are an important number of mast cells on the surface of the airway lumen, this number can be overestimated by washing and brushing techniques which also harvest mast cells from the mucosa. For example,

Guerzon and associates[29] estimated approximately one mast cell for every 10^6 epithelial cells, whereas Patterson and coworkers[30] found 1 per 200 epithelial cells in lung washings. It seems likely that large antigen molecules that are unable to penetrate the mucosa react with the relatively small number of mast cells on the epithelial surface and that chemical mediators released from these mast cells are responsible for opening the epithelial tight junctions. This process allows the antigen to penetrate to the mast cells that are located deep to mucosa in the airway wall.

The change in the epithelial basement membrane is an important histologic feature of the asthmatic lung (Figs. 22–1, 22–2, 22–3). Callerame and colleagues[31] showed

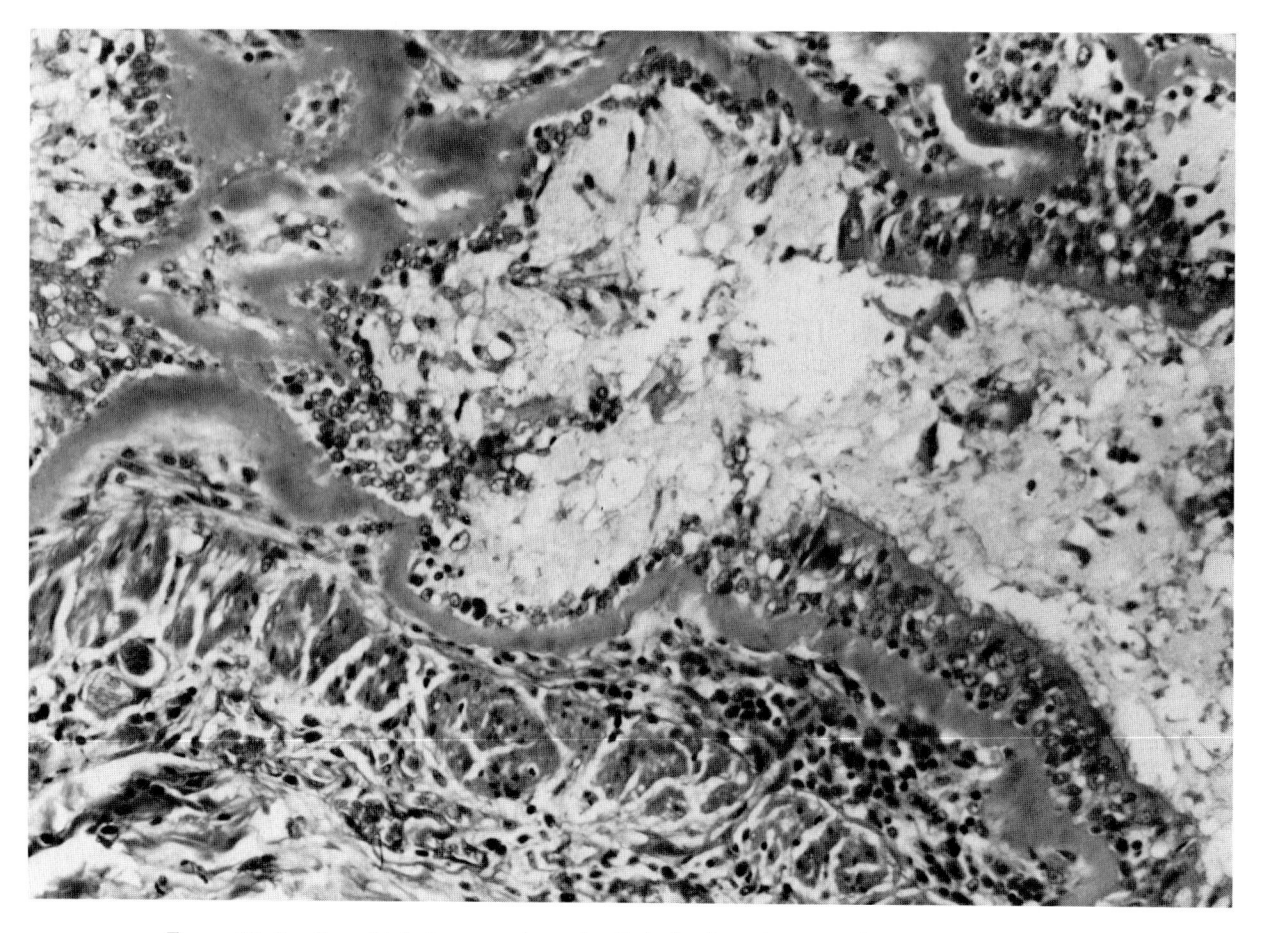

Figure 22–2. Bronchiole from a patient who died of asthma showing inflammatory mucous plug in the airway lumen, disrupted epithelium, and an infiltration of inflammatory cells into the airway wall (H&E, ×40).

that the mean width of the basement membrane from asthmatic patients was 17.5 μm, whereas that from normal subjects was only 7 μm; they attributed the thickening of the basement membrane to the deposition of immunoglobulins. However, recent data on airways inflammation suggest that the basement membrane begins to increase in thickness in association with the increased mitotic activity that heralds the beginning of epithelial repair. This suggests that the increased thickness of the basement membrane may be due to the deposition of type 4 collagen associated with increased epithelial cell turnover in the same way that the basement membrane of the diabetic microvasculature thickens in relation to the increased endothelial cell turnover.[32,33] Curschmann[34] was the first to note that asthmatics had a large number of epithelial cells in their sputum, and this has been amply confirmed by other investigators[35,36] who have demonstrated squamous cells as well as compact clusters of columnar cells known as Creola bodies in the sputum. The loss of the mucosal cells has been attributed to muscle spasm[37] and submucosal edema,[17] but it also seems likely that direct toxic injury to epithelial cells, perhaps by products of the eosinophil,[38] is more important. This increased turnover of the epithelium is also associated with active division of the basal cell layer and the formation of a large number of goblet cells.

Mucous Plugging of the Airways

At autopsy the lungs from patients who die from asthma are hyperinflated and tend not to collapse after the thorax is opened because the segmental and subsegmental airways and the bronchioles are filled with inflammatory mucous plugs (see Fig. 22–2) These plugs are formed by an inflammatory exudate that contains mucus and cellular elements.[22,36] The eosinophilic leukocyte is the cell that tends to predominate in these plugs, but other inflammatory cells and a large number of epithelial cells can also be found. The submucosa shows evidence of an inflammatory reaction which consists of a congested microvasculature and an edematous interstitial space containing the same inflammatory cellular infiltrate as the airways lumen. The reason for the excess mucus in the airways is probably related in part to both increased production and decreased clearance. The machinery for increased production is present in the form of hypertrophy and hyperplasia of the bronchial mucous glands as

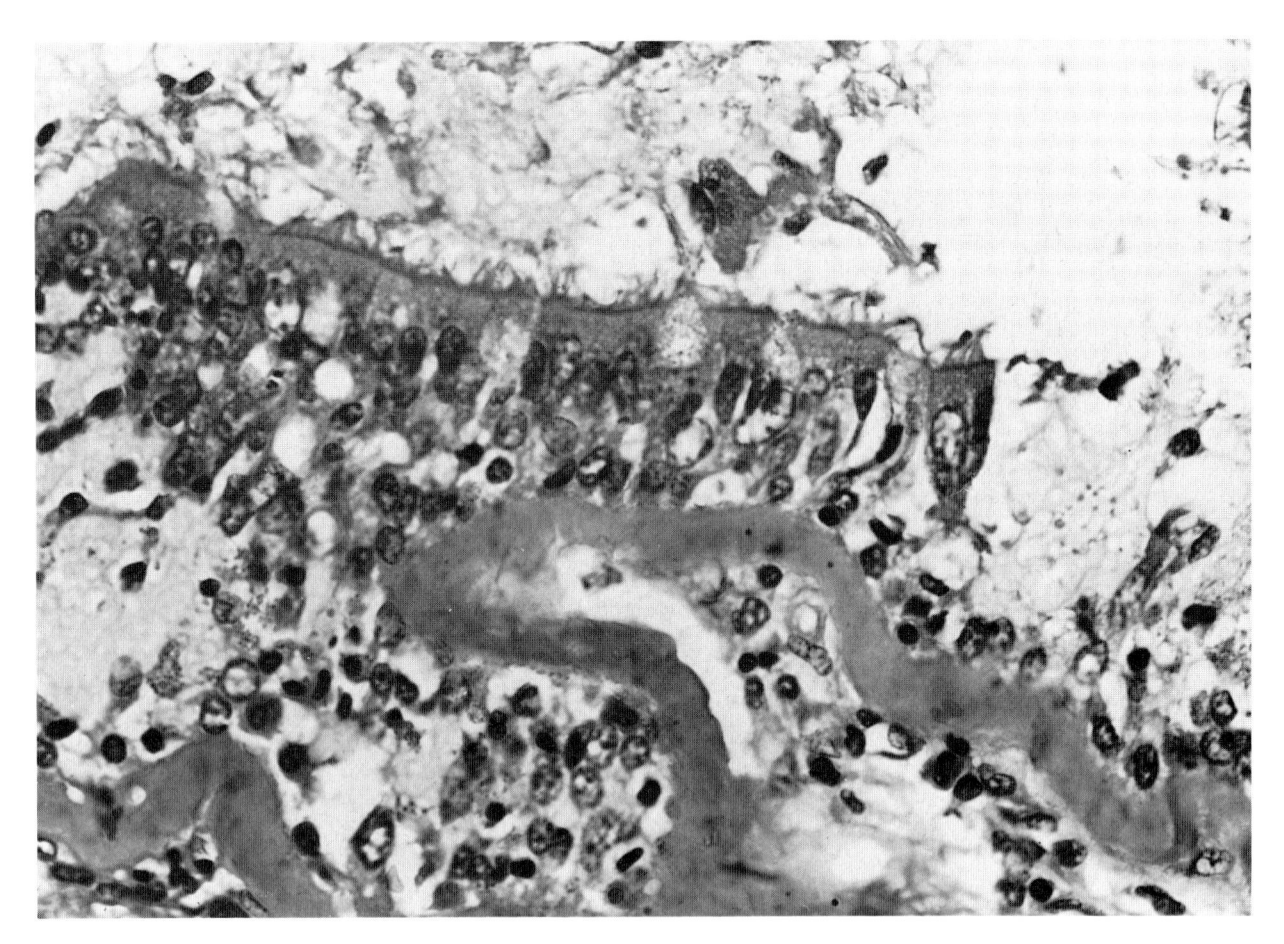

Figure 22-3. High-power view of airway epithelium from a patient with asthma showing disrupted epithelium and thick basement membrane (H&E, ×400).

well as goblet cell metaplasia of the mucosal lining; decreased clearance will result from the disrupted epithelium. The fact that the plugs have a high protein content with much of this protein being albumin[22] shows that the inflammatory exudate[14] contributes to their formation. This indicates that the material occluding the airways may be related to fluid and protein exudation as well as the hypersecretion of mucus.

The nature and source of the fluid that normally lines the airways is a difficult problem to study. It seems possible that the lining fluid emanates largely as a fluid secretion in the distal airways and that its final composition is influenced by water absorption in the more central airways.[39] This concentration of the fluid is necessary to prevent the relatively narrow cross-section of the central airways from being occluded. An increase in the production of fluid in the form of exudate along with an interference with a normal fluid reabsorptive process could greatly increase the amount of fluid in the airways. This could account for the organization and tenacity of the mucous plugs and also contribute to their formation by interfering with mucociliary clearance.

Whether mucous plugging occurs in less severe forms of asthma is not clear. Early bronchographic studies of patients with chronic asthma[40] showed that the airways were often occluded by mucus, but this form of investigation is now known to be dangerous in these patients. The fact that lesser degrees of airways plugging occur is supported by the study of asthmatic sputum in which Curschmann spirals can be identified, but this only provides indirect evidence of the severity of airways obstruction caused by plugging in this disorder.

Chronic Complications of Asthma

The fact that patients with asthma who die of other causes have many of the changes in the airways seen in patients who die in status is of interest. This finding suggests that people who die during a sudden bronchospastic episode probably die because of bronchospasm superimposed on thickened inflamed airways in which the lumen is plugged. Whether these chronic changes in the airway lead to other disease is problematic in that some studies suggest that right ventricular hypertrophy is a problem in 70 percent of cases, whereas others set a figure of only 10 percent. Similarly bronchiectasis is reported as a complication of asthma by some authors, whereas others think it is rare. It is difficult to sort this problem out when, for example, allergic bronchopulmonary aspergillosis is associated with both asthma and bronchiectasis. In this writer's view, it seems likely as in most cases of asthma there is neither bronchiectasis nor cor pulmonale. However, there is no reason that cor pulmonale should not develop in cases in which bronchiectasis is present.

Hypersensitivity Pneumonitis

Many antigens have been associated with hypersensitivity pneumonitis.[41] The majority of these are occupational in nature (Table 22–1), but hypersensitivity pneumonitis has also been described in association with air conditioners,[42] humidified heating systems,[43] and molds growing in floor boards.[44] In every case, a meticulous history is critical in suspecting a diagnosis. Immunologic study, challenge tests with the suspected antigen, and lung biopsy usually provide confirmation of suspicions raised by a careful history. As the materials to which patients are exposed are complex and contain a multitude of antigenic material, it is difficult to be certain about which antigen causes the pneumonitis.

In an experimental study carried out on rabbits, Joubert and associates[45] used a relatively pure antigen (HRP) and found that one major component of this mixture of antigenic materials caused the alveolitis, while other components were responsible for the precipitating antibody in the serum and positive skin tests. This means that the demonstration of positive skin test or precipitating antibody to crude extracts provide evidence of

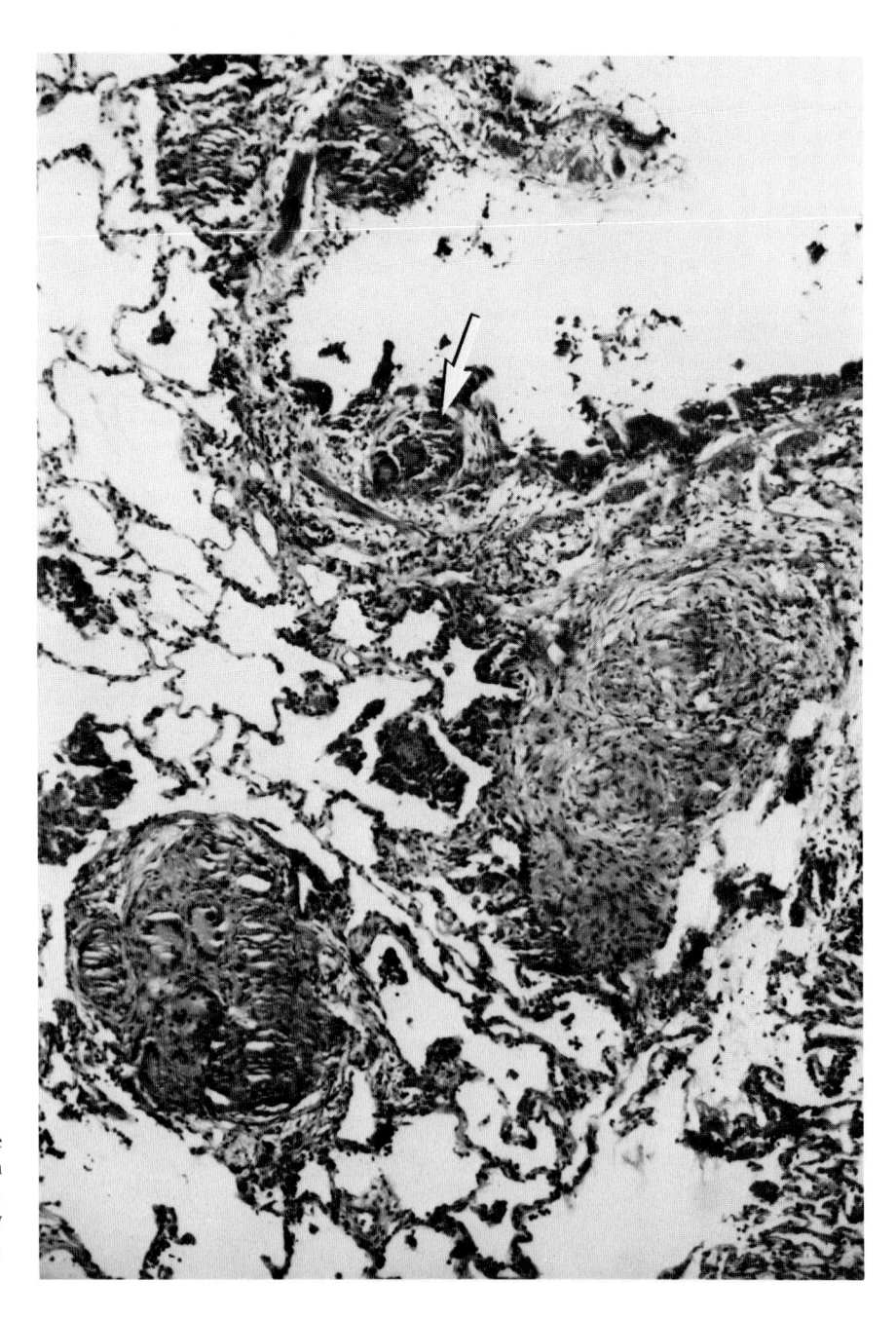

Figure 22–4. Granulomata present in the airway wall (arrow) and parenchyma of a patient with hypersensitivity pneumonitis. There is also an infiltration of inflammatory cells into the airway wall and alveoli (H&E, ×40).

exposure to a material and do not establish that a particular molecule in the crude material is responsible for the lung disease. This suggests that the most effective way of establishing a relationship between a crude mixture of antigens and lung disease is to challenge the patient with an aerosol of the crude material and make objective measurements of the pulmonary response. Unfortunately, it is not possible to be dogmatic about whether this sort of challenge test should be done in every case. In some cases, particularly when the patient's livelihood may be involved, a challenge test may be necessary to establish a firm diagnosis. However, in other cases, a remission of symptoms and signs of disease when the patient leaves an environment may be all that is necessary for satisfactory management of the disease.

Histologic Features of Hypersensitivity Pneumonitis

The histologic appearance of hypersensitivity pneumonitis is stereotyped despite the fact that it can be caused by so many different materials. In general, it is granulomatous inflammatory lesion (Figs. 22–4, 22–5, 22–6) that involves the central portion of the lobule, including the terminal and respiratory bronchioles.[46-53] Bronchiolitis is such an important feature of the disease that Turner-Warwick[41] suggested that it should be called extrinsic allergic bronchioloalveolitis.

In a careful analysis of 60 cases of farmers' lung, (Table 22–2) reported that the common findings were an alveolar interstitial infiltrate consisting of plasma cells, lymphocytes, and occasionally eosinophils in 100 percent of cases; there was a granulomatous interstitial reaction in 70 percent of the cases in which the granulomas tended to be located in the center of the lobules. In about 50 percent of cases, there was a mild form of bronchiolitis obliterans in which connective tissue was observed proliferating in the respiratory bronchioles. Other features of the histology, such as unresolved pneumonia, the presence of alveolar foam cells, and pleural fibrosis, seem more likely to have occurred as a result of the airways obstruction produced by the primary disease. Foreign bodies are commonly found in extrinsic allergic

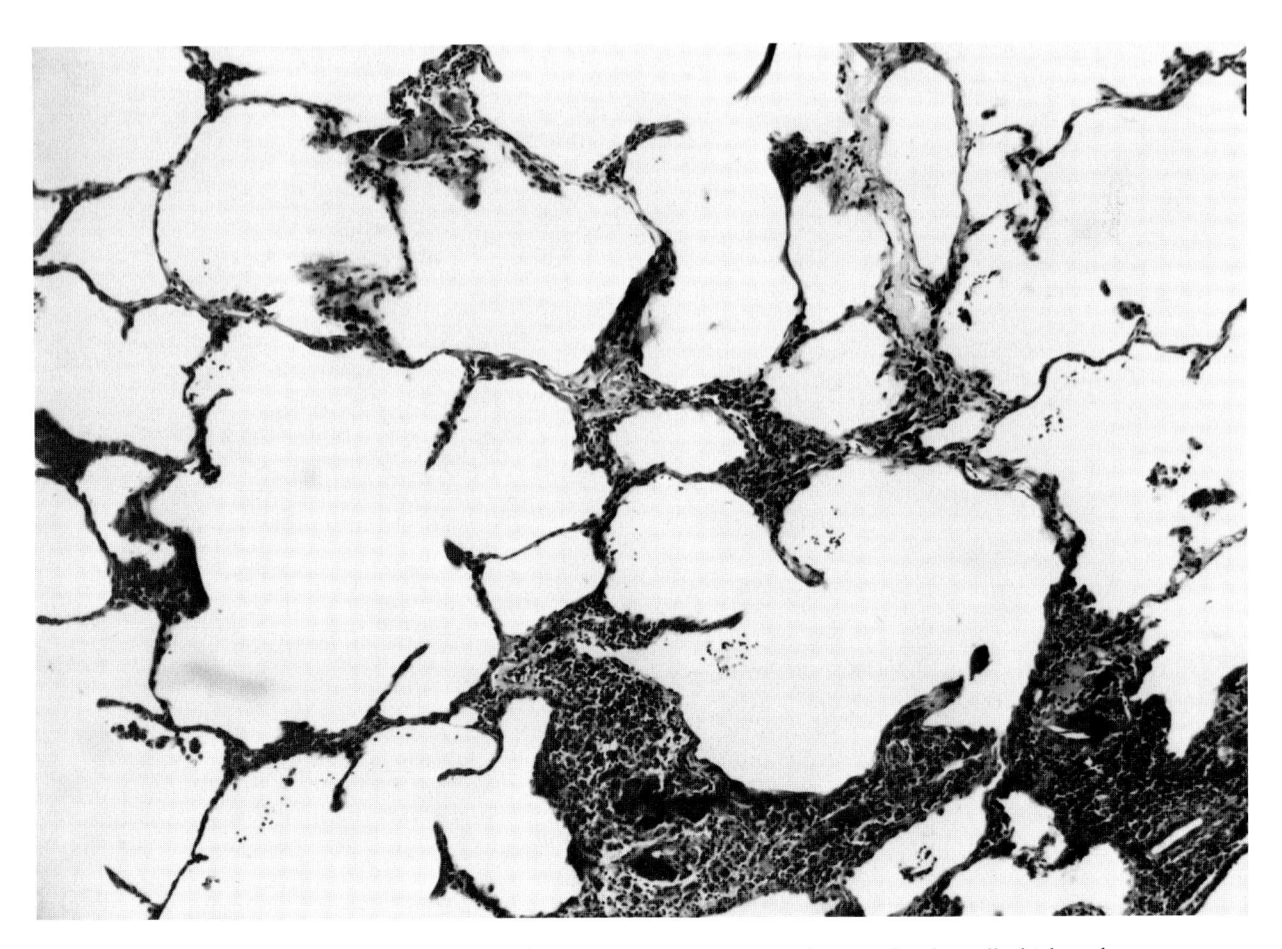

Figure 22–5. From a patient with hypersensitivity pneumonitis showing alveolar walls thickened by an inflammatory infiltrate (H&E, ×40).

Figure 22–6A. Extrinsic allergic alveolitis. A. High-power view of infiltrate in the alveolar wall showing that it consists mainly of lymphocytes.

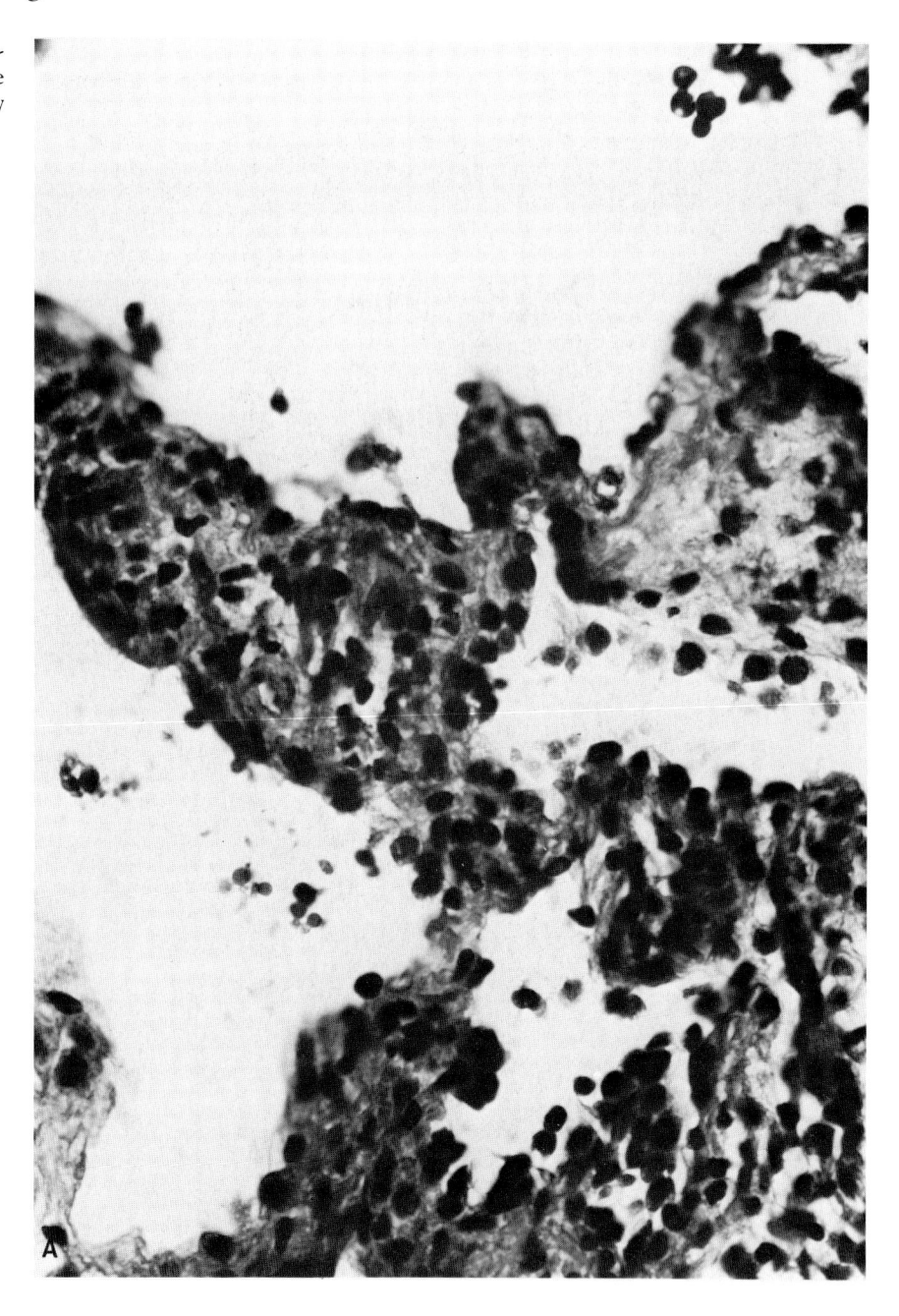

alveolitis, but it is rare to be able to demonstrate the nature of the etiologic agent. Cork dust has been identified within the lesions in suberosis,[54] vegetable fibers in bagassosis,[55] and fungi in maple bark disease. Although these crude materials are the source of the responsible antigens, it is impossible to determine which of the antigens present in the crude material are responsible for different aspects of the disease.

Kawanami and associates[53] reported light and electron microscopic findings in 18 patients who had biopsies for extrinsic allergic alveolitis. Their findings were similar to earlier reports but provided electron microscopic evidence that the primary cell infiltrating the alveolar wall was the lymphocyte (see Fig. 22–6). They also provided good photomicrographs of the granulomas which tended to be poorly formed and showed the deposition of interstitial connective tissue. This latter event was often associated with the formation of masses of loose connective tissue located within the air space which they termed alveolar buds. This probably represents the organization of an exudate that has developed in an area with extensive epithelial damage and is likely a preliminary event in the formation of bronchiolitis obliterans.

These data show that the pathology in hypersensitivity

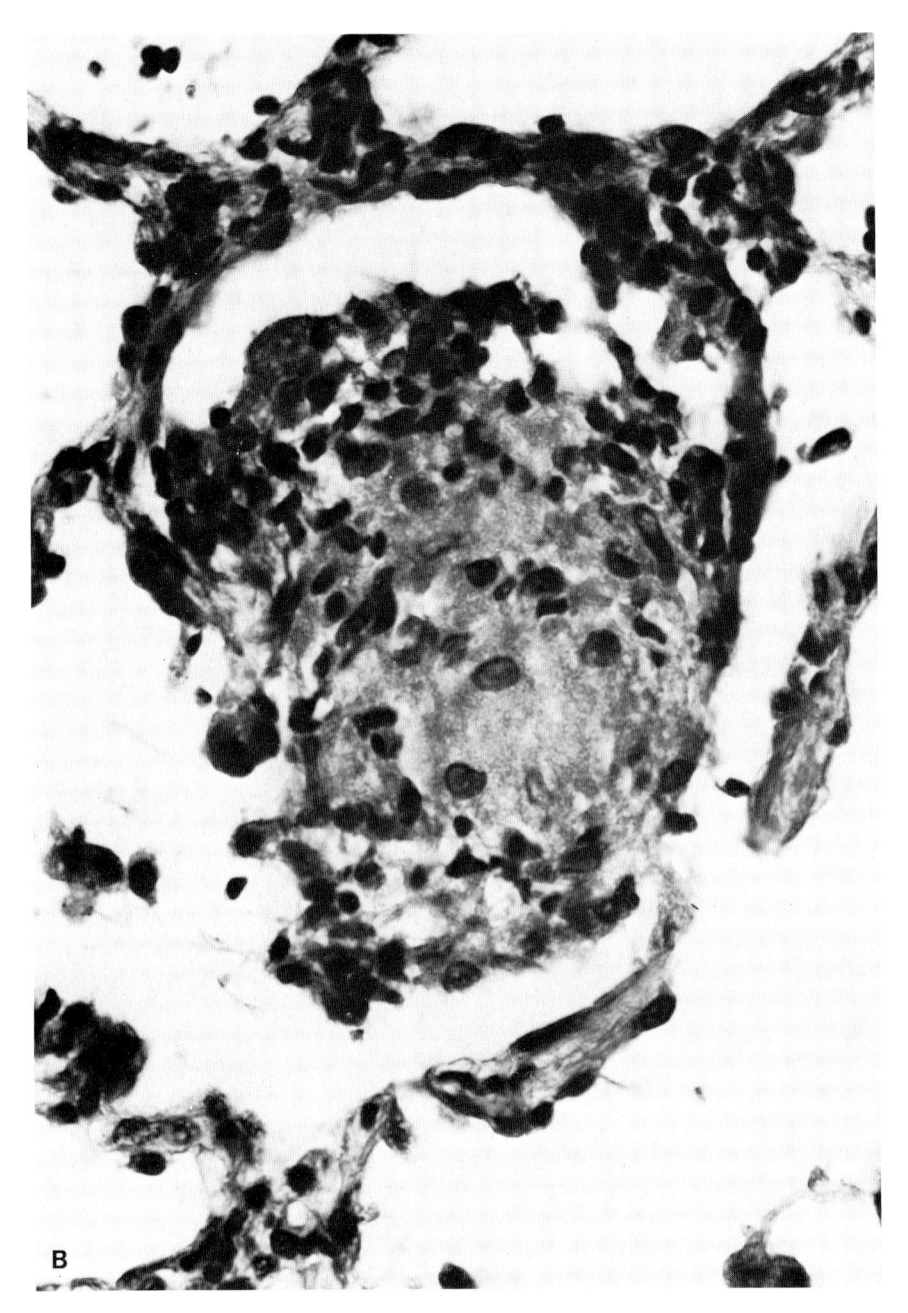

Figure 22–6B. A granuloma formed on the alveolar wall near the area of alveolitis (H&E, both ×400).

pneumonitis are now well enough worked out that the pathologist should be able to suggest a diagnosis on the basis of the histologic findings. When these findings occur and the clinicians are unaware of the possibility of hypersensitivity pneumonitis, the pathologist should suggest that the patient's home and work environment be carefully evaluated.

In recent years, several groups of investigators[57–61] have claimed that this diagnosis can also be established by bronchoalveolar lavage. These claims are seldom supported by a standard assessment of sensitivity, specificity, and calculation of the predictive value of findings on bronchoalveolar lavage, which is thought to be diagnostic of extrinsic allergic alveolitis. The value of this procedure in the diagnosis of lung disease has recently been brought into question,[62] and in the writer's opinion, much more work will be required before bronchoalveolar fluid can be said to reflect the changes in the tissue. This does not mean that bronchoalveolar lavage will not prove to be a useful method of investigation of the pathogenesis of hypersensitivity pneumonitis and other interstitial lung diseases.

Although Seal and associates[48] claimed that the acute phase of extrinsic allergic alveolitis is associated with

Table 22–1. Fungal Antigens

Type of Disease	Source	Specific Agent
Farmers' lung	Moldy hay	Microspora (M.) faeni
Bagassosis	Modly bagasse	T. vulgaris
Mushroom workers' lung	Mushroom composta	Thermoactinomycete
Ventilator pneumonitis	Humidified hot air	M. faeni
Malt workers' lung	Moldy barley	M. faeni
Maple bark strippers' lung	Moldy bark	Cryptostroma cirticule
Suberosis	Moldy cork	Penicillium frequentous
	Avian Antigens	
Pigeon fanciers' lung	Droppings, dust	Pigeon serum
Budgerigar	Droppings, dust	Bugeriga serum
	Mammalian Antigens	
Pituitary snuff	Porcine and bovine pituitary powder	Porcine and bovine pituitary
Rat handlers' lung	Rat urine and serum	Rat serum protein
Fishmeal workers' lung	Fish protein, fishmeal	Fishmeal protein
	Insect Antigens	
Wheat weevil lung	Infested wheat flour	Setophilus grenarius

Table 22–2. Morphologic Features of 60 Cases of Farmers' Lung

Interstitial infiltrate	100%
Granulomas	70%
Unresolved pneumonia	65%
Bronchiolitis obliterans	50%
Foreign bodies	60%

Modified from Reyes et al.[49]

Table 22–3. Histologic Features of Sarcoidosis and Extrinsic Allergic Alveolitis

	Sarcoidosis	Extrinsic Allergic Alveolitis
Alveolitis	Uncommon	100% of cases
Bronchiolitis	Rare	Bronchiolitis obliterans in 50% of cases
Granulomatous	100% of cases located along lymphatics	Centrilobular in position in the airway wall
Foreign bodies	Uncommon	60%

histologic changes similar to those seen in an Arthus reaction, there are few published studies of this early lesion. As the animal studies suggest that changes associated with an Arthus reaction are not responsible for the alveolitis, the early lesions reported in humans should probably be reinvestigated. In any event, most cases come to biopsy in the subacute and chronic phase of the condition in which the major differential diagnosis includes sarcoidosis and the lymphocytic interstitial pneumonias.

Differential Diagnosis

Some criteria that can be used to differentiate extrinsic allergic alveolitis are listed in Table 22–3. The major contentious point is the presence of alveolitis which, in this writer's veiw, is much more common in extrinsic allergic alveolitis than in sarcoidosis. The lesions of extrinsic allergic alveolitis are usually more prominent in the center of the lobule where they involve the luminal and respiratory bronchioles. Sarcoidosis, on the other hand, tracks the lymphatics so that it is prominent at the periphery of the lobule and in the interlobular septa. When found in the airways, sarcoidosis usually follows the lymphatics in the bronchovascular sheath, but the lesions can extend into the airway wall and become endobronchial in some cases. It follows that it is often difficult to separate the two conditions purely on the basis of histology. Therefore, it seems wise to evaluate the clinical story carefully in cases in which there is doubt. Granulomatous lung disease caused by infections with mycobacteria or fungi is different in that the granulomas tend to caseate and the organisms can usually be demonstrated by special stains. However, berylliosis produces a systemic disease that is impossible to separate from sarcoid.

Pathogenesis

Patients with extrinsic allergic alveolitis develop symptoms when they are challenged with the crude extracts of the source of antigens to which they have become allergic. These challenge tests may show an immediate response when the FEV_1 falls significantly within a few minutes after the administration of the aerosol, a delayed response when it falls several hours later, or a combination of both immediate and delayed response. The immediate response is known to be IgE mediated, but the nature of the delayed response is much more controversial. The timing of the late response and the indirect evidence that precipitating antibody was present caused early investigators[63,64] to favor an Arthus reaction as the mechanism that produced the disease. However, a vasculitis consistent with an Arthus reaction has not been a consistent feature of most studies, although some[52] believe it could be a cause of the early lesion. More recently, the experimental models of the disease favored a pathogenesis brought about by delayed-type hypersensitivity[45,65] rather than to an Arthus reaction. Indeed, in the writer's opinion, the development of the granulomatous bronchioloalveolitis typical of the human disease requires particulate antigen and a delayed-type hypersensitivity reaction.

An important feature of extrinsic allergic alveolitis is that it occurs so rarely in relation to the large number of people who are exposed to the antigenic materials thought to cause it. This fact is consistent with the experimental findings in animal models of extrinsic allergic alveolitis in which immunized animals develop disease when first challenged but then tend to improve in the face of repeated challenge.[68-71] This suggests that there is a normal ability to shut down the immune response in the face of repeated challenge and leads to the hypothesis that disease may result in people who have a compromised ability to turn off the immune response. This hypothesis is presently being tested in several laboratories and seems more attractive than the concept that the disease is a simple manifestation of an Arthus or delayed hypersensitivity reaction.

References

1. Hargreave FE: Extrinsic allergic alveolitis. Can Med Assoc J 108:1150–1154, 1973.
2. Porter R, Birch J (eds): *Identification of Asthma*. Edinburgh: Churchill Livingston, 1971.
3. Cockcroft DW, Killian DN, Mellon JA, Hargreave FE: Bronchial reactivity to inhaled histamine: A method and clinical survey. Clin Allergy 7:235–243, 1977.
4. Anderson SD, McEvoy JDS, Bianco S: Changes in lung volumes and airways resistance after exercise in asthmatic subjects. Am Rev Respir Dis 106:30–37, 1972.
5. Deal EC, McFadden ER Jr, Ingram RH Jr, et al.: Role of respiratory heat exchange in production of exercise-induced asthma. J Appl Physiol 46:467–475, 1979.
6. Ishizaka K, Ishizaka T: Biological function of gamma E antibodies and mechanisms of reaginic hypersensitivity. Clin Exp Immunol 6:24–42, 1970.
7. Schellenberg RR: Pathophysiology of allergic diseases. In Devlin, JP (ed): *Pulmonary and Antiallergic Drugs*. New York: John Wiley & Sons, 1985, pp 1–42.
8. Church MK: Biochemical basis of pulmonary and antiallergic drugs. In Devlin JP (ed): Pulmonary and antiallergic drugs. New York: John Wiley & Sons, 1985, pp 43–121.
9. Holtzman MJ, Fabbri ML, O'Byrne PM, et al.: Importance of airways inflammation for hyperresponsiveness induced by ozone. Am Rev Respir Dis 127:686–690, 1983.
10. Hogg JC, Hulbert WC, Armour C, Pare PD: The effect of mucosal inflammation on airways reactivity. In Kay AB, Austen KF, Lichtenstein LM (eds): *Asthma: Physiology, Immunopharmacology and Treatment*. New York: Academic Press, 1985, pp 327–338.
11. Empey DW, Laitinen LA, Jacobs L, et al.: Mechanisms of bronchial hyperreactivity in normal subjects after upper respiratory tract infection. Am Rev Respir Dis 113:131–139, 1976.
12. Orehek J, Massari JP, Gayrard P, et al.: Effect of short-term, low-level nitrogen dioxide exposure on bronchial sensitivity of asthmatic patients. J Clin Invest 57:301–307, 1976.
13. Golden JA, Nadel JA, Boushey HA: Bronchial hyperirritability in healthy subjects after exposure to ozone. Am Rev Respir Dis 118:287–294, 1978.
14. Florey HW: The secretion of mucus and inflammation of mucus membranes. In Florey HW (ed): *General Pathology*. London: Lloyd-Luke, 1962, pp 167–196.
15. Jeffries E, Pare PD, Hogg JC: Measurements of airway edema in allergic bronchoconstriction in the guinea pig. Am Rev Respir Dis 123:687–688, 1981.
16. Dunnill MS: The pathology of asthma. In Porter R, Birch J (eds): *Identification of Asthma*. Edinburgh: Churchill Livingston, 1971, pp 35–46.
17. Dunnill MS: The pathology of asthma, with special reference to changes in the bronchial mucosa. J Clin Pathol 13:27–33, 1960.
18. Daniel EE, Davis C, Jones T, Kannan MS: Control of airway smooth muscle. In Hargreave FE (ed): *Airway Hyperreactivity: Mechanisms and Clinical Relevance*. Mississauga, Ontario, Canada: Astra Pharmaceuticals, 1975, pp 80–107.
19. Szentivanyi A: The beta adrenergic theory of the atropic abnormality in bronchial asthma. J Allergy 42:203–232, 1968.
20. Nadel JA: Structure and function relationships in the airways. Med Thorac 22:231–243, 1965.
21. Richardson JB, Beland J: Nonadrenergic inhibitory nervous system in human airways. J Appl Physiol 41:764–771, 1976.
22. Sanerkin NG, Evans DMD: The sputum in bronchial asthma: Pathognomonic patterns. J Pathol Bacteriol 89:535–541, 1965.
23. Hulbert WC, Walker DC, Jackson A, Hogg JC: Airway permeability to horseradish peroxidase in guinea pigs: The repair phase after injury by cigarette smoke. Am Rev Respir Dis 123:320–326, 1981.
24. Vidruk EH, Hahn HL, Nadel JA, Sampson SR: Mechanisms by which histamine stimulates rapidly adapting receptors in dog lungs. J Appl Physiol 43:397–402, 1977.
25. Michoud MC, Pare PD, Boucher RC, Hogg JC: Airway responses to histamine and methacholine in Ascaris suum-allergic rhesus monkeys. J Appl Physiol 45:846–851, 1978.
26. Holtzman MJ, Sheller JR, DiMeo M, et al.: Effect of ganglionic

blockade on bronchial reactivity in atopic subjects. Am Rev Respir Dis 122:17–25, 1980.

27. Salvato G: Asthma and mast cells of bronchial connective tissue. Experientia 18:330–331, 1962.

28. Salvato G: Mast cells in bronchial connective tissues of man: Their modifications in asthma and after treatment with histamine liberator 48/80. Int Arch Allergy 18:348–358, 1961.

29. Guerzon GM, Pare PD, Michoud MC, Hogg JC: The number and distribution of mast cells in monkey lungs. Am Rev Respir Dis 119:59–66, 1979.

30. Patterson R, Tomita Y, Oh SH, et al.: Respiratory mast cells and basophiloid cells. I. Evidence that they are secreted into the bronchial lumen, morphology, degranulation and histamine release. Clin Exp Immunol 16:223–234, 1974.

31. Callerame ML, Condemi JJ, Bohrod MG, Vaughan JH: Immunologic reactions of bronchial tissues in asthma. N Engl J Med 284:459–464, 1971.

32. Vracko R: Basal lamina layering in diabetes mellitus: Evidence for accelerated rate of cell death and cell regeneration. Diabetes 23:94–104, 1974.

33. Vracko R, Benditt EP: Manifestations of diabetes mellitus: Their possible relationships to an underlying cell defect. Am J Pathol 75:204–224, 1974.

34. Curschmann H: Ueber bronchiolitis exsudativa und ihr Verhaltniss zum asthma nervosum. Dtsch Arch Klin Med 32:1–34, 1882.

35. Cohen RC, Prentice AID: Metaplastic cells in sputum of patients with pulmonary eosinophilia. Tubercle 40:44–46, 1959.

36. Naylor B: The shedding of the mucosa of the bronchial tree in asthma. Thorax 17:69–72, 1962.

37. Houston JC, DeNavasquez S, Trounce JR: A clinical and pathologic study of fatal cases of status asthmaticus. Thorax 8:207–213, 1953.

38. Gleich GJ, Frigas E, Loegering DA, et al.: Cytotoxic properties of eosinophil major basic protein. J Immunol 123:2925–2927, 1979.

39. Boucher RC, Bromberg PA, Gatzy JT: Airway mucosal permeability. In Hargreave FE (ed): *Airway Hyperreactivity: Mechanisms and Clinical Relevance*. Mississauga, Ontario, Canada: Astra Pharmaceuticals, 1980, pp 40–47.

40. Rigler LG, Koucky R: Roentgen studies of pathological physiology of bronchial asthma. AJR 39:353–362, 1938.

41. Turner-Warwick M: Extrinsic allergic bronchiolo alveolitis In Turk J (ed): *Immunology of the Lung*. London: Edward Arnold, 1978, pp 165–190.

42. Pickering CA, Moore WKS, Lacey J, et al.: Investigation of respiratory disease associated with an airconditioning system. Clin Allergy 6:109–118, 1976.

43. Fink JN, Banaszak EF, Theide WH, Barboriak JJ: Interstitial pneumonitis due to hypersensitivity to an organism contaminating a heating system. Ann Intern Med 74:80–83, 1971.

44. Saltos N, Saunders NA, Bhagwandeen SB, Jarvie B: Hypersensitivity pneumonitis in a mouldy house. Med J Aust 2:244–246, 1982.

45. Joubert JR, Ascah K, Moroz LA, Hogg JC: Acute hypersensitivity pneumonitis in the rabbit: An animal model with horseradish peroxidase as antigen. Am Rev Respir Dis 113:503–513, 1976.

46. Dickie HA, Rankin J: Farmer's lung: An acute granulomatous interstitial pneumonitis occurring in agricultural workers. JAMA 167:1069–1076, 1958.

47. Totten RS, Reid DH, Davis HD, Moran TJ: Farmer's lung: Report of two cases in which lung biopsies were performed. Am J Med 25:803–809, 1958.

48. Seal RME, Hapke EJ, Thomas GO, et al.: The pathology of the acute and chronic stages of farmer's lung. Thorax 23:469–489, 1968.

49. Reyes CN, Wenzel FJ, Lawton BR, Emanuel DA: Pulmonary pathology of farmer's lung disease. Chest 81:142–146, 1982.

50. Sutinen S, Reijula K, Huhti E, Karkola P: Extrinsic allergic bronchiolo-alveolitis: Serology and biopsy findings. Eur J Respir Dis 64:271–282, 1983.

51. Emanuel DA, Wenzel FJ, Bowerman CI, Lawton BR: Farmer's lung: Clinical pathologic and immunologic study of 24 patients. Am J Med 37:392–401, 1965.

52. Barrowcliff DF, Arblaster PG: Farmer's lung: A study of an early acute fatal case. Thorax 23:490–500, 1968.

53. Kawanami O, Basset F, Barrios R, et al.: Hypersensitivity pneumonitis in man: Light and electron microscopic studies of 18 lung biopsies. Am J Pathol 110:275–289, 1983.

54. Pimentel JC, Avila R: Respiratory disease in cork workers (suberosis). Thorax 28:409–423, 1973.

55. Wenzel FJ, Emanuel DA, Lawton BR, Magnen GE: Isolation of the causative agent of farmer's lung. Ann Allergy 22:533–540, 1964.

56. Hargreave F, Hinson KF, Reid L, et al.: The radiological appearances of allergic alveolitis to bird sensitivity. Clin Radiol 23:1–10, 1972.

57. Reynolds HY, Fulmer JD, Kazmierowski JA, et al.: Analysis of cellular and protein content of bronchoalveolar lavage fluid from patients with idiopathic pulmonary fibrosis and chronic hypersensitivity pneumonitis. J Clin Invest 59:165–175, 1977.

58. Godard P, Clot J, Jonquet O, et al.: Lymphocyte subpopulations in bronchoalveolar lavages of patients with sarcoidosis and hypersensitivity pneumonitis. Chest 80:447–452, 1981.

59. Hirata T, Nagai S, Ohshima S, Izumi T: Comparative study of T cell subsets and BAL fluids in patients with hypersensitivity pneumonitis and sarcoidosis. Chest 82:232 (abstr), 1982.

60. Hunninghake GW, Gadek JE, Kawanami O, et al.: Inflammatory and immune processes in the human lung in health and disease: Evaluation of bronchoalveolar lavage. Am J Pathol 97:149–206, 1979.

61. Cantin A, Begin R, Boileau R, et al.: Features of bronchoalveolar lavage differentiating hypersensitivity pneumonitis and pulmonary sarcoidosis at time of initial presentation. Clin Invest Med 7:89–94, 1984.

62. Whitcomb ME, Dixon GF: Gallium scanning: Bronchoalveolar lavage and the national debt. Chest 85:719–721, 1984.

63. Parish WE: Farmer's lung. Part I: An immunological study of some antigenic components of mouldy foodstuffs. Thorax 18:83–89, 1963.

64. Pepys J, Jenkins PA, Festenstein GN, et al.: Farmer's lung: Thermophilic actinomycetes as a source of "farmer's lung" hay antigen. Lancet 2:607–611, 1963.

65. Richerson HB, Cheng HF, Bauserman SC. Acute experimental hypersensitivity pneumonitis in rabbits. Am Rev Respir Dis 104:568–575, 1971.

66. Richerson HB: Acute experimental hypersensitivity pneumonitis in the guinea pig. J Lab Clin Med 79:745–757, 1972.

67. Standford RE, Salvaggio JE: Experimental granulomatous pneumonitis: Immunologic, histologic and ultrastructural correlations. Chest 69(suppl):288–290, 1976.

68. Coombs RR, Devey ME, Anderson KJ: Refractoriness to

anaphylactic shock after continuous feeding of cow's milk to guinea pigs. Clin Exp Immunol 32:263–271, 1978.

69. Pare PD, Michoud MC, Boucher RC, Hogg JC: Pulmonary effects of acute and chronic antigen exposure of immunized guinea pigs. J Appl Physiol 46:346–353, 1979.

70. Richerson HB, Seidenfeld JJ, Ratajczak HV, Richards DW: Chronic experimental interstitial pneumonitis in the rabbit. Am Rev Respir Dis 117:5–13, 1978.

71. Andrew DK, Schellenberg RR, Hogg JC, et al.: Physiological and immunological effects of chronic antigen exposure in immunized guinea pigs. Int Arch Allergy Appl Immunol 75: 208–213, 1984.

23 Environmental Lung Disease

A.G. Heppleston

General Considerations

Perspective

Man has mined minerals for millennia and the ill effects on respiration were recognized in olden times. The elder Pliny, who died during the eruption of Vesuvius in 79 A.D., referred to minium (mercuric sulfide) refiners, who enveloped their faces with loose bladders which enabled them to see without inhaling the fatal dust. In his treatise "De re metallica" of 1556 Georgius Agricola (Georg Bauer) emphasized among many other matters the deleterious effects on the lungs of dusts from dry metalliferous mines and advocated the Roman practice for prevention as well as ventilating machines with double shafts. Paracelsus (Philip Theophrastus Bombast von Hohenheim) contributed a major text "Von der Bergsucht und anderen Bergkrankheiten" in 1567 and incriminated inhaled dust as a factor in miner's sickness. The diarist John Evelyn addressed a tract "Fumifugium" to King Charles II in the second year of the Restoration, inveighing against pollution of the atmosphere in London by the "smoake" of "sea-coale" from "New Castle" and reporting that the inhabitants of the city had blackish sputum and were never free from coughs. The prime exposition to date on diseases of workers ("De morbis artificum diatriba") emanated from Bernardino Ramazzini of Modena in 1700 and he is regarded as the father of occupational medicine. He noted that at necropsy the lungs of stonecutters were stuffed with "sharp, rough and corner'd small splinters or particles." From Padua in 1762 came "De sedibus, et causis morborum per anatomen indigatis" by Joannes Baptista Morgagni, who likewise implicated dust inhalation as the cause of disease in stone workers. "The Effects of Arts, Trades and Professions on Health and Longevity" by Charles Turner Thackrah of Leeds appeared in 1832 and emphasized that dust was the great bane of manufacturers; for colliers he recommended the safety lamp and ventilation, for grinders the use of water, and for iron filers magnetic mouthpieces.

It is salutory to recollect the origins of many ideas in regard to the disease in coal workers. Present concepts are greatly indebted to the pioneer pathologic investigations by physicians of the Scottish lowlands in the fourth and fifth decades of the 19th century, beginning with J.C. Gregory in 1831. The magnitude of these contributions must be seen against the restricted amount of material available and the technical limitations for its examination. The essential features of coal worker's pneumoconiosis were identified, confirmation coming a century later from Australia.[1] A brief historical account has already appeared.[2]

The current significance of occupational disorders of the lungs lies in the opportunities still afforded for prevention combined with insights that are provided into basic pathogenetic mechanisms, which could well have applications beyond the present concern. This chapter is devoted mainly to the impact on the respiratory system of aerosols of inorganic matter.

Terminology

The term *aerosol* describes solid particles or liquid droplets that are small enough to form more or less stable suspensions in the atmosphere. Solid particles are customarily referred to as *dust*, which may possess a compact or a fibrous habit, the usual distinction being that fibers exhibit a length/diameter (aspect) ratio of at least 3:1, though this limit is now under closer scrutiny (*see* Disorders due to Asbestos, Asbestosis, Pathogenesis, Fiber Dimensions, below). The finest solid particles are classed as *fumes* which represent condensates from the gaseous state, usually of oxides from hot or boiling metals; aggregation into larger units is common, however. A dispersion of liquid particles large enough to be visible to the naked eye and often formed around solid nuclei constitutes a *mist*, while a *vapor* consists of the gaseous phase of a substance which is normally liquid or solid at 25°C and 760 mmHg, and *gases* exist as molecular suspensions at 25°C and 760 mmHg.

The particles presenting occupational hazards are mostly *minerals*, which may be defined as naturally occurring, crystalline, inorganic compounds or elements. Attention must, however, be concentrated on that fraction of the airborne mineral dust which is *respirable*, that is, capable of reaching the alveolar region. Particle size is the important determinant and for aerodynamic purposes is expressed not as the microscopic but as the equivalent diameter, which denotes the size of a unit density sphere with the same falling speed as the particle in question. The threshold microscopic diameter for unit density spheres is about 10 μm, a lower figure (about 5 μm) applying to denser and irregular compact particles such as those of silica or coal. For fibrous particles, such as asbestos, diameter predominantly determines falling speed and an upper microscopic limit of about 3 μm regulates respirability. *Pneumoconiosis*, a term of Greek derivation introduced by Zenker[3] in 1867, is best defined as the non-neoplastic reaction of the lung to the accumulation of inhaled dust. The appellations pneumoconiosis and silicosis are sometimes used interchangeably, notably in Germany, while on its own pneumoconiosis may be applied to the disease in coal workers. However, pneumoconiosis is a generic term, silicosis and coal worker's disease being particular forms, and the designation anthracosilicosis merely introduces confusion. Most dust hazards are mixtures, though one component may predominate and determine the pulmonary reaction.

Dynamic Aspects

Physical, physiologic, and morphologic factors exert selective effects on the deposition and retention of inhaled particles. The composition of the dust in the lung may differ from that in the atmosphere and the quantity retained constitutes only a tiny proportion of that inhaled. The topic is wide and only an outline can be given.

Pulmonary retention of dust represents the difference between the amount deposited from atmospheric suspension and that subsequently eliminated. While particle composition is a major determinant of the response and is discussed in succeeding sections, other principles have a general connotation.

Deposition

Particles are thrown out of atmospheric suspension by several physical mechanisms, namely, inertial impaction, sedimentation under gravity, diffusion by brownian movement, and interception. Inertia exerts its maximal effect in the nasopharynx and at divisions of major airways where larger compact particles (>10 μm) settle. In the deeper parts of the bronchial tree air flow becomes more turbulent and the overall cross-sectional area of the conducting passages increases, so that sedimentation plays on increasing role. Air movement is minimal or absent in respiratory sections of the bronchiolar tree, so that sedimentation and diffusion become the dominant mechanisms for deposition. On *mathematical* grounds, particles 1 to 2 μm in diameter are the most likely to be deposited in the alveolar region, at about 0.5 μm diffusion more or less counteracts sedimentation and such particles are most likely to be exhaled, while below 0.5 μm deposition increases with decreasing size. Since diameter (<3 μm) is of overriding importance in determining the falling speed of fibrous particles, long thin ones, by escaping impaction and sedimentation, may reach the alveoli; interception, however, plays a larger role. Theoretical predictions are limited by the varying geometry of the airway, respiratory movements, and the lining layers of bronchi and alveoli.

To elucidate the complex *physiologic* factors entails inspiratory and expiratory sampling of clouds or external measurement of radioactivity after inhaling particles labelled with gamma-emitting isotopes. Compact particles 1 to 2 μm in diameter again appear to deposit maximally in alveoli and 0.5 μm- ones minimally with still smaller sizes settling more effectively.

Morphologic observations on deposition are few. Rats inhaling hematite or silica for 1 to 2 hours showed maximal accumulation in ciliated air passages, but acini revealed wide variations in the overall quantity of dust retained and within individual acini the distribution also varied. In rats with preexisting pneumoconiosis due to coal or quartz, brief exposure to hematite led to greater overall deposition and deeper penetration; the pattern of deposition may thus differ in normal and coniotic individuals exposed to compact particles. Short chrysotile fibers inhaled by rats were preferentially deposited at the more proximal bifurcations of respiratory air passages. The electrostatic charge borne by fibers constitutes a neglected factor in this regard.

Clearance

Two phases of particle elimination are recognized, a fast one lasting hours or 1 to 2 days and a slow one extending over weeks or longer, corresponding respectively to clearance from conducting air passages and from alveolar structures, that is, acini.

Mucociliary transport determines the fast phase of clearance, though the rate in humans is subject to wide variations for which mucus viscosity or depth may be responsible. Cigarette smoking in humans (and the donkey) leads to slowing of short- and long-term clearance, probably by impairment of ciliary activity and squamous metaplasia of respiratory epithelium. Mucociliary clearance is accelerated by brief exposure of humans and donkeys to low concentrations of sulfur dioxide but slowed by high or maintained levels.

Extraction procedures quantitate loss by bronchial and lymphatic routes from the acini, but histologic observation establishes the sequence of events and likely mechanisms. With increasing lung burdens of compact particles, the absolute amounts subsequently removed generally rise, probably because dust accumulation simplifies the structure of respiratory airways and so facilitates removal toward the bronchial tree. Lymph node accumulation reflects the total burden of dust in the lungs, though quartz is selectively transported. At low atmospheric concentrations amphibole fibers (see Disorders Due to Asbestos, Mineralogy, Composition and Structure, below) are retained to a much greater degree than chrysotile. Crocidolite exhibits rapid and slow phases of clearance and with survival fibres tend to accumulate in foci subpleurally. It appears that curled chrysotile fibers, offering a larger collision area than straight amphiboles of similar length, deposit more proximally and are removed more easily by mucociliary activity. Histologic observations are needed to elucidate further the disposal of inhaled fibers.

Particle Aggregation and Translocation

Phagocytosis of deposited particles occurs rapidly and aggregation at the apex of the acinus, the critical area, follows the surface route both intra- and extra-cellularly. Even small amounts of dust in humans and animals accumulate thus, implying that bronchiolar elimination is less efficient than alveolar. The double dusting technique[2] permits histologic recognition of particles reaching the lung at widely different times and traces the subsequent movement of one dust in relation to another. Particles from the second exposure soon occurred in lesions derived from the first and mixing was intimate not only in particular lesions but also in individual macrophages throughout them. It made little ultimate difference whether the primary lesions were nonfibrotic or fibrotic. The second dust was evidently incorporated by a regular cycle of cell death, liberation of both dusts and their reingestion by freshly produced macrophages. Isolated histologic preparations thus conceal the dynamic nature of dust lesions. Observations in human beings have confirmed the experimental findings.

To reach the interstitium submicronic particles pass through type I epithelium but larger particles are evidently incorporated into alveolar walls by disintegration of the attenuated epithelium and its reformation over dust lying free or in cells. Fibrosis among dust-laden macrophages crowded into alveolar likewise conveys an interstitial appearance and enables dust lesions to enlarge. From the interstitium particles are translocated in the same cyclical manner through natural openings in lymphatic vessels, while particles or laden macrophages arrested in intrapulmonary lymphoid tissue or the hilar nodes repeat the process, as double dusting experiments indicate. The idea that dust fibrosis of hilar nodes causes lymph stasis and retrograde accumulation of particles in lung parenchyma is not supported by human or experimental evidence irrespective of the nature of the dust. Parenchymal accumulation occurs because the eliminatory capacity of the bronchial and lymphatic routes is overtaxed at the periphery.

Fibers short enough to be ingested completely by macrophages probably undergo transport in the same manner as compact particles, but long ones are likely to be arrested at divisions of respiratory bronchioles there to excite the fibrotic reaction of early asbestosis. Transfer of fibers, some long, from lung to regional nodes is well attested, and a few fibers may enter the bloodstream to be trapped in distant organs. Translocation of inhaled fibers to the peritoneum may follow swallowing after bronchial clearance and penetration of the intestinal wall. In some individuals lymphatic vessels pass from the lower lobes of the lung via the ligamentum pulmonis and oesophageal hiatus to the diaphragmatic plexus and thence to the preoesophageal and coeliac nodes. Fibers could conceivably traverse this route toward the peritoneal serosa. It seems unnecessary to assume retrograde flow from obstruction of lymphatic channels by fibrosed hilar nodes. Dust sometimes collects in the posterior abdominal lymph nodes of coal workers with minimal pulmonary changes.

Macrophage Mobilization

A steady supply of macrophages is required (1) to ingest particles as they progressively accumulate in the lungs, the demand being augmented as laden cells die (particularly under the action of quartz), and (2) to ensure continuous production of the fibrogenic factor (see Disorders Due to Free Silica, Classical Nodular Silicosis, Pathogenesis, Simple Silicosis, The Macrophage Fibrogenic Factor, below). The cell kinetics of murine alveolar walls after inhalation of different dusts suggested that for those of low toxicity (for example, coal), proliferation of immature macrophages from within the walls met the need, while for toxic particles (for example, quartz) the demand for macrophages was such that recruitment of marrow-derived precursors was required. Simple or complex lipids stimulated activity of the mononuclear phagocytic system (see Disorders Due to Free Silica, Classical Nodular Silicosis, Pathogenesis, Complicated Silicosis, below) and marrow monopoiesis was augmented by naturally-derived lung lipid containing a high proportion of dipalmitoyl lecithin (see Disorders Due to Free Silica, Accelerated Silicosis, Pathogenesis, below). The sequence of events thus appears to comprise dust (especially but not exclusively quartz) stimulation of lipid formation by type II cells, circulatory conveyance of lipid to the marrow, acceleration of monopoiesis, and release of monocytes which finally emerge as macrophages into the alveoli. When alveolar macrophages are in high demand, systemic recruitment from the marrow by positive feedback of lipid from the lung may thus be considered to play the dominant role.

Emigration of Monocytes

The capillary endothelium possesses labile junctions, but alveolar epithelium with its tight junctions provides the main obstacle, which silica and probably other dusts evidently overcome by dissolution of type I epithelium. The means of emigration remains speculative, but E-type prostaglandin, which is released from alveolar macrophages by stimuli which include particles, may increase vascular permeability and facilitate emigration. More-

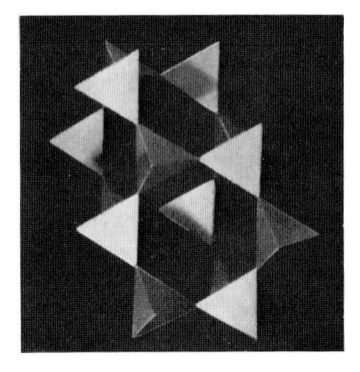

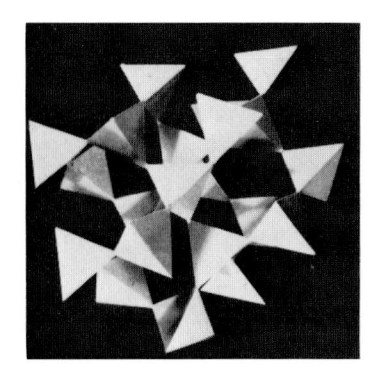

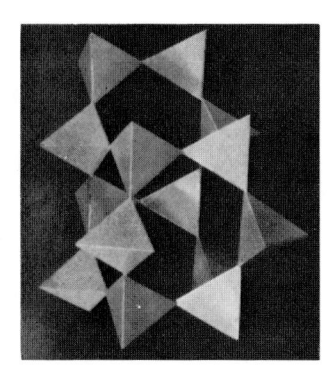

Figure 23–1. Disposition of silicon-oxygen tetrahedra in (from the left) cristobalite, quartz, and tridymite. Courtesy of Dr. Wells and Oxford University Press.

over, chemotactic agents either endogenous, as in the alveolar lining material or products of connective tissue resorption, or exogenous, as with bacterial products notably from *Escherichia coli*, could be involved.

Disorders Due to Free Silica

Mineral Structure

The earth's crust, which is several miles thick, consists largely of silicon and oxygen, the next most common element being aluminium; iron, magnesium, calcium, sodium, and potassium occur in smaller amounts, the remaining elements comprising only 1 to 2 percent of the total. Silicon and oxygen exist in chemical association as *free silica* (often abbreviated to "silica"), while the introduction of various cations into the structure results in the formation of *silicates*, that is, combined silica. The term silica (and hence silicosis) derives from the Latin word *silex* (*silicis*) meaning flint. Free silica constitutes the most common compound and exists in several structural forms based on a standard unit, in which each silicon atom is joined to four outlying oxygen atoms so as to give a tetrahedral arrangement, each oxygen atom being shared with a neighboring atom of silicon. The overall chemical formula is thus SiO_2. If the coordination of the tetrahedria exhibits a regular pattern, the free silica assumes a crystalline form (Fig. 23–1), but if the pattern is irregular the silica is described as amorphous. The latter occurs naturally as diatomite and is formed by vitrification or sublimation. Crystalline silica usually occurs in the stable form of quartz, but under higher temperatures the tetrahedra are rearranged with the formation first of tridymite and then of cristobalite, these latter allotropes being described as metastable. At very high temperature and pressure two further crystalline forms, coesite and stishovite (named after their discoverers), are produced; they were found as natural minerals in the meteor crater of Arizona and have also been synthesized. Coesite possesses the usual tetrahedral structure, but stishovite is peculiar in being octahedrally coordinated so that every silicon atom is joined to six peripherally located atoms of oxygen which are common to adjacent octahedra. Titanium dioxide has the same structure as stishovite. The density of the different structural forms varies, being highest for stishovite next for coesite and diminishing further for the low-temperature, low-pressure crystalline forms through quartz and tridymite to cristobalite. The openness of the structure varies inversely with density and may influence the accessibility of reactive sites under biologic conditions; industrial processes may induce the metamorphosis so that amorphous silica, for example, may be converted into the more active crystalline forms. Cryptocrystalline forms of free silica exist as crystals which may measure no more than 40 nm and which in nature occur as flint or agate.

Classical Nodular Silicosis

Prevalence

In South African gold miners, the annual production rate of silicosis per thousand miners fell as the air-borne dust levels were controlled, and between 1946 and 1967 there was a pronounced reduction in the prevalence of both silicosis and tuberculosis at autopsy, disease often being recognized solely on microscopic examination in the later years.[4] The annual number of reported cases in the United Kingdom is low, but a high prevalence of silicosis occurred in the pottery industry[5] and a Sheffield steel foundry, while until recently the granite industry provided a risk. In the United States silicosis evidently continued to develop in some industries,[6] having previously achieved a prevalence of 32 percent in nonmetallic mineral manufacture with tuberculosis as a prominent complication.[7] Though the overall picture is one of decline, vigilance is still required for several reasons; (1) the ubiquity of silica means that exposure may arise where the exploitation or use of minerals is a recent development, (2) because of the long latent period established industries may continue to provide new cases as in Cornish tin miners,[8] (3) pockets of risk may remain in some industries, and (4) tuberculosis represents a recognized complication. Moreover, silicotic nodules may be present pathologically in the absence of radiologic evidence of disease.[9]

Occupations at Risk

Metalliferous mining notably for gold occurs mainly in Souther Africa, North America, and the USSR. Quarrying for sandstone, granite, or slate, and tunneling, which in coal mines may be described as hard-heading, are recognized sources of exposure, as also are stone cutting, dressing, and cleaning. Foundaries provide another risk, especially cleaning castings (that is, "fettling") and so does boiler scaling. A high risk is currently experienced in the U.S. silica "flour" industries which use crystalline material of respirable size as an abrasive cleaner and filler,[10] while danger may arise in the ceramic industry where crystalline silica forms a variable proportion of the ingredients.

Former sources of exposure, which could recur, included (1) sandblasting in which quartzose sand or crushed flint was employed to clean metal castings or etch glass; (2) metal grinding in the cutlery and sharp-edged tool trade and in foundries where silicon carbide (Carborundum) wheels replaced sandstone; (3) refractories industries engaged in the making of bricks, silica cement, and moulds for castings; and (4) abrasive soap powder in which ground silica or pumice was mixed with anhydrous sodium carbonate and powdered soap.

Pathologic Anatomy

Two forms of the disease may be recognized: simple silicosis, which being the response to dust alone constitutes the essential manifestation, and complicated silicosis in which one or more additional elements participate.

Gross Features

Simple silicosis is typically seen as a hard, nodular lesion measuring up to 5 or 6 mm diameter, many being widely scattered throughout the parenchyma though with a tendency to be larger and more numerous in the upper zones of the lung. The nodules possess a grey color, whose depth depends on the content of carbonaceous pigment, and a concentric pattern of connective tissue notably toward their periphery (Fig. 23–2). Small early lesions are palpable but show little pattern on the cut surface and may be few.

Complicated silicosis appears as a superimposed change, characterized by massive lesions usually measuring several centimeters on cross-section, though the shape is irregular when examined in depth, and some lesions are as small as 1 cm. Massive lesions, which may be single, multiple, or bilateral, are typically located in the upper parts of the lung and somewhat posteriorly; not infrequently lobar fissures are crossed and the pleura may be reached. The cut surface generally shows a conglomeration of hard nodules, more or less defined and fused by connective tissue, which exhibits a variable degree of pigmentation and a concentric or whorled disposition of fibers in the nodular formations (*see* Fig. 23–2). Sometimes evidence of caseous tuberculosis perhaps with cavitation is present in massive lesions and occasionally calcification occurs, particularly toward the edges. Many air passages and blood vessels are obliterated wholly or partly and areas of colliquative necrosis may be seen, the fluid being dark or black. Bullous emphysema may occur around massive lesions as an effect of local lung fixation but the air spaces around nodules are little if at all affected.

The pleura is often thickened and adherent over massive lesions and interlobar fissures may be completely or partially obliterated, but in the simple disease the pleura though a little thickened over subjacent nodules is not usually adherent. The hilar and paratracheal lymph nodes are enlarged, pigmented in shades of grey and diffusely fibrosed (though not always with a nodular pattern) so that they become adherent to each other and neighboring structures, occasionally leading to distortion of major bronchi and pulmonary arteries. Parabronchial or paravascular lymphoid tissue in the lung may also be affected. The right ventricle may show hypertrophy in the complicated disease, but florid cases of silicosis terminating in pulmonary tuberculosis or right heart failure are now rare and for the latter there may be other causes.

Microscopical Features

Simple Silicosis. Simson[11] pioneered investigation of the structure of the silicotic nodule and personal experience confirmed his findings. To understand the microanatomy of dust lesions as well as the acinar architecture demands the three-dimensional approach for which extensive series of sections (20 μm thickness suffices) are required from tissue cubes measuring 1 to 2 cm taken from lungs fixed in distention. The simple silicotic nodule is located in relation to respiratory bronchioles, especially those of the first and second orders and, since this is an expanding lesion, these bronchioles are gradually stenosed, sometimes severely. Pulmonary arterioles normally accompany the bronchioles, the two structures lying in close proximity, so that dust lesions which form primarily around the airway come to enclose the blood vessel secondarily and often excentrically. Histologically, fibrous tissue predominates in the mature nodule and characteristically exhibits three zones (Fig. 23–3). A central islet or group of islets, composed of hyaline connective tissue possessing a whorled pattern, is surrounded by a midzone of concentrically disposed fibers with some cellularity, and the whole is enclosed by an outer zone whose fibers lack regular arrangement and among which lie dust-laden phagocytes. The latter usually contain not only siliceous but also carbonaceous particles derived from the working or urban environment. Many mineral particles in silicotic lesions fail to show birefringence, presumably on account of their small size and the planes of their surfaces. However, the disposition of siliceous material, as revealed by the ash pattern in incinerated preparations, differs in the three zones.[12] The islets contain a variable quantity of finely dispersed dust, while the

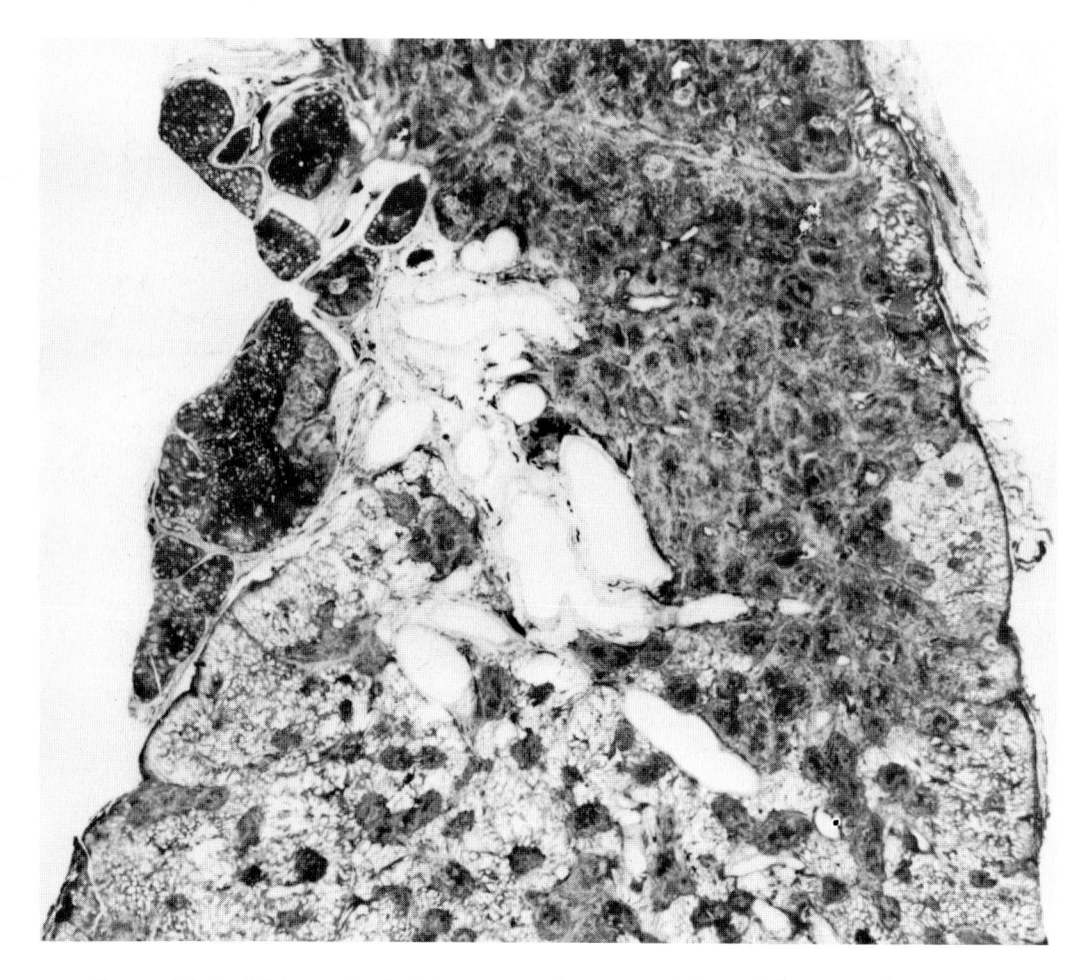

Figure 23–2. Midzone of a whole lung section from a case of classical silicosis in a barytes miner. The upper and middle lobes are occupied by massive fibrosis with a distinctly nodular pattern, while typical nodules occur in the middle and lower lobes. The hilar nodes are enlarged and show nodular fibrosis (×1.2).

midzone is largely particle-free, and the external zone appears as a prominent halo enveloping the whole lesion. The pattern of particles gives the impression that fibrogenesis is initiated at the periphery and that the product accumulates in the interior. Larger nodules are usually made up of two or more islets, progression occurring predominantly by increase in size of existing lesions but also by the formation of new ones,[13] a process that may continue after cessation of exposure. Overall the silicotic nodule exhibits exuberant fibrosis, in that a large amount of connective tissue is formed in proportion to the quantity of siliceous dust and possesses a peculiar arrangement. Since respiratory bronchioles are compressed as fibrosis proceeds, emphysema is not a typical component of the lesion, but if it stabilizes and growth ceases the connective tissue may contract and a minor degree of irregular emphysema may develop. Pulmonary arterioles remain patent and though their walls may show fibrosis the changes are generally minimal.

Complicated Silicosis. The usual appearance is of nodules with typical features embedded in hyaline fibrous tissue bearing particles, many black, lying either free or within macrophages (Fig. 23–4). Pulmonary structures are largely replaced, blood vessels often being stenosed or obliterated by endarteritis in which dust-bearing phagocytes occur, probably as a result of organization of thrombi. Arterial thrombosis may be extensive. Bronchi and bronchioles are deformed and some stenosed partially or completely, patent air passages often showing chronic inflammatory changes that may be high grade. Caseous tuberculosis is uncommon and search of large areas may be needed to discover noncaseous foci, though acid-fast bacilli may lie in softened tissue devoid of cellular components, guinea pig inoculation proving their tuberculous nature. Other areas of softening lack organisms or reaction and are probably ischemic in origin, the consequence of obliterative endarteritis.

Lymph Nodes. The regional lymph nodes in simple or complicated disease exhibit histologic features resembling massive fibrosis. The changes are generally less extensive in simple silicosis and lack as clear a definition of nodular formations as in the lung, a feature attributable to the different distribution and concentration of siliceous particles. Active tuberculosis is rarely evident

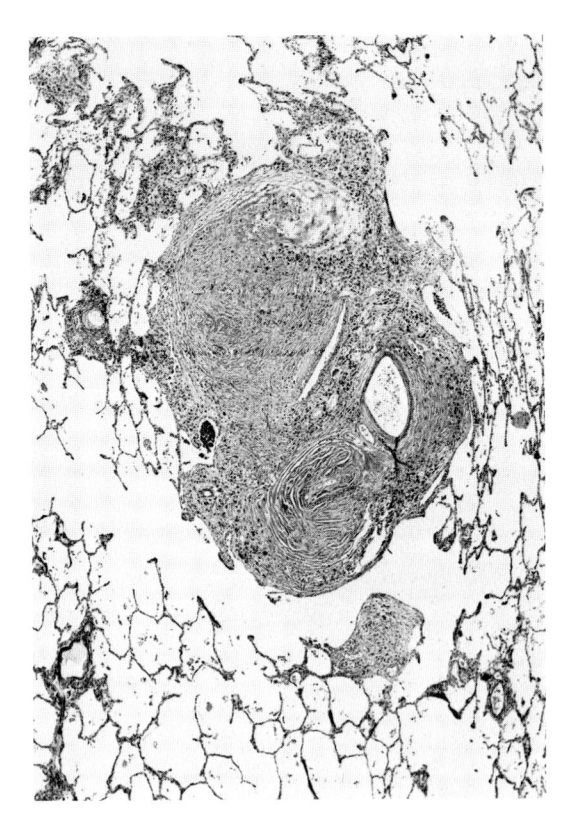

Figure 23–3. Small silicotic nodule having a whorled pattern centrally, being enveloped by concentric fibers, with irregular fibrosis and dust phagocytes lying peripherally. The lesion lies in relation to respiratory bronchioles (H&E, ×25).

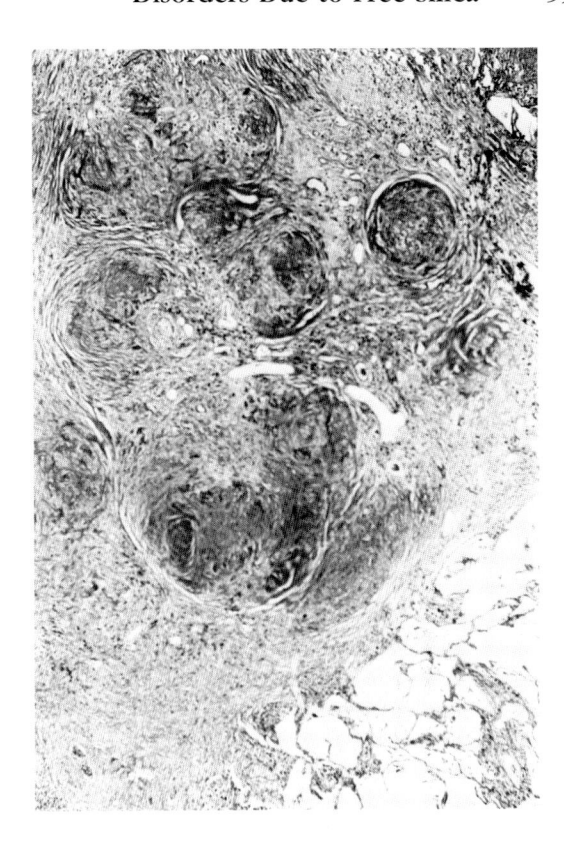

Figure 23–4. Massive silicotic fibrosis, in which nodules are fused by intervening fibrosis (H&E, ×30).

though calcified caseous material may be found. Occasionally the nodes show a peripheral layer of calcification, giving the radiologic "eggshell" appearance, as seen in slate workers; whether it reflects the calcium content of the dust, which could be concentrated from afferent lymph in the peripheral sinus, or is endogenous has not been determined. Rarely, lung nodules are also affected by calcification which may be evident on the x-ray.

Pathogenesis

Simple Silicosis

The Processes Concerned. Human and experimental evidence established that this form of the disease resulted solely from the action of inhaled silica. The histology of nodules does not suggest an infective origin and injection of material from them into guinea pigs failed to detect tubercle bacilli.[13] Rodents, lagomorphs, and monkeys exposed to the inhalation of quartz have repeatedly been shown to develop the disease without the intervention of any other agent.[14,15] Distinct lesions are produced when tuberculous infection is combined with exposure to quartz[16] and pneumococcal pneumonia neither affected nor was affected by the existence of silicosis.[17]

The structure of the established silicotic nodule conveys a static impression that conceals a number of dynamic processes which experimental observations reveal. Inhaled particles, deposited widely over the alveolar surface, gradually accumulate with the aid of macrophages in alveoli around the respiratory bronchioles, notably the first and second orders. Macrophages repeatedly disintegrate under their toxic load and the liberated particles are taken up by fresh generations of these cells which congregate in the same location where fibrous tissue is slowly laid down. To establish the sequence of these events, they had to be examined independently, since under natural conditions of exposure all may be expected to occur simultaneously. The complexity of the in vivo responses necessitated the parallel deployment of in vitro techniques.

Factors Influencing Fibrogenesis. To produce disease a sufficient *quantity of dust* must accumulate, what Mavrogordato called the "effective occupation" of the lungs. Because dust removal proceeds during and after exposure, intratracheal injection has been adopted and the severity of pulmonary fibrosis found to be directly related to the quantity of silica administered as tridymite[18] or quartz.[19] However, when rats inhaled dust mixtures, definite fibrosis developed only when the air-borne and the extracted lung dusts contained 20 percent or more of quartz,[20] though the response was not typically silicotic in form. Moreover, the classical silicotic reaction was generally found in humans only when the

Figure 23–5. Relationship between quartz and total dust contents of the lungs in massive fibrosis. Classical silicosis, as in gold miners, had above 18 percent quartz in the total dust (left of broken line), but the proportion was considerably less in other groups of workers. The division is not, however, sharply defined (from Nagelschmidt[21]).

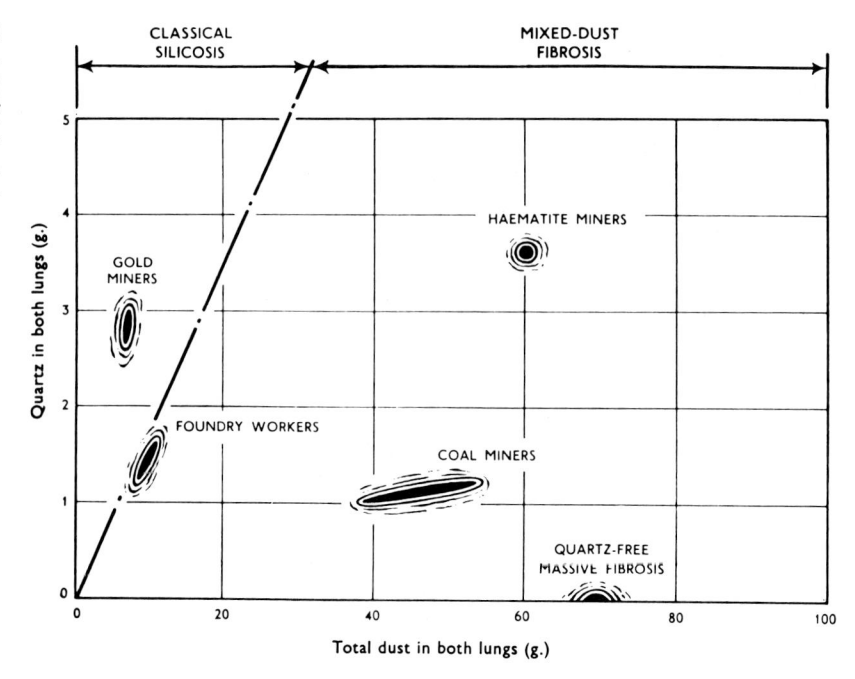

quartz content of the lung dust exceeded 18 percent[21] (Fig. 23–5). Below this proportion silica evidently fails to achieve contact with target cells in a concentration sufficiently high to elicit the customary response.

Particle size and surface area were examined by intratracheal administration of flint (a mixture mainly of cristobalite and quartz) to rats in a range of sizes, first at constant weight and second at constant surface area.[22] The rate at which fibrosis developed as well as its severity were maximal for particles in the 1- to 2-μm range, while smaller ones were less and larger ones least active, although each size fraction dissolved with equal facility. These findings implicated both the size and the surface area of silica particles as relevant in fibrogenesis, though others laid less stress on surface area. The disparities may reflect the shortcomings of the intratracheal route of administration and of the histologic method of grading fibrosis.

The *physical form* of silica is perhaps the most striking property influencing connective tissue formation. Using the same dose of similarly sized duct fractions of high purity intratracheally, the degree of fibrosis and the rate of its development were least with amorphous silica, increasing for quartz and then cristobalite to a maximum with tridymite, even though all forms had corresponding solubilities.[23] It is, however, most unlikely that it will prove possible to test this experimental conclusion by epidemiologic means in humans. Even greater divergencies were found in the tissue responses to the high-pressure, high-temperature forms of silica. With pure samples of comparable surface area administered intraperitoneally, coesite possessed a fibrogenic potency but at a rate only one-tenth that of quartz, while stishovite behaved as a so-called inert dust and induced merely a phagocytic response.[24] Much less fibrosis was obtained in the lung with coesite than with quartz of similar particle size range when given intratracheally.[25] From these results it appears that the fibrogenic action of silica is dependent on surface properties apparently unconnected with solubility, and that surface area alone may not offer a satisfactory explanation.

An echo of the influence of physical form may be suspected from accounts of lung changes in the inhabitants of the Sahara and Negev deserts. Fibrous scars were evident, but no silicotic nodules, mostly in women, and dust accumulation increased with age. The condition resembled simple "anthracosis" and it is possible that silica, weathered in the desert, possessed an amorphous surface unlike freshly fractured quartz, though iron contamination may also have been a factor. That this reaction was not a new phenomenon was established by the detection of similar changes in a 12th Dynasty male Egyptian mummy, who was considered not to have been a stone mason.

Theories of Pathogenesis. Greenhow[26] attributed the pulmonary reaction to *mechanical irritation* by gritty particles to which individuals were exposed occupationally. However, Zenker[3] demonstrated that rounded particles of iron oxide readily gained access to the pulmonary interstitium from atmospheric suspension, while Gardner[27] showed that silicon carbide (Carborundum) inhaled by guinea pigs failed to elicit fibrosis although the particles were as hard as those of the diamond. Imposition of strain on certain crystals leads to the generation of opposite charges on different faces and, subjected to an electrical field, such crystals expand on one axis and contract on another—a property employed in quartz watches. Evans and Zeit[28] introduced this *piezoelectric* effect to account for the generation of fibrous tissue in the presence of free silica, the crystals of which they suggested might be deformed in vivo. Although this theory has never gained acceptance, and has not been followed up, electrical disturbance cannot be dismissed as an element in the silicotic reaction, though if concerned it seems likely to participate in damage to macrophage membranes rather than collagen formation.

A popular view of silicotic fibrogenesis was enshrined in the *silica solubility* hypothesis, which originated with the observations of Gye and Purdy[29] on the toxic and fibrogenic properties of colloidal silica. The tissue reaction to different crystalline forms of silica and to differently sized particles varied despite similar solubilities.[22,23] Further disparities transpired between solubility and fibrogenesis in the lung when the surfaces of different types of silica particles were etched with hydrofluoric acid or sodium hydroxide.[30] The use of diffusion chambers, in which particles are enclosed by plastic rings sealed by membranes of known pore size and then implanted intraperitoneally or subcutaneously, gave no support to the solubility hypothesis. Colloidal silica did not apparently emerge in a concentration or at a rate sufficiently high to induce fibrosis, even though the five samples were fibrogenic on direct introduction into the peritoneal cavity; closer contact was evidently required between silica and cells than diffusion chambers permitted.[31]

The solubility theory of silicosis led to the introduction of compounds or elements which were considered to inhibit fibrogenesis by solubility depression. Kettle[32] claimed success by subcutaneous administration of crystalline silica particles coated with a layer of ferric oxide, but most attention has been devoted to the effect of aluminium.[33,34] A mixture of metallic aluminium and quartz inhaled by rabbits led to a pronounced diminution of fibrosis as compared with control animals exposed only to quartz. Subsequent studies confirmed this conclusion partially or completely in various species and by different routes of administration.[35] Soluble aluminium compounds constituted a later introduction, the hydroxide, hydroxychloride, and chlorhydroxyallantöinate being employed as aerosols alternating with quartz.[35,36] Prevention of silicotic fibrosis was achieved and some therapeutic effect was apparent in established dust lesions, but withdrawal of aluminium prophylaxis was followed by resumption of the fibrogenic action of quartz. It is thought that the beneficial effect of aluminium resides in the slow release of a soluble form which reacts with the silica surface or that substitution of Al ions for Si ions occurs in the SiO_2 lattice rather than an effect on silica solution. Canadian gold miners, at risk from silicosis, received long-term prophylaxis by inhalation of metallic aluminium dust after their working shifts; no ill-effects were observed from the aluminium dust itself and silicosis was eliminated, but credit for the success may largely if not entirely depend on dust suppression measures applied in the mines at the same time.[37] A controlled trial of aluminium therapy in silicotic pottery workers and coniotic coal miners showed no clinical or radiologic benefit. However, the metal and its oxide may not be entirely harmless in some species.

The ability of tuberculous lipid to reproduce the histologic features of the tubercle and the resemblance of tuberculous and silicotic lesions, raised the possibility of a similar mechanism in silicosis.[38] *Phospholipid*, extracted from the lungs of rabbits injected intratracheally with quartz 1 to 20 weeks previously, when given intraperitoneally to other rabbits led to the formation of nodules, some showing extensive necrosis. Unfortunately the experiment failed to include phospholipid extracted from the lungs of control animals. Moreover, lipid extracted from macrophages, obtained from silica-exposed rabbits or guinea pigs, and injected subcutaneously into other animals failed to induce a fibrogenic response,[39] while lipid accumulation in the lungs of rats inhaling quartz was not followed by typical silicotic fibrosis.[40]

Another concept of silicotic fibrogenesis invokes the *membrane effect* exerted by the particles, for the study of which intact macrophages have been employed along with erythrocytes. Since there is a negative surface charge on silica particles and on red cells, simple electrostatic forces are clearly not involved. The toxic effect of silica has been ascribed to hydrogen donation by polymeric silicic acid which was considered to form hydrogen-bonded complexes with the phospholipids of cell membranes.[41] The polymer polyvinylpyridine-N-oxide (PNO) inhibits experimental pneumoconiosis[42,43] and preserves macrophages against the destructive action of silica.[44] The protective effect of PNO was attributed to preferential hydrogen bonding with silicic acid which in consequence was unable to react with biologic membranes which thus remained intact.[41] Lysis of red cells is readily accomplished by silica, whether in crystalline or amorphous form, but is much reduced by PNO. Dispute remains as to whether silica reacts with phospholipids or with proteins. Positively charged tetramethylammonium ions inhibited haemolysis probably by adsorption onto the silica surface, an effect ascribed to the affinity of these ions on the membrane surface for colloidal or particulate mineral.[45] Since silica and titanium dioxide both carry negative charges but only silica is haemolytic, an additional element evidently operates. Lipid peroxidation in membranes is not considered to be responsible for the deleterious effect of quartz. The weight of evidence points to a membrane effect as the primary action of quartz but although its precise nature remains uncertain the reaction almost certainly involves silanol (hydroxyl) groups on the particle surface, since their destruction by heat converts them into siloxane (Si-O-Si) groups and renders the mineral much less active biologically. Difficulties persist in attempting to explain the mechanism of fibrogenesis in physical terms. The theoretical concentrations of surface-OH groups, derived from the spatial orientation of the tetrahedral and octahedral coordinations, were imperfectly related to the estimated values as well as to the relative fibrogenic capacities and the solubilities of the different forms of silica. Electrons may be transferred between membranes and silica particles, for determination of which the electron trap structure and configuration of silanol groups were measured; thermally stimulated luminescence and infrared spectroscopy offered promise, though firm correlations with cytotoxicity and fibrogenicity have yet to be established.[46]

Whatever the ultimate interpretation of the surface effect of silica, the permeability of plasma and intracellu-

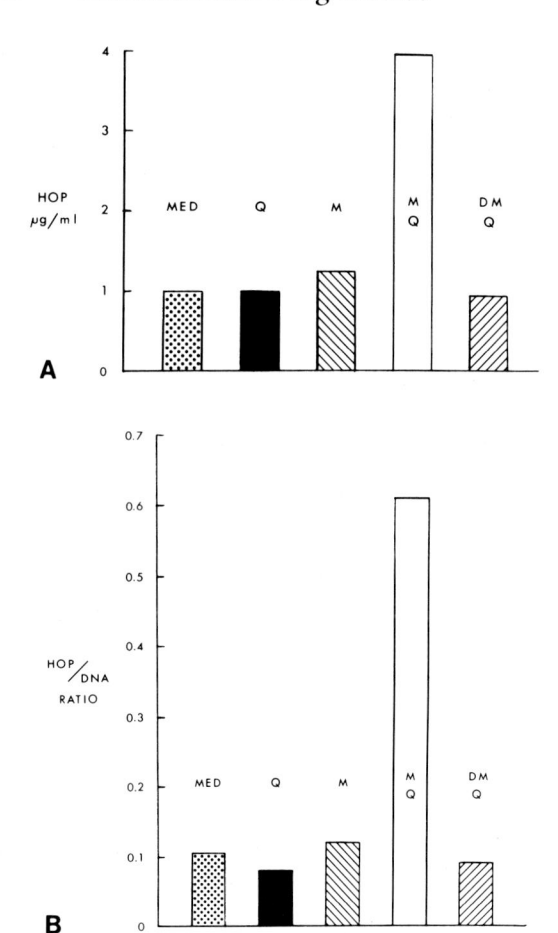

Figure 23–6. Hydroxyproline production by fibroblasts under the influence of the macrophage fibrogenic factor (MFF): (A) absolute values and (B) values relative to DNA. Only viable macrophages treated with quartz (MQ) responded. Fresh medium (MED), quartz particles (Q), and untreated macrophage extract (M) applied directly to fibroblasts had no effect, nor did disintegrated macrophages incubated with quartz (DMQ). From Heppleston.[48]

necessitating cell culture techniques since in vivo or in organ culture the mixed population of cells obscured their interactions. This approach led to the discovery of the macrophage fibrogenic factor (MFF) whose features were later elaborated.[47,48] Relying on a common synthetic maintenance medium (T8), supplemented to encourage both cell survival and hydroxyproline (HOP) formation, rat peritoneal macrophages were first incubated with quartz particles to permit phagocytosis, after which surviving cells were disintegrated and the suspension then centrifuged for separate study of the supernatant and deposit. The supernate replaced the medium of chick embryo fibroblasts grown independently and after intervals of 2 and 4 days their HOP and DNA contents were estimated. Supported by control procedures, several conclusions emerged (Fig. 23–6). (1) The macrophage-quartz extract consistently proved a strong stimulus to HOP formation. (2) Fibroblasts treated directly with particulate quartz or with medium containing dissolved silica failed to produce excess HOP, emphasizing the involvement of the macrophage. (3) No stimulus was obtained with extracts of macrophages disintegrated prior to incubation with quartz, suggesting that simple damage to cell membranes was not sufficient to account for the stimulus to collagen formation by quartz and hence that production of the MFF depended on an essential reaction with other constituents of the macrophage. (4) The disintegration products of untreated macrophages failed to produce a comparable effect and, since this procedure liberated cytoplasmic and lysosomal enzymes, their participation in the collagen response may apparently be eliminated. (5) Protection of cell membranes from damage by allowing macrophages to ingest PNO before addition of dust abolished the stimulus to HOP formation, thereby pointing to a dual effect of quartz, an initial attack on plasma membrane, having penetrated which the particles engage in an intracellular reaction leading to the generation or liberation of the MFF. (6) The residue from the macrophage-quartz interaction, resuspended in medium, was not only devoid of stimulatory capacity but actually depressed HOP formation, suggesting that the factor was soluble or of low molecular weight. (7) Since DNA levels were unaffected by any of the treatments, proliferation of fibroblasts may be excluded and their response was essentially functional. (8) Titanium dioxide, an octahedrally coordinated mineral devoid of fibrogenic ability in vivo, was employed in parallel with quartz but in contrast possessed no stimulatory capacity. (9) Since inhaled quartz comes into contact with alveolar macrophages, which in certain functional respects differ from peritoneal cells,[49,50] they were subjected to the same procedure and again the MFF was produced. (10) In none of the experiments was a humoral or cellular immune mechanism concerned. Confirmatory evidence has come from several laboratories which have preserved the essential aspects of the test system, while further support was provided by means of the diffusion chamber technique (see Disorders Due to Asbestos, Asbestosis, Pathogenesis, Mechanisms of Fibrogenesis, below).

lar membranes increases, as revealed by due penetration from without into the cytoplasm and by release of lysosomal and cytoplasmic enzymes. Particles are taken into macrophages and for a short time the phagolysosomes remain intact but then release their contents into the cytoplasm from which acid hydrolases and cytoplasmic lactate dehydrogenase escape extracellularly. Ultrastructurally, macrophages react similarly to silica in vitro and in vivo, though inhalation of quartz provides a smaller dust burden and permits better visualization of the toxic effects, as by diffusion of acid phosphatase into the cytoplasm.

The Macrophage Fibrogenic Factor. The emphasis on membrane damage by silica diverted attention from other phenomena concerned in phagocytosis and fibrosis. The nature of the connection between the two processes could be examined only when they were allowed to take place independently, a requirement

The mechanism by which the MFF operates has been

studied by Finnish investigators. Incubated with crystalline silica, rat peritoneal macrophages produced a fraction, located in the 20,000-g supernatant, which augmented collagen synthesis in granuloma slices as judged by incorporation of tritiated proline, DNA and RNA levels being unaffected.[51] The factor was believed to act on the polysomes of fibroblasts, whose stability was augmented by preservation of their RNA from degradation,[52] and collagen synthesis was localized to rough endoplasmic reticulum, the protein then being transferred in secretory vesicles to the extracellular fibrillary state.[53] The inhibitory effect of PNO on formation of the fibrogenic factor by macrophages was also confirmed.[54] Fractionation of the medium from treated macrophages by means of gel filtration chromatography and using fibroblasts isolated in culture as the target, disclosed that the silica-liberated MFF was a homogeneous protein of molecular weight 14,300.[55] It proved possible to prepare an antiserum against the purified factor, whose in vitro effect was neutralized, so confirming its protein nature; macrophage RNase activity was also eliminated.[56] Moreover, an antiserum depressed silicotic fibrosis in vivo,[57] the MFF has been identified in silicotic rat lung, and the amino acid composition of the factor established. The MFF may thus be regarded as a soluble protein that adsorbs RNase and so leaves some RNA undegraded. The subsequent sequence of events in fibroblasts was considered to comprise decrease of polysomal RNase, stabilization of RNA, and stimulation of protein synthesis.[56,58] The involvement of macrophage RNase was confirmed by showing it to be greatly decreased in the medium of silica-treated macrophages.[59] On this basis the MFF might appear as a relatively unspecific stimulant of protein synthesis, but some experiments already mentioned suggest that the factor activates elements in fibroblasts that lead to preferential formation of collagen. The biochemical observations establish that formation of the factor is an intracellular and not a surface event.

It is important to assess the significance of the in vitro findings for the intact organism. Human pulmonary fibroses of diverse origin are commonly characterized by a prominent macrophage response at least initially[60] and collagen synthesis is augmented in vivo by silica-treated macrophages.[61] A fibrogenic factor was detected in human rheumatoid synovium by application of extracts to macrophage cultures, the 20,000-g supernatant from which stimulated collagen synthesis in granuloma slices.[51] The use of human monocytes and macrophages for reaction with quartz led to stimulatory activity in the medium when applied to fibroblasts, and a line of human histiocytic lymphoma cells as well as transformed mouse macrophages behaved similarly.[62] Extracts from mouse liver subjected to carbon tetrachloride necrosis stimulated collagen synthesis and collagen proline hydroxylase activity in cultured fibroblasts and the activity resided in cells with the ultrastructural features of macrophages.[63,64] Biologic as well as mineral agents thus provoke generation of the MFF and the mechanism may prove fundamental to fibrogenesis however caused. Other processes nevertheless cooperate in the genesis of connective tissue by silica (see General Considerations, Dynamic Aspects, above, and Disorders Due to Free Silica, Accelerated Silicosis, Pathogenesis, below).

The Immunologic Component. As human silicotic nodules mature, the collagen tends to undergo hyalinization, which was thought to be an antigen antibody precipitate; the earlier evidence, derived from morphologic and humoral changes, has been summarized.[65] More recent observations showed that in some tuberculin-positive individuals exposed to silica the levels of immunoglobulins IgG and IgA were raised but not in tuberculin negative cases, IgM being decreased in both groups.[66] Autoantibodies such as antinuclear factor[67] and rheumatoid factor[68] may also be elevated, though the latter appears to be mainly in cases of Caplan's syndrome (see Disorders Due to Coal Mine and Carbonaceous Dusts, Rheumatoid Pneumoconiosis, Caplan's Syndrome, below). Reports on cell-mediated immunity are at variance, one group reporting no definite changes from control subjects[69,70] and another appreciable alterations in B- and T-cell function.[71] No significant connection has been detected between silicosis and histocompatibility antigens.[72] The idea that familial factors may be concerned requires confirmation. Immunofluorescence failed to identify rheumatoid factor in silicotic lesions.[73] Local accumulation of immune globulin does not necessarily imply production of autoantigen from cells damaged by silica, since antigenic components could originate elsewhere. By analogy with amyloid, the inconstant presence of serum globulin may be attributed to permeation and trapping between the collagen fibers, the sequestration being determined by molecular size and shape as well as the local chemical environment. The configuration of the γ globulin molecule could well be altered nonimmunologically so that it first stimulated formation of rheumatoid factor, then reacted with it, and finally bound complement. Neither in early nor mature silicotic nodules of rats was it possible to demonstrate gamma globulin, whose serum level was unchanged.[74] It may therefore be concluded that if the silicotic nodule contains immune components and there are humoral or cell-mediated counterparts they are secondary events and, as the original in vitro studies showed,[47,48] they play no part in the initiation of fibrogenesis by silica. Consequential immune events may exert an aggravatory role in silicotic fibrosis,[75] but immunologic changes are inconstant and many cases are unaffected.

Complicated Silicosis

The widespread distribution, often fairly symmetrically in each lung, of numerous discrete simple silicotic nodules contrasts with the isolated or restricted occurrence of massive lesions, which may affect only one lung notably in upper posterior zones, although occasionally such lesions develop in lungs containing few, small nodules. The predisposition of silicotic lungs to tuberculous infection is well attested. Early data from South Africa, the United States, and the United Kingdom established the presence of pulmonary tuberculosis in the majority of silicotic individuals and in South Africa the infection was clinically evident from an early stage. Simson and Strachan,[13] in a postmortem experience of almost 5000 black and white workers in South African gold mines, made a correlated histologic and bacteriologic study. They divided silicotic lesions, both nodular and massive, into those thought on naked eye and histologic grounds to be infective as opposed to lesions not so considered. Corresponding lesions (15 to 50 nodules or 1-cm cubes of massive fibrosis or fibrosed hilar lymph nodes per case) from the same series were then prepared for subcutaneous inoculation into guinea pigs and a remarkably close correspondence emerged between the biologic results and the histologic assessment. These authors thus identified two types of silicotic lesions and concluded that one represented the reaction to *dust uninfluenced by any other factor* while, in the other, two elements participated, *dust and infection*. Experimental studies confirmed the involvement of the two components in that infection of guinea pigs with tuberculosis of low virulence plus the administration of quartz led to more extensive fibrosis than either dust or bacilli alone,[16] but this effect was not seen with pneumococcal infection of silicotic rabbits.[17] The occurrence of cases of massive fibrosis without histologic or bacteriologic evidence of tuberculosis does not necessarily imply that infection played no part in their genesis, since it could either have died out or remained inconspicuous. Some 25 percent of apical pulmonary scars with no histologic suggestion of tuberculosis nevertheless contained viable bacilli, while the organism may be recovered from the lung or hilar nodes of exposed rabbits in the absence of overt disease.[76,77] Both quartz and tubercle bacilli stimulated activity of the mononuclear phagocytic system[78] and in combination the system may be so overtaxed that it fails to respond adequately to the infectious component which is allowed to progress. Subtoxic doses of silica were able to potentiate the growth of *Mycobacterium tuberculosis* in cultured macrophages.[79] The available evidence suggests that in complicated silicosis, as in the simple form, the *immunologic* features are nonspecific in character and occupy a position of secondary importance.

Sequelae and Associations

Diagnosis

Clinical recognition of silicosis should rarely be difficult provided the occupational history is not overlooked, which may occur now that the prevalence of the disease is low. Bronchogenic carcinoma needs to be differentiated especially where an isolated massive lesion occurs with little nodulation. Tuberculosis, histoplasmosis, sarcoidosis, microlithiasis alveolaris, and calcified lesions of varicella also enter into consideration.

Difficulty may arise in individuals exposed to silica and developing diffuse fibrosis of interstitial type. Pintar and co-workers,[80] for instance, assumed they were dealing with a diffuse form of silicosis in three foundry workers, whereas the probable explanation is that diffuse interstitial fibrosis occurred first, inhaled silica (identified by energy dispersive x-ray analysis, but whose physical state was unspecified) being subsequently incorporated. Similar problems arise in coal workers (*see* Disorders Due to Coal Mine and Carbonaceous Dusts, Differentiation of Emphysematous and Fibrocystic States in Coal Workers, below).

Sequelae

Tuberculosis and Other Infections. Tuberculosis may progress, cavitate, and disseminate through the lung to dominate the clinical presentation, being more likely to do so in the later stages of the dust disease.[81,82] Overt tuberculosis is much less frequent than formerly. *Mycobacterium kansasii* may occur though the presence of anonymous mycobacteria in the sputum is usually commensal.

The possibility that silica particles favor viral replication arises from in vivo and in vitro observations[83] showing that proliferation of herpes simplex virus is facilitated by the mineral in the presence of a continued supply of macrophages; viruses persisting in these cells might recrudesce under such circumstances. By implication silica retained in the lung might encourage viral infection.

Cor Pulmonale. Only when silicosis is advanced is there sufficient obstruction of the pulmonary arterial system by massive lesions, probably in conjunction with bullous emphysema, to lead to right ventricular hypertrophy and right heart failure.[84] Moreover, cardiovascular or pulmonary causes unrelated to silicosis may primarily be responsible.

Rheumatoid Syndrome and Progressive Systemic Sclerosis. (*see* Disorders Due to Coal Mine and Carbonaceous Dusts, Rheumatoid Pneumoconiosis, below).

Carcinoma of the Lung. Among the numerous cases of silicosis encountered in South Africa, no difference in the prevalence of pulmonary carcinoma was observed between miners with and without silicosis or between miners and nonminers.[85] Negative evidence has also been provided from Great Britain[5] and Switzerland.[86] The explanation may lie in the destructive effect of silica on cells other than macrophages. Epithelial proliferation is not a feature in air spaces adjoining silicotic nodules and it seems likely that regeneration and dysplasia may be prevented by the persisting silica repeatedly destroying epithelium as it attempts to reform. Claims that the risk of lung cancer is raised in silicosis are based not on exposure essentially to silica but on mixed exposures commonly including carcinogens, while the weighty negative evidence is ignored and smoking not adequately considered. A recent account assesses the position in detail.[87]

Other Conditions. Silicosis is not specifically related to bronchitis of the "obstructive" variety, for which cigarette smoking is largely to blame, and though bullous emphysema may develop around massive lesions pneumothorax is almost always prevented or limited by pleural adhesions. Rarely, gross enlargement of hilar lymph nodes may distort and compress the oesophagus.

Diatomite Pneumoconiosis

Nature, Exposure, and Prevalence

Also known as diatomaceous earth or kieselguhr, diatomite represents the siliceous skeletons of unicellular algae of which there are numerous species living in fresh or salt water, each having a characteristic skeletal structure. In the natural deposits, extracted mainly in the United States, Germany, France, and Sweden, the silica is amorphous in type though quartz may constitute a small proportion. Mining is by the open-cast method and the natural material is dried and separated by low heat and cyclones. To remove organic matter diatomite is heated to approximately 1000°C and calcination occurs either in the nonfluxed (straight) or fluxed state, for which sodium carbonate or hydroxide is added. The calcining process alters the physical form of the silica by partial transformation to crystalline cristobalite, which forms 10 to 30 percent of the nonfluxed product but as much as 64 percent of the flux-calcined material, the proportion in the airborne dust being up to 45 percent.

Milling and bagging after cyclone classification into size fractions (the finer being largely respirable in size) provided the main soures of exposure in the manufacturing processes, but dust control measures have proved so effective that even with calcined products containing cristobalite the risks are now minimal, as a follow-up study over 21 years demonstrated.[88] The radiologic prevalence of pneumoconiosis in the industrial processing of calcined diatomite has however been as high as 23 percent in one series and almost 50 percent in another with many cases showing massive type lesions. Quarrying apparently carries no risk, presumably because of the open air conditions, but exposure to diatomite is possible in some of the manufacturing processes, especially its use as a filter in the beverage and pharmaceutical industries where it has largely replaced asbestos. Other applications include the manufacture of insulating components, its use as a filler in various products, as a mild abrasive, and for protection of the surface of iron ingots.

Pathology and Genesis

The intensity of the tissue reaction to diatomite depends on its content of crystalline silica, as was evident experimentally. Exposure of guinea pigs and rats to prolonged inhalation of natural diatomite led to a slowly progressive fibrosis essentially interstitial and focal though without nodule formation, but the response to the calcined product was much more rapid and the initial phagocytic accumulation was followed by proliferation of fibroblasts and pronounced connective tissue formation with some hyalinization, though it did not assume the nodular form of silicosis. Inhalation infection of guinea pigs with tubercle bacilli regressed in control subjects, but exposure to calcined dust simultaneously, before or possibly following the infection, led to its aggravation, spread, and in many animals to death.[89]

Most of the evidence on the pathogenicity of diatomite for humans comes from epidemiologic surveys[90] and pathologic reports are few. Silicosis varying from mild to severe occurred in three kieselguhr workers who were exposed to the natural mineral and who also contracted tuberculosis[91]; the quartz and cristobalite contents of the kieselguhr were considered insufficient to produce the pathologic changes and amorphous silica was blamed, but the content of crystalline silica (15 to 17.5 percent of the lung dust) would nevertheless appear adequate to be causative. Most exposures in humans have involved both natural and calcined earth. The features[89,92] consist in the *gross* of greyish areas of fibrosis with a linear or stellate outline mainly though not exclusively affecting the upper zones of the lung subpleurally, sometimes accompanied by masses of solid fibrosis which may show necrosis but not silicotic nodulation. *Histologically*, laden macrophages accumulate in alveoli around respiratory bronchioles and in the hilar lymph nodes, but the connective tissue reaction is minimal in early lesions. Later collagenous fibrosis and fibroblasts mixed with dust cells overrun some areas of parenchyma and spare others. Small cystic spaces may develop between the fibrous areas especially beneath the pleura. More sold fibrosis also occurs and is generally cellular but the connective tissue is irregularly disposed and lacks the nodular pattern of silicosis (Fig. 23–7). while vessels show endarteritis and there may be ischemic necrosis. Fibrosis affects the hilar nodes. Many dust particles retain their diatomaceous features though fragmentation is usual; some are elongated and others may acquire a ferroprotein coating in a manner analogous to the asbestos body. Pathologically, the fibrous reaction bears a resemblance to asbestosis both in distribution and type, a similarity that could depend on the fibrous aspect of some diatoms, a feature that would also account for the dissimilarity to silicosis. The lung dust contains little quartz.

Submicron Amorphous Silica

The particle sizes of different preparations range from 5 to 40 nm but are uniform in each. They are pure amorphous silica and are prepared by precipitation from sodium or calcium silicates or silicon tetrachloride and appear under different trade names such as Silene, Hi-Sil, Degussa, Aerosil, and Fransil. They are used as fillers, diluents, and carriers of catalysts, as well as in cosmetics and polishes. Although surveys of exposed populations usually showed no evidence of pulmonary disease, granulomatous nodules with interstitial and confluent fibrosis but without classical nodulation have occurred in individuals exposed to submicron amorphous silica produced by vaporization of quartz to obtain elemental silicon, but some crystalline silica remained in the source material and in the lung dust.[93] Interstitial fibrosis and nodulation were attributed to inhalation of amorphous silica fume (<1.0 percent being crystalline in form) in several workers from a silicon factory, some being asymptomatic though functionally there were restrictive features.[93a] Long-term inhalation of 20-nm amorphous silica by rats and guinea pigs caused minimal pulmonary

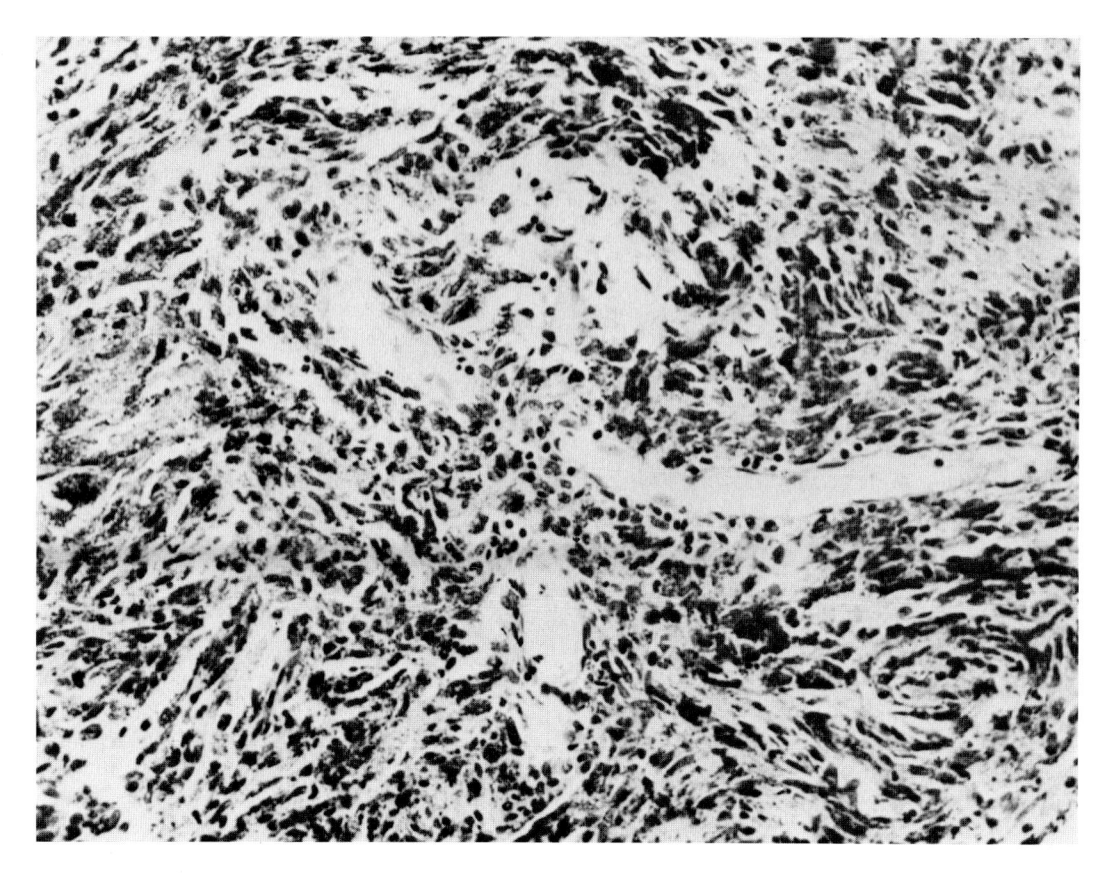

Figure 23-7. Lesion from lung of a worker exposed to calcined diatomite. Irregularly disposed fibrosis occurs among numerous dust-laden macrophages. There is no suggestion of a silicotic pattern (H&E, ×225). Courtesy of Dr. Parkes and Butterworth Scientific Publishers.

fibrosis but little dust was retained in the lungs; tuberculosis in guinea pigs may be encouraged.[94] However, injected into the peritoneum or the lung, submicron amorphous silica was fibrogenic[95], as personal experience also testified. A recent review nevertheless concluded that synthetic amorphous silicas were harmless to humans and animals.[95a] The rather conflicting experimental observations may depend on the state of aggregation of the particles, which while preventing effective pulmonary penetration might not affect injection of suspensions; aggregation could also explain why human disease has not been encountered in some surveys, though contamination with crystalline silica may vitiate interpretation.

Accelerated Silicosis

Occurrence

This term is preferable to the older "acute" silicosis. The disorder commonly develops after a few years' exposure and progresses more speedily than the classical variety (especially with the onset of dyspnea) to a fatal termination. Accelerated disease follows when intense concentrations of quartz in the respirable size range are inhaled usually in confined spaces. It was first encountered in the abrasive soap industry, which utilized finely ground quartzite sand mixed with anhydrous sodium carbonate and soap, many workers being exposed to the mixed dusts; quartz is now considered too abrasive for domestic purposes but it has not been eliminated commercially. Driving tunnels through quartzite rock or sandblasting produced the disease by exposure to silica alone, thus demonstrating that the presence of alkali was not determinative. The condition has been found in copper miners from Cyprus. These sources are for the most part adequately controlled, but sandblasting to clean metal surfaces still produces the requisite conditions (by ejecting sand under high air pressure) in some countries. This operation is proscribed in the United Kingdom and now the European Economic Community, metal grit having replaced sand while coal ash may offer a relatively harmless substitute that has yet to be adequately tested; dust suppression measures and the use of respirators afford other preventive devices. It is from U.S. shipyard sandblasters that accelerated silicosis has most recently been reported[96]; despite availability, protective hoods and respirators were not always worn and high concentrations of silica were experienced during busy periods. Mycobacterial infection was common and half the instances were attributable to atypical varieties such as *Mycobacterium kansasii* and *M. intracellulare*.[97]

Pathology

In the gross the lungs of recent cases show irregular greyish fibrosis lying as strands or as wider areas generally more evident in the upper zones, but true nodule formation is absent or inconspicuous. Other parts of the lung, often adjoining the fibrous formations, are usually consolidated by a firm, pale-pinkish material with a greasy surface. The hilar nodes may be enlarged and partly fibrosed.

The histologic features usually consist of irregularly disposed fibrous tissue, sometimes extensive, sometimes discrete and overrunning a number of adjoining acini, or appearing to be interstitial, but rarely showing nodulation with the classical features. Intervening alveoli though spared fibrosis are often occupied by eosinophilic granular material without organized structure (Fig. 23–8), but this nonfibrous consolidation may extend widely into parenchyma whose architecture is preserved. The intraalveolar material contains neutral mucopolysaccharides and lipid sometimes along with birefringent crystals. Cellular infiltration in the fibrotic areas largely consists of fibroblasts though lymphocytes and plasma cells may also accumulate in alveolar walls. The recognition that inhaled quartz could lead in rats to a condition closely resembling alveolar lipo-proteinosis[40] paralleled the features of human accelerated silicosis in material from Cyprus, demonstrating the association of lipidosis with atypical fibrosis, as American experience in sandblasters confirmed.[98] The lipid nature of the intra-alveolar material was also evident ultrastructurally, as was the paucity of alveolar macrophages and prominence of type II epithelium.[99] Accelerated silicosis with alveolar lipo-proteinosis but no tuberculosis occurred in tombstone sand-blasters, who developed noncaseating granulomas and some acellular nodules with confluence as well as the lipid accumulation which again gave a positive diastase–periodic acid-Schiff (PAS) reaction; energy dispersive x-ray spectrometry revealed elemental silicon in the lung parenchyma.[100] Some cases do nevertheless show tuberculosis which may cavitate. Since pulmonary lavage is now a standard procedure, it may prove possible to remove the lipo-proteinaceous material be repeated treatments, which would convey the additional benefit of extracting admixed silica and thereby discouraging recurrence.

Pathogenesis

In a natural disorder that presents few opportunities for analysis, the experimental approach is unavoidable. Exposed to quartz clouds of fairly high concentration, SPF rats developed extensive pulmonary consolidation which led to death of animals.[40] Histologically the alveoli were filled with granular eosinophilic material devoid of cellular structure, although in the earlier stages vacuolated macrophages were included and the alveolar epithelium was particularly prominent; alveolar septa were not

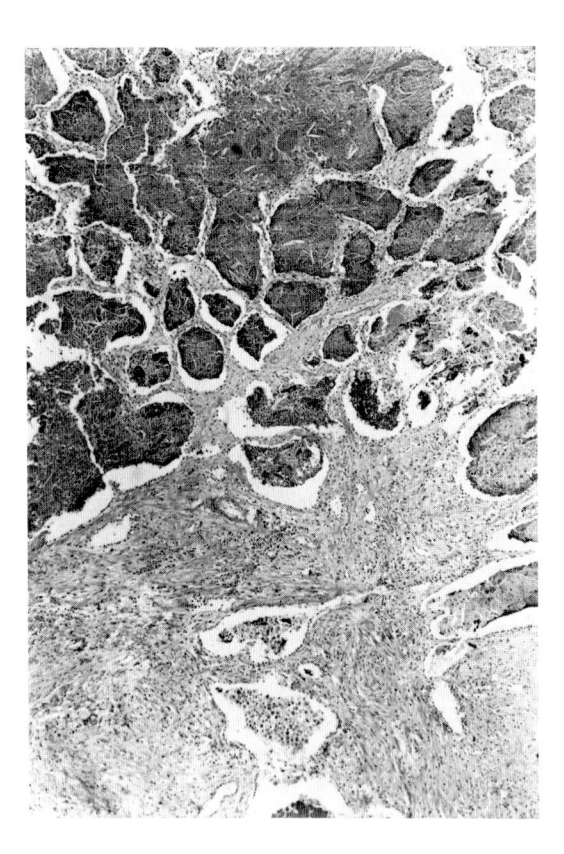

Figure 23–8. Accelerated silicosis in a copper miner. Irregular fibrosis occurs in the lower part of the illustration, while in the upper part alveoli are occupied by diastase resistant, periodic acid Schiff (PAS)-positive material typical of alveolar lipo-proteinosis. (×40). From Heppleston.[48]

fibrosed (Fig. 23–9). The amorphous accumulations contained neutral lipid and phospholipid, protein components and mucosubstances both neutral and acidic, but showed no enzymatic activity though the alkaline phosphatase content of the hyperplastic epithelium was pronounced. In the later stages cellular components became sparse and the epithelium reverted to its usual state, but there was a striking absence of silicotic nodules despite the persistence of silica. Ultrastructurally the initial hyperplasia affected type II cells, the type I epithelium often showing defects and exposing the basement membrane.[101] The alveolar accumulations contained extracellular silica particles but mainly exhibited three components: (1) whole or fragmented osmiophilic lamellar bodies clearly derived from type II cells in which these formations were initially numerous and large, (2) amorphous deposits of high or low osmiophilia, and (3) lamellar structures. The latter assumed the form of a quadratic lattice, though the angle of section often produced the pattern of parallel lamellar arrays with alternating layers of different density (Fig. 23–10). The quadratic or lamellar structure corresponds closely with the liquid-crystalline phase of lipid-water systems obtained in vitro and with the hexagonal formation seen in the human counterpart, both patterns almost certainly

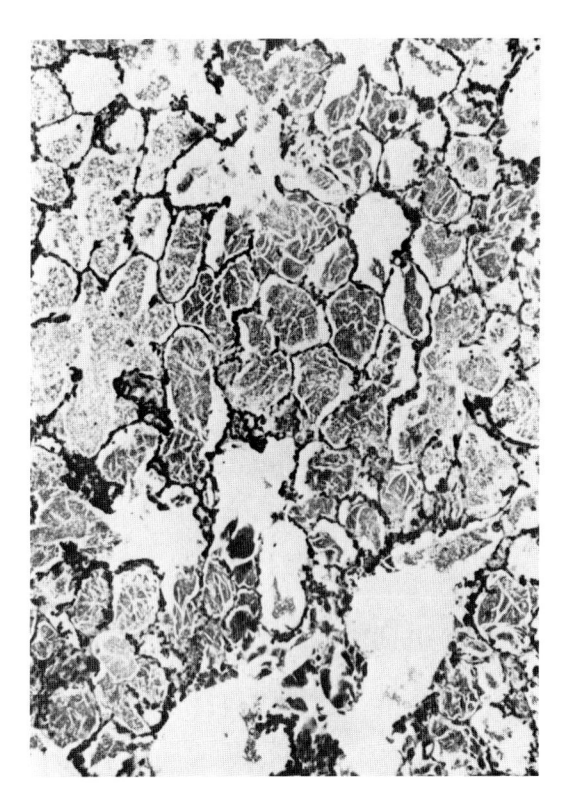

Figure 23–9. Experimental alveolar lipo-proteinosis in a rat after inhaling a high concentration of quartz. The alveoli are largely consolidated but their walls are not thickened (H&E, ×100).

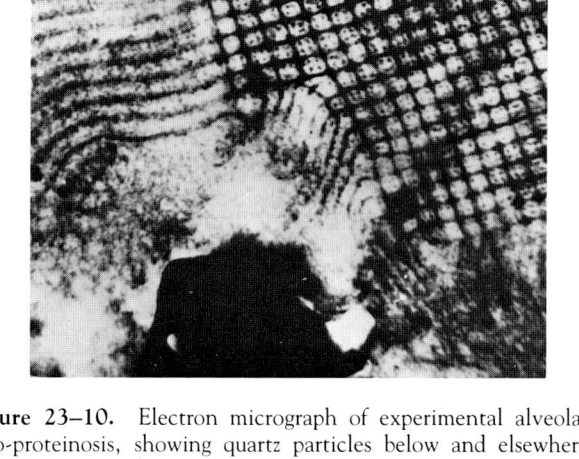

Figure 23–10. Electron micrograph of experimental alveolar lipo-proteinosis, showing quartz particles below and elsewhere lamellar structures typically seen as a quadratic lattice (×60,000). From Heppleston and Young.[101]

being derived from the prominent lipid component of surfactant.

To the massive increase of total lipid phospholipid was the main contributor, in which phosphatidyl choline and particularly the dipalmitate heavily predominated.[102] Protein increase was insignificant by comparison with lipids. Despite alterations in lung fatty acids, those of the plasma showed no abnormality either in total or in proportion following inhalation of quartz, suggesting a local rather than a systematic origin for the pulmonary lipids. The rate of synthesis of dipalmitoyl lecithin in treated animals was treble that in controls, while its rate of decay was doubled. This imbalance meant that retention of phospholipid occurred at a rate approximating to that of the normal synthetic rate. Physical observations on excised lungs and their extracts gave results which conformed to the features of a surface active agent.[103]

An important determinant of the pulmonary response is apparently the rate at which quartz is deposited from atmospheric suspension, a rapid accumulation of larger amounts evoking lipidosis while the slower retention of a smaller quantity permits silicotic nodules to form. Large amounts of lipid, produced by stimulation of type II cells, impair or prevent phagocytosis of quartz and hence production of the MFF. Removal of lipid may be effected by degradation from the action of phospholipases derived from alveolar macrophages and by proximal elimination along the ciliary escalator.

Lung lipids, given intravenously to rats, provoke marrow monopoiesis, thereby suggesting a mechanism for systemic recruitment when destruction of alveolar macrophages, as by silica, greatly augments demand.[104] An integrated scheme designed to embrace the known or conjectured aspects of silicotic fibrogenesis[105] (Fig. 23–11) may well be applicable to diverse pulmonary irritants.

Human Alveolar Lipo-proteinosis

Human alveolar lipo-proteinosis and its relation to silica and other environmental exposures is reviewed in Chapter 20. As with the experimental counterpart, the human disease is predominantly a lipidosis, the change in total protein content being comparatively small. The term proteinosis is accordingly a misnomer, for which lipo-proteinosis should be substituted as a matter of fact and not mere semantics. It is also relevant to hyphenate the term so as not to imply chemical bonding, since the phospholipid-protein attachment in lung surfactant is known to be an artifactual nonspecific complex.[106]

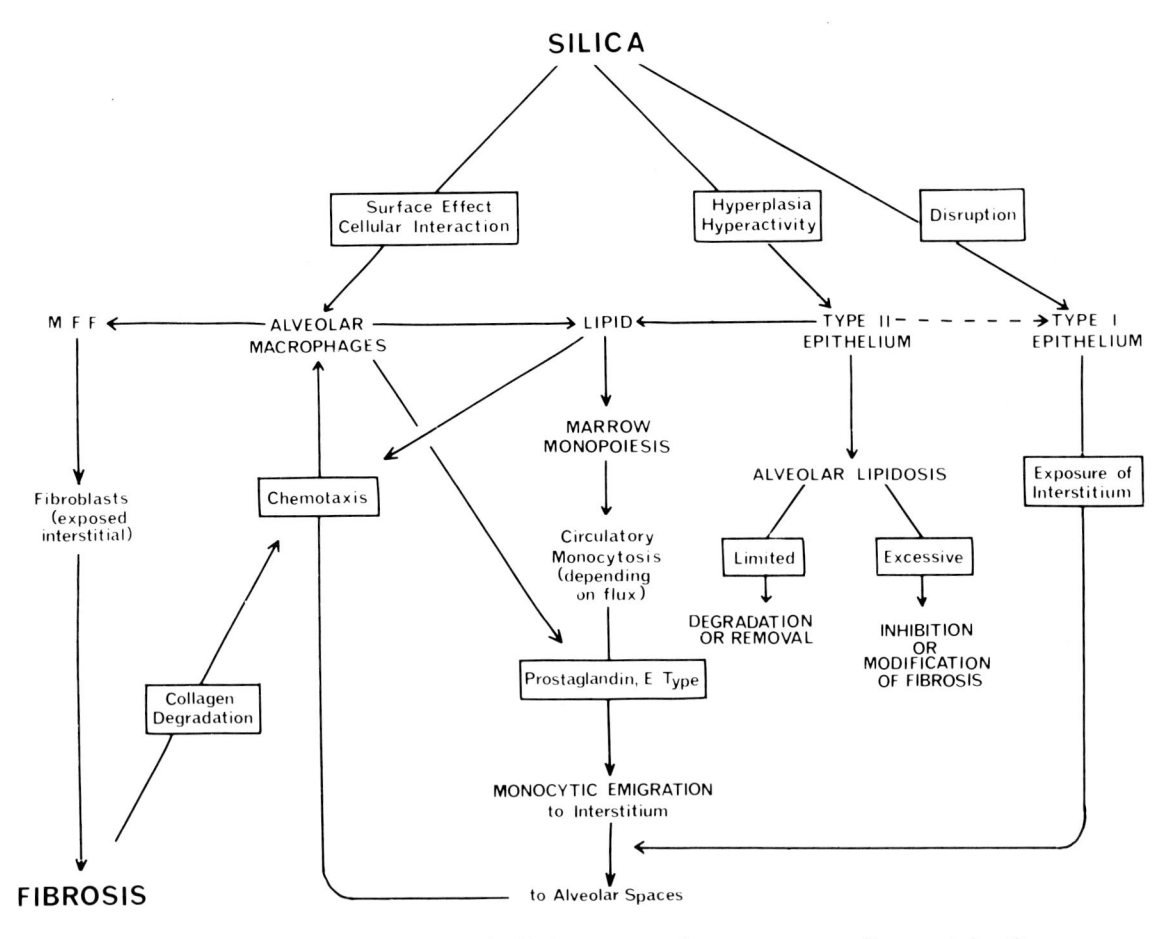

Figure 23–11. Diagram indicating the likely sequence of primary events in fibrogenesis by silica and possibly other irritants. Direct evidence shown by capital letters, inferred evidence by lowercase letters, and mechanisms by enclosures. Secondary events may cooperate.

Disorders Due to Coal Mine and Carbonaceous Dusts

Coal Worker's Pneumoconiosis

Because this form of pneumoconiosis possesses features distinct from those of silicosis, both morphologically and pathogenetically, and because no one component of the dust can be held responsible, it has been accorded a nonspecific designation. The disease in coal workers is the most prevalent variety of pneumoconiosis, but by comparison with underground mining open-cast work carries little risk.

Mineralogy

Airborne dust in coal mines is a mixture of minerals derived both from the actual seam and from the associated rock strata which are inevitably disturbed during extraction. The seams of coal provide most of the airborne dust, but coal itself is not a uniform substance and its composition is to a large extent determined by the position it occupies in the carbonaceous series, that is by its "rank." Peat, brown coal or lignite, bituminous coal, steam coal, and anthracite constitute rising ranks, but the distinctions are not sharp and the spectrum is characterized by increasing contents of carbon and decreasing contents of oxygen. Other properties of coal, mainly technological, have been applied to rank classification but are of no direct significance in pneumoconiosis; rank-related properties may, however, affect the characteristics of the dust produced in mining. Although coal contains inherent mineral matter, much of the mineral, particularly the quartz, content of airborne dust from coal mines is derived from the adjacent noncoal strata.[107] The respirable dust to which face workers were exposed was found to contain a mean of 4.5 percent quartz with a range between 1.8 and 8.6 percent (Welsh collieries falling at the low end), together with higher proportions of kaolin and mica along with smaller quantities of iron, calcium, and magnesium as carbonates.[108] The relative amounts of the different components did not vary in parallel.

Prevalence

The main surveys have been effected in the United Kingdom, the Federal Republic of Germany, and the United States. In 1953 the British National Coal Board initiated a long-term program of Pneumoconiosis Field Research (PFR) in collieries chosen as representative of the different coal fields. The prime object was to establish the relation between the environmental conditions and the development of dust disease, for which the earlier survey of the South Wales coal field by the Medical Research Council[109,110] had paved the way. A recent report[111] demonstrates that since 1960 the prevalence of all categories of coal worker's pneumoconiosis has diminished from 10.8 to 1.9 percent in 1983. The average values conceal a wide range, some coal fields having a higher prevalence notably South Wales where the current figure is 6.2 percent as against 20.7 percent in 1960. Prevalence was greatest in older men both for simple and complicated disease, the latter attaining a current average of 0.1 percent; in South Wales the average was 0.7 percent. A clear correlation of a more or less linear type transpired between mean dust concentration expressed as milligrams per cubic meter and radiologic progression.[112] Moreover, men who at the commencement of the investigation already had radiologic evidence of dust in their lungs not only showed more overall progression but their apparent susceptibility to higher dust concentrations also increased. The results permitted the deduction that a man without initial evidence of dust retention, exposed to a mean dust concentration of 4.3 mg/m^3 over a 35-year period, stood a 3.4 percent chance of ending his working life with radiologic category 2 simple pneumoconiosis. The probabilities of developing category 2 or higher simple pneumoconiosis were estimated according to the mean dust concentration.[113] This is a remarkable achievement when it is remembered that previous surveys of coal worker's pneumoconiosis have had to interpret prevalence in the light of dust levels measured simultaneously with medical assessment, rather than measuring prevalence in terms of levels obtained while the disease was in process of development many years before.

In West Germany, Reisner[114,115] has shown both the cumulative effect of dust exposure on radiologic progression of pneumoconiosis and the differences between individual collieries despite comparable dust exposures. Prevalence of the simple disease has varied between 2 and 40 percent at different mines. It must be stressed that in both these longitudinal studies unexplained colliery-associated variations were detected,[113,115] and it is to this question that current attention is largely devoted. In Pennsylvania[116] the prevalence of simple disease was similar at about 45 percent for workers in both anthracite and bituminous coal mines, but there were more anthracite miners in the higher radiologic categories. Complicated disease was much more frequent among the anthracite miners (14.1 percent) as compared with bituminous miners (2.4 percent). Colorado miners were less affected (4.6 percent) and then only by simple pneumoconiosis.[117] These differences could not be explained by variations in the years spent underground or by differences in smoking habits.

Pathologic Anatomy

As in silicosis, two forms of the disease occur in coal workers, simple pneumoconiosis being the response to coal mine dust alone while in complicated pneumoconiosis other factors cooperate. Modern understanding of the structural features and their genesis derives largely from observations made on workers in the South Wales field which embraces most ranks of coal, the main contributors being Cummins and Sladden,[118] Belt and Ferris,[119] Gough,[120,121] and Heppleston.[122–125] The later accounts achieved the ultimate clarification of the morphological features by reliance only on lungs fixed in expansion so as to preserve the natural anatomic relationships as closely as possible.

Gross Features

Appreciation is best achieved from whole lung sections mounted on paper or preferably between sheets of plastic for durability.

Simple Pneumoconiosis. In the early stages, seen in younger men killed accidentally underground or in older men dying from other conditions after exposure to low dust levels, the pulmonary parenchyma shows small black spots or macules about 2 mm across scattered widely throughout the lung though with a tendency to be larger and more numerous in the upper zones. The dust macules are sharply defined and their borders are rather irregular, but the remainder of the lung appears healthy and the air spaces are of normal size. As more dust accumulates the lesions enlarge and their number may increase, while spaces larger than usual may be seen in and around the macules though the parenchyma otherwise remains clean. At a later stage dust lesions may reach 5 mm across with a scalloped outline and many show air spaces, either peripherally or within their substance, that may be 2 to 3 mm in size (Fig. 23–12). Eventually these dust-related spaces may become large enough to merge with those from neighboring lesions. Up to this stage the macules have been discrete with three to five occupying a lobule (corresponding to the number of acini), but on coalescence their circumscribed form is obscured. Many lesions are impalpable and although others may be felt they are never so firm as silicotic nodules, the fibrous content being inconspicuous and rarely amounting to more than a few short strands with no special orientation. Overall, simple pneumoconiosis in coal workers characteristically appears as discrete black lesions, with a stellate outline, that may be palpable and in some cases show strictly localized enlargement of air spaces, features which afford a macroscopic differentiation from the silicotic nodule. Dust also accumulates in a perilymphatic location, outlining lengths of bronchioles and the accompanying arterial branches, septal venous channels, and forming a mosaic in the pleura.

Complicated Pneumoconiosis. This disorder occurs as a different type of lesion superimposed on simple disease, usually of the more severe grades, though occasionally focal accumulation of dust is only slight. Black massive lesions are hard and may reach several centimeters across though their outline is irregular (Fig. 23–13). Commonly single, though in some cases they are multiple or bilateral, their usual location is in the upper parts of the lung and toward the posterior aspect, sites also favored by tuberculosis. Because of their tendency to increase steadily in size radiologically they are often designated progressive massive fibrosis (PMF). Massive lesions sometimes transgress lobar boundaries and extend to the pleural surface which becomes puckered. Adjacent to an area of PMF or in fairly close proximity, smaller firm lesions 3 to 10 mm in size are often found, perhaps connected to the main lesion and to each other by firm black strands, but they do not resemble simple dust lesions. The cut surface of massive lesions may reveal paler strands of connective tissue with no particular orientation and in many instances fluid resembling India ink and shimmering with cholesterol crystals escapes leaving a ragged cavity without a wall of demarcation. Should such an area of colliquative necrosis erode a patent bronchus in life, a genuine cavity would form and the miner experience the "black spit," which from early times came to be an acknowledged if uncommon clinical feature. Bronchi and large blood vessels are usually inconspicuous. Exceptionally, though formerly encountered more often, a cavity with grey granulomatous walls is located in a massive lesion and raises suspicion of tuberculosis, which may be borne out by caseous foci in adjoining lung or by bronchogenic dissemination. Complicating overt tuberculosis is now rarely met, but bullous or irregular emphysema often surrounds massive lesions and may extend subpleurally. Fibrotic areas up to about 2 cm across, often multiple but distinct from simple macules, are sometimes found in lungs without larger massive lesions and may have a circumscribed or an irregular outline, the latter showing surrounding emphysema apparently of irregular type.

Thickening and adhesion of the *pleura* are common over subjacent massive lesions while interlobar fissures may be wholly or partly obliterated. Widespread pleural adhesion may imply some other cause such as a remote pneumonia. In pure simple pneumoconiosis adhesions are usually absent when the visceral surface shows a polygonal pattern of black lines, especially where septa join the pleura, and small back patches may be interspersed. The *lymph nodes* in the hilar region are black, enlarged, firm, and often adherent to each other as well as to major pulmonary vessels and bronchi, structures which in complicated disease may be invaded by dust fibrosis. Exceptional consequences may then be pulmonary arterial thrombosis with fatal outcome or black spit from bronchial erosion. Pigment deposits are also found in parabronchial and paravascular lymphoid tissue, as well as along the bronchovascular bundles. Honeycomb lung or acquired fibrocystic disease (*see* Differentiation of Emphysermatous and Fibrocystic States in Coal Workers, below) occasionally affects parts of the lung, the cysts

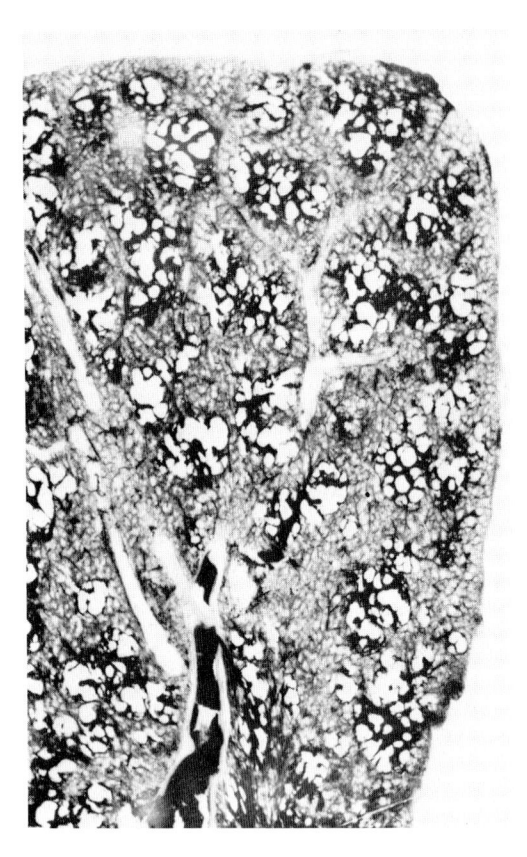

Figure 23–12. Simple coal worker's pneumoconiosis characterized by discrete black dust lesions, in and around which are enlarged air spaces. From a whole lung section (×1.5). From Heppleston.[125]

being enclosed by pigmented connective tissue. A minor degree of bronchiectasis is sometimes present, but when more severe the affected segment or lobe may contain little or no dust. If bronchiectasis precedes dust exposure deposition of dust could be prevented, but in the reverse situation inflammation might mobilize dust and facilitate clearance.

Microscopic Features
Simple Pneumoconiosis. In conventional histologic preparations the fully developed lesion has a stellate border and exhibits three features, a large amount of black or dark-brown dust, a small amount of connective tissue and typically emphysema localized to the immediate vicinity of the dust which encloses the air spaces wholly or partially (Fig. 23–14). The particles occur in small packets, which represent laden macrophages or their remains, though some dust appears to lie extracellularly. The density of dust in the lesions shows some variation, particles usually being closely packed with few other cellular elements but sometimes scattered fibroblasts are evident and macrophages carry a lighter burden. Connective tissue occurs mainly as reticulin and the fibers run irregularly between the dust cells, though collagen fibers are sometimes seen as unpigmented strands. The demarcation of the dust is generally sharp

Figure 23–13. Left upper zone of a coal worker's lung, showing massive fibrosis with central liquefaction necrosis. Simple dust lesions occur elsewhere. Whole lung section (×1.2).

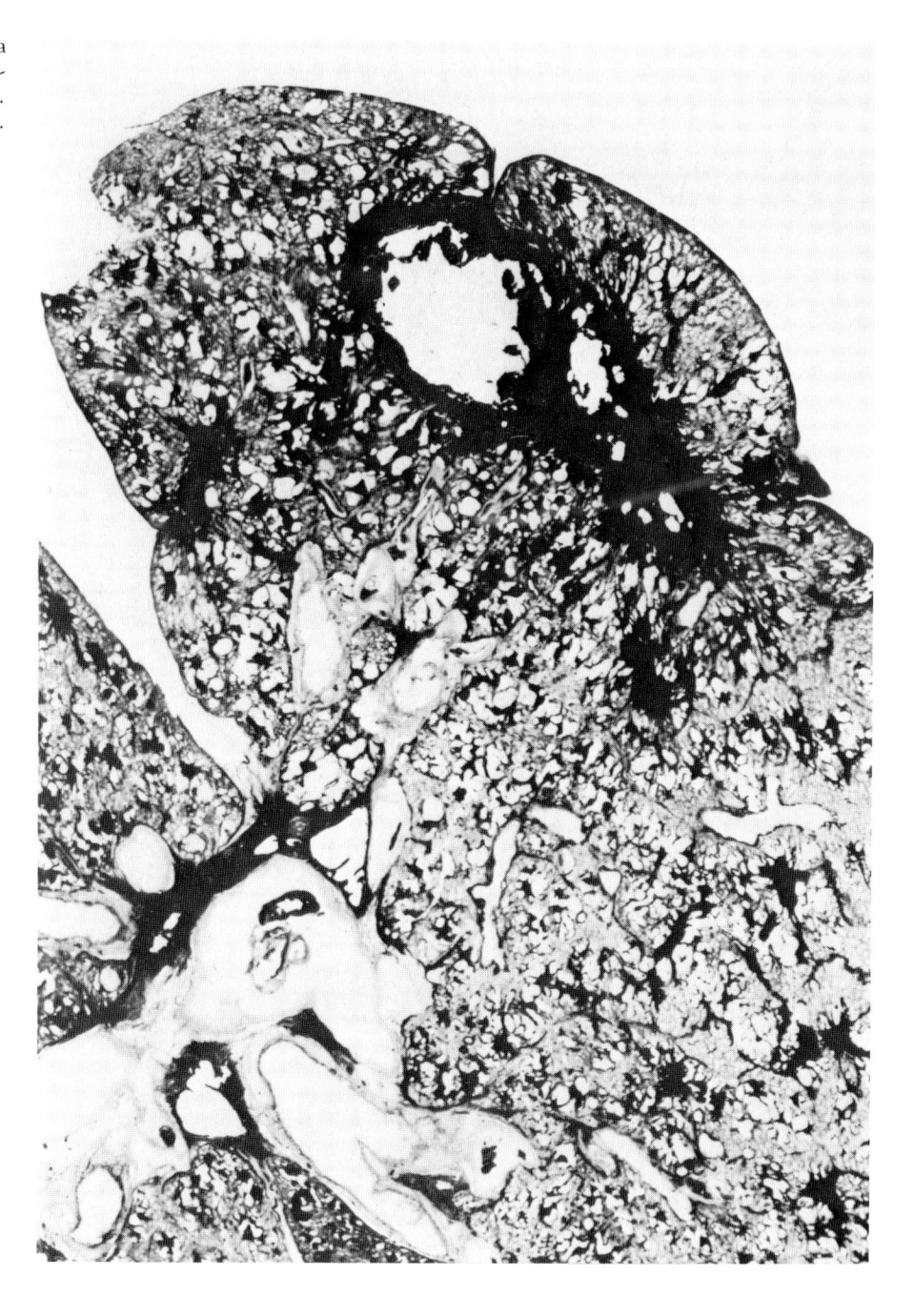

and prolongations extend between the enlarged peripheral air spaces. Smooth muscle fibers lying singly or in small bundles may be found toward the periphery of dust macules without associated emphysematous change but when this is present muscle fibers are few or absent; irrespective of the size of the air spaces elastin fibers are disorganized and fragmented. In contrast to the silicotic nodules, microincineration reveals an ash pattern evenly distributed throughout the macule and birefringent particles are few.

As in silicosis, the microanatomy of the simple dust lesion in coal workers can be appreciated fully only when examined in three dimensions[124] (Fig. 23–15, 23–16). Alveoli surrounding respiratory bronchioles are consolidated by dust which comes to form a dense sheath partly or entirely enclosing all three orders though more particularly the second order. Subdivisions of the pulmonary artery running with the bronchioles are also enveloped but compression is not apparent since they tend to lie peripherally. The adventitia of arterial branches merges with the dust, muscle fibers may be reduced, and the intima often shows a little fibrous thickening. Small, thin-walled vessels pass from the artery into the macule. Bronchioles surrounded by solid or interrupted cylinders of dust often become dilated, a change described as proximal acinar emphysema,[125] whose relation to other forms of emphysema is discussed in Differentiation of Emphysematous and Fibrocystic States in Coal Workers,

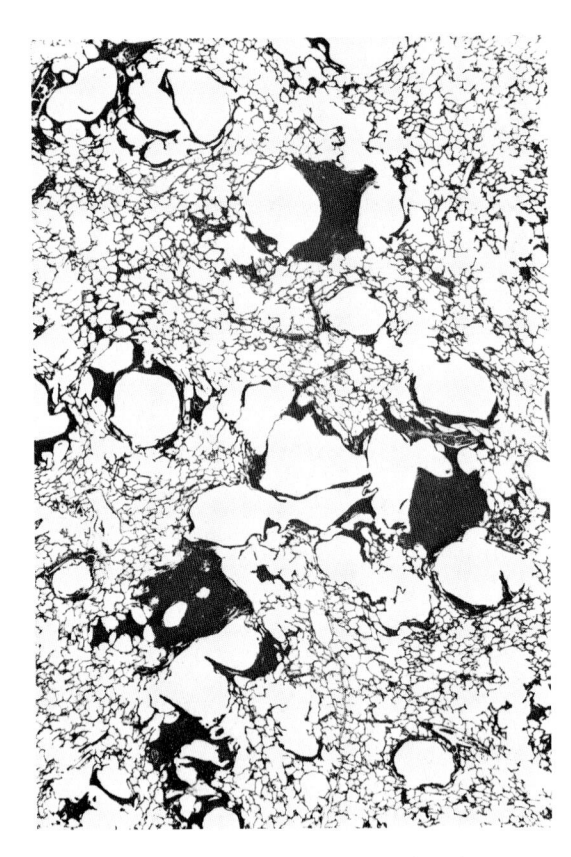

Figure 23–14. Simple dust lesions in a coal worker, comprising dense masses of dust associated with proximal acinar emphysema, situated in normal lung (H&E, ×5).

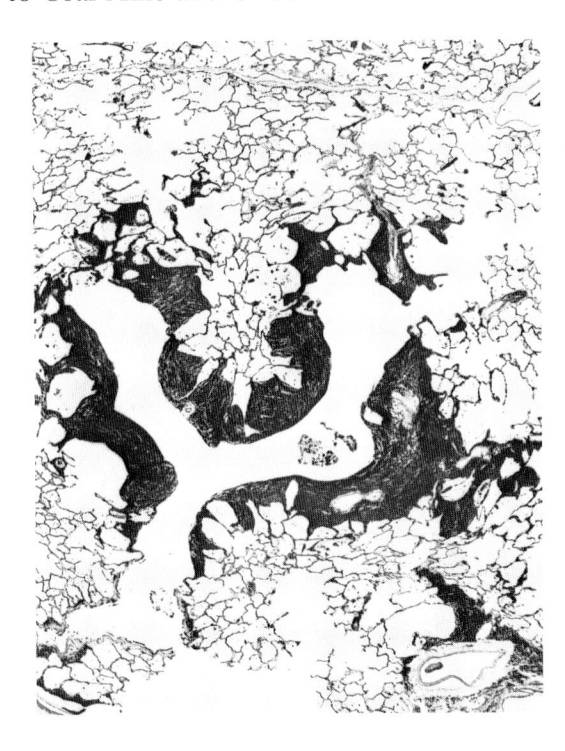

Figure 23–15. Simple dust lesion in a coal worker seen in longitudinal section, extending from the terminal bronchiole to alveolar ducts and sacs beneath the septum. The respiratory bronchioles are dilated where dust and fibrosis have consolidated surrounding alveoli (H&E, ×10).

below. It should be stressed that in simple pneumoconiosis of coal workers there is no evidence of bronchiolar stenosis, the features do not suggest an inflammatory process and disruption of alveolar walls is not a primary event. However, when the disorder reaches an advanced stage the emphysematous spaces belonging to neighbouring acini tend to merge, with disruption of alveolar walls leading to coalescence of lesions, whose circumscribed character is then obscured and it is no longer possible to identify the usual number of acini per lobule (Fig. 23–17). Difficulty may be experienced in reconciling the shape of many dust lesions with the accumulation of dust along the lengths of respiratory bronchioles and in explaining why some enlarged airways appear centrally and others peripherally. When the images of serial sections are transferred to film and projected in rapid sequence, the transition between the different appearances is readily discerned, particular outlines depending on the plane of individual sections.[126] It is evident that in all major respects differences exist between the simple lesions of silicosis and coal worker's pneumoconiosis.

Complicated Pneumoconiosis. This condition has a structure quite distinct from that of simple dust lesions (Fig. 23–18). Connective tissue is much more evident, some appearing pink with Van Gieson's stain though the reaction is less clear in other parts. Fibers have no particular arrangement and bands which may be hyaline course haphazardly through masses of dust. Much of the latter is extracellular and the occurrence of macrophages can only be inferred from the existence of particles in small packets of appropriate size. Electron microscopically, the structure differs according to whether the periphery or the center of a massive lesion is examined. Collagen fibers with the characteristic periodicity lie toward the edge but in the center the organized structure is replaced by amorphous material mixed with particles, while chemical analysis shows that these lesions contain coal, collagen, serum constituents, glycosaminoglycans, and calcium phosphate, though calcification is not usually an overt feature.[127] Small satellite nodules, however, show collagen fibers throughout their substance with occasional fibroblasts and fragments of coal. Fibronectin, a glycoprotein probably important in cell adhesion, occurs in massive lesions from coal workers, as well as in simple disease; asbestotic and silicotic fibrosis also contain it.[128] Colliquative necrosis is common and often extensive but is sometimes microscopic. Loss of connective tissue allows particles to lie loosely in a faint matrix but there is no cellular reaction and the surrounding massive fibrosis merges almost imperceptibly. Occasionally massive lesions contain foci or areas of eosinophilic granular necrosis with little or no pigment and no cellular boundary. Such features raise the possibility of tuberculosis and acid-fast bacilli can sometimes be demonstrated. Frank tuberculosis is not often countered

Figure 23–16. Diagram of the simple coal dust lesion constructed from serial sections. Coal-laden macrophages and irregularly disposed fibrosis ensheath respiratory bronchioles which are dilated to form proximal acinar emphysema; alveolar ducts and sacs remain normal in size. From Heppleston.[125]

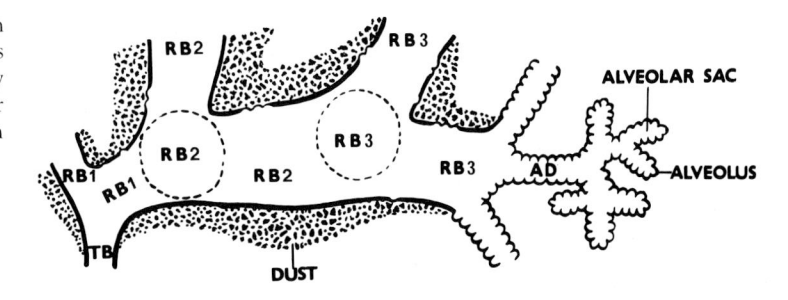

currently, but if softening of caseous material supervenes cavitation may follow. Inflammatory cell infiltration is not usually prominent and, consisting mainly of lymphocytes, appears to be nonspecific.

Vascular changes. Major subdivisions of the pulmonary artery are commonly blocked completely as they enter the massive lesion but in partially occluded vessels the intimal surface is sometimes ulcerated. Around the mass larger arterial branches are generally distorted and stunted. Fibrosis largely replaces the muscle and elastin of the adventitia and media and extends to the intima (Fig. 23–19). Many smaller arteries are totally stenosed, being overrun by fibrosis in which dust cells and vascular channels lie (possibly originating as organized thrombi); their former existence may be evident only after staining for elastin when the crenated or fragmented internal lamina is disclosed. The larger pulmonary arteries leading to massive lesions are sometimes thrombosed and there may be a suggestion of two or three episodes, with organization near the mass. Bronchial arteries are slightly larger and more tortuous than normal, but bronchoarterial anastomoses are not apparently a feature. Intimal fibrosis, perhaps with thrombosis, also affects pulmonary veins. Emphysema of irregular or bullous type especially in relation to massive lesions contributes further to the reduced vascularity. Bronchi suffer a similar fate to

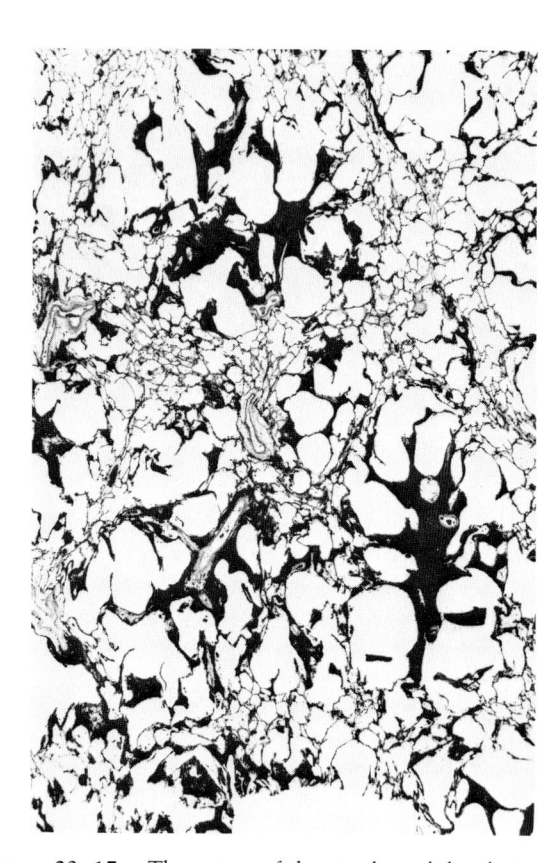

Figure 23–17. The extent of the simple coal dust lesions and the associated emphysematous change has led to confluence, though the discrete form is not obliterated entirely (H&E, ×5). From Heppleston.[125]

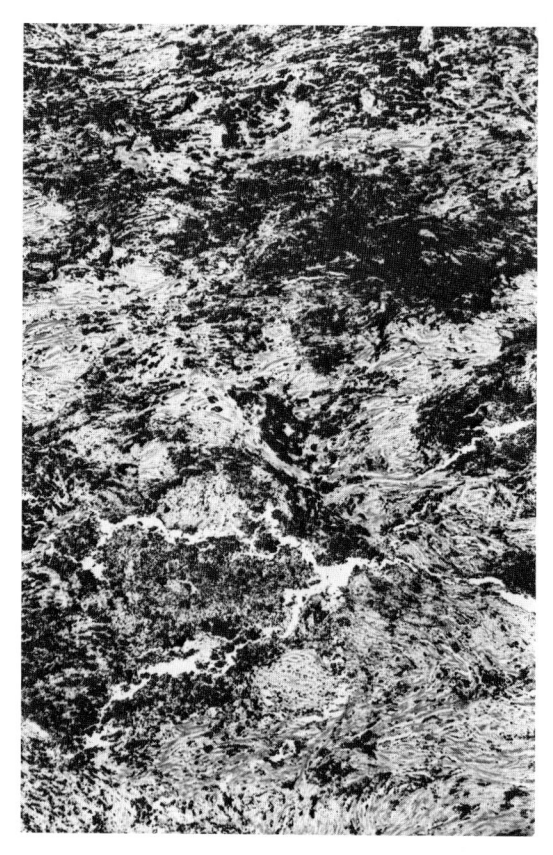

Figure 23–18. Massive fibrosis in a coal worker. Coarse connective tissue mingles irregularly with masses of dust and necrosis is evident in the lower left area (H&E, ×40).

arteries in massive lesions, but it seems that collateral ventilation obviates distal collapse. The avascularity of massive lesions has been confirmed in vivo by perfusion scanning of the lung after intravenous administration of radioiodine-labeled aggregated albumin.

Pigmented Fibrosis. The areas of pigmented fibrosis, ranging from 0.5 to 2 cm or more in size, whether they have an irregular or a smooth outline in the gross, partake of histologic features that are not characteristic of the simple dust lesion but resemble those of massive fibrosis. They do not bear an anatomic relationship to particular sections of the acinus, more than one of which is usually overrun. Strands of dust-bearing connective tissue lie haphazardly between air spaces, many being enlarged and perhaps reaching to septal boundaries. Such changes constitute a source of confusion if the microanatomical features are not borne in mind.

Lymph Nodes. The lymph nodes adjacent to major bronchi and in the hilar region share in the reaction. In simple disease alone pigment, free or in cells, overshadows fibrosis, which is somewhat more evident and more collagenous than in the dust macule. Enlargement and fibrosis, often hyaline, of the nodes are more prominent in complicated disease when adhesions are usual, and the appearances resemble those of massive fibrosis in the lung. Foci of calcification occur in some cases and may represent arrested tuberculosis, possibly the lymph node component of a primary complex.

Graphite and Carbon Pneumoconiosis

Graphite (derived from the Greek word meaning "to write") or black lead occurs as lumps or in amorphous form mined underground and as flake generally taken from outcrops, the principal sources being Korea, Austria, the USSR, China, and Mexico. In each case quartz-containing rock lies adjacent so that most samples of natural graphite contain a small amount of free silica, which is removable by solution in hydrofluoric acid and sodium hydroxide. After drying the graphite is ground and milled to a fine powder. Graphite is widely used in steel manufacture, lubricants, printing, reactors and electrodes, and in "lead" pencils. However, electrodes have been made from coke and anthracite. All processes produce a dusty atmosphere and workers have long been known to be liable to develop radiologic changes.

Both simple and complicated pneumoconiosis occur. Changes were reported in natural graphite workers similar to those of coal workers, including massive fibrosis with nontuberculosis cavitation and focal dust accumulations with localized emphysema.[129,130] Another account reinforced the similarity to coal worker's simple and complicated disease, chemical analysis failing to identify quartz in the lung dust and so permitting the case to be described as nonsilicogenic pneumoconiosis.[131] Closely comparable changes occurred in carbon electrode workers exposed to dense clouds of dust; four men came to autopsy and three showed massive fibrosis, different patients having ischemic necrosis or tuberculosis, though all had simple dust lesions which were severe with localized emphysema in two. Of particular impor-

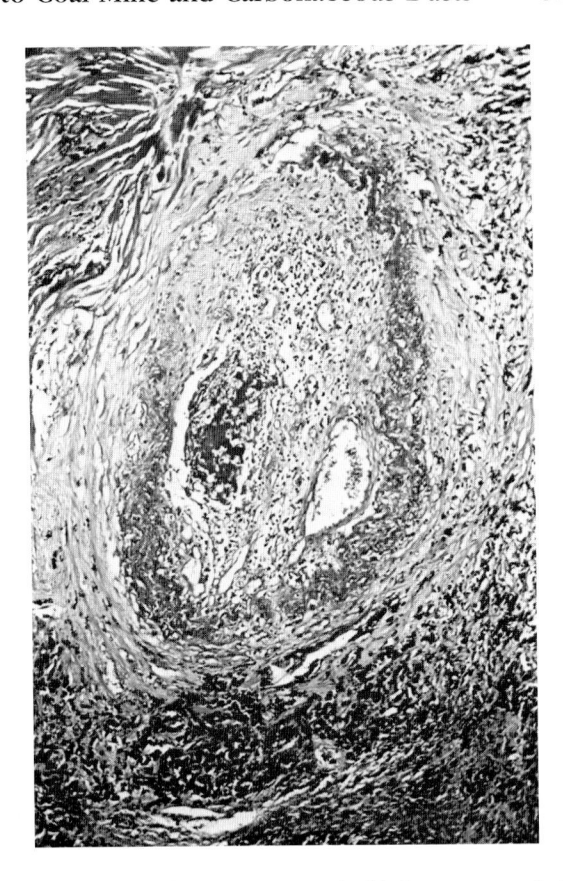

Figure 23–19. Pulmonary artery embedded in a massive lesion from a coal worker. Its lumen is largely obliterated by connective tissue which enmeshes dust-laden cells. The internal elastic lamella is breached (H&E, ×75).

tance was the presence of only traces of quartz in two patients examined chemically.[132] Several other accounts have appeared, including individuals exposed to natural or synthetic graphite, as well as to coal derivatives and soot. In some instances crystalline silica was detected in the lung dust, but in others there was none or only traces, whereas in all cases the pathologic features did not differ essentially from the condition seen in coal workers.

Pathogenesis

Simple Pneumoconiosis

Although the same fundamental processes are concerned in the genesis of dust disease in coal workers as in gold miners, the different composition of the dust greatly affects the balance between the various components of the response. That coal mine dust alone is responsible for simple pneumoconiosis rests on three pieces of evidence. First, the histologic features of the dust macule betray no evidence of a banal inflammatory reaction. Second, large samples of lungs from coal workers examined by biologic and cultural means disclosed no tubercle bacilli in 15 of 17 cases;[133] the presence of organisms in the remaining two workers could well indicate contamination, either because the hilar nodes were for an unaccountable reason minced with the lung or because lesions were not excised individually from lung tissue, which may contain tubercle bacilli in the absence of obvious disease.[76,77] Third, experimental tuberculous infection combined with the administration of carbonaceous dust produced lesions[134,135] that were quite distinct from those developing after inhalation of coal mine dust by rabbits exposed underground.[136]

The sequence of events in the development of the macule is most readily observed experimentally though small lesions encountered in humans suggest a close correspondence. Widespread deposition of dust from inhaled air, phagocytosis, and accumulation around respiratory bronchioles occur in similar fashion to siliceous dust, but disintegration of macrophages is less apparent and fibrosis is much less so, while proximal acinar emphysema is often a feature. Pathogenetic considerations are mainly concerned with these peculiarities.

Quantity of Dust. Dust concentration and duration of exposure are important determinants of dust accumulation in the lungs, though other factors introduce complexities. Overall cumulative dust exposure correlated with radiologic category of simple pneumoconiosis, but the level of abnormality for a given dust exposure showed substantial differences between collieries, high progression at some pits apparently being associated with low dust concentrations and vice versa.[112,137] Moreover for a given level of dust there was no systematic increase of risk in relation to the time worked when long exposures were considered.

The influence of *dust composition* may be examined from two aspects, prospective from airborne dust measurements during life and retrospective from lung dust analyses after death. The original investigation in the South Wales coal field[109] led to the view that simple pneumoconiosis was most prevalent in anthracite miners notably in colliers (that is, coal-face workers) and decreased progressively through the steam coal to the bituminous area, thus sowing the idea that rank of coal affected the incidence and severity of the disease. Subsequent long-term observations indicted that the so-called rank effect was adequately comprehended by measuring the concentration of respirable dust by mass as opposed to particle counts.[112] While some collieries showed risk differences related to coal rank, reflecting differences in mineralogic characteristics, other factors were clearly involved. Of these most attention has focused on the quartz content of airborne dust, but although progression could rise or fall with the quartz percentage, there was no overall effect of the proportion of quartz in the airborne dust.[138] Moreover, neither the quartz exposure, concentration, nor content of the mixed dust sufficed to, explain the observed variations in prevalence when the quartz levels did not exceed 10 percent of the dust.[137] In the latest radiologic survey of 250 British mines, a progressive and fivefold increase in prevalence of pneumoconiosis from low- to high-rank collieries was observed and the suggestion was again made that in the past the highest mass concentrations of respirable dust were experienced in high-rank pits.[139] German evidence also showed a variable risk of disease for comparable dust concentration and the quartz content of the dust failed to explain the differences, lesser risks accompanying high ash and quartz contents and vice versa.[115] On epidemiologic grounds it may therefore be concluded that, where quartz levels in respirable airborne dust fall within the 5 to 10 percent range, the probability of developing simple pneumoconiosis is not explicable in terms of the average quartz content of the respirable dust, though with higher quartz levels, even as much as 20 percent, unusual radiologic changes occurred.[113] Under the latter conditions it might be expected that silicotic features would be evident pathologically.

Characterization of dust extracted from miners' lungs has repeatedly been made. In simple pneumoconiosis encountered in Britain, the mass of dust recovered varied from 2.4 to 44.1 grams per lung, and of the total dust quartz constituted a mean of 3.1 percent.[140] As part of the PFR, the pathologic changes were related to the dust contents.[141] On average about 8 g of dust were recovered of which quartz comprised about 0.3 g and kaolin plus mica about 1.3 g. In percentage terms quartz was <5 percent and kaolin plus mica about 20 percent of the total dust. In another account of PFR material[142] the mean mineral content of the lungs was approximately 1 g for quartz and 2 g for kaolin plus mica, the rank of coal mined being reflected in only slight variations of quartz content. From these observations it is clear that noncoal minerals form a minor part of the lung dust, that quartz is present in only small amounts, and that no lead is forthcoming to account for the different risks of developing simple pneumoconiosis from exposure to coals of different ranks. A comparble situation existed in Cumberland hematite miners; in simple pneumoconiosis of these workers a mean quartz content of 5 percent (range zero to 12.1 percent) was detected in the total lung dust with muscovite contributing 14 percent and hematite 81 percent.[143]

Experimental Analysis of the Quartz Factor. Dusts have customarily been held to be deleterious in accordance with their capacity to induce pulmonary fibrosis and, since this feature is pronounced in silicosis, coal worker's pneumoconiosis is often regarded as a modified quartz effect and experimental studies continue to concentrate on this aspect. It has been suggested that under natural conditions unidentified inhibitory substances, possibly aluminium compounds, combined with the surface of quartz particles to render them inactive, but contamination of quartz surfaces in natural coal mine dusts is probably incomplete.[144] Since PNO abolishes quartz fibrosis, the effect of the polymer on reactions to coal mine dusts might assist interpretation. While some diminution of fibrosis was observed after injection (intraperitoneally or intratracheally) of natural mine dusts, artificial mixtures of coal and quartz, or dusts extracted from colliers' lungs,[145] no substantial therapeutic benefit was derived in monkeys inhaling a mixture containing 40 percent quartz and preventive treatment had no reliable effect.[146] Soluble aluminium compounds administered as aerosols exerted a prophylactic and a therapeutic action on rats exposed to a high concentration of coal mixed with 17 percent quartz but the curative effect diminished as the silica content was reduced.[36] Experimentally, particle size in the 4 to 7 μm range and hence surface area, rather than composition has lately been advanced as a determinant of fibrogenicity by coal mine dusts (Bruch and colleagues, unpublished data).

Specificity of the Dust Macule. The importance attached to the role of quartz in the genesis of the simple dust lesion of coal workers is thus questionable. Where quartz forms only a minor quantity of the lung dust, with a mean as low as 2.2 percent in one series,[140] the major carbonaceous, silicate, or nonsiliceous components deserve more attention. That the latter may partially contaminate quartz surfaces is possible, but once ingested by macrophages the surfaces are likely to be reexposed and a dilution effect must be considered a better explanation. However, the predominant constituents of the dust cannot be regarded merely as a diluent. The distinctive features of the coal macule are basically unaffected by rank of coal mined, whether anthracite, steam, or bituminous, or by workers' employment in coal fields of different countries such as Britain and the United States.[122,123] Hematite pneumoconiosis (*see* Metallic Dusts, Inert Metallic Dusts, Iron, below) differs only in color, and closely comparable changes developed in boiler scalers who are also exposed to a mixed dust probably with a small quartz content.[147] Mention has already been made of the occurrence of indistinguishable lesions in graphite, carbon electrode, and carbon black workers whose lung dust was virtually devoid of quartz and of a graphite worker from whose lung no quartz was recovered, a situation also present in a hematite miner. A primary and dominant role for quartz may thus be reduced to vanishing point and to say that small amounts of quartz may dissolve during prolonged residence in the lung is hardly relevant since the solubility theory of fibrogenesis is discredited and preferential elimination by bronchial or lymphatic routes hardly helps the argument. The simple dust lesion in coal workers and in those exposed to a similar type of hazard may accordingly be regarded as a nonspecific reaction to the accumulation of an excessive quantity of coal or a like mixture, the mineral component of the airborne dust exciting neither a dominant nor a specific contribution. The customarily minimal degree of fibrosis may well be determined by the quality or quantity of the stimulus to generation of the MMF exerted by the dust after ingestion. Where the quartz content of the lung dust somewhat exceeds about 10 percent, the connective tissue component of simple dust lesions may be a little more evident though their basic character remains unaltered, but levels approaching 20 percent introduce the likelihood of a change to the silicotic type of reaction. The development of classical silicosis in those coal workers who have been exposed to highly siliceous dust, as in driving headings, has long been recognized,[122] but is an exceptional occurrence and the nonspecificity of the disease in the great majority of miners is in no way invalidated.

The nonspecific nature of the dust macule may be seen as entertaining peculiar mechanical consequences on local respiratory movements. Elastin within dust aggregates is disorganized or has disappeared from the normal sites in respiratory bronchioles irrespective of the presence of proximal acinar emphysema, so minimizing or eliminating elastic tissue loss as a factor in its genesis. The smooth muscle of respiratory bronchioles may persist in dust macules, when proximal acinar emphysema is not usually encountered, but when the bronchiolar muscle has atrophied or disappeared the localized emphysema then becomes increasingly prominent. A general inverse relationship thus exists between the amount of smooth muscle remaining and the severity of the characteristic emphysema. Atrophy or total loss of muscle in dust foci may be expected to diminish or abolish the normal expiratory shortening and narrowing of respiratory bronchioles caused by the contractile tone of the geodesically disposed fibers. A second mechanical consequence may be visualized by virtue of the consolidation of alveoli around respiratory bronchioles. In effect these complete or partial sleeves of dust and connective tissue prevent inspiratory expansion of affected parenchyma and the traction normally expended on them could well augment the tension to which respiratory bronchioles are subjected directly and which in the normal state serves to dilate and elongate them. The result of such localized disturbances of expiratory and of inspiratory movements would be additive and lead to permanent dilatation of respiratory bronchioles, that is to the development of proximal acinar emphysema due to dust.[125,148] By contrast, the simple silicotic nodule, though forming in the same location as the coal macule, is for much of its existence a progressively expanding lesion which indents respiratory bronchioles to produce stenosis. If silicotic nodules ultimately stabilize, which may not be for years after cessation of exposure, fibrous contraction may ensue and lead to a degree of irregular emphysema around them.

Enzyme involvement in the genesis of proximal acinar emphysema attributable to dust seems unlikely. If macrophage elastase is active, it appears to operate independently of the development of emphysema since elastin fragmentation is seen in lesions without emphysema. Because disruption of alveolar walls is a late feature, local deficiency of alpha$_1$ antiprotease cannot be regarded as having an initiatory role, and since fibrosis overtakes the coat dust aggregates, macrophage collagenase involvement appears insignificant. On the other hand, in consolidated alveoli type II cells are lost and the consequential paucity of surfactant could assist in condensing the macule.

Lipid Involvement. Experimentally, airborne dust from some collieries excites activity in type II epithelial cells as well as in macrophages.[149,150] The effect took the form of lipid accumulation within alveoli that also contained macrophages, but in fewer numbers than after exposure to other mine dusts. In the presence of lipid the dust load per cell was reduced, macrophages were foamy, and aggregation feeble. The variations in response did not appear to correlate with the mineral content of the lung dust but might be connected with the rank of coal. A possible explanation is thereby afforded for the disparities detected epidemiologically between dust composition and prevalence of simple pneumoconiosis (*see* Coal

Worker's Pneumoconiosis, Prevalence, above). Lipid participation constitutes a neglected aspect of the coniotic response and one that could well be relevant to humans; the experimental evidence discussed in Disorders Due to Free Silica, Accelerated Silicosis, Pathogenesis, above, leaves no doubt of its potential importance.

Immunologic Aspects. Antinuclear antibodies were detected in 29 percent and rheumatoid factor in 4 percent of American cases of simple pneumoconiosis.[151] Among British coal workers with simple disease only 9 percent showed antinuclear antibody and 6 percent revealed rheumatoid factor; there was no change as the disease progressed.[152] Cell-mediated immunity has not received the same attention. Findings such as these do not encourage the belief that immunologic factors play a role in simple pneumoconiosis of coal workers and certainly there is no evidence to suggest that they are other than consequential or that they possess diagnostic or prognostic value.

Complicated Pneumoconiosis (Progressive Massive Fibrosis) (PMF)

On pathologic grounds dust alone appears insufficient to account for the development of massive lesions. Simple disease exhibits a symmetric distribution of numerous, discrete lesions throughout the lungs whereas massive fibrosis occurs asymmetrically and may affect only one of a pair of lungs. Massive fibrosis is occasionally seen with little dust elsewhere in the lung. Simple pneumoconiosis may be intense in the absence of massive fibrosis. Hyaline connective tissue is a feature of massive lesions but not of simple macules, while the pattern of dust and connective tissue differs. The shape and distribution as well as the structure of massive lesions argue against collapse of lung tissue affected by simple disease. From the dry weights of normal and diseased lung, the volume of normal lung that a massive lesion would have occupied was calculated and found to be much larger than could be entertained from the size of the whole lung section.[140] Consolidation of tissue is therefore their likely basis. The outstanding question, which remains contentious, revolves around the nature of the additional factor(s) which the inception of massive fibrosis evidently requires.

The Total Dust Factor. The attack rate of progressive massive fibrosis (PMF) was related to the radiologic category of simple disease, being much higher in men with category 2 or 3 than category 1 and also in those miners who reached category 2 when young.[153] However, some cases of PMF have now been found to develop on the basis of category 0 or 1 disease but their cumulative dust exposures were high, suggesting that radiologic regression of simple pneumoconiosis may have occurred (see Clinicopathologic Correlations, Physiologic, below); the attack rate of PMF, moreover, was unaffected by the rank of coal mined.[154] Chemical analysis of affected lungs[155] gave credence to the view that the total quantity of dust, possibly in combination with a higher mineral content, was directly related to the radiologic progression of simple pneumoconiosis.

The Quartz Factor. Irrespective of the size of the massive lesion, its dust content was about double that in the remainder of the lung, showing only simple disease, but the composition of the dust was similar in the two locations; in particular the proportion of quartz was the same at approximately 3 percent.[140] The collagen content of massive lesions did not differ materially from that in the rest of the lung, suggesting that massive lesions comprise other elements, as was subsequently established.[127] The avascularity of massive lesions satisfactorily explains their central amorphous state which may be regarded as a prelude to colliquative necrosis. The situation in hematite workers[143] corresponds with that in coal workers; the quartz content, though somewhat higher at about 5 percent of the lung dust, did not differ in cases of complicated or simple disease. In massive lesions excised form the lungs of ten coal workers the dust concentration proved to be two to three times greater than in the rest of the lung but no different in composition; in abosolute terms the quartz content of lungs with massive lesions was about 1.25 g and that of kaolin and mica approximately 4 g.[141] A later analysis of this material recorded progressive massive fibrosis in lungs from which no quartz was apparently recovered.[142] Selective concentration of quartz is thus not a feature of massive lesions.

The most potent point against the silica contention lies in the occurrence of massive lesions with no detectable quartz in the lung dust both in coal workers and in individuals exposed to purified carbon with indistinguishable pathologic features.[131,132] Massive fibrosis was encountered in a man exposed to nepheline, a feldspar containing no free silica, where the lesion resembled that seen in coal workers in all but color and no free silica was recovered from the lung dust.[156] It is therefore justifiable to conclude that quartz does not play a specific or essential role in the genesis of massive fibrosis in coal workers, as was also evident in regard to simple pneumoconiosis.

The Infective Factor. From early times tuberculosis, often modified in form by the presence of dust, has been advanced as an additional factor in the genesis of massive fibrosis in coal workers. James[157] found bacteriologic (culture and guinea pig inoculation) or histologic evidence of tuberculosis in 40 percent of massive lesions from 245 Welsh coal workers and Rivers and colleagues[133] recovered tubercle bacilli from 35 percent of 118 such lesions from men working in the same coal field. Histologic evidence of active tuberculosis was detected in 47 percent of hematite miners with massive disease.[143] Of particular relevance is James's age-related analysis, which revealed the presence of tubercle bacilli in 88 percent of massive lesions from men under 40 but an incidence of 29 percent in lesions from men of 60 or over, findings that suggested that tuberculosis was concerned in the initiation of massive fibrosis and that with increasing age the infection tended to die out. Whether or not tubercle bacilli were isolated, massive lesions possessed similar histologic appearances, notably in younger and older men between whom percentage recovery of bacilli differed widely. Epidemiologic observations offer a parallel in so far as the rate of progression of massive fibrosis diminished with increasing age.[158] An argument against a tuberculous etiology arose because bacilli were recovered by laryngeal swab during life in only 1.1 percent of cases of massive fibrosis,[159] but this finding entails no serious difficulty since there is little chance for organisms to escape from closed lesions, that is where bronchial communications have been obliterated. In hospital patients, however, tubercle bacilli were recovered by biologic and cultural techniques from the sputum of 7.7 percent of patients,[160] while cultures taken from the bronchus prior to necropsy dissection yielded positive results in 28 percent of massive lesions.[133] The idea that infection occurs after the massive lesion has been established is difficult to envisage, since it would require the development of deeply situated tuberculous foci from blood-borne bacilli in a lesion that is poorly if at all vascularized. Because many examples of massive fibrosis in older men failed to show evidence of tubercle bacilli, other infective agents have been sought. Anonymous mycobacteria were isolated from the sputum of 1 to 2 percent of coal miners with massive fibrosis, but less frequently from nonminers.[161] Many of the recoveries could not be repeated and if they were the organisms sometimes belonged to groups considered to possess low pathogenicity. Anonymous mycobacteria may be more common in the mining environment but identification in the sputum does not necessarily imply infection, and Mycobacterium tuberculosis was actually isolated more frequently than anonymous varieties.[161] A nationwide survey of Britain detected no association between infection by *M. kansasii* and a previous history of coal mining, though there was an apparent connection with exposure to dust of the metal grinding trades.[162] *M. kansasii* has not apparently been isolated from massive lesions themselves, as is the case with *M. tuberculosis*.

Experimental studies encourage the view that coal dust, in contrast to silica, may so alter the tissue response to the presence of tubercle bacilli as to restrict the extent and progression of the disease. Bacillus Calmette-Guérin (BCG) and quartz both stimulated functional activity of the mononuclear phagocytic system,[78] but coal mine dust, being less toxic to macrophages than quartz, is less likely to overtax the macrophage response so that resistance to tuberculosis may be more effective and progression reduced. Infection of guinea pigs with tubercle bacilli of low virulence combined with the administration of coal[134,135] or of hematite[163] led to more extensive fibrosis than bacilli or dust acting alone. As the fibrosis became more severe the bacilli died out,[134] thereby supporting the view that tuberculosis is involved in the inception of massive fibrosis, as in men exposed to dusts with a low free-silica content, and is not just a late phenomenon. Lesions resembling massive fibrosis were obtained in guinea pigs treated with a combination of anthracite mine dust or kaolin and anonymous mycobacteria or vole bacilli, though separately each was relatively harmless.[164] Other experimental observations also lead to the conclusion that mycobacterial infection of the coniotic lung played the dominant role in establishing massive fibrosis.

A neglected aspect of the infective component concerns the possible role of mycobacteriophages. Mutants may resemble atypical mycobacteria or be unrecognizable as such. It is not known whether mycobacteriophages participate in progressive massive fibrosis from which mycobacteria cannot be recovered.

Resistance to the tuberculous concept of massive fibrosis persists despite the evidence adduced. The general decline in prevalence of tuberculosis in developed countries may well be reflected in miners, but differences in the attack rates of mining and nonmining populations cannot exclude a tuberculous factor. Failure of antituberculous chemotherapy may merely reflect inaccessibility of organisms to blood-borne agents or cases that are burnt-out. Although the proportion of reactors to the tuberculin test may be low in some groups, it is high in others. Fritze,[165,166] for instance, recorded epidemiologic observations on nearly 12,000 individuals, comparing miners with nonminers from the Ruhr; the percentage of positive tuberculin reactors rose to over 80 percent at about the age of 50 in miners, but reached less than 60 percent in nonexposed individuals at the same age. Fritze related the frequent and intense reactivity in miners to their high morbidity rate for tuberculosis and stated that their average morbidity rate for the disease was about one hundred times that of Germany as a whole but that pneumoconiotic changes occurred on average 12 to 15 years later than the increase of "contamination" rate. It may fairly be said that the evidence in favor of an infective agent in the genesis of progressive massive fibrosis is too strong to be discounted and no organism other than *M. tuberculosis* has clearly been incriminated. Interpretations of massive fibrosis that fail to give due weight to the infective factor while laboring dust or other factors can only be described as imbalanced.

The Immunologic Factor. Activation of the mononuclear phagocytic system by mycobacteria or their products may be considered as a local or systemic adjuvant effect, though the contribution of the organism may wane when the massive lesion would tend to stabilize. Both in Britain and the United States rheumatoid factor and antinuclear antibodies appeared in the serum of a variable proportion of patients with massive fibrosis,[73,151,152,167] while elevation of IgG and IgA levels was subject to unexplained variations and humoral immune competence was unaffected.[168,169] Antibody levels had no predictive value in the genesis of massive fibrosis.[170] Such findings hardly accord with the idea that mineral particles, especially silica, denature body proteins and render them antigenic.

The existence of IgG and IgA in massive lesions does not necessarily represent an immunologic response since the simultaneous presence of human serum and fibrinogen, suggests exudation. As in silicosis (*see* Disorders Due to Free Silica, Classical Nodular Silicosis, Pathogenesis, Simple Silicosis, The Immunologic Component, above), the development of rheumatoid factor may well be a nonimmunologic process, while the occurrence and level of antinuclear antibodies probably reflects the rate of macrophage demise and tuberculous infection could exert an additive response. The immunologic phenomena are inconstant and often affect a minority of sufferers; moreover they are dependent on preexisting lesions with a prominent fibrotic component. Under these circumstances a primary pathogenetic role cannot be attributed to the immunologic factor in complicated pneumoconiosis of coal workers, though the observed changes may signify a peculiar reactivity on the part of individuals to the presence of dust or infection. However, T and B lymphocyte levels were unrelated to category of pneumoconiosis[171] and, despite earlier claims, no evidence exists to suggest that histocompatibility antigens play a role in determining either simple or complicated disease.[172–174]

Pathologic justification exists for applying the adjective *"progressive"* to massive fibrosis. The restricted distribution of massive lesions as compared with simple disease presupposes a local initiatory factor which is most likely to be infective. Persistence of mycobacteria or their antigenic elements will maintain the inflammatory or "adjuvant" reactions. It is also evident that serum components enter into the composition of massive lesions along with glycosaminoglycans, so that despite ischemia some exudation or transudation occurs. Gradual ischemia may itself contribute replacement fibrosis. Continued exposure may lead to increasing accumulation of dust around a massive lesion where lymphatics and airways are stenosed, while particles situated at the periphery may be evicted into adjacent nonfibrosed alveoli and there initiate further fibrosis, as was observed experimentally in silicotic nodules.[175]

The term *"mixed dust"* lesion encourages confusion. Few occupational exposures are confined to inhalation of a single type of mineral, so that pneumoconiosis in coal or hematite workers could be thus designated. The usual implication is that the "mixed" lesion is larger and more fibrotic than the coal macule and that quartz plays a larger part in its genesis. The isolated fibrotic areas measuring up to 2 cm across (see Coal Worker's Pneumoconiosis, Pathologic Anatomy, Microscopic Features, Pigmented Fibrosis, above) partake of the histologic character of massive fibrosis and may be regarded as entailing the same etiologic considerations. "Mixed dust fibrosis" was encountered pathologically in approximately 1.4 percent of a large series of miners who had worked coal, gold, asbestos and other minerals in South Africa.[176] A significantly higher incidence of active and inactive tuberculosis was found in men with "mixed dust fibrosis" than in those without or than in silica-exposed gold miners. These lesions do not justify a separate identity, especially as they do not possess the characteristic microanatomic features of coal macules and there is no histologic confusion with typical silicotic nodules.

It is perhaps in the employees of *iron and steel foundries* that the use of the term "mixed dust" lesion creates difficulty. The pathology of pneumoconiosis in foundry workers from Switzerland was identified with that of coal workers, free silica forming only a small percentage of the dried lung tissue.[177] In British workers coming to autopsy 94 percent of individuals had pneumoconiosis and 43 percent had tuberculosis, while pneumoconiosis was the main factor causing death in 40 percent[178]; sandblasters developed silicotic-type lesions, and other jobs resulted in what was called "mixed dust fibrosis" which from the illustrations resembled coal worker's pneumoconiosis either as macules, nodules, or massive lesions with indeterminate emphysema. Workers in nonferrous foundries may also be exposed to the risk of pneumoconiosis resembling coal worker's disease.

Clinicopathological Correlations

Despite a voluminous literature, precise functional and pathologic correlation has proved difficult since it is not usually possible to make clinical assessments close to the time when pathologic material becomes available and routine clinical investigations occur at intervals of 4 or 5 years. While pathologists—and clinicians—should tread warily, salient correlations have emerged, though with time patterns may change as disease is affected by dust suppression measures and by personal atmospheric pollution from cigarette smoking, as well as by the occurrence of nonoccupational interstitial lesions (see Differentiation of Emphysematous and Fibrocystic States in Coal Workers, Clinical Correlations, below).

Radiologic

Since the diagnosis of coal worker's pneumoconiosis rests primarily on occupational history and radiology, it is essential to appreciate the qualities of the substance behind the shadow. Focal dust lesions satisfactorily account for the rounded radiologic opacities, also described as pinhead or granular, by superimposition of macular shadows. Differentiation is required from the numerous cause of diffuse, nodular, or reticular radiologic appearances. The mean total dust in the right lung rose from 4.3 to 26.7 g as the x-ray category of simple disease progressed from zero to 3, with mineral and coal contents contributing equally to the radiologic changes, though on a weight basis mineral was about nine times as effective as carbon, probably because of differences in x-ray absorption. Moreover, proximal acinar emphysema tended to increase in parallel with radiologic category and with total dust content while the connective tissue component was not considered to contribute to the radiologic appearances of simple pneumoconiosis.[155] Proximal acinar emphysema, though not capable of recognition radiologically, nevertheless led to a marked degree of overreading.[179] By throwing the macule into better relief, this latter effect would be expected. Fine "p"-type opacities were found to reflect greater dust content, a higher proportion of coal, and an association with emphysema.[180]

Physiologic

A study of lung function from South Wales covered breathlessness, ventilation, diffusion, and perfusion in all the main radiologic categories.[181] Within the range of simple pneumoconiosis no average increase in breathlessness on exertion apparently occurred with increasing radiologic abnormality, but published diagrams showed that in radiologic category 3 the dyspneic index was about double that of the normal for age 55 and clinical dyspnea exceeded that of category B massive fibrosis.

While the mean values for maximum voluntary ventilation (liters per minute) showed little change in relation to degree of simple pneumoconiosis on the radiograph, a scatter diagram disclosed wide variations about the mean with an appreciable number of men, including some in the 45-year age group, showing much reduced values. The maximum voluntary ventilation diminished abruptly with massive fibrosis of increasing severity, while the dyspnoeic index rose. In a group of coal workers with simple pneumoconiosis of the pinhead (p) radiologic type, as opposed to those with micronodular (m) opacities, a defect of gas transfer (diffusing capacity) was later detected in conjunction with a larger physiologic dead space relative to tidal volume,[182,183] a view reinforced by recent evidence on small rounded opacities.[184] Smoking habits could not account for these features and dust-related emphysema was considered to be the likely cause.

Physiologic studies have conveyed to many clinicians the belief that simple coal worker's pneumoconiosis is of little importance in itself and serves primarily to signify the liability to complicated disease. However, a long retrospective analysis[185] indicated progressive impairment of ventilation at radiologic stages earlier than category B massive fibrosis, when substantial disability and premature death were generally expected. These category B cases had already acquired a substantial proportion of their eventual disability while classified as simple pneumoconiosis or category A, and impairment of ventilatory capacity due to pneumoconiosis was sometimes believed to be present before significant radiologic changes were manifest. It was recalled that simple pneumoconiosis may regress radiologically when massive fibrosis develops, presumably as a result of emphysema and fibrosis, and that similar regression can occur with simple disease alone, probably from the same processes.

Much of the evidence on the relation between function and radiology is derived from men whose underground exposures antedated intensive dust suppression measures and some of the contentious aspects may derive from the fact that pneumoconiosis in coal workers is now waning not only in prevalence, but perhaps also in severity. The problem is compounded by the liability of coal workers to develop nonoccupational emphysema and fibrosis (see Differentiation of Emphysematous and Fibrocystic States in Coal Workers, below). Attempts to make morphologic correlation more effective have taken two forms. Hartung[186] developed techniques whereby the mechanical properties of the excised lung could be measured before histologic examination. In morphologically typical cases of simple coal worker's pneumoconiosis with proximal acinar emphysema, in which bronchiolar smooth muscle was lost but bronchiolitis was absent, Hartung[186] was able to demonstrate expiratory bronchiolar collapse (presumably from local loss of lung tension), a much diminished expiratory air thrust, and often greatly raised distensibility along with uneven air distribution, features entirely compatible with dust-related emphysema. On the other hand, pathologic material has been examined in the light of previous radiologic and physiologic findings. In a case control study,[187] the amount of emphysema in simple pneumoconiosis, quantitated in whole lung sections, was much greater in miners than the control group and there was little increase in the presence of massive fibrosis. Functional impairment correlated closely with emphysematous change and pinhead (p or punctiform) shadows exhibited a higher degree of emphysema than the micronodular or nodular types of opacity, an interesting finding in view of the gas transfer results already mentioned. Smoking history was not considered to differ in miners and control subjects. It was subsequently concluded that the presence of emphysema accompanying simple pneumoconiosis was more important in determining impairment of ventilation that was x-ray category.[188] When case selection was minimized, emphysema (assessed macroscopically) was significantly more frequent in coal workers than noncoal workers, after allowing for age and smoking habits, while its severity correlated with the amount of dust in simple lesions.[189] One difficulty may be dispelled when it is remembered that the development of proximal acinar emphysema is apparently influenced by the amount of smooth muscle that persists in the macule. Hence small amounts of dust may lead to proximal acinar emphysema, whereas larger amounts may not, especially if there are natural variations in the quantity of muscle between individuals. No doubt the arguments will continue but skeptical clinicians should engage in similar correlative attempts.

It is reasonable to suggest that the gas transfer defect observed in some cases of simple pneumoconiosis is explicable in terms of the known anatomic changes, that is, enlargement of respiratory bronchioles that are enveloped by dust, so increasing the dead space.[124] The histomechanical observations of Hartung[186] give further credence to the significance of the emphysematous change. Moreover, no study takes separate account of the contribution of proximal acinar emphysema to functional disorder or mortality in complicated pneumoconiosis which usually develops on the basis of the higher radiologic categories of simple disease, that is, with increasing amounts of dust and the likelihood of more severe associated emphysema.

Smoking and Diesel Emissions
Allowance is customarily made for consumption of *cigarettes* in physiologic studies on miners and it might be appropriate to regulate compensation for disability in relation to an individual's propensity for personal pollution, though it is hard to imagine trade unions accepting any such limitation. Smoking by coal miners may be considered from several aspects (for example, bronchitis, emphysema, and particle disposal), but neither the prevalence nor the attack rate of simple pneumoconiosis showed any significant difference between smokers and nonsmokers.[190] Likewise pathologic studies failed to implicate smoking in the genesis of proximal acinar emphysema from dust inhalation in coal workers.[142,191]

Concern has lately arisen about the possible effects of *diesel engine emissions* in coal mines, especially in the United States and Australia. On experimental grounds, such emissions may depress the phagocytic activity of alveolar macrophages and increase the severity of infection by influenza virus, whereas coal dust does not apparently do so; particle clearance may also be impaired. Observations on miners, however, do not suggest deleterious effects and in particular no liability to lung cancer has been found.

Life Expectancy
Two factors affected the rate of dying: the amount of massive fibrosis and the size of the residual volume.[192] It may be suggested that in both cases emphysema could have been a contributor, bullous in the first and proximal acinar in the second place. Miners in the PFR program had a standardized mortality ratio (SMR) of 82 but factors of selection could have been operative,[193] whereas in Wales the SMRs were 115 to 120 for miners and ex-miners without or with simple pneumoconiosis but 195 for the upper categories of massive fibrosis;[194] since nonminers had the lowest SMR simple disease is not exonerated.

Sequelae

Tuberculosis and Other Infections
In a series of 1000 consecutive necropsies on coal workers James (personal communication) attributed death to pulmonary tuberculosis in 87 drawn from 454 cases of massive fibrosis. However, these cases occurred before the antibiotic era and when the general prevalence of infection was higher than now obtains.

In vitro studies suggested that coal dust may predispose to infection by influenza virus through suppression of interferon induction, an effect that may be more pronounced with higher rank coal.[195] Miners may thus be at particular risk to secondary bacterial infections and, while there is no suggestion that these acute phenomena lead to the development of massive fibrosis, interstitial fibrosis may be envisaged as a possible consequence and may lead to diagnostic difficulties.

Cor Pulmonale
Welsh coal workers with massive fibrosis often died from congestive heart failure. Before blaming pneumoconiosis, systemic hypertension, valvular and coronary disease had to be excluded[196] and then it was found that massive fibrosis accounted for cor pulmonale (as judged by the thickness of the right ventricle) in 57 of 136 men but complicated disease could well have contributed materially in other instances. Applying similar criteria to simple disease was more difficult, but, having excluded other pulmonary lesions from 181 cases, cor pulmonale was attributed to pneumoconiosis in 4 instances. Of 546 cases of simple disease occurring in South Wales,[197] 8 died from pulmonary heart disease and in 7 further men no other cause was evident for the right ventricular hypertrophy though death was due to other conditions, but chronic bronchiolitis might also have played a part. Excluding coexisting lesions from the 454 examples of massive fibrosis, 31 individuals showed degrees of right ventricular hypertrophy which increased with the size of the massive lesion and again it could have been a material factor in other cases. However, judged by weight, early evidence of right ventricular hypertrophy was recognized in 34 percent of cases with massive fibrosis and 46 percent of cases of simple disease, but in the presence of marked hypertrophy the proportions were 57 percent and 17 percent, respectively. Right ventricular hypertrophy is thus more frequent and severe in complicated as compared with simple pneumoconiosis and is attributable to vascular stenosis even though emphysema may be absent. None of these studies eliminates simple disease as either the main or a contributory cause of right ventricular hypertrophy and congestive failure, though complicated pneumoconiosis is a major or the sole basis for chronic cor pulmonale in many miners. Pulmonary arterial hypertension occurred in almost one-third of American coal miners in whom physiologic airway obstruction or complicated pneumoconiosis could have been responsible, while a few individuals with simple disease with pinpoint shadows exhibited pulmonary hypertension at rest or on exercise.[198]

Carcinoma of the Lung
In a large necropsy series lung cancer occurred less frequently in coal workers than in the male nonmining population of the same age group and even if selection of material operated it would have tended to increase the observed incidence of lung tumors.[199] Histologically, squamous and anaplastic carcinomas accounted for the great majority of the cases. While early death from pneumoconiosis might have reduced the incidence of lung cancer, there was no indication of an increase. When due allowance was made for age, smoking habits, and atmospheric pollution, the death rate for coal miners in Great Britain from carcinoma of the lung was lower than the national average.[200] The findings in West Germany were similar, taking into consideration age at death and severity of the disease; survival from the time of diagnosis was not affected by pneumoconiosis and miners lived long enough to develop bronchogenic carcinoma, which seldom developed in the presence of severe dust disease.[201] In northwest England, cases of progressive massive fibrosis had the lowest prevalence of carcinoma of the lung and yet the mean age at death was 72.[202] The human evidence has lately been elaborated.[87]

Coal workers with carcinoma of the lung had similar survival rates whether treated surgically or not, and survival time increased as the category of simple pneumoconiosis rose irrespective of treatment.[203] Moreover, miners with category 2 or more simple pneumoconiosis were less likely to die of lung cancer than miners with no pneumoconiosis.[193] Entry of neoplastic cells into the lymphatics may be prevented at the apex of the acinus, that is, where dust primarily collects, and so contribute to the better prognosis.

The occurrence of an excessive rate of lung cancer in gas and coke oven workers[204–206] is attributable not to the effect of dust inhalation but rather to polycyclic aromatic hydrocarbons (present in coal tar fumes and coal distillation products), which may be adsorbed onto particulate matter and so conveyed to the lungs in concentrated form. Tobacco consumption did not account for this excess mortality. A similar situation evidently existed in foundry workers, since, in a British series, bronchogenic carcinoma occurred in over 10 percent at autopsy.[178] Subsequent retrospective cohort studies from Canada, Finland, and elsewhere disclosed significant excesses of lung cancer among iron or steel foundry workers. Although tobacco consumption itself was discounted, the pyrolysis products from the occupation included polycyclic aromatic hydrocarbons.[207]

A significantly high risk of *gastric carcinoma* was detected in coal mining areas, but the equality of risk in both sexes combined with the socioeconomic status negated a connection with exposure to coal mine dust.[208] Although Jacobsen[193] believed that stomach cancer might be related to exposure to coal mine dust, recent evidence from the Netherlands was against this view.[208a] However, further case-control observations are desirable.

Rheumatoid Pneumoconiosis

Immunologic participation in massive fibrosis is inconstant and does not appear to play a primary role, but it assumes importance in coal miners possessing the rheumatoid "diathesis."

Caplan's Syndrome[209]

The original observations, emanating from South Wales, demonstrated that coal workers who were afflicted with rheumatoid arthritis had a greatly increased prevalence of progressive massive fibrosis sometimes with peculiar radiologic features. Approximately one-quarter of these men also showed discrete rounded opacities in their lung radiographs, shadows that were subsequently identified as rheumatoid nodules which may fuse to produce lesions several centimeters across. The recognition of the new syndrome prompted epidemiologic investigation, which demonstrated rheumatoid arthritis in 55 percent of miners with characteristic chest films but in only 3 percent with massive fibrosis; no arthritis was found in miners with and without simple pneumoconiosis.[210] Although the prevalence of rheumatoid arthritis was similar in miners and nonminers, 2.7 percent of men with massive fibrosis had rheumatoid arthritis and in simple pneumoconiosis 0.6 percent were affected.[211] Caplan's syndrome was believed to represent an inherited abnormality of tissue reaction, not restricted to the skeleton, in those with or presumably liable to develop rheumatoid arthritis.

Rheumatoid nodules of the lung tend to develop suddenly and, unlike typical massive fibrosis, they occur throughout the lung fields including the periphery. Radiologically these nodules are much larger than the lesions of simple pneumoconiosis, commonly appear in crops, and tend to progress more rapidly than massive fibrosis in miners without rheumatoid disease, the background of simple disease often being slight. Discrete rheumatoid nodules up to 1.5 cm diameter may be indistinguishable on x-ray examination from silicosis. Rheumatoid arthritis and the lung lesions usually appear contemporaneously, but either manifestation may precede the other by an interval as long as 10 years. Moreover, the lung and joint lesions do not necessarily parallel each other in severity. Corticosteroids and antituberculous chemotherapy convey no obvious benefit. Although coal workers constitute the only community in which a significant association has been demonstrated epidemiologically between occupation and the liability to rheumatoid disease of the lungs, nodules have been reported in association with other dust hazards. Cases were encountered among European gold miners in South Africa and workers exposed to silica in Sweden. Rheumatoid nodules have also been found in individuals exposed to asbestos, the dust of boiler scaling, or after working in a foundry or a chalk mine.

Pathologic Features

The initial description comprised lung lesions from 16 coal miners with rheumatoid arthritis.[212] Nodules, which may be few or numerous, generally measure 5 to 15 mm in diameter and are thus larger than simple dust lesions, which may be scanty and small. A concentric arrangement of alternating light and dark layers characterizes quiescent nodules and histologically these bands consist of collagen, usually necrotic, and extracellular coal dust, though the two components have a less regular arrangement centrally and non-necrotic collagen encloses the whole (Fig. 23–20). Larger lesions, some several centimeters across, are composed of confluent nodules with a fibrous capsule (Fig. 23–21). In the active phase nodules

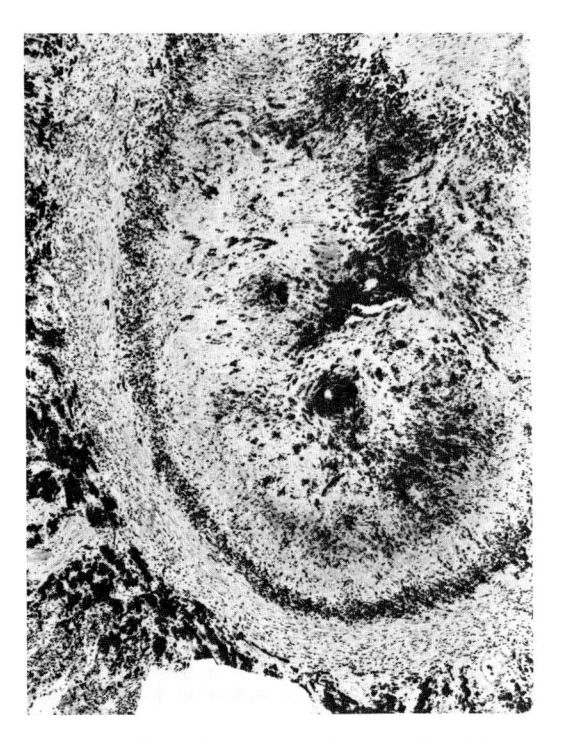

Figure 23–20. Part of a quiescent rheumatoid nodule in a coal worker's lung. The alternate bands of dust and connective tissue are well defined peripherally (H&E, × 40).

Figure 23–21. Rheumatoid pneumoconiosis in a coal worker. Composite lesions affect the right upper lobe, though a few isolated nodules also occur. Zonation can be discerned. From a whole lung section (×1.2).

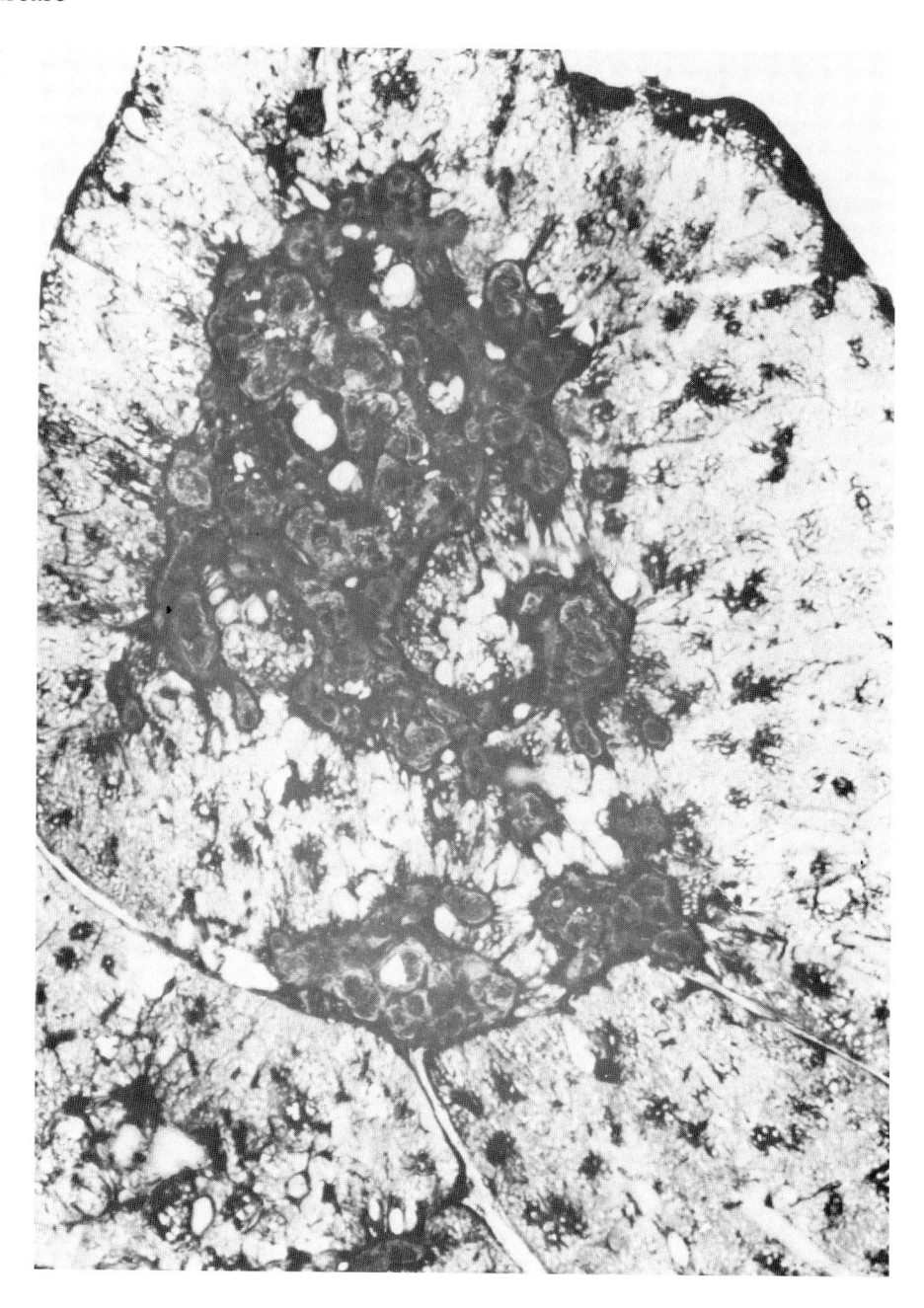

exhibit a peripheral zone of inflammation that wholly or partly encircles the necrotic center (Fig. 23–22). The cellular elements then comprise polymorphs and macrophages, some multinucleated, but compared with subcutaneous nodules palisading is not so prominent a feature. Dust is often collected in the inflammatory zone by the phagocytes and when they disintegrate the liberated particles form the rings typical of the stationary phase. Successive inflammatory episodes evidently account for the concentric layers of dust and of connective tissue laid down during healing. Lymphocytes and plasma cells tend to accumulate around the nodules and these cells also occur in the connective tissue which obliterates the lumina of small peripheral arteries (Fig. 23–23). The inflammatory activity may involve air passages with loss of the necrotic material and the formation of thin-walled cavities which may mimic tuberculosis radiologically. Other rheumatoid nodules undergo calcification. Differentiation from old tuberculosis may be difficult, but the histologic features should prevent confusion with silicotic nodules. Approximately 40 percent of the original material showed evidence of tuberculosis on guinea pig inoculation or histologically, but the peripheral inflammatory zone occurred independently of the presence or absence of biologically identifiable tubercle bacilli; most individuals died from cardiac failure or

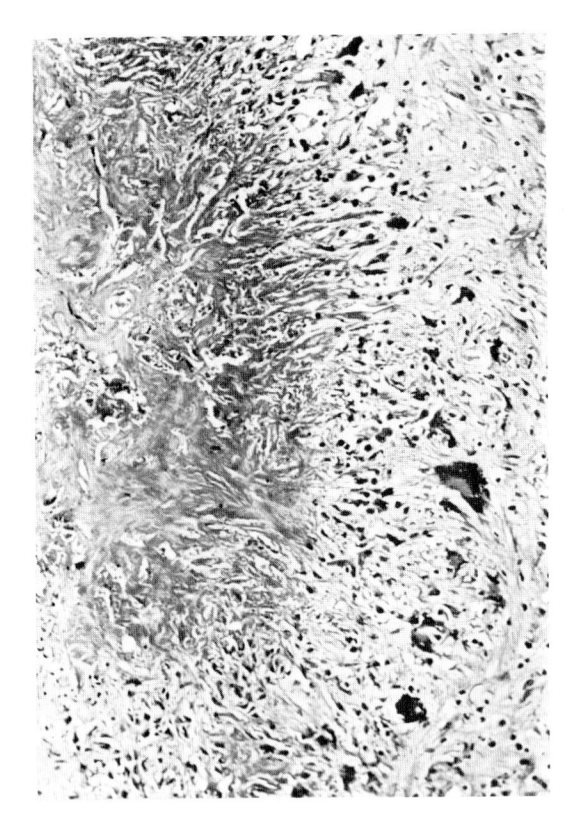

Figure 23–22. Active rheumatoid nodule in a coal worker. The central necrotic collagen is surrounded by a zone of granulation tissue with a tendency to palisading and the presence of giant cells, some of which contain dust (H&E, ×150).

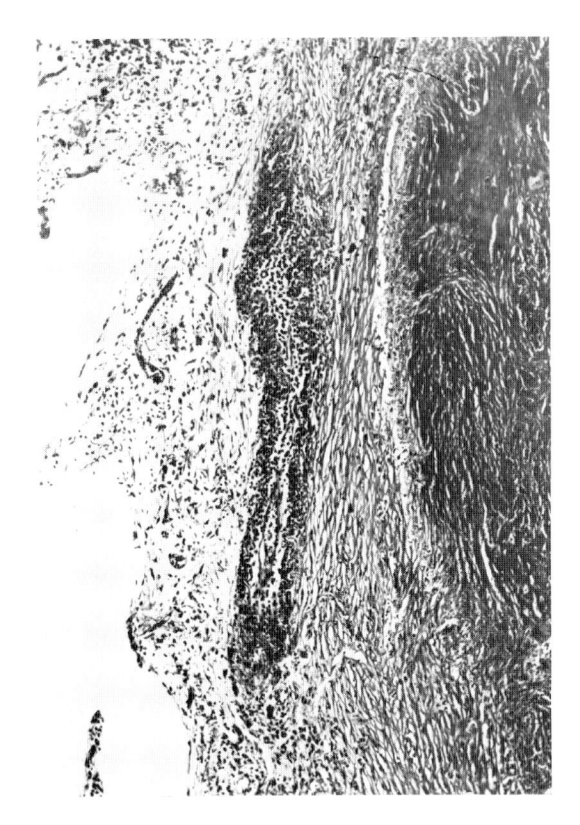

Figure 23–23. Arteriole at the edge of a rheumatoid nodule in a coal worker. The vessel is infiltrated by inflammatory cells, mainly lymphocytes (H&E, ×75).

tuberculosis due to pneumoconiosis, but two succumbed to severe amyloid disease. Nodules are rarely found in the lungs of nonminers with rheumatoid arthritis.

One characteristic of rheumatoid disease is an inflammatory reaction to necrotic collagen, which may be normal to the body part or may be pathologically produced. In pneumoconiosis the collagen may be derived from coexistent simple dust lesions or from foci of complicated disease. In the latter case tuberculosis could well play a part in initiating the lesion but later the rheumatoid reaction may occur in the absence of organisms.

Immunologic Features

The syndrome of rheumatoid pneumoconiosis was expanded by including the radiologic features of small nodules and irregular opacities not previously regarded as rheumatoid in nature.[213] Coal miners without clinical rheumatoid arthritis but possessing typically rheumatoid radiographs were much more likely to exhibit serologic evidence of the rheumatoid factor than nonarthritic miners who had simple or complicated pneumoconiosis. In the presence of arthritis this serologic distinction was not apparent, but some nonarthritic miners with orthodox pneumoconiosis (simple or complicated) did possess the rheumatoid factor.

Titrating sera against heat-aggregated human and rabbit gamma globulins disclosed that rheumatoid factor occurred most frequently and to highest titer in Caplan's syndrome and diminished on both counts as the severity of pneumoconiosis decreased through the complicated and simple grades to the lowest levels in nonminers.[73] Of Caplan's syndrome cases, however, 26 percent failed to show evidence of rheumatoid factor. Histologic localization of the factor and of immunoglobulin was achieved by fluorescence, using labeled aggregated human globulin to detect rheumatoid factor and labelled anti-IgM serum to confirm the specificity of the reaction.[73,214] Rheumatoid factor was identified in 80 percent of characteristic lesions and in 66 percent of cases of progressive massive fibrosis that exhibited prominent peripheral foci of lymphocytes and plasma cells together with obliterative vasculitis, in which plasma cell infiltration was a feature, but in only 18 percent of cases of massive fibrosis without vasculitis. The factor was distributed in plasma cells and the peripheral connective tissue of nodules, while IgM was identified extracellularly in necrotic peripheral areas and in endarteritic vessels.

Rheumatoid factor was stated to occur in a minority of simple dust lesions, but their pathologic nature must be questioned. Silicotic nodules showed no evidence of a reaction. An immunologic overlap might thus exist between massive fibrosis with vasculitis and Caplan's syndrome and it is conceivable that in the former condition the rheumatoid reaction was localized on the collagenous component, possibly under the influence of coal dust, at a later stage than in the established rheumatoid nodule.

Diffuse interstitial fibrosis of the lungs occasionally forms a component of connective tissue disorders, especially rheumatoid disease, which may occur in about 20 percent of cases of diffuse fibrosis,[215,216] and pulmonary involvement is a feature of some cases of systemic sclerosis. Recently it has become apparent that in coal worker's pneumoconiosis and silicosis there is a predisposition to progressive systematic sclerosis and possibly to systematic lupus erythematosus.[96,217-219] How dust disease influences connective tissue disorders is not known though familial or genetic factors may be concerned. In none of the systemic conditions so far reported have rheumatoid nodules been described in the lungs, but interstitial fibrosis may affect miners with rheumatoid arthritis.

Differentiation of Emphysematous and Fibrocystic States in Coal Workers

Emphysema is a generic term embracing more than one species, so that not only may coal workers be afflicted with types that occur in the nonmining population but urban dwellers may develop pigmentation in relation to emphysematous lesions that are not primarily the consequence of an occupational dust hazard. Moreover, miners as well as the population at large are liable to pulmonary fibrosis of multiple etiology; for instance, honeycomb lung developing concurrently with dust exposure becomes heavily pigmented but does not constitute pneumoconiosis. The distinction between occupational and ordinary environmental causation for pigmentation in relation to fibrosis and emphysema depends on the three-dimensional approach.[125]

The Distinction Between Proximal Acinar Emphysema Attributable to Dust and Proximal Acinar Emphysema Due to Inflammation (So-Called Centrilobular Emphysema)

Proximal acinar emphysema attributable to dust is discussed in relation to simple pneumoconiosis of coal and other workers, while emphysema especially the inflammatory type is covered in Chapter 21. In proximal acinar emphysema attributable to dust, disruption of alveolar or bronchiolar walls is not a primary feature, and respiratory bronchioles are not stenosed and are often dilated. By contrast, inflammatory emphysema, although affecting circumscribed areas within the lobule, is characterized by fibrosis and the occurrence of disruption at an early stage. Studied in depth, the inflammatory fibrosis involves terminal and proximal respiratory bronchioles whereas disruption affects mainly respiratory bronchioles of the second and third orders. Severe inflammatory (that is, irregular) emphysema overruns adjacent acini which fuse to form larger spaces, although respiratory bronchioles may be unequally affected by disruption. Fibrosis commonly obscures the identity of first-order respiratory bronchioles, so that the air passage leading to the emphysematous lesions is best described as the parent bronchiole, whose diameter may be normal, reduced, or even enlarged. No parallel exists between the severity of the emphysema and the degree of patency of the parent airway.

In the presence of coal macules the respiratory bronchioles are supported by sleeves of dust-consolidated alveolar tissue and are evidently able to resist the destructive effects of a subsequent bronchiolitis, whose presence may be attested by lymphocytic infiltration. When inflammatory emphysema exists first, collection of particles cannot occur in the characteristic anatomic site because the acinar morphology is grossly deformed and simultaneous operation of bronchiolitis and dust accumulation would achieve the same result. Accordingly coal particles, often borne by phagocytes, come to lie within and around the fibrosed sections of the airway and accumulate in alveoli outside the emphysematous spaces (Fig. 23-24). Naked eye or random histologic preparations may convey a resemblance to simple pneumoconiosis with dust-related emphysema but in-depth examination demonstrates the fundamental differences in architecture. Once the distinction is appreciated a shrewd idea of the diagnosis may be derived from the disposition of dust in relation to spaces; inflammatory proximal acinar emphysema appears as one or two relatively large spaces with a band, often interrupted, of peripheral pigment, whereas the dust-related form occurs as a collection of spaces invested wholly or partially by a greater quantity of dust.

Panacinar Emphysema in Coal Workers

If panacinar emphysema develops in a coal worker whose lungs contain small macules, the only difference from an emphysematous nonminer will be the presence of dust outlining proximal respiratory bronchioles (Fig. 23-25). When macules are larger and dust emphysema is added, dilation of proximal respiratory bronchioles may be exaggerated so that the whole acinus shows a fairly even degree of enlargement. Dust particles are able to aggregate as usual since the pulmonary architecture is preserved at least initially. To distinguish the respective contributions of each process to the total emphysema may be difficult, but the quantity of coal and the degree of distal enlargement may be helpful. When proximal acinar emphysema occurs with a comparatively minor accumulation of coal dust, the initial impression may suggest panacinar emphysema but closer examination reveals the emphasis on respiratory bronchioles with escape of alveolar ducts and sacs.

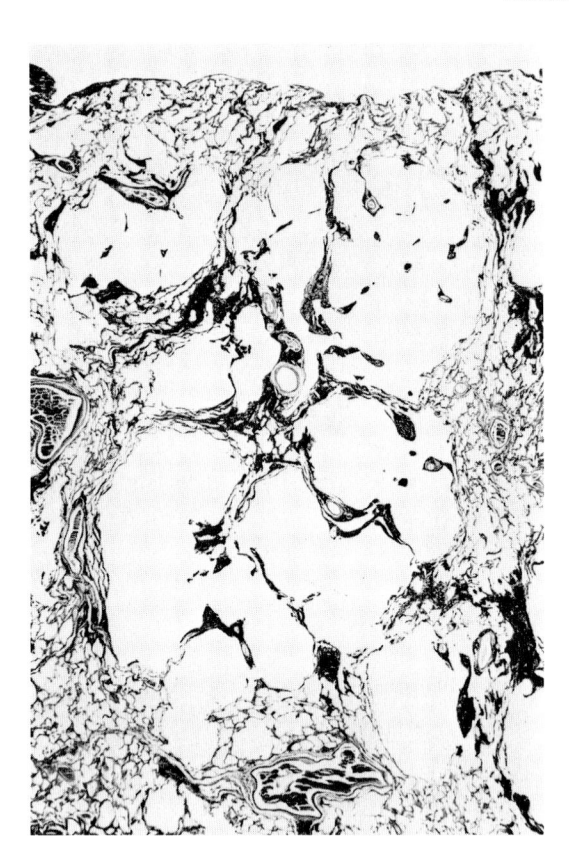

Figure 23–24. Pigmented irregular emphysema in a coal worker. Large intercommunicating spaces, set in normal parenchyma, are bounded in part by coal dust accumulation. All acini of the lobule are affected but parent bronchioles are not obstructed (H&E, ×5). From Heppleston.[125]

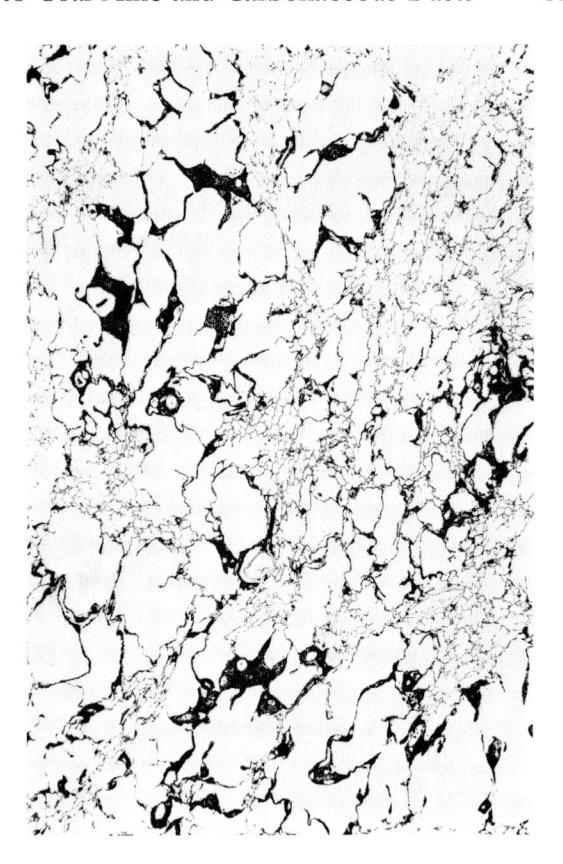

Figure 23–25. Coal worker with panacinar emphysema, the path of an airway being seen in the left upper area (H&E, ×5). From Heppleston.[125]

Fibrocystic Disease of the Lung (Honeycomb Lung)

Honeycombing[220] is not uncommon in coal workers, whose occupation may render them more than usually liable to pulmonary infections (see Coal Worker's Pneumoconiosis, Sequelae, Tuberculosis and Other Infections, above). The features are usually nonspecific but granulomatous states such as the eosinophilic form may rarely be identified. Since fairly extensive tracts of lung are affected, preexisting coal macules will be incorporated and their structure destroyed by a bronchopneumonic exudate, collapse, or interstitial pneumonia as fibrosis supervenes. The interstitial component consequently becomes heavily pigmented and the particles lie either within macrophages or extracellularly. Similar appearances arise if coal dust accumulates during the evolution of interstitial fibrosis into fibrocystic disease when aggregation of dust in the customary manner is prevented. However, in lung parenchyma spared fibrosis, coal macules are able to form so that the two disorders may coexist (Fig. 23–26). Inflammatory emphysema may become so severe in places as to merge into fibrocystic disease and in coal workers both will be pigmented.

Clinical Connotations

The interpretation of certain radiologic appearances in simple pneumoconiosis of coal workers poses a problem. The shadows are classified by size and profusion into three main categories, though recently these have been subdivided into a 12-point scale. Opacities are further separated according to whether they possess a rounded or an irregular outline, the whole being based on the *International Labour Office Classification of Radiographs of Pneumoconiosis* (revised 1980). Attention focused on the irregular shadows that often develop later in the evolution of the disease, though rounded opacities may coexist. Irregular opacities are well recognized in asbestosis and the suspicion arose that coal workers might also be affected by interstitial changes, though the characteristic macules gave rise to the rounded shadows.

Coal workers from South Wales, diagnosed as having simple pneumoconiosis, showed that with the passage of time irregular opacities increased in number while rounded ones apparently regressed.[221] A strong association emerged between the profusion of irregular opacities, the deficit in forced expiratory volume in 1 second (FEV_1), and the increase of emphysema score as gauged from whole lung sections, but cases with rounded opacities did not show the same regularity of progression in FEV_1 deficit. Since rounded opacities depend on dust

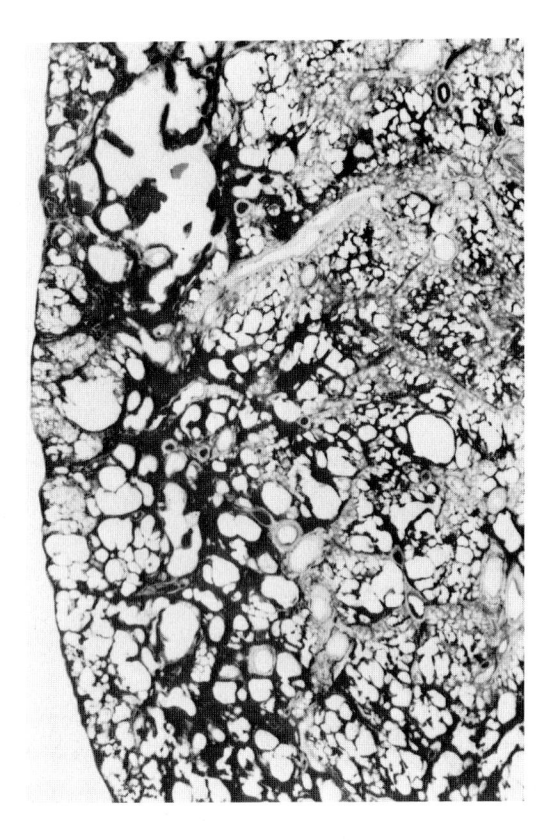

Figure 23–26. Subpleural fibrocystic change in a coal worker, the interstitium being heavily pigmented. Simple dust lesions occur elsewhere. From a whole lung section (×1).

content, their progression would not be expected after dust exposure diminished or ceased, but, if irregular and linear opacities are related to emphysema and parenchymal change, progression might well occur irrespective of dust exposure. Accordingly irregular opacities appear to be a better guide to disablement than rounded ones, dust-impregnated interstitial fibrosis in conjunction with emphysema being the likely basis for the irregular x-ray appearances. Although a gas transfer defect occurred with rounded opacities,[184] irregular ones correlated with lower values for gas transfer and for total lung capacity as well as with the emphysema seen in whole lung sections.[222] Where interstitial disease was identified histologically, the higher scores showed lower gas transfer values. Smoking could not, however, be blamed for the functional or morphologic changes.

The occurrence of interstitial fibrosis in miners with simple pneumoconiosis is not surprising since they are at least as liable as the general population to develop nonindustrial forms of pulmonary fibrosis, which become pigmented secondarily to occupational dust exposure and may progress to honeycombing. The prevalence of different varieties of emphysema or forms of fibrosis in coal workers may alter and it now seems that nonspecific reactions are making interpretation more difficult from both clinical and pathologic standpoints.

Disorders Due to Asbestos

Pliny in the first century A.D. was aware of the properties of "amiantus" (which may now be identified as chrysotile), a mineral mined in Cyprus and described as "the only kind of flax which is not consumed by fire." The term asbestos is derived from the Greek word meaning unquenchable. The material could be woven into garments and it was also used for lamp wicks. However, according to Agricola, amiantus was known to the ancients and Theophrastus probably made the earliest reference to it in the third century B.C., while anthophyllite was used to strengthen earthenware in Finland about 2500 B.C. The fire-resisting and fibrous properties of the mineral were thus apparent from the beginning and they have found increasing application especially over the past one hundred years, starting as an insulator for steam engines.

Mineralogy

Basic Considerations

The substances concerned are fibrous silicates, some naturally occurring inorganic fibers with a crystalline structure and others artificially produced fibers of glass, aluminosilicate, rock or slag wool in which the structure is usually noncrystalline. Other synthetic materials are known as "whiskers," that is, metallic or ceramic filamentary single crystals possessing micron widths and very high tensile strength. The minerals are grouped according to their crystalline structure, in which the cation content varies, and they may crystallize into different *habits* as determined by the shapes of the crystals, the presence of impurities or trace elements, or by other factors. Crystals, single or multiple, may be elongated to form a *fiber* and fibrous minerals are made up of parallel or interlacing aggregates of fibers which are usually separable. The habit concerned here is known as *asbestiform*, in which the fibers have high aspect (length/diameter) ratios, are separable, flexible, and possess high tensile strength. The term asbestos thus includes the asbestiform types of certain hydrated silicate minerals which occur in sufficient quantity to be of commercial value and which fall into two groups, the serpentines and the amphiboles. Serpentines were so named because of markings resembling a serpent's skin in a dull green mineral, while the term amphibole was applied by Haüy in 1801 in allusion to the protean composition. Though generally short, fibers may be 1 to 2 dm long.

Composition and Structure

The chemical composition of the asbestiform minerals is generally given in simplified and approximate form (Table 23–1). Chrysotile, crocidolite, and amosite are the fibrous forms of antigorite, riebeckite, and grünerite, respectively.

The chemical formulae, however, conceal certain physical characteristics. Chrysotile is a layered or sheet silicate, the layers being not flat but repeatedly rolled so as to form a fine tube whose lumen and the spaces between neighboring fibers may contain amorphous material presumed to be a magnesium silicate gel. Chrysotile fibers are accordingly best described as spirals or scrolls, whose ultrastructure (Fig. 23–27) was demonstrated by Yada.[223] A tetrahedrally coordinated silica layer is connected by shared oxygen atoms to an octahedrally coordinated magnesium layer lying externally. The surface of chrysotile fibers is thus formed by brucite [$Mg(OH)_2$] which is acid soluble and has a positive charge from adsorption of hydrogen ions in aqueous media. Because of their peculiar structure chrysotile fibers readily split lengthwise and exhibit longitudinal curvatures (Fig. 23–28). The amphiboles differ in being chain silicates, strong silica chains being bound usually by octahedrally coordinated cations, so that the outer surface is formed by a silica ribbon which is acid resistant and carries a negative charge in aqueous media. The structure of amphiboles is such that cleavages occur at different angles along the length and characteristically straight fibers are produced in a fairly wide range of diameters (see Fig. 23–28). The contrasting molecular orientations may be represented diagrammatically (Fig. 23–29) and the crystallographic arrangements may be portrayed as tetrahedra and octahedra (Fig. 23–30). Although asbestiform minerals are in general resistant to weathering or heat, they do decompose if subjected to high temperatures (varying for the different minerals) as may occur in certain industrial conditions. Whiskers are regarded as the synthetic analogues of asbestos fibers and the graphite whisker may show a scroll structure resembling that of chrysotile.

Sources and Uses of Asbestos

Major chrysotile deposits were discovered in Quebec and in the Urals near Sverdlovsk and have been worked continuously for about one hundred years. Chrysotile also comes from Zimbabwe and China, and in smaller amounts from other countries. Despite the ubiquity and apparent abundance of chrysotile, the amphibole content of the earth's crust is considered to be greater. Crocidolite is found mainly in South Africa (Transvaal and Cape Province) and Australia, amosite being largely confined to South Africa and India. Anthophyllite occurs mostly in Finland but is no longer mined in quantity, while Italy and Korea are sources of tremolite. World production of asbestos has increased enormously during the past 40 years and by 1982 exceeded 4 million tonnes per year, the vast majority being chrysotile.

Asbestos minerals are metamorphic in origin, occurring both superficially and beneath the earth's crust. Chrysotile deposits in Quebec employ open-cast working, while the deeply-located deposits in Zimbabwe and South Africa are exploited mostly by mining along the stratified rocks in which asbestos reefs may be up to 10 feet in depth.

The applications of asbestos minerals are diverse. The largest quantity, mainly in the form of chrysotile but

Table 23–1. The Main Varieties of Asbestos

Group	Type	Empirical Formula
Serpentine	Chrysotile (Greek for "golden")—white asbestos	$Mg_6Si_4O_{10}(OH)_8$
Amphibole	Crocidolite (Greek for "flaky or like the nap of woollen cloth")—blue asbestos	$Na_2Fe'''_3Fe''_2Si_8O_{22}(OH,F)_2$
	Amosite (acronym from Asbestos Mining Organization of South Africa)—brown asbestos	$(MgFe'')_7Si_8O_{22}(OH)_2$
	Anthophyllite (Latin for "clove" in reference to color)	$(MgFe'')_7Si_8O_{22}(OH,F)_2$
	Tremolite (from Tremola in Switzerland)	$Ca_2(MgFe'')_5Si_8O_{22}(OH,F)_2$

including some amphiboles, is consumed by the asbestos cement industry in which the fibers comprise 10 to 15 percent of finished products and act as a reinforcing agent. The products comprise sheets, corrugated roofing, gutters, tiles, drain pipes, and pressure piping, though plastics are emerging as a competitor. A slurry of cement, to which milled fibers of appropriate size have been added, is taken by conveyor to make sheets or to different moulds, the water either drains away or is extruded, and the product is cured slowly in air or quickly in an autoclave. The quartz content of the cement mix may not be negligible. Floor covering absorbs much chrysotile in concentrations of up to 45 percent, again as a reinforcing material and filler in vinyl tiles and cushion vinyls. Insulation and fire protection constitute major uses in various mixes (10 to 100 percent asbestos fibers), which were applied by hand or by spraying onto walls, ceilings, and girders in the construction industry. The larger fibers, especially of chrysotile, are much used in high concentrations for the manufacture of textiles, including conveyor belting and fireproof curtains and clothing, in which carding, mixing with cotton, spinning, and weaving take place. Because of their acid resistance, amphiboles find an application in filtration cloths. Wicks for oil heaters also incorporate asbestos. Asbestos paper is composed mainly of chrysotile and is adopted for insulation layers, engine gaskets, roofing felts, wall coverings and a variety of insulation pads or mats. Automotive products include brake linings and clutch facings along with other heavy duty friction components; up to 70 percent of chrysotile is combined with phenolic resins and even metals, the frictional properties being dependent on the physical and chemical characteristics of the fiber. Asbestos minerals have a role in reinforcing plastic materials and rubber seals (7 to 85 percent mineral) and as filters (30 to 100 percent asbestos) for fluids that include beers, wines, and drugs. Crocidolite was used for respirator masks in World War II. Anthophyllite was mostly exported and served as a filler in rubber and plastics. Tremolite is of little commercial importance but occurs as a contaminant of talc and chrysotile.

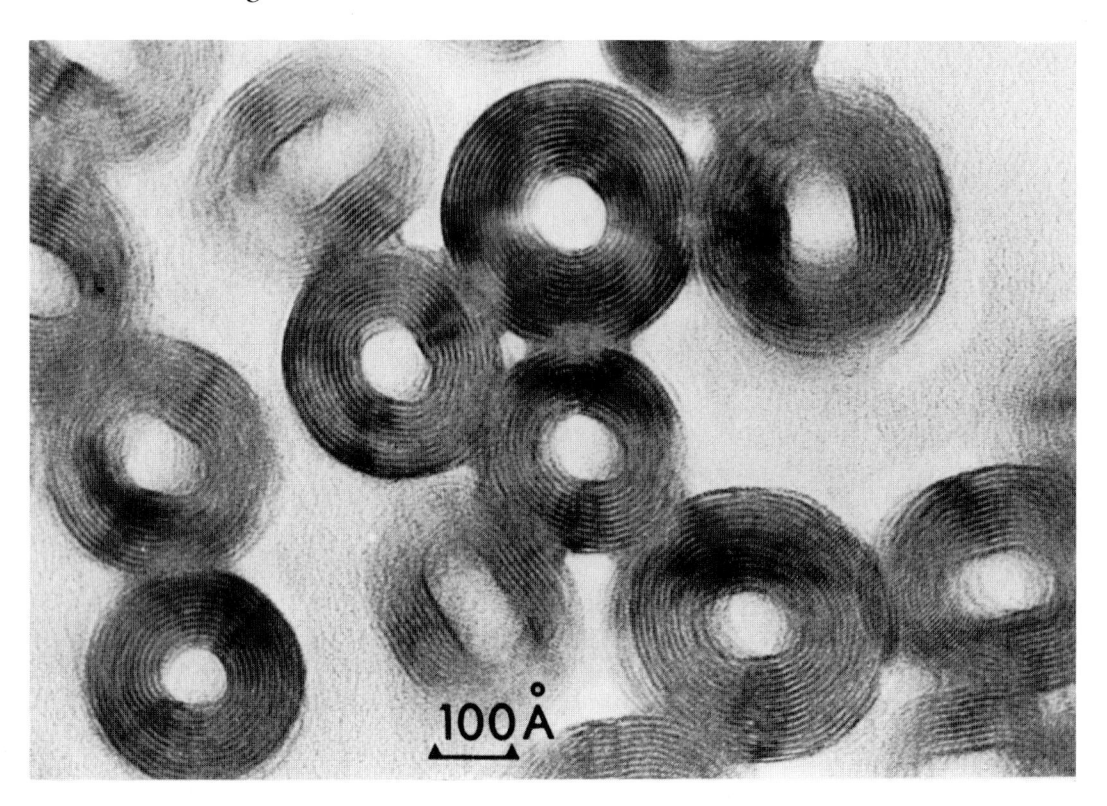

Figure 23–27. Chrysotile fibres in transverse section by transmission electron microscopy (TEM), demonstrating the characteristic scroll pattern. From Yada.[223]

Occupational and Other Sources of Exposure

The industrial applications of the asbestos minerals do not cover the whole field of potential exposures. The occupations at risk are so varied that without detailed enquiry the significance of respiratory disease may be overlooked. Inhalation exposure may be industrial or may come from residence in a specific neighborhood, and may be domestic or related to an urban environment, while ingestion cannot be ignored.

Mining of the ore is probably the least dangerous part of the extraction process, especially in the open-cast recovery of chrysotile where there is no silicosis risk since the serpentine rocks are free from quartz. Extraction of amphiboles involves drilling, blasting, and tunneling and, since it is carried out in relatively confined areas, carries a slight risk of asbestos-related disease. However, because the associated rocks contain quartz silicosis may occur. Ore from the mines occurs as lumps which have to be hand-sorted and then crushed and milled, prior to extraction of the fiber according to quality and size, and finally bagged for transport to the site of application. These latter stages formerly generated large amounts of airborne particles, but enclosure within factories and the use of leakproof polythene bags have virtually eliminated the risk of exposure at the final steps of processing.

An important and continuing source of exposure derives from shipyards. Many vessels were lagged with asbestos cement, the fibers of which gradually loosen and are liberated during repairs, refits, or by breaking down old vessels. The work takes place in a confined atmosphere, so that the potential risks are high and likely to remain so for many years as ships reach the end of their lives. Dismantling buildings insulated or fireproofed with asbestos products constitutes a similar risk and again is likely to continue until all constructions containing fibers have been demolished. In the days of steam locomotives, asbestos lagging was used and exposure occurred to some extent during dismantling. Workers only indirectly involved in these types of operation may also be exposed by virtue of proximity. Fitters, electricians, plumbers, welders, and carpenters (especially in ships), and workers in power stations and boiler houses where lagging and delagging occur, fall into this "neighborhood exposure" category. These descriptions of occupation may not arouse suspicion of industrial exposure unless pursued.

Dust exposure used to be high in the textile industry, largely as a consequence of carding the fibers into lengths and then spinning and weaving them. Enclosure of these processes has greatly reduced the risk but the consequences of dusty conditions may still not be fully revealed. Unusual sources of exposure formerly occurred and may yet produce delayed effects; among such may be mentioned the use of asbestos ropes for grouting and the cleaning of exhaust ventilation ducts and units. However, it appears that cutting asbestos cement products formed by extrusion is practically harmless as the fibers are securely embedded, while grinding brake linings or blowing out brake drums give only low atmospheric contamination and fibers are decomposed by the heat of friction.

Asbestos-related disease has occurred from proximity to mines and dumps or to factories engaged in processing. Restrictions have largely abolished the indiscriminate release of effluent but the possibility of late effects remains. Atmospheric contamination by asbestos in the neighborhood of certain factories may reach 5000 ng/m^3. Domestic exposure formerly occurred as the housewife cleaned contaminated overalls or clothes. Despite some initially disturbing evidence (see Urban Exposure to Asbestos, below), general exposure to asbestos in the urban environment is not apparently of great moment, the concentration usually being less than 10 ng/m^3, and the use of asbestos products in the home carries an insignificant risk since the fibers are captive. However, sanding asbestos vinyl tiles and crumbling of sprayed asbestos insulation could be potential hazards.

Bearing in mind the increasing use of asbestos products and the long latent period between exposure and the development of disease, the problem is likely to persist for many years. The indestructibility of asbestos fibers has, in Thomson's[224] phrase, given them a half-life of infinity. Whether the difficulties will be solved by substituting artificial for natural fibers remains to be seen (see Malignant Mesothelioma, Pathogenesis, Man-made Mineral Fibers, below).

Ingestion constitutes another means of access. Fibers have been discovered in certain natural water supplies and became notorious in the Duluth case (see Malignant Mesothelioma, Pathogenesis, Miscellaneous Factors, Water-Borne Fibers, below). Natural sources, especially in mining regions, may be contaminated, as may beverages (from filters), food, and fluids used as vehicles for drugs.

Asbestosis

The term asbestosis embraces fibrosis of the lungs with or without pleural fibrosis induced by inhalation of minerals of the asbestos group. Plaques of the parietal pleura are considered separately.

Prevalence

The total number of individuals exposed to asbestos is not accurately known, since the usage of asbestos is diverse and employment often intermittent. Defined populations, however, afford a basis on which to gauge prevalence rates. In 1930, Merewether and Price[225] concluded that of 363 asbestos workers examined 26 percent had definite fibrosis attributable to the dust and that obliteration of the functional reserve accounted for the dyspnea. They appreciated the significance of atmospheric concentration of dust and length of exposure in the production of fibrosis, dust suppression measures having a prolongation effect. Some 30 years later the magnitude of the problem was exposed by surveys of exposed populations and the main conclusions have been collated in conference proceedings.[226–229]

Among 17,800 insulation workers from the United States and Canada, a 7 percent prevalence of deaths from asbestosis was found,[230] indicating an extraordinary risk. Workers in an asbestos factory experienced a 12.7 percent death rate from asbestosis.[231] As usual a long interval occurred between first exposure and the development of asbestosis. Since they are mortality statistics these figures disguise the morbidity. Doll and co-workers[232–234] kept an English asbestos textile factory under surveillance for over 25 years, the exposure being mainly to chrysotile but with some crocidolite. Those employees who were exposed before the introduction of the 1931 U.K. Asbes-

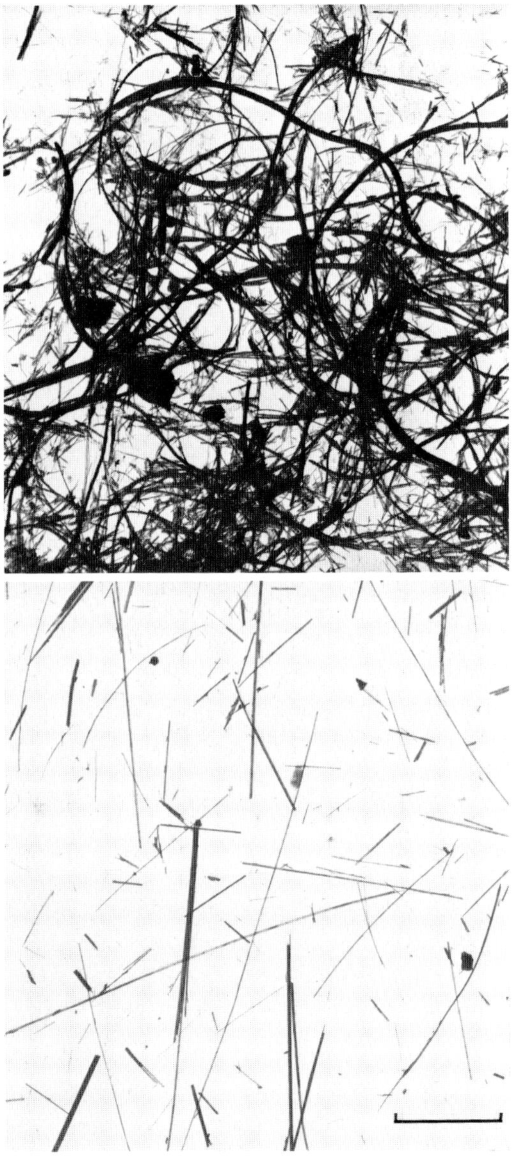

Figure 23–28. Fibres of chrysotile (above) and Cape crocidolite (below) seen longitudinally by TEM. Bar = 10 μm. Courtesy of Dr. Timbrell and Mr. Griffiths.

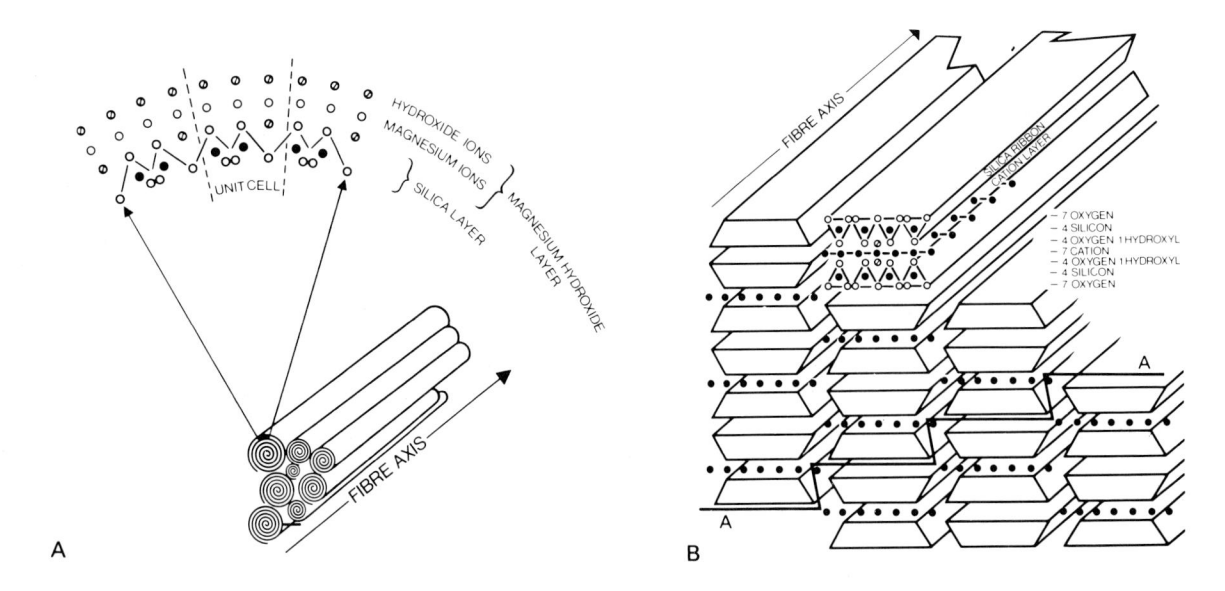

Figure 23–29. Molecular dispositions of (A) chrysolite and (B) amphibole asbestos. Courtesy of Dr. Hodgson.

tos Industry Regulations had a significant excess of deaths from respiratory and circulatory disease associated with asbestosis, but the mortality experience approached the national average in men and women exposed after implementation of the regulations. Mortality increased with age but diminished with reduction in the length of employment. Nonmalignant respiratory disease remained a higher than expected cause of death up to 1974 and cases of asbestosis were occurring up to the end of 1978. A 35-years survey of insulation workers (laggers) in Belfast disclosed that among the excess deaths asbestosis with or without tuberculosis was a contributor though not in the last 10 years of the study.[235] In a London asbestos factory the occurrence of complicating tuberculosis at death from asbestosis fell from 31.3 percent in 1931–1949 to 5.6 percent in 1957–1964.[236] Prospective environmental data, comparable to that obtained for coal workers, are not yet available in regard to asbestos exposures in humans and dose relationships are not therefore as precisely defined, though some would attach less importance to such information, preferring to eliminate asbestos products.

Pathologic Anatomy

The first account of the morphologic changes was given by Murray in 1907[237] though the features had been outlined 7 years earlier. His subject was a male cardroom worker (the sole survivor of ten such individuals) exposed for some 14 years and who at necropsy showed pulmonary fibrosis mainly affecting the lower parts along with pleural adhesions, asbestos spicules being identified histologically. Twenty years elapsed before the next account of a female factory worker whose lungs exhibited diffuse interstitial pneumonia, anthracosis, and tuberculosis.[238] Numerous asbestos bodies were recognized and they gave a positive Prussian blue reaction. For this condition the term asbestosis was introduced.

Gross Features

The appearances differ from those of silicosis and coal worker's pneumoconiosis in that the changes are unevenly distributed throughout the lungs and their outline is often irregular. The lower zones, especially posteriorly, tend to be mainly affected and, though the middle and upper zones may also be involved, some areas generally escape. Early lesions may be detected as small, grey areas of induration, while more extensive disease affects the parenchyma in a patchy manner. A fine, greyish fibrosis may be seen as a subpleural band, a few millimeters to a centimeter deep and of variable length, forming a lace-like network or being more compact. Fibrosis often extends further into the lungs and becomes denser, though linear and ill-defined nodular formations may be seen. A characteristic feature is cyst formation in parenchyma adjacent to but not overrun by fibrosis, giving a honeycomb structure in which the spaces are usually 1 to 3 mm in size but sometimes larger. Again it is customary to find the fibrocystic change in the posterior-basal parts of the lung (Fig. 23–31). A third type of fibrosis takes the form of massive lesions, conventionally considered on radiologic grounds to be 1 cm or more in diameter. The margin of massive fibrosis is usually ill-defined and irregular but may be fairly compact, the lesions measuring up to 10 cm across. A particular feature is their predilection for the lower zones of the lung peripherally or centrally and, though upper zones are not excluded, the distribution contrasts with that of massive fibrosis in coal worker's pneumoconiosis and silicosis. Basal massive fibrosis in gold miners is almost nonexistent. Active tuberculosis is not apparently recorded as occurring in asbestotic massive lesions but necrosis may be seen. Depending on the degree of fibrosis, the lung as a whole may be normal or reduced in size and affected areas are indurated. Rarely, Caplan's syndrome–type lesions of rheumatoid pneumoconiosis are found and partake of the same characteristics as those developing in coal workers. Silicotic nodules of the usual distribution and type may also occur in asbestos cement workers who are exposed to silica and asbestos dusts. Contrary to some assertions, emphysema is uncommon though any nondust type (*see* Differentiation of Emphysematous and Fibrocystic States in Coal Workers, above) may be found in association; the upper zones may appear overaerated in some sufferers. Bronchiectasis is not a notable feature of asbestosis.

The pleura is usually thickened by a chronic nonspecific fibrosis especially over affected lung and adhesion commonly occurs between the visceral and parietal layers, sometimes obliterating fissures. If the pleura overlying fibrocystic disease escapes fibrosis, the lung surface may exhibit a cobbled appearance. Pleural effusion is exceptional, but its formation in established asbestosis may indicate the development of carcinoma, while in workers with little or no clinical evidence of lung fibrosis an effusion may be the presenting feature of mesothelioma. However, benign effusion appears to be a consequence of asbestos exposure.[239,240] The hilar lymph nodes are little enlarged, but some fibrosis may be found as the disease advances and calcification may occur though not apparently in the "eggshell" pattern sometimes seen in silicosis.

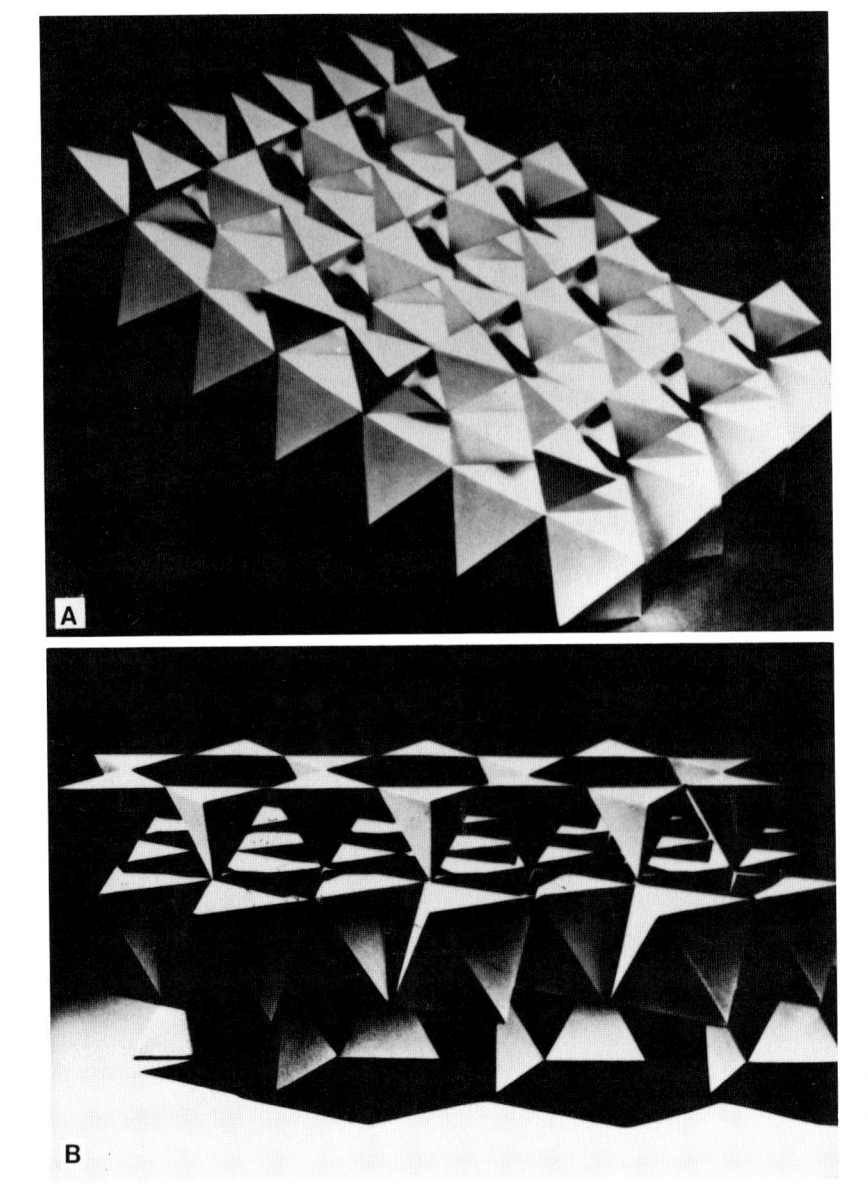

Figure 23–30. Crystallographic patterns of (A) chrysotile forming curved sheets and (B) amphibole asbestos forming straight chains. Courtesy of Dr. Hodgson.

Figure 23–31. Posterobasal portion of lung affected by fibrocystic asbestosis. The demarcation is abrupt. From a whole lung section (×1.2).

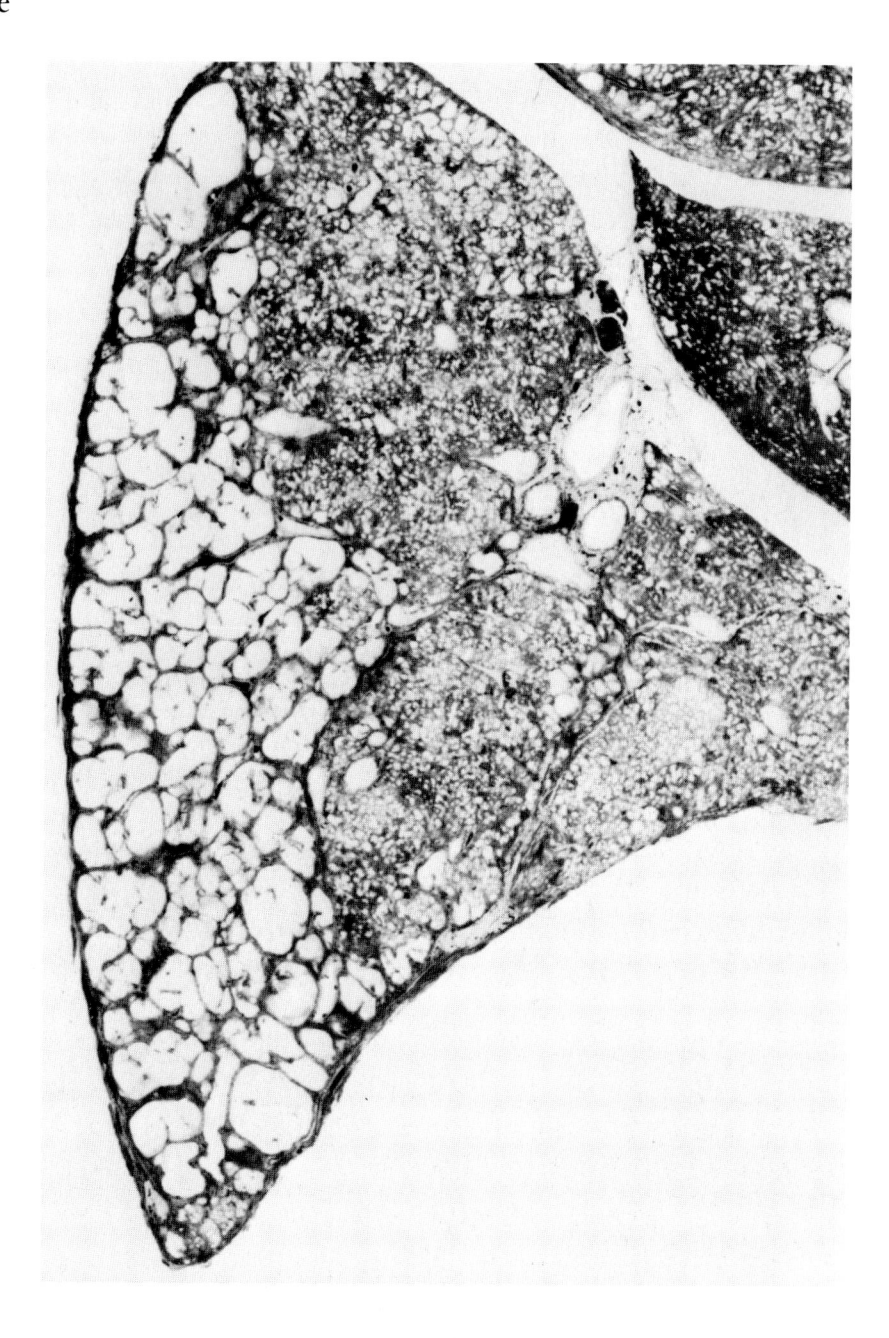

Microscopic Features

As with other forms of pneumoconiosis human evidence on the initial changes is scanty, though small and presumably early lesions occur in lungs with advanced fibrosis elsewhere.

Compared with the lesions induced by silica and coal mine dusts, the initial lesions of asbestosis are less well defined, but still develop in relation to respiratory bronchioles (Fig. 23–32). Asbestos fibers, coated (that is, bodies) and uncoated, collect along with macrophages and a few erythrocytes in alveoli belonging to or abutting on these bronchioles. Many fibers are engulfed by the cells though longer ones, sometimes up to 100 μm long, are often only partially ingested and some fibers and bodies remain extracellularly in the alveoli. Initially these aggregates and the reaction to them do not extend far into the parenchyma, but with increasing exposure further alveoli are occupied and the pattern becomes more diffuse. As alveoli become packed with macrophages, some multinucleated, and fibers, a few fibroblasts and reticulin deposition may be detected. At first the fibrosis appears to line and thicken the alveolar walls but later alveoli are overtaken by organization which becomes collagenous and relatively acellular but which leaves the elastin network relatively intact. A few lymphocytes may be present. These changes may be contrasted with the alveolar consolidation occurring in the discrete coal macule where fibrosis is less but dust more prominent. Peripheral parts of acini are at first spared but with advance of the fibrosis more parenchyma is affected in an irregular manner. Dense tracts of collagen are eventually laid down though fibroblasts are not prominent, macro-

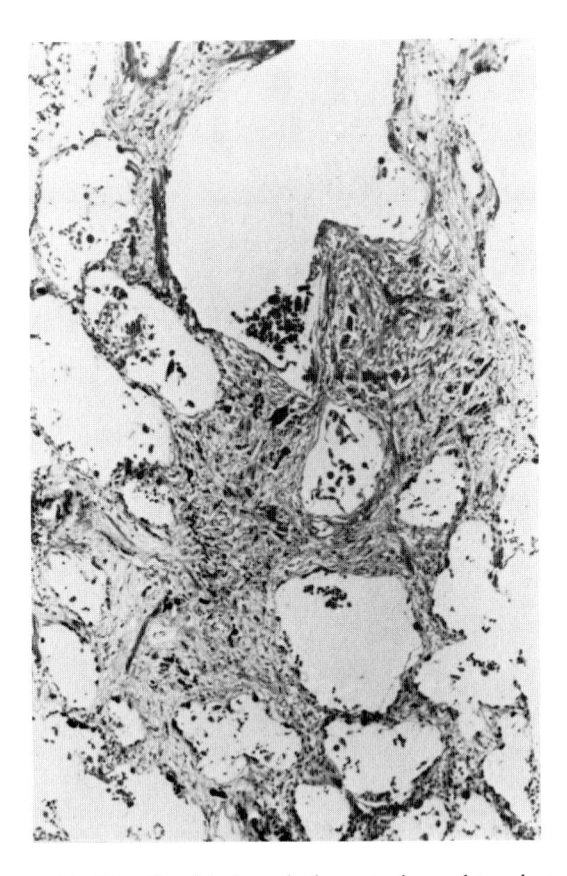

Figure 23-32. Focal lesion of asbestosis, located in relation to respiratory bronchioles and overrunning alveoli. Coated fibers occur in the fibrous tissue and the alveoli (H&E, ×35).

phages become comparatively sparse, and some lymphocytes accumulate. Parenchyma intervening between fibrous bands enlarges to produce the fibrocystic change (Fig. 23-33), the spaces acquiring an epithelial lining of various types, probably arising from type II cell hyperplasia and metaplasia. Some patent alveoli may still be occupied by macrophages containing short fibers or bodies, which may remain outside cells. Such alveoli sometimes possess a prominent epithelial lining, occasionally appearing dysplastic, which gives the appearance of adenomatosis, and the cells may exhibit eosinophilic hyaline bodies similar to those found in the hepatocytes of alcoholics.[241] When the massive stage of asbestosis is reached whole areas of parenchyma are replaced by collagenous fibrosis which may become hyaline while the elastin tends to be fragmented. Fibroblasts are few but lymphocytes are often rather prominent. A concentric arrangement of connective tissue fibers is sometimes seen as are necrosis and calcification though without cellular reaction or histologic evidence of acid-fast bacilli. Endarteritis constitutes a further feature of massive lesions. Asbestos bodies and fragments occur among the connective tissue fibers of diffuse or massive lesions and detection of naked fibers is not difficult. Air spaces packed with asbestos bodies and cells may be enclosed in the fibrosis. Carbonaceous pigmentation also constitutes

a common feature of the fibrotic reaction, the result of incidental exposure, and macules may form in nonfibrosed acini. A terminal pneumonia is sometimes evident.

The pleural fibrosis possesses no special features. Diffuse pleural thickening rarely shows calcification and it is apparently unrecorded in the visceral pleura. Contrary to certain assertions fibrosis does occur in some hilar nodes though it may not be pronounced and only parts may be affected. Asbestos fibers and bodies may be detected in this location and some are long.

Diagnosis of Asbestosis

Compensation for industrial disease requires a firm diagnosis and an assessment of the degree of fibrosis. Apart from the gross changes of asbestosis, evidence should be sought of tuberculosis or neoplasia in lung, mediastinum, pleura, and peritoneum, and of fibrosis or plaques in the pleura. For histologic purposes the International Union Against Cancer (UICC)[242] recommended that blocks of tissue be taken from at least six specific sites: (1) apex of right upper lobe, pleural surface; (2) right middle lobe, lateral pleural surface; (3) right lower lobe, middle of basal surface; (4) left upper lobe, central section; (5) lingula, central section; (6) left lower lobe,

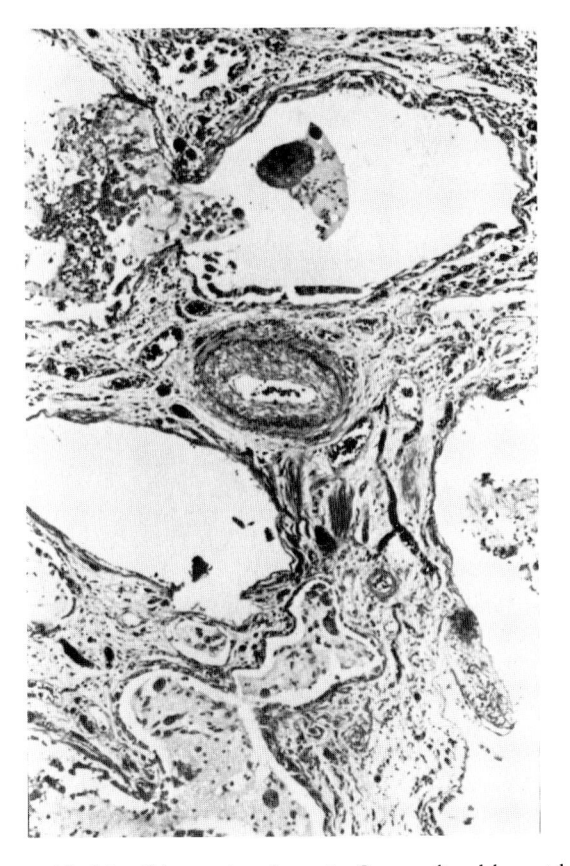

Figure 23-33. Fibrocystic asbestosis. Spaces, lined by epithelium and occupied by mucus (in which macrophages and a giant cell occur), are separated by fibrous tracts which include smooth muscle and an arteriole with intimal thickening (H&E, ×35).

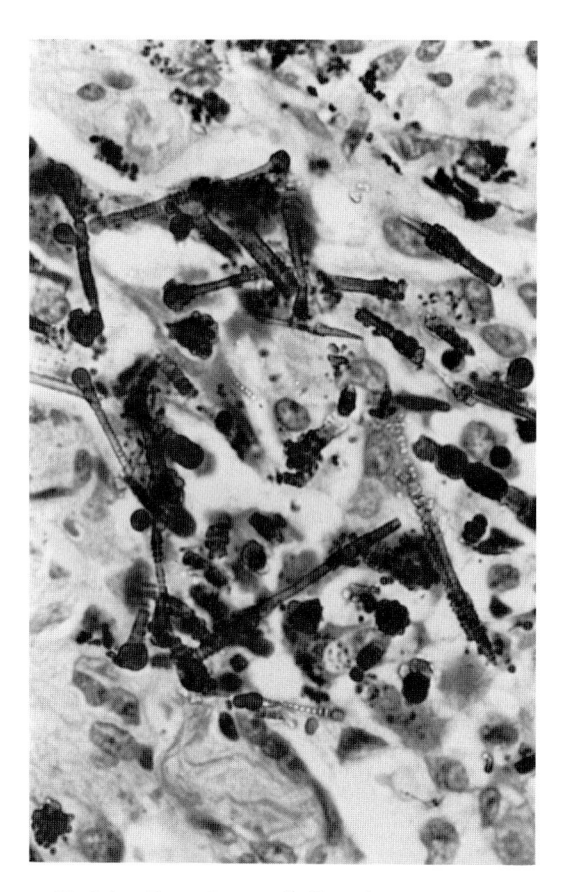

Figure 23–34. Typical coated fibers located in an alveolus along with macrophages (H&E, ×800).

central basal section. In addition sections should be prepared from the hilar lymph nodes and from any other area of abnormal appearance. This latter provision is of particular importance in view of the irregular distribution of the changes which may well affect areas other than those indicated, some of which may escape; moreover, histologic evidence may be found in the absence of obvious gross changes. To grade the extent of fibrosis, both lungs must be considered and the average placed in four categories: nil, less than 25 percent, 25 to 50 percent, and greater than 50 percent. The severity of the fibrosis may be classified similarly: (1) nil; (2) minimal, slight focal reticulin fibrosis around respiratory bronchioles and in related alveoli usually limited to the lower lobes; (3) moderate, greater amount of fibrosis, reticulin and collagenous, with alveolar obliteration and epithelial metaplasia over wider areas; (4) severe, collagenous fibrosis much more extensive, overrunning parenchyma and leading to fibrocystic change or massive lesions. Asbestos bodies on their own indicate only exposure and not necessarily asbestosis. Asbestos workers may also have been exposed to other dusts, so that asbestosis may coexist with evidence of silicosis, siderosis, or coal worker's pneumoconiosis.

Lung biopsy (whether open, by needle, or transbronchial) is rarely justifiable, diagnosis during life being achieved by other means, quite apart from the potential sampling error.

Asbestos Fibers, Uncoated and Coated (Asbestos Bodies).
Marchand[243] first recognized structures that came to be known as asbestos bodies. They are best described as coated fibers to distinguish them from fibers without such an accretion. By light microscoy (Fig. 23–34) coated fibers may be as long as 70 μm or more though the smallest may be less than 1 μm and only be detected electron-optically. They are generally straight but curved or angular forms occur, and the coating assumes a wide variety of shapes (well depicted in older acounts) though commonly appearing as a beaded formation along the fiber with bulbous expansion at one or both ends. The reaction is positive. Bodies are particularly obvious in unstained sections or Van Gieson's preparations.

The structure (Fig. 23–35) of the coating is now well established. Electron microscopical observations on guinea pigs and humans indicated that dense granules, probably of ferritin, accumulated around fibers, mostly ingested by macrophages, as a series of irregular layers. Guinea pigs exposed to different types of asbestos first showed red cell extravasation and lysis with formation of haemosiderin granules, followed by diffusion of an iron-containing product, possibly ferritin, into the cytoplasm of macrophages; if a fiber had also been ingested the ferritin was adsorbed on it.[244,245] Since bodies are formed on fibers containing much or little iron, asbestos itself is an improbable source. If a macrophage contains more than one fiber only the longest is coated.[244] Two or more macrophages may attempt to ingest the longer fiber. In humans the straight, rigid amphibole fibers acquire a coating much more frequently than chrysotile, which is suitable for the formation of bodies only when occurring as straight fiber bundles several microns in length. Presumably the curled shape of long chrysotile fibers is not conducive to phagocytosis so that coating is impaired. The development of the coating experimentally may be summarized as phagocytosis, cytoplasmic accumulation of haemosiderin, intracytoplasmic transport of iron micelles from hemosiderin to the phagosomes, and concentration of micelles around the fiber. The asbestos body thus consists of a central fiber, the hemosiderin-containing coat, and the phagosomal membrane. Uncoated fibers may have undergone phagocytosis but have been released before acquiring a coating, thus remaining available for interaction with cells. The corrugation and beading of the coating and the bulbous ends appear to represent either fracture or uneven deposition of cytoplasmic material onto the fiber, which eventually breaks up leaving coated fragments.

Histochemically, the coating contains not only ferric iron but proteins and acid mucopolysaccharides. Human fibers, studied before and after extraction of iron,[246] first showed deposition of trypsin-digestible proteins, hematoidin, and ferric iron, followed by a layer of hyaluronic acid over which further ferric iron precipitated, the fibers becoming coated only in areas of recent hemorrhage. Experimentally[247] asbestos fibers rapidly acquire a coating of hematoidin, ferric iron, and hyaluronic acid, the latter raising the possibility of an intercellular origin rather than one derived from macrophages. Since only a small proportion of fibers acquire a coating, the appropriate components may not be available in the local environment. A species variability exists in the capacity to produce asbestos bodies, which are most readily formed by guinea pigs and humans. Artificial fibers of glass or ceramic aluminium silicate, or silicon carbide whiskers excite in animals the formation of a coating possessing the same structure. Similar encrustation may also be seen around compact particles, such as coal, in areas where red cells have escaped.

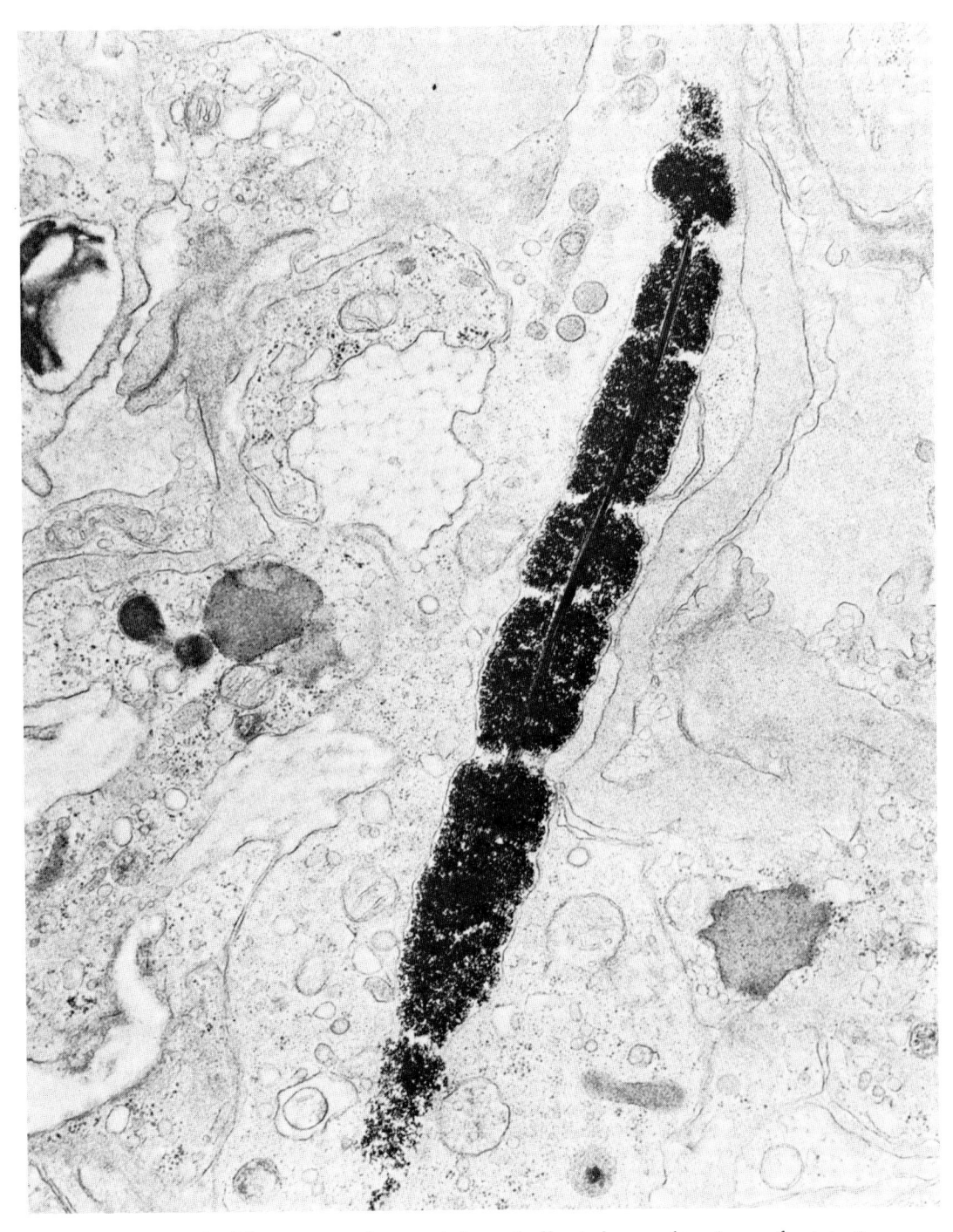

Figure 23–35. Ultrastructure of a coated chrysotile fibre in hamster lung 1 year after injection. The body lies in a septal macrophage and consists of the central fiber, surrounded by finely granular, iron-containing material (black) and enclosed by a phagosomal membrane (×31,300). Courtesy of Dr. Suzuki.

Since the basic component of the fiber coating consists of protein and mucopolysaccharide and the incorporation of inorganic iron is a dependent event, it is appropriate to refer to coated fibers and not to stress one component by describing them as ferruginous bodies, a term better discarded now that the nature of the enclosed fiber can be established precisely. It is apparently the acquisition of a coating that renders the fiber incapable of fibrosis; coated fibers proved much less toxic to human alveolar macrophages than uncoated amosite.[248] The occurrence of iron encrustation on elastin fibers in areas of red cell extravasation, as in pulmonary hypertension from chronic left ventricular failure or mitral stenosis, should not cause difficulty.

Pathogenesis

The physical characteristics of fibers introduce features not encountered in the case of compact particles.

Quantity of Dust

Epidemiology. Fiber concentration and duration of exposure evidently determined the radiologic prevalence of parenchymal abnormality.[249] In a British asbestos textile factory, mainly using chrysotile but with some crocidolite in the past, 6.6 percent of workers had possible asbestosis after an average of 16 years and an exposure to five fibers per cubic centimeter, with radiographic changes being more evident in heavier smokers.[250] In two of H.M. dockyards, the risk of developing nonmalignant asbestos-related lesions of the pleura and lung was related not only to duration, intensity, and time since first exposure but also to smoking habits.[251] Difficulties in relating occupation, exposure, and disease nevertheless remain, since for similar exposures the fibrotic response appears to vary among individuals.

Extraction Procedures. Fiber content may be estimated in lungs where the extent and severity of asbestosis can be graded pathologically. The first step is digestion of lung, ideally by procedures that do not split fiber longitudinally or break them transversely. Drying tissue before maceration fractures some fibers whether coated or not, and to express the number of fibers per gram of dried lung entails drying an adjacent portion of similarly affected tissue to gauge the change in weight.[252] The usual solvents are 40 percent KOH or 5 percent sodium hypochlorite, customarily as commercial bleach, though hydrogen peroxide and formamide are sometimes used. The appropriate technical precautions have been indicated.[252,253] Extracted fibers may be counted in a Fuchs-Rosenthal chamber by phase contrast microscopy, or filtered onto a membrane of known pore size before counting optically on a slide or electron microscopically on a grid. Another procedure involves low-temperature (150°C) ashing of lung tissue in an atmosphere of oxygen. Under these circumstances chrysotile shows no morphologic or crystallographic changes and solution of other minerals in 1N HCl leaves chrysotile unaffected, but higher temperatures may modify chrysotile.[254] Fibers whether coated or not may be examined by transmission electron microscopy (TEM) or scanning electron microscopy (SEM) and characterized by energy dispersive x-ray analysis (EDAX) for elemental structure (Fig. 23–36) and by selected area electron diffraction (SAED) for crystallographic pattern, thereby enabling individual fibers to be identified. X-ray diffractometry (Fig. 23–37) and infrared spectrometry may also be used for crystal recognition. Leaching of magnesium from chrysotile in vivo may vitiate the results of EDAX. Wet digestion and ashing each have their advocates, but dispersion of ashed residues with ultrasonics at high energy is liable to split amphibole and chrysotile fibers longitudinally. Low ultrasonic energy, however, does not affect the crystal structure of asbestos fibers.[255] No one method provides all the information and a combination is desirable.

Pathological Reaction. The fibrotic response is generally assumed to increase in proportion to the quantity of asbestos retained, but not all studies have included uncoated fibers which are the ones retaining biologic activity. For instance, no correlation was found between lung fibrosis and the numbers of asbestos bodies seen histologically.[256] Using the digestive technique in combination with light and electron microscopic counts of uncoated and coated fibers in occupationally exposed individuals, the degree of fibrosis (extent and severity) was graded on the four-point scale.[252] Although considerable variations in fiber content occurred, a general correlation was detected between rising particle counts as the fibrosis progressed from nil to mild and from mild to moderate degrees. By light microscopy the proportion of uncoated fibers was about 70 percent and optically visible fibers comprised 12 to 30 percent of the total count as determined by electron microscopy, which detects fibers with diameters below the limit of optical resolution. A different situation obtained in regard to the most severe degree of fibrosis in which no relationshp was evident between either the total concentration of asbestos particles or the proportion of uncoated fibers and the form the lesion took. Counts were made not only from tissue showing solid fibrosis but also from areas of fibrocystic change, focal lesions, and normally aerated lung, the latter sometimes revealing a surprisingly high concentration of fibers in a range similar to that for advanced fibrosis. Moreover, as far as could be judged from occupational histories, the duration of residence of mineral in the lung was unrelated to the degree of asbestosis, despite epidemiologic suggestions to the contrary. Although exposures were most likely mixed, there was a striking paucity of chrysotile in lung tissue. Being less resistant to attack, some chrysotile might have dissolved or been eliminated during life, thus complicating all postmortem assessments. The different relationship between fiber content and severe asbetosis, including the presence of numerous fibers in nonfibrosed lung, raises the question of complicating factors such as mixed exposures to asbestos and silica or the supervention of a chronic inflammatory state as a consequence of the presence of particles or the fibrosis they induce. Tuberculosis, though formerly common at necropsy, became rare in Britain[236] but in South Africa a 24 percent prevalence of tuberculosis occurred in cases of asbestosis, rising to 40 percent in moderately severe

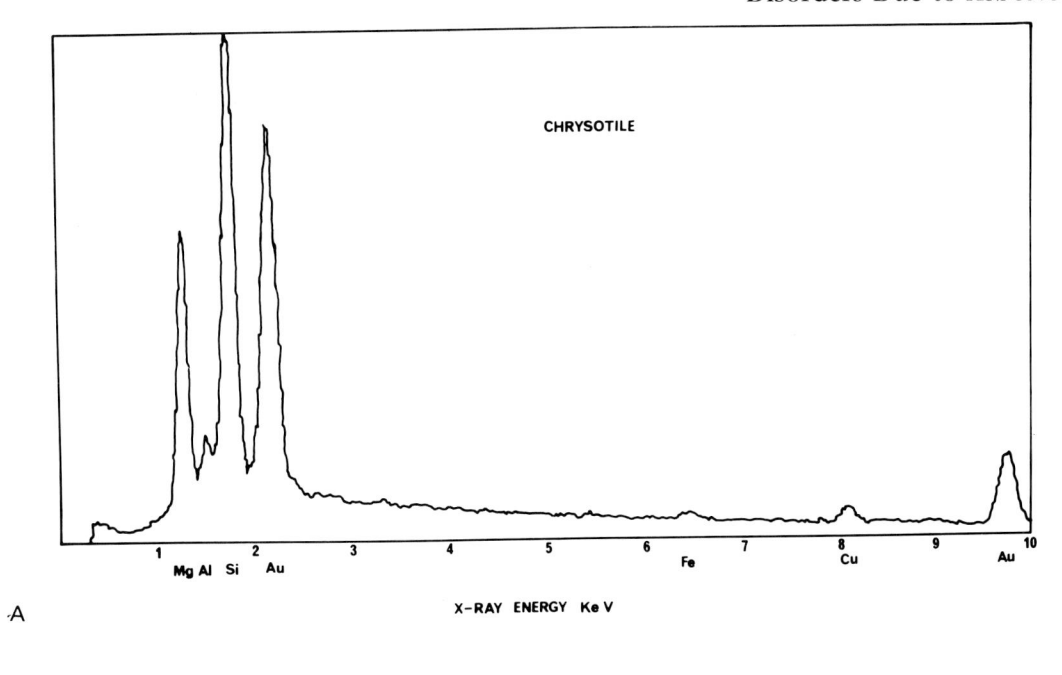

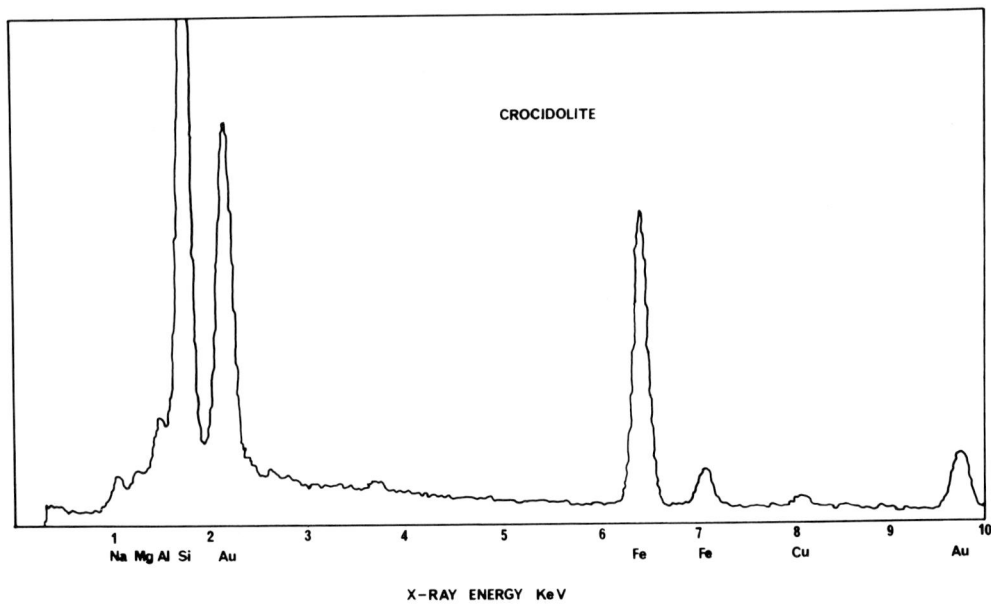

Figure 23–36. Energy-dispersive x-ray spectra of (A) chrysotile and (B) crocidolite by scanning electron microscopy. Peaks (ordinates) indicate individual elements. X-ray emissions are stimulated by the impact of the electron beam on a single small part of the fiber. Gold (Au) and copper (Cu) are derived from the coating and grid, not the mineral.

cases.[257] However, solid and fibrocytic lesions themselves rarely show evidence of specific infection, though nonspecific pulmonary infection accelerates the progression of asbestosis[258] and respiratory infection is common in employees.[257] Bacteriologic examination of massive lesions has not, however, been pursued and, although some may have a raised quartz content, the development of asbestosis under conditions where quartz contamination may be discounted stresses the independent role of fibrous minerals.

Type of Fiber
Sufficient reports are now available for investigators to be confident that all varieties of asbestos possess fibrogenic capacity for humans, whether subjects were engaged in mining and milling or in industrial applications. Related accounts have frequently appeared in the successive conference reports on asbestos-related disease. In the case of chrysotile, progression of asbestosis was sometimes observed after cessation of exposure and disease occasionally appeared first many years after subjects left

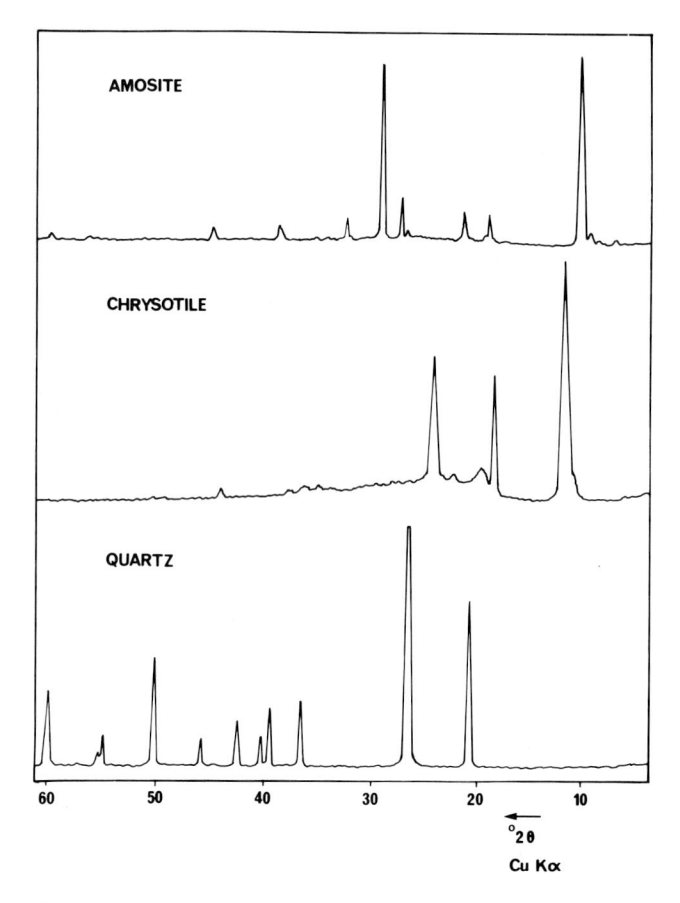

Figure 23–37. X-ray diffraction patterns of amosite, chrysotile, and quartz. Intense peaks (ordinates) reflect regular crystal structure and their positions (abscissae) are fixed for different minerals, thus permitting precise identification.

the mine.[259,260] From the experimental aspect all varieties of the mineral proved capable of inducing fibrosis by inhalation.[261] In rats killed at scheduled times, Canadian chrysotile and anthophyllite were the most fibrogenic, Rhodesian chrysotile and crocidolite proved less active, and amosite gave the least fibrosis. As in humans, progression of asbestosis occurred after the termination of exposure. However, taking surface area into account, the more common types of amphibole were equally fibrogenic (Timbrell and Colleagues, unpublished data). Baboons inhaling asbestos cement dust (36 mg/m³ consisting of 88 percent Portland cement, 10.8 percent chrysotile, and 1.2 percent crocidolite) developed pulmonary fibrosis morphologically similar to asbestosis.[262]

Fiber Dimensions
The importance of fiber length in asbestotic fibrosis was soon appreciated.[16,263] Intratracheal injection and inhalation studies appeared to demonstrate that only particles longer than 20 μm were capable of inducing peribronchiolar fibrosis, the reaction developing sooner as the atmospheric concentration of long fibers increased. In rats and guinea pigs amosite clouds of equal mass concentration led to much greater deposition with fibers of lengths less than 11 μm than with fibers of lengths greater than 11 μm without preferential deposition between lobes, but the subsequent pulmonary reaction proved to be minimal with short fibers and prominent with long ones.[264] Short fibers are readily taken up by macrophages and removal effected by proximal transfer free or intracellularly, via the ciliary escalator, whereas long fibers cannot be totally ingested or removed by this means and hence remain in the vicinity of respiratory bronchioles to induce fibrosis. A discordant claim arose when very short fibers of different varieties of asbestos were shown to be fibrogenic when inhaled by guinea pigs.[265]

In material from mixed human exposures, all fibers were found to be less than 0.5 μm diameter and the proportion shorter than 5 μm long ranged between 70 and 90 percent.[266] Chrysotile, amosite, and crocidolite particles, apparently unaffected physically or chemically by the preparative techniques, were distinguished in lung specimens from cases of asbestosis and mesothelioma.[267] The majority of all these minerals had fiber lengths less than 5 μm with a significant fraction of chrysotile and crocidolite fibers being less than 1 μm long and fibers over 25 μm being very infrequent. Chrysotile occurred mainly as fibrils less than 0.125 μm diameter, crocidolite as fibrils less than 0.25 μm diameter, and amosite as fibers less than 0.375 μm diameter. The amphiboles showed an increase of diameter with increasing length but chrysotile changed little. The aspect ratios for all types were mostly 10:1 or over with chrysotile having the highest ratio. Anthophyllite fibers in Finnish lung specimens had a mean length generally less than 7 μm and a diameter less than 0.7 μm.[268]

The analyses in humans are opposed to most of the experimental findings which emphasize the role of long fibers. During their long residence in the lung fibers may fracture and thereby reduce if not eliminate traces of long ones, but these may well have succeeded in stimulating fibrosis before their disintegration. Short fibers are customarily considered to be eliminated readily by ciliary action, but their massive predominance in human material, as well as in one experimental report,[265] suggests that they should not be dismissed. Short fibers deposited in alveoli are easily ingested by macrophages which may assist their translocation, and toxicity is low. Small quantities may indeed be cleared via conducting airways but larger amounts are likely to accumulate in alveoli related to respiratory bronchioles and there initiate a low-grade progressive reaction. The manner of aggregation then resembles that of coal particles though the fibrogenic potential of fibers is greater. It therefore appears unjustifiable to relegate short fibers to a position of minor significance in the genesis of asbestotic fibrosis and their role may be to maintain the fibrogenic response that long fibers initiated.

Mechanisms of Fibrogenesis
It was natural that solution of the silicon dioxide component of asbestos minerals should be considered but no evidence in its favor has been forthcoming. Being dura-

ble rigid structures, long fibers which are only partially ingested have been thought to disturb the macrophage cytoskeleton mechanically, especially during cellular and respiratory movement, and it is possible that nuclear as well as cytoplasmic structures may be affected, but again there is no firm basis in observation. Short fibers may lie in macrophages without any disturbance being detectable ultrastructurally.

In studying the effect of asbestos fibers on cell membranes, erythrocytes have been used to isolate the surface reaction. Like silica, chrysotile proved strongly hemolytic but amphiboles showed little activity.[269] The magnesium content correlated with lysis and since the silica component of chrysotile varied little its contribution could be ignored for comparative purposes. Removal of the brucite outer layer of chrysotile by acid leaching reduced its activity[270] but hemolysis by silica and glass fiber is independent of magnesium. The lytic potential did not bear a direct relationship with the surface area of asbestos minerals, as was also found with silica. The sialic acid component of membranes imparts a negative charge to which the positively charged chrysotile is attracted. Since hydrogen bonding is not feasible with chrysotile, PNO exerted little protective effect on red cells. The surface charges (zeta potentials) of serpentine and amphibole asbestos, normally similar in magnitude but opposite in polarity, may be altered by leaching or by contact with dipalmitoyl lecithin from the alveolar lining layer, but neither surface charge nor clustering of membrane sialoglycoproteins explains fibrogenesis.

Damage to macrophages, assessed by dye exclusion, showed long fibers to be more deleterious than short ones.[271] Toxicity to peritoneal macrophages and to stable cell lines proved maximal for fibers 10 μm or greater in length and 1.4 μm or less in diameter.[272] Injury to macrophages is reflected by enzyme release. Chrysotile, in contrast to silica, permitted selective release of lysosomal enzymes in a dose-dependent manner, but nonlysosomal lactate dehydrogenase (LDH) did not escape extracellularly though its intracellular level tended to rise.[273] The distinction between lysosomal and cytoplasmic enzyme release has not, however, proved to be absolute.

Membrane changes offer no explanation of the means by which fibrosis is induced. Enzyme release (whether selective or not) or inflammatory mediators of cellular origin seems inadequate to account for fibrogenesis in view of the minimal or absent response of fibroblasts to extracts of disintegrated normal macrophages in vitro[48] and the preservation of cellular architecture for long periods after ingestion of fibers. In paying so much attention to macrophage behavior, the participation of the fibroblast is liable to be obscured and two mechanisms merit consideration. The relatively low toxicity of fibers to macrophages permits longer contact with cell structures or components than in the case of quartz and the less-prominent fibrogenic response could depend on formation of a MFF at a slower rate and in lower concentration. Evidence for the operation of an MFF has indeed been obtained. An extract from macrophages, treated with chrysotile, stimulated the functional activity of fibroblasts.[54] Activation of an MFF by amphibole has also been detected in the same system and attention redirected to the importance of short fibers, whether of amosite or fibrous glass; asbestos fibers applied directly failed to stimulate fibroblasts.[274] An alternative mechanism for fibroblast participation has been termed anchorage dependence. Fibroblasts grown in suspension culture along with glass fibers 200 μm long and 0.6 μm in diameter showed maximum growth but none was obtained when the length was 20 μm or less. Fibroblasts were anchored to the glass fibers and linear extension evidently stimulated cellular division.[275] To establish an anchorage effect requires the deployment of cell kinetic techniques to measure cell proliferation and collagen estimation to assess functional activity, but the MFF may still be implicated. Implantation of chrysotile and peritoneal macrophages within diffusion chambers into the peritoneal cavity of syngeneic mice led to greater fibrosis than macrophages alone, the maximal response occurring at 2 to 4 weeks and then slowly subsiding to control levels.[276] Only the smallest dose of quartz evoked corresponding fibrosis, presumably by permitting better cell survival, but hematite had no effect nor did minerals alone. These findings not only reemphasize the role of the macrophage in fibrogenesis and the release of a diffusible factor acting on fibroblasts but also focus on the necessity for macrophage recruitment to sustain the response.

Evidence of lipid participation in the in vivo reaction to inhaled fibers is scanty, though, as with silica,[101,102] chrysotile led to hyperplasia of type II alveolar epithelial cells and to an increase of surfactant in the lung lavage fluid, with the physical behavior of excised lungs conforming.[277] Inhalation of ground glass fiber induced alveolar lipo-proteinosis.[278] A qualitative correspondence evidently exists between compact and fibrous particles in this regard though quantitative differences may transpire. If lipid accumulation assumes sufficient proportions the effect could be to isolate cells from fibers.

The Immunologic Component
Antinuclear antibodies and rheumatoid factor were detected in the sera of only a minority of British patients,[279] though elevated levels occurred in American asbetotics.[280] Other studies suggest the formation of surface antigen-antibody complexes on macrophages. Significant rises of secretory IgA and serum IgA, IgG, IgM, and IgE occurred in affected individuals and also of non-organ-specific autoantibodies.[281] Impairment of cellular immunity has been claimed,[281–284] but depression of response by lymphocytes proved variable among series.

Although some of the immunologic findings achieved statistical significance, the responses were not universal and sometimes affected a minority of cases. The development of immunologic features in serum, cells, or lesions is dependent on preexisting changes of a fibrotic nature where continued demise of macrophages may be expected. Others[285] concur that serologic changes (antinuclear antibodies and rheumatoid factor) in asbestosis are probably a consequence of the pulmonary lesions and not evidence of an autoimmune mechanism in pathogenesis, as may well be true of the cellular phenomena. The immunologic features might signify a peculiar reactivity to the accumulation of dust or a liability to the development of infection and the prevalence of histocompatibility antigens has again been examined. HLA-B8, encountered in a variety of immunologically mediated disorders,[286] has not yet been connected with the pneumoconiosis and the present position is that HLA phenotypes at the A, B, or C loci bear no consistent relationship to the development of asbestosis and are thus devoid of diagnostic value.[287]

Clinical Correlations

Radiologic

The early diffuse interstitial changes may not be detected on the radiograph and when opacities appear they have often been antedated by physiologic evidence of lung involvement. At first the appearances take the form of small, irregularly shaped opacities classified under the 1980 ILO scheme into three categories according to size and profusion, and distinguished from the small, rounded opacities seen in coal workers. The distribution of the changes varies with the anatomic location of the disease.

Physiologic

The pattern is essentially that of restrictive lung disease, the result of diffuse fibrosis and not specific for asbestosis. Lung volumes, especially the vital capacity and functional residual capacity, are reduced and air flow is diminished. Diffusing capacity is generally depressed on account of the smaller lung volume and inhomogeneity of ventilation-perfusion relationship. Impaired gas transfer may be evident though initially exercise elicitation may be needed. Emphysema is not generally encountered in asbestosis. Pulmonary hypertension may, however, be evident from an early radiologic stage and before lung function is affected[288]; periarterial fibrosis, originating in lymphatics, is believed to account for the hypertension.

Compared with coal worker's pneumoconiosis, functional-morphologic relationships in asbestosis have received less attention, largely because the pathological reaction is much more pronounced and easier to interpret. Overall asbestosis exhibits a weaker correlation between dust exposure and radiologic appearances and a stronger one between lung function and mortality, than coal worker's disease.

Clinical and Pathologic Diagnosis

Other causes of diffuse interstitial fibrosis or honeycomb lung, whether local or systemic in origin, must be excluded and the possible coexistence of other forms of pneumoconiosis should not be overlooked. Diffuse pleural thickening is not necessarily attributable to asbestos exposure and may be the result of empyema, hemothorax, or tuberculosis.

Nonspecific interstitial fibrosis, alone or with progression to honeycombing, in individuals exposed to asbestos poses a diagnostic problem greater than in coal workers (see Disorders Due to Coal Mine and Carbonaceous Dusts, Differentiation of Emphysematous and Fibrocystic States in Coal Workers, Clinical Connotations, above). Compared with compact particles, fibers lead to a simple dust lesions which is less clearly demarcated and thus comes to resemble the pattern of a patchy and diffuse interstitial fibrosis, onto which cystic changes may be grafted. The presence of fibers, coated or uncoated, in the lesion does not constitute conclusive evidence of an occupational origin, since nonspecific interstitial fibrosis could incorporate fibers already in the lung and, by interfering with translocation, might accumulate fibers subsequently inhaled. The problem may prove insoluble on morphologic grounds but, although not decisive, a history of asbestos exposure tends to bias the interpretation. Irrespective of occupational exposure, a negative indication may sometimes be derived from comparison of fiber counts in digests of fibrosed tissue and of normal parenchyma taken from the same lung; if the fiber concentration in normal parenchyma corresponds to that expected in lungs from the nonindustrial, urban population of the area and the concentration in fibrosed tissue is of a similar order, the fibrosis may reasonably be regarded as having a nonspecific origin. Minor degrees of interstitial fibrosis may not justify such labor.

Sequelae

Tuberculosis and Other Infections

The decline in tuberculosis as a complication of asbestosis in Whites probably reflects the changing prevalence of infection in the general population and, though massive asbestosis may involve a tuberculous component, there is no reason to believe that asbestosis or exposure to the dust constitute a predisposing factor, in contrast to silicosis.

Serpentine and amphibole asbestos possess the ability to depress the induction of interferon by influenza virus in monkey kidney cells, an effect that PNO counteracts.[289,290] Application to the in vivo situation demands caution, but the implication remains that asbestos accumulation in the lung with or without fibrosis may predispose to viral infection which in turn could facilitate bacterial complications.

Cor Pulmonale

Advanced disease may terminate in respiratory failure or chronic cor pulmonale from vascular obliteration, but many sufferers succumb to a superimposed infection.

Carcinoma of the Lung

The suspicion that pulmonary carcinoma might bear a peculiar relationship with asbestosis was raised 50 years ago.[291,292] Up to 1963 the annual totals for deaths from asbestosis in Great Britain increased, a thoracic neoplasm occurring in over 50 percent of males dying with asbestosis.

Prevalence. The longest cohort study concerned an asbestos textile factory using chrysotile plus a little crocidolite.[232–234] With an exposure of 20 years or more, including 5 years or over prior to the enforcement of the U.K. Asbestos Industry Regulations of 1931, the prevalence of carcinoma of the lung and pleura was significantly greater than expected; in the group with the longest and most intense exposure the risk was over 15 times that experienced by the general population. Following implementation of the Regulations, the risk was greatly reduced but, despite hopes to the contrary, the latest account still records a highly significant excess of deaths from carcinoma of the bronchus among employees. Similar evidence was provided by another cohort study of a London asbestos factory that produced mainly textiles and insulation products from crocidolite, amosite, and chrysotile.[293,294] Asbestos cement workers also experienced an excess risk from respiratory cancer but it was confined to those who had moderate or high cumulative exposures.[295] The evidence from these and other investigations leaves no doubt of the consistent excess mortality from lung cancer. Neither of the two groups of asbestos fiber seems to carry a special risk, with excess lung cancers occurring in chrysotile miners, millers, and textile workers, anthophyllite miners, and amosite factory workers. Dust levels and duration of exposure correlate in a linear manner with lung cancer SMRs of miners and manufacturing employees.

Experimental Evidence. The proportion of SPF rats developing malignant lung tumors was more or less the same after inhalation of UICC samples of Canadian chrysotile, crocidolite, amosite, and anthophyllite, although retention of chrysotile was much less than that of the amphiboles.[261]

Smoking. Asbestos workers who smoked apparently had a risk of dying from bronchogenic carcinoma 92 times that of men who neither worked with asbestos nor smoked.[296] Asbestos exposure alone did not apparently increase greatly the risk to men who did not smoke cigarettes regularly. The view gained ground that the combination of asbestos exposure and smoking had a multiplicative or synergistic rather than an additive effect. With low or mild exposure to asbestos smoking had no effect on the SMR for lung cancer, but the ratio was significantly elevated in those who smoked and were heavily exposed.[297] In Finnish anthophyllite miners and millers the relative risks of lung cancer were 1 for nonsmokers not exposed to asbestos, 1.6 for nonsmoking asbestos workers, 12 for nonexposed smokers, and 19 for smoking workers; the findings were explicable as a multiplicative or promotor effect.[298] The current overall position may be worse in that, compared with nonexposed nonsmokers, asbestos exposure alone caused a 5-fold increase in the death rate from lung cancer, smoking alone an 11-fold rise, and smoking with exposure a 53-fold rise.[299] The import of such figures is plain. Although a role for chrysotile had been doubted, it is now evident that nonsmoking miners experienced a greater rise of incidence as exposure increased than did smokers.[300]

Morphologic Peculiarities. The neoplasm is located predominantly in the lower part of the lung and tends to be situated peripherally and to involve the pleura, when differentiation from mesothelioma is required. This predilection for the lower lobe[301] is the reverse of the situation in the nonindustrial population and the distribution of the carcinoma corresponds with that of asbestosis, which probably coexists in all cases. Where asbestosis is not recorded the evidence is usually radiologic, which constitutes too insecure a basis to detect mild or even moderate degrees of fibrosis, such as is revealed by histologic examination. Asbestosis may thus be considered as a precursor of neoplasia in the lung and it seems likely that the hyperplastic or dysplastic epithelium (with abnormal nuclei) which comes to line persisting spaces, whether cystic or not, merges into neoplasia. Experimentally malignant epithelial changes were noted in areas of fibrosis, which was greater in rats with lung tumors.[261] As might be expected, an excess of adenocarcinoma has been reported both in humans[301] and animals[261] but anaplastic and squamous varieties occur in humans and squamous varieties also in rats, no doubt developing from epithelium that had first undergone metaplasia. The frequency of different histologic varieties is, however, influenced by the source of material, whether biopsy, surgical, or necropsy and mixed sources (for example, see Kannerstein and Churg[256]) may not be the most reliable indicators; necropsy provides the most extensive information and if all or most asbestos workers were so examined case selection would be avoided.

Fiber Content of the Lung. Since carcinoma customarily arises in asbestotic lung, the fiber content corresponds. Concern arose over the possible role of asbestos contamination of the urban atmosphere as a factor in the genesis of pulmonary carcinoma in the nonindustrial population. Using matched control subjects, the concentrations of asbestos bodies were similar in the presence not only of pulmonary but also of gastrointestinal carcinoma,[302] but no account was taken of uncoated fibers which form the great majority and probably retain their biologic activity. Taking cognizance of both coated and uncoated fibers by light microscopy, the range of total fibers, though varying widely, was similar in control subjects and lung cancer cases, 57 percent of both having less than 10,000 fibers per gram dried lung with high counts being less frequent in the cancer series and amphibole consituting most of the fibers. It was therefore concluded that urban asbestos pollution probably did not contribute to the overall incidence of lung cancer for which cigarette smoking was blamed.[303] This remains the present position.

Cocarcinogenesis. Such a role for asbestos fibers remains sub judice, but is mentioned in Malignant Mesothelioma, Pathogenesis, Mechanisms, below.

Carcinoma of the Gastrointestinal Tract and Other Sites

The possibility that malignant neoplasms of the alimentary system might be more frequent that expected in asbestos workers arose from epidemiologic investigations and the increase appeared to be proportional to the degree of asbestos exposure. In recent accounts, chrysotile, amosite, and mixtures including crocidolite have all been implicated.[230,304–306] Smoking does not appear to affect the risk to asbestos workers of developing gastrointestinal carcinoma. It seems wise to treat the evidence with some reserve, since histologic distinction has not always been achieved between peritoneal involvement in primary mesothelioma and secondary carcinoma from the gastrointestinal tract. The idea that carcinoma of the ovary might be more frequent in asbestos workers is not established, some of the reported cases proving to be mesotheliomata on histologic examination. Laryngeal carcinoma has also been connected with asbestos exposure, the risk allegedly being confined to smokers and increasing with cigarette consumption. However, a large retrospective study revealed that asbestos exposure was not more common in cases of laryngeal carcinoma than in those with cysts, polyps, or inflammatory lesions, or in individuals with a macroscopically normal larynx.[307] Neoplasia of the hemopoietic system appears to be another complication of asbestos exposure.[308–310]

Pleural Plaques

Morphology

Gross Features
These lesions are distinct from the fibrous thickening and adhesion of the visceral and parietal surfaces of the pleura that are virtually universal in asbestosis and which may also follow infections or hemothorax. A feature of plaques is in fact the absence of conventional adhesions which may nevertheless occur elsewhere. Plaques occur almost exclusively on the parietal surface, are frequently bilateral and symmetric, and show a predilection for certain sites. The apices and costophrenic angles are spared, while an anterior location is exceptional. Characteristically plaques are multiple, elongated, and lie posteriorly and laterally over the lower thoracic cage, especially in the region of the seventh to tenth ribs, whose direction they follow, though bridges between plaques are common as are irregular extensions. The anterolateral and upper parts of the thoracic cage may also be affected as may the pleural surface of the pericardium. The tendinous portion of the diaphragm posterolaterally is a favorite location though the muscular portion is generally spared.

Plaques, likened to sugar icing (*Zuckerguss*), appear as sharply defined, abruptly elevated areas of irregular, often elongated outline and between them the pleura may appear normal or slightly thickened. The surface is typically smooth and shiny, having a greyish-white color when thin and being ivory or cream colored when thick (up to 1 cm). In size they range from a few millimeters to 10 cm or more on the diaphragm. Sometimes, however, the surface is mammillated, though still smooth (Fig. 23–38). Plaques strip easily from the ribs and intercostal muscles, but diaphragmatic ones are firmly adherent. Plaques possess a leathery consistency that permits them to bend, but when heavily calcified they are brittle. On section plaques possess a laminated texture and calcification tends to lie centrally.

Microscopic Features
Avascular, coarse collagen is arranged in interweaving bundles which lie more or less parallel to the surface and

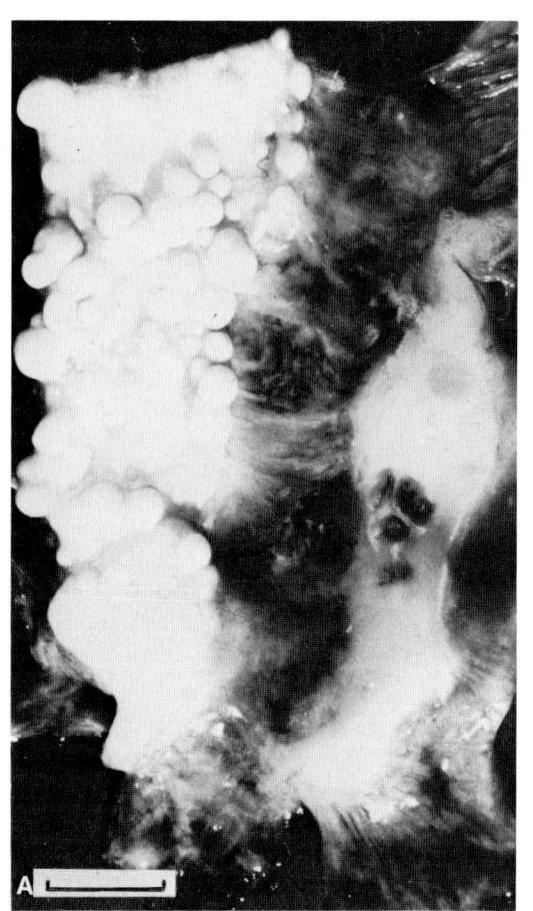

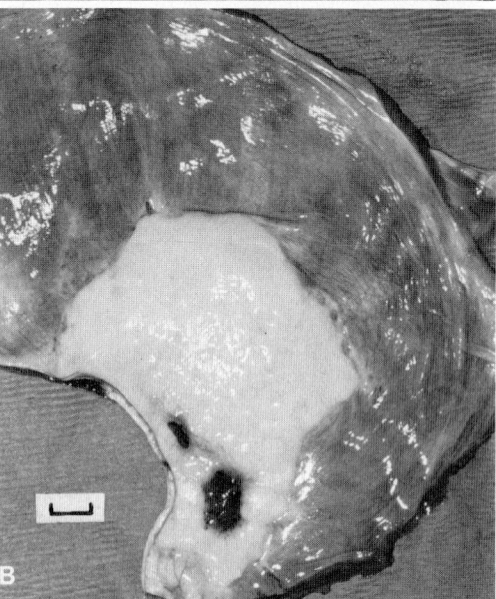

Figure 23–38. Parietal pleural plaques. A. On the thoracic cage, showing mammillated and flattened surfaces with fine fibrous strands bridging the intercostal space shown vertically (courtesy of Prof. Meurman). B. On the diaphragm, where the surface is smooth. Courtesy of Dr. Roberts. Bars = 1 cm.

terminate abruptly at the margin (Fig. 23–39); in nodular lesions a whorled pattern is seen. The connective tissue may, however, take the elastin stain. Fibrocyte nuclei are few and occur mostly at the periphery, but although granulation tissue is not evident lymphocytes and plasma cells may be found deep to the plaque along with fibroblasts. The latter component suggests that plaque formation originates from the deeper aspects, but the normal connective tissue of the pleura, both collagen and elastin, continues unbroken beneath the plaque. It must also be emphasized that plaque formation takes place beneath the mesothelial lining layer which in well-preserved instances forms a simple surface covering. Plaques may thus be described more precisely as being extrapleural in location. Since growth of a plaque is slow and nonexudative and mesothelial cells evidently play no part in its formation, the absence of pleural adhesions is understandable. Calcification varies widely among cases, sometimes being light and focal and at others heavy and extensive. The deposit occurs as fine granules between the collagen fibers, readily demonstrable by conventional stains, and does not extend beyond the boundaries of the plaque. It is generally considered that the calcification is dystrophic in nature and it is more common in older individuals irrespective of sex. The pseudoelastic fibers may also show calcification.

Electron microscopy confirms the collagenous structure of plaques though fibers with normal periodicity may be wider than usual. In fibrous zones electron-dense particles are scattered between the fibers and appear as solid or laminated structures up to 0.5 μm while others have a needle-like exterior or appear as acicular crystals. These particles represent incipient calcification with electron diffraction patterns of whitlockite or apatite, respectively.[311] In calcified zones the fibrohyaline tissue is the seat of extensive invasion by apatite, which is deposited along the collagen fibers. Phosphorus is increased in the calcified zone, as are acid mucopolysaccharides.

Asbestos bodies have been sought in pleural plaques with little or no success by light microscopy.[312,313] Applying alkali digestion and phase-contrast microscopy, a tenfold increase occurred in plaques when the total lung fiber (mostly amphibole) concentration was greater than 20,000 fibers per gram.[303] In cases with no history of industrial exposure to asbestos, the fiber content of the plaque was much less than that of the lung but the two were not correlated and coated fibers were absent or scanty.[314] By electron microscopy after low-temperature ashing in activated oxygen under reduced pressure and weak acid extraction to remove calcium, numerous, small (0.1 to 2.0 μm) chrysotile fibers were demonstrated in two exposed individuals; fiber concentration was much higher in the calcified than the fibrous parts of the plaques, though the relationship to lung content varied and there amphiboles predominated.[311] The predominance of amphibole in the lung is now accepted, though in plaques chrysotile may be found alone or may coexist with amphibole.[315,316]

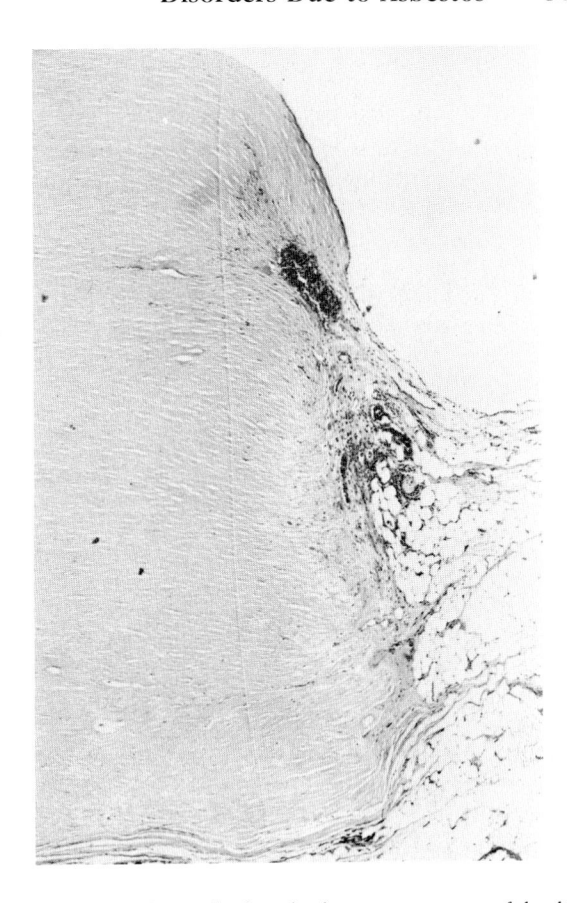

Figure 23–39. Parietal pleural plaque consisting of hyaline collagen fibers in parallel array, covered by mesothelium and lying on adipose tissue. Lymphocytes have collected at the edge which is abrupt (H&E, ×35). Courtesy of Dr. Whitwell.

Occurrence

In a Finnish necropsy series, among which anthophyllite-exposed individuals occurred, the overall frequency of plaques was almost 40 percent with some 70 percent of cases being bilateral and cases being more frequent among males than females.[312] In addition, the frequency of plaques was higher in the urban than the rural population. The necropsy prevalence was 12.3 percent in an urban population, some of whom were probably exposed occupationally.[313] Environmental exposure in proximity to anthophyllite, crocidolite, amosite, and chrysotile mines has also been associated with a raised prevalence of pleural plaques, but nonexposed groups provided few or no examples. In Bulgaria pleural plaques were endemic among the population where tobacco was grown and where the soil contained anthophyllite, tremolite, and sepiolite.[317] There is thus a clear relationship between the development of pleural plaques and exposure to all forms of asbestos fiber, though on present evidence it is not necessarily the only cause. A higher prevalence of plaques, whether calcified or not, occurred in smokers and ex-smokers than in nonsmokers.[251] The lesion is as a rule asymptomatic and plaques may precede or follow pleural effusion in which erythrocytes and lymphocytes may occur.[318]

Pathogenesis

The genesis of plaques is generally regarded as unknown. Thomson[319] proposed that inhaled asbestos fibers gravitated inferiorly and laterally and, being sharp, penetrated the soft structures of the lung to reach the pleura which was irritated mechanically during its constant movement. It is difficult to visualize how such a mechanism would account for the localization of plaques to particular parts of the parietal pleura and allow the visceral layer to escape.

A peculiar anatomic feature, however, permits an explanation. Scattered lymphatic stomata were found to open onto the parietal pleura.[320] If fibers penetrate the visceral layer, either passively under respiratory movement or actively by cellular transport, their concentration in the pleural space could well be determined by drainage toward the stomata. Obstruction of the latter by uncoated rather than coated fibers, presumably short ones which lay extracellulary rather than in macrophages, could lead to local accumulation with backup to extend over ribs and diaphragm, there to excite a fibrotic reaction in the parietal pleura and beneath the mesothelium. Mesothelium may well be capable of responding to the accumulation of fibrous minerals by generation of a macrophage type of fibrogenic factor, since in culture mesothelial cells resemble macrophages in their response to quartz[321] and macrophages react with both quartz and asbestos fibers. Compact particles do not appear to possess the same ability as fibers to penetrate the pleura. Respiratory movements may be invoked to give the connective tissue its typical orientation and smooth surface. The occurrence of plaques in agricultural communities may relate to soil constituents, but only electron microscopic examination of plaques for fiber content will establish whether they are universally the result of exposure to fibrous minerals, that is, irrespective of known asbestos exposure.

Plaques are distinct from mesotheliomata and there is no evidence of a transition between them, though they may coexist.

Malignant Mesothelioma

Occurrence and Prevalence

Although instances of this uncommon neoplasm occur in individuals with no known exposure to fibrous minerals, König[322] from Germany and Wagner and co-workers[323] from South Africa alerted epidemiologists to the likely magnitude of the problem. The South African cases came from the northwestern Cape Province where crocidolite was mined by men and cobbed by women and children, who played on the dumps from mines and mills; the exposure thus comprised occupational and environmental groups. Despite early resistance to the diagnosis by a few pathologists, numerous reports establishing the connection between asbestos exposure and mesothelioma have since appeared, the most reliable being case control studies. Mesothelioma occurred mainly in processing and manufacturing industries or shipyards rather than in mining or milling and most exposures were to mixed types of asbestos. The neoplasm affects the pleura, peritoneum, pericardium, and tunica vaginalis, though the association with asbestos almost entirely concerns the first two sites; cases of primary pericardial mesothelioma following exposure to asbestos have recently been recorded.[324–326]

In North America the annual incidence of malignant mesothelioma was 6.5 to 7.0 cases per million males 45 years old or over,[327] the estimated annual incidence in different accounts ranging from 1 to 6 cases per million population with the necropsy rate being about 0.25 percent. Over 7 percent of all deaths or 17.5 percent of cancer deaths in asbestos insulation workers were due to mesothelioma with peritoneal cases being nearly double the pleural ones,[230] while in England the rate was 7.3 percent of all deaths in male asbestos factory workers and it was predicted that mortality from mesothelioma will rise by up to 11 percent of the total mortality in the present decade before declining as the population at risk diminishes.[328] In the United States, the estimated annual number of asbestos-related cancer deaths is now over 8000 and expected to rise.[329] However, considerable epidemiologic difficulties lie in the way of establishing the true prevalence of mesothelioma in exposed populations. A characteristically long interval elapses between the beginning of exposure and development of the neoplasm, ranging from 3.5 to 53 years, according to the English mesothelioma registry, the mean being 37.4 years and 85 percent of neoplasms occurring over 25 years from first exposure.[330] In a few cases exposure has been both brief and distant, one case, for example, developing a mesothelioma 30 years after an exposure of 6 months.[331] Other problems arise from familiar causes, unreliability of death certification, necropsy statistics, histologic diagnosis including failure to distinguish carcinoma of the lung from mesothelioma, and sometimes the inadequate employment of cohort studies. Perhaps the best hope lies with the more confined dockyard populations. The risk of developing mesothelioma in shipyard workers with pleural plaques has been estimated as 1 in 377 per year.[332] The dockyard problem will persist for some decades, since shipbreaking and repair has released and will continue to release amphiboles, especially crocidolite, from vessels constructed after World War II.

Nonoccupational exposure to asbestos was recognized as being sufficient to lead to mesothelioma in the area where crocidolite was mined and by residence near a textile factory or in the same house as a worker.[323,333] Female household contacts experienced a relative risk factor of 10.[334] In a survey of domestic exposure 35 percent of 678 family contacts of amosite factory workers showed x-ray film abnormalities, amounting to asbestosis in 17 percent, and five cases of pleural mesothelioma were identified.[335] In France the proportions of mesothelioma cases who had experienced occupational, paraoccupational, and unknown asbestos exposure were 77 percent, 3 percent, and 20 percent, respectively.[336]

Pathologic Anatomy

The morbid anatomy of mesothelioma is covered in Chapter 26. The national mesothelioma panels afford diagnostic support, but difficulties may remain on account of disagreement even among experienced histopathologists. Needle biopsy may not only be unreliable because of the small sample but may encourage dissemination of the neoplasm, as may open thoracotomy or laparotomy; diagnosis may nevertheless depend on the latter. If for clinical reasons fluid has to be aspirated from the pleural cavity, cytology may prove useful, though by that time the diagnosis has usually been established on other grounds. The effusion may contain neutrophil granulocytes with cytoplasmic inclusions, such as occur in rheumatoid arthritis.

Distinction between diffuse mesothelioma and adenocarcinoma or bronchioloalveolar carcinoma may be achieved by indirect immunohistochemical techniques, keratin proteins predominantly characterizing mesotheliomas and carcinoembryonic antigen characterizing carcinomas.[337,338] Other investigators found that carcinoembryonic antigen and β_1 pregnancy-specific glycoprotein within the tumor strongly contraindicated mesothelioma.[339] Cytoplasmic surfactant-specific apoprotein has been found in some cases of bronchioloalveolar carcinoma.[340] Identification of α_1 antichymotrypsin may serve to differentiate reactive from malignant mesothelium.[341]

Pathogenesis

Quantity of Dust

Epidemiologic Evidence. The occurrence of domestic and environmental cases suggests that comparatively small amounts of asbestos are sufficient to produce mesotheliomata. Data are, however, vague since exposures often occurred many years previously when dust levels were not recorded systematically. The mesothelioma rate shows some evidence of dose dependence in terms of length and intensity of exposure.[328]

Pathologic Evidence. Dose relationships rely on lung dust analysis by extraction procedures. By light microscopy a wide range of total fiber content was found in 36 cases of mesothelioma; 2 cases without known asbestos exposure had zero or occasional fibers, while exposed individuals varied between 154,000 and 684 million fibers per gram dry weight and uncoated fibers accounted for 50 to 80 percent of the total.[331] In control cases counts ranged from nil to almost 8 millions per gram dry lung and thus overlapped extensively with the mesothelioma series, in which the proportion of coated fibers was higher. No relationship was discernible between total fiber count and the latent period of mesothelioma. In another study,[303] total fiber estimations by light microscopy ranged from zero to 70 million per gram dried lung, but in cases with a history of asbestos exposure the level was over 20,000 in all but one case. On the other hand, 71 percent of control material had less than 20,000 fibers and 57 percent less than 10,000. Of particular interest were housewives who developed mesothelioma after exposures of 0.5 to 5 years making gas masks or sacks in the first and second world wars; fiber counts lay between 300,000 and 57 millions and were almost all amphibole.

Few estimations have been made of the fiber content in the tumor itself. In three cases of pleural mesothelioma, low-termperature ashing revealed fiber concentrations of 1.2 to 18.3 millions per gram, the ratio to the content of adjacent lung varying from 0.008 to 1.07.[254] A peculiar feature of these cases was the enrichment of chrysotile content in the tumor and of amphibole in the lung from mixed exposures. Low concentrations of uncoated fibers were detected in mesotheliomata (less than 100,000 per gram dry weight) but no coated fibers; tumor and lung concentrations were not apparently related.[253]

These analyses reflect cumulative dust retention in the lung over many years and do not necessarily indicate the dose of fiber required to initiate tumor formation. Concurrence between epidemiologic and pathologic findings is nevertheless apparent in that a very low pulmonary concentration of fibers occurs in cases whose exposure was both brief and very distant. In other cases no clear dose-response relationship can yet be discerned.

Pathologic Reaction in the Lung

One series of 36 mesotheliomata included 20 with asbestosis, 6 of which were of moderate or severe degree and in which the more severe fibrosis predominated in peritoneal as opposed to pleural tumors[331]; the pulmonary fiber content tended to reflect the grade of asbestosis.[252] Among 100 cases, 23 had developed asbestosis and in 14 the disorder was of moderate or severe degree; the fiber counts in the lungs of asbestotic patients varied greatly, with considerable overlap between the grades though the means rose in parallel.[303] A lack of correlation thus emerges between the occurrence and severity of asbestosis and the development of mesothelioma, for which a different pathogenesis may therefore be suspected.

Type of Fiber

The Advisory Committee on Asbestos Cancers[342] concluded that in the induction of mesothelioma all commercial types of asbestos may be responsible with one exception. Among Finnish anthophyllite miners no example of mesothelioma was discovered despite a follow-up reaching 40 years[343] and that remains the current position (K. Karkola, personal communication, 1984). The risk of mesothelioma appears to be greatest with crocidolite, less with amosite, and least with chrysotile; the risk for chrysotile is likely to remain much lower than for crocidolite.[344] Chrysotile is now considered to be a rare cause of pleural mesothelioma, while a role in peritoneal tumors is doubtful. Such differences could be related to the proportion of fibers with small aerodynamic diameters. Chrysotile, crocidolite, and amosite can be identified in the lungs of affected individuals.[267] North American experience suggested that mesothelioma was particularly associated with the presence of amosite in the lung,[345] while amphiboles seemed to lead preferentially to peritoneal tumors.[346] Tremolite was held responsible for mesothelioma in humans[347] and when injected intrapleurally into rats led to tumors.[348] Tremolite has been identified as a not uncommon contaminant of commercially used chrysotile, as well as of talc (see Disorders Due to Other Silicates, and So Forth, below). After inhaling tremolite, rats developed fibrosis and frequently carcinoma of the lung, together with an occasional mesothelioma; the latter, however, was almost universal following intraperitoneal administration.[348a] A role for chrysotile in the genesis of human mesothelioma thus appears even more dubious.

Crocidolite has been incriminated in the genesis of mesothelioma among workers in English and Canadian factories that made gas mask filters or canisters during World War II, with the English cases being almost all women.[349-351] The exposures were short and the latent period at least 20 years, the English survey revealing not only a considerable excess of mesothelioma but also of bronchial carcinoma. The risk of mesothelioma from crocidolite exposure was evidently much greater than for chrysotile in the Canadian experience.

Attention has lately focused on diffuse pleural mesothelioma restricted to a remote region of Anatolia in Turkey. Over 7 years there were 36 deaths from this cause confined to a particular village with 575 inhabitants, but no cases occurred in neighboring villages.[352] No environmental or occupational sources of fibers were identified. In two villages 50 percent of deaths were due to mesothelioma whereas other villages in the vicinity escaped. The mesothelioma cases now total 185 and affected villages are being relocated. Contamination of drinking water has been discounted.[353] Zeolite minerals of fibrous habit having tetrahedral linkages in a three-dimensional network (mordenite, erionite, and chabazite—complex silicates with a general formula $(NaCaBa)_{1-2} (SiAl)_5O_{10}nH_2O$) and most being less than 0.25 μm diameter) have been identified in the soil, local volcanic rock, building stones, street dust, and lungs of the inhabitants of one small village. It is suggested that these fibers are the causative agents in a disease which has an annual incidence 942 times greater than expected.[354] However, chrysotile and tremolite have lately been detected in environmental samples from affected villages but not from those escaping disease, though all samples contained erionite; lung tissue of mesothelioma cases contained 90 percent of fibrous erionite along with a small proportion of tremolite.[355] The precise etiology is thus sub judice, but fibrous zeolite and asbestos may both be concerned since erionite proved carcinogenic in the peritoneum of mice[356] and the pleura of rats.[357] Inhaled erionite, having a very small diameter, was highly effective in producing mesotheliomas relatively quickly in rats.[358]

To isolate the particle effect, fibers were applied to the pleura[359,360] and revealed a range of carcinogenicity which in decreasing order was superfine chrysotile, crocidolite, amosite, anthophyllite, Canadian chrysotile. Inhalation experiments produced far fewer mesotheliomas than lung cancers, but UICC chrysotile and crocidolite were equally effective, amosite and anthophyllite less so.[261] The experimental response to tremolite is indicated above.

Fiber Dimensions

The recovery of minerals from the lungs of individuals with mesothelioma showed the fibers to be both short and narrow. The diameter of most was less than 0.4 μm, that is, below the limit of optical resolution, and few fibers longer that 5 μm were observed.[252] Another study showed that fibers less than 5 μm long predominated, those over 25 μm being very infrequent, while diameters were mostly less than 0.25 μm.[267]

When fibrous glass was applied to the pleura the incidence of neoplasms varied with particle size.[361] The highest probability of malignancy was obtained with fibers 1.5 μm or less in diameter and greater than 8 μm in length. Carcinogenicity evidently depended on both fiber dimension and durability. Asbestos minerals behaved similarly.[362]

Man-made Mineral Fibers

The unique properties of asbestos produce conflict between its use and its ill-effects on health, and the search for artificial fibers aims to retain the first and diminish or abolish the second. The fibers are made from glass, natural rock, or fusible slag, which are all amorphous silicates of boron, aluminium, and calcium with trace elements of no apparent biologic significance. Fibers occur in three ranges of diameter; continuous filaments are much too wide to enter the respiratory parenchyma but insulation wool and special-purpose fibers possess diameters that make them respirable. Unlike asbestos fibers, man-made mineral fibers (MMMF) do not split longitudinally but may break transversely.

There was no evidence of an increased risk of malignant respiratory disease 20 to 30 years after the onset of exposure to fibers having median diameters within the respirable range.[363,364] A large retrospective survey of MMMF plants in seven European countries failed to establish a clear cancer risk though the issue was suggestive, but smoking histories were not available.[365] Pathologically no pulmonary changes could be attributed to fibrous glass in workers with exposures of up to 32 years[366] and experimentally glass wool and fiber-glass plastic proved nonfibrogenic, but diffuse interstitial pulmonary fibrosis has developed after exposure to fiberglass[367] and rock wool.[368] Moreover, recent evidence indicates that fibrous glass is capable of stimulating production of the MFF[274] and is fibrogenic when inhaled by baboons.[369] Man-made mineral fibers may, like asbestos fibers, acquire a ferroprotein coating. The ability of glass fibers within particular size ranges to induce malignancy after direct application to mesothelial surfaces[359,361,362,370] nevertheless emphasizes the need for caution. Introduction of fibers into the pleural cavity is not comparable to inhalation exposure and the commercial employment of fibers with diameters of 1 μm or less is relatively recent and much higher airborne dust levels may be observed. The commercial application of whiskers, that is, metallic and ceramic filamentary single crystals with their micron-sized widths, poses another problem for the future. Alumina fiber (aluminium oxide with about 4 percent silica, used in high-temperature insulation and including fibers with dimensions that permit alveolar penetration) provoked minimal fibrosis but no tumors on long-term inhalation by rats, in contradistinction to chrysotile.[371]

Miscellaneous Factors

Trace Metals. Contamination of asbestos by traces of metals such as nickel and chromium has been considered as a factor in carcinogenesis, but animal experiments demonstrated that it was unnecessary to invoke such a hypothesis either in regard to mesothelioma or to carcinoma of the lung.[261,359,360] Removal of the brucite layer from chrysotile greatly diminished the incidence of mesothelial tumors in animals,[270] but a role for magnesium cannot be deduced since magnesium-free crocidolite is also carcinogenic.

Oils and Waxes. It has also been suggested that contamination of asbestos with natural oils or waxes or with oils from fiber preparation could contribute to carcinogensis, as might diphenoquinone from plastic storage bags. Benzene extraction of oil from UICC samples did not, however, affect their carcinogenicity to the pleura.[359]

Smoking. Epidemiologic follow-up in one group for over 20 years showed that cigarette smoking had little or no effect on death rates for mesothelioma,[372] a situation which contrasts with that of lung cancer and to a lesser extent with asbestosis. No association was detected between smoking and deaths from mesothelioma among asbestos factory workers.[373]

Water-Borne Fibers. Fibrous minerals are found in water supplies and beverages. The tailings from an iron ore mine in Minnesota were dumped into Lake Superior and the potable water of Duluth and other municipalities was found to be contaminated with amphibole fibers, sometimes indistinguishable from amosite and other fibers.[374] In about 60 percent of necropsies on individuals from the Duluth area with long-term oral intake, amphibole fiber has been detected in lung, liver, and intestine by means of selected area electron diffraction and energy dispersive x-ray analysis.[375] The air of the district did not contain appreciable numbers of amphibole fibers which presumably gained access through the intestinal mucosa. Chrysotile occurred in the lungs of both Duluth and control subjects. Earlier reports suggested that water-borne asbestos fibers, sometimes derived from asbestos cement pipes, did not lead to excess deaths from cancer of the lung or digestive tract, but the follow-up periods were probably not long enough. On the contrary, in the San Francisco Bay area, the incidence of alimentary cancers was related significantly to the chrysotile content of the drinking water.[376] It is as yet impossible to predict with confidence the consequences of oral intake in humans, as the latest experience in Duluth attests.[377] Assurance may possibly be derived from animal studies. Duluth tap water or reservoir sediment, the plant tailings and amosite fed to rats over their life span failed to augment the incidence of malignant neoplasms.[378] Moreover, rats fed large quantities of UICC chrysotile, crocidolite, or amosite for periods up to 25 months and followed for life exhibited no gastrointestinal abnormalities or excess malignant neoplasms, while the cytokinetics of the intestinal mucosa was unaffected by amosite ingestion.[379] Nevertheless chrysotile was apparently able to penetrate the intestinal mucosa of the rat, while in a baboon fed chrysotile and crocidolite, fibers were recovered from blood and viscera.[380]

Mechanisms

The cellular reactions to asbestos fibers are evidently not determined by chemical composition, but physical characteristics assume importance in carcinogenesis irrespective of whether fibers occur naturally or are man-made. Dimensions are clearly significant and so apparently is durability. Penetration of the pleura presumably depends on the fineness of fibers, whose diameter is generally much less than that of compact particles.

Injected intratracheally, chrysotile led to a pronounced increase in the labeling index of visceral mesothelium,[381] suggesting augmented proliferative activity, but the whole range of cell kinetic techniques has yet to be applied to mesothelium in situ under particle stimulation. Hamster embryo cells exposed to chrysotile in culture did, however, show dose-related chromosomal aberrations possibly affecting the G2 phase,[382] while chromosomal alterations were induced in human lymphocytes.[383] Furthermore, amphiboles and chrysotile elevated sister chromatid exchange in hamster cells.[384,385] Whether such abnormalities indicate neoplastic potential is unknown as is the influence of genetic constitution on individual liability to mesothelioma. Anchorage dependence offers a possible explanation for neoplasia as for fibrosis, there being a parallel between this phenomenon and the size of fibers inducing mesotheliomata by pleural application.[386] An apparent anomaly lies in the difference between the ranges in length and diameter of chrysotile, crocidolite, and amosite fibers recovered from the lungs of mesothelioma patients[267] and the optimum dimensions for experimental carcinogenicity to the pleura. Promotion of fibrosis in the pleura by a macrophage fibrogenic factor (*see* Pleural Plaques, Pathogenesis, above) may contribute the mesenchymal component of mesothelioma, the mesothelial element deriving from a proliferative response which could correspond to that of pulmonary epithelium in carcinoma arising in asbestotic lungs.

Fibrous dusts proved more effective than compact ones in adsorbing and encouraging transport of polycyclic aromatic hydrocarbons into rat liver microsomes,[387] while chrysotile enhanced DNA binding of the metabolic products of such carcinogens.[388] Chrysotile though not amosite evidently promoted benzo(a)pyrene carcinogenesis in the respiratory tract of hamsters.[389] These observations raise the question of cocarcinogenesis which might also bear on carcinoma of the lung in asbestosis where cigarette smoke could provide the carcinogen.

Unlike the plaque, mesothelioma affects visceral and parietal layers of the pleura and, since asbestos fibers are likely to reach the pleura or peritoneum in many more individuals than develop the tumor, other factors, as yet unknown, may be concerned in its genesis.

Urban Exposure to Asbestos

The development of mesothelioma after slight exposure to asbestos and the occurrence of neighborhood cases raised the suspicion that urban environmental contamination might place the general population at risk and led to the search for asbestos in lungs from random necropsies. Attention was initially directed to the readily recognizable coated fiber and, on the basis of lung smears, Thomson[224] first disclosed asbestos inhalation as an urban hazard in Cape Town and others subsequently confirmed the frequent occurrence of asbestos bodies in the lungs of city-dwellers from several countries with positive cases amounting to between 18 and 48 percent. In one area more than half the cases with numerous asbestos bodies had in fact been exposed at work although they formed part of a routine necropsy series and other studies confirmed the occupational or domiciliary (including cosmetics) source of asbestos bodies.

All these reports were, however, confined to coated fibers, whereas the potential danger lies with uncoated fibers which, on evidence already cited, form the great majority of particles in the lung. In control cases from Tyneside, England a history of definite or probable occupational exposure was obtained in 41 percent of subjects,[331] while in a report from Liverpool the number of fibers in control subjects was probably related to the individual's work,[303] both series relying on total fiber (uncoated plus coated) counts. It is not easy to assess the magnitude of the risk of mesothelioma from urban exposure, but in the Tyneside area it was estimated that fewer than 50 cases of mesothelioma occurred over a 12-year period, representing less than 0.1 percent of persons apparently at risk as judged by the asbestos content of control lungs. While these conclusions suggest that the population at large is not exposed to an appreciable risk of mesothelioma from urban exposure to asbestos, vigilance should be maintained. Austrian evidence on mortality from cancer of the lung (and of the stomach) among the urban population is reassuring.[390]

Comparative Responses to the Principal Minerals

Table 23–2 separates the main components of the tissue reactions and indicates the similarities and contrasts between silica, coal, and asbestos.

Disorders Due to Other Silicates, and So Forth

Although particular minerals tend to occur in more or less concentrated deposits, their exploitation inevitably involves admixed or adjacent minerals of different types so that exposure to pure airborne dust is exceptional. In many instances the contaminating minerals constitute minor components but in other cases the mixture is both complex and variable.

Talc

Composition, Uses, and Risks

Talc is a hydrated magnesium silicate with the empiric formula $3MgO.4SiO_2.H_2O$ and it consists of a trioctahedral layer of magnesium hydroxide between two weakly held sheets of linked silica tetrahedra, the composite layers forming stacks. The particles thus possess a plate-like structure of polygonal outline and are strongly birefringent. Although possessing chemical affinities with chrysotile, talc is structurally dissimilar. It is important to distinguish talc itself from commercial talc which contains other minerals formed simultaneously and in intimate association. The contaminants principally comprise chlorite, magnesite, and dolomite though calcite, quartz, chrysotile, anthophyllite, and tremolite are common, the serpentine and amphiboles assuming the asbestiform habit.[391,392] The latter give rise to the so-called fibrous talcs. Elemental substitutions, in particular aluminium, iron, and nickel, may occur in natural talcs. High-grade nonasbestiform talc occurs in Italy, the Pyrenees, China, and India. The commercial talcs of New York State possess a variable composition in which tremolite,

Table 23—2. Primary and Secondary Responses to Compact and Fibrous Minerals

	Silica	Coal	Asbestos
Fibrous lung lesions	Sharply defined: typical structure, fibrosis exuberant	Sharply defined: typical structure, fibrosis minor	Ill-defined: nonspecific, fibrosis moderate
Pleural plaques	Exceptional or incidental	Exceptional	Characteristic
Fibrogenicity	High	Low	Low or moderate
	MFF	?MFF	MFF: possibly plus anchorage
Cytotoxicity	Severe: nonselective	Variable: nonselective	Mild: relatively selective
Lipidosis	Severe under appropriate conditions	Slight or moderate	Nil or mild
Carcinogenicity	None to lung or pleura	None to lung or pleura	Characteristic in lung and pleura
Infection	Promotion of mycobacterial growth	Liability to mycobacterial infection	Reduced resistance to viral attack
	Encouragement of virus replication	Reduced resistance to viral attack	

Abbreviation: MFF, macrophage fibrogenic factor.

anthophyllite, or serpentine may predominate, while the quartz content may be high and may even average 7.5 percent.[393] Talc from Vermont, by contrast, contains no asbestos or minimal amounts of tremolite and traces of quartz. In the United Kingdom a very limited amount of talc is recovered from Shetland, but it contains much magnesite. Soapstone constitutes a rock containing talc and other minerals.

The industrial and other applications of talc depend on its chemical inertness, laminar structure conferring high slip (nonadherence) and hence lubricating properties, high absorption, and refractoriness with low conductivity. Accordingly talc, especially high grade, is much used as a filler and extender for paints and in the pharmaceutical and cosmetic industries; for the latter quartz must not be present and the particle size such that talc will not penetrate much beyond the nose. Plastics and asphalt are also filled with talc. Ceramic insulators employ talc, as well as the pottery industry. The lubricant properties of talc find use in rubber moulding and extrusion and in keeping separate the layers of rolled roofing felt. Its heat resistance is utilized in filling mould castings, and its color is used to whiten sacks, ropes, and string. Glass moulds are dusted with talc; chocolate, rice, and chewing gum are polished with it, and paper filled with it, and it is also a vehicle for pecticides. Consumer products using talc have been shown to contain chrysotile, tremolite, and anthophyllite.

Although the rubber and roofing industries provide sources of exposure, the main risks arise in mining by open or underground methods and in milling. Correlated studies of environmental exposure, x-ray films, and pathology are few; Kleinfeld's long-term observations[394] and the National Institute of Occupational Safety and Health (NIOSH) report[395] constitute the best evidence, but dose-response relationships have not been clearly established.

Pathology and Pathogenesis

Talc pneumoconiosis was first recognized by Thorel in 1896[396] but decades elasped before other studies appeared. McLaughlin and co-workers[397] reported the first case from Great Britain and reviewed the literature.

Gross Features
Pleural adhesions are usual and, where the fiber content of the dust is high, hyaline plaques with calcification may affect the parietal layer. On section the lung may show irregularly disposed fibrosis of interstitial type, perhaps with a honeycomb structure, often most evident basally or subpleurally (Fig. 23–40). Widely scattered and ill-demarcated nodules are a feature of some cases but such lesions are not as indurated as silicotic nodules and generally lack a concentric pattern of connective tissue; however, if the dust contained a high proportion of quartz silicotic nodules may develop. Large, greyish, fibrotic masses occasionally occur and may be the seat of ischemic necrosis.[398]

Microscopic Features
The histologic changes are influenced by the composition of the dust and the amount retained. *Asbestiform talc* leads to lesions resembling those of asbestosis, that is, to focal fibrosis originating in relation to respiratory bronchioles, cellular interstitial fibrosis perhaps with cyst formation, or even solid fibrosis. Coated tremolite fibers, reacting strongly with Perls's reagent, may be seen among the connective tissue, and polarized light reveals numerous birefringent particles of talc (Fig. 23–41) free or in macrophages both interstitially and in alveoli. As the fibrosis progresses endarteritis develops. The response to *nonasbestiform talc* tends to differ in that with relative short exposure small foci of cellular fibrosis adjacent to bronchioles predominate, while after longer exposure the fibrosis becomes diffuse and confluent with many mutlinucleated giant cells containing dust (Fig. 23–42) and endarteritis.[399] Granulomatous lesions of so-called foreign body type may also be seen, consisting of macrophages, some multinucleated, with birefringent particles.[398,400] Poorly developed nodules of essentially silicotic type may occur where quartz exposure was high.

These lesions—focal fibrosis, diffuse interstitial fibrosis, ill-defined nodules, and granulomata—cannot be regarded as specific for talc and to establish the causal connection on pathologic grounds ideally requires chemical analysis, but, the occurrence of birefringent particles offers a good lead, though seen end-on they appear as needles. Electron microscopy may be needed to identify talc particles and the newer techniques of energy dispersive x-ray analysis along with x-ray crystallography firmly establish their nature.

Talc may also reach the lung via the bloodstream, since it forms a vehicle for medicaments intended to be ingested but which may be injected intravenously by drug addicts. The "talcosis" that results has loosely been designated "junkie's lung." Differentiation between the inhalation and injection routes has been postulated on the basis of the larger particle size of injected talc,[401] but surface size does not determine respirability. The aerodynamic size of talc particles is small, being determined by thickness. Hence penetration of talc particles to the alveoli is as readily achieved as that of long, thin fibers, both of which are too large to be cleared by macrophages or other means and thus remain to induce tissue changes. Cellulose, similarly administered, also leads to pulmonary granulomatosis.

Pathogenesis
Talc alone, that is, apart from contaminating fibers or quartz, was claimed to be nonfibrogenic or at most to produce a mild peribronchiolar reaction, while calcining converted talc to cristobalite, which induced fibrosis as did long tremolite fibers and talc mixed with quartz. This view was refuted by inhalation experiments in which rats were exposed to Italian talc[402,403] which had a mean particle size of 25 μm and a purity of 92 percent; chlorite and carbonate minerals were minor impurities, quartz amounted to no more than 1 percent, and asbestiform minerals were not detected. Comparison with control and other rats concurrently exposed to chrysotile showed that the extent of the fibrosis was similar for the

two dusts; small amounts of talc were effective and there was some evidence of progression after exposure.

Nonasbestiform talc may therefore be accepted as a fibrogenic agent in animals and humans, the lesions evidently proceeding through a granulomatous phase in the same location as other compact particles of relatively low fibrogenicity. Whether the occurrence of massive fibrosis depends on a complicating factor such as infection is unknown. Asbestiform talc produces lesions that reflect the fibrous component, while nodular fibrotic lesions probably depend on a high quartz content. The pathogenesis may accordingly be determined by the dominant component of the dust and it may be suggested that three forms of lesion are distinguishable depending on the talc, fiber, or quartz contents.

Morbidity and Mortality

The longitudinal studies of Kleinfeld and recent observations[404] demonstrate impairment of lung function in asbestiform talc miners and millers with over 15 years of exposure, while radiologically the prevalence of pleural thickening and calcification is greater than in coal or chrysotile workers. Cosmetic (nonasbestiform) talc induces no detectable changes in lung function. However, despite pathologic evidence of focal and diffuse fibrosis, radiologic changes and functional disturbance may be absent.[399]

As causes of death in 108 talc workers, pneumoconiosis and its complications (including cor pulmonale) and malignancy of the "lung and pleura" figured prominently[394]; the observed deaths from pulmonary and pleural neoplasms were significantly greater than expected (though data on cigarette smoking were not available) but there was no increase in gastrointestinal malignancy. Asbestiform talc miners and millers experienced significant rises in SMR for bronchogenic carcinoma, chronic nonmalignant respiratory disease, and respiratory tuberculosis[405]; the rise in SMR for bronchogenic carcinoma was much higher than cigarette smoking was thought likely to have produced, while tremolite and anthophyllite were considered the prime etiologic factors. No connection has been established between talc the mineral and mesothelioma. In nonasbestiform talc miners from Italy respiratory deaths were higher than expected, but lung cancer and cardiovascular deaths were reduced; deaths from respiratory disease (notably silicosis) were higher in miners than millers who had experienced much lower dust concentrations and a lower proportion of quartz.[406] Cosmetic grade talc was not considered to be carcinogenic in humans, a view that animal experiments have borne out.

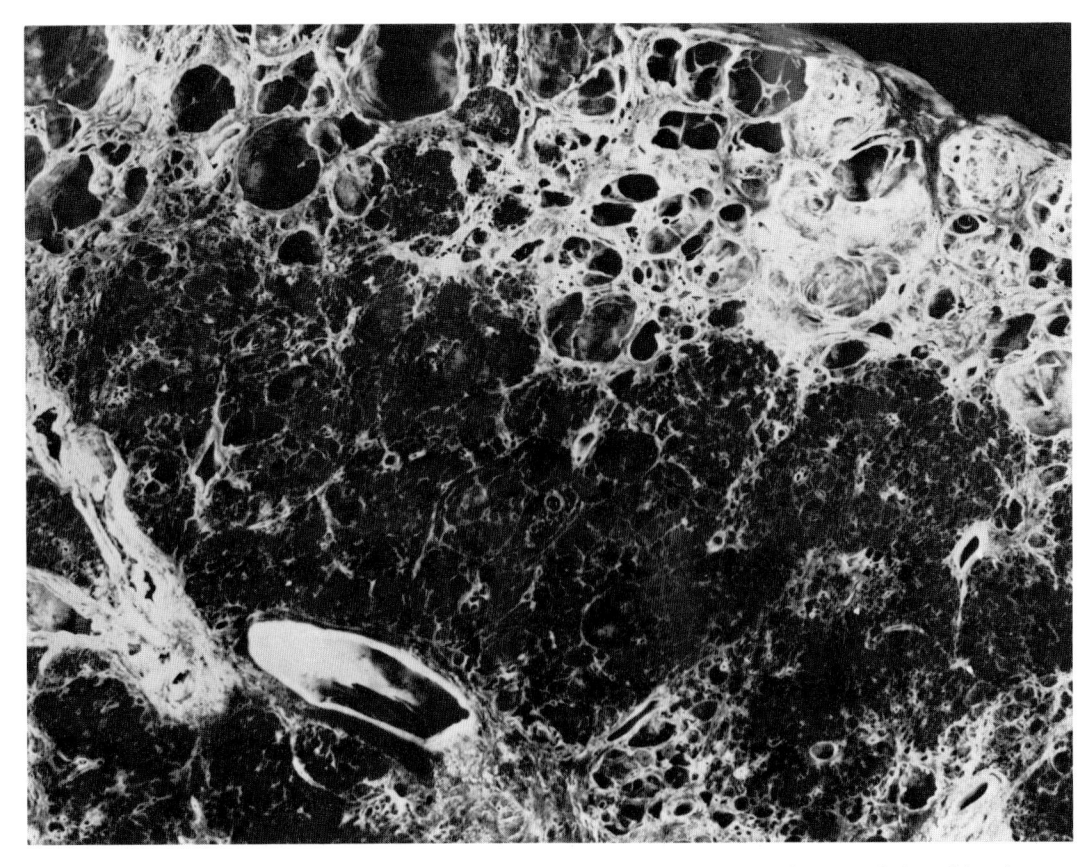

Figure 23–40. Fibrocystic reaction to asbestiform talc, occurring mainly as a subpleural band (above) in the left lower lobe. From a whole lung section (×1.5). Courtesy of Dr. Seal.

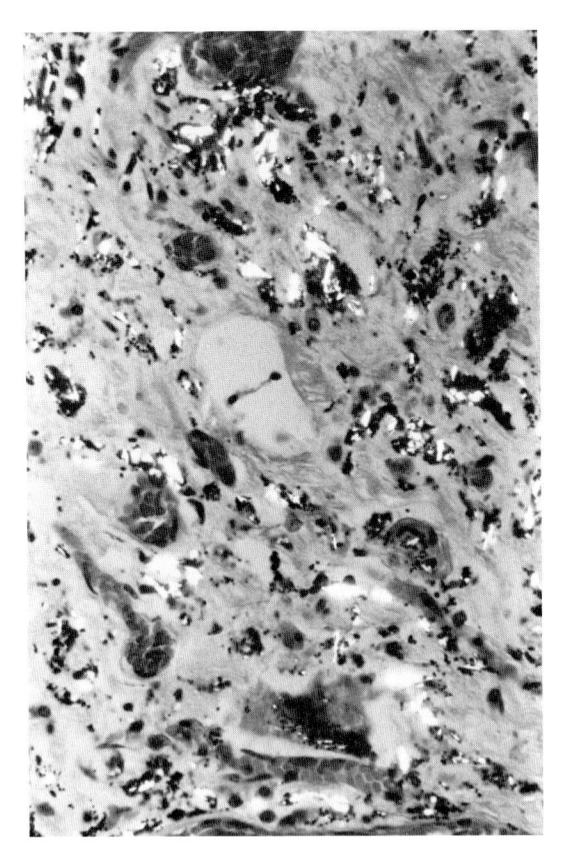

Figure 23–41. Birefringent particles of talc, mostly within macrophages which also contain carbonaceous particles, in a fibrous tract of asbestiform talcosis (H&E, ×300).

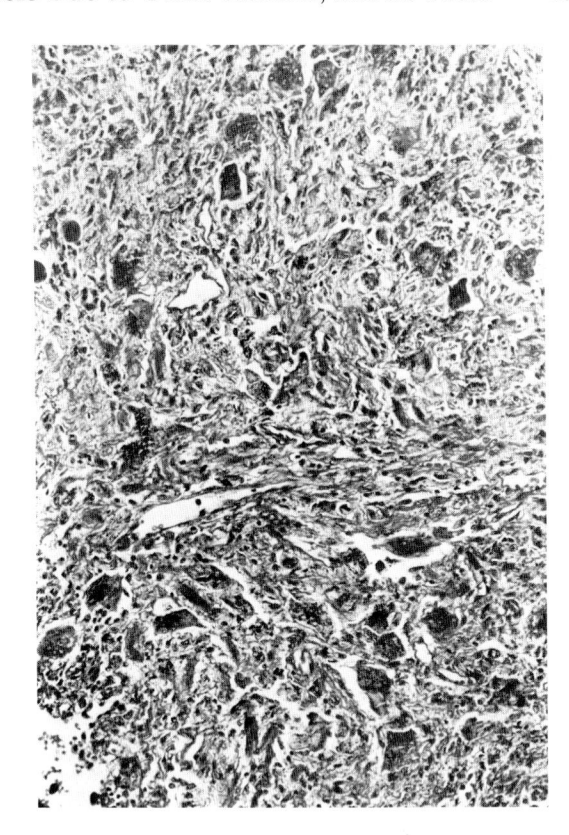

Figure 23–42. Pulmonary granulomatous lesion with numerous, multinucleated giant cells and fibrosis in nonasbestiform talcosis (H&E, ×150). Courtesy of Dr. Craighead.

Kaolin

Composition, Uses, and Risks

Otherwise known as china clay, the principal mineral of kaolin is kaolinite, a hydrated aluminium silicate [$Al_2O_3(SiO_2)_2.(H_2O)_2$] possessing a hexagonal, plate-like, nonfibrous structure and measuring 0.1 μm thick and up to 15 μm across. It is produced in several countries, notably England and United States. Cornish kaolin is abstracted by high-pressure jets of water applied to the walls of open pits, recovered by differential sedimentation to remove contaminants, and then dried either in kilns or by spraying. However, not all the quartz may be removed.

Kaolin finds application as a filler in paper, the surface of which may be coated, and in ceramics, where it is used in the production of china ware, among others. The mineral is also used as a filler in paints, plastic, and rubber, is a component of refractories, and serves as a vehicle for insecticides, cosmetics, and pharmaceuticals, as well as being a mild abrasive in tooth paste.

The dust hazard is encountered mainly in the china clay industry after drying of the product, when cleaning, bagging, and loading for transport tend to release the dust. Exposure is possible in the manufacturing applications of the clay, while in the ceramic industry crystalline silica may also be present. Radiologic evidence of pneumoconiosis occurred in 9 percent of Cornish kaolin-processing workers, including 2 percent with massive fibrosis and 5.4 percent with category 2 or 3 simple disease; in one subgroup high concentration of dust and prolonged exposure were important factors in leading to a prevalence of 23 percent.[407]

Pathology and Pathogenesis

Few instances of kaolin pneumoconiosis have come to autopsy or biopsy.[408–410] The pleura was usually adherent and thickened, the hilar nodes being enlarged, dark, and fibrosed. Grey nodular lesions up to 5 or 6 mm across occurred mostly in the upper zones of the lung and firm greyish massive lesions were also encountered, while tuberculosis cavitation has been recognized. Histologically the discrete lesions resemble coal dust macules in that dust-laden macrophages are enmeshed by reticulin and collagen fibers; although some lesions are more fibrous, the connective tissue pattern is irregular and unlike that of silicotic nodules. Dust-laden cells also occur in the alveoli and though diffuse interstitial fibrosis has been reported it may well be coincidental as in coal workers. The massive lesions consist of collagen and reticulin in which are embedded accumulations of kaolin, mostly extracellular, and there is a strong resemblance to the massive lesions of coal workers.

Lung dust analyses revealed mainly kaolin but some mica and amorphous silica although no quartz[409]; however, EDAX and x-ray diffractometry identified kaolinite but silica was not found.[410] While kaolin, like coal mine dust, did not lead to nodular pulmonary fibrosis experimentally, the conjunction with mycobacteria produced extensive lesions which regressed however.[164,411,412] Since kaolin pneumoconiosis resembles the disease in coal workers, similar pathogenetic factors evidently operate. In the reported cases quartz played no part.

Shale

The widespread occurrence of oil shales, that is, rocks containing organic compounds, renders this type of mineral an important potential substitute or supplement for natural oil or gas in producing fossil energy. Rich deposits of oil shale occur in the western United States (Colorado, Utah, and Wyoming) and in Estonia. The sedimentary rock of the United States contains layers rich in kerogen, a high molecular weight organic material which when thermally decomposed yields a dark, viscous oil that is then refined.[413,414] Estonian shale contains 37 percent organic substances, 12 percent silica (of which 42 percent is quartz and 58 percent silicates), calcium, aluminium, and iron; oil shale dust, however, has a free silica content of 3 to 4 percent.[415] Both raw and spent shale contained 9 percent quartz.[414] Extraction is by underground mining but open-cast methods may be developed. Dust concentrations may be high and the particles are largely of respirable size. Opportunities exist for atmospheric pollution by both raw and processed shale, but since this is a relatively new industry the risks are not fully known.

Küng[415] observed coniotic fibrosis of the lungs and hilar lymph nodes in oil shale workers. Discrete foci of cellular fibrosis occurred around airways and vessels, along with "perifocal" emphysema, diffuse interstitial changes, bronchitis, and bronchiolitis. The lung lesions were not severe but the hilar nodes were sclerosed and in some cases silicotic nodules occurred. A small oil shale industry formerly existed in Scotland, mainly involving mining, and in four men who developed pneumoconiosis, two cases were established by necropsy and one by lobectomy.[416] Black massive lesions up to 4.5 cm across, one with liquefaction necrosis, were encountered along with pigmented lesions resembling coal macules, and two cases also had squamous carcinoma of the lung. Many particles were birefringent. Dust extracted from the lungs had 66 to 91 percent ash made up of kaolin and mica with a small amount of free silica, the proportions corresponding with those of the natural shale. The exposure is thus similar to that of kaolin workers and the pneumoconiosis resembles that seen in coal workers.

Experimentally, oil shale dust proved to be mildly fibrogenic by intratracheal injection into rats, but the ash was more active.[415] Inhalation studies with hamsters and American raw and retorted shale produced a minimal macrophage response which was greater after injection, but fibrosis was not mentioned in these short-term observations.[417] Long-term inhalation by rats and monkeys of raw or spent shale led to accumulation of pigment-laden macrophages in the parenchyma with an inflammatory reaction but no indication of progressive fibrosis or of carcinogenesis.[414]

Preliminary population studies in Estonia do not suggest a particular liability of oil shale workers to pulmonary or gastric carcinoma though skin cancer is a hazard.[418] Up to 1984 silicosis emerged as the greatest risk to oil shale workers in the United States, with pneumoconiosis of coal worker's type constituting a lesser and lung cancer a very small risk. Scottish oil shale workers experienced an excess of deaths from cancer of the skin but not of the lung, while the prevalence of simple and complicated pneumoconiosis was low.

Fuller's Earth

Composition, Uses, and Risks

Fulling is the name given to the process of removing grease from wool to cleanse and thicken it, and the material used is a clay mineral with adsorbent properties which has an approximate empiric formula of $(AlFeMg)_4Si_8O_{22}(OH)_4$, though the proportions of the three associated metals are variable. This compound is known as montmorillonite and fuller's earth is the calcium derivative, which in the lump looks like olive-green soap. Deposits occur in England, the United States, and Germany, extraction being by open-case quarrying followed by milling, drying, and grinding. This natural soapy fuller's earth may be "activated" by soda ash to give a greater swelling ability. In English material impurities are few, quartz rare, and the crystals are very small, while the quartz content may be greater in U.S. deposits.

Although formerly important in the British woollen industry, fuller's earth now serves as a base for cosmetic and pharmaceutical powders, and its adsorbent properties are used to decolorize lubricating, technical, and edible oils. It also finds application as a bonding agent in foundry moulds, a filler and a stabilizer of emulsion paints, and as a mud in oil well drilling.

Dust generation seems to be associated particularly with mining and bagging, but there appears to be no risk from secondary processes in industry or when fuller's earth is used as a cosmetic.

Pathology and Pathogenesis

All patient's coming to autopsy were exposed to fuller's earth from Surrey, England.[419–421]

Small nodules two or more millimeters in diameter occupy mainly the upper zones of the lung where some confluence may occur. They are round, firm, and black but not hard like silicotic nodules. Pleural adhesions may be seen and the hilar nodes appear black. The lesions lie in relation to respiratory bronchioles and consist of dust-laden macrophages among which reticulin fibers run irregularly. Many particles are birefringent.

X-ray and electron diffraction of extracted or in situ dust showed it to consist of montmorillonite along with feldspar, but no kaolin or mica was detected.[421] The structure of the lesion bears a strong similarity to that of the coal dust macule and presumably arises in a similar manner. In these cases there was no evidence of tuberculosis or of massive fibrosis. This variety of pneumoconiosis is rare, requires prolonged and intense exposure, and is unlikely to affect life expectancy or introduce complications.

Bentonite

The term bentonite derives from Fort Benton in Wyoming, where a major deposit of montmorillonite, mainly in the sodium form, is located. The clay originates by devitrification of volcanic ash deposited in water and the free silica content varies from less than 1 percent to over 24 percent.[422] Mining is open-cast but milling occurs indoors. The crushed clay is dried after which bagging and loading create most dust, settled or airborne specimens of which contain appreciable amounts of cristobalite. It is not certain whether the latter occurs in the parent material or is formed by thermal conversion during drying. Bentonite clays possess great water-retaining properties and the extracted product is used as lubricant in oil-well drilling, ceramics, foundry mould bonding, and as a carrier for insecticides and fungicides.

Minimal to advanced radiologic silicosis was found in 14 cases and one lung biopsy disclosed a silicotic reaction.[422] Tuberculosis consitutes a complication and the disease may be totally disabling. Although bentonite itself has been regarded as innocuous, there is no doubt that the risk depends on the free silica content.

Micas and Sillimanites

Minerals of the mica group exist as sheet-like lattices which characteristically cleave into thin layers. They are complex silicates of potassium and aluminium (muscovite or white mica); magnesium, aluminium, iron and potassium (biotite); magnesium and aluminium (phlogopite); or aluminium and potassium (sericite), which is fibrous in form. Muscovite comes from India, Africa, and the United States and its heat and electrical resistances enable it to be used as a window in stoves and as an electrical insulator; when crushed it serves similar uses to talc. Biotite acts as a filler and coating agent, while phlogopite is employed as a high-temperature electrical insulator.

Radiologic evidence of pneumoconiosis occurred in 17 percent of men exposed to pulverized mica though the dust contained almost no free silica; radiologic silicosis was encountered in 3 percent of workers in pegmatite, a mixture of mica, quartz, and feldspar (aluminium silicates with potassium, sodium, or calcium).[423] Pigmented fibrosis (diffuse and massive) and biotite occurred in the lungs of a rubber worker, but other causes could not be excluded.[424] Exposure to muscovite led to ill-defined nodules up to 15 mm across together with smaller, circumscribed lesions, especially in the basal regions of the lungs; mineral crystals lay between collagen fibers, while histiocytes and foreign body giant cells were also present.[425] Experimentally mica induced focal dust cell granulomata, reticulin, and some collagenous fibrosis in rats. The particles are birefringent. Sericite achieved a transitory notoriety when it was proposed as the casual agent in silicosis.

Silicate pneumoconiosis has recently been described in farm workers,[426] zoo animals,[427] and horses,[428] In the former, birefringent particles accumulated focally in macrophages, occupying alveoli in relation to respiratory airways and exciting slight to severe fibrosis. X-ray analysis identified mostly silicates of the mica group in lung and soil samples along with some silica and the silicates may have come from pesticides or the soil itself. Birefringent particles of mica and illite were also identified in the simple pneumoconiosis of mammals and birds as well as in air samples from the zoo, but cristobalite was blamed for the disease in horses. It is premature, however, to suggest that simple pneumoconiosis is likely to be widespread in humans residing in desert or semidesert climates.

The sillimanites are aluminium silicates with a fibrous form used to make temperature-resistant refractories such as sparking plugs. No acceptable case of human disease has apparently resulted from handling sillimanite and experimental evidence supports its inertness.

Nepheline

Reference (see Disorders Due to Coal Mine and Carbonaceous Dusts, Coal Worker's Pneumoconiosis, Pathogenesis, Complicated Pneumoconiosis, The Quartz Factor, above) has been made to Barrie and Gosselin's[156] case, in which simple dust deposits and massive fibrosis occurred in a man exposed to the feldspar albite, which is a silicate of sodium, potassium, and aluminium used for glazing and filling. This rock contained no free silica and the pulmonary reaction differed from that in coal workers only in its grey color. Nepheline syenite, with which free silica is incompatible, comes mainly from Ontario and 14 individuals engaged in milling developed radiologic pinhead mottling and areas of conglomeration.[429] The disease was confirmed pathologically in four cases, forming small and large aggregates of dust with reticulin fibrosis. Further cases are not anticipated since dust levels have been much reduced.

Volcanic Ash

The opportunity to study volcanic ash that had recently been airborne was grasped when Mount St. Helens erupted in May 1980. The principal mineral components of the ash comprised volcanic glass or pumice and crystalline feldspar and orthopyroxene, with crystalline silica as quartz, tridymite, or cristobalite forming 1 to 3 percent of bulk samples and 1 to 2 percent of respirable fractions,[430] though another analysis of respirable dust gave a crystalline silica content of about 7.2 percent, 4.2 percent being cristobalite and 3 percent quartz.[431] Given intratrechally to rats, ash led to mononuclear accumulation without much toxicity and a limited linear fibrosis in a minority of animals along with moderate lipo-proteinosis; quartz by comparison induced nodular lesions that fibrosed and lipo-proteinosis.[432] The lymph nodes of rats given ash showed numerous microgranulomata whereas quartz led to pronounced fibrosis. Longer survival after injection of ash containing 7.2 percent crystalline silica indicated that the granulomatous and fibrotic reaction persisted, while heavily exposed humans developed either a giant-cell granuloma or an interstitial reaction.[433] No biochemical or histologic changes were detected in normal rats or rats with elastase-induced emphysema followed for up to a year after brief inhalation of fine volcanic ash, sulfur dioxide, or both combined.[433a] Individuals caught in the heavy fallout mostly died from asphyxia, the inhaled ash with mucus forming occlusive plugs in the upper airways.[434] The preliminary results thus raise the possibility of a pneumoconiosis risk from volcanic ash, but the consequences to humans of long-term exposure to low concentrations are not only unknown but seem unlikely to be realized.

Fly Ash

Fly ash is the particulate material emitted with the effluent from coal-fired power stations and, since as much as 5 million tons may be dispersed into the atmosphere annually in the United States, concern grew about the general environmental effects of the ash whether alone or in combination with gaseous pollutants. The only biologic approach was experimental.

Silicon is the major element in fly ash (collected by high-volume sampling) along with aluminum, iron, calcium, magnesium, and other elements, the main compound being an aluminosilicate.[435] Long-term exposure of monkeys to low particle concentrations (comparable to urban experience) of respirable size indicated no functional disturbances and no serious morphologic abnormalities, the only histologic feature being the formation of small alveolar aggregates of dust-laden macrophages. Chronic inhalation studies of respirable fly ash in rats led to small lung burdens and no microscopic changes apart from an increase in lung macrophages; an increase of colony-forming units from lavaged macrophages was held to indicate local recruitment.[436] Trace elements in fly ash could pose special problems though chronic inhalation experiments in hamsters suggested that nickel enrichment did not enhance the pathogenicity of fly ash.[437] Monkeys and guinea pigs exposed to prolonged inhalation of fly ash and sulfur dioxide revealed no adverse effects, which were confined to accumulation of dust-bearing macrophages in lung and nodes.[438] Sulfur dioxide thus possesses no apparent enhancing effect on fly ash. The idea that, in humans fly ash might lead to honeycomb lung[439] is unjustified, since in the case reported asbestos fibers, a known cause, were also indentified; this account illustrates the danger of attributing the fibrocystic state to particulate matter that probably accumulated coincidentally [see Disorders Due to Coal Mine and Carbonaceous Dusts, Differentiation of Emphysematous and Fibrocystic States in Coal Workers, Fibrocystic Disease of the Lung (Honeycomb Lung), above]. To date the position is reassuring so far as the fibrotic reaction to the particles is concerned but carcinogenicity requires longer to explore in view of the presence of radioactive elements (alpha-emitters) in fly ash.[440]

Fuel ash after pulverization is widely used in road works, concretes, and building blocks, and consists mostly of glass particles with a crystalline element of up to 30 percent which includes quartz, but cell studies do not suggest toxicity.

Silicon Carbide

Also known as Carborundum, silicon carbide is much used as an artificial abrasive of remarkable hardness, capable of resisting solution by hydrofluoric acid which dissolves silica. Ground carbon (as petroleum coke) and silica with sawdust are first fused in an electric furnace and then ground, sieved, or elutriated before bonding with materials that used to contain crystalline silica though silica-free substitutes or self-bonding are now available. Radiologic evidence of pneumoconiosis has been reported in silicon carbide workers, but dust compositions were lacking and quartz participation cannot be eliminated. However, exposure of animals to high concentrations of Carborundum failed to induce pulmonary fibrosis.[27] Quartz may be inhaled from materials used in its manufacture and iron or quartz particles may be generated from employment of the abrasive, but pneumoconiosis rarely arises and there is no firm evidence to incriminate silicon carbide itself.

Nonsiliceous Dusts

Cement

Cement is used on an enormous scale and several raw materials enter into its manufacture. The basis is limestone or chalk to which is added clay or shale, together with gypsum plus a small amount of sand or quartz dust. The raw materials are crushed and ground, and mixed in appropriate proportions for calcination in rotary kilns to eliminate moisture and form clinker of calcium silicates and aluminates with very little quartz. To control setting gypsum is added to the clinker before grinding to a fine powder. Blast furnace slag may also be used for direct production of cement. Radiologic surveys of numerous employees in several countries have disclosed no abnormalities apart from the occasional development of nodules in men exposed to higher quartz contamination. Being hygroscopic, cement dust probably forms aggregates in the upper respiratory tract and these are too large to penetrate to the alveolar level; moreover, the quartz particles in raw dust are relatively large.

Gypsum

Gypsum, a hydrated calcium sulphate, is a well-known and long-used building material and an important component of cement. It is extracted by open-cast working or underground mining in the United States, Europe, and Russia, and the associated strata may contribute a small amount of quartz. Crushing and calcining are deployed to produce plasters and plaster board as well as to make surgical casts. Gypsum is virtually devoid of effect in human beings and does not induce fibrosis experimentally. Small nodular lesions in the radiograph indicate silicosis of mild degree.

Limestone

A calcareous material, limestone commonly contains a small proportion of quartz, though rarely this is as much as 15 percent. Workers in pure limestone do not develop pneumoconiosis, but when there is a siliceous component a disabling pneumoconiosis may follow.

Metallic Dusts

In this category are included not only metals but also their inorganic compounds, mostly oxides. Inhaled in particulate form some metals lead to serious consequences, but others are harmless and have acquired the designation of "nuisance" dusts because their high atomic numbers confer radio-opacity and they thus require differentiation from other nodular shadows, an exercise in which the occupational history assumes importance. The situation may, however, be complicated when fibrogenic particles such as quartz contaminate inert dusts.

Beryllium Disease

The deleterious effects of beryllium compounds whether as dusts or fumes are not confined to the lungs and may indeed be restricted to the skin, so that it is prefereable to refer to beryllium disease rather than to beryllium pneumoconiosis in order to convey the systemic nature of the disorder.

Composition and Uses

The source of the metal and its compounds is beryl (Greek *beryllos*) ore, beryllium aluminium silicate with the empirical formula $3BeO \cdot Al_2O_3 \cdot 6SiO_2$, mined in South America, Southern Africa, Australia, and India. Bertrandite, a hydrated beryllium silicate $[Be(OH)_2Si_2O_7]$, occurs in Utah and is mined for its BeO content. Extraction as the oxide is effected by treatment of the milled ore with either sulfuric acid or sodium silicofluoride followed by calcination. Beryllium is usually employed as an alloy with copper which is greatly strengthened and becomes nonmagnetic, though for particular industrial purposes other types of alloy are needed and contain less beryllium than the basic form. Extraction and the manufacture of master and industrial alloys as well as machining and drilling create dust and fume, as may reclamation of nonferrous scrap metals. Beryllium was formerly used extensively as a phosphor of zinc and magnesium beryllium silicate in fluorescent lighting tubes and led to recognition of a particularly hazardous form of occupational exposure. The phosphor dust containing beryllium oxide escaped during coating and also from accidental breakage of tubes, but manufacture was abolished some 30 years ago. The hardness, strength, and corrosion resistance of the metal make it invaluable in metallurgic technology, the lightness of the particles of metal or compounds rendering them easily airborne. Nonferrous alloys form the basis of integrated circuits and are used in atomic reactors and space capsule heat shields. Beryllium metal is employed in x-ray tubes and there may be a risk from rocket exhausts since it has been used in the propellant. Because of its stability and high thermal conductivity the oxide is employed in ceramics and in jet engine blades.

The Risks

General acceptance of the beryllium hazard is largely to the credit of Dr. Harriet L. Hardy, who in 1952 instituted the Beryllium Case Registry in the United States. She had to overcome official public health and industrial denials of the harmfulness of beryllium exposure combined with obstructive legal stratagems, despite evidence to the contrary from Europe and Russia as well as the United States itself.[441] Up to the end of 1977, the Registry had 887 cases on file, of which 631 were classified as chronic, 212 as acute, and 44 as acute becoming chronic; 46 percent of patients were known to have died.[442] Fluorescent tube manufacture provided the early cases, but in the period 1973–1977, when 55 cases were added, tubes still accounted for 31 percent, with metal products, especially alloys, contributing 45.5 percent and extraction plus smelting 12.7 percent. Beryllium disease is thus a continuing occupational hazard and stress should be laid on the long latent period, since of the cases reported in the final 5-year period over half were first exposed before 1950, as well as on the relatively recent exposures and the current use of beryllium especially in electronics and nuclear productions.

The prevalence, let alone the attack rate, of beryllium disease is difficult to estimate since the size of the populations at risk is unknown and many cases are believed to be undiagnosed; moreover, the beryllium contents of the lungs and viscera have not always been available. Both sexes are equally vulnerable though at first females predominated because of their employment in fluorescent lamp manufacture. Hardy emphasizes not only the systemic character of the disease but also that the illness is both job and dose related. With better environmental control the latent period of beryllium disease is apparently lengthening and its severity diminishing. Laboratory work has led to development of the disease.[443] Those not directly employed in the preparation or application of beryllium or its compounds, including even office staff, have been affected; neighborhood and domestic cases from contaminated clothing have also occurred. The risk from atmospheric contamination by beryllium in the effluent from coal-burning power stations is unknown.

Pathology

The pulmonary manifestations take two forms. The acute variety consists of a chemical pneumonitis, though the upper respiratory tract is also affected, arising from fumes or dusts and it is customary to confine the term to cases of less than 1 year in duration. Chronic disease may follow acute or be insidious with a long latent period and takes the form of a fibrosing granuloma.

Acute Type

Grossly the lungs are heavy, consolidated, and retain their shape. A fibrinous exudate may be seen on the pleura. The cut surface appears pink or greyish and a frothy exudate may be expressed. The mucosa of the main airways is reddened and the hilar nodes enlarged. Histologically the pneumonitis is extensive and bilateral, showing pronounced oedema and exudation with hyperaemia and some diapedesis. The exudate, however, exhibits peculiarities in that there is a striking paucity of polymorphs while plasma cells, lymphocytes, and macrophages fill alveolar spaces and infiltrate their walls and the adventitia of arterioles and bronchioles. Strands of fibrin run between the cells. The reaction may be pronounced around arterioles, and endarteritis may occur and thrombosis follow. Acute bronchitis and bronchiolitis are sometimes so severe that the smaller lumina are occluded by exudate and desquamated epithelial cells. In some cases the distribution of the changes is patchy, macrophages predominate and organization may follow, but granulomas are not a feature.[444,445] The hilar nodes show reactive changes. Recovery is usually complete, the only residue being a minor degree of fibrosis. Acute pneumonitis is now a rare event.[442]

Chronic Type

The changes assume an entirely different character. The pleura is thickened and usually adherent, while the surface of the lung may appear cobbled. On section the lungs show considerable fibrosis with which cyst formation may be associated. Small, firm nodules, a few millimeters in diameter, may also be detected. The hilar nodes are somewhat enlarged and usually show areas of fibrosis. These features are not specific.

The microscopic appearances assume two main forms, a diffuse interstitial pneumonitis and discrete granulomatous lesions. The diffuse change affects most alveolar walls, many of which are much thickened by accumulation of lymphocytes, plasma cells, and mononuclear cells with connective tissue formation, while capillaries are inconspicuous. In consequence alveolar spaces are distorted and reduced in size, though macrophages and giant cells may be found in the lumina. More common, however, are the noncaseating granulomata, which consist of epithelioid cells, including typical Langhans giant cells especially in the larger lesions, surrounded by lymphocytes and plasma cells, located interstitially, subpleurally, and around vessels and airways. Rarely larger than a millimeter, the granulomata are widely distributed and while some are essentially cellular others show fibrosis without particular pattern and are evidently more mature (Fig. 23–43). The lesions sometimes become confluent and larger areas of fibrosis are then seen with the cellular response peripherally. Interspersed between the fibrotic areas enlarged spaces may develop giving a honeycomb structure, the cysts showing the usual variety in epithelial lining. Nodular, hyaline, fibrotic lesions measuring several millimeters across and sometimes showing central necrosis with calcification are also a feature in about 40 percent of cases and may predominate[445]; the whorled pattern of the fibrosis resembles that of the silicotic nodule though the other changes are peculiar to beryllium disease. A diffuse interstitial fibrosis is present in approximately half the cases and presumably derives from the diffuse pneumonitis; granulomata may be incorporated. Endarteritis obliterans occurs in areas of more severe fibrosis. The hilar nodes exhibit similar granulomata with hyalinization and fibrous nodules also form. Granulomata may also be found occasionally in distant lymph nodes, spleen, liver and bone marrow, kidneys, and muscle. Skin granulomata may follow traumatic introduction of beryllium compounds and may also follow inhalation and precede clinical pulmonary involvement.

Inclusion bodies within giant cells and occasionally epithelioid cells are a characteristic finding and assume three forms.[446] Asteroid bodies, now known to be composed of microfilaments and microtubules, are relatively uncommon; laminated conchoidal (Schaumann) bodies composed of calcium and mucoprotein and up to 50 μm across are frequent but not invariable, as are birefringent plate-like crystals (appearing as spicules when seen end-on) probably of calcite up to 10 μm long occurring singly or in clumps mostly within conchoidal bodies. Extrusion of the latter places them extracellularly and they may then provoke a foreign body–type giant cell reaction. The presence of inclusions has no diagnostic value, since they occur in sarcoidosis, histoplasmosis and tuberculosis. Histologic classification of chronic beryllium disease based on the predominance of the interstitial cellular infiltration, granuloma formation and prominence of conchoidal bodies[445] is of uncertain prognostic value since extent of the disease is likely to be determinant.

The beryllium granuloma and the lesion of sarcoidosis bear strong resemblances, so much so that no fundamental differences have been found by conventional microscopy, including enzyme histochemistry, or ultrastructurally. Most epitheliod cells of beryllium granulomata possess numerous large membrane-limited vesicles, prominent Golgi complexes but relatively small mitochondria, features that are shared with the epithelioid cell of sarcoidosis and of the zirconium-induced granuloma[447–449] and that suggest a secretory role. The tuberculosis epithelioid cell typically exhibits abundant rough endoplasmic reticulum, large mitochondria, many free ribosomes, and smaller vesicles; such cells may be in a synthetic phase which gradually converts to the vesicular or storage form, though these relationships are debated. Tissue analysis for beryllium provides important confirmatory evidence and may be of diagnostic value in biopsy material from the minority of dubious cases. The element has been detected in lung, hilar, and other lymph nodes, liver, skin, and other tissues by spectrographic methods. The technique favored for specificity and sensitivity is a modified Morin fluorometric procedure and a level of 0.02 μg/g has been found only in exposed individuals, that is, not in sarcoidosis or normal urban subjects.[442] However, the beryllium content does not necessarily parallel the severity of the disease and the element may be irregularly distributed in the lungs. In beryllium disease the hilar nodes are less affected and the distribution of the changes is more limited than in sarcoidosis.

Hypercalciuria is a feature of beryllium disease, as of sarcoidosis, and stone formation may occur; calcium is apparently absorbed from the gut and osteosclerosis may follow.[441] Hyperuricaemia also characterizes some cases of beryllium disease (and sarcoidosis) and correlates with its severity, though interstitial pneumonitis and fibrosis are more characteristic of beryllium disease.

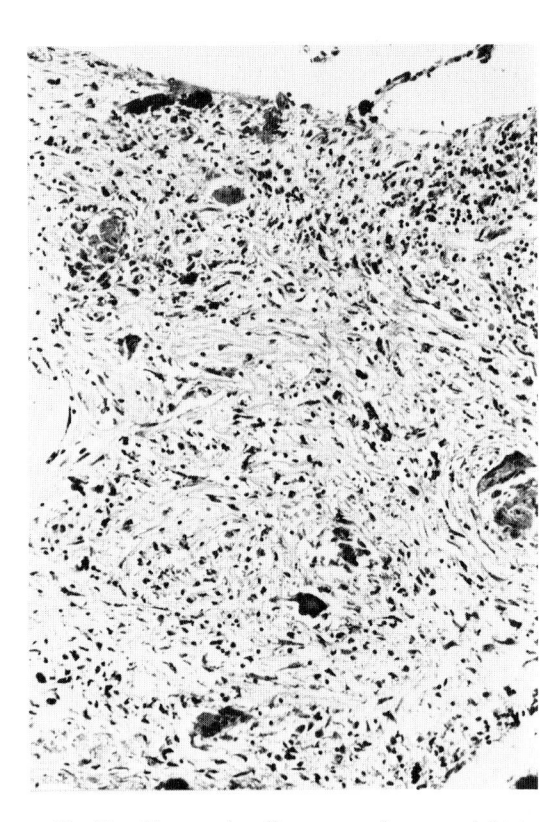

Figure 23–43. Human beryllium granuloma, exhibiting ill-defined follicles in which multinucleated giant cells occur (H&E, ×150).

Pathogenesis

Beryllium and its compounds may be handled safely with a dose level of 2–5 μg/m^3 for a 40-hour week, but higher levels and duration, particle size, and solubility determine the severity of the response.[441] The acute disorder is considered to be chemically induced[450] and chronic disease has been reproduced experimentally[451] but development of this phase seems to involve an immunologic component. The Kveim reaction is, however, negative and tuberculin reactivity is unaffected. Blast transformation of lymphocytes in the presence of BeSO$_4$ occurred in 71 percent of patients with chronic disease (despite steroid therapy) and serum IgA levels were elevated in almost 50 percent of cases.[452] A classical delayed hypersensitivity reaction to beryllium compounds was obtained in guinea pigs and there was good correlation with the presence of migration inhibition factor,[453] an association that also occurred in patients with experimentally induced beryllium granulomata of the skin.[454] Human and experimental evidence thus suggests a type IV hypersensitivity response in the chronic condition, and the beryllium lymphocyte transformation test appears to be a sensitive and reliable adjunct to diagnosis and a means of population screening.[455,456] Caution is necessary, however, in using the Curtis cutaneous patch test which may induce hypersensitivity. The low apparent attack rate of beryllium disease may indicate individual susceptibility.

Complications

Cor pulmonale, respiratory failure and pneumothorax are well known and the first two often prove fatal, but there is no predisposition to tuberculosis. Renal failure from nephrolithiasis is occasionally encountered. In animals beryllium salts proved to be rachitogenic, possibly through inactivation of alkaline phosphatase.

The most serious consequence of beryllium exposure to emerge is neoplasia. Beryllium compounds proved carcinogenic to three species of animal including primates by injection or inhalation, leading to osteosarcoma and pulmonary carcinoma.[457] Exposed humans experienced a significantly increased risk of neoplastic and non-neoplastic respiratory disease and of heart disease, notably lung cancer among long exposed individuals in whom cigarette smoking and other factors seemed unlikely to be responsible.[458] A cohort[459] provided results consistent with those of other epidemiologic studies demonstrating that beryllium is carcinogenic to the lung. No one histologic type of bronchogenic carcinoma predominated though a deficit of squamous carcinoma occurred.[460] How beryllium acts is uncertain, though it is known to augment infidelity of DNA synthesis. Experimental evidence, based on pulmonary aryl hydrocarbon hydroxylase activity, suggested that beryllium did not serve as a cocarcinogen by affecting the metabolism of carcinogenic polycyclic hydrocarbons in the lung.[461]

Aluminium

Uses and Risks

Because of its lightness and strength metallic aluminium forms an important component of alloys such as Duralumin, but it is also employed in a finely divided state for the manufacture of explosives and fireworks (hence the commercial term "pyro"), as a spreader for paints, and in wrapping foils and refractories. The oxide, alumina (Al_2O_3), occurs in crystalline form as corundum, but for making artificial abrasives bauxite is the raw material, the ore being obtained in the United States, Brazil, and elsewhere. Aluminium is obtained by smelting or electrolytic extraction of bauxite. Artificial corundum (emery) is made from the calcined and crushed raw material, mixed with coke to reduce oxides and iron turnings to remove impurities, by fusion in an electric furnace with carbon electrodes at a temperature of about 2000°C.[462] During the fusion process dense white fumes are evolved and consist largely of alumina and amorphous silica, which may be concentrated in the fines. The atmosphere also contains bauxite dust, some particles of which are respirable in size. All elements in the fume were also present in the lung ash from exposed workers, with high proportions of alumina and silica.[463] Aluminium metal used as a powder assumes two forms according to the method of preparation, a granular type made from molten metal and a flake type produced by stamping the cold metal. Granular aluminium has a particle size mostly beyond the respirable range while flake aluminium is largely of respirable size. Separation of flake particles is assisted by the addition of stearine, a mixture of fatty acids, or mineral oil. During and after World War II stearine was unobtainable in Germany and a mineral wax was substituted; partial replacement by mineral oil also occurred for a time in Britain. Around these periods pulmonary fibrosis was ascribed to aluminium dust[464–468] but cases still occur.[469]

Pathology

Pulmonary changes resulting from employment in the alumina abrasive industry were first recognized by Shaver, the condition becoming eponymous, and in one of his later accounts[470] reported 35 well-established cases with 10 deaths, 9 in patients who had experienced bilateral pneumothorax. Accounts of the pathologic changes soon followed.[471,472] Aluminium dust led to similar lung lesions.

Grossly, the lungs were sometimes shrunken, the pleura thickened, adherent, and often pebbled, with surface bullae an almost invariable feature. The cut surface revealed grey pigmentation with dark bands and masses of fibrous tissue, generally affecting central areas; the bands were 2 to 4 cm wide and finer tracts extended centrally and peripherally where irregular zones of coarse emphysema occurred. No fibrous nodules were detected. The hilar nodes were pigmented and slightly enlarged but not fibrosed.

Microscopically, the fibrosis had a diffuse distribution, obliterating much of the normal architecture and incorporating dust-laden phagocytes. Adjacent alveolar walls showed fibrous thickening and fibroblasts along with mononuclear cells, and lymphocytes might be evident. Alveolar spaces contained dust cells, sometimes numerous, and giant cells surrounding crystal clefts could be prominent. Parenchyma intervening between fibrous strands often showed enlarged spaces and bronchiolectasis, the spaces having a lining of cuboidal cells sometimes with squamous metaplasia. Endarteritis obliterans was a frequent occurrence, while lipidosis and tuberculosis affected individual cases. No silicotic nodules were found in the lungs or hilar lymph nodes, where dust-laden phagocytes accumulated along with a small amount of connective tissue. Aurine staining has been employed to identify aluminium in the tissues.

Pathogenesis

Fibrosis has mostly occurred from exposure to flake aluminium, in the preparation of which oil has replaced stearine in whole or in part. Contact between tissues and the metal was believed to be prevented by a surface layer of inert alumina in the case of granular aluminium, while stearine was considered to prevent oxidation of the flakes but mineral oil or wax was thought to be more readily removed and so expose the metal. Granular and stearine-containing aluminium were nonreactive with water, but in the presence of oil the metal reacted vigorously; granular aluminium proved weakly fibrogenic in rats, whereas the flake was strongly fibrogenic irrespective of whether stearine or oil or neither was present.[473] The protective effect of stearine was not therefore established, as was also apparent in a patient in whom a stearine-containing powder was held responsible for pulmonary fibrosis.[474]

The role of aluminium thus appears doubtful, especially since human cases of pulmonary fibrosis are few despite a large work force, while the experimental findings depend on big doses and the granular material has a large particle size. Moreover, a species difference exists in the fibrogenicity of metallic aluminium and hydrated alumina. The silica in the fume from abrasive manufacture is amorphous, any crystalline forms undergoing temperature conversion into a glassy state, fine particles of which were found not to be fibrogenic in the lungs of rats and guinea pigs.[475] If the participation of aluminium and silica is open to question, an alternative explanation is required. The pathologic features suggest pigmentation of fibrocystic disease of the lung of nonspecific type (in which pneumothorax may be a feature) rather than pneumoconiosis. Accordingly it may be suggested that affected individuals have developed patchy consolidation or collapse with organization as a result of banal and probably unrecorded infections (to which the occupational environment may have contributed) and that aluminium and other particulates have been incorporated incidentally. Alternatively or additionally the fatty content of flake material may excite a lipid reaction and progress to honeycombing. The aluminium powders employed in the treatment of silicosis corresponded with the granular type.

Aluminium has recently come under suspicion as a lung carcinogen.[476]

Hard-Metal Disease

Possessing extreme hardness and heat resistance, tungsten carbide (that is, hard-metal) is employed extensively in the machine tool industry, in bearings and alloys, dental and other drills. It is produced by blending finely divided tungsten and carbon in an electric furnace in an atmosphere of hydrogen and then milling with 5 to 25 percent cobalt which serves as a matrix for the crystals of tungsten carbide. To this mixture may be added other metals such as titanium, tantalum, or vanadium according to the desired properties. After adding wax, the mixture is pressed into ingots prior to fusing (sintering) in an electric furnace.[477] The particle size of all constituents is 1 to 2 μm,[478] but few exposed individuals develop respiratory disease.

Several accounts of pathology have appeared,[477–483] the gross and microscopical features suggesting a diffuse fibrosis with no suggestion of silicosis or sarcoidosis. The disorder assumes the form of a chronic interstitial pneumonitis in which dust-laden phagocytes, lymphocytes, and plasma cells, and sometimes mast cells, are enmeshed by widespread though patchy fibrosis. Cystic spaces may develop in uninvolved parenchyma and be lined by cuboidal epithelium. Type II alveolar epithelial cells become hyperplastic and sometimes multinucleated. The alveoli contain macrophages which may be multinucleate and particles thought to be tungsten carbide sometimes appear in these cells. Tungsten, cobalt, and titanium have been found in the lungs of a few individuals.

Because tungsten and tantalum in particulate form proved relatively harmless to animals' lungs but cobalt was more irritant, leaving an obliterative bronchiolitis and focal pneumonitis, the latter element has been held responsible for the pulmonary fibrosis in humans, though there was no correlation between the severity of the disease and the cobalt content of the lung.[478] As with aluminium, the features suggest nonspecific fibrocystic disease and the same question must be asked, that is, whether hard-metal disease is a distinct entity or another example of pigment accumulating in diffuse interstitial fibrosis from an unrelated cause. No certain answer is possible without controlled epidemiological observations. A restrictive syndrome with low diffusing capacity developed and cor pulmonale followed.[478] Cobalt but not tungsten induced symptoms on inhalation and a sensitivity phenomenon was suggested, especially as cobalt alone proved toxic to leucocytes from sufferers.[484]

Nickel

Nickel ore comes mainly from Ontario, though smaller deposits are located in the USSR, Cuba, New Caledonia, Norway, and elsewhere. The metal has wide applications in the chemical industry and in metallurgy, being used for plating, alloys (notably stainless steel), storage batteries, resins, pigments, and as a catalyst. The ore is refined either by smelting and electrolytic separation or by the Mond process in which carbon monoxide reacts with the impure nickel powder to form nickel carbonyl [$Ni(CO)_4$] as a vapor. The latter is then heated at 180°C to release the carbon monoxide and deposit the highly purified nickel.

From a large refinery in Wales—the original Mond works—where Canadian ore was and is processed, five cases of diffuse interstitial fibrosis were reported, two developing honeycomb lung and dying with cor pulmonale, these changes being regarded as infective rather than industrial in origin.[485] Of these five patients, three developed squamous and one alveolar cell carcinoma; excess Ni and Cu were present in the lungs of two patients but arsenic was not detected.

Inhaled nickel increased the susceptibility of mice to subsequent pulmonary infection by inhibiting the activity of cilia and the ability of alveolar macrophages to ingest and kill *Staphylococcus pyogenes*, the immunologic response also being inhibited.[486] Nickel fibrogenesis could therefore arise mainly from macrophage involvement and impaired defense against bacteria, so accounting for the fibrotic and cystic changes.

Of deaths in Welsh nickel workers 35 percent were due to cancer of the lung or nose.[487] The risk for nasal cancer in this refinery was several hundred times the national average and for lung cancer 6 to 11 times, but with improved industrial conditions these risks were eliminated.[488] Norwegian nickel workers likewise experienced a persistent high risk of nasal and lung cancer,[489] as did Canadian refiners in respect of the lung.[490] Lung cancer mortality proved to be two to four times higher in USSR nickel refiners than in the general population.[491] However, no firm evidence of a special liability to develop lung cancer has yet been detected in men exposed to metallic nickel or nickel oxide.[492] In Wales, dust from the calcination process may have been responsible rather than gaseous nickel carbonyl; suspicion now rests on the subsulfide (Ni_3S_2) but soluble compounds cannot be eliminated. Arsenic and cobalt figured among the metals to which workers were also exposed, but an etiologic role for arsenic is now discounted. Of the lung cancers reported in nickel workers most have been squamous or small cell in type. Experimental evidence established nickel compounds as carcinogens in various species and by different routes of administration. Only weakly soluble nickel compounds proved carcinogenic and all histologic types of neoplasm were induced. The increased frequency of chromosomal aberrations in lymphocytes from nickel workers suggested a mutagenic effect, while in hamsters the carbonyl and divalent salts proved teratogenic.[493,494] Nickel may be one of the carcinogens in tobacco smoke and $Ni(CO)_4$ inhibits induction of benzo(a)pyrene hydroxylase in the lung,[495] thus preventing degradation of the hydrocarbon, present in tobacco smoke, to an inactive form.

Chromium

The prime mineral ore is chromite ($Cr_2O_3 \cdot FeO$) which comes from southern Africa, Russia, and Turkey and is used largely in the production of chromate cement and refractory brick. However, the main risks occur in chromate and chrome pigment producers, dye manufacturers, and chromate spray painters. Being poorly susceptible to oxidation, the metal forms corrosion-resistant alloys and is used for plating.

The South African mineral almost always contains less than 1 percent quartz and the radiologic appearances in workers were considered to be a benign pneumoconiosis, a view substantiated experimentally by the reaction in rats' lungs.[496] Human material shows focal aggregatons of black pigment, in which birefringent particles may occur, along with some fibrosis; severer manifestations comprise interstitial fibrosis with honeycombing and epithelial metaplasia. Neoplasia constitutes the main concern, the lung cancer rate in American chromate workers being estimated as 15 to 28 times the normal rate.[497,498] In Britain, carcinoma of the lung proved to be an occupational hazard in chromate-producing factories and smoking was unlikely to be responsible for the relative excess mortality of 3.6.[499] In a follow-up study a significant excess of deaths from lung cancer was again detected but the risk had diminished, probably as a result of modifications to the plant and working environment.[500] Experience in Japan confirms these conclusions, showing a rate 49 times that expected for lung cancer whilst failing to incriminate smoking.[501] Most neoplasms are squamous or anaplastic in type. Exposure to trivalent chromium as in ferrochromium manufacture does not appear to increase the risk of lung cancer.[502] Moreover, lung cancer mortality was not apparently elevated in the population exposed to the exhaust from a ferrochromium factory.[503]

The results of animal experiments aimed at carcinogenesis have been disappointing, whether by injection (intratracheal and intravenous) or inhalation techniques. Current evidence tends to implicate the weakly soluble hexavalent compounds of chromium, as opposed to the trivalent compounds, in the genesis of neoplasia, but the mechanisms are unknown.[504] Contact with chromate leads to perforation of the nasal septum and to skin sensitization especially in cement workers.

Inert Metallic Dusts

Titanium

The metal is used mainly in aircraft manufacture and its alloys possess great strength and corrosion resistance. Titanium dioxide, being chemically indifferent, is used in the dye industry and the annual world production is over 2 million tons. Grinding the ore produces high atmospheric levels of dust in the respirable size range but few reports of pulmonary involvement have appeared. Three workers showed pigment-bearing phagocytes in alveoli and dense accumulations of particles were located in relation to some vessels and airways but connective tissue increase in alveolar septa and subpleural areas was slight.[505] The lymph nodes contained dust without reactive changes. By electron microscopy particles resembling those of the native mineral were present in the lysosomes of macrophages and x-ray fluorescence spectrometry demonstrated high titanium contents as compared with control subjects. Application of energy dispersive x-ray analysis to lysosomal material confirmed the presence of titanium particles but also indicated the presence of silicon and aluminium.[506] There is no reason to suspect that titanium dioxide itself is fibrogenic. In vitro studies showed it to be nontoxic to macrophages and incapable of liberating the fibrogenic factor.[48] An extensive sarcoid-like granulomatous reaction has been attributed to titanium but appears to be another example of incorporation of inert particles by an independent lesion.

Iron

The principal ores are hematite (Fe_2O_3) and magnetite (Fe_3O_4). The former comes mainly from Canada but also from Cumberland in the United Kingdom, and Spain, while the latter occurs as a major deposit in Sweden, but the larger sources are contaminated by a little quartz. The dust from Cumberland contains a small portion of quartz and a larger amount of muscovite, but hematite forms the major component.[144] Apart from mining and crushing ores, exposure to particulate iron or its oxides with minimal or absent contamination may be experienced in steel rolling and grinding, electric arc and oxyacetylene welding, silver and glass polishing with ferric oxide (rouge or crocus), cleaning and dressing iron castings, boiler scaling, and the extraction and use of emery, which is obtained largely from Turkey and is second in hardness only to diamond. Iron ores are also used in the production of pigments. Mining, foundry work, and scaling of boilers burning coal may entail a silica risk.

The lesions of hematite worker's pneumoconiosis, recognized in England over 50 years ago[507,508] resemble those in coal workers, the only distinction lying in the reddish-brown color imparted by the dust. Simple pneumoconiosis occurs as macules, developed around respiratory bronchioles which may be affected by proximal acinar emphysema. Fibrosis is minimal, usually of reticulin irregularly dispersed among laden phagocytes. Complicated pneumoconiosis also affects some cases, is located preferentially though not exclusively in the upper parts of the lung and posteriorly, and may occur as single, multiple, or bilateral masses, which may show necrosis of ischemic or tuberculous origin. Firm, fibrous nodules may be seen in the vicinity of massive lesions and both consist of irregularly disposed tracts of connective tissue lying between masses of dust most of which is extracellular. Pulmonary arteries within massive lesions show changes ranging from intimal fibrosis or fibroelastosis to fibrosis of media and adventitia, many vessels being occluded by vascularized connective tissue containing hematite-laden macrophages, possibly indicating thrombosis with recanalization, as in coal workers. Many arterioles are identifiable only by remains of the internal elastic lamina. Veins are similarly affected. Incinerated preparations viewed by incident light show the hematite as brilliant orange-red particles, which do not, however, give a positive Perls's reaction for iron, although the reaction is positive in the cytoplasm of macrophages. Lymphatic involvement is invariable and deposits of hematite, free or in cells, lie along bronchovascular bundles, venules, and in the pleura. The hilar nodes are the seat of dust accumulation and in complicated disease irregular fibrosis becomes prominent, as may adhesions between nodes and neighboring bronchi and vessels. Inhaled experimentally pure iron oxide is nonfibrogenic.

The Cumbrian necropsy study suggested that hematite miners experienced a greater incidence of *lung carcinoma* than comparable nonminers.[508] Retrospective epidemiologic enquiry in the same population disclosed a prevalence of lung cancer significantly higher (70 percent) than expected for underground but not surface workers[509]; similar indications came from France. No evidence, human or experimental, exists to incriminate iron oxides in carcinogenesis[510] and, as quartz too may be exonerated, blame attaches to the high level of airborne radon daughter products in three of the six haematite mines, as also obtained in Cornish tin mines.[511] Radioactivity was likewise implicated when the ore mined was mainly magnetite.[512] Welding, which involves exposure to several metallic oxides and gases, led to excess mortality from lung cancer.[513]

In workers other than miners exposure is virtually to pure iron and this is usually referred to as *siderosis*. Radiologically, the prevalence of arc-welder's siderosis has varied between 7 and 30 percent. Zenker[3] first described the pathological features in two individuals exposed to the inhalation of iron oxide in making matches and grinding glass. On the pleura brick-red macules and lines are prominent. Macules also characterize the cut surface and resemble those produced by coal in size and distribution; lymphatics in lobular septa may also be outlined. Microscopically, the particles are held in macrophages which accumulate as usual in relation to respiratory bronchioles, especially those of the first and second orders. The Prussian blue reaction of the particles is negative. Fibrosis is minimal and confined to reticulin disposed irregularly between the phagocytes, while proximal acinar emphysema is insignificant or absent. Silver may also be inhaled by polishers and this metal is deposited on the elastin of arteries and airways to give it a blackish color which dilute KCN removes.

Occupational siderosis is unlikely to be confused with pulmonary hemosiderosis which occurs in primary and secondary forms. The primary type may be an isolated lesion or form part of Goodpasture's syndrome (*see* p. 303). Secondary haemosiderosis follows chronic passive hypertension from raised pulmonary venous pressure commonly the consequence of chronic left ventricular failure or mitral stenosis. The lesions assume a similar pattern, though the hemosiderin gives a positive Prussian blue reaction and the elastic fibers show iron encrustation and may excite a foreign body reaction.

Zirconium

The element occurs in combination with silica as zircon ($ZrO_2.SiO_2$) which has pronounced refractory properties and is thus used in ceramics, including electrical insulators, and in alloys notably for jet propulsion purposes. Dust is generated during processing and there may be a quartz risk in milling and separation.

From the clinical and experimental aspects there is no evidence to suggest that industrial dusts are other than inert. However, some zirconium compounds produce granulomata and chronic interstitial pneumonitis in a variety of animals by inhalation[514,515]; the ultrastructural features of the granuloma are similar to those of the sarcoid and beryllium granulomata.[449] Caution is therefore necessary before dismissing zirconium compounds as harmless, especially as they are known to produce granulomata in the skin after application as deodorants.

Tin

Smelting of tin may have neolithic origins and Cornwall, England was an important source in olden times and there is still some production in this region. Most of the ore, principally tin oxide (cassiterite) but including sulfides, comes from Africa, South America, southeast Asia, and China. Underground mining in quartz-containing rock still continues though most mineral being alluvial is obtained by dredging. Mining may entail exposure to quartz, but unloading and milling of ore, its calcination and smelting give rise to dust of tin oxide. The metal forms alloys with ease and is pliable.

Tin miners may contract silicosis but stannosis occurs in individuals employed in extraction.[516–518] The only positive clinical finding was dense radiologic nodulation. The peritoneal reaction in guinea pigs showed little evidence of connective tissue formation. In seven necropsy cases,[518] soft black and dark grey macules, 2 to 5 mm across, were uniformly distributed within the lung and the fibrous septa were also pigmented. The dust foci consisted of laden macrophages collected around respiratory bronchioles; the connective tissue reaction varied and might be lacking, while dust-related emphysema was not a feature. Dust cells also occurred in alveoli and in relation to lymphatics. The tin oxide content ranged from 0.5 to over 3 g per lung, but the quartz content was minimal. X-ray diffraction and x-ray emission microanalysis confirmed the nature of the particles. Stannosis is accordingly a further example of a benign pneumoconiosis since it contributes neither to morbidity nor to mortality, but the risk of carcinoma from mine radiations[8] remains.

Antimony

The metal is used in alloys for accumultors, electrodes, and printer's type, whilst the oxide serves as a pigment for paints and enamels, plastics, and rubber. Antimony also has medicinal uses and was employed as a cosmetic. The usual ore is stibnite, the sulfide (Sb_2S_3), which is associated with quartz and is mined in South Africa, China, Mexico, Bolivia, and Europe. United Kingdom deposits are not now worked and all the ore is imported mostly from South Africa to be smelted and refined on Tyneside in the largest European plant to produce the metal and the white trioxide.[519] In the United States smelting takes place in Texas and Pennsylvania.[520] The chief risk arises in smelting, when antimony oxide particles less than 1 μm diameter are produced, and in bagging.

Radiographic evidence of pneumoconiosis occurred in 16.8 percent of men employed in the English plant, but the condition did not cause measurable respiratory disability, and histologic evidence indicated that the dust accumulated focally in macrophages and was not fibrogenic.[519] Progressive massive fibrosis has not been encountered in antimony process workers. Experimentally fibrosis was not produced in the lungs by the ore or the trioxide.[520] X-ray spectrophotometry serves to detect and quantitate antimony in the lungs of employees, thus going beyond conventional radiography; the method is also applicable to tin workers. Mining, however, may entail a risk of silicosis. No convincing evidence yet exists to implicate antimony in lung carcinogenesis.

Barium

Barytes or barite ($BaSO_4$) constitutes the principal ore and witherite ($BaCO_3$) a subsidiary ore. Barytes comes from the United States, Germany (Federal Republic), Russia, Ireland, Italy, and other countries; U.K. production is now minimal. Other minerals are usually associated. In the United Kingdom barytes was ground and then leached into grades of purity, and the better grades dried, pulverized, and bagged, while the third grade was raked manually as it was dried and bagged again by hand.[521] The latter process produced considerable dust. Mining may involve exposure to free silica but there is little risk from open cast workings. Barytes finds application in drilling mud for oil exploration, as a filler or extender for paper, textiles, leather, linoleum, and rubber, as well as in ceramics and glass; the electronic and chemical industries use barytes and other compounds of barium widely. The insolubility and radio-opacity of barium sulphate have long rendered it valuable as a diagnostic agent.

In baritosis discrete grey macules occur throughout the lungs but fibrosis is confined to reticulin formation and massive fibrosis is not a feature. Experimentally barium sulfate proved to be inert in the lungs.[522] X-ray diffraction affords firm identification of the mineral. Radiologically there may be a "snowstorm" appearance, but the changes regress slowly after employment ceases, and there are no functional disturbances. Silicosis constitutes the main risk in barytes miners and the disease may be severe.

Cerium

Cerium is the most common of the rare earth group of elements which have high atomic numbers. It is used as a polishing agent for lenses and glassware, in ceramics and alloys, and to increase brilliance in carbon arc rods and tracer bullets. Although radiologic changes occurred in men working with carbon arc lamps, no fibrosis was detected in animals after intratracheal injection or inhalation.[523] Human material has shown nonspecific chronic bronchiolitis and focal septal sclerosis.

Effects of Fumes

While dusts and fumes have different origins (*see* General Considerations, Terminology, above), both form particles whose size ranges overlap and in the extraction processes of a metal for instance both types of particle may be produced. While individual fume particles lie in the smaller submicron range, aggregation into larger units is not uncommon.

Cadmium

Because of its resistance to corrosion, cadmium is employed in alloys and electroplating, in alkaline accumulators and atomic reactors (where it absorbs neutrons), and in photovoltaic cells, as well as a pigment. It is a by-product of the extraction of zinc, and so comes from North and South America, USSR, and Australia. Fumes of the oxide are generated when the metal is heated and welding thus constitutes a hazard. Urban atmospheric contamination probably arises from smelters and coal-burning power stations. Pulmonary effects usually follow exposure to fumes though dust particles may also be inhaled. The subject of cadmium toxicity was surveyed.[524]

In acute poisoning from fresh fume, symptoms are delayed for several hours. Recovery is usual but the fatality rate may be 15 to 20 percent.[525] The lungs are enlarged and the alveoli filled by proteinaceous fluid with numerous macrophages and red cell extravasation; alveolar walls are swollen by fluid and contain neutrophils, lymphocytes, and fibroblasts. The alveolar epithelium undergoes necrosis and repair by proliferation of type II cells follows, so that the alveolar lining becomes cuboidal. Death has followed from renal cortical necrosis.

Chronic poisoning usually follows prolonged low-level exposures which may be intermittent. The principal pulmonary change appears to be the development of emphysema without chronic bronchitis,[526–528] but from the descriptions it is difficult to identify the type in modern terms. However, in personal cases (provided by Dr. J. D. Heppleston) the emphysema assumed a circumscribed form with fibrosis of parent bronchioles, and conformed to the irregular inflammatory type. Since emphysema is common in the population at large and surveys of cadmium workers do not always take account of smoking habits or include control subjects, it is difficult to establish a causal relationship between occupation and disease, especially as some workers exhibit no evidence of lung damage.[529] Even the detection of cadmium in the lung may be inconclusive since other causes for the emphysema could operate. Cadmium accumulates in emphysematous lungs, to which state cigarette smoking predisposes, and though the smoke contains small amounts of cadmium other irritants are also present in greater proportion. However, an aerosol of cadmium chloride led to the development of circumscribed emphysema experimentally.[530] Chronic interstitial pneumonia has also been found in cadmium welders. Chronic exposure to cadmium fume or cadmium oxide led to a significantly raised mortality from lung cancer and also prostatic cancer.[531] Proteinuria is a feature of chronic cadmium poisoning and renal fibrosis may develop,[525,532] while the urinary β_2 microglobulin is raised after exposure to cadmium oxide irrespective of the presence of proteinuria.[533] Osteomalacia affected Japanese women consuming cadmium-contaminated rice and water (*itai-itai* disease. . . . it hurts—it hurts).

Metal and Polymer Fume Fever

No pathologic changes are recorded in metal fume fever since the acute condition remits spontaneously within a day or two and chronic effects are unknown. The condition assumes the form of an acute febrile illness resembling influenza or even malaria, developing a few hours after exposure to fumes (often generated by welding) mainly from zinc, copper, and magnesium though nickel, manganese and other metals are sometimes the cause. Accordingly the names brass founder's ague, copper fever, welder's ague, brass fever, and Monday fever have been attached. The last term refers to the resistance that soon develops and as easily disappears, but whether it signifies sensitization is unknown. The occupations generating fumes include smelting and galvanizing with zinc, welding or cutting of galvanized iron, brass foundries producing zinc fume and copper fume from the molten metal. Diagnosis depends on the occupational history, but care is needed to distinguish the more serious acute cadmium poisoning which is symptomatically similar but more protracted.

The features of polymer fume fever resemble those of metal fume fever, the fumes being generated by degradation of the polymer polytetrafluoroethylene (Teflon, Fluon) under the influence of heat above 300°C, though dusts formed when the products are machined in the cold are also responsible.[534,535] Smoking contaminated cigarettes appears to determine the onset by virtue of the high burning temperature. Polytetrafluoroethylene is widely used in the manufacture of plastics and resins. Experimentally type I pneumocytes are particularly vulnerable.

Rare Sources of Fumes

Vanadium ores occur in South Africa, Russia, the United States, and Peru, while dusts from oil-fired boilers[536,537] and from the deposit on heat exchangers of gas turbines[538] contain vanadium. Mining and milling may produce quartz dust, but the association of vanadium with uranium in carnotite involves radioactive products. Vanadium forms a major component of high-speed steel, to which is imparted a degasifying and deoxidizing action. In steel alloys vanadium confers fatigue and temperature resistance. Vanadium pentoxide, which acts as a catalyst in making sulfuric acid, is toxic.[539] In the chemical industry vanadium compounds are widely used as catalysts. The effects of inhalation are acute bronchitis and pneumonitis, but no chronic state is known to ensue in humans or animals.

Osmium occurs as a natural alloy with iridium. Although the metal is innocuous, osmium tetroxide is highly irritant and causes acute conjunctivitis with a halo around lights and tracheobronchitis but the effects are transient.[540]

The deleterious effect of *mercury* exposure was known to Ramazzini and the vapor may, after a delay of a few hours, lead to trancheobronchitis and pneumonitis. The reaction takes the form of diffuse alveolar damage with mononuclear infiltration and edema of alveolar septa, interstitial proliferation of fibroblasts and formation of hyaline membranes composed of fibrin and cell organelles. Accompanying the parenchymal reaction is an acute necrotizing bronchiolitis, the lumina being occupied by desquamated cells, exudate, and mucus. This obstruction is thought to act as a check-valve and to be responsible for the interstitial emphysema and pneumothorax. Regeneration of epithelium is an early feature and by 3 weeks interstitial fibrosis has occurred and some honeycombing may be evident, whilst epithelial hyperplasia may appear atypical. Resolution is usual though patchy pulmonary fibrosis may remain.[541–544] Disease of the central nervous system is a consequence of poisoning by organic compounds of mercury (as at Minamata and in Iraq), while the treatment of fur with mercuric nitrate in hat making led to mental changes and the phrase "mad as a hatter" (*Alice's Adventures in Wonderland*), though the connection has been questioned.

Manganese is used as an alloy for hardening steel and is incorporated with bronze to resist corrosion in marine constructions and mining machinery. The oxide acts as a bleaching agent and other salts serve as dyes or oxidizing agents. It occurs as the oxide in various ores mined in a number of countries. Chronic manganese poisoning is seen in miners and millers. The central nervous system is affected and Parkinsonism is a common sequel, dopamine being decreased in the corpus striatum and melanin in the substantia nigra being reduced; L-dopa treatment confers benefit. Workers handling manganese dioxide (80 percent of the particles being below 0.2 μm in diameter) in the manufacture of the permanganate, experienced a high rate of pneumonitis which tended to be prolonged though permanent changes were not evident.[545] Manganese dioxide given intratracheally to rats induced an intense interstitial infiltration with mononuclear cells and numerous dust phagocytes, but the reaction eventually subsided.[546] It seems likely that these changes would now be described as interstitial pneumonia of a rather mild type. Manganese is an essential element in plant and animal nutrition.

Arsenic. Exposure to fumes and dusts in the smelting of arsenic-bearing ores[547] or the manufacture of inorganic arsenical pesticides,[548] now largely superseded, led to an increased liability to lung cancer.

Irritant Gases

Industrial risks from gases arise by asphyxiation, as from carbon monoxide or methane in coal mining, or by irritation, as from oxides of nitrogen. Since particular features are produced only by irritants, asphyxiants are not considered.

Oxides of Nitrogen

Several combinations exist. Nitrous oxide (N_2O) constitutes the nonirritant anesthetic gas, while nitric oxide (NO) is slowly oxidized in air to nitrogen dioxide (NO_2). The latter polymerizes to the tetroxide (N_2O_4) which soon dissociates, so that these two forms occur in equilibrium as a heavy reddish-brown gas with an unpleasant smell and irritating properties.

Nitrogen dioxide arises from the burning of fossil fuels and from several industrial processes. *Welding* by oxyacetylene or electric arc produces NO_2 by high-temperature combination of atmospheric oxygen and nitrogen and by ultraviolet irradiation from the arc, but the concentration rises to toxic levels only in confined and ill-ventilated spaces such as ship hulls. Shielding of the electrode and welds with inert gases largely overcomes this risk. Welding and cutting may also produce fume from the metal and lead to siderosis (*see* Metallic Dusts, Inert Metallic Dusts, Iron, above) or metal fume fever (*see* Effects of Fumes, Metal and Polymer Fume Fever, above). *Ensilage* is the means by which grass or green crops are preserved for winter cattle feed. Modern practice employs tower silos at a controlled temperature. Both carbon dioxide and NO_2 are quickly formed, the former by bacterial action on carbohydrates and the latter by enzyme conversion of plant nitrates, probably derived from fertilizers, to nitrites which in the acid environment left by carbohydrate decomposition proceed through nitrous acid (HNO_2) to NO_2. Since CO_2 and NO_2 are heavier than air, they accumulate on top of the silage, especially in depressed pockets, and the levels may be dangerous within days and may persist for months if the tower is unopened. The oxygen concentration, moreover, is low. A man entering the tower to shovel out the silage may thus be exposed to high concentrations of gases and be so rapidly overcome as to prevent escape; gases may even be evident immediately outside the silo. The condition has received the designation of silo filler's disease and prevention is usually achieved by blowing air into the top of the tower before entering. *Mining* operations entailing nitroexplosives constitute a further source of NO and NO_2 and the concentrations reach toxic levels where ventilation is poor as in tunneling. The gases travel as a bolus so the maximum exposure is brief. Work at the coal face carries no detectable risk because of ventilation, and return to the face after shot-firing is delayed to permit dispersal of gases. The *chemical* industry provides a risk from spillage in the manufacture of nitric acid when fumes arise as the acid reacts with organic material such as paper and wood. Acid cleaning of metals also gives rise to NO_2.

The lesions caused by NO_2 are described in Chapter 16. The gas proved useful in studying pulmonary epithelial dynamics.

Ozone

Ozone is a highly reactive form of oxygen. It occurs at high altitudes and has been detected in aircraft cockpits; it is produced by lightning and high-tension discharges and, in association with nitrogen and sulfur dioxides, forms a constituent of photochemical smog. Ozone is produced from atmospheric oxygen by ultraviolet rays during electric arc welding with a shield of inert gas and it serves as a bleaching or sterilizing agent. Pulmonary function is adversely affected, as is the ability of macrophages to kill bacteria, production of interferon by respiratory epithelium is inhibited, while fibroblastic cells and connective tissue appear in the respiratory parenchyma. The clinical features and lesions of ozone toxicity are oxygen poisoning described in Chapter 16.

Sulfur Dioxide

Combustion of impurities present in coal or oil products leads to general pollution of the urban atmosphere by sulfur dioxide, while industrially it may arise in refrigeration, paper production, preservation of fruit, and refining of oil. Chronic exposure causes damage to the inanimate and animate alike—limestone buildings corrode and the bronchi are irritated. Deaths in London from chronic bronchitis and indeed from all causes correlated with rises in atmospheric concentration of sulfur dioxide (amounting to about 25 percent more than background level) and of black suspended matter (amounting to about 20 percent more than background level).[549] Moreover, morbidity was estimated to rise by 80 percent with the high levels of pollution experienced in the industrial northeast of England.[550] Mortality and morbidity from chronic bronchitis among the adult population of other cities likewise paralleled atmospheric pollution by sulfur dioxide and particulate matter,[551,552] while chronic occupational exposure to sulfur dioxide significantly affected the prevalence of chronic bronchitis.[553] As air pollution increased, a highly significant rise occurred in lower respiratory tract infections in children.[554] Implementation of the U.K. Clean Air Act of 1956 has led to an amelioration of respiratory disorder and there has been no repetition of the disastrous London "smog" of December 1952. High concentrations of sulfur dioxide are acutely irritant and precipitate removal from the source. The growth of different species of lichen provides an indication of the degree of atmospheric pollution by sulfur dioxide.

Long-term exposure of monkeys to sulfur dioxide induced functional and histologic changes (bronchiolitis and alveolitis but little fibrosis).[555] Production of mucus in the trachea was increased and its flow diminished in rats inhaling sulfur dioxide over a prolonged period.[556] Sulfuric acid mist, especially of small particle size, proved a more potent irritant and caused functional deterioration along with focal thickening, connective tissue increase, and epithelial hyperplasia in bronchiolar walls of monkeys.[557]

Other Gases

Chlorine is extensively employed in the chemical and pharmaceutical industries and it serves as a disinfectant. It is conveyed in liquid form under pressure with obvious risks. The element is thought to act as an oxidant and by liberation of hydrochloric acid[558]; in toxic concentration it gives rise to pulmonary edema with alveolar hyaline membranes as well as to upper respiratory irritation, while secondary infection may occasionally cause bronchopneumonia. Survivors of accidental exposure do not apparently suffer long-term effects.[559]

Phosgene ($COCl_2$) may arise in the chemical industry and in welding with a gas shield; it was employed as a weapon in World War I. Fatality has ensued from stripping paint with methylene chloride[560] and the gas may arise from fire extinguishers employing carbon tetrachloride.[561] The manifestations resemble those of chorine poisoning and arise from capillary damage. Fluid exudate fills the alveoli and fibrinous hyaline membranes form while bronchiolar epithelium is destroyed and infection may supervene. Pleural effusion may be a concomitant. Experimentally phosgene led to chronic pneumonitis with maximum damage to respiratory bronchioles,[562] but a chronic counterpart in man has not been convincingly established.

Ammonia forms a major ingredient of fertilizers and explosives, and it is used in the manufacture of plastics, in oil-refining and refrigeration. The gas is a powerful irritant and accidental exposure to high concentration may quickly result in asphyxia from laryngeal edema, while in less severe cases pulmonary edema develops with loss of respiratory epithelium. The latter regenerates though disability may persist for many months.[563] Bronchiolar damage and fibrosis with honeycombing could conceivably result. Obliterative bronchiolitis with consequent bronchiectasis may follow acute ammonia exposure.

Radioactive Particles

Radiations may reach the lung by inhalation, external application, or the vascular route. In human beings alpha particles (positively charged helium nuclei) and beta particles (negatively charged electrons) are inhaled occupationally or unintentionally, while electromagnetic radiations (x-rays and gamma rays) are used therapeutically or diagnostically by delivery to the exterior of the thorax, though orally administered radioiodine is blood-borne.[564] The main environmental concern is with particulate radiation, but electromagnetic radiations also exert their effects by ionization and the two forms may be considered together. In both cases the energy is derived from atoms that are naturally unstable or deliberately rendered so by fission. However, alpha particles and neutrons, possessing greater mass than beta-particles, penetrate tissues less readily but ionize more intensely (i.e., high linear-energy-transfer radiation) and so tend to cause greater cell damage for a particular energy level. The range of alpha particles in air is about 36 mm and in unit density tissue 45 μm. Radiobiology is now so vast a subject that only the main pulmonary effects can be outlined. Although the fundamental mechanisms of cell damage have yet to be elucidated, it is believed that radiations particularly affect the S (synthetic) and G_2 (postsynthetic) phases of the cell cycle. In general, sensitivity to radiation depends on the rate of cell division, though exceptions are recognized.

Exposure

Radiations are encountered *naturally* from cosmic rays, soil, and rocks, and internal radionuclides, which together contribute about two-thirds of the total body dose. The remaining third is derived very largely from *medical* sources, with less than 1 percent each coming from fallout, consumer products, and so on; occupation and radioactive waste contribute a small fraction of 1 percent in Great Britain. The principal risks of radiation exposure come from nuclear explosions, diagnostic radiology and radiotherapy, and from the occupations of mining uranium and associated metals together with the application of luminous paint to dials. Work in processing plutonium and in nuclear shipyards represents a risk which at present is debated, but the enormous longevity of plutonium dioxide, with its half-life of 24,000 years, must constantly be borne in mind, especially in the disposal of nuclear reactor waste.

Uranium mining deserves special mention since it provided the first evidence of occupational risk. For 400 years the metalliferous miners of Schneeberg on the Saxon or northern slope of the Erzgebirge are known to have suffered an excessive respiratory mortality, though it is only about 100 years since the condition was shown to be malignant. At first regarded as lymphosarcoma, Schmorl[565] later identified the lesion as bronchogenic carcinoma, a finding which Pirchan and Šikl[566] confirmed. A similar risk was recognized in the uranium miners of Joachimsthal on the southern side of the Erzgebirge in Czechoslovakia over 50 years ago by Löwy[567] and the association has latterly been detected in the United States.

Uranium occurs as a compound oxide with vanadium and potassium (carnotite) and as an oxide in pitchblende, the ores being mined by underground and open-cast methods in Canada, the United States, Australia, South Africa, Zaire, Czechoslovakia, and the USSR. The ore is milled and extracted as a uranate, termed yellowcake, in which form it is packed into drums to be taken to the site of use, mainly atomic energy production. Uranium ores occur in quartz-bearing rock, so that silicosis may also be a risk.

Uranium-238 gives rise to the longest decay chain known and its daughters have achieved equilibrium in the ores.[568] After passage through several solid elements, it becomes radium-226 which decays to the gas radon-222 and then to the radon daughters, which are short-lived, alpha-emitting isotopes of polonium, before ending as stable lead. At some stages of the decay process, beta particles are also emitted. The toxicity of uranium is considered to arise from two sources; radon and its daughters leak through the rocks and are liberated as mining proceeds, the gases having least chance to escape from underground workings, while the ore dusts contain long-lived radionuclides. Thorium may occur along with uranium and contribute to the alpha activity. Radon decay products readily condense on molecules of water vapor or on respirable dust particles; from the latter the radiation dose, largely of alpha particles, delivered to the lungs may be 20 times greater than that from radon.[569]

Pneumonitis

The features of human radiation pneumonitis are described on p. 278. Low level inhalation of $^{239}PuO_2$ by mice led to type II cell damage with discharge of lamellar bodies and massive secondary uptake by alveolar macrophages, while in rats interstitial fibroblasts increased, though in both species endothelium was spared.[570] Higher dose rates generated interstitial pneumonitis and diffuse fibrosis with epithelial metaplasia.

Neoplasia

In the light of Schmorl's observations, Peller[571] found a greatly increased mortality from lung cancer among miners in Joachimsthal as well as in Schneeberg, reaching 44 percent according to Šikl[572] who also demonstrated that silicosis was as frequent as cancer though no relationship was detected between them. In uranium miners from the Colorado plateau, the mortality from respiratory cancer was proportional to the calculated cumulative exposure to radiation and the excess ranged from 3 to 38 times the expected.[573] Cigarette smoking contributed to the risk but was not the sole factor.[574] A dose-response relationship was also established in Czechoslovak uranium miners and smoking was excluded as a major causal agent in producing the excess of lung cancer cases.[575] Furthermore, nonmalignant respiratory disease among whites approached lung cancer in importance as a cause of death in U.S. uranium miners, probably as a result of diffuse radiation damage.[569] However, the alpha emitters ^{210}Po and ^{210}Pb are concentrated in cigarette smoke and tend to accumulate at the bifurcations of segmental bronchi.[576] Histologically, the lung cancer assumed mainly the small cell, undifferentiated (oat cell) type, while epidermoid carcinoma diminished in frequency.[577,578] Further evidence incriminating atmospheric alpha particles in the genesis of lung cancer came from the fluorspar (CaF_2, used as a flux in the manufacture of steel and aluminium, and as a source of fluorine) miners of Newfoundland, in whom the death rate from this cause was 29 times that expected, for which rise smoking could not apparently be blamed nor was a relation to pneumoconiosis detected.[579] Water percolating into the mine was shown to contain radon daughters but the ore itself was not radioactive and no arsenic was present. External irradiation for ankylosing spondylitis proved to be carcinogenic for the lung[580] and suggestive evidence comes from survivors of atomic explosions[581] and x-ray technologists.[582] Radon daughters are believed to be responsible for the excess of lung cancer in hematite miners from Cumberland (*see* Metallic Dusts, Inert Metallic Dusts, Iron, above), in Swedish lead/zinc and iron ore miners,[583] and in Cornish tin miners.[8] Radiation pneumonitis is not known to be followed by secondary lung cancer, probably because survival is too short.

Numerous long-term experimental studies have been performed with β-γ and α emitters inhaled by several species.[584,585] The peak tumor incidence for α emitters follows doses of about 10 Gy, but β-γ emitters may well produce a greater effect.[586] Tumors of several histologic types developed, adenocarcinoma being the most common followed by bronchioloalveolar, epidermoid, and mixed adenoepidermoid carcinoma; metastasis was frequent. Hemangiosarcoma frequently occurred in dogs inhaling β-γ emitters and in rats exposed to α emitters. In contrast to human experience, oat cell carcinoma has not been induced in animals by radionuclides. The value of animal experiments is believed to lie in relating dose and dose rate to pulmonary response and in measuring clearance rates and the energy exposures of individual cells. Pulmonary lavage has proved effective in removing α particles deposited in the lung.[587,588] In baboons nearly 60 percent of the initial lung burden was thus recovered and up to a further 30 percent was lost by accelerated natural clearance following lavage. Moreover, lavage itself left no permanent ultrastructural changes and largely abolished plutonium pneumonitis and diminished fibrosis. Application in humans is now feasible, but the effect on neoplasia is not yet known. Chelation offers a further possibility of removing plutonium from the body.

As a generalization, animals receiving high levels of radionuclides develop fatal radiation pneumonitis while neoplasms arise from exposure to low levels, which are nevertheless greater than most human exposures. Although the cumulative dose of radiation required for carcinogenesis or genetic effects in humans is unknown, few consider that the risk will be abolished as dosage diminishes and the ALARA ("as low as reasonably achievable") concept is hardly reassuring. The lifetime risk of lung cancer to the general population from exposure to radon and its decay products has been estimated as 0.12 percent compared with the overall risk of 4 percent, largely attributable to cigarette smoking.[589]

Prediction of Risks from Atmospheric Pollutants

Human Evidence

Epidemiologic studies constitute the ultimate basis on which to judge the harmfulness of a dust hazard. To establish a deleterious effect and unravel the interplay of different factors may take decades, during which many employees suffer disability or death. Justification thus exists for animal experimentation in an attempt to anticipate the effects of human exposure and take preventive action. Since minerals are indispensable to 20th century human existence, attention must concentrate on dust suppression measures and on attempts to identify individuals who may be particularly susceptible to dust-related disorders. The latter constitutes a task for the future, but genetically determined or connected influences afford no apparent leads.

Experimental Evidence

In Vivo

Injection of particles by various routes has frequently been adopted in assessing their fibrogenic capacity, as the foregoing accounts exemplify. Such techniques possess the advantage of relatively short duration and are also applicable to carcinogenesis, but by overriding or eliminating the natural mechanisms of pulmonary deposition and clearance they suffer in comparison with inhalation experiments. These require elaborate apparatus, especially for the study of asbestos with its risk to operators of neoplasia from small doses, and only studies employing atmospheric concentrations of particles resembling fairly closely those experienced by humans are acceptable. Differences among animal species and between them and humans in respect of anatomy, posture, and fibrogenic or carcinogenic capacity also need to be borne in mind when making deductions from inhalation studies. Injection experiments serve best as a screening procedure to select for inhalation studies those dusts which appear to be deleterious.

Problems raised by animal studies may be exemplified. To identify the activity of the quartz component in mixed dusts as from coal mines, an intraperitoneal injection test of fibrogenicity was devised in West Germany.[590] Penetration of the dust to the lymph nodes was considered to depend on cytotoxicity but not on the quartz content, while the fibrogenic response did correlate with the quartz content and was PNO sensitive. If other constituents of coal mine dust (whose proportions may vary from one sample to another) determine penetration, the amount of quartz in the primary and secondary sites could well vary. The occurrence of so-called quartz-typical areas separate from the remainder of the dust reaction in the nodes is difficult to explain. In vivo assessment of cytotoxicity might be gauged by quantitation of alveolar macrophages lavaged from the lung after administration of dust. Theoretically the procedure could reflect macrophage recruitment, but cells destroyed by particles will not be detected nor will macrophages residing interstitially at the time of lavage, while lipid feed-back to the marrow[104] also requires consideration. The immunologic status merits further scrutiny, since athymic mice injected intraperitoneally with quartz developed lymph node lesions sooner and more extensively than normal mice.[591]

In Vitro

As a rapid substitute for in vivo observations, the injurious effect of particles has been gauged by their effects on cell membranes, that is, hemolytic capacity and cytotoxicity, the latter being measured by cell death and enzyme release from macrophages or macrophage-like cell lines. These responses have been outlined in regard to quartz and asbestos, but it was thought that the predictive value would lie with mixed dusts such as that from coal mines where the composition varies. Wide colliery-associated variations were found in the probability of developing the higher radiologic categories of simple pneumoconiosis quite apart from the quartz content of the respirable dust.[113] For such problems it was hoped that the in vitro methods could provide an answer, but the results, which were recently reviewed,[592] were not encouraging. In general no particular role for quartz was detected in cytotoxicity experiments and these correlated poorly with haemolytic activity. Disparities between cytotoxicity and hemolysis also exist in respect of fibrous minerals. A similarly poor correlation is apparent between fibrogenicity, lytic ability, and toxicity where prediction is most desirable, that is, for mixed dusts. Cell lines were thought to afford standardization, but have proved too unstable and hence are not reliable. The current European consensus is that, for coal mine dusts, epidemiologic evidence correlates poorly with dust composition and tests of cell toxicity, though the relationship between lung fibrogenicity and composition is somewhat better. Furthermore, in vitro study with macrophages ignores the interplay of type II epithelium and its lipid secretion as well as the important factor of macrophage recruitment. A means of overcoming some of these difficulties may be afforded by adaptation of the in vitro technique, by which the MFF was discovered, for quantitative assay of fibrogenicity directly on fibroblasts instead of inferring fibrogenic capacity from cytotoxic behavior.[593]

An area where in vitro study is potentially valuable lies in the assessment of respiratory defence against gaseous pollutants. Lavaged alveolar macrophages were maintained in direct contact with the atmosphere, and their morphology (by optical microscopy, TEM, and SEM), bactericidal activity and viability subsequently measured.[594–596] By this means the effects of oxygen, ozone, NO_2, tobacco smoke, automobile exhaust gases, and paraquat have been examined.

The prediction of carcinogenic risks from the results of in vitro tests demands caution, especially with negative findings. Fiber length plays a role in toxicity, fibrogenicity, and carcinogenicity, but under natural conditions the reaction time is much longer and occurs at lower concentrations than in culture. Cytotoxicity is measured in cells of the mononuclear phagocytic system or in abnormal cell lines, whereas neoplasia arises in epithelium or mesothelium and the nature of the changes leading to that state is unknown, though in asbestos-related carcinoma of the lung fibrosis appears to be a prerequisite of which no in vitro procedure can take account. It is thus desirable to concentrate attention on the target cells—fibroblasts, epithelium, and mesothelium—rather than rely on the indirect approach.

Chronic Bronchitis and Dust Exposure

The pathology of chronic bronchitis is covered in Chapter 21, but the evidence incriminating occupation as a factor in its genesis requires mention. Accepting the Medical Research Council's criteria for the clinical recognition of chronic bronchitis, the PFR program, in its long-term survey of British coal mines, established a statistically significant association between increasing exposure to airborne dust and rising prevalence of chronic bronchitis.[597] Furthermore, bronchitis contributed to the loss in FEV_1 over and above the reduction anticipated from the effects of dust exposure, smoking, age, and physique.[598] Coal workers in Yugoslavia and Utah provided similar evidence. These conclusions were amplified by European studies on the epidemiology of chronic bronchitis in a range of dusty occupations and, though the prevalence varied widely, prominence was given to the factors of smoking followed by dust exposure and age.[599,600] Experience among asbestos workers, gold miners, and coke workers corresponded. Nevertheless, dust exposure had a greater effect than smoking on symptoms and on the reduction of FEV_1 in British coal workers.[601] The degree of ventilatory impairment from "industrial" bronchitis is usually insufficient to amount to serious disability. Smoking, however, does not appear to determine the development of simple pneumoconiosis in coal workers, in whom the main variable is exposure to airborne dust. Neither pneumoconiosis nor lung dust content is related to the dimensions of bronchial mucous glands; dust exposure contributes to their enlargement but smoking is the main determinant.[602,603]

The difficulty in making a clinical distinction between the effects of inhaled dust on the bronchial tree and on alveolar structures has to some extent been resolved by adoption of the flow-volume curve to assess dysfunction in peripheral airways. Conventional ventilatory tests rely on measurement of the FEV_1, forced vital capacity, and total airways resistance, which mainly reflect pressurized flow in larger air passages, but are usually little affected by changes in peripheral airways resistance. It is, however, in relation to respiratory bronchioles that the simple coal dust lesion develops[124] and simple pneumoconiosis of coal workers would not overall be expected to have a major effect on ventilatory capacity as measured by standard methods. When flow-volume curves were obtained from coal workers it transpired that nonsmokers afflicted with bronchitis predominantly exhibited loss of peak flow and of flow at high lung volumes, while smoking disturbed both peak flow and flow at all lung volumes.[604,605] These physiologic changes related to the duration of underground exposure but not to increase of radiologic category. Occupation may therefore be blamed in nonsmokers who have had long exposure to dust (whether in coal mining or other industrial processes) and who exhibit symptoms and minor degrees of physiologic obstruction to the main air passages.

Pathogenetically the dust factor in "occupational" bronchitis probably relates to particles of a size in the upper part of or above the respirable range. Whilst the smaller particles induce disease in parenchymal structures, the larger-sized fractions, especially above 10 μm which are likely to be inhaled by mouth breathing during exertion, will deposit preferentially in the main conducting airways, there to exert a long-continued, low-level irritation. However, flow-volume curves may not be sufficiently sensitive to measure the functional state in the respiratory portion of the bronchiolar tree where airflow is minimal and diffusion dominant.

Byssinosis

Lung disease in flax and hemp workers was known to Ramazzini and it is from the Greek word for flax that the term byssinosis is derived. Mechanization in the 19th century brought the condition into prominence among cotton workers in Lancashire, England and flax workers in Ulster, though the same manifestation was subsequently experienced in the United States and other countries. Byssinosis affects some employees in the cotton, flax, or hemp industries and differs from disorders already considered in being provoked by organic material.

Exposure

The capsule or boll (i.e., cotton fruit) consists of pericarp and lint (that is, long seed hairs) which constitute the *cotton* fibers from which textiles are made. After picking, the lint is separated from the seed by suction in a gin and then taken to the mill where bales are opened and the cotton cleaned in the blowing room to separate fibers and remove impurities. Carding, a combing process, follows and serves to extract further dirt and to align the fibers whilst removing shorter ones. Dust is particularly liable to be generated in the blowing and carding rooms, especially during cleaning the machines. Twisting the fibers into strands, spinning, and weaving are much less dusty operations. *Flax* fibers, from which linen is manufactured, are long and have to be separated from the rest of the stem by decomposition, a process known as retting, which employs bacteria in slow-flowing water, exposure on the ground to dew and fungi, or chemical digestion in tanks. The stems are next crushed and beaten to separate fibers, while in the mill the bales are hand-separated and machine-combed to remove dust and shorter fibers before being carded. Separation and straightening of fibers is achieved by drawing prior to spinning, either wet or dry. Combing, carding, and dry spinning produce the most dust. Soft *hemp* undergoes similar treatment to isolate the fiber for rope or yarn manufacture.

The Syndrome

Symptoms do not develop for several years, averaging 20 years in Lancashire cotton workers. The characteristic complaints are tightness in the chest and reversible breathlessness, experienced initially on the first day of the working week (hence the "Monday" feeling) though later on other days as well. A peculiarity is that symptoms take a few hours to develop after a weekend off work. Removal from the dusty atmosphere relieves the symptoms.

Functionally, a fall in forced expiratory volume in 1 second (FEV_1), measured under controlled conditions during a shift at the beginning of the working week, and which is greater than 10 percent or 200 ml is generally regarded as diagnostic provided confounding factors can be eliminated. Annual decrements in ventilatory values have been detected, but ex-cotton and ex-flax workers had only a slight reduction of lung function when compared with nontextile workers, an effect to which shorter stature perhaps from social and nutritional deprivation may have contributed.[606] Whether the disorder evolves into a specific chronic phase has been argued, though large-scale surveys of former textile workers failed to disclose evidence of permanent ill effects.[606] Some employees never develop clinical manifestations of airway obstruction.

The prevalence of all grades of byssinosis is in general determined by dust concentration and length of exposure.[607,608] It was estimated that about 10 percent of workers exposed to 0.5 mg/m^3 over a working life of 40 years will develop symptoms.[607] Despite earlier suggestions to the contrary, cotton textile workers did not have an excess of respiratory deaths,[609,610] as was also the case among flax workers.[611] Moreover, lung cancer appeared to be less frequent in cotton preparation and processing operatives.[610,612] A longitudinal study of workers from entering the industry to development of the syndrome and their subsequent fate has, however, yet to be performed and combined with pulmonary morphometry.

Allowing for concentration of dust and duration of exposure, cigarette smoking by cotton and flax workers augmented the risk of developing byssinosis and its severity.[607,608,611] Up to 10 years after cessation of employment a progressive loss of ventilatory capacity (FEV_1) occurred among persistent smokers with byssinosis, though some nonsmokers with the disorder were similarly affected; longer than 10 years away from dust, smokers retained this effect but nonsmokers had no excess decrement.[613] Cotton workers also experienced chronic bronchitis (mucus hypersecretion) not related to dust exposure, though smoking played an aggravating role.[607,608] Other studies revealed a higher prevalence of chronic bronchitis in cotton textile workers as compared with control subjects.

Pathology

Morphometric analysis applied at the gross and microscopic levels to patients with byssinosis from Lancashire disclosed emphysema in 16, inflammatory proximal acinar (centrilobular) disease in 10, and 6 with panacinar emphysema; the extent of lung involvement ranged from 6 to 40 percent.[614] Excessive fibrosis, honeycombing, and granuloma formation were absent. Lobar and segmental bronchi exhibited muscular hypertrophy and glandular hyperplasia, but the features were nonspecific.[615] Furthermore, in particular individuals there was no clear distinction between byssinosis and chronic bronchitis on morphologic or morphometric grounds, while smoking had no apparent structural effect. The peroxidase-antiperoxidase technique demonstrated that fewer interstitial plasma cells contained IgA in byssinotics as compared with normal individuals or chronic bronchitics. The evidence thus excluded allergic bronchiolo-alveolitis and extrinsic asthma. The pulmonary vasculature was normal for age and the ventricular weights paralleled those in control specimens.

Lung specimens from 44 American textile workers and a large control group, all of whose smoking habits were known, were also subjected to point counting.[616] In respect to "centrilobular" (inflammatory proxmal acinar) emphysema, significant increases of frequency and extent occurred in smokers, but not between cotton and noncotton workers. The volume of bronchial mucous glands and bronchiolar goblet cell metaplasia were, however, unaffected by smoking. Excluding cigarette smokers, these two histologic features were significantly related to cotton exposure. Another autopsy study from the United States, comprising 282 active and retired textile workers and many control subjects, detected no statistical evidence that exposure to cotton dust led to emphysema, interstitial fibrosis, or cor pulmonale.[617] Occupation affected neither the prevalence nor the severity of emphysema, though smoking habits were incompletely known, while neoplastic and non-neoplastic disorders of the lung were not increased among employees.

Emphysema in cotton workers may thus be attributed to cigarette smoking rather than to cotton dust, a conclusion now supported by physiologic evidence,[618] while bronchitic changes may be blamed on the industrial element. The lesions in pulmonary parenchyma and conducting airways could well be determined by particle size, smaller particles from cigarette smoke penetrating to and damaging the former while the larger cotton fibers impinge mostly on the latter inducing a form of industrial bronchitis. Removal from the dusty atmosphere would be expected to benefit bronchitic but not emphysematous changes, which on present evidence should not be regarded as occupational. These morphologic studies were assailed by epidemiologists, but the firm findings cannot be gainsaid and they serve to indicate directions for future clinical observation.

Pathogenesis

In the absence of a distinct morphologic base for byssinosis, functional interpretations have been explored extensively, but the mechanisms are still imperfectly understood and the precise causal agent(s) remain elusive.

Airborne dust in the mills is a complex mixture consisting of cotton fibers (cellulose) of various lengths, fragments derived from the bracts (thin brittle leaves around the stem of the cotton bolls and the most abundant component of respirable raw cotton dust) and pericarp of the seed head, along with contaminating bacteria and fungi plus inorganic material from soil. The range of organic compounds is thus wide. The symptoms resemble delayed asthma but not immediate asthma and are, therefore, unlikely to result from IgE-mediated hypersensitivity. Three principal mechanisms have been advanced.

1. Nonallergic *histamine release* in the lung might explain the rapid onset of symptomatic and functional changes in normal individuals inhaling cotton dusts or aqueous extracts, while the first-day response of workers might reflect histamine accumulation over the rest period. As with histamine aerosols, the functional effect of challenge inhalation of hemp dust was promoted or inhibited by appropriate drugs.[619]

Human lung tissue treated with extracts of cotton bracts in vitro released histamine,[620] and platelets behaved similarly when exposed to mill dust.[621] Moreover, blood histamine levels were elevated in cotton or flax workers, whether asymptomatic or byssinotic, especially after a rest period.[622] Though mast cells come under suspicion, the site of histamine release has not been determined nor the chemical compounds responsible, while the timing of the response in normal humans differed from that seen occupationally. Purified aqueous extracts of cotton bracts induced airway constriction in healthy volunteers and, unlike histamine, the maximum response was subject to a delay; the effect occurred in the absence of endotoxin.[623] The possible involvement of other mediators which induce smooth muscle contraction, such as SRS-A, leukotrienes, or other arachidonic acid metabolites, including prostaglandin and thromboxane, has lately received attention.[624,625] The releasing agents in cotton dust and bracts appear to be of plant rather than bacterial origin and they may operate via macrophages, platelets, or polymorphonuclear neutrophils attracted to the lung.

2. *Antigen-antibody complexes.* Allergic hypersensitivity might develop from formation in the lungs of complexes between antigens in cotton or flax dust and precipitating IgG antibodies. However, no true precipitating antibodies were detected in preshift sera from textile workers or control subjects collected on Monday when examined by gel diffusion and immunoelectrophoresis against aqueous extracts from cardroom dust, bract, stems, leaves, or lint.[626] Nevertheless, anticomplementary activity in serum and decreased FEV_1 were found in normal subjects exposed to cotton dust from closed bolls with bracts intact, and appeared to be independent of endotoxin.[627] If a type III response is concerned in byssinosis, features of extrinsic allergic bronchioloalveolitis might be expected but such is not the case.

3. *Endotoxins.* The cell walls of gram-negative bacteria contaminating cotton contain a toxic lipopolysaccharide, whose effects include histamine release and reduced FEV_1. In Lancashire cotton mills a disparity transpired between dust concentration and symptoms, but their correlation with the level of atmospheric Gram-negative bacteria was highly significant.[628] In American[629] and Swedish[630] cotton mills, symptoms or decrement in FEV_1 related better to the number of airborne Gram-negative bacteria than to dust levels. Chemically retted flax gives rise to dust free of organisms and apparently does not lead to byssinosis. Steamed cotton diminished the "Monday" decrement of FEV_1,[631] while water washing of cotton reduced airborne endotoxin and bronchoconstriction.[632] Cotton dust may activate complement by the classical and alternative pathways, though not necessarily by endotoxin.[633] Proteolytic enzymes of cotton dust itself are the latest agents to be suspected of causing tissue damage.

Although histamine release may be a late effector mechanism, other agents promoting contraction of smooth muscle appear to mimic better the natural disorder, whilst doubts remain about the role of endotoxin. The outstanding lead centers on the bracts of the cotton plant. To date there is no evidence for HLA antigen involvement in susceptibility to byssinosis and the disorder may prove to be multifactorial in origin. Unfortunately no animal model of byssinosis exists.

References

1. Badham C, Taylor HB: *The Lungs of Coal, Metalliferous and Sandstone Miners and Other Workers in New South Wales. Chemical Analysis and Pathology. Studies in Industrial Hygiene No. 19.* Annual Report of the Department of Public Health, New South Wales, 1936.

2. Heppleston AG: Pigmentation and disorders of the lung. In Wolman M, (ed). *Pigments in Pathology.* New York: Academic Press, 1969, pp 33–73.

3. Zenker FA: Über Staubinhalationskrankheiten der Lungen. Dtsch Arch Klin Med 2:116–172, 1867.

4. Webster I: Silicosis in South African gold mines. The Leech 39:36, 1969.

5. Meiklejohn A: Silicosis in the Potteries. Some observations based on seven hundred and fifty necropsies. Br J Indust Med 6:230–240, 1949.

6. Ayer HE: The proposed ACGIH mass limits for quartz; review and evaluation. Am Indust Hyg Assoc J 30:117–125, 1969.

7. Trasko VM: Some facts on the prevalence of silicosis in the United States. Arch Indust Health 14:379–386, 1956.

8. Fox AJ, Goldblatt P, Kinlen LV: A study of the mortality of Cornish tin miners. Br J Indust Med 38:378–380, 1981.

9. Craighead JE, Vallyathan NV: Cryptic pulmonary lesions in

workers occupationally exposed to dust containing silica. J Am Med Assoc 244:1939–1941, 1980.

10. Banks DE, Morring KL, Boehlecke BA et al.: Silicosis in silica flour workers. Am Rev Respir Dis 124:445–450, 1981.

11. Simson FW: Reconstruction models showing the moderately early simple silicotic process and how it affects definite parts of the primary unit of the lung. J Pathol Bacteriol 40:37–44, 1935.

12. Belt TH: Silicosis of the spleen: A study of the silicotic nodule. J Pathol Bacteriol 49:39–44, 1939.

13. Simson FW, Strachan AS: Silicosis and tuberculosis. Observations on the origin and character of silicotic lesions as shown in cases occurring on the Witwatersrand. Publ South Afr Inst Med Res 6:367–406, 1935.

14. Gardner LU: Studies on experimental pneumonokoniosis VIII. Inhalation of quartz dust. J Indust Hyg 14:18–38, 1932.

15. Heppleston AG: The disposal of dust in the lungs of silicotic rats. Am J Pathol 40:493–506, 1962.

16. Gardner LU: Experimental pneumoconioses. In: Lanza AJ (ed): *Silicosis and Asbestosis*. New York: Oxford University Press, pp 257–345, l938.

17. Vorvald AJ, Delahant AB, Dworski M: Silicosis and type III pneumococcus pneumonia: An experimental study. J Indust Hyg Toxicol 22:64–78, 1940.

18. Attygalle D, King EJ, Harrison CV, Nagelschmidt G: The action of variable amounts of tridymite, and of tridymite combined with coal, on the lungs of rats. Br J Indust Med 13:41–50, 1956.

19. Chvapil M, Holuša R: Zusammenhang der Dosis von Quarzstaub mit der Grösse der Entzündungsreaktion der Lungen. Int Arch Gewerbepath Gewerbehyg 21:369–378, 1965.

20. Ross HF, King EJ, Yoganathan M, Nagelschmidt G: Inhalation experiments with coal dust containing 5 percent, 10 percent, 20 percent and 40 percent quartz: Tissue reactions in the lungs of rats. Ann Occup Hyg 5:149–161, 1962.

21. Nagelschmidt G: The relation between lung dust and lung pathology in pneumoconiosis. Br J Indust Med 17:247–259, 1960.

22. King EJ, Mohanty GP, Harrison CV, Nagelschmidt G. The action of flint of variable size injected at constant weight and constant surface into the lungs of rats. Br J Indust Med 10:76–92, 1953.

23. King EJ, Mohanty GP, Harrison CV, Nagelschmidt G. The action of different forms of pure silica on the lungs of rats. Br J Indust Med 10:9–17, 1953.

24. Strecker FJ: Histophysiologische Untersuchungen zur "silikotischen Gewebsreaktion" im Intraperitonealtest und zur Gewebswirkung von Coesit und Stischowit. Beitr Silikose-Forsch Sb6:55–83, 1965.

25. Charbonnier J, Collet A, Daniel-Moussard H, Martin JC: Étude par test trachéal du pouvoir fibrosant d'une coesite synthétique. Beitr Silikose-Forsch Sb6:85–92, 1965.

26. Greenhow EH: Stone-worker's pulmonary disease. Specimen of collier's lung. Specimen of potter's lung. Trans Pathol Soc Lond 17:24–27, 34–36, 36–38, 1866.

27. Gardner LU: Studies on the relation of mineral dusts to tuberculosis III. The relatively early lesions in experimental pneumokoniosis produced by carborundum inhalation and their influence on pulmonary tuberculosis. Am Rev Tuberc 7:344–347, 1923.

28. Evans SM, Zeit W: Tissue responses to physical forces II. The response of connective tissue to piezoelectrically active crystals. J Lab Clin Med 34:592–609, 1949.

29. Gye WE, Purdy WJ: The poisonous properties of colloidal silica. I and II. Br J Exp Pathol 3:75–85, 86–94, 1922.

30. Engelbrecht FM, Yoganathan M, King EJ, Nagelschmidt G: Fribrosis and collagen in rats' lungs produced by etched and unetched free silica dusts. Arch Ind Health 17:287–294, 1958.

31. Heppleston AG, Ahlquist KA, Williams D: Observations on the pathogenesis of silicosis by means of the diffusion chamber technique. Br J Indust Med 18:143–147, 1961.

32. Kettle EH: The interstitial reactions caused by various dusts and their influence on tuberculous infection. J Pathol Bacteriol 35:395–405, 1932.

33. Denny JJ, Robson WD, Irwin DA: The prevention of silicosis by metallic aluminium I. Can Med Assoc J 37:1–11, 1937.

34. Denny JJ, Robson WD, Irwin DA: The prevention of silicosis by metallic aluminium II. Can Med Assoc J 40:213–228, 1939.

35. Policard A, Letort M, Charbonnier J, et al.: Recherches expérimentales concernant l'inhibition de l'action cytotoxique du quartz au moyen de substances minérales, notamment de composés de l'aluminium. Beitr Silikose-Forsch (Pneumokon) 23:1–58, 1971.

36. Le Bouffant L, Daniel H, Martin JC. The therapeutic action of aluminium compounds on the development of experimental lesions produced by pure quartz or mixed dust. In Walton WH (ed): *Inhaled Particles IV*. Oxford: Pergamon Press, 1977, pp 389–401.

37. Dix WG: Aluminum powder and silicosis prevention. Can Mining J 92:35–42, 1971.

38. Fallon JT: Specific tissue reaction to phospholipids: A suggested explanation for the similarity of the lesions of silicosis and pulmonary tuberculosis. Can Med Assoc J 36:223–228, 1937.

39. Webster I, Henderson CI, Marasas LW, Keegan DJ: Some biologically active substances produced by the action of silica and their possible significance. In: Davies CN (ed): *Inhaled Particles and Vapours II*. Oxford: Pergamon Press, 1967, pp 111–119.

40. Heppleston AG, Wright NA, Steward JA: Experimental alveolar lipo-proteinosis following the inhalation of silica. J Pathol 101:293–307, 1970.

41. Nash T, Allison AC, Harington JS: Physico-chemical properties of silica in relation to its toxicity. Nature 210:259–261, 1966.

42. Schlipköter H-W, Brockhaus A: Die Wirkung von Polyvinylpyridin auf die experimentelle Silikose. Dtsch Med Wochenschr 85:920–923, 1960.

43. Schlipköter H-W, Brockhaus A: Die Hemmung der experimentellen Silikose durch subcutane Verabreichung von Polyvinylpyridin-N-oxyd. Klin Wochenschr 39:1182–1189, 1961.

44. Beck EG, Bruch J, Brockhaus A: Die Beeinflussung der cytotoxischen Quarzwirkung an Mäusefibroblasten (Strain L) durch Polyvinylpyridin-N-oxyd (P204). Z Zellforsch 59:568–576, 1963.

45. Depasse J: Mechanism of the haemolysis by colloidal silica. In Brown RC, Gormley IP, Chamberlain M, Davies R (eds): *The In Vitro Effects of Mineral Dusts*. London: Academic Press, 1980, pp 125–130.

46. Kriegseis W, Biederbick R, Boese J, et al.: Investigations into the determination of the cytotoxicity of quartz dust by physical methods. In Walton WH (ed): *Inhaled Particles IV*. Oxford: Pergamon Press, 1977, pp 343–357.

47. Heppleston AG, Styles JA: Activity of a macrophage factor in collagen formation by silica. Nature 214:521–522, 1967.

48. Heppleston AG: Cellular reactions with silica. In: Bendz G, Lindqvist I (eds): *Biochemistry of Silicon and Related Problems*

(*Nobel Foundation Symposium 40*). New York: Plenum Press, 1978, pp 357–379.

49. Leu RW, Eddleston ALWF, Hadden JW, Good RA: Mechanism of action of migration inhibitory factor (MIF) I. Evidence for a receptor for MIF present on the peritoneal macrophage but not on the alveolar macrophage. J Exp Med 136:589–603, 1972.

50. Simon LM, Robin ED, Phillips JR, et al.: Enzymatic basis for bioenergetic differences of alveolar versus peritoneal macrophages and enzyme regulation by molecular O_2. J Clin Invest 59:443–448, 1977.

51. Aalto M, Potila M, Kulonen E: The effect of silica-treated macrophages on the synthesis of collagen and other proteins in vitro. Exp Cell Res 97:193–202, 1976.

52. Aho S, Kulonen E: Effect of silica-liberated macrophage factors on protein synthesis in cell-free systems. Exp Cell Res 104:31–38, 1977.

53. Lehtinen P, Kulonen E: Subcellular targets of the soluble SiO_2-liberated macrophage factors in experimental granulation tissue. Biochem Biophys Acta 564:132–140, 1979.

54. Aalto M, Turakainen H, Kulonen E: Effect of SiO_2-liberated macrophage factor on protein synthesis in connective tissue in vitro. Scand J Clin Lab Invest 39:205–213, 1979.

55. Aalto M, Kulonen E: Fractionation of connective tissue activating factors from the culture medium of silica-treated macrophages. Acta Pathol Microbiol Scand Sect C 87:241–250, 1979.

56. Aalto M, Viljanen M, Kulonen E: Neutralization of the fibrogenic silica-released macrophage factor by antiserum. Exp Pathol 22:181–184, 1982.

57. Aho SA, Lehtinen PA, Viljanen MK, Kulonen EI: Antifibrogenic effects of antiserum against the macrophage RNase. Am Rev Respir Dis 127:180–184, 1983.

58. Aho S, Kulonen E: Involvement of ribonuclease in the interactions of macrophages and fibroblasts in experimental silicosis. Experientia 36:29–30, 1980.

59. Aho S, Lehtinen P, Kulonen E: Effects of purified macrophage RNases on granuloma fibroblasts with reference to silicosis. Acta Physiol Scand 109:275–281, 1980.

60. Heppleston AG: Pulmonary repair and fibrosis. In Glynn LE (ed): *Handbook of Inflammation*, vol 3. *Tissue Repair and Regeneration*. Amsterdam: Elsevier/North Holland, 1981, pp 393–456.

61. Kulonen E, Potila M: Macrophages and the synthesis of connective tissue components. Acta Pathol Microbiol Scand Sect C 88:7–13, 1980.

62. Aalto M, Kulonen E. Rönnemaa T, et al.: Liberation of a fibrogenic factor from human blood monocytes, ascites cells, cultured histiocytes and transformed mouse macrophages by treatment with SiO_2. Scand J Clin Lab Invest 40:311–318, 1980.

63. McGee J O'D, O'Hare RP, Patrick RS: Stimulation of the collagen biosynthetic pathway by factors isolated from experimentally-injured liver. Nature New Biol 243:121–123, 1973.

64. Shaba JK, Patrick RS, McGee J O'D: Collagen synthesis by mesenchymal cells isolated from normal and acutely-damaged mouse liver. Br J Exp Pathol 54:110–116, 1973.

65. Vigliani EC, Pernis B: Immunological aspects of silicosis. Adv Tuberc Res 12:230–279, 1963.

66. Cocarla AA, Gabor S, Milea M, Suciu I: Serum immunoglobulins in workers exposed to silicogenic risk with tuberculin negative test and hyperergia. J Hyg Epidemiol Microbiol Immunol 21:374–380, 1977.

67. Jones RN, Turner-Warwick M, Ziskind M, Weill H: High prevalence of antinuclear antibodies in sandblasters' silicosis. Am Rev Respir Dis 113:393–395, 1976.

68. Unge G, Mellner Ch: Caplan's syndrome—a clinical study of 13 cases. Scand J Resp Dis 56:287–291, 1975.

69. Schuyler MR, Ziskind M, Salvaggio J: Cell-mediated immunity in silicosis. Am Rev Respir Dis 116:147–151, 1977.

70. Schuyler MR, Ziskind MM, Salvaggio J: Function of lymphocytes and monocytes in silicosis. Chest 75:340–344, 1979.

71. Dauber JH, Finn DR, Daniele RP: Immunologic abnormalities in anthracosilicosis. Am Rev Respir Dis 113(abstr):94, 1976.

72. Gualde N, Leobardy J de, Serizay B, Malinvaud G: HL-A and silicosis. Am Rev Respir Dis 116:334–336, 1977.

73. Wagner JC, McCormick JN: Immunological investigations of coalworkers' disease. J R Coll Physicians Lond 2:49–56, 1967.

74. Jones JH, Heppleston AG: Immunological observations in experimental silicosis. Nature 191:1212–1213, 1961.

75. Burrell R: Immunological aspects of silica. In: Dunnom DD (ed): *Health Effects of Synthetic Silica Particulates*. Philadelphia: American Society for Testing and Materials Special Technical Publication 732, 1981, pp 82–92.

76. Opie EL, Aronson JD: Tubercule bacilli in latent tuberculous lesions and in lung tissue without tuberculous lesions. Arch Pathol 4:1–21, 1927.

77. Heppleston AG: Quantitative air-borne tuberculosis in the rabbit. The course of human type infection. J Exp Med 89:597–610, 1949.

78. Conning DM, Heppleston AG: Reticulo-endothelial activity and local particle disposal: A comparison of the influence of modifying agents. Br J Exp Pathol 47:388–400, 1966.

79. Allison AC, Hart PD'A: Potentiation by silica of the growth of Mycobacterium tuberculosis in macrophage cultures. Br J Exp Pathol 49:465–476, 1968.

80. Pintar K, Funahashi A, Siegesmund KA: A diffuse form of pulmonary silicosis in foundry workers. Arch Pathol 100:535–538, 1976.

81. Chatgidakis CB: Silicosis in South African white gold miners. A comparative study of the disease in its different stages. S Afr J Adv Med Sci 9:383–392, 1963.

82. Jones JG, Owen TE, Corrado HA: Respiratory tuberculosis and pneumoconiosis in slate workers. Br J Dis Chest 6:138–143, 1967.

83. du Buy H: Effect of silica on virus infections in mice and mouse tissue culture. Infect Immunol 11:996–1002, 1975.

84. Chatgidakis CB: A study of the state of the heart in the white South African gold miner. S Afr J Adv Med Sci 10:132–138, 1964.

85. Irvine LG: *Report of Miners' Phthisis Medical Bureau, 1935–1938*. Pretoria: Government Printer, Union of South Africa, 1939.

86. Rüttner JR, Heer HR: Silikose und Lungenkarzinom. Schweiz Med Wochenschr 99:245–249, 1969.

87. Heppleston AG: Silica, pneumoconiosis, and carcinoma of the lung. Am J Indust Med 7:285–294, 1985.

88. Cooper WC, Jacobson G: A 21-year radiographic follow-up of workers in the diatomite industry. J Occup Med 19:563–566, 1977.

89. Vorwald AJ, Durkan TM, Pratt PC, Delahant AB: Diatomaceous earth pneumoconiosis. In *Proceedings Ninth International Congress Industrial Medicine*. Bristol: John Wright, 1949, pp 725–741.

90. Cooper WC: Effects of diatomaceous earth on human health. *Report to Ad Hoc Technical Committee Diatomaceous Earth Producers*. Denver: Johns-Manville, 1977, pp 1–15.

91. Einbrodt HJ, Grussendorf J: Kieselguhr and its toxic effect on the human system. Staub 33:273–276, 1973.

92. Dutra FR: Diatomaceous earth pneumonconiosis. Arch Environ Health 11:613–619, 1965.

93. Vitums VC, Edwards MJ, Niles NR, et al.: Pulmonary fibrosis from amorphous silica dust, a product of silica vapor. Arch Environ Health 32:62–68, 1977.

93a. Brambilla C, Brambilla E, Rigaud D, et al.: Pneumoconiose aux fumées de silice amorphe. Étude minéralogique et ultrastructurale de 6 cas. Rev Fr Mal Resp 8:383–391, 1980.

94. Schepers GWH, Delahant AB, Fear EJ, Schmidt JG: The biological action of Degussa submicron amorphous silica dust (Dow Corning silica) IV. Arch Indust Health 16:363–379, 1957.

95. Policard A, Collet AJ: Toxic and fibrosing action of submicroscopic particles of amorphous silica. Arch Indust Hyg Occup Med 9:389–395, 1954.

95a. Ferch H: Zur gewerbehygienischen Unbedenklichkeit: pulverförmige amorphe synthetische Kieselsäuren. Staub-Réinhalt Luft 45:236–239, 1985.

96. Ziskind M, Weill H, Anderson AE, et al.: Silicosis in shipyard sandblasters. Environ Res 11:237–243, 1976.

97. Bailey WC, Brown M, Buechner HA, et al.: Silico-mycobacterial disease in sandblasters. Am Rev Respir Dis 110:115–125, 1974.

98. Buechner HA, Ansari A: Acute silico-proteinosis. Dis Chest 55:274–284, 1969.

99. Hoffman EO, Lamberty J, Pizzolato P, Coover J: The ultrastructure of acute silicosis. Arch Pathol 96:104–108, 1973.

100. Suratt PM, Winn WC, Brody AR, et al.: Acute silicosis in tombstone sandblasters. Am Rev Respir Dis 115:521–529, 1977.

101. Heppleston AG, Young AE: Alveolar lipo-proteinosis: An ultrastructural comparison of the experimental and human forms. J Pathol 107:107–117, 1972.

102. Heppleston AG, Fletcher K, Wyatt I: Changes in the composition of lung lipids and the "turnover" of dipalmitoyl lecithin in experimental alveolar lipo-proteinosis induced by inhaled quartz. Br J Exp Pathol 55:384–395, 1974.

103. Heppleston AG, McDermott M, Collins MM: The surface properties of the lung in rats with alveolar lipo-proteinosis. Br J Exp Pathol 56:444–453, 1975.

104. Civil GW, Heppleston AG: Replenishment of alveolar macrophages in silicosis: Implication of recruitment by lipid feed-back. Br J Exp Pathol 60:537–547, 1979.

105. Heppleston AG. Silicotic fibrogenesis: A concept of pulmonary fibrosis. Ann Occup Hyg 26:449–462, 1982.

106. Shelley SA, L'Heureux MV, Balis JU: Characterization of lung surfactant: Factors promoting formation of artificial lipid-protein complexes. J Lipid Res 16:224–234, 1975.

107. Nagelschmidt G: The composition of the air-borne dusts at the coal face in certain mines. In *Chronic Pulmonary Disease in South Wales Coalminers. II—Environmental Studies.* Medical Research Council, Special Report Series No. 244. London: His Majesty's Stationary Office, 1943, pp 95–124.

108. Dodgson J, Hadden GG, Jones CO, Walton WH: Characteristics of the airborne dust in British coal mines. In Walton WH (ed): *Inhaled Particles III*. Old Woking, Surrey, England: Unwin, 1971, pp 757–781.

109. Medical Research Council. *Chronic Pulmonary Disease in South Wales Coalminers. I.—Medical Studies.* Special Report Series No 243. London: His Majesty's Stationary Office, 1942, pp 1–222.

110. Medical Research Council: *Chronic Pulmonary Disease in South Wales Coalminers. II—Environmental Studies.* Special Report Series No. 244. London: His Majesty's Stationary Office, 1943, pp 1–222.

111. National Coal Board: *Medical Service. Annual Report 1983–84.* London: National Coal Board.

112. Jacobsen M, Rae S, Walton WH, Rogan JM: The relation between pneumoconiosis and dust-exposure in British coal mines. In Walton WH (ed): *Inhaled Particles III*. Old Woking, Surrey, England: Unwin, 1971, pp 903–917.

113. Jacobsen M: New data on the relationship between simple pneumoconiosis and exposure to coal mine dust. Chest 78 (suppl):408S–410S, 1980.

114. Reisner MTR: Results of epidemiological studies of pneumoconiosis in West German coal mines. In Walton WH (ed): *Inhaled Particles III*. Old Woking, Surrey, England: Unwin, 1971, pp 921–929.

115. Reisner MTR, Robock K: Results of epidemiological, mineralogical and cytotoxicological studies on the pathogenicity of coal-mine dusts. In Walton WH (ed): *Inhaled Particles IV*. Oxford, Pergamon Press, 1977, pp 703–715.

116. Morgan WKC, Reger R, Burgess DB, Shoub E: A comparison of the prevalence of coal workers' pneumoconiosis and respiratory impairment in Pennsylvania bituminous and anthracite miners. Ann NY Acad Sci 200:252–259, 1972.

117. Morgan WKC, Burgess DB, Jacobson G, et al.: The prevalence of coal workers' pneumonconiosis in U.S. coal miners. Arch Environ Health 27:221–226, 1973.

118. Cummins SL, Sladden AF: Coal-miner's lung. An investigation into the anthracotic lungs of coal miners in South Wales. J Pathol Bacteriol 33:1095–1132, 1930.

119. Belt TH, Ferris AA: Histology of coalminers' pneumokoniosis. In *Chronic pulmonary disease in South Wales coalminers. I.—Medical Studies.* Medical Research Council, Special Report Series No. 243. London: His Majesty's Stationery Office, 1942, pp 203–222.

120. Gough J: Pneumoconiosis in coal trimmers. J Pathol Bacteriol 51:277–285, 1940.

121. Gough J: Pneumoconiosis in coal workers in Wales. Occup Med 4:86–97, 1947.

122. Heppleston AG: The essential lesion of pneumokoniosis in Welsh coal workers. J Pathol Bacteriol 59:453–460, 1947.

123. Heppleston AG: Coal workers' pneumoconiosis. Pathological and etiological considerations. Arch Indust Hyg Occup Med 4:270–288, 1951.

124. Heppleston AG. The pathological anatomy of simple pneumokoniosis in coal workers. J Pathol Bacteriol 66:235–246, 1953.

125. Heppleston AG: The pathological recognition and pathogenesis of emphysema and fibrocystic disease of the lung with special reference to coal workers. Ann NY Acad Sci 200: 347–369, 1972.

126. Heppleston AG. Cinephotography of serial sections. Technic for demonstration of microanatomy in depth. Lab Invest 4:374–381, 1955.

127. Wagner JC, Wusteman FS, Edwards JH, Hill RJ: The composition of massive lesions in coal miners. Thorax 30:382–388, 1975.

128. Wagner JC, Burns J, Munday DE, McGee J O'D: Presence of fibronectin in pneumoconiotic lesions. Thorax 37:54–56, 1982.

129. Gloyne SR, Marshall G, Hoyle C: Pneumoconiosis due to graphite dust. Thorax 4:31–38, 1949.

130. Harding HE, Oliver GB: Changes in the lungs produced by natural graphite. Br J Indust Med 6:91–99, 1949.

131. Rüttner JR, Bovet P, Aufdermaur M: Graphit, Carborund, Staublunge. Dtsch Med Wochenschr 77:1413–1415, 1952.

132. Watson AJ, Black J, Doig AT, Nagelschmidt G: Pneumoconiosis in carbon electrode makers. Br J Indust Med 16:274–285, 1959.

133. Rivers D, James WRL, Davies DB, Thomson S: The prevalence of tuberculosis at necropsy in progressive massive fibrosis of coalworkers. Br J Indust Med 14:39–42, 1957.

134. Zaidi SH, Harrison CV, King EJ, Mitchison DA: Experimental infective pneumoconiosis. IV. Massive pulmonary fibrosis produced by coal-mine dust and isoniazid-resistant tubercle bacilli of low virulence. Br J Exp Pathol 36:553–559, 1955.

135. King EJ, Yoganathan M, Harrison CV, Mitchison DA: Experimental infective pneumoconiosis. V. Massive fibrosis of the lungs produced by coal-mine dust and Mycobacterium tuberculosis var muris (vole bacillus). Arch Ind Health 16:380–392, 1957.

136. Heppleston AG: Changes in the lungs of rabbits and ponies inhaling coal dust underground. J Pathol Bacteriol 67:349–359, 1954.

137. Hurley JF, Burns J, Copland L, et al.: Coalworkers' simple pneumoconiosis and exposure to dust at 10 British coal mines. Br J Indust Med 39:120–127, 1982.

138. Walton WH, Dodgson J, Hadden GG, Jacobsen M: The effect of quartz and other non-coal dusts in coalworkers' pneumoconiosis. Part 1. Epidemiological studies. In: Walton WH (ed): *Inhaled Particles IV*. Oxford: Pergamon Press, 1977, pp 669–689.

139. Bennett JG, Dick JA, Kaplan YS, et al.: The relationship between coal rank and the prevalence of pneumoconiosis. Br J Indust Med 36:206–210, 1979.

140. Nagelschmidt G, Rivers D, King EJ, Trevella W: Dust and collagen content of lungs of coal-workers with progressive massive fibrosis. Br J Indust Med 20:181–191, 1963.

141. Davis JMG, Ottery J, le Roux A: The effect of quartz and other non-coal dusts in coalworkers' pneumoconiosis. Part II. Lung autopsy study. In Walton WH (ed): *Inhaled Particles IV*. Oxford: Pergamon Press, 1977, pp 691–700.

142. Davis JMG, Chapman J, Collings P, et al.: Autopsy Studies in Coalminers' Lungs. Technical Memo 79/9. Edinburgh: Institute Occupational Medicine, 1979.

143. Faulds JS, Nagelschmidt G: The dust in the lungs of haematite miners from Cumberland. Ann Occup Hyg 4:255–263, 1962.

144. Kriegseis W, Scharmann A: Specific harmfulness of respirable dusts from West German coal mines. V. Influence of mineral surface properties. Ann Occup Hyg 26:511–525, 1982.

145. Schlipköter H-W, Hilscher W, Pott F, Beck EG: Investigations on the aetiology of coal workers' pneumoconiosis with the use of PVN-oxide. In Walton WH (ed): *Inhaled Particles III*. Old Woking, Surrey, England: Unwin, 1971, pp 379–389.

146. Weller W: Long-term test on rhesus monkeys for the PVNO therapy of anthracosilicosis. In Walton WH (ed): *Inhaled Particles IV*. Oxford: Pergamon Press, 1977, pp 379–386.

147. Harding HE, Massie AP: Pneumoconiosis in boiler scalers. Br J Indust Med 8:256–264, 1951.

148. Heppleston AG: The pathogenesis of simple pneumokoniosis in coal workers. J Pathol Bacteriol 67:51–63, 1954.

149. Heppleston AG, Civil GW, Critchlow A: The effects of duration and intermittency of exposure on the elimination of air-borne dust from high and low rank coal mines. In Walton WH (ed): *Inhaled Particles III*. Old Woking, Surrey, England: Unwin, 1971, pp 261–270.

150. Civil GW, Heppleston AG, Casswell C: The influence of exposure duration and intermittency upon the pulmonary retention and elimination of dusts from high and low rank coal mines. Ann Occup Hyg 17:173–185, 1975.

151. Lippmann M, Eckert HL, Hahon N, Morgan WKC: Circulating antinuclear and rheumatoid factors in coal miners. Ann Intern Med 79:807–811, 1973.

152. Soutar CA, Turner-Warwick M, Parkes WR: Circulating antinuclear antibody and rheumatoid factor in coal pneumoconiosis. Br Med J 3:145–147, 1974.

153. Cochrane AL: The attack rate of progressive massive fibrosis. Br J Indust Med 19:51–64, 1962.

154. Shennan DH, Washington JS, Thomas DJ, et al.: Factors predisposing to the development of progressive massive fibrosis in coal miners. Br J Indust Med 38:321–326, 1981.

155. Rivers D, Wise ME, King EJ, Nagelschmidt G: Dust content, radiology and pathology in simple pneumoconiosis of coalworkers. Br J Indust Med 17:87–108, 1960.

156. Barrie HJ, Gosselin L: Massive pneumoconiosis from a rock dust containing no free silica. Nepheline lung. Arch Environ Health 1:109–117, 1960.

157. James WRL: The relationship of tuberculosis to the development of massive pneumokoniosis in coal workers. Br J Tuberc Dis Chest 48:89–96, 1954.

158. Cochrane AL, Carpenter RG, Clarke WG, et al.: Factors influencing the radiological progression rate of progressive massive fibrosis. Br J Indust Med 13:177–183, 1956.

159. Cochrane AL, Cox JG, Jarman TF: Pulmonary tuberculosis in the Rhondda Fach. A survey of a mining community. Br Med J 2:843–853, 1952.

160. Kilpatrick GS, Heppleston AG, Fletcher CM: Cavitation in the massive fibrosis of coalworkers' pneumoconiosis. Thorax 9:260–272, 1954.

161. Marks J: Anonymous mycobacteria and the pneumoconiosis of coal-miners. Beitr Silikose-Forsch Sb5:261–265, 1963.

162. British Thoracic and Tuberculosis Association: Opportunist mycobacterial pulmonary infection and occupational dust exposure: An investigation in England and Wales. Tubercle 56:295–310, 1975.

163. Byers PD, King EJ: Experimental infective pneumoconiosis with Mycobacterium tuberculosis (var. muris) and haematite by inhalation and by injection. J Pathol Bacteriol 81:123–134, 1961.

164. Byers PD, King EJ: Experimental infective pneumoconiosis with coal, kaolin and mycobacteria. Lab Invest 8:647–664, 1959.

165. Fritze E: Some epidemiological aspects in coal-miners' dust-exposure. 16th International Congress Occupational Health, Tokyo, 1969, pp 685–686.

166. Fritze E: Zur Tuberkulinsensitivität von Staubbelasteten Kohlenbergarbeiten und von niemals staubexponierten Bevölkerungsgruppen des Ruhrgebiets. Int Arch Occup Environ Health 35:201–215, 1975.

167. Pearson DJ, Mentnech MS, Elliott JA, et al.: Serologic changes in pneumoconiosis and progressive massive fibrosis of coal workers. Am Rev Respir Dis 124:696–699, 1981.

168. Hahon N, Morgan WKC, Petersen M: Serum immunoglobulin levels in coal workers' pneumoconiosis. Ann Occup Hyg 23:165–174, 1980.

169. Robertson MD, Boyd JE, Collins HPR, Davis JMG: Serum immunoglobulin levels and humoral immune competence in coalworkers. Am J Indust Med 6:387–393, 1984.

170. Boyd JE, Robertson MD, Davis JMG: Auto-antibodies in coalminers: Their relationship to the development of progressive massive fibrosis. Am J Indust Med 3:201–208, 1982.

171. Robertson MD, Boyd JE, Fernie JM, Davis JMG: Some

immunological studies on coalworkers with and without pneumoconiosis. Am J Indust Med 4:467–476, 1983.

172. Heise ER, Mentnech MS, Olenchock SA, et al.: HLA-A1 and coalworkers' pneumoconiosis. Am Rev Respir Dis 119:903–908, 1979.

173. Wagner MMF, Darke C: HLA-A and B antigen frequencies in Welsh coalworkers with pneumoconiosis and Caplan's syndrome. Tissue Antigens 14:165–168, 1979.

174. Soutar CA, Coutts I, Parkes WR, et al.: Histocompatibility antigens in coal miners with pneumoconiosis. Br J Indust Med 40:34–38, 1983.

175. Heppleston AG, Morris TG: The progression of experimental silicosis. The influence of exposure to "inert" dust. Am J Pathol 46:945–958, 1965.

176. Goldstein B, Webster I: Mixed dust fibrosis in mine workers. In Walton WH (ed): *Inhaled Particles III*. Old Woking, Surrey, England: Unwin, 1971, pp 705–711.

177. Rüttner JR: Foundry workers' pneumoconiosis in Switzerland (anthracosilicosis). Arch Indust Hyg Occup Med 9:297–305, 1954.

178. McLaughlin AIG, Harding HE: Pneumoconiosis and other causes of death in iron and steel foundry workers. Arch Indust Health 14:350–378, 1956.

179. Rossiter CE, Rivers D, Bergman I, et al.: Dust content, radiology and pathology in simple pneumoconiosis of coalworkers (further report). In Davies CN (ed): *Inhaled Particles and Vapours II*. Oxford: Pergamon Press, 1967, pp 419–434.

180. Ruckley VA, Fernie JM, Chapman JS, et al.: Comparison of radiographic appearances with associated pathology and lung dust content in a group of coalworkers. Br J Indust Med 41:459–467, 1984.

181. Gilson JC, Hugh-Jones P: *Lung Function in Coalworkers' Pneumoconiosis*. Medical Research Council Special Report Series No. 290. London: Her Majesty's Stationary Office, 1955.

182. Cotes JE, Deivanayagam CN, Field GB, Billiet L: Relation between type of simple pneumoconiosis (p or m) and lung function. In Walton WH (ed): *Inhaled Particles III*. Oxford: Pergamon Press, 1971, pp 633–641.

183. Cotes JE, Field GB: Lung gas exchange in simple pneumoconiosis of coal workers. Br J Indust Med 29:268–273, 1972.

184. Musk AW, Cotes JE, Bevan C, Campbell MJ: Relationship between type of simple coalworkers' pneumoconiosis and lung function. A nine-year follow-up study of subjects with small rounded opacities. Br J Indust Med 38:313–320, 1981.

185. Lyons JP, Campbell H: Evolution of disability in coalworkers' pneumoconiosis. Thorax 31:527–533, 1976.

186. Hartung W, Einbrodt HJ: Lokalisation und Art der Staubablagerungen in der Lunge und ihre funktionelle Bedeutung. Beitr Silikose-Forsch Sb6:379–394, 1965.

187. Ryder R, Lyons JP, Campbell H, Gough J: Emphysema in coal workers' pneumoconiosis. Br Med J 3:481–487, 1970.

188. Lyons JP, Ryder R, Campbell H, Gough J: Pulmonary disability in coal workers' pneumoconiosis. Br Med J 1:713–716, 1972.

189. Cockcroft A, Seal RME, Wagner JC, et al.: Post-mortem study of emphysema in coalworkers and non-coalworkers. Lancet 2:600–603, 1982.

190. Jacobsen M, Burns J, Attfield MD: Smoking and coalworkers' simple pneumoconiosis. In Walton WH (ed): *Inhaled Particles IV*. Oxford: Pergamon Press, 1977, pp 759–771.

191. Lyons JP, Ryder RC, Seal RME, Wagner JC: Emphysema in smoking and non-smoking coal workers with pneumoconiosis. Bull Eur Physiopathol Respir 17:75–85, 1981.

192. Oldham PD, Rossiter CE: Mortality in coalworkers' pneumoconiosis related to lung function: A prospective study. Br J Indust Med 22:93–100, 1965.

193. Jacobsen M: Dust exposure, lung diseases, and coalminers' mortality. PhD thesis, University of Edinburgh, 1976.

194. Cochrane AL, Haley TJL, Moore F, Hole D: The mortality of men in the Rhondda Fach 1950–1970. Br J Indust Med 36:15–22, 1979.

195. Hahon N: Effect of coal rank on the interferon system. Environ Res 30:72–79, 1983.

196. Wells AL: Cor pulmonale in coal-workers' pneumoconiosis. Br Heart J 16:74–78, 1954.

197. James WRL, Thomas AJ: Cardiac hypertrophy in coalworkers' pneumoconiosis. Br J Indust Med 13:24–29, 1956.

198. Lapp NL, Seaton A, Kaplan KC, et al.: Pulmonary hemodynamics in symptomatic coal miners. Am Rev Respir Dis 104:418–426, 1971.

199. James WRL: Primary lung cancer in South Wales coalworkers with pneumoconiosis. Br J Indust Med 12:87–91, 1955.

200. Goldman K: Mortality of coal miners from carcinoma of the lung. Br J Indust Med 22:72–77, 1965

201. Schimanski P, Rosmanith J: Über den Zusammenhang von Bronchialkrebs und Anthrako-Silikose. Beitr Silikose-Forsch (Pneumokon) 26:59–109, 1974.

202. Rooke GB, Ward FG, Dempsey AN, et al.: Carcinoma of the lung in Lancashire coalminers. Thorax 34:229–233, 1979.

203. Goldman K: Prognosis of coal miners with carcinoma of the lung. Thorax 20:170–174, 1965.

204. Doll R, Vessey MP, Beasley RWR, et al.: Mortality of gas workers—final report of a prospective study. Br J Indust Med 29:394–406, 1972.

205. Christian HA: Cancer of the lung in employees of a public utility. A fifteen-year-study (1946–1960). J Occup Med 4:133–139, 1962.

206. Hurley JF, Archibald RMcL, Collings PL, et al.: The mortality of coke workers in Britain. Am J Indust Med 4:691–704, 1983.

207. Palmer WG, Scott WD: Lung cancer in ferrous foundry workers: A review. Am Indust Hyg Assoc J 42:329–340, 1981.

208. Creagan ET, Hoover RN, Fraumeni JF: Mortality from stomach cancer in coal mining regions. Arch Environ Health 28:28–30, 1974.

208a. Swaen GHM, Aerdts CWHM, Sturmans F, et al.: Gastric cancer in coal miners: A case-control study in a coal mining area. Br J Indust Med 43:627–630, 1985.

209. Caplan A: Certain unusual radiological appearances in the chest of coal-miners suffering from rheumatoid arthritis. Thorax 8:29–37, 1953.

210. Miall WE, Caplan A, Cochrane AL, et al.: An epidemiological study of rheumatoid arthritis associated with characteristic chest X-ray appearances in coal-workers. Br Med J 2:1231–1236, 1953.

211. Miall WE: Rheumatoid arthritis in males. Ann Rheum Dis 14:150–158, 1955.

212. Gough J, Rivers D, Seal RME: Pathological studies of modified pneumoconiosis in coal-miners with rheumatoid arthritis (Caplan's syndrome). Thorax 10:9–18, 1955.

213. Caplan A, Payne RB, Withey J: A broader concept of Caplan's syndrome related to rheumatoid factors. Thorax 17:205–212, 1962.

214. De Horatius RJ, Abruzzo JL, Williams RC: Immunofluorescent and immunologic studies of rheumatoid lung. Arch Intern Med 129:441–446, 1972.

215. Doctor L, Snider GL: Diffuse interstitial pulmonary fibrosis associated with arthritis. Am Rev Respir Dis 85:413–422, 1962.

216. Popper MS, Bogdonoff ML, Hughes RL: Interstitial rheumatoid lung disease: A reassessment and review of the literature. Chest 62:243–249, 1972.

217. Erasmus LD: Scleroderma in gold miners on the Witwatersrand, with particular reference to pulmonary manifestations. S Afr J Lab Clin Med 3:209–231, 1957.

218. Rodnan GP, Benedek TG, Medsger TA, Cammarata RJ: The association of progressive systemic sclerosis (scleroderma) with coal miners' pneumoconiosis and other forms of silicosis. Ann Intern Med 66:323–334, 1967.

219. Günther G, Schuchardt E: Silikose und progressive Sklerodermie. Dtsch Med Wochenschr 95:467–468, 1970.

220. Heppleston AG: The pathology of honeycomb lung. Thorax 11:77–93, 1956.

221. Lyons JP, Ryder RC, Campbell H, et al.: Significance of irregular opacities in the radiology of coal workers' pneumoconiosis. Br J Indust Med 31:36–44, 1974.

222. Cockcroft AE, Wagner JC, Seal RME, et al.: Irregular opacities in coal workers' pneumoconiosis—correlation with pulmonary function and pathology. Ann Occup Hyg 26:767–787, 1982.

223. Yada K: Study of chrysotile asbestos by a high resolution electron microscope. Acta Crystallog 23:704–707, 1967.

224. Thomson JG: Asbestos and the urban dweller. Ann NY Acad Sci 132:196–214, 1965.

225. Merewether ERA, Price CW: *Report on Effects of Asbestos Dust on the Lungs and Dust Suppression in the Asbestos Industry*. London: His Majesty's Stationery Office, 1930.

226. Whipple HE, Van Reyen P: *Biological effects of asbestos*. Ann NY Acad Sci 132:1–765, 1965.

227. Bogovski P, Gilson JC, Timbrell V, Wagner JC: *Biological Effects of Asbestos*. IARC Scientific Publication No. 8. Lyon: International Agency for Research on Cancer, 1973, pp 1–346.

228. Gravatt CC, LaFleur PD, Heinrich KFJ: *Proceedings of Workshop on Asbestos: Definitions and Measurement Methods*. Washington, DC: National Bureau of Standards, U.S. Department of Commerce, 1978, pp 1–496.

229. Selikoff IJ, Hammond EC: Health hazards of asbestos exposure. Ann NY Acad Sci 330:1–814, 1979.

230. Selikoff IJ, Hammond EC, Seidman H: Mortality experience of insulation workers in the United States and Canada, 1943–1976. Ann NY Acad Sci 330:91–116, 1979.

231. Nicholson WJ, Langer AM, Selikoff IJ: Epidemiological evidence on asbestos. In: Gravatt CC, LaFleur PD, Heinrich KFJ (eds): *Proceedings of Workshop on Asbestos: Definitions and Measurement Methods*. Washington, DC: National Bureau of Standards, U.S. Department of Commerce, 1978, pp 71–90.

232. Knox JF, Holmes S, Doll R, Hill ID: Mortality from lung cancer and other causes among workers in an asbestos textile factory. Br J Indust Med 25:293–303, 1968.

233. Peto J, Doll R, Howard SV, et al.: A mortality study among workers in an English asbestos factory. Br J Indust Med 34:169–173, 1977.

234. Peto J: Lung cancer mortality in relation to measured dust levels in an asbestos textile factory. In Wagner JC (ed): *Biological Effects of Mineral Fibres*. IARC Scientific Publication No. 30. Lyon: International Agency for Research on Cancer, 1980, pp 829–836.

235. Elmes PC, Simpson MJC: Insulation workers in Belfast. A further study of mortality due to asbestos exposure (1940–75). Br J Indust Med 34:174–180, 1977.

236. Smither WJ: Secular changes in asbestosis in an asbestos factory. Ann NY Acad Sci 132:166–181, 1965.

237. Murray HM: In *Report of Departmental Commission on Compensation for Industrial Diseases*, Cd 3496. London: His Majesty's Stationery Office, 1907, pp 127–128.

238. Cooke WE, McDonald S: Pulmonary asbestosis. Br Med J 2:1024–1026, 1927.

239. Robinson BWS, Musk AW: Benign asbestos pleural effusion: Diagnosis and course. Thorax 36:896–900, 1981.

240. Epler GR, McLoud TC, Gaensler EA: Prevalence and incidence of benign asbestos pleural effusion in working population. JAMA 247:617–622, 1982.

241. Kuhn C, Kuo TT: Cytoplasmic hyalin in asbestosis. Arch Pathol 95:190–194, 1973.

242. U.I.C.C. Report and recommendation of the working group on asbestos and cancer. Br J Indust Med 22:165–171, 1965.

243. Marchand F: Über eigentümliche Pigmentkristalle in den Lungen. Verh Dtsch Pathol Gesell 10:223–228, 1906.

244. Botham SK, Holt PF: The mechanism of formation of asbestos bodies. J Pathol Bacteriol 96:443–453, 1968.

245. Botham SK, Holt PF: Development of asbestos bodies on amosite, chrysotile and crocidolite fibres in guinea-pig lungs. J Pathol 105:159–167, 1971.

246. Governa M, Rosanda C: A histochemical study of the asbestos body coating. Br J Indust Med 29:154–159, 1972.

247. Governa M, Rosanda Vadalà C: Histochemical study of asbestos fibre coating in experimental carrageenin granulomas. Br J Indust Med 30:248–252, 1973.

248. McLemore TL, Roggli V, Marshall MV, et al.: Comparison of phagocytosis of uncoated versus coated asbestos fibers by cultured human pulmonary alveolar macrophages. Chest 80:39S–42S, 1981.

249. Irwig LM, Du Toit RSJ, Sluis-Cremer GK, et al.: Risk of asbestosis in crocidolite and amosite mines in South Africa. Ann NY Acad Sci 330:35–52, 1979.

250. Berry G, Gilson JC, Holmes S, et al.: Asbestosis: A study of dose-response relationships in an asbestos textile factory. Br J Indust Med 36:98–112, 1979.

251. McMillan GHG, Pethybridge RJ, Sheers G: Effect of smoking on attack rates of pulmonary and pleural lesions related to exposure to asbestos dust. Br J Indust Med 37:268–272, 1980.

252. Ashcroft T, Heppleston AG: The optical and electron microscopic determination of pulmonary asbestos fibre concentration and its relation to the human pathological reaction. J Clin Pathol 26:224–234, 1973.

253. Morgan A, Holmes A: Concentrations and dimensions of coated and uncoated asbestos fibres in the human lung. Br J Indust Med 37:25–32, 1980.

254. Le Bouffant L: Investigation and analysis of asbestos fibers and accompanying minerals in biological materials. Environ Health Perspect 9:149–153, 1974.

255. Spurny KR, Opiela H, Weiss G: On the milling and ultrasonic treatment of fibres for biological and analytical applications. In Wagner JC (ed): *Biological Effects of Mineral Fibres*. IARC Scientific Publ No. 30. Lyon: International Agency for Research on Cancer, 1980, pp 931–933.

256. Kannerstein M, Churg J: Pathology of carcinoma of the lung associated with asbestos exposure. Cancer 30:14–21, 1972.

257. Webster I: Asbestos exposure in South Africa. In Shapiro HA (ed): *Pneumoconiosis, Proceedings International Conference Johannesburg 1969*. Cape Town: Oxford University Press, 1970, pp 209–212

258. Elder JL: Asbestosis in Western Australia. Med J Aust 2:579–583, 1967.

259. Becklake MR, Liddell FDK, Manfreda J, McDonald JC: Radiological changes after withdrawal from asbestos exposure. Br J Indust Med 36:23–28, 1979.

260. Rubino GF, Newhouse M, Murray R, et al.: Radiological changes after cessation of exposure among chrysotile asbestos miners in Italy. Ann NY Acad Sci 330:157–161, 1979.

261. Wagner JC, Berry G, Skidmore JW, Timbrell V: The effects of the inhalation of asbestos in rats. Br J Cancer 29:252–269, 1974.

262. Goldstein B, Webster I, Rendall R, Skikne MI: The effect of asbestos-cement dust inhalation on baboons. Environ Res 16:216–225, 1978.

263. Vorwald AJ, Durkan TM, Pratt PC: Experimental studies of asbestosis. Arch Ind Hyg Occup Med 3:1–43, 1951.

264. Timbrell V, Skidmore JW: Significance of fibre length in experimental asbestosis. In Holstein, Anspach (eds): *Biologische Wirkungen des Asbestes*. Dresden: Deutsches Zentralinstitut Arbeitsmed, 1968, pp 52–56.

265. Holt PF, Mills J, Young DK: Experimental asbestosis with four types of fibers: Importance of small particles. Ann NY Acad Sci 132:87–97, 1965.

266. Sebastien P, Fondimare A, Bignon J, et al.: Topographic distribution of asbestos fibres in human lung in relation to occupational and non-occupational exposure. In Walton WH (ed): *Inhaled Particles IV*. Oxford: Pergamon Press, 1977, pp 435–444.

267. Pooley FD, Clark N: Fiber dimensions and aspect ratio of crocidolite, chrysotile and amosite particles detected in lung tissue specimens. Ann NY Acad Sci 330:711–716, 1979.

268. Timbrell V: Deposition and retention of fibres in the human lung. Ann Occup Hyg 26:347–369, 1982.

269. Harington JS, Miller K, Macnab G: Hemolysis by asbestos. Environ Res 4:95–117, 1971.

270. Morgan A, Davies P, Wagner JC, et al.: The biological effects of magnesium-leached chrysotile asbestos. Br J Exp Pathol 58:465–473, 1977.

271. Robock K, Klosterkötter W: Biological action of different asbestos dusts with special respect to fibre length and semiconductor properties. In Walton WH (ed): *Inhaled Particles III*. Old Woking, Surrey, England: Unwin, 1971, pp 465–474.

272. Chamberlain M, Brown RC, Davies R, Griffiths DM: In vitro prediction of the pathogenicity of mineral dusts. Br J Exp Pathol, 60:320–327, 1979.

273. Davies P, Allison AC, Ackerman J, et al.: Asbestos induces selective release of lysosomal enzymes from mononuclear phagocytes. Nature 251:423–425, 1974.

274. Aalto M, Heppleston AG: Fibrogenesis by mineral fibres: An in vitro study of the roles of the macrophage and fibre length. Br J Exp Pathol 65:91–99, 1984.

275. Maroudas NG: Growth of fibroblasts on linear and planar anchorages of limiting dimensions. Exp Cell Res 81:104–110, 1973.

276. Bateman E, Emerson RJ, Cole PJ: A study of macrophage-mediated initiation of fibrosis by asbestos and silica using a diffusion chamber technique. Br J Exp Pathol 63:414–425, 1982.

277. McDermott M, Wagner JC, Tetley T, et al.: The effects of inhaled silica and chrysotile on the elastic properties of rat lungs: Physiological, physical and biochemical studies of lung surfactant. In Walton WH (ed): *Inhaled Particles IV*. Oxford: Pergamon Press, 1977, pp 415–425.

278. Lee KP, Barras CE, Griffith FD, Waritz RS: Pulmonary response to glass fiber by inhalation exposure. Lab Invest 40:123–133, 1979.

279. Turner-Warwick M, Parkes WR: Circulating rheumatoid and antinuclear factors in asbestos workers. Br Med J 3:492–495, 1970.

280. Lange A: An epidemiological survey of immunological abnormalities in asbestos workers. Environ Res 22:165–175, 176–183, 1980.

281. Kagan E, Solomon A, Cochrane JC, et al.: Immunological studies of patients with asbestosis. II. Studies of circulating lymphoid cell numbers and humoral immunity. Clin Exp Immunol 28:268–275, 1977.

282. Kagan E, Solomon A, Cochrane JC, et al.: Immunological studies of patients with asbestosis. I. Studies of cell-mediated immunity. Clin Exp Immunol 28:261–267, 1977.

283. Campbell MJ, Wagner MMF, Scott MP, Brown DG: Sequential immunological studies in an asbestos-exposed population. II. Factors affecting lymphocyte function. Clin Exp Immunol 39:176–182, 1980.

284. Wagner MMF, Campbell MJ, Edwards RE: Sequential immunological studies on an asbestos-exposed population. I. Factors affecting peripheral blood leucocytes and T Lymphocytes. Clin Exp Immunol 38:323–331, 1979.

285. Toivanen A, Salmivalli M, Gabor M: Pulmonary asbestosis and autoimmunity. Br Med J 1:691–692, 1976.

286. Bach FH, Van Rood JJ: The major histocompatibility complex—genetics and biology. N Engl J Med 295:927–936, 1976.

287. Turner-Warwick M: HLA phenotypes in asbestos workers. Br J Dis Chest 73:243–244, 1979.

288. Tomasini M, Chiappino G: Hemodynamics of pulmonary circulation in asbestosis: Study of 16 cases. Am J Indust Med 2:167–174, 1981.

289. Hahon N, Eckert HL: Depression of viral interferon induction in cell monolayers by asbestos fibers. Environ Res 11:52–65, 1976.

290. Hahon N, Booth JA, Eckert HL: Antagonistic activity of poly (4-vinylpyridine-N-oxide) to the inhibition of viral interferon induction by asbestos fibres. Br J Indust Med 34:119–125, 1977.

291. Wood WB, Gloyne SR: Pulmonary asbestosis. A review of one hundred cases. Lancet 2:1383–1385, 1934.

292. Lynch KM, Smith WA: Pulmonary asbestosis III: Carcinoma of the lung in asbesto-silicosis. Am J Cancer 24:56–64, 1935.

293. Newhouse ML: A study of the mortality of workers in an asbestos factory. Br J Indust Med 26:294–301, 1969.

294. Newhouse ML, Berry G, Wagner JC, Turok ME: A study of the mortality of female asbestos workers. Br J Indust Med 29:131–141, 1972.

295. Alies-Patin AM, Valleron AJ: Mortality of workers in a French asbestos cement factory 1940–1982. Br J Indust Med 42:219–225, 1985. (Includes other references.)

296. Selikoff IJ, Hammond EC, Churg J: Asbestos exposure, smoking and neoplasia. JAMA 204:106–112, 1968.

297. Berry G, Newhouse ML, Turok M: Combined effect of asbestos exposure and smoking on mortality from lung cancer in factory workers. Lancet 2:476–479, 1972.

298. Meurman LO, Kiviluoto R, Hakama M: Combined effect of asbestos exposure and tobacco smoking on Finnish anthophyllite miners and millers. Ann NY Acad Sci 330:491–495, 1979.

299. Selikoff IJ, Hammond EC: Asbestos and smoking. JAMA 242:458–459, 1979.

300. McDonald JC, Liddell FDK, Gibbs GW, et al.: Dust exposure and mortality in chrysotile mining, 1910–1975. Br J Indust Med 37:11–24, 1980.

301. Whitwell F, Newhouse ML, Bennett DR: A study of the histological cell types of lung cancer in workers suffering from asbestosis in the United Kingdom. Br J Indust Med 31:298–303, 1974.

302. Churg AM, Warnock ML: Numbers of asbestos bodies in urban patients with lung cancer and gastrointestinal cancer and in matched controls. Chest 75:143–149, 1979.

303. Whitwell F, Scott J, Grimshaw M: Relationship between occupations and asbestos-fibre content of the lungs in patients with pleural mesothelioma, lung cancer and other diseases. Thorax 32:377–386, 1977.

304. Schneiderman MA: Digestive system cancer among persons subjected to occupational inhalation of asbestos particles: A literature review with emphasis on dose response. Environ Health Perspect 9:307–311, 1974.

305. Miller AB: Asbestos fibre dust and gastrointestinal malignancies. Review of the literature with special regard to a cause/effect relationship. J Chron Dis 31:23–33, 1978.

306. Newhouse ML, Berry G: Patterns of mortality in asbestos factory workers in London. Ann NY Acad Sci 330:53–60, 1979.

307. Newhouse ML, Gregory MM, Shannon H: Etiology of carcinoma of the larynx. In: Wagner JC (ed): *Biological Effects of Mineral Fibres.* IARC Scientific Publ No. 30. Lyon: International Agency for Res on Cancer, 1980, pp 687–695.

308. Gerber MA: Asbestosis and neoplastic disorders of the hematopoietic system. Am J Clin Pathol 53:204–208, 1970.

309. Kagan E, Jacobson RJ, Yeung KY, et al.: Asbestos-associated neoplasms of B cell lineage. Am J Med 67:325–330, 1979.

310. Maguire FW, Mills RC, Parker FP: Immunoblastic lymphadenopathy and asbestosis. Cancer 47:791–797, 1981.

311. Le Bouffant L, Martin JC, Durif S, Daniel H: Structure and composition of pleural plaques. In Bogovski P, Gibson JC, Timbrek V, Wagner JC (eds): *Biological Effects of Asbestos.* IARC Scientific Publication No. 8. Lyon: International Agency for Research on Cancer, 1973, pp 249–257.

312. Meurman L: Asbestos bodies and pleural plaques in a Finnish series of autopsy cases. Acta Pathol Microbiol Scand suppl 181:1–107, 1966.

313. Roberts GH: The pathology of parietal pleural plaques. J Clin Pathol 24:348–353, 1971.

314. Jones AW, Broadbent MV, Burton G: The asbestos fibre content of lungs and pleural plaques. J Pathol 139:468, 1983.

315. Churg A: Asbestos fibers and pleural plaques in a general autopsy population. Am J Pathol 109:88–96, 1982.

316. Warnock ML, Prescott BT, Kuwahara TJ: Numbers and types of asbestos fibers in subjects with pleural plaques. Am J Pathol 109:37–46, 1982.

317. Burilkov T, Michailova L: Asbestos content of the soil and endemic pleural asbestosis. Environ Res 3:443–451, 1970.

318. Hillerdal G: Non-malignant asbestos pleural disease. Thorax 36:669–675, 1981.

319. Thomson JG: The pathogenesis of pleural plaques. In Shapiro HA (ed): *Pneumoconiosis, Proceeding International Conference Johannesburg 1969.* Cape Town: Oxford University Press, 1970, pp 138–141.

320. Wang N-S: The preformed stomas connecting the pleural cavity and the lymphatics in the parietal pleura. Am Rev Respir Dis 111:12–20, 1975.

321. Aalto M, Kulonen E, Penttinen R, Renvall S: Collagen synthesis in cultured mesothelial cells. Response to silica. Acta Chir Scand 147:1–6, 1981.

322. König J: Über die Asbestose. Arch Gewerbepath Gewerbehyg 18:159–204, 1960.

323. Wagner JC, Sleggs CA, Marchand P: Diffuse pleural mesothelioma and asbestos exposure in the North Western Cape Province. Br J Indust Med 17:260–271, 1960.

324. Kahn EI, Rohl A, Barrett EW, Suzuki Y: Primary pericardial mesothelioma following exposure to asbestos. Environ Res 23:270–281, 1980.

325. Roggli VL: Pericardial mesothelioma after exposure to asbestos. N Eng J Med 304:1045–1047, 1981.

326. Beck B, Konetzke G, Ludwig V, et al.: Malignant pericardial mesotheliomas and asbestos exposure: A case report. Am J Indust Med 3:149–159, 1982.

327. McDonald AD, McDonald JC: Malignant mesothelioma in North America. Cancer 46:1650–1656, 1980.

328. Newhouse ML, Berry G: Predictions of mortality from mesothelial tumours in asbestos factory workers. Br J Indust Med 33:147–151, 1976.

329. Nicholson WJ, Perkel G, Selikoff IJ: Occupational exposure to asbestos: Population at risk and projected mortality—1980–2030. Am J Indust Med 3:259–311, 1982.

330. Greenberg M, Davies TAL: Mesothelioma register 1967–68. Br J Indust Med 31:91–104, 1974.

331. Ashcroft T: Epidemiological and quantitative relationships between mesothelioma and asbestos on Tyneside. J Clin Pathol 26:832–840, 1973.

332. Edge JR: Incidence of bronchial carcinoma in shipyard workers with pleural plaques. Ann NY Acad Sci 330:289–294, 1979.

333. Newhouse ML, Thompson H: Mesothelioma of pleura and peritoneum following exposure to asbestos in the London area. Br J Indust Med 22:261–269, 1965.

334. Vianna NJ, Polan AK: Non-occupational exposure to asbestos and malignant mesothelioma in females. Lancet 1:1061–1063, 1978.

335. Anderson HA, Lilis R, Daum SM, Selikoff IJ: Asbestosis among household contacts of asbestos factory workers. Ann NY Acad Sci 330:387–399, 1979.

336. Bignon J, Sebastien P, Di Menza L, Payan H: French mesothelioma register. Ann NY Acad Sci 330:455–466, 1979.

337. Wang N-S, Huang S-N, Gold P: Absence of carcinoembryonic antigen-like material in mesothelioma. Cancer 44:937–943, 1979.

338. Corson JM, Pinkus GS: Mesothelioma: Profile of keratin proteins and carcinoembryonic antigen. Am J Pathol 108:80–87, 1982.

339. Gibbs AR, Harach R, Wagner JC, Jasani B: Comparison of tumour markers in malignant mesothelioma and pulmonary adenocarcinoma. Thorax 40:91–95, 1985.

340. Singh G, Katyal SL, Torikata C: Carcinoma of type II pneumocytes. Immunodiagnosis of a subtype of "bronchiol-oalveolar carcinomas." Am J Pathol 102:195–208, 1981.

341. Herbert A, Gallagher PJ: Interpretation of pleural biopsy specimens and aspirates with the immunoperoxidase technique. Thorax 37:822–827, 1982.

342. Report of Advisory Committee on Asbestos Cancers. Br J Indust Med 30:180–186, 1973.

343. Meurman LO, Kiviluoto R, Hakama M: Mortality and morbidity among the working population of anthophyllite asbestos miners in Finland. Br J Indust Med 34:105–112, 1974.

344. McDonald JC, Liddell FKD: Mortality in Canadian miners and millers exposed to chrysotile. Ann NY Acad Sci 300:1–9, 1979.

345. McDonald AD, McDonald JC, Pooley FD: Mineral fibre

content of lung in mesothelial tumours in North America. Ann Occup Hyg 26:417–422, 1982.

346. Peto J, Seidman H, Selikoff IJ: Mesothelioma mortality in asbestos workers: Implications for models of carcinogenesis and risk asessment. Br J Cancer 45:124–135, 1982.

347. Yazicioglu S, Ilcayto R, Balci K, Sayli BS, Yorulmaz B: Pleural calcification, pleural mesotheliomas, and bronchial cancers caused by tremolite dust. Thorax 35:564–569, 1980.

348. Wagner JC, Chamberlain M, Brown RC, et al.: Biological effects of tremolite. Br J Cancer 45:352–360, 1982.

348a. Davis JMG, Addison J, Bolton RE, et al.: Inhalation studies on the effects of tremolite and brucite dust in rats. Carcinogenesis 6:667–674, 1985.

349. Jones JSP, Smith PG, Pooley FD, et al.: The consequences of exposure to asbestos dust in a wartime gas-mask factory. In Wagner JC (ed): *Biological Effects of Mineral Fibres*. IARC Scientific Publication No. 30. Lyon: International Agency for Research on Cancer, 1980, pp 637–653.

350. Wignall BK, Fox AJ: Mortality of female gas mask assemblers. Br J Indust Med 39:34–38, 1982.

351. McDonald AD, McDonald JC: Mesothelioma after crocidolite exposure during gas mask manufacture. Environ Res 17:340–346, 1978.

352. Baris YI, Sahin AA, Ozesmi M, et al.: An outbreak of pleural mesothelioma and chronic fibrosing pleurisy in the village of Karain/Urgüp in Anatolia. Thorax 33:181–192, 1978.

353. Baris YI, Artvinli M, Sahin AA: Environmental mesothelioma in Turkey. Ann NY Acad Sci 330:423–432, 1979.

354. Artvinli M, Baris YI: Malignant mesotheliomas in a small village in the Anatolian region of Turkey: An epidemiological study. J Natl Cancer Inst 63:17–22, 1979.

355. Rohl AN, Langer AM, Moncure G, et al.: Endemic pleural disease associated with exposure to mixed fibrous dust in Turkey. Science 216:518–520, 1982.

356. Suzuki Y, Kohyama N: Malignant mesothelioma induced by asbestos and zeolite in the mouse peritoneal cavity. Environ Res 35:277–292, 1984.

357. Maltoni C, Minardi F, Morisi L: Pleural mesotheliomas in Sprague-Dawley rats by erionite: First experimental evidence. Environ Res 29:238–244, 1982.

358. Wagner JC: The risk assessment of asbestos carcinogenicity in the normal population. Animal to human correlations. In *Fibrous Dusts, VDI Colloquium*. Düsseldorf: Vereins Deutscher Ingenieure Berichte No. 475, 1983, pp 305–308.

359. Stanton MF, Wrench C: Mechanisms of mesothelioma induction with asbestos and fibrous glass. J Natl Cancer Inst 48:797–821, 1972.

360. Wagner JC, Berry G, Timbrell V: Mesotheliomata in rats after inoculation with asbestos and other minerals. Br J Cancer 28:173–185, 1973.

361. Stanton MF, Layard M, Tegeris A, et al.: Carcinogenicity of fibrous glass: Pleural response in the rat in relation to fiber dimension. J Natl Cancer Inst 58:587–603, 1977.

362. Stanton MF, Layard M: The carcinogenicity of fibrous minerals. In Gravatt CC, La Fleur PD, Heinrich KFJ (eds): *Proceedings Workshop on Asbestos: Definitions and Measurement Methods*. Washington, DC: National Bureau of Standards, U.S. Department of Commerce, 1978, pp 143–150.

363. Enterline PE, Henderson V: The health of retired fibrous glass workers. Arch Environ Health 30:113–116, 1975.

364. Bayliss DL, Dement JM, Wagoner JK, Blejer HP: Mortality patterns among fibrous glass production workers. Ann NY Acad Sci 271:324–335, 1976.

365. Simonato L, Fletcher AC, Cherrie J, et al.: The man-made mineral fiber European historical cohort study. Extension of the follow-up. Scand J Work Environ Health 12 (suppl 1): 34–47, 1986.

366. Gross P, Harley RA, Davis JMG: The lungs of fiber glass workers: Comparison with the lungs of a control population. In *Occupational Exposure to Fibrous Glass*. Washington: Department of Health, Education and Welfare Publication (NIOSH) 76-151, 1976, pp 249–263.

367. Murphy GB: Fiber glass pneumoconiosis. Arch Environ Health 3:704–710, 1961.

368. Ciaccia A, Pusinanti F, Beltrami A, Fasano E: Pneumoconiosi da fibre di lana di roccia. Riv Pat Clin Tuberc e Pneumol 49:305–333, 1978.

369. Goldstein B, Rendall REG, Webster I: A comparison of the effects of exposure of baboons to crocidolite and fibrous glass dusts. Environ Res 32:344–359, 1983.

370. Pott F, Huth F, Friedrichs KH: Results of animal carcinogenesis studies after application of fibrous glass and their implications regarding human exposure. In *Occupational Exposure to Fibrous Glass*. Washington, DC: Department of Health, Education and Welfare Publication (NIOSH) 76-151, 1976, pp 183–191.

371. Pigott GH, Gaskell BA, Ishmael J: Effects of long term inhalation of alumina fibres in rats. Br J Exp Pathol 62:323–331, 1981.

372. Hammond EC, Selikoff IJ, Seidman H: Asbestos exposure, cigarette smoking and death rates. Ann NY Acad Sci 330:473–490, 1979.

373. Berry G, Newhouse ML, Antonis P: Combined effect of asbestos and smoking on mortality from lung cancer and mesothelioma in factory workers. Br J Indust Med 42:12–18, 1985.

374. Langer AM, Maggiore CM, Nicholson WJ, et al.: The contamination of Lake Superior with amphibole gangue minerals. Ann NY Acad Sci 330:549–572, 1979.

375. Carter RE, Taylor WF: Identification of a particular amphibole asbestos fiber in tissues of persons exposed to a high oral intake of the mineral. Environ Res 21:85–93, 1980.

376. Conforti PM, Kanarek MS, Jackson LA, et al.: Asbestos in drinking water and cancer in the San Francisco bay area: 1969–1974 incidence. J Chron Dis 34:211–224, 1981.

377. Sigurdson EE, Levy BS, Mandel J, et al.: Cancer morbidity investigations: Lessons from the Duluth study of possible effects of asbestos in drinking water. Environ Res 25:50–61, 1981.

378. Hilding AC, Hilding DA, Larson DM, Aufderheide AC: Biological effects of ingested amosite asbestos, taconite tailings, diatomaceous earth and Lake Superior water in rats. Arch Environ Health 36:298–303, 1981.

379. Bolton RE, Davis JMG, Lamb D: The pathological effects of prolonged asbestos ingestion in rats. Environ Res 29:134–150, 1982.

380. Kaczenski JH, Hallenbeck WH: Migration of ingested asbestos. Environ Res 35:531–551, 1984.

381. Bryks S, Bertalanffy FD: Cytodynamic reactivity of the mesothelium. Arch Environ Health 23:469–472, 1971.

382. Lavappa KS, Fu MM, Epstein SS: Cytogenetic studies on chrysotile asbestos. Environ Res 10:165–173, 1975.

383. Valerio F, De Ferrari M, Ottaggio L, et al.: Cytogenetic effects of Rhodesian chrysotile on human lymphocytes in vitro. In Wagner JC (ed): *Biological Effects of Mineral Fibres*. IARC Scientific Publication No. 30. Lyon: International Agency for Research on Cancer, 1980, pp 485–489.

384. Livingston GK, Rom WN, Morris MV: Asbestos-induced

sister chromatid exchanges in cultured Chinese hamster ovarian fibroblast cells. J Environ Pathol Toxicol 4:373–382, 1981.

385. Babu KA, Nigam SK, Lakkad BC, et al.: Effect of chrysotile asbestos (AP-I) on sister chromatid exchanges in Chinese hamster ovary cells. Environ Res 24:325–329, 1981.

386. Maroudas NG, O'Neill CH, Stanton MF: Fibroblast anchorage in carcinogenesis by fibres. Lancet 1:807–809, 1973.

387. Lakowicz JR, Bevan DR: Effects of adsorption of benzo(a)pyrene to asbestos and non-fibrous mineral particulates upon its rate of uptake into phospholipid vesicles and rat liver microsomes. In Brown RC, et al. (eds): *The In Vitro Effects of Mineral Dusts*. London: Academic Press, 1980, pp 169–175.

388. Daniel FB, Beach CA, Hart RW: Asbestos-induced changes in the metabolism of polycyclic aromatic hydrocarbons in human fibroblast cell cultures. In Brown RC, et al. (eds): *The In Vitro Effects of Mineral Dusts*. London: Academic Press, 1980, pp 255–262.

389. Miller L, Smith WE, Berliner SW: Tests for effect of asbestos on benzo(a)pyrene carcinogenesis in the respiratory tract. Ann NY Acad Sci 132:489–500, 1965.

390. Neuberger M, Kundi M, Friedel HP: Environmental asbestos exposure and cancer mortality. Arch Environ Health 39:261–265, 1984.

391. Hamer DH, Rolle FR, Schelz JP: Characterization of talc and associated minerals. Am Indust Hyg Assoc J 37:296–304, 1976.

392. Rohl AN, Langer AM, Selikoff IJ, et al.: Consumer talcums and powders: Mineral and chemical characterization. J Toxicol Environ Health 2:255–284, 1976.

393. Weiss B, Boettner EA: Commercial talc and talcosis. Arch Environ Health 14:304–308, 1967.

394. Kleinfeld M, Messite J, Zaki MH: Mortality experiences among talc workers: A follow-up study. J Occup Med 16:345–349, 1974.

395. National Institute of Occupational Safety and Health technical report. *Occupational Exposure to Talc Containing Asbestos*. Department of Health, Education and Welfare (National Institute of Occupational Safety and Health Publication No. 80-115. Washington, DC: Occupational Safety and Health Administration, 1980.

396. Thorel C: Die Specksteinlunge. Beitr Pathol Anat 20:85–101, 1896.

397. McLaughlin AIG, Rogers E, Dunham KC: Talc pneumoconiosis. Br J Indust Med 6:184–194, 1949.

398. Hunt AC: Massive pulmonary fibrosis from the inhalation of talc. Thorax 11:287–294, 1956.

399. Vallyathan NV, Craighead JE: Pulmonary pathology in workers exposed to nonasbestiform talc. Hum Pathol 12:28–35, 1981.

400. Kleinfeld M, Giel CP, Majeranowski JF, Messite J: Talc pneumoconiosis. A report of six patients with postmortem findings. Arch Environ Health 7:101–115, 1963.

401. Abraham JL, Brambilla C: Particle size for differentiation between inhalation and injection pulmonary talcosis. Environ Res 21:94–96, 1980.

402. Wagner JC, Berry G, Cooke TJ, et al.: Animal experiments with talc. In Walton WH (ed): *Inhaled Particles IV*. Oxford: Pergamon Press, 1977, pp 647–652.

403. Wagner JC, Berry G, Hill RJ, Skidmore JW: An animal model for inhalation exposure to talc. In Lemen R, Dement JM (eds): *Dusts and Disease*. Park South, IL: Pathotox Publications, 1979, pp 389–392.

404. Gamble J, Fellner W, DiMeo MJ: Respiratory morbidity among miners and millers of asbestiform talc. In Lemen R, Dement JM (eds): *Dusts and Disease*. Park Forest South, IL: Pathotox Publications, 1979, pp 307–316.

405. Brown DP, Dement JM, Wagoner JK: Mortality among miners and millers occupationally exposed to asbestiform talc. In Lemen R, Dement JM (eds): *Dusts and Disease*. Park Forest South, IL: Pathotox Publications, 1979, pp 317–324.

406. Rubino GF, Scansetti G, Piolatto G, Romano CA: Mortality study of talc miners and millers. J Occup Med 18:186–193, 1976.

407. Sheers G: Prevalence of pneumoconiosis in Cornish kaolin workers. Br J Indust Med 21:218–225, 1964.

408. Lynch KM, McIver FA: Pneumoconiosis from exposure to kaolin dust: Kaolinosis. Am J Pathol 30:1117–1127, 1954.

409. Hale LW, Gough J, King EJ, Nagelschmidt G: Pneumoconiosis of kaolin workers. Br J Indust Med 13:251–259, 1956.

410. Lapenas D, Gale P, Kennedy T, et al.: Kaolin pneumoconiosis: Radiologic, pathologic and mineralogic findings. Am Rev Respir Dis 130:282–288, 1984.

411. Attygalle D, Harrison CV, King EJ, Mohanty GP: Infective pneumoconiosis I. Br J Indust Med 11:245–259, 1954.

412. Schmidt KG, Lüchtrath H: Die Wirkung von frischem und gebranntem Kaolin auf die Lunge und das Bauchfell von Ratten. Beitr Silikose-Forch Heft 58:1–37, 1958.

413. Decora AW, Kerr RD: Processing use, and characterization of shale oil products. Environ Health Perspect 30:217–223, 1979.

414. MacFarland HN, Coate WB, Disbennett DB, Ackerman LJ: Long-term inhalation studies with raw and processed shale dusts. Ann Occup Hyg 26:213–226, 1982.

415. Küng VA. Morphological investigations of fibrogenic action of Estonian oil shale dust. Environ Health Perspect 30:153–156, 1979.

416. Seaton A, Lamb D, Brown WR, et al.: Pneumoconiosis of shale miners. Thorax 36:412–418, 1981.

417. Holland LM, Smith DM, Thomas RG: Biological effects of raw and processed oil shale particles in the lungs of laboratory animals. Environ Health Perspect 30:147–152, 1979.

418. Purde M, Rahn M: Cancer patterns in the oil shale area of the Estonian SSR. Environ Health Perspect 30:209–210, 1979.

419. Campbell AH, Gloyne SR: A case of pneumonokoniosis due to the inhalation of fuller's earth. J Pathol Bacteriol 54:75–80, 1942.

420. Tonning HO: Pneumoconiosis from fuller's earth. Report of a case with autopsy findings. J Indust Hyg Toxicol 31:41–45, 1949.

421. Sakula A: Pneumoconiosis due to fuller's earth. Thorax 16:176–179, 1961.

422. Phibbs BP, Sundin RE, Mitchell RS: Silicosis in Wyoming bentonite workers. Am Rev Respir Dis 103:1–17, 1971.

423. Dreessen WC, Dallavalle JM, Edwards TI, et al.: *Pneumoconiosis Among Mica and Pegmatite Workers*. Washington, D.C., U.S. Public Health Service, Public Health Bulletin No. 250, 1940.

424. Vorwald AJ: Diffuse fibrogenic pneumoconiosis. Indust Med Surg 29:253–258, 1960.

425. Davies D, Cotton R: Mica pneumoconiosis. Br J Indust Med 40:22–27, 1983.

426. Sherwin RP, Barman ML, Abraham JL: Silicate pneumoconiosis of farm workers. Lab Invest 40:576–582, 1979.

427. Brambilla C, Abraham J, Brambilla E, et al.: Comparative pathology of silicate pneumoconiosis. Am J Pathol 96:149–170, 1979.

428. Schwartz LW, Knight HD, Whittig LD, et al.: Silicate pneumoconiosis and pulmonary fibrosis in horses from the Monterey-Carmel peninsula. Chest 80:82S–85S, 1981.

429. Holness L: Nepheline syenite pneumoconiosis. Occup Health Ontario 2:21–31, 1981.

430. Fruchter JS, Robertson DE, Evans JC, et al.: Mount St. Helens ash from the 18 May 1980 eruption: Chemical, physical, mineralogical, and biological properties. Science 209:1116–1125, 1980.

431. Green FHY, Bowman L, Castranova V, et al.: Health implications of the Mount St. Helens eruption: Laboratory investigations. Ann Occup Hyg 26:921–933, 1982.

432. Sanders CL, Conklin AW, Gelman RA, et al.: Pulmonary toxicity of Mount St. Helens volcanic ash. Environ Res 27:118–135, 1982.

433. Green FHY, Vallyathan V, Mentnech MS, et al.: Is volcanic ash a pneumoconiosis risk? Nature 293:216–217, 1981.

433a. Raub JA, Hatch GE, Mercer RR, Grady M, Hu P-C: Inhalation studies of Mt. St. Helens volcanic ash in animals II. Environ Res 37:72–83, 1985.

434. Eisele JW, O'Halloran RL, Reay DT, et al.: Deaths during the May 18, 1980, eruption of Mount St. Helens. N Engl J Med 305:931–936, 1981.

435. MacFarland HN, Ulrich CE, Martin A, et al.: Chronic exposure of cynamolgus monkeys to fly ash. In Walton WH (ed): *Inhaled Particles III*. Old Woking, Surrey England: Unwin, 1971, pp 313–326.

436. Raabe OG, Tyler WS, Last JA, et al.: Studies of the chronic inhalation of coal fly ash by rats. Ann Occup Hyg 26:189–211, 1982.

437. Wehner AP, Dagle GE, Milliman EM: Chronic inhalation exposure of hamsters to nickel-enriched fly ash. Environ Res 26:195–216, 1981.

438. Alarie Y, Kantz RJ, Ulrich CE, et al.: Long-term continuous exposure to sulfur dioxide and fly ash mixtures. Arch Environ Health 27:251–253, 1973.

439. Golden EB, Warnock ML, Hulett LD, Churg AM: Fly ash lung: A new pneumoconiosis? Am Rev Respir Dis 125:108–112, 1982.

440. Chakarvarti SK, Nagpaul KK: Determination of the uranium content in some Indian coal and fly ash samples. Health Phys 30:358–361, 1980.

441. Hardy HL: Beryllium disease: A clinical perspective. Environ Res 21:1–9, 1980.

442. Sprince ML, Kazemi H: U.S. beryllium case registry through 1977. Environ Res 21:44–47, 1980.

443. McCallum RI, Rannie I, Verity C: Chronic pulmonary berylliosis in a female chemist. Br J Indust Med 18:133–142, 1961.

444. Vorwald AJ: Medical aspects of beryllium disease. In: Stokinger HE (ed): *Beryllium—Its Industrial Hygiene Aspects*. London: Academic Press, 1966, pp 167–200.

445. Freiman DG, Hardy HL: Beryllium disease. Hum Pathol 1:25–44, 1970.

446. Jones Williams W: A histological study of the lungs in 52 cases of chronic beryllium disease. Br J Indust Med 15:84–91, 1958.

447. Jones Williams W, Fry E, James EMV: The fine structure of beryllium granulomas. Acta Pathol Microbiol Scand 80 (suppl 233): 195–202, 1972.

448. James EMV, Jones Williams W: Fine structure and histochemistry of epithelioid cells in sarcoidosis. Thorax 29: 115–120, 1974.

449. Black MM, Epstein WL: Formation of multinucleate giant cells in organized epithelioid cell granulomas. Am J Pathol 74:263–274, 1974.

450. Stokinger HE, Spiegl CJ, Root RE, et al.: Acute inhalation toxicity of beryllium. Arch Indust Hyg Occup Med 8:493–506, 1953.

451. Vorwald AJ, Reeves AL, Urban ECJ: Experimental beryllium toxicity. In Stokinger HE (ed): *Beryllium—Its Industrial Hygiene Aspects*. London: Academic Press, 1966, pp 201–234.

452. Deodhar SD, Barna B, Van Ordstrand HS: A study of the immunologic aspects of chronic berylliosis. Chest 63:309–313, 1973.

453. Marx JJ, Burrell R: Delayed hypersensitivity to beryllium compounds. J Immunol 111:590–598, 1973.

454. Henderson WR, Fukuyama K, Epstein WL, Spitler LE: In vitro demonstration of delayed hypersensitivity in patients with berylliosis. J Invest Dermatol 58:5–8, 1972.

455. Williams WR, Jones Williams W: Comparison of lymphocyte transformation and macrophage migration inhibition tests in the detection of beryllium hypersensitivity. J Clin Pathol 35:684–687, 1982.

456. Jones Williams W, Williams WR: Value of beryllium lymphocyte transformation tests in chronic beryllium disease and in potentially exposed workers. Thorax 38:41–44, 1983.

457. Groth DH: Carcinogenicity of beryllium: Review of the literature. Environ Res 21:56–62, 1980.

458. Wagoner JK, Infante PF, Bayliss DL: Beryllium: An etiologic agent in the induction of lung cancer, nonneoplastic respiratory disease, and heart disease among industrially exposed workers. Environ Res 21:15–34, 1980.

459. Mancuso TF: Mortality study of beryllium industry workers' occupational lung cancer. Environ Res 21:48–55, 1980.

460. Smith AB, Suzuki Y: Histopathologic classification of bronchogenic carcinomas among a cohort of workers occupationally exposed to beryllium. Environ Res 21:10–14, 1980.

461. Jacques A, Witschi H: Beryllium effects on aryl hydrocarbon hydroxylase in rat lung. Arch Environ Health 27:243–247, 1973.

462. Finlay GR: In Vorwald AJ (ed): *Pneumoconiosis: Sixth Saranac Symposium*. New York: Hoeber, 1950, pp 493–497.

463. Jephcott CM: Chemical aspects of Shaver's disease. In Vorwald AJ (ed): *Pneumoconiosis: Sixth Saranac Symposium*. New York: Hoeber, 1950, pp 489–493.

464. Goralewski G: Die Aluminiumlunge—eine neue Gewerbeerkrankung. Z Ges Inn Med 21/22:665–673, 1947.

465. Goralewski G: Die Aluminiumlunge: Eine klinische Studie. Arbeitsmed Heft 26:1–68, 1950.

466. Mitchell J: Pulmonary fibrosis in an aluminium worker. Br J Indust Med 16:123–125, 1959.

467. Mitchell J, Manning GB, Molyneux M, Lane RE: Pulmonary fibrosis in workers exposed to finely powdered aluminium. Br J Indust Med 18:10–20, 1961.

468. Jordan JW: Pulmonary fibrosis in a worker using an aluminium powder. Br J Indust Med 18:21–23, 1961.

469. Cataldi R, De Palma M, Valente T, Bonsignore AD: Su due casi di fibrosi polmonare da ossido di alluminio. Med Lavoro 72:318–322, 1981.

470. Shaver CG: Pulmonary changes encountered in employees engaged in the manufacture of alumina abrasives. Clinical and roentgenologic aspects. Occup Med 5:718–724, 1948.

471. Riddell AR: Pulmonary changes encountered in employees engaged in the manufacture of alumina abrasives. Pathologic aspects. Occup Med 5:710–717, 1948.

472. Wyatt JP, Riddell ACR: The morphology of bauxite-fume pneumoconiosis. Am J Pathol 25:447–465, 1949.

473. Corrin B: Aluminium pneumoconiosis I and II. Br J Indust Med 20:264–267, 268–276, 1963.

474. McLaughlin AIG, Kazantzis G, King E, et al.: Pulmonary fibrosis and encephalopathy associated with the inhalation of aluminium dust. Br J Indust Med 19:253–263, 1962.

475. Gross P, Westrick ML, McNerny JM: Glass dust: a study of its biological effects. Arch Ind Health 21:10–23, 1960.

476. Giovanazzi A, D'Andrea F: Cause di morte fra i lavoratori di un impianto di riduzione elettrolitica di allumina. Med Lavoro 72:277–282, 1981.

477. Bech OA, Kipling MD, Heather JC: Hard metal disease. Br J Indust Med 19:239–252, 1962.

478. Coates EO, Watson JHL: Diffuse interstitial lung disease in tungsten carbide workers. Ann Intern Med 75:709–716, 1971.

479. Lundgren KD, Öhman H: Pneumokoniose in der Hartmetallindustrie. Virchows Arch 325:259–284, 1954.

480. Güthert H, Einbrodt HJ, Heuer W: Weitere Untersuchungen zur Hartmetallexposition beim Menschen. Int Arch Gewerbepath Gewerbehyg 21:379–391, 1965.

481. Coates EO, Watson JHL: Pathology of the lung in tungsten carbide workers using light and electron microscopy. J Occup Med 15:280–286, 1973.

482. Baudouin J, Jobard P, Moline J, et al.: Fibrose pulmonaire interstitielle diffuse: Responsabilité des métaux durs. Nouv Presse Med 4:1353–1355, 1975.

483. Davison AG, Haslam PL, Corrin B, et al.: Insterstitial lung disease and asthma in hard metal workers. Thorax 38:119–128, 1983.

484. Coates EO, Sawyer HJ, Rebuck JW, et al.: Hypersensitivity bronchitis in tungsten carbide workers. Chest 64:390, 1973.

485. Jones Williams W: The pathology of the lung in five nickel workers. Br J Indust Med 15:235–242, 1958.

486. Gardner DE: Dysfunction of host defences following nickel inhalation. In Brown SG, Sunderman FW (eds): *Nickel Toxicology*. London: Academic Press, 1980, pp 121–124.

487. Doll R: Cancer of the lung and nose in nickel workers. Br J Indust Med 15:217–223, 1958.

488. Doll R, Matthews JD, Morgan LG: Cancers of the lung and nasal sinuses in nickel workers: A reassessment of the period of risk. Br J Indust Med 34:102–105, 1977.

489. Andersen A, Høgetveit AC, Magnus K: A follow-up study among Norwegian nickel workers. In Brown SG, Sunderman FW (eds): *Nickel Toxicology*. London: Acacemic Press, 1980, pp 31–32.

490. Chovil A, Sutherland RB, Halliday R: Respiratory cancer in a cohort of nickel sinter plant workers. Br J Indust Med 38:327–333, 1981.

491. Saknyn AV, Shabynina NK: Epidemiology of malignant tumours in nickel refineries. Gig Tr Prof Zabol 9:25–29, 1973. (In Russian)

492. Cox JE, Doll R, Scott WA, Smith S: Mortality of nickel workers: Experience of men working with metallic nickel. Br J Indust Med 38:235–239, 1981.

493. Boysen M, Waksvik H, Solberg LA, et al.: Histopathological follow-up studies and chromosome analysis in nickel workers. In Brown SG, Sunderman FW (eds): *Nickel Toxicology*. London: Academic Press, 1980, pp 35–38.

494. Sunderman FW, Shen SK, Reid MC, Allpass PR: Teratogenicity and embryotoxicity of nickel carbonyl in Syrian hamsters. In Brown SG, Sunderman FW (eds): *Nickel Toxicology*. London: Academic Press, 1980, pp 113–116.

495. Sunderman FW: Recent research on nickel carcinogenesis. Environ Health Perspect 40:131–141, 1981.

496. Sluis-Cremer GK, Du Toit RSJ: Pneumoconiosis in chromite miners in South Africa. Br J Indust Med 25:63–67, 1968.

497. Baetjer AM: Pulmonary carcinoma in chromate workers. Arch Ind Hyg Occup Med 2:487–504, 505–516, 1950.

498. Mancuso TE, Hueper WC: Occupational cancer and other health hazards in a chromate plant: A medical appraisal. I. Lung cancers in chromate workers. Indust Med Surg 20:358–363, 1951.

499. Bidstrup PL, Case RAM: Carcinoma of the lung in workmen in the bichromates-producing industry in Great Britain. Br J Indust Med 13:260–264, 1956.

500. Alderson MR, Rattan NS, Bidstrup L: Health of workmen in the chromate-producing industry in Britain. Br J Indust Med 38:117–124, 1981.

501. Ohsaki Y, Abe S, Kimura K, et al.: Lung cancer in Japanese chromate workers. Thorax 33:372–374, 1978.

502. Axelsson G, Rylander R, Schmidt A: Mortality and incidence of tumours among ferrochromium workers. Br J Indust Med 37:121–127, 1980.

503. Axelsson G, Rylander R: Environmental chromium dust and lung cancer mortality. Environ Res 23:469–476, 1980.

504. Norseth T: The carcinogenicity of chromium. Environ Health Perspect 40:121–130, 1981.

505. Elo R, Määttä K, Uksila E, Arstila AU: Pulmonary deposits of titanium dioxide in man. Arch Pathol 94:417–424, 1972.

506. Määttä K, Arstila AU: Pulmonary deposits of titanium dioxide in cytologic and lung biopsy specimens. Lab Invest 33:342–346, 1975.

507. Stewart MJ, Faulds JS: The pulmonary fibrosis of haematite miners. J Pathol Bacteriol 39:233–253, 1934.

508. Faulds JS. Haematite pneumoconiosis in Cumberland miners. J Clin Pathol 10:187–199, 1957.

509. Boyd JT, Doll R, Faulds JS, Leiper J: Cancer of the lung in iron ore (haematite) miners. Br J Indust Med 27:97–105, 1970.

510. Stokinger HE: A review of world literature finds iron oxides noncarcinogenic. Am Indust Hyg Assoc J 45:127–133, 1984.

511. Duggan MJ, Soilleux PJ, Strong JC, Howell DM: The exposure of United Kingdom miners to radon. Br J Indust Med 27:106–109, 1970.

512. Edling C: Lung cancer and smoking in a group of iron ore miners. Am J Indust Med 3:191–199, 1982.

513. Beaumont JJ, Weiss WS: Lung cancer among welders. J Occup Med 23:839–844, 1981.

514. Prior JT, Cronk GA, Ziegler DD: Pathological changes associated with the inhalation of sodium zirconium lactate. Arch Environ Health 1:297–300, 1960.

515. Brown JR, Mastromatteo E, Horwood J: Zirconium lactate and barium zirconate. Acute toxicity and inhalation effects in experimental animals. Am Ind Hyg Assoc J 24:131–136, 1963.

516. Oyanguren H, Haddad R, Maass H: Stannosis I. Environmental and experimental studies. Indust Med Surg 27:427–431, 1958.

517. Schuler P, Cruz E, Guijon C, et al.: Stannosis II. Clinical study. Indust Med Surg 27:432–435, 1958.

518. Robertson AJ, Rivers D, Nagelschmidt G, Duncumb P: Stannosis. Benign pneumoconiosis due to tin oxide. Lancet 1:1089–1093, 1961.

519. McCallum RI, Day MJ, Underhill J, Aird EGA: Measurement of antimony oxide dust in human lungs in vivo by X-ray spectrophotometry. In Walton WH (ed): *Inhaled Particles III*. Old Woking, Surrey, England: Unwin, 1971, pp 611–618.

520. Cooper DA, Pendergrass EP, Vorwald AJ, et al.: Pneumoconiosis among workers in an antimony industry. Am J Roentgenol 103:495–508, 1968.

521. Doig AT: Baritosis: A benign pneumoconiosis. Thorax 31:30–39, 1976.

522. Huston J, Wallach DP, Cunningham GJ: Pulmonary reaction to barium sulphate in rats. Arch Pathol 54:430–438, 1952.

523. Heuck F, Hoschek R: Cer-pneumoconiosis. Am J Roentgenol 104:777–783, 1968.

524. Mennear JH (ed): *Cadmium Toxicity*. New York: Marcel Dekker, 1979.

525. Bonnell JA: Cadmium poisoning. Ann Occup Hyg 8:45–50, 1965.

526. Baader EW: Chronic cadium poisoning. Indust Med Surg 21:427–430, 1952.

527. Lane RE, Campbell ACP: Fatal emphysema in two men making a copper cadmium alloy. Br J Indust Med 11:118–122, 1954.

528. Smith JP, Smith JC, McCall AJ: Chronic poisoning from cadmium fume. J Pathol Bacteriol 80:287–296, 1960.

529. De Silva PE, Donnan MB: Chronic cadmium poisoning in a pigment manufacturing plant. Br J Indust Med 38:76–86, 1981.

530. Snider GL, Hayes JA, Korthy AL, Lewis GP: Centrilobular emphysema experimentally induced by cadmium chloride aerosol. Am Rev Respir Dis 108:40–48, 1973.

531. Lemen RA, Lee LS, Wagoner JK, Blejer HP: Cancer mortality among cadmium production workers. Ann NY Acad Sci 271:273–279, 1976.

532. Adams RG, Harrison JF, Scott P: The development of cadmium-induced proteinuria, impaired renal function, and osteomalacia in alkaline battery workers. Q J Med 38:425–443, 1969.

533. Stewart M, Hughes EW: Urinary β_2 microglobulin in the biological monitoring of cadmium workers. Br J Indust Med 38:170–174, 1981.

534. Challen PJR, Sherwood RJ, Bedford J: "Fluon" (polytetrafluorethylene): A preliminary note on some clinical and environmental observations. Br J Indust Med 12:177–178, 1955.

535. Harris DK: Some hazards in the manufacture and use of plastics. Br J Indust Med 16:221–229, 1959.

536. Williams N: Vanadium poisoning from cleaning oil-fired boilers. Br J Indust Med 9:50–55, 1952.

537. Lees REM: Changes in lung function after exposure to vanadium compounds in fuel oil ash. Br J Indust Med 37:253–256, 1980.

538. Browne RC: Vanadium poisoning from gas turbines. Br J Indust Med 12:57–59, 1955.

539. Zenz C, Berg BA: Human responses to controlled vanadium pentoxide exposure. Arch Environ Health 14:709–712, 1967.

540. McLaughlin AIG, Milton R, Perry KMA: Toxic manifestations of osmium tetroxide. Br J Indust Med 3:183–186, 1946.

541. Teng CT, Brennan JC: Acute mercury vapor poisoning. Radiology 73:354–361, 1959.

542. Tennant R, Johnston HJ, Wells JB: Acute bilateral pneumonitis associated with the inhalation of mercury vapour. Conn Med 25:106–109, 1961.

543. Hallee TJ: Diffuse lung disease caused by inhalation of mercury vapor. Am Rev Respir Dis 99:430–436, 1969.

544. Milne J, Christophers A, De Silva P: Acute mercurial pneumonitis. Br J Indust Med 27:334–338, 1970.

545. Lloyd Davies TA: Manganese pneumonitis. Br J Indust Med 3:111–135, 1946.

546. Lloyd Davies TA, Harding HE: Manganese pneumonitis. Further clinical and experimental observations. Br J Indust Med 6:82–90, 1949.

547. Tokudome S, Kuratsune M: A cohort study on mortality from cancer and other causes among workers at a metal refinery. Int J Cancer 17:310–317, 1976.

548. Mabuchi K, Lilienfeld AM, Snell LM: Cancer and occupational exposure to arsenic: A study of pesticide workers. Prev Med 9:51–77, 1980.

549. Martin AE, Bradley WH: Mortality, fog and atmospheric pollution. Monthly Bull Minist Health Publ Health Lab Service 19:56–72, 1960.

550. Davies D: Power stations and pollution. Br J Dis Chest 56:171–175, 1962.

551. Petrilli FL, Agnese G, Kanitz S: Epidemiologic studies of air pollution effects in Genoa, Italy. Arch Environ Health 12:733–740, 1966.

552. Higgins ITT: Effects of sulfur oxides and particulates on health. Arch Environ Health 22:584–590, 1971.

553. Skalpe IO: Long-term effects of sulphur dioxide exposure in pulp mills. Br J Indust Med 21:69–73, 1964.

554. Douglas JWB, Waller RE: Air pollution and respiratory infection in children. Br J Prev Soc Med 20:1–8, 1966.

555. Alarie Y, Ulrich CE, Busey WM, et al.: Long-term continuous exposure to sulfur dioxide in Cynomolgus monkeys. Arch Environ Health 24:115–128, 1972.

556. Lightowler NM, Williams JRB: Tracheal mucus flow rates in experimental bronchitis in rats. Br J Exp Pathol 50:139–149, 1969.

557. Alarie Y, Busey WM, Krumm AA, Ulrich CE: Long-term continuous exposure to sulfuric acid mist in Cynomolgus monkeys and guinea pigs. Arch Environ Health 27:16–24, 1973.

558. Kramer CG: Chlorine. J Occup Med 9:193–196, 1967.

559. Beach FXM, Sherwood Jones E, Scarrow GD: Respiratory effects of chlorine gas. Br J Indust Med 26:231–236, 1969.

560. Gerritsen WB, Buschmann CH: Phosgene poisoning caused by the use of chemical paint removers containing methylene chloride in ill-ventilated rooms heated by kerosene stoves. Br J Indust Med 17:187–189, 1960.

561. Seidelin R: The inhalation of phosgene in a fire extinguisher accident. Thorax 16:91–93, 1961.

562. Gross P, Rinehart WE, Hatch T: Chronic pneumonitis caused by phosgene. Arch Environ Health 10:768–775, 1965.

563. Walton M: Industrial ammonia gassing. Br J Indust Med 30:78–86, 1973.

564. Rall JE, Alpers JB, Lewallen CG, et al.: Radiation pneumonitis and fibrosis: A complication of radioiodine treatment of pulmonary metastases from cancer of the thyroid. J Clin Endocrinol Metab 17:1263–1276, 1957.

565. Schmorl G: Die Bergkrankheit der Erzbergleute in Schneeberg in Sachsen ("Schneeberger Lungenkrebs"). II. Pathologisch-anatomischer Teil. Z Krebsforsch 23:376–384, 1926.

566. Pirchan A, Šikl H: Cancer of the lung in the miners of Jáchymov (Joachimstal). Am J Cancer 16:681–722, 1932.

567. Löwy J: Über die Joachimstaler Bergkrankheit. Med Klin 25:141–142, 1929.

568. Jammet H, Mechali D, Dousset M: Uranium toxicity with special reference to its radiation hazards. In Shapiro HA (ed): *Pneumoconiosis. Proceedings International Conference Johannesburg 1969*. Cape Town: Oxford University Press, 1970, pp 547–550.

569. Archer VE, Gillam JD, Wagoner JK: Respiratory disease mortality among uranium miners. Ann NY Acad Sci 271:280–293, 1976.

570. Heppleston AG, Young AE: Population and ultrastructural

changes in murine alveolar cells following ^{239}PuO$_2$ inhalation. J Pathol 146:155–166, 1985.

571. Peller S: Lung cancer among mine workers in Joachimsthal. Hum Biol 11:130–143, 1939.

572. Šikl H: The present status of knowledge about the Jachymov disease (Cancer of the lungs in the miners of the radium mines). Acta Unio Int Cancr 6:1366–1375, 1950.

573. Archer VE, Brown MC: American uranium miners and lung cancer. In Shapiro HA (ed): *Pneumoconiosis. Proceedings International Conference Johannesburg* 1969. Cape Town: Oxford University Press, 1970, pp 569–571.

574. Archer VE, Wagoner JK, Lundin FE: Uranium mining and cigarette smoking effects on man. J Occup Med 15:204–211, 1973.

575. Ševc J, Junz E, Plaček V: Lung cancer in uranium miners and long-term exposure to radon daughter products. Health Phys 30:433–437, 1976.

576. Winters TH, Di Franza JR: Radioactivity in cigarette smoke. N Engl J Med 306:364–365, 1982.

577. Saccomanno G, Archer VE, Auerbach O, et al.: Histologic types of lung cancer among uranium miners. Cancer 27:515–523, 1971.

578. Archer VE, Saccamanno G, Jones JH: Frequency of different histologic types of bronchogenic carcinoma as related to radiation exposure. Cancer 34:2056–2060, 1974.

579. de Villiers AJ, Windish JP: Lung cancer in a fluorspar mining community. I. Radiation, dust, and mortality experience. Br J Indust Med 21:94–109, 1964.

580. Smith PG, Doll R: Mortality among patients with ankylosing spondylitis after a single treatment course with X-rays. Br Med J 284:449–460, 1982.

581. Cihak RW, Ishimaru T, Steer A, Yamada A: Lung cancer at autopsy in A-bomb survivors and controls, Hiroshima and Nagasaki, 1961–1970. I. Autopsy findings and relation to radiation. Cancer 33:1580–1588, 1974.

582. Miller RW: Late radiation effects: Status and needs of epidemiological research. Environ Res 8:221–233, 1974.

583. Axelson O, Sundell L: Mining, lung cancer and smoking. Scand J Work Environ Health 4:46–52, 1978.

584. Hahn FF, Benjamin SA, Boecker BB, et al.: Comparative pulmonary carcinogenicity of inhaled beta-emitting radionuclides in beagle dogs. In Walton WH (ed): *Inhaled Particles IV*. Oxford: Peragamon Press, 1977, pp 625–635.

585. Dagle GE, Sanders CL: Radionuclide injury to the lung. Environ Health Perspect 55:129–137, 1984.

586. International Commission on Radiological Protection Task Group. Biological effects of inhaled radionuclides. Ann ICRP 4:1–108, 1980.

587. Brightwell J, Ellender M: Removal of macrophages and plutonium dioxide particles by bronchopulmonary lavage. In Sanders CL, Schneider RP, Dagle GE, Ragan HA, (eds): *Pulmonary Macrophage and Epithelial Cells*. Springfield, VA: Energy Research and Development Administration (CONF-760927), 1977, pp 463–474.

588. Nolibé D, Metivier H, Masse R, Lafuma J: Therapeutic effect of pulmonary lavage in vivo after inhalation of insoluble radioactive particles. In Walton WH (ed): *Inhaled Particles IV*. Oxford: Pergamon Press, 1977, pp 597–612.

589. Evans RD, Harley JH, Jacobi W, et al.: Estimate of the risk from environmental exposure to radon-222 and its decay products. Nature 290:98–100, 1981.

590. Bruch J, Hilscher W, Kramer U: Pathogenicity to animals of fine dusts from Ruhr mines. In Walton WH (ed): *Inhaled Particles IV*. Oxford: Pergamon Press, 1977, pp 373–377.

591. Zaidi SH, Hilscher B, Hilscher W, et al: Vergleichende morphometrische und autoradiographische Untersuchungen quarzinduzierter Läsionen bei nu/nu Mäusen und Kontrollmäusen. Silikosebericht Nordrhein-Westfalen 12:187–192, 1979.

592. Heppleston AG: Pulmonary toxicology of silica, coal and asbestos. Environ Health Perspect 55:111–127, 1984.

593. Heppleston AG, Kulonen E, Potila M: In vitro assessment of the fibrogenicity of mineral dusts. Am J Indust Med 6:373–386, 1984.

594. Voisin C, Aerts C, Jakubczak E, Tonnel AB: La culture cellulaire en phase gazeuse. Un nouveau modèle expérimental d'étude in vitro des activités des macrophages alvéolaires. Bull Eur Physiopathol Respir 13:69–82, 1977.

595. Voisin C, Aerts C, Jakubczak E, et al.: Effets du bioxyde d'azote sur les macrophages alvéolaires en survie en phase gazeuse. Un nouveau modèle expérimental pour l'étude in vitro de la cytotoxicité des gas nocifs. Bull Eur-Physiopathol Respir 13:137–144, 1977.

596. Voisin C, Aerts C: Le macrophage alvéolaire en culture en phase gazeuse, indicateur biologique en toxicologie des gaz: Application à l'étude de la cytotoxicité du bioxyde d'azote (NO$_2$). Bull Acad Natl Med 168:755–760, 1984.

597. Rae S, Walker DD, Attfield MO: Chronic bronchitis and dust exposure in British coalminers. In Walton WH (ed): *Inhaled Particles III*. Old Woking, Surrey, England: Unwin, 1971, pp 883–894.

598. Rogan JM, Attfield MD, Jacobsen M, et al.: Role of dust in the working environment in development of chronic bronchitis in British coal miners. Br J Indust Med 30:217–226, 1973.

599. Deutsche Forschungsgemeinschaft: *Research Report—Chronic Bronchitis and Occupational Dust Exposure*. Boppard: Harald Boldt Verlag KG, 1978, pp 1–503.

600. Minette A: *Epidemiology of Chronic Bronchitis*. Industrial Health and Medicine Series—No. 20. Luxembourg: Commission of the European Communities—ECSC, 1979, pp 1–43.

601. Jacobsen M: Smoking and disability in miners. Lancet 2:740, 1980.

602. Ryder RC, Lyons JP, Campbell H, Gough J: Bronchial mucous gland status in coal workers' pneumoconiosis. Ann NY Acad Sci 200:370–380, 1972.

603. Douglas AN, Lamb D, Ruckley VA: Bronchial gland dimensions in coalminers: Influence of smoking and dust exposure. Thorax 37:760–764, 1982.

604. Hankinson JL, Reger RB, Morgan WKC: Maximal expiratory flows in coalminers. Am Rev Respir Dis 116:175–180, 1977.

605. Hankinson JL, Reger RB, Fairman RP, et al.: Factors influencing expiratory flow rates in coal miners. In Walton WH (ed): *Inhaled Particles IV*. Oxford: Pergamon Press, 1977, pp 737–752.

606. Elwood PC, Sweetnam PM, Elwood JH, Campbell M: Respiratory symptoms and lung function in ex-cotton and flax workers. In Elwood PC (ed): *New Light on Byssinosis*. Cardiff: Medical Research Council Epidemiology Unit, 1985, pp 95–127.

607. Fox AJ, Tombleson JBL, Watt A, Wilkie AG: A survey of respiratory disease in cotton operatives. Part II. Br J Indust Med 30:48–53, 1973.

608. Berry G, Molyneux MKB, Tombleson JBL: Relationships between dust level and byssinosis in Lancashire cotton mills. Br J Indust Med 31:18–27, 1974.

609. Berry G, Molyneux MKB: A mortality study of workers in Lancashire cotton mills. Chest 79:11S–15S, 1981.

610. Merchant JA, Ortmeyer C: Mortality of employees of two cotton mills in North Carolina. Chest 79:6S–11S, 1981.

611. Elwood PC, Thomas HF, Sweetnam PM, Elwood JH: Mortality of flax workers. Br J Indust Med 39:18–22, 1982.

612. Henderson V, Enterline PE: An unusual mortality experience in cotton textile workers. J Occup Med 15:717–719, 1973.

613. Rooke GB, Dempsey AN, Hillier VF, et al.: Observations on byssinotics diagnosed in the United Kingdom between 1974 and 1980. In Elwood PC (ed): *New Light on Byssinosis*. Cardiff: Medical Research Council Epidemiology Unit, 1985, pp 69–94.

614. Edwards C, Macartney J, Rooke G, Ward F: The pathology of the lung in byssinotics. Thorax 30:612–623, 1975.

615. Edwards CW, Carlile A: The pathology of byssinosis in Lancashire cotton workers. In Elwood PC (ed): *New Light on Byssinosis*. Cardiff: Medical Research Council Epidemiology Unit, 1985, pp 33–47.

616. Pratt PC, Vollmer RT, Miller JA: Epidemiology of pulmonary lesions in nontextile and cotton textile workers: A retrospective autopsy analysis. Arch Environ Health 35:133–138, 1980.

617. Moran TJ: Emphysema and other chronic lung disease in textile workers: An 18-year autopsy study. Arch Environ Health 38:267–277, 1983.

618. Honeybourne D, Pickering CAC: Physiological evidence that emphysema is not a feature of byssinosis. Thorax 41:6–11, 1986.

619. Bouhuys A: Byssinosis. Airway responses caused by inhalation of textile dusts. Arch Environ Health 23:405–407, 1971.

620. Hitchcock M, Piscitelli DM, Bouhuys A: Histamine release from human lung by a component of cotton bracts. Arch Environ Health 26:177–182, 1973.

621. Ainsworth SK, Neuman RE, Harley RA: Histamine release from platelets for assay of byssinogenic substances in cotton mill dust and related materials. Br J Indust Med 36:35–42, 1979.

622. Noweir MH: Studies on the etiology of byssinosis. Chest 79:62S–67S, 1981.

623. Buck MG, Wall JH, Schachter EN: Airway constrictor response to cotton bract extracts in the absence of endotoxin. Br J Indust Med 43:220–226, 1986.

624. Mundie TG, Ainsworth SK: Byssinosis: In vitro release of prostaglandin and thromboxane from lung tissue and polymorphonuclear leukocytes induced by cotton dust and bract extracts. Environ Res 38:400–406, 1985.

625. Mundie TG, Ainsworth SK. Byssinosis: Thromboxane release from human platelets by cotton dust and bract extracts. Arch Environ Health 40:165–169, 1985.

626. Kutz SA, Mentnech MS, Olenchock SA, Major PC: Immune mechanisms in byssinosis. Chest 79:56S–58S, 1981.

627. Olenchock SA, Mull JC, Boehlecke BA, Major PC: Cotton dust and complement in vivo. Chest 79:53S–55S, 1981.

628. Cinkotai FF, Lockwood MG, Rylander R: Airborne microorganisms and prevalence of byssinotic symptoms in cotton mills. Am Indust Hyg Assoc J 38:554–559, 1977.

629. Rylander R, Imbus HR, Suh MW: Bacterial contamination of cotton as an indicator of respiratory effects among card room workers. Br J Indust Med 36:299–304, 1979.

630. Haglind P, Lundholm M, Rylander R: Prevalence of byssinosis in Swedish cotton mills. Br J Indust Med 38:138–143, 1981.

631. Merchant JA, Lumsden JC, Kilburn KH, et al.: Intervention studies of cotton steaming to reduce biological effects of cotton dust. Br J Indust Med 31:261–274, 1974.

632. Petsonk EL, Olenchock SA, Castellan RM, et al.: Human ventilatory response to washed and unwashed cottons from different growing areas. Br J Indust Med 43:182–187, 1986.

633. Mundie TG, Boackle RJ, Ainsworth SK: In vitro alternative and classical activation of complement by extracts of cotton mill dust: A possible mechanism in the pathogenesis of byssinosis. Environ Res 32:47–56, 1983

24 Disorders of the Vascular System

Donald Heath
Paul Smith

Introduction

Diseases of the heart may affect the lungs and diseases of the lungs may affect the heart; the anatomic pathway through which this relationship is effected is the pulmonary vasculature. The pulmonary circulation operates at a pressure of only one-sixth of that of systemic circulation; therefore, the pulmonary arterial vessels have a different histologic structure than their systemic counterparts. Being initially thinner and less muscular, they react in a striking fashion to an elevated intravascular pressure.

However, there is no one form of hypertensive pulmonary vascular disease. The histopathology of pulmonary hypertension is dependent on the reason for the raised pressure. Hence this chapter begins with an account of the causes of pulmonary arterial hypertension. It then considers the pathology of the two extremes of the spectrum of hypertensive pulmonary vascular disease: plexogenic pulmonary arteriopathy and vascular disease in the lung secondary to chronic hypoxia. Consideration is also given to the pathology of pulmonary venous hypertension. The concept of dietary pulmonary hypertension in animals due to pyrrolizidine alkaloids is described, followed by a consideration of the role of drugs in inducing primary pulmonary hypertension. Next the pathology of clinically unexplained pulmonary hypertension with its three major causes—primary pulmonary hypertension, pulmonary veno-occlusive disease, and recurrent pulmonary thromboembolism—is covered. Pulmonary fibrosis is a common association of many diseases of the lung, and its effects on the pulmonary blood vessels are considered. Parasitic disease of the pulmonary circulation and congenital anomalies of the pulmonary vasculature are also described. Finally, the effects on the pulmonary circulation of diminished pressure and flow and of emboli are considered.

Causes of Pulmonary Arterial Hypertension

Many diseases are associated with a raised pulmonary arterial pressure, but it is possible to group them on the basis of a shared main factor responsible for the production of pulmonary hypertension.[1] Although the precise pathophysiologic mechanism by which the common underlying factor operates is often poorly understood, distinct groups may be recognized.

Pretricuspid Shunts

Pretricuspid shunts occur between the right and left atria, allowing a large left-to-right flow of blood to enter the systemic venous stream before it enters the right ventricle. Examples are high atrial septal defects such as those of secundum or sinus venosus type.[2] The natural history of this type of shunt is that it predisposes to a long period of high pulmonary blood flow before the onset of significant pulmonary arterial pressure as late as middle age. Pretricuspid shunts may lead to plexogenic pulmonary arteriopathy. Another congenital anomaly leading to this hemodynamic situation is anomalous pulmonary venous drainage into systemic veins or the right atrium.[3]

Post-tricuspid Shunts

When there is a large defect between the left ventricle or aorta and the right ventricle or pulmonary arteries, the direct transmission of systemic blood pressure into the pulmonary circulation leads to pulmonary arterial hypertension. In these diseases, which almost exclusively comprise congenital cardiac anomalies, pulmonary hypertension is present from birth, and this has implications for the structure of the pulmonary trunk in these cases. The form of pulmonary vascular disease which develops in these cases is plexogenic pulmonary arteriopathy. The congenital cardiac anomalies that give rise to post-tricuspid shunts are numerous, and severe pulmonary vascular disease may develop in ventricular septal defect,[4] single ventricle,[5] wide patent ductus arteriosus,[6] aortopulmonary septal defect,[7] Eisenmenger's complex,[8] cardioaortic fistula,[9] and persistent truncus arteriosus.[10] Rarely post-tricuspid shunts are acquired, such as in rupture of an aortic aneurysm into one of the main pulmonary arteries[11] or rupture of the interventricular septum following a myocardial infarction.[12]

Chronic Pulmonary Venous Hypertension

Any disease leading to a sustained elevation of blood pressure in the left atrium or pulmonary veins will lead to pulmonary arterial hypertension and characteristic histopathologic changes in the pulmonary arteries, pulmonary veins, and lung parenchyma. Mitral stenosis is the most common cause; usually this is rheumatic in etiology, but very rarely it may be congenital.[13] Mitral incompetence will have a similar effect; hence, pulmonary hypertension may complicate, in addition to chronic rheumatic heart disease, "floppy" mitral valve, bacterial endocarditis, and trauma.[1] Tumors of the left atrium and compression of the large pulmonary veins by a mediastinal granuloma are other rare causes of pulmonary arterial hypertension secondary to pulmonary venous hypertension. Chronic left ventricular failure due to myocardial ischemia or some other rare myocardial disease such as amyloidosis or sarcoidosis are other main causes.

Chronic Hypoxia

Persistent chronic alveolar hypoxia will induce pulmonary hypertension. The most common conditions by far to elevate pulmonary arterial pressure by this means are chronic bronchitis and emphysema, kyphoscoliosis and other thoracic deformities, and the Pickwickian syndrome. Such oddities as chronic hypoxia secondary to enlarged adenoids will also induce pulmonary hypertension. Finally, millions of people live at high altitude, and the diminished barometric pressure of their mountain habitat leads to a decreased partial pressure of oxygen in the alveolar spaces. Most of these native highlanders are chronically hypoxic and have a mild degree of pulmonary hypertension, although they are healthy. Only a few develop chronic mountain sickness (Monge's disease) when the degree of elevation of the pulmonary arterial pressure may become somewhat greater.

Pulmonary Fibrosis

Massive pulmonary fibrosis as seen in the pneumoconioses may lead to significant pulmonary vascular obstruction and pulmonary hypertension by engulfing the pulmonary arteries and arterioles.[14] Sometimes, as in hematite lung, characteristic industrial dust accumulates in and around the affected blood vessels.[15] Interstitial fibrosis of the lung and honeycomb lung are characterized by their own form of pulmonary vascular disease[16] irrespective of the underlying cause, in which an early stage of muscularization is followed by one of fibrous ablation. The causes of fibrosing alveolitis which may lead to this form of vascular disease are numerous. They include rheumatoid disease, sarcoidosis, the Hamman-Rich syndrome, and various industrial diseases such as berylliosis. Various granulomatous diseases may involve the walls of the pulmonary arteries or even lead to their occlusion; the best-known example is sarcoidosis.

Recurrent Pulmonary Embolism

Descriptions are given elsewhere in this chapter of the classic medical emergency of massive pulmonary thromboembolism and the equally well-known red infarcts of lung produced by a combination of smaller thromboemboli and pulmonary venous hypertension. A third variant of pulmonary thromboembolism is the condition in which showers of silent, small thromboemboli impact into the muscular pulmonary arteries and pulmonary arterioles leading to the development of a significant degree of pulmonary arterial hypertension.[17]

Many other varieties of emboli will, however, give rise to pulmonary hypertension. They include fat, right atrial myxoma (Fig. 24–1)[18] bilharzial ova, and amniotic fluid.[19] In fact the pulmonary circulation is the great filter of the body, and the patient histopathologist will find all manners of emboli impacted in the small pulmonary arteries, ranging from bone marrow to megakaryocytes (Fig. 24–2). Iatrogenic emboli include air and other gases[20] introduced during operations and a variety of investigations and cotton-fiber emboli.[21] Gas-induced embolism, however, is more likely to give rise to a medical emergency than pulmonary hypertension; the latter condition is of interest only to the histologist.

Primary Pulmonary Hypertension

Sometimes severe pulmonary hypertension develops in the absence of heart or lung disease or any of the predisposing causes of a raised pulmonary arterial pressure listed in this chapter. The clinical condition of unexplained pulmonary hypertension may be produced by three pathologic entities: plexogenic pulmonary arteriopathy (when the clinical condition is one of primary pulmonary hypertension), pulmonary veno-occlusive disease (when the brunt of the disorder falls on the pulmonary veins rather than the pulmonary arteries), and recurrent pulmonary thromboembolism. Plexogenic pulmonary arteriopathy is not pathognomonic of primary pulmonary hypertension, but also constitutes the pulmonary vascular disease associated with congenital cardiac shunts and liver disease.

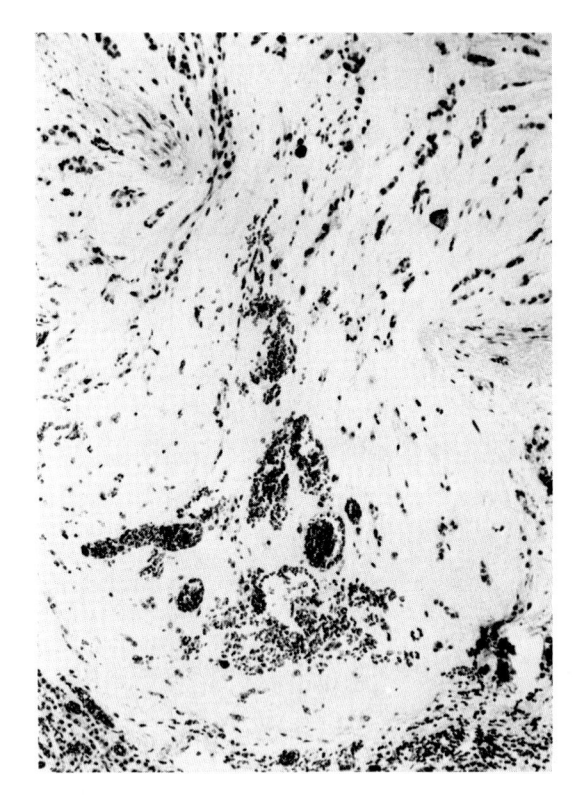

Figure 24–1. Transverse section of a muscular pulmonary artery from a woman aged 38 years with a myxoma of the right atrium. An embolus from the tumor has impacted in the vessel. It consists largely of amorphous myxoid material containing scanty myxoma cells. The raised intravascular pressure brought about by the multiple emboli has ruptured the vessel so that the myxomatous tissue has escaped into the surrounding lung parenchyma. Such appearances can mimic the invasiveness of malignancy (H&E, ×96).

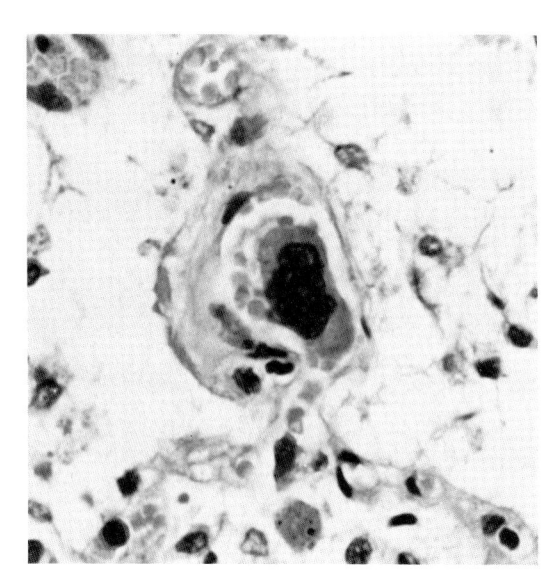

Figure 24–2. Transverse section of a pulmonary arteriole from a man who died following traumatic injury. The vessel contains a megakaryocyte embolus derived from the bone marrow (H&E, ×600).

Diet

Pulmonary hypertension may be dietary in origin. So far this has been demonstrated only in animals, and the substances incriminated have been pyrrolizidine alkaloids derived from species of Crotalaria and Senecio such as *C. spectabilis*,[22] *C. fulva*,[23] and *S. jacobaea*.[24] In one case, there was a suspicion that a case of primary pulmonary hypertension in humans was associated with ingestion of *C. laburnoides*.[25] An epidemic of primary pulmonary hypertension in Europe which began in 1967 was considered on epidemiologic grounds to be the result of the ingestion of an anorexigen, aminorex fumarate. Experimental confirmation of this in animals, however, was never obtained.

Hepatic Disease

As noted elsewhere in this chapter (*see* Pulmonary Circulation in Liver Disease, below) both cirrhosis of the liver and portal vein thrombosis can very rarely give rise to severe pulmonary hypertension based on plexogenic pulmonary arteriopathy.

Parasites

The impaction of ova of Schistosoma into the pulmonary arteries with subsequent granulomatous and immunologic reactions can lead to pulmonary hypertension. The possible implication of filariasis in an epidemic of primary pulmonary hypertension in Sri Lanka is much more controversial.

Developmental Anomalies

These constitute a rare but interesting group of causes of pulmonary hypertension. In unilateral absence of a pulmonary artery, pulmonary hypertension may ensue in the absence of a congenital cardiac shunt, the cause of the elevation of pulmonary arterial pressure being the pumping of all the blood into one lung with the probable additional factor of hyperreactive pulmonary arteries to this stimulus. Multiple stenoses of pulmonary arteries will also elevate pulmonary arterial pressure. In the scimitar syndrome, the pulmonary arteries in the base of the right lung supplied by systemic arteries are exposed to high blood pressure and show hypertensive changes. A variety of congenital malformations involving the left atrium or pulmonary veins, such as congenital stenosis of pulmonary veins and cor triatriatum, give rise to pulmonary venous hypertension and secondary elevation of pulmonary arterial pressure.

Postoperative Pulmonary Hypertension

Pulmonary hypertension may follow overgenerous anastomotic operations for the relief of such congenital anomalies as Fallot's tetrad which may in effect create significant post-tricuspid shunts.

Plexogenic Pulmonary Arteriopathy

Morphology

Plexogenic pulmonary arteriopathy is the form of hypertensive pulmonary vascular disease that complicates pre- and post-tricuspid congenital cardiac shunts, rare cases of cirrhosis of the liver and portal vein thrombosis, and classic primary pulmonary hypertension. It represents one extreme of the spectrum of pulmonary vascular disease and is of particular interest to the histopathologist, for its histologic components include the whole gamut of vascular responses to pulmonary hypertension. Its designation arose from a meeting of a working party of the World Health Organization on primary pulmonary hypertension in 1973, in recognition of the fact that this form of vascular disease has the potential for the formation of plexiform lesions, although they are not present in every case.

The lesions of plexogenic pulmonary arteriopathy are complex, but they can be graded according to increasing degree of severity and complexity of histopathologic change.[26] These grades are based on the relation of the histologic changes to a progressively falling level of pulmonary blood flow.[27] Their histopathologic features are as follows:

1. Medial hypertrophy of muscular pulmonary arteries and muscularization of pulmonary arterioles.
2. Further medial hypertrophy with cellular intimal proliferation.
3. Acellular intimal fibrosis in small muscular pulmonary arteries and arterioles that may be occlusive.
4. Generalized and localized dilation and thinning of pulmonary arteries with the formation of plexiform lesions.
5. Chronic dilation of pulmonary vessels with rupture of some to cause hemorrhage and hemosiderosis.
6. Fibrinoid necrosis.

This grading system is of value in that it enables one to express succinctly a complex collection of changes, without recourse to detailed descriptions or morphometry which are likely to be too time-consuming for the pathologist without a special interest in this field. It applies only to plexogenic pulmonary arteriopathy and must not be used in cases of pulmonary arterial hypertension induced by hypoxia, recurrent pulmonary thromboembolism, pulmonary venous hypertension, or pulmonary veno-occlusive disease, all of which have a pathology peculiar to them. Although fibrinoid necrosis is involved in the formation of plexiform lesions, it has been given a higher (and thus later) grade number than dilation lesions. The reason for this is that each successive grade is based on a progressive fall in level of pulmonary blood flow; hence a case with well-developed fibrinoid necrosis follows rather than precedes the formation of plexiform lesions. The histopathology of each of the grades, speculation on their pathogenesis, and discussion of their clinical importance are as follows.

Grade 1. This grade is characterized by muscularization of the pulmonary vasculature so that the muscular pulmonary arteries show medial hypertrophy with a ratio of medial thickness to external diameter that may exceed 20 percent, in contrast to normal value of around 5 percent (Fig. 24–3). Pulmonary arterioles have a thick media of smooth muscle which is sandwiched between internal and external elastic laminae so that the vessels resemble systemic arterioles (Fig. 24–4). Their percentage medial thickness may exceed 25 percent. In disease where pulmonary hypertension is present from birth, as in post-tricuspid congenital cardiac shunts such as the ventricular septal defect, these muscular vessels represent a persistence of the thick-walled, muscular, fetal pulmonary arteries into adult life. In contrast, in atrial septal defect of septum secundum types, or other forms of pretricuspid congenital cardiac shunt characterized by a long period of high pulmonary blood flow before the onset of pulmonary hypertension, the pulmonary arteries are initially thin walled and the pulmonary arterioles devoid of a muscular media. As pulmonary hypertension supervenes, there is associated medial hypertrophy of the muscular pulmonary arteries and muscularization of the

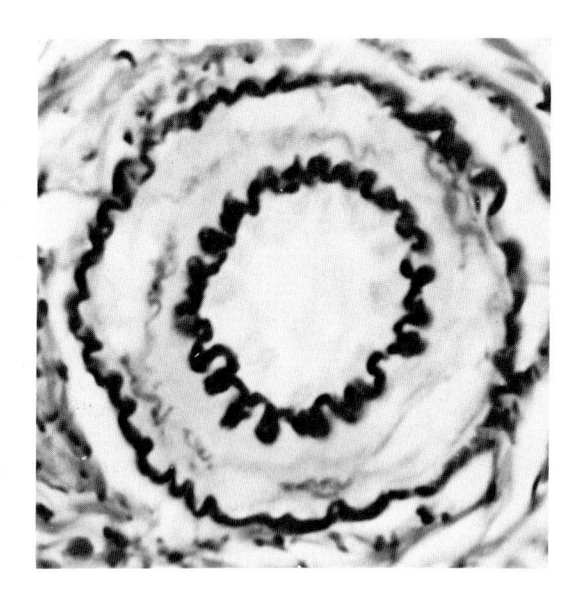

Figure 24–3. Transverse section of a muscular pulmonary artery from a male infant of 18 months with a large ventricular septal defect. If shows pronounced medial hypertrophy. The crenated elastic laminae are consistent with some degree of collapse or constriction [elastic Van Gieson (EVG), ×600].

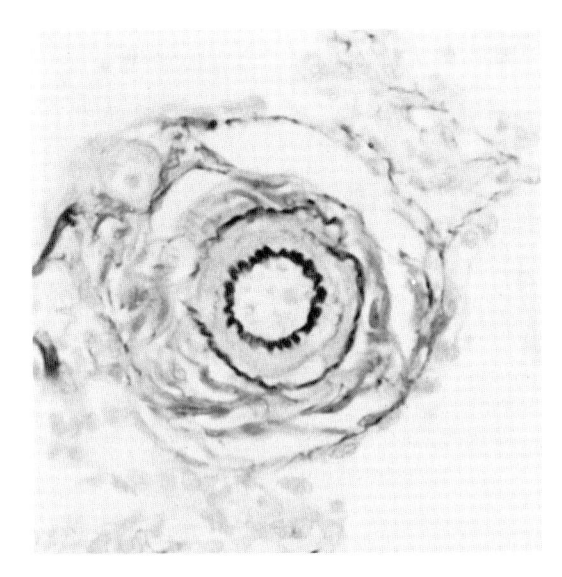

Figure 24-4. Transverse section of a pulmonary arteriole from the same case as Fig. 24-3. The vessel is muscularized and has a thick media of circularly oriented smooth muscle sandwiched between two elastic laminae. It resembles a systemic arteriole (EVG, ×600).

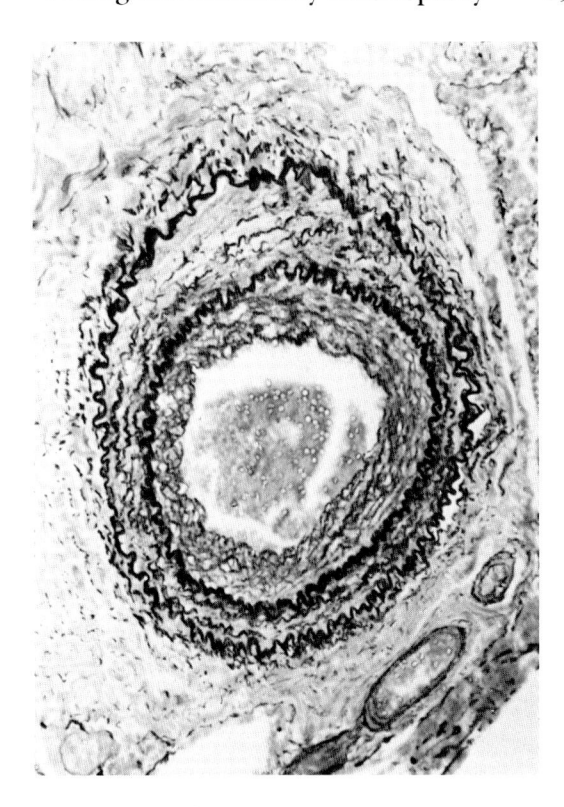

Figure 24-5. Muscular pulmonary artery in slightly oblique section from a 12-year-old girl with ventricular septal defect. There is an intimal proliferation of fine elastic and collagen fibers (EVG, ×165).

pulmonary arterioles. In this way, the appearances come to resemble those of post-tricuspid shunts seen in infancy.

Grade 2. In this grade, there is a cellular intimal proliferation. The endothelial cells play but a small part because, after showing early evidence of increased metabolic activity in response to the raised intravascular pressure, they die and desquamate. Most of the cellular intimal proliferation is due to myofibroblasts between the endothelium and the internal elastic lamina.

Grade 3. The hallmark of this grade is the appearance of collagen in the intimal proliferation (Fig. 24-5). The intimal fibrosis may be mild or lead to vascular occlusion. There may be considerable variation in a single case. In plexogenic pulmonary arteriopathy, fibrous tissue is commonly laid down in concentric rings, giving it an onion-skin appearance[28] (Fig. 24-6). In its early stages, concentric-laminar intimal proliferation is largely composed of collagen, but later elastic tissue is also deposited as fine concentric fibrils. Sometimes the elastic fibers are coarser and are laid down as discrete bands separating zones composed largely of collagen (Fig. 24-7); this suggests that the intimal fibroelastosis is deposited in episodes rather than as a continuous process. In some arteries, the deposition of elastic tissue may be extreme, forming a dense black ring when stained by the elastic Van Gieson technique (Fig. 24-8). The lumen may be almost totally obliterated, but a small endothelial-lined channel usually persists. Fibrosis affects predominantly the pulmonary arterioles and the smaller muscular pulmonary arteries. Large muscular and elastic arteries show atherosclerosis rather than fibrosis. Concentric-laminar intimal fibrosis can usually be distinguished from fibrosis

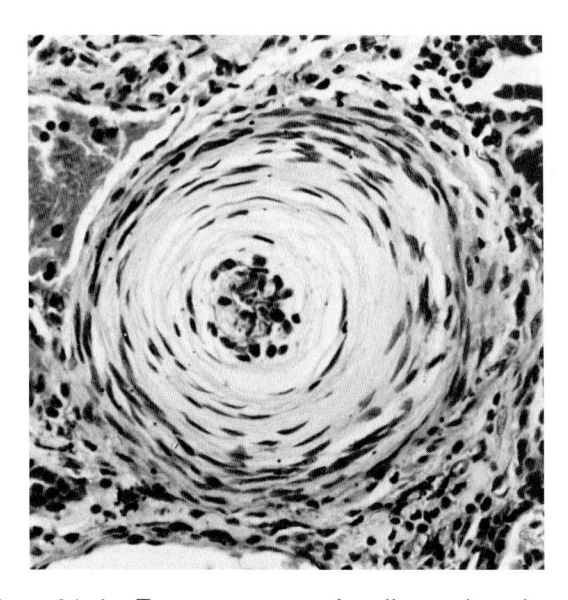

Figure 24-6. Transverse section of small muscular pulmonary artery from a 26-year-old woman with aortopulmonary septal defect. The vessel is almost totally occluded by a concentric, laminar intimal proliferation. The nuclei of the myofibroblasts are arranged in concentric rings, creating the typical onion-skin appearance (H&E, ×322).

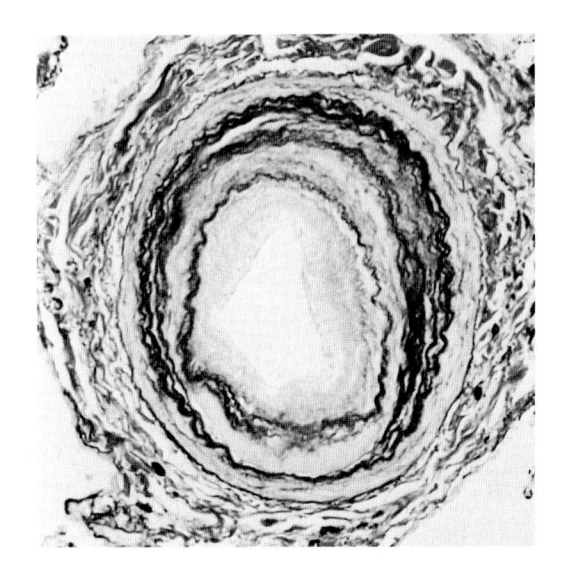

Figure 24–7. Transverse section of a muscular pulmonary artery from a 19-year-old girl with double outlet right ventricle and ventricular septal defect. The intima contains a concentric laminar fibroelastosis in which the collagen and elastin fibers are separated into discrete bands suggesting different episodes of fibrogenesis of the intima (EVG, ×168).

due to age change, which is acellular, often eccentrically situated, and lacking in significant quantities of elastic tissue. Furthermore, the intimal fibrosis of plexogenic pulmonary arteriopathy is usually seen in young subjects. In grade 3, the media of both pulmonary arteries and arterioles reach the limits of their capacity to hypertrophy.

Grade 4. Generalized and localized thinning of the pulmonary arterial tree heralds the onset of grade 4. It involves both pulmonary arteries free of intimal proliferation (Fig. 24–9) and those involved by fibrosis. Dilated vessels free of intimal proliferation can constitute a diagnostic pitfall, since they may be misinterpreted as being of normal thickness and hence inconsistent with hypertensive pulmonary vascular disease (*see* Fig. 24–9). In arterioles and small arteries affected by intimal fibrosis, dilation occurs at, or distal to, the areas of fibrotic occlusion, whereas in medium-sized vessels, it is usually seen proximal to this occlusion.

In addition to the generalized dilation of the pulmonary vasculature, there are localized changes in the smaller pulmonary arterial vessels which are collectively referred to as 'dilatation lesions'. The most characteristic of these is the plexiform lesion from which the term plexogenic pulmonary arteriopathy is derived. Plexiform lesions develop when a segment of a muscular pulmonary artery (Fig. 24–10) or an arteriolar side branch immediately proximal to a zone of fibrotic occlusion (Fig. 24–11) undergoes pronounced dilation to form an expanded sac with very thin walls containing little, if any, smooth muscle. Fibrous tissue from the occluded segment often extends into the opening of this sac, but the bulk of its lumen is occupied by cellular elements in which there is a tortuous series of capillaries and vascular

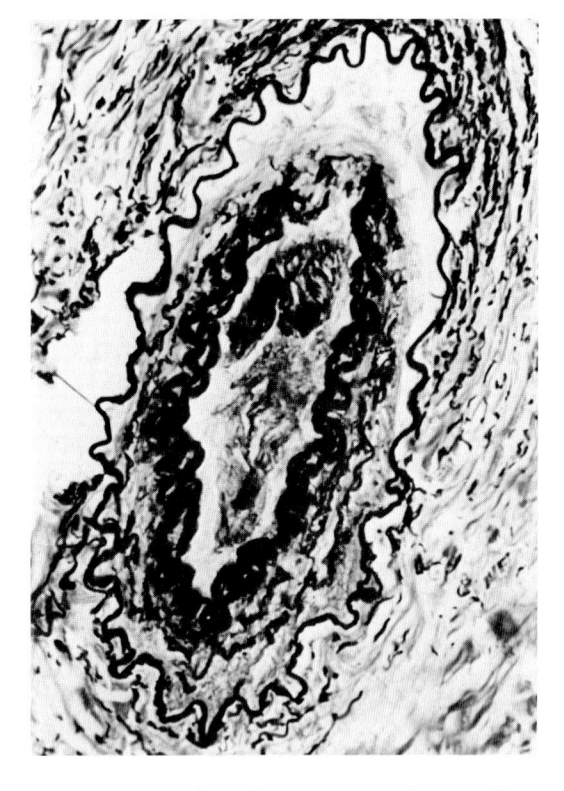

Figure 24–8. Muscular pulmonary artery from a 22-year-old woman with primary pulmonary hypertension. There is a thick media of smooth muscle with intense elastosis of the intima which occludes the lumen. There is pronounced crenation of the internal and external elastic laminae (EVG, ×375).

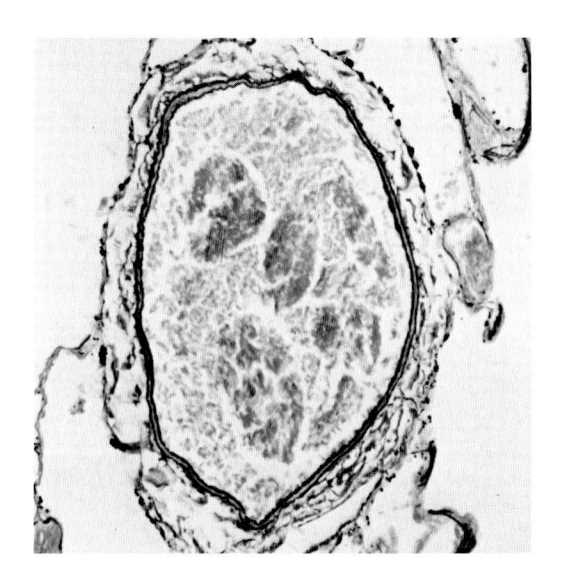

Figure 24–9. Transverse section of a muscular pulmonary artery from the same patient as in Figure 24–8. Dilation of the vessel has caused thinning of the media so that it resembles a normal pulmonary artery (EVG, ×150).

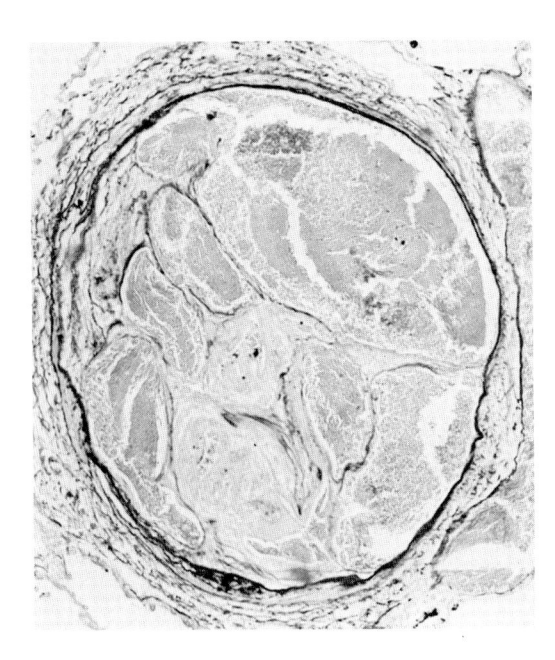

Figure 24-10. Muscular pulmonary artery in transverse section from the same patient as in Figure 24-9. The vessel is dilated so that the media is thin and in places atrophic. It contains an organizing plexiform lesion consisting of strands of fibroelastic tissue separating vascular sinuses (EVG, ×108).

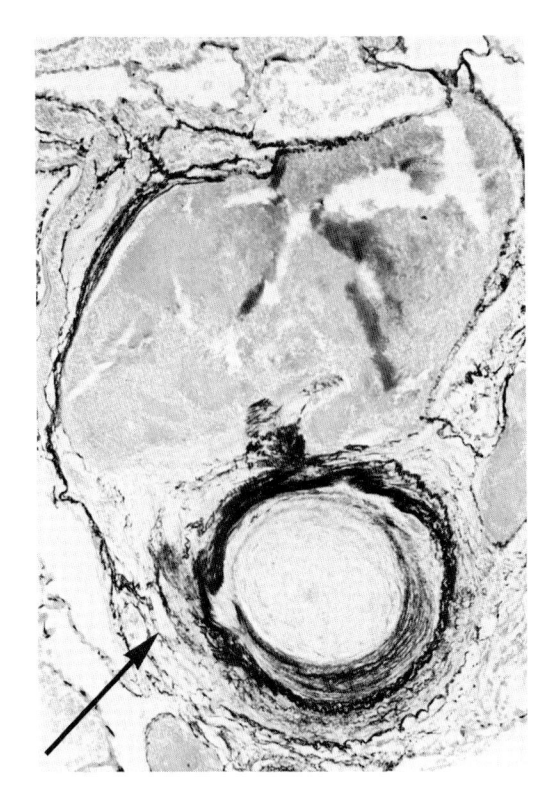

Figure 24-11. Muscular pulmonary artery from 24-year-old Indian man with plexogenic pulmonary arteriopathy complicating portal vein thrombosis. The vessel is occluded by concentric laminar, intimal fibroelastosis. A side branch is dilated into a large balloon-like sac or dilatation lesion. The arterial media distant from the dilatation lesion consists of compact smooth muscle, but near the origin of the sac, it becomes paler and looser (arrow). In this region, cells from the media appear to be spreading into the cavity of the sac, perhaps representing an early stage in the formation of a plexiform lesion (EVG, ×96).

sinuses (Figs. 24-12 through 24-15). The lesion resembles a vascular plexus, hence its designation. The distal part of the sac may lead into several dilated thin-walled channels which terminate as capillaries that pass to the alveolar walls.

In the early stages of their development, plexiform lesions are cellular, consisting of numerous, plump cells, resembling endothelium, lining vascular sinuses (*see* Fig. 24-13). In the walls of the sinuses, there are rounded cells and small quantities of collagen. The media of the parent artery often contains a focus of fibrinoid necrosis adjacent to, and extending into, the wall of the dilated sac. There is also commonly thrombosis of the vascular sinuses but not of the dilated vessels distal to them. More advanced plexiform lesions contain large quantities of collagen (*see* Fig. 24-14), suggesting that the natural history of these lesions is toward progressive fibrosis. The fibrous tissue is laid down in the septa between the sinuses and may encroach upon the latter (*see* Fig. 24-15). The areas of fibrinoid necrosis and thrombosis undergo organization to form large masses of collagen. Finally, elastic fibers become deposited. These organized plexiform lesions may appear different from the younger ones but can still be recognized as dilated sacs containing irregular bands of fibroelastic tissue in which a plexus of vascular channels persists. They must not be mistaken for organized thromboemboli.

Often associated with plexiform lesions are vein-like branches of muscular pulmonary arteries which represent the extreme of vascular dilation in which the muscular media is all but absent. They are grossly dilated with wide, patent lumens frequently forming a convoluted cluster around the periphery of an obstructed pulmonary artery (Fig. 24-16). They are believed to form a collateral circulation to the alveolar capillaries and have been misinterpreted as arteriovenous anastomoses. Serial sections have demonstrated conclusively that they are arterial in nature and end as pulmonary capillaries.[29]

The third type of dilation lesion is rare and consists of a dilated vessel containing numerous thin-walled sinuses resembling an angioma.[30] Such angiomatoid lesions occur in lateral branches of pulmonary arteries proximal to segments of fibrous occlusion of a parent vessel. They are derived from a proliferation of capillaries in the wall of the parent vessel that pass into the dilated side branch and form the angiomatoid mass before passing distally as capillaries which ramify in all directions to end in capillary walls.

Grade 5. At this stage, some of the highly dilated, thin-walled vessels (described previously), which ramify throughout the lung, rupture to liberate blood into the alveolar spaces and interstitium. The histologic appear-

694   Disorders of the Vascular System

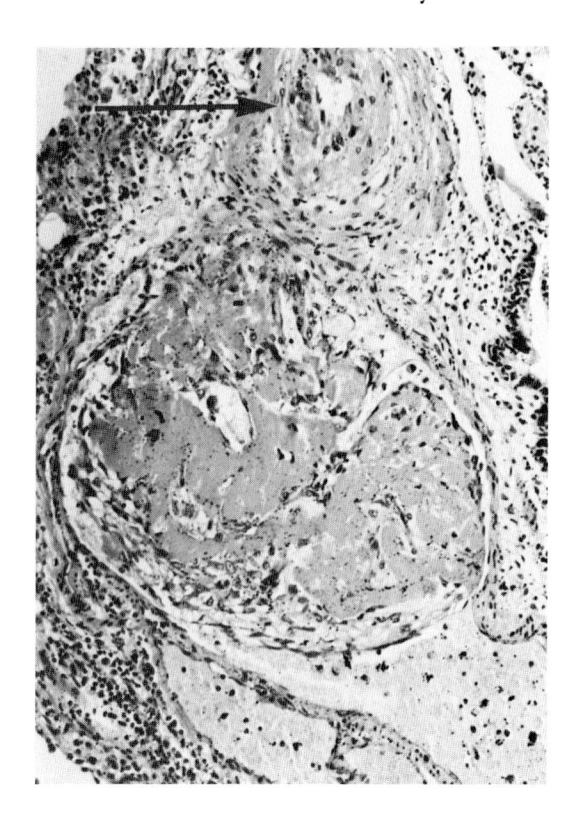

Figure 24–12. A plexiform lesion from a 12-year-old girl with cor triloculare biatriatum. A dilated side branch extends from an occluded parent pulmonary artery (arrow). This dilatation lesion contains a tortous series of vascular sinuses. The acellular material within many of the sinuses is fibrin (H&E, ×96).

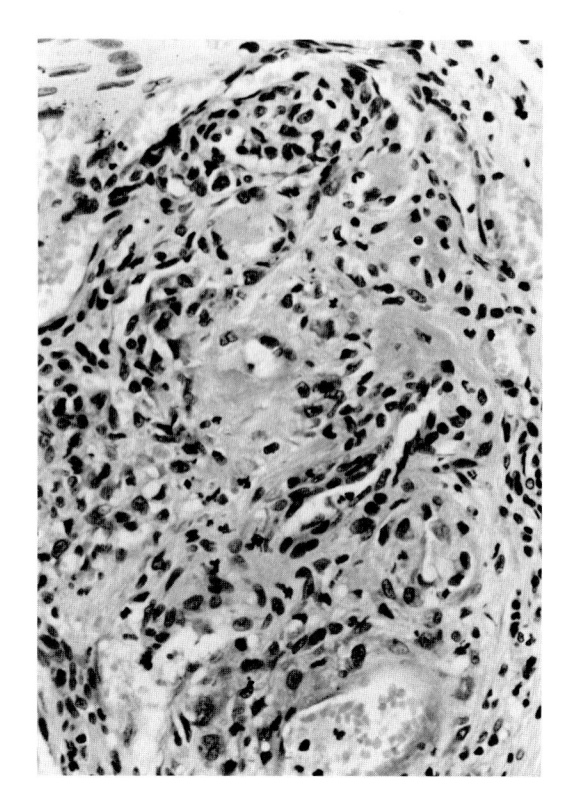

Figure 24–13. Same patient seen in Figure 24–12, showing detail of an early plexiform lesion. The vascular sinuses are lined by plump cells with rounded cells in the interstitial tissues forming the septa. The material between the cells consists largely of fibrin with only a few collagen fibers (H&E, ×285).

ances are, therefore, those of a highly vascular lung containing foci of pulmonary hemorrhage and macrophages. In long-standing cases, hemosiderin is formed. Many pulmonary arteries become rigidly dilated as a result of combined medial and intimal sclerosis (Fig. 24–17).

Grade 6. The final phase of plexogenic pulmonary arteriopathy is necrotizing arteritis which, like its counterpart in the systemic circulation, appears to be caused by a severe and sudden elevation of intravascular pressure. It is usually patchy in distribution with some muscular pulmonary arteries and pulmonary arterioles being severely affected while others are completely spared. Fibrinoid necrosis occurs earlier as a focal change inducing plexiform lesions, but its full, widespread form is the final stage of this type of hypertensive pulmonary vascular disease. The media becomes swollen with loss of nuclear detail. It stains intensely and homogeneously with eosin, the tinctorial reaction resembling that of fibrin (Fig. 24–18). There is frequently mural thrombosis closely adherent to the endothelium. Consequent to this damage, there is an infiltration into the intima and media of neutrophil polymorphs, the lesion then being called necrotizing arteritis (Fig. 24–19). Older lesions undergo organization of granulation tissue, and the healing involves the adventitia as well as the media often causing fragmentation of the external elastic lamina (Fig. 24–20). Sometimes the entire vessel becomes overrun by granulation tissue which may assume the form of a dumbbell-shaped mass with nodules in the intima and adventitia linked by a connecting bar in the media.

Longitudinal Muscle in Pulmonary Arteries

Fasciculi of longitudinally oriented smooth muscle fibers are commonly found in muscular pulmonary arteries in hypertensive pulmonary vascular disease of any severity.[31] This is a nonspecific change which is not related to the underlying cause of the pulmonary hypertension. Hence it is not restricted to plexogenic pulmonary arteriopathy but occurs also, for example, in chronic alveolar hypoxia.[32] The longitudinal muscle may be deposited as small bundles or as a complete ring round the circumference of the vessel (Fig. 24–21). Within these bundles, small fasciculi are usually separated from one another by an anastomosing network of fine elastic fibers. Longitudinal muscle is usually most prominent in the outer media adjacent to the adventitia (*see* Fig. 24–21). In hypertensive pulmonary vascular disease associated with states of chronic hypoxia, the longitudinal muscle commonly occurs in the intima. Under these circumstances,

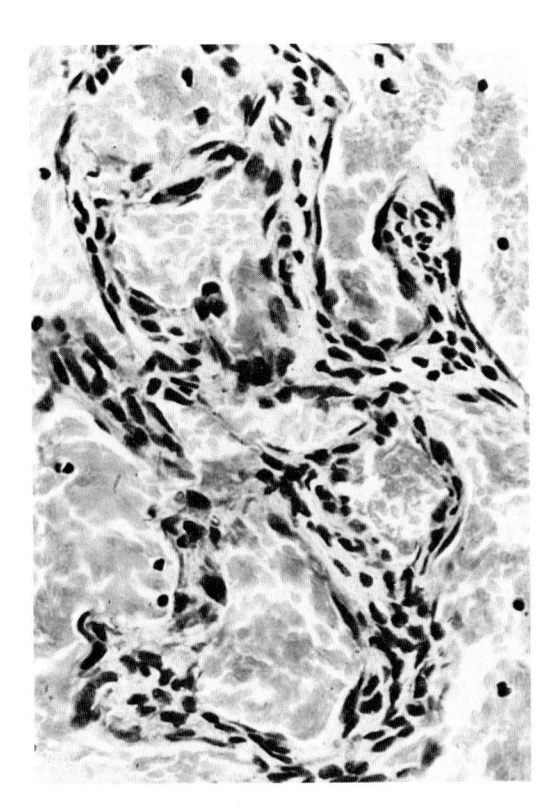

Figure 24–14. Detail of an organizing plexiform lesion from a 22-year-old woman with primary pulmonary hypertension. The distinction between vascular sinuses and septa is clearly seen, the whole resembling a vascular plexus. Although most of the cells lining the sinuses are rounded, some are now elongated. The septa contain elongated myofibroblasts embedded in a matrix of ground substance and collagen. There is no fibrin evident (H&E ×275).

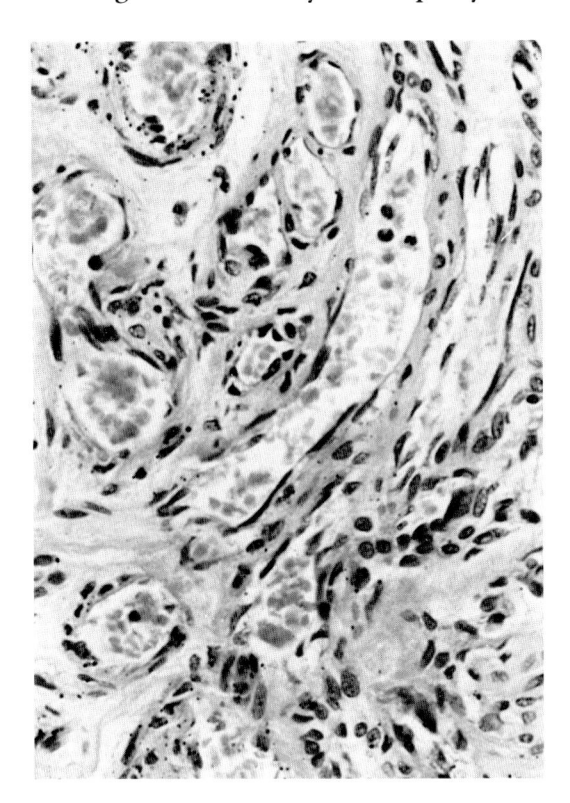

Figure 24–15. Detail of an organized plexiform lesion from a 25-year-old man with patent ductus arteriosus and pulmonary hypertension. All the cells lining the vascular sinuses are elongated. The septa contain myfibroblasts and amorphous elastic tissue (H&E ×375).

care has to be exercised not to confuse such vessels with bronchial arteries, which normally possess a thick band of longitudinal muscle in their intima.

Pathogenesis of Vascular Changes

Hypertrophy and Hyperplasia of Smooth Muscle

Hypertrophy of vascular smooth muscle follows sustained increased vascular tone and renders the pulmonary arterial tree capable of more forceful vasoconstriction.[33] This increases pulmonary vascular resistance. Under the electron microscope, the hypertrophied smooth muscle cell in the arterial wall shows an increased volume of cytoplasm mainly filled with myofilaments. Mitochondria, which are normally perinuclear in position, extend between the myofilaments in the form of long chains which also contain numerous free ribosomes and glycogen granules (Fig. 24–22). The ground substance between smooth muscle cells is more extensive and is thought to be secreted by the smooth muscle.

The process of muscularization of pulmonary arterioles has been studied in experimental animals in which pulmonary hypertension has been induced by pyrrolizidine alkaloids[34] or exposure to hypoxia.[35,36] First, the preexisting smooth muscle cells in the pulmonary arterioles hypertrophy. They are situated between the endothelium and the single elastic lamina of the vessel and, in the distal part of the arteriole, are normally so thin as to be invisible on light microscopy. Hypertrophy is succeeded by hyperplasia so that the number of muscle cells increases. It is not certain whether they arise from division of existing cells or whether they migrate from more proximal muscular regions of the arterial tree, but there is autoradiographic evidence to suggest that local division does occur.[37] Whatever the mechanism, these new muscle cells are metabolically active and contain extensive rough endoplasmic reticulum, free ribosomes, Golgi complexes, and numerous mitochondria.[35] Their myofilaments are scanty and restricted to the periphery of the cell. Within a few weeks these immature smooth muscle cells undergo maturation (Fig. 24–23). Initially there is a single elastic lamina external to the muscle representing the original lamina of the arteriole. After about 1 month, elastin is deposited in the endothelial basement membrane to create a new, internal elastic lamina (see Fig. 24–23). This can often be seen under the

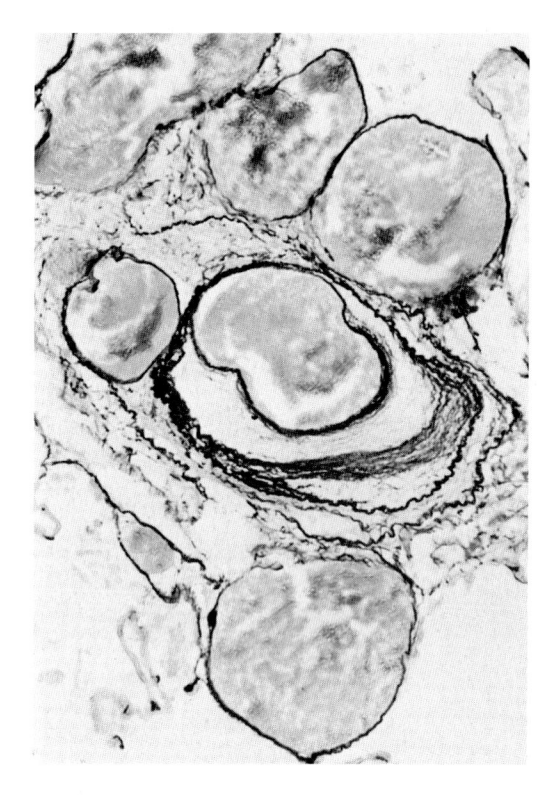

Figure 24–16. Muscular pulmonary artery from the patient illustrated in Figure 24–11 showing intimal fibroelastosis. It is surrounded by several dilated vessels which resemble veins but are in fact entirely arterial in nature being derived from the artery which they surround (EVG, ×150).

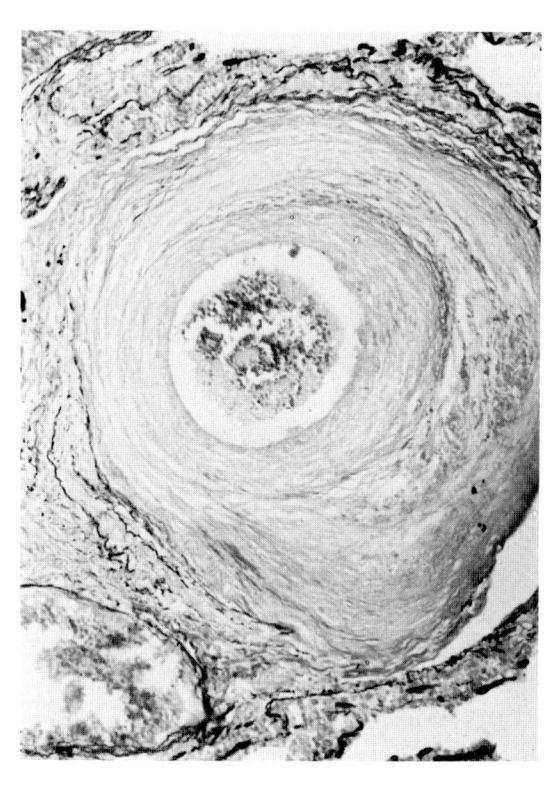

Figure 24–17. Transverse section of a muscular pulmonary artery from the patient illustrated in Figs. 24–12 and 24–13 showing a profuse concentric intimal fibrosis. The media is atrophic and disrupted and has been lost over much of its circumference (EVG, ×150).

light microscope as a thin, rather tenuous, lamina lining the inner aspect of the media of the newly muscularized arteriole (Fig. 24–24).

Intimal Proliferation

The ultrastructure of the cells that proliferate in the intima showed them to resemble smooth muscle cells.[38,39] Thus, they contain bundles of parallel myofilaments, focal condensations, and attachment points and are surrounded by a basal lamina (Figs. 24–25, 24–26). However, they differ in several respects from the normal smooth muscle of the media. In particular their myofilaments are shorter and less numerous, and both attachment points and focal condensations are atypical in that they consist of large, irregular areas of indeterminate shape, often divorced from the myofilaments instead of being intimately attached to them.

Also mitochondria are more numerous, and there is a prominent zone of both rough and smooth endoplasmic reticulum in the perinuclear zone (see Fig. 24–25).[39] Similar cells have been described in the intima of pulmonary arteries in cases of congenital cardiac septal defects with pulmonary hypertension.[40] Identical cells appeared in the intima of pulmonary arteries of dogs with experimentally induced pulmonary hypertension[41] and appeared to have migrated from the media and hence from smooth muscle. A similar observation was made in human pulmonary arteries.[38] On these grounds, it seems most likely that the source of intimal cells is from medial smooth muscle, especially in view of the fact that they are similar to the cells that produce intimal fibrosis in renal arteries and arterioles in systemic hypertension[42] and the cells that migrate into the intima after endothelial damage[43,44] or experimental atherosclerosis.[45–47] In all these studies except one,[45] the origin of the intimal cells has been traced to the media. Indeed there is evidence that medial smooth muscle is multifunctional and is responsible for producing all the connective tissue elements of normal as well as diseased arteries.[48]

Although the intimal cells are probably derived from smooth muscle, their ultrastructural appearances are not entirely typical of that type of cell. In fact they share the features both of smooth muscle and fibroblast, sometimes equally, sometimes with the features of one type of cell predominantly[49]; therefore, they are referred to here as myofibroblasts. This term was originally proposed by Gabbiani and colleagues[50] to describe contractile fibroblasts in proliferating granulation tissue. However, they are similar to the cells referred to as myointimal cells that invade the intima of systemic arteries during systemic

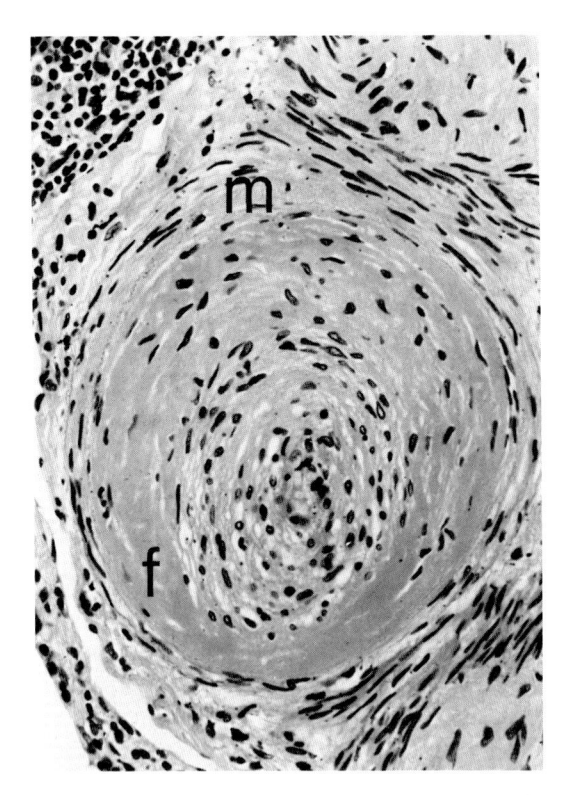

Figure 24–18. Transverse section of a muscular pulmonary artery from a 12-year-old girl with cor triloculare biatriatum. There is a striking concentric laminar, intimal fibrosis which has occluded the vessel. The media (m) is thin and atrophic, and internal to it is a broad zone of fibrin (f) which has a smudgy amorphous appearance. This is a feature of fibrinoid necrosis (H&E, ×285).

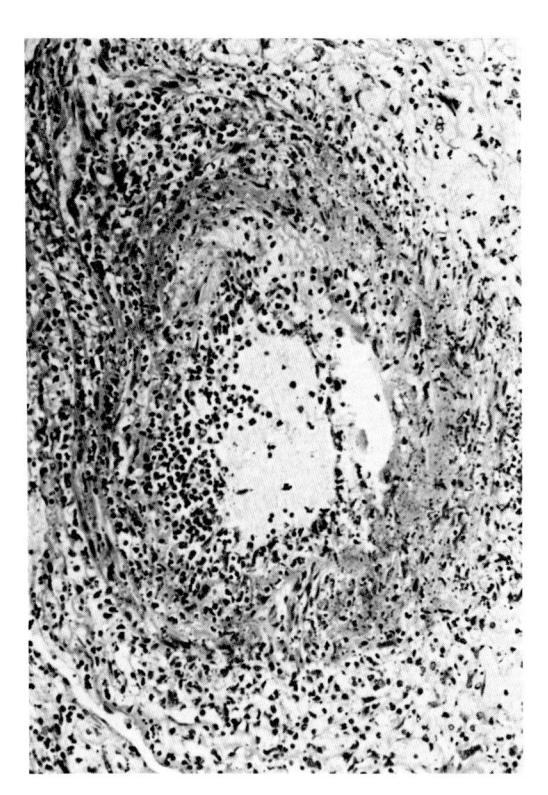

Figure 24–19. Transverse section of a muscular pulmonary artery from the same patient as Figure 24–18, showing acute necrotizing arteritis. The vessel is infiltrated with fibrin and shows some necrosis of its media. These changes are associated with an intense infiltrate of neutrophil polymorphs (H&E, ×150).

hypertension or following endothelial damage. They are also similar to those that form intimal fibrosis in pulmonary arteries. Thus, although some workers refer to them as smooth muscle,[38,51] the term myofibroblast embodies both their muscular origin as well as their important role in the secretion of ground substance and collagen. It seems likely that smooth muscle cells and fibroblasts are interchangeable given the right stimuli, and the myofibroblast is simply an intermediate form.

Dilated Vein-Like Branches of Pulmonary Arteries

Under the electron microscope, vein-like side branches of pulmonary arteries can be seen to contain finely attenuated smooth muscle cells.[39] Although greatly stretched, these cells have all the normal cytologic features of vascular smooth muscle. The elastic laminae, however, are fragmented, and the external lamina is absent for much of its circumference. The internal elastic lamina consists merely of disjoined clumps of elastin in which the fibers are arranged haphazardly, often with frayed edges. These appearances suggest that the vessels are distended to such an extent that the elastic laminae become ruptured, thus providing their resemblance to pulmonary veins.[39]

The Plexiform Lesion

Electron microscopy of the plexiform lesion reveals that the proliferation which forms within the dilated sac has three components: a plexus of vascular channels lined by cuboidal cells, a mixed population of cells between the channels, and an acellular matrix.[39] The cells lining the vascular channels superficially resemble endothelial cells and until recently have been generally assumed to be so. Ultrastructurally, however, they differ from normal endothelium in that they lack a basement membrane, micropinocytotic vesicles, caveolae, and Weibel-Palade bodies. Instead their cytoplasm contains numerous 10 nm filaments arranged in a haphazard fashion (Fig. 24–27). Many of the cells between the sinuses are myofibroblasts indentical to those forming intimal fibrosis. This is hardly surprising in view of the close juxtaposition of plexiform lesions and occlusive intimal fibroelastosis. Other cells resemble the sinus-lining cells in that they contain an abundance of 10-nm filaments arranged in whorls or as an interlacing network. A third type of cell in this location is the fibroblast with its typical profusion of open rough endoplasmic reticulum. The

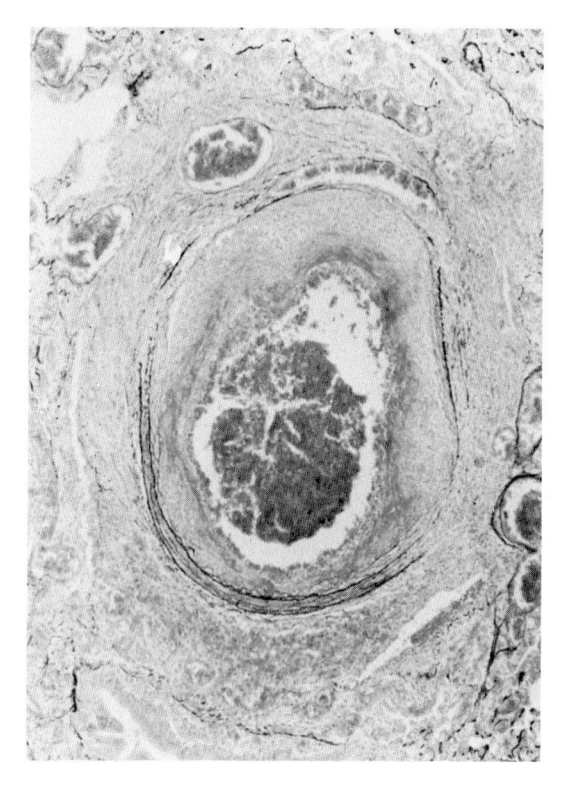

Figure 24–20. Healing necrotizing arteritis in a muscular pulmonary artery. The media is necrotic and disrupted with fragmentation of its elastic laminae. The lumen contains a mural thrombus. Surrounding the vessel is granulation tissue which in places has infiltrated the media (EVG, ×66).

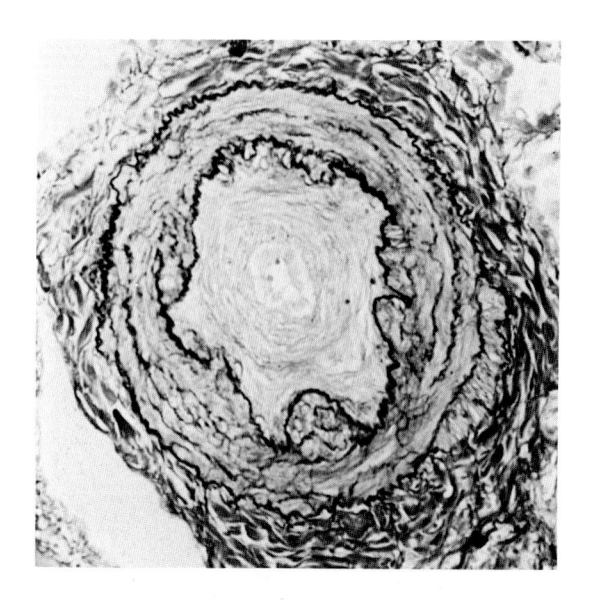

Figure 24–21. Transverse section of a hypertrophied muscular pulmonary artery from a girl of 18 years with primary pulmonary hypertension. The vessel is occluded by concentric intimal fibrosis. There are large nodules of longitudinally oriented smooth muscle projecting from the inner aspect of the media. There is a similar nodule in the adventitia. (EVG, ×117).

acellular component consists of a mass of amorphous or faintly fibrillary ground substance in which are embedded variable numbers of collagen fibers.

From these observations, it seems that the plexiform lesion is not composed of endothelium but of connective tissue elements probably derived from vascular smooth muscle. The nature of the cells containing numerous microfilaments is unknown, and they have been designated simply fibrillary cells. These cells are identical to those comprising the cardiac myxoma and the so-called papillary tumor of heart valves.[52] Similar cells are also found in the normal heart and great vessels and have been termed subendothelial vasoformative reserve cells.[53] Fibrillary cells may, therefore, be these vasoformative reserve cells which have accumulated within dilatation lesions. Alternatively they may be derived from altered smooth muscle in a manner similar to myofibroblasts. Whatever their origin, they are clearly an important component of plexiform lesions since they line the vascular channels as well as contribute to the stroma. They may be responsible for secreting the mucopolysaccharide ground substance in the same manner as their counterparts do in the cardiac myxoma. As plexiform lesions age, they become less cellular. It is likely that fibrillary cells become converted first to myofibroblasts and then to fibroblasts. The fibroblasts then convert the lesion into an acellular fibroelastic scar.

There remains the question of the role of fibrinoid necrosis in the pathogenesis of the plexiform lesion, since fibrinoid necrosis is commonly associated with them.[28] In the ultrastructural study described previously, fibrin was observed inside the cytoplasm of fibrillary cells or else apparently in the process of being phagocytosed by them.[39] Also, if early plexiform lesions are stained for light microscopy using special techniques to demonstrate fibrin, the cells lining the sinuses can be seen to contain numerous, small globules of fibrin (Fig. 24–28).[39] This presents the interesting possibility that plexiform lesions develop as a response to fibrin accumulating within a dilated sac. It seems likely that a focus of fibrinoid necrosis forms in a side branch proximal to a segment of fibrotic occlusion (Fig. 24–29). The high intravascular pressure causes this weakened vessel to dilate to form a sac or microaneurysm. Mural thrombus forms in the sac adjacent to the zone of fibrinoid necrosis (see Fig. 24–29). This stimulates fibrillary cells and myofibroblasts to accumulate within the sac, the former cells surrounding and ingesting the fibrin and thrombus. Other fibrillary cells and myofibroblasts secrete an extensive matrix of ground substance. In this way, the typical plexiform arrangement of vascular channels and stroma is built up. Once the fibrin has been removed, the lesion ages into a fibroelastic scar after the transformation of the multipotential fibrillary cells into myofibroblasts and eventually fibroblasts. Plexiform lesions do not occur in mitral stenosis, although fibrinoid necrosis of pulmonary arteries may occur in this condition.[28] The reason may lie in

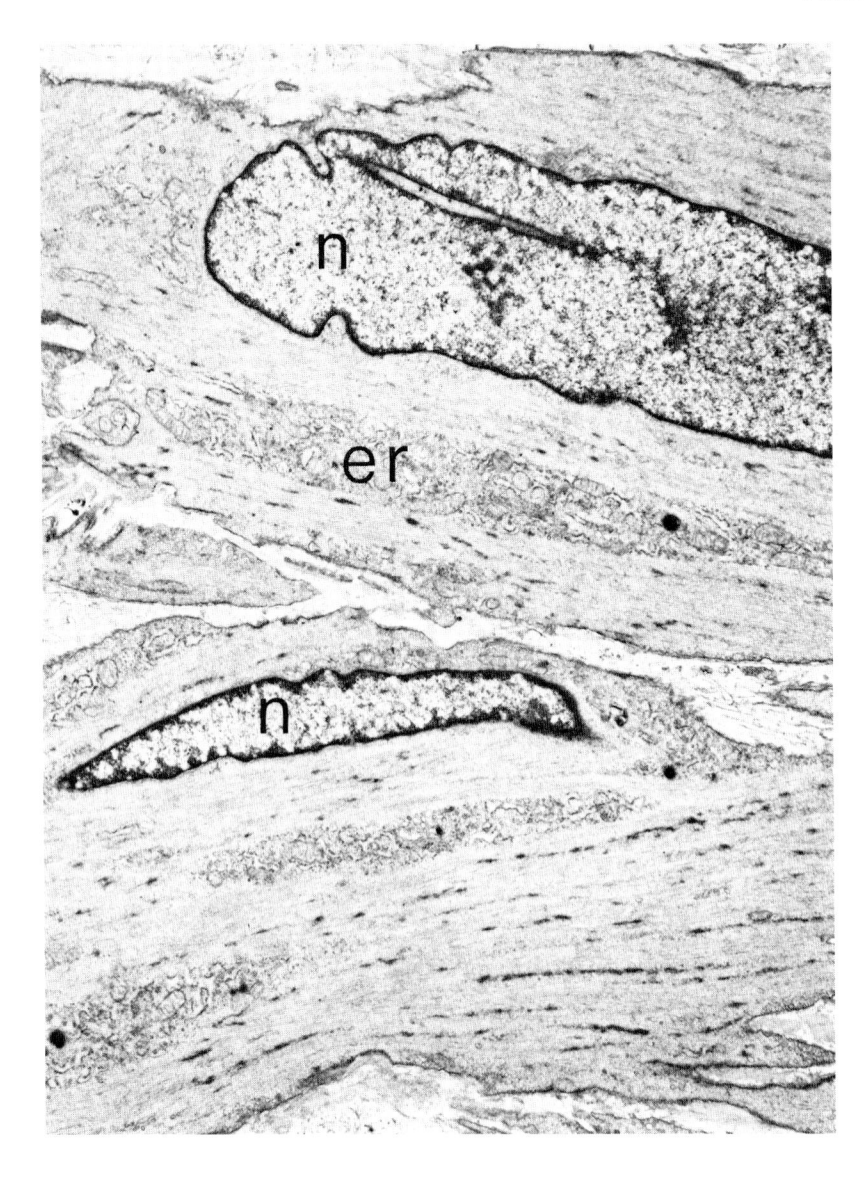

Figure 24–22. Pulmonary trunk from a rat subjected to a reduced barometric pressure of 380 mmHg for 4 weeks. Two hypertrophied smooth muscle cells from the media are shown. Apart from their nuclei (n), the bulk of the cytoplasm is occupied by longitudinally aligned myofilaments in which there are many dense bodies. The myofilaments are interrupted in places by cigar-shaped accumulations of mitochrondria, rough and smooth endoplasmic reticulum, and free ribosomes (er) (EM), [electron micrograph ×7,500].

the fact that dilated arterial branches do not occur in this form of pulmonary vascular disease. The absence of dilatation lesions in mitral stenosis may be related in some way to the presence of pulmonary venous hypertension. Thus, it can be postulated that if dilated sacs do not occur, neither do plexiform lesions.

Necrotizing Arteritis

The nature and origin of fibrinoid necrosis have been extensively studied in the renal arteries of animals with experimentally induced systemic hypertension. The process consists of a leakage of plasma and finely fibrillary fibrin into the subintima and inner media.[54,55] Later the fibrin adopts the crystalline-striated appearance of fibrinoid.[54,56] There is little or no necrosis of muscle, and the fibrin originates from the blood by passing through ruptures in the endothelium.[54–57] Carbon particles injected into the blood were closely associated with these fibrinous deposits.[55]

In the pulmonary circulation, the origin of fibrinoid necrosis is the same.[58,59] The high intravascular pressure creates small splits in the endothelium through which blood plasma passes into the subendothelial space, often distending it (Fig. 24–30). The fibrin then becomes precipitated as lens-shaped crystalline structures with a fine cross-banding of 20.8 nm periodicity.[59] It is usually held up by the internal elastic lamina (Fig. 24–31) but may pass through fenestrae into the media which it traverses until it is once again held up by the external lamina. The pattern of fibrinoid necrosis can thus adopt a picture of radial spokes joining two concentric rings of fibrin.[28] This is best demonstrated using special stains for fibrin such as picro-Mallory or Martius's scarlet blue. Since fibrinoid necrosis is dependent on the passage of fibrinogen into the media and not on the death of smooth muscle cells, the term fibrinoid necrosis is a misnomer. A more precise term is fibrinous vaculosis.[60] Fibrinoid necrosis may be the sole lesion in a hypertensive pulmonary artery, but it is frequently complicated by an infiltrate of neutrophil polymorphs (see Fig. 24–31). These cells may invade the media in response to cellular

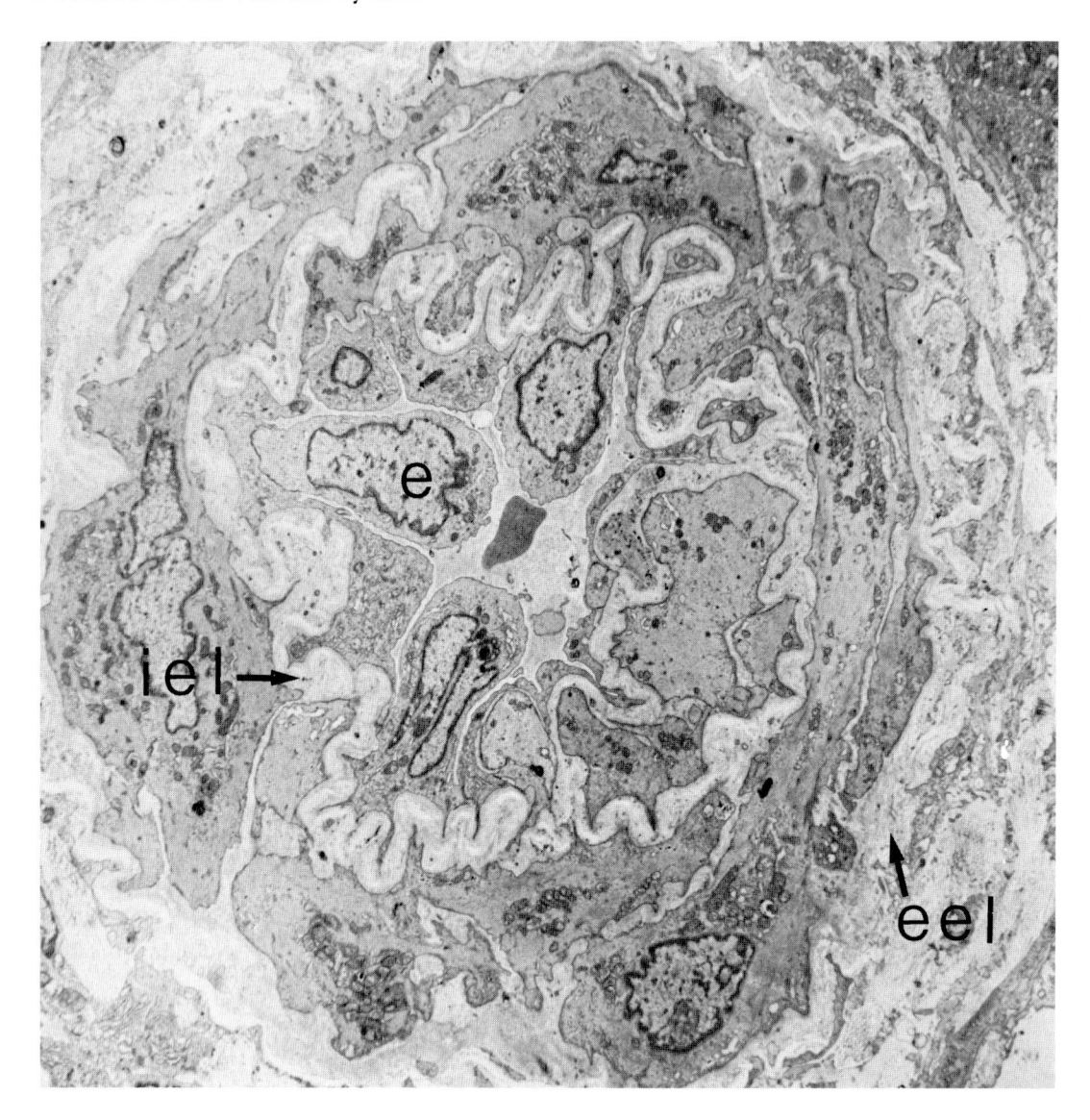

Figure 24–23. Muscularized pulmonary arteriole from a rat fed on a diet containing powdered C. *spectabilis* seeds for 26 weeks. The external elastic lamina (eel) represents the original elastic lamina of the arteriole. Internal to this is a new layer of circularly oriented smooth muscle cells. Beneath the endothelium (e) is a newly formed internal elastic lamina (iel). Note that in places this branches to surround totally some of the smooth muscle cells (EM, ×3700).

necrosis, or when this is absent, they may be attracted by chemotactic factors released from the breakdown of fibrin.

Clinical Associations

Incidence in Congenital Cardiac Shunts

Plexogenic pulmonary arteriopathy develops only in those cases of congenital cardiac shunt in which critical levels of pulmonary arterial pressure and flow are reached and exceeded. In post-tricuspid shunts, such as a ventricular septal defect, the magnitude of the shunt is proportional to the size of the defect and to the difference in pressure between the two ventricles during systole. Associated stenosis of the pulmonary valve increases the resistance to outflow from the right ventricle and diminishes the size of the left-to-right shunt. Conversely, stenosis of the aortic valve raises left ventricular systolic pressure and increases the shunt of blood into the right ventricle. At birth there is normally a rapid fall in pulmonary vascular resistance as the ductus arteriosus closes and the pulmonary arteries dilate, but in the presence of a large post-tricuspid septal defect, this fall in pulmonary vascular resistance and pressure may be delayed for several weeks.[61] Only when the resistance finally starts to decline does the left-to-right shunt increase; this delay probably explains why such infants do not usually develop symptoms during the first four weeks.⁶¹ As the shunt subsequently increases in magnitude, the child becomes vulnerable to developing pulmonary edema. This is partly the consequence of the heightened pulmonary blood flow leading to a transudate of plasma through the dilated pulmonary arteries and partly the effect of left ventricular failure.

In most children, these early symptoms regress over a period of a few months. In some cases, this is due to spontaneous closure of the defect either by apposition of a cusp of the tricuspid valve⁶² or by overgrowth of muscle and fibrous tissue. Even if such closure is incomplete, it may be sufficient to reduce the extent of the shunt below dangerous levels. Sometimes the area of the defect remains constant while the heart is growing, thereby gradually reducing its relative size. In other cases, the outflow tract from the right ventricle undergoes stenosis.⁶³ Only in a minority of children is the flow of blood to the lung reduced by an increase in pulmonary vascular resistance. Initially this helps to reduce the pulmonary blood flow from the high levels reached during the first few months of life. However, as hypertensive pulmonary vascular disease develops and progresses, the vascular resistance increases leading to congestive cardiac failure. Thus, what commences as a life-saving process ends as a life-threatening one.

Severe pulmonary arterial hypertension occurs in only a small proportion of cases of posttricuspid shunt. Thus, in a survey of 1500 cases of ventricular septal defect of all sizes,⁶⁴ between 20 and 25 percent were found to close spontaneously, 50 percent persisted merely as a small defect, 5 percent of patients developed infundibular stenosis, and 5 percent died in early childhood. Only 5 percent ultimately died from the effects of plexogenic pulmonary arteriopathy. The evolution of these advanced vascular lesions takes years. In a group of patients dying with ventricular septal defect complicated by pulmonary hypertension, the youngest age at which dilatation lesions occurred was 2½ years.⁶⁵

In cases of pretricuspid shunt exemplified by a high atrial septal defect, the physiologic basis for the development of plexogenic pulmonary arteriopathy is different.⁶⁶ Here the major factor which influences the magnitude of left-to right shunt is the distensibility of the two ventricles as they fill with blood during diastole. At birth the thickness of the ventricles is similar, and their distensibilities do not differ appreciably; as a result, there is little or no shunting of blood through the atrial defect.⁶⁶ However, once right ventricular pressure falls, the wall of the right ventricle becomes thinner relative to the left while its distensibility becomes relatively greater. As a result, a left-to right shunt develops through the atrial defect, thereby increasing the pulmonary blood flow.⁶⁶ Although this causes a degree of enlargement of the right ventricle, it does not lead to significant pulmonary arterial hypertension for many years, often until adulthood. This means that the normal postnatal regression of muscle in the pulmonary arteries and arterioles can take place, and the elastic tissue configuration of the pulmonary trunk changes from the fetal to the adult type. Hence, in these patients, the pulmonary vascular resistance is normal or reduced and their pulmonary arterial

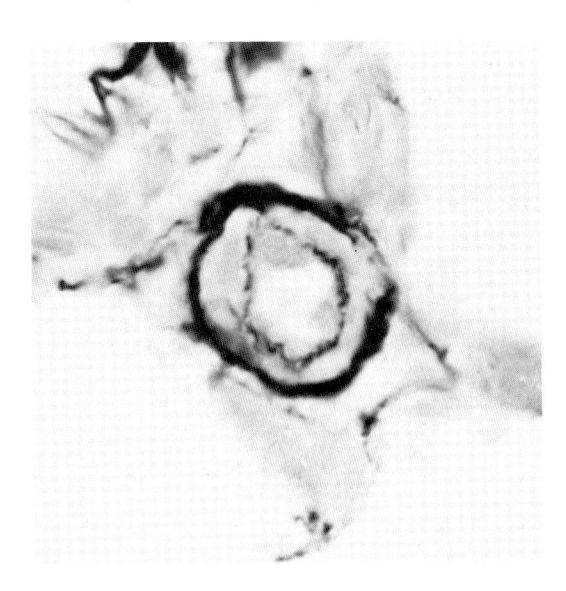

Figure 24–24. Muscularized pulmonary arteriole from a rat subjected to a reduced barometric pressure of 380 mmHg for 4 weeks. The original thick elastic lamina can be seen externally, while the internal elastic lamina is thin and less distinct. Between them is a newly formed layer of smooth muscle (EVG, ×600).

pressure is normal.⁶⁷ They are thus generally asymptomatic, although a few may develop mild exertional dyspnea. Serious pulmonary hypertension is usually delayed until the fourth decade,⁶⁸,⁶⁹ only rarely occurring early in adult life.⁶⁷ The pulmonary vascular disease that it promotes is plexogenic in nature.

Pulmonary Hemodynamics

In cases of post-tricuspid shunt such as ventricular septal defect, the level of pulmonary arterial pressure rises with progressive severity of plexogenic pulmonary arteriopathy.²⁷ Thus, the pulmonary arterial mean pressure is in the range of 40 to 70 mmHg in patients with grade 1 changes, and 50 to 80 mmHg in those with grade 3, but shows a sharp increase to 80 to 100 mmHg in cases with higher grades of plexogenic pulmonary arteriopathy.

The relation to pulmonary blood flow is obviously in the reverse direction. Thus, patients with early grades of change have an abnormally high pulmonary blood flow as described previously. Those with grade 4 lesions usually have a pulmonary blood flow that is either normal or diminished below normal. In grades 5 and 6, the flow is invariably lower than normal.

The pulmonary vascular resistance is only slightly elevated in grade 1 pulmonary vascular disease. By grade 3, there is a modest increase in resistance to approximately three times normal, but in grade 5, the vascular resistance has increased to as much as seven to nine times the normal value. These trends are similar in cases of pretricuspid shunt, but the relationship is even steeper. This is largely because grade 1 in these cases is

Figure 24–25. Detail of a myofibroblast. The central region of cytoplasm is occupied by numerous mitochrondria, free ribosomes, and rough endoplasmic reticulum with dilated cisternae such as one sees in active fibroblasts. The periphery of the cells is occupied by parallel myofilaments, dense bodies, and microvesicles which are features of smooth muscle (EM, ×25,000).

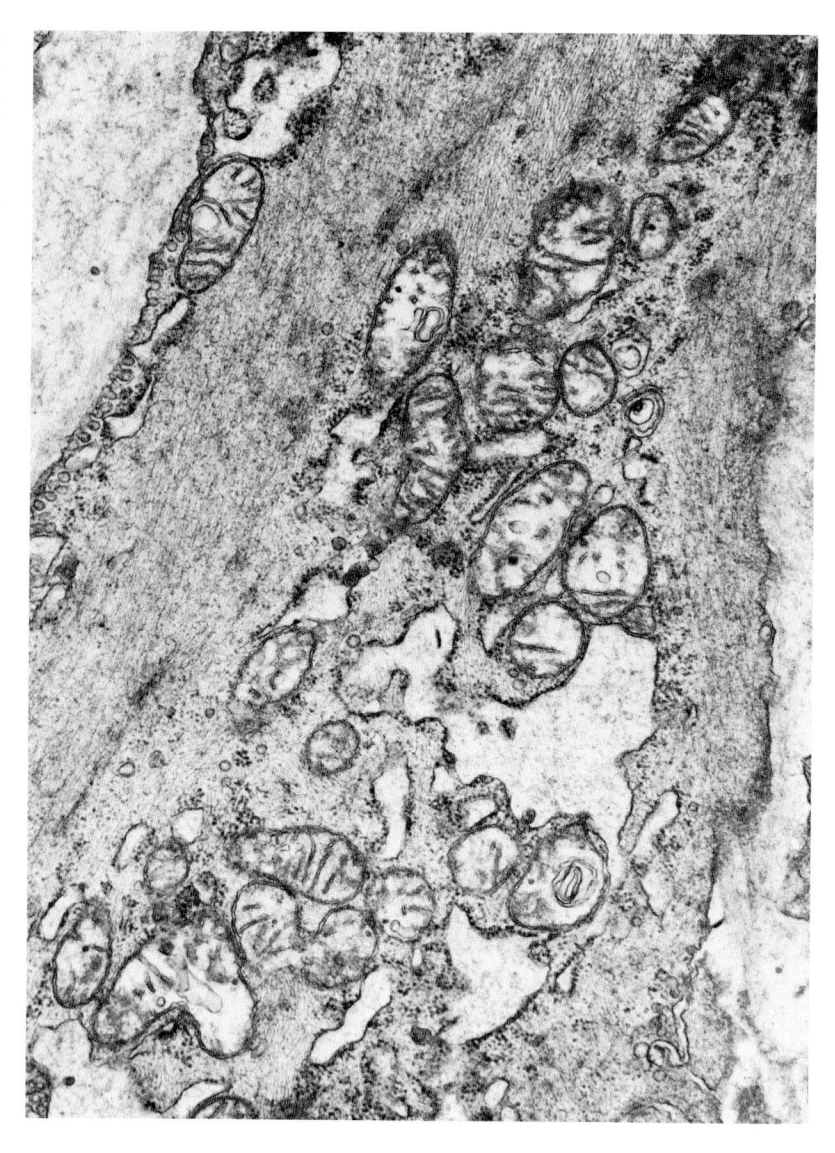

associated with a normal pulmonary vascular resistance and high blood flow. The highest pulmonary arterial pressures and resistances are encountered in grade 6 in which the pulmonary vascular resistance may be in the order of 15 times normal.

In the patients from whom the above data were obtained, the effects of breathing 100 percent oxygen were compared with the histologic grade of plexogenic pulmonary arteriopathy.[27] In general the effect of oxygen is to cause vasodilation which lowers the pulmonary arterial pressure and increases the blood flow. In grade 1, the pressure is frequently reduced to normal as is the pulmonary vascular resistance. However, with increasing grades of severity, the reduction in vascular resistance fails to reach normality. Thus in grade 5, the residual pulmonary vascular resistance after breathing oxygen is still five times greater than normal.

The relation between the grade of vascular change and pulmonary hemodynamics indicates that pulmonary vascular resistance in these patients is determined by the structural changes in the pulmonary arteries and arterioles. Furthermore, the effect of breathing oxygen suggests that these changes comprise two components. The first of these is a reversible muscular change leading to vasoconstriction. The second is an irreversible change based on vascular occlusion. Thus, the early grades are largely muscular in nature and should be reversed if the cause of the pulmonary hypertension is removed. Grade 3 is also largely muscular but with associated intimal fibrosis. This grade should also be reversible, although perhaps not totally so if the intimal fibrosis is extensive. In grades 4 to 6, intimal fibrosis is occlusive and causes damage to the media in the form of generalized dilation, fibrinoid necrosis, or localized dilatation lesions. One would not expect such lesions to be reversible. These considerations are of great practical value when deciding whether closure of a congenital cardiac defect will reverse the pulmonary hypertension which it has caused.

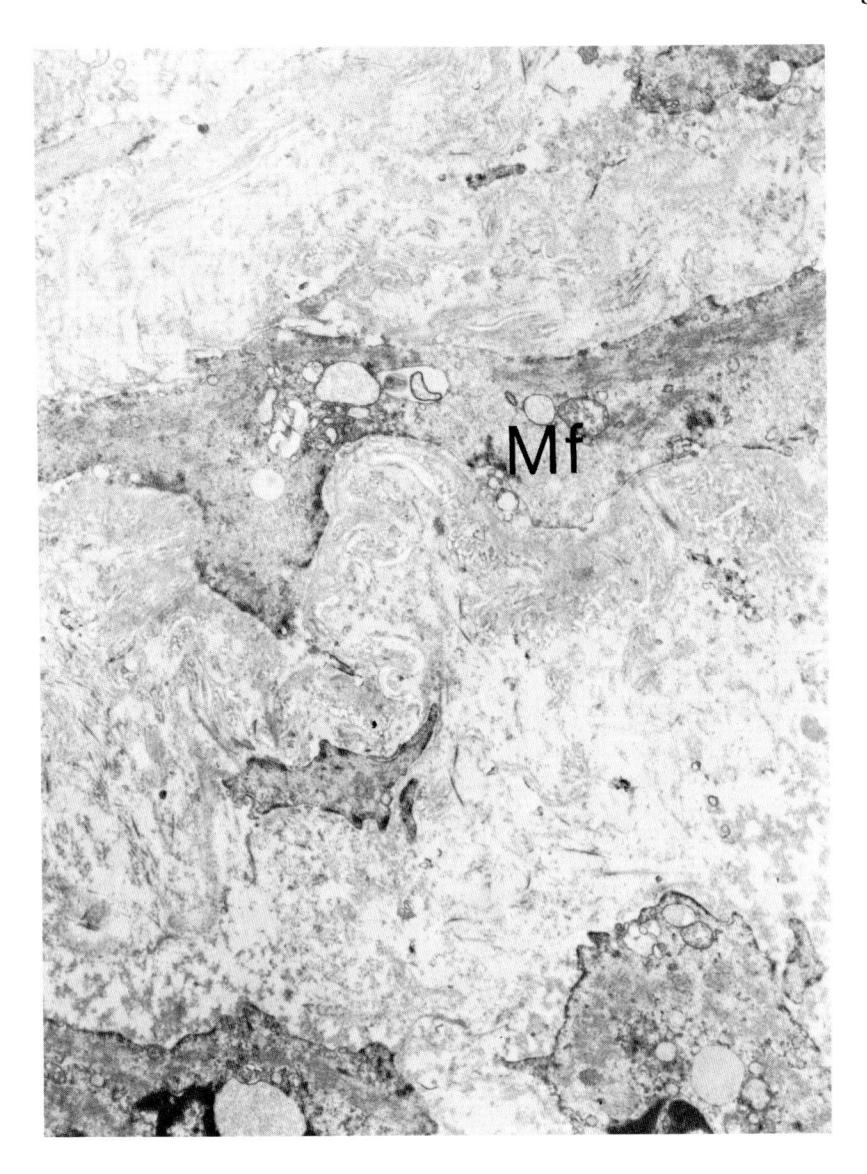

Figure 24–26. Concentric laminar intimal fibrosis in a muscular pulmonary artery from a case of plexogenic pulmonary arteriopathy. Myofibroblasts (Mf) containing scanty myofilaments are arranged in layers. Between these layers are large deposits of ground substance in which there is a haphazard arrangment of collagen and elastic fibers (EM, ×7500).

Relation to Closure of Septal Defects

In recent years, advances in cardiac surgery enabled congenital cardiac defects to be rectified with minimal immediate mortality. However, the long-term prognosis following such operations is not necessarily good. For example, cases of severe pulmonary arterial hypertension with ventricular septal defect may develop a reversal of the shunt. In this situation, the defect is acting like a safety valve, permitting blood entering the right ventricle to by-pass the pulmonary vasculature. Closure of the defect in these circumstances would divert all the blood through the lungs, thereby further increasing the pulmonary arterial pressure rather than alleviating it. From the theoretic considerations presented in the preceding section, one might envisage an exacerbation of pulmonary hypertension in those grades of plexogenic pulmonary arteriopathy that are irreversible.

The effect of the grade of vascular change on the immediate reversibility of pulmonary hypertension has been tested in 32 patients with ventricular or atrial septal defect.[70] In these patients, the pulmonary arterial pressure was monitored on the operating table before and after closure of the cardiac defect. The grade of plexogenic pulmonary arteriopathy was determined from lung biopsy specimens. It was found that in 23 of 24 patients with grades 1 to 3, the pulmonary hypertension was reversible. In these patients, the systolic pulmonary arterial pressure fell immediately to less than 50 mmHg. Thus, in these patients, the pulmonary hypertension was largely the result of a high blood flow which was alleviated once the shunt was closed. In all four patients with grade 5 hypertensive pulmonary vascular disease, there was no fall in pulmonary arterial pressure, the systolic pressure exceeding 50 mmHg following closure of the defect. Grade 4 represented an intermediate situation since, in three of four cases, there was a fall in pulmonary arterial blood pressure after operation. Nevertheless, the systolic pressure was still in excess of 50 mmHg. In these patients, changes in the pulmonary

Figure 24–27. Part of a plexiform lesion from the same patient illustrated in Figure 24–26. A fibrillary cell is shown which contains a profusion of randomly aligned, 10-nm-thick filaments. The fibrillary cell lines a vascular channel (c) in which there are clumps of fibrin (f) (EM, ×25,000).

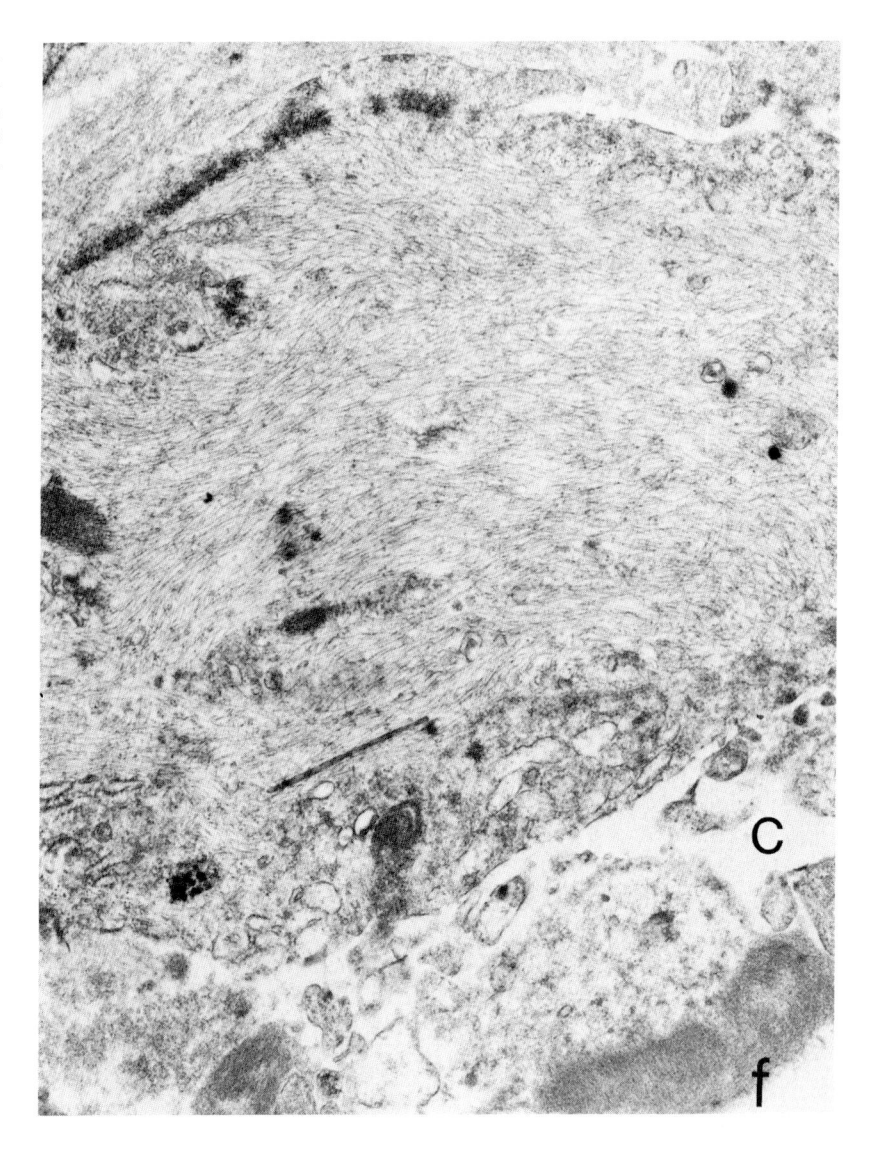

vasculature had created a permanently high resistance so that pulmonary hypertension persisted after the shunt had been removed. Thus, the immediate reversibility of pulmonary hypertension after closure of a cardiac defect correlates well with what one might anticipate from structural changes in the pulmonary arteries.

What the above study does reveal is whether the reversibility or irreversibility of pulmonary hypertension is permanent. In two long-term follow-up studies, 13 patients were studied for up to 4 years after closure of an atrial septal defect.[71,72] The patients ranged in age from 6 to 48 years, with a mean age of 34 years. Three of these patients had a pulmonary vascular resistance in excess of 750 dynes/s/cm^{-5} before the operation and showed an increase in resistance afterward which in one patient was measured 4 years after closure to the defect. All the remaining patients had lower pulmonary vascular resistances before operation, and all but one of these showed a fall in resistance to the normal range up to 3 years later.

These studies strongly suggest that hypertensive pulmonary vascular disease involutes completely if it is in its early stages, whereas in its later stages, it continues to progress regardless of whether or not the shunt is stopped. One can speculate that in the former instance, the pulmonary arteries show hypertrophy and muscularization only, whereas in the latter case, there is extensive intimal fibrosis and dilatation lesions.

Similar data for ventricular septal defect have been derived by Dushane.[73] He studied 36 patients who underwent surgery after the age of 2½ years. He found that the pulmonary vascular resistance increased in some patients, whereas it decreased substantially in others. Those who experienced dyspnea before operation generally developed an increased pulmonary vascular resistance after operation. However, their initial resistances were similar to those of many other patients who did not have clinical symptoms and who showed either a moderate increase or reduction in pulmonary vascular resist-

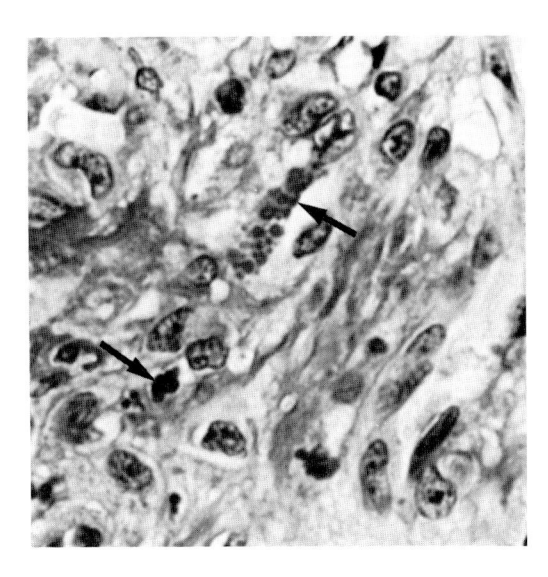

Figure 24–28. Detail of an early plexiform lesion stained to demonstrate fibrin. Globules of fibrin can be seen within the cytoplasm of some of the cells (arrow) Martius's scarlet blue, ×744).

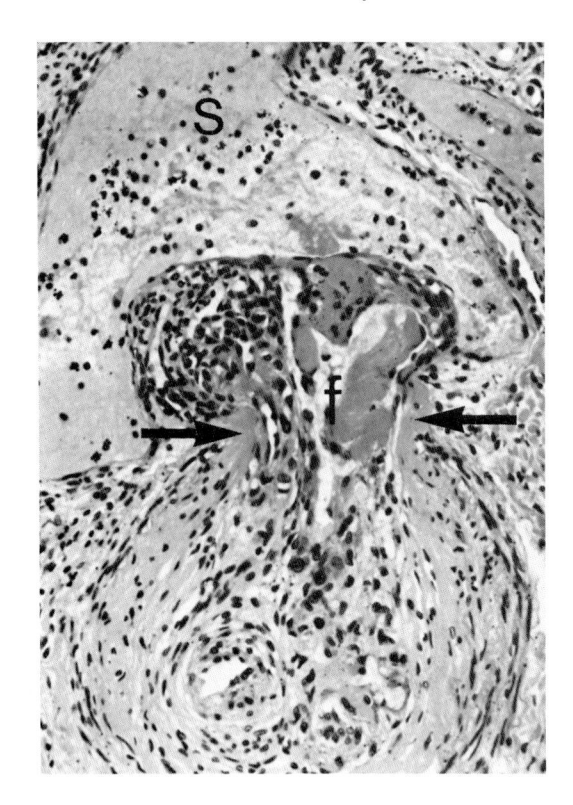

Figure 24–29. An early plexiform lesion that demonstrates how these structures may develop. A muscular pulmonary artery is almost totally occluded by intimal fibrosis, but there is a focus of fibrinoid necrosis in the media (arrow). This acts as the origin for a large dilated sac (s). Adjacent to the fibrinoid necrosis is a clump of intravascular fibrin (f) adherent to it. Extending from the parent vessel into the sac is a plexiform arrangement of rounded cells which surround the fibrin. The plexiform lesion may therefore develop as an attempt to engulf and remove the fibrin which collects within the sac (H&E, ×186).

ance after operation. It is therefore impossible to set any upper limit of pulmonary vascular resistance below which an operation is likely to ameliorate the pulmonary hypertension and above which an operation should not be performed. In a similar investigation into the effects of closure of a ventricular septal defect, in all but 1 of 25 patients a decrease in pulmonary arterial resistance occurred after operation.[74] Such studies emphasize the difficulties in deciding whether closure of a cardiac defect will be advantageous or deleterious. Clearly patients with a pulmonary arterial systolic pressure approaching systemic levels and who are cyanosed should not be recommended for surgery. Those with a lower pulmonary arterial pressure, a high pulmonary blood flow, and low vascular resistance stand a good chance of permanent reversibility of their pulmonary hypertension after operation. However, those patients between these two extremes present a prognostic problem. It is in these cases that the pathologist can offer helpful advice from lung biopsy specimens.

Effects of Hypertension on Elastic Pulmonary Arteries

Time of Onset of Pulmonary Hypertension

The changes that normally occur in the elastic tissue configuration of the media of the pulmonary trunk after birth have been described in Chapter 2. In general there is a progressive fragmentation and reduction in density of elastic fibers associated with a relative reduction in medial thickness.[75] In cases of pulmonary arterial hypertension, it is possible to determine whether the raised pressure has been present from infancy or acquired later in life by examination of the pattern of the elastic tissue in the media of the pulmonary trunk. Thus, when pulmonary hypertension complicates a pretricuspid congenital cardiac shunt, such as a high atrial septal defect or such conditions as mitral stenosis, the raised pulmonary arterial pressure occurs after the transition from an aortic to an adult pulmonary elastic tissue configuration has occurred. Hence an adult elastic tissue pattern is indicative of acquired pulmonary hypertension[75] (Fig. 24–32). On the other hand, when pulmonary hypertension complicates a post-tricuspid cardiac shunt, such as a ventricular septal defect, the raised pressure is present from birth and the elastic tissue in the pulmonary trunk fails to fragment. Thus, an aortic configuration of elastic tissue in the pulmonary trunk is indicative of pulmonary hypertension present from infancy (Fig. 24–33).

Figure 24–30. Muscular pulmonary artery of a rat in which advanced hypertensive pulmonary vascular disease was induced by oral administration of powdered C. *spectabilis* seeds. The vessel shows fibrinous vasculosis in which the subendothelial space is grossly distended by an accumulation of plasma protein and dark, crystalline clumps of fibrin (f). This has gained entry to the vessel from the lumen (l) through small ruptures in the endothelium (e) which do not appear on this field (EM, ×7500).

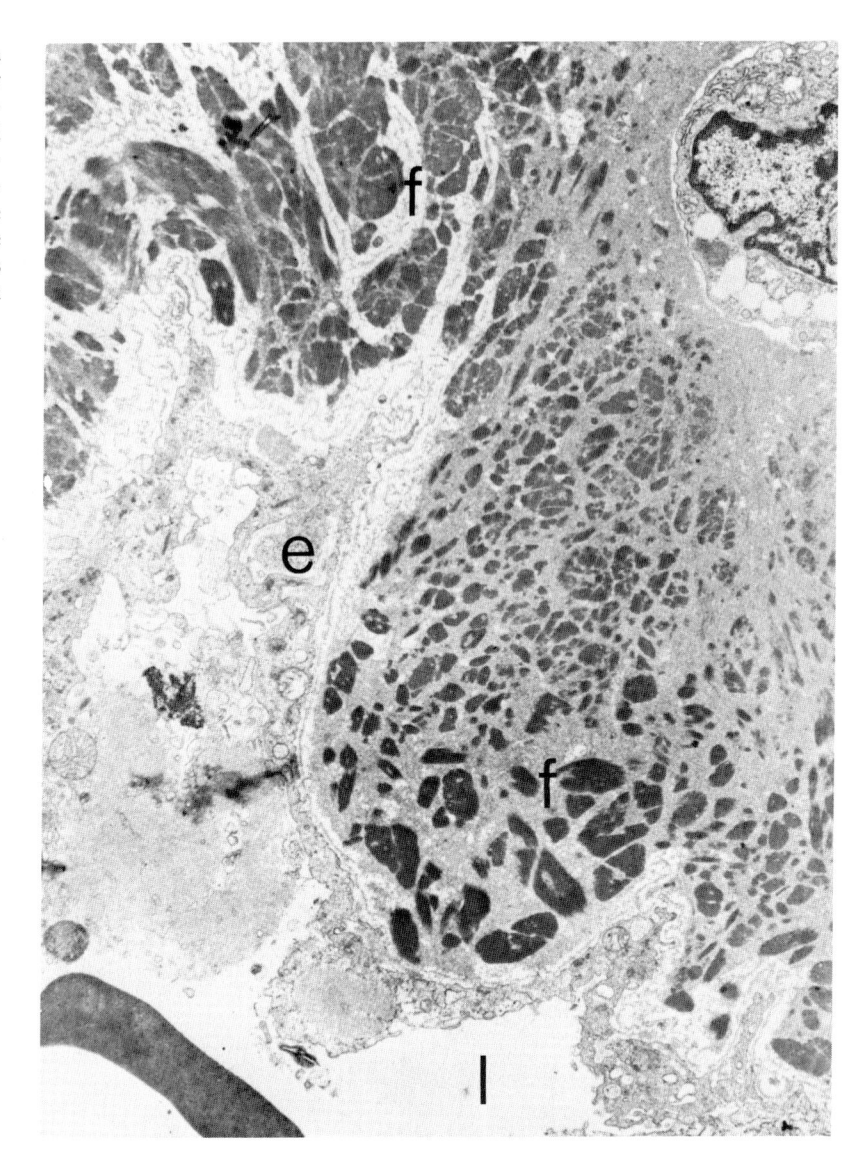

The Pulmonary Trunk at High Altitude

These concepts of elastic tissue variants in the pulmonary trunk were applied to the native highlanders of the Andes by Saldaña and Arias-Stella.[76,77] People who live at high altitude have a mild degree of pulmonary hypertension throughout their lives due to the hypoxia inherent in this environment which causes pulmonary vasoconstriction. In highlanders it is possible to identify a "persistent" variety of elastic tissue pattern in which only partial fragmentation of the elastic laminae occurs, so that there are long, continuous elastic fibers interspersed among shorter, fragmented ones.[76] This incomplete fragmentation may be attributed to the mild pulmonary hypertension present from birth in these populations. Saldaña and Arias-Stella[76] found that the age at which the aortic configuration was lost depended on the altitude at which the subject lived, for this in turn determined the degree of pulmonary hypertension. Thus at altitudes between 4030 and 4530 m, the aortic configuration persisted to the age of 9 years followed by the persistent pattern that remained for the rest of adult life. At lower altitudes, in the range of 3440 to 3830 m, the aortic configuration was lost at age 3 years, followed by the persistent configuration until 55 years of age when there was a gradual change to the adult pattern.[76] In native highlanders, the medial thickness of the pulmonary trunk relative to that of the aorta is greater than that at sea level.[77] People who ascend to high altitude later in life would show the adult type of elastic tissue configuration typical of acquired pulmonary hypertension.

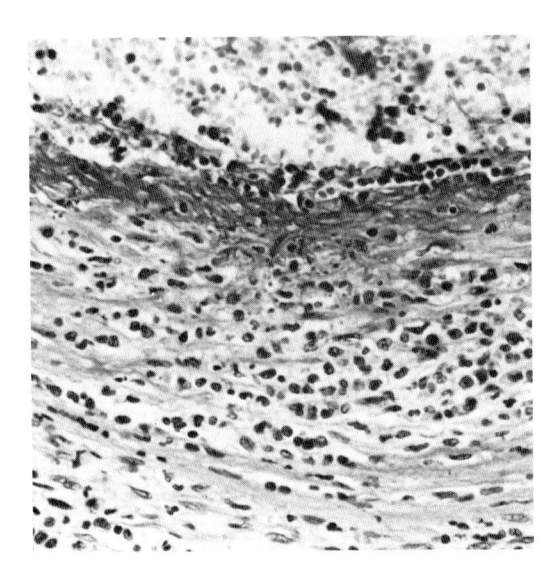

Figure 24–31. Segment of muscular pulmonary artery with necrotizing arteritis, which has been stained to demonstrate fibrin. Note that the darkly staining fibrin is confined to a narrow layer immediatley beneath the endothelium (Martius's scarlet blue, ×285).

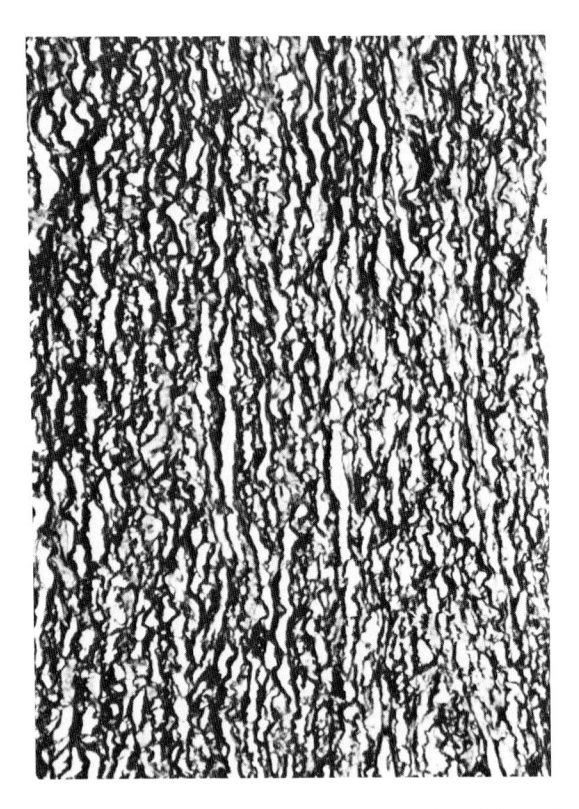

Figure 24–33. Transverse section of the media of the pulmonary trunk from a case of ventricular septal defect. The elastic fibers are long, broad, and parallel. They form a series of laminae as in the aorta. This is the fetal, "aortic" elastic tissue configuration seen in neonates or in cases of pulmonary arterial hypertension present from birth (EVG, ×150).

Cystic Medial Degeneration

The muscle, elastic tissue, and collagen fibers of the pulmonary trunk are embedded in a ground substance of proteoglycans. The acid mucopolysaccharide components can be demonstrated metachromatically with toluidine blue or positively with alcian blue. In cases of severe pulmonary arterial hypertension, the quantity of this ground substance becomes excessive, forming islands between the elastic laminae. There is a tendency for cysts to form within these deposits, presenting the appearance of cystic medial degeneration identical to that which occurs in the aorta (Figs. 24–34, and 24–35). As in the aorta, cystic medial degeneration of the pulmonary trunk can lead to dissecting aneurysm or, more rarely, rupture of the vessel. Saccular aneurysms can also occur.[28]

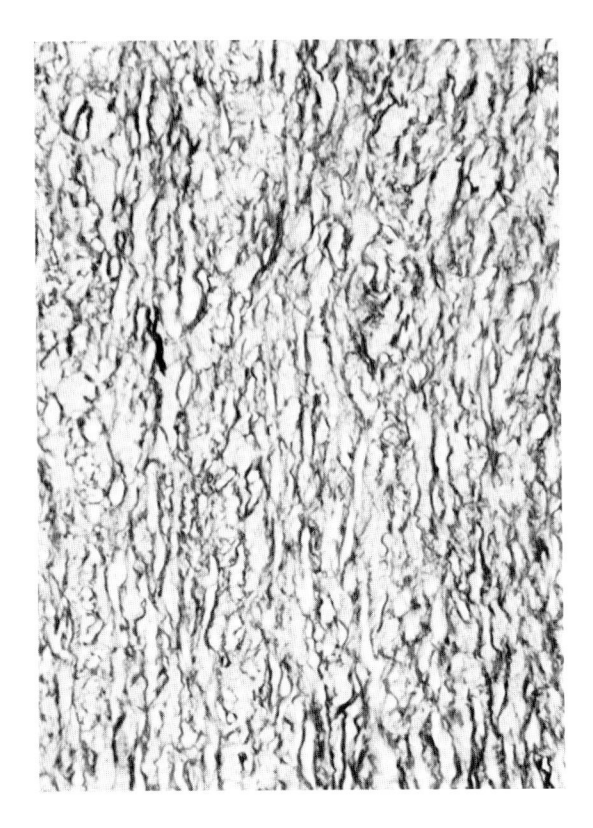

Figure 24–32. Transverse section of part of the media of the pulmonary trunk from a case of rheumatic mitral stenosis with pulmonary arterial hypertension. Most of the elastic fibers are short and irregular, many consisting of fine wispy strands. This is the adult elastic tissue configuration seen in acquired pulmonary hypertension (EVG, ×150).

Atherosclerosis

Atherosclerosis of the pulmonary trunk and the intrapulmonary elastic arteries is commonly associated with all forms of pulmonary arterial hypertension. The lesions

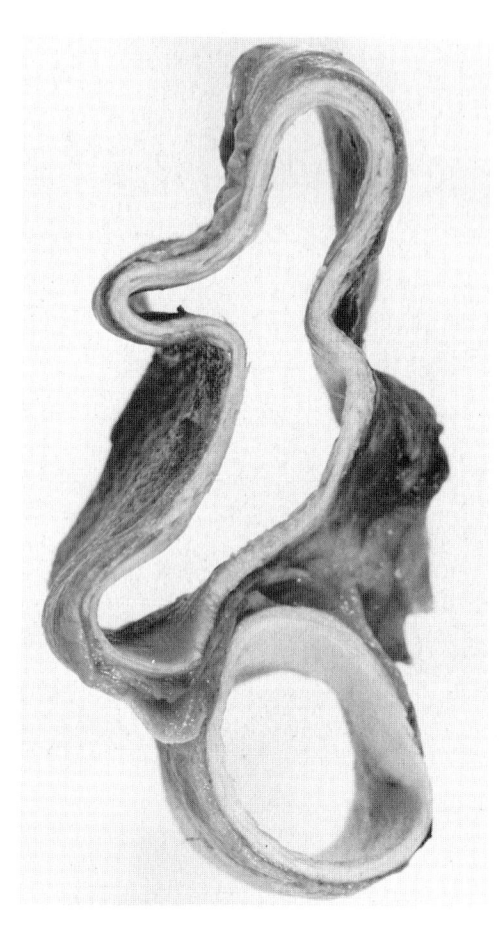

Figure 24–34. Pulmonary trunk and aorta from a case of plexogenic pulmonary arteriopathy complicating portal vein thrombosis occurring in a 24-year-old Indian man. The pulmonary trunk, at the top, has become distended to several times its normal diameter. This is due to a combination of severe pulmonary arterial hypertension superimposed upon cystic medial degeneration (×1.7)

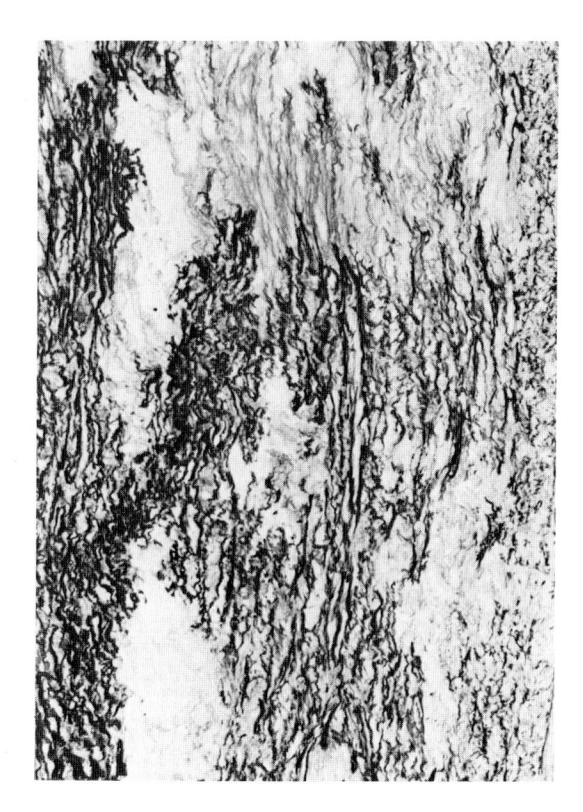

Figure 24–35. Histology of the pulmonary trunk shown in Figure 24–34. There is extensive fragmentation and dissolution of the elastic laminae with the formation of large focal areas devoid of elastin. There areas contain deposits of acid mucupolysaccharide (EVG, ×66).

have the same macroscopic and histologic appearances as those in the systemic circulation. In the pulmonary trunk and its main branches, the atheroma presents as raised plaques (Fig. 24–36), but in the smaller intrapulmonary elastic arteries, it may also be deposited as a generalized intimal thickening involving the whole circumference of the vessel. Histologically atheroma consists of numerous lipid-laden cells embedded within a matrix of fine collagen and elastic fibers (see Fig. 24–36). As the lesions age, the collagen fibers become thicker and denser. In a study of the incidence of pulmonary atherosclerosis in congenital heart disease, in all but 1 of 16 patients dying after the age of 3½ years with pulmonary arterial hypertension present from birth, there was atherosclerosis of elastic pulmonary arteries.[78] This change was also found in all 21 cases of acquired pulmonary hypertension in patients who were 20 years of age or older.[78] Pulmonary atherosclerosis is in no way pathognomonic of pulmonary hypertension. It occurs commonly as an aging process in middle-aged and elderly subjects who die from disease unassociated with a raised pulmonary arterial pressure. However, the atherosclerosis associated with pulmonary hypertension occurs at a much earlier age and is often more extensive than that which is a consequence of aging.

Pulmonary Venous Hypertension

Any disease that is associated with chronic pulmonary venous hypertension leads to characteristic pathologic changes in the pulmonary capillaries, lung parenchyma, and pulmonary arteries and veins.[79] Such diseases include conditions in which the elevated pressure in the pulmonary veins is present from birth and in which there may or may not be an associated congenital cardiac septal defect. The former group includes mitral atresia with single ventricle, and the latter group congenital mitral stenosis or incompetence, cor triatriatum, congenital stenosis of pulmonary veins, and constrictive endocardial sclerosis. Most cases of pulmonary venous hypertension are acquired in later life. By far the most common example is rheumatic mitral stenosis, but other examples involving the mitral valve include rheumatic incompetence, ischemic heart disease causing rupture of its chordae tendineae or papillary muscle dysfunction, "floppy" mitral valve, and bacterial endocarditis.[1] Rarer causes include mediastinitis constricting pulmonary veins and chronic left ventricular failure due to myocardial disease.

The earliest effects of pulmonary venous hypertension appear to be on the pulmonary capillaries. The thickness of the basement membrane increases from 10 nm to between 15 to 30 nm and may reach 50 nm.[80] Sometimes this thickened basal lamina is split to enclose disintegrating fragments or extravasated erythrocytes undergoing diapedesis.[81] There is frequently subendothelial deposition of a hyaline ground substance of mucopolysaccharides.[80] The endothelial cells of the pulmonary capillaries become swollen and edematous and develop vacuoles up to 400 nm in diameter.[81] The swollen endothelial cytoplasm may project into the capillary lumen, and it accumulates protein, fat, and hemosiderin.

Interstitial edema develops in the alveolar-capillary wall and is more common in the collagen-containing portions. With persistence of edema in the alveolar walls, there is proliferation of reticulin and elastic fibrils,[82] so that the alveolar capillaries become embedded in dense connective tissue.[81] Type I pneumonocytes are lost from the linings of the alveolar walls and are replaced by type II cells, corresponding to the "cuboidal cell metaplasia" seen on light microscopy.[83] Pulmonary macrophages and desquamated granular pneumonocytes accumulate in the alveolar spaces. The permeability of the interendothelial junctions of the pulmonary capillaries appears to be dependent upon intraluminal pressure. Alveolar epithelium rather than capillary endothelium seems to be the critical barrier to the entry of water and solutes into the alveolar spaces. A perfusion pressure greater than 50 mmHg is required to bring about leakage of horseradish peroxidase (HRP) or hemoglobin into alveolar spaces, but lower pressures will allow their escape through interendothelial junctions to enter the interstitial space of the alveolar septum.[84]

Pulmonary edema in mitral stenosis and other states of chronic pulmonary venous hypertension can be demonstrated radiologically.[85] It may show as transient basal horizontal lines which appear when the mean left atrial pressure exceeds 24 mmHg[86] and which are due to edema of connective tissue septa and distension of pulmonary lymphatics. The degree of distension of pulmonary lymphatics in mitral stenosis has been assessed histologically.[87] Persistent lines are due to the deposition of hemosiderin in the fibrous tissue septa between the secondary lobules.[88]

Under the influence of sustained elevation of pressure in the pulmonary capillaries and veins, the capillaries in the lung substance become congested and distended. Fragments of extravasated erythrocytes pass through their thickened basal laminae and are then engulfed by macrophages to give rise to accumulations of siderophages which may be demonstrated clearly by Perls' stain (Fig. 24–37). In this condition of pulmonary hemosiderosis, ferric salts encrust the reticulin and elastic

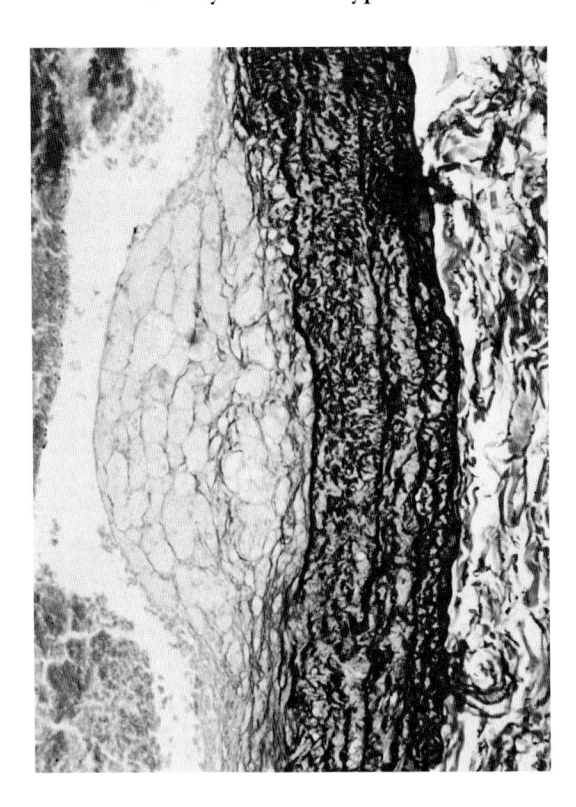

Figure 24–36. Large plastic pulmonary artery from a 22-year-old woman with primary pulmonary hypertension. The vessel is cut in transverse section and contains an atheromatous plaque in its intima. This comprises pale, lipid-laden macrophages enmeshed in a fine network or elastic fibers (EVG ×144).

fibrils of the pulmonary blood vessels and lung parenchyma and may provoke a giant cell reaction. Studies[89] have revealed no direct relation between the occurrence and degree of pulmonary hemosiderosis and the level of blood pressure in either the pulmonary arteries or veins.

There is a gradual change from pulmonary hemosiderosis to siderofibrosis. Hyperplasia of granular pneumonocytes is joined by an increase of reticulin fibers in the alveolar-capillary walls and then by interstitial pulmonary fibrosis. As this is allied with the rusty discoloration of deposition of ferric salts, the condition known to classic pathology as brown induration of lung results. This developing fibrosis in the lung parenchyma is associated with a hyperplasia of mast cells in the lung.[90]

Ossification in the alveolar spaces in mitral stenosis is not infrequent.[91–93] The nodules of lamellar bone possibly develop on the basis of persistent clumps of fibrin in the alveolar ducts and spaces. They may become several millimeters in diameter and provoke little or no tissue reaction. Much rarer is the remarkable disease microlithiasis alveolaris pulmonum in which calcification occurs around foci of alveolar exudate to form numerous microliths or calcospherites (Fig. 24–38). These are uniform in size and consist largely of stratified concre-

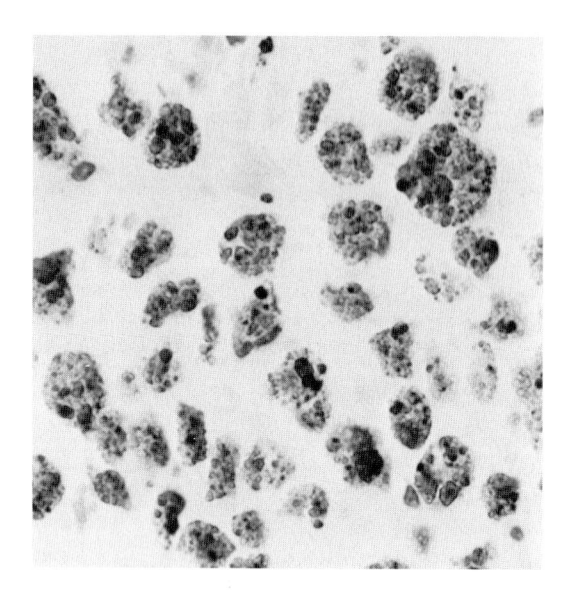

Figure 24–37. Pulmonary hemosiderosis from a long-standing case of mitral stenosis. Numerous alveolar macrophages contain ingested erthrocytes and granules of hemosiderin derived from their intracellular digestion (H&E, ×600).

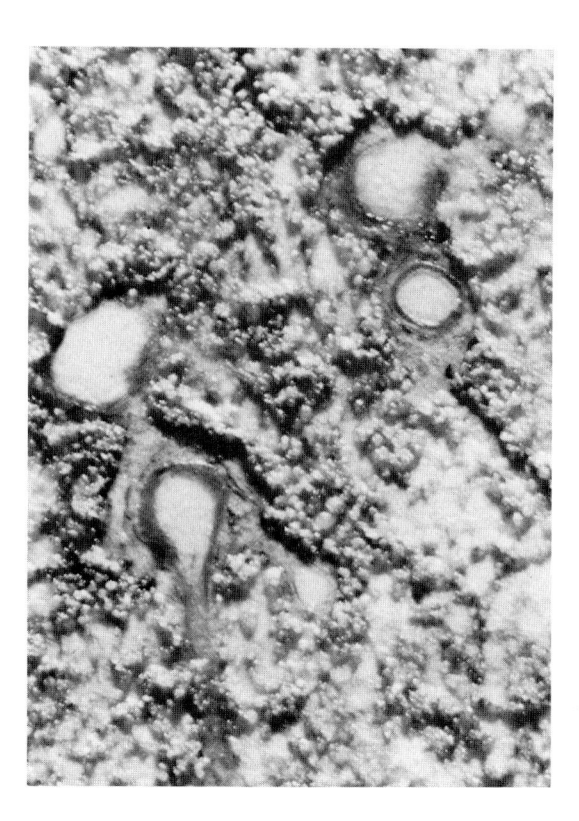

Figure 24–38. Gough-Wentworth lung preparation from a 50-year-old woman with rheumatic mitral stenosis. Numerous spherical concretions within the alveoli give the lung an appearance and feel resembling sandpaper. This is a typical example of microlithiasis alveolaris pulmonum (×2).

tions of calcium phosphate which can be dissolved in hydrochloric acid to leave an organic envelope which contains iron.[94] Each microlith, up to 750 µm in diameter, contains up to 15 rings of calcium phosphate. The calcospherites produce miliary opacities in the chest radiograph and render the lungs stony hard. Gough-Wentworth sections of lung in this condition resemble sandpaper (see Fig. 24–38).

Changes in Pulmonary Blood Vessels

Sustained pulmonary venous hypertension becomes associated with pulmonary arterial hypertension, and hence structural changes occur in both pulmonary arteries and veins. The elastic tissue pattern in the elastic pulmonary arteries is usually of the adult pulmonary type since pulmonary venous and arterial hypertension are usually acquired long after infancy. However, in the rarer cases (such as congenital mitral stenosis) in which these hemodynamic disturbances are present from birth, the elastic tissue configuration will be of aortic type. The elevated pulmonary arterial pressure leads to medial hypertrophy in the muscular pulmonary arteries.[95] Longitudinal muscle is frequently found in the media adjacent to the intima or adventitia. At the same time, there is muscularization of the pulmonary arterioles.

The small pulmonary arteries often show severe intimal fibrosis, probably due to the activity of myofibroblasts. The proliferation may assume a concentric or crescentic form, but it does not have the onion-skin appearance seen in plexogenic pulmonary arteriopathy. Mucopolysaccharides are sometimes prominent in the media and may account for a significant proportion of the medial thickness. The adventitia is usually thick and fibrous.

When the pulmonary arterial hypertension complicating mitral stenosis is severe or shows unusually rapid elevation, the muscular pulmonary arteries may show fibrinoid necrosis with rings of fibrin held up at their elastic laminae, the so-called fibrinoid vasculosis.[60] Necrotizing arteritis has been reported in mitral stenosis by a number of authors.[91,96] Earlier workers[83,97] reported it but regarded it as rheumatic vasculitis rather than being related to a high pulmonary arterial pressure.

Plexiform lesions do not occur in mitral stenosis, although their predisposing condition, fibrinoid necrosis, is found in this disease. Plexiform lesions will develop, however, in such conditions as mitral atresia combined with large congenital cardiac shunts such as a common ventricle or patent ductus arteriosus.[70] Hence pulmonary venous hypertension in itself does not prevent the development of plexiform lesions. The illustrations supporting the claim of Tandon and Kasturi[98] that they had seen dilatation lesions in four patients with mitral stenosis have been regarded as unconvincing.

Pulmonary veins, like pulmonary arteries, respond to an elevation in their intraluminal pressure.[79] The muscle of the vein wall becomes hypertrophied and confined to

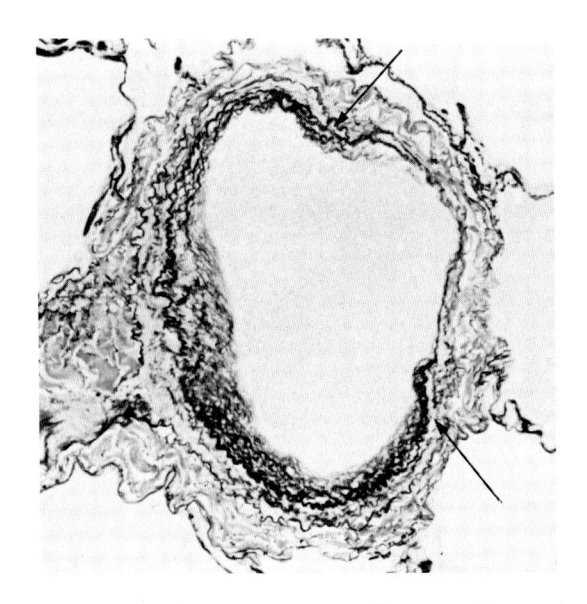

Figure 24–39. Pulmonary vein in mitral stenosis. For two-thirds of its circumference, the vessel has a distinct media sandwiched between two elastic laminae (arrows), an appearance sometimes referred to as arterialization. The laminae are less smooth and continuous than in muscular pulmonary arteries. The intima contains acellular fibrosis (EVG, ×150).

a distinct muscular media delineated by inner and outer elastic laminae (Fig. 24–39). Thus, the appearance of an arterial media is simulated, a process which has come to be called arterialization. Significant intimal proliferation, exceeding that expected of age change, takes place (Fig. 24–40). The cells responsible are very likely myofibroblasts which, lying in the veins in the absence of pronounced pulsation, lose their myofibrils and undergo transition into fibroblasts. The ultrastructural changes shown by pulmonary arteries in mitral stenosis include an infiltration of the subendothelial zone with a hyaline material similar to that which occurs in the capillaries.[80] With further rises of pressure, intracytoplasmic vacuolation and deposition of hemosiderin are found in the endothelial cells. Myofibroblasts with myofibrils in their cytoplasm are found in the subendothelial zone and come to lie enmeshed in a hyaline material between elastic fibrils which is related to ground substance and which the myofibroblasts secrete. The myofibroblasts give rise to frank smooth muscle cells in the intima. Should fibrinoid necrosis supervene, muscle cells begin to disintegrate with disappearance of the intracytoplasmic fibrillar structure, clarification of the cytoplasm, and nuclear breakdown.

Variations in Histopathology with Site in Lung

With increasing elevation of pulmonary arterial and venous pressures in mitral stenosis, the upper portions of the lungs tend to become more perfused. Postmortem angiographs show dilation of the pulmonary arteries or no change in their size in the upper parts of the lungs, whereas those in the lower parts are narrowed.[99] Histologic examination reveals that the muscular pulmonary arteries in the lower lobes and lingula are more severely hypertrophied than those in the apices.[79, 99–102] Medial hypertrophy in the pulmonary veins is also more prominent in the lower lobes. Pulmonary congestion and edema, dilation of lymphatics, and pulmonary hemosiderosis are maximal in the posterior part of the upper lobe in which the pulmonary arterial narrowing is minimal.[99]

Relation of Pathologic Changes to Clinical and Radiologic Features

In a study of histopathology of biopsy specimens of lingula in 20 patients with mitral stenosis, Jordan and colleagues[103] found medial hypertrophy of pulmonary arteries and muscularization of pulmonary arterioles when the pulmonary vascular resistance exceeded only 260 dynes/s/cm^{-5}/m^{2}BSA. There was no linear relation between the severity of medial hypertrophy and the height of pulmonary vascular resistance. The presence of pulmonary hemosiderosis was not related to the height of the pulmonary venous pressure. Radiologic evidence of enlargement of the main pulmonary arteries was found to be an indication of the presence of pulmonary arterial hypertension and associated hypertensive pulmonary vascular disease but not of its degree. Horizontal lines on the chest radiograph were related to the presence of alveolar fibrosis. The relation between structural changes in the alveolar wall and respiratory function was poor. Diffusing capacity was more closely related to pulmonary vascular disease than to changes in the alveolar walls. The severity and duration of dyspnea were related to the grade of hypertensive pulmonary vascular disease.

Regression of Pulmonary Vascular Lesions after Mitral Valvotomy

When mitral valve obstruction is removed, there is usually an immediate fall in pulmonary vascular resistance and pulmonary arterial pressure.[104] There is little evidence regarding the long-term effects of mitral valvotomy on the structural changes in the pulmonary arteries and veins in mitral stenosis as described previously. In one case, a lung biopsy specimen showed medial hypertrophy and intimal fibrosis, whereas 11 years later following mitral valvotomy, the muscularity had returned to almost normal while the intimal fibrosis had regressed.[105] In the same way, the arterialization of pulmonary veins had been reported as resolving over the period of a decade.[51] It is improbable that necrotizing arteritis or the pulmonary hypertension associated with it would be reversible.

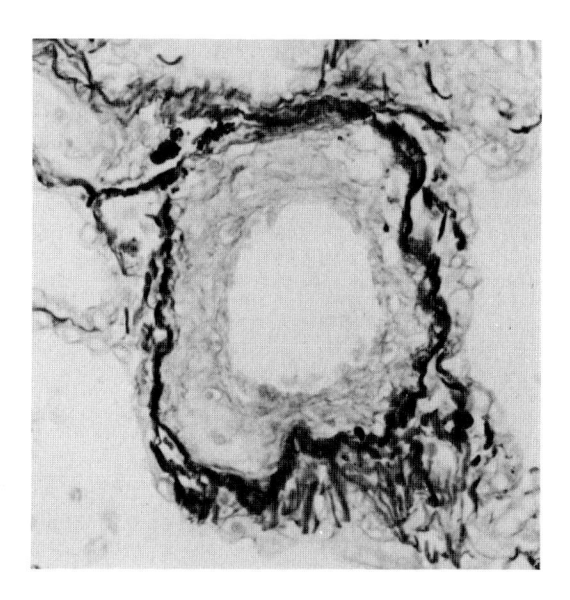

Figure 24–40. Small pulmonary vein in mitral stenosis showing pronounced intimal proliferation of acellular fibrosis (EVG, ×375).

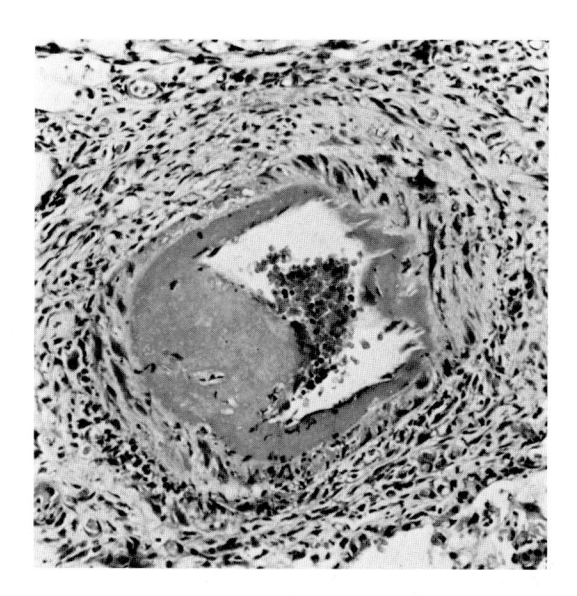

Figure 24–41. Transverse section of a muscular pulmonary artery from a rat which had been feed seeds of the plant C. spectabilis for 100 days. The vessel shows a healing necrotizing arteritis in which there is an infiltration of neutrophil polymorphs and lymphocytes into the adventitia and media. The adventitia is also infiltrated with granulation tissue. A large mural thrombus is adherent to the intima, but there is no intimal fibrosis (H&E, ×150).

Dietary Pulmonary Hypertension

Pulmonary hypertension and associated hypertensive pulmonary vascular disease can be induced in animals by pyrrolizidine alkaloids derived from plants. To date neither alkaloids nor any other chemical substance has proved to cause pulmonary vascular disease in humans, although the anorexigen aminorex fumarate has been suspected of being an etiologic factor in an epidemic of primary pulmonary hypertension that occurred in western Europe. However, studies in animals have established the concept of dietary pulmonary hypertension.

Pyrrolizidine Alkaloids

Crotalaria spectabilis

The first agent which was found to induce pulmonary hypertension when ingested orally was the leguminous plant *C. spectabilis*, which is common in India, Australia, Central America, and Florida. It is commonly referred to as rattlebox due to the noise made by the seeds in their pods. The pyrrolizidine alkaloid monocrotaline is present in the leaves and in a higher concentration in the seeds. Rats fed on them develop pulmonary arteritis,[106] right ventricular hypertrophy, and medial hypertrophy of muscular pulmonary arteries.[107] Quantitative investigations[108] have shown that powdered seeds of *C. spectabilis* at a concentration of 0.1 percent in the diet of rats produced right ventricular hypertrophy, medial hypertrophy of muscular pulmonary arteries, muscularization of pulmonary arterioles, and in about one-third of the animals, a necrotizing arteritis (Fig. 24–41). These changes occurred after a latent period of 36 days. They were associated with an increase in the thickness of the media of the pulmonary trunk[109] and a fourfold elevation of the mean pulmonary arterial blood pressure.[110] When injected intraperitoneally into rats, monocrotaline induces the same pulmonary vascular changes.[111] Prolonged administration of lower doses of the seeds will also give rise to necrotizing arteritis and vascular lesions not found in humans, such as cartilaginous metaplasia in elastic pulmonary arteries.[112] There are also extensive parenchymal lesions such as interstitial and intra-alveolar fibrosis, hemosiderosis, osseous nodules (Fig. 24–42), and a proliferation of the bronchiolar epithelium.[112] The alkaloid induced muscular hyperplasia in the walls of pulmonary veins, and this may induce pulmonary venous hypertension and the parenchymal lesions just described.

Crotalaria fulva

C. fulva is common in the West Indies where it is frequently prepared as a bush tea for consumption by the indigenous population for medicinal and social purposes. This decoction, and one from a related plant *C. retusa*, causes hepatic veno-occlusive disease which was once very common in Jamaica but is now on the decline following a program of health education. The active principle of *C. fulva* is the pyrrolizidine alkaloid fulvine

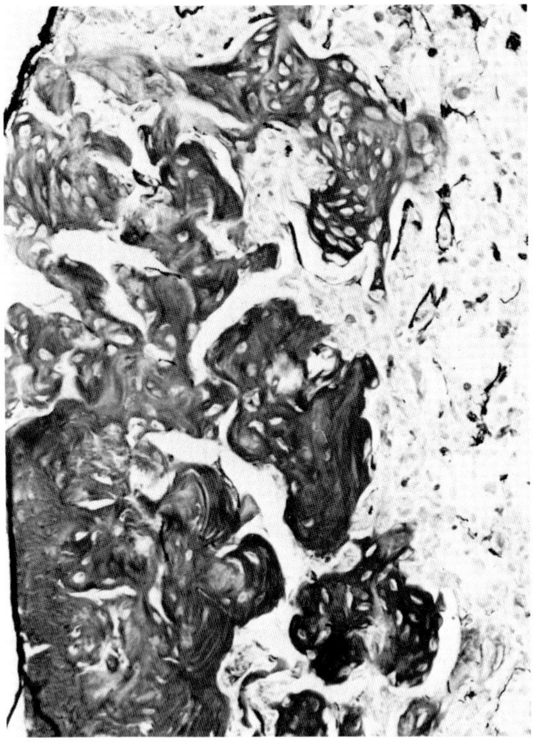

Figure 24-42. An aggregate of osseous nodules in the lung parenchyma adjacent to the pleura in a rat fed on C. spectabilis seeds for 100 days. The nodules consist of a lamellar bone and are the product of organization of intra-alveolar fibrinous transudate (EVG, ×150).

which is chemically similar to monocrotaline. When it is administered to rats,[113] many die within 3 weeks from acute hepatic necrosis. Those that survive develop hypertensive pulmonary vascular disease of the type that occurs with monocrotaline.

Senecio jacobaea

This is the common ragwort plant which farmers have long recognized as being toxic to cattle. Its seeds and foliage contain several pyrrolizidine alkaloids including seneciphylline, senecionine, jacobine, jaconine, jacoline, and jacozine. It is available in some healthfood stores in a dried, chopped form which is made into an infusion taken to cure a plethora of ailments. When this plant was administered in a concentration of 5 to 10 percent by weight to the diet of rats, they developed hypertensive pulmonary vascular disease and died in congestive cardiac failure.[114]

Crotalaria laburnoides

This is a common wild plant in East Africa. Its seeds will induce hypertensive pulmonary vascular disease and congestive cardiac failure in rats.[115] In a case of plexogenic pulmonary arteriopathy in a 19-year-old Tanzanian, an interesting feature of the clinical history was the possibility that he had been given a herbal remedy by a witch doctor before attending the University Hospital in Dar-es-Salaam. There was no proof, however, that the young African had developed his pulmonary vascular disease as a result of ingesting C. laburnoides.

The Mode of Action of the Pyrrolizidine Alkaloids

The mechanism by which the pyrrolizidine alkaloids induce pulmonary hypertension is unclear. Monocrotaline is stable and relatively unreactive, but there is evidence that it is metabolized in the liver to produce a reactive pyrrole derivative.[116] This derivative induced pulmonary arterial hypertension when injected into rats[117] and also pronounced swelling of endothelial cells in the pulmonary capillaries and arterioles with superimposed thrombosis in rats and monkeys.[118] It has been suggested that this endothelial swelling increases pulmonary vascular resistance sufficiently to lead to hypertensive pulmonary vascular disease.[118] Large edematous endothelial vesicles protruding into the alveolar capillaries[119] were also thought to be sufficiently occlusive to exaggerate the increase in pulmonary vascular resistance, but microscopical studies by Kay and associates[120] suggested that they were not numerous enough to obstruct significantly the capillary bed with its enormous reserve capacity.

The pyrrolizidine alkaloids also affect pulmonary veins. Thus, C. spectabilis seeds increase the size of the fibromuscular pads in the pulmonary veins of the rat.[108,112] These obstruct the lumens of veins and may thus elevate the pulmonary venous blood pressure. Indeed prolonged administration of C. spectabilis seeds induces a histopathology typical of a chronic exudation of plasma into the lung parenchyma, including the intra-alveolar fibrosis, hemosiderosis, and osseous nodules referred to previously. The similarity between these lesions and those produced by mitral stenosis is striking. Histologic examination of the pulmonary arteries and veins of rats poisoned with fulvine suggests that this alkaloid causes constriction of both classes of vessel.[121] Hence pyrrolizidine alkaloids appear to induce both pulmonary arterial and venous hypertension.

It has been suggested that vasoconstriction induced by pyrrolizidine alkaloids may be mediated by mast cells secreting serotonin. This hypothesis is based on the observation that mast cells proliferate following administration of monocrotaline[122] or C. spectabilis[123] to rats. It would explain the latent period between administration of the alkaloids and the development of pulmonary hypertension. However, it does not stand up to experimental testing since the level of blood serotonin in rats given C. spectabilis is not elevated.[124] The hyperplasia of mast cells is probably a response to the exudative changes in the lung since, as discussed in the preceding section, it also occurs in mitral stenosis.

In conclusion, the precise mechanism by which the pyrrolizidine alkaloids induce pulmonary arterial hypertension is not known. They may in some way directly stimulate vascular smooth muscle to contract, although opposing this notion is the observation that the smooth muscle relaxant cinnarizine fails to counteract the influence of monocrotaline.[125] Alternatively their effect on the vascular endothelium may be important. Whatever its cause, the pulmonary vascular disease induced by pyrrolizidine alkaloids is usually progressive and fatal unless small doses are administered for a limited period when reversible, purely muscular changes ensue.[126]

Anorexigens

An epidemic of primary pulmonary hypertension occurred in West Germany, Switzerland, and Austria following the marketing in these countries of a new appetite suppressant, 2-amino, 5 phenyl, 2-oxazoline, usually called aminorex fumarate. It is an alpha-type sympathicomimetic drug. It was introduced in the Swiss market in November 1965 under the name of Menocil. Two years later Gurtner and colleagues,[127] at the University Medical Clinic in Berne, reported a significant increase in the incidence of primary pulmonary hypertension. They found that in a series of patients studied by cardiac catheterization between the years 1955 and 1966, the incidence of primary pulmonary hypertension was 0.87 percent, but between 1967 and 1968, the incidence rose to 15.4 percent. Gurtner refuted the suggestion that this sudden 20-fold increase in the disease was due to chance or improved diagnosis; he noticed that many of the patients with the disease since 1967 had taken aminorex fumarate to lose weight, and he postulated that this drug was the cause.

Similar increases in the incidence of primary pulmonary hypertension were found in every clinical center in Switzerland[128] and also in Austria[129] and Germany.[130] In each of these countries, aminorex was available to the public. Clinical signs appeared in these patients 6 to 12 months after starting to take the drug. They comprised exertional dyspnea, reduced exercise tolerance, syncope, and right ventricular failure.[131] The histopathology of these cases was that of plexogenic pulmonary arteriopathy.[132-135] Following these observations, Menocil was taken off the market in October 1968, and since then there has been a decline in the incidence of primary pulmonary hypertension. However, there was a three- to fivefold increase in primary pulmonary hypertension in Switzerland that was not associated with the ingestion of aminorex.[136] Thus, there may have been other unrecognized environmental factors tending to increase the recorded incidence of primary pulmonary hypertension at the same time that aminorex was marketed.

Attempts to induce hypertensive pulmonary vascular disease in animals by feeding them aminorex met with total lack of success. Prolonged and heavy dosage of aminorex to rats and beagles did not produce pulmonary hypertension or pulmonary vascular disease.[133] Aminorex also had no effect in patas monkeys[137] and calves.[138] To exclude the possibility that obesity was an important etiologic factor, Smith and Heath[139] gave aminorex to rats which were also fed on a diet rich in fat, but even after 154 days, there was no evidence of hypertensive pulmonary vascular disease.

Pharmacologists have demonstrated transient rises in pulmonary arterial blood pressure and resistance in rats or dogs given injections of aminorex, but their significance has been challenged. In one study, the pulmonary arterial pressure rose to 30 to 40 mmHg with a small residual elevation which persisted more than one hour afterward.[140] These authors concluded that aminorex has cardiovascular effects similar to norepinephrine but differs from it in that aminorex induces a greater increase in pulmonary vascular resistance.

The outcome of these and numerous other animal experiments is that no one has been able to demonstrate a persistent, high pulmonary blood pressure or hypertensive pulmonary vascular disease in animals given aminorex. Nevertheless, there is still the strong epidemiologic evidence incriminating the drug as a cause of pulmonary hypertension in humans. This conflicting evidence has not been reconciled. Epidemiologists can claim that a lack of response in animals does not exclude any influence in humans. Experimentalists can claim that the clinical evidence against aminorex is purely circumstantial. The clarity of such arguments in recent years has been blurred by misinterpretation and imprecise terminology. Thus, acute and mild elevation of pulmonary arterial pressure following administration of aminorex to animals has been equated with the severe pulmonary vascular disease produced by pyrrolizidine alkaloids. Also many cases in the epidemic were diagnosed as primary pulmonary hypertension when there was no evidence of plexogenic pulmonary arteriopathy. These patients should be referred to as having unexplained pulmonary hypertension since many of them are still alive.

In the wake of the aminorex controversy, several other anorexigenic drugs were incriminated as inducers of pulmonary hypertension, although on scanty evidence. Foremost among these were phenmetrazine, phentermine, and chlorphentermine. The last two of these drugs have been administered to rats but have shown no evidence of inducing hypertensive pulmonary vascular disease or right ventricular hypertrophy.[141-142] Although chlorphentermine does not induce pulmonary hypertension in rats, it is responsible for pronounced alveolar phospholipidosis in these animals.[143]

Unexplained Pulmonary Hypertension

In some patients, the cause of pulmonary arterial hypertension remains unexplained even following detailed clinical and physiologic studies. The clinical diagnosis in such cases should be one of unexplained pulmonary hypertension since the underlying pathology may be one of three distinct entities (Table 24-1). These are plexogenic pulmonary arteriopathy, pulmonary veno-occlusive disease, and recurrent pulmonary thromboembolism.

Table 24–1. Pathologic Entities of Unexplained Pulmonary Hypertension

> Primary plexogenic pulmonary arteriopathy
> Recurrent pulmonary thromboembolism
> Pulmonary veno-occlusive disease

Table 24–2. Causes of Plexogenic Pulmonary Arteriopathy

> Congenital intracardiac shunts, both pre- and post-tricuspid
> Rare cases of cirrhosis of the liver and portal vein thrombosis
> Primary pulmonary hypertension

Primary Pulmonary Hypertension

Plexogenic pulmonary arteriopathy occurs most typically in large congenital cardiac shunts but also rarely in cases of cirrhosis of the liver or portal vein thrombosis (Table 24–2). Rarely plexogenic pulmonary arteriopathy develops in the absence of heart or liver disease and the clinical condition is then termed primary pulmonary hypertension. The light and electron microscopy of this plexiform variety of vascular disease have been described; suffice it to confirm that in patients with primary pulmonary hypertension, one finds medial hypertrophy of elastic and muscular pulmonary arteries together with muscularization of pulmonary arterioles. Longitudinally orientated smooth muscle is frequently found in the intima and adventitia of these vessels. Intimal fibrosis is often widespread and severe and of the concentric-laminar, onion-skin variety. Dilatation lesions, and in particular plexiform lesions, are numerous; indeed it is upon the identification of these structures that an unequivocal diagnosis of plexogenic pulmonary arteriopathy and thus primary pulmonary hypertension depends. Fibrinoid necrosis is also very characteristic. Thrombi may form in vessels affected by necrotizing arteritis and may give rise to emboli which pass to more distal vessels. With the passage of time, such emboli become organized and recanalized to lead to septa within the lumina of affected vessels (Fig. 24–43). Such appearances can be confused with those of recurrent pulmonary thromboembolism or with aging plexiform lesions.

Primary pulmonary hypertension is a rare disease. In 1951 Dresdale and colleagues[144] collected 39 cases, and by 1956 Wood[145] had seen the condition 17 times. In 1957, 25 cases were reported in three papers in one issue alone of the *British Heart Journal*.[146–148] A survey of the world literature in 1971 revealed reports of a total of 602 cases diagnosed as such from 260 publications.[149] There was a transient but striking increase in the incidence of the disease in Europe between the years 1965 and 1970 associated with an increase in the use of the anorexigen aminorex.

The factors that have been implicated in the etiology of primary pulmonary hypertension are numerous and diverse, suggesting that the term probably encompasses a heterogeneous group of diseases.[150] The situation is confused by the fact that the condition is often misdiagnosed. Thus one series of 110 cases verified histologically was selected from a total of 156 cases which had been diagnosed clinically, and sometimes pathologically, as primary pulmonary hypertension.[149] The most frequent condition misdiagnosed as such was recurrent pulmonary thromboembolism.

The majority of patients with primary pulmonary hypertension are young adults or children. Of the series of 110 cases,[149] 39 were young children, with an average age of 5.1 years. The remainder had a mean age of 33 years. In infants the pulmonary hypertension is likely to be present from birth, whereas in adults it is acquired, as indicated by an adult elastic tissue configuration in the pulmonary trunk.[151] In young adults, the disease is four times more common in women. This is in contrast to recurrent pulmonary thromboembolism which is only twice as common in women. It has been suggested that nonfatal amniotic fluid embolism to the lung may be implicated in the etiology.[148] Certainly in a minority of cases, primary pulmonary hypertension follows soon after, or is exacerbated by, pregnancy or delivery, but so also are other forms of pulmonary vascular disease.[149] Furthermore, this explanation excludes cases involving men and children.

Recurrent pulmonary thromboembolism is frequently cited as a cause of primary pulmonary hypertension.[148,152,153] In part this may be due to misdiagnosis, but the histopathology of primary pulmonary hypertension and recurrent pulmonary embolism are sufficiently distinct to enable one to distinguish between them even in their advanced stages. Furthermore, a thromboembolic origin does not explain the high incidence of the disease in children in whom thromboembolism is rare.

Bronchopulmonary anastomoses were found in two of the patients described by Wade and Ball[150] who thought that they might be responsible for elevating the pulmonary arterial blood pressure. This seems unlikely, for in bronchiectasis, extensive bronchopulmonary anastomoses may develop in the absence of pulmonary hypertension. They are more likely to be the result of vascular occlusion characteristic of plexogenic pulmonary arteriopathy.

Some cases of primary pulmonary hypertension are familial. Reports on a familial predisposition to the disease were made by Clark and colleagues[154] and later by Fleming.[155] The latter report assumed an even greater interest when the father remarried and the disease appeared in the second family.[156] Such a distribution is best explained by an autosomal dominant trait, although a recessive form of inheritance has also been suggested following a study of one family in which only one generation was affected.[157] However, the parents of this family were not examined and may have had a mild form of the disease.[156] It is thus possible that the mode of inheritance, even when apparently restricted to one generation, could be interpreted as an autosomal domi-

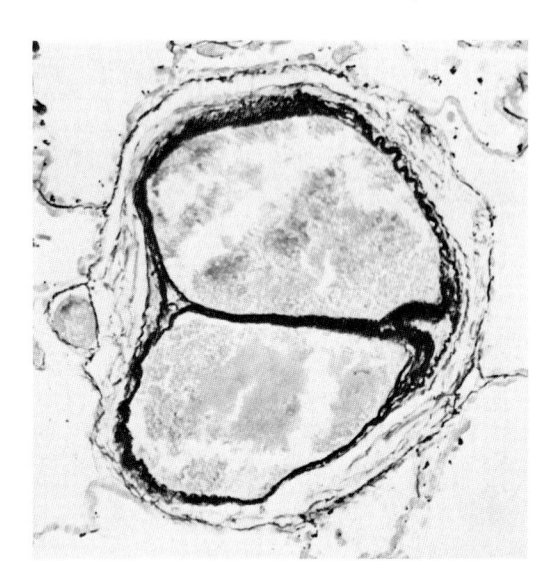

Figure 24-43. Muscular pulmonary artery from a 22-year-old woman with primary pulmonary hypertension. The media is atrophic, and the lumen of the vessel is divided into two by a transverse septum of elastic tissue. Such appearances are the result of reduced pulmonary blood flow which predisposes to thrombosis with subsequent organization and recanalization (EVG, ×150).

nant trait with varying expression. An alternative view is that familial primary pulmonary hypertension is not confined to a single gene locus, but is polygenic and influenced by environmental factors.

The notion that primary pulmonary hypertension is an autoimmune disease is suggested by the fact that the histologic changes often progress to fibrinoid necrosis and necrotizing arteritis. These conditions are sometimes associated with Raynaud's phenomenon and one of the collagen diseases such as scleroderma or rheumatoid disease.[150] Fibrinoid necrosis in primary plexogenic pulmonary arteriopathy is almost certainly an expression of a severe elevation of pulmonary arterial pressure in the same manner as in congenital cardiac shunts.

These associations are interesting but do not reveal the nature of the stimulus that causes vasconstriction in primary pulmonary hypertension. Normally the smooth muscle of the media contracts in response to increased distension of the vessel brought about by elevation of intravascular blood pressure. These altered hemodynamics elevating pulmonary arterial pressure form the assumed origin of the pulmonary vascular disease in congenital cardiac shunts, but this cannot apply to the primary form of the disease. Neither is there evidence of any primary occlusion of the muscular pulmonary arteries or arterioles. The initiating factor for the disease appears to be pulmonary vasoconstriction, but the stimulus for this remains obscure. Of the various known natural vasoactive substances, none is sufficiently potent to initiate such an intense vasoconstriction. Hypoxia is a well-recognized and powerful pulmonary arterial vasoconstrictor, but even this stimulus fails to induce the advanced lesions and severe hypertension which occur in primary pulmonary hypertension. Furthermore, hypoxia acts predominantly on the pulmonary arterioles effecting a pronounced muscularization. In some cases of primary pulmonary hypertension, changes in arterioles may be minimal, suggesting that the vasoconstriction occurs mainly at the level of the muscular pulmonary arteries. It is possible, however, that prior exposure to hypoxia initiates some change in the pulmonary vasculature which renders it abnormally vasoreactive. The authors studied the lungs of a 22-year-old woman who had died from primary pulmonary hypertension based on plexogenic pulmonary arteriopathy. She had been born and spent her early childhood at high altitude in Peru before moving to sea level. Perhaps the sustained exposure to hypoxia in infancy induced some structural or physiologic changes in her pulmonary arterial tree which predisposed to the later development of plexogenic pulmonary arteriopathy. Such a hypothesis demands the presence of other genetic or environmental factors since most people born at high altitude do not develop primary pulmonary hypertension.

An environmental factor to be kept in mind is diet. The effects of the pyrrolizidine alkaloids on the pulmonary vasculature of animals and the possible role of aminorex fumarate in an epidemic of primary pulmonary hypertension in Western Europe have been described. In the latter instance, the human disease occurred in only a proportion of people who took the drug, suggesting that any causal relationship must involve another predisposing factor. Nevertheless, one should be alert to the possibility that dietary substances may be involved in some cases to primary pulmonary hypertension.

Pulmonary Veno-Occlusive Disease

The brunt of this disease occurs in the pulmonary veins, and for this reason, it is called pulmonary veno-occlusive disease.[158,159] The condition is characterized by intimal fibrosis of the pulmonary veins and venules, the collagen being deposited in a loose, irregular fashion within vessels ranging from large pulmonary veins to minute venules (Figs. 24-44, 24-45), often occuding them. The intimal proliferation differs from that associated with aging in that the latter in veins is acellular, compact, and often hyalinized. It resembles age-change fibrosis, however, in being commonly eccentric, forming discrete pads or rings of unequal thickness so that the narrowed lumen becomes displaced to one side. It is common for pulmonary veins to contain two or more lumens which are separated by septa of loose fibrous tissue containing scanty fibroblasts (see Fig. 24-45). Longitudinal sections of such vessels show a tortuous series of channels running through the intimal fibrosis so that the appearances resemble those of an organized recanalized thrombus. This impression is especially marked in the larger veins in which the collagen may be deposited in bundles of varying density and at various angles to the circumference incorporating several endothelial-lined channels (see Fig. 24-45). Such an appearance is similar to the so-called colander lesion of an organized thrombus.

Unexplained Pulmonary Hypertension 717

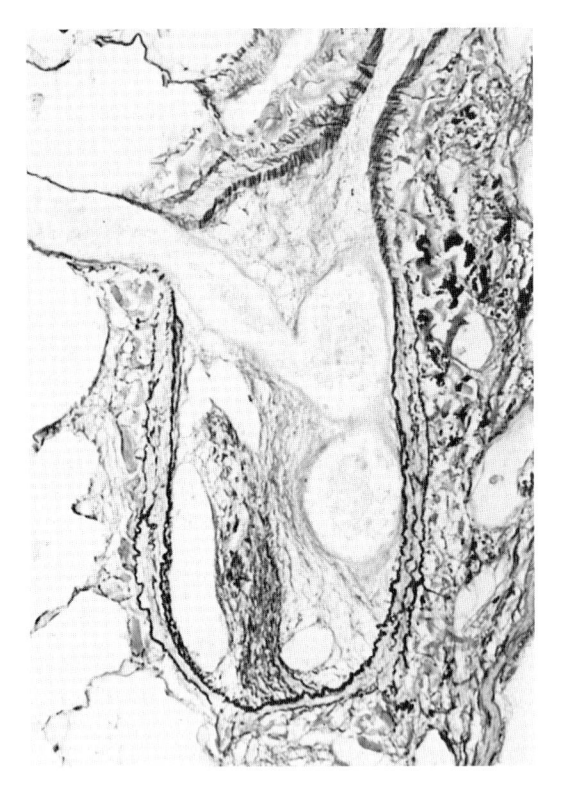

Figure 24–44. Transverse section of a pulmonary vein from a 34-year-old woman with pulmonary veno-occlusive disease. The vessel shows arterialization with a distinct media sandwiched between two elastic laminae which are thinner and less regular than in muscular pulmonary arteries. The lumen contains a colander lesion consisting of a loose, irregular deposit of collagen and scanty elastic fibers in which there are several vascular channels. These appearances are reminiscent of organized, recanalized thrombus (EVG, ×165).

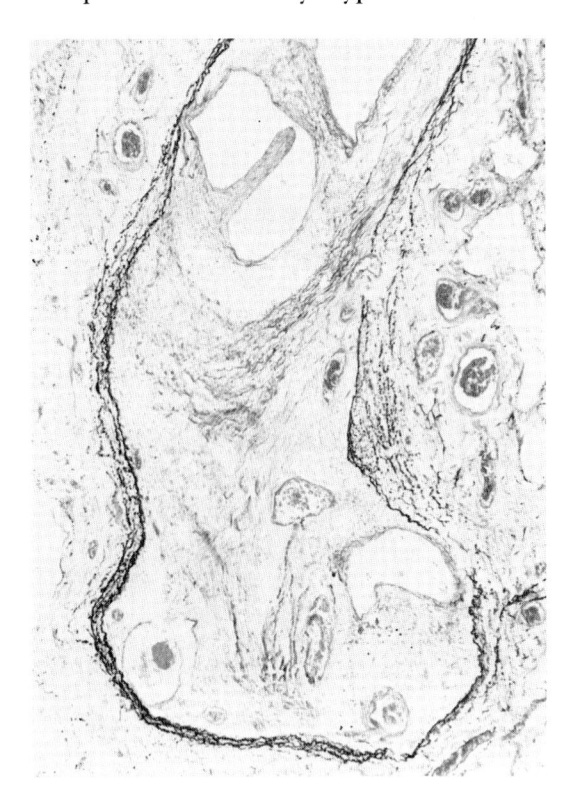

Figure 24–45. Longitudinal section of a large pulmonary vein in a case of pulmonary veno-occlusive disease. The intimal fibrosis is largely collagenous and of haphazard orientation. Several vascular channels pass through the fibrosis so that the vessel contains multiple lumens (EVG, ×41).

As in the case of mitral stenosis the obstruction to the venous outflow from the lung leads to arterialization of pulmonary veins. They develop a thick media of smooth muscle sandwiched between internal and external elastic laminae and as such mimic muscular pulmonary arteries (see Fig. 24–44). Careful examination, however, reveals that the thickness of the media is uneven and the elastic laminae are incomplete and rather ragged in appearance, so that such vessels can usually be distinguished from arteries. Also in common with mitral stenosis, there are changes in the pulmonary arterial tree. Initially these consist of medial hypertrophy of muscular pulmonary arteries and muscularization of pulmonary arterioles (Fig. 24–46). Intimal fibrosis may also occur in the pulmonary arteries, but this is of a loose, irregular nature like that in the pulmonary veins. It may also resemble recanalized thrombus, especially in the elastic pulmonary arteries in which it forms a tortuous series of endothelial-lined channels separated by a web like arrangement of fibroelastic septa.[160] It is seldom occlusive. In more advanced cases, the pulmonary arteries may become dilated[160] or develop fibrinoid necrosis.[161] The authors have not seen plexiform lesions in pulmonary veno-occlusive disease.

Striking changes frequently occur in the lung parenchyma. These are consistent with a chronic exudation of plasma from grossly distended alveolar capillaries (Fig. 24–47). Thus, there are foci of pulmonary hemorrhage and hemosiderosis, the latter sometimes forming encrustations of the elastic laminae. Alveolae contain numerous hemosiderin-laden macrophages and a fibrinous transudate. Organization of this transudate leads to intra-alveolar and interstitial pulmonary fibrosis (Figs. 24–47, 24–48). The thickened alveolar walls become lined by a prominent epithelium of hyperplastic type II cells resembling the histologic picture of fibrosing alveolitis (see Fig. 24–48). Spicules of osseous metaplasia may develop in the lung parenchyma. The edematous changes in the lung, and particularly the edema of connective tissue septa, will frequently be demonstrated on radiographs of the chest. This is often of considerable clinical significance in that a differential diagnosis can be made from primary pulmonary hypertension. However, only half the cases of pulmonary veno-occlusive disease have an elevated pulmonary wedge pressure.[160]

The resemblance of the intimal fibrosis affecting the

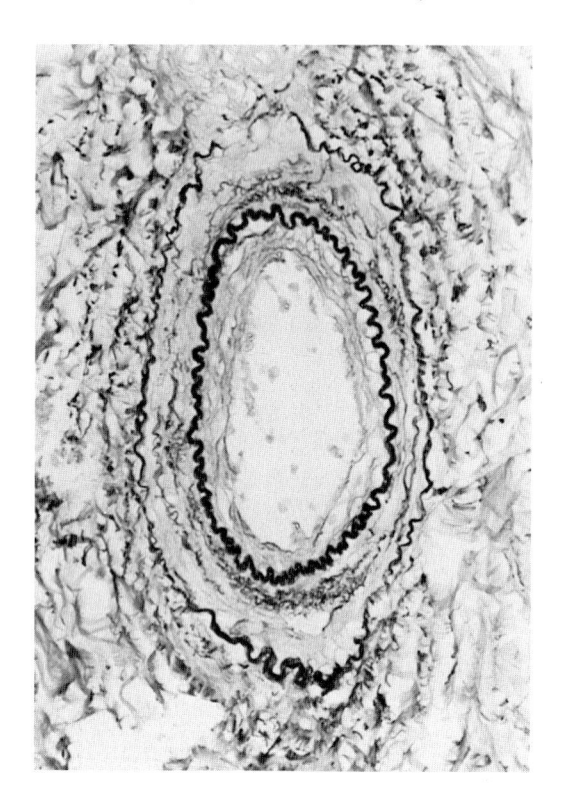

Figure 24-46. Transverse section of a small muscular pulmonary artery from a case of pulmonary veno-occlusive disease. The media is hypertrophied whereas the intima contains a loose, collagenous fibrosis (EVG, ×300).

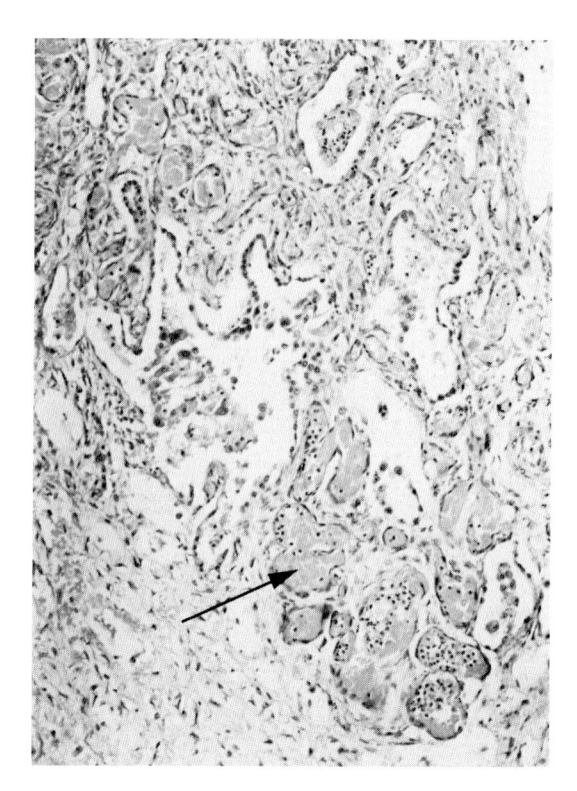

Figure 24-47. Lung parenchyma from a 34-year-old woman with pulmonary veno-occlusive disease. It shows the effects of chronic venous hypertension. Groups of capillaries are grossly distended with blood to form angioma-like masses (arrow). Much of the lung architecture is obliterated by intra-alveolar and interstitial fibrosis, and surviving alveoli are lined by a cuboidal epithelium of hyperplastic granular pneumonocytes (H&E, ×96).

pulmonary veins to organized thrombus of thromboembolus is so great that many believe the lesions to be thrombotic in origin. However, no satisfactory explanation for such thrombosis has yet been put forward. Brown and Harrison,[159] noted an increased platelet adhesiveness in their patient and thought that it might be of etiological significance, but coagulation studies in another patient were normal.[162]

Frequently it is possible to find a history of an infection. Thus some authors have referred to a previous illness resembling influenza[163] or chest infections.[161] In one case, there were raised serologic levels for toxoplasmosis,[164] but these were not high enough to be diagnostic. In another case,[158] histologic examination of the lymph nodes failed to show lymphohistiocytic medullary reticulosis, which might be anticipated if toxoplasmosis were involved. In a case of a 39-day-old infant, the mother gave a history of upper respiratory tract infection during the second trimester of pregnancy, suggesting that the disease may have been acquired in utero.[165]

The possibility that pulmonary veno-occlusive disease may have an immunologic etiology has been considered.[166] A case of pulmonary veno-occlusive disease occurring in a 33-year-old woman showed electron-dense ultrastructural deposits in the alveolar capillary basement membranes. Immunoglobulin and complement were demonstrated in a similar situation by immunofluorescence microscopy. It was suggested that immune complexes may have caused thrombotic occlusion of the small pulmonary venules. However, the electron-dense deposits were similar in appearance to extravasated erythrocytes occurring in mitral stenosis.[81] Extravasation of erythrocytes is a typical feature of pulmonary veno-occlusive disease.

Recurrent Pulmonary Thromboembolism

In this condition, showers of small, clinically silent emboli lodge in the pulmonary arterial tree over a period of months or years. They are two small to cause infarction or suddenly to embarrass the action of the right ventricle. Instead there is a gradual occlusion of the pulmonary arterial bed which is sufficiently extensive to significantly increase pulmonary vascular resistance so that pulmonary arterial hypertension ensues with hypertrophy of the right ventricle. Thromboemboli impacted in the elastic pulmonary arteries are organized and recanalized

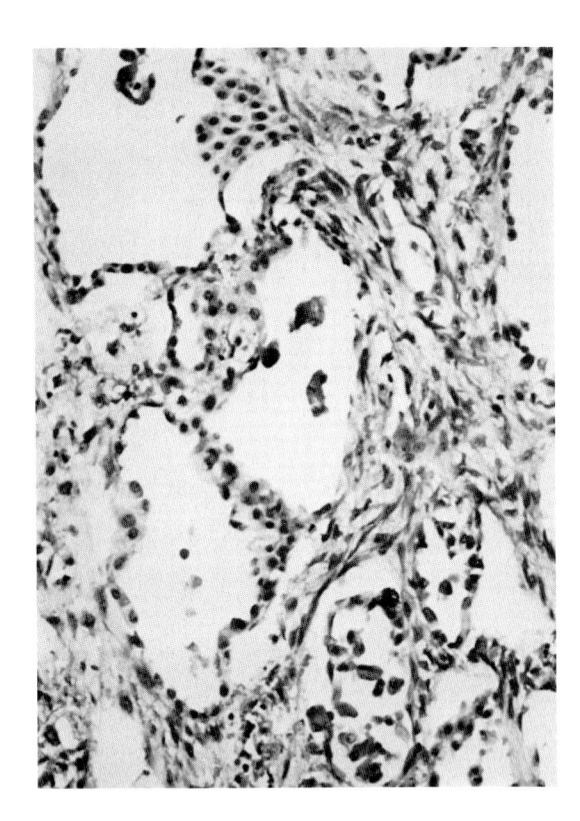

Figure 24-48. Fibrosing alveolitis in a patient with pulmonary veno-occlusive disease. The alveolar septa are thickened by fibrous tissue and lined by a continuous epithelium of hyperplastic granular pneumonocytes. The alveolar spaces contain a mixture of hemosiderin-laden macrophages and desquamated granular pneumonocytes (H&E, ×168).

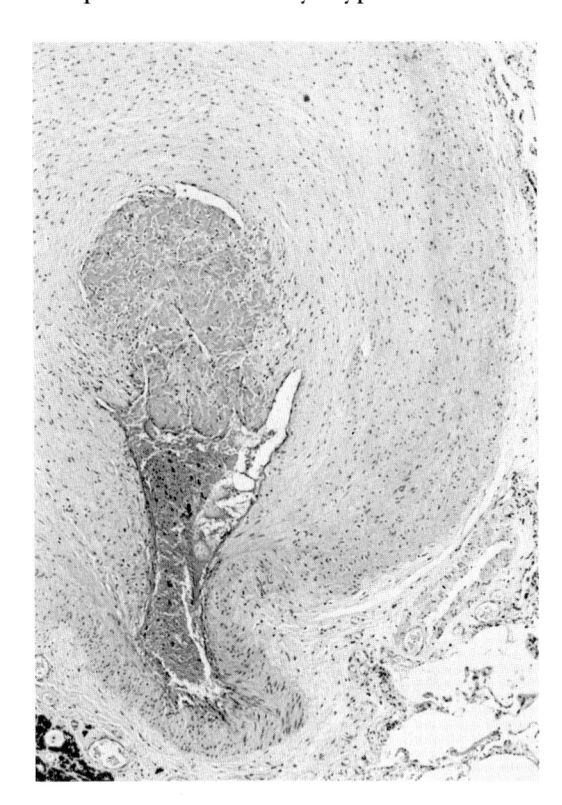

Figure 24-49. Transverse section of an elastic pulmonary artery from a 72-year-old woman with recurrent pulmonary thromboembolism complicated by pulmonary hypertension. The vessel has been sectioned near the origin of a lateral branch. The intima is greatly thickened by fibrous tissue which has formed from organized thromboembolus. The residual lumen is occluded by recent thrombus which shows early invasion by granulation tissue at its periphery (H&E, ×53; Figs. 24-50 through 24-53 are from the same patient).

to form a web of fibrous septa enclosing numerous vascular channels. As the lesions age, the walls of these channels develop extensive deposits of elastic tissue. At first they are lined merely by endothelium, but later smooth muscle forms in them so that these recanalization channels look like muscular pulmonary arteries embedded in fibroelastic tissue within the lumen of an elastic pulmonary artery. The obstruction to blood flow causes medial hypertrophy proximally, and the abrupt thinning of the wall of the major pulmonary artery distal to the organized embolus can be detected by the naked eye. Intimal fibrosis and atherosclerosis may form in the vessels proximal to the embolus.

Muscular pulmonary arteries are the site of impaction and subsequent organization of numerous emboli. In sections of a case of recurrent pulmonary thromboembolism, some emboli are recent and consist of thrombus invaded by fibroblasts at its periphery (Fig. 24-49). Most are older and completely converted into fibrous tissue which shrinks to produce mural pads or eccentric intimal fibrosis with recanalization (Figs. 24-50, and 24-51). The formation of multiple recanalization channels leads to the production of colander lesions, the name of which is derived from a supposed similarity to the culinary instrument (Fig. 24-52). The internal elastic lamina may fragment and elastic tissue extend into the intimal fibrous tissue. These occlusive intimal lesions lead to pulmonary arterial hypertension to which the pulmonary circulation responds by medial hypertrophy of muscular pulmonary arteries and muscularization of pulmonary arterioles (see Fig. 24-51). There may also be intimal fibrosis in both classes of vessel which is a consequence of pulmonary hypertension and not organization of emboli. However, these hypertensive vascular lesions seldom progress beyond a state of intimal fibrosis, and dilatation lesions never occur. Pulmonary arterioles may also contain organized thrombus with one or more recanalization channels. The walls of these channels may develop circularly oriented smooth muscle between two elastic laminae and thus resemble muscularized arterioles inside an existing elastic lamina (Fig. 24-53). Pulmonary veins are normal.

Pulmonary thromboembolism is a common event, and in one investigation,[167] a thorough search of the lungs in 263 necropsies revealed that 51.7 percent of subjects had pulmonary emboli. Therefore, it is curious that pulmonary hypertension due to recurrent pulmonary thrombo-

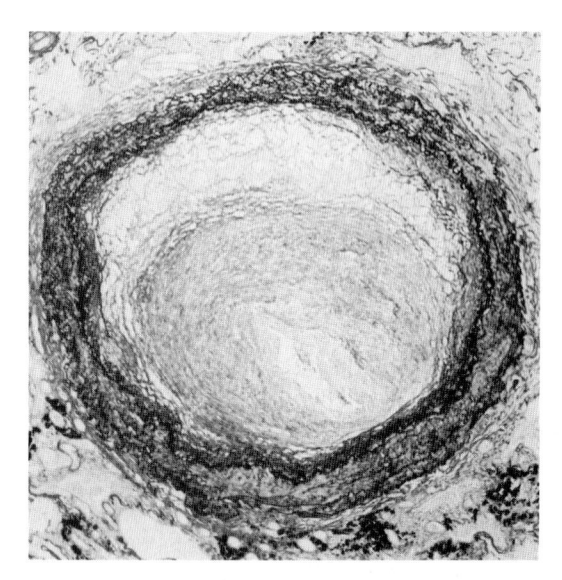

Figure 24–50. Transverse section of an elastic pulmonary artery which is occluded by organized thromboembolus. The intimal proliferation consists largely of collagen which is arranged into discrete zones suggesting several episodes of embolism. There is a small, eccentrically situated recanalization channel (EVG, ×38).

embolism is so rare. This may be due in part to the speed with which emboli are normally removed. Victims of this disease may have an abnormality of their pulmonary vascular endothelium with deficient fibrinolysis.

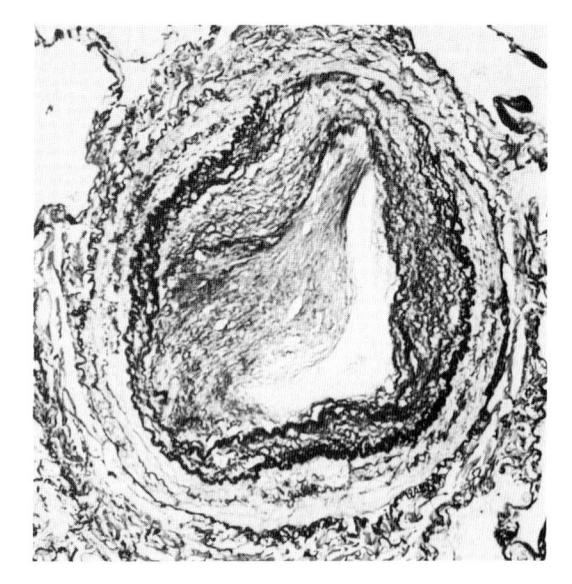

Figure 24–51. Transverse section of a muscular pulmonary artery from a case of recurrent pulmonary thromboembolism. The media is hypertrophied, while the intima contains an eccentric fibrosis comprising collagen and fine elastic fibrils. Part of this fibrosis froms an intimal cushion which reduces the lumen to a slit (EVG, ×138).

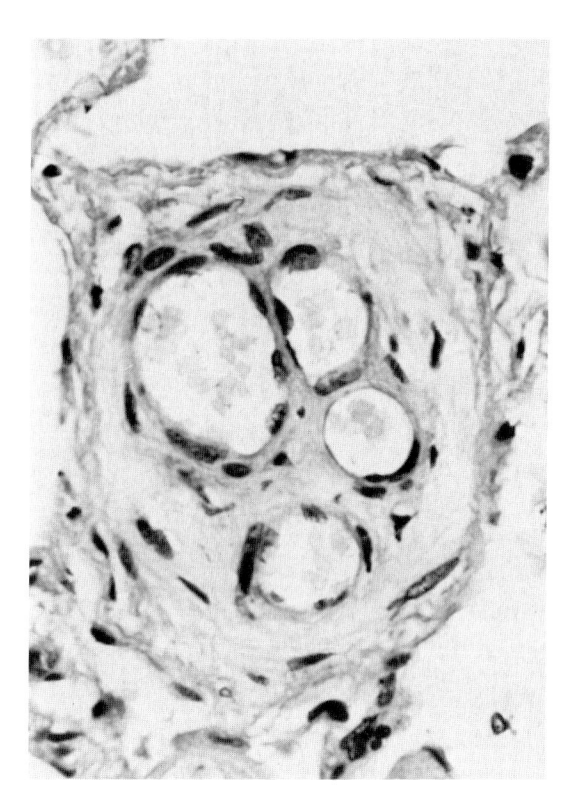

Figure 24–52. Transverse section of a small muscular pulmonary artery containing a colander lesion. Recanalization of organized thromboembolus has created several lumens, each of which has become lined endothelium (H&E, ×540).

The lungs have a great capacity for the removal of thromboemboli, and this is especially pronounced in the canine lung. Thus several hundred milliliters of fresh blood clot can be injected intravenously into dogs over a period of several months without any rise in pulmonary arterial blood pressure.[168] Thrombi which have aged for two or three weeks before entering the lungs are removed more slowly, and in humans the process of removal of pulmonary thromboemboli from elastic pulmonary arteries takes about four weeks.[169] In the majority of cases of recurrent pulmonary thromboembolism, there is no evidence of systemic venous thrombi. It has been suggested that the basis for the occlusion of the lung circulation lies not in excessive numbers of emboli, but in an inability of the lung to deal with them rapidly enough.[168,170] So far, however, there is no direct evidence of inadequate fibrinolytic activity in the blood of these patients, although the possibility exists that the defect is in the pulmonary vascular endothelium.

Differential Diagnosis of Unexplained Pulmonary Hypertension

The clinical distinctions among the three forms of unexplained pulmonary hypertension do not come within the scope of this book. Suffice it to say that a precise clinical diagnosis is in many cases either impossible or prone to

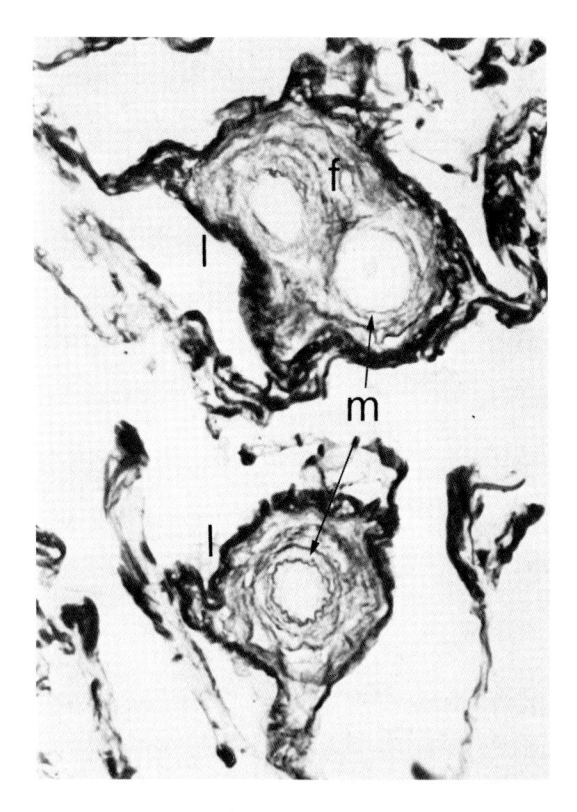

Figure 24–53. Two pulmonary arterioles showing recanalization of organized thromboembolus. New smooth muscle has formed around the recanalization channels. The vessels thus consist of the original arteriolar elastic lamina (l) internal to which is a layer of loose fibrous tissue (f) lined by one or two rings of circularly oriented smooth muscle (m) which have developed internal and external elastic laminae of their own (EVG, ×375).

error. Pulmonary veno-occlusive disease can sometimes be distinguished when it produces radiologic signs of pulmonary edema and venous hypertension, but they are not always present. The difficulty in making a correct diagnosis of primary pulmonary hypertension based on plexogenic pulmonary arteriopathy even when lung tissue is available for histologic examination is well known. In a histologic study[149] of 156 cases collected from 51 medical centers throughout the world in which a diagnosis of primary pulmonary hypertension had been made and in which both clinical and necropsy examinations had already been performed before the cases had been reported in the literature, the diagnoses was incorrect in no fewer than 46 instances. Conditions incorrectly labeled primary pulmonary hypertension were recurrent thromboembolism in 31 cases, pulmonary veno-occlusive disease in 5 cases, chronic pulmonary venous hypertension in 5 cases, and sarcoidosis, schistosomiasis, and chronic bronchitis with emphysema in isolated instances. The pathologic diagnosis is especially difficult where small quantities of lung tissue are available as in biopsy specimens.

One difficulty is the distinction among the intimal reactions of pulmonary blood vessels in the three forms of unexplained pulmonary hypertension. In plexogenic pulmonary arteriopathy, the intimal fibrosis of pulmonary arteries is of the concentric-laminar, onion-skin type in contrast to the loose, irregular fibrosis typical of the other two forms. The identification of plexiform lesions will give a positive diagnosis of plexogenic pulmonary arteriopathy. Recognition of plexiform lesions is easy if they are young and cellular, but the web-like, septate arrangement of aging lesions can be confused with organized thrombus or thromboemboli. Thrombosis of the small muscular pulmonary arteries can also occur in plexogenic pulmonary arteriopathy, adding to the difficulty in distinguishing this condition from recurrent pulmonary thromboembolism. In general, however, fresh or organizing thrombi are uncommon in plexogenic pulmonary arteriopathy, whereas in recurrent thromboembolism, they are more common and tend to affect larger vessels including elastic pulmonary arteries.

Pulmonary Circulation in Liver Disease

Arterial Oxygen Desaturation

Two main disturbances of the pulmonary circulation may occur in liver disease. The first is oxygen unsaturation of systemic arterial blood, and the second is the development of severe pulmonary arterial hypertension and associated plexogenic pulmonary arteriopathy. The most likely explanation for the desaturation is a shunt that allows poorly oxygenated venous blood to bypass the alveolar capillary bed of the lung. The bypasses which have been proposed are intrapulmonary arteriovenous shunts and portapulmonary venous anastomoses. Direct communications between pulmonary arteries and veins have been demonstrated in lungs from cirrhotic patients into which plastic beads or radiopaque media have been injected.[171–174] These abnormal vascular channels usually occur on the pleural surface where they may resemble spider nevi as more commonly observed on the skin. However, some workers[175] have been unable to detect any significant pulmonary arteriovenous shunt at all in the cirrhotic patients they have investigated.

The authors' work[176] involving the injection of barium sulphate suspension into rats rendered cirrhotic by repeated exposure to carbon tetrachloride vapor suggests that the unsaturation of systemic arterial blood is more likely to be due to the flow of blood from portal to pulmonary veins. The portal vein communicates via the coronary and short gastric veins with the periesophageal plexus, which connects with a network of mediastinal veins some of which penetrate the pleura and drain directly into the alveolar capillaries. Other branches of the mediastinal venous plexus, in rats at least, terminate directly in the large extrapulmonary veins. Similar portapulmonary venous anastomoses have been demonstrated in cirrhotic human cadavers.[177] It seems probable that as a result of portal hypertension, unsaturated sys-

Figure 24–54. Coronal section of the heart a 24-year-old man who died in congestive cardiac failure after a five-year history of severe pulmonary arterial hypertension complicating cavernomatous transformation of the portal vein. There is gross hypertrophy of the right ventricle (r) such that its thickness exceeds that of the left (l). The weight of the right ventricle was 290 gm in contrast to a left ventricular weight of 121 g. Histology of the pulmonary vasculature showed plexogenic pulmonary arteriopathy and is illustrated in Figs. 24–11, 24–16, 24–34, and 24–35 (natural size).

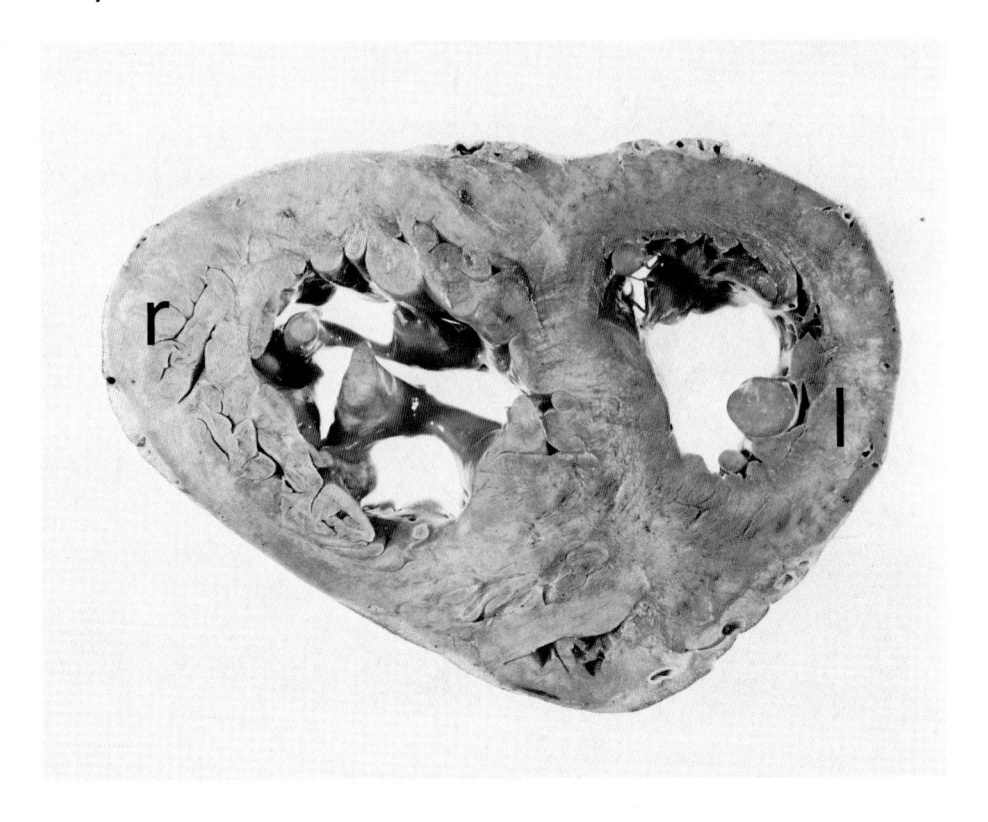

temic venous blood leads directly into large pulmonary veins creating unsaturation of systemic arterial blood with the development of cyanosis. Desaturation has been demonstrated in patients with cirrhosis,[175] and similar shunts have been confirmed in humans.[178] The functional significance of the alternative vascular pathway with flow from the mediastinal venous plexus directly into the pulmonary capillaries is much less obvious. The combined perfusion by both pulmonary arterial and portal venous blood increases capillary blood flow, but it seems unlikely that this would interfere with oxygenation unless such flow increased tremendously.

Pulmonary Hypertension in Hepatic Disease

Severe pulmonary hypertension is rarely associated with cirrhosis of the liver and portal vein thrombosis which has been recognized for 30 years.[179] At first it was regarded as a chance combination of liver disease and primary pulmonary hypertension, but now there have been so many examples of this association reported[180–187] as to suggest a causal relationship.

At cardiac catheterization, there is severe pulmonary arterial hypertension, sometimes exceeding 70 mmHg, and a great elevation of pulmonary vascular resistance, even beyond 4500 dynes/s/cm^{-5}. The pulmonary wedge pressure remains normal. Cardiac output and plasma volume tend to be increased.

Cases of severe pulmonary hypertension complicating alcoholic cirrhosis[186] and cavernomatous transformation of the portal vein[187] (Fig. 23–54) are convincing that the type of hypertensive pulmonary vascular disease complicating liver disorders is plexogenic pulmonary arteriopathy. The pathogenesis of pulmonary hypertension and structural changes in the pulmonary arteries is complex. The increase in blood volume characteristic of cirrhosis may lead to slight hypertension[188] but is hardly likely to produce great elevations of pulmonary arterial pressure and plexogenic pulmonary arteriopathy. Increases in blood flow are also unlikely to be responsible. In cases of portal vein thrombosis, thromboemboli may reach the pulmonary arterial tree via anastomoses between the portal and systemic veins. This has led some authors[179,181,189] to postulate that pulmonary hypertension is embolic in origin. However, the type of vascular disease found in cirrhosis of the liver is plexogenic pulmonary arteriopathy, a condition which can be clearly distinguished from recurrent pulmonary thromboembolism. Very few cases of cirrhosis or portal vein thrombosis develop pulmonary hypertension. Great difficulty is also found in producing elevation of pulmonary arterial pressure in animals in which liver disease has been produced experimentally. Thus, pulmonary hypertension was not induced in rats in which cirrhosis was induced by carbon tetrachloride[176] or in rats which survived for a year following partial ligation or total occlusion of the portal vein.[190] In clinical cases also, there is no obvious relation

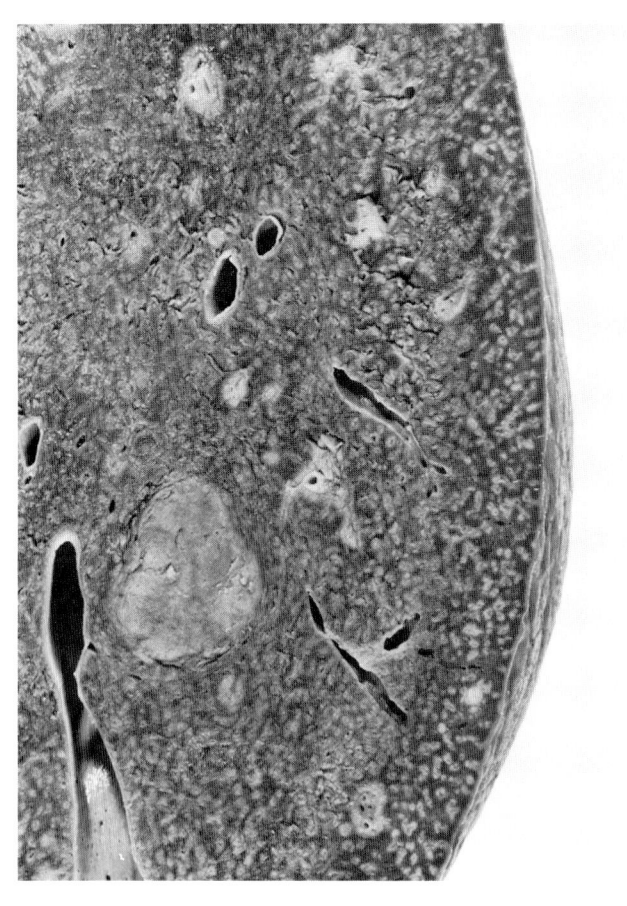

Figure 24–55. Cut surface of the liver from the same patient as in Figure 24–54. There is a "nutmeg" pattern typical of congestive cardiac failure. There is an oval area of adenomatous hyperplasia which has compressed the surrounding liver parenchyma (natural size).

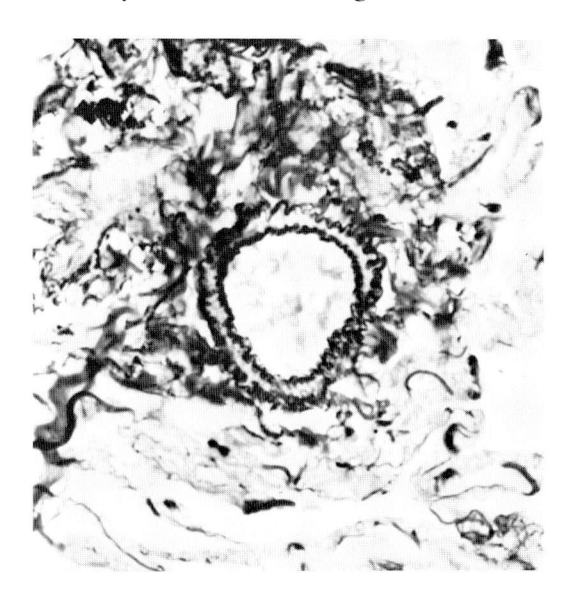

Figure 24–56. Muscularized pulmonary arteriole from a 35-year-old Aymara Indian man living at La Paz, Bolivia, at an altitude of 3800 m above sea level (EVG, ×412).

between the severity of liver disease and the tendency to develop pulmonary hypertension.[191]

It is conceivable that the elevation of pulmonary arterial pressure in these cases is the result of pulmonary vasoconstriction induced by dietary factors or metabolites from the intestine no longer detoxified by the diseased liver. Pyrrolizidine alkaloids may affect both the liver and the pulmonary circulation.[192] Thus, fulvine causes both veno-occlusive disease of the liver and pulmonary hypertension. Metabolites from the intestine which are normally inactivated by the hepatic cells may fail to be detoxified by the diseased liver in a minority of cases and give rise to pulmonary vasoconstriction and plexogenic pulmonary arteriopathy when carried to the lungs. Ligation of the portal vein in experimental rats did not lead to elevation of blood estrogen levels[190] to suggest that they were responsible for the pulmonary vasoconstriction. Nodules of adenomatous hyperplasia are often to be found in the liver in cases of cavernomatous transformation of the portal vein (Fig. 24–55). Although such nodules have always being regarded as innocent, they are conceivably a source of metabolites capable of inducing pulmonary arteries to constrict.

Pulmonary Vasculature at High Altitude

Native highlanders of the Andes show a mild elevation of pulmonary arterial pressure[193] which is greater in children and exaggerated on exercise. The hypertension is associated with muscularization of the terminal portions of the pulmonary arterial tree[194] (Fig. 24–56). Studies in La Paz, Bolivia (3800 m),[195] suggest that such muscularization is more evident in Quechua and Aymara Indians, who exhibit natural acclimatization[196] than in mestizos and Caucasians long resident in that city. Since the pulmonary hypertension is based on muscularization, it is not surprising that it is reversible. Immediate partial reversibility on inhalation of oxygen is almost certainly due to relief of hypoxic vasoconstriction. Long-term reversibility of the residual pulmonary hypertension, however, is likely to be due to regression of muscle in the terminal portions of the pulmonary arterial tree. Age-change intimal proliferation occurs in the small pulmonary blood vessels of highlanders just as it does in lowlanders (Fig. 24–57), and such a thick layer of intimal fibrosis might well impede the long-term reversibility of pulmonary hypertension on descent to sea level.

Indigenous mountain animals which are adapted in a Darwinian sense, rather than acclimatized, to high altitude do not show muscularization of the terminal portions of their pulmonary arterial tree.[196] As a result they do not develop pulmonary hypertension. Heath and co-workers have found the small pulmonary arteries to

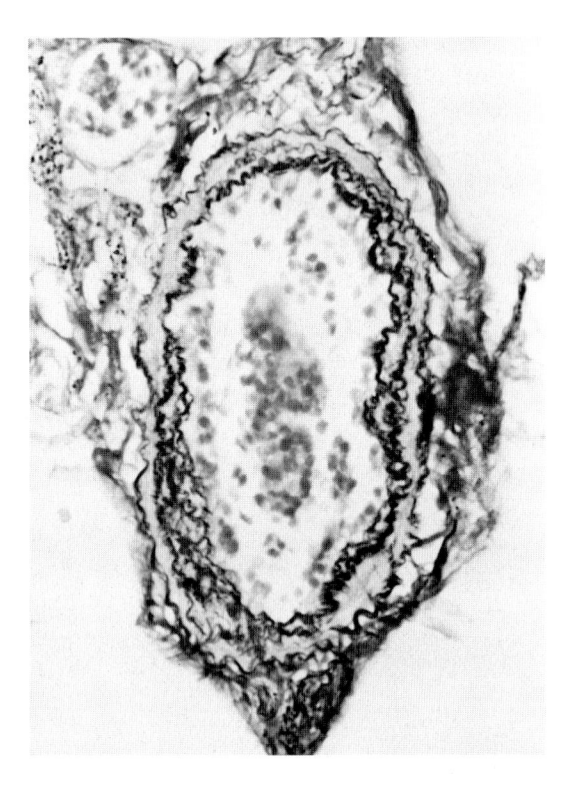

Figure 24–57. Transverse section of a muscular pulmonary artery from a 70-year-old mestizo Indian man from La Paz. The media is of normal thickness, and the intima contains small pads of fibroelastic tissue consistent with aging (EVG, ×412).

be thin-walled in the llama (*Lama glama*),[197,198] the alpaca, and the mountain-viscacha (*Lagidium peruanum*),[199] although these animals are born and live all their lives exposed to significant hypobaric hypoxia. (The structure of the pulmonary trunk of the highlander has been considered elsewhere in this chapter.)

A minority of highlanders in the Andes develops alveolar hypoventilation which leads to an increased degree of arterial oxygen unsaturation and an exaggeration of pulmonary hypertension. They are said to have chronic mountain sickness or Monge's disease, and their clinical features have been subjected to intense investigation.[200] This condition is thought by some to be due to a loss of acclimatization, but others regard the alveolar hypoventilation as an expression of aging at high altitude. Subjects with Monge's disease develop high levels of hemoglobin exceeding 23 gm/dl and may be so cyanosed as to be called cardiac negroes.

The pulmonary vasculature of some calves taken up to graze in highland pastures around Salt Lake City is unduly sensitive to hypobaric hypoxia. These animals show an exaggeration of the normal pulmonary hypertension of cattle at high altitude and develop congestive cardiac failure which presents as edema of the brisket. This gives the disease its name of brisket disease.[201]

Pulmonary Arteries in Emphysema

In emphysema two major factors have a profound effect on the pulmonary circulation. One is chronic alveolar hypoxia which induces pulmonary vasoconstriction. The other is the formation of abnormal air spaces in the lung with the obliteration of lung tissue and its included pulmonary capillaries. There are now available both macroscopic and histologic methods of tissue morphometry which allow one to determine with some accuracy the remaining internal surface area of the lung and the surviving numbers of alveolar spaces. If at the same time one weighs the right ventricle by the method of Fulton and associates,[202] it is possible to relate the loss of internal surface area, with its included capillary bed, to the degree of sustained elevation, if any, of the pulmonary arterial pressure as assessed by the mass of the right ventricular myocardium. Hicken and colleagues, using the mean linear intercept, geometric, and linear dimensions methods, suggest that there is little or no relation between the weight of the right ventricle and the extent of loss of lung substance[203] or the degree of loss of internal surface area of alveolar spaces[204] due to emphysema. Such results suggest that the basis for the elevation of pulmonary arterial pressure in emphysema is not loss of capillary bed but pulmonary vascular disease.

There are four aspects of the histopathologic features found in the pulmonary vasculature in emphysema: development of longitudinal muscle in pulmonary arteries and aterioles; lack of significant hypertrophy of the media of circularly oriented smooth muscle in the muscular pulmonary arteries; lack of occlusive intimal proliferation; and muscularization of the pulmonary arterioles.[205]

Longitudinal muscle may develop in the intima of muscular pulmonary arteries and pulmonary arterioles as small fasciculi. These may become exaggerated to form a thicker, continuous band of longitudinal muscle (Fig. 24–58). Anastomosing elastic fibrils separate these muscle fibers from one another. Finally intimal fibrosis develops to obliterate the longitudinal muscle so that the observer, unaware of the earlier muscular stages of the process, might dismiss the intimal change as nonspecific intimal fibroelastosis (Fig. 24–59). Such intimal changes are almost certainly due to myofibroblasts which have the capacity not only for the formation of smooth muscle but can also secrete collagen and elastin and thus give rise to the characteristic intimal proliferation seen in pulmonary emphysema. Longitudinal muscle occurs in cases of emphysema with or without right ventricular hypertrophy,[205] and hence it is not related to the development of pulmonary hypertension. Previous studies[31] on the formation of longitudinal muscle in pulmonary arteries suggest that this orientation is a reaction to the combined stimulus of raised pulmonary arterial pressure and repeated longitudinal stretch. This view agrees with the observations that longitudinal muscle is to be found in pulmonary arteries distorted around the abnormal air spaces of centrilobular[206] or bullous emphysema.[207]

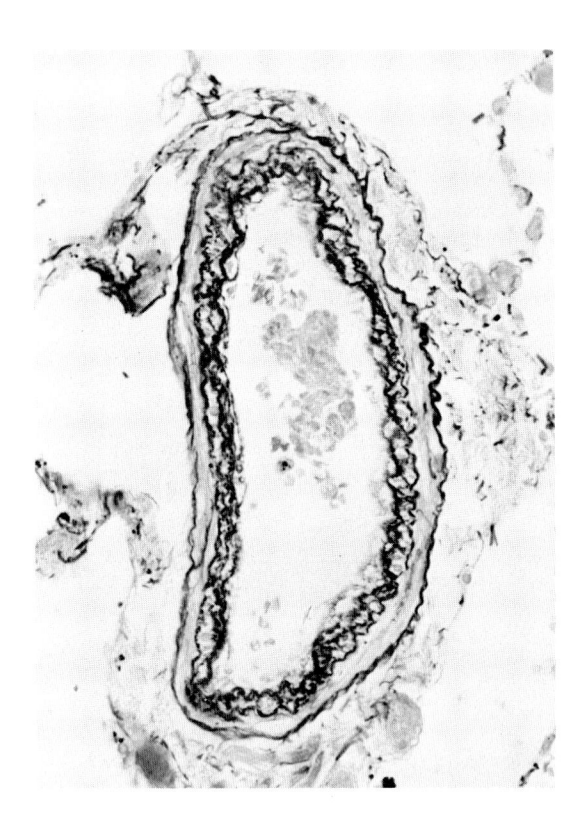

Figure 24–58. Transverse section of a muscular pulmonary artery from a 46-year-old man with centrilobular emphysema. The media is of normal thickness, and the intima contains anastomosing elastic fibers in the interstices of which are longitudinally oriented smooth muscle cells (EVG, ×300).

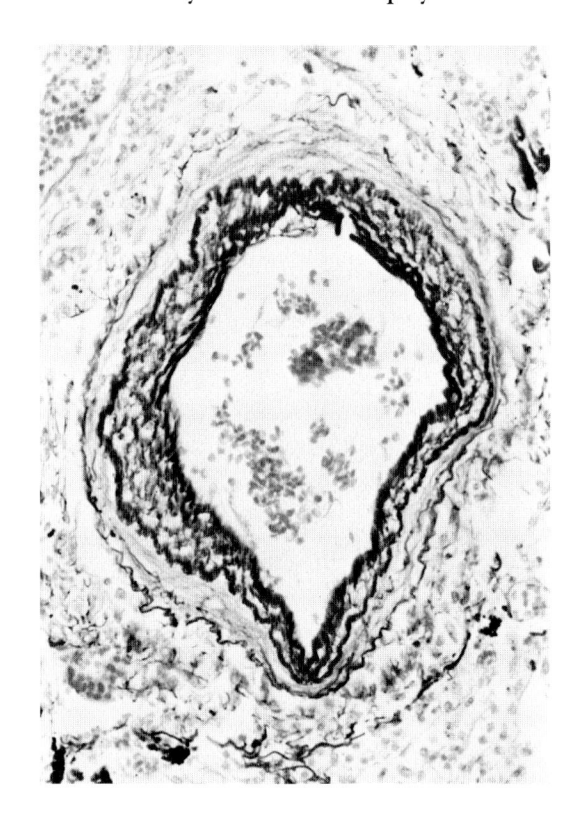

Figure 24–59. Muscular pulmonary artery from a 48-year-old man with panacinar emphysema. The media shows only a mild degree of hypertrophy. The initmal layer consists of anastomosing elastic fibers, but the smooth muscle cells have become converted into fibrous tissue. Such appearances may represent an aging phenomenon within the intimal longitudinal muscle (EVG, ×300).

In emphysema the muscular pulmonary arteries do not commonly show the pronounced medial hypertrophy that characterizes the pulmonary vascular disease of congenital cardiac shunts, left atrial hypertension, or primary pulmonary hypertension. This is almost certainly a reflection of the fact that usually the degree of pulmonary hypertension in emphysema is less severe and sustained than in the cardiac conditions listed previously.

The intimal fibrosis which occurs in the pulmonary arteries in emphysema is also mild compared with that which develops in congenital cardiac anomalies or mitral stenosis. It incorporates far less elastic tissue than is found in plexogenic pulmonary arteriopathy, and the degree of obstruction of vessels is less (see Fig. 24–59). The appearances suggest that this intimal proliferation is not important in elevating pulmonary vascular resistance in emphysema and certainly does not form an organic basis for irreversible pulmonary hypertension.

The important vascular change in the lung in emphysema seems to be muscularization of pulmonary arterioles, so that these vessels come to resemble systemic arterioles with a distinct muscular media sandwiched between two elastic laminae (Fig. 24–60). There is a close relation between the development of such muscularized pulmonary arterioles and right ventricular hypertrophy in emphysema, suggesting that they represent the organic basis for the increased pulmonary vascular resistance in this disease.[205]

Hypoxic Hypertensive Pulmonary Vascular Disease

This muscularization of the terminal portions of the pulmonary arterial tree occurs in all states of chronic hypoxia irrespective of etiology. It has thus been reported in healthy Quechua and Aymara Indians living at high altitude in Peru and Bolivia,[195] and in sufferers of Monge's disease,[196] the pickwickian syndrome, and thoracic deformities such as kyphoscoliosis. This association led to the introduction of the concept of hypoxic hypertensive pulmonary vascular disease, having the histologic features just described.[208]

Studies of experimental rats exposed to hypobaric hypoxia[209,210] confirm that hypoxic muscularization of the terminal portions of the pulmonary arterial tree is highly reversible together with the associated pulmonary hypertension. The results of such experiments, instructive as they are, should not be applied uncritically to

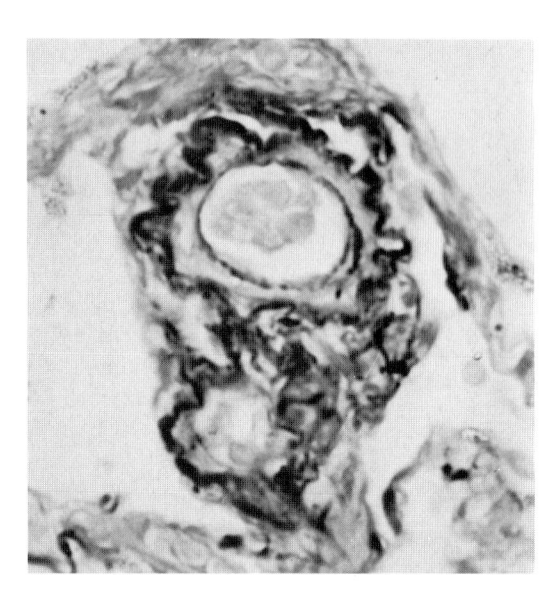

Figure 24–60. Transverse section of a muscularized pulmonary arteriole from a patient with pulmonary emphysema. The vessel consists of an outer, original elastic lamina internal to which is a layer of circularly oriented smooth muscle lined by a new, thin internal elastic lamina. Below the vessel is a precapillary which also shows a pad of smooth muscle in its wall (EVG, ×804).

human disease and in particular to the pulmonary vascular lesions of emphysema. In emphysema the vascular disease in the lungs includes an element of intimal proliferation probably due to myofibroblasts. Although this intimal hyperplasia is not so florid and occlusive as that occurring with congenital cardiac septal defects, it is nevertheless present. Attempts have been made to bring about a reversal of the increased pulmonary vascular resistance which accompanies the sustained hypoxia of chronic airflow obstruction by long-term oxygen therapy. Such treatment of based on the idea that relief from hypoxia may relax the constricted terminal portions of the pulmonary arterial tree and thereby in the long-term cause regression of the hyperplasia of smooth muscle. Although one can accept that premise, it seems unlikely that oxygen will stop the activity of myofibroblasts or lead to a regression of their secretions, namely collagen and elastin.

Other Vascular Lesions in Emphysema

Exceptionally a severe and sustained pulmonary hypertension in emphysema will be associated with fibrinoid necrosis of pulmonary arteries.[211] Pulmonary thrombi are common in the disease and frequently undergo organization and recanalization. The capillary blood vessels which bring about this recanalization are often derived from the vasa vasorum which originate from bronchial arteries, and thus they effect bronchopulmonary anastomoses.

Chemoreceptor Tissue and Pulmonary Circulation

Glomic tissue is found in various sites throughout the body such as the carotid bodies, the aorticopulmonary bodies including the so-called glomus pulmonale, and the glomus jugulare. These structures are sensitive to changes in the pressure of oxygen and carbon dioxide in the blood as well as its pH. In addition foci of glomic tissue have been described in association with pulmonary venules. Argyrophilic cells with an ultrastructure similar to that of the carotid bodies are found scattered throughout the bronchial mucosa. They occur either singly as Feyrter cells or in corpuscular groups termed neuroepithelial bodies.

The Carotid Bodies

These organs are of interest in cardiopulmonary pathology in that they show alterations in size and histologic appearance in states of chronic hypoxemia induced by many forms of lung disease. They form typically ovoid, pedunculated organs which arise from the bifurcations of both common carotid arteries. Usually there is one carotid body within the bifurcation, but sometimes there may be two cartoid bodies on one side and one on the other, each receiving a blood supply through its own glomic artery.[212] Glomic arteries may also originate from either the internal or external carotid arteries or the ascending pharyngeal artery.

The carotid body is easily dissected free and can then be weighed. In one series,[213] the average weight of the right carotid body was 12.9 mg; that of the left was 11.3 mg. In another series of 57 subjects with normal cardiac weights, the mean weight of both carotid bodies combined was 18.0 mg, with an estimated upper limit of normal of 30 mg.[212]

Under conditions of chronic hypoxemia, the carotid bodies enlarge. They were found to be larger in the Quechua Indians of Cerro de Pasco, a mining town in the Peruvian Andes at an altitude of 4330 m above sea level, than in mestizos living in Lima at sea level.[214] A similar increase in size of the carotid bodies with altitude has also been found in animals such as cattle which like humans have to acclimatize.[215] Since the enlargement of the carotid bodies at high altitude is associated with the hypobaric hypoxia, it is not surprising that a similar increase in their size occurs in those patients with emphysema with chronic alveolar hypoxia.[213,216] Here the enlargement of the carotid bodies is not related either to the type or the severity of emphysema, but to the presence of hypoxemia and right ventricular hypertrophy.[216]

Hypoxia does not appear to be the sole factor responsible for the hyperplasia of glomic tissue, as some patients with systemic hypertension and left ventricular hypertrophy in the absence of emphysema also had enlarged carotid bodies.[216] This association was later confirmed in a series of 100 routine necropsies from which it transpired that left ventricular hypertrophy due to other causes such as aortic stenosis was not associated with enlargement of the carotid bodies, suggesting that in some way systemic hypertension causes the glomic hyperplasia.[212]

Histology of the Carotid Body

The carotid body consists of several ovoid lobules of glomic tissue separated by an acellular collagenous stroma (Fig. 24–61). The whole structure is enclosed by an ill-defined capsule of loose collagenous and adipose tissue. Each lobule contains many clusters of glomic cells which are usually spherical, but some may be ovoid or cord-like (see Fig. 24–61). The parenchymal tissues comprise chief (type I) and sustentacular (type II) cells. The former has three variants designated by the appearance of their rounded nuclei as light, dark, and pyknotic. Sustentacular cells are elongated, and it has been suggested that they are related to Schwann cells. They are more numerous at the periphery of each cell cluster where they separate the chief cells from the blood capillaries and form a thin envelope around each cell cluster.

When the carotid body undergoes hyperplasia, either

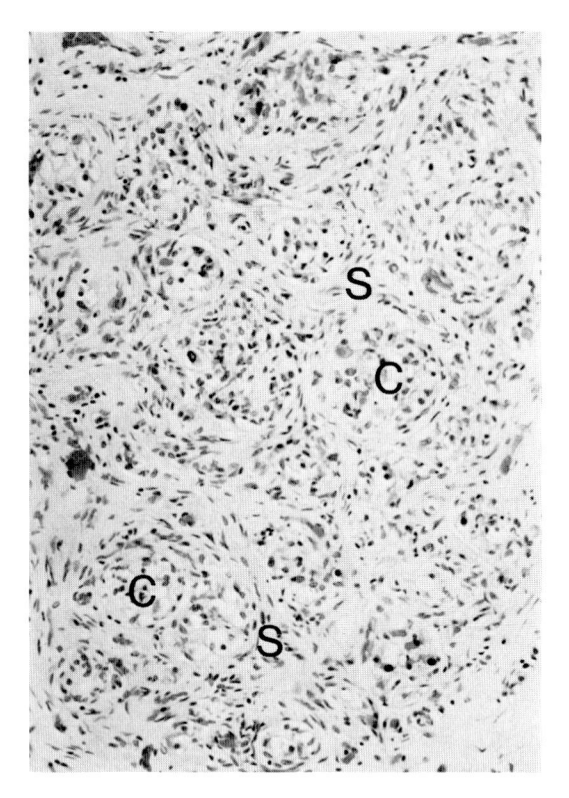

Figure 24–62. Hyperplastic carotid body at the same magnification as Figure 24–61 from a woman of 80 years with systemic hypertension. A lobule is greatly enlarged and only part of it is shown. The arrangement of glomic tissue into cell clusters is accentuated by the hyperplastic sustentacular cells (s) which form a thick envelope to each cell cluster. Chief cells (c) are restricted to the center of the clusters and are atrophic (H&E, ×150).

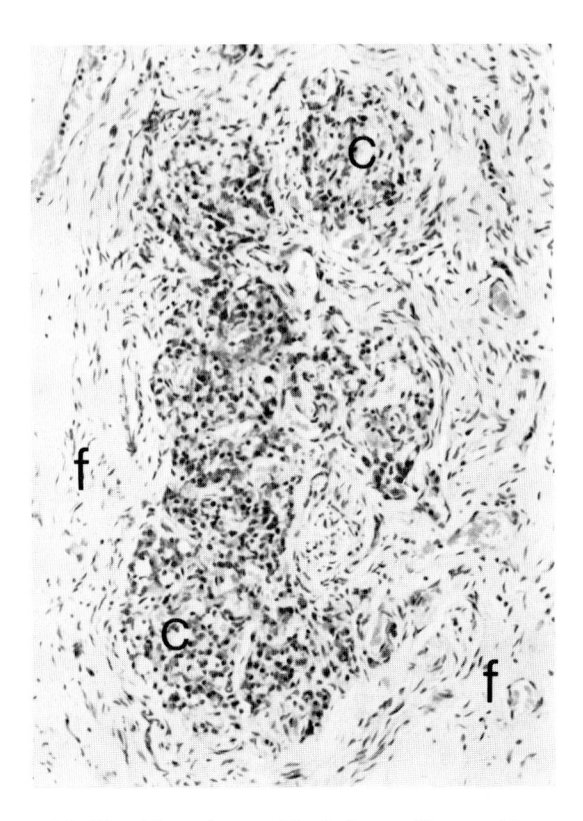

Figure 24–61. Normal carotid body from a 57-year-old woman. An entire lobule of glomic tissue is shown which is surrounded by a fibrous stroma (f) containing fibrocytes and blood vessels. The glomic tissue is organized into roughly circular cell clusters consisting predominantly of chief cells (c). Elongated sustentacular cells are inconspicuous (H&E, ×150).

in response to hypoxemia or systemic hypertension, the lobules enlarge greatly (Fig. 24–62), but the cell clusters remain the same size: they are simply more numerous.[212,217] The two types of glomic cells do not proliferate to the same degree. In the hyperplastic carotid body of the high-altitude guinea pig, the qualitative impression is that the light cells are disproportionately more numerous.[215] However, in a quantitative investigation[212] of human hyperplastic carotid bodies, the sustentacular cells underwent hyperplasia, increasing from the normal value of 39 percent of the cell population to 55 percent of the cells. So intense is the hyperplasia of sustentacular cells that is can be detected without recourse to measurement (see Fig. 24–62). The sustentacular cells are larger and broader than normal and form a thick rind to the cell cluster which sometimes appears to compress and obliterate the chief cells within it.[217]

Ultrastructurally the most characteristic feature of the chief cells of the carotid body is the possession of numerous secretory vesicles which resemble neurosecretory granules and consist of a central dense core surrounded by a clear halo and a limiting membrane. These granules contain catecholamines which are thought to be released by hypoxemia. In guinea pigs at high altitude, the central core of the granules becomes smaller, and the halo widens so that it is transformed into a microvacuole.[218] This change may represent increased secretion of catecholamine in response to hypoxia, thereby stimulating an increase in respiration. Another possibility is that the vacuolation of the granules in chief cells represents secretion of a hormone. The chief cells share many ultrastructural and biochemical properties with the amine precurser uptake and decarboxylation series of cells, many of which have been shown to secrete polypeptide hormones.[219]

It may seem self-evident that the carotid body enlarges at high altitude and in emphysema in reponse to the stimulus of chronic hypoxia. However, several observations are inconsistent with this hypothesis. Native highlanders and patients with chronic hypoxemia show an impaired hypoxic drive.[220] The carotid body undergoes hyperplasia in patients with systemic hypertension in which there is no hypoxemia. Finally, it is not the bioamine-containing chief cell which proliferates in carotid body hyperplasia but the sustentacular cell. Indeed chief cells appear to be ablated by the hyperplastic sustentacular cells, and this may explain the reduced hypoxic drive in these subjects. On these grounds, it seems necessary to postulate an underlying factor common to systemic hypertension, cor pulmonale due to pulmonary emphysema and residence at high altitude which is associated with proliferation of sustentacular cells. The common denominator may be sodium and water retention.[217] Honig and Schmidt[221] showed that stimulation of the carotid body increases renal sodium excretion due to the inhibition of renal tubular sodium absorption, and section of the carotid sinus nerves in cats prevents this natriuresis. They also found that the carotid bodies of rats with spontaneous systemic hypertension were significantly larger than those of age-matched, normotensive control subjects. It is thus conceivable that the carotid body secretes a substance that corrects the tendency to develop edema by inhibiting sodium reabsorption in the renal tubules. There is evidence that such a circulating substance exists,[222] but it is not known whether it is produced by the carotid bodies.

The Glomus Pulmonale

According to Krahl,[223] there is a glomus associated with each branchial arch and its derivatives. Thus the glomus jugulare is situated on the second arch, the carotid bodies on the third, and the aorticopulmonary bodies on the fifth arch which fails to persist. Krahl suggested that there is also a glomus associated with the sixth arch which becomes the pulmonary trunk. This structure he designated the glomus pulmonale and suggested that it had a chemoreceptor function in association with the pulmonary circulation. Edwards and Heath[224] confirmed the existence of this structure as a nodule of glomic tissue just distal and caudal to the bifurcation of the pulmonary trunk, but disputed that it is a true glomus pulmonale receiving its blood supply from the pulmonary trunk. It seems more likely that the artery supplying this glomic tissue is one of the intertruncal branches of the coronary arteries which passes up between the ascending aorta and the pulmonary trunk.[224,225] Edwards and Heath[226] traced the blood supply to this glomus by serial sections in a 32-week-old stillborn and also by latex injection studies in rats. Both studies confirmed that it receives a systemic arterial blood supply from the intertruncal arteries. It is, therefore, most probably one of the coronary groups of aorticopulmonary bodies which is situated in the adventitia of the pulmonary trunk.

Pulmonary Venous Glomic Tissue

In some subjects, there are small nodules of glomic tissue associated with the pulmonary venules.[227] They measure about 1 mm in diameter and are found close to pulmonary venules up to 100 μm in diameter. Such multiple nodules of glomic tissue were first described by Korn and colleagues[228] who regarded them as neoplastic. However, they can be found occasionally in routine sections of lung taken at necropsy.[227] At present their functional significance is unknown.

Feyrter Cells and Neuroepithelial Bodies

If the bronchial mucosa is stained with silver salts using a technique to demonstrate argyrophilia, darkly staining cells will be found scattered diffusely among the epithelial cells of bronchi and bronchioles either singly or in small groups. These are collectively referred to as pulmonary agryrophil cells, although the single cells are termed Feyrter cells and the groups of cells neuroepithelial bodies. Histologically and ultrastructurally, the two cells are identical, and it is likely that they have the same function whatever that may be.

Feyrter cells have been described in various species including rats, rabbits, guinea pigs, hamsters, and humans. In the rat, they are common during the neonatal period, but their density falls off rapidly during the first weeks of life.[229] They are also common in the human infant.[230] This suggests that they may be chemoreceptors which mediate the changes in the lung during the transition to extrauterine life. They bear a close similarity to the chief cells of the carotid body in that they contain numerous dense core vesicles (Fig. 24–63), indistinguishable from those of the carotid body.[229,230] Moreover, these vesicles show a reduction in their cores to form microvacuoles in response to hypoxia in the same manner as occurs in the carotid body chief cell.[229] The possible effector response of such chemoreceptors is unclear. Conceivably any effect of argyrophil cells on the tone of the bronchial smooth muscle, especially at birth, could through dilation or constriction of bronchioles affect the degree of oxygenation in the alveolar spaces and thus the degree of constriction of the terminal portions of the pulmonary arterial tree. Whatever their function, they undoubtedly respond to hypoxia and are more numerous in rabbits native to high altitude than in

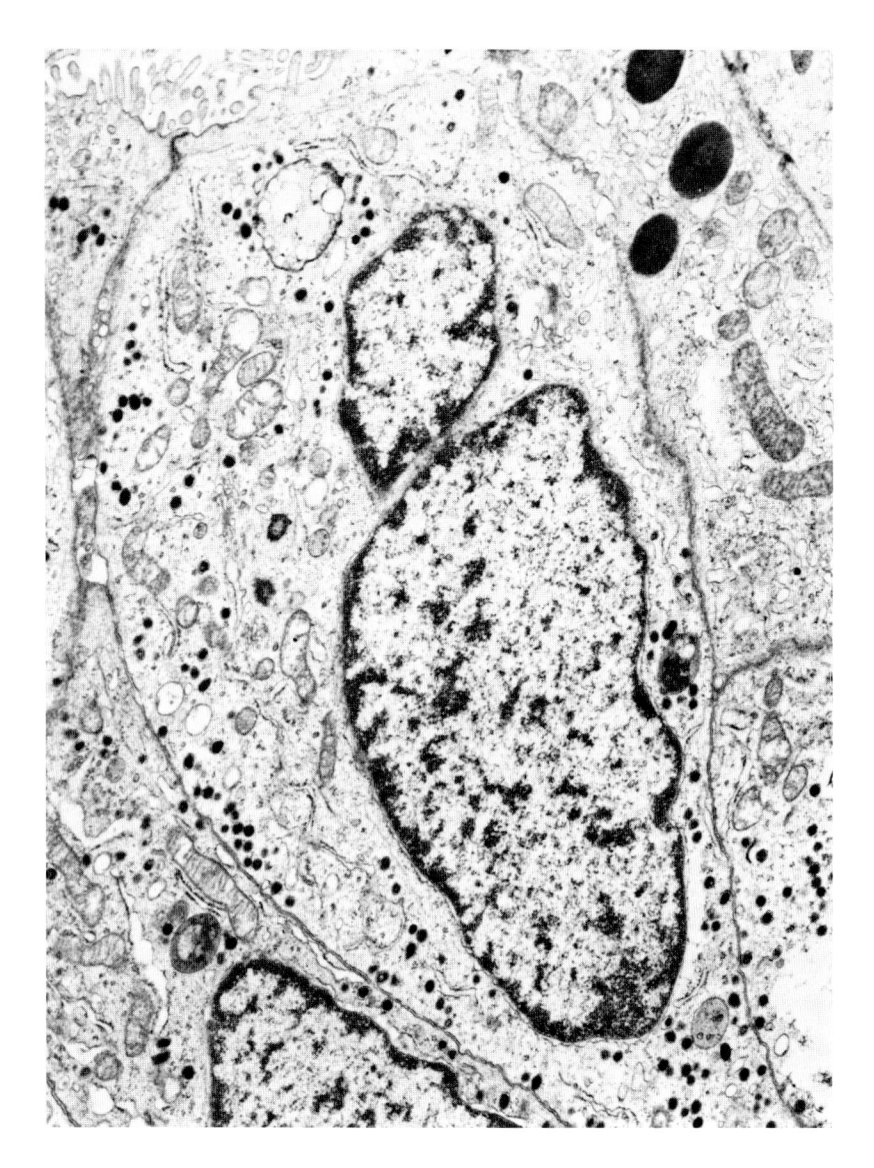

Figure 24–63. Part of a neuroepithelial body from the bronchus of a rabbit. A whole Feyrter cell is shown with parts of adjacent ones to the left and lower right. In addition to a large central nucleus and several mitochondria, the cells contain numerous, dark, spherical granules measuring 120 nm in diameter. These are the dense-core vesicles which resemble neurosecretory granules. This ultrastructural appearance is identical to that of the chief cells in the carotid body (EM, ×12,500).

sea level representatives of the same species.[231] To the practicing pathologist, however, their importance lies more in the possibility that they represent the cell of origin of tumorlets of lung, the bronchial carcinoid tumor, and oatcell carcinoma.

Vasculature of the Lung in Pulmonary Stenosis

When pulmonary stenosis is associated with a defect of the atrial or ventricular septum, the magnitude of the pulmonary blood flow and of the pressure in the pulmonary artery varies greatly from case to case and may be reduced, normal, or increased. The hemodynamic situation determines the structural changes, if any, that take place in the pulmonary vasculature.

With diminished pulmonary flow and pressure, the media of the pulmonary trunk is thin, being half or less of the medial thickness of the aorta.[75] The elastic fibrils of the media are either very thin or clumped together to form irregularly shaped masses. In Fallot's tetrad, the pulmonary trunk is commonly smaller and narrower than the aorta, but sometimes it is dilated due to the turbulence of the blood which vibrates the wall of the vessel and makes it more distensible.[232,233] The media of the muscular pulmonary arteries is thin, and these vessels are commonly dilated.[234,235] This atrophic state of the media has even been reported in infants with pulmonary stenosis or atresia suggesting that the thinning may even have commenced before birth.[236] Dilation of the pulmonary arteries results in complete filling of the vasculature

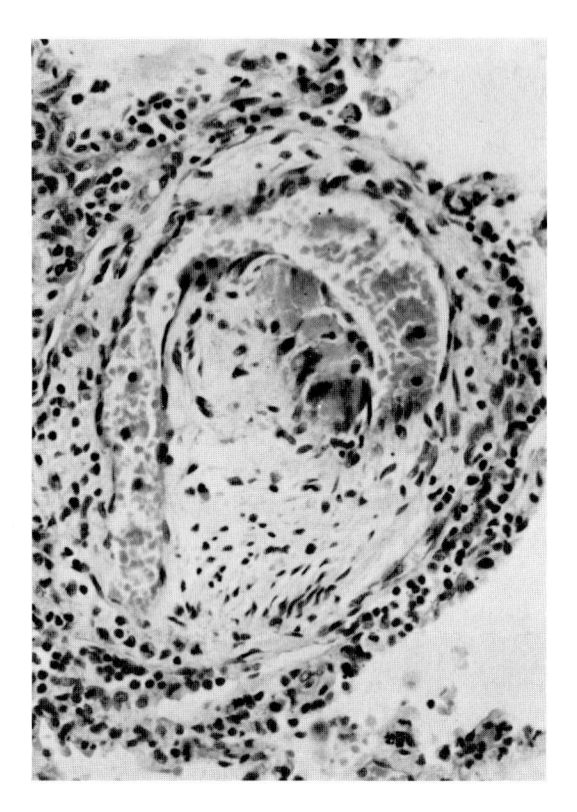

Figure 24-64. Transverse section of a muscular pulmonary artery from a case of tricuspid atresia. The lumen of the vessel contains a thrombus which is undergoing organization by granulation tissue. There is early recanalization with the formation of a crescentic lumen lined by prominent endothelial cells (H&E, ×292).

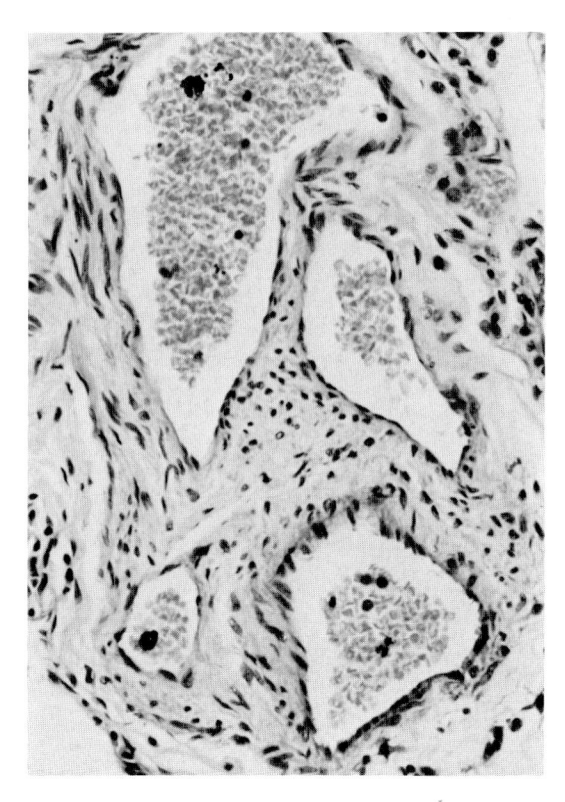

Figure 24-65. Muscular pulmonary artery from the same patient as in Figure 24-64 showing a colander lesion in which there are several recanalization channels lined by endothelium. These show the early development of smooth muscle in their walls (H&E, ×277).

which leads to a moss-like appearance in postmortem angiograms. Diminished flow and pressure in Fallot's tetrad become associated with increased blood viscosity due to polycythemia. This combination of factors predisposes to thrombus formation in the pulmonary blood vessels.[234,237,238] It is seen most prominently when pulmonary flow is less than 2.5 L/min/m² of body surface area.[238] Thrombosis in cyanotic congenital heart disease of this type is more common in adolescents and adults. The thrombi undergo organization into nodular, crescentic, and concentric forms (Fig. 24-64). They frequently become recanalized by thin-walled, endothelium-lined channels to form colander lesions (Fig. 24-65, 24-66). In severe congenital anomalies such as pulmonary or tricuspid atresia, as many as three-quarters of pulmonary blood vessels in a section may be involved by fresh or organizing thombi.

When the pulmonary blood flow in pulmonary stenosis is normal, the media of the pulmonary trunk is of normal thickness and has a normal elastic tissue pattern. The muscular pulmonary arteries are of normal medial thickness, and there is little or no evidence of thrombosis. When pulmonary stenosis is associated with a high pulmonary flow and pulmonary hypertension, the media of the pulmonary trunk may be as thick as that of the aorta. The elastic tissue pattern of the media is of aortic type, consistent with the presence of pulmonary hypertension from birth. In cases of Fallot's tetrad and allied congenital cardiac anomalies with pulmonary stenosis, the pulmonary arteries may become subjected to pulmonary hypertension due to an overgenerous improvement in the blood supply to the lung as a result of an anastomotic operation or total correction of the anomaly. The lungs of patients dying within a few days of an anastomotic operation for Fallot's tetrad usually show congestion and distension of blood vessels, with pulmonary edema and even rupture of capillaries with hemorrhage.[239] If the patient survives an overgenerous anastomosis to develop pulmonary hypertension, he shows initially increased medial thickness of muscular pulmonary arteries.[240] Even plexogenic pulmonary arteriopathy may develop, especially after the Potts and Waterston operations. The Blalock-Taussig operation carries less risk of the complication of pulmonary hypertension. After a total surgical correction of this congenital cardiac anomaly, there may be immediate pulmonary congestion and edema or later development of pulmonary hypertension.[241]

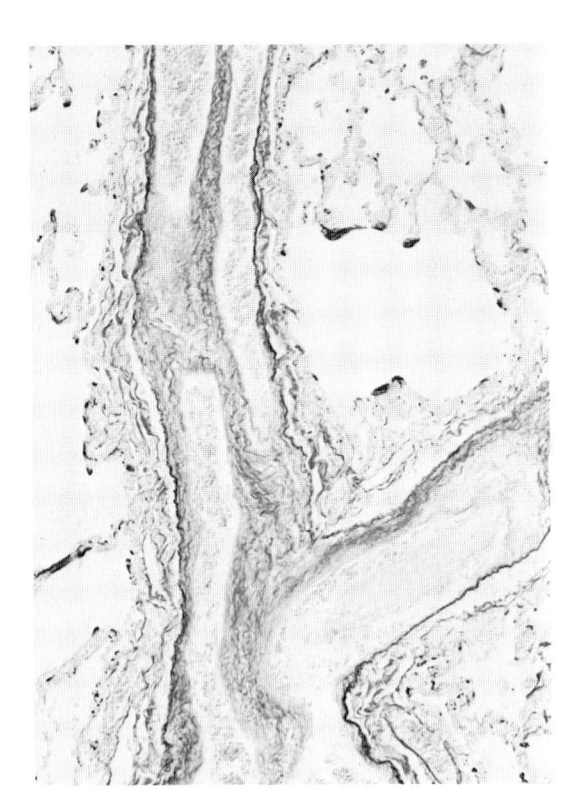

Figure 24–66. Longitudinal section through a large muscular pulmonary artery from the same patient as in Figures 24–64 and 24–65 containing a colander lesion. A web-like arrangement of fibrous septa divides the lumen into several separate channels. The media of the vessel is atrophic (EVG, ×132).

Parasites of the Pulmonary Circulation

Schistosomiasis

The human pulmonary circulation may become infested by helminthic parasites. One of these is the trematode Schistosoma which is a cause of severe pulmonary hypertension and congestive cardiac failure in many tropical and subtropical areas. Three species of these blood flukes live and copulate in veins. The adult *S. mansoni* wedges in the tributaries of the portal vein, especially in the walls of the colon; it is prevalent in Egypt and East Africa. *S. japonicum* lives in the veins of the small intestine; it is distributed throughout China, Japan, and the Far East. *S. haematobium* inhabits the veins of the urinary bladder. It is a scourge in many tropical countries but is especially common in Egypt. The adult male of this species is 13 mm long; the female, 20 mm, lies in the gynecophoric canal of the male. Copulation in the vesical veins leads to the production of ova, 130 μm in length, with a terminal spine. *S. mansoni* in the tributaries of the portal vein produces ova 140 μm long with a lateral spine. The eggs, voided by the two species in the urine or feces, respectively, swell and burst, liberating ciliated larvae called miracidia. These enter certain species of fresh water snails to form free-swimming cercariae which are highly infectious for humans. They enter the body through the skin or the mucous membranes of the mouth and pharynx and then burrow into systemic capillaries and small venules to enter the blood stream as metacercariae. Thus, they are carried once again to the veins of the colon, small intestine, or urinary bladder in which they take up permanent residence, depending on which species of Schistosoma is involved.

It is at this point that the pulmonary circulation may become involved, for ova laid by the females in these veins lack the protective coating of mucopolysaccharide found around the adult flukes. As a result, they stimulate a delayed hypersensitivity reaction with accumulation of epithelioid cells and dense fibrosis. Eggs may escape from these nodular, granulomatous areas to reach the liver, in which they bring about pipe-stem cirrhosis, and then to the lung, in which they impact in the pulmonary arterioles. Here the ova lead to pulmonary vascular disease which is far more complex than simply the result of mere impaction into pulmonary arteries with resultant progressive vascular obstruction. The obstruction is soon exaggerated by a granulomatous reaction, probably allergic in nature, around the egg[242–244] (Fig. 24–67). This

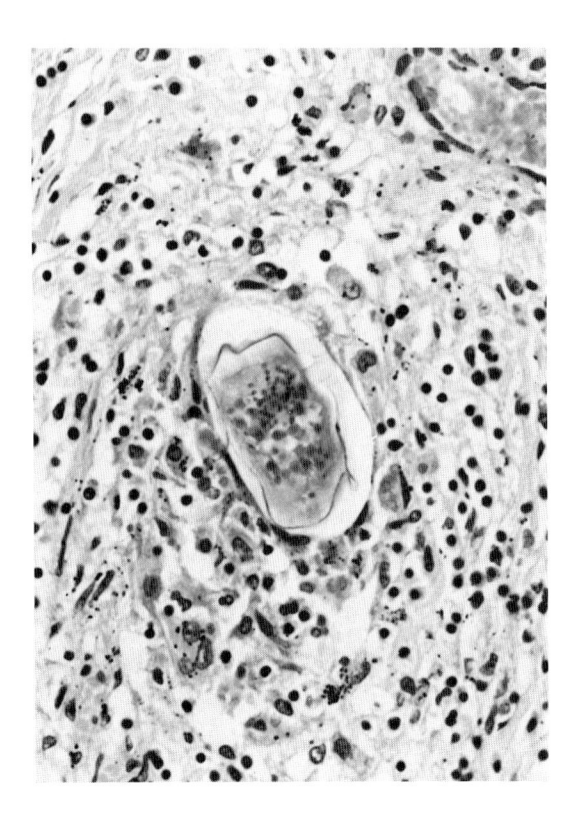

Figure 24–67. Pulmonary schistosomiasis. An ovum of *S. mansoni* is enclosed by a florid granulomatous reaction consisting of macrophages and epithelioid cells. This is surrounded by collagenous fibrosis which is infiltrated by lymphocytes, plasma cells, and eosinophil polymorphonuclear leukocytes (H&E, ×375).

comprises foreign body giant cells, eosinophils, and mononuclears, often with calcified remains of ova. This granulomatous reaction may be in the lumen, where it may provoke surrounding thrombosis, or it may penetrate the media of the pulmonary artery[245,246] (Fig. 24–68). A third component, in addition to pulmonary vascular obstruction and granulomatous reaction, is fibrinoid necrosis which is usually accepted by histopathologists as a manifestation of hypersensitivity or hypertension (Fig. 24–69). In pulmonary bilharzia, the fibrinoid necrosis is probably partly an allergic reaction to the foreign proteins of the ova[243–245] and partly a reaction by vasoconstriction to the severely raised pulmonary arterial pressure.

The most striking and classic histopathologic change in the lung in schistosomiasis is the angiomatoid lesion.[242,243,247] This probably arises in the same way as the dilatation lesions of plexogenic pulmonary arteriopathy. In bilharzia the occlusion of the muscular pulmonary arteries is due to the granulomatous reaction around the ova rather than to intimal fibroelastosis. Careful reconstruction of these bilharzial lesions show them to be identical in structure to the classic plexiform lesion.[248,249] Rarely Schistosoma ova have been observed in the angiomatoid lesions.[242]

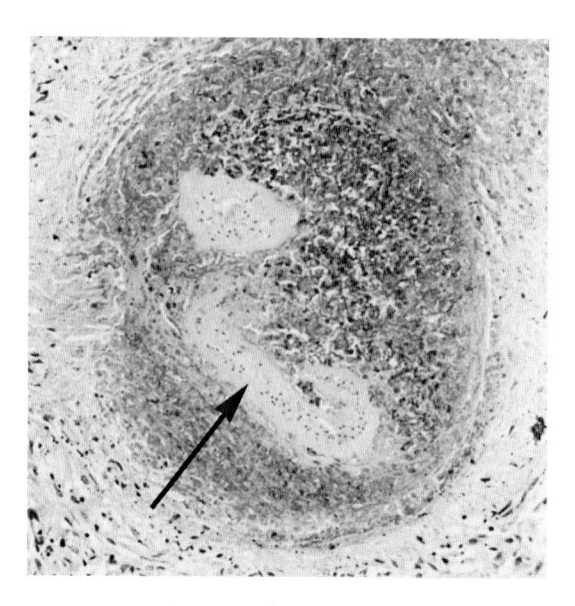

Figure 24–69. Pulmonary schistosomiasis with fibrinoid necrosis is a muscular pulmonary artery. The media is indistinct and amorphous (arrow) and is surrounded by an acute inflammatory exudate (H&E, ×150).

Filaria

The role of filariasis in the production of pulmonary vascular disease is far more controversial. During the period 1967 to 1972, there was an increased frequency of unexplained pulmonary hypertension in Sri Lanka.[250,251] The cases of primary pulmonary hypertension reported were unusual in that a disproportionately large number of men were affected, the severity of the pulmonary hypertension was unusual, and there was a frequent association with eosinophilia. These unusual clinical features and the occurrence of most cases on the southwest coastal border of the island where *Wuchereria bancrofti* infestation was endemic led Obeyesekere and co-workers[250,251] to suspect that filariasis was involved in the etiology of the elevated pulmonary arterial pressure.

In tropical pulmonary eosinophilia, the filarial worms are not confined to the lymphatic system but are found in the lungs as well as in the liver and spleen. It is believed that this condition represents hypersensitivity to a specific filarial antigen, so that while adult worms produce microfilariae, the so-called *Microfilaria nocturna*, they are destroyed rapidly in the blood. It has been postulated that many of these microfilariae are destroyed continually in the lung, leading to widespread blockage of pulmonary arterioles and capillaries and thus leading to severe pulmonary hypertension. These views are refuted by other observers who believe the cases to be examples of primary pulmonary hypertension with an underlying histopathology of plexogenic pulmonary arteriopathy.

Filarial worms are known to cause pulmonary hypertension in animals. *Brugia buckleyi* leads to right ventricular hypertrophy in the Ceylon wild hare.[252] The nematode *Dirofilaria immitis* may give rise to pulmonary

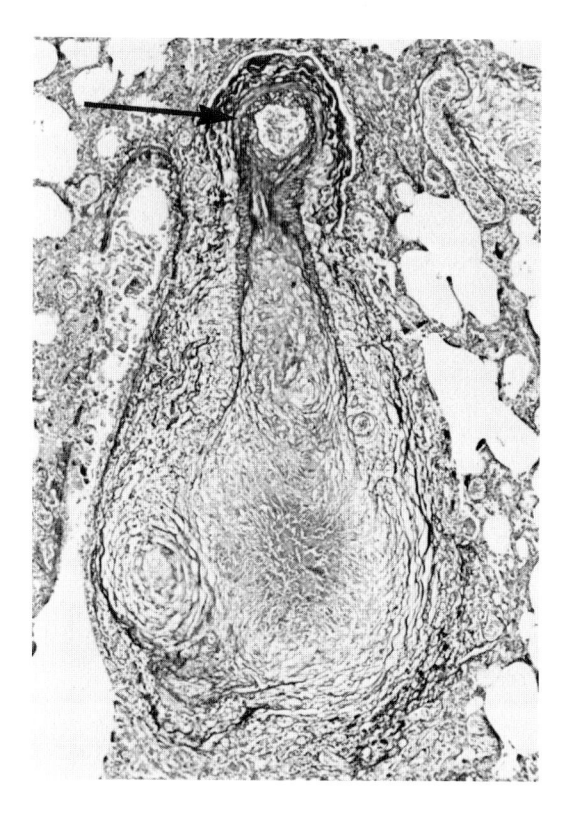

Figure 24–68. A pulmonary granuloma in schistosomiasis. A lateral branch containing several schistosomal granulomas arises from a parent vessel (arrow). These are associated with an intense fibrotic reaction. The media of the artery has been obliterated and replaced by collagen, so the granulomas are situated extravascularly (EVG, ×60).

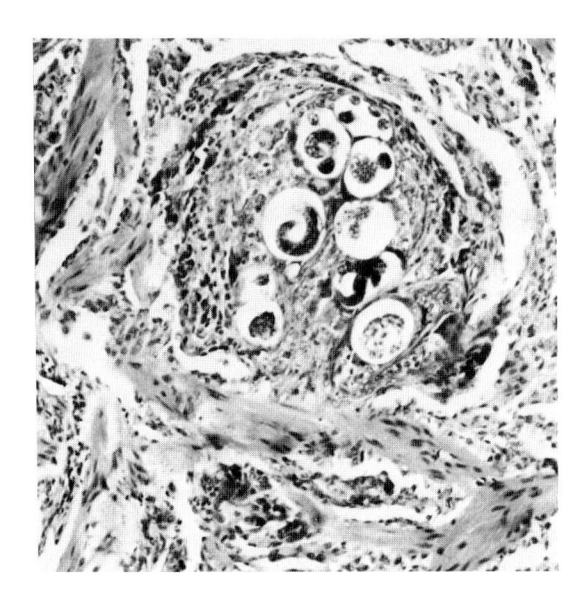

Figure 24-70. Lung of a cat infested with the nematode worm *A. abstrusus*. Extravasated ova showing various stages of development are surounded by a granuloma consisting of macrophages and epithelioid cells. Note the hyperplastic smooth muscle in the surrounding lung parenchyma (H&E, ×150).

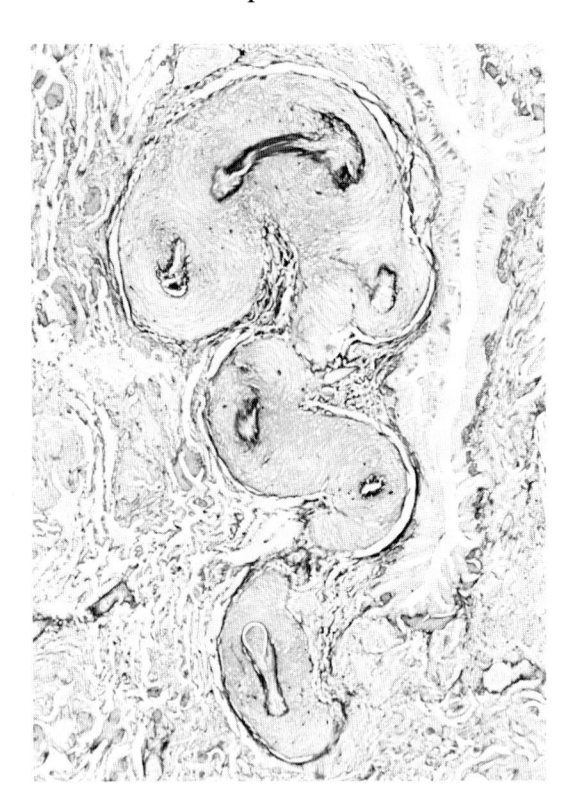

Figure 24-71. Muscular pulmonary artery from a cat infested with *A. abstrusus*. The media of the vessel is grossly thickened and tortuous. Such hypertrophy and hyperplasia of vascular smooth muscle is thought to be due to chemical substances released from the worms rather than to physical obstruction to the vessel (EVG, ×60).

hypertension in dogs. A lung mite *Pneumonyssus simicola* has been reported to enter the pulmonary arteries of monkeys and bring about pathologic changes in them.[253]

Cat Lung Worm

Cats may become infested with lung worm *Aelurostrongylus abstrusus* and develop pulmonary vascular disease as a result. The adult worms live in the pulmonary arteries and terminal bronchioles and deposit eggs there (Fig. 24-70). This nematode parasite has a complex life cycle involving snails and mice or birds as paratenic hosts. The lung worms induce pulmonary hypertension with gross muscular thickening of the pulmonary arteries by hypertrophy and hyperplasia (Fig. 24-71), which is probably a response to toxic substances derived from the worms, the eggs, or first stage larvae.[254] At the same time there is pronounced hyperplasia of smooth muscle in the lung parenchyma and bronchial tree as well as in the vasculature (*see* Fig. 24-70)

Developmental Anomalies

Pulmonary Trunk

The earliest blood supply to the developing lungs comes from paired segmental arteries arising from the dorsal aorta caudal to the aortic arches,[255] but later it comes from the developing main pulmonary arteries which arise from the sixth aortic arches.[256] The development of the sixth arch has been considered in detail.[257] It receives ventral and dorsal buds but also a pulmonary postbranchial plexus derived from arteries arising from the dorsal aortae in the vicinity of the primary lung bud. (The development of the pulmonary vasculature is considered in Chapters 1 and 2.)

The pulmonary trunk may show congenital idiopathic dilation, perhaps as a forme fruste of Marfan's syndrome.[258] Conversely it may show congenital stenosis immediately above the pulmonary valve which must be distinguished from degenerative calcified rings in the pulmonary trunk of the elderly.[51] Stenosis of the bifurcation of the pulmonary trunk has been described and designated coarctation of the pulmonary artery.[259] Atresia may reduce the pulmonary trunk to a cord-like structure when it is commonly associated with components of Fallot's tetrad or stenosis of peripheral pulmonary arteries.

In persistent truncus arteriosus, the spiral septum fails to develop so that the primitive vessel remains as a single artery with a single semilunar valve (Fig. 24-72). There are anatomic variants.[260] In the first three of the four types, the pulmonary trunk or pulmonary arteries arise

Figure 24–72. Persistent truncus arteriosus of type III. A common arterial trunk from the heart gives rise both to systemic arterial vessels (A) and pulmonary arteries (P).

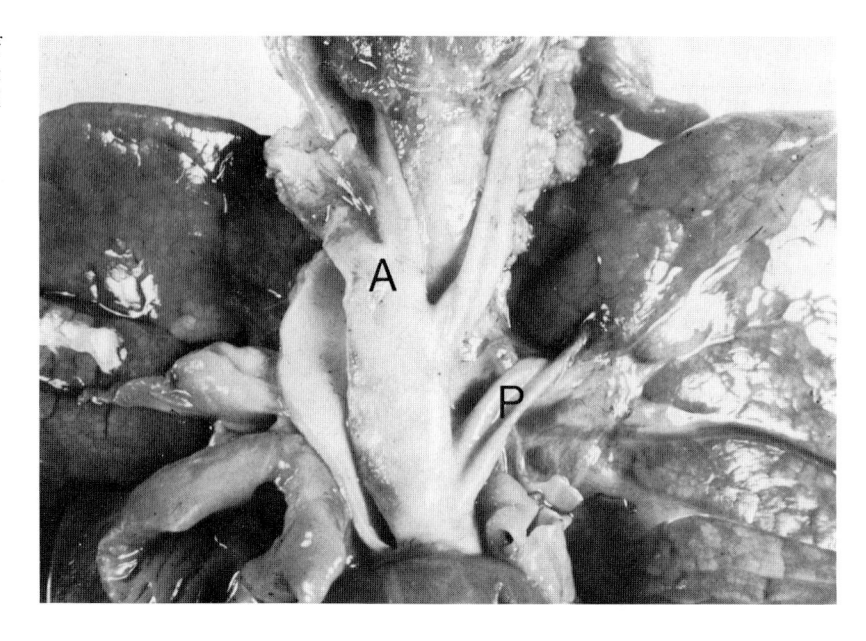

from the truncus (see Fig. 24–72). If large enough, they allow the development of pulmonary hypertension and plexogenic pulmonary arteriopathy. In the fourth type, the blood supply to the lungs is through the bronchial arteries, and there is no elevation of pulmonary arterial pressure. Aortopulmonary septal defect may be regarded as a partial form of persistent truncus arteriosus, the defect representing a focal absence of the truncoconal septum. This uncommon congenital condition is associated with patent ductus arteriosus only in about a tenth of the cases.[261] Like the persistent truncus, the aortopulmonary septal defect acts like a post-tricuspid shunt, elevating pulmonary arterial pressure and leading to plexogenic pulmonary arteriopathy.

The coronary arteries may originate from the pulmonary trunk, the most common variant being origin of the left coronary artery from the pulmonary trunk which leads to serious ischemia of the left ventricle in infancy.[262] In these patients, a retrograde flow occurs from the aorta, through the right coronary artery, which becomes enlarged, into the left coronary artery with the anomalous origin into the pulmonary trunk. Anomalous origin of the right coronary artery is more likely to allow survival to adult life, but origin of both coronary arteries from the pulmonary trunk is rapidly fatal.[263]

Pulmonary Arteries

The major pulmonary arteries may have an anomalous origin from the pulmonary arterial system, the aorta, or its branches. They may also be subject to stenosis or atresia. The right pulmonary artery may arise below and to the left of the left pulmonary artery so that the left vessel has to cross in front of its right partner on its way to supply the left lung. Such crossed pulmonary arteries[264] are of no functional significance. Exceptionally the left pulmonary artery arises from its right counterpart proximal to its branches[265] and passes back to the left lung, pressing down on the right main bronchus. It then courses behind the trachea and in front of the esophagus. This vascular sling does not exert untoward hemodynamic effects but has some clinical significance in obstructing the right bronchus.

Very rarely the pulmonary trunk continues as a single pulmonary artery to supply one of the lungs, the other receiving an anomalous systemic supply originating from the ascending aorta or aortic arch by way of the ductus arteriosus or the innominate artery. Such unilateral absence of a pulmonary artery may involve either lung, but the pulmonary trunk is more likely to continue as the right pulmonary artery.[266] There is often pulmonary hypertension in the lung receiving the normal pulmonary arterial supply; this may occur because the lung is exposed to the entire cardiac output from fetal life when the pulmonary arteries are normally thick walled.[267] The minority of patients developing pulmonary hypertension may be composed of subjects with hyperreactive pulmonary arteries. Sometimes pulmonary hypertension develops in the other lung due to its systemic blood supply.

Sometimes a lobe, or part of a lobe, of a lung does not communicate with the bronchial tree and has the structure of a hamartoma. This abnormal sequestration of lung, which usually involves the left lower lobe, is supplied by one or more arteries that arise from either the lower thoracic or abdominal aorta.[268,269] The surrounding lung has a normal pulmonary arterial supply. Some authorities[270] regard the anomalous arteries as the primary abnormality leading to the sequestration, whereas others[271] consider the arterial supply secondary. Sequestrations of lung may be intralobar or extralobar, and the latter may take the form of a cyst in the diaphragm[272] (Fig. 24–73). The arteries supplying a sequestration of lung are subjected to systemic blood pressure and show hypertensive changes such as atheroma,[273] plexiform lesions[274] and necrotizing

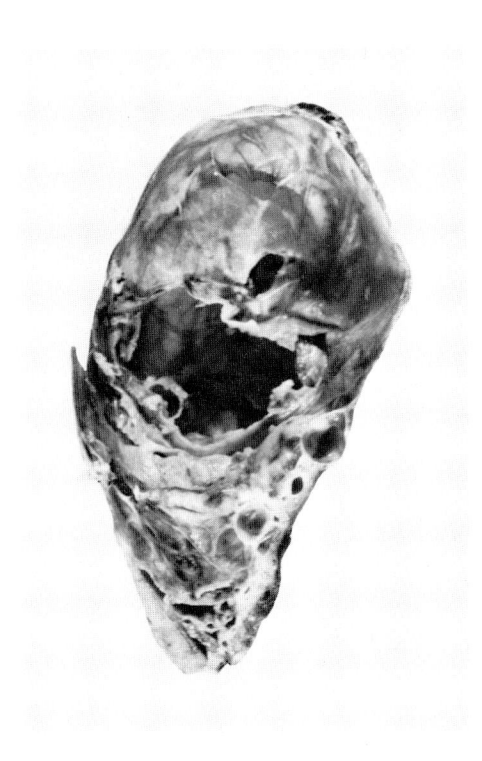

Figure 24–73. Extralobular sequestration of lung presenting as a cyst in the diaghram (×2).

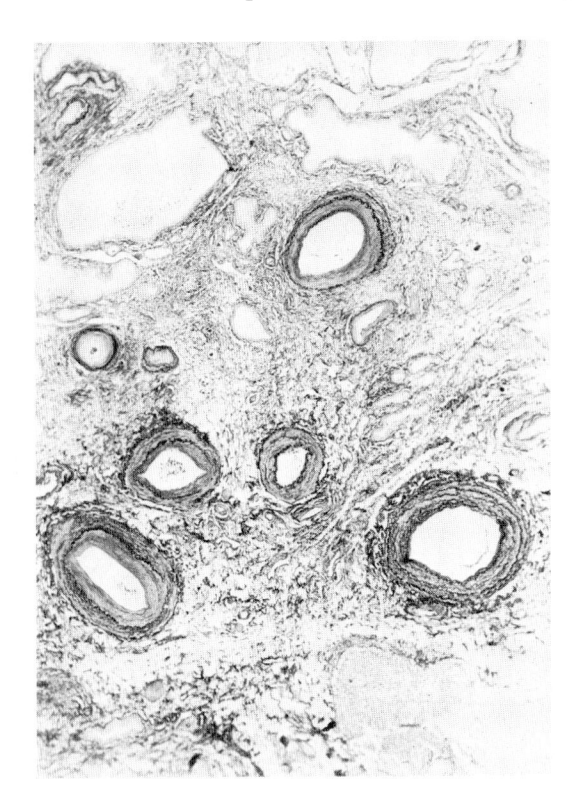

Figure 24–74. Extralobular sequestration of lung from the same patient seen in Figure 24–73. Arteries supplying the sequestration are derived from the systemic circulation and have developed an elastic media despite their small diameter. They more closely resemble elastic pulmonary arteries than systemic vessels, although their have retained a thick media. Several vessels are affected by intimal fibrosis (EVG, ×60).

arteritis.[272] On arising from the aorta, the anomalous arteries are elastic but more distally become muscular. On entering the sequestration, they become thick walled and tortuous and may show a combination of histologic features normally associated with systemic and pulmonary arteries; for this reason, they are sometimes called hybrid arteries (Fig. 24–74).

Congenital stenosis of the pulmonary arteries in the lung substance constitutes a rare cause of pulmonary hypertension.[275] Four variants based on the local or diffuse nature of the stenosis are recognized. The stenoses are due to medial thickening and intimal proliferation in involved segments of vessels and, being associated with congenital rubella,[276] are found with other forms of congenital cardiac anomaly such as coarctation of the aorta.

Pulmonary Veins

Since the lungs are derived by division of the foregut, they share with it a blood supply from the splanchnic plexus. This plexus drains into systemic pre- and postcardinal veins, the umbilicovitelline system, hepatic sinusoids, and so on. Hence the primordia of the lungs drain at first not into the heart but into a wide variety of veins throughout the body, making possible all manner of congenital abnormalities of the pulmonary venous system. Only later does an outpouching from the heart called the common pulmonary vein extend into that part of the splanchnic plexus related to the lungs.

In the condition of anomalous pulmonary venous drainage, the pulmonary veins drain into the right atrium or systemic or portal veins (Fig. 24–75). It is said to be partial when part of the pulmonary venous drainage is into the left atrium, and total when none of the drainage is normal. Other congenital cardiac anomalies are commonly associated with anomalous pulmonary venous drainage.[277] Anatomic sites receiving anomalous pulmonary veins include the left innominate vein, right atrium, coronary sinus, right superior vena cava, portal vein (see Fig. 24–75), ductus venosus, inferior vena cava, and hepatic vein. In total anomalous pulmonary venous drainage, all the blood returning to the heart in systemic and pulmonary veins drains into the right atrium from which it passes either into the right ventricle and pulmonary circulation or through an atrial septal defect into the left atrium and thence into the systemic circulation. There is a high pulmonary blood flow, and this leads to pulmonary arterial hypertension. However, in part the pulmonary hypertension found in this condition is also related to pulmonary venous obstruction due to kinking

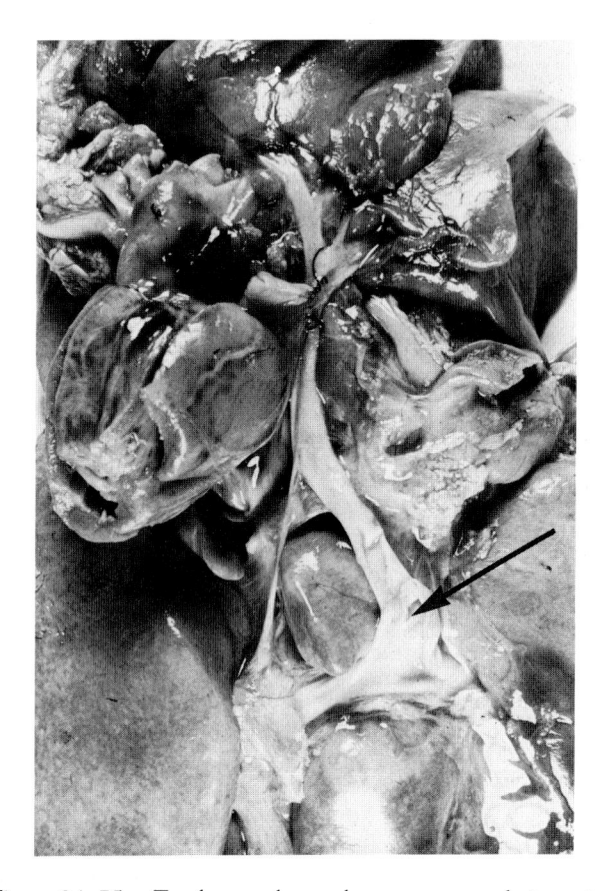

Figure 24-75. Total anomalous pulmonary venous drainage in which the pulmonary veins drain directly into the hepatic portal vein (arrow).

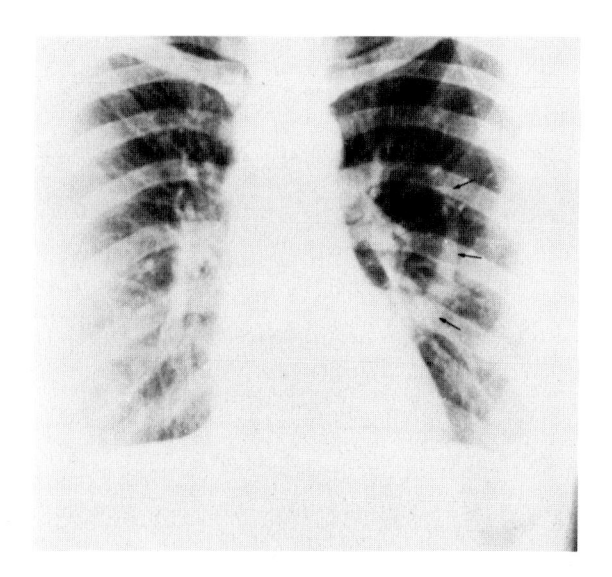

Figure 24-76. Chest radiograph from a case of the scimitar syndrome. The anomalous pulmonary vein (arrows) can be seen as a crescent-shaped shadow in the right lung field.

of the long anomalous veins or to stenotic lesions in them or by pressure of contiguous structures on them.

Cor triatriatum is thought to be a malformation of the pulmonary venous system brought about by failure of the common pulmonary vein to become absorbed by differentiated growth into the left atrium. Hence there is an accessory atrial chamber connected to the left atrium by an opening, and the pulmonary veins drain into this chamber.[278] The hemodynamic and pathologic effects of the condition are like those of mitral stenosis.

In the scimitar syndrome, a bilobar right lung with a systemic arterial supply occurs in association with anomalous pulmonary venous drainage.[279] The anomalous veins can be recognized on a chest radiograph as a crescent-shaped shadow resembling a scimitar, hence the name of the syndrome (Fig. 24-76). The right upper lobe is supplied by pulmonary arteries, but the right lower lobe is supplied by systemic arteries from the descending aorta. The pulmonary arteries in the right lower lobe may develop hypertensive changes including plexiform lesions.[280]

Stenosis of pulmonary veins with normal connections is common. The severity of the condition varies so that in some patients only one or a few veins are involved, whereas in others the condition may be widespread throughout the lungs.[281,282] The stenoses are due to localized fibrous proliferation and are usually restricted to the venoatrial junction[283] (Fig. 24-77). The condition brings about pulmonary venous and arterial hypertension and the histopathologic changes in the lungs associated with these hemodynamic disturbances.

Arteriovenous fistula of the lung is sometimes erroneously referred to as a cavernous hemangioma. It consists of a distended, thin-walled artery leading to a labyrinth of dilated vessels which in turn drain into efferent veins.[284] The fistulae in a lung may be so small as to resemble telangiectases or so large as to replace an entire lobe by a pulsating mass of vessels.[285] The vessels forming the substance of the fistula are cavernous, blood-filled spaces linked to one another and frequently show severe intimal fibrosis and contain organizing thrombi. Structurally they are more akin to pulmonary veins than arteries. Patients with this disease frequently show vascular nevi on the lips, face, and soft palate, indicating that this condition is a manifestation of Rendu-Osler-Weber's disease. The shunting of a large flow of deoxygenated blood into the pulmonary veins brings about cyanosis, finger clubbing, and polycythemia.[285] Such fistulae lead to systolic murmurs and thrills over the chest and produce worm-like shadows on the chest radiographs.

Pulmonary Vasculature in Fibrosis of the Lung

When pulmonary fibrosis affects primarily the alveolar walls, it is termed interstitial or fibrosing alveolitis. The initial effect is on the pulmonary capillaries, although with progression of the disease, the pulmonary arterioles

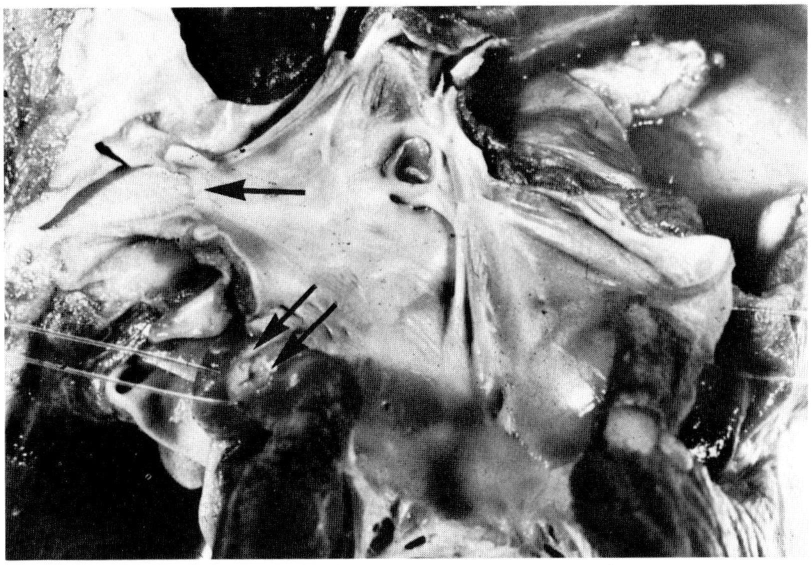

Figure 24–77. Congenital stenosis of pulmonary veins. The left atrium has been opened to show the origins of the pulmonary veins which are compressed by large fibrous pads (single arrow). One vein has been cut transversely to show its thickened wall and narrow lumen (double arrow).

and muscular pulmonary arteries become secondarily involved. On the other hand, fibrosis may obliterate large areas of lung parenchyma with its associated vasculature including even large conducting elastic arteries and substantial pulmonary veins.

Interstitial pulmonary fibrosis frequently leads to an impaired diffusing capacity for oxygen in the lung. This has been shown to be due to a combination of a reduced volume of blood in the alveolar capillaries and fibrous thickening of the alveolar-capillary wall, which increases the distance across which oxygen has to diffuse from the alveolar space to the pulmonary capillary.[286,287] During the last few years, this second factor has been referred to as alveolar-capillary block, but the influence of this feature on oxygenation of the blood should not be overemphasized, for oxygen is a readily diffusable gas. Inadequate perfusion of the pulmonary capillary bed is probably a more potent factor in the genesis of impaired pulmonary diffusing capacity. When interstitial pulmonary fibrosis progresses to honecomb lung by dilation of bronchioles, another factor is introduced, namely, inequality of ventilation-perfusion ratios and the development of abnormal anatomic shunts.[288,289] At first oxygen saturation is normal at rest but falls on exercise, so that the patient is cyanosed only on exertion. With progression of the disease, however, cyanosis and dyspnea occur even at rest. In honeycomb lung, the dilation of the terminal bronchioles interferes with diffusion of oxygen to the alveolar spaces, and this alveolar hypoxia induces pulmonary hypertension and muscularization of the pulmonary arterioles. Later intimal fibrosis leads to the partial obstruction or occlusion of many of the pulmonary arteries, and thus becomes the dominant feature of the pulmonary vascular disease associated with fibrosis of the lung.

Interstitial Pulmonary Fibrosis

In this condition, there is often associated muscularization of pulmonary arterioles and medial hypertrophy of muscular pulmonary arteries which lead to right ventricular hypertrophy. When progression to honeycomb lung occurs, hypoxic hypertensive pulmonary vascular disease becomes more pronounced.[16] Since the muscularization of the pulmonary arterioles appears to be induced by alveolar hypoxia in honeycomb lung, the entire pulmonary arterial tree is involved and, therefore, occurs both in honeycombed and in noncystic areas of lung. However, certain vascular lesions develop only in areas of lung showing cystic dilation of terminal bronchioles. These include the development of a prominent layer of longitudinally oriented smooth muscle which is indistinguishable from that occurring in emphysema and probably has the same etiology, namely distortion and longitudinal stretching or arteries around cystic spaces. Frequently this intimal longitudinal muscle becomes converted gradually into an acellular intimal fibrosis that splints the medial smooth muscle, which undergoes atrophy and even fibrous replacement. The final stage of this process is fibrous ablation of the entire media with framentation of the elastic laminae. The lumen of the vessel becomes filled with fibroelastic tissue. Thus, in honeycomb lung, there are two stages in the development of pulmonary vascular disease: an initial stage of muscularization followed by fibrous atrophy and ablation. This is in contrast to pulmonary emphysema in which vascular changes in the lung are mainly muscular, with intimal fibrosis being a late and relatively mild development.

Honeycomb lung is not always associated with pulmonary arterial hypertension, and in some cases of several

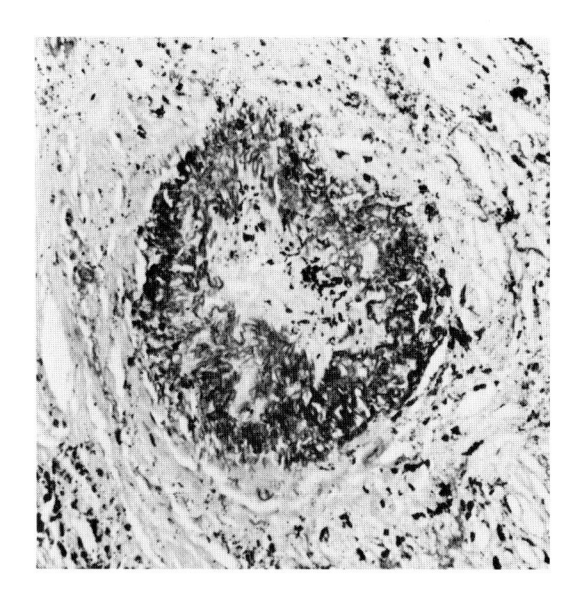

Figure 24–78. Muscular pulmonary artery within an area of dense fibrosis in a case of hematite lung. It has become engulfed by the fibrous tissue so that all that remains of it is a fibroelastic scar. EVG, ×165).

years' duration with pronounced intimal changes in the pulmonary vasculature, there is no right ventricular hypertrophy.[16] This may be due to the formation of a collateral circulation bypassing the obstructed segments of the pulmonary arterial tree. Such thin-walled, dilated anastomotic vessels can sometimes be seen on histologic sections, and a plexus of such vessels about 50 μm in diameter has been demonstrated radiographically.[290,291] Scleroderma can also cause interstitial pulmonary fibrosis, and honeycomb change, and pulmonary vascular disease similar or identical to that described previously. Although Naeye[292] considered these changes to be characteristic for scleroderma, it seems more likely that they are simply an expression of honeycomb lung.

Massive Pulmonary Fibrosis

This form of lung fibrosis occurs in the pneumoconioses due to prolonged inhalation of silica, asbestos, or talc by workers such as miners, sand blasters, and asbestos workers. The pneumoconioses are characterized by large areas of dense, acellular, fibrous tissue which lead to widespread obliteration of the lung architecture. The effect of this fibrosis on the pulmonary blood vessels varies depending on whether they are embedded within the fibrous tissue or are in relatively normal lung adjacent to the fibrosis. The small pulmonary arteries and veins engulfed in fibrosis develop severe intimal fibroelastosis. This intimal proliferation is rigid and causes atrophy of the medial smooth muscle. The surrounding fibrous tissue encroaches on muscular pulmonary arteries, fragmenting first of all the external elastic lamina and then the internal elastic lamina. Any remaining smooth muscle is destroyed and replaced by fibrous tissue. At this stage, the elastic laminae can still be recognized as discontinous fragmented rings, but as more elastic tissue is deposited, they become indistinguishable from the generalized fibroelastic reaction. Finally, the fibrosis invades the lumen of the vessel, completely obliterating it, a process which may be aided by organization of thrombus. At this final stage, muscular pulmonary arteries and small veins appear simply as fibroelastic scars engulfed by fibrous tissue (Fig. 24–78).

Elastic pulmonary arteries are not readily ablated by massive pulmonary fibrosis, but in coal miners' pneumoconiosis, they become dilated and atheromatous.[14] Acid mucopolysaccharide accumulates within the media of these large vessels, which thus stains metachromatically with toluidine blue. It may even progress to cystic medial degeneration. Elastic arteries, which pass close to fibrotic lymph nodes filled with silica particles, may become ulcerated and subject to episodes of thrombosis.[14]

The pulmonary vascular disease associated with the pneumoconioses is often characterized by the presence of specific dust or fibers, but the most easily demonstrable particles should not be too readily accepted as the cause of the lung fibrosis and vascular lesions. Thus, although hematite lung can produce an intense and massive pulmonary fibrosis with pronounced obliterative pulmonary vascular disease[15] (see Fig. 24–78), it is not the aggregations of iron sesquioxide which cause the damage, despite their prominence and the large numbers of siderophages which give the lung a rusty coloration. Rather the silica dust inhaled with the hematite ore is the active principal which promotes the fibrotic reaction and a vascular disease.[15] Pulmonary blood vessels that are distorted around areas of fibrosis but not engulfed by it show intimal longitudinal muscle similar to that found in honeycomb lung and pulmonary emphysema (Fig. 24–79). Its etiology is probably similar since it is believed to form in response to elongation and stretching of muscular pulmonary arteries around fibrous nodules in the lung. With the passage of time, the intimal longitudinal muscle is replaced by fibrous tissue, including fine elastic fibrils which can be misinterpreted as nonspecific if one does not appreciate that it was preceded by a purely muscular change. These intimal fibromuscular changes extend into the pulmonary arterioles that may also show muscularization of their media, suggesting that some degree of pulmonary hypertension follows the obliteration of the pulmonary vascular bed.

Granulomatous Pulmonary Vascular Disease

Diseases such as tuberculosis and sarcoidosis may involve the pulmonary vasculature to give rise to what is termed granulomatous pulmonary arteritis. Very rarely syphilis of the lung may involve the pulmonary circulation. In pulmonary tuberculosis, elastic pulmonary arteries adjacent to areas of caseation may show caseous

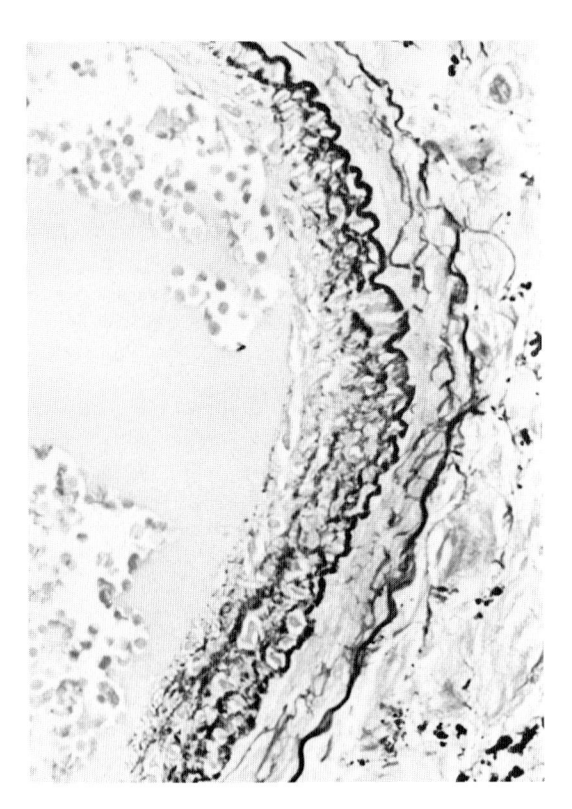

Figure 24–79. Part of a transverse section of a muscular pulmonary artery from a case of hematite lung. The vessel was situated in an area adjacent to dense fibrosis. Its media is of normal thickness, but the intima contains longitudinally oriented smooth muscle cells separated by anastomosing elastic fibers. (EVG, ×412).

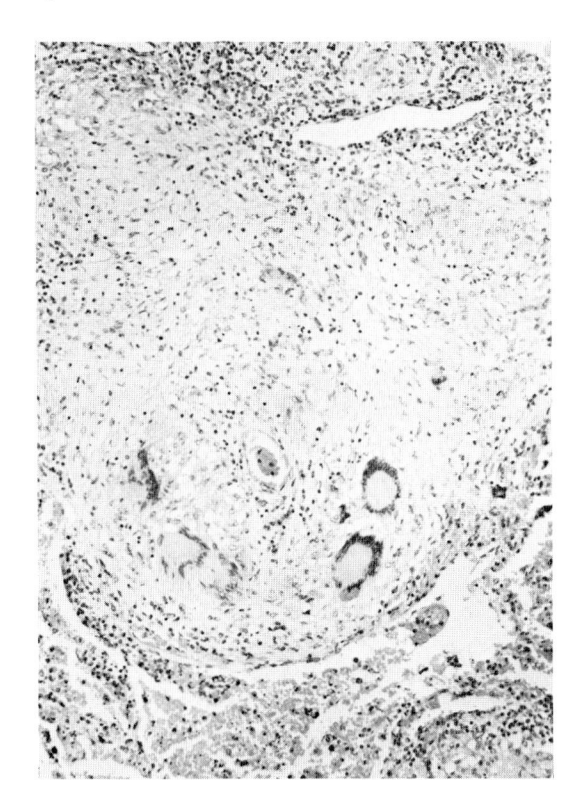

Figure 24–80. A sarcoid granuloma which has invaded a muscular pulmonary artery. Most of the media of the vessel is replaced by collagen, lymphocytes, and multinucleated giant cells of Langhans type (H&E, ×96).

necrosis of their media. Muscular pulmonary arteries may be engulfed in such necrotic areas showing caseous destruction of the media with fragmentation and dissolution of their elastic laminae. In elastic pulmonary arteries which lie near tuberculous cavities, the media may become eroded so that aneurysms of Rasmussen form. They may rupture into the cavities leading to massive pulmonary hemorrhage. There are frequently inflammatory changes in the pulmonary blood vessels in tuberculosis. This is usually lymphocytic, but occasionally there may be epithelioid cell granulomas containing Langhans giant cells in their walls. Sometimes these granulomas in the media have a dumbbell appearance, with part outside the vessel and part in the lumen, the two components being connected by a narrow waist which passes through a defect in the media. In areas of extensive pulmonary fibrosis, the pulmonary blood vessels show changes similar to those described for the pneumoconioses.

Sarcoid granulomas can develop adjacent to, and eventually envelop, pulmonary arteries and veins, but they are usually less destructive than those of tuberculosis due to the absence of caseous necrosis. The granulomas usually lie in the adventitia but may extend to infiltrate the media, forming a focal granulomatous arteritis consisting of lymphocytes, plasma cells, and multinucleated giant cells (Fig. 24–80). The granulomas may rupture elastic laminae and invade the intima where they provoke an intense, obliterative intimal fibrosis which is probably in part thrombotic in origin (Fig. 24–81).

Pulmonary syphilis may develop as an acute interstitial pneumonia, diffuse interstitial fibrosis, gross scarring, or gumma formation. When it involves the smaller pulmonary arteries, it produces changes similar to those in pulmonary tuberculosis, with gummatous necrosis of the media and occlusion of the lumen by fibrosis. Beyond such gummatous areas, the muscular pulmonary arteries show intimal fibrosis infiltrated by lymphocytes and plasma cells, the so-called endarteritis obliterans, typical of syphilis in many organs. Such changes are not specific, and the condition cannot be diagnosed with certainty unless gummas or spirochetes can be demonstrated in the lungs. When syphilis involves the pulmonary trunk, it induces a chronic inflammatory infiltrate in the vicinity of the vasa vasorum. Occlusion of these vessels by fibrosis leads to focal necrosis of the media with loss of muscle and disruption of the elastic tissue. As a consequence, the media may be weakened sufficiently for a fusiform aneurysm to develop.

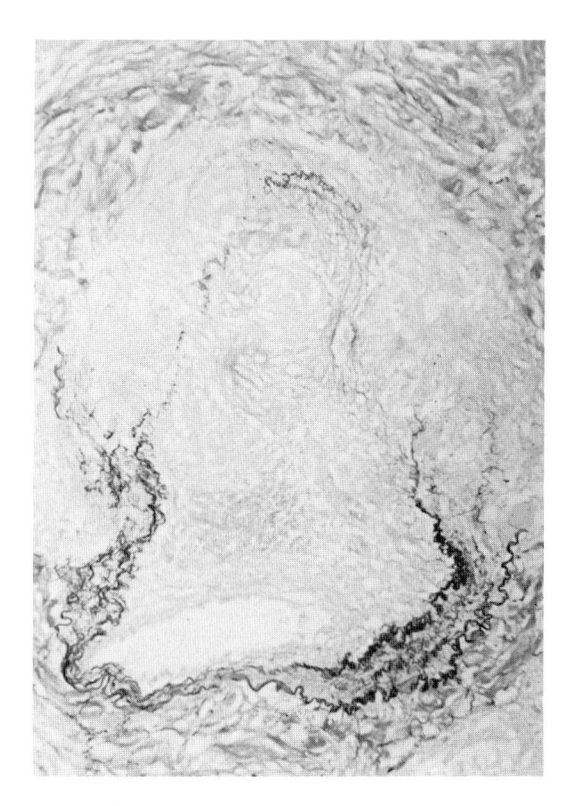

Figure 24–81. Invasion of a muscular pulmonary artery by a sarcoid granuloma. For half of its circumference, the artery has lost its media and elastic laminae. These are replaced by granulomatous tissue and collagen which has also invaded and obliterated the lumen (EVG, ×120).

Pulmonary Embolic Disease

The capillary bed of the lung acts as a filter for particulate matter of any description which either gains entry into, or is formed within, the systemic venous system. Thus a wide variety of emboli may be found in the pulmonary arterioles and capillaries at necropsy. The most common by far are thromboemboli and these shall be considered before briefly describing the other forms.

Origin and Incidence

Most thrombi originate within the deep veins of the leg, particularly those of the calf muscles. This has been confirmed using intravenous injections of fibrinogen labeled with radioiodine.[293] Such thrombi tend to propagate proximally into the inferior vena cava. Other sites of phlebothrombosis are the iliac, prostatic, and utero-ovarian veins. Rarely a mural thrombus may form in the right side of the heart in response to right atrial fibrillation or damage to the ventricular endocardium. Pulmonary thromboemboli may also on occasion originate from the mesenteric veins or those in the neck and arms.

Thromboembolism is rare in children, but it is not clearly established whether its incidence increases linearly with age. It appears to be more common in cold weather. There is an unusually low incidence of the condition in people with blood type O,[294] and it is more prevalent in people with the surface antigen HLA-Cw4.[295] Other predisposing factors include obesity, surgical shock, congestive cardiac failure, and malignant disease, especially of the pancreas. Immobolization of the affected limb is an important localized predisposing factor.

Pulmonary thromboembolism is a common condition that may pass undetected both clinically and at necropsy. Morrell and Dunnill[167] performed a painstaking survey of its incidence in 263 necropsies. They carefully examined the right lungs of these patients for evidence of thromboemboli, while the left lungs were examined routinely by the service pathologist. The latter diagnosed pulmonary thromboemboli in 11.8 percent of patients, whereas the more exhaustive studies of Morrell and Dunnill revealed a prevalence of no less than 51.7 percent. Even so, they suspected that their screening failed to detect all the cases. They also found that emboli of various ages commonly occurred together, indicating the recurrent nature of the condition.

The Fate of Pulmonary Thromboemboli

Because pulmonary thromboemboli occur so commonly, the lungs appear to have evolved an effective means of disposing of them. Thus several hundred milliliters of fresh blood clot can be injected intravenously into dogs repeatedly over a period of months with no rise in pulmonary arterial pressure.[168] Even large, fresh thrombi injected into dogs are removed from the lungs within 6 weeks.[296–298] If the thrombi have aged for a few weeks before being liberated into the circulation, however, their removal from the lungs proceeds more slowly.[299,300] In humans, removal of emboli from the lobar arteries takes approximately 4 weeks.[169]

Small pulmonary thromboemboli are rapidly removed by fibrinolysins, which are normally present in the intima of pulmonary arteries.[301] When emboli are larger or older, they tend to undergo organization instead. As a result, they become reduced to patches of intimal fibrosis with concomitant recanalization and restoration of blood flow.

The clinical and pathologic effects of pulmonary thromboembolism depend on the size of the thrombus or thrombi reaching the lungs. Thus large emboli induce the syndrome of acute, massive pulmonary embolism; a smaller embolus may induce pulmonary infarction; recurrent pulmonary thromboembolism occurs when numerous, small, clinically silent emboli impact in small pulmonary arteries over a protracted period of time.

Massive Pulmonary Embolism

The syndrome of massive pulmonary embolism is a familiar complication of trauma or surgery which presents as an acute emergency. It is created by a large thromboembolus, usually from the veins of the legs or inferior vena cava, lodging at the bifurcation of the pulmonary trunk or its major branches (Fig. 24–82). It thus presents a drastic obstruction to the pulmonary arterial blood flow. However, in order to be fatal, more than half of the pulmonary bed must be occluded. Thus sudden occlusion of one of the major branches of the pulmonary trunk by a balloon induces no clinical disturbances.[302] In normal subjects, this procedure creates a slight increase in pulmonary arterial pressure of about 5 mmHg.[302] If, however, there is preexisting pulmonary arterial hypertension, occlusion of a major pulmonary artery can lead to a dramatic increase in pulmonary arterial blood pressure. This situation can occur when there has been occlusion of part of the pulmonary arterial tree by previous episodes of thromboembolism. This effect is probably due to the fact that the right ventricle is hypertrophied and capable of more forceful contraction when its outlet is obstructed. Nevertheless, even in these cases, the obstruction to blood flow may be so severe that the right ventricle is unable to deliver a sufficient volume of blood to fill the left ventricle. As a result, the patient loses consciousness and may die in acute right ventricular failure.

A massive pulmonary thromboembolus is a common finding at postmortem. It is usually readily distinguishable from postmortem clot since it is much drier and paler and often bears lines of Zahn on its surface (*see* Fig. 24–82). It is also usually narrower than the artery in which it is found, often forming a coiled mass at the bifurcation of the pulmonary trunk. Fresh thrombus arriving at the lungs can be difficult to distinguish from postmortem clot. Nevertheless, it should have the shape of a systemic vein, and careful examination may reveal the imprints of venous valves on its surface. Mortality is too rapid for the vascular changes of infarction to occur, and apart from the presence of the embolus, the only pathologic findings are a dilated right atrium, bulging of the pulmonary trunk, and a variable degree of collapse and edema of the lung. Older, small emboli or infarcts in the lung may attest to previous episodes of thromboembolism. If massive thromboemboli do not cause death, they undergo organization. The end result of this process is the formation of fibroelastic webs and septa traversing the lumen of the major pulmonary arteries.[28]

Pulmonary Infarction

Pulmonary infarction may ensue when a embolus lodges in a lobar artery or one of its branches. However, only in a minority of such patients does infarction take place. This is due to the rapid establishment of a collateral circulation either from the bronchial arteries or adjacent pulmonary arteries. Thus, frequently following obstruction of a pulmonary artery, all that occurs is congestion of the capillary bed with blood flowing in from patent branches in the surrounding lung. Following recanalization of the embolus, the blood flow and appearance of the lung return to normal. Sometimes what is known as incipient infarction may occur. In this situation, the

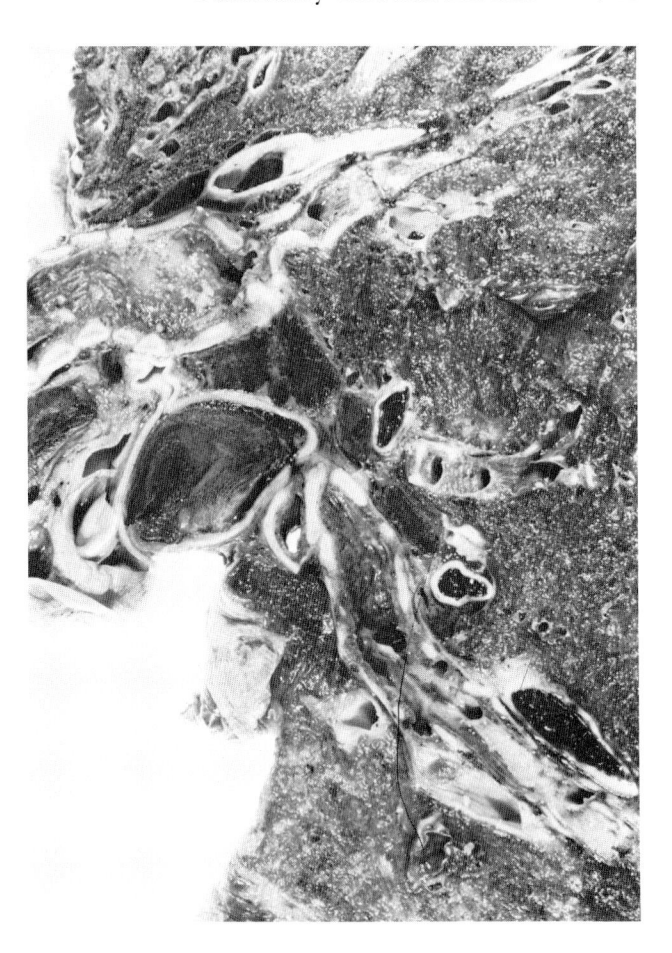

Figure 24–82. Slice through the left lung of a 58-year-old man who died as a consequence of massive pulmonary thromboembolism. The main branch of the left pulmonary artery is occluded by antemortem laminated thromboembolus. The smaller branches of the artery contain postmortem gelatinous blood clot.

collateral circulation is insufficient to prevent the capillaries from becoming engorged with sluggishly flowing blood. As a result, there is capillary damage without necrosis of the lung parenchyma. Plasma fluid and red blood cells leak into the alveoli, but later, as a more efficient collateral supply is established, these changes regress with complete resolution.

A true infarct results when the alveolar walls undergo necrosis, and the bronchial arterial collateral supply leads to hemorrhage into the alveoli. As a result, a red or hemorrhagic infarct of the lung develops. Macroscopically such infarcts are conical with the base of the cone in contact with the pleural surface. The lower lobes are more commonly affected and may involve two pleural surfaces at the costophrenic margin. In this situation, they are not conical but wedge-shaped with a convex inner surface directed toward the hilum. A fibrinous pleurisy frequently forms over the affected visceral pleura.

The histology of pulmonary infarcts reveals alveolar spaces stuffed with blood. The alveolar walls show coagulative necrosis with preservation of their architecture. Bronchi may be spared owing to their bronchial arterial supply. In older infarcts, the red cells disintegrate and hemosiderin-laden macrophages appear. Organization proceeds from the periphery and reduces the necrotic tissue to a small linear scar. Pulmonary infarcts may sometimes become infected, either secondarily from the airways, or from the septic embolus. In these instances, a purulent abscess may form in the lung which liquefies the necrotic tissue.

The pathogenesis of pulmonary infarction is poorly understood. It is difficult to induce in animals by ligating the arterial supply to the lung.[168] Furthermore, the presence or absence of a bronchial arterial supply has little bearing on its genesis. Factors which seem to be important in its pathogenesis, in addition to pulmonary arterial obstruction, include an increased pulmonary venous pressure, a diminished local ventilation due to pulmonary collapse, binding of the chest, pleural effusion or bronchial obstruction, and pulmonary edema or pulmonary infection. These factors would certainly explain the predilection for the lower lobes since such patients are generally nursed sitting upright. In this position, the venous pressure is higher at the lung bases as is the incidence of pulmonary infections and infusions. There is a high incidence of pulmonary infarction in patients with cardiac disease.

Recurrent Pulmonary Thromboembolism

In this condition, showers of small thromboemboli lodge in the smaller radicles of the pulmonary arterial tree over a protracted period of time. The histopathologic features of this disease and its induction of pulmonary arterial hypertension are described in detail in the section of unexplained pulmonary hypertension.

Nonthrombotic Pulmonary Embolism

Fat emboli in the lungs are a common finding at postmorten in people who died several hours or days after traumatic injury. They may also occur as a sequel to bone fractures, crush injuries to subcutaneous tissues, or surgical operations. Fat embolism is also a complication of fatty change and necrosis in the liver caused by hepatic poisoning. Fat emboli consist of droplets of neutral fat in the arterioles and capillaries of the lung. They can be demonstrated using conventional lipid stains on frozen sections. Small and nonwidespread fat emboli are largely asymptomatic and are readily broken down by serum lipases and removed from the lungs. However, extensive fat embolism may prove fatal.

Bone marrow emboli also originate from traumatic injury to the skeleton, especially following cleavage of the sternum for heart surgery.[28] Fragments of bone marrow enter damaged systemic veins and are carried to the lungs. They are generally larger than fat emboli, consisting of small clumps of hemopoietic or adipose tissue which obstruct muscular pulmonary arteries. They are asymptomatic and a common incidental finding at postmortem. Sometimes only megakaryocytes escape into the circulation and lodge in the pulmonary arterioles and precapillaries (see Fig. 24–2). Megakaryocyte emboli soon fragment into platelets which are dispersed.

Air embolism has been recognized for many years as a complication of surgery to the head and neck or fracture of the skull.[28] It may also occur accidentally during intravenous infusions, intrauterine injection of soapy solutions, or during insufflation of the fallopian tubes.[255] Air becomes sucked into partly collapsed large veins, whereupon air bubbles lodge in the pulmonary capillary bed. If the volume of air is small or is introduced gradually, it has no ill effect producing localized and transient interruptions to capillary blood flow. Large volumes may be fatal, although death may be delayed for several hours. The condition can be detected at postmortem by the presence of a frothy mass inside the pulmonary artery which may extend into the right side of the heart. Air emboli within the lungs are difficult to detect unless they are opened under water.

Amniotic fluid embolism is a clinical and pathologic entity which may afflict women during or soon after childbirth. Clinically it is characterized by dyspnea, cyanosis, and the rapid development of shock. It is often fatal. Partial detachment of the placenta, rupture of the myometrium, or cervical tears may permit amniotic fluid to enter the venous system while uterine contractions facilitate its passage.[28] The emboli do not consist solely of fluid but contain epithelial squames, fetal hair, meconium, mucin, and occasionally chorionic villi.[28]

Small trophoblast emboli in the lungs are a common and asymptomatic complication of pregnancy. Rarely they may be much larger and cause pulmonary infarction or even death. This severe form of trophoblastic embolism is sometimes encountered in cases of hydatidiform mole.

Tumor emboli from many systemic malignancies enter the pulmonary vasculature and lodge in the smaller radicles of the pulmonary arterial tree. Most degenerate, but a few survive to grow into hematogenous metastases. Rarely they may produce hemodynamic disturbances. A case in point is the atrial myxoma which usually develops in the left atrium but less commonly develops in the right.[18] Multiple fragments of this neoplasm can impact in the pulmonary arteries creating a sufficient obstruction to blood flow as to cause pulmonary hypertension. The raised pulmonary arterial pressure can rupture the affected arteries and sqeeze the myxomatous material through the defect into the alveolar spaces (see Fig. 24–1). This can mimic the appearances of neoplastic invasion.

Foreign Body Embolism

When foreign material is introduced into the systemic veins, it forms foreign body emboli in the lungs. A wide variety of such bodies has been described by Barrett[303] and includes shrapnel, mercury droplets, intravenous needles, pins, and tubing. Cotton fibers are commonly introduced into systemic veins during medical procedures. On arrival in the lungs, the fibers lodge in small pulmonary arteries and arterioles and set up a foreign body granulomatous reaction.[304] The fibers are best viewed using crossed polaroid filters since they are birefringent. This technique reveals that the fibers have a hollow central core which may appear as a split in longitudinal section.

Cotton wool fibers are commonly introduced into the circulation during cardiac catheterization. Contamination of the catheter probably occurs during its storage in gamgee tissue. Bottles or bags of intravenous fluid are commonly changed at the bedside, and the cotton fibers from clothing and bedding may contaminate them. Fibers can also be introduced by syringe needles either by direct contamination or indirectly from the skin following the classic preinjection sterilization by swabs of alcohol. Jaques and Mariscal[305] found a direct correlation between the amount of intravenous fluid administered and the number of cotton fibers per unit area of lung.

Experiments with animals have shown that cotton fibers first become encased in a mass of platelets and plasma proteins which become adherent to the endothelium.[21,306] Within an hour, polymorphs accumulate around the fibers, but this is transient and they are rapidly replaced by monocytes. The monocytes change into epitheloid cells and foreign body giant cells to form a granuloma enclosing the fibers. This occurs over a period extending from 16 hours to 3 weeks.[21] During this cellular reaction, the fibers rupture the internal elastic lamina and migrate through the media into the adventitia or the alveoli. Within a month of impaction, the vast majority of cotton fibers are extravascular forming granulomatous nodules in the parenchyma. Although these become fibrous with the passage of time, occasional giant cells can be detected up to a year later. Following extrusion of the granulomas, the defects in the arterial walls are repaired in the absence of hemorrhage, and the vascular system returns to normal.[21,306] Cotton fiber embolism is asymptomatic and does not induce pulmonary hypertension even when large numbers of fibers are injected into rats.[21] The patient pathologist will encounter them frequently in routine sections of the lung.

Foreign body embolism is becoming increasingly common among drug addicts due to their practice of crushing tablets for intravenous injection. Some tablets contain microcrystalline cellulose as a filler which embolizes in the lungs. Tomashefski and coworkers[307] described a group of patients who had extensive pulmonary emboli following injection of pentazocine tablets. Histology of their lungs showed large numbers of foreign body granulomas in the parenchyma with thrombosis and dilation of muscular pulmonary arteries associated with destruction of their elastic laminae.

References

1. Harris P, Heath D: *The Human Pulmonary Circulation*, 3rd ed. Edinburgh: Churchill Livingstone, 1986.

2. Heath D, Whitaker W: The small pulmonary vessels in atrial septal defect. Br. Heart J. 19:327–332, 1957.

3. Whitaker W: Total pulmonary venous drainage through a persistent left superior vena cava. Br Heart J 16:177–188, 1954.

4. Heath D, Brown JW, Whitaker W: Muscular defects in the ventricular septum. Br Heart J 18:1–7, 1956.

5. Heath D: Cor triloculare biatriatum. Circulation 15:701–712, 1957.

6. Whitaker W, Heath D, Brown JW: Patent ductus arteriosus with pulmonary hypertension. Br Heart J 17:121–137, 1955.

7. Fleming HA: Aorto-pulmonary septal defect with patent ductus arteriosus and death due to rupture of dissecting aneurysm of the pulmonary artery into the pericardium. Thorax 11:71–76, 1956.

8. Brown JW, Heath D, Whitaker W: Eisenmenger's complex. Br Heart J 17:273–284, 1955.

9. Brown JW, Heath D, Whitaker W: Cardioaortic fistula. A case diagnosed in life and treated surgically. Circulation 12:819–826, 1955.

10. Hicken P, Evans D. Heath D: Persistent truncus arteriosus with survival to the age of 38 years. Br Heart J 28:284–286, 1966.

11. Heath D, Parker RL, Edwards JE: Rupture of an aortic aneurysm into the pulmonary artery. Br J Clin Pract 12:701–707, 1958.

12. Shillingford JP, Kay JM, Heath D: Perforation of interventricular septum following myocardial infarction. Am Heart J 80:562–569, 1970.

13. Walton KW, Heath D: Iron encrustation of the pulmonary vessels in patent ductus arteriosus with congenital mitral valvular disease. Br Heart J 22:440–444, 1960.

14. Wells AL: Pulmonary vascular changes in coal-worker's pneumoconiosis. J Pathol Bacteriol 68:573–587, 1954.

15. Heath D, Mooi W, Smith P: The pulmonary vasculature in haematite lung. Br J Dis Chest 72:88–94, 1978.

16. Heath D, Gillund TD, Kay JM, Hawkins CF: Pulmonary vascular disease in honeycomb lung. J Pathol Bacteriol 95:423–477, 1968.

17. Goodwin JF, Harrison CV, Wilcken DEL: Obliterative pulmonary hypertension and thrombo-embolism. Br Med J i: 701–777, 1963.

18. Heath D, Mackinnon J: Pulmonary hypertension due to myxoma of the right atrium. With special reference to the behavior of myxoma in the lung. Am Heart J 68:227–235, 1964.

19. Steiner PE, Lushbaugh CC: Maternal pulmonary embolism by amniotic fluid as a cause of obstetric shock and unexpected deaths in obstetrics. JAMA 117:1245–1254, 1340–1345, 1941.

20. Barnard PJ: Pulmonary arteriosclerosis due to oxygen, nitrogen and argon embolism. Arch Pathol 63:322–232, 1957.

21. Johnston B, Smith P, Heath D: Experimental cotton-fibre pulmonary embolism in the rat. Thorax 36:910–916, 1981.

22. Kay JM, Heath D: *Crotalaria spectabilis, The Pulmonary Hypertension Plant*. Springfield, Ill: Charles C Thomas, 1969.

23. Kay JM, Heath D, Smith P, et al.: Fulvine and the pulmonary circulation. Thorax 26:249–261, 1971.

24. Burns J: The heart and pulmonary arteries in rats fed on *Senecio jacobaea*. J Pathol 106:187–194, 1972.

25. Heath D, Shaba J, Williams A, et al.: A pulmonary hypertension-producing plant from Tanzania. Thorax 30:399–404, 1975.

26. Heath D, Edwards JE: The pathology of hypertensive pulmonary vascular disease. A description of 6 grades of structural changes in pulmonary arteries. Circulation 18:533–547, 1958.

27. Heath D, Helmholz HF, Burchell HB, et al.: Graded pulmonary vascular changes and haemodynamic findings in

cases of atrial and ventricular septal defects and patent ductus arteriosus. Circulation 18:1155–1166, 1958.

28. Wagenvoort CA, Heath D, Edwards JE: *The Pathology of the Pulmonary Vasculature.* Springfield, Il: Charles C Thomas, 1964.

29. Wagenvoort CA: The morphology of certain vascular lesions in pulmonary hypertension. J Pathol Bacteriol 78:503–511, 1959.

30. Brewer DB, Heath D: Pulmonary vascular changes in Eisenmenger's complex. J Pathol Bacteriol 77:141–147, 1959.

31. Heath D: Longitudinal muscle in pulmonary arteries. J Pathol Bacteriol 85:407–412, 1963.

32. Hasleton PS, Heath D, Brewer DB: Hypertensive pulmonary vascular disease in states of chronic hypoxia. J Pathol Bacteriol 95:431–440, 1968.

33. Smith P, Heath D, Padula F: Evagination of smooth muscle cells in the hypoxic pulmonary trunk. Thorax 33:31–42, 1978.

34. Smith P, Heath D: Evagination of vascular smooth muscle cells during the early stages of Crotalaria pulmonary hypertension. J Pathol 124:177–183, 1978.

35. Smith P, Heath D: Ultrastructure of hypoxic hypertensive pulmonary vascular disease. J. Pathol 121:93–100, 1977.

36. Meyrick B. Reid L: The effect of continued hypoxia on rat pulmonary arterial circulation. An ultrastructural study. Lab Invest 38:188–200, 1978.

37. Meyrick B, Reid L: Hypoxia and incorporation of ^{3}H-thymidine by cells of the rat pulmonary arteries and alveolar wall. Am J Pathol 96:51–70, 1979.

38. Balk AG, Dingemans KP, Wagenvoort CA: The ultrastructure of the various forms of pulmonary arterial intimal fibrosis. Virchows Arch [A] 382:139–150, 1979.

39. Smith P, Heath D: Electron microscopy of the plexiform lesion. Thorax 34:177–186, 1979.

40. Hatt PY, Rouiller, CH, Grosgogeat Y: Les ultrastructures pulmonaires et le regime de la petite circulation. II. Au cours de cardiopathies congenitales comportant une augmentation du debit sanguin intrapulmonaire. Pathol Biol 7:515–544, 1959.

41. Esterly JA, Glagov S, Ferguson DJ: Morphogenesis of intimal obliterative hyperplasia of small arteries in experimental pulmonary hypertension. An ultrastructural study of the role of smooth muscle cells. Am J Pathol 52:325–347, 1968.

42. Spiro D, Lattes RG, Wiener J: The cellular pathology of experimental hypertension. I. Hyperplastic arteriosclerosis. Am J Pathol 47:19–49, 1965.

43. Buck RC: Intimal thickening after ligature of arteries. Circ Res 9:418–426, 1961.

44. Poole JCF, Cromwell SB, Benditt EP: Behavior of smooth muscle cells and formation of extracellular structures in the reaction of arterial walls to injury. Am J Pathol 62:391–414, 1971.

45. Haust MD, More RH, Movat HZ: The role of smooth muscle cells in the fibrogenesis of arteriosclerosis. Am J Pathol 37:377–389, 1960.

46. Thomas WA, Jones R, Scott RF, et al.: Production of early atherosclerotic lesions in rats characterized by proliferation of "modified smooth muscle cells." Exp Mol Pathol 2(suppl):40–61, 1963.

47. Parker F, Odland GF: A light microscopic, histochemical and electron microscopic study of experimental atherosclerosis in rabbit coronary artery and a comparison with rabbit aorta atherosclerosis. Am J Pathol 48:451–481, 1966.

48. Wissler RW: The arterial medial cell, smooth muscle or multifunctional mesenchyme? J Atheroscler Res 8:201–213, 1968.

49. Smith P, Heath D: The ultrastructure of age-associated intimal fibrosis in pulmonary blood vessels. J Pathol 130:247–253, 1980.

50. Gabbiani G, Hirschel BJ, Ryan GB, et al.: Granulation tissue as a contractile organ. A study of structure and function. J Exp Med 135:719–734, 1972.

51. Wagenvoort CA, Wagenvoort N: *Pathology of Pulmonary Hypertension.* New York: John Wiley & Sons, 1977.

52. Stovin PGI, Heath D, Khaliq U: Ultrastructure of the cardiac myxoma and the papillary tumour of heart valves. Thorax 28:273–285, 1973.

53. Stein AA, Mauro J, Thibodeau L, Alley R: The histogenesis of cardiac myxomas: Relation to other proliferative diseases of subendothelial vasoformative reserve cells. In SC Sommers (ed): *Pathology Annual*, vol 4. London: Butterworths, 1969.

54. Hüttner I, Jellinek H, Kerényi T: Fibrin formation in vascular fibrinoid change in experimental hypertension. An electron microscopic study. Exp Mol Pathol 9:309–321, 1968.

55. Goldby FS, Beilin LJ: How an acute rise in arterial pressure damages arterioles. Electron microscopic changes during angiotensin infusion. Cardiovasc Res 6:569–584, 1972.

56. Wiener J, Spiro D, Lattes RG: The cellular pathology of experimental hypertension. II. Arteriolar hyalinosis and fibrinoid change. Am J Pathol 47:457–485, 1965.

57. Koletsky S, Rivera-Velez JM, Pritchard WH: Experimental renal hypertension. Origin of high blood pressure and vascular disease. Arch Pathol 78:24–30, 1964.

58. Mercow L, Kleinerman J: An electron microscopic study of pulmonary vasculitis induced by monocrotaline. Lab Invest 15:547–564, 1966.

59. Heath D, Smith P: The electron microscopy of "fibrinoid necrosis" in pulmonary arteries. Thorax 33:579–595, 1978.

60. Lendrum AC: Fibrinous vasculosis. J Clin Pathol 8:180, 1955.

61. Hoffman JIE, Rudolf AM: The natural history of ventricular septal defects in infancy. Am J Cardiol 16:634–653, 1965.

62. Bloomfield DK: The natural history of ventricular septal defects in patients surviving infancy. Circulation 29:914–955, 1964.

63. Keith JD, Rose V, Collins G, Kidd BSL: Ventricular septal defect. Incidence, morbidity and mortality in various age groups. Br Heart J 33(suppl): 81–87, 1971.

64. Keith JD: In Kidd BSL, Keith JD (eds); *The Natural History and Progress in Treatment of Congenital Heart Defects.* Springfield, IL: Charles C Thomas, 1971.

65. Wagenvoort CA, Neufeld HN, Dushane JW, Edwards JE: The pulmonary arterial tree in ventricular septal defect. A quantitative study of anatomic features in fetuses, infants and children. Circulation 23:740–748, 1961.

66. Harris P, Heath D: *The Human Pulmonary Circulation*, 2nd ed. Edinburgh: Churchill Livingstone, 1977.

67. Evans JR, Rowe RD, Keith JD: The clinical diagnosis of atrial septal defect in children. Am J Med 30:345–356, 1961.

68. Campbell M, Neill C, Suzman S: The prognosis of atrial septal defect. Br Med J i:1375–1383, 1957.

69. Markham P, Howitt G, Wade EG: Atrial septal defect in the middle-aged and elderly. QJ Med 34:409–426, 1965.

70. Heath D, Helmholz HF, Burchell HB, et al.: Relation between structural changes in the small pulmonary arteries and the immediate reversibility of pulmonary hypertension following closure of ventricular and atrial defects. Circulation 18:1167–1174, 1958.

71. Reeve R, Selzer A, Popper RW, et al.: Reversibility of

pulmonary hypertension following cardiac surgery. Circulation 33(suppl)107–114, 1966.

72. Beck W, Swan HJC, Burchell HB, Kirklin JW: Pulmonary vascular resistance after repair of atrial septal defects in patients with pulmonary hypertension. Circulation 22:938–946, 1960.

73. Dushane JW: In Langford-Kidd BS, Keith JD (eds): *The Natural History and Prognosis in Treatment of Congenital Heart Defects.* Springfield, IL: Charles C Thomas, 1971.

74. Hallidie-Smith KA, Hollman A, Cleland WP, et al.: Effects of surgical closure of ventricular septal defects upon pulmonary vascular disease. Br Heart J 31:246–260, 1969.

75. Heath D, Wood EH, Dushane JW, Edwards JE: The structure of the pulmonary trunk at different ages and in cases of pulmonary hypertension and pulmonary stenosis. J Pathol Bacteriol 77:443–456, 1959.

76. Saldaña M, Arias-Stella J: Studies on the structure of the pulmonary trunk. III. The evolution of the elastic configuration of the pulmonary trunk in people native to high altitudes. Circulation 27:1094–1100, 1963.

77. Saldaña M, Arias-Stella J: Studies on the structure of the pulmonary trunk. III. The thickness of the media of the pulmonary trunk and ascending aorta in high-altitude natives. Circulation 27:1101–1104, 1963.

78. Heath D, Wood EH, Dushane JW, Edwards JE: The relation of age and blood pressure to atheroma in the pulmonary arteries and thoracic aorta in congenital heart disease. Lab Invest 9:259–272, 1960.

79. Heath D, Edwards JE: Histological changes in the lung in diseases associated with pulmonary venous hypertension. Br J Dis Chest 53:8–18, 1959.

80. Hatt PY, Rouiller C: Les ultrastructures pulmonaires et le régime de la petite circulation. I. Au cours du rétrécissement mitral serré. Pathol Biol 6:1371–1397, 1958.

81. Kay JM Edwards FR: Ultrastructure of the alveolar-capillary wall in mitral stenosis. J Pathol 111:239–245, 1973.

82. Coalson JJ, Jacques WE, Campbell GS, Thompson WM: Ultrastructure of the alveolar-capillary membrane in congenital and acquired heart disease. Arch Pathol 83:377–391, 1967.

83. Parker F, Weiss S: The nature and significance of the structural changes in the lungs in mitral stenosis. Am J Pathol 12:573–598, 1936.

84. Szidon JP Pietra GG, Fishman AP: The alveolar-capillary membrane and pulmonary edema. N Engl J Med 286:1200–1204, 1972.

85. Shanks SC, Kerley P (ed): *A textbook of X-Ray Diagnosis by British Authors.* London:Lewis, 1951.

86. Rossall RE, Gunning AJ: Basal horizontal lines on chest radiographs; Significance in heart disease. Lancet i:604–606, 1956.

87. Heath D, Hicken P: The relation between left atrial hypertension and lymphatic distension in lung biopsies. Thorax 15:54–58, 1960.

88. Fleishner FG, Reiner L: Linear x-ray shadows in acquired pulmonary hemosiderosis and congestion. N Engl J Med 250:900–905, 1954.

89. Heath D, Whitaker W: The relation of pulmonary haemosiderosis to hypertension in the pulmonary arteries and veins in mitral stenosis and congenital heart disease. J Pathol Bacteriol 72:531–542, 1956.

90. Heath D, Trueman T, Sukonthamarn P: Pulmonary mast cells in mitral stenosis. Cardiovasc Res 3:467–471, 1969.

91. Hicks JD: Acute arterial necrosis in the lungs. J Pathol Bacteriol 65:333–343, 1953.

92. Whitaker W, Black A, Warrack AJN: Pulmonary ossification in patients with mitral stenosis. J Fac Radiol 7:29–34, 1955.

93. Galloway BW, Epstein EJ, Coulshed N: Pulmonary ossific nodules in mitral valve disease. Br Heat J 23:297–307, 1961.

94. Sharp ME, Danino EA: An unusual form of pulmonary calcification: 'Microlithiasis alveolaris pulmonum.' J Pathol Bacteriol 65:389–399, 1953.

95. Heath D, Whitaker W: The pulmonary vessels in mitral stenosis. J Pathol Bacteriol 70:291–298, 1955.

96. Symmers W St C: Necrotizing pulmonary arteriopathy associated with pulmonary hypertension. J Clin Pathol 5:36–41, 1952.

97. Elkeles A, Glynn LE: Disseminated parenchymatous ossification in the lungs associated with mitral stenosis. J Pathol Bacteriol 58:517–522, 1946.

98. Tandon HD, Kasturi J: Pulmonary vascular changes associated with isolated mitral stenosis in India. Br Heart J 37:26–36, 1975.

99. Harrison CV: IV. The pathology of the pulmonary vessels in pulmonary hypertension. Br J Radiol 31:217–226, 1958.

100. Doyle AE, Goodwin JF, Harrison CV, Steiner RE: Pulmonary vascular patterns in pulmonary hypertension. Br Heart J 19:353–365, 1957.

101. Ferencz C, Dammann JF: Significance of the pulmonary vascular bed in congenital heart disease. V. Lesions of the left side of the heart causing obstruction of the pulmonary venous return. Circulation 16:1046–1056, 1957.

102. Gough J: The lungs in mitral stenosis. In Harrison CV (ed): *Recent Advances in Pathology*, 7th ed. London:Churchill Livingstone, 1960.

103. Jordan SC, Hicken P, Watson DA, et al.: Pathology of the lungs in mitral stenosis in relation to respiratory function and pulmonary haemodynamics. Br Heart J 28:101–107, 1966.

104. Dalen JE, Matloff JM, Evans GL, et al.: Early reduction of pulmonary vascular resistance after mitral valve replacement. N Engl J Med 277:387–394, 1967.

105. Ramirez A, Grimes ET, Abelmann WH: Regression of pulmonary vascular changes following mitral valvuloplasty. An anatomic and physiologic case study. Am J Med 45:975–982, 1968.

106. Lalich JJ, Mercow L: Pulmonary arteritis produced in rats by feeding *Crotalaria spectabilis*. Lab Invest 10:744–750, 1961.

107. Turner JH, Lalich JJ: Experimental cor pulmonale in the rat. Arch Pathol 79:409–418, 1965.

108. Kay JM, Heath D: Observations on the pulmonary arteries and heart weight of rats fed on *Crotalaria spectabilis* seeds. J Pathol Bacteriol 92:385–394, 1966.

109. Heath D, Kay JM: Medial thickness of pulmonary trunk in rats with cor pulmonale induced by ingestion of *Crotalaria spectailibis* seeds. Cardiovasc Res 1:74–79, 1967.

110. Kay JM, Harris P, Heath D: Pulmonary hypertension produced in rats by ingestion of *Crotalaria spectabilis* seeds. Thorax 22:176–179, 1967.

111. Hayashi Y, Hussa JF, Lalich JJ: Cor pulmonale in rats. Lab Invest 16:875–881, 1967.

112. Smith P, Kay JM, Heath D: Hypertensive pulmonary vascular disease in rats after prolonged feeding with *Crotalaria spectabilis* seeds. J Pathol 102:97–106, 1970.

113. Kay JM, Heath D, Smith P, et al.: Fulvine and the pulmonary circulation. Thorax 26:249–261, 1971.

114. Burns J: The heart and pulmonary arteries in rats fed on *Senecio jacobaea*. J Pathol 106:187–194, 1972.

115. Heath D, Shaba J, Williams A, et al.: A pulmonary hyper-

tension producing plant from Tanzania. Thorax 30:399–404, 1975.

116. Mattocks AR: Toxicity of pyrrolizidine alkaloids. Nature 217:723–728, 1968.

117. Chesney CF, Allen JR, Hsu I: Right ventricular hypertrophy in monocrotaline pyrrole treated rats. Exp Mol Pathol 29:257–268, 1974.

118. Chesney CF, Allen JR: Monocrotaline-induced pulmonary vascular lesions in non-human primates. Cardiovasc Res 7:508–518, 1973.

119. Valdivia E, Sonnad J, Hayashi U, Lalich JJ: Experimental interstitial pulmonary oedema. Angiology 18:378–383, 1967.

120. Kay JM, Smith P, Heath D: Electron microscopy of Crotalaria pulmonary hypertension. Thorax 24:511–526, 1969.

121. Wagenvoort CA, Wagenvoort N, Dijk HJ: Effect of fulvine on pulmonary arteries and veins of the rat. Thorax 29:522–529, 1974.

122. Takeoka O, Angevine DM, Lalich JJ: Stimulation of mast cells in rats fed various chemicals. Am J Pathol 40:545–554, 1962.

123. Kay JM, Gillund TD, Heath D: Mast cells in the lungs of rats fed on *Crotalaria spectabilis* seeds. Am J Pathol 51:1031–1044, 1967.

124. Kay JM, Crawford N, Heath D: Blood 5-hydroxytryptamine in rats with pulmonary hypertension produced by ingestion of *Crotalaria spectabilis* seeds. Experientia 24:1149–1150, 1968.

125. Kay JM, Smith P, Heath D, Will JA: The effects of phenobarbitone, cinnarizine and zoxazolamine on the development of right ventricular hypertrophy and hypertensive pulmonary vascular disease in rats treated with monocrotaline. Cardiovasc Res 10:200–205, 1976.

126. Hislop A, Reid L: Arterial changes in *Crotalaria spectabilis*-induced pulmonary hypertension in rats. J Exp Pathol 55:153–163, 1974.

127. Gurtner HP, Gertsch M, Salzmann C, et al.: Haufen sich die primar vascularen Formen des chronischen Cor pulmonale? Schweiz Med Wochenschr 98:1579–1589, 1695–1707, 1968.

128. Rivier JL: Hypertension artérielle pulmonaire primitive. Schweiz Med Wochenschr 100:143–145, 1970.

129. Kaindl F: Primare pulmonare hypertension. Wein Zeit Inn Med 50:451–453, 1969.

130. Lang E, Haupt EJ, Köhler JA, Schmidt J: Cor pulmonale durch Appetitzügler? Munch Med Wochenschr 111:405–412, 1969.

131. Gurtner HP: Hypertensive pulmonary vascular disease. Some remarks on its incidence and etiology. Proc Eur Soc Study Drug Tox 12:81, 1971.

132. Jornod J, Widgren S, Fischer G: Etude anatomo-clinique d'un cas d'hypertension artérielle pulmonaire chez une jeune femme. Schweiz Med Wochenschr 100:151–154, 1970.

133. Kay JM, Smith P, Heath D: Aminorex and the pulmonary circulation. Thorax 26:262–270, 1971.

134. Obiditsch-Mayer L: Lingulabiopsien bei Patienten mit primärer pulmonaler Hypertonie. Wien Zeit Inn Med 50:486–489, 1969.

135. Widgren S, Kapanci Y: Pulmonary hypertensive disease in connection with Menocil intake. In Blankart R (ed): *Obesity, Circulation Anorexigens.* Berne: Hans Huber, 1974, pp 231–237.

136. Blankart R: Epidemiologische Untersuchungen zur Haufung der pulmonalen Hypertonie in den Jahren 1967–1969. In Blankart R (ed) *Obesity, Circulation Anorexigens.* Berne: Hans Huber, 1974, pp 187–201.

137. Smith P, Heath D, Kay JM, et al.: Pulmonary arterial pressure and structure in the patas monkey following prolonged administration of aminorex fumarate. Cardiovasc Res 7:30–38, 1973.

138. Byrne-Quinn E, Grover RF: Aminorex (Menocil) and amphetamine: Acute and chronic effects on pulmonary and systemic haemodynamics in the calf. Thorax 27:127–131, 1972.

139. Smith P, Heath D: Aminorex and the pulmonary circulation of rats fed on a high fat diet. Arzneim Forsch 24:1277–1229, 1974.

140. Kraupp O, Stülinger W, Roberger G, Turnheim K: Die Wirkung von Aminorex (Menocil) auf die Hamodynamik des keinen und grossen Kreislaufs bei i. v. Darreichung am Hund. Naunyn Schmiedeberg Arch Exp Pathol Pharmacol 264:389–405, 1969.

141. Hasleton PS, Kay JM, Heath D: Phentermine resinate and the pulmonary vasculature of the rat. Arzneim Forsch 27:2112–2113, 1977.

142. Heath D, Smith P, Hasleton PS: The effects of chlorphentermine on the rat lung. Thorax 28:551–558, 1973.

143. Smith P, Heath D, Hasleton PS: Effects of prolonged administration of chlorphentermine on the rat lung. Pathol Eur 9:273–287, 1974.

144. Dresdale DT, Schultz M, Michtom RJ: Primary pulmonary hypertension. Am J Med 11:686–705, 1951.

145. Wood P: *Diseases of the Heart and Circulation.* London: Eyre & Spottiswode, 1956.

146. Evans W, Short DS, Bedford DE: Solitary pulmonary hypertension. Br Heart J 19:93–116, 1957.

147. Heath D, Whitaker W, Brown JW: Idiopathic pulmonary hypertension. Br Heart J 19:83–92, 1957.

148. Shepherd JT, Edwards JE, Burchell HB, et al.: Clinical, physiological and pathological considerations in patients with idiopathic pulmonary hypertension. Br Heart J 19:70–82, 1957.

149. Wagenvoort CA, Wagenvoort N: Primary pulmonary hypertension. A pathologic study of the lung vessels in 156 clinically diagnosed cases. Circulation 42:1163–1184, 1971.

150. Wade G, Ball J: Unexplained pulmonary hypertension. QJ Med J 26:83–120, 1957.

151. Heath D, Edwards JE: Configuration of elastic tissue of pulmonary trunk in idiopathic pulmonary hypertension. Circulation 21:59–62, 1960.

152. Castleman B, Bland EF: Organized emboli of the tertiary pulmonary arteries. An unusual case of cor pulmonale. Arch Pathol 42:581–589, 1946.

153. Barnard PJ: Thrombo-embolic primary pulmonary hypertension. Br Heart J 16:93–100, 1954.

154. Clark RC, Coombs CF, Hadfield G, Todd AT: On certain abnormalities congenital and acquired, of the pulmonary artery. QJ Med 21:51–70, 1927.

155. Fleming H: Primary pulmonary hypertension in eight patients including a mother and her daughter. Aust Ann Med 9:18–28, 1960.

156. Thompson P, McRae C: Familial pulmonary hypertension. Evidence of autosomal dominant inheritance. Br Heart J 32:758–760, 1970.

157. Hood WB, Spencer H, Lass RW, Daley R: Primary pulmonary hypertension. Familial occurrence. Br Heart J 30:336–343, 1968.

158. Heath D, Segel N, Bishop J: Pulmonary veno-occlusive disease. Circulation 34:242–248, 1966.

159. Brown CH, Harrison CV: Pulmonary veno-occlusive disease. Lancet 2:61–65, 1966.

160. Thadani U, Burrow C, Whitaker W, Heath D: Pulmonary veno-occlusive disease. QJ Med 173:133–159, 1975.
161. Heath D, Scott O, Lynch J: Pulmonary veno-occlusive disease. Thorax 26:633–674, 1971.
162. Rosenthal A, Vawter G, Wagenvoort CA: Intrapulmonary veno-occlusive disease. Am J Cardiol 31:78–83, 1973.
163. Brewer DB, Humphreys DR: Primary pulmonary hypertension with obstructive venous lesions. Br Heart J 22:445–448, 1960.
164. Stovin PGI, Mitchinson MJ: Pulmonary hypertension due to obstruction of the intrapulmonary veins. Thorax 20:106–113, 1965.
165. Wagenvoort CA, Losekoot G, Mulder E: Pulmonary veno-occlusive disease of presumably intrauterine origin. Thorax 26:429–434, 1971.
166. Corrin B, Spencer H, Turner-Warwick M, et al.: Pulmonary veno-occlusion — an immune complex disease? Virchows Arch [A] 364:81–91, 1974.
167. Morrell MT, Dunnill MS: The post mortem incidence of pulmonary embolism in a hospital population. Br J Surg 55:347–352, 1968.
168. Marshall R: In *Pulmonary Embolism*. Springfield, IL: Charles C Thomas 1965, pp 61–66.
169. Poe ND, Swanson LA, Dore EK, Taplin GV: The course of pulmonary embolism. Am Heart J 73:582–589, 1967.
170. Goodwin JF. In Sasahara AA, Stein M (eds): *Pulmonary Embolic Disease*. New York: Grune & Stratton, 1965.
171. Karlish AJ, Marshall R, Reid L, Sherlock S: Cyanosis with hepatic cirrhosis. Thorax 22:555–561, 1967.
172. Hales MR: Multiple small arteriovenous fistulae of the lungs. Am J Pathol 32:927–943, 1956.
173. Rydell R, Hoffbauer FW: Multiple pulmonary arteriovenous fistulas in juvenile cirrhosis. Am J Med 21:450–460, 1956.
174. Bertholet P, Walker JG, Sherlock S, Reid L: Arterial changes in the lungs in cirrhosis of the liver — Lung spider nevi. N Engl J Med 274:291–298, 1966.
175. Fritts HW Jn, Hardewig A, Rochester DF, et al.: Estimation of pulmonary arteriovenous shunt-flow using intravenous injections of T-1824 dye and Kr[85]. J Clin Invest 39:1841–1850, 1960.
176. Khaliq SU, Kay JM, Heath D: Porta-pulmonary venous anastomoses in experimental cirrhosis of the liver in rats. J Pathol 107:167–174, 1972.
177. Calabresi P, Abelmann WH: Porto-caval and porto-pulmonary anastomoses in Laennec's cirrhosis and in heart failure. J Clin Invest 36:1257–1265, 1957.
178. Mellemgaard K, Winkler K, Tygstrup N, Georg J: Sources of venoarterial admixture in portal hypertension. J Clin Invest 42:1399–1405, 1963.
179. Mantz FA, Craige E: Portal axis thrombosis with spontaneous portacaval shunt and resultant cor pulmonale. Arch Pathol 52:91–97, 1951.
180. Murray JF, Dawson AM, Sherlock S. Circulatory changes in chronic liver disease. Am J Med 24:358–367, 1958.
181. Naeye RL: "Primary" pulmonary hypertension with coexisting portal hypertension. Circulation 22:376–384, 1960.
182. Kerbel NC: Pulmonary hypertension and portal hypertension. Can Med Assoc J 87:1022–1026, 1962.
183. Cohen N, Mendelow H: Concurrent "active juvenile cirrhosis" and "primary pulmonary hypertension" Am J Med 39:127–133, 1965.
184. Lal S, Fletcher E: Pulmonary hypertension and portal venous system thrombosis. Br Heart J 30:723–725, 1968.
185. Senior RM, Britton RC, Turino GM, et al.: Pulmonary hypertension associated with cirrhosis of the liver and with portacaval shunts. Circulation 37:88–96, 1968.
186. Segel N, Kay JM, Bayley TJ, Paton A: Pulmonary hypertension with hepatic cirrhosis. Br Heart J 30:575–578, 1968.
187. Saunders JB, Constable TJ, Heath D, et al.: Pulmonary hypertension complicating portal vein thrombosis. Thorax 34:281–283, 1979.
188. Segel N, Bayley TJ, Paton A, et al.: The effects of synthetic vasopressin and angiotensin on the circulation in cirrhosis of the liver. Clin Sci 25:43–55, 1963.
189. Owen WR, Thomas WA, Castleman B, Bland EF: Unrecognized emboli to the lungs with subsequent cor pulmonale. N Engl J Med 249:919–926, 1953.
190. Kibria G, Smith P, Heath D, Sagar S: Observations on the rare association between portal and pulmonary hypertension. Thorax 35:945–949, 1980.
191. Lunseth JH, Olmstead EG, Abboud F: A study of heart disease in one hundred eight hospitalized patients dying with portal cirrhosis. Arch Intern Med 102:405–413, 1958.
192. Kay JM, Heath D, Smith P, et al.: Fulvine and the pulmonary circulation. Thorax 26:249–261, 1971.
193. Peñaloza D, Sime F, Banchero N, Gamboa R: Pulmonary hypertension in healthy man born and living at high altitudes. Med Thorac 19:449–460, 1962.
194. Arias-Stella J, Saldaña M: The terminal portion of the pulmonary arterial tree in people native to high altitudes. Circulation 28:915–925, 1963.
195. Heath D, Smith P, Rios Dalenz J, et al.: The small pulmonary arteries in some natives of La Paz, Bolivia. Thorax 36:599–604, 1981.
196. Heath D, William DR: *Man at High Altitude*, 2nd ed. Edinburgh: Churchill Livingstone, 1981.
197. Heath D, Castillo Y, Arias-Stella J, Harris P: The small pulmonary arteries of the llama and other domestic animals native to high altitude. Cardiovasc Res 3:75–78, 1969.
198. Heath D, Smith P, Williams D, et al.: The heart and pulmonary vasculature of the llama (*Lama glama*). Thorax 29:463–471, 1974.
199. Heath D, Williams D, Harris P, et al.: The pulmonary vasculature of the mountain-viscacha (*Lagidium peruanum*). The concept of adapted and acclimatized vascular smooth muscle. J Comp Pathol 92:293–301, 1981.
200. Peñaloza D, Sime F: Chronic cor pulmonale due to loss of altitude acclimatization (chronic mountain sickness). Am J Med 50:728–743, 1971.
201. Hecht HH, Lange RL, Carnes WH, et al.: Brisket disease. I. General aspects of pulmonary hypertensive heart disease in cattle. Trans Assoc Am Phys 72:157–172, 1959.
202. Fulton RM, Hutchinson EC, Morgan Jones A: Ventricular weight in cardiac hypertrophy. Br Heart J 14:413–420, 1952.
203. Hicken P, Heath D, Brewer D: The relation between the weight of the right ventricle and the percentage of abnormal air space in the lung in emphysema. J Pathol Bacteriol 92:519–528, 1966.
204. Hicken P, Brewer D, Heath D: The relation between the weight of the right ventricle and the internal surface area and number of alveoli in the human lung in emphysema. J Pathol Bacteriol 92:529–546, 1966.
205. Hicken P, Heath D, Brewer DB, Whitaker W: The small pulmonary arteries in emphysema. J Pathol Bacteriol 90:107–114, 1965.
206. Dunnill MS: An assessment of the anatomical factor in cor pulmonale in emphysema. J Clin Pathol 14:246–258, 1961.

207. Liebow AA: Summary: Biochemical and structural changes in the aging lung. In Cander L, Moyer JH (eds) *Aging of the Lung. Perspectives.* New York: Grune and Stratton, 1964, p 97.

208. Hasleton, PS, Heath D, Brewer DB: Hypertensive pulmonary vascular disease in states of chronic hypoxia. J Pathol Bacteriol 95:431–440, 1968.

209. Abraham AS, Kay JM, Cole RB, Pincock AC: Haemodynamic and pathological study of the effect of chronic hypoxia and subsequent recovery on the heart and pulmonary vasculature of the rat. Cardiovasc Res 5:95–102, 1971.

210. Heath D, Edwards C, Winson M, Smith P: Effects on the right ventricle, pulmonary vasculature and carotid bodies of the rate of exposure to, and recovery from, simulated high altitude. Thorax 28:24–28, 1973.

211. Dunnill MS. Fibrinoid necrosis in the branches of the pulmonary artery in chronic non-specific lung disease. Br J Dis Chest 54:355–358, 1960.

212. Smith P, Jago R, Heath D: Anatomical variation and quantitative histology of the normal and enlarged carotid body. J Pathol 137:287–304, 1982.

213. Heath D, Edwards C, Harris P: Postmortem size and structure of the human carotid body. Thorax 25:129–140, 1970.

214. Arias-Stella J: Human carotid body at high altitudes. From the proceedings of the 69th meeting of the American Association of Pathologists and Bacteriologists, San Francisco, Cal, 1969.

215. Edwards C, Heath D, Harris P, et al.: The carotid body in animals at high altitude. J Pathol 104:231–238, 1971.

216. Edwards C, Heath D, Harris P: The carotid body in emphysema and left ventricular hypertrophy. J Pathol 104:1–13, 1971.

217. Heath D, Smith P, Jago R: Hyperplasia of the carotid body. J Pathol 138:115–127, 1982.

218. Edwards C, Heath D, Harris P: Ultrastructure of the carotid body in high altitude guinea pigs. J Pathol 107:131–136, 1971.

219. Pearse AGE: The cytochemistry and ultrastructure of polypeptide hormone-producing cells of the APUD series and the embryologic, physiologic and pathologic implications of the concept. J Histochem Cytochem 17:303–313, 1969.

220. Severinghaus JW, Bainton CR, Carcelan A: Respiratory insensitivity to hypoxia in chronically hypoxic man. Respir Physiol 1:308–334, 1966.

221. Honig A, Schmidt M: Kidney function during carotid chemoreceptor stimulation. Influence of unilateral renal nerve section. In Lichardus B, Schrier RW, Ponec J (eds): *Hormonal Regulation of Sodium Excretion.* Amsterdam: Elsevier/North Holland, 1980.

222. Poston L, Sewell RB, Wilkinson SP, et al.: Evidence for a circulating sodium transport inhibitor in essential hypertension. Br Med J 282:847–849, 1981.

223. Krahl VE: In de Reuck AVS, O'Connor M (eds): *Ciba Foundation Symposium on Pulmonary Structure and Function.* London: Churchill Livingstone, 1962.

224. Edwards C, Heath D: Microanatomy of glomic tissue of the pulmonary trunk. Thorax 24:209–217, 1969.

225. Becker AE: MD thesis, Laboratory of Pathological Anatomy, University of Amsterdam, 1966.

226. Edwards C, Heath D: Site and blood supply of the intertruncal glomera. Cardiovasc Res 4:502–508, 1970.

227. Edwards C, Heath D: Pulmonary venous glomic tissue. Br J Dis Chest 66:96–100, 1972.

228. Korn D, Bensch K, Liebow A, Castleman B: Multiple minute pulmonary tumours resembling chemodectomas. Am J Pathol 37:641–672, 1960.

229. Moosavi H, Smith P, Heath D: The Feyrter cell in hypoxia. Thorax 28:729–741, 1973.

230. Lauweryns JM, Peuskens JC, Cokelaere M: Argyrophil, fluorescent, and granulated (peptide and amine producing?) AFG cells in human infant bronchial epithelium. Light and electron microscopic studies. Life Sci 9:1417–1429, 1970.

231. Taylor W: Pulmonary argyrophil cells at high altitude. J Pathol 122:137–144, 1977.

232. Roach MR: An experimental study of the production and time course of poststenotic dilation in the femoral and carotid arteries of adult dogs. Circ Res 13:537–551, 1963.

233. Roach MR: Changes in arterial distensibility as a cause of post stenotic dilatation. Am J Cardiol 12:802–815, 1963.

234. Best PV, Heath D: Pulmonary thrombosis in cyanotic congenital heart disease without pulmonary hypertension. J Pathol Bacteriol 75:281–291, 1958.

235. Wagenvoort CA, Nauta J, Van der Schaar PJ, et al.: Vascular changes in pulmonic stenosis and tetralogy of Fallot in lung biopsies. Circulation 36:924–932, 1967.

236. Naeye RL: Perinatal changes in the pulmonary vascular bed with stenosis and atresia of the pulmonary valve. Am Heart J 61:586–592, 1961.

237. Rich AR: A hitherto unrecognized tendency to the development of widespread pulmonary vascular obstruction in patients with congenital pulmonary stenosis (Tetralogy of Fallot). Bull Johns Hopkins Hosp 82:389–395, 1948.

238. Heath D, DuShane JW, Wood EH, Edwards JE: The aetiology of pulmonary thrombosis in cyanotic congenital heart disease with pulmonary stenosis. Thorax 13:213–217, 1958.

239. Ferenz C: The pulmonary vascular bed in tetralogy of Fallot II. Changes following a systemic-pulmonary arterial anastomosis. Bull Johns Hopkins Hosp 106:100–118, 1960.

240. Fragoyannis S, Kardalinos A: Congenital heart disease with pulmonary ischemia. A study of the pulmonary vascular lesions before and after systemic pulmonary anastomosis. Am Heart J 63:335–345, 1962.

241. Kinsley RH, McGoon DC, Danielson GK, et al.: Pulmonary arterial hypertension after repair of tetralogy of Fallot. J Thorac Cardiovasc Surg 67:110–120, 1974.

242. Shaw AFB, Ghareeb AA: The pathogenesis of pulmonary schistosomiasis in Egypt with special reference to Ayerza's disease. J Pathol Bacteriol 46:401–424, 1938.

243. Marchand EJ, Marcial-Rojas RA, Rodriguez R, et al.: The pulmonary obstruction syndrome in *Schistosoma mansoni* pulmonary endarteritis. Arch Intern Med 100:965–980, 1957.

244. Garcia-Palmieri N: Cor pulmonale due to *Schistosoma mansoni.* Am Heart J 68:714–715, 1964.

245. De Faria JL: Pulmonary vascular changes in schistosomal cor pulmonale. J Pathol Bacteriol 68:589–602, 1954.

246. Chaves E: The pathology of the arterial pulmonary vasculature in Manson's schistosomiasis. Dis Chest 50:72–77, 1966.

247. Al-Naaman YD, Shamma AH, Damluji SF, El-Sayed HM: Angiologic manifestation of cardiopulmonary schistosomiasis "Bilharziasis." Angiology 17:40–45, 1966.

248. Brewer DB: Fibrous occlusion and anastomosis of the pulmonary vessels in a case of pulmonary hypertension associated with patent ductus arteriosus. J Pathol Bacteriol 70:299–310, 1955.

249. Naeye RL: Advanced pulmonary vascular changes in

schistosomal cor pulmonale. Am J Trop Med Hyg 10:191–199, 1961.

250. Obeyesekere I, De Soysa N: "Primary" pulmonary hypertension, eosinophilia, and filariasis in Ceylon. Br Heart J 32:524–536, 1970.

251. Obeyesekere I, Peiris D: Pulmonary hypertension and filariasis. Br Heart J 36:676–681, 1974.

252. Dissanaike AS, Paramananthan DC: On Brugia (Brugiella subgen. nov.) buckelyi n. sp., from the heart and blood vessels of the Ceylon hare. J Helminth 35:209–220, 1961.

253. Woodard JC: Acarous (*Pneumonyssus simicola*) arteritis in rhesus monkeys. J Am Vet Med Assoc 153:905–909, 1968.

254. Hamilton JM: Pulmonary arterial disease of the cat. J Comp Pathol 76:133–145, 1966.

255. Spencer H: *Pathology of the Lung*, 3rd ed. Oxford: Pergamon Press, 1977.

256. Congdon ED: Transformation of the aortic arch system during the development of the human embryo. Contr Embryol (Carnegie Inst Wash) 14:47–110, 1922.

257. Pool PE, Vogel JHK, Blount SG: Congenital unilateral absence of a pulmonary artery. Am J Cardiol 10:706–732, 1962.

258. Edwards JE: Congenital pulmonary vascular disorders. In Moser KM (ed): *Pulmonary Vascular Diseases*. New York: Marcel Dekker, 1979, pp 527–571.

259. Søndergaard T: Coarctation of the pulmonary artery. Dan Med Bull 1:46–48, 1954.

260. Collett RW, Edwards JE: Persistent truncus arteriosus: Classification according to anatomical types. Surg Clin North Am 29:1245–1270, 1949.

261. Neufeld HN, Lester RG, Adams P, et al.: Aorticopulmonary septal defect. Am J Cardiol 9:12–25, 1962.

262. Keith JD: The anomalous origin of the left coronary artery from the pulmonary artery. Br Heart 21:149–161, 1959.

263. Alexander RW, Griffith GC: Anomalies of the coronary arteries and their clinical significance. Circulation 14:800–805, 1956.

264. Jue KL, Raghib G, Amplatz K, et al.: Anomalous origin of the left pulmonary artery from the right pulmonary artery; Report of 2 cases and review of the literature. AJR 95:598–610, 1965.

265. Niwayama G: Unusual vascular ring formed by the anomalous left pulmonary artery with tracheal compression. Am Heart J 59:454–461, 1960.

266. Caudill DR, Helmsworth JA, Daoud G, Kaplan S: Anomalous origin of left pulmonary artery from ascending aorta. J Thorac Cardiovasc Surg 57:493–506, 1969.

267. Anderson RC, Char F, Adams P Jr: Proximal interruption of a pulmonary arch (absence of one pulmonary artery); Case report and a new embryologic interpretation. Dis Chest 34:73–86, 1958.

268. Pryce DM, Sellors TH, Blair LG: Intralobular sequestration of lung associated with an abnormal pulmonary artery. Br J Surg 35:18–29, 1947.

269. Salvioni D, Goldin RR: Intralobular pulmonary sequestration. Dis Chest 37:122–124, 1960.

270. Pryce DM: Lower accessory pulmonary artery with intralobar sequestration of lung: Report of seven cases. J Pathol Bacteriol 58:457–467, 1946.

271. Abbey-Smith R: A theory of the origin of intralobar sequestration of the lung. Thorax 11:10–24, 1956.

272. Heath D, Watts GT: The significance of vascular changes in an accessory lung presenting as a diaphragmatic cyst. Thorax 12:142–147, 1957.

273. Johnston DG: Inflammatory and vascular lesions of bronchopulmonary sequestration. Am J Clin Pathol 26:636–644, 1956.

274. Ostrow PT, Salyer WR, White JJ, et al.: Hypertensive pulmonary vascular disease in intralobar sequestration. Am J Pathol 70:33a–34a, 1973.

275. D'Cruz IA, Agustsson MH, Bicoff JP, et al.: Stenotic lesions of the pulmonary arteries. Clinical and hemodynamic findings in 84 cases. Am J Cardiol 13:441–450, 1964.

276. Rowe RD: Maternal rubella and pulmonary artery stenoses. Pediatrics 32:180–185, 1963.

277. Burroughs JT, Edwards JE: Total anomalous pulmonary venous connection. Am Heart J 59:913–931, 1960.

278. Loeffler E: Unusual malformation of the left atrium: Pulmonary sinus. Arch Pathol 48:371–376, 1949.

279. Halasz NA, Halloran KH, Liebow AA: Bronchial and arterial anomalies with drainage of the right lung into the inferior vena cava. Circulation 14:826–846, 1956.

280. Neill CA, Ferencz C, Sorbiston DC, Sheldon H: The familial occurrence of hypoplastic right lung with systemic arterial supply and venous drainage "Scimitar syndrome". Bull Johns Hopkins Hosp 107:1–21, 1960.

281. Reye RDK: Congenital stenosis of the pulmonary veins in their extrapulmonary course. Med J Aust 1:801–802, 1951.

282. Edwards JE: Congenital stenosis of pulmonary veins. Pathologic and developmental considerations. Lab Invest 9:46–66, 1960.

283. Shermann FE: Stengel WF, Bauersfeld SR: Congenital stenosis of pulmonary veins at their atrial junctions. Am Heart J 56:908–919, 1958.

284. Lindskog GE, Liebow AA, Kausel H, Janzen A: Pulmonary arteriovenous aneurysm. Ann Surg 132:591–606, 1950.

285. Whitaker W: Cavernous haemangioma of the lung. Thorax 2:58–64, 1947.

286. McNeill RS, Rankin J, Forster RE: The diffusing capacity of the pulmonary membrane and the pulmonary capillary blood volume in cardio-pulmonary disease. Clin Sci 17:465–482, 1958.

287. Bates DV, Varvis CJ, Donevan RE, Christie RV: Variations in the pulmonary capillary blood volume and membrane diffusion component in health and disease. J Clin Invest 39:1401–1412, 1960.

288. Finley TN, Svenson EW, Comroe JH Jr: The cause of arterial hypoxaemia at rest in patients with alveolar-capillary block syndrome. J Clin Invest 41:618–622, 1962.

289. Arndt H, King TK, Briscoe WA: Diffusing capacities and ventilation: perfusion ratios in patients with the clinical syndrome of alveolar capillary block. J Clin Invest 49:408–422, 1970.

290. Turner-Warwick M: Precapillary systemic-pulmonary anastomoses. Thorax 18:255–237, 1963.

291. Livingstone JL, Lewis JG, Reid L, Jefferson KE: Diffuse interstitial pulmonary fibrosis. A clinical radiological and pathological study based on 45 patients. QJ Med 33:71–103, 1964.

292. Naeye RL: Pulmonary vascular lesions in systemic scleroderma. Dis Chest 44:374–379, 1963.

293. Kakkar VV, Nicolaides AN, Renney JTG, et al.: ^{125}I-labelled fibrinogen test adapted for routine screening for deep-vein thrombosis. Lancet i:540–542, 1970.

294. Jick H, Shone D, et al.: Venous thromboembolic disease and ABO blood type. Lancet i:539–542, 1969.

295. Riedel M, Ivaskova E, Sajdlova H: HLA and venous thromboembolism. Tissue Antigens 18:280–281, 1981.

296. Allison PR, Dunnill MS, Marshall R: Pulmonary embolism. Thorax 15:273–283, 1960.

297. Hume M, Glenn WWL, Grillo T: Behavior in the circulation of the radioactive pulmonary embolus and its application to the study of fibrinolytic enzymes. Ann Surg 151:507–516, 1960.

298. Wessler S, Frieman DG, Ballon JD, et al.: Experimental pulmonary embolism with serum-induced thrombi. Am J Pathol 38:89–101, 1961.

299. Freiman DG, Wessler S, Lertzman M: Experimental pulmonary embolism with serum-induced thrombi aged in vivo. Am J Pathol 39:95–102, 1961.

300. Marshall R, Sabiston DC, Allison PR, et al.: Immediate and late effects of pulmonary embolism by large thrombi in dogs. Thorax 18:1–9, 1963.

301. Todd AS: The histological localization of fibrinolysin activator. J Pathol Bacteriol 78:281–283, 1959.

302. Harris P, Segel N, Bishop JM: The relation between pressure and flow in the pulmonary circulation is normal subjects and in patients with chronic bronchitis and mitral stenosis. Cardiovasc Res 2:73–83, 1968.

303. Barrett NR: Foreign bodies in the cardiovascular system. Br J Surg 37:416–445, 1950.

304. Heath D, Mackinnon J: Cotton wool granuloma of pulmonary artery. Br Heart J 24:18–20, 1962.

305. Jaques WE, Mariscal GG: A study of the incidence of cotton emboli. Bull Int AM Mus 32:63–72, 1951.

306. Von Glahn WC, Hall JW: The reaction produced in pulmonary arteries by emboli of cotton fibres. Am J Pathol 25:575–593, 1949.

307. Tomashefski JF, Hirsch CS, Jolly PN: Microcrystalline cellulose pulmonary embolism and granulomatosis. A complication of illicit intravenous injections of pentazocine tablets. Arch Pathol Lab Med 105:89–93, 1981.

25 Consequences of Aspiration and Bronchial Obstruction

Joanne L. Wright

Aspiration

Inhalation of foreign and/or infected material into the lung is a common cause of atelectasis, pneumonia, and lung abscess. The most common predisposing condition in adults is alcoholism; others applicable to all ages include loss of consciousness or neurologic damage, seizures, drugs, vomiting, and gastroesophageal reflux or other motility disorders (Table 25–1). Involved areas depend on anatomy and the position of the subjects. The posterior segments of the upper lobes or superior segments of the left lower lobe are involved when the subject is recumbent, basal segments of the lower lobes when upright, and the anterior segment of the middle lobe if the patient is prone or inclined forward, such as occurs in vomiting.[1,2] Lesions depend to a large part on the nature of the material inhaled, varying from mild bronchiolitis, to hemorrhagic pulmonary edema, to pneumonia, to granulomatous inflammation (Table 25–2).

Foreign Body Aspiration

Aspiration of a foreign body large enough to occlude partially a segmental or subsegmental airway is common in both children and adults. Symptoms may be minimal in children, or there may be varying degrees of cough and choking; in adults the dramatic "café coronary" of sudden death may result. After an asymptomatic period, signs of prolonged retention are manifested.[3] These signs, including cough, hemoptysis, and purulent sputum, are most likely due to complications, including bronchiectasis and infection, rather than the foreign body itself. There is an inflammatory reaction in the walls of the airway, and because of obstruction, lipid-filled macrophages accumulate to produce obstructive pneumonia (see Obstructive Pneumonia, below). Radiologically 50 percent of larger foreign bodies are opaque. Features of atelectasis, bronchiectasis, pneumonia, and lung abscess may be present. Initial therapy consists of removal of the material, which in 99 percent of patients may be performed by bronchoscopy.[3] In other cases, large foreign bodies may result in obstructive stenosis or overinflation. The Holzknecht sign, consisting of inspiratory retraction of the mediastinum and heart into the affected chest cavity, may be observed in cases of either stenosis or valvular obstruction and guides the bronchoscopist to the site of the body. Obstructive overinflation purportedly results because valvular action by the foreign body allows airflow into but not out of the affected lung segment.[3]

Aspiration of Gastric Acid

Vomiting with aspiration of gastric contents occurs frequently and is probably the most common cause of diffuse alveolar damage. Gastric acid can cause extensive injury to the bronchioles and alveoli. Mendelson[4] originally described the clinical findings of aspiration occurring in women during labor and established an experimental model. This model has been thoroughly explored, with various acid concentrations used to produce mild bronchiolitis,[5] necrotizing bronchiolitis,[6] and diffuse alveolar damage[7] (Fig. 25–1). Clinical findings depend on the severity of the reaction. These can be profound, and shock, hypoxia, and death may occur within a short period. Cough, cyanosis, wheezing, fever, tachypnea, and dyspnea are common symptoms in less fulminating cases.

Table 25-1. Cause of Aspiration

Central Nervous System–Related Aspiration
    Loss of consciousness
    Alcoholic stupor
    Neurologic damage
    Seizures
    Drugs (narcotic or non-narcotic)
    Debilitation
    Anesthesia

Gastrointestinal Related Aspiration
    Vomiting
    Gastrointestinal reflux
    Achalasia
    Esophageal dysmotility
    Fistula to respiratory tract
    Nasogastric intubation
    Swallowiing difficulties

Table 25-2. Results of Aspiration

Foreign Bodies	Gastric Contents	Lipid Materials
Death from anoxia	Acid	Granulomatous response
Obstructive overinflation	Bronchiolitis	
Obstructive airway stenosis	Hemorrhagic edema	
Atelectasis	Diffuse alveolar damage	
Obstructive pneumonia	Food particles	
	Granulomatous response	

Aspiration of Lipid Material (Exogenous Lipid Pneumonia)

The types of lipid aspirated include contrast medium, milk, mineral oil, or liquid paraffin. Unusual sources of lipid, actually inhaled as an aerosol, include hair spray propellant,[8] Guyanan blackfat tobacco smoke,[9] oil mist used in steel rolling,[10] and the products of burning fats.[10]

Radiologically an early finding is the presence of acinar filling[11] and fibroblastic proliferation with interstitial fibrosis subsequently producing streaky nodular infiltrates.[12]

The reaction to the oils is fairly similar, and four stages have been described.[13] The initial stage is a hemorrhagic bronchopneumonia. This stage is followed by an intense macrophagic infiltrate with cells filled with oil droplets in the alveoli and often in the draining lymph nodes (Fig. 25–2). Weill and colleagues[11] described methods using fluorescence microscopy with benzpyrene staining for the identification of oil droplets both in sputum and lung biopsy material. The third stage is characterized by fibroblastic proliferation resulting in bands of collagen surrounding pools of oil. Vascular obliteration is prominent in this stage, and bronchiolar obliteration and ectasia are present (Fig. 25–3). The final stage consists of dense fibrous obliteration with the lipid pools still recognizable; this is the classic paraffinoma (Fig. 25–4). In stages three and four, the lipid pools can be mistaken for alveoli. Inspection of the walls, however, should reveal macrophages, giant cells, or no cells at all; pneumonocytes are never present. The fibroblastic response of mineral oil aspiration has been used as a model for investigation of pulmonary fibrosis.[14]

Although mineral oil does not predispose to infection, there have been reports of colonization of the droplets by atypical mycobacterium, the oil apparently enhancing the growth of the bacilli.[15,16]

Atelectasis

Atelectasis (Fig. 25–5) is defined as a state of collapsed peripheral gas-exchange regions of the lung with resultant loss of volume. Table 25–3 shows the various mechanisms that result in atelectasis. Direct lung compression, decreased alveolar surface tension, and inability to expand the lung reduce the ability of the deflated lung to reinflate. Airway obstruction, however, reduces ventilation to the lung followed by absorption of resident gases; collateral ventilation is important in this mechanism (see below) since it would provide some incoming air and total resorption would not occur. Atelectasis is common in both children and adults, and airflow obstruction is the most likely primary event in both age groups, although etiologies of the obstruction may be different (see Table 25–3).

In early pediatric literature, infection was a common cause of atelectasis. James[17] reviewed 854 children with documented atelectasis and found 18.9 percent due to pertussis, 17.2 percent to upper respiratory tract infection, 13.8 percent to "sinobronchitis" (defined as purulent nasal discharge with bronchitis), 13.7 percent to pneumonia, 13.6 percent to lower respiratory tract infections, 6.5 percent to asthma, and 6.1 percent to tuberculosis. Although the ratio of infective lesions is different today, it is important to recognize these associations.[18]

In general there is no overall propensity for a certain area of lung to be atelectatic. Some causes have a propensity for particular lobar involvement; asthma, cystic fibrosis, and tuberculosis involve the right lung more often than the left, whereas respiratory tract infections cause predominately left lower lobe atelectasis, and postintubation atelectasis affects the right upper lobe.[18] Multiple areas of atelectasis are seen in measles, pertussis, and sinobronchitis.[17] The majority of atelectatic areas re-expand within 3 months. Recurrent atelectasis is most common in patients with chronic diseases such as asthma and cystic fibrosis. Patients with persistent atelectasis accounted for 10.6 percent of James' cases[17] and were caused by tuberculosis and sinobronchitis; more recent studies[18] have incriminated cystic fibrosis.

In adults bronchogenic carcinoma is an important cause of bronchial obstruction and should be strongly suspected in recurrent atelectasis. In contrast to the

Atelectasis   753

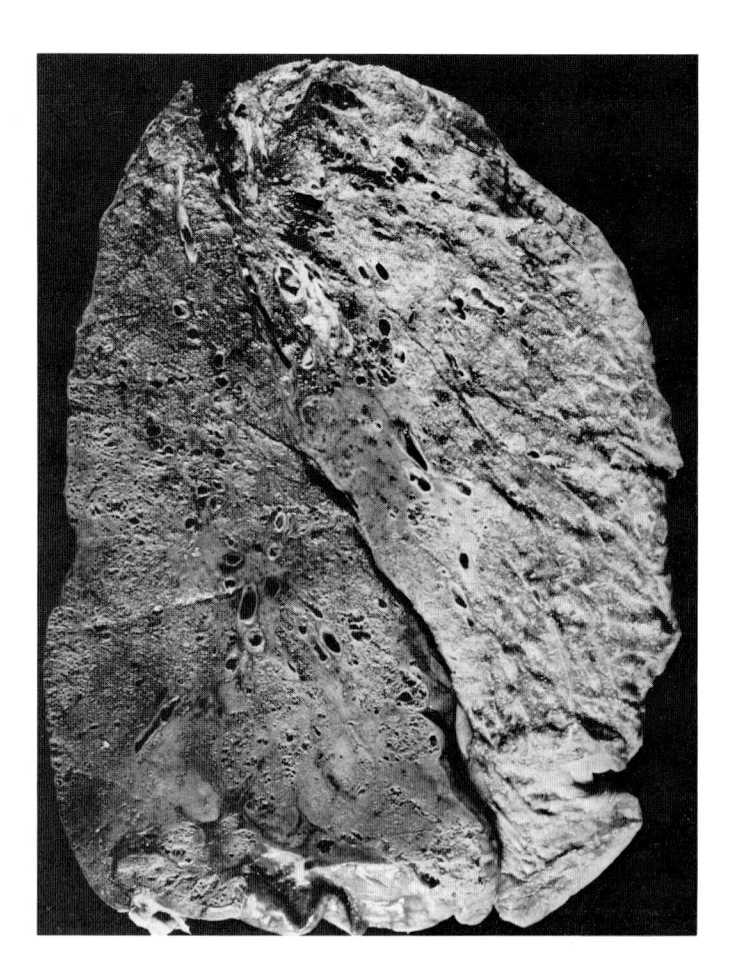

Figure 25–1. Gross photograph of lung showing the homogenous lung parenchyma of diffuse alveolar damage after aspiration of gastric contents.

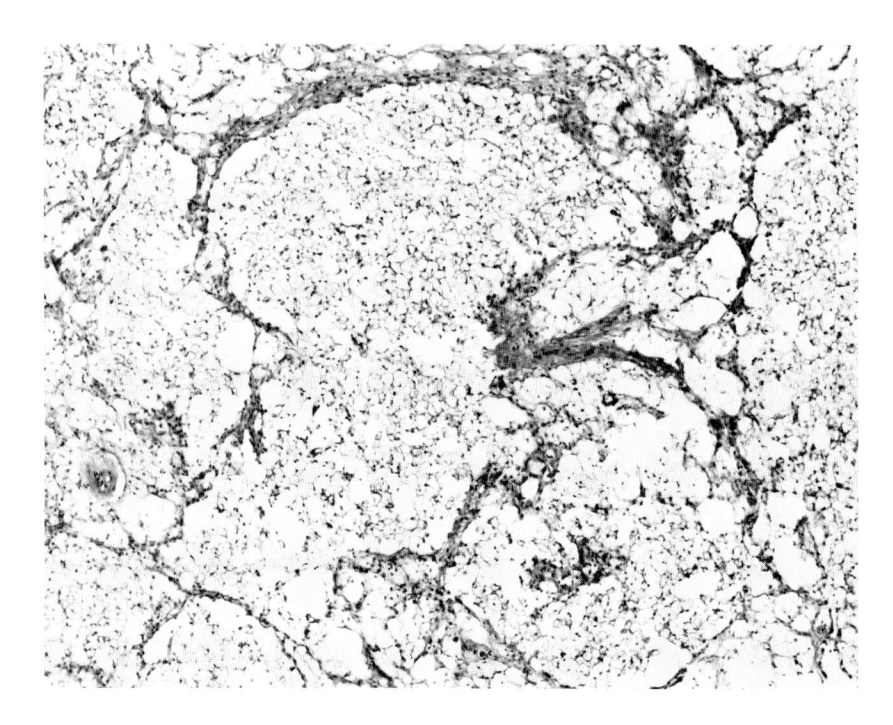

Figure 25–2. Alveoli filled by lipid-laden macrophages in early stage of inhalation lipid pneumonia. There is little fibroblastic response (H&E, ×64).

Figure 25–3. The third phase of inhalation lipid pneumonia with large pools of lipid partially surrounded by macrophages and multinucleated giant cells. A fibroblastic response is present in this stage (H&E, ×160).

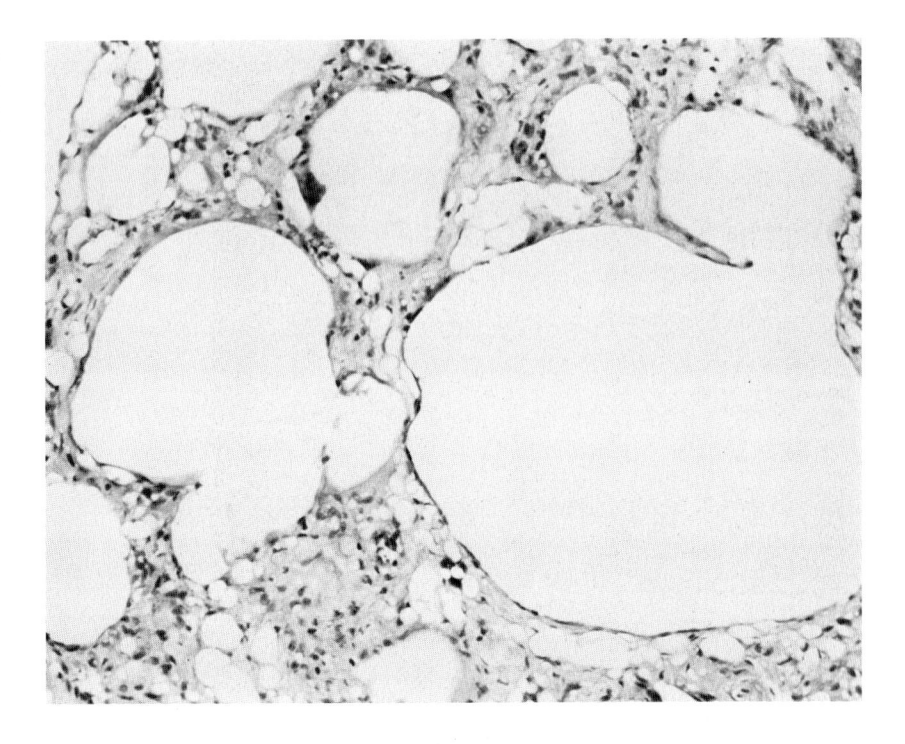

Pathophysiology

Occlusion of a bronchus is followed by resorption of air from alveoli. The partial pressure of gas in the lung is 760 mmHg, and the partial pressure of gases in the end capillary mixed venous blood is 706 mmHg (O_2 40; CO_2 46; H_2O 47; N_2 573); thus, the alveolar gas is easily resorbed since the diffusion gradients of O_2 and N_2 are directed toward the bloodstream. Resorption is rapid when atelectasis occurs as the patient is receiving high concentrations of oxygen. In this setting, N_2 concentration in the capillary blood is low, and since oxygen is

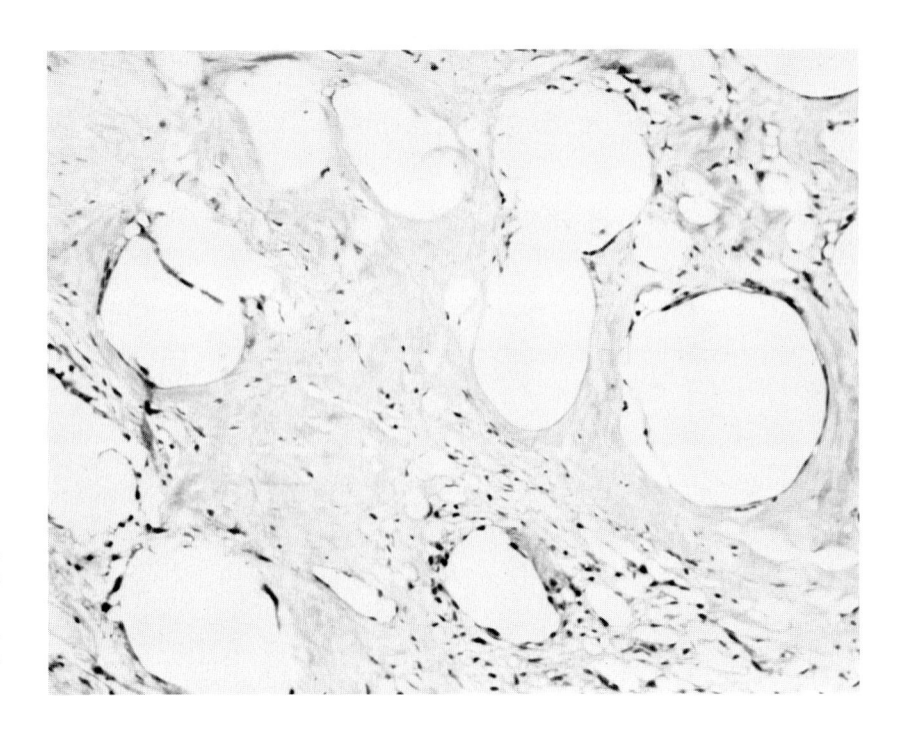

Figure 25–4. Dense collagen surrounds lipid pools. The macrophage response is much less prominent than that seen in the earlier stages. This represents the final stage in inhalation lipid pneumonia and is the classic paraffinoma (H&E, ×160).

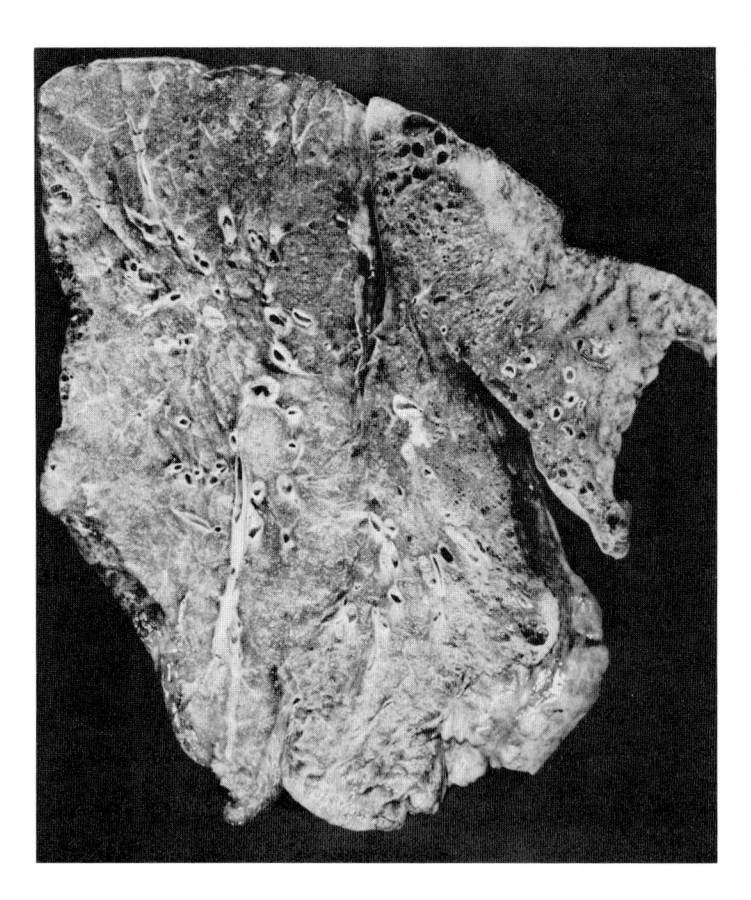

Figure 25–5. Gross photograph showing chronic atelectasis of the lower lobe in an alcoholic.

much more soluble than nitrogen, the gas is resorbed easily.

Atelectasis compromises lung mechanics, gas exchange, hemodynamics, and host defenses.[18] Lung compliance is reduced in accordance with the LaPlace law which states that a critical closing pressure is related directly to the surface tension, and inversely to the radius of the sphere. The tendency for an alveolus to collapse is greater when its internal diameter is decreased; therefore, a greater effort is needed for it to inflate. Levine and Johnson[19] investigated differences in compliance in lungs atelectatic for various lengths of time. They found that higher pressures were needed to inflate the lungs that were atelectatic for the longest time, but once inflated, all lungs deflated in a similar fashion. Although the amount of surfactant was slightly decreased in atelectatic lungs, these results were interpreted cautiously by the authors, who suggested that surfactant activity did not appear to be decreased. Berezovsky and associates[20] showed disturbed release of osmophilic granules in type II cells in biopsy specimens of lungs with long-term atelectasis, with only "dyscirculatory" changes present in atelectasis of short duration.

Changes in blood flow appear to be directly related to the extent of the lung collapsed. The alveolar hypoxia produces pulmonary vasoconstriction with associated increase in pulmonary vascular resistance, thus shunting blood away from the affected areas.[21] Unfortunately this becomes less effective as large amounts of lung are collapsed, and eventually intrapulmonary shunt is produced resulting in hypoxemia. This was demonstrated by Marshall[22] who showed that approximately 50 percent atelectasis could be compensated for.

Changes in pulmonary defense mechanisms are important when considering complications of atelectasis (see Bronchiectasis, below). Experimental data suggest that the hypoxic lung removes and kills some bacteria less effectively than a normoxic lung.[23] Drinkwater and co-workers[24] showed decreased clearance of *Streptococcus pneumoniae* in atelectasis. Since there was also stimulation of cellular phagocytosis and bactericidal activity in these lungs, the authors stressed the importance of mucociliary clearance. This is in accordance with early experimental data that showed that bronchiectasis did not develop in atelectatic lobes unless infection associated with bronchial obstruction was present.[25,26]

Clinical Findings

Clinical findings may relate to the atelectasis, its etiology, or its complications. The most common signs in children include cough, tachypnea, rhonchi, fever, and chest pain. If complications such as pneumonia, abscess, or bronchiectasis arise, fever may be pronounced, and the cough may produce sputum, often purulent and occa-

Table 25–3. Causes of Atelectasis

> Airway obstruction
> > Tumors
> > Infections
> > Aspirated foreign body
> > Mucous plugs (asthma, cystic fibrosis)
> > Extrinsic pressure (lymph nodes, neoplasm)
> > Infiltration of wall (sarcoid, amyloid)
>
> Compression of lung
> > Pneumothorax, effusion
> > Neoplasm
> > Localized emphysema
>
> Decreased alveolar surface tension
> > Adult respiratory distress syndrome
> > Hyaline membrane disease
>
> Inability to expand lung
> > Weak respiratory muscles
> > Pain
> > Obesity, scoliosis
> > Central nervous system depression
>
> Miscellaneous
> > Thromboembolism

sionally associated with hemoptysis.[18] Importantly there may be no clinical signs, and the chest radiograph provides the diagnosis.

Radiology

Changes in chest radiograph are variable.[27] Alveolar alterations depend on whether the affected lung is air filled or fluid filled; if the lung is fluid filled, density is increased. The adjacent lung shows compensatory overinflation with the spreading of vascular shadows and a rather oligemic appearance. This situation can be differentiated from air trapping since the former reduces in volume on expiration. Vascular alterations in the affected lung occur when it collapses to two-thirds its normal volume, and the vessels then show crowding. Bronchi may be reorientated with normally nonvisable bronchi easily identifiable. If the bronchi contain air and the alveoli contain fluid, an air bronchogram is present. The position and shape of fissures may change and can appear as different markings depending on whether air or fluid is present in alveoli. The mediastinum may shift in position; this is seen more commonly in cases of lower lobe collapse as opposed to upper lobe collapse. In upper lobe collapse, the paratracheal stripe and the superior vena cava shadow become obliterated. Rib approximation is difficult to assess but when present suggests lower lobe collapse. The diaphragm may be elevated, particularly in upper lobe collapse, whereas in lower lobe collapse, the diaphragm markings may be partially obscured.

Pathology

Atelectasis is associated with minimal morphologic changes, even in its chronic phase. There may be small collections of macrophages within the alveoli on light microscopy, and electron micrographs show type II cells with numerous and irregular osmophilic granules.[20]

Special Types of Atelectasis

Right Middle Lobe Atelectasis (Middle Lobe Syndrome)

Chronic or recurrent atelectasis of the right middle lobe was first described in 1937 by Brock and associates,[28] but the term middle lobe syndrome was not established until 11 years later when Graham and co-workers[29] described collapse due to lymphadenopathy that was not only caused by tuberculosis, as Brock had thought, but by a multiplicity of causes.

The anatomy of the middle lobe appears to be a major factor accounting for its propensity to collapse.[30] The bronchus is surrounded by a collar of lymph nodes receiving drainage from large amounts of the lung parenchyma. The bronchus has a sharp take-off, is narrow, and does not divide immediately into segmental bronchi, but it is very long, making it vulnerable to compression. Compression is not always present, however; Culiner[31] demonstrated a lack of bronchial obstruction in nine patients studied bronchographically and pathologically. Perhaps more important is the isolation of the middle lobe from collateral ventilation, particularly when a complete minor fissure is present. Support for this theory was provided by Inners and colleagues[32] who measured middle lobe collateral ventilation in healthy volunteers. They found a high resistance and a long-time constant in this lobe when compared with the upper lobes; they suggested that these were due to a greater ratio of pleural to nonpleural surface in the middle lobe. Time constant is defined as the product of airway resistance and compliance; the longer the time constant, the longer the lung takes to empty or fill. When collateral ventilation is inadequate, atelectasis may occur by resorption of gas in obstructed alveoli and by impairment of removal of airway secretions. The latter occurs because the cough mechanism depends on the compression of alveolar gas by increasing intrapleural pressure; this increases the airway pressure and therefore aids in expelling airway mucus.

Clinically there is a classic quartet associated with middle lobe collapse: cough, pain, hemoptysis, and recurrent pneumonia. In a study of 99 patients, 77 percent had recurrent pneumonia, 52 percent had pain which was primarily pleuritic in nature, and 42 percent had recurrent hemoptysis.[33] A dry hacking cough was almost universal. Radiologically the typical signs of middle lobe collapse[27] are present and consist of obscuration of the right heart border and a flattened triangular density with

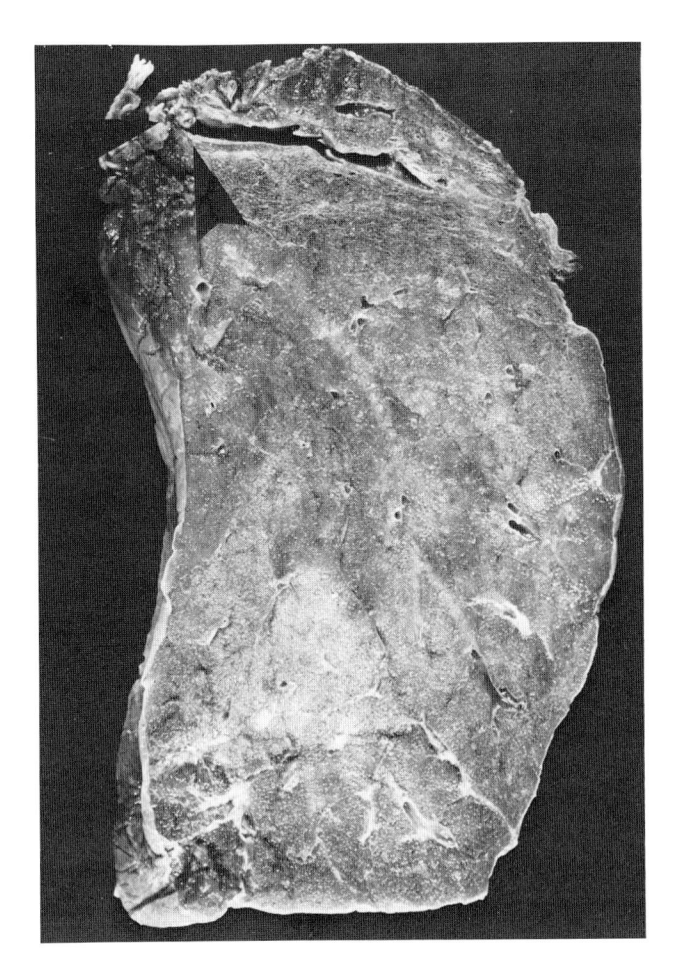

Figure 25–6. Gross photograph of the middle lobe showing a broncholith firmly impacted in the lumen of an airway (arrow). Note the distal airway dilation.

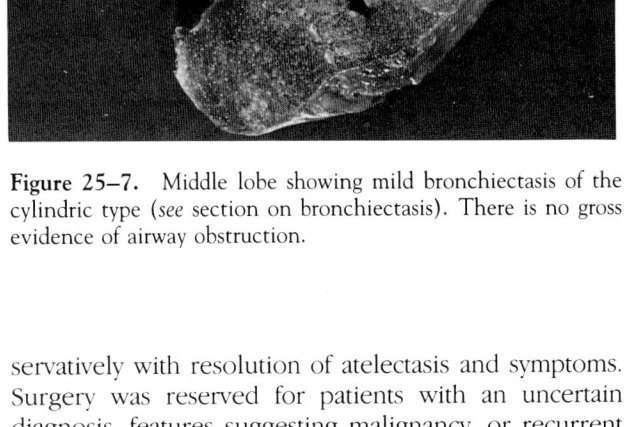

Figure 25–7. Middle lobe showing mild bronchiectasis of the cylindric type (*see* section on bronchiectasis). There is no gross evidence of airway obstruction.

the apex at the hilum. Bronchographic abnormalities are present at least 70 percent of the time.[34]

Pathology

In a review of the literature, Wagner and Johnston[34] found that 47 percent of right middle lobe atelectasis were associated with benign parenchymal inflammation, 15 percent were due to bronchiectasis, and 9 percent were due to tuberculosis (Figs. 25–6, 25–7). The morphologic features of middle lobe syndrome are therefore varied and represent etiologic pathology rather than any specific feature of atelectasis. A surprising 24 percent of collapse were associated with neoplasm, the majority (22 percent) malignant (Fig. 25–8). Bertelsen and colleagues[35] considered that in patients with a previously normal radiograph, middle lobe atelectasis was a sign of potential malignancy, findings in conflict with early observations by Brock[28] who suggested that neoplasia in the middle lobe was a rare phenomenon.

Treatment is related to the etiology. In Albo and Grimes's study,[33] 54 of 99 patients were managed conservatively with resolution of atelectasis and symptoms. Surgery was reserved for patients with an uncertain diagnosis, features suggesting malignancy, or recurrent or persistent disease.

Rounded Atelectasis

Rounded atelectasis is an unusual form of peripheral lung parenchymal collapse. It has many synonyms including folded lung, atelectatic pseudotumor, pleuroma, and shrinking pleuritis. A review of several studies[36–39] shows that most patients were men (55 of 56), had been exposed to asbestos (51 of 56), and many were cigarette smokers. Although the majority of patients were asymptomatic, occasional presenting complaints of cough and pleural chest pain were found. Pulmonary function tests were generally within normal limits.

The lesion is generally found on chest radiograph and has a predisposition to the right lower lobe (18 of 40). It appears as a rounded or lobulated mass lesion with

Figure 25–8. Surgical specimen of middle lobe shows a carcinoid tumor compressing one of the segmental bronchi.

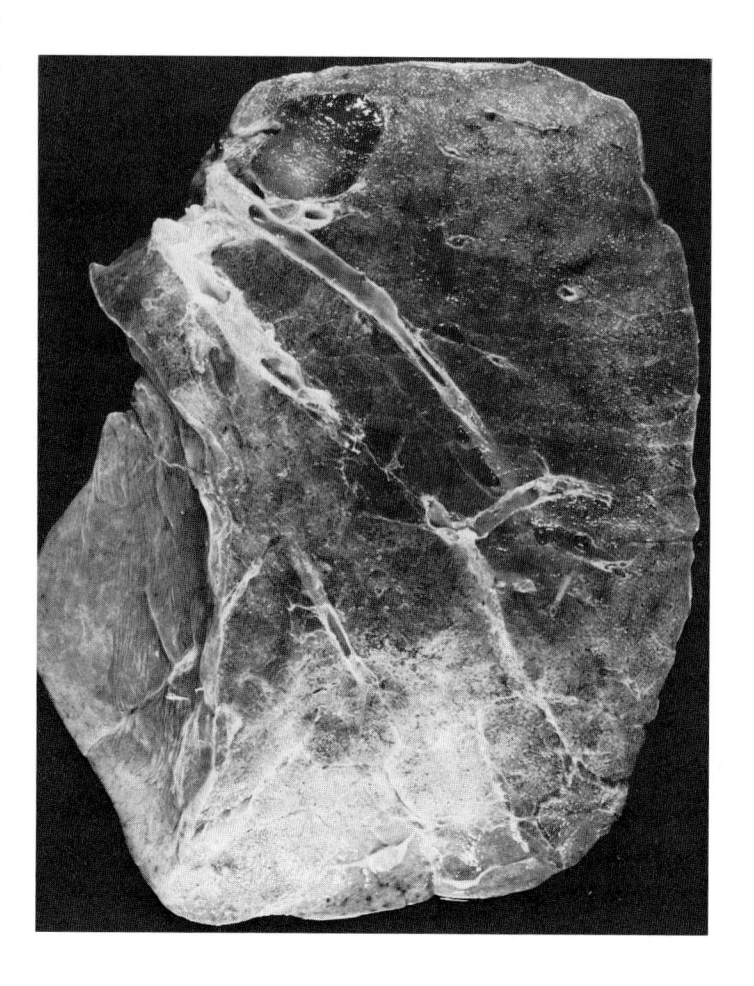

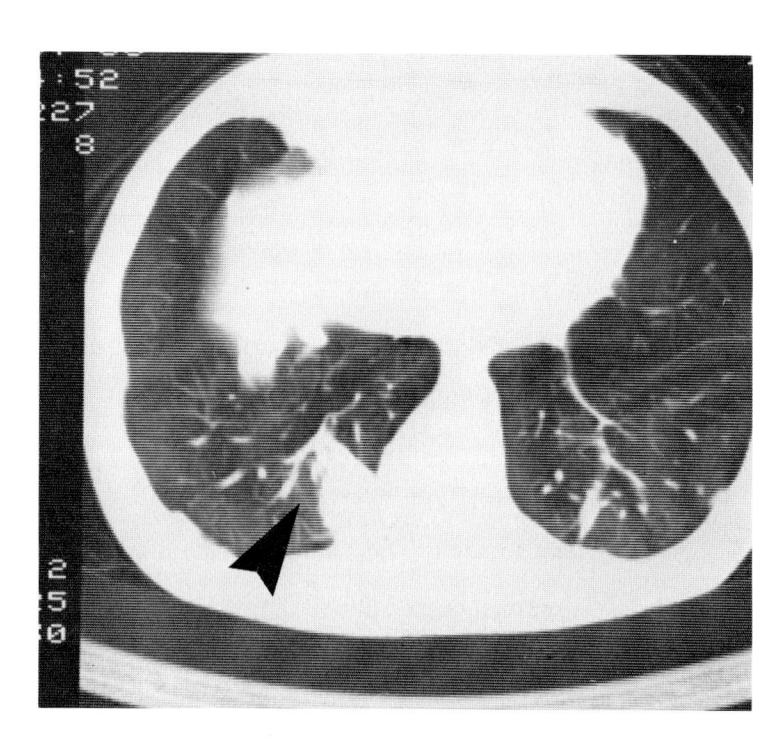

Figure 25–9. Chest CT of an asbestos worker showing rounded atelectasis. Note the pleural-based density with adjacent lung forming a "comet tail" (arrow).

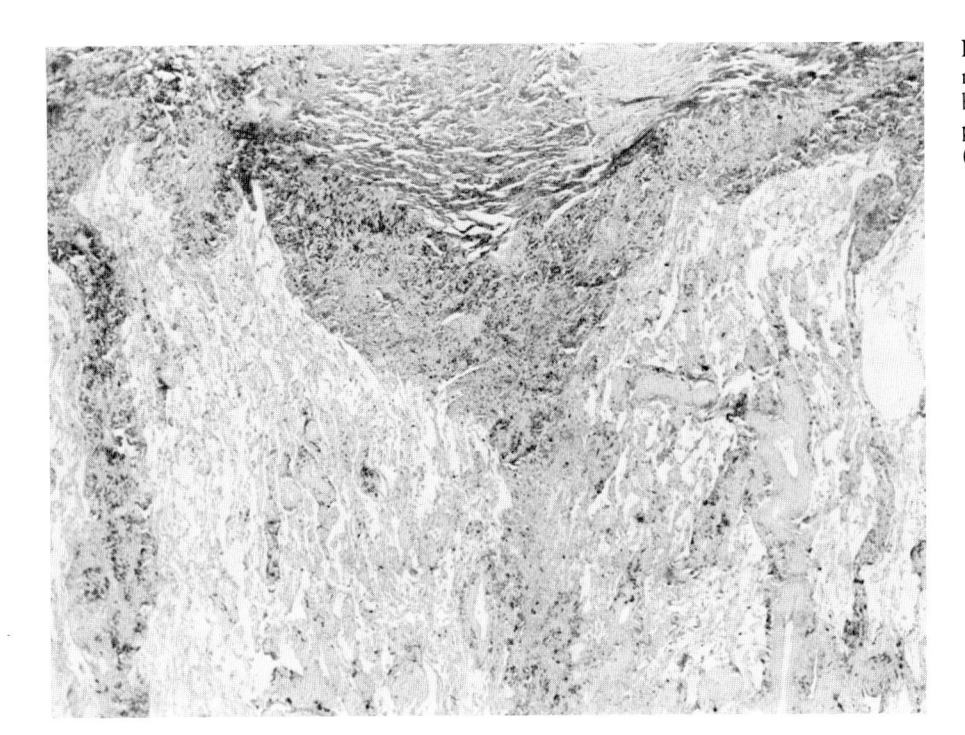

Figure 25–10. Rounded atelectasis in a man exposed to asbestos. The thick bands of fibrous tissue radiate from the pleural surface into the underlying lung (H&E, ×24).

adjacent pleural thickening.[36,40] Although usually solitary, bilateral lesions have been reported.[40] The lobe may be reduced in size, and wedge-shaped areas of atelectasis are noted extending from a margin of the lesion.[39] The characteristic feature is seen best on lateral tomograms and consists of a comet-like tail formed by the vessels and bronchi curling into the mass from below. The adjacent lung may be hyperinflated, and an air bronchogram can be seen centrally. Computed tomography (CT) is apparently specific and can be used to differentiate this lesion from both malignant mesothelioma and lung carcinoma.[41] Doyle and Lawler[40] reported several distinguishing features including (1) peripheral rounded mass, most dense at the periphery, and not completely surrounded by lung; (2) the lesion forms an acute angle with the pleura which also shows scarring; and (3) at least two sharp margins are formed by adjacent curving lung, while the vessels and bronchi curl inward causing blurring of the central margin (Fig. 25–9).

Two different mechanisms have been suggested for rounded atelectasis. Hanke and Kretzchmar[39] initially suggested it was due to the mechanical influence of pleural effusion. They postulated that the pleural effusion caused atelectasis, followed by formation of a cleft between the atelectatic and aerated segment. The lung tilts at the cleft and becomes fixed in this position by fibrin deposition followed by contraction and inward curling of the segment. This concept was challenged by Schneider and colleagues[42] who failed to find free fluid in a group of collected cases, but it was supported by Mintzer and Cugell[38] and Smith and Schillaci,[43] who reported cases of rounded atelectasis in association with effusion in patients with and without asbestos exposure. The marked association of rounded atelectasis and asbestos exposure prompted Dernevik and colleagues[36] to suggest that it was due to an irritative effect of the asbestos fibers on the pleura, perhaps in a manner analogous to the postulated formation of pleural plaques. The pleural fibrotic reaction causes pleural shrinkage with folding of the lung, hence the synonym shrinking pleuritis.

Many early cases of rounded atelectasis required thoracotomy for confirmation of diagnosis; at surgery, the atelectatic lung would often inflate immediately after pleural incision. Because of the sensitivity and specificity of CT, the current trend is toward observation, with surgery reserved for symptomatic or unusual cases.

Pathologic features are nonspecific, and this lesion represents a surgical and radiologic rather than a pathologic diagnosis. The pleura is thickened and fibrotic, generally without a mesothelial reaction. The underlying lung parenchyma is relatively unremarkable (Fig. 25–10).

Pneumonia

There are two basic types of pneumonia associated with bronchial obstruction: pneumonia due to the consequences of the material aspirated, and pneumonia due to interference with the mucociliary escalater.

Figure 25–11. Multiple vegetable particles are surrounded by a mixed inflammatory infiltrate (H&E, ×64).

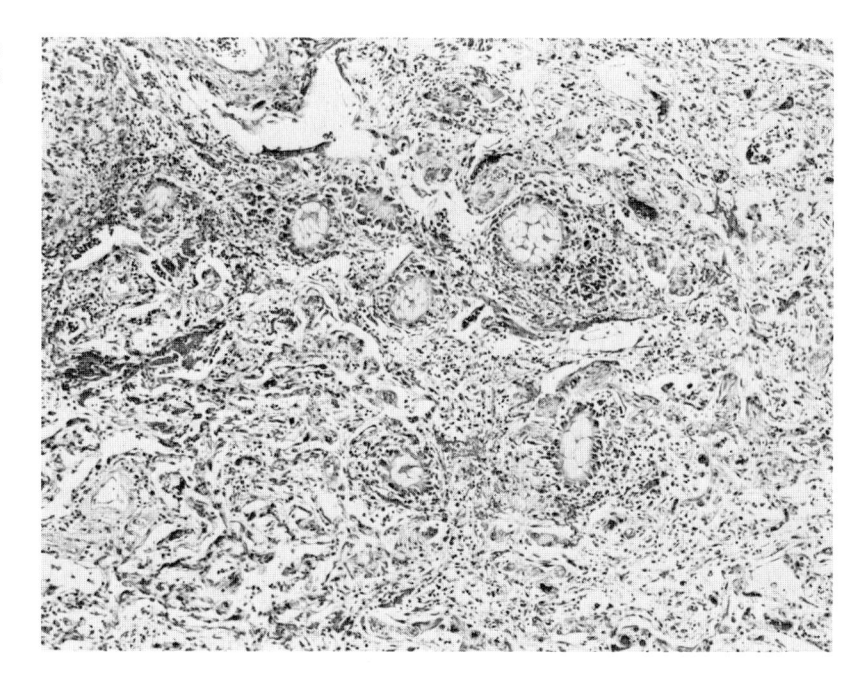

Aspiration Pneumonia

Damage to airways and lung parenchyma because of the aspiration of material is a common condition and a major source of morbidity and mortality. The causes are summarized in Table 25–1. (Various other aspects of aspiration are discussed in Chapters 13 and 16. In a large study of patients in a mental institution, 25 percent of autopsies showed aspiration pneumonia.[44]

Clinical Findings

There may be a previous history of vomiting. In a large review series of Le Frock and associates[45] dyspnea and cough were the common symptoms, and tachypnea and cyanosis with rales, rhonchi, and wheezes were the most frequent physical findings. Low-grade fever may occasionally occur.

Radiology

There are areas of consolidation that may be unilobar or multilobar, either unilateral or bilateral.[46] The junction between normal and abnormal lung is often abrupt, and the lesions have the appearance of a diffuse air space process (nonhomogeneity, air space nodules, air bronchogram, and rapid evolution) with minimal atelectasis. If severe emphysema is present, the consolidation surrounds the cysts, making their walls visible and simulating a lung abscess.

Pathology

Fluid aspirated from the oropharynx or gastrointestinal tract contains a myriad of substances including bacteria, foreign material, cells, saliva, and gastric juice. Aspiration of bacterial-contaminated fluids results in deposition of the organisms on the mucosa of bronchi and bronchioles and in the alveoli. *Streptococcus pneumoniae* and *Klebsiella pneumoniae* characteristically involve the subpleural parenchyma and result in an initial hemorrhagic edema. Alveolar air is replaced by a fluid and cellular (neutrophils and macrophages) exudate, resulting in areas of consolidation. Vascular necrosis results in areas of parenchymal necrosis, which may form abscesses. Massive vascular involvement can yield gangrene. Foreign material such as meat or vegetable fibers can often be recognized (Fig. 25–11). In early stages, they are surrounded by a neutrophilic response, which, as the lesions become chronic, are replaced by macrophages and giant cells (Fig. 25–12). Small areas of fibrosis and granulomas can give a micronodular or miliary appearance.

Microbiologic cultures are often mixed, and both aerobes and anaerobes may be present. Bartlett and co-workers[47] stress the importance of anaerobic culture in aspiration pneumonia as they found anaerobes present in 50 of 54 cases. Gram-negative enteric and Pseudomonas strains are common when aspiration pneumonia occurs in hospital.[47]

Obstructive (Endogenous Lipid, Golden) Pneumonia

Although bronchogenic carcinoma is the most frequent cause, any condition associated with bronchial obstruction can result in obstructive pneumonitis with lipid accumulation. In early investigations, De Navasquez and Haslewood[48] found lipid accumulations in carcinoma, tuberculosis, abscess formation, and bronchiectasis. They

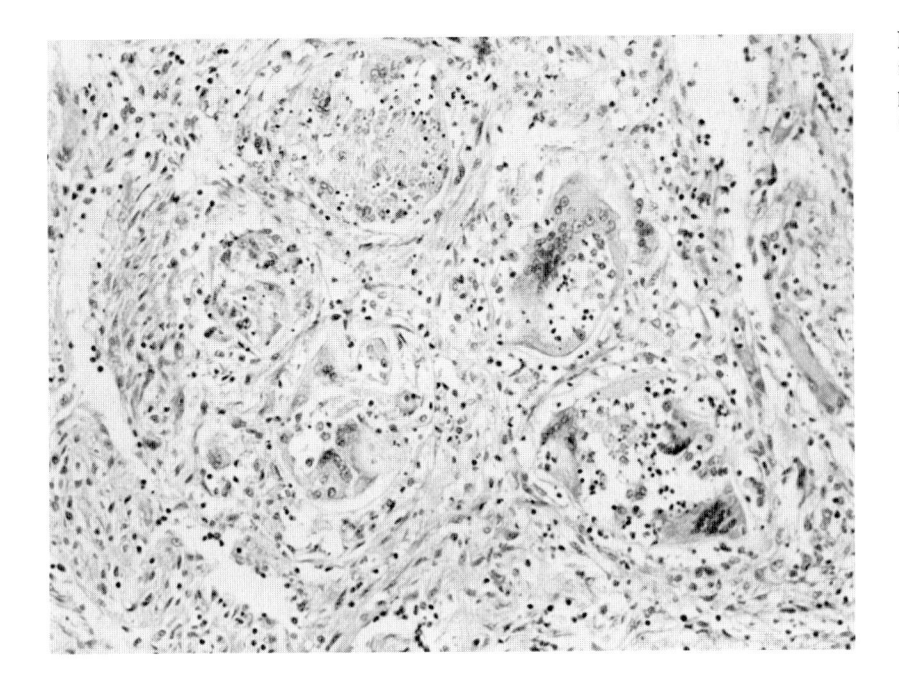

Figure 25–12. Granulomatous inflammation in chronic aspiration. Fragmented aspirated particles are surrounded by multinucleate cells (H&E, ×160).

postulated that the lipid was either derived from the tumors or from degenerating lung. It is now thought that the lipid represents surfactant material secreted by the type II pneumonocytes.[49] Cholesterol clefts may be either derived from this material or formed from cellular membrane and plasma cholesterol products.

Clinical Findings

Clinical findings are related to the etiology of the obstruction and may include cough, fever, and dull or pleuritic chest pain.

Radiology

There is a combination of atelectasis and consolidation which may have an irregular pattern.[46] Cavitation may also be present, and lymphadenopathy and pleural effusion can also occur.

Pathology

Grossly the affected area is firm with irregular margins and has a characteristic yellow coloration responsible for the synonym golden pneumonia (Fig. 25–13). The alveolar spaces are filled with foamy histiocytes. Alveolar walls are often thickened, and there can be marked type II cell hyperplasia (Fig. 25–14). Cholesterol clefts are often present, and these may be partially surrounded by multinucleated giant cells.

There is a rare, apparently separate, entity of lipid pneumonia without obvious obstruction or other etiology. Radiologic features are again atelectasis and consolidation, but the process appears to extend along a pleural base, similar to an infarct.[12] Complications such as abscess, pleural fibrosis, and bronchiectasis are similar to

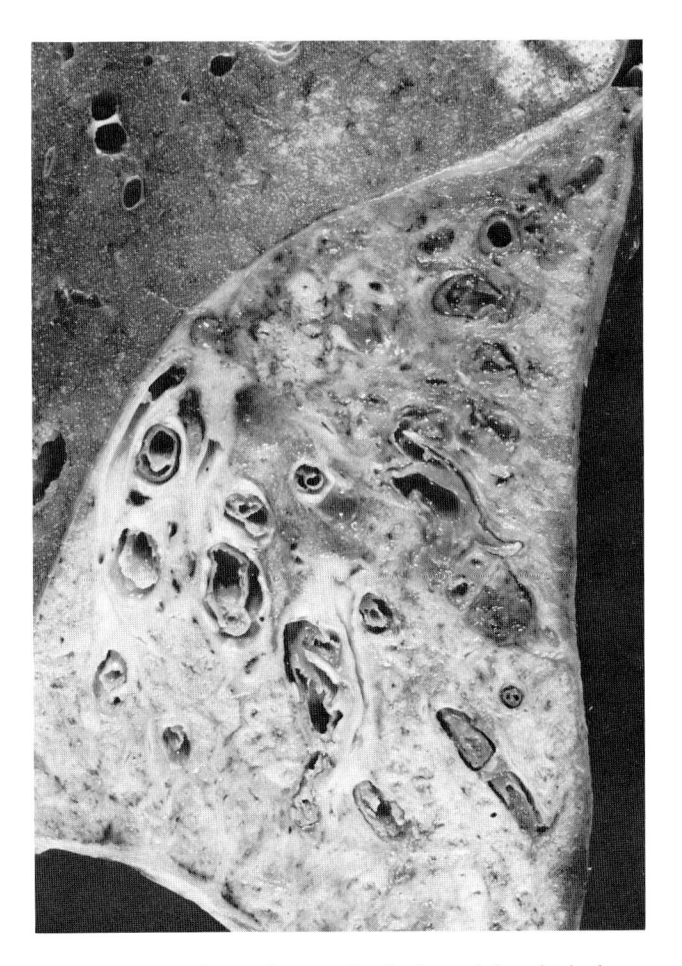

Figure 25–13. Gross photograph of a lower lobe which shows massive consolidation and bronchiectasis. The lobe has a distinct yellow coloration. The lower lobe bronchus was completely obstructed by a squamous cell carcinoma.

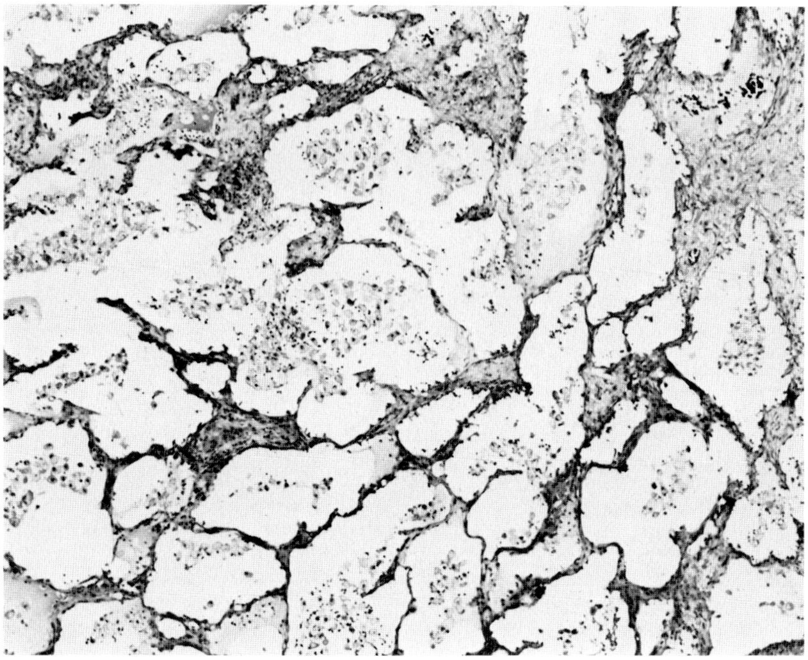

Figure 25-14. Microscopic section taken from Figure 25-13 displays numerous histiocytes within alveoli. There is prominent type II pneumonocyte hyperplasia, and the alveolar walls are irregularly thickened (H&E, ×64).

lipid accumulations with obstructive pneumonia. Clinically there is a marked male predominance with a wide age range.[50] The majority of patients complain of chest pain and cough, and hemoptysis was present in 50 percent. The pathologic features have been described by Lawler,[50] who reviewed 50 such cases. The lesion was often confined to a single lobe, usually the upper or middle, and appeared grossly as a firm, well-demarcated grey-yellow area of consolidation. Microscopic examination revealed alveoli filled with foamy macrophages with associated interstitial fibrosis. Reduplication of elastic fibers and giant cell phagocytosis of elastic fibers could also be identified.

It has been postulated that the lesion is a hypersensitivity phenomenom, or that it is an area of incomplete infarction. Interestingly there is a similar entity in the Hawaiian feral mongoose that may be caused by a viral infection.[51]

Lung Abscess

Lung abscess may result from many causes including aspiration, bronchial obstruction, septic emboli, trauma, and bacterial pneumonia (synpneumonic). It is commonly due to aspiration in patients with poor dental hygiene[52] and in alcoholics (see Chapter 13). In the early literature, lung abscess was frequently (51 percent of 1149 cases) traced back to operative procedures such as tonsilectomy or tooth extraction, either under local or general anesthesia.[1] The importance of poor dental hygiene was also stressed; in one study, carious teeth and infected gums were found in 84 percent of 74 patients in whom an immediate etiology for the abscess was not apparent. In Brock's own series of 276 cases, 14 percent were due to malignancy, 22.5 percent were postoperative, and a further 18 percent had dental sepsis.

Lung abscesses due to aspiration tend to be polymicrobial and are a mixture of anaerobes and aerobes[52] (Fig. 25-15). Although the majority of the organisms are standard oral flora, uncommon organisms such as Legionella and Actinomyces are occasionally identified (Figs. 25-16, 25-17). Proper bacteriologic diagnosis with both aerobic and anerobic cultures is extremely important.

Radiologically, the lesions are poorly marginated and consist of thick-walled irregular cavities. An air-fluid level is common, and there may be surrounding consolidation[2] (Fig. 25-18). Pulmonary gangrene is suggested when a large solitary mass of mecrotic material, surrounded by air, remains in the cavity.[46] Abscesses from septic emboli tend to be multiple and are often subpleural. Abscesses complicating bacterial penumonia (synpneumonic abscesses) occur with a variety of organisms including Staphlococci, Klebsiella, *Streptococcus pneumoniae*, and Pseudomonas. Klebsiella and Staphlococci may cause marked destruction. Cavitating neoplasms, the major radiologic differential diagnosis, have become more common than the early literature suggested, and this can be related to the rising incidence of lung cancer. Squamous cell carcinoma is particularly prone to cavitation. Abscesses can also form in lung parenchyma made atelectatic by airflow obstruction by the tumor.

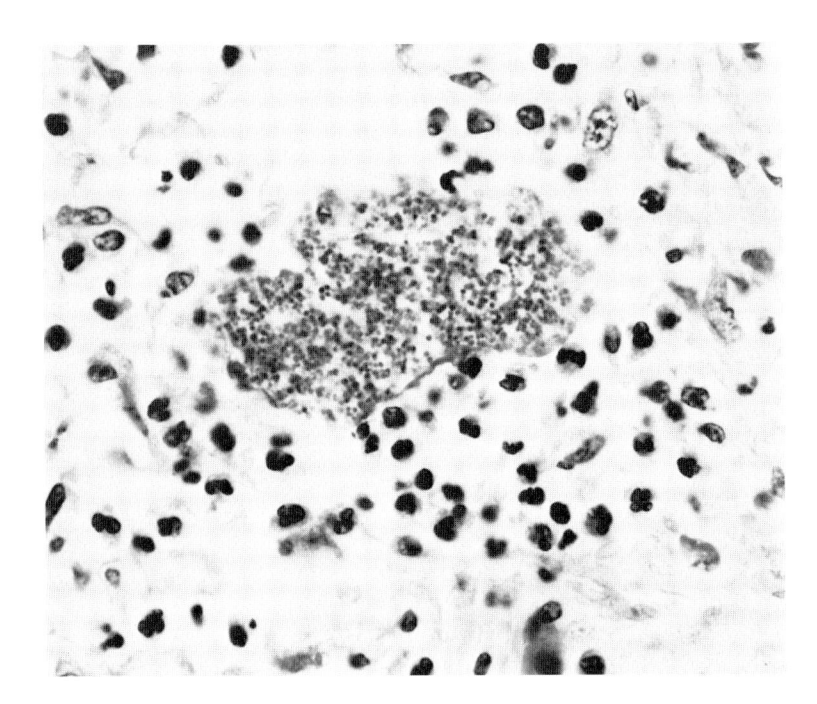

Figure 25–15. Clusters of gaffkya (*Micrococcus tetragena*). This is a common organism inhabiting the mouth and upper respiratory tract (H&E, ×640).

Bronchiectasis

Bronchiectasis is a well-recognized sequel to bronchial obstruction, and other forms of bronchiectasis are discussed elsewhere in detail (*see* Chapter 21).

Pathophysiology

The pathophysiology of bronchiectasis is not completely understood. Three theories have been proposed: traction on the airway from adjacent parenchymal collapse, weak-

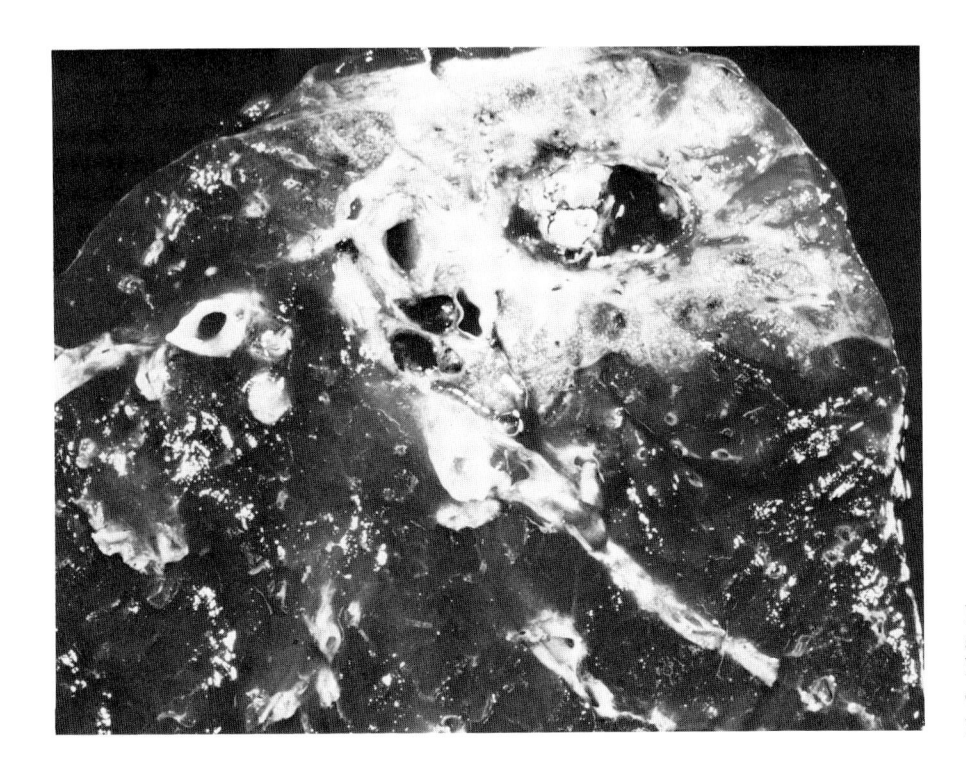

Figure 25–16. Surgical specimen showing actinomycotic abscess cavity. Note the presence of sulfur granules in cavity. Patient was an alcoholic with poor dentition.

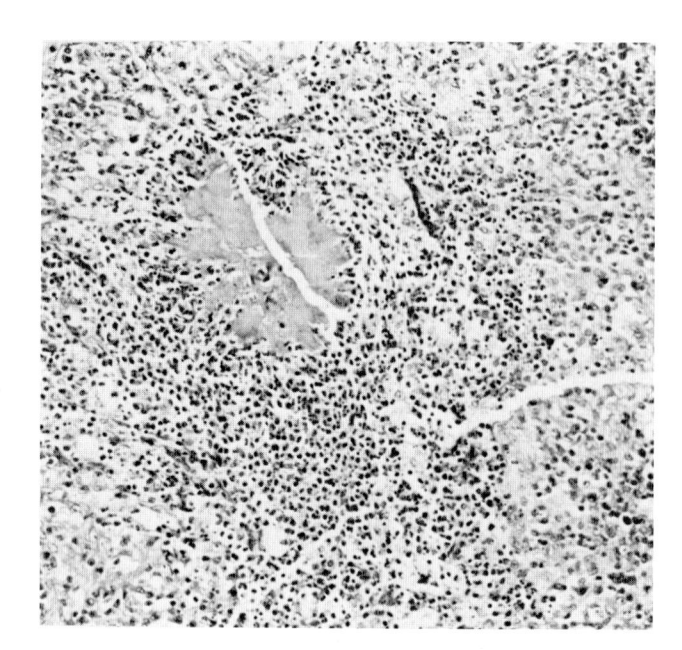

Figure 25–17. Microscopic section from lung abscess in elderly man with poor dentition. The cluster of actinomyces shows the classic eosinophilic fringe (*Hoeppli splendori* effect) and is situated in a pool of pus (H&E, ×160).

ening of the wall from inflammation, and bulging of the wall by pressure from retained secretions. The latter two probably form the basis for the production of bronchial dilation and deformation.[53]

Tannenberg and co-workers[25] and Cheng[26] performed early experiments relating to bronchiectasis. In their animal models, neither chronic atelectasis nor bronchial ligation resulted in bronchiectasis unless there was a superadded infection. These data provided evidence against the theory of traction and supported the importance of inflammation and inspissation. Tanneberg[25] postulated the inflammatory response caused damage to the bronchial nerves, vessels, or both, resulting in inhibition of muscular contraction and impairment of secretion elimination.

Although the importance of obstruction due to tumor (Fig. 25–19) or foreign body aspiration (Fig. 25–20) should not be underestimated, the majority of cases of bronchiectasis in which the etiology can be deduced are post–lower respiratory tract infection. Glauser and associates[54] found 69 percent of cases in their study were postinfective, whereas Fernald[55] reported previous pneumonia in two-thirds of patients studied. Pertussis has enjoyed a resurgence in incidence, particularly in the United Kingdom, because of the decline in childhood vaccinations.[57] The pathologic lesion is a necrotizing bronchitis resulting in atelectasis,[58] and it is not surprising that such an infection should produce bronchiectasis. Similar pathology is seen in some cases of mycoplasma, and it has been suggested that this too may represent a pathogen in the production of bronchiectasis.[59]

Tuberculosis was one of the original etiologic agents identified in bronchiectasis, both because of associated

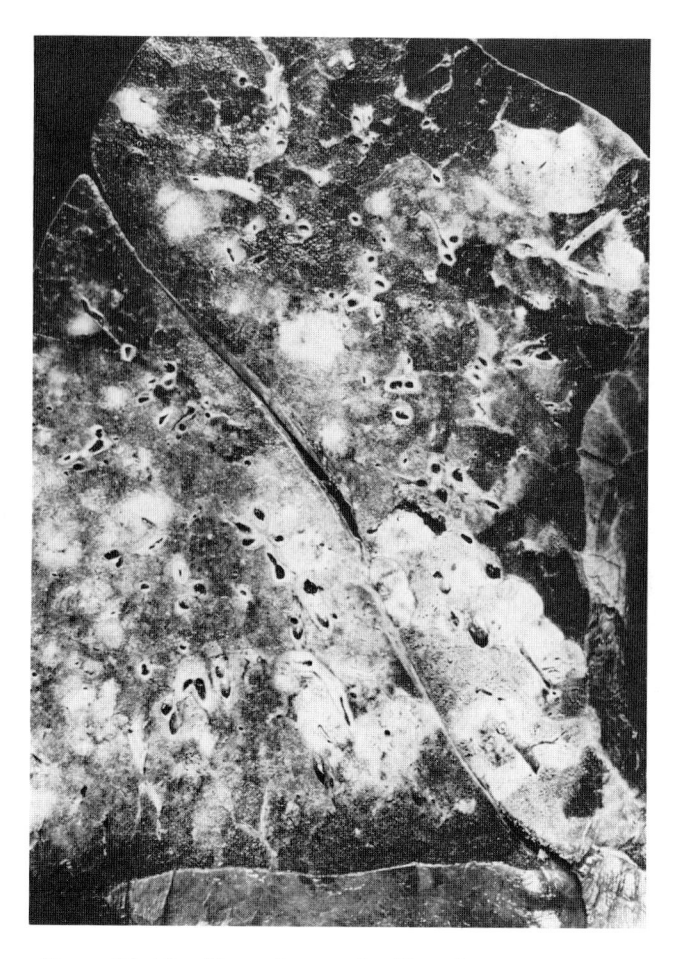

Figure 25–18. Gross photograph of lung from a young man who survived near-drowning but died with sepsis. Lung shows numerous abscesses in various stages of evolution.

lymphadenitis with extrinsic bronchial compression and direct airway necrosis. Although there has been a decrease in tuberculosis in the North American population, the increased number of immigrants from developing countries has resulted in a sharp increase in incidence rates.[53]

Treatment and Prognosis

In the early literature, bronchiectasis was treated by surgical removal of the diseased tissue. Today, because of antibiotics, the trend has switched to total medical management. The best solution probably lies somewhere between the two extremes.

Medical management consists of antibiotic therapy for active infections only; there is no evidence that long-term antibiotic coverage aids in the therapy of bronchiectasis not associated with cystic fibrosis.[53] Aggressive physiotherapy is applied to remove mucous plugs and prevent stagnation of secretions. Bronchoscopy is helpful for management in evaluating extent of disease, and for removal of tenacious mucous plugs.[59]

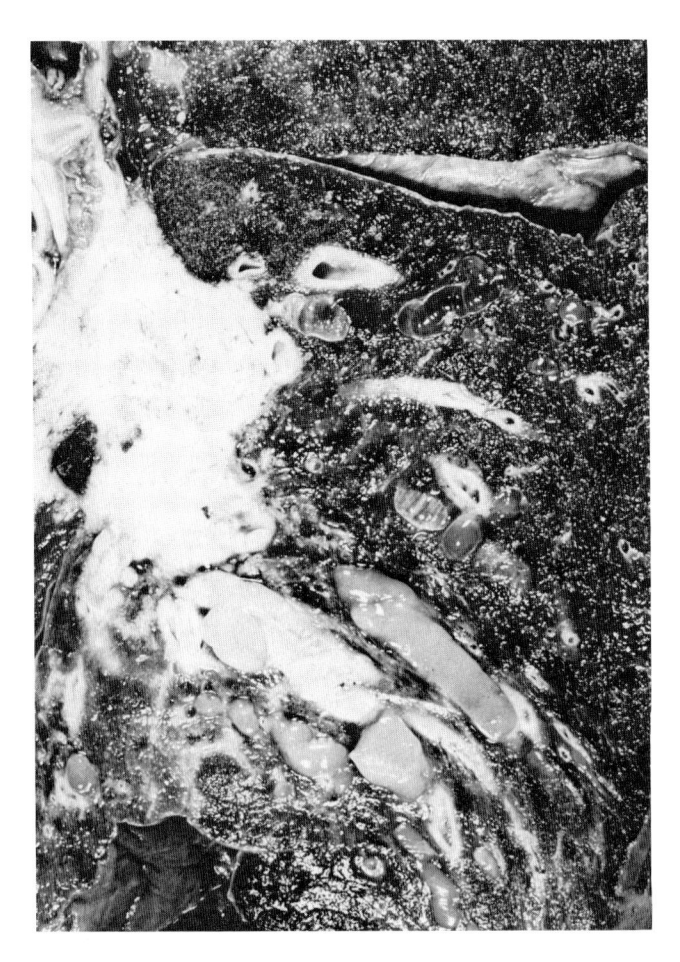

Figure 25–19. Cylindric bronchiectasis distal to obstructing neoplasm. Note the marked mucous plugging.

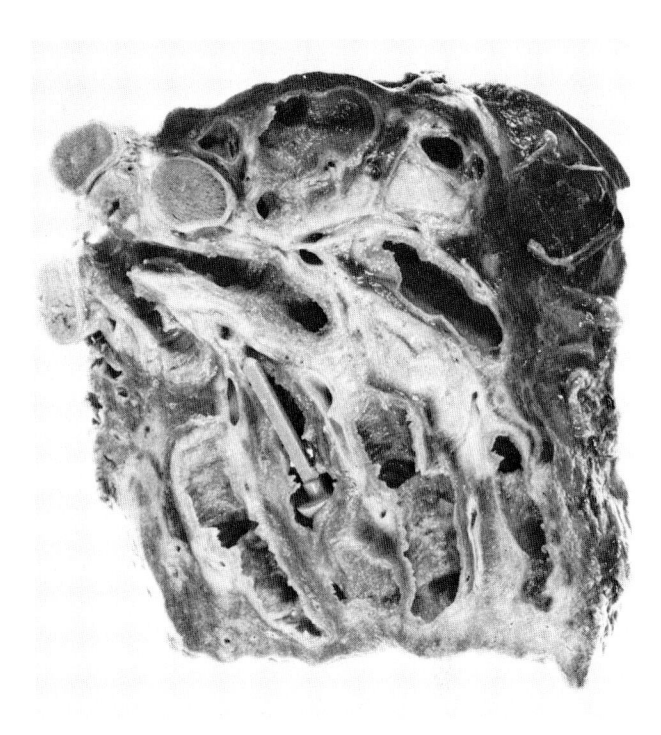

Figure 25–20. Severe bronchiectasis in a young male adult. The cause was a plastic toy, most likely inhaled during childhood. Note the massively enlarged hilar lymph nodes.

Field[57,59,60] has presented an excellent long-term follow-up on childhood bronchiectasis. Field found a tendency for symptoms to improve and remain stable in adolescence and adulthood. Wilson and Dekker,[61] proponents for surgical management, stress that active, although minimal, disease which is present often shows marked postresection progression, and for this reason, they would agree that surgery should be delayed until the full extent of the disease is present. These authors[61] have provided a list of indications for surgery:

1. Localized disease producing severe symptoms, such as sputum or cough that interfere with a normal life pattern.
2. Threatening hemorrhage from a demonstrated source.
3. Resectable disease of significant severity associated with failure to thrive.
4. Resectable disease that acts as a source for repeated lower respiratory tract infections.
5. Unstable disease with progression, or extension of resectable disease.
6. Not totally resectable disease associated with failure to thrive.
7. Not totally resectable disease associated with disabling or life-threatening symptoms such as hemorrhage and severe recurrent infections.

Not surprisingly prognosis depends to a large measure on the extent and severity of the disease. Patients with severe abnormalities of pulmonary function have a higher mortality than those with lesser abnormalities.[62] Field[60] has shown that those patients with symptoms tend to do poorly, and hemoptysis should suggest worse disease. In contrast, post-tuberculous bronchiectasis has a relatively good prognosis in the absence of secondary infection.

In Wilson and Decker's series,[61] 87 cases were classified as surgical candidates (28 subsequently had resections); in the patients without surgery, symptomatology remained unchanged or became progressively severe. Another surgical group consisted of patients whose operations were classed as curative, intermediate, or salvage. Curative cases had localized unilateral disease, whereas intermediate cases had less localized disease, and surgery was performed to reduce symptoms. Salvage operations were performed in 13 patients who had severe bilateral disease in an effort to reduce the disease sufficiently so that medical management would be effective. In the first two groups, all patients were either cured or their symptoms improved. Even in the salvage group, 77 percent improved, but the remainder were unchanged. A major review by Lewiston[53] has compared the outcome of medical and surgical therapy in seven studies. Although a sound comparison cannot be made because of the nature of the studies, improvement appears greater in the group who received surgical therapy.

A further factor, often ignored, is the quality of life enjoyed by bronchiectatic patients. Ellis and colleagues[62] addressed this question in a study of 116 patients treated with surgical and medical therapy. Although 77 percent of the surviving patients had no physical disability as assessed by work record, interviews of the spouses found that 46 percent found the patients' cough distasteful, and 29 percent had sexual difficulties. These data indicate that social problems are a significant factor in the lives of patients with bronchiectasis.

References

1. Brock RC: Studies in lung abscess. Part V. The aetiology of lung abscess. Guys Hosp Rep. 96:141–167, 1947.

2. Fraser RG, Pare JAP: Pneumonia caused by anaerobic organisms. In Fraser RG, Pare JAP (eds): *Diagnosis of Diseases of the Chest*, 2nd ed. Philadelphia: WB Saunders, 1978.

3. Kassay D: Observations on one hundred cases of bronchial foreign body. Arch Otolaryngol 71:42–58, 1960.

4. Mendelson CL: The aspiration of stomach contents into the lungs during obstetric anesthesia. Am J Obstet Gynecol 52:191–205, 1946.

5. Baile EM, Wright JL, Pare PD, Hogg JC: The effect of acute small airway inflammation on pulmonary function in dogs. Am Rev Respir Dis 126:298–301, 1982.

6. Winternitz MC, Smith GH, McNamara FP: Effect of intrabronchial insufflation of acid. J Exp Med 32:199–204, 1920.

7. Wynne JN: Aspiration pneumonitis. Clin Chest Med 3:25–34, 1982.

8. Wright JL, Cockroft DW: Lung disease in hairspray abuse Arch Pathol Lab Med 105:363–366, 1981.

9. Miller GJ, Ashcroft MT, Beadnell HMSG, et al.: The lipoid pneumonia of blackfat tobacco smokers in Guyana. Q J Med 40(160):457–470, 1971.

10. Stein DA, Bradley BL: Lipid pneumonia with diffuse interstitial infiltrates. Texas Med 80:50–51, 1984.

11. Weill H, Ferrans VJ, Gay RM, Ziskind MM: Early lipoid pneumonia. Am J Med 36:370–376, 1964.

12. Genereux GP: Lipids in the lungs: Radiologic-pathologic correlation. J Can Assoc Radiol 21:1–15, 1970.

13. Spencer H: *Pathology of the Lung*, 3rd ed. Toronto: Pergamon Press, 1977.

14. Eckert H, Jerochin S, Winsel K: Ultrastructural and autoradiographical investigations of early changes in experimental lung fibrosis. Z Erkr Atmungsorgane 152:37–41, 1979.

15. Hutchins GM, Boitnott JK: Atypical mycobacterial infection complicating mineral oil pneumonia. JAMA 240:539–541, 1978.

16. Greenberger PA, Katzenstein A-L A: Lipid pneumonia with atypical mycobacterial colonization. Association with allergic bronchopulmonary aspergillosis. Arch Intern Med 143: 2003–2005, 1983.

17. James U, Brimblecombe FSW, Wells JW: The natural history of pulmonary collapse in childhood. Q J Med 25:121–136, 1956.

18. Redding GJ: Atelectasis in childhood. Pediatr Clin North Am 31:891–905, 1984.

19. Levine BE, Johnson RP: Effects of atelectasis on pulmonary surfactant and quasi-static lung mechanics. J Appl Physiol 20:859–864, 1965.

20. Berezovsky ME, Albats EI, Klembovsky AI, Sergeev VM: The alveolar wall structure in obstruction atelectasis in children. Arkh Patol 44:31, 1979.

21. Glasser SA, Domino KB, Lindgren L, et al.: Pulmonary blood pressure and flow during atelectasis in the dog. Anesthesiology 58:225–231, 1983.

22. Marshall BE: Importance of hypoxic pulmonary vasoconstriction with atelectasis. Ad Shock Res 8:1–12, 1982.

23. Harris GD, Johanson WG Jr, Pierce AK: Determinants of lung bacterial clearance in mice after acute hypoxia. Am Rev Respir Dis 116:671–677, 1977.

24. Drinkwater DC Jr, Wittnich C, Mulder DS, et al.: Mechanical and cellular bacterial clearance in lung atelectasis. Ann Thorac Surg 32:235–242, 1981.

25. Tannenberg J, Pinner M: Atelectasis and bronchiectasis: An experimental study concerning their relationship. J Thorac Surg 2:571–613, 1942.

26. Cheng K-K: The experimental production of bronchiectasis in rats. J Pathol Bacteriol 67:89–98, 1954.

27. Proto AV, Tocino I: Radiographic manifestations of lobar collapse. Semin Roentgenol 15:117–173, 1980.

28. Brock RC, Cann RJ, Dickinson JR: Tuberculous mediastinal lymphadenitis in childhood; Secondary effects on the lungs. Guys Hosp Rep 87:295–317, 1937.

29. Graham EA, Burford TH, Mayer JH: Middle lobe syndrome. Postgrad Med 4:29–34, 1948.

30. Brock RC: *Anatomy of the Bronchial Tree*. Oxford, London: 1946.

31. Culiner M: The right middle lobe syndrome: A nonobstructive complex disease. Dis Chest 50:57–66, 1966.

32. Inners CR, Terry PB, Traystman RJ, Menkes HA: Collateral ventilation and the middle lobe syndrome. Am Rev Respir Dis 118:305–310, 1978.

33. Albo RJ, Grimes OF: The middle lobe syndrome: A clinical study. Dis Chest 50:509–518, 1966.

34. Wagner RB, Johnston MR: Middle lobe syndrome. Ann Thorac Surg 35:679–686, 1983.

35. Bertelsen S, Struve-Christensen E, Aasted A, Sparup J: Isolated middle lobe atelectasis: Aetiology, pathogenesis, and treatment of the so-called middle lobe syndrome. Thorax 35:449–452, 1980.

36. Dernevik L, Gatzinsky P, Hultman E, et al.: Shrinking pleuritis with atelectasis. Thorax 37:252–258, 1982.

37. Hillerdal G, Hemmingsson A: Pulmonary pseudotumours and asbestos. Acta Radiol Diag 21:615–620, 1980.

38. Mintzer RA, Cugell DW: The association of asbestos-induced pleural disease and rounded atelectasis. Chest 81:457–459, 1982.

39. Hanke R, Kretzschmar R: Round atelectasis. Semin Roentgenol 15:174–182, 1980.

40. Doyle TC, Lawler GA: CT features of rounded atelectasis of the lung. Am J Roentgenol 143:225–228, 1984.

41. Libshitz HI: Malignant pleural mesothelioma: The role of computed tomography. J Comput Tomog 8:15–20, 1984.

42. Schneider HJ, Felson B, Gonzalez LL: Rounded atelectasis. AJR 134:225–232, 1980.

43. Smith LS, Schillaci RF: Rounded atelectasis due to acute exudative effusion. Spontaneous resolution. Chest 85:830–832, 1984.

44. Polednak AP: Postmortem bacteriology and pneumonia in a mentally retarded population. Am J Clin Pathol 67:190–195, 1977.

45. LeFrock JL, Clark TS, Davies B, Klainer AS: Aspiration pneumonia: A ten-year review. Am Surg 45:305–313, 1979.

46. Genereux GP, Stilwell GA: The acute bacterial pneumonias. Semin Roentgenol 15:9–16, 1980.

47. Bartlett JG, Gorbach SL, Finegold SM: The bacteriology of aspiration pneumonia. Am J Med 56:202–207, 1974.

48. De Navasquez S, Haslewood GAD: Endogenous lipoid pneumonia with special reference to carcinoma of the lung. Thorax 9:35–37, 1954.

49. Corrin B, King E: Experimental endogenous lipid pneumonia and silicosis. J Pathol 97:325–330, 1969.

50. Lawler W: Idiopathic cholesterol pneumonitis. Histopathology 1:385–395, 1977.

51. Hayashi T, Stemmermann GN: Lipid pneumonia in the Hawaiian feral mongoose. J Pathol 108:205–210, 1972.

52. Schacter EN: Suppurative lung disease: Old problems revisited. Clin Chest Med 2:41–45, 1981.

53. Lewiston NJ: Bronchiectasis in childhood. Pediatr Clin North Am 31:865–878, 1984.

54. Glauser EM, Cook CD, Harris GBC: Bronchiectasis: A review of 187 cases. Acta Pediatr Scand (Suppl) 165:1–15, 1966.

55. Fernald GW: Bronchiectasis in childhood: A 10-year survey of cases treated at North Carolina Memorial Hospital. NC Med J 39:368–372, 1978.

56. Avery ME, Frantz ID III: Whooping cough in the United States and Britain. N Engl J Med 309:108–109, 1983.

57. Field CE: Bronchiectasis in childhood. I,II,III Pediatrics 4:21–45, 231–247, 355–371, 1949.

58. Davis AL. Bronchiectasis. In Fishman AP (ed): *Pulmonary Diseases and Disorders*. New York: McGraw-Hill, 1980.

59. Field CE: Bronchiectasis: A long-term follow-up of medical and surgical cases from childhood. Arch Dis Child 36:587–603, 1961.

60. Field CE: Bronchiectasis: Third report on a follow-up study of medical and surgical cases from childhood. Arch Dis Child 44:551–561, 1969.

61. Wilson JF, Decker AM: The surgical management of childhood bronchiectasis: A review of 96 consecutive pulmonary resections in children with nontuberculous bronchiectasis. Ann Surg 195:354–363, 1982.

62. Ellis DA, Thornley PE, Wightman AJ, et al.: Present outlook in bronchiectasis: Clinical and social study and review of factors influencing prognosis. Thorax 36:659–664, 1981.

26 Diseases of the Pleura

Andrew Churg

Pleural Effusion, Pleural Biopsy, and Empyema

Pleural effusion refers to fluid, either serous or sanguinous, within the pleural space, whereas empyema refers to pus within the pleural space. The distinction is usually obvious, but in some instances, particularly in tuberculous disease, pus may be thin and watery and separation from exudative effusion may be difficult.[1] Some authors classify empyema as one end of a continuous spectrum of pleural effusions.[2]

The etiologies of pleural effusion are legion; a partial list is presented in Table 26–1. The exact frequency with which various causes of effusion are seen depends on the nature of the patient population and the specialty of the physician. To the internist or general practitioner, congestive heart failure is by far the most common cause of pleural effusion, as indeed it is in the population as a whole; in a referral center, neoplasms tend to dominate the list.[3] Obvious cases of congestive heart failure are not usually biopsied, so that in biopsy series neoplasms and infections account for the majority of cases.[4–7] Together, cardiac failure, tuberculosis, and neoplasms account for about 75 percent of effusions.[8] Hemorrhagic effusions are associated with trauma, surgical procedures, tuberculosis, pulmonary infarctions, and neoplasms; the latter cause the vast majority of spontaneous hemorrhagic effusions.[8]

For the pathologist examining pleural biopsies or cytologic preparations of pleural fluid, only a limited number of morphologic etiologies of effusion can be diagnosed. These include neoplasms, infections, especially tuberculosis, sarcoid, and to a limited extent, collagen vascular diseases and hypersensitivity reactions.

Leff and co-workers[9] have summarized data obtained in various fashions on the incidence of pleural effusions and specific types of malignancy. They found that metastases from carcinoma of the breast produced 26 to 49 percent of malignant effusions, lung primaries 10 to 24 percent, ovarian neoplasms 6 to 17 percent, and lymphomas 13 to 24 percent. They note that about 50 percent of women with breast cancer will have an effusion related to metastases some time during their course. In more recent studies based on pleural biopsy, cytology, or both[4–6, 10] there appears to be an increase in the number of effusions associated with lung cancer relative to breast cancer: in 361 patients, breast cancer caused 19 percent of effusions, lung cancer 38 percent, ovarian cancer 9 percent, and lymphoma 10 percent (Table 26–2). These figures may reflect progressive increase in the number of cases of lung cancer in the population. Needle biopsy alone provided a positive diagnosis of malignancy in 51 percent of 622 patients,[4,5,7] with a range from 34 to 69 percent. Cytologic examination alone produced a positive diagnosis in 54 percent of 1683 patients known to have a malignant effusion.[4,5] Salyer and co-workers[5] note that in their own series, the combination of cytologic examination and pleural biopsy yielded a diagnosis rate in excess of 90 percent. Van Hoff and LiVolsi[7] point out that the yield of pleural biopsies, both for benign and malignant underlying disease, can be somewhat improved with repeated biopsies because the pathologic processes may be widely but discretely scattered over the pleura; this is quite obviously true of granulomatous diseases. An example of a pleural biopsy positive for malignancy is shown in Figure 26–1. In difficult cases, pleuroscopy may also improve the yield by allowing direct visualization of the lesion to be biopsied.[11]

Konikov and associates[10] have examined the survival of patients with a positive cytologic diagnosis of pleural malignancy; their mean survival for 140 patients was 2.2 months. Patients with lung cancer had a mean survival of 2.6 months, those with breast cancer 6.1 months, ovarian cancer 7.2 months, and lymphoma 2.0 months; the latter

Table 26–1. Causes of Pleural Effusion

> Transudative effusions
>   Cardiac failure
>   Renal failure
>   Nephrotic syndrome
>   Cirrhosis
>   Superior vena cava syndrome
>   Meig's syndrome
> Exudative effusions
>   Infections
>   Bacterial
>   Viral
>   Tuberculous
>   Fungal
>   Collagen vascular diseases
>   Pulmonary infarctions
>   Neoplasms
>   Intra-abdominal processes
>   Acute pancreatitis
>   Subphrenic abscess
>   Abdominal surgery
> Eosinophilic effusions
>   Idiopathic
>   Drug sensitivity
>   Pneumonia
>   Pulmonary infarction
>   Pneumothorax
> Hemorrhagic effusions
>   Neoplasms
>   Tuberculosis
>   Pulmonary infarctions
>   Trauma
>   Surgical procedures
>   Pneumothorax

Table 26–2. Primary Sites of Malignancy Producing Pleural Effusion in Needle Biopsy Series

Site	Konikov et al.[10]	Salyer et al.[5]	Frist et al.[4]	Van Hoff and LiVolsi[7]	Total
Breast	43	11	14	1	69 (19%)
Lung	35	42	11	49	137 (38%)
Ovary	31		3		34 (9%)
Lymphoma	18	11	1	5	35 (10%)
Miscellaneous including gut, uterus, cervix, kidney, soft tissue sarcomas and mesothelioma	29	31	13	11	84 (23%)

figure would probably be considerably improved with current treatment methods. Occasional individuals with breast cancer survived to 3 and 4 years, while the longest survival for lung cancer patients was 11 months.

After cardiac failure, infection is the next most frequent cause, overall, of pleural effusion; in general the infection is pulmonary, but spread from other infectious foci within the chest, for example, vertebral osteomyelitis, and from intra-abdominal infections, especially subphrenic abscess, may cause both effusion and empyema (*see below*). Bacterial pneumonias that extend to the pleura commonly produce effusion which may or may not be sterile, depending on concurrent antibiotic therapy.[2,8] Effusion is seen in approximately 20 percent of viral and mycoplasma pneumonias.[12] Pleural biopsy in bacterial, viral, and mycoplasma pneumonias is as a rule unrewarding when examined histologically; the biopsies commonly demonstrate fibrin deposition and a variable infiltrate of inflammatory cells, and proliferating mesothelial cells, but not bacteria or viral inclusions.

Pleural effusions accompanying fungal infections are relatively infrequent. In patients with acute coccidioidomycosis, pleuritic chest pain is present in up to 70 percent, radiographic blunting of the costophrenic angle is seen in 20 percent, and 2 to 6 percent develop substantial effusions. The latter are generally associated with a pulmonary infiltrate on the affected side extending to the pleura. Pleural biopsy will demonstrate the organisms.[13] Pleural involvement may also be seen in cryptococcal infection. Salyer and Salyer[14] found organisms in pleura in 7 of 37 patients, most of whom were debilitated or immunosuppressed; Young and co-workers[15] reviewed the literature and were only able to find a total of 30 cases. In about half the diagnoses was made histologically. In pleural effusion produced by *Histoplasma capsulatum*, histologic examination of the pleura shows typical granulomas[16] containing the organisms. Aspergillus infection is a rare cause of pleural effusion,[17] and blastomycosis as a rule does not produce pleural effusion.[18]

In the past, tuberculosis was a very comon cause of pleural effusions, and, despite the decrease in the incidence of tuberculosis in the population, tuberculous effusions are still encountered quite frequently. Because tuberculous effusion is associated with primary infection, it was previously considered to be a disease of adolescents and young adults[1,19]; with continued increase in the number of susceptible individuals, tuberculous effusion is now also frequent in older adults. In four recent biopsy series totaling 845 patients, tuberculosis produced 167 effusions (20% of total)[4–7] as shown in Table 26–3.

Clinically the disease presents with fever, chest pain, and dyspnea; sputum is not produced and cough is absent or minimal. Radiographic examination frequently fails to show a tuberculous focus within the pulmonary parenchyma, hence the older term "primary" pleural effusion, but the disease is nonetheless considered to result from rupture of a small subpleural granuloma into the pleural space or from dissemination of myobacteria via pleural lymphatics during the primary infection.[1,2,8]

Thoracentesis yields a fluid which may be hemorrhagic and contains predominantly lymphocytes. Needle biopsy of the pleura is an excellent method of establishing the diagnosis (Fig. 26–2); in the first three series cited above, granulomas were found in pleura in 64 percent of patients with proven tuberculous effusion (*see* Table 26–3). Culture of the needle biopsy specimen was posi-

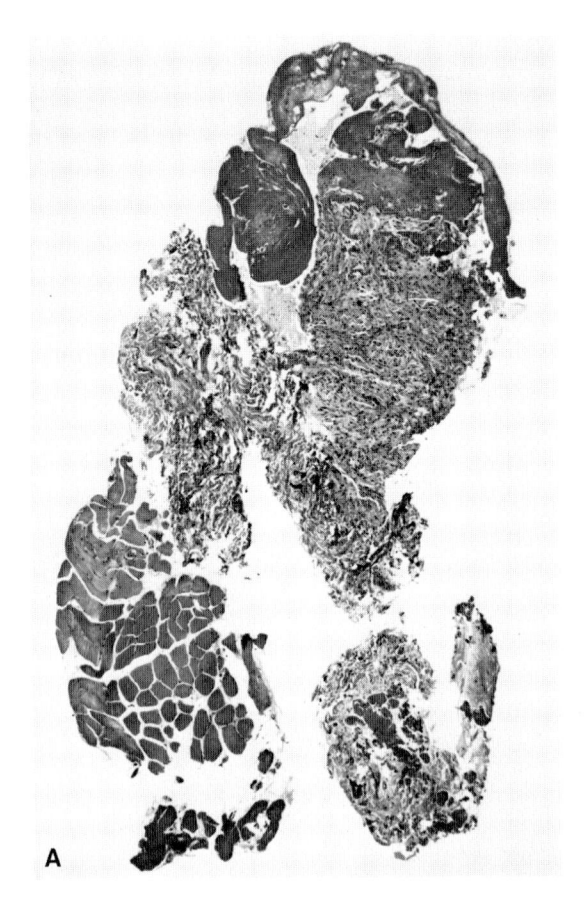

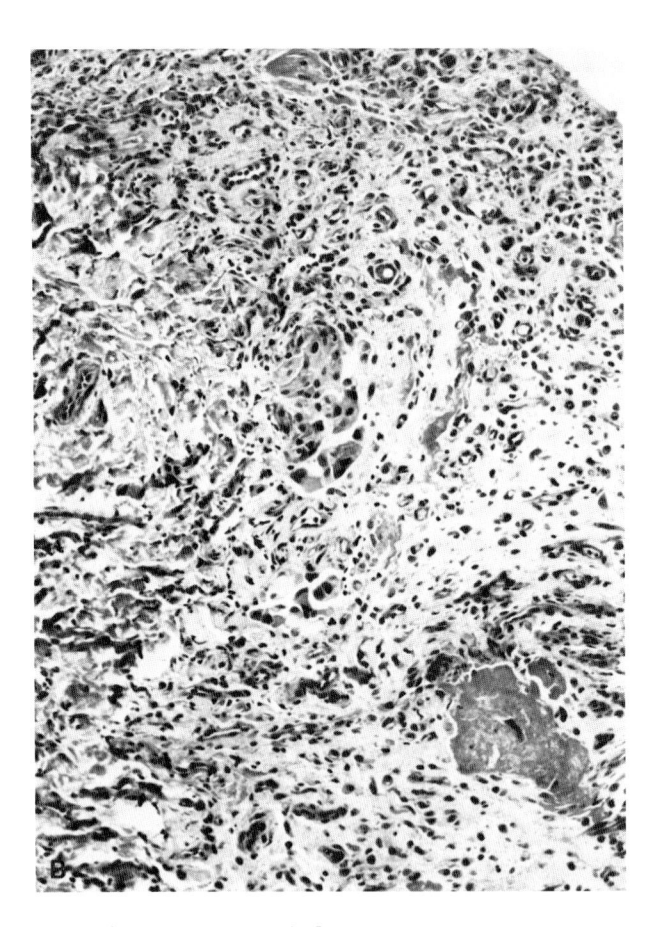

Figure 26–1. Pleural needle biopsy showing metastatic breast carcinoma. A. Lower-power view demonstrating skeletal muscle bundles and fibrous tissue containing inflammatory cells and tumor cells. The skeletal muscle bundles are a normal finding in this type of biopsy, but the pleura itself should normally be represented by only a single layer of mesothelial cells (×40). B. Higher-power view showing tumor cells with inflammatory cells and desmoplastic reaction (×160).

tive in 80 to 100 percent of the patients with histologic evidence of tuberculosis.[6,7] One patient in the series of Van Hoff and LiVolsi[7] and one in the series of Scerbo and colleagues[6] had a positive culture despite a nonspecific histologic appearance. In both these series the diagnostic yield was improved by repeated biopsy.

Table 26–3. Results of Pleural Biopsy for Tuberculous

	No. Patients with Proven TB/No. Patients in Biopsy Series	No. Positive Histologic Diagnoses/No. Suspected Cases	No. Positive Cultures of Biopsy
Van Hoff and LiVolsi(7)	52/245 (21%)	32/52 (61%)	33/52 (63%)
Scerbo et al.[6]	49/163 (31%)	35/49 (71%)	12/16 (80%)
Frist et al.[4]	10/166 (6%)	4/10 (40%)	ND
Salyer et al.[5]	56/271 (21%)	ND	ND
	167/845 (20%)	71/111 (64%)	

Abbreviations: ND, not determined; TB, tuberculosis.

Tuberculous effusion tends to be a self-limited disease which disappears with hospitalization; however, it is important to diagnose and treat patients with tuberculous effusion, because up to 65 percent will subsequently develop another focus of tuberculosis if left untreated.[2]

Sarcoidosis is a relatively rare cause of pleural effusion. Sharma[20] reports effusion in eight patients with sarcoidosis; needle biopsy showed granulomas in only two and nonspecific reactions in the other six. Only 2 of the 245 patients undergoing needle biopsy in the series of Van Hoff and LiVolsi[7] were considered clinically to have sarcoidosis.

Pleural effusion is a common occurrence in some of the collagen vascular diseases, especially lupus and rheumatoid arthritis. Needle biopsy may show rheumatoid nodules in the latter group[7,21] but this is a rare finding. Recently Halla and co-workers[22] have shown that effusions from patients with rheumatoid arthritis and lupus contain immune complexes. In theory, immunohistochemical examination of pleural biopsies from patients with these diseases should demonstrate granular deposits of immune complexes; however, the phenomenon in

Figure 26–2. Tuberculous effusion. A. Chest radiograph of a Vietnamese immigrant who presented with chest pain and a moderate right-sided effusion. B and C. Low and high-power views of pleural needle biopsy from this patient showing caseating granulomas. Stains for acid-fast organisms were positive (B ×64, C ×160).

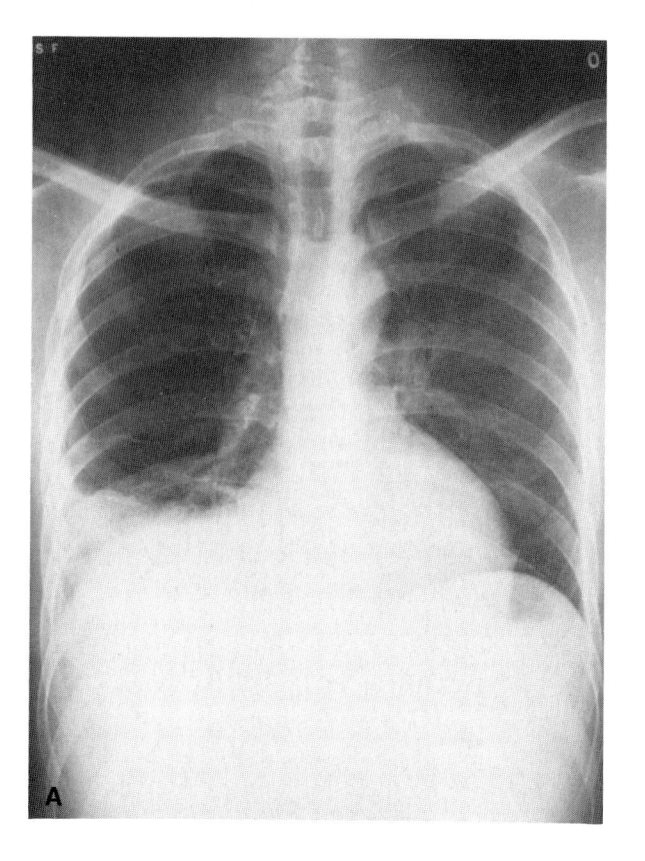

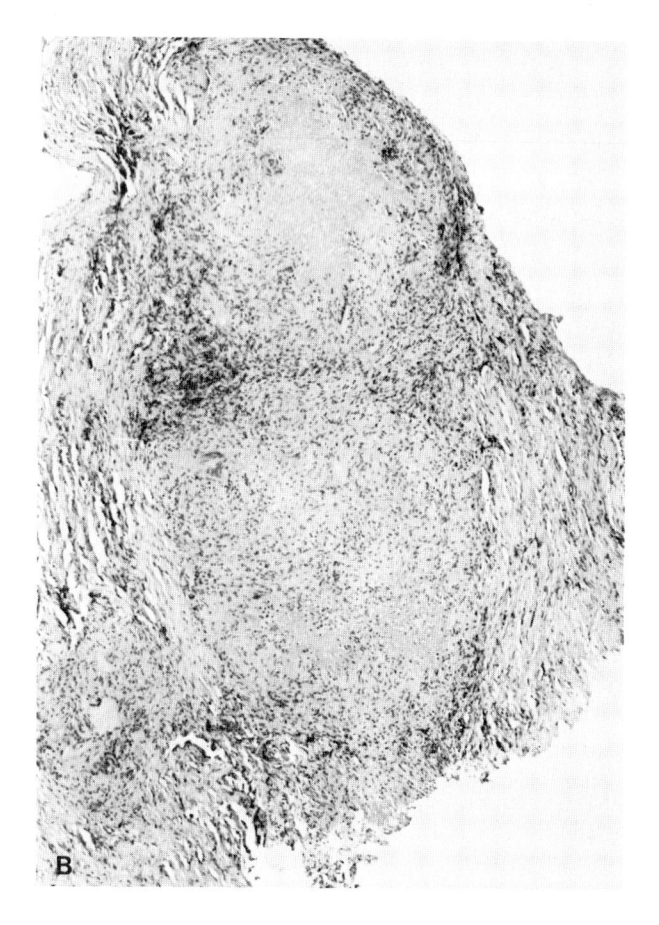

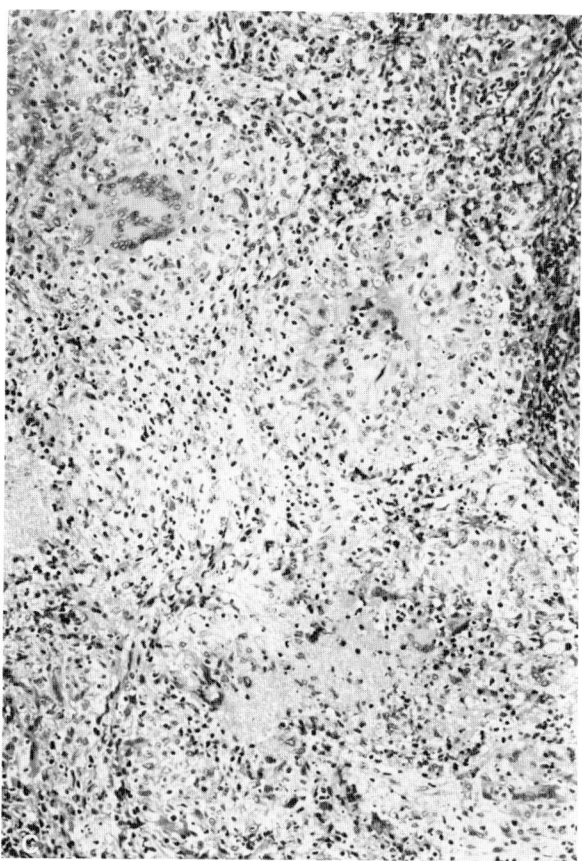

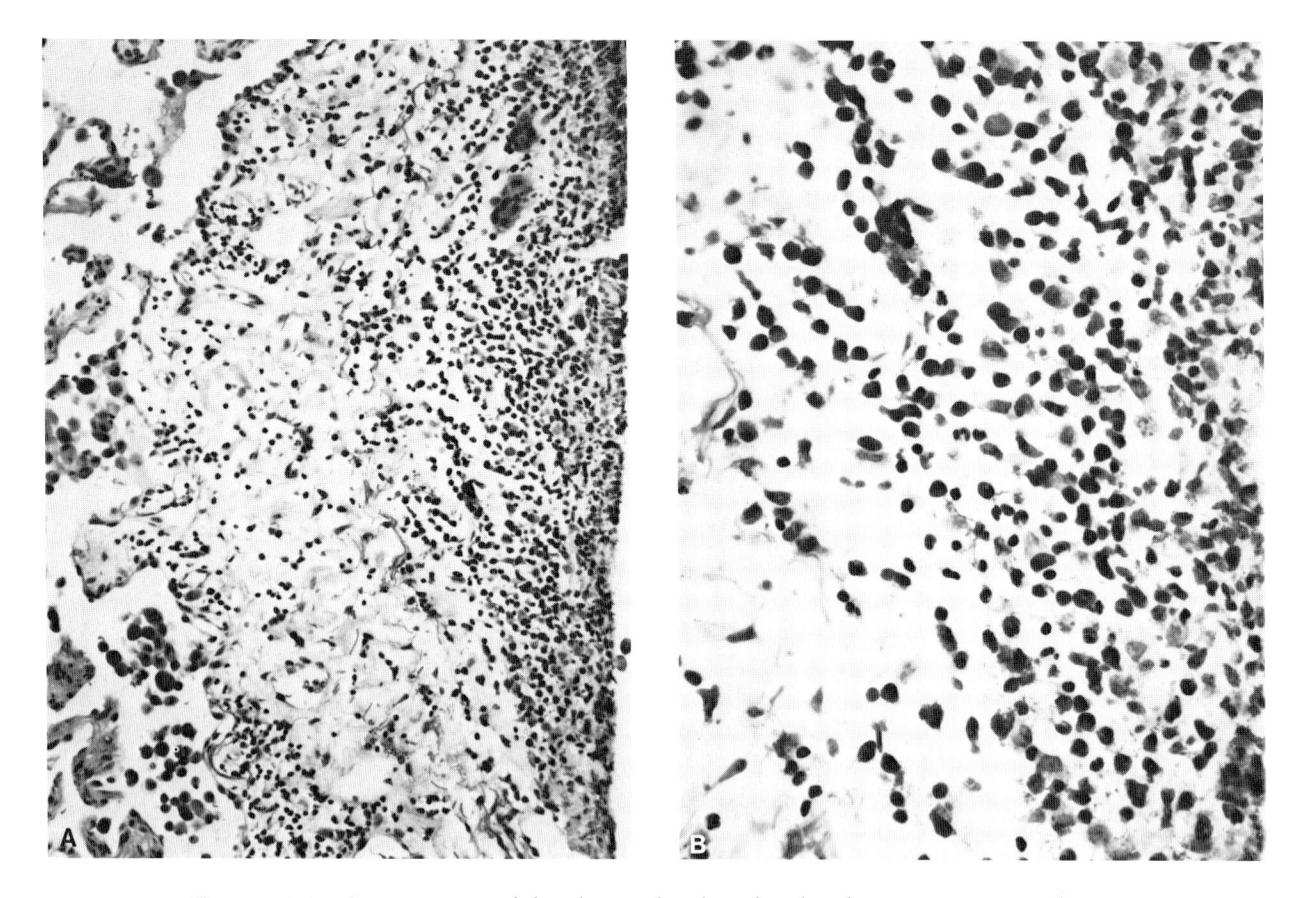

Figure 26–3. Reactive eosinophilic pleuritis found in the pleural resection specimen from a young adult with spontaneous pneumothorax. A. Low-power view of inflammatory reaction in the pleura. Note the giant cells (×64). B. High-power view showing numerous eosinophils (×160).

the pleural fluid is not limited to patients with collagen diseases[22] and the specificity of such a finding in a biopsy at this point is uncertain.

Pleural effusions may contain large numbers of eosinophils. In some instances eosinophils constitute as much as 94 percent of the white cells.[23] Campbell and Webb[23] reviewed 101 cases of eosinophilic effusion, and found that the largest group (28 percent) were of unknown cause, followed by pneumonia (24 percent), trauma, especially pneumothorax (16 percent), known hypersensitivity (14 percent), infarcts (6 percent), and malignancies (6 percent). Seventy-five percent of the patients had blood eosinophilia at the time of the effusion. The patient with 94 percent eosinophilia proved to have histoplasmosis. The histologic counterpart of eosinophilic pleural effusion is the disease described by Askin and colleagues[24] as "reactive eosinophilic pleuritis." The histologic picture is that of an intense histiocytic infiltration of the pleura admixed with eosinophils, giant cells, and other inflammatory cells (Fig. 26–3). The lesions described by Askin and associates[24] were found in specimens from 22 of 57 patients with spontaneous pneumothorax. Both the clinical setting and the histologic appearance are suggestive of eosinophilic granuloma, but none of their patients had clinical or radiographic evidence of eosinophilic granuloma either at presentation or up to 5 years afterward, nor were the typical Langerhans cells of eosinophilic granuloma seen by electron microscopy. The lesion appears to be a nonspecific reaction of the pleura to injury.

Any of the organisms which can produce pleural effusion may also cause empyema. At present, empyema is a relatively uncommon disease; over the period 1935 to 1957, the incidence of pneumoccocal empyema declined by a factor of approximately 8, and of streptococcal empyema by a factor of 2 to 3; staphylococcal empyema also declined initially, but since the early 1950s has slowly increased in frequency.[25] Whereas in past years the major cause of empyema was underlying spontaneous pulmonary infection, at present a large fraction of the cases seen in adults are iatrogenic or secondary to trauma. At the University of Florida Hospitals, 72 patients with empyema were seen during the 10-year period 1960 to 1970. Exactly half of these patients developed their empyema as a result of an underlying pyogenic pneumonia, and the majority of those patients were either immunosuppressed or debilitated from severe extrapulmonary disease. Tuberculosis accounted for five other cases. In the remaining 31 patients, empyema was the result of trauma, thoracotomy, cardiovascular sur-

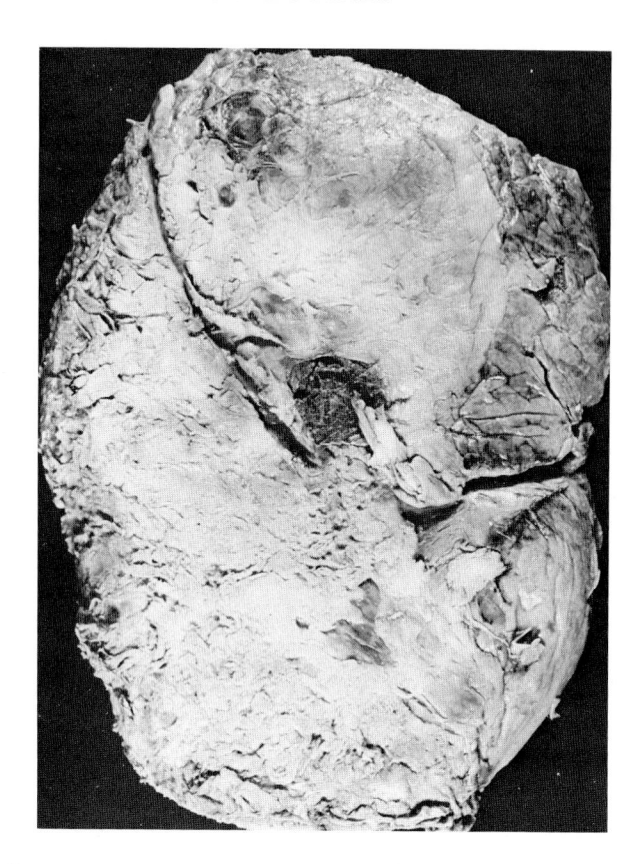

Figure 26–4. Gross appearance of empyema. Note the shaggy exudate on the pleural surface. The patient was an elderly man with an abscess and empyema behind an obstructing carcinoma.

gery, or esophageal surgery. The overall mortality was 25 percent.[26] The incidence of tuberculous empyema, which in the past accounted for a substantial fraction of cases, has also declined considerably. Tuberculous empyema accounted for 7 percent of the cases in the series of Emerson and co-workers,[26] 10 percent of the cases of Vianna and colleagues,[27] and 2.6 percent of the cases reported by LeRoux[28]; the latter figure is artificially low because of local referral practices.

Prior to the days of antibiotics, any nontuberculous infectious effusion was likely to result in empyema; pneumococcal pneumonia, for example, was accompanied by effusion in about 10 percent of cases[8] and almost all of these patients developed empyema. At present the incidence of effusion in pneumoccocal pneumonia is unchanged, but empyema occurs in less than 1 percent of patients.[29] Empyema now occurs in settings in which there is massive direct spread of purulent material into the pleural space. These settings include staphylococcal pneumonia, which produces abscesses liable to rupture, gram-negative pneumonias which are generally necrotizing and are complicated by empyema in 20 to 25 percent of cases, extension from intra-abdominal infections, either hematogenously or through the diaphragm, and extension from nonpulmonary intrathoracic infections such as vertebral osteomyelitis[30] and infected surgical sites (Fig. 26–4).

Currently about 75 percent of nonsurgical empyemas involve anerobes, and anaerobic species are the only organisms cultured in about 50 percent of cases.[31] These empyemas are almost always the result of extension from anerobic pneumonias; aspiration is responsible for about 70 percent of such cases.[31] Fungal empyemas are rare and are usually seen in association with aspiration of actinomyces,[32] in immunosuppressed patients, or patients with old tuberculous disease,[17] and in up to 3 percent of cases of cavitary coccidioidomycosis.[13] Staphylococcal empyema remains a serious problem in infants, and children. Over the years 1934 to 1958, the incidence of empyema in children hospitalized for pneumonia at the Harrient Lane Home in Baltimore dropped from 10 to 2 percent, but then rose to 14 percent. Ninety-two percent of the empyemas in the period 1955 to 1958 were caused by staphylococci, as opposed to 13 percent before the antibiotic era.[33] The mortality of this disease was initially reported as 25 to 100 percent, but is now steady at about 10 percent.[33,34]

The exact treatment of empyema depends on the infecting organism, extent of disease, and response to antibiotic therapy; closed tube drainage is commonly used, and open drainage or procedures such as thoracoplasty are less common to rare. Chronic empyema, especially that caused by mycobacteria, may produce a fibrothorax and require decortication.[1,35,36]

Hemothorax

Hemothorax is defined as blood in the pleural cavity. The distinction between hemothorax and sanguinous effusion may be difficult; a concentration of hemoglobin in the pleural fluid greater than 25 percent that in the blood is considered to indicate a hemothorax.[2] The common cause of hemothorax is trauma; spontaneous hemothorax is relatively rare, but may be seen occasionally with pleural neoplasms, with rupture of a dissecting aneurysm of the aorta, and in patients receiving anticoagulant therapy. Small amounts of bleeding accompanying pneumothorax (hemopneumothorax) are not uncommon. Massive hemothorax may cause shock as well as respiratory impairment.

The major complications of hemothorax are infection and organization of the blood clot to form a fibrothorax. Mesothelial tissue normally produces fibrinolysins[37] and blood is normally removed from the pleural space. Hemothorax fails to resolve in 5 to 10 percent of patients[2,8,38] and instead organizes, eventually producing a pleural peel. In such cases decortication is usually necessary to restore pulmonary function.

Chylothorax

Chylothorax is used to describe a chylous pleural effusion. This condition is rare and is generally associated with trauma or with surgical procedures which disrupt the thoracic duct. In the past, spontaneous chylothorax was seen most commonly in tuberculosis[2,8]; at present chylothorax is found in association with lymphomas and carcinomas in the mediastinum. Chylothorax is extremely common in lymphangioleiomyomatosis. Corrin and associates[39] report an incidence of 61 percent for 62 patients in the literature. The effusion results from involvement of the thoracic duct by lymphangioleiomyomatosis.

Fibrothorax, Pleural Fibrosis, and Pleural Plaques

Fibrothorax refers to the formation of a thick collagenous peel which binds the parietal and visceral pleurae and effectively immobilizes a portion or the whole of the affected lung. Pulmonary function tests reveal decreased lung volumes, decreased capillary volumes, and decreased diffusing capacity; if there is no underlying parenchymal disease, many of the physiologic changes can be at least partially reversed by decortication.[8,40]

Pathologically the appearance of a fibrothorax is not indicative of etiology: the lesion consists of dense fibrous tissue which often obliterates the original line of the visceral pleura and extends down into the interlobular septae and is also adherent to the parietal pleura (Fig. 26–5). Calcification or ossification may occur in long-standing cases and produce spectacular and bizarre radiographic appearances.

In the past, fibrothorax was generally seen in cases of organizing hemothorax, organizing empyema, and sometimes as a result of the treatment of tuberculosis by plombage therapy. Tuberculous empyema was a particularly common cause of fibrothorax, but identical lesions could be found complicating chronic empyema caused by other bacteria. Collapse therapy in the form of extrapleural pneumolysis and plombage was attempted with a variety of agents including paraffin, gauze, pectoral muscle, air, lucite, and methyl methacrylate, and other plastics[41,42]; escape of some of these materials into the pleural space provoked a severe inflammatory reaction and eventual fibrothorax.

Currently, fibrothorax secondary to empyema or hemothorax is a rare event and is commonly prevented by early decortication. Fibrosis of the pleura is in itself a very nonspecific finding caused by a wide variety of processes; however, severe fibrosis with splinting of the lung is more commonly seen either with drug therapy or exposure to mineral fibers. Treatment with practolol may produce severe pleural fibrosis requiring decortication.[43] A number of mineral fibers have been shown to induce fibrosis of both the visceral and parietal pleurae, and the formation of pleural plaques; these minerals include asbestos, talc (probably as a result of contamination with asbestos), and more recently, the fibrous silicate erionite.[44,45] A requirement for the development of mineral fiber-induced pleural disease appears to be inhalation of long, thin fibers; the exact mineral type is probably of less importance. Asbestos-induced pleural lesions may be seen with occupational or environmental exposure.[44–46] A distinguishing feature from infectious, especially tuberculous, pleural fibrosis, or plaques, is the tendency for asbestos-induced disease to be bilateral, sometimes symmetric, and preferentially distributed over the lower lobes and diaphragm. Tuberculous pleural disease is more commonly unilateral or markedly asymmetric and frequently more or equally severe toward the apex. As a rule, asbestos induced pleural fibrosis or plaques cause no or minimal respiratory impairment in the absence of parenchymal asbestosis, but on occasion severe fibrosis functionally equivalent to fibrothorax occurs, necessitating decortication.[47] Asbestos-induced pleural disease is discussed at length in Chapter 23.

Pneumothorax

Pneumothorax is defined as the presence of air in the pleural space. Pneumothorax can be divided into traumatic, iatrogenic, and spontaneous cases; the latter are further subdivided into secondary spontaneous pneumothorax, when there is known disease in the underlying lung, and primary spontaneous pneumothorax, when there is normal or essentially normal underlying lung. A list of the causes of pneumothorax is presented in Table 26–4.

Traumatic pneumothorax is seen in accidents or events which result in either trauma to the lung or disruption of the integrity of the chest wall or sometimes the diaphragm and intestines. Iatrogenic pneumothorax is seen

Table 26–4. Diseases and Conditions Associated with Pneumothorax

Trauma
Iatrogenic Causes
  Thoracotomy
  Closed pulmonary or pleural biopsy
  Mechanical ventilation
  Acupuncture

Secondary Spontaneous Pneumothorax
  Emphysema
  Asthma
  Sarcoidosis
  Eosinophilic granuloma
  Usual interstitial pneumonia
  Collagen diseases
  Pneumoconioses
  Necrotizing infections, especially tuberculosis
  Malignant neoplasm, primary or secondary
  Pulmonary infarction
  Connective tissue disorders
  Esophageal rupture
  Hyaline membrane disease of the newborn
  Meconium aspiration
  Transient tachypnea of the newborn
  Catamenial pneumothorax

Primary Spontaneous Pneumothorax
  Idiopathic or sporadic
  Familial

776 Diseases of the Pleura

Figure 26–5. Fibrothorax. A. Chest radiograph showing changes of fibrothorax which developed as a result of a tuberculous empyema more than 20 years in the past. B. Example of a decortication specimen showing thick fibrous pleural peel. C. Microscopic appearance of fibrothorax. Note dense collagen with scanty inflammatory cells (×64).

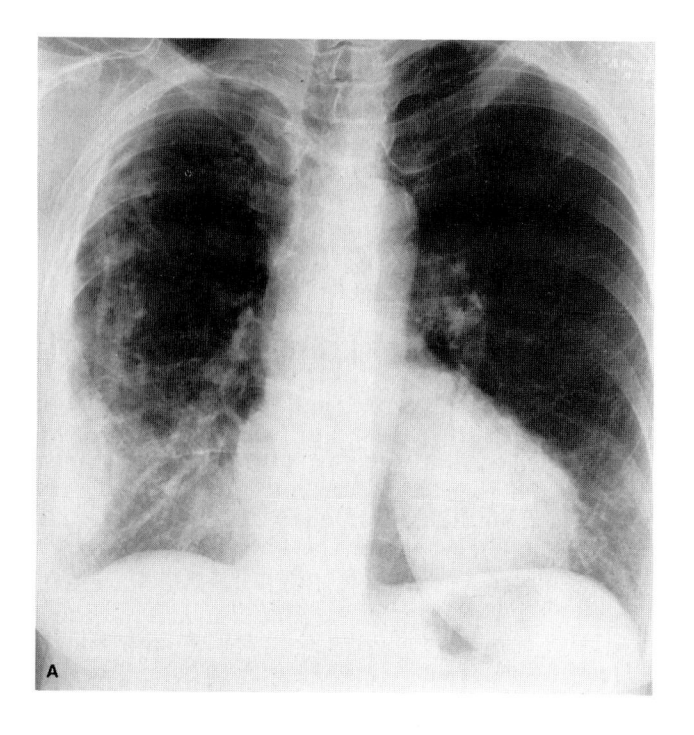

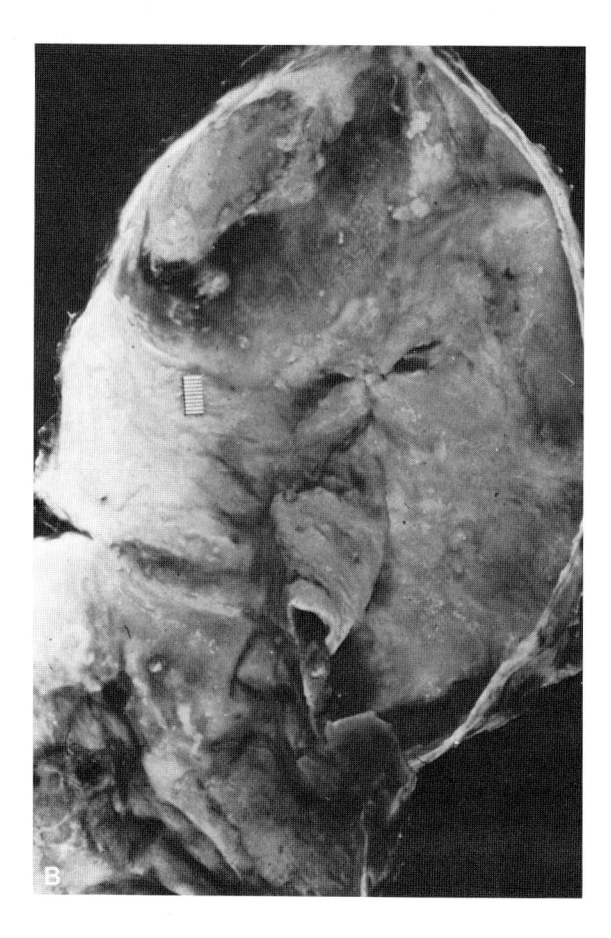

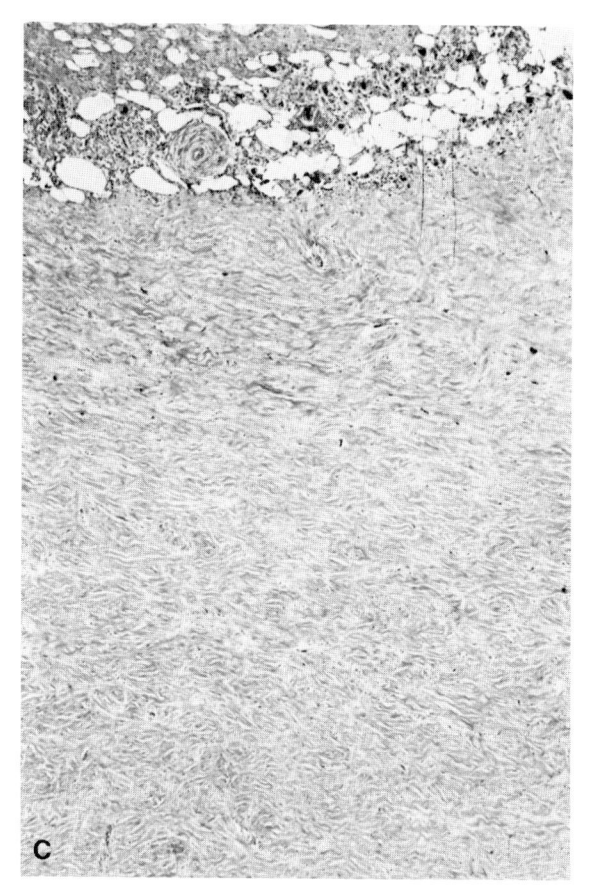

invariably with thoracotomy, and with variable frequency after percutaneous biopsy procedures. Gaensler[48] cites values as high as 51 percent of cutting needle biopsies, 43 percent of trephine needle biopsies, and 5.5 percent of transbronchial biopsies. Mechanical ventilation is another frequent iatrogenic cause of pneumothorax. The normal pleura will tolerate pressures up to about 80 cm of water,[2] but the diseased lung is frequently much more fragile; 3 to 5 percent of patients treated by intermittent positive pressure ventilation[2] and approximately one-sixth of patients treated by more than 8 cm of positive end-expiratory pressure develop pneumothorax. Acupuncture is another more unusual iatrogenic cause of pneumothorax. The pathological findings in these cases reflect the disease, if any, in the underlying lung; the clinical features are those of spontaneous pneumothorax with the addition of changes produced by the underlying lung disease. Hemothorax may complicate any of the situations listed above.

A detailed history of the observation and understanding of pneumothorax is presented in Killen and Gobbel[49] and a brief resume by Mark and Lindskog.[50] Spontaneous pneumothorax was first described and named by Itard in 1803 and more clearly described by Lannec in 1819 (cited in Mark[50]), who suggested that the process might be related to emphysematous bullae. Throughout the 19th century and the first third of the 20th century, spontaneous pneumothorax was believed to result almost invariably from tuberculosis; Biach[51] in 1880 reported 918 cases, of which 715 were thought to be associated with tuberculosis. Until the 1930s, patients presenting with spontaneous pneumothorax were generally treated as if they did have tuberculosis. In 1932 Kjaergaard[52] showed that in fact most cases of spontaneous pneumothorax in apparently healthy individuals were not of tuberculous etiology, and it is presently accepted that tuberculosis-related spontaneous pneumothorax accounts for no more than 3 percent of hospital admissions for pneumothorax.

Spontaneous pneumothorax accounts for 0.3 to 0.8% of hospital admissions[53]; summary of a large number of cases reveals that about 70 percent are of the primary variety.[49] The accuracy of this figure is difficult to determine since it is weighted in one direction by series from military installations where the typical young male patient who develops primary spontaneous pneumothorax is overrepresented, and in the other direction by inclusion of a number of older series containing a considerably larger number of cases of tuberculosis than would be seen currently. Even in civilian populations, however, it is clear that primary pneumothorax is a disease of males; the overall proportion varies from about 3:1 to 6:1 and the bulk of cases in both males and females occur between the ages of 20 and 40.[2,49,50,54,55] Estimates of the incidence of primary spontaneous pneumothorax range from 2.4 to 17.8 per 100,000 persons per year. This figure is undoubtedly an underestimate because there are many apparently subclinical cases. In approximately 1600 patients from 18 different reports collected by Killen and Gobbel,[49] primary pneumothorax accounted for 72 percent of the total, and secondary pneumothorax for 28 percent. There is no doubt that some cases of secondary pneumothorax are also subclinical,[56] but the incidence is likely much lower than in primary disease, since persons with secondary pneumothorax and severe underlying lung disease are likely to suffer respiratory embarrassment from even a fairly small pneumothorax. Johnston and Dovnarsky[2] state that over the age of 40, two-thirds of the patients with spontaneous pneumothorax have underlying pulmonary disease.

Breakdown of cases of secondary pneumothorax by cause is also somewhat difficult, in part because the older literature includes not only the disproportionate number of active tuberculous cases mentioned above, but tends to include inactive tuberculosis which has left extensive scarring. Thus, in the same 18 series collected by Killen and Gobbel,[49] 51 percent of cases are associated with chronic airflow obstruction, largely emphysema, 23 percent with active tuberculosis, 15 percent with "pulmonary fibrosis," and 7 percent with pneumonia and lung abscess. The report of Carr and co-workers,[57] which is included above, is probably more representative: 54 percent of cases are caused by emphysema, 22 percent by fibrosis of various etiologies, and 7 percent by pneumoconioses; no cases associated with tuberculosis are present. Green[58] agrees that chronic airflow obstruction accounts for about half the cases of secondary pneumothorax.

Despite its frequency in collected series of pneumothorax patients, pneumothorax occurs in less than 1 percent of all cases of chronic bronchitis and emphysema[2,49,59] but bullous emphysema may be complicated by pneumothorax in as many as 25 percent of cases. Infiltrative lung disease in which there is parenchymal fibrosis, cyst formation, or honeycombing is also complicated by pneumothorax. Pneumothorax is associated with eosinophilic granuloma in 15 percent[59] to 44 percent[49] of cases and is a common presenting complaint. The incidence of pneumothorax in sarcoidosis varies from 0 to 4 percent (average 2 percent) of cases in large series[20]; as a rule this phenomenon is seen late in the disease, but rare cases of early disease presenting as pneumothorax have been reported.[60] Pneumothorax is seen overall in about 5 percent of cases of interstitial fibrosis, whether of the idiopathic usual interstitial pneumonia type, interstitial pneumonia associated with collagen disease, or pneumoconiosis[59]; among these diseases the incidence appears to be higher in those, for example, scleroderma, that tend to progress frequently and rapidly to honeycombing. Lymphangioleiomyomatosis has a high rate of pneumothorax, and particularly of repeated pneumothorax. Carrington and colleagues[59] report an incidence of 39 percent for 61 cases in the literature, and 4 of their own patients had 25 episodes.

Infectious diseases which produce necrosis or cavitation are also relatively common causes of secondary pneumothorax. Fishberg[61] cites pneumothorax rates of 0.73 to 13 percent for patients in hospital who have tuberculosis, and Wilder's[56] figures are 1 to 3 percent. More than 90 percent of these patients have cavitary disease. In some instances several months may elapse between the onset of pneumothorax and its clinical discovery.[56] Rupture of tuberculous foci into the pleural space may produce empyema as well as pneumothorax; this is also true of infections with Staphylococcus, Klebsiella, Pseudomonas, Actinomyces, Nocardia, and Coccidiodes.[2]

Malignant neoplasms occasionally produce a pneumothorax; Dines and colleagues[62] recorded 10 instances in 1143 patients at the Mayo Clinic. The pneumothorax may occur without treatment or as a result of treatment, and on rare occasions may be the first indication that a neoplasm is present. Pneumothorax has been reported with bronchogenic carcinoma, metastatic soft tissue sarcomas, lymphomas, metastatic germ cell tumors, and metastatic osteosarcomas.[62–64]

Pneumothorax is a fairly common event in newborn infants. It has been reported that some form of pulmonary air leak is seen in 27 percent of newborns with hyaline membrane disease, 41 percent of those with meconium aspiration, and 10 percent of those with transient tachypnea of the newborn, as well as in apparently healthy infants.[65] Lastly there are diseases defined entirely by the presence of pneumothorax; these include primary spontaneous pneumothorax and catamenial pneumothorax, in both of which by definition the incidence of pneumothorax is 100 percent. Catamenial pneumothorax consists of spontaneous pneumothorax, almost always on the right side, coincident with menstrual flow. Shearin and co-workers[66] summarize 32 cases in the literature, and note that their 11 cases constitute 6 percent of pneumothoraces in women under 50 years old in their institution.

Clinical and Radiographic Features

Both clinical and radiographic findings depend on presence or absence of coexistent pulmonary disease. As mentioned above, some patients are asymptomatic and the process may be discovered incidentally. The vast majority of patients present with chest pain and dyspnea; the latter tends to be most severe in those with the largest pneumothoraces. Hemoptysis, weakness, and syncope may also occur, particularly in patients with hemopneumothorax. Physical examination typically reveals a hyperresonant percussion note on the affected side and breath sounds are diminished or absent. Pulmonary function tests reveal decreased lung volumes and decreased compliance and usually hypoxemia with widening of the alveolar-arterial oxygen difference. Bilateral pneumothorax is found in only about 2 percent of patients.[2,58]

Roentgenographic examination usually clearly reveals the pneumothorax separating the lung from the chest wall; in those without adhesions or other underlying lung disease, the margin of the lung appears as a thin outwardly convex line (Fig. 26–6A). In emphysematous patients with large bullae, physical examination may be misleading and roentgenographic examination required to determine the diagnosis.[67]

Etiology and Pathogenesis: Secondary Pneumothorax

It is clear from studies of patients on artificial respiration that many different disease processes may weaken the structure of the pulmonary parenchyma and pleura.[2,68] Conceptually, these may be divided into diseases that produce increased intrapulmonary pressure, diseases that produce thin or thick-walled cysts, and diseases that produce actual destruction of parenchyma. The first two factors probably operate together in most instances. It is possible to produce pneumothorax from high pressure alone in relatively normal lungs, for example, in asthma, but more typically pneumothorax is seen in the context of chronic airflow obstruction in patients with emphysema who have both high intrapulmonary pressures and weakened pulmonary tissues.[67] Large thin-walled bullae similarly have little mechanical strength. Infiltrative lung diseases such as usual interstitial pneumonia, sarcoid, and eosinophilic granuloma most commonly are associated with pneumothorax when honeycombing is present; it is probable that even relatively thick-walled revised air spaces may rupture because of local air trapping. Early eosinophilic granuloma has also been shown to be associated with the formation of small cysts,[69] a feature that probably accounts for the high incidence of pneumothorax in this disease.

The presence of pneumothorax with miliary tuberculosis or with early sarcoidosis, both relatively uncommon events, has been considered to represent fusion and necrosis of subpleural granulomas with rupture into the pleural space.[20,60,70] Rupture of cavitary lesions or lesions undergoing necrosis into the pleural space is more easily understandable as a cause of pneumothorax in patients with cavitary tuberculosis,[56] other necrotizing infections, and malignant neoplasms,[62,64] particularly when the latter undergo rapid necrosis as a result of chemotherapy.[63] In all of these diseases the lesion probably involves the pleura directly. Cavitation of infarcts with subsequent pneumothorax is a rare event[71] which probably occurs by a similar mechanism.

The mechanism of catamenial pneumothorax remains unexplained. Shearin and co-workers[66] have reviewed 32 cases and examined the various theories offered in the literature. Almost all of the patients have presented with right-sided pneumothorax, although two of Shearin and associates'[66] patients had subsequent left-sided pneumothoraces. A morphologic abnormality was detected in 78 percent of women undergoing thoracotomy; these abnormalities included pleural or diaphragmatic endometriosis in 30 percent, bullae, blebs, or cysts in 48 percent, and diaphragmatic fenestrations in 22 percent. Eleven of the group of 32 patients were thought to have pelvic endometriosis. How these features relate to pneumothorax is unclear; if the blebs are of the sort seen in primary spontaneous pneumothorax, the association with menstrual flow is unexplained. A better possibility is that they result from pleural endometriosis, and that hormonal changes in the endometrial tissue cause necrosis of the underlying pleura. It has also been suggested,[72]

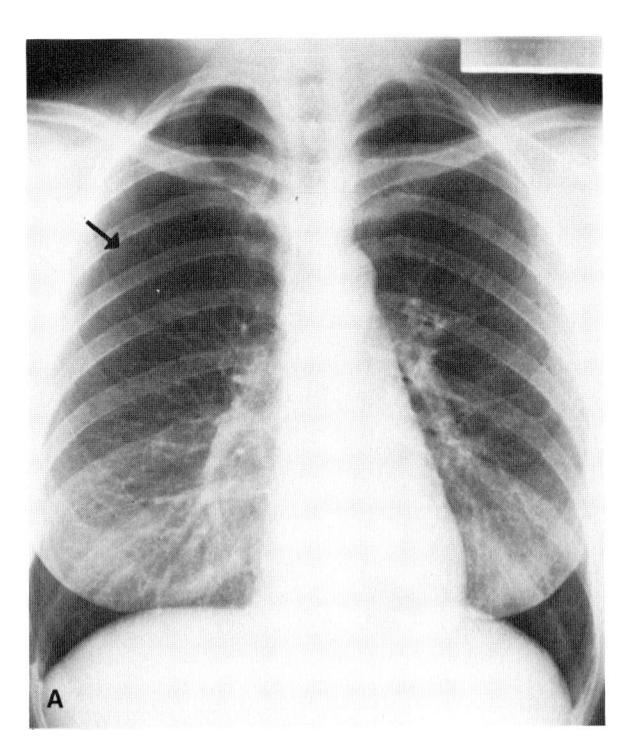

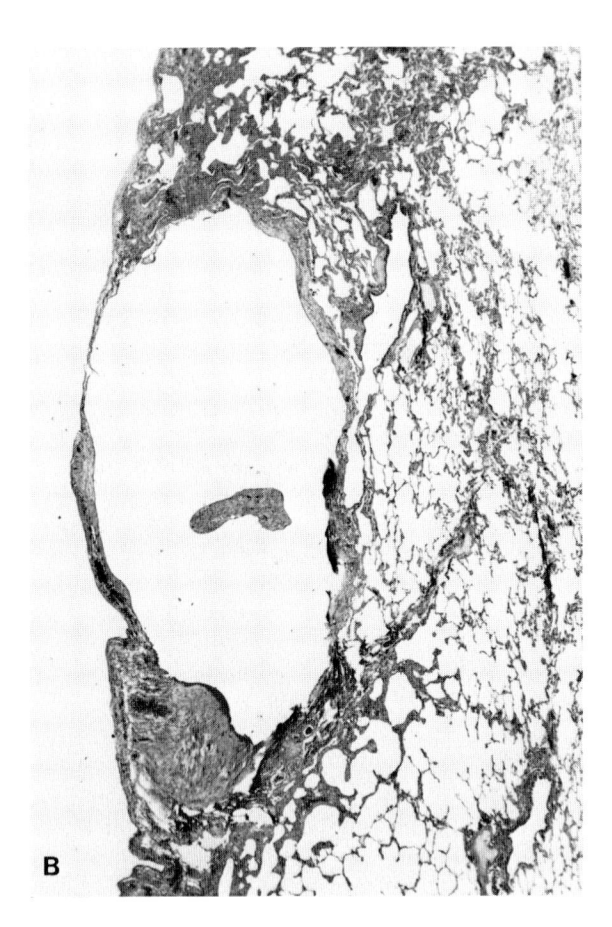

Figure 26–6. Primary spontaneous pneumothorax in a young woman. A. Chest radiograph of a young woman with multiple episodes of spontaneous pneumothorax. The partly collapsed lung is identifiable as a fine convex line in the upper right lung field (arrow). B. Low-power micrograph of specimen from the same patient showing subpleural bleb with fibrous walls and surrounding fibrous reaction in lung tissue (×20).

that air enters the vagina and gains access to the peritoneal cavity through the uterus and fallopian tubes and to the pleural cavity through the diaphragmatic defects. Such an explanation, even if correct, would only account for a small portion of cases.

Etiology and Pathogenesis: Primary Pneumothorax

The mechanism of primary pneumothorax has been the subject of considerable debate. Any explanation must consider not only the fact of pneumothorax itself, but the findings that the majority of cases occur between the ages of 20 and 40, that there is a male predominance varying from 3:1 to 5:1,[2,50,54,55] and that there is a tendency for such persons to be of a tall, thin physique.[55,73,74]

The most commonly offered explanation is that the pneumothorax itself results from the rupture of small apical blebs, although in large series such blebs are not invariably found: Ohata and Suzuki,[75] Mark and Lindskog,[50] and Saha and co-workers,[55] for example, report blebs in only two-third of their 67 patients. Kjaergaard's[52] original report describes and illustrates the presence of such blebs, although many of them appear to be bullae (rather than blebs) of Reid type 1 (see below) and were probably associated with underlying emphysema. A more interesting and convincing argument is produced by Baronofsky and colleagues[76] who performed bilateral thoracotomies in 26 consecutive patients (23 males, 3 females) presenting with unilateral pneumothorax. Bilateral apical blebs were found in 25 of the 26 patients.

The pathologic findings in wedge resections have been described by Lichter and Gwynne[74] and Glenn and associates,[41] and my own observations of pathologic material are similar (Fig. 26–6B). Lichter and Gwynne[74] described the presence of small apical cysts ranging in size from 0.2 to 1 cm and surmounting an area of fibrosis measuring up to about 2 × 3 cm. There were generally not associated adhesions. The cysts were sometimes lined by mesothelial cells, and sometimes had a bare fibrous lining. The underlying tissue showed variable degrees of emphysema or air space enlargement, scarring, infiltration by chronic inflammatory cells, metaplastic change in air space lining cells, and the deposition of pigment. The bronchi or bronchioles which were present frequently were obstructed by mucus. The small arteries demonstrated marked thickening of their walls. I have observed this last phenomenon at a relatively great distance from the area of scarring and inflammation, and also noted focal loss of elastic tissue in such vessels. Lichter and Gwynne[74] concluded, and the present author agrees, that most if not all of the changes observed were secondary to inflammation. Most recently Ohata and Suzuki[75] examined 126 cases histologically and 54 of these by scanning electron microscopy. They concluded that in three-fourths of the patients under age 40, the "blebs" were Reid type 2 bullae (or blebs, if small), that is, bullae with broad necks situated on a shallow but wide region of overinflated lung from which they are not clearly demarcated, whereas only 40 percent of the bullae in those over 40 were type 2. The remainder were either giant bullae or type 1 bullae; that is, those with a narrow neck and sharply demarcated from the underlying lung parenchyma. These findings again suggest a fairly distinctive, if entirely nonspecific, set of morphologic findings associated with the entity of spontaneous pneumothorax in young adults.

The origin of these blebs is uncertain and have been the source of much speculation. Although they are sometimes casually described as "congenital,"[58,77] this is probably a rare event. Roentgenographic series of patients with primary spontaneous pneumothorax have shown an incidence of about 15 percent of blebs[49,77]; similar blebs are almost never found in radiographs of comparable persons without pneumothorax.[49] It is remotely possible that the so-called apical cap is the end state of bleb disease where rupture has not occurred and the bleb has disappeared, but in my experience apical caps are not associated with blebs at autopsy, even in young people, and the finding of blebs at all in such persons at autopsy is very rare.

Lichter and Gwynne[74] suggest that the underlying process is a subclinical nontuberculous infection which affects the apices preferentially. The pathologic findings are certainly consistent with such a process but there is no other evidence to suggest its correctness.

Hofer[78] has shown experimentally that repeated injection of air into the pleural space of rats results first in proliferation of mesothelial cells and, within 4 days, in the formation of "neomembranes" composed of fibroblasts and collagen and variably covered with mesothelium. Some of Hofer's illustrations show the formation of cyst-like spaces by these membranes. If such a hypothesis were to account for bleb formation in humans, one would then have to determine a separate cause for the initiating air leak; a more useful conclusion from these experiments is that some of the pathologic findings could be the result of the pneumothorax rather than the cause.

The tall thin body habitus associated with this condition has also attracted attention. Withers and colleagues[79] have suggested that rapid growth of relatively tall lungs toward the end of adolescence may not be accompanied by adequate vascular growth, thus accentuating the already existing relative ischemia of the apices and causing bleb formation as a degenerative phenomenon. Glenn and co-workers[41] have surmised that air trapping of unknown etiology forms the blebs and that the relative ischemia of the region leads to their rupture.

A more intriguing notion related to body habitus is that the very weight of tall lungs causes damage. Vater and co-workers[80] have calculated the effects of lung shape and size on stresses within the lung; they point out the internal stress and surface pressure are most closely related to lung weight and proportional to lung height but not to shape. Distortion of the lung by gravity causes higher negative intrapleural pressures at the apex and more alveolar distention with possible rupture of alveolar walls and formation of thin-walled blebs.[81] Careful measurements confirm not only that young men with spontaneous pneumothorax have a median height 3 inches taller than average,[81] but that they have longer chests and greater height to width ratios than matched control subjects.[54] In young women, however, similar studies have shown only diminished anteroposterior diameters compared to control subjects. Although this hypothesis is attractive, one has to question why the same phenomenon does not occur in persons with tall and broad lungs, since weight rather than shape is of importance.

One additional hypothesis which is raised by these observations is that the pneumothoraces and blebs result from a genetic defect in connective tissue. Documented genetic defects of this sort such as Marfan's syndrome and Ehlers-Danlos syndrome are associated with spontaneous pneumothorax; and there are also families in which spontaneous pneumothorax is common. Sharpe and colleagues[82] have recently found an association with HLA antigens A_2B_{40} and also with the antitrypsin phenotype M_1M_2 in one such family.

Therapy and Prognosis

A number of different therapeutic modalities are recommended, ranging from observation to suction to pleurodesis, either by instillation of irritating materials or by thoracotomy with pleurectomy or abrasion. The exact choice of therapy depends on the clinical situation. Patients with severe underlying respiratory disease may tolerate even a small pneumothorax badly[67,71] and require immediate placement of a large suction tube, followed by thoracotomy if permanent reexpansion of the lung does not occur. Healthy young patients with small pneumothoraces can be observed or treated by placement of a small catheter with flutter valve.[83] The recurrence rate for this type of treatment in various series varies from 10 to 60 percent with 20 percent generally accepted as the best estimate[49,50,55]; about one-fourth of the recurrences are on the contralateral side. Large pneumothoraces or recurrent pneumothoraces may be treated by instillation of a sclerosing agent such as nitrogen mustard, quinacrine, or tetracycline, or by thoracotomy. The latter approach almost invariably is successful in preventing further recurrences.[41]

Hemopneumothorax

Pneumothorax may be accompanied by blood in the pleural space, and is then referred to as hemopneumothorax. Hemopneumothorax is most commonly a result of trauma. Fluid is said to accompany spontaneous pneumothorax in as many as one-fourth of patients[2] but significant accumulation of blood is relatively uncommon. The etiology is thought to be tearing of thin-walled blood vessels in adhesions as the escaped air pushes the lung away from the chest wall; these vessels are of systemic origin and consequently at systemic pressure. Clinically, spontaneous hemopneumothorax is accompanied by pain, dyspnea, and, when bleeding becomes significant, weakness, syncope, or shock. Chest roentgenograph shows an air fluid level in addition to pneumothorax. Massive hemopneumothorax has a 25 percent mortality without surgical intervention[84]; accumulations of blood of less than 1000 cc can usually be drained and the patient treated by closed suction.

Systemic Effects of Pleural Disease

The syndrome of inappropriate secretion of antidiuretic hormone may be seen with conditions that produce mass lesion on the pleura. These include loculated empyema[85] and some tumors, especially mesothelioma.[86] Although some tumors, particularly bronchogenic carcinoma, produce and secrete antidiuretic hormone (ADH), the syndrome in the pleura appears to be a mechanical phenomenon, possibly related to stretching of vagal receptors in the visceral pleura and release of ADH from the pituitary.[86,87] The mesothelioma analyzed by Perks and co-workers[86] did not contain immunoreactive ADH, but the hormone was present in the serum and urine in increased concentration.

Large pleural tumors may sometimes be associated with hypoglycemia.[88,89]

Tumors of the Pleura: Mesotheliomas

The nature of tumors which appear to originate in the pleura has been a matter of considerable historical controversy. Klemperer and Rabin[90] popularized the use of the term mesothelioma for primary pleural tumors, and were the first to suggest the currently accepted division of such neoplasms into localized and diffuse forms. Despite numerous subsequent reports indicating the accuracy of their observations, the existence of primary mesothelial tumors is still occasionally questioned in the more modern literature.[91] Brief historical reviews of the problems of histogenesis and nomenclature are provided by Spencer,[92] Selikoff and Lee,[93] and extensive detailed reviews by Klemperer and Rabin[90] and Stout and Murray.[94]

Until the work of Klemperer and Rabin[90] was accepted, four different theories of the origin of supposed primary pleural neoplasms were considered[94]: (1) that all of the neoplasms were actually metastases. Although occult primary tumors of viscera or soft tissue have always been a problem, large number of pleural tumors without any other apparent primary have now been examined, making this hypothesis unlikely; (2) that they arose from endothelial cells of the pleural or chest wall capillaries or larger vessels; (3) that they arose from rests of lung deposited in the parietal pleura during embryogenesis. There was, in fact, essentially no scientific support for these latter theories; (4) that they were actually derived from mesothelial cells. Tissue culture studies were of great importance in explaining the origin of tumors which appeared to be epithelial in some areas and mesenchymal in others. Maximov showed that explants of normal pleura could produce fibroblastic cells, whereas Young demonstrated that, with irritation, cells of the pleura formed squamous-like epithelia as well as glandular structures (reviewd by Stout and Murray[94]). Stout and Murray[94] grew explants of a spindled cell type mesothelioma in tissue culture and found the formation of sheets of epithelial-like cells which very much resembled normal mesothelium. In the modern era, electron microscopic studies of a variety of benign and malignant mesothelial tumors have shown that some are ultrastructurally similar to normal mesothelial cells[95,96]; the diagnostic usefulness of electron microscopy should not, however, be overrated (*see below*). Finally, epidemiologic studies linking malignant mesothelioma with exposure to asbestos have reinforced the concept that specific types of primary pleural tumors do exist.

Localized Mesotheliomas

The pleural origin of these tumors was first clearly proposed by Klemperer and Rabin.[90] They have been reported under a wide variety of names: the current literature uses fibrous mesothelioma, benign fibrous mesothelioma, and submesothelial fibroma in addition to localized mesothelioma; in the older literature they were regarded variously as benign neural tumors, benign mesenchymal tumors (fibroma, leiomyoma) and as sarcomas (fibrosarcoma, myxosarcoma, "giant sarcoma of the visceral pleura").[90,97] More than 80 percent of these tumors are definitely benign (*see* Table 26–1), but malignant forms do exist. Localized mesotheliomas are not associated with smoking, nor has asbestos been implicated in the etiology of either the benign or malignant forms.

Benign Forms

Series of reports of localized mesothelioma have shown a wide age range, running from childhood to the eighth decade; however, most of the tumors in children and adolescents have proved to be malignant. The actual age range for the benign tumors appears to be from about 20 to 70 or 80 years with a mean of 40 to 50 years. The sex incidence is roughly equal.[97-101] In some instances tumor has been known to be present from radiographs for several years before surgical removal.

Twenty-five to 50 percent of the patients are asymptomatic at the time of discovery of the tumor. Cough, chest pain, and dyspnea are common in the symptomatic patients. Clubbing and hypertrophic osteoarthropathy have been reported in as many as 20 percent of patients[101]; other systemic signs such as fever and weight loss are less common. An interesting variant is the small number of patients who present with hypoglycemia. Fewer than 20 examples of this phenomenon have been reported,[99,102] almost invariably in association with extremely large tumors. Assay for insulin in these mesotheliomas has been unrewarding, and, most likely, the tumors cause hypoglycemia by consuming large amounts of glucose.[102]

Chest radiographs reveal sharply circumscribed rounded or lobulated masses which may be situated peripherally in contact with the pleura, may be associated with a fissure, or may be buried in the pulmonary parenchyma (Fig. 26–7A).

On gross examination, the tumors range from 2 to 30 cm and may weigh as much as 3000 g. In a collected series of 168 tumors (Table 26–5), 38 percent arose from the visceral pleura, 11 percent from the parietal pleura, 2 percent arose in a fissure, and 16 percent were intrapulmonary but almost always in contact with the visceral pleura. The remaining tumors were attached to several sites on the visceral and parietal pleurae. The majority of intrapleural tumors are pedunculated and are usually attached to the pleura by a fine fibrous band (see Fig. 26–7A); the sessile tumors, although circumscribed, tend to infiltrate lung locally (Fig. 26–7C). This is also true of the intrapulmonary tumors. The cut surfaces are commonly white with a whorled appearance; small foci of hemorrhage and areas of softening as well as cysts are occasionally observed, but the presence of large amounts of hemorrhage or necrosis is usually indicative of a malignant tumor.

Microscopically, the majority of tumors are remarkably similar and show a variable combination of three histologic patterns (Fig. 26–7C through F). The collagenized pattern consists of dense relatively acellular fibrous tissue in which slit-like spaces are present; the spaces are lined by thin cells with elongated nuclei. Somewhat larger but similar cells are present in the stroma. Rarely the fibrous stroma forms storiform patterns. The collagenized pattern was the predominant one in 23% of the tumors reported by Dalton and co-workers.[99] Thirty percent of their tumors had areas virtually identical to hemangiopericytoma, the second common pattern. Such areas are similar in appearance to hemangiopericytoma of the lung or soft tissue, even to the presence of leaf-like vascular channels. The third pattern, found to some extent in 65 percent of the tumors reported by Dalton and co-workers,[99] has been referred to as "cellular"[99,101]; the cells are rounded to spindled, uniform, and densely packed. When mitotic activity is present at all in a localized benign mesothelioma, it is usually found in the cellular areas. The distinction between the three patterns is not always sharp, and continuous transitions from one to another are easy to demonstrate.

Where the broad-based tumors project into lung it is common to find structures which appear to be broad-based papillae. Rare truly papillary variants of localized benign mesothelioma have been reported by Foster and Ackerman[100] and Yesner and Hurwitz.[103] Glenn and colleagues[41] believe that the papillary tumors are actually post-inflammatory pseudotumors. Occasionally in these tumors one finds what initially appears as a biphasic pattern with epithelial nests and stromal cells, as well as transitions between the one and the other; however, it is clear that most such nests represent entrapped alveolar epithelium.

The histogenesis of the benign localized mesotheliomas, as well as the malignant forms, remains a source of argument between those who believe they arise from mesothelial cells, and those who believe, as did Klemperer and Rabin,[90] that they arise from undifferentiated submesothelial cells, hence the name "submesothelial fibroma." Modern studies have failed to resolve the issue. Motomiya and co-workers[104] demonstrated that hyaluronic acid, a substance known to be produced by benign mesothelial cells and malignant mesotheliomas, was present in a benign mesothelioma; dermatan sulfate and heparin sulfate were also found. This might be taken as evidence in favor of a mesothelial origin, but hyaluronic acid is produced by a variety of mesenchymal tumors in which there is no reason to

Table 26–5. Localized Mesothelioma

Series	Total Cases	Visceral Pleura	Parietal Pleura	Intra-pulmonary	Origin in Fissure	Benign	Recurrence Considered Benign	Malignant
Stout and Hamadi[109]	8			5		5		3
Clagett et al.[98]	24			6		20		4
Foster and Ackerman[100]	18	7	4	5	1	18		0
Okike et al.[101]	60	29	9	8	3	52	1	8
Sharifker and Kaneko[97]	18					18		0
Dalton et al.[99]	40	28	5	3	—	32		8
	168	64	18	27	4	145	1	23

Table 26–6. Fibrous Mesothelioma—Electron Microscopic Studies

Series	Cases	Observations	Conclusions
Osamura[105]	1	Epithelial and mesenchymal cells	Mesothelial origin
Kawai et al.[95]	6	Primitive mesenchymal cells	Cells with minimal mesothelial differentiation, similar to rat fetal pleura
Hernandez and Fernandez[106]	2	Identical to fibroblasts	Submesothelial origin
Wang[96]	2	Nonspecific, more like fibroblasts	Submesothelial origin

postulate a mesothelial origin. Electron microscopic examination (Table 26–6) has also been confusing; some authors have reported cells forming lumen-like spaces and possessing microvilli,[105] features of mesothelial cells, or intracytoplasmic filaments, microvilli, and basement membranes,[95] features considered consistent with fetal mesothelial cells. On the other hand, Hernandez and Fernandez,[106] Kay and Silverberg,[107] and Wang[96] showed only spindled mesenchymal cells with features similar to those of fibroblasts.

As a rule the localized benign mesothelioma is easily separated on histologic grounds from the malignant version. Eighty-six percent of the 168 cases listed in Table 26–5 were considered benign. A high mitotic index, extensive hemorrhage and necrosis, and recurrence were generally predictive of malignant behavior. Utley and associates[108] reported three recurrent localized tumors after 5, 13, and 16 years; all appeared to behave benignly. However, in the 168 tumors listed above, only one benign recurrence was noted, whereas more than half the malignant tumors recurred locally. Glenn and colleagues[41] suggested that some recurrent tumors, especially those with broad initial attachments to lung, are curable by more extensive surgery and should be considered variants of benign mesothelioma. It should also be appreciated that, while most of the malignant variants are obvious histologically, a small proportion of cellular tumors that are not otherwise histologically malignant may cause death from local recurrence or metastases.[99]

The differential diagnosis of this neoplasm is generally not a problem: the only point of confusion is separation from a benign hemangiopericytoma when the tumor is intraparenchymal. This distinction is often not histologically feasible, but is also not of prognostic or therapeutic importance.

Malignant Localized Mesothelioma

This category appears to contain a wide histologic range of tumors; clearly some of the intrapulmonary tumors, such as those reported by Stout and Hamadi,[109] have little to recommend the name mesothelioma and today would probably be regarded as primary pulmonary sarcomas. The remaining group have the common features of gross pedunculation or sessile attachment to the visceral pleura such as is seen with benign localized mesothelioma. Hemorrhage and necrosis are common both grossly and histologically, and many, but not all, of the tumors are histologically malignant (Fig. 26–8). The histologic descriptions range from tumors with features of diffuse mesothelioma[101] to tumors resembling malignant variants of benign mesothelioma[99] to sarcomas which might be otherwise called synovial sarcoma, malignant fibrous histiocytoma, or fibrosarcoma.[110] The clinical features are not greatly different from those of the benign form if the tumor has not metastasized at the time of presentation, but Okike and colleagues[101] noted that none of the malignant tumors they observed were associated with hypertrophic osteoarthropathy. The prognosis appears to be uniformly poor for tumors considered to be malignant at initial excision; recurrence and dissemination of tumors initially thought to be benign may not occur for 5 to 10 years.

Malignant Mesothelioma

Demographic and Clinical Features

In the general population, malignant mesothelioma is a rare tumor; recent studies have found incidence rates in North America of 2.2 to 2.8/million population/year.[111,112] The incidence rates in Canada are about half those in the United States. Rates for men are generally four to five times the rates for women.[112] Mesothelioma accounts for approximately 1 in 1000 to 1 in 10,000 unselected autopsies.[113] The incidence of mesothelioma has increased steadily over the past four decades, partly because of improved diagnosis, but also because of the increase in tumors related to asbestos exposure. The figures cited above apply to the combination of pleural and peritoneal mesotheliomas; because of their common etiology, and clinical and pathological features, these tumors are usually grouped together. Collected series show that upward of 80 percent of mesotheliomas originate in the pleura.

The median age at presentation in most series is approximately 60, and few cases are seen under the age of 30; however, clinically and histologically typical mesotheliomas have been reported in children and adolescents.[111,112,114] Males are more commonly affected than females; the sex ratio in various reports ranges from 2:1 to 6:1.[111,112,115] Mesothelioma is not related to cigarette smoking. The most common presenting complaints for patients with pleural mesothelioma are chest pain and

784   Diseases of the Pleura

Figure 26–7A–C. Localized benign fibrous mesothelioma. A. Chest radiograph of a patient with a localized fibrous mesothelioma showing huge sharply circumscribed mass on the right side. B. Gross photograph of resected mass. Note the lobulation and apparent encapsulation as well as the fine pedicle (arrow) which connected mass to pleura. C. Low-power light micrograph of a localized fibrous mesothelioma which has a broad attachment to underlying lung. Note the peculiar papillary formations at the point of contact with lung tissue (×20).

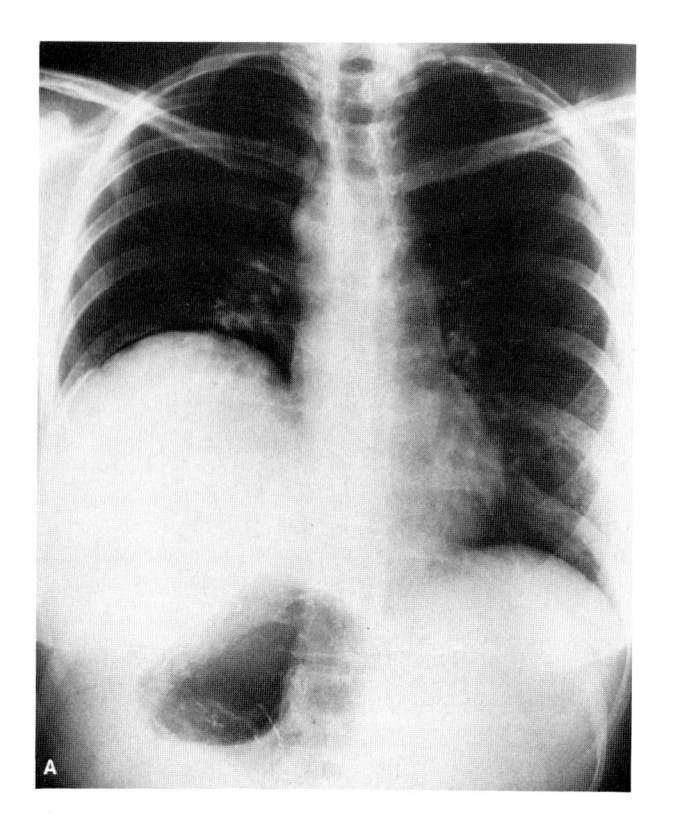

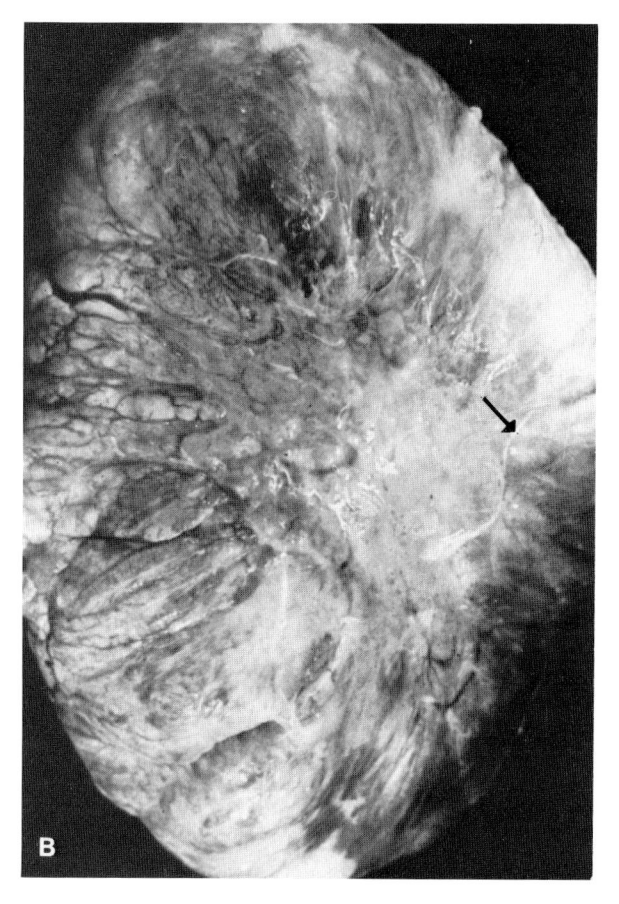

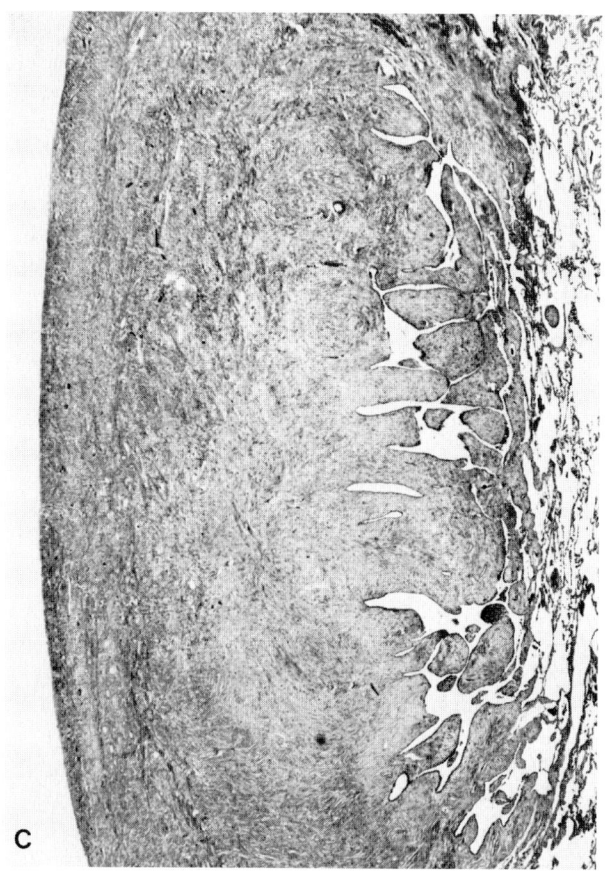

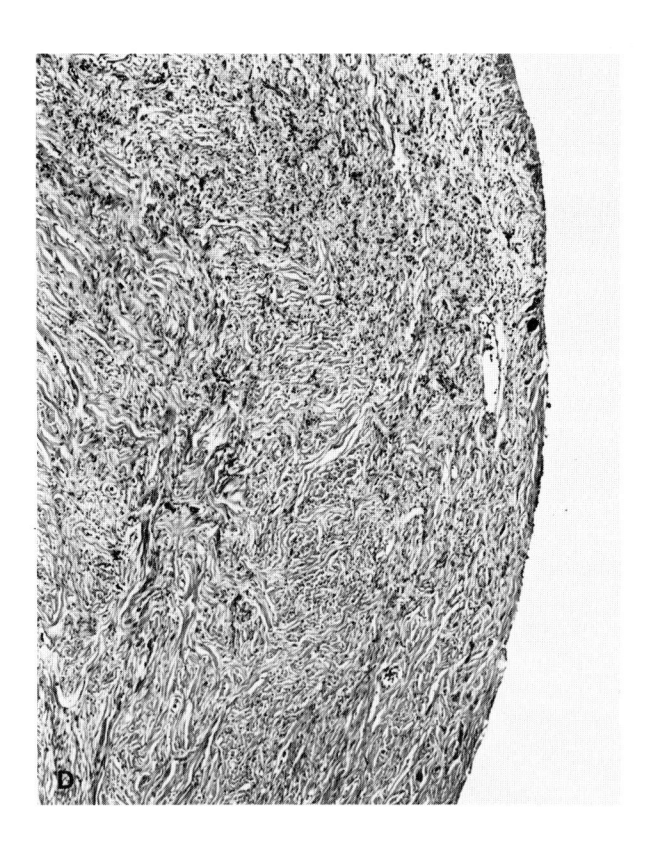

Figure 26–7D–F. D. Low-power light micrograph of another localized fibrous mesothelioma showing sharp circumscription of the tumor (×40). E. Higher-power view showing one of the typical patterns of fibrous tissue with slit-like spaces, characteristic of this neoplasm (×160). F. Another field of the same tumor illustrating a cellular area with a hemangiopericytoma-like pattern (×160).

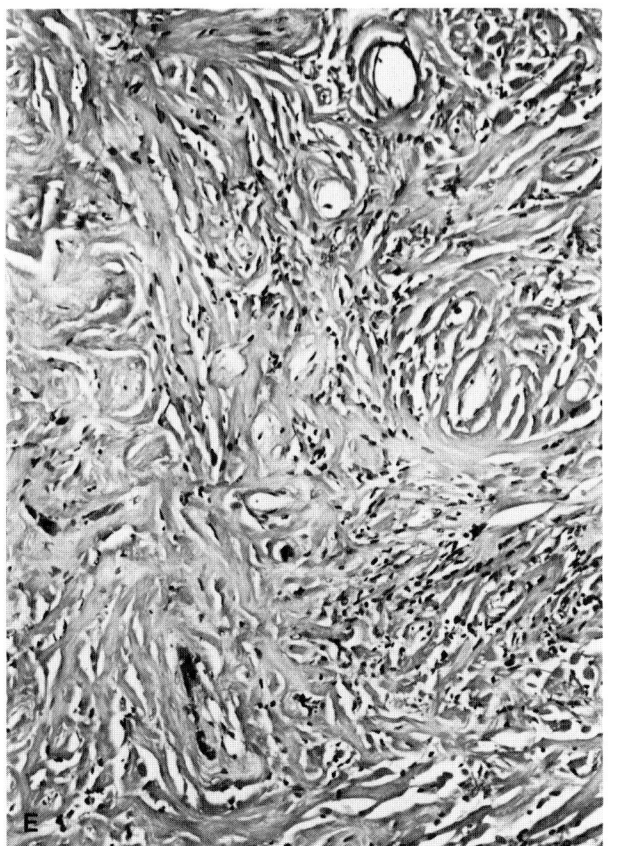

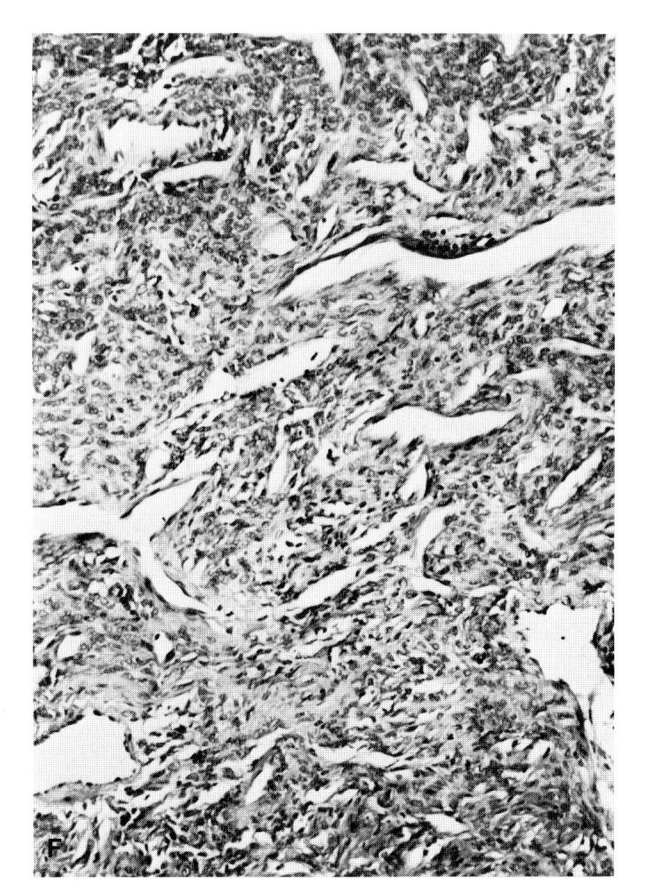

Figure 26–8. Malignant variety of localized fibrous mesothelioma. Light micrographs of a sharply circumscribed lobulated tumor mass developing in the pleura of a 50-year-old woman. The cellularity of the tumor is apparent at low power. Note the resemblance of B to the benign form of the tumor shown in 26-7F. C. Shown are numerous mitoses and cellular atypicality (A ×40, B ×160, C ×400).

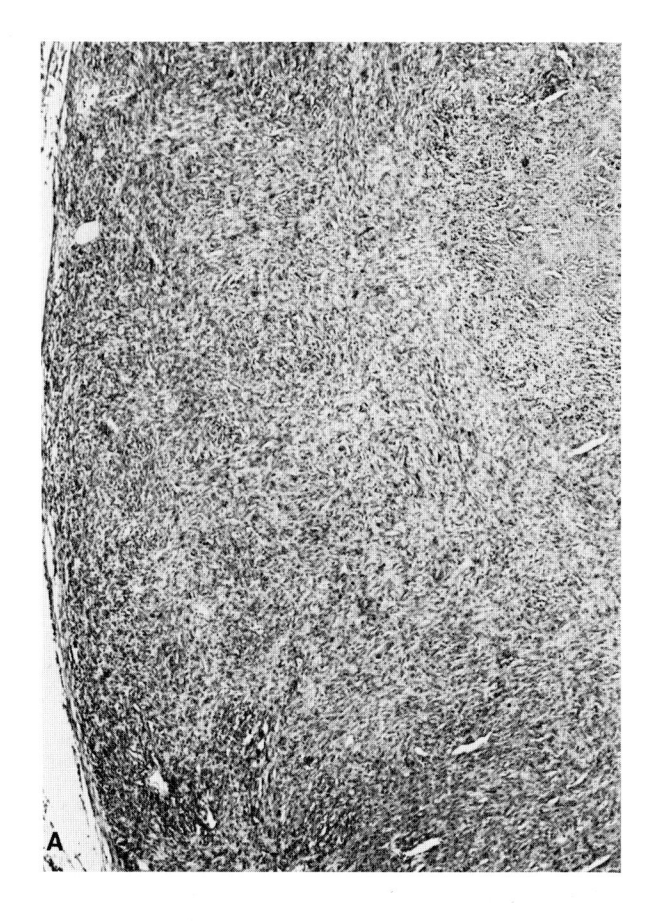

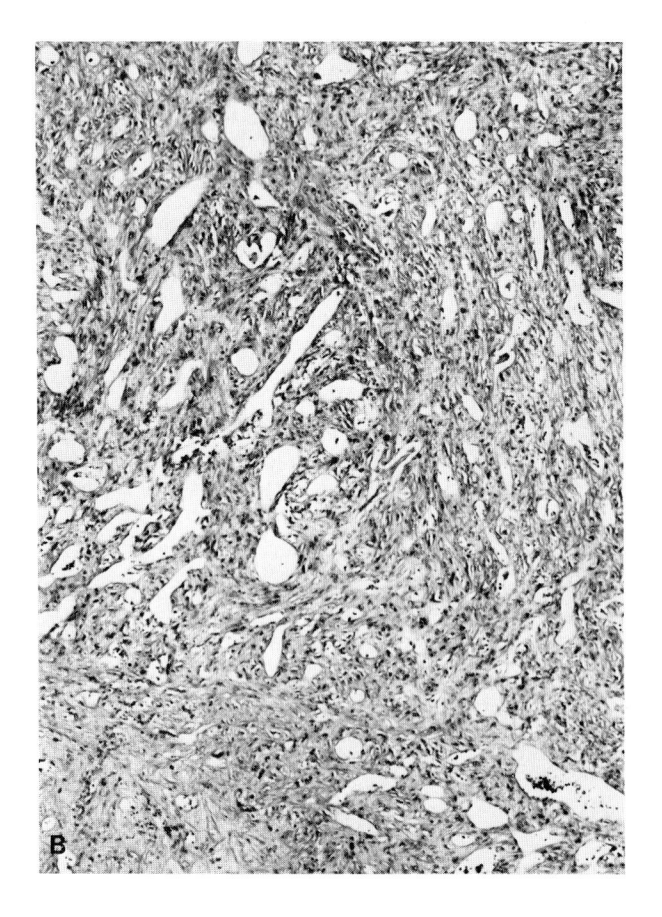

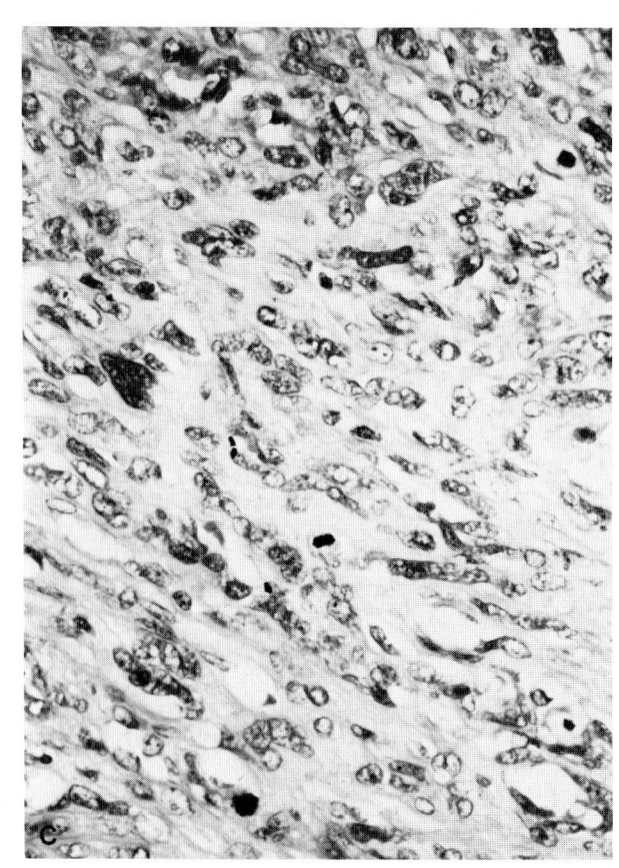

dyspnea; peritoneal tumors may present with a palpable mass, ascites, pain, and weight loss. Clubbing, hypertrophic osteoarthropathy, and hypoglycemia may also be seen with malignant mesothelioma but less commonly than is the case for benign localized mesothelioma. In the typical case of pleural mesothelioma, physical examination reveals little except dullness over the affected hemothorax; enlarged cervical nodes may be seen late in the disease, at which time contraction of the chest wall is also observed. Bowel obstruction is usually a late complication of peritoneal mesothelioma.

Radiographically, several different appearances are found. Effusion is extremely common; after drainage of the effusion, the pleura may be seen to be diffusely thickened, or nodular (Fig. 26–9A, B). Less commonly, an apparently solitary circumscribed mass is seen and may mimic an intrapulmonary process[93,111,115,116]. Other radiographic features of asbestos exposure may also be present. Elmes and Simpson[115] found pleural plaques in 37 of 150 cases of pleural mesothelioma and 3 of 14 cases of peritoneal mesothelioma; evidence of asbestosis was present in nine and five of these patients. The relatively high incidence of asbestosis in these patients with peritoneal mesothelioma correlates with the observation that peritoneal mesothelioma tends to be seen in patients with very heavy asbestos exposure.[93]

Thoracentesis reveals that the pleural effusion is serosanguinous or overtly bloody in 25 to 50 percent of patients[111,115] and may occasionally be quite gelatinous. This latter finding reflects the presence of large quantities of glycosaminoglycan, especially hyaluronic acid, which is secreted by mesothelial cells. Quantification of hyaluronic acid levels in pleural effusion has been suggested as a diagnostic procedure (reviewed in Legha and Muggia[111]); probably only very high levels (greater than 0.8 g/ml)[117] are diagnostic, since inflammatory and nonmesothelial neoplastic conditions can also cause an increase in pleural fluid hyaluronic acid.

Epidemiology

The epidemiological features of malignant mesothelioma are considered in detail in Chapter 23, and only a few salient features will be covered here. This topic is briefly reviewed by Becklake[118] and in more detail by Kannerstein and co-workers[113] and Selikoff and Lee.[93]

The association of malignant mesothelioma with exposure to asbestos was first brought to attention by the report of Wagner and colleagues[119] in a report that has predicted many of the salient epidemiologic associations. A portion of the patients had occupational exposure, but another significant portion had nonoccupational (in retrospect, usually quite substantial) exposure, for example, playing, as a child, on an asbestos mine tailings. The tumor was initially found in persons exposed to one particular type of asbestos, crocidolite, from one particular location, the northwestern Cape Province; subsequently it has been shown that other types of asbestos also produce mesothelioma, but crocidolite is particularly carcinogenic. The time between exposure and the appearance of the tumor was typically many years. Numerous subsequent studies have confirmed the relationships just listed.[93,118]

The bulk (80 to 90 percent) of tumors are pleural, but persons with heavy occupational exposure are prone to develop peritoneal tumors.[93,116] In some workers with heavy exposure, mesothelioma now accounts for 10 to 14 percent of deaths, a fraction almost comparable to that caused by bronchogenic carcinoma. The tumor may appear from 15 to 60 years after initial exposure to asbestos; the mean latent period is approximately 30 to 40 years.[93,118] Men are more likely to have a history of occupational exposure than women; in the recent report by McDonald and McDonald[112] on mesotheliomas in North America, an occupational history of exposure could be found in about half the males but only 5 percent of females. A large number of the occupational cases appear to result from shipyard work during World War II. Women who have mesothelioma are likely to give a history of family contact, usually in the form of a relative who worked in the asbestos industry and wore work clothes home[120]; in rare instances several members of such a family have developed mesothelioma.[121] Anderson and colleagues[122] examined 326 family contacts of asbestos workers. Chest radiograph abnormalities were found in 35 percent, and 17 of 70 deaths were caused by mesotheliomas.

In animals, mesothelioma can be induced by inhalation of asbestos, or by intrapleural injection of asbestos, a method that produces a high yield of tumors.[123,124] In humans, exposure to different types of fiber appears to produce different incidence rates of mesothelioma; crocidolite is probably the most dangerous, followed by amosite and then chrysotile.[112,125,126] Churg and co-workers[127] have reported a patient in whom mesothelioma developed after instillation of asbestos and fiberglass into the pericardium.

In animals many other types of fiber will induce mesothelioma when instilled into the pleural or pericardial cavity; fibers that have been found to be effective include fibrous glass, synthetic aluminum silicate, nemalite, and the clay attapulgite (palygorscite). Granular forms of the same dusts are ineffective.[123,124] Stanton and co-workers[128] have shown that carcinogenicity in this system is a reflection of fiber size and aspect ratio (length/width ratio) and postulated that induction of mesothelioma is related to the physical parameters of the mineral, rather than the chemical type. The prediction that any long thin high aspect ratio fiber might induce mesothelioma has been recently confirmed in reports from Turkey.[129] These studies demonstrated that in certain villages in Turkey where mesothelioma is endemic, no asbestos is mined or used, but the soil contains the fibrous noasbestos mineral, erionite.

It should be emphasized that by no means all mesotheliomas in humans are definitely related to asbestos or erionite exposure, and this is particularly true in women.[130] Individual cases with histories of radiation, insufflation of paraffin as therapy for tuberculosis, and exposure to other dusts such as glass have been reported.[130,131] Whether these are actually specific etiologic

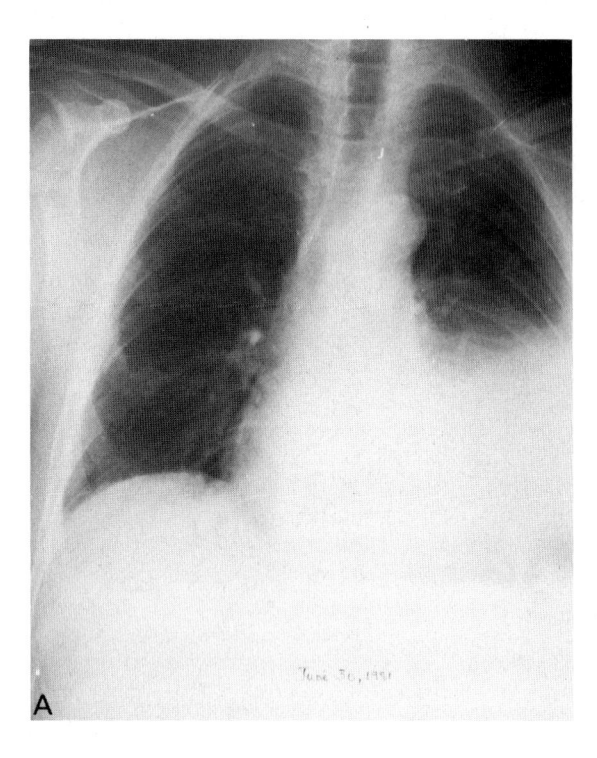

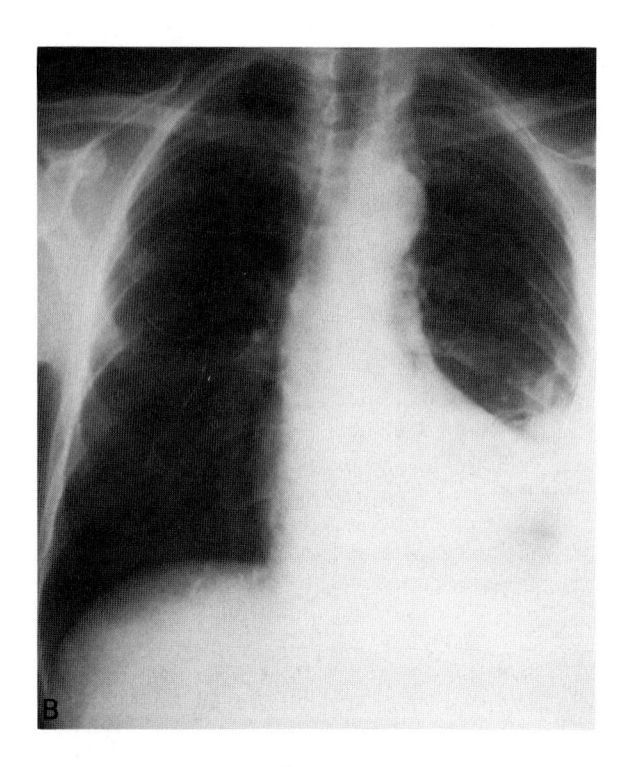

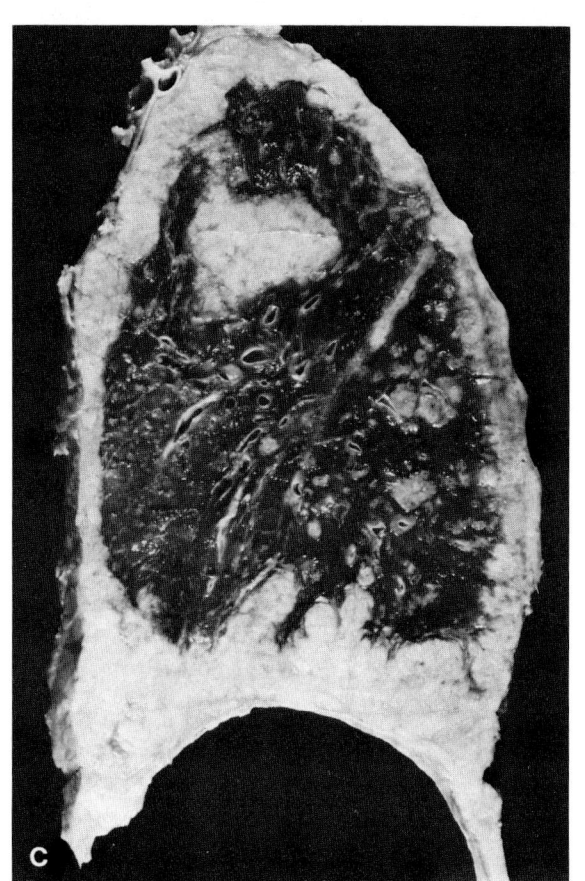

Figure 26-9A-C. Malignant mesothelioma. A and B. Chest radiographs of a 49-year-old man with a history of asbestos exposure who presented with a pleural effusion shown in A. After drainage of the effusion (B) tumor masses involving the pleura were visible. C. Autopsy specimen from the same patient showing tumor encasing lung. This mode of growth is typical of malignant mesothelioma but is sometimes mimicked by adenocarcinoma of the lung.

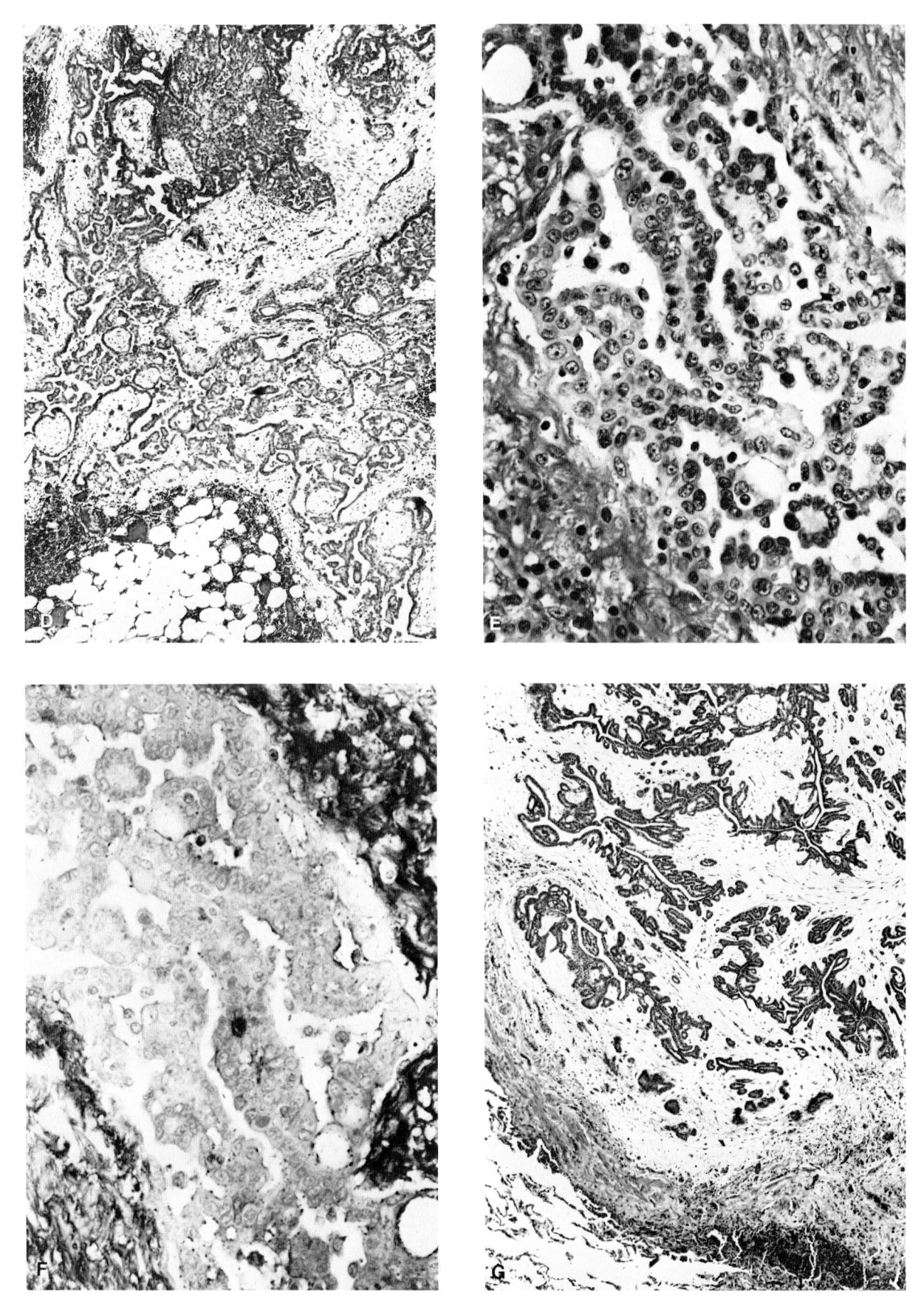

Figure 26–9D–G. D through H. Variants of tubulopapillary type of epithelial mesothelioma. The tumor illustrated in D through F is a peritoneal tumor developing in an insulation worker with asbestos exposure; the tumor shown in G and H is a pleural mesothelioma developing in an electrician with a history of asbestos exposure. In F is shown a droplet of colloidal iron positive material in the cytoplasm of one of the tumor cells. The material disappeared with hyaluronidase indicating that it was hyaluronic acid, a finding characteristic of malignant mesothelioma (D ×20, E ×400, F ×400, G ×40).

790   Diseases of the Pleura

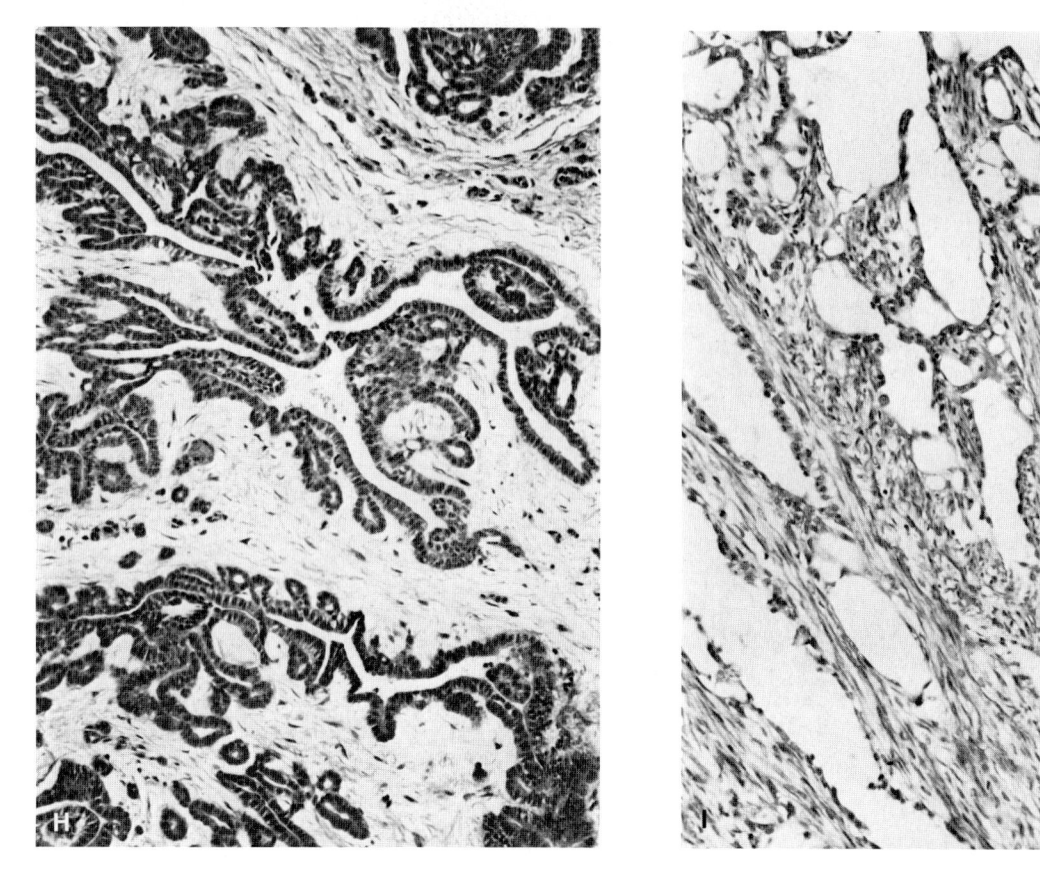

Figure 26–9H, I. H. A higher power view of F (×160). I. Mixed epithelial and sarcomatous mesothelioma showing so-called adenomatoid type of epithelial component (×160).

ported.[130,131] Whether these are actually specific etiologic agents or merely sporadic cases with accidentally suggestive histories remains to be determined. Other cases have no clearly defined etiology.

Pathologic Features

Detailed descriptions of the pathological features of malignant mesothelioma have been published by Churg and Selikoff,[132] Hourihane[133,134] McCaughey,[135] Kannerstein and Churg,[136] and Kannerstein and colleagues.[137] The major problem in diagnosis is the ability of certain other neoplasms metastatic to the pleura or peritoneum to mimic malignant mesothelioma microscopically, and sometimes grossly.[137] For this reason it is necessary to make use of every possible diagnostic technique, including gross and microscopic appearances, clinical findings, and histochemical reactions. A number of newer immunohistochemical and electrophoretic techniques have also been proposed for this purpose and are discussed in Analysis of Glycosaminoglycans, below.

Gross Appearances

The gross appearance of mesothelioma is often characteristic. The neoplasm tends to surround viscera, particularly in the thorax where one lung is commonly encased by hard white tumor at autopsy (Fig. 26–9C). Sometimes, particularly at an earlier stage of disease, the tumor appears as multiple nodules or plaques studded over the pleura and diaphragm. Usually by the time of diagnosis tumor appears on both parietal and visceral pleurae, but there is some evidence that tumor may first develop on the parietal surface.[132] At autopsy the pleural tumor may show extensive growth into the mediastinum with compression of the vascular structures. Tumor also frequently spreads into the underlying lung, particularly along interlobular septae, and sometimes by invasion of the bronchial tree in the hilum.[134] Spread through the diaphragm and into the chest wall, particularly along needle or surgical tracts, is common. It should be remembered that peripheral adenocarcinomas of the lung may also spread in a similar fasion leading to encasement of the lung (see Figure 19–11B).

The gross appearance of the peritoneal tumors is similar; the neoplasm may appear as diffuse nodules over

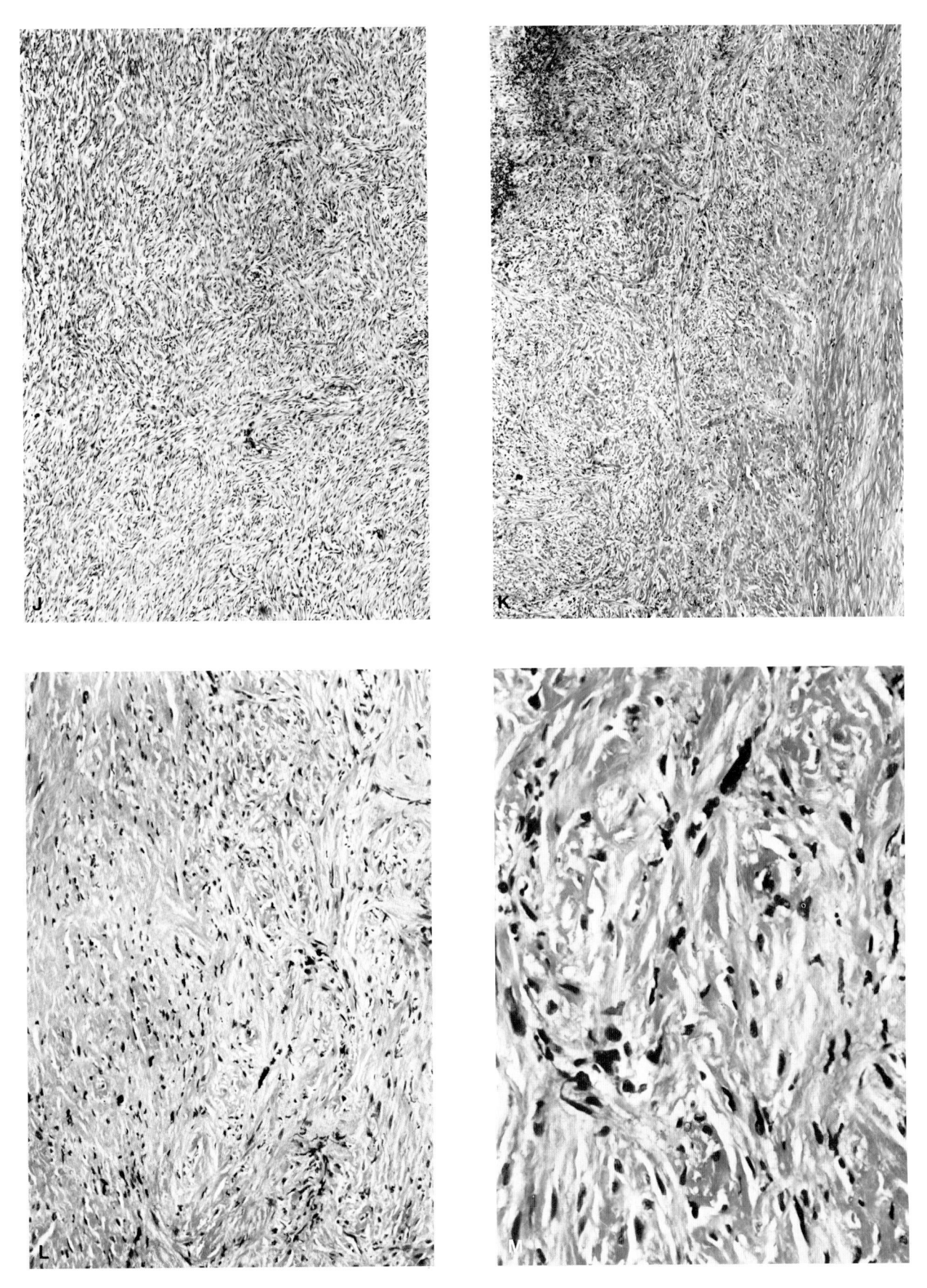

Figure 26–9J–M. Sarcomatous mesothelioma. Note the extremely cellular low power appearance with the suggestion of storiform areas in J, and the transition to densely collagenized sparsely cellular areas in K. In L and M are shown the sparsely cellular areas at higher power. This pattern of tumor growth (so-called desmoplastic mesothelioma) can be mistaken for reactive change, particularly if the cells are cytologically bland (J and K ×40, L ×160, ×400).

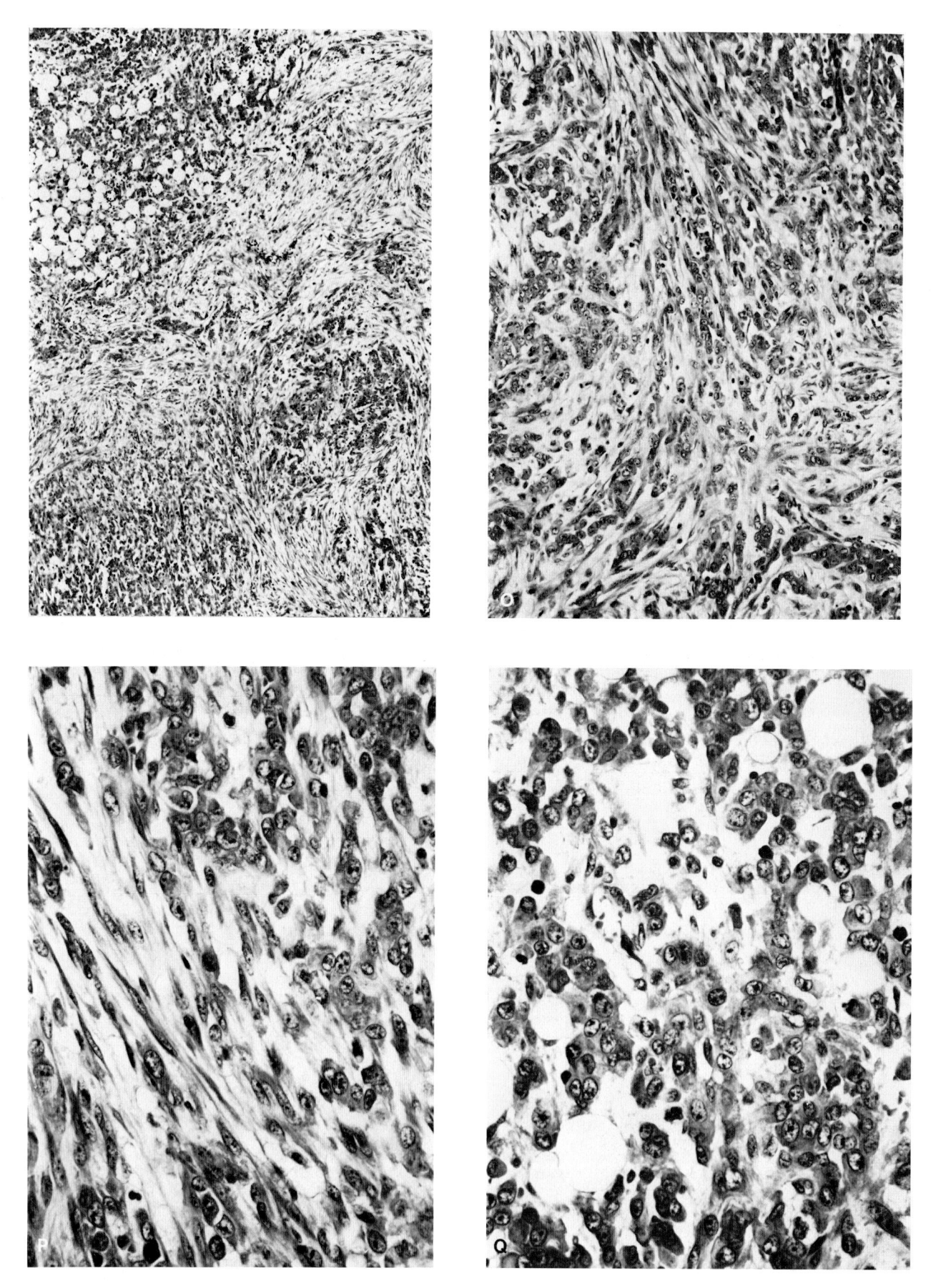

Figure 26–9N–Q. Example of a mixed epithelial and sarcomatous mesothelioma. A low power view of the tumor is shown in N. O and P illustrate transitions between the spindled and epithelial components. In Q is shown a purely epithelial area composed of cells that resemble ordinary reactive mesothelial cells. Some epithelial mesotheliomas are entirely of this latter pattern (N ×40, O ×160, P and Q ×400).

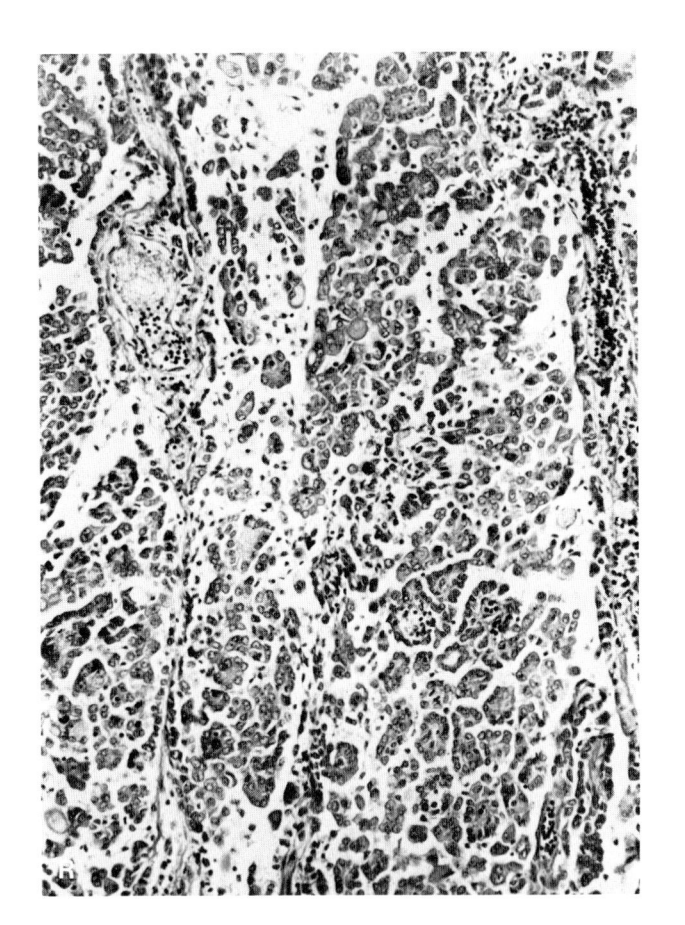

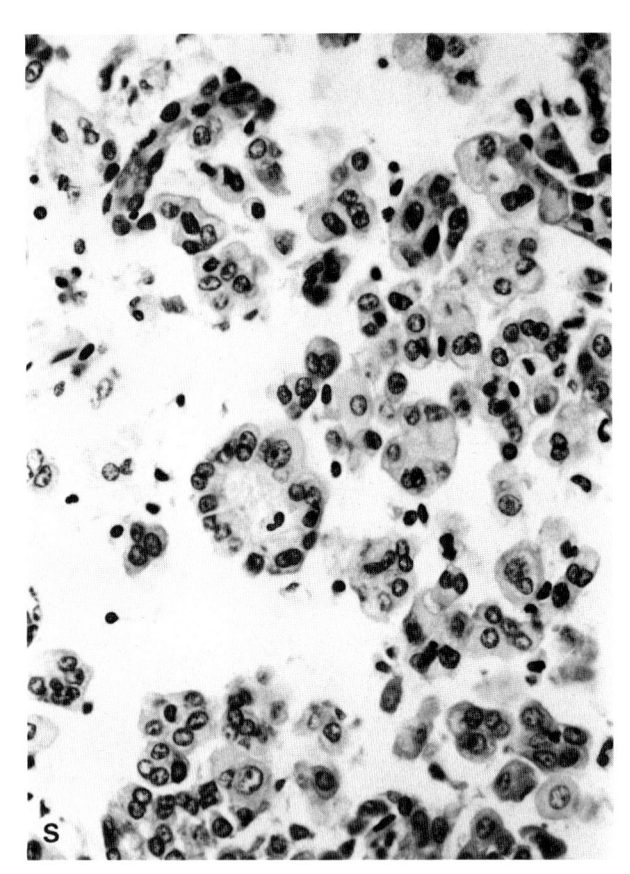

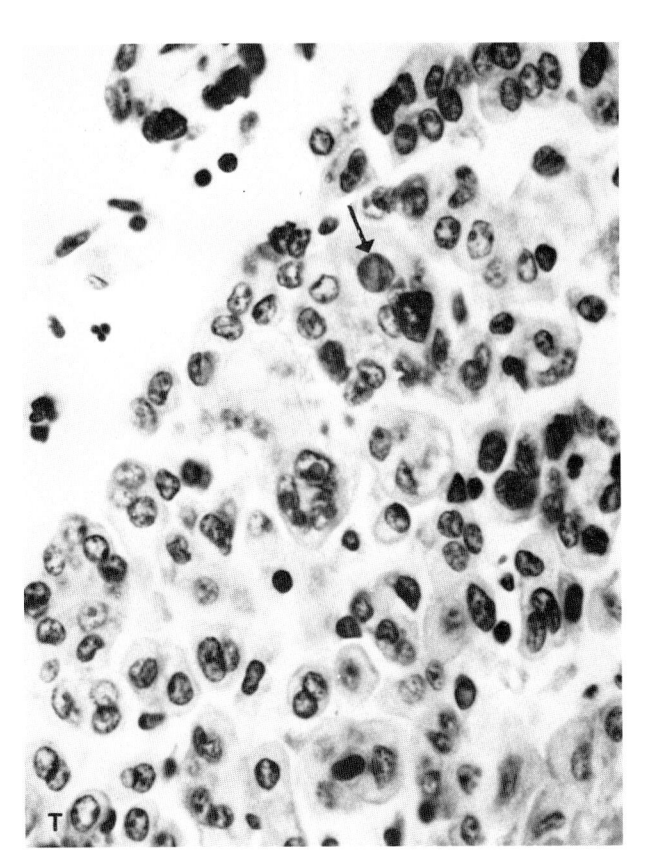

Figure 26–9R–T. Example of an adenocarcinoma mimicking a tubulopapillary mesothelioma. This tumor appeared as a diffuse neoplasm without any obvious primary in the abdomen of a young male. Note the resemblance to tubulopapillary mesothelioma in R and S. T illustrates a periodic acid-Schiff stain showing a droplet of mucin (arrow), a finding that establishes the diagnosis of adenocarcinoma (R ×64, S ×160, T ×400).

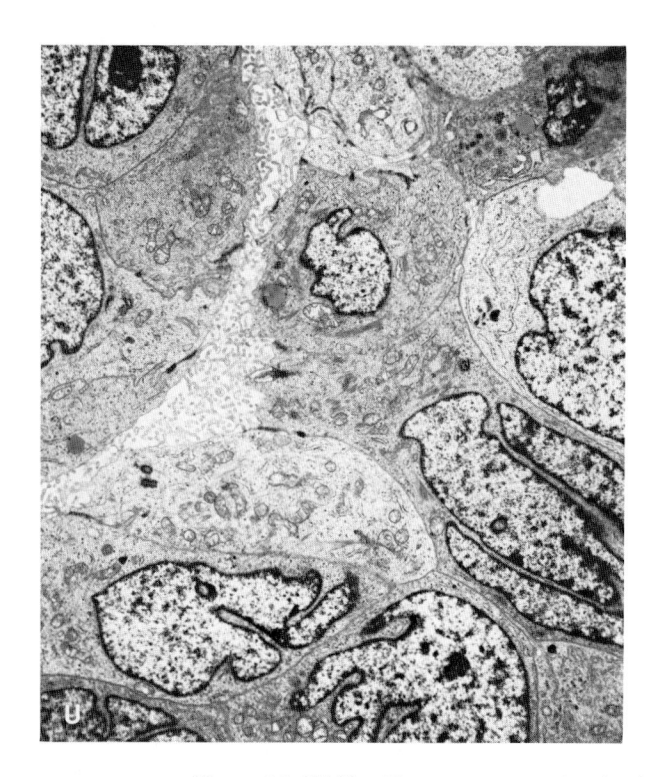

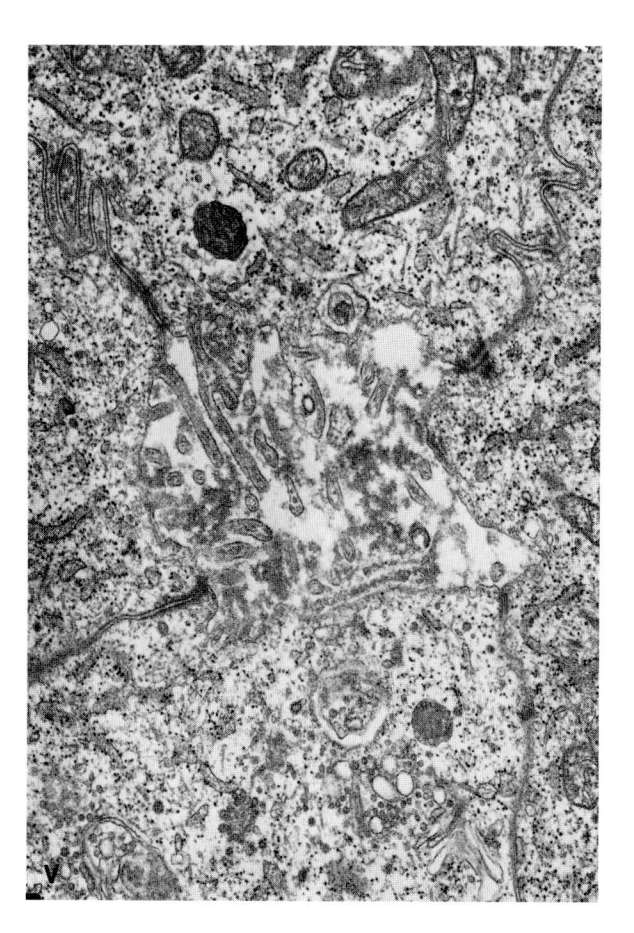

Figure 26–9U,V. Electron micrographs of malignant mesothelioma. All are taken from the same tumor. U shows a low-power view of an epithelial area. The cells are connected by well-formed junctions but are otherwise fairly nondescript (×2000). V illustrates a lumen formed by four tumor cells. Note the numerous long microvilli and the junctional complexes bordering the lumen. It has been claimed that long microvilli are a diagnostic feature of mesothelioma (see text, Malignant Mesothelioma, Pathologic Features, Ultrastructure) but this figure should be compared to Figure 19–11F (×12,000).

the peritoneum, simulating disseminated carcinoma, or as plaques, or as massive aggregates of tumor encasing bowel, liver, and spleen.[138]

Microscopic Appearances

The diversity of patterns which may be seen microscopically in malignant mesothelioma is remarkable, considering that all of the neoplasms are thought to derive from a single cell line.[138] In general one can divide mesotheliomas into epithelial, sarcomatous, and mixed types. Legha and Muggia[111] summarized the classification of pleural tumours from 382 patients in 9 different reports and found that 54.5 percent were epithelial, 21.5 percent sarcomatous, and 24 percent mixed. Kannerstein and Churg[138] found that of 82 cases of peritoneal mesothelioma, 75 percent were epithelial, 24 percent mixed, and only 1 percent sarcomatous. The histologic patterns of pleural and peritoneal tumors are similar and they will be considered together.

The most characteristic form of epithelial mesothelioma is the so-called tubulopapillary variant (Fig. 26–9D through H). In this pattern the tumor forms branching tubules and papillae lined by flattened to cuboidal cells; columnar cells are uncommon and are more characteristic of adenocarcinoma. The cell cytoplasm may be vacuolated; sometimes the appearance is that of a signet ring cell. Aggregates of multiple vacuolated cells can produce an adenomatoid or lacy pattern (Fig. 26–9I).

Another rather different type of epithelial tumor is composed of large cells with copious eosinophilic cytoplasm and very sharp cell borders. In some instances these cells are arranged in pavement-like sheets, and in other cases resemble aggregates of large polygonal mesothelial cells such as are commonly found in reactive pleural effusions (see Fig. 26–9Q). These cells may also be vacuolated. In my experience, such cells are often separated by periodic acid-Schiff (PAS)–positive material which may represent basement membrane. Mitoses may

Table 26-7. Inflammatory Mesothelial Reaction Vs. Mesothelioma[a]

Reaction	Neoplasm
Cells relatively small	Cells large with large nuclei
Nucleoli inconspicuous	Prominent eosinophilic nucleoli
Tubules/clefts scanty and connected to surface	Numerous deep epithelial-lined tubules and clefts
Single cells/nests of cells not found deep to surface	Single cells/nests of cells well away from surface
Cells do not form heaped-up papillae	Cells form heaped-up papillae
Mitoses often present	Mitoses often present

[a] Based on the results of Hourihane,[133] Kannerstein et al.[137] and on unpublished data of Churg.

Table 26-8. Histochemical Staining Reactions of Carcinoma and Mesothelioma

Stain	Mesothelioma	Adenocarcinoma
PAS (diastase digested)	Negative	Positive
Colloidal iron or alcian blue	+	+ or −
Colloidal iron or alcian blue predigested with hyaluronidase	−	If + before digestion then remains positive

Abbreviations: PAS, periodic acid-Schiff.

be extremely infrequent. Psammoma bodies may be present in the papillary tumors, but not in the numbers seen in carcinoma.[135,137]

At the other end of the histologic spectrum are the sarcomatous tumors (Fig. 26–9J through M). These are generally composed of spindled cells which resemble fibroblasts; in contrast to the epithelial forms, mitoses are usually readily apparent. Collagen production is usually marked; in some tumors the collagenous stroma makes up almost the whole of the neoplasm, and the cellular component is represented by single entrapped cells. This latter pattern has been referred to as "desmoplastic,"[139] and may occasionally be seen with epithelial or mixed mesotheliomas, as well as with sarcomatous tumors.[140] Care must be taken not to mistake such patterns for benign reactions. In other sarcomatous tumors, variable numbers of giant cells are present, and the author has seen such tumors with storiform areas indistinguishable from malignant fibrous histiocytoma. Other differentiated mesenchymal components such as cartilage[141] are rarely found.

The mixed types of mesothelioma show variable combinations of epithelial and mesenchymal elements, and sometimes clearly transitional cell forms are present (Fig. 26–9N through Q). Many tumors contain numbers of poorly differentiated cells which may be vaguely epithelial or mesenchymal; as the histologic appearance becomes more and more unlike the forms just described, definitive diagnosis on the basis of histology becomes progressively more difficult. Extremely anaplastic mesotheliomas with high mitotic rates, although uncommon, do occur.

In some instances the question posed by microscopic examination is not the mesothelial origin of a proliferative process, but its neoplastic or inflammatory nature. A number of differential features are listed in Table 26–7. In the author's experience, inflammatory mesothelial reactions do not "invade" the stroma, and the finding of deep tubules or collections of cells should arouse suspicion of a neoplasm. Although inflammatory reactions may produce sheets of cells, irregular papillary masses are probably an indicator of malignancy. Cytologic criteria are also helpful, but it should be remembered that intense mesothelial reactions may be characterized by a marked mitotic rate.

Histochemical Reactions

The value of a rather simple set of histochemical stains in the diagnosis of mesothelioma cannot be overemphasized. Adenocarcinomas usually secrete neutral or slightly acidic mucins, whereas mesotheliomas produce highly acidic mucopolysaccharides, particularly hyaluronic acid. Separation of adenocarcinoma and mesothelioma can therefore be accomplished by utilizing the scheme shown in Table 26–8.

By definition, tumors that form PAS-positive mucins (see Fig. 26–9R through T) are classified as carcinoma[132,137,142]; mesothelioma produces hyaluronic acid which stains with alcian blue or colloidal iron and can be removed by predigestion with hyaluronidase (see Fig. 26–9F). A number of cautions must be applied to the interpretation of these reactions. The PAS-positive material must be droplets of mucin and not merely granular debris in the cytoplasm, since the latter probably are lysosomes. Similarly, the colloidal iron must stain droplets in the cytoplasm and not merely stroma; the stroma of many types of tumor contains hyaluronic acid. According to Kannerstein and colleagues,[142] about half of the carcinomas they examined contained colloidal iron–positive droplets; however, this material could not be removed by pretreatment with hyaluronidase. The use of mucicarmine as a differential stain is not recommended since mesotheliomas show a variable reaction depending on the exact technique used.[142,143] Histochemical techniques are primarily of use in separating the epithelial mesotheliomas from carcinoma; sarcomatous tumors rarely if ever demonstrate cytoplasmic droplets, although most have strong stromal staining.

A drawback to the use of the histochemical techniques just described is the water-lability of hyaluronic acid. About 50 percent of otherwise acceptable cases of mesothelioma show no staining reaction at all,[132,137,142] presumably because of leaching of hyaluronic acid. Poorly differentiated tumors also appear to secrete hyaluronic acid less frequently than well-differentiated tumors.

Ultrastructure

Despite claims to the contrary,[96,144-146] the ultrastructural features of malignant mesothelioma are basically nonspecific, reflecting differentiation toward a secretory type epithelial cell or a fibroblastic mesenchymal cell, and various intermediate or poorly differentiated variants.[146] The well-differentiated epithelial mesotheliomas are composed in part of nests or aggregates of cells surrounded by a basement membrane. The "apical" poles of such cells demonstrate microvilli which may be quite numerous and long.[145] Intercellular and intracellular lumina are commonly formed (see Fig. 26–9U, V). The cells are linked by numerous well-formed desmosomes; occasional cells have large numbers of tonofilament bundles in the cytoplasm. The rough endoplasmic reticulum and Golgi apparatus are prominent, and glycogen particles as well as lipid are usually present.[96,144,145] Even in the best differentiated tumors, cells that show only some of these features, or that show no differentiating features, are common.[146]

At the other end of the spectrum are the tumors composed of spindled cells which, for all intents and purposes, are ultrastructurally indistinguishable from fibroblasts. These elongated cells are sometimes linked by small junctions of the zonula adherens type, and may interdigitate when closely packed.[147] Some tumors produce collagen. The cell cytoplasm contains short strands of anastomosing rough endoplasmic reticulum of the type seen in a variety of mesenchymal tumors. The giant cells sometimes found in these tumors are similar in structure to those found in malignant fibrous histiocytoma, giant cell tumors of bone, and other related neoplasms (Churg, unpublished data).

Suzuki and co-workers[146] have examined the ultrastructure of several tumors of mixed light microscopic pattern, and have shown that both epithelial and mesenchymal cells are present at the electron microscope level. Of greater interest was their finding of mesenchymal-type cells in four of eight tumors where the light microscopic histology was that of a purely epithelial tumor. Bolen and Thorning[148] have recently reported a spindled mesothelioma in which the cells had many ultrastructural features of mesenchymal cells but also formed intracellular lumina. These findings provide strong support for the histologic and tissue culture observations that tumors derived from mesothelium may produce cells of two different appearances.

Although descriptions of the ultrastructure of mesothelioma have been reasonably consistent, attempts to find features of diagnostic significance appear, to me, to have ignored the fact that the fine structure of epithelial cells in a malignant mesothelioma is not really different from the structure of the cells of many secretory adenocarcinomas, for example, those of breast, colon, or lung; and that the structure of the spindled cells could equally well be found in a fibrosarcoma or malignant fibrous histiocytoma. Attempts to use the electron microscope for diagnosis of mesothelioma have produced rather vague statements to the effect that the overall collection of features is somehow specific[96,144,146,149] or that certain features, such as number of microvilli[150] or length of microvilli,[145] are specific. Similarly, claims that the presence of fibroblastic cells are diagnostic of mesothelioma[144] must be questioned, since carcinomas with spindled components are present in a number of organs, especially lung, and also since non-neoplastic fibroblasts are commonly found at the ultrastructural level in a variety of tumors. Warhol and co-workers[151] have attempted to overcome this problem by quantitative estimation of microvillous length and intermediate filament content. They found that mesotheliomas had a mean microvillous length/diameter ratio of about 12 compared to about 5 for adenocarcinomas; and that the intermediate (tonofilament) content of mesotheliomas was much higher than was true of carcinomas. They also suggested that the presence of basal rootlets under microvilli was against a diagnosis of mesothelioma. However, in my experience these criteria do not always work (see Fig. 29–9V and Fig. 19–11F) and are usually only obvious in tumors which are so well differentiated that the diagnosis is not in doubt. Overall, the present author believes that ultrastructural examination is far inferior to the faster and less expensive histochemical stains or to immunohistochemical stains.

Immunohistochemical Techniques

Wang and co-workers[152] were the first to suggest that, using immunohistochemical techniques, mesotheliomas do not stain for carcinoembryonic antigen (CEA) while adenocarcinomas do. Other authors have examined this staining and generally confirmed these findings (Table 26–9); however, the distinction is not entirely clear-cut, because according to the experience of Holden and Churg[153] and that of Corson and Pinkus,[154] some mesotheliomas will stain weakly for CEA. Staining for keratin has also been advanced as a means of separating these tumors. Corson and Pinkus[154] and Said and co-workers[155] claim that mesotheliomas are strongly positive for keratin while adenocarcinomas stain weakly or not at all (see Table 26–9). However, both these studies were performed with the same home-grown antiserum; when Holden and Churg[153] examined keratin staining using commercial antisera, most cases of both mesothelioma and adenocarcinoma stained poorly and there was no usable distinction between the two tumors.

Table 26–9. Results of Immunohistochemical Staining for CEA and Keratin

Series	CEA		Keratin	
	Adenoca	Mesothelioma	Adenoca	Mesothelioma
Corson and Pinkus[154]	20/20	9/20	11/20	9/20
Said et al.[155]	6/6	0/8	0/6	8/8
Holden and Churg[153]	18/18	8/22	13/18	10/22
Whitaker et al.[158]	22/26	0/43		
Kwee et al.[159]	16/25	0/37		

Abbreviations: CEA, carcinoembryonic antigen.

The scientific rationale for this approach is peculiar, since both epithelial and mesothelial cells contain keratins, and furthermore keratin is poorly preserved by formalin fixation. It is likely that the results obtained by Corson and Pinkus[154] and Said and colleagues[155] reflect use of an antisera that happens to cross-react strongly with a mesothelial keratin.[156] A reasonably safe conclusion at this point is that, using formalin-fixed, paraffin-embedded material and commercial antisera, strong diffuse staining for CEA favors a carcinoma and a total lack of staining for CEA is good evidence against a carcinoma, but that staining for keratin is not useful.

Singh and associates[157] have produced an antiserum that stains mesothelial cells in culture; this system has apparently not been tried on tissue.

Analysis of Glycosaminoglycans

Waxler and co-workers[160] have utilized electrophoresis of glycosaminoglycans extracted from mesotheliomas and carcinomas and claimed that mesotheliomas will yield only or almost entirely hyaluronic acid in this system, while carcinomas show a variety of glycosaminoglycans. The author's experience does not bear this out: qualitatively both mesotheliomas and carcinomas yield all types of glycosaminoglycans, although quantitatively the mesotheliomas contain statistically greater amounts of hyaluronic acid than adenocarcinomas.[161] These techniques essentially represent more sensitive variants of the standard immunohistochemical staining reactions.

Patterns of Spread

Mesotheliomas spread by contiguous growth, or by hematogenous and lymphatic metastases; clinically death usually results from local disease. Mesothelioma commonly spreads into adjoining viscera and body walls as described in Gross Appearances, above. At one time it was believed that the presence of metastases mitigated against the diagnosis of mesothelioma. However, more recent studies[113,138,162,163] have shown that metastases are present in about half the cases of both pleural and peritoneal mesothelioma. Lymph nodes within the thoracic or abdominal cavities are most commonly involved; pleural tumors may also metastasize to supraclavicular or cervical nodes, and abdominal tumors to inguinal nodes. Favored sites of visceral metastases include lungs, liver, pleura, bone, adrenal, and heart. Law and co-workers[164] claim that the epithelial tumors tend to spread locally, while sarcomatous tumors more commonly have distant metastases; however, Elmes and Simpson[115] suggest that the reverse is true.

Differential Diagnosis

A number of different tumors metastatic to pleura or peritoneum commonly mimic mesothelioma.[137] The most common differential problem is with adenocarcinomas, particularly of lung; as mentioned and illustrated in Chapter 19, adenocarcinomas may even spread over the surface of the lung in a fashion identical to mesothelioma. Gastrointestinal cancers, particularly stomach cancers, may also produce diagnostic problems. However, all of these are usually resolved by staining with PAS, and it is probably unwise to render a diagnosis of mesothelioma at any time without at least a PAS stain. In the peritoneal cavity, papillary adenocarcinomas of the ovary may be difficult to separate from mesothelioma; mucin stains can again be helpful. Kannerstein and colleagues[139] suggest that ovarian carcinomas have smaller cells than mesothelioma, and that the nuclei are more hyperchromatic. Foyle and colleagues[165] discuss separation of mesothelioma and papillary ovarian carcinomas. Psammoma bodies in large numbers favor a carcinoma. Thymoma, renal cell carcinoma, and metastatic thyroid carcinoma may also occasionally resemble mesothelioma.[137] In my opinion, the histologic distinction between sarcomatous mesothelioma and some metastatic fibrosarcomas or malignant fibrous histiocytomas is not feasible, and reference must be made to the clinical history. Autopsy is often valuable in ruling out an occult primary tumor.

Diagnostic Procedures

The use of the needle biopsy to diagnose mesothelioma should be avoided because of the necessity for observing a sufficiently large area to find a characteristic pattern. Histochemical and immunohistochemical stains similarly may only be focally positive and useful areas may not be present in a needle biopsy.

Problem cases in North America can be referred to the Canadian or U.S. Mesothelioma Reference Panels.

Therapy and Prognosis

The course of most patients with malignant mesothelioma is one of rapid progression: the mean survival of 267 patients from eight different series summarized by Legha and Muggia[111] was 12.5 months from the onset of symptoms; 75 percent of the patients were dead within a year of diagnosis. Certain patients fare somewhat better. Antman[166] has summarized five series of 331 patients who underwent surgical resection; survivals were 47 percent at 1 year, 28 percent at 2 years, and 8 percent at 5 years. Whether these figures reflect extent of spread at time of diagnosis or some other factor relating to tumor aggressiveness is unclear, but there is some evidence that histologic pattern can be correlated with prognosis. Elmes and Simpson[115] found that, in a series of 237 patients, those whose tumors showed a purely epithelial pattern had a mean survival of 18 months, those with a mixed pattern a survival of 11 months, and those with purely sarcomatous components a survival of 8 months. About one-third of the epithelial and mixed tumors demonstrated extensive spread at autopsy, compared to about half the sarcomatous tumors. The more favorable prognosis of epithelial tumors has also been noted by other investigators.[163,164,167] Sarcomatous tumors of the desmoplastic type appear to have particularly poor survival.[140] Death usually results from respiratory failure, cardiac embarrassment, or

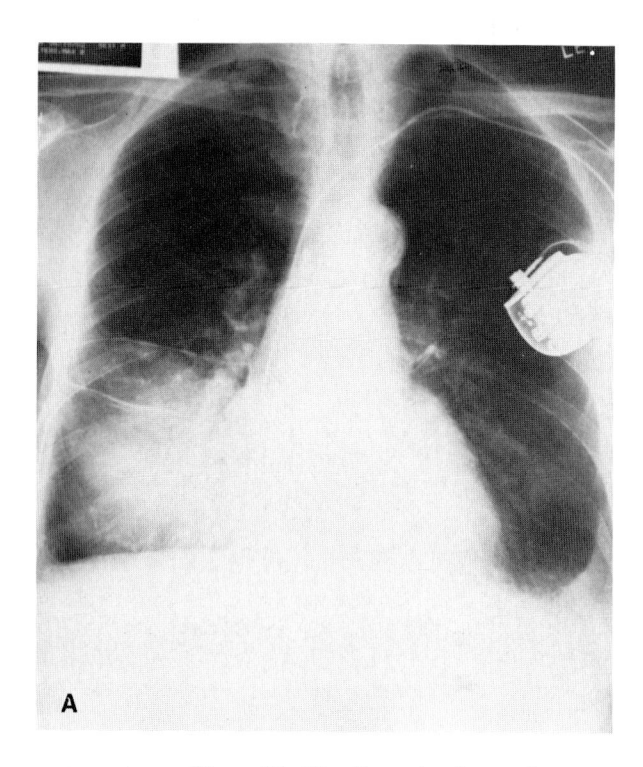

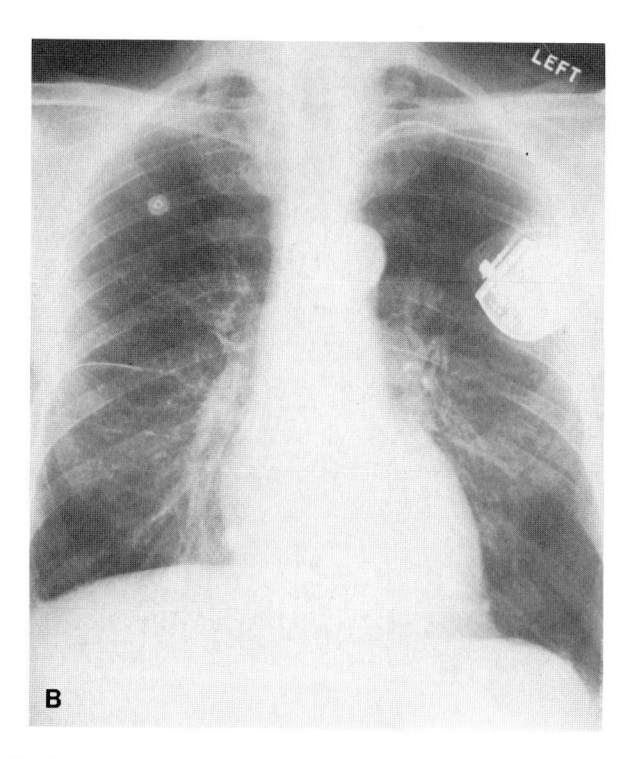

Figure 26–10. Example of a pseudotumour caused by fluid accumulation in a fissure in a patient with congestive failure. In (A) a mass-like lesion appears to be present; in (B) several days later the mass has disappeared after diuresis.

bowel obstruction, and is only rarely related to metastatic disease.[168]

Radiation and chemotherapy have been applied to mesothelioma with modest success. Adriamycin-containing regimes seem to be most effective, with response rates up to 40 percent. In the series of Antman and co-workers,[168] the medial survival was 15 months for those treated with chemotherapy and 8.5 months for those not treated with chemotherapy. Similar results were reported by Yap and co-workers.[169] Occasional patients have prolonged survivals, sometimes exceeding 5 years, with or without chemotherapy.[168,170,171]

Miscellaneous Rare Tumors and Pseudotumors

So-called "phantom tumors" are produced by collections of fluid in the interlobar fissures; phantom tumors are generally found in patients with heart failure and disappear when the patient is dehydrated[2] (Fig. 26–10). Pleural plaques and granulomas have been reported as examples of radiographic pseudotumors[172]; occasionally plaques may even simulate metastatic malignancies.[173]

Lipomas may occur in the chest wall, intrathoracically, or in the pulmonary parenchyma. Krause and Ross[174] reviewed 80 cases; of these, two-thirds protruded into the pleural space, and 20 percent were located in the mediastinum. In some instances, the tumors were dumbbell-shaped and extended from subcutaneous to intrapleural location through the interspaces between the ribs. Most likely, all of these tumors arise from the intercostal fat, or possibly from the immediately subpleural fat; they are probably not actually tumors derived from mesothelial cells.

Squamous cell carcinomas occasionally are found as primary pleural neoplasms, almost invariably in association with chronic draining sinuses or long-standing empyemas.[175] Most of the sarcomas arising in the pleura appear to have been reported as malignant variants of localized mesothelioma ("giant sarcoma of pleura"), but rare cases of large localized tumors recognized as specific types of sarcoma have been reported.[176] Smith and Opipari[177] claim to have identified the first primary melanoma of the pleura; given the known propensity of primary melanomas to regress, and their tendency to widespread metastases, this report must be interpreted with caution.

References

1. Langston HT, Barker WL, Graham AA: Pleural tuberculosis. J Thorac Cardiovasc Surg 54:511, 1967.

2. Johnston RF, Dovnarsky JH: Pleural diseases. In Fishman AP (ed): *Pulmonary Diseases and Disorders*. New York: McGraw-Hill, 1980, p 1357.

3. Tinney WS, Olson AM: The significance of fluid in the pleural space. J Thorac Surg 14:248, 1945.

4. Frist B, Kahan AV, Koss LG: Comparison of the diagnostic

values of biopsies of the pleura and cytologic evaluation of pleural fluids. Am J Clin Pathol 72:48, 1979.

5. Salyer WR, Eggleston JC, Erozan US: Efficacy of pleural needle biopsy and pleural fluid cytopathology in the diagnosis of malignant neoplasm involving the pleura. Chest 67:536, 1975.

6. Scerbo J, Keltz H, Stone DJ: A prospective study of closed pleural biopsies. JAMA 218:377, 1971.

7. Van Hoff DD, LiVolsi V: Diagnostic reliability of needle biopsy of the parietal pleura. A review of 272 biopsies. Am J Clin Pathol 64:200, 1975.

8. Green RA: Pleural inflammation and pleural effusion. In Baum GL (ed): *Textbook of Pulmonary Disease.* Boston: Little, Brown, 1965, p 668.

9. Leff A, Hopewell PC, Costello J: Pleural effusion from malignancy. Ann Intern Med 88:532, 1978.

10. Konikov N, Bleisch V, Piskie V: Prognostic significance of cytologic diagnoses of efffusions. Acta Cytol 10:335, 1966.

11. Weissberg D, Kaufman M, Zurkowski Z: Pleuroscopy in patients with pleural effusion and pleural masses. Ann Thoracic Surg 29:205, 1980.

12. Fine NL, Smith LR, Sheedy PF: Frequency of pleural effusions in mycoplasma and viral pneumonias. N Engl J Med 283:790, 1970.

13. Drutz D, Catanzara A: Coccidioidomyocosis. Am Rev Respir Dis 117:559, 727, 1978.

14. Salyer WR, Salyer DC: Pleural involvement in cryptococcosis. Chest 66:139, 1974.

15. Young EJ, Hirsch DD, Fainstein V, Williams TW: Pleural effusions due to Cryptococcus neoformans: A review of the literature and report of two cases with cryptococcal antigen determinations. Am Rev Respir Dis 121:743, 1980.

16. Silverman FN, Schwarz J, Lahey ME, Carson RP: Histoplasmosis. Am J Med 19:410, 1955.

17. Krakowa P, Rowinska E, Halweg H: Infection of the pleura by *Aspergillus fumigatus.* Thorax 25:245, 1970.

18. Varkey B, Lohaus G, Rose HD, Sohnle PG: Blastomycosis: Clinical and immunologic aspects. Chest 77:789, 1980.

19. Roper WH, Waring JJ: Primary serofibrinous effusion in military personnel. Am Rev Tuber 71:616, 1955.

20. Sharma OP: Sarcoidosis. Unusual pulmonary manifestations. Postgrad Med 61:67, 1977.

21. Tserkezoglou A, Metakidis S, Papastamatiou-Tsimara H, Zoitopoulos M: Solitary rheumatoid nodule of the pleura and rheumatoid pleural effusion. Thorax 33:769, 1978.

22. Halla JT, Schronenloher RE, Volkanis JE: Immune complexes and other laboratory features of pleural effusions. A comparison of rheumatoid arthritis, systemic lupus erythematosus, and other diseases. Ann Intern Med 92:748, 1980.

23. Campbell GD, Webb WR: Eosinophilic pleural effusion. Am Rev Respir Dis 90:194, 1964.

24. Askin FB, McCann BG, Kuhn C: Reactive eosinophilic pleuritis. Arch Pathol Lab Med 101:187, 1977.

25. Finland M, Jones WF, Barnes MW: Occurrence of serious bacterial infections since introduction of antibacterial agents. JAMA 170:2188, 1959.

26. Emerson JD, Boruchow IB, Daicoff GR, et al.: Empyema. J Thorac Cardiovasc Surg 62:697, 1971.

27. Vianna NJ: Nontuberculous bacterial empyema in patients with and without underlying diseases. JAMA 215:69, 1971.

28. LeRoux BT: Empyema thoracis. Br J Surg 52:89, 1965.

29. Sanford JP: Pneumonias caused by gram-positive bacteria. In Fishman AP (ed): *Pulmonary Diseases and Disorders.* New York: McGraw-Hill, 1980, p 1130.

30. Bloom R, Yeager H, Garagusi VF: Pleuropulmonary complications of thoracic vertebral osteomyelitis. Thorax 35:156, 1980.

31. Green SL: Anaerobic pleuro-pulmonary infections. Postgrad Med 65:62, 1979.

32. Rabin CB, Janowitz HD: Actinomyces in putrid empyema. J Thorac Surg 19:355, 1950.

33. Ravitch MM, Fein R: The changing picture of pneumonia and empyema in infants and children. JAMA 175:1039, 1961.

34. Stiles QR, Lindesmith GG, Tucker BL, et al.: Pleural empyema in children. Ann Thorac Surg 10:37, 1970.

35. Okano T, Walkup HE: Chronic purulent tuberculous empyema and pulmonary tuberculosis treated by decortications and resections. J Thorac Cardiovasc Surg 43:752, 1962.

36. Samson PC: Empyema thoracis. Essentials of present day management. Ann Thorac Surg 11:210, 1971.

37. Porter JM, Ball AP, Silver D: Mesothelial fibrinolysis. J Thorac Cardiovasc Surg 62:725, 1971.

38. Tuttle WM, Langston HT, Crowley RT: The treatment of organizing hemothorax by pulmonary decortication. J Thorac Surg 16:117, 1947.

39. Corrin B, Liebow AA, Friedman PJ: Pulmonary lymphangiomyomatosis. Am J Pathol 79:348, 1973.

40. Siebens AA, Storey CF, Newman MM, et al.: The physiologic effects of fibrothorax and the functional results of surgical treatment. J Thorac Surg 32:53, 1956.

41. Glenn WWL, Liebow AA, Lindskog GF: *Thoracic and Cardiovascular Surgery with Related Pathology,* 3rd ed. New York: Appleton-Century-Crofts, 1975.

42. Wilson DA: Extrapleural pneumolysis with lucite plombage. J Thorac Surg 17:111, 1948.

43. Hall DR, Morrison JB, Edwards FR: Pleural fibrosis after practolol therapy. Thorax 33:822, 1978.

44. Anderson HA, Selikoff IJ: Pleural reactions to environmental agents. Fed Proc 37:2496, 1978.

45. Baris YI, Artvinli M, Sahin AA: Environmental mesothelioma in Turkey. Ann NY Acad Sci 330:423, 1979.

46. Burilkov T, Michailova L: Asbestos content of the soil and endemic pleural asbestosis. Environ Res 3:443, 1970.

47. Wright PH, Hanson A, Kreel A, Capel LH: Respiratory function after asbestos pleurisy. Thorax 35:31, 1980.

48. Gaensler EA: Open and closed lung biopsy. In Sachner MA (ed): *Diagnostic Techniques in Pulmonary Disease, Part II.* New York: Marcel Dekker 1980, pp. 579–683.

49. Killen DA, Gobbel WG: *Spontaneous Pneumothorax.* Boston: Little, Brown, 1968.

50. Mark JBD, Lindskog GE: Spontaneous pneumothorax with special emphasis on treatment. Conn Med 25:479, 1961.

51. Biach A: Zur Aetiologie des Pneumothorax. Wien Med Wochenschr 30:131, 1980.

52. Kjaerjaard H: Spontaneous pneumothorax in the apparently healthy. Acta Med Scand 43(suppl):1, 1932.

53. Myerson RM: Spontaneous pneumothorax. A clinical study of 100 consecutive cases. N Engl J Med 238:461, 1948.

54. Peters RM, Peters BA, Benirschke SK, Friedman PJ: Chest dimensions in young adults with spontaneous pneumothorax. Ann Thorac Surg 25:193, 1978.

55. Saha SP, Arrants JE, Kosa A, Lee WH: Management of spontaneous pneumothorax. Ann Thorac Surg 19:561, 1975.

56. Wilder RJ, Beacham EG, Ravitch MM: Spontaneous

pneumothorax complicating cavitary tuberculosis. J Thorac Cardiovasc Surg 43:561, 1962.

57. Carr DT, Silver AW, Ellis FE: Management of spontaneous pneumothorax: With special reference to prognosis after various kinds of therapy. Mayo Clin Proc 38:103, 1963.

58. Green RA: Pneumothorax. In Baum GL (ed): *Textbook of Pulmonary Diseases.* Boston: Little, Brown, 1965, p 688.

59. Carrington CB, Cugell DW, Gaensler EA, et al.: Lymphangioleiomyomatosis. Am Rev Respir Dis 116:977, 1977.

60. Fein A, Gupta R, Goodman P: Spontaneous pneumothorax as a presenting pulmonary manifestation of early sarcoidosis. Chest 77:455, 1980.

61. Fishberg M: *Pulmonary Tuberculosis*, 4th ed. Philadelphia: Lea & Febiger, 1932, p 108.

62. Dines D, Cortese D, Brenham M, et al.: Malignant pulmonary neoplasms predisposing to spontaneous pneumothorax. Mayo Clin Proc 48:541, 1973.

63. Schulman P, Cheng E, Cvitkovic E, Golbey R: Spontaneous pneumothorax as a result of intensive cytotoxic chemotherapy. Chest 75:194, 1979.

64. Yeung K-Y, Bonnet JD: Bronchogenic carcinoma presenting as spontaneous pneumothorax. Cancer 39:2286, 1977.

65. Madansky DL, Lawson EE, Chernick V, Taeusch HW: Pneumothorax and other forms of pulmonary air leak in newborns. Am Rev Respir Dis 120:729, 1979.

66. Shearin RPN, Hepper NGG, Payne WS: Recurrent spontaneous pneumothorax concurrent with menses. Mayo Clin Proc 49:98, 1974.

67. George RB, Herbert SJ, Shames JM, et al.: Pneumothorax complicating pulmonary emphysema. JAMA 234:389, 1975.

68. Zwillich CW, Pierson DJ, Creagh CE, et al.: Complications of assisted ventilation. A prospective study of 354 consecutive episodes. Am J Med 57:161, 1974.

69. Brody AR, Kanich RE, Graham WG, Craighead JE: Cyst wall formation in eosinophilic granuloma. Chest 66:576, 1974.

70. Peiken AS, Lamberta F, Seriff NS: Bilateral recurrent pneumothoraces: A rare complication of miliary tuberculosis. Am Rev Respir Dis 110:512, 1974.

71. Hall FM, Salzman EW, Ellis BI, Kurland GS: Pneumothorax complicating aseptic cavitating pulmonary infarction. Chest 72:232, 1977.

72. Kovarik JL, Toll GD: Thoracic endometriosis with recurrent spontaneous pneumothorax. JAMA 196:595, 1966.

73. Forgacs P: Stature in simple pneumothorax. Guys Hosp Rep 118:199, 1969.

74. Lichter I, Gwynne JF: Spontaneous pneumothorax in young subjects. Thorax 26:409, 1971.

75. Ohata M, Suzuki H: Pathogenesis of spontaneous pneumothorax with special reference to the ultrastructure of emphysematous bullae. Chest 77:771, 1980.

76. Baronofsky KD, Warden HG, Kaufman JL, et al.: Bilateral therapy for unilateral spontaneous pneumothorax. J Thorac Surg 34:310, 1957.

77. Aust JB: Spontaneous pneumothorax. Postgrad Med 29:368, 1961.

78. Hofer W: Zum problem des sog. idiopathischen Spontanpneumothorax. Virchows Arch [A] 347:95, 1969.

79. Withers JN, Fishback PV, Kiehl PV, Hannon JL: Spontaneous pneumothorax: Suggested etiology and comparison of treatment method. Am J Surg 108:772, 1964.

80. Vater DL, Matthews FL, West JB: Effect of shape and size of lung and chest wall on stresses in the lung. J Appl Physiol 39:9, 1975.

81. Anonymous: Spontaneous pneumothorax and apical lung disease. Br Med J 2:573, 1971.

82. Sharpe IK, Ahmad A, Braun W: Familial spontaneous pneumothorax and HLA antigens. Chest 78:264, 1980.

83. Anonymous: Spontaneous pneumothorax. Br Med J 1:526, 1975.

84. Deaton WR, Johnston FR: Spontaneous hemopneumothorax. J Thorac Cardiovasc Surg 43:413, 1962.

85. Petty BG, Smith CR: The syndrome of inappropriate section of antidiuretic hormone associated with anaerobic thoracic empyema. Am Rev Respir Dis 115:685, 1977.

86. Perks, WH, Crow JC, Green M: Mesothelioma associated with the syndrome of inappropriate secretion of antidiuretic hormone. Am Rev Respir Dis 117:789, 1978.

87. Petty BG: Pleural masses and the syndrome of inappropriate secretion of antidiuretic hormone. Am Rev Respir Dis 118:627, 1978.

88. Maier HC, Barr D: Intrathoracic tumors associated with hypoglycemia. J Thorac Cardiovasc Surg 44:321, 1962.

89. Miller DR, Bolinger RE, Janigan D, et al.: Hypoglycemia due to nonpancreatic mesodermal tumors. Ann Surg 150:684, 1959.

90. Klemperer P, Rabin CB: Primary neoplasms of the pleura. Arch Pathol 11:385, 1931.

91. Willis RA: *Pathology of Tumors*, 4th ed. London: Butterworths, 1967.

92. Spencer H: *Pathology of the Lung*, 3rd ed. London: Pergamon Press, 1977.

93. Selikoff IJ, Lee DKH: *Asbestos and Disease*. New York: Academic Press, 1978, p 189.

94. Stout AP, Murray MR: Localized pleural mesothelioma. Arch Pathol 34:951, 1942.

95. Kawai T, Mikata A, Torikata C, et al.: Solitary (localized) pleural mesothelioma. Am J Surg Path 2:365, 1978.

96. Wang NS: Electron microscopy in the diagnosis of pleural mesotheliomas. Cancer 31:1046, 1973.

97. Scharifker D, Kaneko M: Localized fibrous "mesothelioma" of pleura (submesothelial fibroma). Cancer 43:627, 1979.

98. Clagett OT, McDonald JR, Schmitt KW: Localized fibrous mesothelioma of the pleura. J Thorac Surg 24:213, 1952.

99. Dalton WT, Zolliker AS, McCaughey WTE, et al.: Localized primary tumors of the pleura. An analysis of 40 cases. Cancer 44:1465, 1979.

100. Foster EA, Ackerman LV: Localized mesothelioma of the pleura. Am J Clin Pathol 34:349, 1969.

101. Okike N, Bernatz PE, Woolner LB: Localized mesothelioma of the pleura—benign and malignant variants. J Thorac Cardiovasc Surg 75:363, 1978.

102. Nelson R, Burman SO, Kiani R, et al.: Hypoglycemia associated with benign pleural mesothelioma. J Thorac Cardiovasc Surg 69:306, 1975.

103. Yesner R, Hurwitz A: Localized pleural mesothelioma of epithelial type. J Thorac Surg 26:325, 1953.

104. Motomiya M, Endo M, Arai H, et al.: Biochemical characterization of hyaluronic acid from a case of benign, localized, pleural mesothelioma. Am Rev Respir Dis 111:775, 1975.

105. Osamura RY: Ultrastructure of localized fibrous mesothelioma of the pleura. Cancer 39:139, 1977.

106. Hernandez FJ, Fernandez BB: Localized fibrous tumors of pleura: A light and electron microscopic study. Cancer 34:1667, 1974.

107. Kay S, Silverberg SG: Ultrastructural studies of a malignant fibrous mesothelioma of the pleura. Arch Pathol 92:449, 1971.

108. Utley JR, Parker JC, Hahn RS, et al.: Recurrent benign fibrous mesothelioma of the pleura. J Thorac Cardiovasc Surg 65:830, 1973.

109. Stout AP, Himade GM: Solitary (localized) mesothelioma of the pleura. Ann Surg 133:50, 1951.

110. Kerr WF, Nohl HC: Recurrence of "benign" intrathoracic fibromas. Thorax 16:180, 1961.

111. Legha SS, Muggia FM: Pleural mesothelioma: Clinical features and therapeutic implications. Ann Intern Med 87:613, 1977.

112. McDonald AC, McDonald JC: Malignant mesothelioma in North America. Cancer 46:1650, 1980.

113. Kannerstein M, Churg J, McCaughey WTE: Asbestos and mesothelioma: A review. Pathol Annu 1978, pp. 81–129.

114. Grundy GW, Miller RW: Malignant mesothelioma in childhood. Cancer 30:1216, 1972.

115. Elmes PC, Simpson MJC: The clinical aspects of mesothelioma. Q J Med 45:427, 1976.

116. Ellis K, Wolff M: Mesotheliomas and secondary tumors of the pleura. Semin Roentgenol 12:303, 1977.

117. Rasmussen KN, Faber V: Hyaluronic acid in 247 pleural fluids. Scand J Respir Dis 48:366, 1967.

118. Becklake MR: Asbestos-related diseases of the lung and other organs: Their epidemiology and implications for clinical practice. Am Rev Respir Dis 114:187, 1976.

119. Wagner JC, Sleggs CA, Marchand P: Diffuse pleural mesothelioma and asbestos exposure in the Northern Western Cape Province. Br J Indust Med 17:260, 1960.

120. Vianna NJ, Polan AK: Non-occupational exposure to asbestos and malignant mesothelioma in females. Lancet 1978.

121. Risberg B, Nickels J, Wagernark J: Familial clustering of malignant mesothelioma. Cancer 45:2422, 1980.

122. Anderson HA, Lilis R, Daum SM, et al.: Household-contact asbestos neoplastic risk. Ann NY Acad Sci 271:310, 1976.

123. Pott F, Huth F, Friedrichs KH: Tumorigenic effect of fibrous dusts in experimental animals. Environ Health Perspect 9:313, 1974.

124. Wagner JC, Berry G, Timbrell: Mesotheliomatas in rats after innoculation with asbestos and other materials. Br J Cancer 28:173, 1973.

125. McDonald AD, McDonald JC: Mesothelioma after crocidolite exposure during gas mask manufacture. Environ Res 17:340, 1978.

126. Newhouse ML: The geographical pathology of mesothelial tumors. J Occup Med 19:480, 1977.

127. Churg A, Warnock M, Bensch KG: Mesothelioma arising after direct application of asbestos to a mesothelial surface. Am Rev Respir Dis 118:419, 1978.

128. Stanton MF, Layard M, Tegeris A, et al.: Carcinogenicity of fibrous glass: Pleural response in the rate in relation to fiber dimension. Natl Cancer Inst J 58:587, 1977.

129. Artvin M, Baris YI: Malignant mesotheliomas in a small village in the Anatolian region of Turkey: An epidemiologic study. J Natl Cancer Inst 63:17, 1979.

130. Hirsch A, Brochard P, DeCremoux H, et al.: Features of asbestos-exposed and unexposed mesothelioma. Am J Indust Med 3:413, 1982.

131. Maurer R, Egloff B: Malignant peritoneal mesothelioma after cholangiography with thorotrast. Cancer 36:1381, 1975.

132. Churg J, Selikoff IJ: Geographic pathology of pleural mesothelioma. In Liebow AA (ed): *The Lung*. Baltimore: Williams & Wilkins, 1968, p 284.

133. Hourihane DO: A biopsy series of mesotheliomata, and attempts to identify asbestos within some of the tumors. Ann NY Acad Sci 132:647, 1965.

134. Hourihane DO: The pathology of mesotheliomata and an analysis of their association with asbestos exposure. Thorax 19:268, 1964.

135. McCaughey WTE: Criteria for diagnosis of diffuse mesothelial tumors. Ann NY Acad Sci 132:603, 1965.

136. Kannerstein M, Churg J: Desmoplastic diffuse malignant mesothelioma. Prog Surg Pathol 1:19, 1980.

137. Kannerstein M, McCaughey WTE, Churg J, Selikoff IJ: A critique of the criteria for the diagnosis of diffuse malignancy mesothelioma. Mt Sinai J Med 44:485, 1977.

138. Kannerstein M, Churg J: Peritoneal mesothelioma. Hum Pathol 8:83, 1977.

139. Kannerstein M, Churg J, McCaughey WTE, Hill DP: Papillary tumors of the peritoneum in women: Mesothelioma or papillary carcinoma. Am J Obstet Gynecol 127:806, 1977.

140. Cantin R, Al-Jabi M, McCaughey WTE: Desmoplastic diffuse mesothelioma. Am J Surg Pathol 6:215, 1982.

141. Goldstein B: Two malignant pleural mesotheliomas with unusual histological features. Thorax 34:375, 1979.

142. Kannerstein M, Churg J, Magner D: Histochemical studies in the diagnosis of mesothelioma. In J C, Timbrell V, Wagner JC (eds): *Biological Effects of Asbestos*. Lyon: International Agency for Research on Cancer Scientific Publications, No. 8, 1973, p 62.

143. Whitwell P, Rawcliffe RM: Diffuse malignant pleural mesothelioma and asbestos exposure. Thorax 26:6, 1971.

144. Davis JMG: Ultrastructure of human mesotheliomas. J Natl Cancer Inst 52:1715, 1974.

145. MacKay B, Osbourne BM, Wilson RA: Ultrastructure of lung neoplasms. In Straus MJ (ed): *Lung Cancer. Clinical Diagnosis and Treatment*. New York: Grune & Stratton, 1977, p 71.

146. Suzuki Y, Churg J, Kannerstein M: Ultrastructure of human malignant diffuse mesothelioma. Am J Pathol 85:241, 1976.

147. Kay S, Silberberg SG: Ultrastructural studies of a malignant fibrous mesothelioma of the pleura. Arch Pathol 92:449, 1971.

148. Bolen JW, Thorning D: Mesotheliomas. A light and electron microscopical study concerning histogenetic relationships between the epithelial and the mesenchymal variants. Am J Surg Pathol 4:451, 1980.

149. Stoebner P, Bernaudin J-F, Adnet J-J, Basset F: Problemes du diagnostic ultra-structural des cancers pleuraux. A propos de 125 cas. Rev Fr Mal Respir 7:265, 1979.

150. Dionne GP, Wang N-S: A scanning electron microscopic study of diffuse mesothelioma and some lung carcinomas. Cancer 40:707, 1977.

151. Warhol MJ, Hickey WF, Corson JM: Malignant mesothelioma: Ultrastructural distinction from adenocarcinoma. Am J Surg Pathol 6:307, 1982.

152. Wang N-S, Huang S-N, Gold P: Absence of carcinoembryonic antigen-like material in mesothelioma. Cancer 44:937, 1979.

153. Holden JK, Churg A: Immunohistochemical staining for keratin and CEA in the diagnosis of mesothelioma. Am J Surg Pathol 8:277, 1984.

154. Corson JM, Pinkus JS: Mesothelioma: Profile of keratin proteins and carcinoembryonic antigen. Am J Pathol 108:80, 1982.

155. Said JW, Nash G, Tepper G, Banks-Schlegel S. Keratin proteins and carcinoembryonic antigen in lung carcinoma. Hum Pathol 14:70, 1983.

156. Wu YJ, Parker LM, Binder NE, et al.: The mesothelial keratins: A new family of cytoskeletal proteins identified in

cultured mesothelial cells and nonkeratinizing epithelia. Cell 31:693, 1983.

157. Singh G, Whiteside TL, Dekker A: Immunodiagnosis of mesothelioma. Use of antimesothelial cell serum in an indirect immunofluorescence assay. Cancer 43:2288, 1979.

158. Whitaker D, Sterrett GF, Shilkin KB: Detection of tissue CEA-like substance as an aid in the differential diagnosis of malignant mesothelioma. Pathology 14:255, 1982.

159. Kwee WS, Vedhuizen RW, Godling RP, et al.: Histologic distinction between malignant mesothelioma, benign pleural lesion, and carcinoma metastases. Virchows Arch [A] 397:287, 1982.

160. Waxler B, Eisenstein R, Battifora H: Electrophoresis of tissue glycosaminoglycans as an aid in the diagnosis of mesotheliomas. Cancer 44:221, 1979.

161. Chiu B, Churg A, Tengblad A, et al.: Analysis of glycosaminoglycans in the diagnosis of malignant mesothelioma. Cancer 54:2195, 1984.

162. Roberts GH: Distant visceral mestastases in pleural mesothelioma. Br J Dis Chest 70:246, 1976.

163. Wanebo JH, Martini N, Melamed MR, et al.: Pleural mesothelioma. Cancer 38:2481, 1976.

164. Law MR, Hodson ME, Heard BE: Malignant mesothelioma of the pleura: Relation between the histological type and clinical behaviour. Thorax 37:810, 1982.

165. Foyle A, Al-Jabi M, McCaughey WTE: Papillary peritoneal tumors in women. Am J Surg Pathol 5:241, 1981.

166. Antman KH: Malignant mesothelioma. N Engl J Med 303:200, 1980.

167. Butchart EG, Ashcroft T, Bamsley WC, Holden MP: Pleuropneumonectomy in the management of diffuse malignant mesothelioma of the pleura. Thorax 31:15, 1976.

168. Antman KH, Blum RH, Greenberger JS, et al.: Multimodality therapy for malignant mesothelioma based on a study of natural history. Am J Med 68:356, 1980.

169. Yap B-H, Benjamin RS, Burgess MA, Bodey GP: The value of adriamycin in the treatment of diffuse malignant pleural mesothelioma. Cancer 42:1692, 1978.

170. Chahinian AP, Suzuki Y, Mandel EM, Holland JF: Diffuse pulmonary malignant mesothelioma. Response to Doxorubicin and 5-Azacytidine. Cancer 42:1687, 1978.

171. Fischbein A, Suzuki Y, Selikoff IJ, Bekesi JG: Unexpected longevity of a patient with malignant pleural mesothelioma. Cancer 42:1999, 1978.

172. Tivenius L: Benign pleural lesions simulating tumour. Thorax 18:39, 1963.

173. Funahashi A, Kumar UN, Varkey B: Multiple pleural plaques simulating metastatic lung tumor. Postgrad Med 61:262, 1977.

174. Krause LG, Ross CA: Intrathoracic lipomas. Arch Surg 84:82, 1962.

175. Ruttner JR, Heinzl S: Squamous-cell carcinoma of the pleura. Thorax 32:497, 1977.

176. Duhig JT: Solitary rhabdomyosarcoma of the pleura. J Thorac Surg 37:236, 1959.

177. Smith S, Opipari MI: Primary pleural melanoma. J Thorac Cardiovasc Surg 75:827, 1978.

27 Diagnostic Cytology

Geno Saccomanno
Linda Ferrell

Sputum Cytology

The state of the art of sputum cytology is currently sufficiently accurate, cost-effective, and time-saving to be used as a screening test in most patients suspected of having lung cancer. This is particularly true in patients who are cigarette smokers and have some clinical signs or symptoms that make neoplasia a strong possibility. The value of cytologic examination of sputum in patients at high risk for lung cancer is questioned by some studies, but indications are accumulating that morbidity and mortality are improved. The high-risk patient is older than age 45 and smokes at least one pack of cigarettes a day.

Another value of sputum cytology is the importance of determining tumor cell type when the sputum is positive. First, it is usually possible to determine the cell type (squamous, small, large-cell undifferentiated, adenocarcinoma) and even grade the degree of differentiation of the squamous cell cancers. Generally, carcinoma in situ, when present even in small bronchi, can be readily diagnosed with sputum cytology because the lesion does not obstruct the bronchus. As the lesion becomes larger, it may obstruct the bronchus, thus preventing shed cells from being carried into the sputum mucous stream. As the tumor becomes larger, it invades surrounding alveoli and adjacent respiratory bronchioles and may then be found in the sputum sample.

The epithelium of the tracheobronchial tree is lined by ciliated tall columnar cells and nonciliated goblet cells. Reserve cells and granular cells are also present, but their numbers are small. The granular cells are increased in cases with tumor, but the explanation for this increase is unknown. All of these cells are exfoliated into the tracheobronchial tree, and make up a portion of the sputum.

The goblet cells have a dual role. These cells secrete mucins which provide the vehicle of the mucous blanket. The amount of mucus varies, and the amount is increased by hyperplasia and hypertrophy of the submucous glands of the tracheobronchial tree and by goblet cell metaplasia. Since the turnover of all respiratory cells is estimated to be about 30 days, there must be an active multiplication of these cells. It is difficult to believe that these cells have such a rapid turnover, however, particularly since one rarely sees mitotic figures in the cells, either in sputum smears or in sections of these structures. The abundance of these cells in sputum samples, however, is strong evidence that these cells replicate rather rapidly.

The product of this constant shedding of cells provides large numbers of cells which ultimately are mixed with squamous cells of pharynx and mouth. All of these components of sputum show varying degrees of degeneration. Some are rather well preserved, others are fragmented; some are shrunken, whereas others are swollen.

Bacterial, fungal, viral, and parasitic infections of the tracheobronchial tree stimulate the production of a variety of cells. Polymorphonuclear leukocytes are seen in acute inflammation of the lung and bronchial tree; eosinophils are seen in asthma and allergies. Basophils are rarely seen in patients with neoplasia. Lymphocytes are always seen, but are more numerous in viral infections. These inflammatory cells abound in active respiratory infections, but disappear equally rapidly with recovery. Polymorphonuclear leukocytes persist in chronic bronchitis. Intensive treatment with antibiotics reduces their number, but rarely to a marked degree. The reduction of these inflammatory cells is helpful in cases in which one is searching for tumor cells.

Other irritants, including carcinogens and in many instances bacterial infections, elicit focal squamous cell metaplasia, usually at the bifurcation of bronchi and bronchioles. The squamous cell metaplasia produced by infection is transitory, lasting slightly longer than the

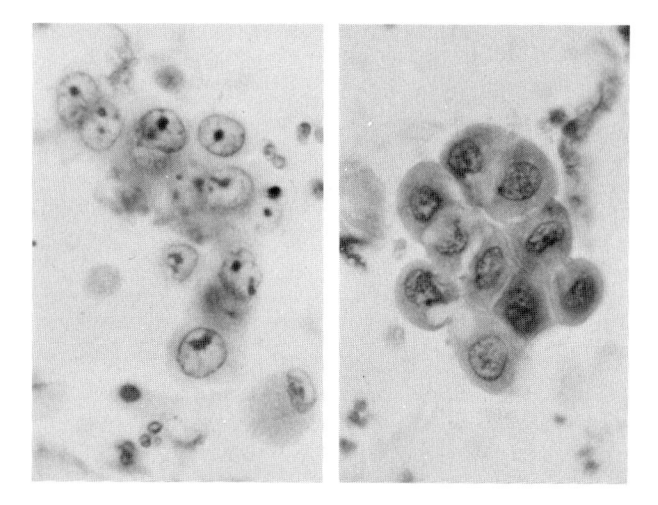

Figure 27–1. Young histiocytes (×600).

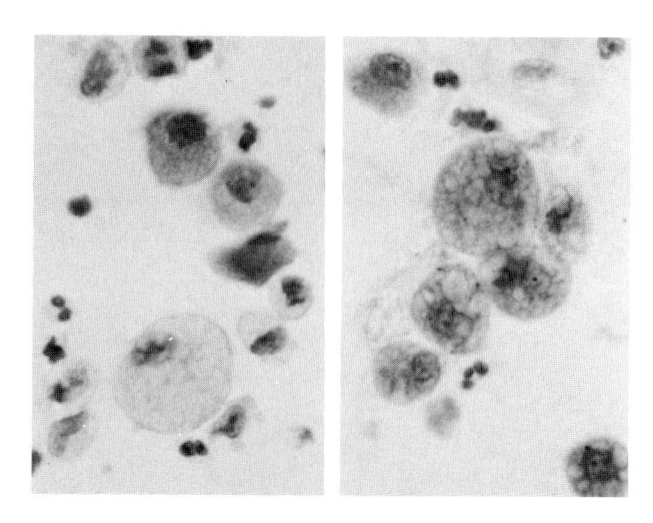

Figure 27–2. Fat-laden histiocytes (×600).

infection. Squamous cell metaplasia occurring during an infection usually shows minor degrees of atypia, but rarely causes marked atypical changes. These cells readily disappear with the inflammation. The squamous metaplastic cells that persist may be due to carcinogenic affect.

Initially areas of epithelial atypia are small, but with time may become larger as the cells become more and more atypical. Some of the early malignant lesions (carcinoma in situ) have been found to extend for several centimeters. In any event, cells shed from these areas (be it a single lesion or multiple lesions) find their way into the sputum samples.

Therefore, the sputum sample of lung origin will show a variety of cells—normal, inflammatory, metaplastic squamous, and neoplastic. The sputum sample is a good index of the activity and products of the respiratory system.

Cellular Elements Found in Sputum, Bronchial Brushing, Lavage, and Washing

Exfoliated cells, both benign and malignant, present diagnostic pitfalls that require careful study to determine their exact origin and correct identification. Some benign normal habitants of the respiratory tree simulate tumor cells.

The histiocytes are the first of these cells which are sometimes seen in abundance. Histiocytes arise from circulating blood cells. The cells undergo transformation from the time they are released in the tracheobronchial tree mucous blanket to their ultimate removal. Young histiocytes (Fig. 27–1) show prominent vesicular nuclear material with sharply defined nuclear membrane and little identifiable cytoplasm that is clear of any material. The nucleus is rounded to kidney-shaped, depending on how the cell is oriented on the slide. If it is kidney-shaped, it will show a small cleft along the hilus of the cellular concavity; this feature readily identifies these as young histiocytes. Once the histiocytes begin to accumulate phagocytized material—be it fat (Fig. 27–2), carbonaceous material (Fig. 27–3, left), or blood pigment (Fig. 27–3, right)—the cell's cytoplasm increases in size, and the cells are easy to identify. The significance of histiocytes in sputum in patients with clinical disease is poorly understood and merits more research.

Lymphocytes, monocytes, and plasma cells are rather easy to identify, but often it is difficult to determine if these are benign or malignant. Plasma cells are rarely seen as neoplastic cells in sputum unless there is extensive myeloma, not only in the lung but in other organs. It is usually not a diagnostic problem at this time because in most cases the diagnosis has already been established.

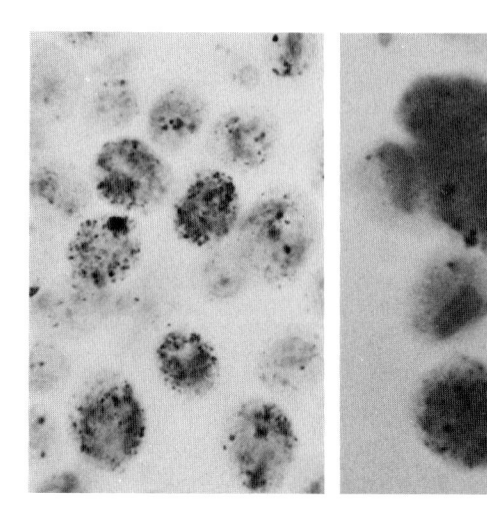

Figure 27–3. Left: Histiocytes with carbon (×600). Right: Histiocytes with blood pigment (×600).

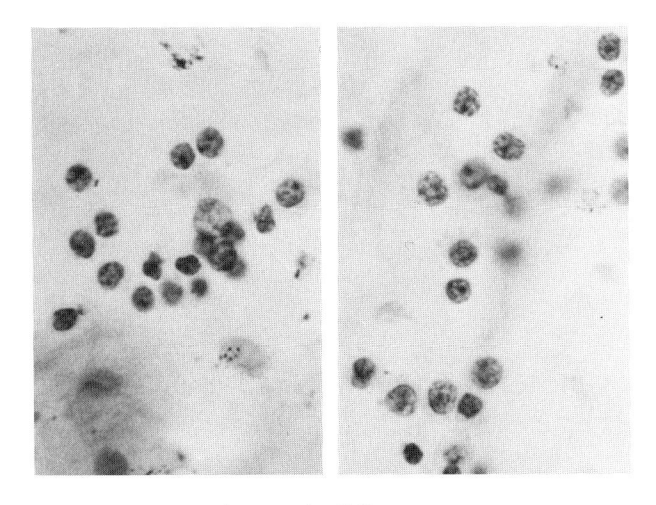

Figure 27–4. Lymphocytes (×600).

Monocytic leukemia diagnosed from sputum is probably not a diagnostic problem because the hematologic route of diagnosis long precedes the increase of these cells in sputum.

The lymphocytes observed in sputum, however, deserve particular attention. Usually many normal-appearing lymphocytes are found in the sputum in both primary pulmonary and systemic lymphomas. Any time a large number of lymphocytes is noted in sputum, one should consider the possible diagnosis of lymphoma. The cells in the normal size range measure 8 to 9 μm in diameter, have a large nuclear/cytoplasmic ratio, and have barely recognizable bluish cytoplasm along one border. In malignant lymphoma, larger lymphocytic cells are admixed with the regular-sized lymphocytes. The nuclei are usually hyperchromatically stained, and the nuclear material is coarse (Fig. 27–4). One must always have a good clinical history since these cells are sometimes difficult to differentiate from small-cell carcinomas. An understanding of the cytology of oat cells found in sputum also helps to separate these two entities. In addition, small-cell carcinomas are usually seen in patients with a rapid clinical course. Lymphocytic lymphomas, which are diagnosed by hematologic examination, do not always run an acute course. Occasionally a primary tumor of the lung may be a lymphoma, and cells expectorated in sputum may be the first clue.

Degenerated tumor cells arise from two sources. These fragments of cells are sometimes the product of necrotic tumor that evacuates into the bronchial tree (Fig. 27–5), or they are from degenerated tumor cells that fragment and degenerate after they have been shed from tumor surface by exfoliation. The material seen in cytology specimens varies in amount and may be seen in sample smears which also show well-preserved tumor cells.

When tumor cell fragments are seen, they consist of nuclear debris. The cytoplasm is usually not attached and probably degenerates more readily leaving no telltale residuum. The nuclear debris fragments are usually coal black or very hyperchromatically stained and stand out conspicuously. They may vary in size and shape, but are usually round and most often measure less than 10 μm in diameter with many of the fragments measuring less than 5 μm in diameter. Occasionally, a sputum sample will show a fine granular background which should also be suspect of neoplasm. When one becomes accustomed to the granular background seen in positive cytology, one learns to suspect this background even when tumor cells are not present. It is a cardinal policy to request good aerosol sputum samples from patients who show nuclear debris or granular background on a sputum smear. Usually a good aerosol sputum sample will confirm the suspicious nuclear debris as representing the product of neoplasia.

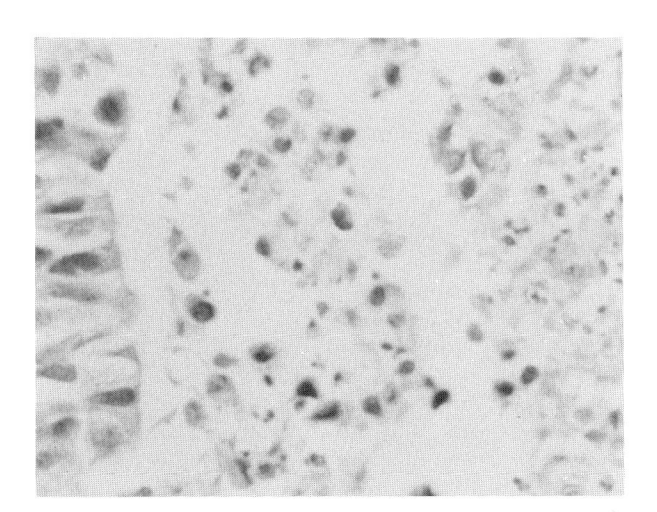

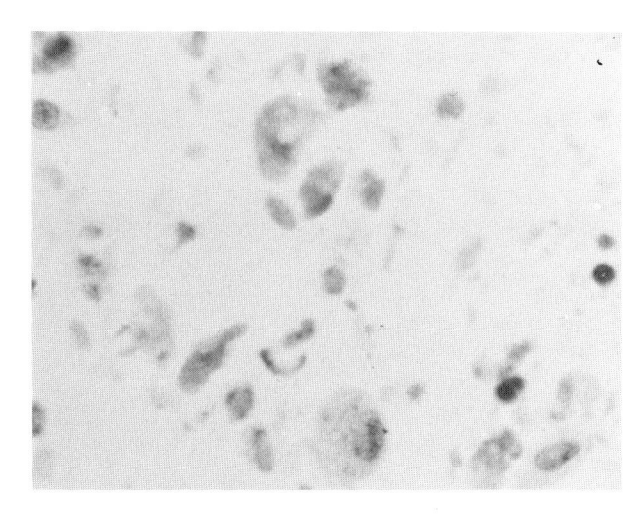

Figure 27–5. Nuclear debris from tumor cells. Left: Tissue (×400). Right: Cytology (×400).

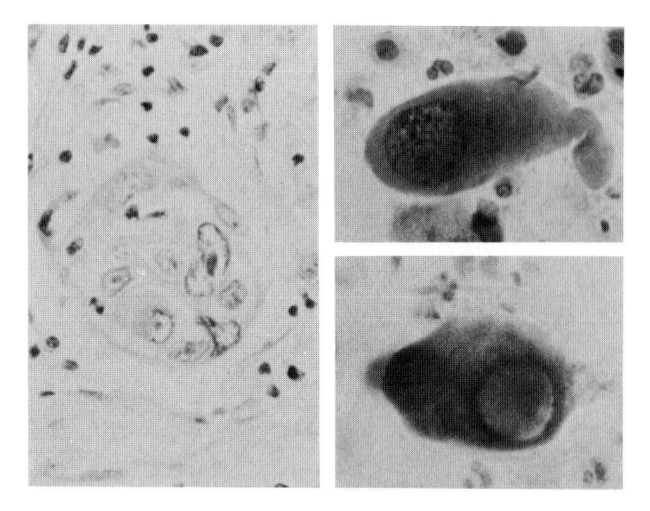

Figure 27-6. Keratinizing epidermoid carcinoma (WHO-IA). Left: Tissue (×400). Right: Cytology (×600).

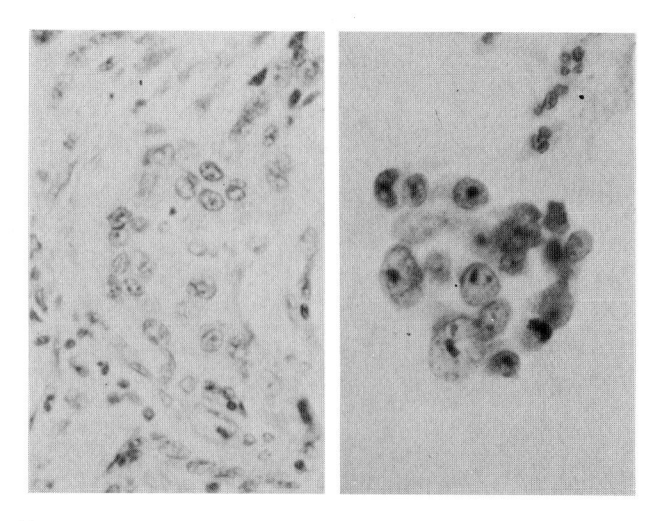

Figure 27-7. Squamous carcinoma (WHO-IB). Left: Tissue (×400). Right: Cytology (×600).

Primary Carcinomas of the Lung—Histology and Cytology

A general and detailed study of the clinical behavior and histology of primary lung carcinomas is presented elsewhere. The presentation here will be limited to a general discussion and correlation of cytologic and histologic data. This correlation adds considerably to the understanding of the clinical behavior of lung tumors. Only consideration of the more common lung tumors will be presented here: epidermoid tumors, small-cell tumors, adenocarcinoma, and bronchioloalveolar tumors.

Epidermoid carcinomas of the lung were divided by the World Health Organization into three cell types. The first is keratinizing epidermoid carcinoma (WHO-IA; Fig. 27-6) that is composed histologically of mature squamous cells showing foci of keratin or epithelial pearls and intercellular bridges. There are several variants such as clear cell, large-cell undifferentiated (which is frequently placed in a separate subgroup), and adenosquamous cell carcinoma. Generally the clinical behavior is the same in all of these lesions. The cells found in these lesions of the lung show some variations, but the cells are usually keratinizing. Some of the cells are larger than 50 μm in diameter and, in some cases, may reach even larger dimensions seen in the keratinizing squamous tumors. Some of the cells may be smaller than 40 to 50 μm, may not be orangeophilic, and may even be vacuolated, as is sometimes noted in the large-cell undifferentiated and adenosquamous carcinomas.

The second group of epidermoid carcinomas (designated WHO-IB; Fig. 27-7) are those that do not show epithelial pearls or keratinization but do show intercellular bridges. These tumors are more basophilically stained, and the cells are more uniform. The cells vary from 25 to 50 μm and almost always appear to be regular, hyperchromatically stained, and single, although they rarely may be found in clusters. The cell size is the most important characteristic of these lesions. Often the histology of the lesions will show considerable variation in degree of differentiation. Some areas will fulfill all the characteristics of the undifferentiated squamous cell group. Equally important, if one is to identify these specific groups of tumors cytologically from sputum samples, one must study many cells and, if necessary, many samples.

The third group of lesions in the epidermoid group are the most undifferentiated squamous cell carcinomas (WHO-IC; Fig. 27-8). It is of utmost importance to have as much data available as possible on these cases. The clinical history, including the duration of the disease, the

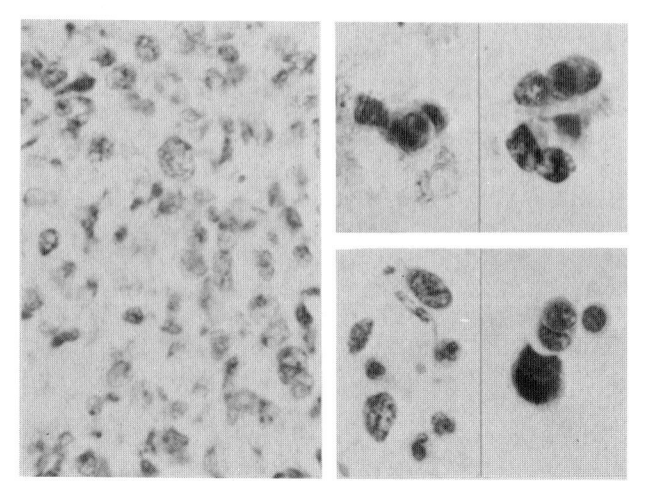

Figure 27-8. Squamous carcinoma (WHO-IC). Left: Tissue (×600). Right: Cytology (×600).

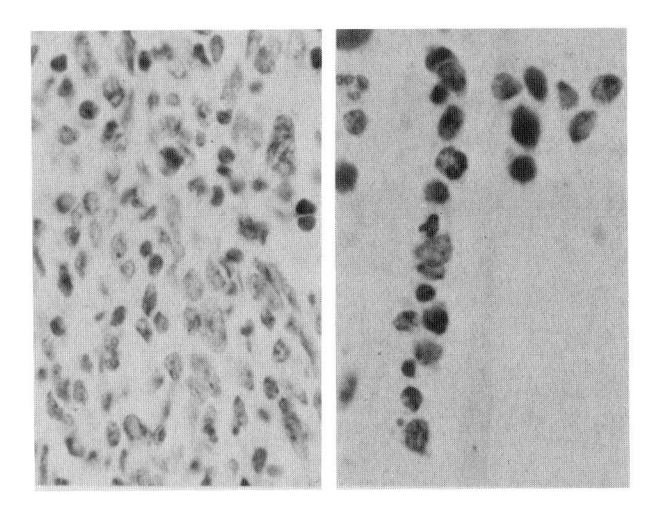

Figure 27-9. Small-cell carcinoma (WHO-IIA). Left: Tissue (×600). Right: Cytology (×600).

Figure 27-11. Bronchioloalveolar adenocarcinoma (WHO-IIIB). Left: Tissue (×100). Middle: Tissue (×600). Right: Cytology (×600).

cytology, and the histology, is to be studied carefully to separate these lesions from the small-cell cancers of the lung. The histology of these undifferentiated cells may be mistaken for the IB cancers. Since the behaviors of the IB and IC carcinomas are essentially the same, the clinical approach to these lesions does not vary. However, one must study these in detail so that the commonly made error of calling these small-cell carcinomas is not made. Histologically these tumors are composed of tightly packed, undifferentiated, hyperchromatically stained cells that may or may not form sheets. Frequently, the supporting stroma is scanty. Cytologically, the cells are small (10 to 35 μm in diameter) and do not show "Indian file" arrangement; careful review will reveal rare cells that exceed 35 μm in diameter. Small-cell carcinomas rarely show cells of this size. Electron microscopy studies sometimes may be helpful if numerous secretory granules are found.

Small-cell carcinomas of the lung (WHO-IIA, IIB, IIC; Fig. 27-9) really should be one group because, histologically, all these lesions show the same characteristics if enough sections are made of the tumors; all these lesions reveal varying numbers of secretory granules on electron microscopy studies. Cytologically, these are uniformly small, hyperchromatic cells which rarely exceed 20 μm in greatest diameter. The cells are usually round, single, or in loose clusters supported by thin sheets of fine mucus. Variation in nuclear size is common. Often the cells line up in Indian file. These cells may be confused with lymphoblastic leukemic cells, but primary leukemic lesions of the lung are very rare. The cells of leukemia are usually larger and frequently associated with systemic disease.

The adenocarcinomas of the lung (Fig. 27-10) vary considerably, histologically and cytologically. If the lesions originate in the proximal bronchial tree, they may reveal a predominately papillary or glandular pattern; if the lesions originate peripherally (Fig. 27-11), there is less stroma and there are alveolar spaces with tumor cells lining them.

Generally the cytology of these tumors consists of single cells and clusters of cells. Occasionally only single cells are present, and in other cases, all of the cells are clustered sheets as if the whole lining of alveolar spaces is shed into the sample. The cells vary considerably in size, measuring 15 to 65 μm in diameter. Usually the cells have basophilic cytoplasm which may be vacuolated. Often the nuclei reveal a coarse nuclear material and prominent eosinophilic nucleoli.

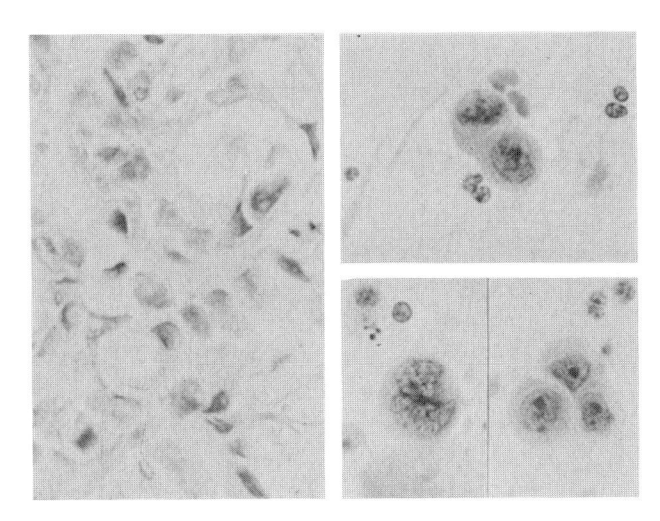

Figure 27-10. Bronchogenic adenocarcinoma (WHO-IIIA-1). Left: Tissue (×600). Right: Cytology (×600).

Differentiation of Carcinoma In Situ Vs. Invasive Carcinoma of the Lung

The differentiation between carcinoma in situ and invasive carcinoma relates only to epidermoid carcinomas. The development and identification of invasive carcinoma and carcinoma in situ in other neoplasias of the lung have not been reported at this time. Since many of the lung neoplasias are epidermoid carcinomas, this is worthy of analysis, because it seems that carcinoma in situ may be amenable to hematoporphyrin derivative for localization and treatment.

The authors' experience has indicated that the diagnosis of carcinoma in situ of the lung is more difficult to make than that of the cervix, but nonetheless can be correctly made in the majority of early lung cancers. The cytologic features of carcinoma in situ are regularity of the cytologic pattern with absence of nucleoli and lack of cells with basophilic cytoplasm. The features of invasive neoplasia of the lung show marked cellular pleomorphism and prominent nucleoli in some of the malignant cells; often a portion of the cells will have basophilically stained cytoplasm. On serial sectioning of tissue sections, these cases frequently will show some degree of superficial invasion if the cytology was unquestionably malignant with mixed cytologic features of both in situ and invasive qualities.

Nearly all nonradiologically visible lesions of the lung are localized to the immediate area with no regional nodal metastasis—not even intrapulmonary parenchyma nodal metastasis. These lesions are amicable to surgical excision or hematoporphyrin derivative treatment. Naturally if hematoporphyrin is found to be an effective treatment in any reasonable number of the early lung lesions that can be localized, then this will be the preferred modality of treatment. If response is noted in localized premalignant lesions treated with hematoporphyrin, prevention in this manner may be forthcoming also.

Metastatic Carcinoma

The lungs are frequently subject to metastasis from tumors in other parts of the body. This is probably due to the massive capillary bed that is housed in the lung and constantly filters the body's circulating blood.

Occasionally tumor cells from distant origins are found in abundance in sputum samples without radiologic evidence of metastasis in the lung. The authors have seen rare cases in which, after death, no microscopic metastases were found in the lung. This suggests that some tumors allow tumor cells to transgress the capillary bed and the alveolar cells but not form a nidus of tumor growth. Most often when tumor cells are found in sputum, tumor metastasis is visible on radiographs, or microscopic lesions are demonstrable on histologic examination.

The sputum slides showing metastatic tumor cells are usually different from primary lung lesions. They are commonly free from abundant inflammatory cells and cellular or nuclear debris. The tumor cells are often single or in clusters (breast), lie free in a clear field (bladder and pancreas), or may be in a bed of partially necrotic or degenerate cells in which the nuclei are fragmented and degenerated. Metastatic breast tumor cells are often rolled in a small ball-like mass (Fig. 27–12). Some of the cells are paired or single.

Tumors of the pancreas or primary liver tumor cells often are paired, but may be single, frequently showing prominent, acidophilic, round nucleoli indicating rapid growth of these tumors. The cytoplasm is often abundant and basophilic. When the cells are single, they tend to be rounded (Fig. 27–13). Tumors of the urinary bladder, ureter, and renal pelvis are in sheets or paired cells with bland vesicular nuclei in varying degrees of

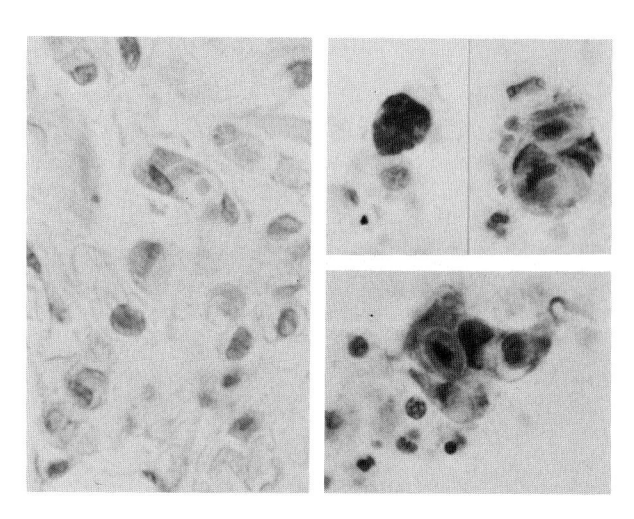

Figure 27–12. Adenocarcinoma of the breast metastatic to lung. Left: Tissue (×600). Right: Cytology (×600).

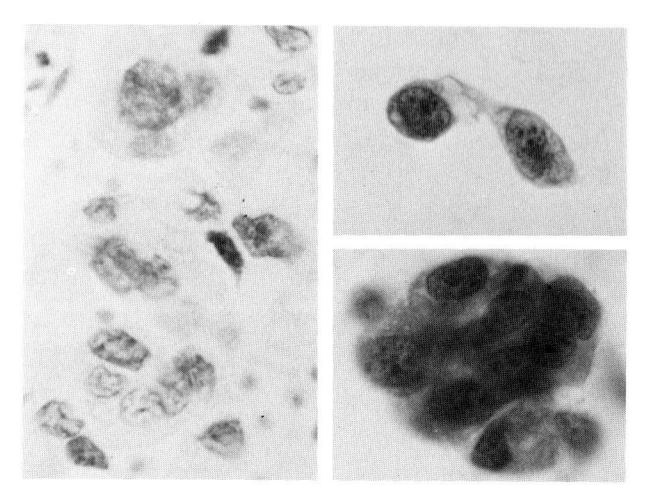

Figure 27–13. Adenocarcinoma of pancreas metastatic to lung. Left: Tissue (×600). Right: Cytology (×600).

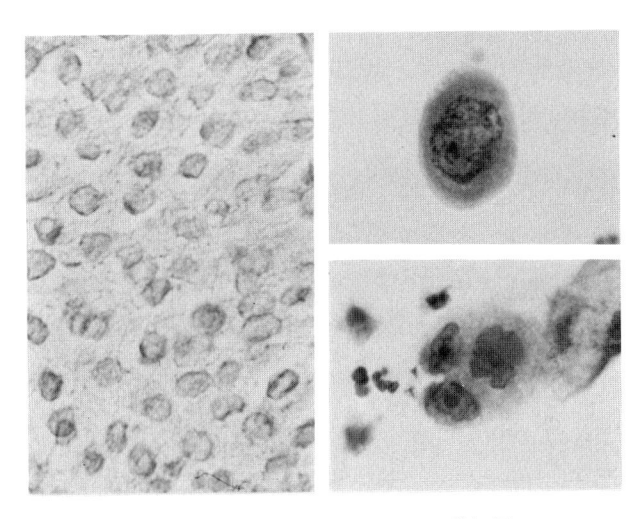

Figure 27–14. Transitional cell carcinoma of bladder metastatic to lung. Left: Tissue (×600). Right: Cytology (×600).

hyperchromasia with abundant bluish cytoplasm (Fig. 27–14).

Cytopathology of Fine Needle Aspiration Biopsy

Although the principles of cytology obtained from sputum and cytology from fine needle aspiration are the same, some practical differences exist. The following section lists what may be encountered in fine needle aspirations; emphasis will be placed on non-neoplastic disease, and supplementary information is provided to that just discussed.

Normal Findings

The cell types from normal lung include epithelial cells, macrophages, lymphocytes, blood elements, and occasionally mesothelial cells. Bronchiolar cells can be identified by their columnar appearance, eccentrically placed round to ovoid nuclei, and the presence of the terminal bar and cilia (Fig. 27–15). Many nuclei will contain small chromocenters as seen on Papanicolaou (PAP) stain (see Fig. 27–15A). Cilia are blue-green on PAP, red on Wright's stain (see Fig. 27–15B). Goblet cells and cuboidal-shaped cells (Fig. 27–16) possibly representative of reserve cells or cells from terminal airways can also be seen.

Macrophages are commonly seen in lung aspirates from any type of lesion. Macrophages in general have an eccentric, folded or round nucleus, often containing a small nucleolus. The cytoplasm is often blue-green and foamy on PAP, but may be paler and contain microvacuoles as seen in lipoid pneumonia, or it may contain hemosiderin or anthracotic pigment (Fig. 27–17). Multinucleate (Fig. 27–18) and binucleate cells are relatively common.

Mesothelial cells are less commonly observed, but when present, they usually occur in monolayer sheets in a honeycomb pattern rather than singly or in small clusters as seen in pleural fluid specimens. They still maintain fairly uniform nuclei with small nucleoli and evenly distributed chromatin. In addition, Bonfiglio[1] has noted that many will have a groove along the long axis of the nucleus.

Tissues such as skeletal muscle, connective tissue, cartilage, and skin can contaminate a lung aspirate. These elements can usually be readily recognized if one looks for specific identifying features. Skeletal muscle usually aspirates as squared-off blocks of tissue which stain orange on PAP and blue on Wright's stain. Cross-striations and bland nuclei within the muscle fragments are fea-

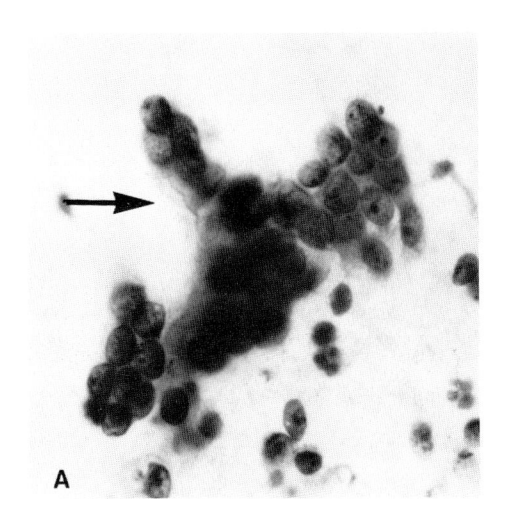

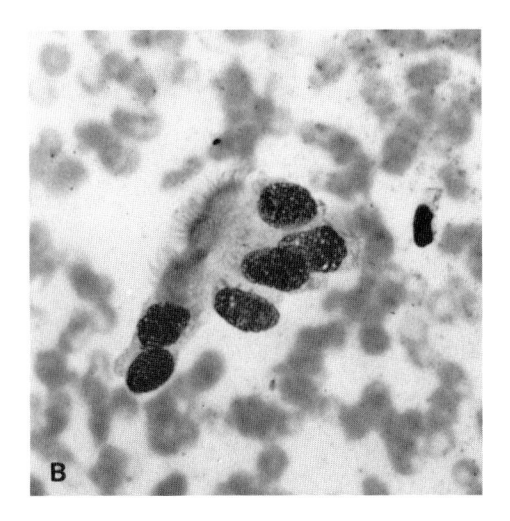

Figure 27–15. Normal ciliated epithelial cells (arrow shows ciliated surface). A. Papanicolaou (PAP) smear (×500). B. Wright's stain (×500).

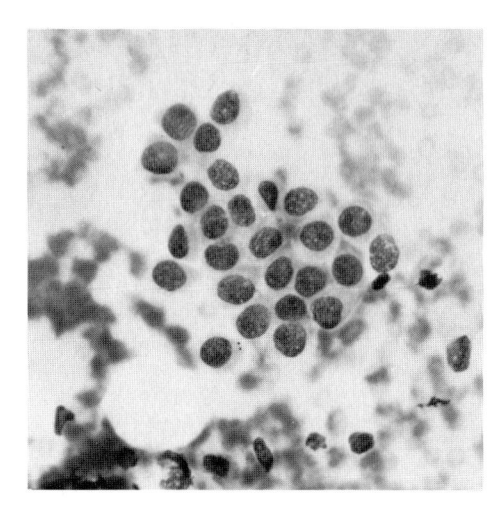

Figure 27–16. Cuboidal epithelial cells with round regular nuclei and a moderate amount of cytoplasm (Wright-Giemsa, ×325).

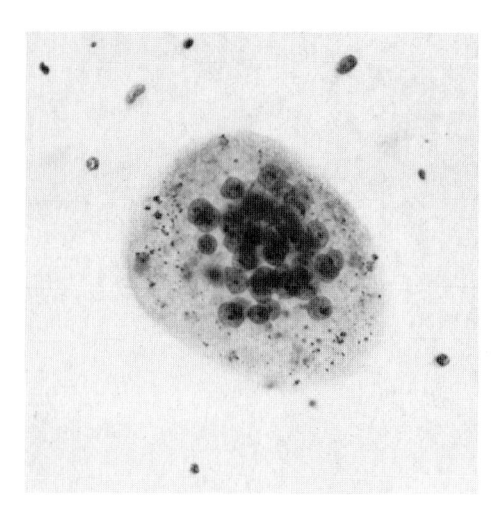

Figure 27–18. Multinucleated giant cell of macrophage type containing anthracotic cytoplasmic pigment (PAP, ×500).

tures to note (Fig. 27–19). Cartilage stains pale blue to green on PAP, bright blue to pink on Wright's stain. Lacunae-containing nuclei can be identified. Incidental cartilage should be differentiated from a pulmonary hamartoma.

Reactive or Inflammatory Changes

A variety of processes can cause alterations in the normal cellular elements that must not be confused with neoplasm. Acute or chronic infections are occasionally

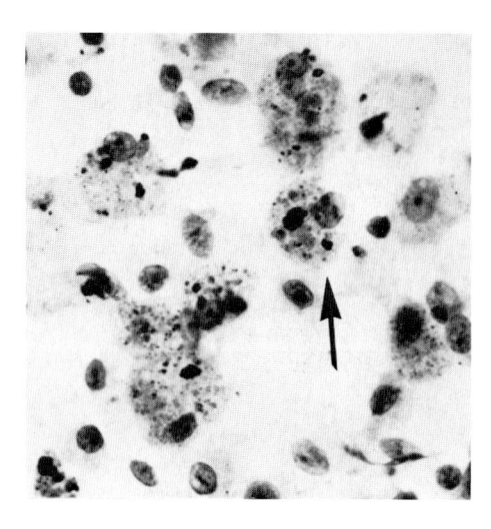

Figure 27–17. Numerous pigmented macrophages (arrow) containing anthracotic pigment. Note typical round to oval nucleus and foamy, ill-defined cytoplasm (PAP, ×500).

biopsied using fine needle aspiration to obtain culture material. In such instances, bacteria or viral inclusions may be seen. *Pneumocystis carinii* can also be aspirated in this manner. The alveolar exudate appears as blue-green to orange-green, finely vacuolated material on PAP stain (Fig. 27–20A). The outlines of the organisms can be identified within this exudate. For confirmation of the diagnosis, the slide can be destained and then restained by a silver methenamine method (Fig. 27–20B). This same stain also works well for other fungal organisms, but many times fungi can be seen on PAP or Wright's stain without the use of special stain (Fig. 27–21). Abscesses, bacterial or fungal, may mimic neoplasia on radiographs, but if the lesion is adequately sampled centrally, the typical inflammatory pattern of neutrophils, lymphocytes, and mononuclear cells should predominate.

Granulomatous lesions may show large numbers of multinucleate histiocytes and macrophages, but the presence of multinucleated cells, especially if they contain carbon pigment (*see* Fig. 27–18), are not pathognomonic of granulomas. A mononuclear or lymphocytic background may be present. In addition, granulomatous lesions often demonstrate a variable amount of necrotic debris. If this combination of giant cells and necrotic tissue is present, special stains for acid-fast and fungal organisms should be done.

Atypical reactive epithelial or mesothelial changes can be seen as part of or surrounding all chronic inflammatory processes as well as other lung disorders. These reactive or reparative cells are usually arranged in large or small sheets and may show enlarged and irregular nuclei, often with prominent nucleoli (Fig. 27–22). Such atypical cells may be numerous, especially if the biopsy material is obtained from the periphery of the lesion. These cellular changes may be especially alarming in instances of chemotherapy or irradiation history. Such cases may be difficult to distinguish from a well-differen-

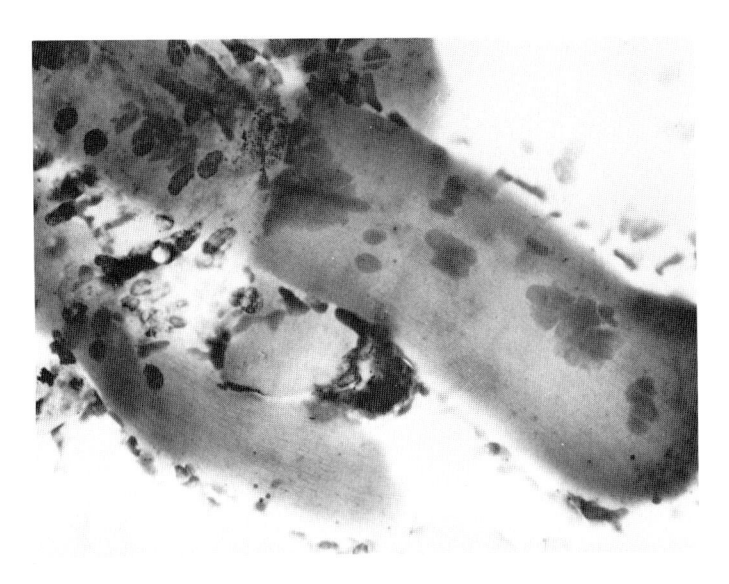

Figure 27-19. Skeletal muscle with squared-off appearance, striations, and bland nuclei (PAP, ×325).

tiated adenocarcinoma or a mesothelioma. Thus, care must be taken to sample such lesions thoroughly, both centrally and peripherally at different sites. This type of problem may defy definitive diagnosis by fine needle aspiration, requiring close clinical follow-up of the mass or thoracotomy in order to exclude a neoplastic process.

Neoplasia

The cytology on fine needle aspiration specimens of most pulmonary tumors is somewhat similar to that seen on brush, wash, or sputum specimens, except that fine needle aspiration usually yields many more and better preserved cells. In addition, since small fragments of tissue are also aspirated, there is some similarity to histologic sections as well. A more extensive sampling of numerous areas within the tumor is also usually done, which may account for the diagnosis of more carcinomas with both glandular and squamous components than usually seen on transbronchial tissue biopsies. Cells are less likely to be distorted by crushing (as in tissue biopsies) and more readily show evidence of cohesion; both features are especially helpful in distinguishing small-cell carcinoma from lymphoma.

Squamous Carcinoma

To make a diagnosis of squamous carcinoma, one of the three following findings must be present: individual cell keratinization, intercellular bridges, or keratin pearls.

Moderately to well-differentiated squamous carcinomas demonstrate isolated keratinized forms with a glassy appearance or orangeophilia on PAP, or a dense, bright blue appearance on Wright-Giemsa stain. Many cells may be anucleate (Fig. 27–23). Pseudocannibalism (cells

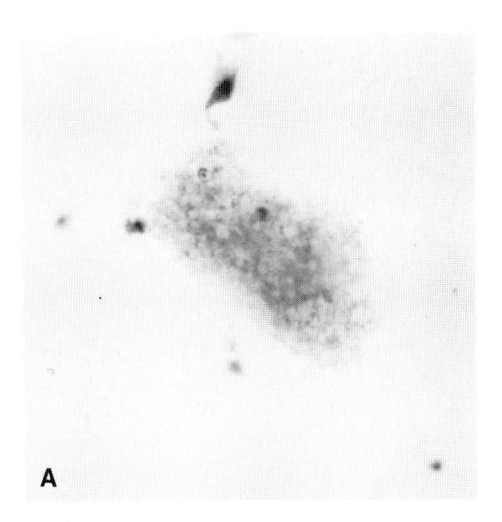

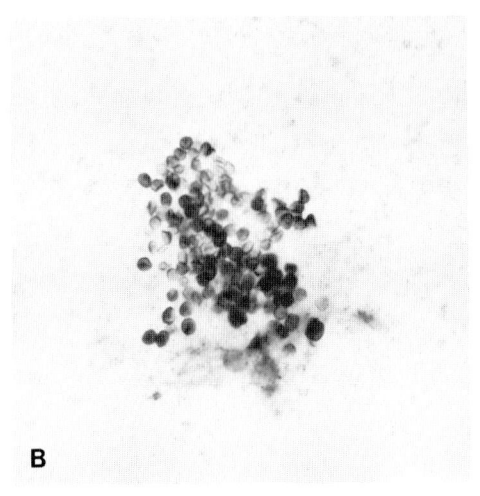

Figure 27-20. A. *Pneumocystis* pneumonia can be suspected on PAP stain by the presence of blue-green to orange-green, finely vacuolar material (PAP, ×500). B. It is confirmed by use of silver stain which shows the typical, small, round organisms (methenamine silver, ×500).

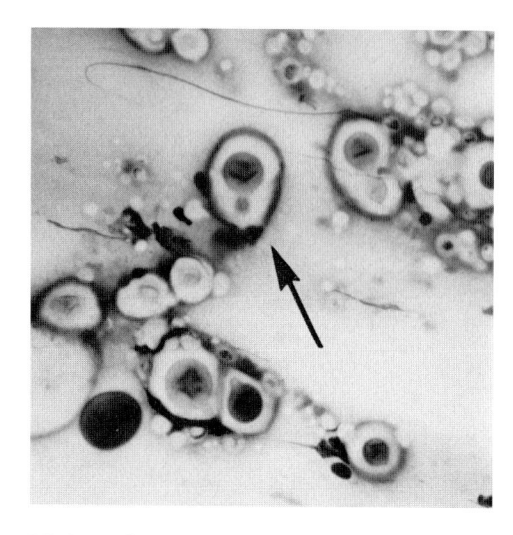

Figure 27–21. *Cryptococcus neoformans* in an immunosuppressed patient. Note halo around the organisms indicative of the capsule and the presence of budding (arrow) (Wright-Giemsa, ×325).

within cells) and keratin pearls may also be found. Elongate, spindled, and pleomorphic forms with hyperchromatic nuclei are common (see Fig. 27–23). The nuclear/cytoplasmic ratio may be only moderately increased.

Poorly differentiated lesions show more isolated cells or small syncytial groups with less nuclear pleomorphism, a higher nuclear/cytoplasmic ratio, and cyanophilic cytoplasm on PAP stain. Evidence of keratinization may be difficult to find in such cases, but cells with distinct cytoplasmic borders (Fig. 27–24) or cytoplasmic rings (Fig. 27–25) suggest squamous differentiation. The nuclear chromatin is often coarsely granular rather than densely hyperchromatic, and nucleoli can be found, although they are not present in most cells.

Adenocarcinoma

Acinar groups or glandular aggregates of cells are important features of adenocarcinomas. A side-by-side arrangement of the cells and an eccentrically placed nucleus in an elongated cell are typical of glandular and columnar differentiation (Fig. 27–26). Papillary configurations can also be seen (Fig. 27–27). The cytoplasm is usually cyanophilic and finely to coarsely vacuolated with fairly ill-defined borders (Fig. 27–28). Cytoplasmic eosinophil-

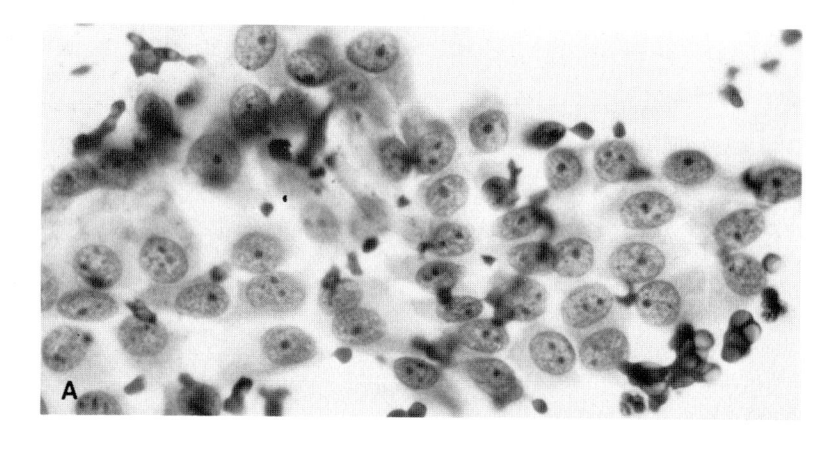

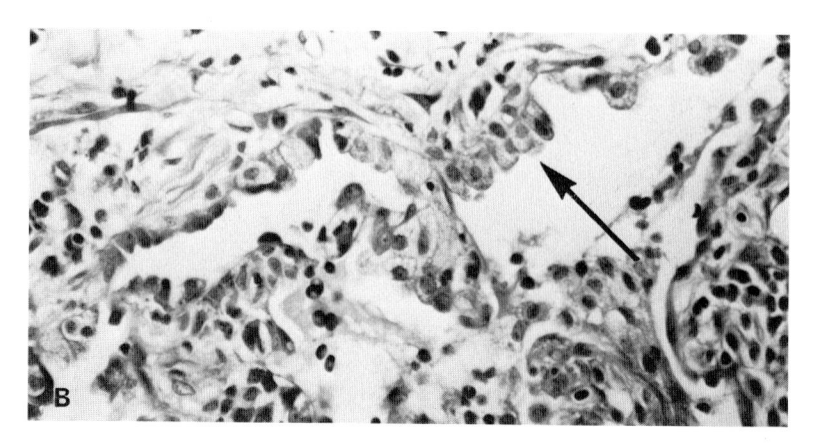

Figure 27–22. A. Reactive alveolar lining cells can form fairly uniform sheets. Nuclei are round to oval, regular, with small nucleoli and finely granular chromatin. Cytoplasm can be somewhat dense or foamy, simulating well-differentiated adenocarcinoma (PAP, ×400). B. Tissue section from same case with reactive alveolar lining cells (arrow) [hematoxylin and eosin (H&E), ×325].

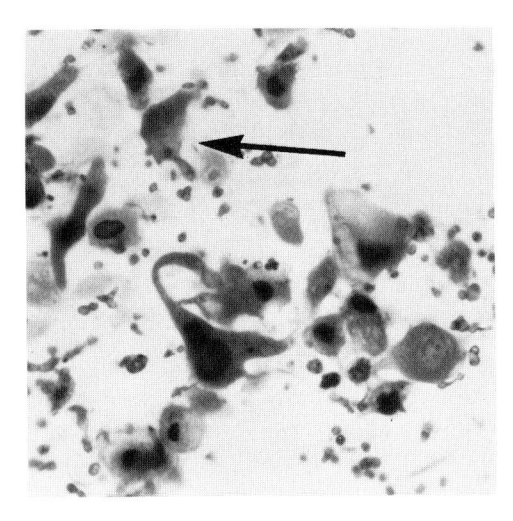

Figure 27–23. Well-differentiated keratinizing squamous cell carcinoma demonstrating nuclear and cytoplasmic pleomorphism. Note anucleate form (arrow) (PAP, ×325).

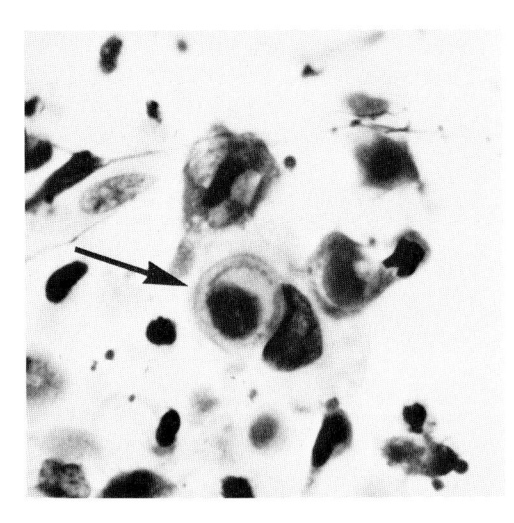

Figure 27–25. Squamous carcinoma. Note nuclear pleomorphism and cell with cytoplasmic ringing (arrow) (PAP, ×640).

ia and eosinophilic necrotic debris can be seen, however, and must not be confused with squamous differentiation. Well-differentiated tumors, especially bronchioloalveolar adenocarcinomas (Fig. 27–29), can produce large amounts of mucin, which can be identified on PAP stain (Fig. 27–30) as streaks of acellular material and on Wright-Giemsa stain as a blue-staining background substance.

In more poorly differentiated lesions, the nuclear/cytoplasmic ratio is often greatly increased and large nucleoli (so-called macronucleoli) are present in most cells (Fig. 27–31). Some of these nucleoli can be as large as an erythrocyte. Multiple nucleoli within one nucleus are fairly common. Poorly differentiated adenocarcinomas can be difficult to distinguish from large-cell undifferentiated lesions. Mucicarmine or periodic acid-Schiff (PAS)-diastase positivity for intracellular mucins can be helpful in differentiating between the two.

Small-Cell Carcinoma

The cells of this tumor type are often arranged in small syncytia (Fig. 27–32) on a background of necrotic cellular debris. The cells have very scant cytoplasm (less than poorly differentiated adenocarcinoma or large-cell) and irregular nuclei that usually vary considerably in size (two to five times that of erythrocytes), all within one lesion. Nuclear molding, or the distortion of nuclear shapes in adjacent cells due to crowding, can be seen within the cell groups. The chromatin is rather coarse, and nucleoli are not prominent or are absent. In the intermediate type, nuclei can be bigger, cytoplasm can be more abundant, and nucleoli more frequent. However, no large nucleoli are seen. The cells in these tumors are fragile and easily distorted by the smearing technique (Fig. 27–33), thus accounting for the strands of bluish nuclear debris seen on the smears.[1]

Large-Cell Carcinoma

This classification should be reserved for those tumors that are undifferentiated and do not show features of small-cell carcinoma. These tumors will usually be composed of fairly large cells with ill-defined cytoplasmic borders, markedly increased nuclear/cytoplasmic ratio, and prominent large nucleoli as in poorly differentiated adenocarcinoma (Fig. 27–34). Nuclear chromatin is usually finely granular. There may be less nuclear overlapping[1] and no evidence of secretory activity as seen in adenocarcinoma. Single nucleoli may be more common (as opposed to multiple nucleoli) in large-cell carcinoma than in adenocarcinoma. The background of necrotic debris seen in small-cell carcinoma is often present (Fig. 27–35).

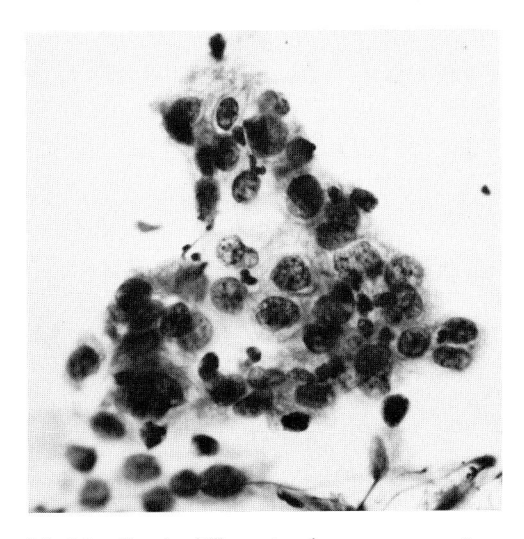

Figure 27–24. Poorly differentiated squamous carcinoma with coarse nuclear chromatin, increased nuclear/cytoplasmic ratio, distinct cell borders, and lack of prominent nucleoli (PAP, ×325).

Figure 27–26. Moderate- to well-differentiated adenocarcinoma. A. Note vacuolization (arrow) (PAP, ×325). B. Side-by-side arrangements (lower left) (Wright-Giemsa, ×325).

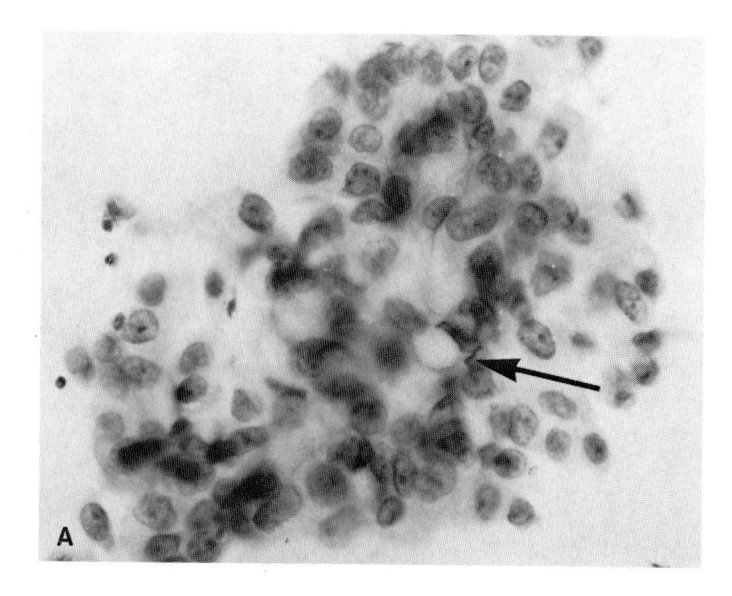

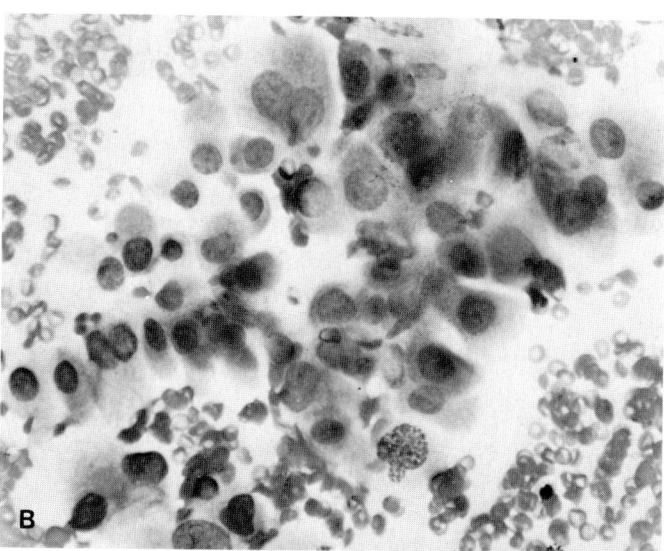

Mixed Adenosquamous Carcinoma

Definite glandular and squamous components must be seen as previously described. These lesions are probably more frequently seen on cytologic preparations than on histologic sections because of the better sampling compared with bronchial biopsy and because of better cytologic criteria for diagnosis on well-prepared smears.[1]

Carcinoid Tumors

The cells of a typical carcinoid tumor have regular, uniform, round to oval nuclei, "salt and pepper" chromatin, and inconspicuous nucleoli on PAP stain (Fig. 27–36). The cytoplasm may be moderate in amount, oval to columnar, basophilic to amphophilic. The cells may be single, arranged in sheets or acini, or even side by side. Mitoses and necrosis are usually not seen. Atypical carcinoids may show much more nuclear variability in size and shape, simulating small-cell carcinomas. However, nuclear molding is not as prominent, and no necrotic background should be seen as with small-cell anaplastic carcinoma.[1]

Bronchial Gland Tumors

Adenoid cystic carcinoma characteristically shows a cellular specimen with the presence of diagnostic metachromatic "hyaline" balls on Wright-Giemsa stain (Fig. 27–37). Pleomorphic adenomas also show abundant metachromatic stroma (Fig. 27–38), but not arranged in balls.[2] Mucoepidermoid tumors might be considered in a central lesion with fairly bland squamous components and goblet cells.

Sarcoma

Sarcomas primary to the lung are rare, but a specimen with scant cellularity, spindle cells with hyperchromatic nuclei and bizarre forms, and mitoses should suggest

Figure 27–27. Well-differentiated adenocarcinoma. Papillary configuration with columnar cells lining the fibrovascular stroma (PAP, ×200).

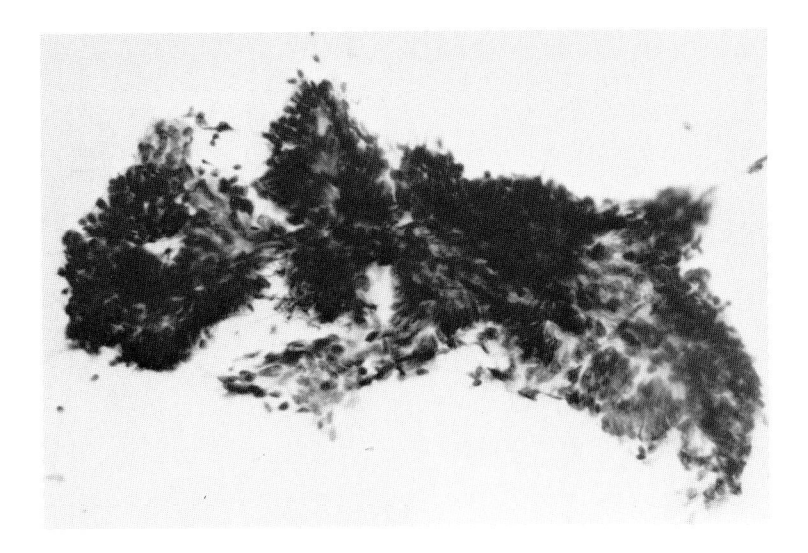

such a diagnosis. A history of previous sarcoma, such as Ewing's sarcoma, osteosarcoma, or chondrosarcoma, is also important as these can metastasize to the lung.

Lymphoma

Some primary lymphomas may be difficult to diagnose on fine needle aspiration because of the problems of differentiating such lesions from lymphocytic interstitial lung disease, pseudolymphoma, and lymphomatoid granulomatosis. The identification of Dutcher bodies, the PAS-diastase–resistant intranuclear inclusions seen in some lymphomas, can be helpful diagnostic findings. Large-cell lymphomas with their monotonous pattern of large, atypical, single lymphoid cells are not as much of a problem. Hodgkin's disease can often be identified because of the heterogeneous cellular infiltrate, including plasma cells, eosinophils, normal-appearing lymphocytes, and Reed-Sternberg cells. However, to subclassify for staging, histology is needed. In general lymphocytic lesions result in single cells on aspiration, although some cells may be crushed together (Fig. 27–39). Sheets or syncytial aggregates do not generally occur, although germinal centers will have a tendency to clump (see Fig. 27–39) because the reticular cells hold the lymphoid cells together. The background shows numerous, small, blue blobs with Wright-Giemsa stain. These are cytoplasmic fragments of the lymphocytes and could be mistaken for platelets by the unaware pathologist. The two can be differentiated by the presence of red granules in the platelets.

Mesothelioma

These tumors are pleural based (radiographic appearance is helpful) and may show either a fibrous, epithelial, or mixed pattern. The epithelial component usually looks mesothelial, except the cells are generally bigger or look similar to well-differentiated adenocarcinoma. Features include round nuclei containing prominent nucleoli and abundant cytoplasm (Fig. 27–40). Acinar groups may also be present, but mesotheliomas probably show more flat sheets of cells and less variation in nuclear size than adenocarcinomas. The cells are negative for neutral mucin and positive for hyaluronic acid (negative staining using colloidal iron with hyaluronidase digestion).

Fibrous mesotheliomas, on the other hand, show a spindle cell pattern (Fig. 27–41). The nuclei, in general, have a bland, finely granular chromatin pattern lacking nucleoli. The specimen is likely to be scant because of the fibrous nature of the tumor. A proteinaceous background substance, probably representing connective tissue acidic mucins (myxoid material), can be seen as a lightly staining blue fluid on Wright-Giemsa preparations. Peroxidase-CEA and keratin studies are sometimes helpful in differentiating mesothelioma and carcinoma.

Others

Pulmonary hamartoma is a benign tumor characterized by a mixture of mesenchymal tissue[3] such as cartilage, fat, connective tissue with a fibromyxomatous appearance,

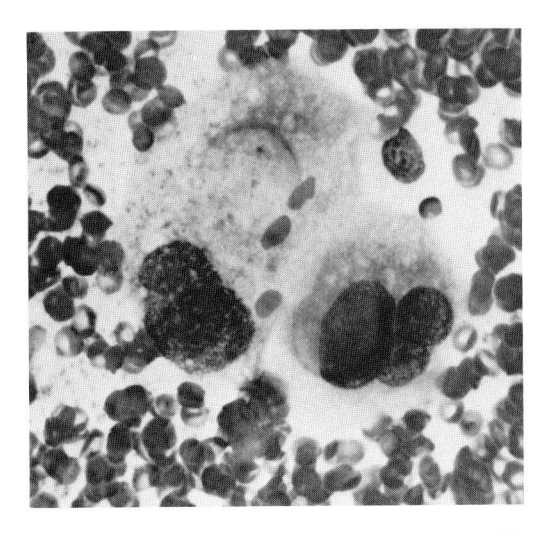

Figure 27–28. Poorly differentiated adenocarcinoma. Note eccentric nuclei and abundant, foamy, ill-defined cytoplasm (Wright-Giemsa, ×500).

816   Diagnostic Cytology

Figure 27–29. Bronchioloalveolar adenocarcinoma. Sheets of "macrophage-like" cells with a honeycomb pattern and irregular nuclear features (PAP, ×640).

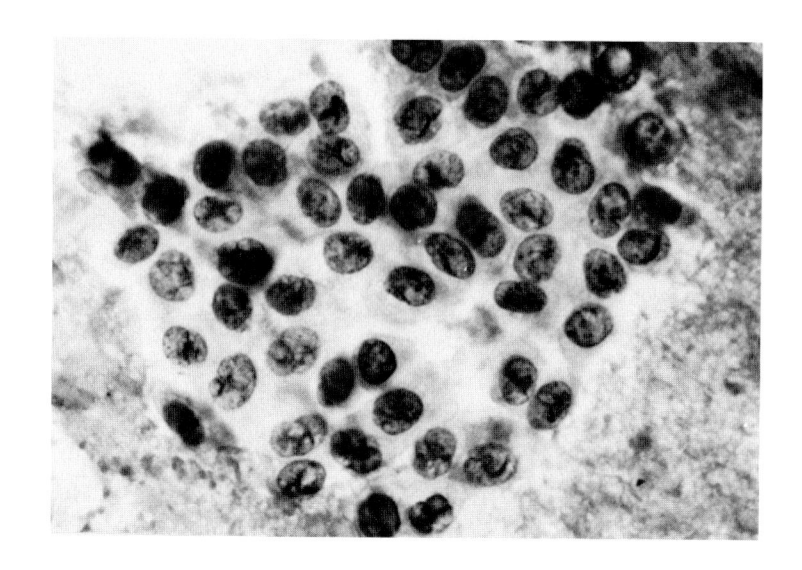

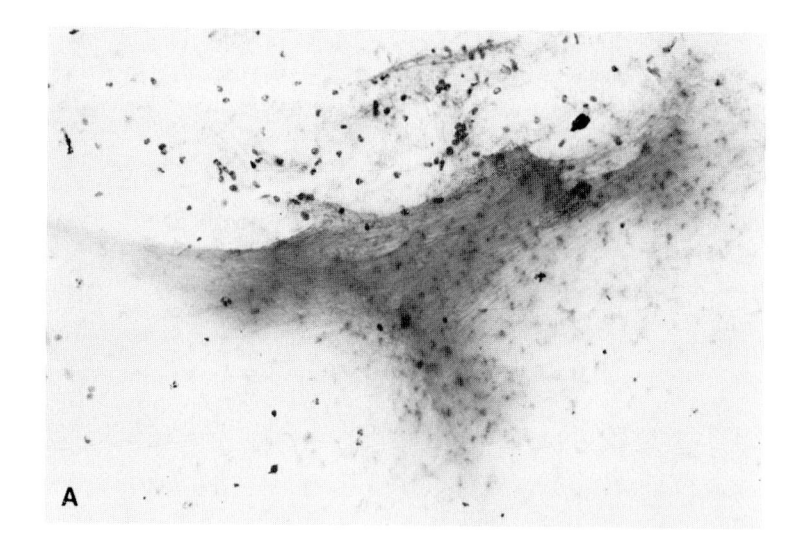

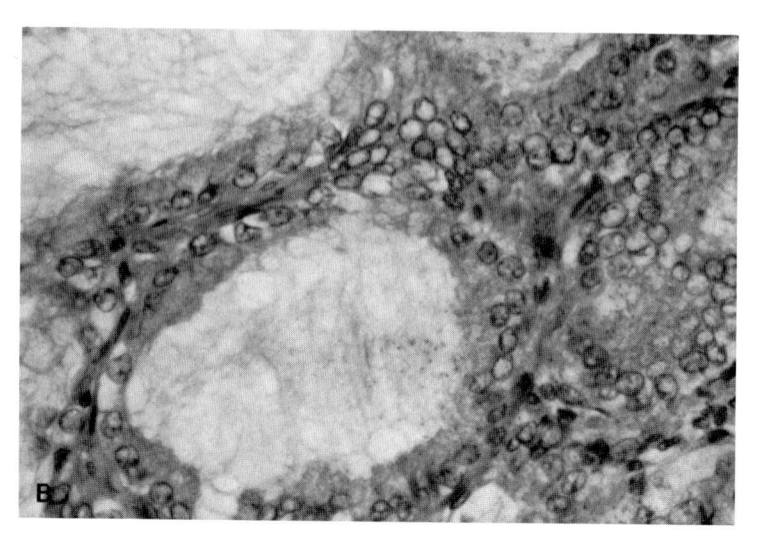

Figure 27–30. A. Mucin on PAP smear from bronchioloalveolar carcinoma. B. Histology section from same tumor showing mucin pools surrounded by columnar cells.

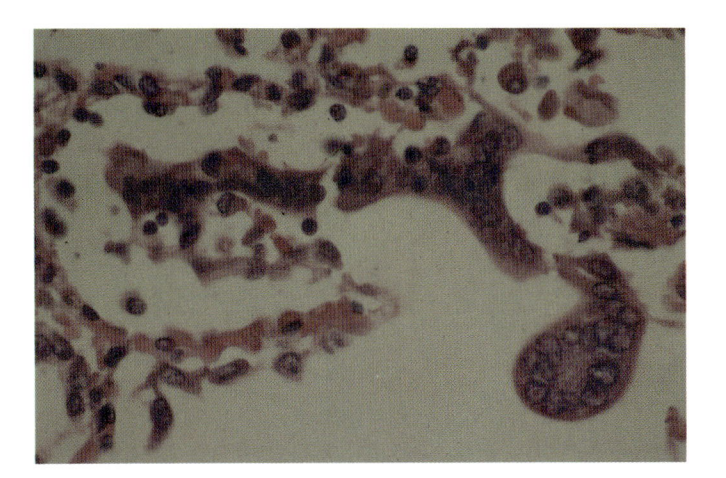

Plate 1.

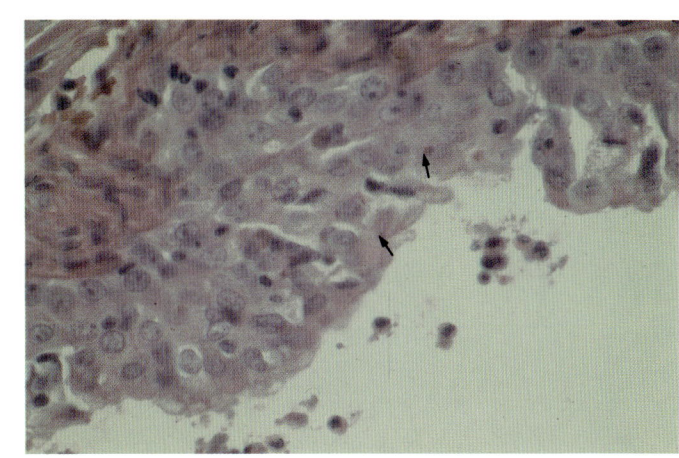

Plate 2.

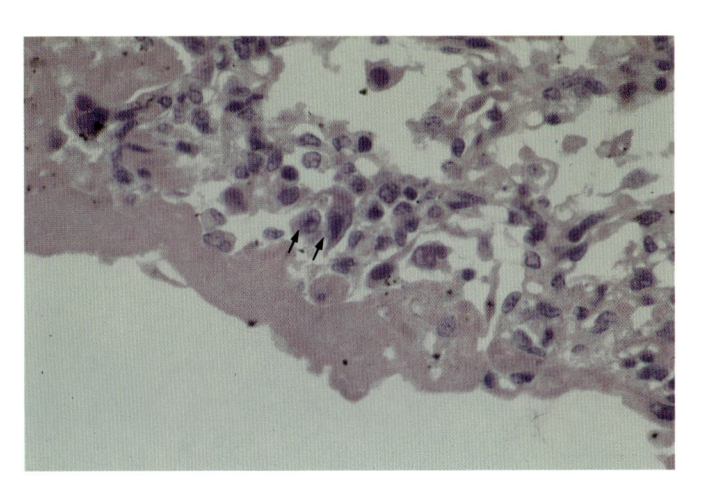

Plate 3.

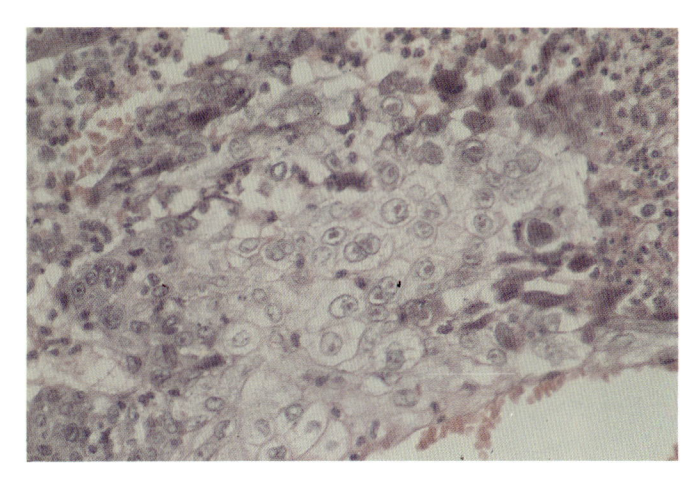

Plate 4.

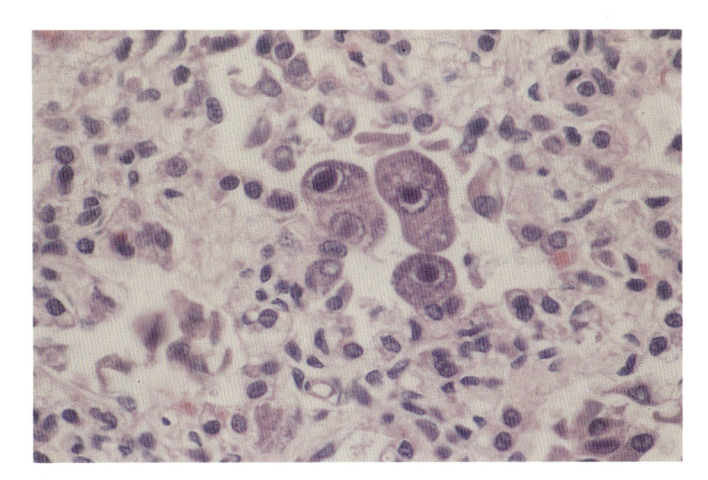

Plate 5.

Plate 1. Multinucleated giant cells in measles. Note intranuclear inclusions (H&E, ×816).

Plate 2. Respiratory syncytial virus cytoplasmic inclusions (arrows) (H&E, ×652).

Plate 3. Intranuclear inclusion in two cells (arrows) and several smudge cells in adenovirus (H&E, ×860).

Plate 4. Herpetic Cowdry A nuclear inclusions (H&E, ×800).

Plate 5. Cytomegalovirus-infected cells with nuclear and cytoplasmic inclusions (H&E, ×830).

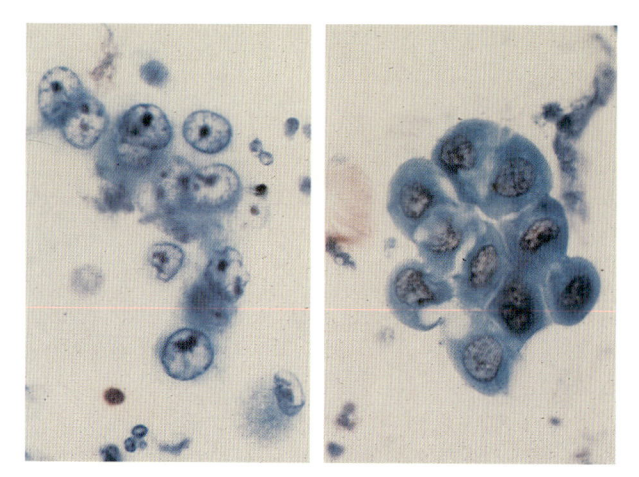

Figure 27–1.

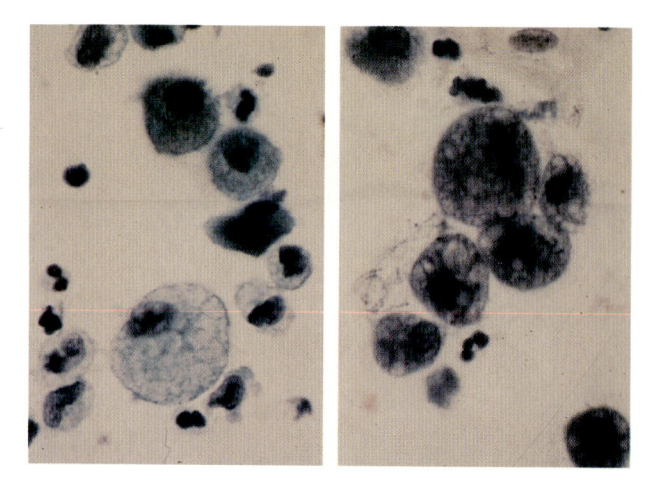

Figure 27–2.

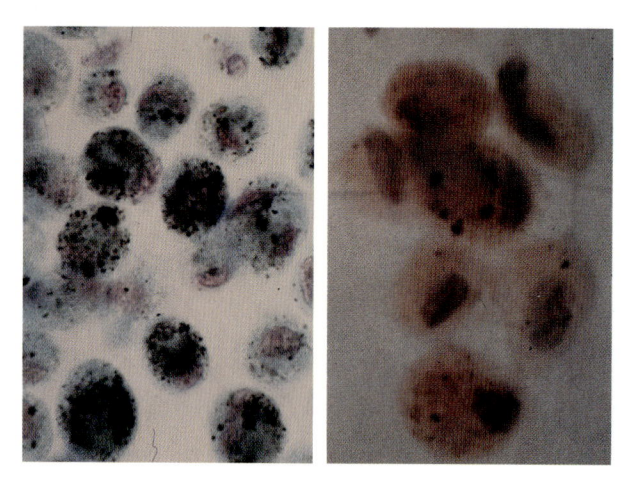

Figure 27–3.

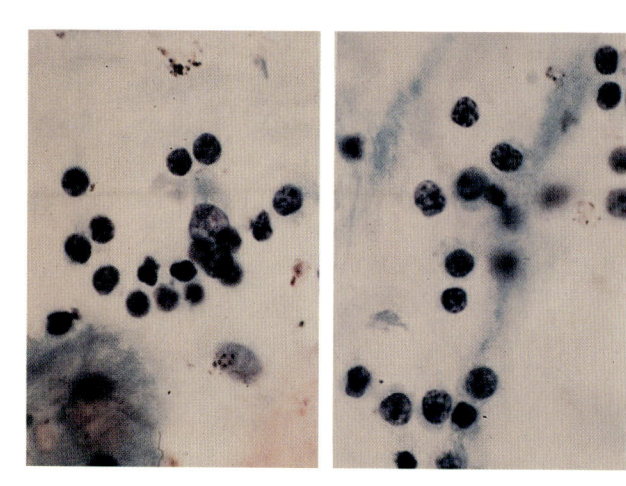

Figure 27–4.

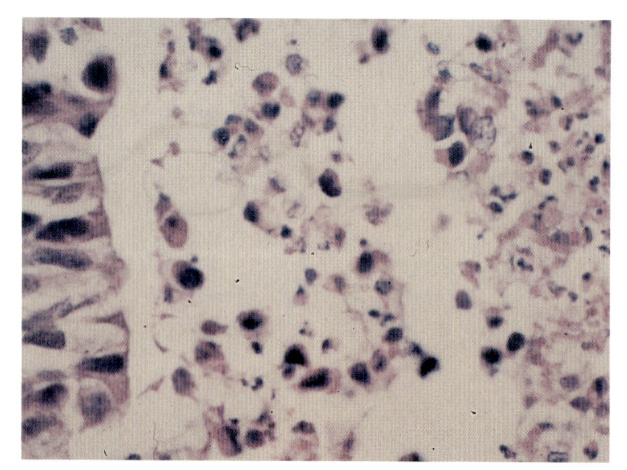

Figure 27–5A.

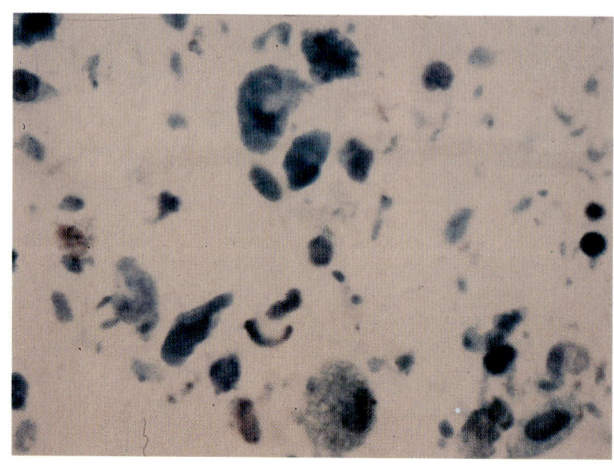

Figure 27–5B.

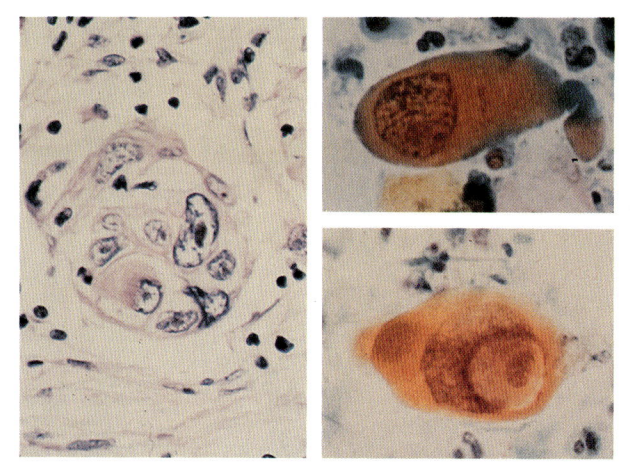

Figure 27–6.

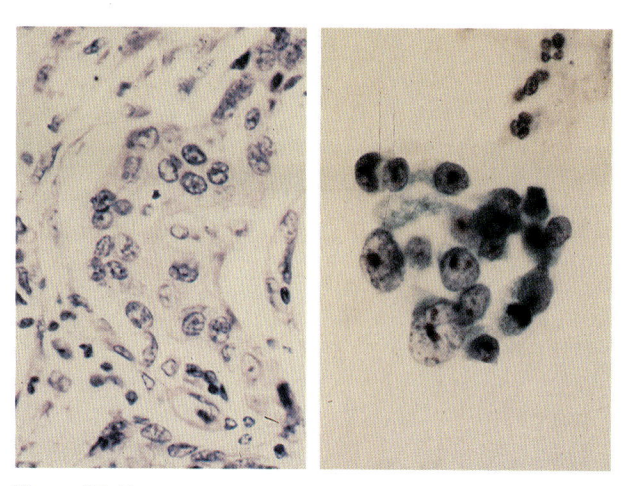

Figure 27–7.

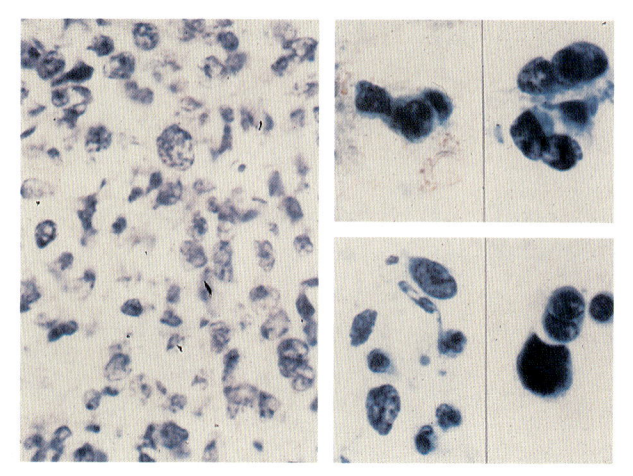

Figure 27–8.

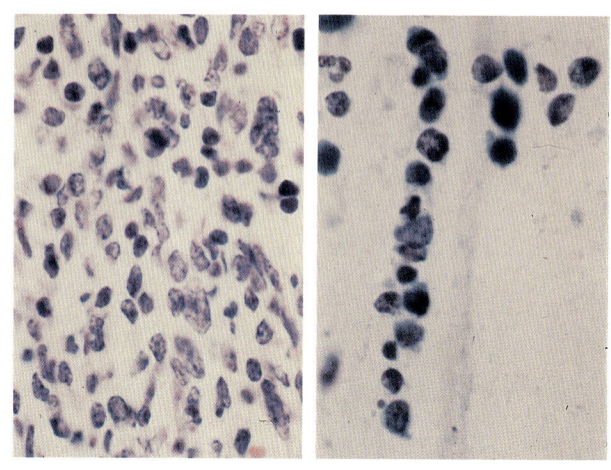

Figure 27–9.

Figure 27–1. Young histiocytes (×600).

Figure 27–2. Fat-laden histiocytes (×600).

Figure 27–3. Left: Histiocytes with carbon (×600). Right: Histiocytes with blood pigment (×600).

Figure 27–4. Lymphocytes (×600).

Figure 27–5. Nuclear debris from tumor cells. Left: Tissue (×400).

Figure 27–6. Keratinizing epidermoid carcinoma (WHO-IA). Left: Tissue (×400). Right: Cyotology (×600).

Figure 27–7. Squamous carcinoma (WHO-IB). Left: Tissue (×400). Right: (×600).

Figure 27–8. Squamous carcinoma (WHO-IC). Left: Tissue (×600). Right: (×600).

Figure 27–9. Small-cell carcinoma (WHO-IIA). Left: Tissue (×600). Right: (×600).

Figure 27–10. Bronchogenic adenocarcinoma (WHO-IIIA-1). Left: (×600). Right: (×600).

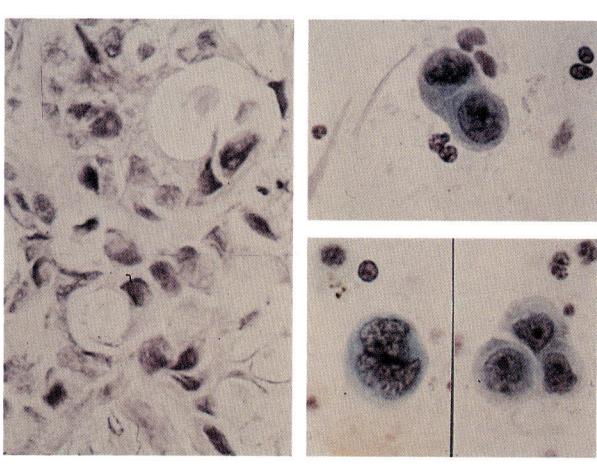

Figure 27–10.

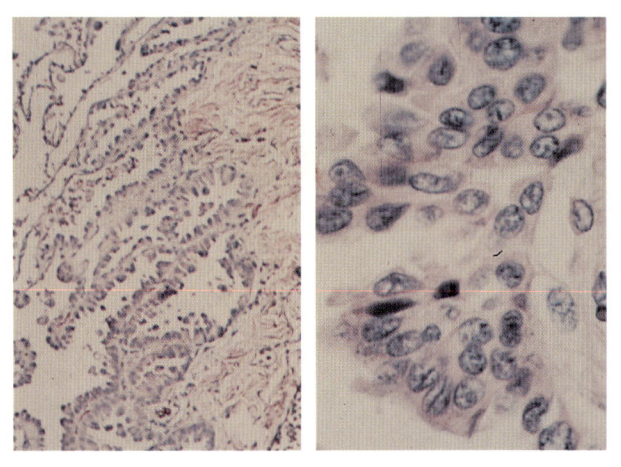

Figure 27–11A.   Figure 27–11B. 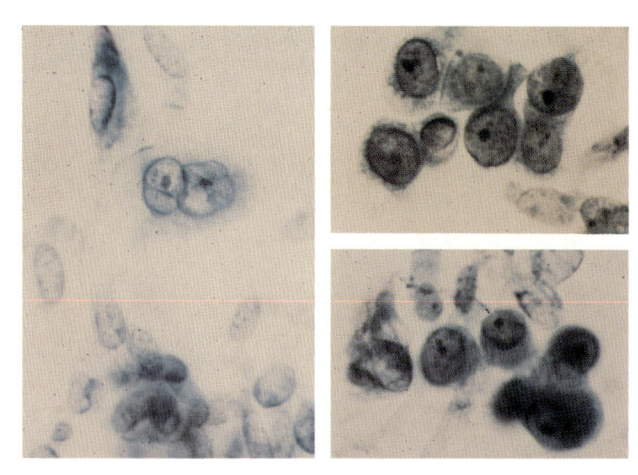   Figure 27–11C.

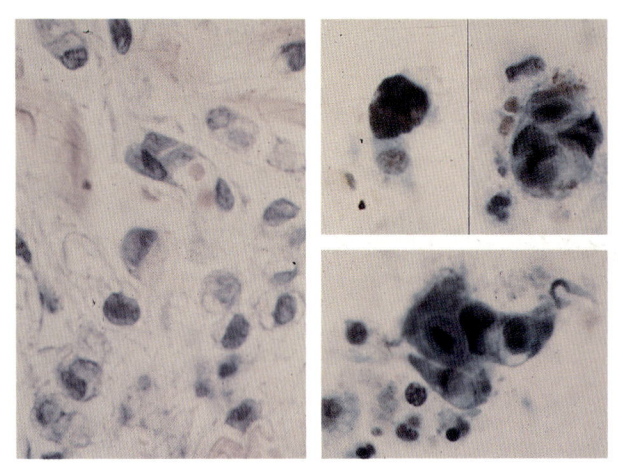

Figure 27–12. 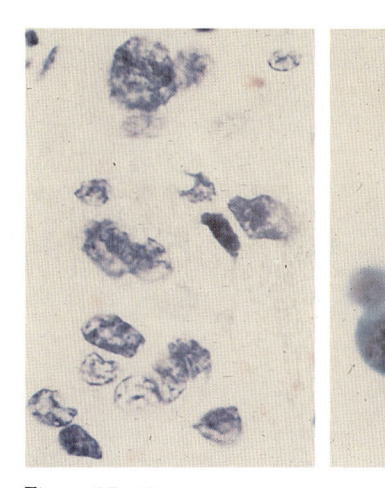 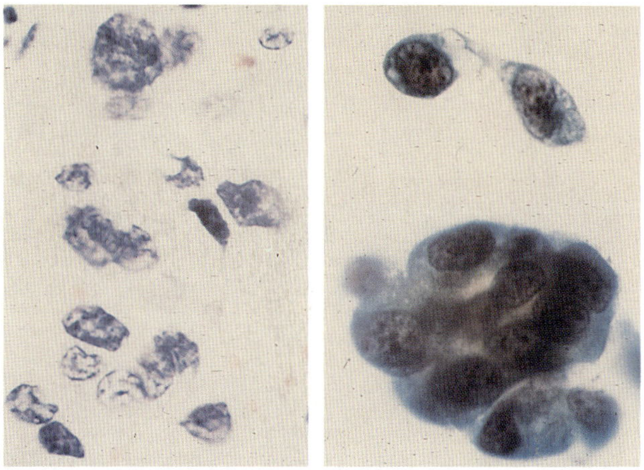   Figure 27–13.

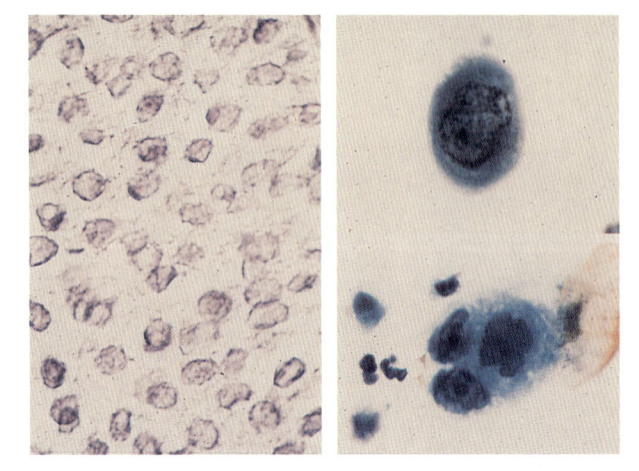

Figure 27–14.

Figure 27–11. Bronchioloalveolar adenocarcinoma (WHO-IIIB). A. Tissue (×100). B. Tissue (×600). C. Cytology (×600).

Figure 27–12. Adenocarcinoma of the breast metastatic to lung. Left: Tissue (×600). Right: Cytology (×600).

Figure 27–13. Adenocarcinoma of pancreas metastatic to lung. Left: Tissue (×600). Right: Cytology (×600).

Figure 27–14. Transitional cell carcinoma of bladder metastatic to lung. Left: Tissue (×600). Right: Cytology (×600).

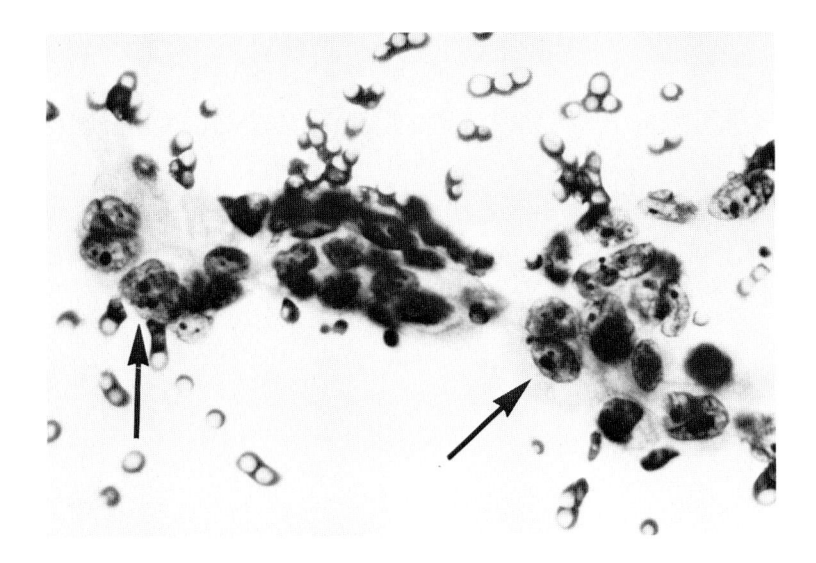

Cytopathology of Fine Needle Aspiration Biopsy 817

Figure 27–31. Poorly differentiated adenocarcinoma. Note prominent nucleoli within many cells (arrows). Cells in center have scanter cytoplasm (PAP, ×500).

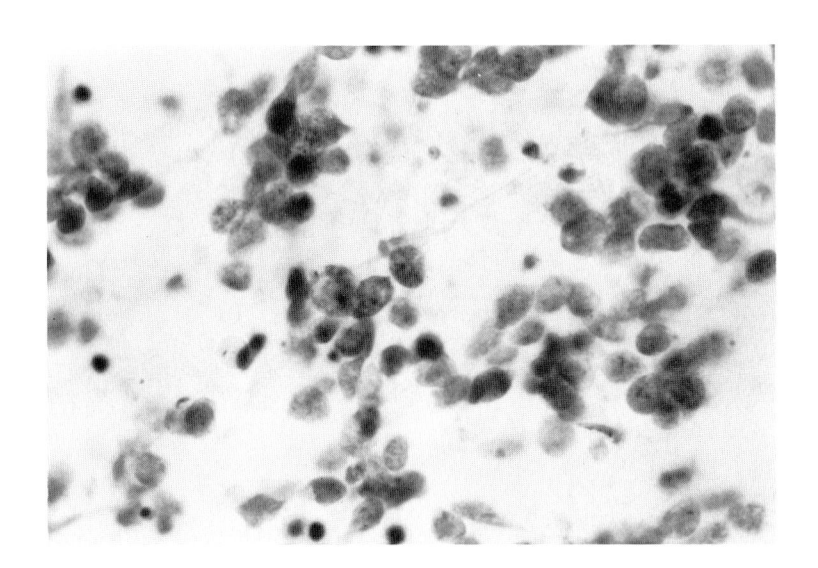

Figure 27–32. Small cell anaplastic carcinoma. Syncytial groups of cells with dark staining, irregularly shaped nuclei and scant to absent cytoplasm (PAP, ×500).

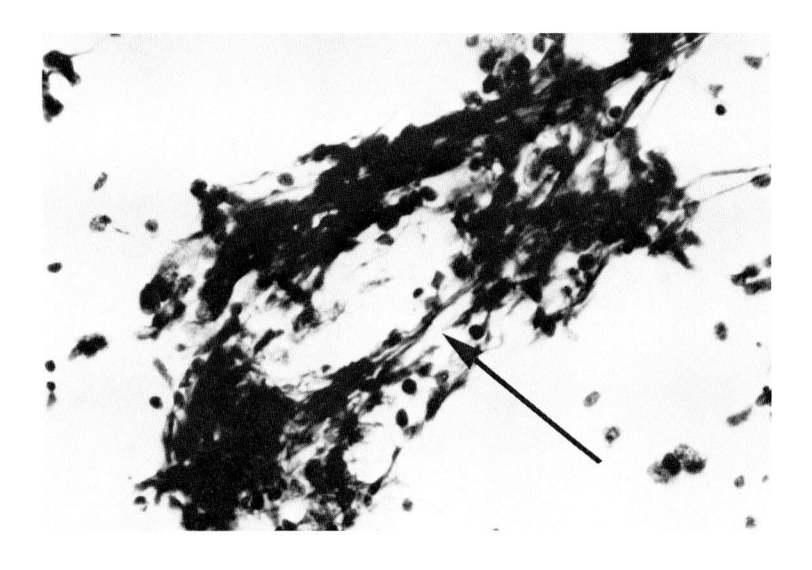

Figure 27–33. Small-cell anaplastic carcinoma, streaks of nuclear material (arrow) (PAP, ×325).

818   Diagnostic Cytology

Figure 27–34. Large-cell carcinoma. Cells show a moderate amount of ill-defined cytoplasm, nuclei with finely granular chromatin, and prominent nucleoli (PAP, ×500).

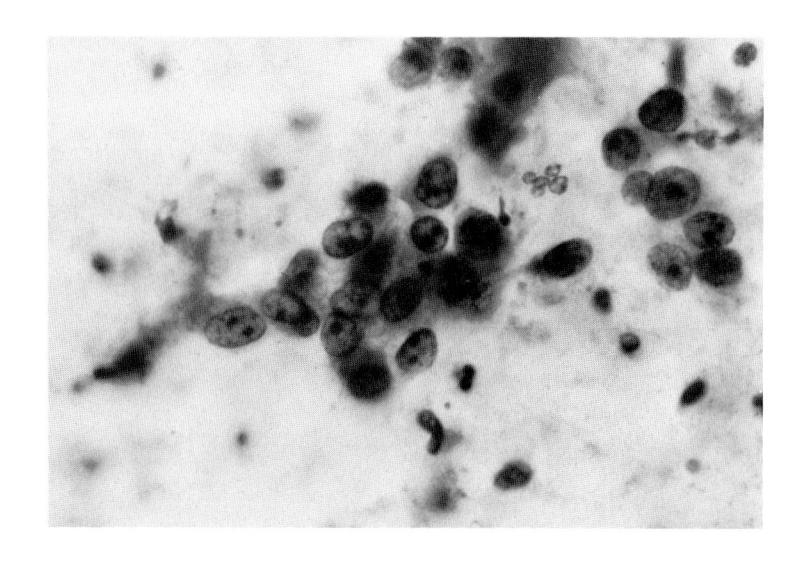

Figure 27–35. Large-cell carcinoma. Cells have large nuclei and ill-defined cytoplasm. Necrotic background is common (center) (Wright-Giemsa, ×325).

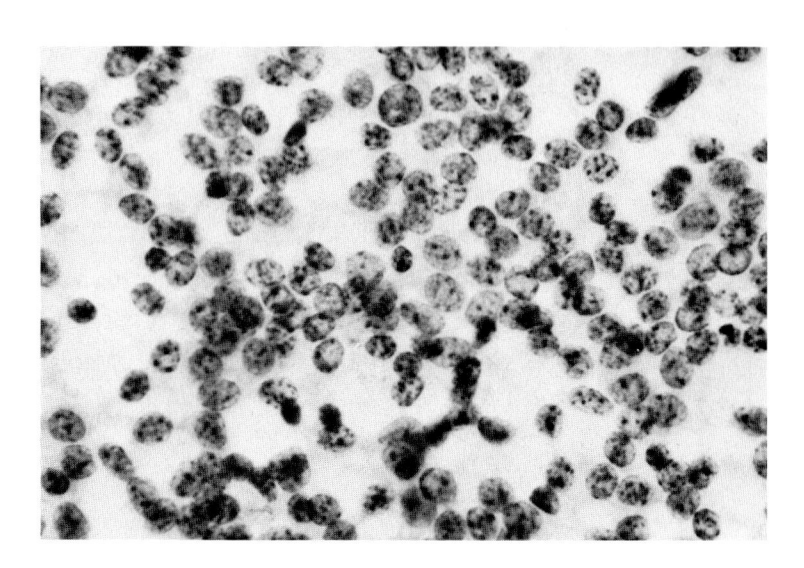

Figure 27–36. Carcinoid tumor. Round to oval nuclei show typical "salt and pepper" chromatin pattern (PAP, ×500).

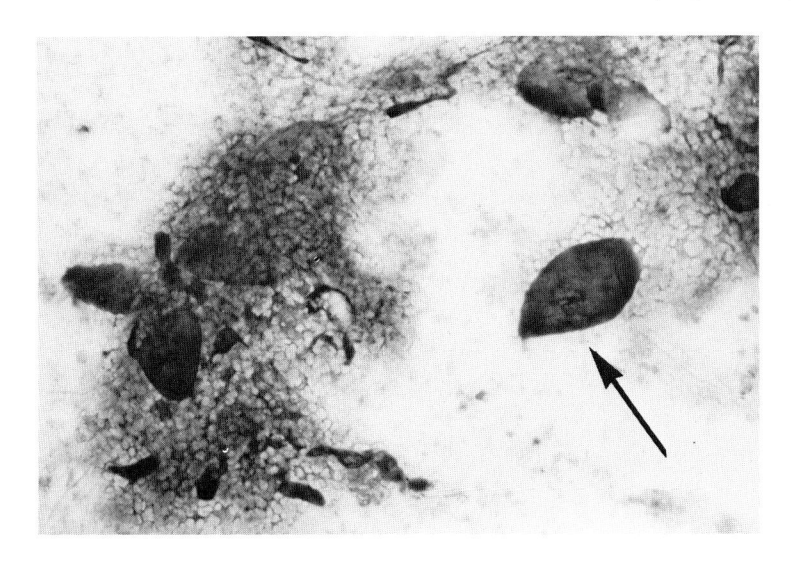

Figure 27-37. Adenoid cystic carcinoma. The hyaline stromal balls are the dense rounded structures, metachromatic on Wright-Giemsa stain (arrow) (Wright-Giemsa, ×125).

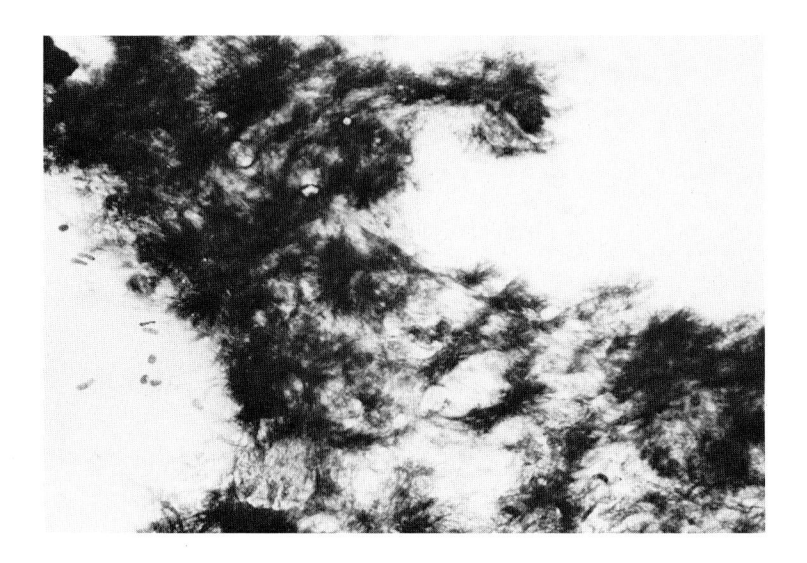

Figure 27-38. Pleomorphic adenoma. Abundant metachromatic stroma (Wright-Giemsa, ×125).

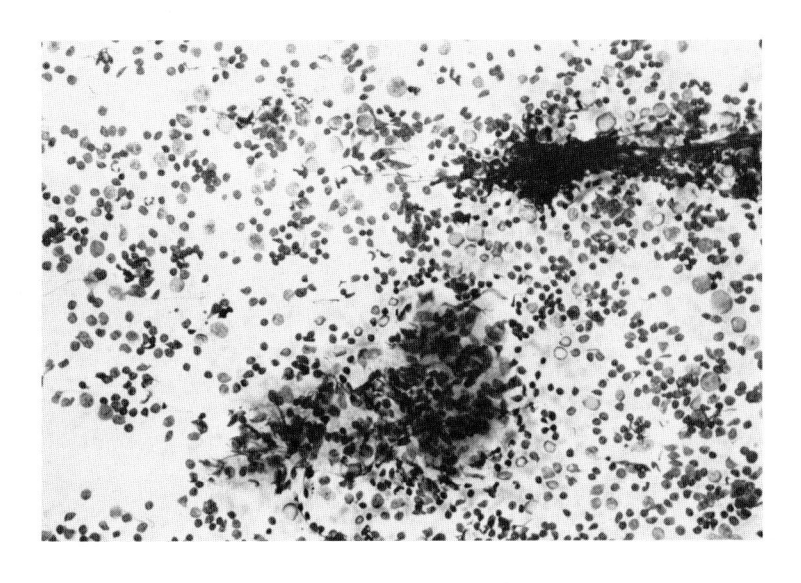

Figure 27-39. Lymphoid tissue from reactive process showing aggregate of germinal center cells (center) and lymphoid crush (upper right). The rest of the cells are single (Wright-Giemsa, ×160).

820   Diagnostic Cytology

Figure 27–40. Mesothelioma, epithelial type. Note large, round to oval nuclei with prominent nucleolus and abundant cytoplasm (PAP, ×325).

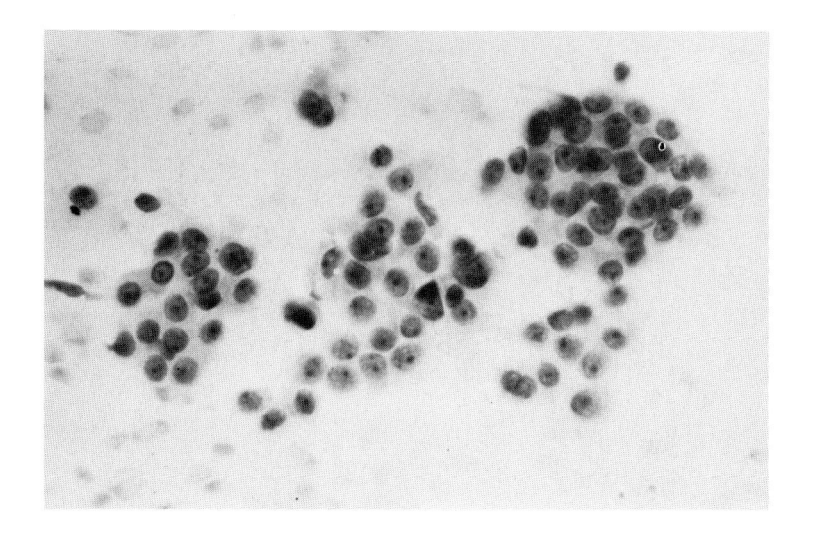

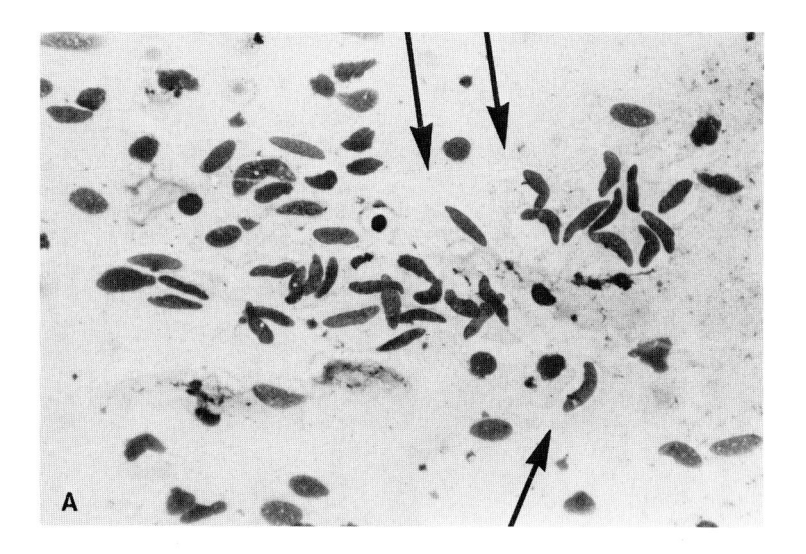

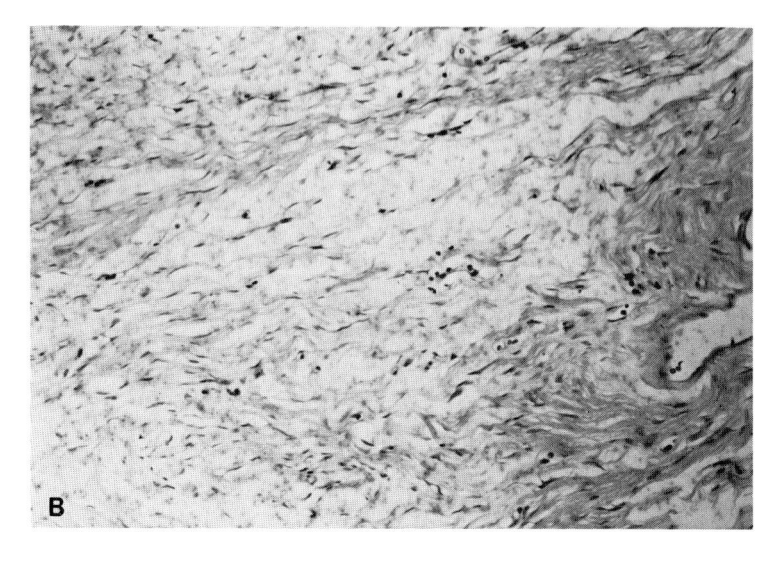

Figure 27–41. A. Fibrous mesothelioma. Spindle cells with finely granular chromatin and elongate cytoplasm, blue on Wright-Giemsa, here white in contrast to granular background (arrows). Note debris in background (blue staining on Wright-Giemsa) that probably represents myxoid connective tissue material (Wright-Giemsa, ×325). B. Tissue section, same case. Spindle cells embedded in myxoid and collagenous stroma (H&E, ×125).

Figure 27–42. Pulmonary hamartoma. A. Cartilaginous matrix (PAP, ×125). B. Myxoid spindle cell stroma (left) and bland epithelial cells (right) (PAP, ×325). C. Spindle cell stroma (metachromatic on Wright-Giemsa), scattered bland epithelial cells, and cartilaginous matrix (arrow) (PAP, ×160).

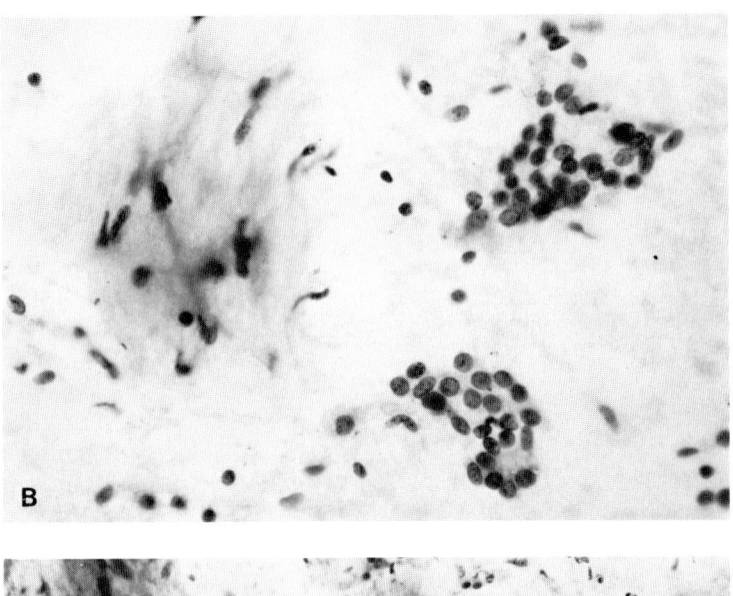

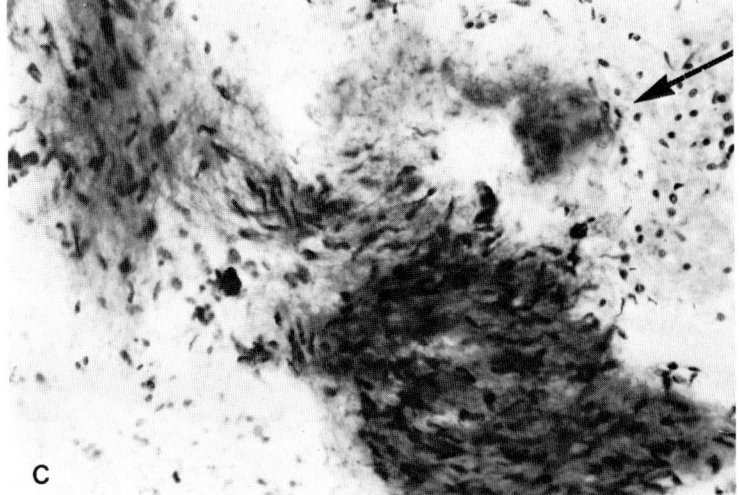

and small bland epithelial cells of bronchiolar and alveolar type (Fig. 27–42). On radiographs, these tumors are generally well defined and usually less than 4 cm in diameter. Wright-Giemsa stains of aspirated material are useful because the cartilage stains bright to dark blue and the stroma stains bright pink. Since these connective tissue elements may not aspirate well using a beveled needle, the Rotex needle may be better for sampling.

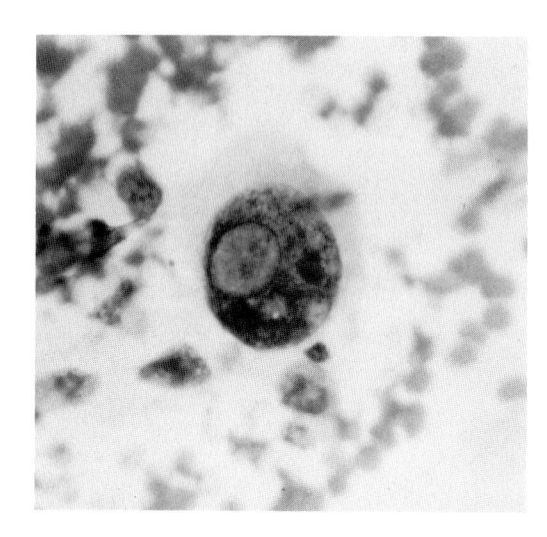

Figure 27–43. Metastatic melanoma. Large tumor cell with intranuclear inclusions (PAP, ×500).

Metastatic Tumors

The cytology of these tumors corresponds to the primary lesion; thus, histologic sections of the original tumor are helpful in the determination of whether a lesion represents a metastasis or second primary in the lung. Special stains for melanin, lipids, or mucins may be done in order to confirm a diagnosis of melanoma, renal cell carcinoma, or adenocarcinoma, respectively. In the case of melanoma, the presence of intranuclear inclusions (Fig. 27–43) and predominance of numerous single cells may suggest the diagnosis, especially in the absence of visible melanin. Metastatic breast adenocarcinoma may show cytoplasmic granularity and, rarely, the presence of pink cytoplasmic inclusions on Wright's stain.[2]

References

1. Bonfiglio TA: *Cytopathologic Interpretation of Transthoracic Fine-Needle Biopsies*. New York: Masson, 1983.
2. Linsk JA, Franzen S: *Clinical Aspiration Cytology*. Philadelphia: JB Lippincott, 1983.
3. Perez-Atayde AR, Seiler MW: Pulmonary hamartoma: An ultrastructural study. Cancer 53:485–492, 1984.

Additional Reading

Auffermann W, Bocking A: *Early Detection of Precancerous Lesions in Dysplasias of the Lung by Rapid DNA Image Cytometry*. Anal Quant Cytol Histol 7(3):218, 1985.

Broghamer WL Jr, Richards ME, Biscopink RJ, Faurest SH: Pulmonary cytologic examination in the identification of the second primary carcinoma of the lung. Cancer 56(11):2664, 1985.

Covell JL, Feldman PS: Fine needle aspiration diagnosis of aspiration pneumonia (Phytopneumonitis). Acta Cytol 28:77–80, 1984.

Greenberg SD: *Recent Advances in Pulmonary Cytopathology*. Hum Pathol 14(10):901, 1983.

Harrow EM, Oldenburg FA, Smith AM: Transbronchial needle aspiration in clinical practice. Thorax 40(10):756, 1985.

Kato H, Konaka C, Ono J, et al.: *Cytology of the Lung: Techniques and Interpretation*. New York: Igaku-Shoin, 1983.

Katzenstein AA, Askin FB: *Surgical Pathology of Non-Neoplastic Lung Disease. Major Problems in Pathology*, vol 13. Philadelphia: WB Saunders, 1982.

McDowell EM, Trump BF: Histogenesis of preneoplastic and neoplastic lesions in tracheobronchial epithelium. Surv Synth Pathol Res 2:235, 1983.

Moloo Z, Finley RJ, Lefcoe MS, et al.: Possible spread of bronchogenic carcinoma to the chest wall after a transthoracic fine needle aspiration biopsy (a case report). Acta Cytol 29:167–170, 1984.

Risse EKJ, van't Hof MA, Laurini RN, Vooijs PG: Sputum cytology by the Saccomanno method in diagnosing lung malignancy. Diag Cytopathol 1(4):286, 1985.

Saccomanno G: *Carcinoma In Situ of the Lung: Its Development, Detection, and Treatment*. Semin Resp Med 4:156, 1982.

Schumann GB, DiFiore K, Johnston JL: Sputum cytodiagnosis of disseminated histiocytic lymphoma: A case report. Acta Cytol 27:262, 1983.

Silverman JF, Finley JL, Park HK, et al.: Fine needle aspiration cytology of bronchioloalveolar-cell carcinoma of the lung. Acta Cytol 29:887–894, 1985.

Silverman JF, Johnsrude IS: Fine needle aspiration cytology of granulomatous cryptococcosis of the lung. Acta Cytol 29: 157–161, 1985.

Silverman JF, Weaver MD, Shaw R, Newman WJ: Fine needle aspiration cytology of pulmonary infarct. Acta Cytol 29:162–166, 1985.

Strobel SL, Keyhani-Rofagha S, O'Toole RV, Jahman BJ: Non-aspiration-needle smear preparations of pulmonary lesions. A comparison of cytology and histology. Acta Cytol 29:1047–1052, 1985.

Tanaka T, Yamamoto M, Tamura T, et al.: Cytologic and histologic correlation in primary lung cancer. A study of 154 cases with resectable tumors. Acta Cytol 29:49–56, 1985.

Truong LD, Underwood RD, Greenberg SD, McLarty JW: Diagnosis and typing of lung carcinomas by cytopathologic methods. A review of 108 cases. Acta Cytol 29:379–384, 1985.

Yesner R: *Small Cell Tumors of the Lung*. Am J Surg Pathol 8:775, 1983.

Index

Acid-fast bacteria, special stains, 102
Acid maltase deficiency, see Pompe's disease
Acinus
   anatomy and histology, 23–29
   blood supply to, 24–25
   branching variability and complexity, 28
   quantitative anatomy, 54
Acquired immunodeficiency syndrome (AIDS), 247, 308
   Kaposi's sarcoma in lung with, 258
Actinomyces, special stains, 102
Actinomycosis, 210–212
Adenocarcinomas
   development of, 320–321
   fine needle aspiration biopsy, 812–813
   mixed, 352
   survival by histologic subtype, 358, 360
Adenoid cystic carcinoma, 377, 381
Adenoid cystic sarcoma, 814, 819
Adenomatoid malformations, congenital, 121–125
Adenosquamous carcinoma, 352, 354
   mixed, 814
Adenovirus infections
   diffuse alveolar damage in, 163
   of lower respiratory tract, 159–165
Adrenocorticotropic hormone (ACTH), in lung cancer, 354
Adult respiratory distress syndrome (ARDS), 129, 268–279, 425
   bronchiolitis obliterans in, 447
   and diffuse alveolar damage, 269
   drug-related, 505
   hyaline membrane formation, 269–270, 271
   noxious gases and fumes, 276–277
   pneumonocyte proliferation, 270–271
   preclinical and clinical phases, 269–275
Aerobic bacteria, pneumonia caused by, 196–203
Aerosols, 58–59
   defined, 591
Agenesis, pulmonary, 115, 116
Aging lung, 54
   changes occurring in, 555–556
   emphysema-like conditions in, 555–556
Air embolism, in fine needle aspiration, 112
Airflow, see also Chronic airflow obstruction
   mucous gland enlargement, 533
   viral infections and, 174–176
Air pollutants

   human and experimental evidence, 667–668
   photochemical reactions of, 57
   prediction of risks from 667–668
Air space
   exudates in infiltrative lung disease, 431
   flooding in interstitial space, 267
Airways
   anatomy and histology, 14–23
   bacterial infections, 186–190
   casting techniques, 98
   changes in chronic bronchitis, 533–535
   classification, 14
   conducting, 51–53
   fibrosis in, 521
   Horsfield-Cumming model, 52
   inflammation in asthma, 578, 580
   intrauterine development of, 1–2
   and lung parenchyma, 519–520
   models of, 52
   nonciliated, clearance from, 60
   protection provided by, 58
   quantitative anatomy, 51–53
   resistance, partitioning of, 520
   smoking and epithelium changes, 318
   transitional and respiratory zones, 53
   Weibel's model, 52
   zone categories, 51–53
Alagille's syndrome, 117
Alcoholism
   and atelectasis, 752, 755
   Proteus bacteria in, 196
Allescheria boydii, 237
Alternaria, 232
Aluminum, uses and risks, 658
Aluminum disorders, pathology and pathogenesis, 658
Alveolar proteinosis, 479–482, 606
   in immunocompromised patient, 251–253
Alveolar wall
   anatomy and histology, 26–29
   cell types, 31
   interstitial space, 263, 267
   tissue loss in aging lung, 555
Alveolitis
   cryptogenic fibrosing, 440
   extrinsic allergic, 584, 586
Alveolus, 2, 7; see also Diffuse alveolar injury
   in aging lung, 555
   capillary dysplasia in neonate, 117
   duct anatomy and histology, 25

   macrophage as defense mechanism, 60–62
   septal amyloidosis, 492
   surface complexity decrease, 555
Amine precursor uptake and decarboxylation cells, 21
Aminorex fumarate, in pulmonary hypertension, 714
Ammonia disorders, 665
Amniotic fluid, 116
   "infection syndrome," 134
Amosite asbestos, 627
Amphibole asbestos, 627, 630
Amyloidosis, 489–493
   of hilar lymph nodes, 493
   multisystemic or systemic, 493
   primary and multisystemic, 489–493
Anaerobic infections, 203–205
Anasarca, fetal, 121
Anatomy
   general features, 11–13
   and histology, 11–50
   normal, 12–50
   quantitative, 51–55
Angiitis (vasculitis), 283–302
   clinical features, 284
   defined, 283
   drug-related, 506
   histologic features, 285, 290
   and polyarteritis, 290
   sites of involvement, 289
   treatment and prognosis, 290
Angioimmunoblastic lymphadenopathy, 77
Angiokeratoma, see Fabry's disease
Angiotension converting enzyme (ACE) in sarcoidosis, 464
Ankylosing spondylitis, pulmonary involvement in, 462
Anomalous venous return, in neonate infant and child, 117
Anorexigens, in pulmonary hypertension, 714
Anthrax, cutaneous vs. inhaled, 210
Antibodies, for microbiologic diagnosis, 102
Anticoagulant therapy, 112
Antidiuretic hormone, and pleural disease, 781
Antigen-antibody complexes, in byssinosis, 670
Antigens, 64
   in hypersensitivity pneumonitis, 582–583
Antiglomerular basement membrane disease (AGBMD), 303–305

Antimony disorders, 661–662
Antitrypsin, abnormalities in familial emphysema, 544–546
Aortopulmonary lymph nodes, 63
Arsenic fumes, 663
Arterial anomalies, in neonate infant and child, 117, 136
Arterial oxygen desaturation, in liver disease, 721–722
Arteries, pulmonary
  developmental anomalies of, 734–735
  dilated vein-like branches of, 697
  elastic, 32, 36, 705–708
  in emphysema, 724–726
  hypertension effects, 705–708
  longitudinal muscle in, 694
  postnatal growth, 8–9
  quantitative anatomy, 54
Arteriograms, in postmortem examination, 97
Arterioles, pulmonary, 34
Arteriopathy, plexogenic pulmonary, 700
Arteritis, necrotizing, 699
Asbestiform minerals, composition and structure, 626
Asbestos
  bodies, 634–636
  cellular mechanisms, 647
  comparative responses to, 648
  habits and fibers, 626
  main varieties of, 627
  molecular dispositions, 627, 630
  occupational and other sources of exposure, 628–629
  sources and uses, 627
  uncoated and coated fibers, 634–636
  urban exposure to, 648
  workers, rounded atelectasis in, 757–759
Asbestos disorders, 626–648
  malignant mesothelioma, 644–647, 787–790
  mineralogy, 626–629
  pleural plaques, 642–644
Asbestosis, 629–642
  clinical correlations and sequelae, 640–642
  diagnosis of, 633–636
  dust quantity and fiber type, 636–638
  epidemiology and pathologic reaction, 636–637
  extraction procedures, 636
  fibrocystic, 630, 632
  fibrogenesis mechanisms, 638–639
  focal lesions, 632–633
  gross and microscopic features, 630–633
  immunologic component, 639–640
  lung cancer prevalence and morphology, 640–641
  pathogenesis of, 636–640
  prevalence and pathologic anatomy, 629–636
  radiologic and physiologic correlations, 640
Aspergillosis, 232–234
Aspiration, 751–752
  and bronchial obstruction, 751–767
  causes and results, 752
  foreign body, 751
  of gastric acid, 751
  of lipid material, 752
  lung abscess and, 762
  pneumonia, 760
Asthma, 577–581
  airways inflammation and mast cells, 578–580
  and bronchocentric granulomatosis, 296, 299

childhood, 176
chronic airflow obstruction in, 562
complications, 581
drug-related, 505
mucous plugging of airways, 580–581
pathology of, 577
smooth muscle spasm in, 578
Atelectasis, 752–759
  causes of, 752–756
  pathophysiology and clinical findings, 754–755
  radiology and pathology, 756
  right middle lobe, 756–757
  rounded, 757–759
  special types of, 756–759
Atherosclerosis, of pulmonary trunk, 707–708
Autopsy, 95–100; see also Examination
  for emphysema, 96
  lung inflation during, 95
  microbiologic diagnosis, 101–102
  vs. open lung biopsy, 259
  slicing methods, 95–96
  special procedures, 96–98
Axoneme, structure of, 16

Bacteremia
  in burn patients, 199
  with lobar pneumonia, 192
Bacterial infections, 185–220
  actinomycosis, 210–212
  acute tracheobronchitis, 186
  of airways, 186–190
  anaerobic, 203–205
  anthrax, 210
  brucellosis, 209–210
  diptheria, 186–187
  gram-negative aerobic, 196–203
  nocardia, 212
  plague, 205–207
  pneumococcal pneumonia, 190–192
  pseudomycosis, 214–215
  routes of, 185–186
  staphylococcal pneumonia, 193–196
  streptococcal pneumonia, 192–193
  syphilis, 212–214
  tularemia, 207–209
  unusual variants of lung abscess, 214–215
  whooping cough, 187–190
Barium disorders, 662
Basal cell hyperplasia, 318
BCG (bacillus Calmette-Guérin) infection, 223
Behçet's syndrome, pulmonary involvement in, 462
Benign clear-cell tumor, 405–407, 408
Bentonite disorders, 653
Beryllium
  composition of, 655
  uses and risks, 655
Beryllium disease, 655–657
  complications of, 657
  pathology and pathogenesis, 656–657
Beta-hemolytic streptococcal pneumonia, 192–193
Beveled needle, 109
Bilateral pulmonary hypoplasia etiology of, 116
Biopsy, see also Fine needle aspiration
  diagnostic yield and long-term consequences, 255–260
  handling and diagnostic limitations, 67–78
  in immunocompromised patients, 255–260
  invasive, 256

open and transbronchial, 67–77
Birds, host for chlamydia, 183
Blastomas
  and carcinosarcomas, 385–392
  as epithelial tumors, 391
Blastomycosis
  etiology and histopathology, 231–232
  granulomatous inflammation in, 234
  morphologic features, 235
  North American, 230–232
Bleeding diathesis, 112
Blending vessel, for sputum processing, 106–107
Blood
  clearance by, 62–63
  dyscrasias, 308
  monocytes, 60–61
Blood vessels
  development of, 2–3
  in pulmonary venous hypertension, 710–711
Blue boater syndrome, 553
Blue bodies, intra-alveolar, 499–500
Bubonic plague, 206
Bochdalek's hernia, 138
Bombesin, enolase and, 356
Bone marrow transplants, 174
Bone meal, anthrax from, 210
Bordetella pertussis, 187–188
Botryomycosis, 214–215
Breast carcinoma, pleural biopsy showing, 769, 771
Breathing difficulty, see Dyspnea
Bronchi
  anatomy and histology, 14–20
  arteries and veins, 3, 33, 563
  brushing and cytology, 108, 804
  congenital anomalies, 115
  diptheria of, 188
  endocrine cells, histochemistry of, 23
  gland tumors, aspiration of, 814, 819
  lavage and exfoliative cytology, 108
  measles-induced inflammation, 153
  mucosal anatomy and histology, 15
  neoplasms and salivary gland tumors, 378–379
  submucosal bony metaplasia, 502
Bronchial amyloidosis, 565
Bronchial atresia, 547
Bronchial obstruction, 751–767
  arteries and veins, 563
  lung abscess and, 762
Bronchiectasis, 558–562, 763–766
  airway lesions, 560
  classification of, 559
  clinical features, 561
  congenital, 116, 561
  cylindrical, 559
  gross and microscopic lesions, 559–560
  parenchymal and other lesions, 560–561
  pathophysiology, 763–764
  saccular, 559
  treatment and prognosis, 764–766
  varicose, 559
Bronchioles
  anatomy and histology, 22–23
  mucosal lining and epithelium, 25–26
Bronchiolitis, 521–529
  airway size distribution, 521, 525
  cryptogenic obliterative, 527–528
  in immunocompromised patient, 256
  respiratory, 159–160, 524–525
  rheumatoid, 526–527
  sequelae, 521–526
  special forms of, 526–529

Bronchiolitis obliterans
   chronic airflow obstruction in, 528–529
   drug-related, 504
   etiology and differential diagnosis, 445–447
   and organizing pneumonia, 71, 74, 444–448
   spectrum of, 529
Bronchioloalveolar carcinoma
   cell types found in, 349
   intravascular sclerosing, 385
   pathological features, 343–349
   prognosis and survival, 359
   radiographic abnormalities, 352
Bronchitis, 148; see also Chronic bronchitis
   acute, 186
   viral infections and, 174
Bronchitis obliterans, 127, 130
Bronchocentric granulomatosis, 296–300
Bronchogenic carcinoma, 311–360; see also Lung cancer
Bronchograms, in postmortem examination, 97
Bronchopneumonia, pneumococcal, 190
Bronchopulmonary dysplasia, 124, 127, 129
   complications and long-term prognosis, 133
   etiology, 130
   evolution of, 128
   variant form, 132, 133
Bronchoscopy, fine needle aspiration vs., 112
Brucellosis, 209–210
Brushings, bronchial, 108
Bullae and blebs in emphysema, 549–550
Burn patients, pseudomonas bacteremia in, 199
Byssinosis, 668–670
   exposure sources, 668
   pathogenesis of, 670
   syndrome and pathology, 669

Cadmium fumes, lung disorders due to, 662–663
Calcification, 496–500
   dystrophic and metastatic, 496–498
   lesions and histologic features, 495
   metastatic, 496–498, 505
Calcitonin, in lung cancer, 355
Calcium oxalate, in giant cell granulomas, 500
Campbell-Williams syndrome, 116
Canalicular phase, of lung development, 1, 3
Cancer, see Lung cancer
Candida, typical yeasts, 239
Candidiasis, 235–237
Capillaries, pulmonary, 34
Caplan's syndrome, 621
Carbonaceous dust, 607–626
Carbon pneumoconiosis, 613
Carborundum disorders, 654
Carcinogens
   in cigarette smoke, 312
   dose-response relationship, 317
   lung cancer after exposure to, 316
Carcinoid tumors, 362–373
   central and peripheral, 365–369
   fine needle aspiration biopsy, 814, 818
   high-grade, 369, 374
   histogenesis and ultrastructure, 362
   prognosis, 369–371
   small-cell carcinoma relation to, 331–335
   substances produced by, 362–365
   types of, 364
   unusual variants, 373

Carcinoma, see also Bronchogenic carcinoma
   diagnostic cytology, 808
   invasive, 808
   metastatic, 808
   mucoepidermoid, 376, 380
   pathologic staging problems, 83
   transbronchial biopsy, 73
Carcinosarcomas, blastomas and, 385–392
Cardiac atrophy, chronic airflow obstruction and, 563
Cardiac shunts, congenital, 700
Cardiovascular disease, 308
Cardiovascular system, 32–39
   chronic airflow obstruction and, 562–563
Carotid bodies, and pulmonary circulation, 726–728
Cartilage atrophy, in chronic bronchitis, 534–535
Catecholamines, in lung cancer, 356
Cat lung worm, 733
Cattle, brucellosis from, 209
Cell-mediated immunity, 64–65
Cellular infiltrates, and epithelial proliferation in lung disease, 429–430
Cement disorders, 654
Centrifuge tube, for sputum processing, 107
Centrilobular emphysema, 539, 540
   in coal workers, 624
   morphology and associations, 541–542
   with panacinar emphysema and chronic airflow obstruction, 547
Cerium disorders, 662
Chemicals, ingestion of, 277–278
Chemodectoma, 373
   minute pulmonary, 377–379
Chemoreceptor tissue, and pulmonary circulation, 726–729
Chemotherapy, 277–278
Chest, see Thorax
Chiba needle, 109
Chickenpox, see Varicella zoster
Chilaiditi's syndrome, 138
Child, 115–146
   acute tracheobronchitis in, 186
   adenomatoid malformation, 121–123
   bronchogenic cysts in, 120–121, 122
   bronchopulmonary sequestration in, 118–120
   congenital anomalies, 115–117
   Hemophilus influenzae in, 197
   histoplasmosis in, 225
   pulmonary lymphangiectasis, 123, 126
   respiratory syncytial virus, 151–159
   staphylococcal pneumonia in, 196
   varicella zoster in, 167
   vascular anomalies, 117–135
Chlamydia
   pneumonitis, 134, 138
   types of, 182–183
Chlorine gas, 665
Cholestasis, in child, 117
Chondrosarcoma, 384
Chorionic gonadotrophin, in lung cancer, 355
Chromium disorders, 660
Chronic airflow obstruction, 519–575
   alterations in other organs, 562–564
   asthma, 562
   bronchial amyloidosis, 565
   in bronchiectasis, 558–562
   bronchiolitis, 521–529
   in chronic bronchitis, 529–538
   defined, 519
   diseases associated with, 519
   in emphysema, 538–555

emphysema-like conditions, 555–557
   immotile cilia syndrome, 566–567
   lesions in peripheral airways, 521–526
   panacinar with centrilobular emphysema, 547
   relapsing perichondritis, 565–566
   tracheal stenosis, 565
   tracheobronchomegaly, 565
   tracheobronchopathica osteoplastica, 564–565
   viral infections and, 174–176
Chronic bronchitis, 529–538
   airway changes in, 533–535
   bronchial wall pits and airway lesions, 535
   and dust exposure, 668
   emphysema and, 535–536
   epidemiology, etiology and pathogenesis, 537–538
   mucous gland enlargement, in, 537
   muscle increase and cartilage atrophy, 534–535
Chrysotile asbestos, 627, 630, 637
Churg-Strauss syndrome, 289–290, 478
Chylothorax, 774–775
Cigarette smoking
   airway epithelium changes, 318
   and bronchogenic carcinoma, 311–313
   and coal worker's pneumoconiosis, 619
   number and depth of inhalation, 312
Cigar smoking, lung cancer mortality, 312
Cilia, 15–17
   as defense mechanism, 59–60
Circulation, pulmonary
   carotid bodies and, 726–728
   chemoreceptor tissue and, 726–729
   Feyrter cells and neuroepithelial bodies, 728
   glomus pulmonale and venous glomic tissue, 728
   in liver disease, 721–723
   parasites of, 731–733
   schistosomiasis and filaria, 731–732
Classical nodular silicosis, 594–602
   diagnosis and sequelae, 602
   gross and microscopic features, 595–597
   pathologic anatomy and pathogenesis, 595–602
   prevalence and occupations at risk, 594–595
   sequelae and associations, 602
Clear-cell tumor, benign, 405–407, 408
Coagulation disorders, 112
Coal dust, 607–626
   comparative responses to, 648
   simple lesion diagram, 612
Coal workers
   acinar and panacinar emphysema in, 624
   emphysematous and fibrocystic states in, 624–626
   fibrocystic disease in, 625
Coal worker's pneumoconiosis, 607–621
   dust quantity and composition, 614
   gross and microscopic features, 608–613
   life expectancy factors, 620
   mineralogy and prevalence, 607–608
   pathologic anatomy and pathogenesis, 608–618
   radiologic and physiologic correlations, 618–619
   sequelae, 618–621
   simple and complicated, 608–613
   vascular changes, 612–613
Coccidioidomycosis, 227–228
Colds, 148
Collagen vascular disease, 451–462

Collagen vascular disease *(cont.)*
  diffuse pulmonary hemorrhage (DPH) with, 305–306
  DPH and nephropathy without, 306–307
  pleural effusion in, 771
  pleuropulmonary lesions in, 456
Collapsed lung, *see* Atelectasis
Complicated pneumoconiosis
  gross and microscopic features, 609–613
  immunologic factors, 617–618
  quartz and infective factors, 616–617
  total dust factor, 616
Conchoidal bodies, 500
Congenital anomalies
  of lower espiratory tract, 115–117
  in neonate, infant and child, 115–117
Congestion, chronic passive from mitral steosis, 501
Connective tissue, 3–4
  postnatal development, 9
  skeleton, 29
Cor pulmonale
  asbestosis sequelae, 640
  chronic airflow obstruction and, 562
  pneumoconiosis sequelae, 620
  silicotic sequelae, 602
Coronavirus, 159
Corpora amylacea, 502, 503
Corynebacteria, 186
Coxiella infections, 183–184
Crocidolite asbestos, 627, 637
Crotalaria, in pulmonary hypertension, 712–713
Croup (laryngotracheobronchitis), 156
Cryoglobulinemia
  essential mixed, 462
  pulmonary involvement in, 462
Cryptococcosis, 228–230
  identification of organisms, 229
  in immunocompromised patient, 231
Cushing's syndrome, and carcinoid tumors, 365, 375
Cutis laxa, 117
Cylindroma, 377–378
Cystic fibrosis, in newborn, 139–140
Cysts
  bronchogenic, in neonates, 120, 122
  subpleural, 140
Cytology, *see also* Diagnostic cytology
  diagnostic techniques, 105–114
  expoliative techniques, 105–109
  sputum collection, 105–106
Cytomegalovirus infections
  epidemiology and morphology, 172–174
  inclusions and virions, 175, 176
  in lung abscess, 173
  of respiratory tract, 172–174
Cytoplasm, outpouchings and desmosomes, 328, 330
Cytoxic drugs, in diffuse alveolar damage/ interstitial pneumonia, 251

Deer fly, tularemia from, 207
Defense mechanisms, 57–66
Dental plaque, actinomycosis in, 211
Deposition, physiologic and morphologic factors, 592
Desquamative interstitial pneumonia (DIP), 435–444
  background and clinical features, 435–436
  vs. crytogenic fibrosing alveolitis, 440
  histology and differential diagnosis, 440–443

  pathogenesis and gross morphology, 436–437
  steroid response, 445
  treatment of, 444
Developmental anomalies
  in arterial hypertension, 689
  of arteries and veins, 734–736
  of pulmonary trunk, 733–734
Diabetes, 124
Diagnosis, *see* Microbiologic diagnosis
Diagnostic cytology, 803–822
  primary carcinomas, 806–807
Diaphragm disorders, 116, 564
  in newborn, 138–139
Diatomite pneumoconiosis, 603–604
  exposure and prevalence, 603
Diesel emissions, and coal worker's pneumoconiosis, 619–620
Dietary pulmonary hypertension, 712–714
  from anorexigens, 714
  pyrrolizidine alkaloids in, 712–713
Diffuse alveolar damage (DAD)
  acute stage, 269–270
  chemical ingestion and, 277–278
  diagnosis of, 71, 74
  drugs causing, 251, 277, 503
  etiology, 275–279
  experimentally induced, 273
  honeycomb lung stage, 272
  in immunocompromised patient, 248–251
  liquid aspiration in, 276
  paraquat lung and, 278
  proliferative phase, 271, 274
  pulmonary edema and, 263–282
  repair phase, 269, 272
  vs. UIP, 274
Diffuse pulmonary hemorrhage (DPH), 303–310
  from acute long injury, 308
  from blood dyscrasias, 308
  from cardiovascular disease, 308
  classification of, 304
  with collagen vascular diseases, 305–306
  from drug reactions, 308
  in immunocompromised patient, 255
  and nephropathy without collagen vascular disease or immunologic abnormality, 306–307
  SLE-associated, 306
  tumor-induced, 308
Dilated vein-like branches, in plexogenic pulmonary arteriopathy, 697
Diphtheria, 186–187
Dirofilariasis, 241–243
  distribution and life cycle, 243
Distal acinar emphysema, 547–549
Distant metastasis, staging in lung cancer, 81, 83
Dog heartworm disease, *see* Dirofilariasis
Dogs, parainfluenza in, 157
Down's syndrome, pulmonary hypoplasia in, 116
Drowning, 276
Drug abusers, staphylococcal pneumonia in, 195
"Drug lung," 71
Drug reactions, 502–506
  histologic patterns, 503–504
  primary and secondary, 502
Drugs, 503
  clinical pathologic pulmonary syndromes, 505–506
Ductus arteriosus, persistent patency of, 126
Dusts, 607–626
  coal mine and carbonaceous, 607–626

  defined, 591
  emphysema due to, 540
  exposure and chronic bronchitis, 668
  macule specificity in pneumoconiosis, 615
  proximal acinar emphysema due to, 542, 624
  quantity factor, 597, 614
Dwarfism, 139
Dynein arms, structure of, 16–18
Dysplasia, 121
Dyspnea, and infiltrative lung disease, 425
Dysproteinemia, in lymphocytic interstitial pneumonia, 449

Echinococcal cysts, 112
Ectopic hormone syndromes, in carcinoid tumors, 364–365
Edema
  ARDS pathophysiology and phases, 269–275
  from chemotherapeutic agents, 278
  classification of, 267–279
  and diffuse alveolar injury, 263–282
  elevated interstitial oncotic pressure, 268
  high altitude, 279
  increased microvascular pressure, 267–268
  lowered interstitial hydrostatic pressure, 268
  low plasma oncotic pressure, 268
  microvascular damage, 268
  neurogenic, 279
  noxious gases and fumes, 276–277
  safety factors to prevent, 267
  smoke inhalation, 277
  specific drugs causing, 278
  uncertain etiology, 279
Ehlers-Danos syndrome, 117
Electron microscopy
  in open lung biopsy, 69
  in postmortem examination, 97
Embolic disease, 740–743
  origin and incidence, 740
Embolism
  massive, 740–741
  nonthrombotic and foreign body, 742–743
Emphysema, 112, 538–555
  age-sex incidence, 552–553
  with bronchial and/or bronchiolar atresia, 547
  bronchiolar lesions in, 526
  bullae and blebs, 549–550
  chronic airflow obstruction in, 538–555
  and chronic bronchitis, 535–536
  classification of, 539–540
  in coal workers, 624–626
  definition and recognition, 538–540
  diagnosis of, 69
  etiology and pathogenesis, 554–555
  examination for, 96
  increased frequency in aging lung, 556
  irregular, 540, 549
  mucous gland enlargement in, 535
  NHLBI workshop definition, 557–558
  panacinar, 540–549
  prevalence and clinicopathologic correlations, 550–554
  pulmonary arteries in, 724–726
  pulmonary interstitial, 120
  vascular lesions in, 724–726
Emphysema-like conditions, 555–557
Empyema, 769–774
  incidence and pathology, 773–774
Endocrine syndromes, in lung cancer spread, 354–356

Index

Endothelium, 40
  metabolic functions of, 39, 41
  specialization and pavement patterns, 36–39
Endotoxins, in byssinosis, 670
End-stage lung disease, *see* Honeycomb lung
Enolase, and bombesin, 356
Ensilage disorders, 664
Enteric cysts, 120
Environmental lung disease, 591–685
  aggregation and translocation, 593
  asbestos, 626–648
  atmospheric pollutants, 667–668
  byssinosis, 668–670
  coal worker's pneumoconiosis, 607–621
  deposition and clearance, 592
  dynamic aspects of, 592–593
  free silica disorders, 594–606
  from coal mine and carbonaceous dusts, 607–626
  fumes and gases, 662–665
  macrophage mobilization and monocyte emigration, 593
  metallic dusts, 655–662
  perspective and terminology, 591–592
  radioactive particles, 665–667
  rheumatoid pneumoconiosis, 621–624
  silicate disorders, 648–655
Eosinophilia, in chronic bronchitis, 534
Eosinophilic pneumonia, 474–479
  chronic, 475–478
  syndromes, 474–479
  treatment of, 479
Eosinophils, in pleural effusions, 773
Epidermoid carcinomas
  histology and cytology, 806–807
  pathological features, 324–330
Epithelium
  cell types, 26–27
  development of, 2
  gas-exchanging, 3
  in infiltrative lung disease, 430
  necrosis and proliferation, 430
Escherichia coli, 197
Evagination, muscular, 34
Examination, 95–100
  of lung resection specimens, 79–93
  special procedures, 96–98
Exfoliative cytology, 105–109
  bronchial brushings and lavages, 108
  sputum collection, 105–106
Extra-alveolar interstitial space, 264–265, 266
  fluid movement in, 267
Extrauterine transition disorders, 123–132

Fabry's disease, 494
Familial emphysema, with antitrypsin abnormalities, 544–546
Farber's disease, 495
Farmers' lung, morphologic features, 586
Fascitis, eosinophilic, 459
Fetoproteins, in lung cancer, 356
Feyrter cells, 21, 728
Fibrobullous disease
  and ankylosing spondylitis, 462
  in coal workers, 624–626
Fibrogenesis, factors in simple silicosis, 597–598
Fibromas, intrapulmonary, 383
Fibrosarcoma, 384
Fibrosis, pulmonary, 688
  bronchoalveolar lavage in, 109
  in bronchopulmonary dysplasia, 131
  diagnosis of, 75–77
  diffuse interstitial, 624
  drug-related, 503, 506
  interstitial and massive, 737–738
  "progressive," 618
  vasculature in, 736–739
Fibrothorax, 775–776
Filaria, 732
Filariasis, 478
Filter cigarettes, 313
Fine needle aspiration
  air-dried smears, 111
  contraindications and complications, 112
  cytopathology of, 809–822
  diagnostic accuracy, 113
  dry vs. saline specimens, 111
  equipment for, 109
  localization of lesion, 111–112
  of neoplasms, 811–822
  normal findings, 809
  pneumothorax complication, 112
  practical considerations, 109–113
  reactive or inflammatory changes, 810
  slide arrangement, 110
  smearing techniques, 110–111
  techniques and indications, 109–112
Fistulas, in neonate infant and child, 117
Flax and hemp workers, lung disease in, 668
Fluorescent antibody techniques, in viral infections, 148
Fly ash disorders, 654
Foamy exudate, interstitial pneumonia with, 251
Foreign body, embolism and aspiration, 742, 751
Francisella tularensis, 297
Free radicals, 57
Free silica disorders, 594–606
  accelerated silicosis, 604–606
  diatomite pneumoconiosis, 603–604
  human alveolar lipo-proteinosis, 606
  mineral structure, 594
Friedlander's bacillus, 196
Fuller's earth
  composition of, 652
  disorders, 652–653
  uses and risks, 652
Fume fever, metal and polymer, 663
Fumes, 662–663
  defined, 591
  rare sources, of, 663
Fungal antigens, and lung disease, 586
Fungal diseases, invasive, 232–238
Fungal infections
  coccidioidomycosis, 227–228
  cryptococcosis, 228–230
  granulomatous, 224–232
  histoplasmosis, 224–226
  sporotrichosis and paracoccidiodis, 232
Fungemia, 237
Fungi, special stains, 102
Fungus balls, 237–238

Gangrene, pulmonary, 214
Gaseous injury, protection from, 57
Gases, 664–665
Gas-exchanging epithelium, development of, 3
Gastric acid aspiration, 751
Gastrointestinal tract, asbestosis sequelae, 641–642
Gaucher's disease, 493
Genetic factors, in lung cancer incidence, 314
Geography, and lung cancer incidence, 313–314
Gestation, branching interaction, 3–4
Ghon's focus, in primary pulmonary tuberculosis, 221–222
Giant cell carcinoma, 351, 353
Giant cell interstitial pneumonia, 448–449
Glial heterotopia, in neonate infant, 117
Globoid leukoystrophy, *see* Krabbe's disease
Glomerular enlargement, chronic airflow obstruction and, 564
Glomerulonephritis, diffuse pulmonary hemorrhage differentiated from, 305
Glomus pulmonale, and pulmonary circulation, 728
Glycogenosis, *see* Pompe's disease
Glycosaminoglycans, in malignant mesothelioma, 797
Goats, brucellosis from, 209
Goblet cells, 18, 19
  in bronchioloalveolar tumor, 346
  in chronic bronchitis, 533
  in sputum cytology, 803
Golden pneumonia, 760–762
Gold mining, nodular silicosis and, 594–595
Goodpasture's syndrome, 303–305
Graft rejection, 174
Gram-negative aerobic bacteria, pneumonia caused by, 196–203
Gram-positive cocci, pneomonia caused by, 190–192
Granular cell tumors, 407–408
Granulomas
  diagnosis of, 73
  eosinophilic, 470–473
  in infiltrative lung disease, 431
  necrotizing and non-necrotizing, 102, 253
Granulomatosis, 283–302
  allergic angiitis and, 289–290
  angiitis and, 283–302
  bronchocentric, 296–300
  clinical features, 284
  defined, 283
  histologic features, 285
  histopathology, 290
  lymphomatoid, 292–296
  necrotizing sarcoid, 468–470
  sites of involvement, 289
  treatment and prognosis, 290
Graphite and carbon pneumoconiosis, 613
Gross anatomy, 11–14
Gummas, in pneumonia of syphilis, 213–214
Gypsum disorders, 655

Hairy cell leukemia, mycobacterial infections with, 253, 255
Hamartoma, 121, 403–405
  fine needle aspiration biopsy, 815, 821
  vs. neoplasms, 405, 406
Hand-Schüller-Christian disease, 470
Hard-metal disease, 659
Hemangiomas
  in neonate infant, 117, 119
  sclerosing, 401, 404
Hemangiopericytoma, 384, 386
Hemodialysis, metastatic calcification in, 497
Hemodynamics, in plexogenic arteriopathy, 701–702
Hemophilus influenzae, 197–198
Hemopneumothorax, 781
Hemoptysis, 303
Hemorrhage
  drug-related, 505
  in fine needle aspiration, 112
  immune complex-induced, 257
  in neonate infant, 132

828 Index

Hemopneumothorax, 781
Hemothorax, 774–775
Hepatic disease
  and arterial hypertension, 689
    pulmonary circulation in, 721–723
    pulmonary hypertension in, 722–723
Herbicides, and DAD, 278
Hermansky-Pudlak syndrome, pulmonary involvement in, 494
Hernia, diaphragmatic, 116, 138
Herpes infections, 134
Herpes simplex, 165–167
  cytoplasmic virion, 170
  hemorrhagic necrosis with hyaline membranes, 167
  leukocyte reaction and nuclear dust, 168
  nuclear inclusions, 169
  pneumonitis, 165
  tracheal ulcers due to, 165–166
Heterotopia
  bone ossification, 500
  lung and adrenal cortex, 117
High altitude
  pulmonary edema due to, 279
  pulmonary trunk and vasculature at, 706, 723
Higher bacteria, pneumonias caused by, 210–214
Hilar lymph nodes, amyloidosis, of, 493
Histaminase, in lung cancer, 355
Histamine, release in byssinosis, 670
Histiocytes, in sputum cytology, 804
Histiocytic lymphoma, 395, 399
Histiocytoma, malignant fibrous, 384, 387
Histiocytosis X, *see* Eosinophilic granuloma
Histology, 11-50; *see also* Cytology
Histoplasma capsulatum, 226
Histoplasmomas, 225
Histoplasmosis, 224–226
  acute pulmonary, 224–225
  chronic and disseminated, 225, 227
  classification of, 225
  epidemic, 225
  identification of organisms, 226
Hodgkin's disease, 256, 398
Honeycomb lung, 129, 434
  causes and classification, 434
  in coal workers, 625
  in end-stage disease, 69–72
Hormones, from lung cancers, 354–356
Horseshoe lung, 115
Horsfield-Cumming model, of airways, 52
Humoral immunity, 64
Hyaline membrane disease, 124, 128, 269
  collapse pattern, 129
Hydrostatic pressure
  microvascular, 266
  pulmonary edema due to, 268
Hypereosinophilic syndrome, 479
Hypersecretion, of mucus, 529–538
Hypersensitivity pneumonitis, 582–587
  drug-related, 503–505
Hypertension, pulmonary, 112
  causes of, 687–690
  dietary, 712
  drug-related, 506
  effects on elastic arteries, 705–708
  in hepatic disease, 722–723
  onset time of, 705
  persistent, 136–139
  postoperative, 690
  primary, 688, 715
  unexplained, 714–721
  venous, 708–711
Hypoplasia, 4, 6, 115

Hypoxemic respiratory failure, 269, 276
Hypoxia, chronic, 688
Hypoxic hypertensive pulmonary vascular disease, 725–726

Idiopathic pulmonary hemosiderosis (IPH), 307–308
Immotile cilia syndrome, 566–567
Immune complex-induced hemorrhage with systemic lupus, 257
Immunity
  cell-mediated, 64–65
  humoral, 64
Immunoblastic sarcoma, 395–396
Immunocompromised patient, 247–262
  alveolar proteinosis in, 251–253
  chronic interstitial pneumonia in, 248–251
  cryptococcosis in, 231
  diffuse alveolar damage in, 71, 248–251
  necrotizing and non-necrotizing pneumonias and granulomas, 253
  organizing pneumonia in, 248–251
  pathologic reaction patterns, 247–255
  pulmonary infiltrates in, 248
  tracheobronchitis/bronchiolitis in, 253
  transbronchial biopsy, 74
  tumors in, 255
Immunofluorescent techniques, in microbiologic diagnosis, 102
Immunoglobulins, respiratory, 64
Immunologic lung disease, 577–588
  asthma, 577–581
  extrinsic, 577–588
  hypersensitivity pneumonitis, 582–587
Immunologic response, 63–64
  abnormal, 306–308
  in silicosis, 601
  in simple pneumoconiosis, 616
Immunoperoxidase techniques, in microbiologic diagnosis, 102
Immunosuppressed patients, survival data for lung biopsy, 260
Inert metallic dusts, lung disorders due to, 660–662
Infant
  adenomatoid malformation, 121–123
  bronchogenic cysts, 120, 122
  bronchopulmonary sequestration in, 118–120
  congenital anomalies of lower respiratory tract, 115–117
  extrauterine transition disorders, 123–132
  hemorrhage in, 132
  meconium aspiration in, 132–133, 136
  tachypnea (wet lung), 124
  vascular anomalies in, 117–135
Infantile gangliosidosis, pulmonary involvement in, 495
Infarction, pulmonary, 741–742
Infections, *see also* Bacterial infections; Viral infections
  in complicated pneumoconiosis, 616–617
  in immunocompromised patient, 74
  in neonate, 133
  transbronchial biopsy, 73–74
Infiltrative lung disease, 425–507
  acute vs. chronic, 425
  air space exudates, 431
  calcification and ossification, 496–502
  capillary and pericytes, 430
  causes and classification, 426
  cellular infiltrates and epithelial proliferation, 429–430
  definitions and terms, 425

  distribution of lesions, 429
  drug reactions, 502–506
  granulomas and necrosis, 431
  morphologic approach to, 428–434
  and renal tubular acidosis, 495
  scarring and honey combing, 431–434
  structures and special stains, 434
Inflammation
  bronchiolar, 521–525
  granulomatous, 65
  proximal acinar emphysema due to, 624
Inflammatory pseudotumor, 398, 403
Inflation fixation, in open lung biopsy, 67–68
Influenza, 149–151
  with bronchiolitis, 149
  diffuse alveolar damage in, 150
  hemophilus, 197–198
  pneumonia, 151, 152
  syndrome, 148
Inhalation
  anthrax, 210
  lipid pneumonia, 752, 754
  of particles, protection from, 58
Interalveolar pores, anatomy and histology, 29
Interstitial emphysema, 120, 130, 134
Interstitial pneumonia
  chronic, 74–77
  cytoxic drugs causing, 251
  desquamative interstitial, *see* Desquamative interstitial pneumonia
  diagnosis of, 69, 71, 72, 74
  with foamy exudate, 251
  giant cell and lymphocytic, 448–451
  in immunocompromised patient, 248–251
  usual interstitial pneumonia, *see* Usual interstitial pneumonia
Interstitial space, 263–267
  air space flooding in, 267
  alveolar and extra-alveolar, 263–265
Intimal proliferation, in plexogenic pulmonary arteriopathy, 696–697
Intra-alveolar blue bodies, 499–500
Intrabronchial lipoma, 379, 382
Invasive fungal diseases, 232–238
  Allescheria boydii, 237
  aspergillosis, 232–234
  candidiasis, 235–237
  mucormycosis (phycomycosis), 235
  mycetomas (fungus balls), 237–238
  Torulopsis glabrata, 237
Iron ore disorders, 660–661
Iron oxides, 314
Irritant gases, 664–665

Juvenile rheumatoid arthritis, 454, 459

Kaolin
  composition of, 651
  uses and risks, 651
Kaolin disorders, 651–652
Kaposi's sarcoma, 394
Kennel cough, 157
Kidney anlargement, chronic airflow obstruction and, 564
Klebsiella pneumoniae, 196
Kohn, pores of, *see* Interalveolar pores
Krabbe's disease, pulmonary involvement in, 495
Kultschitzky cells, 21

L-dopa decarboxylase, 355

Large-cell carcinoma, 349–352
  fine needle aspiration biopsy, 813, 818
Larynx
  closure during swallowing, 58
  diphtheria of, 188
Lavage, 804–805
  bronchial, 108
Left ventricular hypertrophy, chronic airflow obstruction and, 563
Legionella, 201–203
  immunity to, 203
  pneumonia from, 201–202
Leiomyomas, 392–394
  metastasizing, 392–394
  solitary, 381
Leiomyosarcoma, 384
Letterer-Siwe disease, 472
Limestone disorders, 655
Lipid pneumonia, exogenous and endogenous, 752, 760–762
Lipids
  aspiration of, 752
  in simple pneumoconiosis, 615
Lipogranulomatosis, see Farber's disease
Lipomas, 379–380
  in chest wall, 798
Lipo-proteinosis, human alveolar, 606
Liquid aspiration, 276
Liver disease, see Hepatic disease
Lobar obstruction, pathologic staging problem, 86
Lobar pneumonia, pneumococcal, 190–191
Löffler's syndrome, 474–475
Longitudinal muscle, in pulmonary arteries, 694
Lower respiratory tract
  adenovirus infections, 159–165
  congenital anomalies of, 115–117
  infections in children, 157
  protection provided by, 59
  radiologic findings, 148
  viral infections of, 148
Lung, 1–10
  abscess, 203, 214, 762
  acute injury, 308
  aging and overinflation, 555–557
  anatomy and histology, 11–50
  asbestos fiber content of, 641
  changes occurring with age, 555–556
  circulatory system, 32–39
  cytology techniques, 105–114
  defense mechanisms, 57–66
  drug reactions in, 502–506
  embryonal development, 1
  fine needle aspiration, 109–113
  intrauterine growth, 1, 4–6
  lymphoid system, 39–42, 357
  morphometric data, 52
  nerves in, 42–44
  normal anatomy, 12–50
  paper-mounted sections, 98–99
  pleura, 44
  postnatal growth, 7–9
  primary and secondary sarcomas of, 383–394
  pseudoglandular phase, 1
  quantitative anatomy, 51–55
  resection, 79–83
  saccular development, 1, 6
  structure, 14, 97
  tumors and tumor-like lesions of, 398–408
  uncommon and secondary tumors of, 360–411
Lung cancer
  age-adjusted incidence in various countries, 313
  asbestosis sequelae, 460–641
  cigarette smoke and, 311–313
  classification of common types, 321–322
  clinical manifestations, 352–360
  "constitutional hypothesis," 311–312
  defined, 311
  endocrine and neuroendocrine substances produced by, 354–356
  epidemiology, 311–317
  in ex-cigarette smokers, 313
  genetic and socioeconomic factors, 314–316
  geography and air pollution factors, 313–314
  histogenesis and development, 317–321
  histologic types and secular trends, 322–323
  incidence by sex and smoking, 54, 311, 324
  in situ vs. invasive, 808
  intrapulmonary effects, 353
  mortality rates, 312–313
  Naruke mode mapping diagrams (modified), 80
  origin of, 317
  pathologic features, 321–324
  pneumoconiosis sequelae, 620–621
  prognosis and survival, 358–360
  radiographic abnormalities, 352
  signs and symptoms, 355
  silicotic sequelae, 602
  socioeconomic factor, 314–316
  spread patterns in, 356–357
  staging of, 79–83, 359
  survival by stage and cell type, 358, 360, 361
  ultrastructural features, 342
  urban/rural differences, 313
Lung disease, see also Pulmonary disorders
  environmental, 591–685
  extrinsic immunologic, 577–588
  fungal antigens in, 586
  infiltrative, 425–507
  interstitial, 109
Lymph
  clearance and damage, 62, 63
  proliferation in lung tumors, 394–398
Lymphangiectasis, 120, 123, 126
Lymphangioleiomyomatosis, 482–488
Lymphangitic carcinoma, 411
Lymphatic system, anatomy and histology, 39–42
Lymph nodes, 62, 87
  intrapulmonary, 394
  in silicosis, 596–597
Lymphocytes
  immune reactions by, 64
  in sputum cytology, 804–805
Lymphocytic interstitial pneumonia, 449–451
Lymphocytic lymphoma, 77, 394
Lymphocytic small-cell carcinoma, 335
Lymphoid proliferations, diagnosis of, 74, 77
Lymphoma, 295, 394–398
  diagnosis of, 73
  fine needle aspiration biopsy, 815, 819
  secondary involvement of lung, 398
Lymphomatoid granulomatosis, 292–296
  extrapulmonary involvement, 293
  prognosis and treatment, 293–294
  vascular infiltration in, 295–297

MacLeod's syndrome, 123, 547
Macrophages
  anatomy and histology, 30–32
  fibrogenic factor in silicosis, 600
  mobilization and monocyte emigration, 593
  secretory products of, 36
Maduromycosis, 237
Malignant mesothelioma, 783–798; see also Mesothelioma
  asbestos-related, 787–790
  vs. carcinomas, 795
  demographic and clinical features, 783–787
  diagnostic procedures, 797
  dust quantity and fiber type, 645–646
  epidemiology and pathology, 787–798
  epithelial and sarcomatous, 789–792
  fine needle aspiration biopsy, 815, 820
  glycosaminoglycan analysis, 797
  histochemistry and ultrastructure, 795–796
  inflammatory mesothelial reaction vs., 795
  mixed, 792, 795
  occurrence and prevalence, 644
  pathologic reaction in lung, 645
  rate and pseudotumors, 798
  spread patterns, 797
  therapy and prognosis, 797
Manganese fumes, 663
Man-made mineral fibers, malignancy of, 646
Mast cells, in asthma, 578–580
Measles (rubeola), 151–156
  complications and morphology, 151–156
  diffuse alveolar damage in, 155
  hyperplastic epithelial changes in, 154
  intranuclear inclusion, 156
  pneumonia, 151
Meconium aspiration, in neonate infant, 132–133, 136
Mediastinal invasion, pathologic staging problem, 86
Mediastinum, lymph nodes, 63
Melanoma
  fine needle aspiration biopsy, 822
  malignant, 408
Melioidosis, 200–201
Membrane effect, in silicotic fibrogenesis, 599
Men smokers, lung cancer mortality of, 312
Mercury fumes, 663
Mesenchymal tumors, benign and malignant, 379–394
Mesothelial cells, 44
Mesotheliomas, 781–783; see also Malignant mesotheliomas
  asbestos-related, 644–647
  dust quantity and fiber type, 645–646
  fibrous, 783–786
  localized, 781–783
  occurrence and prevalence, 644
  pathologic reaction in lung, 645
Metabolism, inborn errors of, 493–495
Metal and polymer fume fever, 663
Metallic dusts, 655–662
Mica disorders, 653
Microbiologic diagnosis, 101–103
Microlithiasis, pulmonary alveolar, 498
Microvasculature, 263
  damage due to edema, 268
  fluid movement across, 265–267
  shock-induced injury, 278
Middle lobe syndrome, 756–757
Miliary tuberculosis, 222, 223
Milk products, brucellosis from, 209
Minerals
  compact and fibrous, 648
  comparative responses to, 648

Minerals (cont.)
  hazardous, 592
Mist, defined, 592
Mitral valvotomy, regression of pulmonary vascular lesions after, 711
Mixed connective tissue disease, pulmonary involvement in, 460
Mixed dust lesions, 618
Monocytes, 60
  emigration and macrophage mobilization 593
  in sputum cytology, 804
Montmorillonite disorders, 653
Morphometric data, 52
Motor innervation, 43–44
Mounier-Kuhn syndrome, 116, 565
Mucociliary clearance, 59–60
Mucormycosis (phycomycosis), 235, 238
Mucous glands
  adenoma, 379, 382
  airflow obstruction, 533
  anatomy and histology, 18–20
  bronchi proportion, 533
  enlargement, 529–533, 535–537
  measurement of, 530–533
  in smokers and nonsmokers, 536–537
  tracheobronchial, enlargement of, 529–533
  volume proportion of, 532–533
Mucus
  cell types, 17–19
  secretion and hypersecretion, 17–18, 529–538
Murine toxin, 206
Mycetomas (fungus balls), 237–238
Mycobacterial infections, 221–223
Mycoplasma, 181–182
Myoblastomas, granular cell, 407–408
Myoepithelial cells, 19
Myofibroblasts, 696, 702

Nasal protection, 58
Needle aspiration, see Fine needle aspiration
Neonate, see Infant
Neoplasms, 121; see also Tumors
  fine needle aspiration biopsy, 811–822
  radiation-induced, 666
Nepheline disorders, 653
Nephropathy, 306–308
Nerves, 42–44
Neural tumors, 381–383
Neuroendocrine system, 21, 354
Neuroepithelial bodies, and pulmonary circulation, 728, 729
Neurofibromatosis, 488
Neurogenic pulmonary edema, 279
Neurolemma, 383
Neuron-specific enolase, 356, 364
Neurosecretory granules, in small-cell carcinoma, 331, 333
Newborn, see also Neonate and specific conditions
  accessory diaphragm in, 139
  cystic fibrosis in, 139–140
  diaphragm disorders in, 138–139
  persistant pulmonary hypertension in, 136–137
  vascular disorders in, 136–140
Nickel disorders, 659
Niemann-Pick disease, pulmonary involvement in, 493–494
Nitrofurantoin, 278
Nitrogen oxide disorders, 664
Nitrogen oxides, 57
  inhalation of, 277

Nocardia, 102, 212
Nodes
  ossification of, 501–502
  staging problems, 80, 83–86
Nodular parenchymal amyloidosis, 489–492
Nodular silicosis, 594–602
  classical, 594–602
  diagnosis and sequelae, 602
  prevalence and occupations at risk, 594–595
Noncardiogenic pulmonary edema, drug related, 505
Noncaseating granuloma, with Hodgkin's disease, 256
Nonciliated airways, clearance from 60
Noncoughing patients, sputum collection from, 106
Nonendocrine syndromes, in lung cancer spread, 353–354
Non-neoplastic disease
  bronchoalveolar lavage in, 108–109
  lung resection for, 89–93
Nonsiliceous dusts, 654–655
Nonsmokers, 312
Nonthrombotic pulmonary embolism, 742
North American blastomycosis, 230–232
Noxious gases and fumes, inhalation of, 276 277
Nucleic acid sandwich hybridization, 149

Oat cell
  carcinoma, 335
  in sputum cytology, 805
Obstruction, see Chronic airflow obstruction
Obstructive pneumonia, 760–762
Occupational hazards, 316, 595, 628
Oils and waxes, in asbestos contamination, 647
Oncotic pressure, in microvasculature, 266, 268
Open lung biopsy, 67–72
  vs. autopsy, 259
  in immunocompromised patients, 259–260
  inflation fixation in, 67–68
  nonspecific or unreliable diagnoses, 69–71
  site of, 69
  specific and nonspecific diagnoses, 69, 259
  vs. transbronchial biopsy, 74
  yield of, 71
Oral cavity, Klebsiella pneumoniae, 196
Organizing pneumonia, 193, 271
  bronchiolitis obliterans and, 71, 444–448
  in immunocompromised patient, 248–251
Oropharynx, diphtheria involving, 186
Osler-Weber-Rendu syndrome, 117
Osmium fumes, 663
Osmotic pressure, in microvasculature, 267
Ossification, 496–502
  disseminated nodular, 501
  dystrophic and tracheobronchial, 500–502
  lesions and histologic features, 495
Ossifying pneumonia, 500, 501
Overinflation
  acquired obstructive, 557
  and chronic airflow obstruction, 556–557
  congenital and compensatory, 123, 556–557
Oxygen, inhalation of, 276, 277
Ozone, 57, 277, 664

Panacinar emphysema, 539, 540, 542–547
  in coal workers, 624
  incidental, 547

  in young subjects, 546
Panbronchiolitis, diffuse, 528
Pancoast's tumor, 328, 353, 359
Paper-mounted lung sections, 98–99
Papillary tumors, 360, 363
Paracoccidioidosis, 232
Paraesophageal lymph nodes, 63
Paragangliomas, possible true, 373
Paraquat lung, 278
Parainfluenza, 156–157, 161
Paraneoplastic syndromes, in lung cancer spread, 353–356
Parasites, 689, 731–733
Parathyroid hormone, in lung cancer, 355
Paratracheal lymph nodes, 63
Parenchyma, 489–492, 560–561
Particles
  aggregation and translocation, 593
  deposition and clearance, 58, 61, 592
  inhaled, 58
Patch organizing pneumonia, 445, 450
Peptic ulceration, chronic airflow obstruction and, 564
Peptides, 354–356
Periarteritis nodosa and polyarteritis, 479
Peribronchiolar fibrosis, 131
Perichondritis, relapsing, 565–566
Pericytes, capillary and endothelium, 430
Perinatal pneumonia, 133–134
Peripheral airways, 521–526, 535
Peripheral nodule, without definitive diagnosis, 58
Pertussis, toxic factors, 189–190
Petroleum workers, lung cancer mortality in, 316
Phagocytes, 60
Phantom tumors, 798
Phosgene disorders, 665
Phycomycosis, 235
Picornaviruses, 159
Piezoelectric effect, in simple silicosis, 598
Pigmented fibrosis, in coal worker's pneumoconiosis, 613
Pipe smokers, lung cancer mortality ratios, 312
Pittsburg pneumonia, 203
Plague, 205–207
  plaque dental, actinomycosis in, 211
  pneumonia, 207
Plasma cell, 20
  granuloma, 398–402
  in sputum cytology, 804
Plasmacytoma, 398
Plastic workers, nitrogen oxide inhalation by, 277
Pleomorphic adenoma, 814, 819
Pleura
  anatomy and histology, 44
  biopsy, 769–774
  effusion, 769–774
  fibrosis of, 775
  lymphatic system, 39–41
  plaques, 642–644
  pneumococcal infection of, 192
  tumors of, 781–798
Pleural diseases, 769–802
  rare and pseudotumors, 798
  systemic effects of, 781
Pleurisy, 452
Pleuritis, drug-related, 506
Pleuropulmonary disease, 451, 456
Plexogenic pulmonary arteriopathy, 690–705; see also Hypertension, pulmonary
  causes of, 715
  clinical associations, 700–705

Index

in congenital cardiac shunts, 700–701
hemodynamics and septal defects, 701–705
muscularization and intimal proliferation, 695–696
necrotizing arteritis in, 699
vascular changes in, 695–700
Pneumatocele, 120
Pneumococcal infection, 190–192
Pneumoconiosis
coal worker's, 607–621
defined, 592
diatomite, 603–604
graphite and carbon, 613
rheumatoid, 621–624
Pneumocystitis, 239–241
Pneumonocytes
membranous and granular, 26–27
staining and lavage, 102, 108
Pneumonia, 759–762
adenovirus, 159
anaerobic necrotizing, 203, 204
aspiration and obstructive, 760–762
beta-hemolytic streptococcal, 192–193
and bronchial obstruction, 759–762
chronic interstitial, 248–251
coccidioidal, 227–228
eosinophilic, 475–478
herpes simplex, 165
from higher bacteria, 210–214
in immunocompromised patient, 248–251
influenza, 151, 152
from Legionella, 201–202
measles, 151
mycoplasma, 181–182
necrotizing and non-necrotizing, 253
nocardial, 212
perinatal, 133–134
plaque, 207
staphylococcal, 193–196
syndrome, 148
of syphilis, 213
tularemic, 208–209
varicella zoster, 171
Pneumonitis
acute lupus, 305
radiation, 278, 666
Pneumothorax, 775–780
traumatic and iatrogenic, 775
Pollutants, prediction of risks from, 667–668
Polyarteritis nodosa, 290
Polymer fume fever, 663
Polymyositis-dermatomyositis, 460–461
Pompe's disease, pulmonary involvement in, 495
Pontiac fever, 201
Posterolateral diaphragm hernia, 138
Postinfarction subpleural cysts, 140
Postnatal lung growth, 7–9
Postoperative pulmonary hypertension, 690
Poultry, host for chlamydia, 183
Pretricuspid and post-tricuspid shunts, 687
Progressive systemic sclerosis, *see* Scleroderma
Proteinosis, alveolar, 479–482
Proteus, 196, 198
Protozoal infections, 239, 243
dirofilariasis, 241–243
pneumocystis pneumonia, 239–241
Proximal acinar emphysema, 540–542
dust-induced, 542, 624
Pseudolymphoma, 394–398
Pseudomonal infections
melioidosis, 200–201
pneumonia, 198–200
Pseudomonas, 198–200

Pseudomycosis, 214–215
Pseudotumors, 798
Psittacosis, 183
Pulmonary hypertension
causes of, 687–690
dietary origins, 689
fibrosis and embolism, 688
hepatic disease and, 689
parasites and developmental anomalies, 689
postoperative, 690
pretricuspid and post-tricuspid shunts, 687
primary, 688
Pulmonary trunk
cystic medial degeneration of, 707
developmental anomalies of, 733–734
at high altitude, 706
sarcomas of, 384–385
Pyrrolizidine alkaloids, 712–713

Q fever, 183–184
Quantitative anatomy, 51–55
Quartz factor, in pneumoconiosis, 614, 616

Rabbit, tularemia from, 207
Radiation
diffuse alveolar damage from, 251
neoplasms, 666
pneumonitis, 71, 278
Radioactive particles, 665–667
Ragwort, in pulmonary hypertension, 713
Rare tumors, 798
Ray fungi, 210
Reid index, for mucous gland sizing, 530–532
Relapsing perichondritis, 565–566
Renal tubular acidosis, infiltrative lung disease and, 495
Resection, lung, 79–93
Respirable particles, defined, 592
Respiratory distress syndrome, 124, 129
Respiratory syncytial virus, 151–159
Respiratory tract
adenovirus infections, 159–165
airways, 53
bronchiolitis, 525, 527
brucellosis in, 210
chlamydia, 182–183
chronic airflow obstruction, 174–176
Coxiella infections, 183–184
cytomegalovirus infections, 172–174
immunoglobulins, 64
lower, 59
mycoplasma, 181–182
protection provided by, 59
viral infections of, 148–179
Reticulosis, polymorphic or malignant midline, 293
Rhabdomyomatous dysplasia, 115, 117
Rhabdomyosarcoma, 385
Rheumatoid arthritis, 451–453
lymphoid hyperplasia in, 453, 458
pleuropulmonary involvement in, 451–453
pulmonary lesions in, 456, 457
silicotic sequelae, 602
Right middle lobe atelectasis, 756–757
Rodents, plague from, 206
Rotex needle, 109, 111
Rounded atelectasis, 757–759
in asbestos worker, 751–759
Rubella, and pulmonary hypoplasia, 117
Rubeola, *see* Measles

Saccular bronchiectasis, 559
Salivary gland tumors, 376–379
Sarcoid granulomatosis, necrotizing, 290–292, 468–470
Sarcoidosis, 463–470
bronchoalveolar lavage in, 109
classic pulmonary, 463–467
honeycombing and granulomas, 464–467
nodular pulmonary, 468
pulmonary variants, 468–470
transbronchial biopsy, 73
vascular involvement in, 466, 467
Sarcomas
fine needle aspiration biopsy, 814
primary and secondary, 383–394
of pulmonary trunk, 384–385
sclerosing vascular, 385, 388
Scarring
carcinoma, 320–321
in infiltrative lung disease, 431–432
irregular emphysema and, 549, 551
Schaumann bodies, 500
Schistosomiasis, 731–732
Scimitar syndrome, in neonate infants, 116, 117
Scleroderma
pulmonary involvement in, 456–459
silicotic sequelae, 602
Screw-type needle, 109, 111
Senile amyloid deposition, 492–493
Sensory receptors, 43
Septal amyloidosis, diffuse alveolar, 492
Septal defects, 703–705
Septicemia, 199, 206
Sequestration
bronchopulmonary, 118–120
intralobar and extralobar, 118–120
Serous cells, 19
Serpentine asbestos, 626–627
Shale disorders, 622
Shingles, *see* Varicella zoster
Shock, microvascular injury due to, 278
Short-rib syndrome, 139
Shunts, pre- and post-tricuspid, 687
Silica
comparative responses to, 648
solubility hypothesis, 599
submicron amorphous, 603–604
Silica disorders, 594–606, 648–655
Silicon carbide disorders, 654
Silicosis
accelerated, 604–606
classical nodular, 594–602
complicated, 595–602, 609–618
lymph nodes in, 596–597
simple, 595–601
solubility theory, 599
Sillimanite disorders, 653
Silo workers, nitrogen oxide inhalation by, 277
Sjögren's syndrome, pulmonary involvement in, 460
Small airways disease, 521–526
Small-cell carcinoma, 330–337
development of, 320–321
fine needle aspiration biopsy, 813, 817
histology and cytology, 807
mixed types, 337–339
prognosis and survival, 358–359
subtypes in various sites, 337
survival by histologic subtype, 358, 360
Small-granule cells, 21
Smog, 57
Smokers and smoking, 311–313, 324
asbestosis and lung cancer, 641

Smokers and smoking (cont.)
  emphysema incidence in, 553
  and mesothelioma, 647
  mucous gland enlargement in, 536–537
Smooth muscle
  hypertrophy and hyperplasia of, 695
  spasm in asthma, 578
Solitary endocrine cells, 21
Sporotrichosis, 232
Sputum
  cellular elements found in, 804–805
  collection and preservation, 105–106
  cytology, 803–804
  early morning specimens, 106
  staining procedure, 108
Squamous carcinoma, see also Lung cancer
  development of, 317–318
  fine needle aspiration biopsy, 811–812
  in situ and early, 318–320
  in pleura, 798
  small-cell, 330
  survival by histologic subtype, 358, 360
Staccato cough, 134
Staging, of lung cancer, 79–83
Staphylococcal pneumonia, 193–196
Stature, lung changes with, 54
Stenosis
  in neonate infant and child, 117–118
  vasculature in, 729–730
Steroid hormones, 354–356
Stillbirth, 121
Streptococcal pneumonia, 190, 192
Subcarinal lymph nodes, 63
Submucosal glands, 2, 153
Subpleural cysts, 140
Sugar tumors, 405
Sulfur dioxide disorders, 664
Sulfur granules, in actinomycosis, 211
Surface epithelium, papillary tumors of, 360, 363
Surfactant, secretion of, 27–28
Swallowing, protection during, 58
Swine, brucellosis from, 209
Swyer-James syndrome, 123, 547
Syphilis, 212–214
  pneumonia of, 213
  tracheobronchial, 213
Systemic lupus erythematosis (SLE), 305, 455, 459
  drug-induced, 503, 506
  immune complexes and tissue injury, 257, 456

Tachypnea, in neonate infant, 124, 134
Talc, uses and risks, 648–649
Talc disorders, 648–650
Talcosis, 74
Teratoma, intrapulmonary, 408
Thoracopulmonary region, malignant small-cell tumor of, 392
Thoracotomy, fine needle aspiration vs., 112
Thromboembolism, recurrent pulmonary, 718–721
Ticks, tularemia from, 207
Tin ore disorders, 661
Tissue, complexity and hypoplasia, 6–7
Titanium disorders, 660

Tonsils, 196
  diphtheria involving, 186
Toxic agents
  lung cancer after exposure to, 316
  in pertussis, 189–190
Trace metals, in asbestos contamination, 647
Trachea, 408–410
  diphtheria of, 188
  stenosis of, 213, 565
  ulcers from herpes simplex, 165–166
Tracheobronchial tree, branching pattern of, 59, 60
Tracheobronchiomegaly, 116, 565
Tracheobronchitis, 165, 186, 253
Tracheopathia osteoplastica, 502, 564
Transbronchial biopsy, 73–77
  in immunocompromised patients, 258
Transitional airways, 53
Transitional cell carcinoma, 809
Tremolite asbestos, 627
Tropical eosinophilia, 478–479
Tuberculosis, 221–223
  asbestos and, 640
  chronic and generalized, 222
  classification and histopathology, 221–223
  granulomatous inflammation in, 222–224
  pleural effusions from, 770–771
  pneumoconiosis sequelae, 620
  silicotic sequelae, 602
Tuberous sclerosis, 482–488
Tubular parainfluenza, cytoplasmic inclusion, 158, 161
Tubulopapillary mesothelioma, 789, 794
Tularemia, 207–209
Tumorlets, 366–369
Tumor-like lesions, 398–408
Tumors, 311–423
  cell types, 112, 805
  cytologic diagnosis, 105
  in immunocompromised patient, 255
  lymphoproliferative processes, 394–398
  metastatic, 808
  uncommon, 360–423
Tungsten carbide disease, 659

Unexplained pulmonary hypertension, 714–721
Unilateral hyperlucent lung, 123; see also MacLeod's syndrome and Swyer-James syndrome
Upper airway, protection provided by, 58
Upper respiratory tract, viral infections of, 148
Uranium mining, 665–666
Urban exposure, to asbestos, 648
Urbanization, and lung cancer mortality, 316
Urinary tract infections, 197
Usual interstitial pneumonia (UIP), 435–444
  vs. cryptogenic fibrosing alveolitis, 440
  drug-related, 503
  in immunocompromised patient, 251
  steroid response, 445
  synonyms of, 435

Vaccination, 186–188
Valley fever, acute, 227

Vanadium fumes, 663
Varicella zoster, 167–172
Varicose bronchiectasis, 559
Vascular system disorders, 687–750
  coal worker's pneumoconiosis, 612
  collagen disease, 451–462
  dietary pulmonary hypertension, 712–714
  lesions, 112, 724–726
  in newborn, 117–140
  parasites and developmental anomalies, 731–736
  plexogenic pulmonary arteriopathy, 690–705
  pulmonary embolic disease, 740–743
  pulmonary fibrosis, 736–739
  pulmonary venous hypertension, 708–711
  unexplained pulmonary hypertension, 714–721
Vasculitis, see Angiitis
Veins
  anomalies of, 735–736
  chronic airflow obstruction and, 563
  development of, 2–3
  glomic tissue, 728
  and venules, 35
Venograms, in postmortem examination, 97
Veno-occlusive disease, pulmonary, 716–718
Venous hypertension, 708–711
  chronic, 688
Ventrifuge tube, for sputum processing, 107
Viral infections
  and chronic airflow obstruction, 174–176
  clinical syndromes, 148
  herpes simplex, 165–167
  in immunocompromised patient, 253, 254
  influenza, 149–151
  microscopic techniques, 148
  pneumonia, 134, 149
  of respiratory tract, 148–179
  varicella zoster, 167–172
Viruses, "gold standard" for identification, 148
Visceral pleural invasion, pathologic staging problems, 83
Vocal chords, true and false, 58
Volcanic ash disorders, 653–654

Washing, cellular elements found in, 804–805
Water-borne fibers, in asbestos contamination, 647
Wegener's granulomatosis, 284–289
Weibel's model, of airways, 52
Weight loss, chronic airflow obstruction and, 563–564
Welding disorders, 664
Well-differential lymphocytic lymphoma, 394–395
Wheezing, drug-related, 505
White lung, of congenital syphilis, 214
Whooping cough, 189–190
Women smokers, lung cancer mortality of, 312
Woolsorters' disease, 210

Zirconium disorders, 661
Zoonosis, 207